Children with Disabilities

Children with Disabilities

Eighth Edition

edited by

Mark L. Batshaw, M.D.
Children's National Medical Center
George Washington University
School of Medicine and Health Sciences
Washington, D.C.

Nancy J. Roizen, M.D.
University Hospitals Rainbow Babies and Children's Hospital
Division of Developmental-Behavioral Pediatrics and Psychology
Case Western Reserve University School of Medicine
Cleveland, Ohio

and

Louis Pellegrino, M.D.
Department of Pediatrics
Center for Development, Behavior, and Genetics
Upstate Golisano Children's Hospital
SUNY Upstate Medical University
Syracuse, New York

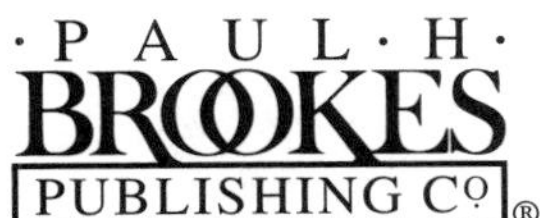

Baltimore • London • Sydney

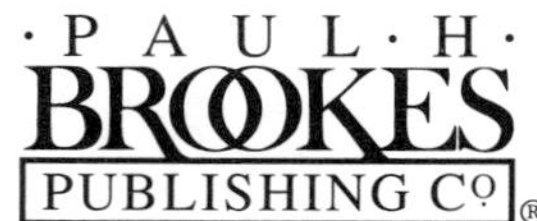

Paul H. Brookes Publishing Co.
Post Office Box 10624
Baltimore, Maryland 21285-0624
USA
www.brookespublishing.com

Typeset by Progressive Publishing Solutions, York, Pennsylvania.
Manufactured in the United States of America by
Sheridan Books, Inc., Chelsea, Michigan.

Appendix C, Commonly Used Medications, which appears in the back matter and in the book's online materials, provides information about numerous drugs frequently used to treat children with disabilities. This appendix is in no way meant to substitute for a physician's advice or expert opinion; readers should consult a medical practitioner if they are interested in more information.

The publisher and the authors have made every effort to ensure that all of the information and instructions given in this book are accurate and safe, but they cannot accept liability for any resulting injury, damage, or loss to either person or property, whether direct or consequential and however it occurs. Medical advice should only be provided under the direction of a qualified health care professional.

The vignettes presented in this book are composite accounts that do not represent the lives or experiences of specific individuals, and no implications should be inferred. In all instances, names and identifying details have been changed to protect confidentiality.

Library of Congress Cataloging-in-Publication Data

Names: Batshaw, Mark L., 1945- editor. | Roizen, Nancy J., editor. | Pellegrino, Louis, editor.
Title: Children with disabilities / edited by Mark L. Batshaw, M.D., Nancy J. Roizen, M.D., and Louis Pellegrino, M.D.
Description: Eighth edition. | Baltimore : Paul H. Brookes Publishing Co., [2019] | Includes bibliographical references and index.
Identifiers: LCCN 2018048552 (print) | LCCN 2018059190 (ebook) | ISBN 9781681253213 (epub) | ISBN 9781681253220 (pdf) | ISBN 9781681253206 (hardcover)
Subjects: LCSH: Developmental disabilities. | Developmentally disabled children—Care. | Children with disabilities—Care.
Classification: LCC RJ135 (ebook) | LCC RJ135 .B38 2019 (print) | DDC 618.92/8588—dc23
LC record available at https://lccn.loc.gov/2018048552

British Library Cataloguing in Publication data are available from the British Library.

2023 2022 2021 2020 2019
10 9 8 7 6 5 4 3 2 1

Contents

About the Online Companion Materials

All readers can access Online Companion Materials, which supplement and expand upon the content, the knowledge, and the resources offered in this text.

Please visit **http://downloads.brookespublishing.com/children-with-disabilities-8e** to access the following:

- Appendices A, B, and C in digital form
- Appendix D, a resource directory of national organizations, federal agencies, information sources, self-advocacy and accessibility programs, and support groups that provide assistance to families and professionals
- Study questions and extension activities for every chapter to help readers check and expand their knowledge of key concepts
- Letters from Andrew Batshaw, spanning all eight editions of the book

About the Online Companion Materials for Faculty

Attention instructors! Online Companion Materials are available to help you teach a course using *Children with Disabilities, Eighth Edition.*

Please visit **http://downloads.brookespublishing.com/children-with-disabilities-8e** to access the following:

- Customizable PowerPoint presentations for every chapter, totaling over 450 slides
- All original illustrations from the book, downloadable for easy use in your PowerPoint presentations, tests, handouts, and other course purposes
- Study questions for every chapter to help students check their knowledge of key concepts
- Extension activities for class use, group projects, and homework to help students apply the information from the text
- A test bank with more than 200 multiple-choice, fill-in-the-blank, and essay questions for instructors to use and adapt in course exams
- Extended case studies to enrich discussions of how concepts are interconnected
- Sample syllabi from various fields to help you determine what chapters and sequence best suits the needs of your course
- Letters from Andrew Batshaw, spanning all eight editions of the book
- Appendix D: Childhood Disabilities Resources, Services, and Organizations

About the Editors

Mark L. Batshaw, M.D., holds the "Fight for Children" Chair of Academic Medicine and is Chief Academic Officer, and Physician-in-Chief at the Children's National Medical Center (CNMC) in Washington, D.C. He is also Professor of Pediatrics at George Washington University School of Medicine and Health Sciences in Washington, D.C.

Dr. Batshaw is a board-certified neurodevelopmental pediatrician who has treated children with developmental disabilities for more than 40 years. In 2006, Dr. Batshaw received both the Capute Award for notable contributions to the field of children with disabilities by the American Academy of Pediatrics and the Distinguished Research Award from The Arc. In 2015, he received the C. Anderson Aldrich Award in Child Development from the American Academy of Pediatrics.

Before moving to Washington in 1998, Dr. Batshaw was Physician-in-Chief of Children's Seashore House, the child development and rehabilitation institute of The Children's Hospital of Philadelphia. He is a graduate of the University of Pennsylvania and the University of Chicago Pritzker School of Medicine. Following pediatric residency at the Hospital for Sick Children in Toronto, he completed a fellowship in developmental pediatrics at the Kennedy Krieger Institute at The Johns Hopkins Medical Institutions.

Dr. Batshaw continues to pursue his research on innovative treatments for inborn errors of metabolism, including gene therapy. He has published more than 150 articles, chapters, and reviews on his research interests and the medical aspects of caring for children with disabilities. Dr. Batshaw was the founding editor-in-chief (1995–2001) of the journal *Mental Retardation and Developmental Disabilities Research Reviews*.

Dr. Batshaw lives in Washington, D.C. He and his wife Karen, a novelist, have three children and nine grandchildren.

Nancy J. Roizen, M.D., is Chief of the Division of Developmental-Behavioral Pediatrics and Psychology at University Hospitals Rainbow Babies and Children's Hospital in Cleveland and Professor of Pediatrics, Case Western Reserve University. She is certified in neurodevelopmental disabilities and developmental-behavioral pediatrics.

Dr. Roizen received her B.S. and M.D. degrees from Tufts University. After completing an internship in pediatrics at Massachusetts General Hospital, she did a residency in pediatrics at The Johns Hopkins Hospital. Her fellowships were in neurodevelopmental disabilities at the Kennedy Krieger Institute and in developmental and behavioral pediatrics at University of California, San Francisco. She was then a staff physician at the Child Development Center at Oakland Children's Hospital for 8 years, followed by 16 years as Chief of the Section of Developmental Pediatrics at University of Chicago. Next, at SUNY Upstate Medical University, she was Vice Chair for Education for the Department of Pediatrics and Chief of the Division of Neurosciences for 4 years. Next stop was the Cleveland Clinic, where she was the Chief of the Department of Developmental Pediatrics and Physiatry for 2 years. Dr. Roizen has published 125 articles, books, reviews, and chapters on research and the clinical aspects of children with developmental disabilities, including those with Down syndrome, toxoplasmosis, and velocardiofacial syndrome.

Dr. Roizen lives in Shaker Heights, Ohio, with her husband. They have two children and one granddaughter.

Louis Pellegrino, M.D., is Associate Professor of Pediatrics at SUNY Upstate Medical University, in Syracuse, New York. He is the director of the Child Development Program in the Center for Development, Behavior, and Genetics at Upstate Golisano Children's Hospital in Syracuse, New York.

Dr. Pellegrino is board-certified in neurodevelopmental disabilities and developmental-behavioral pediatrics and has been working with children with developmental disabilities for over 25 years. He is a graduate of the University of Connecticut School of Medicine, received his pediatric residency training at Upstate

Medical University, and completed a fellowship in developmental pediatrics at the University of Rochester.

Dr. Pellegrino was a co-editor of the sixth edition of *Children with Disabilities* and is the author of *The Common Sense Guide to Your Child's Special Needs: When to Worry, When to Wait, What to Do* (Paul H. Brookes Publishing Co., 2012), a companion volume to *Children with Disabilities* that was written for caregivers.

Dr. Pellegrino lives in Syracuse, New York, with his wife Joan, an accomplished medical geneticist and fellow author in this book. They have two children: Elizabeth, who is studying science writing and creative nonfiction, and Nicholas, who is studying computer science. Dr. Pellegrino is an avid gardener who loves all things green and growing.

Contributors

Nicholas Ah Mew, M.D.
Pediatric Geneticist, Rare Disease Institute
Children's National Medical Center
Assistant Professor of Pediatrics
George Washington University School of Medicine and Health Sciences
111 Michigan Avenue NW, Suite 1950
Washington, DC 20010

Nickie N. Andescavage, M.D.
Neonatologist
Children's National Medical Center
Assistant Professor of Pediatrics
George Washington University School of Medicine and Health Sciences
111 Michigan Avenue NW
Washington, DC 20010

Laura Gutermuth Anthony, Ph.D.
Associate Professor
Division of Child and Adolescent Psychiatry
Department of Psychiatry
University of Colorado School of Medicine
Children's Hospital of Colorado
Mail Stop A036/B130
13123 East 16th Avenue
Aurora, CO 80045

Virginia W. Berninger, Ph.D.
Educational Psychologist
Professor Emeritus of Educational Psychology
University of Washington
Seattle, WA 98195

Elizabeth Berry-Kravis, M.D., Ph.D.
Pediatric Neurology
Professor
Rush University Medical Center
1725 West Harrison, Suite 718
Chicago, IL 60612

Marisa Birkmeier, PT, DPT, PCS
Physical Therapist
Assistant Professor
George Washington University School of Medicine and Health Sciences
2000 Pennsylvania Avenue NW
Second Floor, Suite 215
Washington, DC 20006

Mackenzie E. Brown, D.O.
Fellow in Pediatric Rehabilitation Medicine
Children's National Medical Center
111 Michigan Avenue NW
Washington, DC 20010

Justin M. Burton, M.D.
Pediatric Physiatrist
Attending Physician, Pediatric Rehabilitation Medicine
Children's National Medical Center
Assistant Professor of Pediatrics
George Washington University School of Medicine and Health Sciences
111 Michigan Avenue NW
Washington, DC 20010

Gabrielle Sky Cardwell, B.A.
Clinical Research Assistant
Children's National Medical Center
111 Michigan Avenue NW
Washington, DC 20010

Thomas D. Challman, M.D., FAAP
Medical Director and Neurodevelopmental Pediatrician
Geisinger-Bucknell Autism & Developmental Medicine Center
120 Hamm Drive, 2nd Floor, Suite 2A
Lewisburg, PA 17837

Eric M. Chin, M.D.
Fellow, Neurology and Developmental Medicine
Kennedy Krieger Institute
707 North Broadway
Baltimore, MD 21205

Robin P. Church, Ed.D.
Senior Vice President for Education
Associate Professor of Education
Kennedy Krieger Institute
The Johns Hopkins University
3825 Greenspring Avenue
Baltimore, MD 21211

Elissa Batshaw Clair, Ed.S., M.Ed., NCSP
School Psychologist
Special School District
12110 Clayton Road
St. Louis, MO 63131

Catherine Larsen Coley, PT, DPT, PCS,
Physical Therapist and Pediatric Clinical Specialist
Division of Physical Medicine and Rehabilitation
Children's National Medical Center
111 Michigan Avenue NW
Washington, DC 20010

Laurie S. Conklin, M.D.
Pediatric Gastroenterologist
Children's National Medical Center
Assistant Professor of Pediatrics
George Washington University School of Medicine and Health Sciences
111 Michigan Avenue
Washington, DC 20010

Denice Cora-Bramble, M.D., M.B.A.
Chief Medical Officer and Executive Vice President
Ambulatory and Community Health Services
Children's National Medical Center
Professor of Pediatrics
George Washington University School of Medicine and Health Sciences
111 Michigan Avenue NW
Washington, DC 20010

Heather de Beaufort, M.D.
Pediatric Ophthalmologist
Children's National Medical Center
Assistant Professor
George Washington University School of Medicine and Health Sciences
111 Michigan Avenue NW
Washington, DC 20010

Dewi Frances T. Depositario-Cabacar, M.D.
Pediatric Neurologist
Children's National Medical Center
Assistant Professor, Neurology and Pediatrics
George Washington University School of Medicine and Health Sciences
111 Michigan Avenue NW
Washington, DC 20010

Larry W. Desch, M.D.
Medical Director of Developmental Pediatrics
Associate Professor of Clinical Pediatrics
Chicago Medical School, Rosalind Franklin University
Advocate Hope Children's Hospital
4440 West 95th Street
Oak Lawn, IL 60453

Lina Diaz-Calderon, M.D.
Pediatric Gastroenterology Fellow
Children's National Medical Center
111 Michigan Avenue
Washington, DC 20010

Peggy S. Eicher, M.D.
Medical Director, Center for Pediatric Feeding and Swallowing
St. Joseph's Children's Hospital
703 Main Street
Paterson, NJ 07503

Barbara L. Ekelman, Ph.D.
Adjunct Associate Professor of Psychology
Case Western Reserve University
11635 Euclid Avenue
Cleveland, OH 44106

Sarah H. Evans, M.D.
Pediatric Physiatrist
Chief of the Division of Rehabilitation Medicine
The Children's Hospital of Philadelphia
3401 Civic Center Boulevard
Philadelphia, PA 19104

Olanrewaju O. Falusi, M.D.
Associate Medical Director of Municipal and Regional Affairs, Child Health Advocacy Institute
Assistant Program Director, Community Health Track
Children's National Medical Center
Assistant Professor of Pediatrics
George Washington University School of Medicine and Health Sciences
2233 Wisconsin Avenue, Suite 317
Washington, DC 20007

Melissa Fleming, M.D.
Pediatric Physiatrist
Children's National Medical Center
Assistant Professor of Pediatrics
George Washington University School of Medicine and Health Sciences
111 Michigan Avenue NW
Washington, DC 20010

William Davis Gaillard, M.D.
Chief of Child Neurology, Epilepsy, and Neurophysiology
Children's National Medical Center
Professor of Neurology and Pediatrics
George Washington University School of Medicine and Health Sciences
111 Michigan Avenue NW
Washington, DC 20010

Satvika Garg, Ph.D.
Occupational Therapist
Children's National Medical Center
111 Michigan Avenue NW
Washington, DC 20010

Virginia C. Gebus, RN, MSN, APN, CNSC
Nutritionist
Children's National Medical Center
111 Michigan Avenue NW
Washington, DC 20010

Angelo P. Giardino, M.D., Ph.D., M.P.H.
Wilma T. Gibson Presidential Professor
Chair, Department of Pediatrics
University of Utah School of Medicine
Chief Medical Officer, Primary Children's Hospital
81 North Mario Capecchi Drive
Salt Lake City, UT 84113

Marianne M. Glanzman, M.D.
Attending Physician, Developmental and Behavioral Pediatrics
The Children's Hospital of Philadelphia
Clinical Professor of Pediatrics, Perelman School of Medicine
3550 Market Street, 3rd floor
Philadelphia, PA 19104

Monika Goyal, M.D., M.S.CE
Assistant Professor of Pediatrics and Emergency Medicine
Children's National Medical Center
George Washington University
111 Michigan Avenue NW
Washington, DC 20010

Andrea Gropman, M.D.
Pediatric Neurologist, Geneticist, and Neurodevelopmental Pediatrician
Chief, Division of Neurogenetics and Developmental Pediatrics
Children's National Medical Center
Professor in Neurology and Pediatrics
George Washington University School of Medicine and Health Sciences
111 Michigan Avenue NW
Washington, DC 20010

Mary A. Hadley, B.S.
Senior Executive Assistant
Children's National Medical Center
111 Michigan Avenue NW
Washington, DC 20705

Alexander H. Hoon, Jr., M.D., M.P.H.
Neurodevelopmental Pediatrician
Director, Phelps Center for Cerebral Palsy and Neurodevelopmental Medicine
Kennedy Krieger Institute
Associate Professor of Pediatrics
The Johns Hopkins University School of Medicine
801 North Broadway
Baltimore, MD 21205

Tara L. Johnson, M.D.
Assistant Professor
Developmental Neurologist
Arkansas Children's Hospital
1 Children's Way
Little Rock, AR 72202

Peter B. Kang, M.D.
Chief, Division of Pediatric Neurology
Professor of Pediatrics
University of Florida College of Medicine
P.O. Box 100296
Gainesville, FL 32610

Susan Keller, M.L.S., M.S.-HIT
Research Librarian
Children's National Medical Center
111 Michigan Avenue NW
Washington, DC 20010

Michael E. Kelley, Ph.D.
Pediatric Psychologist
Professor and Executive Director
Scott Center for Autism Treatment
Florida Institute of Technology
150 West University Boulevard
Melbourne, FL 32901

Lauren Kenworthy, Ph.D.
Neuropsychologist
Director, Center for Autism Spectrum Disorders
Children's National Medical Center
Professor of Pediatrics
George Washington University of Medicine and Health Sciences
15245 Shady Grove Road, Suite 350
Rockville, MD 20850

Monisha S. Kisling, M.Sc.
Genetic Counselor
Children's National Medical Center
111 Michigan Avenue NW, Suite 1950
Washington, DC 20010

Eyby Leon, M.D.
Pediatric Geneticist
Rare Disease Institute
Children's National Medical Center
Assistant Professor of Pediatrics
George Washington University School of Medicine and Health Sciences
111 Michigan Avenue
Washington, DC 20010

Barbara A. Lewis, Ph.D., CCC-SLP
Professor of Communication Sciences
Case Western Reserve University
11635 Euclid Avenue
Cleveland, OH 44106

M.E.B. Lewis, Ed.D.
Visiting Assistant Professor, School of Education
The Johns Hopkins University
2800 North Charles Street
Baltimore MD 21218

Toby M. Long, Ph.D., PT, FAPTA
Professor, Georgetown University
Director, Georgetown University Certificate in Early Intervention
Georgetown University
Center for Child and Human Development
3300 Whitehaven Street NW, Suite 3000
Washington, DC 20007

Erin MacLeod, Ph.D., RD, LD
Metabolic Dietitian
Rare Disease Institute
Children's National Medical Center
111 Michigan Avenue NW
Washington, DC, 20010

Lewis H. Margolis, M.D., M.P.H.
Associate Professor
Gillings School of Global Public Health
Department of Maternal and Child Health
University of North Carolina
135 Dauer Drive
Chapel Hill, NC 27599

Brian K. Martens, Ph.D.
Professor of Psychology
Syracuse University
Department of Psychology
430 Huntington Hall
Syracuse, NY 13244

Margaret B. Menzel, M.S., CGC
Genetic Counselor
Fetal Medicine Institute
Children's National Medical Center
111 Michigan Avenue NW, Suite M3119
Washington DC 20010

Shogo John Miyagi, Ph.D., Pharm.D., BCPPS
Fellow, Pediatric Clinical Pharmacology
Clinical Pharmacist
Children's National Medical Center
111 Michigan Avenue NW, M3.5-R102
Washington, DC 20010

Katherine Myers, D.O., M.P.H.
Developmental/Behavioral Pediatrician
UH Rainbow Babies and Children's Hospital
Assistant Professor of Pediatrics
Case Western Reserve University School of Medicine
W.O. Walker Building
10524 Euclid Avenue
Cleveland, Ohio 44106

Scott M. Myers, M.D.
Neurodevelopmental Pediatrician
Geisinger Health System
Clinical Assistant Professor of Pediatrics
Temple University School of Medicine
100 North Academy Avenue
Danville, PA 17822

Judith Owens, M.D., M.P.H.
Developmental/Behavioral Pediatrician
Director, Center for Pediatric Sleep Disorders
Boston Children's at Waltham
Professor of Neurology
Harvard Medical School
9 Hope Avenue
Waltham, Massachusetts 02453

Mitali Y. Patel, D.D.S.
Program Director, Pediatric Dentistry
Children's National Medical Center
111 Michigan Avenue NW
Washington, DC 20010

Joan E. Pellegrino, M.D.
Pediatric Geneticist
Associate Professor of Pediatrics
SUNY Upstate Medical University
750 East Adams Street
Syracuse, NY 13210

Deborah Potvin, Ph.D.
Neuropsychologist, Center for Autism Spectrum Disorders
Children's National Medical Center
Assistant Professor Pediatrics
George Washington University School of Medicine and Health Sciences
15245 Shady Grove Road, Suite 350
Rockville, MD 20850

Cara E. Pugliese, Ph.D.
Clinical Psychologist
Children's National Medical Center
Assistant Professor of Pediatrics
George Washington University School of Medicine and Health Sciences
111 Michigan Avenue NW
Washington, DC 20010

Khodayar Rais-Bahrami, M.D.
Neonatologist
Director, Neonatal-Perinatal Medicine Fellowship Program

Children's National Medical Center
Professor of Pediatrics
George Washington University School of Medicine and Health Sciences
111 Michigan Avenue NW
Washington, DC 20010

Allison B. Ratto, Ph.D.
Neuropsychologist, Center for Autism Spectrum Disorders
Children's National Medical Center
Assistant Professor Pediatrics
George Washington University School of Medicine and Health Sciences
15245 Shady Grove Road, Suite 350
Rockville, MD 20850

Sarah Risen, M.D.
Neurodevelopmental Pediatrician
Assistant Professor
Baylor College of Medicine
Texas Children's Hospital
6701 Fannin Street, Suite 1250
Houston TX 77030

Henry S. Roane, Ph.D.
The Gregory S. Liptak Professor of Child Development
Department of Pediatrics
SUNY Upstate Medical University
750 East Adams Street
Syracuse NY 13202

Adelaide S. Robb, M.D.
Distinguish Endowed Chair of Psychiatry and Behavioral Sciences
Children's National Medical Center
Professor of Psychiatry and Pediatrics
George Washington University School of Medicine and Health Sciences
111 Michigan Avenue NW
Washington, DC 20010

Angela McCaffrey Rosenberg, PT, DrPH, BCC
President, Inside Out Leadership, Inc.
Faculty, University of Arizona
Retired Associate Professor, University of North Carolina

Dimitrios A. Savva, Pharm.D.
Pediatric Pharmacy Resident
University of Maryland School of Pharmacy
20 North Pine Street
Baltimore MD 21201

Joseph Scafidi D.O.
Pediatric Neurologist
Associate Professor of Neurology and Pediatrics
Children's National Medical Center
Associate Professor of Neurology and Pediatrics
George Washington University School of Medicine and Health Sciences
111 Michigan Avenue NW
Washington, DC 20010

Erik Scheifele, D.M.D.
Chief, Division of Oral Health
Children's National Medical Center
111 Michigan Avenue NW
Washington, DC 20010-2970

Catherine Scherer, D.O.
Developmental/Behavioral Pediatrician
UH Rainbow Babies and Children's Hospital
Clinical Assistant Professor, Pediatrics
Case Western Reserve School of Medicine
10524 Euclid Avenue, Suite 3150
Cleveland, OH 44106

Rhonda L. Schonberg, M.S., CGC
Genetic Counselor, Rare Disease Institute
Children's National Medical Center
Clinical Instructor
George Washington University School of Medicine and Health Sciences
111 Michigan Avenue NW
Washington, DC 20010

Scott C. Schultz, M.D.
Pediatric Physiatrist
Associate Director of Physical Medicine and Rehabilitation
Children's Hospital
200 Henry Clay Avenue
New Orleans, LA 70118

Neelam Kharod Sell, M.D.
Developmental Behavioral Pediatrician
The Milestones Center
628 Shrewsbury Avenue
Tinton Falls, NJ 07701

Bruce K. Shapiro, M.D.
The Arnold J. Capute, M.D., M.P.H. Chair in Neurodevelopmental Disabilities
Vice President, Training
Kennedy Krieger Institute
Professor of Pediatrics
The Johns Hopkins University School of Medicine
707 North Broadway
Baltimore, MD 21205

Billie Lou Short, M.D.
Chief, Division of Neonatology
Children's National Medical Center
Professor of Pediatrics

George Washington School of Medicine
and Health Sciences
111 Michigan Avenue NW
Washington, DC 20010

Kara L. Simpson, M.S., CGC
Genetic Counselor
Children's National Medical Center
111 Michigan Avenue NW, #1950
Washington, DC 20010

William E. Sullivan, Ph.D.
Postdoctoral Associate
SUNY Upstate Medical University
600 E. Genesee Street, Suite 130
Syracuse, NY 13202

Anupama Rao Tate, D.M.D. M.P.H.
Pediatric Dentist
Children's National Medical Center
Associate Professor of Pediatrics
George Washington University School of Medicine
and Health Sciences
111 Michigan Avenue NW
Washington DC 20010

Shruti N. Tewar, MBBS, M.P.H.
Developmental/Behavioral Pediatrician
Clinical Assistant Professor
University of Iowa Stead Family Children's Hospital
100 Hawkins Drive, 209-A CDD
Iowa City, IA 52242-1011

Melissa K. Trovato, M.D.
Pediatric Physiatrist
Director of Inpatient Rehabilitation
Kennedy Krieger Institute
Assistant Professor
The John Hopkins University School of Medicine
707 North Broadway
Baltimore, MD 21205

Lisa Tuchman, M.D.
Chief, Division of Adolescent and Young Adult
Medicine
Center for Translational Science, Children's
Research Institute
Children's National Medical Center
Associate Professor of Pediatrics
George Washington University School of Medicine
and Health Sciences
111 Michigan Avenue NW
Washington, DC 20010

Renee M. Turchi, M.D., M.P.H.
Section Chief, General Pediatrics
Medical Director, The Center for Children with
Special Health Care Needs
St. Christopher's Hospital for Children
Clinical Professor of Pediatrics and Community
Health and Prevention
Drexel University School of Public Health
3601 A Street
Philadelphia, PA 19134

Johannes N. van den Anker, M.D., Ph.D., FCP
Division Chief of Clinical Pharmacology
Vice Chair of Experimental Therapeutics
Children's National Medical Center
Evan and Cindy Jones Professor of Pediatrics and
Pharmacology
George Washington University School of Medicine
and Health Sciences
111 Michigan Avenue NW
Washington, DC 20010

H. Barry Waldman, D.D.S., M.P.H., Ph.D.
Distinguished Teacher Professor
Department of General Dentistry
School of Dental Medicine
Stony Brook University
Stony Brook, NY 11794

Miriam Weiss, CPNP-PC
Nurse Practitioner
Children's National Medical Center
111 Michigan Avenue NW
Washington, DC, 20010

Susan E. Wiley, M.D.
Developmental/Behavioral Pediatrician
Cincinnati Children's Hospital Medical Center
Professor, Department of Pediatrics
University of Cincinnati College of Medicine
3333 Burnet Avenue ML 4002
Cincinnati, OH 45229

Michaela L. Zajicek-Farber, M.S.W., LCSW-C,
BCD, Ph.D.
Social Worker
Associate Professor
National Catholic School of Social Service
The Catholic University of America
Shahan Hall #112
620 Michigan Avenue NE
Washington, DC 20064

Tesfaye Getaneh Zelleke, M.D.
Pediatric Neurologist
Children's National Medical Center
Associate Professor of Neurology and Pediatrics
George Washington University School of Medicine
and Health Sciences
111 Michigan Avenue NW
Washington, DC 20010

A Personal Note to the Reader

As it enters its eighth edition, *Children with Disabilities* has continued to evolve. The first edition was derived from lectures I gave for a special education course at The Johns Hopkins University School of Education in Baltimore in 1978. The book contained 23 chapters, and I authored or co-authored virtually all of them. When I started writing the first edition, I was 3 years out of my neurodevelopmental disabilities fellowship training program, and I thought I knew everything about developmental disabilities! I also considered myself an expert in my own children's development, having just welcomed into our family our third child, Andrew (Drew).

With this new edition of the book, the number of chapters and pages has basically tripled since its inception, and I have authored but a few chapters. I have recognized the need for additional help and counsel and have brought on two valued colleagues, Dr. Louis Pellegrino and Dr. Nancy J. Roizen, to coedit the book with me. Lou directs the Child Development Program in the Center for Development, Behavior, and Genetics at Upstate Golisano Children's Hospital in Syracuse, New York. My friendship with Nancy, Division Chief of Pediatric Developmental and Behavioral Psychology at University Hospitals Rainbow Babies and Children's Hospital in Cleveland, Ohio, dates back to our training together at Hopkins. Based on our individual areas of expertise, we divided the book up. I took the sections As Life Begins, The Child's Body: Physiology, and Outcomes; Lou focused on Developmental Assessment and Developmental Disabilities; and Nancy edited the sections on Associated Disabilities and Interventions.

The book has also become somewhat of a family affair. My daughter Elissa, a special education teacher and school psychologist, authored the chapter on Special Education Services and contributed to the chapter on Racial and Ethnic Disparities. And Drew has continued his autobiographical letters concerning the effect of attention-deficit/hyperactivity disorder on his life, with him now being a successful executive in a start-up company and father to Mika and Gia.

It has been both personally and professionally very rewarding to develop this book over the past 40 years. Many of those rewards have come from the students, colleagues, and parents who have shared with me their thoughts and advice about the book. It is my hope that *Children with Disabilities* will continue to fill the needs of its diverse users for many years to come.

Mark L. Batshaw

Preface

One of the first questions asked about a subsequent edition of a textbook is, "What's new?" The challenge of determining what to revise, what to add, and, in some cases, what to delete is always significant in preparing a new edition in a field that is changing as rapidly as developmental disabilities. Since the publication of the seventh edition in 2013, advances in the fields of neuroscience and genetics have greatly enhanced our understanding of the brain and inheritance. This creates opportunities for treatments previously not thought possible for some children with developmental disabilities. Genomic sequencing is now used routinely (and sometimes recreationally), gene therapy is being used to correct birth defects, and the brain can be probed noninvasively by functional imaging techniques.

The need to examine and explain this advanced knowledge and its significance for children with disabilities has necessitated an increase in the depth and breadth of the subjects covered in the book. Yet, although the book is now more expansive and has several new chapters, we have worked hard to ensure that it retains its clarity and cohesion. Its mission continues to be to provide the individual working with and caring for children with disabilities the necessary background to understand different disabilities and their treatments, thereby enabling affected children to reach their full potential.

THE AUDIENCE

Since it was originally published, *Children with Disabilities* has been used by students in a wide range of disciplines as a medical textbook addressing the impact of disabilities on child development and function. It has also served as a professional reference for special educators, general educators, physical therapists, occupational therapists, speech-language pathologists, psychologists, child-life specialists, social workers, pediatric residents and medical students, psychiatrists, neurologists, pediatric nurses and nurse practitioners, advocates, and other practitioners who provide care for children with disabilities. Finally, as a family resource, parents, grandparents, siblings, and other family members and friends have used the book. They have found useful information on the medical and rehabilitative aspects of care for the child with developmental disabilities.

FEATURES FOR THE READER

We have been told that the strengths of previous editions of this book have been the accessible writing style, the clear illustrations, and the up-to-date information and references. We have dedicated our efforts to retaining these strengths and building on them with the addition of new features to highlight the application of content to evidence-based practice. Some of the features you will find in the eighth edition include the following.

- *Learning goals:* Each chapter begins with learning outcomes to orient you to the key content of that particular chapter.
- *Thought questions:* Questions have been crafted to "prime" the reader for what he or she should be thinking about while reading the chapter.
- *Case studies:* Most chapters include one or more situational examples to help bring alive the conditions and issues discussed in the chapter.
- *Key terms:* As key medical terms pertaining to a specific chapter are introduced in the text, they appear in boldface type at their first use; definitions for these terms appear in the Glossary (Appendix A).
- *Illustrations and tables:* More than 200 drawings, photographs, radiographs, imaging scans, and tables reinforce important concepts and provide ways for you to more easily understand and remember the material you are reading.
- *Summary:* Each chapter closes with a final section that in a bulleted list summarizes its key elements and provides you with an abstract of the covered material.
- *References:* The reference list accompanying each chapter can be considered more than just a list of the literature cited in the chapter. These citations

include review articles, reports of study findings, research discoveries, and other key references that can help you find additional information. We have tried to keep the majority of the references within 5 years of the book's publication so they are recent and relevant, although classic research is often still relevant and included.

- *Interdisciplinary boxes:* New to this edition, chapters include special boxes that summarize the role of specific disciplines relevant to the chapter's content. This feature emphasizes the interprofessional nature of caring for children with developmental disabilities.
- *Evidence-based practice boxes:* This new feature acknowledges the importance of evidence-based practice by summarizing the results of current research relevant to the topic and providing a "take-away message" so readers can apply the information to practice.
- *Appendices:* In addition to the Glossary, there are two other helpful appendices: 1) Syndromes and Inborn Errors of Metabolism, a mini-reference of pertinent information on inherited disorders causing developmental disabilities, and 2) Commonly Used Medications, to describe indications and side effects of medications often prescribed for children with disabilities.
- *Web site:* We have created a web site specific for *Children with Disabilities* that has additional content, including the following: 1) a resource directory of a wide range of national organizations, federal agencies, information sources, self-advocacy and accessibility programs, and support groups that can provide assistance to families and professionals; 2) a bank of 250 test questions for instructors; and 3) study questions and extension activities for every chapter. This content will be continuously updated.

CONTENT

In developing this eighth edition, we have aimed for a balance between consistency with the text that many of you have come to know so well and appreciate in its previous editions and innovation in exploring the new topics that demand our attention. All chapters have been substantially revised, and many have been rewritten to include an expanded focus on the psychosocial, rehabilitative, and educational interventions, as well as to provide information discovered through educational, medical, and scientific advances since 2013.

Seven new chapters have been added, including the following.

- Chapter 7: The Senses: The World We See, Hear, and Feel
- Chapter 11: Child Development
- Chapter 28: Sleep Disorders
- Chapter 30: Interdisciplinary Education and Practice
- Chapter 38: Pharmacological Therapy
- Chapter 42: Racial and Ethnic Disparities

The new chapters focus on recently gained knowledge that is transforming our understanding of the causes and treatment of developmental disabilities.

The chapters are grouped into seven parts and organized to help guide readers through the breadth of content. Each part is detailed next.

Part I: The book starts with a section titled As Life Begins, which addresses what happens before, during, and/or shortly after birth to cause a child to be at increased risk for a developmental disability. The concepts and consequences of genetics, environmental influences, prenatal diagnosis, newborn screening, neonatal complication, and prematurity are explained.

Part II: The next section of the book, The Child's Body: Physiology, covers embryonic and fetal development, the sensory systems, the brain and central nervous system, muscles, bones and nerves, and the gastrointestinal tract—how they develop and work, and what can go wrong.

Part III : The third section covers Developmental Assessment. It includes chapters on typical and atypical development, diagnosing developmental disabilities, assessing physical disabilities, and neurocognitive and behavioral assessment.

Part IV: As its title implies, the fourth section, Developmental Disabilities, provides comprehensive descriptions of the major developmental disabilities and genetic syndromes that cause disabilities. This section includes chapters on intellectual disability, Down syndrome and fragile x syndrome, inborn errors of metabolism, speech and language disorders, autism spectrum disorder, attention-deficit/hyperactivity disorder, specific learning disabilities, cerebral palsy, epilepsy, acquired brain injury, and chronic diseases with related developmental disabilities.

Part V: The fifth section addresses Associated Disabilities, those disorders that occur more commonly in individuals with developmental disabilities. Chapters include discussions on visual deficits, hearing impairment, behavioral/mental health issues, sleep disorders and feeding disorders.

Part VI: The sixth section focuses on Interventions. It contains chapters on interdisciplinary care, early intervention and special education services, (re)habilitative services, oral health care, behavioral therapy, assistive technology, family assistance, medication, and complementary health approaches.

Part VII: The final section is directed at Outcomes. This section concentrates on transition to adulthood, the effect of health care systems on outcomes, and health care disparities and their effect on outcomes in children with developmental disabilities.

THE CONTRIBUTORS AND REVIEW PROCESS

For contributors to this edition, we chose educators, physicians, dentists, psychologists, social workers, genetic counselors, occupational and physical therapists, speech-language pathologists, and other health care professionals who are experts in the areas they write about. Many are colleagues from Children's National Medical Center in Washington, D.C. Each chapter in the book has undergone editing at Paul H. Brookes Publishing Co. to ensure consistency in style and accessibility of content. Once the initial drafts were completed, each chapter was sent for peer review by major clinical and academic leaders in the field and was revised according to their input.

A FEW NOTES ABOUT TERMINOLOGY AND STYLE

As is the case with any book of this scope, the editors and contributors make decisions about the use of particular words and the presentation style of information. We would like to share with you some of the decisions we have made for this book.

- *Categories of intellectual disability:* This book uses the American Psychiatric Association's categories according to the term *intellectual disability* (i.e., mild, moderate, severe, profound) when discussing medical diagnosis and treatment, and uses the categories that the American Association on Intellectual and Developmental Disabilities (formerly the American Association on Mental Retardation) established in 1992 (i.e., requiring limited, intermittent, extensive, or pervasive support) when discussing educational and other interventions, thus emphasizing the capabilities rather than the impairments of individuals with intellectual disability.
- *"Typical" versus "normal":* Recognizing diversity and the fact that no one type of person or lifestyle is inherently "normal," we have chosen to refer to the general population of children as "typical" or "typically developing," meaning that they follow the natural continuum of development.
- *Person-first language:* We have tried to preserve the dignity and personhood of all individuals with disabilities by consistently using person-first language, speaking, for example, of "a child with cerebral palsy," instead of "a cerebral palsied child." In this way, we are able to emphasize the person, not define him or her by the condition.

As you read this eighth edition of *Children with Disabilities,* we hope you will find that the text continues to address the frequently asked question, "Why this child?" and to provide the medical background you need to care for children with developmental disabilities.

Acknowledgments

We would like to thank our colleagues at Paul H. Brookes Publishing Co., Inc., for their great help. Jolynn Gower served as Acquisitions Editor, Liz Gildea as Associate Editor, and Stephanie Henderson as Editorial Assistant, providing developmental oversight and management of the project. Nicole Schmidl managed the production of the book, and Janet Wehner managed the production of the online content. We also would like to acknowledge Nancy Peterson, who helped organize this project as well as contributed to its editorial development.

A book such as *Children with Disabilities* is best understood with illustrations that help to explain medical concepts. Expert medical illustrators are crucial in this effort. Elaine Kasmer and Lynn Reynolds have contributed to this endeavor in previous editions, and Catherine Twomey has created new illustrations for this eighth edition. We deeply acknowledge their important contributions.

We thank previous contributors whose work on the seventh edition laid an excellent foundation for this text: Kruti Acharya, George Acs, Stephen Baumgart, Donna Bernhardt Bainbridge, Michelle L. Bestic, Michael J. Bina, Pamela Buethe, Philippa Campbell, Marilyn Cataldo, Michael F. Cataldo, Taeun Chang, Iser G. DeLeon, Nienke P. Dosa, Patrick C. Friman, Chrysanthe Gaitatzes, Brooke E. Geddie, Arlene Gendron, James Gleason, Rebecca M. Haesler, Gilbert R. Herer, Susan L. Hyman, SungWoo Kahng, Robert Keating, Brendan Lanpher, Susan E. Levy, Michelle Huckaby Lewis, Marijean M. Miller, Jocelyn J. Mills, Jerome Paulson, Steven P. Perlman, Adré J. du Plessis, Vincent Schuyler, Peter J. Smith, Sheela Stuart, Adrienne S. Tedeschi, Frances Tolley, Betty R. Vohr, Patience H. White, Amanda Yaun, and Michelle H. Zimmer. Finally, many of our colleagues reviewed and edited the manuscript for content and accuracy, and we would like to acknowledge their efforts.

Why me?
Why me?
Why do I have to do so much more than others?
Why am I so forgetful?
Why am I so hyperactive?
And why can't I spell?
Why me? O'why me?

I remember when I almost failed first grade because I couldn't read. I would cry hour after hour because my mother would try to make me read. Now I love to read. I couldn't write in cursive but my mother helped me and now I can. I don't have as bad a learning disability as others. At lest I can go to a normal school. I am trying as hard as I can (I just hope it is enough). My worst nightmare is to go to a special school because I don't want to be treated differently.

I am getting to like working. I guess since my dad is so successful and has a learning disability, it helps make me not want to give up. Many people say that I am smart, but sometimes I doubt it. I am very good at math, but sometimes I read a number like 169 as 196, so that messes things up. I also hear things incorrectly, for instants entrepreneur as horse manure (that really happened). I guess the reason why a lot of people don't like me is because I say the wrong answer a lot of times.

I had to take medication, but then I got off the medication and did well. Then in 7th grade I wasn't doing well but I didn't tell my parents because I thought they would just scream at me. My dad talked to the guidance counselor and found out. It wasn't till a week ago that I started on the medication again; I have been doing fine since than. As I have been getting more organized, I have had more free time. I guess I feel good when I succeed in things that take hard work.

This is my true story . . .

Andrew Batshaw

Andrew Batshaw
1989 (age 12)

Twenty-eight years ago, I wrote the first letter that appears in this book. I was 12, a child on the cusp of becoming a teenager, and grappling (emotionally, socially, and intellectually) with my learning disability. I felt like its victim. I was scared and ashamed. I was unsure if I'd have the opportunities that others had, and even worse, unsure if I'd be able to live what I imagined was a normal life. Fortunately for me, I was born with not just a learning disability but also many advantages. I am naturally hopeful, curious, and smart, and I was born into a loving family with the means and knowledge to support me.

I am now 40 years old and living a life that my 12-year-old self would have found extraordinary. I am enjoying a time of stability, growth, and powerful impact. My wife and I are thrilled to be celebrating our 13th wedding anniversary this year. Our children, Gia and Mika, are now older and more independent at 10 and 8; they are healthy, bright, and beautiful. I have satisfying relationships including long-term friendships with people I met around the time I wrote that first letter. On the work front, I have found my home: I am proud to serve as the CTO and a co-founder of Waggl, a 60-person company that provides an innovative real-time feedback platform for employees. I am so proud to have built an organization where employees love to work and where we improve the work lives of hundreds of thousands of people every year. In my role, I get to lead not just the technology of the company but also its culture and how we grow as an organization.

Right now, my eldest daughter Gia is nearing the age that I was when I wrote my first letter, and I am nearing the age that my father was. Over the last several years, my daughters have been learning to read, write, and spell. I have found myself occasionally feeling anxious that they might also have learning disabilities and that they, too, would struggle as I did through much of their childhood. When I sat down to read with them in the early days, it often brought back painful memories. Sometimes when they were frustrated sounding out an unknown word, it was as if I were back at the living room table with my mother, looking at a word, trying as hard as I could to figure it out, and failing. When my youngest, Mika, came home one day and said without concern, "I think I am in the easiest spelling group," I immediately thought of being sorted into reading groups in second grade and wondering why I was in the group with the kids who were always struggling in class. When she has trouble sitting still and focusing on what we are discussing, I can't help but wonder, "Does she have ADHD, or is that normal behavior for a second-grader?" Both of their teachers have reassured us that they are doing well, and are learning and focused in class. So, I am happy to say that there aren't any real indications that either daughter inherited my disability. Even so, I sometimes think, what if they did?

I've imagined that Andrew from 1989 was my child. What would I do for him now? I don't think I could replicate what my mom did for me—devoting herself with heroic patience, time, and energy to support me academically—but I could arrange for daily support. I would enroll him in a regular private school to allow him more individualized attention than public school could offer (but respect his wishes not to go to a specialized school). Like my father, I would share my childhood struggles with Andrew. I would share the letters I have written over the years about my disability to help him understand the kind of journey that is ahead of him and how much better things get. I would give him tools for working with his feelings of frustration and inadequacy, and I would teach him to meditate. I would encourage him to pursue nonacademic interests to give him a variety of experiences of success.

And . . . I would sit him down and read his letter "Why Me?" . . . look him straight in the eye and say, "I know this is hard right now, and that you are struggling. You may not believe this, but this struggle will serve you. You are worried that you may not be able to live a normal life. This struggle will help you live an **extraordinary** life. Why you? Because someday you will transcend this disability. In that process, you will learn things that will make you successful . . . and, even more importantly, will help you make this world a better place."

Andrew Batshaw
2018

Dedicated to all of the families we have been honored to serve
and to the health care professionals we have taught
so they could expertly care for children with disabilities

PART I

As Life Begins

CHAPTER 1

The Genetics Underlying Developmental Disabilities

Mark L. Batshaw, Eyby Leon, and Monisha S. Kisling

Upon completion of this chapter, the reader will

- Know about the human genome and its implication for the origins of developmental disabilities
- Be able to explain how errors in cell division can cause genetic syndromes
- Know about Mendelian inheritance
- Recognize the importance of mutations and genetic variation
- Understand the ways that genes can be affected by the environment in which they reside, i.e., epigenetics
- Know about genetic testing for the origins of developmental disability
- Be aware of novel genetic treatment approaches

Whether we have brown or blue eyes is determined by genes passed on to us from our parents. Other traits, such as height and weight, are affected by genes and by our environment both before and after birth. In a similar manner, genes alone or in combination with environmental factors can place children at increased risk for many developmental disorders, including birth defects such as meningomyelocoele (spina bifida). In the case of meningomyelocoele, a maternal nutritional deficiency of folic acid can markedly increase the risk of the genetic disorder. Disorders associated with developmental disabilities have a spectrum of genetic and environmental origins. Some disorders are purely genetic, such as Tay-Sachs disease (a progressive neurologic disorder) and result from a defect in a **single gene,** while others like Down syndrome (see Chapter 15), result from a chromosomal error, in which an extra chromosome containing hundreds of genes exists. Other developmental disorders result from purely environmental exposures, including prenatal viral infections such as cytomegalovirus and teratogenic agents like alcohol and thalidomide (see Chapter 2). There are also conditions in which genes are affected by their environment, leading to epigenetic disorders such as fragile X syndrome and Angelman syndrome.

As an introduction to the topics discussed in the other chapters of this volume, this chapter describes the human cell and explains chromosomes and genes. It also reviews and provides illustrations and examples of the errors that can occur in the processes of **meiosis** (reductive cell division) and **mitosis** (cell replication), summarizes inheritance patterns of single-gene disorders, and presents the concept of epigenetics. Furthermore, this chapter discusses innovative treatments that manipulate or use an understanding of the child's genome to improve an outcome. It is important to understand that while these disorders are individually rare, genetic alterations underlie almost half of developmental disabilities. Medical treatment is increasingly available for a number of these disorders, though often at great cost.

CASE STUDY

Katy developed typically until she was 2 years old, when she started to have episodes of vomiting and lethargy after high-protein meals. Her parents became very concerned because their older son, Andrew, had died in infancy after an episode of lethargy and seizures was followed by coma, although no specific diagnosis had been made. After extensive testing by a genetic specialist, Katy was discovered to have a specific mutation or error in the gene that codes for ornithine transcarbamylase (OTC), an enzyme that prevents the accumulation of toxic ammonia in the body and brain. The OTC gene is located on the X chromosome; since girls have two X chromosomes, when one X has the mutation, there is a second normal copy to mitigate the defect. As a result, girls are less likely to be affected by X-linked disorders than boys, and, when affected, they generally have less severe symptoms. After Katy was diagnosed with OTC deficiency, her specialist tested DNA that was extracted before Andrew's death and found that he too carried this mutation. Katy was placed on a low-protein diet and given a medicine to provide an alternate pathway to rid the body of ammonia, and she has done well. Now age 7, she appears to have a mild nonverbal learning disability resulting from her prior metabolic crises; if Katy had been left untreated, she would probably not be alive.

Thought Questions:

How often do we miss a genetic diagnosis as a cause of developmental disabilities? Could earlier diagnosis and treatment improve outcomes in many of these cases?

GENETIC DISORDERS

The human body is composed of approximately 100 trillion cells. There are many cell types: nerve cells, muscle cells, white blood cells, liver cells and skin cells, to name a few. All cells, with the exception of the red blood cell, are divided into two compartments: a central, enclosed core—the **nucleus**—and an outer area—the **cytoplasm** (Figure 1.1). The red blood cell differs insofar as it does not have a nucleus. The nucleus houses **chromosomes,** structures that contain the genetic code—DNA (**deoxyribonucleic acid**), which is organized into hundreds of

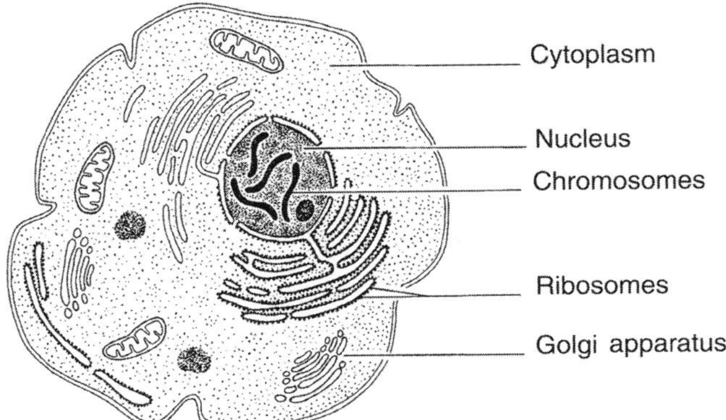

Figure 1.1. An idealized cell. The genes within chromosomes direct the creation of a product on the ribosomes. The product is then packaged in the Golgi apparatus and released from the cell.

genes (units of heredity) in each chromosome. There are 23 pairs of chromosomes and about 20,000 protein-coding genes that collectively make up the human **genome.** These genes are responsible for our physical attributes and for the biological functioning of our bodies. Under the direction of the genes, the products that are needed for the organism's development and functions, such as waste disposal and the release of energy, are made in the cytoplasm. The nucleus contains the blueprint for the organism's growth and development, and the cytoplasm manufactures the products needed to complete the task.

When there is a defect within this system, the result may be a genetic disorder, often causing developmental disabilities. These disorders take many forms. They include the addition of an entire chromosome in each cell (e.g., Down syndrome), the loss of an entire chromosome in each cell (e.g., Turner syndrome), and the loss or deletion of a significant portion of a chromosome (e.g., Cri-du-chat syndrome). There can also be a **microdeletion** of a number of closely spaced or contiguous genes within a chromosome (e.g., chromosome 22q11.2 deletion syndrome, also called velocardiofacial syndrome [VCFS]). Microdeletions may have varied expression depending on stochastic (randomly determined) and environmental processes, as well as on genetic effects, with these factors potentially acting alone or in combination (Bertini et al., 2017). Finally, there can be a defect within a single gene (e.g., phenylketonuria) or altered expression of the gene (e.g., Rett syndrome). This chapter discusses each of these types of genetic defects.

CHROMOSOMES

Each organism has a fixed number of chromosomes that directs the cell's activities. In each human cell, there are normally 46 chromosomes. Each chromosome contains many genes, but some chromosomes have more (e.g., 500–800 gene loci in chromosomes 1, 19, and X) and others have fewer (50–120 in chromosomes 13, 18, 21, and Y). The 46 chromosomes are organized into 23 pairs. Typically, one chromosome in each pair comes from the mother and the other from the father. Egg and sperm cells, unlike all other human cells, each contains only 23 chromosomes. During conception, these **germ cells** (i.e., sperm and eggs) fuse to produce a fertilized egg with the full complement of 46 chromosomes.

Among the 23 pairs of chromosomes, 22 are termed **autosomes.** The 23rd pair consists of the X and Y chromosomes and are called the **sex chromosomes.** The Y chromosome, which is involved in male sex determination and development, is one-third to one-half the size of the X chromosome, has a different shape, and has far fewer genes. Two X chromosomes determine the child to be female; an X and a Y chromosome determine the child to be male.

CELL DIVISION AND ITS DISORDERS

Cells have the ability to divide into daughter cells that contain genetic information that is identical to the information from the parent cell. The prenatal development of a human being is accomplished through cell division, differentiation into different cell types, and movement of cells to different locations in the body. There are two kinds of cell division: **mitosis** and **meiosis.** In mitosis, or nonreductive division, 2 daughter cells, each containing 46 chromosomes, are formed from 1 parent cell. In meiosis, or reductive division, 4 daughter cells, each containing only 23 chromosomes, are formed from 1 parent cell. Although mitosis occurs in all cells, meiosis takes place only in the germ cells.

The ability of cells to continue to undergo mitosis throughout the life span is essential for proper bodily functioning. Cells divide at different rates, however, ranging from once every 10 hours for skin cells to once a year for liver cells. This is why a skin abrasion heals in a few days but the liver may take a year to recover from hepatitis. By adulthood, some cells, including neurons and muscle cells, appear to have a significantly decreased ability to divide. This limits the body's capacity to recover after medical events, such as strokes, or from traumatic injuries.

One of the primary differences between mitosis and meiosis can be seen during the first of the two meiotic divisions. During this cell division, the corresponding chromosomes line up beside each other in pairs (e.g., both copies of chromosome 1 line up together). Unlike in mitosis, however, they intertwine and may "cross over," exchanging genetic material. This adds variability. Although this crossing over (or recombination) of the chromosomes may result in disorders (e.g., deletions), it also allows for the mutual transfer of genetic information, reducing the chance that siblings end up as exact copies (clones) of each other. Some of the variability among siblings can also be attributed to the random assortment of maternal and paternal chromosomes during the first of the two meiotic divisions.

Throughout the life span of the male, meiosis of the immature sperm produces **spermatocytes** with 23 chromosomes each. These cells will lose most of their cytoplasm, sprout tails, and become mature sperm. This process is termed spermatogenesis. In the female, meiosis forms oocytes that will ultimately become mature eggs in a process called oogenesis. By the time a girl is born, her body has produced all of the approximately 2 million eggs she will ever have.

A number of events that adversely affect a child's development can occur during meiosis. When chromosomes divide unequally, a process known as **nondisjunction** occurs; as a result, 1 daughter egg or sperm contains 24 chromosomes and the other 22 chromosomes. Meiotic nondisjunction, particularly in oogenesis, is the most common mutational mechanism in humans responsible for chromosomally atypical fetuses. Usually, these cells do not survive, but occasionally they do and can lead to the child being born with too many chromosomes (e.g., Down syndrome) or too few (e.g., Turner syndrome). Notably, the most commonly found **trisomy** in miscarriages is trisomy 16, and embryos with trisomy 16 are never carried to term (Nussbaum, McInnes, & Willard, 2016). The chromosome 16 contains so many genes important for normal development that its disruption is incompatible with life. Conversely, trisomies 13, 18, and 21 are the most commonly observed full trisomies at birth (Mai et al., 2013). However, even in these conditions, the vast majority of embryos with the defect do not survive.

The majority of fetuses carrying chromosomal abnormalities are spontaneously aborted. Among those children who survive these genetic missteps, **intellectual disability,** unusual (dysmorphic) facial appearances, and various congenital organ malformations are common. In the general population, chromosomal errors causing disorders occur in 6–9 per 1,000 of all live births. In children who have intellectual disability, however, the prevalence of chromosomal abnormality increases, being responsible for 20% of the cases (Martin & Ledbetter, 2017). It is also clear that as the woman ages, the risk of errors in meiosis increases, as is typified by Down syndrome.

Chromosomal Gain: Down Syndrome

The most frequent chromosomal abnormality is unequal division of non-sex chromosomes, and the most common clinical consequence is trisomy 21, or Down syndrome (Nussbaum, McInnes, & Willard, 2016; also see Chapter 15). Nondisjunction can occur during either mitosis or meiosis but is more common in meiosis (Figure 1.2). When nondisjunction occurs during the first meiotic division, both copies of chromosome 21 end up in one cell. Instead of an equal distribution of chromosomes among cells (23 each), 1 daughter cell receives 24 chromosomes and the other receives only 22. The cell containing 22 chromosomes is unable to survive. However, the egg (or sperm) with 24 chromosomes occasionally can survive. After fertilization with a sperm (or egg) containing 23 chromosomes, the resulting embryo contains 3 copies of chromosome 21, or trisomy 21. The child will be born with 47 rather than 46 chromosomes in each cell and will thus have Down syndrome (Figure 1.3).

The majority of individuals with Down syndrome (approximately 95%) have trisomy 21. This trisomy results from nondisjunction during meiosis in oogenesis in 90% of the cases and from nondisjunction during spermatogenesis in 10% (Nussbaum, McInnes, & Willard, 2016). This disparity is partially due to the increased rate of autosomal nondisjunction in egg production, but also to the lack of viability of sperm with an extra chromosome 21. Another 3%–4% of individuals acquire Down syndrome as a result of **translocation** (discussed later) and 1%–2% acquire it from **mosaicism** (some cells being affected and others not; this is also discussed later).

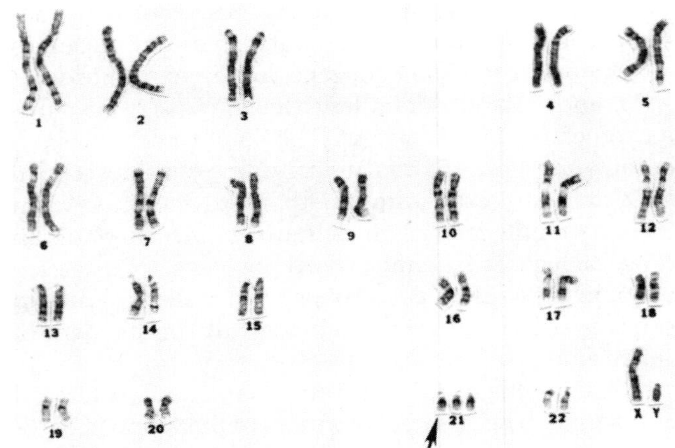

Figure 1.3. Karyotype of a boy with Down syndrome (47, XY). Note that the child has 47 chromosomes; the extra one is a chromosome 21.

Chromosomal Loss: Turner Syndrome

Turner syndrome is the only disorder in which a fetus can survive despite the loss of an entire chromosome. Even so, more than 99% of the 45,X conceptions appear

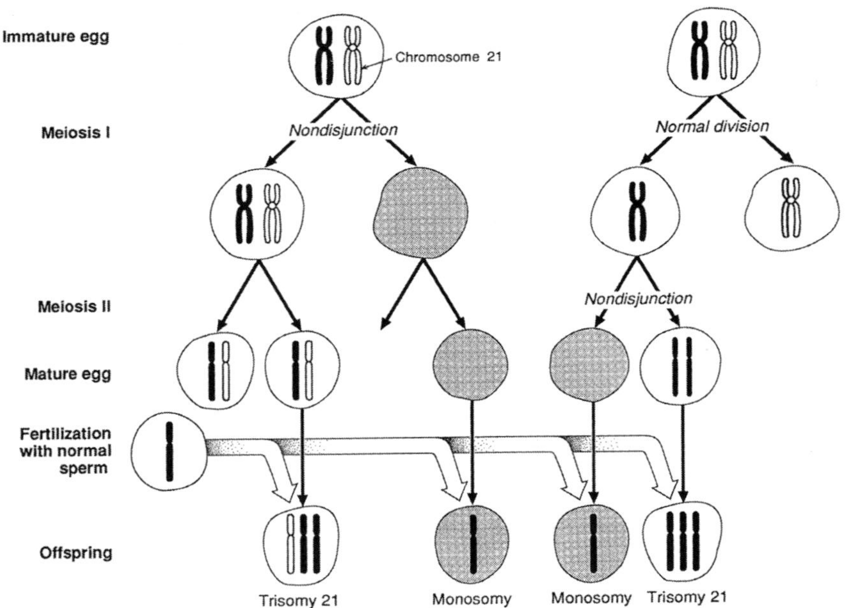

Figure 1.2. Nondisjunction of chromosome 21 in meiosis. Unequal division during meiosis I or meiosis II can result in trisomy or monosomy.

to be miscarried (Hook & Warburton, 2014). Females with Turner syndrome (1 in every 5,000 live births) have a single X chromosome and no second X or Y chromosome, for a total of 45, rather than 46, chromosomes. In contrast to Down syndrome, 80% of individuals with **monosomy** X conditions are affected by meiotic errors in sperm production; these children usually receive an X chromosome from their mothers but no sex chromosome from their fathers.

Girls with Turner syndrome typically have short stature, a webbed neck, a broad "shield-like" chest with widely spaced nipples, and nonfunctional ovaries. Twenty percent have obstruction of the left side of the heart, most commonly caused by a **coarctation** of the **aorta.** Unlike children with Down syndrome, most girls with Turner syndrome develop typically. They do, however, have visual–perceptual impairments that predispose them to develop nonverbal learning disabilities (Table 1.1; Hong & Reiss, 2014). Human growth hormone injections have been effective in increasing height in girls with Turner syndrome, and **estrogen** supplementation can lead to the emergence of secondary sexual characteristics; however, these girls remain infertile.

Mosaicism

In mosaicism, cells in the same individual have different genetic makeups (Nussbaum, McInnes, & Willard, 2016). For example, a child with the mosaic form of Down syndrome may have trisomy 21 in skin cells but not in blood cells. or the individual may have trisomy 21 in some, but not all, brain cells. Children with mosaicism often appear as though they have a particular condition (in this example, Down syndrome); however, the physical/organ and cognitive impairments may be less severe. Usually mosaicism occurs when some cells in a trisomy conception lose the extra chromosome via nondisjunction during mitosis. Mosaicism also can occur if some cells lose a chromosome after a normal conception (e.g., some cells lose an X chromosome in mosaic Turner syndrome). Mosaicism is present in only 5%–10% of all children with chromosomal abnormalities.

Translocations

A relatively common dysfunction in cell division, translocation can occur during mitosis and meiosis when the chromosomes break and then exchange parts with other chromosomes. Translocation involves the transfer of a portion of one chromosome to a completely different chromosome. For example, a portion of chromosome 21 might attach itself to chromosome 14 (Figure 1.4). If this occurs during meiosis, 1 daughter cell will then have 23 chromosomes but will have both a chromosome 21 and a chromosome 14/21 translocation. Fertilization of this egg, by a sperm with a cell containing the normal complement of 23 chromosomes, will result in a child with 46 chromosomes. This includes two copies of chromosome 21, one chromosome 14/21, and one chromosome 14. This child will have Down syndrome because of the functional trisomy 21 caused by the translocation.

Deletions

Another somewhat common dysfunction in cell division is deletion. Here, part, but not all, of a chromosome is lost. Chromosomal deletions occur in two forms: visible deletions and microdeletions. Those that are large enough to be seen through the microscope are called visible deletions. Those that are so small that they can only be detected at the molecular level are called microdeletions and can be identified by a test called chromosomal microarray.

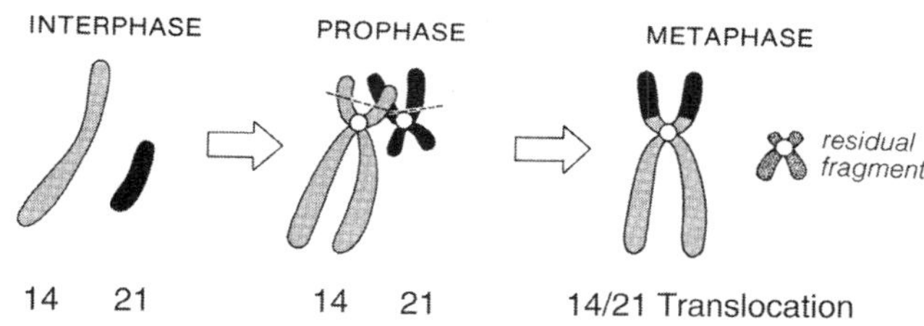

Figure 1.4. Translocation. During **prophase** of meiosis in a parent, there may be a transfer of a portion of one chromosome to another. In this figure, the long arm of chromosome 21 is translocated to chromosome 14, and the residual fragments are lost.

Table 1.1. Neurocognitive deficits in Turner syndrome

Intellectual function	Typical but 5–10 points below siblings; verbal IQ > performance IQ
Visual spatial	Deficits in spatial orientation
Math	Difficulties with calculation
Executive function	Impairment in attention, processing speed, working memory, cognitive flexibility, and planning
Social	Impairments in face recognition and social reciprocity
Behavior	Overall risk of attention-deficit/hyperactivity disorder and dyscalculia; equivocal evidence for autism

Source: Hong and Reiss (2014).

Cri-du-chat ("cat cry") syndrome is an example of a visible chromosomal deletion in which a portion of the short arm of chromosome 5 is lost. Cri-du-chat syndrome affects approximately 1 in 50,000 children, causing microcephaly and an unusual facial appearance with a round face, widely spaced eyes, **epicanthal folds,** and low-set ears. Children with the syndrome have a high-pitched cry and intellectual disability (Cerruti Mainardi, 2006).

Examples of **microdeletion syndromes** (also called **contiguous gene syndromes** because they involve the deletion of a number of adjacent genes) include Smith-Magenis syndrome, Williams syndrome, and VCFS (Weischenfeldt, Symmons, Spitz, & Korbel, 2013). Smith-Magenis is caused by a microdeletion in the short arm of chromosome 17, Williams syndrome by a deletion in the long arm of chromosome 7, and VCFS by a deletion in the long arm of chromosome 22. Children with Smith-Magenis syndrome have feeding difficulties, hypotonia, distinctive facial features, self-injurious behavior, and intellectual disability. Children with Williams syndrome likewise have intellectual disability with a distinctive facial appearance, but they also have cardiac defects and a unique cognitive profile with apparent expressive language skills beyond what would be expected based on their cognitive abilities. Children with VCFS syndrome may have a cleft palate, a congenital heart defect, a characteristic facial appearance, and/or a nonverbal learning disability. Cognitive problems are often present, and many affected children satisfy the criteria for a diagnosis of autism.

Frequency of Chromosomal Abnormalities

In total, approximately 25% of eggs and 3%–4% of sperm have an extra or missing chromosome, and an additional 1% and 5%, respectively, have a structural chromosomal abnormality (Hassold, Hall, & Hunt, 2007). As a result, 10%–15% of all conceptions have a chromosomal abnormality. Somewhat more than 50% of these abnormalities are trisomies, 20% are monosomies, and 15% are **triploidies** (69 chromosomes). The remaining chromosomal abnormalities are composed of structural abnormalities and **tetraploidies** (92 chromosomes). It may therefore seem surprising that more children are not born with chromosomal abnormalities. The explanation is that more than 95% of fetuses with chromosomal abnormalities do not survive to term. In fact, many are lost very early in gestation, even before a pregnancy may be recognized.

GENES AND THEIR DISORDERS

The underlying problem with the previously mentioned chromosomal disorders is the presence of too many or too few genes resulting from extra or missing chromosomal material. Genetic disorders can also result from an abnormality in a single gene. As noted above, there are about 20,000 genes in the human genome. This is quite remarkable given that the fruit fly has approximately 13,000 genes, the round worm 19,000 genes, and a simple plant 26,000 genes. It was previously thought that each gene regulated the production of a single protein. Now it is known that the situation is much more complex; single genes in humans code for multiple proteins, giving humans the combinational diversity that lower organisms lack. Humans can produce approximately 100,000 proteins from less than one-quarter of that many genes. However, it must be acknowledged that the chimp shares 99% of the human genome. Having now examined the genome of innumerable organisms, the minimum number of genes necessary for life appears to be approximately 300; all living organisms share these same 300 genes.

The mechanism by which genes act as blueprints for producing specific proteins needed for body functions is as follows. Genes are composed of various lengths of DNA that, together with intervening DNA sequences, form chromosomes. DNA is formed as a **double helix,** a structure that resembles a twisted ladder (Figure 1.5). The sides of the ladder are composed of sugar and phosphate molecules, whereas the "rungs" are made up of four chemicals called **nucleotide bases: cytosine** (C), **guanine** (G), **adenine** (A), and **thymine** (T). Pairs of nucleotide bases interlock to form each rung: cytosine bonds with guanine, and adenine bonds with thymine. The sequence of nucleotide bases on a segment of DNA (spelled out by the four-letter alphabet C, G, A, T) make up an individual's genetic code. Individual genes range in size, containing from 1,500 to more than 2 million nucleotide–base pairs. Overall, there are approximately 3.3 billion base pairs in the human genome, but only about 1% encode genes that serve as a blueprint for protein production. It should also be noted that all genes are not "turned on" or expressed at all times. Some are only active during fetal

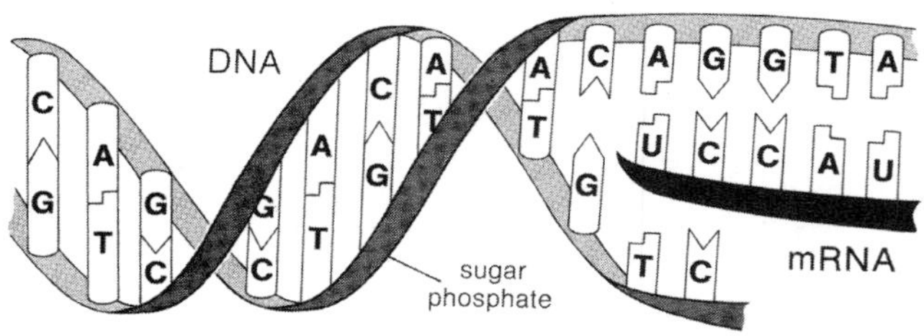

Figure 1.5. Deoxyribonucleic acid (DNA). Four nucleotides (C, cytosine; G, guanine; A, adenosine; T, thymine) form the genetic code. On the mRNA molecule, uracil (U) substitutes for thymine. The DNA unzips to transcribe its message as mRNA.

life (e.g., the fetal hemoglobin gene), and it is hoped that some are never expressed (e.g., oncogenes, which have the potential to cause cancer). The turning on and off of genes usually follows a carefully developmentally regulated process, but it can also be influenced by the environment. Regulation of gene expression plays a particularly important role during fetal development; as a result, problems involving gene expression during fetal development can be particularly devastating. The way gene expression is regulated involves a number of structural changes to the DNA and its architecture without altering the actual nucleotide sequence of the DNA. This process is termed *epigenetics* and is a cause of a number of genetic syndromes that are associated with developmental disabilities.

Transcription

The production of a specific protein begins when the DNA comprising that gene unwinds and the two strands (the sides of the ladder) unzip to expose the genetic code (Jorde, Carey, & Bamshad, 2015). The exposed DNA sequence then serves as a template for the formation, or **transcription** (the writing out), of a similar nucleotide sequence called **messenger ribonucleic acid** (mRNA; Figure 1.6). In all RNA, the nucleotides are the same as in DNA except that uracil (U) substitutes for thymine (T). In most genes, coding regions (**exons**) are interrupted by noncoding regions (**introns**). During transcription, the entire gene is copied into a pre-mRNA, which includes exons and introns. During the process of RNA splicing, introns are removed and exons are joined to form a contiguous coding sequence. In its entirety, the part of the human genome formed by exons is called the **exome.** As might be expected, errors or mutations may occur during transcription; however, a proofreading enzyme generally catches and repairs these errors. If not corrected, however, transcription errors can lead to the production of a disordered protein and a disease state.

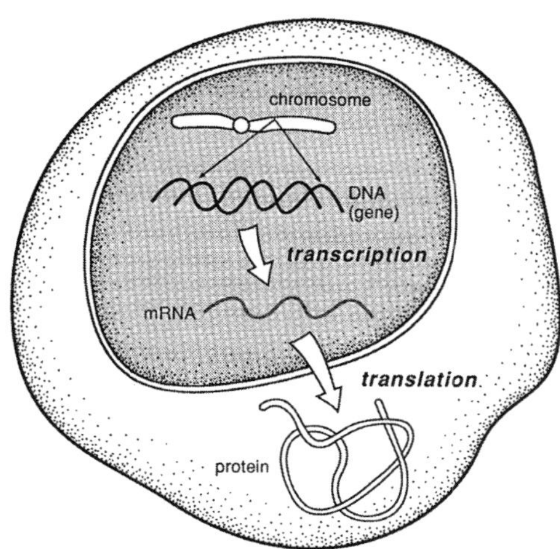

Figure 1.6. A summary of the steps leading from gene to protein formation. Transcription of the DNA (gene) onto mRNA occurs in the cell nucleus. The mRNA is then transported to the cytoplasm, where translation into protein occurs.

Translation

Once transcribed, the single-stranded mRNA detaches and the double-stranded DNA zips back together. The mRNA then moves out of the nucleus into the cytoplasm, where it provides instructions for the production of a protein, a process termed **translation** (Figure 1.7). The mRNA attaches itself to a **ribosome.** The ribosome moves along the mRNA strand, reading the message in three-letter "words," or **codons,** such as GCU, CUA, and UAG. Most of these triplets code for specific **amino acids,** the building blocks of proteins. As these triplets are read, another type of RNA, transfer RNA (tRNA), carries the requisite amino acids to the ribosome, where they are linked to form a protein.

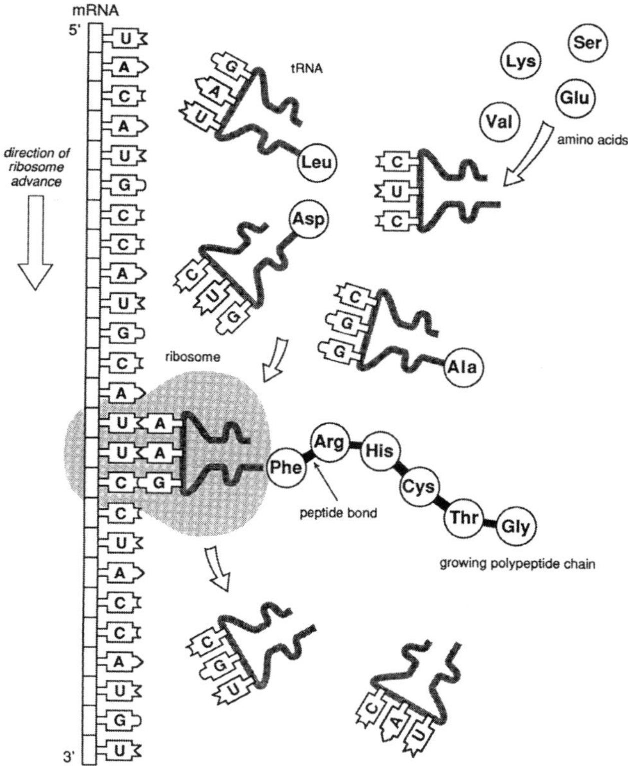

Figure 1.7. Translation of mRNA into protein. The ribosome moves along the mRNA strand assembling a growing polypeptide chain using tRNA–amino acid complexes. In this example, it has already assembled six amino acids (phenylalanine [Phe], arginine [Arg], histidine [His], cystine [Cys], threonine [Thr], and glycine [Gly]) into a polypeptide chain that will become a protein.

Certain triplets, termed *stop codons,* instruct the ribosome to terminate the sequence by indicating that all of the correct amino acids are in place to form the complete protein, for example, thyroid hormone.

Once the protein is complete, the mRNA, ribosome, and protein separate. The protein is released into the cytoplasm and is either used by the cytoplasm or prepared for secretion into the bloodstream. If the protein is to be secreted, it is transferred to the **Golgi apparatus** (Figure 1.1), which packages it in a form that can be released through the cell membrane and carried throughout the body.

Mutations

An abnormality at any step in the transcription or translation process can cause the body to produce a structurally abnormal protein, reduced amounts of a protein, or no protein at all. When the error occurs in the gene itself, thus disrupting the subsequent steps, that mistake is termed a *mutation.* The likelihood of mutations occurring increases with the size of the gene. In sperm cells, the point mutation rate also increases with paternal age. Although most mutations occur spontaneously, they can be induced by radiation, toxins, and viruses. Once they occur, mutations become part of a person's genetic code. If they are present in the germline, they can be passed on from one generation to the next.

Point Mutations

The most common type of mutation is a single base pair substitution (Jorde et al., 2015), also called a **point mutation.** Because there is redundancy in human DNA, many point mutations have no adverse consequences. Depending on where in the gene they occur, however, point mutations are capable of causing a **missense mutation** or a **nonsense mutation** (Figure 1.8). A missense mutation results in a change in the triplet code that substitutes a different amino acid in the protein chain. For example, in most cases of the inborn error of metabolism, **phenylketonuria** (PKU), a single base substitution causes an error in the production of phenylalanine hydroxylase, the enzyme necessary to metabolize the amino acid **phenylalanine.** The result is an accumulation of phenylalanine that can cause brain damage (see Chapter 16). In a nonsense mutation, the single base pair substitution produces a stop codon that prematurely terminates the protein formation. In this case, no useful protein is formed. **Neurofibromatosis-1** (NF1) is an example of a disorder commonly caused by a nonsense mutation. In NF1 a tumor suppressor, neurofibromin, is not formed. As a result, multiple benign neurofibroma tumors form on the body and in the brain. Children with NF1 also have a high incidence of attention-deficit/hyperactivity disorder (Friedman, 2014).

Insertions and Deletions

Mutations can also involve the insertion or deletion of one or more nucleotide bases. As one example, insertion of nucleotides in the fukutin gene (expressed in muscle, brain, and eyes) can affect its function when associated with other mutations and cause Fukuyama congenital muscular dystrophy (Saito, 2012). In contrast, a common mutation in another inherited muscle disease, Duchenne muscular dystrophy, usually involves a deletion in the dystrophin gene (see Chapter 9).

Base additions or subtractions may also lead to a **frame shift** in which the three-base-pair reading frame is shifted. All subsequent triplets are misread, often leading to the production of a stop codon and a nonfunctional protein. Certain children with Tay-Sachs disease have this type of mutation. Other mutations

	Missense Mutation	Nonsense Mutation	Frame shift Mutation
DNA	AAG AGT GTA CGT TTC TCA CAT GCA	AAG AGT GTA CGT TTC TCA CAT GCA	AAG AGT GTA CGT* TTC TCA CAT GCA
mRNA	UUC UCA CAU GCA	UUC UGA CAU GCA	UUC UGA CAU GCA
Amino acid	Phe Ser His Arg	Phe Ser His Arg	Phe Ser His Arg
Mutation	A/T for G/C	C/G for G/C	A/T inserted
DNA	AAG AGT ATA CGT TTC TCA TAT GCA	AAG ACT ATA CGT TTC TGA TAT GCA	AAG AGA TGT ACG* TTC TCT ACA TGC
mRNA	UUC UCA UAU GCA	UUC UGA CAU GCA	UUC UCU ACA UGC
Amino acid	Phe Ser Tyr Arg	Phe Stop codon — —	Phe Ser Thr Cys

*note that this is same sequence, shifted right

Figure 1.8. Examples of point mutations: Missense mutation, nonsense mutation, and frame shift mutation. The shaded areas mark the point of mutation.

can affect regions of the gene that regulate transcription but that do not actually code for an amino acid. These areas are called promoter and enhancer areas. They help turn other genes on and off and are very important in the normal development of the fetus. A mutation in a transcription gene leads to **Rubinstein-Taybi syndrome,** which is associated with multiple congenital malformations and severe intellectual disability (Spena, Gervasini, & Milani, 2015). Mutations in a transcription gene also may result in a normal protein being formed but at a much slower rate than usual, leading to an enzyme or other protein deficiency. An example is **Cornelia de Lange syndrome,** in which patients have a mutation in the NIPBL gene that codes for the developmentally important cohesin-loading protein, delangin. Affected children manifest growth delay, a dysmorphic appearance including confluent eyebrows, limb impairments, and intellectual disability.

Selective Advantage

The **incidence** of a genetic disease in a population depends on the difference between the rate of mutation production and that of mutation removal. Typically, genetic diseases enter populations through mutation errors. Natural selection, the process by which individuals with a selective advantage survive and pass on their genes, works to remove these errors. For instance, because individuals with sickle cell disease (an **autosomal recessive** inherited blood disorder) historically have had a decreased life span, the gene that causes this disorder would have been expected to be removed from the gene pool over time. Sometimes natural selection, however, favors the individual who is a carrier of one copy of a mutated recessive gene. In the case of sickle cell disease, unaffected carriers (called heterozygotes) who appear clinically healthy actually have minor differences in their hemoglobin structure that make it more resistant to a malarial parasite (López, Saravia, Gomez, Hoebeke, & Patarroyo, 2010). In Africa, where malaria is endemic, carriers of this disorder have a selective advantage. This selective advantage has maintained the sickle cell trait among Africans. Northern Europeans, for whom malaria is not an issue, rarely carry the sickle cell gene at all; this mutation has presumably died out via natural selection in this population (Jorde et al., 2015).

Single Nucleotide Polymorphisms

Despite the more than 3 billion base pairs in the genetic code, people of all races and geography share a 99.9% genetic identity (Ridley, 2006). Although this is quite remarkable, that 0.1% difference means there are about 3 million DNA sequence variations, also called **single nucleotide polymorphisms** (SNPs). This genetic variation is the basis of evolution, but it can also contribute to health, unique traits, or disease. One SNP involved in muscle formation, if present, makes individuals much more likely to become "buff" if they weight lift; another SNP is associated with perfect musical pitch. There is an SNP that makes individuals more susceptible to adverse effects from certain medications because it leads to slower metabolism of drugs by the liver. There also are SNPs that place people at greater risk for developing Alzheimer's disease and an inflammatory bowel disease called Crohn's disease (Uniken Venema, Voskuil, Dijkstra, Weersma, & Festen, 2016). Knowledge of these SNPs, as well as candidate disease genes, allows a better understanding of certain genetic conditions, which can lead to the development of novel treatments.

Single-Gene (Mendelian) Disorders

Gregor Mendel (1822–1884), an Austrian monk, pioneered our understanding of single-gene defects. While cultivating pea plants, he noted that when he bred two differently colored plants—yellow and green—the **hybrid** offspring all were green rather than mixed in color. Mendel concluded that the green trait was **dominant,** whereas the yellow trait was **recessive** (from the Latin word for "hidden"). However, the yellow trait sometimes appeared in subsequent generations. Later, scientists determined that many human traits, including some birth defects, are also inherited in this fashion. They are referred to as **Mendelian traits.**

Table 1.2 indicates the prevalence of some common single-gene disorders associated with developmental disabilities. Approximately 1% of the population has a known single-gene disorder. These disorders can be transmitted to offspring on the autosomes or on the X chromosome. Mendelian traits may be either dominant or recessive. Thus, Mendelian disorders are characterized as being **autosomal recessive, autosomal dominant,** or **X-linked**.

Autosomal Recessive Disorders Among the currently recognized Mendelian disorders, over 1,000 are inherited as autosomal recessive traits (McKusick-Nathans Institute of Genetic Medicine & The National Center for Biotechnology Information, 2017). For a child to have a disorder that is autosomal recessive, he or she must carry an abnormal gene on both copies of the relevant chromosome. In the vast majority of cases, this means that the child receives an abnormal copy from both parents. The one exception is uniparental disomy, which is discussed in the next section.

Table 1.2. Prevalence of genetic disorders

Disease	Appropriate prevalence
Chromosomal disorders	
Down syndrome (trisomy 21)	1/850
Klinefelter syndrome (47, XXY)	1/600
Trisomy 13	1/12,000–1/20,000
Trisomy 18	1/6,000–8,000
Turner syndrome (45, X)	1/2,500–1/4,000 females
Single-gene disorders	
Duchenne muscular dystrophy	1/3,300 males
Fragile X syndrome	1/3,000–1/4,000 males; 1/8,000 females
Neurofibromatosis type I	1/3,000
Phenylketonuria	1/5,000 to 1/10,000
Tay-Sachs disease	1/3,600 Ashkenazi Jews
Mitochondrial inheritance	
Leber hereditary optic neuropathy	Rare 1/30,000–1/50,000
MERRF	Rare (< 1/100,000)
MELAS	Rare, unknown

Sources: Nussbaum, McInnes, and Willard (2016) and Adam, Ardinger, Pagon, Wallace, Bean, Stephens, and Amemiya (1993–2018).

Key: MELAS, mitochondrial encephalomyelopathy, lactic acidosis, and stroke-like episodes; MERRF, myoclonic epilepsy and ragged red fibers.

Tay-Sachs disease is an example of an autosomal recessive condition. It is caused by the absence of an enzyme, hexosaminidase A, which normally metabolizes a potentially toxic product of nerve cells (Kaback & Desnick, 2011). In affected children, this product cannot be broken down and is stored in the brain, leading to progressive brain damage and early death.

Alternate forms of the gene for hexosaminidase A are known to exist. The different forms of a gene, called **alleles,** include the normal gene, which can be symbolized by a capital "A" because it is dominant, and the mutated allele (in this example, carrying Tay-Sachs disease), which can be symbolized by the lowercase "a" because it is recessive (Figure 1.9). Upon fertilization, the embryo receives two genes for hexosaminidase A, one from the father and one from the mother. The following combinations of alleles are possible: **homozygous** (carrying the same allele) combinations, AA or aa, and **heterozygous** (carrying alternate alleles) combinations, aA or Aa. Because Tay-Sachs disease is a recessive disorder, two abnormal recessive genes (aa) are needed to produce a child who has the disease. Therefore, a child with aa would be homozygous for the Tay-Sachs mutation (i.e., have two copies of the mutated gene and manifest the disease), a child with aA or Aa would be heterozygous and a healthy carrier of the Tay-Sachs mutation, and a child with AA would be a healthy noncarrier.

If two heterozygotes (carrying alternate alleles) were to have children (aA × Aa or Aa × aA), the following combinations could occur: AA, aA or Aa, or aa (Figure 1.9). According to the law of probability, each pregnancy would carry a one in four chance of the child

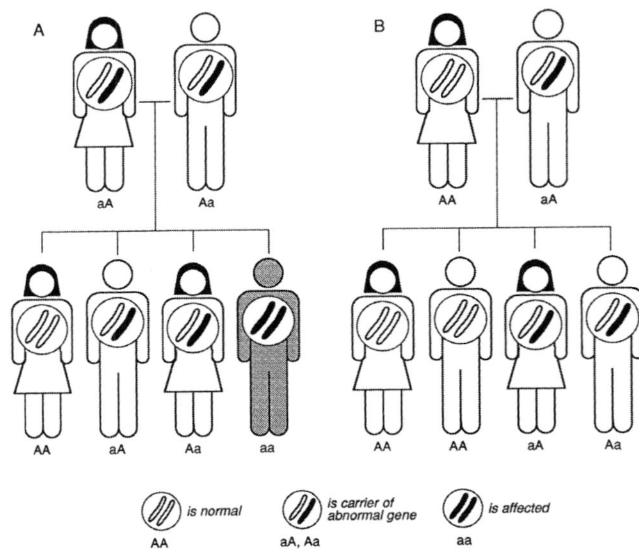

Figure 1.9. Inheritance of autosomal recessive disorders. Two copies of the abnormal gene (aa) must be present to produce the disease state: A) Two carriers mating will result, on average, in 25% of the children being affected, 50% being carriers, and 25% noncarriers; B) A carrier and a noncarrier mating will result in 50% noncarriers and 50% carriers and no children will be affected.

being a noncarrier (AA), a one in two chance of the child being a carrier (aA or Aa), and a one in four risk of the child having Tay-Sachs disease (aa). If a carrier has children with a noncarrier (aA × AA), each pregnancy carries a one in two chance of the child being a carrier (aA, Aa), a one in two chance of the child being a noncarrier (AA), and virtually no chance of the child having the disease (Figure 1.9). Siblings of affected children, even if they are carriers, are unlikely to produce children with the disease because this can only occur if they have children with another carrier, which is an unlikely occurrence in these rare diseases except in cases of intermarriage.

The one in four risk when two carriers have children is a probability risk. This does not mean that if a family has one affected child the next three will be unaffected. Each new pregnancy carries the same one in four risk; the parents could, by chance, have three affected children in a row or five unaffected children. In the case of Tay-Sachs disease, carrier screening is used to identify at-risk couples and prenatal diagnosis to provide information about whether the fetus is affected (see Chapter 3).

Because it is unlikely for a carrier of a rare condition to have children with another carrier of the same disease, autosomal recessive disorders are quite rare in the general population, ranging from 1 in 2,000 to 1 in 200,000 or fewer births (McKusick-Nathans Institute of Genetic Medicine & The National Center for Biotechnology Information, 2017). When a union occurs within an extended family, also called consanguinity (e.g., cousin marriage; Figure 1.10) or when unions among ethnically, religiously, or geographically isolated populations occur, the incidence of these disorders increases markedly. Some ethnic populations have higher carrier frequency than others; for example, carrier frequency for cystic fibrosis in people of Northern European background is 1 in 28, but for Asians, the carrier frequency is 1 in 118 (Ong et al., 2017).

Like Tay-Sachs disease, certain other autosomal recessive disorders are caused by mutations that lead to an enzyme deficiency of some kind. In most cases, there are a number of different mutations within the gene that can produce the same disease. Because these enzyme deficiencies generally lead to biochemical abnormalities involving either the insufficient production of a needed product or the buildup of toxic materials, **developmental disabilities** or early death may result (see Chapter 16). Autosomal recessive disorders affect males and females equally, and there tends to be clustering in families (i.e., more than one affected child per family). However, a history of the disease in past generations rarely exists unless there has been intermarriage.

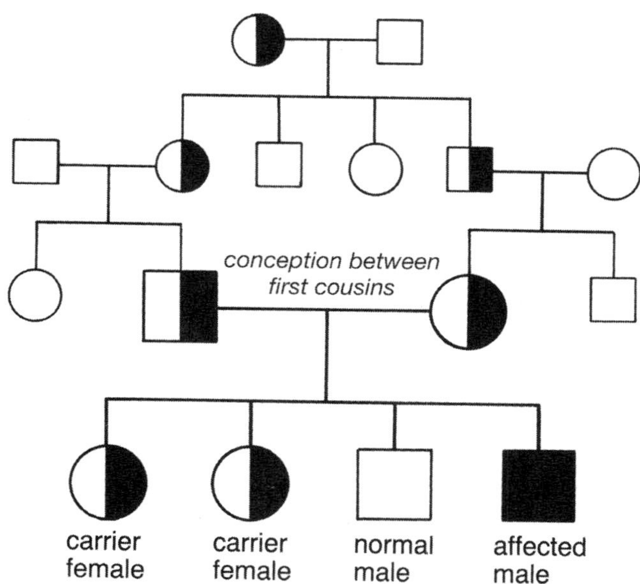

Figure 1.10. A family tree illustrating the effect of consanguinity (in this case, a marriage between first cousins) on the risk of inheriting an autosomal recessive disorder. The chance of both parents being carriers is usually less than 1 in 300. When first cousins conceive a child, however, the chance of both parents being carriers rises to 1 in 8. The risk, then, of having an affected child increases almost 40-fold.

Autosomal Dominant Disorders Over 1,000 autosomal dominant disorders have been identified, the most common ones having a frequency of 1 in 200 births (Youngblom et al., 2016). Autosomal dominant disorders are quite different from autosomal recessive disorders in mechanism, incidence, and clinical characteristics (Table 1.3). Because autosomal dominant

Table 1.3. Comparison of autosomal recessive, autosomal dominant, and X-linked inheritance patterns

	Autosomal recessive	Autosomal dominant	X-linked
Type of disorder	Enzyme deficiency	Structural abnormalities	Mixed
Examples of disorder	Tay-Sachs disease	Achondroplasia	Fragile X syndrome
	Phenylketonuria (PKU)	Neurofibromatosis	Muscular dystrophy
Carrier expresses disorder	No	Yes	Sometimes
Increased risk in other family members from intermarriage/consanguinity	Yes	No	No

disorders are caused by a single abnormal allele, individuals with the **genotypes** Aa or aA are both affected to some degree.

To better understand this, consider NF1, the neurological disorder discussed previously. Suppose *a* represents the normal recessive gene and *A* indicates the mutated dominant gene for NF1. If a person with NF1 (aA or Aa) has a child with an unaffected individual (aa), there is a one in two risk, statistically speaking, that the child will have the disorder (aA or Aa) and a one in two chance he or she will be unaffected (aa; Figure 1.11). An unaffected child will not carry the abnormal allele and therefore cannot pass it on to his or her children.

Autosomal dominant disorders affect men and women with equal frequency. They tend to involve physical impairments (tumors in the case of NF1) rather than enzymatic defects. In affected individuals, there is often a family history of the disease; however, approximately half of affected individuals represent a new mutation. Although individuals with a new mutation will risk passing the mutated gene to their offspring, their parents are unaffected and at no greater risk than the general population of having a second affected child. In some cases, a mutation occurs early in the development of eggs and sperm. This is called germline, or gonadal, mosaicism and is estimated to occur approximately 1.3% of the time. If gonadal mosaicism is present in a parent, theoretically two siblings can be affected with the same condition and neither parent appears to be affected (Rahbari et al., 2015). There can also be partial penetrance of the gene, which produces a less severe disorder (e.g., in NF1 or tuberous sclerosis), or a delayed onset form of the disease (e.g., in Huntington disease).

X-Linked Disorders Unlike autosomal recessive and autosomal dominant disorders, which involve genes located on the 22 non-sex chromosomes (autosomes), X-linked (previously called sex-linked) disorders involve mutant genes located on the X chromosome. X-linked disorders primarily affect males (Genetics Home Reference, 2017a). The reason for this is that males have only one X chromosome; therefore, a single dose of the abnormal gene causes disease. Because females have two X chromosomes, a single recessive allele usually does not cause disease provided there is a normal allele on the second X chromosome (Figure 1.12). Approximately 1,000 X-linked disorders have been described, including Duchenne muscular dystrophy and hemophilia (McKusick-Nathans Institute of Genetic Medicine & The National Center for Biotechnology Information, 2017). Carrier mothers in two-thirds of the cases pass on these disorders from one generation to the next; one-third of these cases represent new mutations.

As an example of an X-linked disorder, children with Duchenne muscular dystrophy develop a

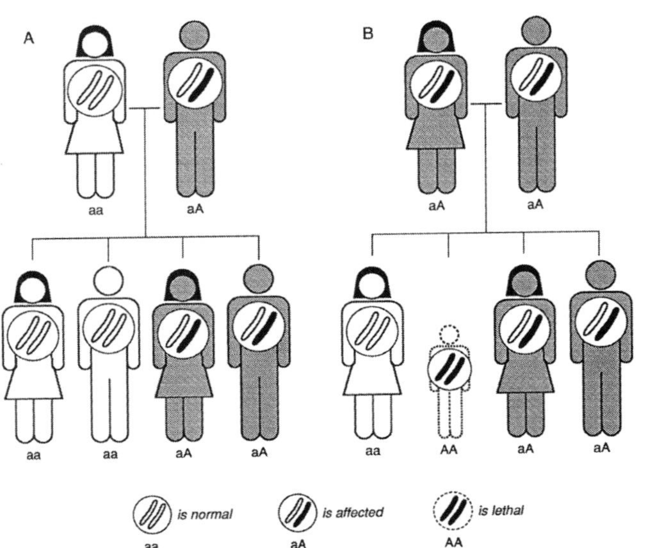

Figure 1.11. Inheritance of autosomal dominant disorders. Only one copy of the abnormal gene (A) must be present to produce the disease state: A) If an affected person conceives a child with an unaffected person, statistically speaking, 50% of the children will be affected and 50% will be unaffected; B) If two affected people have children, 25% of the children will be unaffected, 50% will have the disorder, and 25% will have a severe (often fatal) form of the disorder as a result of a double dose of the abnormal gene.

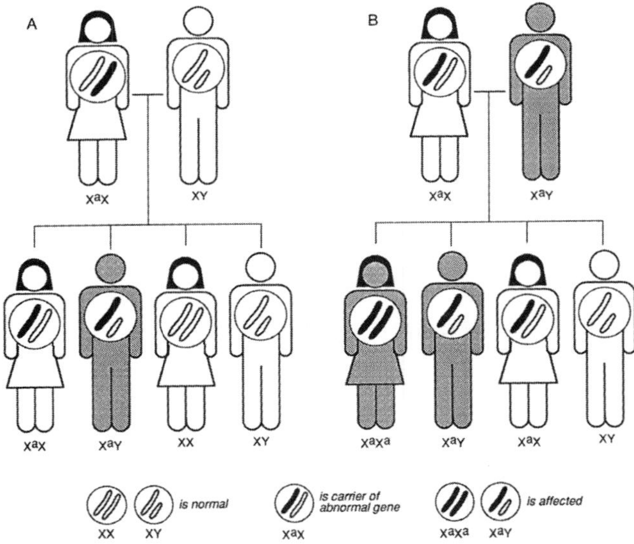

Figure 1.12. Inheritance of X-linked disorders: A) A carrier woman has a child with an unaffected man. Among the female children, statistically speaking, 50% will be carriers and 50% will be unaffected. Among the male children, 50% will be affected and 50% will be unaffected; B) A carrier woman has a child with an affected man. Of the female children, 50% will be carriers and 50% will be affected. Of the male children, statistically speaking, 50% will be unaffected and 50% will be affected.

progressive muscle weakness (Bushby et al., 2010a, 2010b; Suthar & Sankhyan, 2017). The disease results from a mutation in the dystrophin gene (located on the X chromosome), the function of which is to ensure stability of the muscle cell membrane. Because the disease affects all muscles, eventually the heart muscle and the diaphragmatic muscles needed for circulation and breathing respectively are impaired. Dystrophin is also required for typical brain development and function, so affected boys may have cognitive impairments.

In fact, approximately 10% of males with intellectual disability and 10% of females with learning disabilities are affected by X-linked conditions (Inlow & Restifo, 2004). Males are more than twice as likely to have intellectual disability than females. This finding is attributable to a combination of factors: first, X-linked disorders affect males disproportionately more than females, and second, there is an unusually large number of genes residing on the X chromosome that are critical for normal brain development, nerve cell function, learning, and memory. Up to 10% of all known genetic errors causing intellectual disability are on the X chromosome despite the X chromosome containing only 4% of the human genome.

The mechanism for passing an X-linked recessive trait to the next generation is as follows: Women who have a recessive mutation (Xa) on one of their X chromosomes and a normal allele on the other (X) are carriers of the gene (XaX). Although these women are usually clinically unaffected, they can pass on the abnormal gene to their children. Assuming the father is unaffected, each female child born to a carrier mother has a one in two chance of being a carrier (i.e., inheriting the mutant Xa allele from her mother and the normal X allele from her father; Figure 1.12). A male child (who has only one X chromosome), however, has a one in two risk of having the disorder. This occurs if he inherits the X chromosome containing the mutated gene (XaY) instead of the normal one (XY). A family tree frequently reveals that some maternal uncles and male siblings have the disease. X-linked disorders are never passed from father to son because boys inherit their Y chromosome from their father and their X chromosome from their mother.

Occasionally, females are affected by X-linked diseases. This can occur if the woman has adverse **lyonization** (inactivation of one of the X chromosomes) or if the disorder is X-linked "dominant." Regarding the former mechanism, the geneticist Mary Lyon questioned why women have the same amount of X chromosome–directed gene product as men instead of twice as much, as would be predicted from their genetic makeup. Dr. Lyon postulated that early in embryogenesis, one of the two X chromosomes in each cell is inactivated, making every female fetus a mosaic. This implied that some cells would contain an active X chromosome derived from the father, whereas others would contain an active X chromosome derived from the mother. This "lyonization" hypothesis was later proven to be correct. In most instances, the cells in a woman's body have a fairly equal division between maternally and paternally derived active X chromosomes. In a small fraction of women, however, the distribution is very unequal. If the normal X chromosome is inactivated preferentially in cells of a carrier of an X-linked disorder, the woman will manifest the disease, although usually in a less severe form than the male. An example is OTC deficiency, the disorder Katy had in this chapter's opening case study (see also Chapter 16).

The second mechanism for a female to manifest an X-linked disorder is if the disorder is transmitted as X-linked dominant. Although most X-linked disorders are recessive, a few appear to be dominant. One example is Rett syndrome (Chahrour & Zoghbi, 2007; Liyanage & Rastegar, 2014; Matijevic, Knezevic, Slavica, & Pavelic, 2009; Percy, 2008). It appears that in this disorder, the presence of the mutated transcription gene *MECP2* on the X chromosome of a male embryo nearly always leads to lethality. When it occurs in one of the X chromosomes of the female, however, it is compatible with survival but results in a syndrome marked by microcephaly, developmental regression, intellectual disability, and autism-like behaviors. That is why virtually all children with Rett syndrome are girls.

Mitochondrial Inheritance

Each cell contains several hundred mitochondria in its cytoplasm (Figure 1.1). Mitochondria produce the energy needed for cellular function through a complex process termed **oxidative phosphorylation.** It has been proposed that mitochondria were originally independent microorganisms that invaded our bodies during the process of human evolution and then developed a symbiotic relationship with the cells in the human body. They are unique among cellular **organelles** (the specialized parts of a cell) in that they possess their own DNA, which is in a double-stranded circular pattern rather than the double-helical pattern of nuclear DNA and contains genes that are different from those contained in nuclear DNA (Figure 1.13). Most of the proteins necessary for mitochondrial function are coded by nuclear genes, and disorders caused by abnormalities in these genes are most often inherited in an autosomal recessive manner. Certain mitochondrial functions, however, are dependent on genes encoded on the mitochondrial DNA. A mutation in

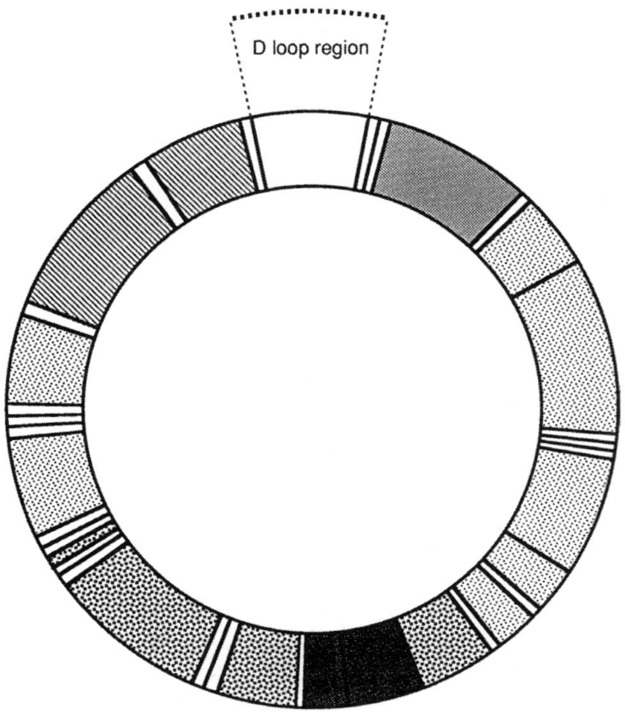

Figure 1.13. Mitochondrial DNA genome. The genes code for various enzyme complexes involved in energy production in the cell. The displacement loop (D loop) is not involved in energy production. (This figure was published in *Medical genetics*, revised 2nd edition, by Jorde, L.B., Carey, J.C., & Bamshad, M.J., et al., p. 105, Copyright C.V. Mosby [2001]; adapted by permission.) (*Key:* ▨ Complex I genes [NADH dehydrogenase], ▩ Complex III genes [ubiquinol: cytochrome c oxidoreductase], □ tRNA genes, ▦ Complex IV genes [cytochrome c oxidase], ■ Complex V genes [ATP synthase], ▧ ribosomal RNA genes.)

a mitochondrial gene can result in defective energy production and a disease state, particularly affecting organs with high energy demands, such as the heart, skeletal muscle, and brain (Gorman, 2016). An example of a disorder with mitochondrial inheritance is mitochondrial encephalomyelopathy, lactic acidosis, and stroke-like episodes (MELAS), a progressive neurological disorder marked by episodes of stroke and dementia. Other disorders with mitochondrial inheritance can lead to blindness, deafness, or muscle weakness. There are hundreds of mitochondrial diseases, some of which have clear genetic causes, while others do not. Every cell contains many mitochondria, but not every mitochondrion may carry a given mutation. In many disorders that are inherited through the mitochondrial genome, there is great clinical variability based on the **heteroplasmy** or the mix of different mitochondrial genomes within a single individual. There may be significant variability among specific tissues in an individual; some organs or tissues may be affected by the mitochondrial disorder and others may not.

Because eggs, but not sperm, contain cytoplasm, mitochondria are inherited from one's mother. As a result, mitochondrial DNA disorders are passed on from generally unaffected mothers to their children, both male and female (Figure 1.14). Men affected by a mitochondrial disorder cannot pass the trait to their children. In some cases, a mother with significant heteroplasmy may have only mild effects of a disease but may pass on only mutated mitochondrial genomes to a child. In that case, a child would have a homoplasmic mitochondrial mutation and would have a much more severe clinical course.

Trinucleotide Repeat Expansion Disorders

There has been an increased recognition that **copy number variability** accounts for several developmental disabilities (Sansović, Ivankov, Bobinec, Kero, & Barišić, 2017). One particular type of copy number variation is the trinucleotide repeat expansion (triplet repeat disorder), which has been linked to a number of disorders that do not follow typical Mendelian inheritance. Trinucleotide repeat disorders result from problems in recombination and replication during meiosis. Certain genes have highly repetitive sequences of trinucleotides. These repetitive sequences may expand (or contract) in size during meiosis. Once the repetitive sequence reaches a certain size threshold, it may interfere with the function of the gene and lead to a clinically apparent disorder. The expansion length is linked to the phenotype, with the longer expansions often presenting with earlier and more severe clinical signs and symptoms.

The first triplet repeat disorder discovered was fragile X syndrome, the most common inherited cause of intellectual disability. Boys and girls with fragile X syndrome have a phenotype that includes

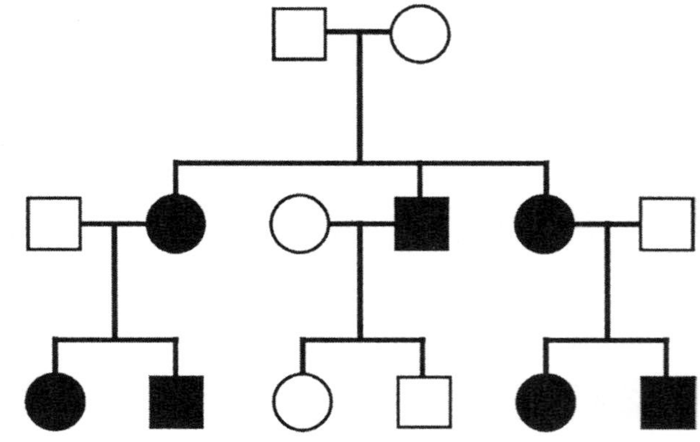

Figure 1.14. Mitochondrial inheritance. Because mitochondria are inherited exclusively from the mother, defects in mitochondrial disease will be passed on from the mother to her children, as illustrated in this pedigree.

a characteristic physical appearance, cognitive skills impairments, and impaired adaptive behaviors (Chonchaiya, Schneider, & Hagerman, 2009; Schneider, Hagerman, & Hessl, 2009; also see Chapter 15). Many affected children satisfy the criteria for the diagnosis of autism. The prevalence of fragile X syndrome (the full mutation) for males is about 1 in 3,600. The prevalence of the full mutation in females is estimated to be at least 1 in 4,000 to 1 in 6,000. Fragile X syndrome arises from an expansion of the number of cytosine-guanine-guanine (CGG) trinucleotide repeats occurring within the fragile X mental retardation protein (*FMR1*) gene. Inheritance of the instability in CGG regions leads to expansion from the normal number of repeats (6–40) to a premutation state (50–200 repeats) or from a premutation state to full mutation (>200 repeats). The stability of the CGG repeat depends upon the length of the repeat, as well as the sex of the individual passing on the mutation. The increased risk of CGG expansion from one generation to another is a phenomenon termed **anticipation.** Anticipation leads to an increasingly severe clinical phenotype in successive generations. When a child is suspected of having fragile X syndrome, the diagnosis can be confirmed by detecting the number of trinucleotide repeats in FMR1 using a clinically available molecular genetic blood test (Collins et al., 2010). There is a correlation between the number of trinucleotide repeats and the severity of disease. Other trinucleotide repeat disorders include myotonic dystrophy and Huntington's disease.

EPIGENETICS

The diagnostic evaluation of children with intellectual disability and other developmental disabilities has become increasingly complex in recent years due to a number of newly recognized genetic mechanisms and the availability of sophisticated methods to diagnose them. It has been appreciated that changes in gene expression can occur by mechanisms that do not permanently alter the DNA sequence (Urdinguio, Sanchez-Mut, & Esteller, 2009), a phenomenon termed **epigenetics.** Epigenetic mechanisms are important regulators of biological processes because they include genome reprogramming during embryogenesis (Kumar, 2008). Epigenetic modification, which is important in developmental processes, may have long-term effects on learning and memory formation. Epigenetic impairments may result from dysfunction of certain enzymes, genomic imprinting, and triplet repeat copy number variation. A number of conditions causing developmental disabilities, including fragile X syndrome, Rett syndrome, Rubinstein-Taybi syndrome, Prader-Willi syndrome, and VCFS, can be attributed to disruptions in epigenetic function. It is interesting to note that virtually all epigenetic disorders have been found to have a high incidence of symptoms consistent with autism spectrum disorder or other neurodevelopmental disorders (Moss & Howlin, 2009). In addition, the risk of epigenetic disorders has been found to be increased in pregnancies assisted by *in vitro* fertilization (Lazaraviciute, Kauser, Bhattacharya, Haggarty, & Bhattacharya, 2014).

According to Mendelian genetics, the **phenotype,** or appearance of an individual should be the same whether the given gene is inherited from the mother or the father. This is not always the case, however, because of **genomic imprinting.** This is an epigenetic phenomenon in which the activity of the gene is modified depending upon the sex of the transmitting parent (Genetics Home Reference, 2017b). Most autosomal genes are expressed in both maternal and paternal alleles. However, imprinted genes show expression from only one allele (the other is silenced or used differently), and this is determined during production of the egg or sperm. Imprinting implies that the gene carries a "tag" placed on it during spermatogenesis or oogenesis. This is most often accomplished by adding methyl groups to the DNA, affecting the expression of the methylated genes. Imprinted genes are important in development and differentiation, and if expression from both alleles is not maintained, disturbances in development can result (Soellner et al., 2017).

The first human imprinting disorder discovered was Prader-Willi syndrome. It is caused by a paternal deletion in chromosome 15 or by maternal uniparental disomy in which both chromosome 15s come from the mother. It can also result if both copies of chromosome 15 are imprinted as if they came from the mother regardless of the actual parent of origin (Conlin et al., 2010; Driscoll, Miller, Schwartz, & Cassidy, 2017). Prader-Willi syndrome is characterized by severe hypotonia and feeding difficulties in early childhood, followed by an insatiable appetite and obesity by school age. It features significant motor and language delays in the first 2 years of life; borderline to moderate intellectual disability; and severe behavioral problems, including compulsive and hording behaviors. Many affected children satisfy the criteria for the diagnosis of autism (Driscoll et al., 2017; Goldstone, Holland, Hauffa, Hokken-Koelega, & Tauber, 2008). Other examples of imprinted neurogenetic disorders include Angelman syndrome and Beckwith-Wiedemann syndrome (Dan, 2009; Gurrieri & Accadia, 2009; Soellner et al., 2017).

GENETIC TESTING

Genetic tests have been developed for many of the roughly 7,000 rare diseases identified, including all those described in this chapter. Most tests look at single genes and are used to diagnose rare genetic disorders, such as fragile X syndrome and Duchenne muscular dystrophy. In addition, some genetic tests look at rare inherited mutations of otherwise protective genes that are responsible for some hereditary breast and ovarian cancers. An increasing number of tests are being developed to look at multiple genes that may increase or decrease a person's risk for developing common diseases, such as cancer or diabetes. In addition, pharmacogenetic tests may be used to help identify genetic variations that influence a person's response to medicines. Here, we will focus on genetic testing used in diagnosing causes of developmental disabilities.

There are three types of genetic testing currently being used to detect genomic-based causes of developmental disabilities: **chromosomal microarray analysis, next-generation sequencing,** and **whole-exome/genome sequencing.** Chromosomal microarrays use probes to test for known DNA sequences and can identify disorders where the specific genetic abnormality is caused by a microdeletion or microduplication, as seen in Williams syndrome or chromosome 15q duplication syndrome. Microarrays cannot be used to identify mutations (alterations of a single nucleotide, such as a point mutation) in a gene. In general, a chromosomal microarray is the first-line test recommended for a child presenting with developmental delays or autism (see Box 1.1). The second type of genetic testing, next-generation sequencing, allows detection of mutations in single genes, such as *NF1* associated with neurofibromatosis type 1, or *CFTR*, in which two mutations are needed to cause cystic fibrosis. The final approach is whole-exome/genome sequencing and may be used in a case where no genetic cause has been identified for the child's phenotype. Whole-exome sequencing is typically utilized when a child's clinical history is suspicious for a genetic condition based on the presence of multiple congenital anomalies, developmental delays, or other undiagnosed issues. Here, exome sequencing (sequencing the entire exome) can help identify alterations in genes all at once rather than looking at

BOX 1.1 EVIDENCE-BASED PRACTICE

Autism and Genetic Testing

Autism spectrum disorder (ASD) is a highly variable group of neurodevelopmental conditions. There is evidence that children with ASD more commonly have medical issues and/or physical differences and dysmorphic features. Because of this high level of variability, the genetic workup may differ depending on the child's clinical issues. Stratification of children with ASD can help to determine what type of genetic testing might be most appropriate for a patient. The general recommendation is that chromosomal microarray (CMA) is the first-line test for a child with ASD.

Tammimies et al. (2015) reported molecular diagnostic yields for CMA and whole-exome sequencing (WES) in a population of 258 children with ASD stratified by clinical features, including number and type of physical anomalies. Each child was classified as having essential, equivocal, or complex ASD based on their morphology score. The main outcomes measured were the clinical differences, the yield of molecular diagnosis from CMA and WES, and the differences in the diagnostic yields between the three categories

Most of the patients had essential autism (approximately 70%), while approximately 20% had equivocal autism and approximately 10% were classified as complex. Of the 258 subjects, the WES diagnostic yield was 8.4% and the CMA yield was 9.3%. In children who received both tests, the diagnostic yield was 15.8%. In children with complex ASD, the molecular diagnostic yield was near 35% when both CMA and WES were performed. Age at diagnosis with ASD was also significantly older for this complex group. In the children with essential autism, the diagnostic yield was much lower when using both CMA and WES.

Points to Remember

- CMA should still be considered the first-line test for children with autism. A medical genetics evaluation should be completed **prior** to ordering any genetic testing.
- Medical genetics evaluation might help identify patients more likely to achieve a molecular diagnosis with genetic testing; complex patients might benefit from WES if properly counseled by a medical geneticist and genetic counselor.
- Patients with complex medical issues receive later diagnoses of autism; it is important to be aware of these symptoms and provide an autism evaluation when features are first noted.

each gene individually. It does this by selecting the approximately 180,000 exons that constitute about 1% of the human genome (or approximately 30 million base pairs) and then sequencing the DNA using a high-throughput DNA sequencing technology. This technique has been used to identify genetic variants seen in autism. Exome sequencing, however, is only able to identify those variants found in the coding region of genes that affect protein function. It is not able to identify structural and non-coding variants associated with disease; this can be found using whole-genome sequencing. Presently, whole-genome sequencing is typically not utilized in the clinical setting due to the high costs and time associated with sequencing full genomes. In addition to these challenges, our understanding of much of our genome is still in its infancy. As our knowledge continues to grow, clinicians will be able to more accurately interpret results and provide appropriate genetic counseling for families.

There are many other types of genetic tests available for specific disorders. For example, some inborn errors of metabolism can be identified by detecting the accumulation of specific compounds in blood, urine, or other tissue samples. Testing for methylation patterns on DNA samples detects certain epigenetic disorders. Other genetic disorders may be detected radiologically. The decision about which tests are most appropriate for a specific patient is complex, and physicians with expertise in medical genetics can help guide testing and interpret results. While some tests, such as karyotype analysis to detect large chromosome abnormalities or rearrangements (like those seen in Down syndrome and Klinefelter syndrome), are no longer commonly used during evaluation of a child with developmental delay, they may be appropriate depending on a child's clinical presentation. For example, a girl referred for mild developmental delays, short stature, webbed neck, and a heart defect should first undergo a karyotype to evaluate for Turner syndrome; microarray and next-generation sequencing would not be the most appropriate initial tests for this patient. Medical geneticists and genetic counselors can help determine the correct test for a patient based on utility and cost effectiveness. They can also ensure that the patient is properly consented and understands the implications of these complex analyses (see Box 1.2).

ENVIRONMENTAL INFLUENCES ON HEREDITY

The particular genes that a person possesses determine his or her genotype, and the expression of the genes results in the physical appearance of traits—that is, the phenotype of the individual. For some traits and clinical disorders, however, the same genotype can produce quite different phenotypes depending on environmental influences. In terms of traits, bright parents tend to have bright children and tall parents tend to have tall children; however, the interaction of genetics with the prenatal and postnatal environments allows for many possible outcomes. For example, it has been found that, as a result of an increased protein intake during childhood, Asians who grow up in the United States are significantly taller than their parents who grew up in Asia. Disorders that have both genetic and environmental influences include diabetes, meningomyelocele, cleft palate, and pyloric stenosis (Au, Ashley-Koch, & Northrup, 2010). Considering the example of PKU, an affected child will develop intellectual disability if the PKU is not treated early but will have typical development if it is treated with a diet low in phenylalanine from infancy (Feillet et al., 2010; also see Chapter 16).

BOX 1.2 INTERDISCIPLINARY CARE

What Is a Genetic Counselor?

Genetic counselors are health care professionals with specialized, master's-level training in human genetics. They are an excellent resource for both patients and providers of children with rare diseases and developmental disabilities, as they are able to explain complex genetic ideas while also providing psychosocial support. Genetic counselors can guide patients on how inherited diseases might affect them or their families, analyze family histories, and help determine what kind of genetic testing might be most appropriate for a patient. In a pediatric setting, genetic counselors work alongside medical geneticists and are often the patient's point of contact within their team of genetic care providers. Genetic counselors also work with pregnant women, cancer patients, and people with more common conditions such as heart disease, diabetes, and Alzheimer's disease. Genetic counselors also meet with couples planning a pregnancy to help determine risks for future children. For more information or to find a genetic counselor, please visit www.nsgc.org.

GENETIC THERAPIES

A range of approaches is being used to treat genetic disorders. In the case of inborn errors of metabolism, treatment has focused on either replacing the deficient product of the defective enzyme (e.g., in thyroid hormone deficiency) preventing the accumulation of toxic material because the enzyme does not break it down or replacing the defective enzyme (see Chapter 16). Preventing accumulation of toxic metabolites often relies on dietary manipulation (e.g., PKU) or stimulation of an alternate pathway around the enzyme block (urea cycle disorders). In a few cases, enzyme replacement therapy is available (e.g., in Gaucher disease). Here the missing or defective enzyme is given intravenously at intervals to correct the metabolic defect. Bone marrow transplantation (e.g., in sickle cell disease) or liver transplantation (e.g., in OTC deficiency) has been used to correct other genetic disorders by replacing the organ that is producing the defective product with an organ that can produce a normal one. While these approaches to genetic disorders have improved outcomes in a number of disorders, they represent only a fraction of all the genetic causes of developmental disabilities and their cost can be up to $500,000 per year.

More recently, the concepts of exon skipping, gene therapy, and gene editing have been advanced and are in clinical trials. In **exon skipping,** a form of RNA splicing is used to cause cells to "skip" over faulty sections of the genetic code, leading to a truncated but still functional protein despite the genetic mutation (Kole & Krieg, 2015). The first exon skipping drug was approved in 2016 for use in a subgroup of individuals with Duchenne muscular dystrophy who have a specific mutation. In **gene therapy,** copies of the normal gene are infused most commonly using a virus transporter in order to "replace" the defective gene. At the writing of this edition, the only approved gene therapy drugs are for cancer and HIV, although gene therapy clinical trials for several single gene defects causing developmental disabilities are currently in process. **Gene editing** is a form of gene therapy in which a technology called CRISPR/Cas9 is used to cut the gene at the point of the mutation and to replace it with a corrected gene sequence. The first successful case of gene editing in an embryo in the United States was reported in 2017 (Ma et al., 2017). Researchers targeted and edited a gene associated with cardiac disease at the level of the embryo. Although gene editing technology is available, many ethical considerations exist around this type of practice. Some argue that gene editing of an embryo allows prevention of serious genetic diseases, while others express concerns around creating "designer babies" or selecting traits such as desirable physical characteristics or gender.

SUMMARY

- Each human cell contains a full complement of genetic information encoded in genes contained in 46 chromosomes.
- The unequal division of the reproductive cells, the deletion of a part of a chromosome, the mutation in a single gene, or the modification of gene expression can each lead to developmental disabilities.
- There are numerous genetic tests available to diagnose many of these genetic disorders.
- Early identification may lead to improved outcome as a result of therapies that are now available for certain rare genetic disorders associated with developmental disabilities.

ADDITIONAL RESOURCES

National Library of Medicine (NLM): http://www.nlm.nih.gov

Genetic Alliance: http://www.geneticalliance.org

Online Mendelian Inheritance in Man (OMIM): http://www.ncbi.nlm.nih.gov/omim

Additional resources can be found online in Appendix D: Childhood Disabilities Resources, Services, and Organizations (see About the Online Companion Materials).

REFERENCES

Adam, M. P., Ardinger, H. H., Pagon, R. A., Wallace, S. E., Bean, L. J. H., Stephens, K., Amemiya, A. (Eds.). (1993–2018). *GeneReviews* [Internet]. Retreived from https://www.ncbi.nlm.nih.gov/books/NBK1116/

Au, K. S., Ashley-Koch, A., & Northrup, H. (2010). Epidemiologic and genetic aspects of spina bifida and other neural tube defects. *Developmental Disabilities Research Reviews, 16*(1), 6–15.

Batshaw, M., Roizen, N. J., & Lotrecchiano, G. R. (Eds.). (2013). *Children with disabilities* (7th ed.). Baltimore, MD: Paul H. Brookes Publishing Co.

Bertini, V., Azzar‡, A., Legitimo, A., Milone, R., Battini, R., Consolini, R., & Valetto, A. (2017). Deletion extents are not the cause of clinical variability in 22q11.2 deletion syndrome: Does the interaction between DGCR8 and miRNA-CNVs play a major role? *Frontiers in Genetics, 8*(47), 1–13.

Bushby, K., Finkel, R., Birnkrant, D. J., Case, L. E., Clemens, P. R., Cripe, L., . . . Constantin, C. (2010a). Diagnosis and management of Duchenne muscular dystrophy, Part 1: Diagnosis, and pharmacological and psychosocial management. *Lancet Neurology, 9*(1), 77–93.

Bushby, K., Finkel, R., Birnkrant, D. J., Case, L. E., Clemens, P. R., Cripe, L., . . . Constantin, C. (2010b). Diagnosis and management of Duchenne muscular dystrophy, Part 2:

Implementation of multidisciplinary care. *Lancet Neurology, 9*(2), 177–189.

Cerruti Mainardi, P. (2006). Cri du chat syndrome. *Orphanet Journal of Rare Disease, 5*(1), 33.

Chahrour, M., & Zoghbi, H. Y. (2007). The story of Rett syndrome: From clinic to neurobiology. *Neuron, 56*(3), 422–437.

Chonchaiya, W., Schneider, A., & Hagerman, R. J. (2009). Fragile X: A family of disorders. *Advances in Pediatrics, 56,* 165–186.

Collins, S. C., Coffee, B., Benke, P. J., Berry-Kravis, E., Gilbert, F., Oostra, B., . . . Warren, S. T. (2010). Array-based FMR1 sequencing and deletion analysis in patients with a fragile X syndrome-like phenotype. *Public Library of Science, 5*(3), e9476.

Conlin, L. K., Thiel, B. D., Bonnemann, C. G., Medne, L., Ernst, L. M., Zackai, E. H., . . . Spinner, N. B. (2010). Mechanisms of mosaicism, chimerism, and uniparental disomy identified by single nucleotide polymorphism array analysis. *Human Molecular Genetics, 19*(7), 1263–1275.

Dan, B. (2009). Angelman syndrome: Current understanding and research prospects. *Epilepsia, 50*(11), 2331–2339.

Driscoll, D. J., Miller, J. L., Schwartz, S., & Cassidy, S. B. (1998, updated 2017). Prader-Willi syndrome. In M. P. Adam, H. H. Ardinger, R. A. Pagon, S. E. Wallace, L. J. H. Bean, K. Stephens, & A. Amemiya (Eds.), *GeneReviews*. Retrieved from https://www.ncbi.nlm.nih.gov/books/NBK1330/

Feillet, F., van Spronsen, F. J., MacDonald, A., Trefz, F. K., Demirkol, M., Giovannini, M., . . . Blau, N. (2010). Challenges and pitfalls in the management of phenylketonuria. *Pediatrics, 126*(2), 333–341.

Friedman J. M. (2014). Neurofibromatosis 1. *GeneReviews*. University of Washington, Seattle. Retrieved from https://www.ncbi.nlm.nih.gov/books/NBK1109/

Genetics Home Reference (2017a). *Inheriting genetic conditions*. National Library of Medicine: Bethesda, MD. Retrieved from https://ghr.nlm.nih.gov/primer/inheritance/riskassessment

Genetics Home Reference (2017b). *What are genomic imprinting and uniparental disomy?* National Library of Medicine: Bethesda, MD. Retrieved from https://ghr.nlm.nih.gov/primer/inheritance/updimprinting

Goldstone, A. P., Holland, A. J., Hauffa, B. P., Hokken-Koelega, A. C., & Tauber, M. (2008). Recommendations for the diagnosis and management of Prader-Willi syndrome. *Journal of Clinical Endocrinology and Metabolism, 93*(11), 4183–4197.

Gorman, G. S. G. (2016). Mitochondrial diseases. *Nature Reviews. Disease Primers, 2,* 16080. https://doi.org/10.1038/nrdp.2016.80

Gurrieri, F., & Accadia, M. (2009). Genetic imprinting: The paradigm of Prader-Willi and Angelman syndromes. *Endocrine Development, 14,* 20–28.

Hassold, T., Hall, H., & Hunt, P. (2007). The origin of human aneuploidy: Where we have been, where we are going. *Human Molecular Genetics, 16*(2), R203–R208.

Hong D. S., Reiss A. L. (2014). Cognitive and neurological aspects of sex chromosome aneuploidies. *The Lancet. Neurology, 13*(3), 306–318.

Hook, E. B., & Warburton, D. (2014). Turner syndrome revisited: Review of new data supports the hypothesis that all viable 45, X cases are cryptic mosaics with a rescue cell line, implying an origin by mitotic loss. *Human Genetics, 133*(4), 417–424.

Inlow, J. K., & Restifo, L. L. (2004). Molecular and comparative genetics of mental retardation. *Genetics, 166*(2), 835–881.

Jorde, L. B., Carey, J. C., & Bamshad, M. D. (2015). *Medical genetics* (5th ed.). Philadelphia, PA: Mosby Elsevier.

Kaback, M. M., & Desnick, R. J. (1999, updated 2011). Hexosaminidase A deficiency. In M. P. Adam, H. H. Ardinger, R. A. Pagon, S. E. Wallace, L. J. H. Bean, K. Stephens, & A. Amemiya (Eds.), *GeneReviews*. Retrieved from https://www-ncbi-nlm-nih-gov.proxygw.wrlc.org/books/NBK1218/

Kole, R., & Krieg, A. M. (2015). Exon skipping therapy for Duchenne muscular dystrophy. *Advanced Drug Delivery Review, 87,* 104–107. doi:10.1016/j.addr.2015.05.008

Kumar, D. (2008). Disorders of the genome architecture: A review. *Genome Medicine, 2*(3–4), 69–76.

Lazaraviciute, G., Kauser, M., Bhattacharya, S., Haggarty, P., & Bhattacharya, S. (2014). A systematic review and meta-analysis of DNA methylation levels and imprinting disorders in children conceived by IVF/ICSI compared with children conceived spontaneously. *Human Reproduction Update, 20*(6), 840–852. https://doi.org/10.1093/humupd/dmu033

Liyanage, V. R. B., & Rastegar, M. (2014). Rett syndrome and MeCP2. *NeuroMolecular Medicine, 16*(2), 231–264. https://doi.org/10.1007/s12017-014-8295-9

López, C., Saravia, C., Gomez, A., Hoebeke, J., & Patarroyo, M. A. (2010). Mechanisms of genetically-based resistance to malaria. *Gene, 467*(1–2), 1–12.

Ma, H., Marti-Gutierrez, N., Park, S.-W., Wu, J., Lee, Y., Suzuki, K., . . . Mitalipov, S. (2017). Correction of a pathogenic gene mutation in human embryos. *Nature, 548*(7668), 413–419. https://doi.org/10.1038/nature23305

Mai, C. T., Kucik, J. E., Isenburg, J., Feldkamp, M. L., Marengo, L. K., Bugenske E. M., . . . Kirby, R. S. (2013). Selected birth defects data from population-based birth defects surveillance programs in the United States, 2006 to 2010: Featuring trisomy conditions. *Birth Defects Research (Part A) Clinical and Molecular Teratology, 97,* 709–725.

Martin, C. L., & Ledbetter, D. H. (2017). Chromosomal microarray testing for children with unexplained neurodevelopmental disorders. *Journal of the American Medical Association, 317*(24), 2545–2546.

Matijevic, T., Knezevic, J., Slavica, M., & Pavelic, J. (2009). Rett syndrome: From the gene to the disease. *European Neurology, 61*(1), 3–10.

McKusick-Nathans Institute of Genetic Medicine & The National Center for Biotechnology Information. (2017). *Online Mendelian Inheritance in Man* (OMIM). Retrieved from http://www.ncbi.nlm.nih.gov/omim/

Moss, J., & Howlin, P. (2009). Autism spectrum disorders in genetic syndromes: Implications for diagnosis, intervention, and understanding the wider autism spectrum disorder population. *Journal of Intellectual Disability Research, 53*(10), 852–873.

Nussbaum, R. L., McInnes, R. R., & Willard, H. F. (2016). *Thompson & Thompson genetics in medicine* (8th ed.). Philadelphia, PA: Elsevier.

Ong, T., Marshall, S. G., Karczeski, B. A., Stemen, D. L., Cheng, E., & Cutting, G. R. Cystic fibrosis and congenital absence of the vas deferens. (2001, updated 2017). In M. P. Adam, H. H. Ardinger, R. A. Pagon, S. E. Wallace, L. J. H. Bean, K. Stephens, & A. Amemiya (Eds.), *GeneReviews* [Internet]. Retrieved from https://www.ncbi.nlm.nih.gov/books/NBK1250/

Percy, A. K. (2008). Rett syndrome: Recent research progress. *Journal of Child Neurology, 23*(5), 543–549.

Rahbari, R., Wuster, A., Lindsay, S. J., Hardwick, R. J., Alexandrov, L. B., Al Turki, S., . . . Hurles, M. E. (2015). Timing, rates and spectra of human germline mutation. *Nature Publishing Group, 48*(2). https://doi.org/10.1038/ng.3469

Ridley, M. (2006). *Genome: The autobiography of a species in 23 chapters*. New York, NY: HarperCollins.

Saito, K. (2012). Fukuyama congenital muscular dystrophy. *GeneReviews*. Seattle, WA: University of Washington. Retrieved from https://www.ncbi.nlm.nih.gov/books/NBK1206/

Sansović, I., Ivankov, A.-M., Bobinec, A., Kero, M., & Barišić, I. (2017). Chromosomal microarray in clinical diagnosis: a study of 337 patients with congenital anomalies and developmental delays or intellectual disability. *Croatian Medical Journal, 58*(3), 231–238. Retrieved from https://www.ncbi.nlm.nih.gov/pmc/articles/PMC5470123/

Schneider, A., Hagerman, R. J., & Hessl, D. (2009). Fragile X syndrome: From genes to cognition. *Developmental Disabilities Research Reviews, 15*(4), 333–342.

Soellner, L., Begemann, M., Mackay, D. J. G., Grønskov, K., Tümer, Z., Maher, E. R., . . . Eggermann, T. (2017). Recent advances in imprinting disorders. *Clinical Genetics, 91*(1), 3–13. https://doi.org/10.1111/cge.12827

Spena, S., Gervasini, C., & Milani, D. (2015). Ultra-rare syndromes: The example of Rubinstein-Taybi syndrome. *Journal of Pediatrics Genetics, 4*(3), 177–186.

Suthar, R., & Sankhyan, N. (2017). Duchenne muscular dystrophy: A practice update. *Indian Journal of Pediatrics, 85*(4), 276–281. https://doi.org/10.1007/s12098-017-2397-y

Tammimies, K., Marshall, C. R., Walker, S., Kaur, G. K., Thiruvahindrapuram, B., Lionel, A. C., . . . Fernandez, B. A. (2015). Molecular diagnostic yield of chromosomal microarray analysis and whole-exome sequencing in children with autism spectrum disorder. *Journal of the American Medical Association, 314*(9), 895–903.

Uniken Venema, W. T., Voskuil, M. D., Dijkstra, G., Weersma, R. K., & Festen, E. A. (2016). The genetic background of inflammatory bowel disease: From correlation to causality. *The Journal of Pathology, 241*(2), 146–158. https://doi.org/10.1002/path.4817

Urdinguio, R. G., Sanchez-Mut, J. V., & Esteller, M. (2009). Epigenetic mechanisms in neurological diseases: Genes, syndromes, and therapies. *Lancet Neurology, 8*(11), 1056–1072.

Weischenfeldt, J., Symmons, O., Spitz, F., & Korbel, J. O. (2013). Phenotypic impact of genomic structural variation: Insights from and for human disease. *Nature Reviews Genetics, 14*(2), 125–138.

Youngblom, E., Pariani, M., & Knowles, J. W. (2014, updated 2016). Familial hypercholesterolemia. Prader-Willi syndrome. https://www.ncbi.nlm.nih.gov/books/NBK174884/

CHAPTER 2 Environmental Exposures

Shruti N. Tewar

Upon completion of this chapter, the reader will be able to

- Explain the history of environmental exposures in childhood
- Discuss individual environmental toxicants from the perspectives of epidemiology, mechanism of toxicity, and effect on brain development
- Describe screening and prevention strategies for environmental toxicant exposure
- Understand how environmental toxicants influence epigenetic changes and impact development
- Discuss the societal financial implications and cost of environmental toxicant exposure
- Describe prevention and public policy regarding environmental exposures

The world has undergone incredible advances over the last two centuries, beginning with the Industrial Revolution, which drove changes in agriculture, transportation, and manufacturing and led to urbanization. This industrialization also necessitated the large-scale production of chemicals to build stronger, better materials used in manufacturing with diverse applications. Today, there are more than 80,000 chemicals in commercial use; unfortunately, roughly 1,000 of these have been identified as toxins. Some are teratogenic, leading to physical malformations due to *in utero* exposures, and others are neurotoxic, resulting in developmental disabilities from postnatal exposure. The twentieth century was marked by a number of catastrophes caused by environmental toxins that have affected children and led to developmental disabilities. In addition, low-level exposures to a number of environmental toxicants have been shown to be associated with low birth weight, preterm births, failure to thrive, asthma, obesity, cognitive impairments, learning disabilities, and other neurodevelopmental disorders, including attention-deficit/hyperactivity disorder (ADHD) (Baghurst et al., 1992; Bellinger, Stiles, & Needleman, 1992; Lanphear et al., 2005).

CASE STUDY

Jaylen is a 6-year-old boy. At a well-child visit, his mother shared her concern that he is struggling at

Acknowledgments: I am very grateful to Dr. Mirko von Elstermann, Biomedical Sciences Librarian at the University of Iowa's Hardin Library for the Health Sciences, for his support in finding relevant toxicant literature.

school. He is very active and cannot sit and participate in learning like most children in his class. He can sing the ABCs but cannot identify letters or write his first and last name. Jaylen's birth and early development were uncomplicated per parent report, with developmental milestones achieved on time. His lead levels at 12 months and 24 months were less than 5 mcg/dL (normal). However, he was screened again at 4 and 5 years of age for lead poisoning due to concerns about lead contamination in the drinking water. His venous lead levels were 28 mcg/dL at 4 years and 25 mcg/dL at 5 years of age, both elevated. While the local municipality addresses the lead contamination in the drinking water, since Jaylen's lead level is greater than 15 mcg/dL, his pediatrician has recommended switching to bottled water with plans to monitor his lead levels every 3 months until they are below the reference range of 5 mcg/dl.

Thought Questions:

What other professionals will need to be involved in Jaylen's health and development going forward? What are some long-term effects of lead poisoning? Are they reversible once the lead level returns to an acceptable range?

A HISTORICAL PERSPECTIVE

As more and more chemicals were invented and produced on a large scale, there was an increased awareness of the potentially toxic effects of these chemicals to the human population, especially to young children and women of childbearing age. The most devastating of these toxic exposures have been lead, methylmercury, thalidomide, and isocyanate gas:

- Lead (in the form of lead paint) was the first identified environmental toxin to affect children, described in 1904 by an Australian pediatrician, J. Lockhart Gibson (Gibson, 2005). Affected children presented clinically with severe anemia, paralysis, blindness, and occasionally death. In 2015, a state of emergency was declared in Genesee County, Michigan, when extremely high lead levels were detected in the water supply for the city of Flint after the city switched its water supply source without using adequate measures to prevent corrosion and leaching from lead pipes. As a result, the children living in Flint who were exposed to the untreated water were noted to have significantly elevated lead levels after the switch (Hanna-Attisha, LaChance, Sadler, & Champney Schnepp, 2015).
- In 1956, methylmercury poisoning was identified as the cause of sensory disturbances, ataxia, dysarthria, constriction of the visual field, auditory disturbances, and tremor in individuals eating contaminated fish from Minamata Bay, Japan (Harada, 1995). Furthermore, when pregnant women ate the fish, their fetuses were found to be poisoned by the methylmercury and to have sustained extensive brain damage.
- In 1961, thalidomide, which was used to treat morning sickness in pregnant women, was found to induce severe limb defects (phocomelia) in the fetus (Neil, 2015). Over 10,000 children were born with a range of severe and debilitating malformations.
- In 1984, a leak at a pesticide plant in Bhopal, India, led to over 500,000 people being exposed to methyl isocyanate gas. It affected more than 200,000 children, causing respiratory, neurologic, psychiatric, and ophthalmic symptoms (Mishra et al., 2009). For women who were pregnant at the time, more than one-half of their progeny were still born or did not survive the first 30 days of life, and several children were born with birth defects (Varma, 1987).

As a result of these tragedies, the role of environmental toxins on child health and development became more prominently recognized.

THE DEVELOPING BRAIN AND TOXIC EXPOSURE

Environmental toxins affect the brain and body of children through multiple routes; they are ubiquitous in air, dust particles, water, and contact surfaces. Some of the common routes of exposure are through ingestion, inhalation, skin contact, and placental transfer. The fetus is particularly susceptible to environmental exposures, beginning with conception and continuing during the rapid phase of cell differentiation, proliferation, and migration (see Chapter 6). The placenta does not provide a significant barrier against environmental toxins. In fact, in the case of methylmercury, the fetus was found to be exposed to even larger doses than the mother (Ramirez, Cruz, Pagulayan, Ostrea, & Dalisay, 2000). Additionally, the fetus may lack critical enzymes necessary to metabolize and rid the body of certain toxins, such as pesticides including isocyanate (Chen, Chang, Tao, & Lu, 2015). Younger children also have a greater risk for toxic exposure due to higher hand-to-mouth activity, increased absorption rates, and an immature blood-brain barrier. Furthermore, their bodies are not efficient at removing some of the toxins, leading to accumulation in the body over time.

TIMING OF VULNERABILITY TO ENVIRONMENTAL TOXINS

The effects of environmental toxins vary based on the timing of the exposure during fetal development. In the first and second trimesters, environmental toxins can interfere with cell migration, differentiation, and proliferation through placental transfer. This can lead to physical deformities as well as impact brain development. As examples, thalidomide is teratogenic in the first trimester during the period of limb formation, whereas methyl mercury and polychlorinated biphenyls (PCBs) affect synaptogenesis (see Chapter 8) throughout pregnancy. Although environmental exposure to toxins does not cause physical defects after birth, it can significantly affect postnatal brain development. In this context, lead exposure interferes with pruning and myelination in the brain, which continues throughout early childhood.

SPECIFIC NEUROTOXICANTS

The following section describes specific neurotoxicants and their effects on fetal and child development, including lead, tobacco, mercury, alcohol, polychlorinated biphenyls, and endocrine disruptors. Table 2.1 summarizes these neurotoxicants, their common adverse effects, and recommendations for evaluation, prevention, and management.

Lead

Lead is the most commonly studied and best known neurotoxicant. It is commonly found in pipes, storage batteries, weights, ammunition, cable covers, paints, dyes, ceramic glazes, and caulk. Although it has been known to be neurotoxic since the early 1900s, lead-containing paint was not banned for interior use until 1978 and lead as an additive to gasoline was only removed in 1996 in the United States. Since then, the amount of lead released into the environment has been significantly reduced. However, lead that falls to the ground as dust; chipping lead paint from buildings and bridges; leaching of lead from landfills; disposal of lead containing products in landfills; industrial activities, such as ore mining, battery production, or ammunition manufacturing; and the corrosion of lead pipes can all result in the seepage of lead into the ground water.

Children are most commonly exposed to lead by eating foods or water contaminated with lead, or by ingesting or inhaling lead dust particles or paint chips. Lead poisoning can lead to a multitude of health problems, including anemia, kidney damage, neurocognitive impairments, and peripheral neuropathy. Young children are at a higher risk for lead toxicity due to increased hand-to-mouth behaviors, higher respiratory rates, and increased absorptive capacity compared with older children and adults. There are multiple studies demonstrating the neurotoxic effects of lead on brain development (Bellinger et al., 1992; Braun, Kahn, Froehlich, Auinger, & Lanphear, 2006; Lanphear et al., 2005).

Increasingly, the effects on brain development of even low levels of lead exposures have been identified; no amount of lead exposure is deemed safe in children. Low-level lead exposure has been associated with an increased risk of cognitive impairment, impairments in memory, ADHD, and learning difficulties (Canfield et al., 2003; Evens et al., 2015; Jusko et al., 2008; Kim et al., 2010; Mason, Harp, & Han, 2014). Lanphear and colleagues (2005) demonstrated that an increase of blood lead concentration from less than 1 μg/dL to 10 μg/dL was associated with a 6.9-point decrease in IQ. While a 5-point change in IQ may not seem very large for an individual child, a 5-point decrease in the mean population IQ can have a substantial impact. It results in a 57% increase in children with an IQ less than 70 (Gilbert & Weiss, 2006) and an increased need for special education and other supports.

Animal studies have shown that lead disrupts neurotransmission, synaptogenesis, synaptic trimming, and myelination (Baranowska-Bosiacka et al., 2017; Gassowska et al., 2016; Lidsky & Schneider, 2006; Neal & Guilarte, 2010; Toscano & Guilarte, 2005). Lead also has been shown to alter gene expression within the brain, leading to inflammatory damage (Kidd, Anderson, & Schneider, 2008; Raciti & Ceccatelli, 2017; Schneider, Anderson, Kidd, Sobolewski, & Cory-Slechta, 2016).

In 2012, the Centers for Disease Control and Prevention (CDC) concluded that there is no safe level of lead exposure. **Chelation therapy**, a medical procedure to remove heavy metals from the body, is recommended when blood lead levels are greater than or equal to 45 μg/dL. Chelation therapy, however, does not reverse existing neurocognitive defects. Prevention of lead exposure is the best recommendation to protect against its effects on the developing brain.

Tobacco Smoke

Maternal smoking of tobacco during pregnancy and postnatal environmental tobacco exposure are associated with several adverse health outcomes in children. The effect of tobacco on the fetus is related to its active ingredient, nicotine, which crosses the placenta into the fetal circulation. Nicotine decreases

Table 2.1. Specific neurotoxicants, common adverse effects, and recommendations

Neurotoxicant	Common adverse effects	Recommendations
Lead	Low level exposure: Nausea, vomiting, anemia, abdominal pain, constipation, developmental delay, cognitive deficits, ADHD High lead levels: altered mental status, seizures, difficulty walking, coma and death	Lead monitoring, screening, and abatement Blood lead > 5 mcg/dL – 45 mcg/dL: close monitoring Blood lead > 45 mcg/dL: chelation
Tobacco smoke	Low birth weight Preterm labor and birth Increased risk of SUID, asthma, allergies, ADHD, intellectual disability, sleep problems, behavioral problems	Reduce secondhand smoke exposure Pregnant women should quit smoking
Methyl mercury	Sensory disturbances of vision, hearing, and touch Tremors Brain damage Microcephaly Cerebral palsy Seizures Cognitive impairment	Women who are pregnant, nursing, and of childbearing age and young children should avoid predatory fish with high mercury content in diet
Alcohol	Atypical facial features Microcephaly Short stature Cognitive deficits, attention and memory deficits, executive function deficits, cognitive impairment Speech and language disorders Learning disabilities Vision and hearing impairments	No alcohol consumption during pregnancy
Pesticides	Developmental delay Cognitive deficits ADHD Delayed social development and autism-like behaviors Respiratory problems Childhood cancers	Limit indoor and outdoor pesticide use Use comprehensive pest management Monitor water sources for high pesticide content in agricultural communities
Polychlorinated biphenyls (PCBs)	Low birth weight Cognitive delays Attention problems and impulsivity Obesity Decreased immunity Childhood cancers Delayed social skills with autism-like behaviors	Dispose of PCB-containing products safely Women who are pregnant, nursing, and of childbearing age and young children should avoid farm-raised salmon
Endocrine disruptors	Obesity Cognitive deficits ADHD Sex-specific changes in hormone levels Anxiety Social skill deficits	Choose BPA-free and/or phthalate-free plastics Avoid heating plastic containers with food

Key: ADHD, attention-deficit/hyperactivity disorder; SUID, sudden unexplained infant death; BPA, bisphenol A.

oxygen delivery, increases resistance to blood flow, and decreases the nutrient supply. Fetal exposure to nicotine has been shown to cause atypical cell proliferation, differentiation, and synaptic activity in the brain (Ino, 2010). The result is an increased risk of low birth weight (<2,500 gm) and preterm births. Maternal smoking also has been shown to affect brain development and vision. Furthermore, fetal exposure increases the risk of obesity, hypertension, asthma, and impaired lung function in children and adolescents up to 18 years of age (Banderali et al., 2015; Clifford, Lang, & Chen, 2012; Weng, Redsell, Swift, Yang, & Glazebrook, 2012).

Postnatally, second-hand smoke exposure is associated with an increased risk of sudden infant death syndrome (SIDS), neurodevelopmental and behavioral disorders such as ADHD, conduct disorder, intellectual disability, sleep disruption, and respiratory disorders such as asthma and allergies (Banderali et al., 2015; Froehlich et al., 2009; Hughes et al., 2017; Poole-Di Salvo, Liu, Brenner, & Weitzman, 2010; Zhou et al., 2014).

Mercury

Mercury is released into the environment from rock, burning of fossil fuels, and incineration of consumer products containing mercury (e.g., electronic devices, batteries, light bulbs, and thermometers). Mercury is toxic in both its elemental and inorganic forms. The elemental form gets vaporized and can be inhaled, and the inorganic form is converted by naturally occurring biologic processes into organic methylmercury, which is highly toxic.

Methylmercury can be concentrated in the aquatic food chain; as such, human consumption of seafood is a major route of exposure. Methyl mercury crosses the placental barrier easily, and because the fetal blood-brain barrier is not fully developed, prenatal exposure can result in severe brain damage, microcephaly, seizures, cerebral palsy, and cognitive impairment (Boucher et al., 2012; Debes, Weihe, & Grandjean, 2016; Grandjean, Weihe, Debes, Choi, & Budtz-Jorgensen, 2014; Harada, 1995). Low levels of methylmercury exposure have been associated with decrements in IQ and deficiencies in visual spatial processing, memory, attention, and language (Boucher et al., 2012; Grandjean et al., 2014). The mechanism of action for methylmercury neurotoxicity is dependent on the timing and dose of exposure and includes widespread damage to the blood-brain barrier, neuronal cell damage/death, interference with neuronal migration, and alterations in brain neurotransmitters (Antunes dos Santos et al., 2016). Currently, it is believed that the benefits of eating fish and other seafood outweigh the risks of methylmercury toxicity. It is recommended, however, that young children and women of childbearing age avoid fish that may contain high levels of mercury (U.S. Food & Drug Administration, 2017a).

Ethylmercury is a metabolite of thimerosal, a mercury-containing chemical used as a preservative in multidose vials of some vaccines. After the publication of a fraudulent (and subsequently retracted) article (Murch, 2004) purporting a linkage between thimerosal in the MMR vaccine and autism, many parents became concerned about giving vaccines to their children. Subsequently, numerous epidemiologic studies have shown there to be no evidence that thimerosal in vaccines is linked to autism (American Academy of Pediatrics, 2013). There is, in fact, a robust body of peer-reviewed, scientific studies done in the United States and other countries supporting the safety of thimerosal-containing vaccines (U.S. Food & Drug Administration, 2017b; World Health Organization, 2006). Currently, with the use of single-dose vials, all routinely recommended vaccines for infants in the United States are available as thimerosal-free preparations or contain less the 1 μg mercury/dose of thimerosal. Evidence-based practice Box 2.1 presents a discussion of thimerosal in vaccines and autism.

BOX 2.1 EVIDENCE-BASED PRACTICE

Vaccines and Autism

Ethylmercury is a metabolite of thimerosal, a mercury-containing chemical used as a preservative in multidose vials of some vaccines. Ethylmercury is different from methylmercury, which is associated with long-term neurologic effects of mercury poisoning. Since the publication of a fraudulent study in 1998, questions have been raised regarding the relationship between autism and vaccines, particularly the measles, mumps, rubella (MMR) combination vaccine. Parents have also raised concerns about too many vaccines overwhelming the immune system when given simultaneously.

These concerns have been shown to be invalid. The preservative thimerosal was never present in the MMR vaccine even though it was used in other vaccines in the 1990s. Furthermore, the American Academy of Pediatrics examined the available studies and published evidence that vaccines including the MMR were not associated with or caused autism and that children with delayed immunizations showed no benefits of delaying immunizations in the first year of life (American Academy of Pediatrics, 2013).

Application to Practice

- Clinicians should be aware of available evidence refuting the link between vaccines and autism.
- Clinicians should discuss the importance of vaccines and provide appropriate education to vaccine hesitant parents. It is important to revisit this discussion multiple times if necessary at each clinical encounter.
- Clinicians should be aware of resources and educational materials that can be shared with families about the safety of vaccines.

Alcohol

Alcohol is a known **teratogen,** and prenatal exposure to alcohol has been associated with a range of physical and neurodevelopmental disabilities covered under the umbrella term of **fetal alcohol spectrum disorders** (**FASD**; Williams & Smith, 2015). Findings of FASD include atypical facial features (i.e., a thin upper lip and smooth surface rather than a vertical groove between the base of the nose and the border of the upper lip), microcephaly, short stature, attention and memory difficulties, executive function impairments, and cognitive impairments, including intellectual disability, speech and language difficulties, learning disabilities, and vision or hearing problems (Flak et al., 2014; Glass et al., 2017; Gross et al., 2017).

No amount of alcohol is considered safe during pregnancy. FASDs are entirely preventable developmental disorders. Despite this, in the United States 1 in 10 pregnant women reported alcohol use and 1 in 33 reported binge drinking in the past 30 days per data collected by the CDC from 2011–2013 using the Behavioral Risk Factor Surveillance System (Tan, Denny, Cheal, Sniezek, & Kanny, 2015). A recent study looking at the worldwide prevalence of FASD reported a significantly high prevalence in South Africa, Croatia, and Italy (Roozen et al., 2016).

Prenatal alcohol exposure interferes with neuronal migration, brain organization, brain growth, and synaptic formation (Derauf, Kekatpure, Neyzi, Lester, & Kosofsky, 2009; Hendrickson et al., 2017; Jacobson et al., 2017; Jarmasz, Basalah, Chudley, & Del Bigio, 2017; Wozniak et al., 2017). Guidelines for evaluating and diagnosing FASD were recently revised and published by the American Academy of Pediatrics (Hagan et al., 2016; Hoyme et al., 2016).

Marijuana and Opioids

Statistics published from the National Survey of Drug Use and Health in 2014 indicated that 27 million people ages 12 or older had used an illicit drug in the past 30 days, equivalent to 10.2% of the U.S. population (CBHSQ, 2015). Common illicit drugs used include **marijuana** and hashish, nonmedical use of pain relievers and stimulants such as methamphetamines, tranquilizers, cocaine, heroin, inhalants, sedatives, and hallucinogens (LSD and Ecstasy). This section focuses on marijuana and opioids.

Marijuana policy is rapidly evolving in many states across the United States, with 30 states and the District of Columbia having laws broadly legalizing marijuana in some form at the time of the writing of this chapter. Eight states and the District of Columbia have expansive laws legalizing marijuana for recreational use. Marijuana, often referred to as cannabis, is derived from the plant *Cannabis sativa.* It can be consumed in many forms, including smoking, vaping using e-cigarettes, hash oil, and edible products. The psychoactive properties of cannabis are due to the compound Δ-9-tetrahydrocannabinol (THC), which leads to both pleasurable and concerning effects, including relaxation, euphoria, heightened perception, sociability, sensation of time slowing, increased appetite, and decreased perception of pain, as well as paranoia, anxiety, irritability, impaired short-term memory, poor attention and judgement, and poor coordination and balance. Physiologic effects include tachycardia, hypertension, dry mouth and throat, and conjunctival injection (eye redness). There are also synthetic cannabinoids marketed as herbal mixtures and sold for recreational purposes under the names of Spice, K2, or Kronic.

Because of decriminalization and legalization of cannabis in certain states, the perception of marijuana being harmful has lessened, and, combined with the ease of access, rates of use have increased over the past several years. In 2015, 21% of youth reported using marijuana one or more times within the past 30 days (Kann et al., 2016). Marijuana readily crosses the placenta and is present in breast milk in pregnant and breastfeeding mothers (Baker et al., 2018; Grant, Petroff, Isoherranen, Stella, & Burbacher, 2018). Children born with prenatal exposure to marijuana are at increased risk for problems in the neonatal period, difficulty with emotional regulation after birth, and being a victim of domestic violence (Crume et al., 2018; Eiden, Schuetze, Shisler, & Huestis, 2018; Victor, Resko, Ryan, & Perron, 2018). Several studies have shown that long-term adolescent cannabis use may be associated with a decline in IQ (Hadland, Knight, & Harris, 2015), although a recent systematic review and metaanalysis did not find a strong correlation (Scott et al., 2018).

Recreational marijuana should not be confused with "medical marijuana" or cannabidiol, which does not have the psychoactive properties of THC and is being evaluated for the management of certain neurological conditions including refractory epilepsy, dystonia, spasticity, and central pain. While there are also trials underway for its use in developmental and behavioral conditions, including autism, ADHD, and anxiety disorders, there is no evidence to support its use for treatment of these conditions at this time.

Given the substantial increase in unintentional pediatric exposures, more commonly due to oral ingestions and subsequent hospital visits after recreational use of marijuana in certain states, several states have passed regulations to prevent these exposures with requirements for warning labels, dosing regulations, packaging requirements, rules about edibles, and educational campaigns. As clinicians and health care providers, it is important to screen for marijuana exposure and its associated risk factors and to provide education that makes the point that decriminalization of marijuana does not necessarily mean it is safe.

Due to the rising opioid epidemic, children are at risk for prenatal and secondhand exposure to opioids. In several longitudinal studies, children born to mothers with opioid or polysubstance use during pregnancy had lower levels of cognitive functioning, lower birth weight, and decreased brain volumes compared to non-drug-exposed peers (Nygaard, Moe, Slinning, & Walhovd, 2015; Nygaard et al., 2018; Nygaard, Slinning, Moe, & Walhovd, 2017).

Pesticides

A **pesticide** is any substance or mixture of substances intended for preventing, destroying, repelling, or mitigating unwanted insects, plants, molds, and rodents. U.S. pesticide usage totaled more than 1.1 billion pounds in 2012, accounting for 20% of the pesticide usage in the world (Atwood & Paisley-Jones, 2017). Pesticides contain both active and inert ingredients, either of which can be toxic to human health. However, U.S. law currently does not require manufacturers to disclose the content and percentage of inert ingredients.

The most common source of pesticide exposure for children is in food, but pesticides are also present in the air, dust, soil, indoor and outdoor surfaces, and certain water sources. Pesticides can cross the placental barrier and be present in breast milk. Some of the major classes of pesticides include organophosphates, carbamates, pyrethroids, and organochlorines. Organochlorine pesticides such as dichlorodiphenyltricholorethane (DDT), aldrin, dieldrin, and chlordane can remain in the environment for a very long time and tend to accumulate in the food chain. These pesticides are labelled *persistent toxic substances* and are banned for agricultural and domestic use in Europe, North America, and many countries in South America; however, DDT is still used to control malaria in some low-resource countries.

Organophosphate pesticides are widely used in agriculture yet are known to be neurotoxicants, especially for children. The risk to children is higher because the dose exposure is greater per kilogram of body weight and children have lower levels of enzymes to remove some of the organophosphates. High-dose exposure to pesticides can lead to systemic health problems, including permanent damage to major organ systems and even death. Low-level chronic exposure is noted to have a multitude of adverse neurodevelopmental and health outcomes. Prenatal exposure to organophosphates has been associated with decreased IQ and social-emotional responsiveness, developmental delay, and autistic behaviors (Bouchard et al., 2011; Braun et al., 2014; Eskenazi et al., 2014; Eskenazi et al., 2008; Munoz-Quezada et al., 2013; Rowe et al., 2016; Shelton et al., 2014; Stein et al., 2016). Exposure to pesticides during childhood has been associated with cognitive impairments, ADHD, childhood cancers, and respiratory problems (Bouchard, Bellinger, Wright, & Weisskopf, 2010; Chen, Chang, Tao, & Lu, 2015; Raanan et al., 2015; Richardson et al., 2015; Wagner-Schuman et al., 2015).

The U.S. Environmental Protection Agency (EPA) regulates the pesticide use in food (i.e., grains, fruits, and vegetables) and sets standards for allowable pesticide residue in food under the Food Quality Protection Act. Under this provision, since 2007 the EPA has cancelled or restricted the use of several pesticides, including carbamates, several organophosphates, methyl parathion, and acephate.

Polychlorinated Biphenyls

PCBs are a group of industrial chemicals used in electronics, plasticizers, plastics, rubber products, pigments, dyes, carbonless copy paper, and pesticides. Manufacturing of PCBs was banned in the United States in 1979, but they are still present in products and materials produced before that time. They are released into the environment by improper disposal of hazardous waste or PCB-containing products, resulting in soil and water contamination. PCBs do not readily breakdown in the environment and can accumulate in the food chain due to their high lipid solubility. Fish are the most likely source of PCBs for humans. Farm-raised salmon may be high in PCBs and should be avoided by young children and women who are pregnant, nursing, or planning to become pregnant.

PCB ingestion has been associated with an increased risk of cancer, reduced immunity, decreased birth weight, and endocrine disruption. Low-level prenatal or postnatal exposure to PCBs has been associated with cognitive delays, behavior disorders, attention problems and impulsive behaviors, obesity, and autistic behaviors (Berghuis, Soechitram, Hitzert, Sauer, & Bos, 2013; Braun et al., 2014; Casas et al., 2015; Delvaux et al., 2014; Eubig, Aguiar, & Schantz, 2010; Tang-Peronard et al., 2014).

Endocrine Disruptors

Endocrine disruptors are chemicals that interfere with the function of the endocrine system. They can mimic, block, or alter the synthesis, metabolism, or excretion of hormones and thereby interfere with the action or concentration of hormones produced in the body. Under this umbrella, several chemicals have been noted to have endocrine-disrupting properties, including phthalates, PCBs, bisphenol A (BPA), DDT, perfluorinated compounds (PFCs), and organochlorine pesticides.

Bisphenol A is an industrial chemical used in the manufacturing of polycarbonate plastics. These plastics are used in metal food can linings, reusable water bottles, sports safety equipment, thermal paper receipts, and adhesives. Phthalates are a group of chemicals called plasticizers that are used to make plastics more flexible and harder to break. Both BPA and phthalates can leach out of products and be ingested. Exposure to phthalates and BPA can also occur through skin absorption, inhalation, and mouthing. Both BPA and phthalates can cross the placental barrier and influence the neurodevelopment of the fetus.

Exposure to endocrine disruptors at certain stages of brain and body development can have profound and lasting effects. Prenatal exposure to BPA in animal models has been shown to alter expression of genes coding for estrogen receptors and the dopamine transporter. BPA also disrupts signaling pathways in lipid metabolism and alters serum gonadal hormones, leading to sex-specific effects on the developing fetus (Alyea & Watson, 2009; Ishido, Masuo, Terasaki, & Morita, 2011; Masuo & Ishido, 2011).

Prenatal and early childhood BPA exposure is associated with inattention, impulsivity, ADHD, disruptive behaviors, anxiety, and impairments in working memory (Braun et al., 2017; Evans et al., 2014; Perera et al., 2016; Tewar et al., 2016). Prenatal exposure to phthalates is associated with cognitive impairments, including lower IQ, inattention, hyperactivity, and poor social communication (Braun, 2017; Ejaredar, Nyanza, Ten Eycke, & Dewey, 2015). Oftentimes children are exposed to multiple endocrine disruptors simultaneously during sensitive periods of development, placing them at greater risk for significant impairments. Evidence-Based Practice Box 2.2 presents a discussion of endocrine-disrupting chemicals and neurodevelopment.

Congenital Infections

In addition to environmental toxicants, several biologic agents, including bacteria and viruses, have been identified to be teratogenic depending on the timing of exposure during pregnancy. Prenatal infections, commonly known as **TORCH,** which includes **T**oxoplasmosis, **O**ther (i.e., syphilis, varicella-zoster, and parvovirus B19), **R**ubella, **C**ytomegalovirus, and

BOX 2.2 EVIDENCE-BASED PRACTICE

Endocrine-Disrupting Chemicals and Neurodevelopment

Endocrine-disrupting chemicals (EDCs) are a class of compounds that can increase the risk of disease throughout the lifespan by altering or interfering with the homeostasis of hormones or other signaling components of the endocrine system. Humans may be exposed to a mixture of EDCs simultaneously, and because the developing brain of the fetus and young child is more vulnerable to the effects of EDCs, this is of particular concern for this age group.

Braun (2017) has examined and summarized available epidemiological studies on the effects of early-life exposure to EDCs, particularly bisphenol A (BPA), phthalates, triclosan, and perfluoroalkyl substances (PFAS), on childhood neurobehavioral disorders and obesity. Review of available epidemiological studies shows that prenatal BPA and phthalate exposure is associated with adverse neurobehavioral outcomes, including ADHD, autism, cognitive deficits, and emotional problems but not the risk of obesity or being overweight. In contrast, prenatal PFAS exposure has been associated with low birth weight and increased risk of obesity or being overweight in children but not neurobehavioral deficits.

Application to Practice

- Clinicians should be aware of exposures to EDCs and their role in neurodevelopment.
- Clinicians can help identify and reduce exposure to BPA by promoting a balanced diet, the use of BPA-free plastics, reducing consumption of canned or packaged foods, and avoiding heating food in plastic containers to reduce leaching of BPA.

Herpes infections, account for 2%–3% of congenital anomalies. The American College of Obstetricians and Gynecologists recommends that pregnant women be screened for rubella and syphilis. However, universal screening for TORCH is not recommended due to the low yield and high costs.

More recently, the emergence of Zika virus (ZIKV) in the Americas and other regions has highlighted the importance of congenital infections in developmental disabilities. ZIKV is a vector-borne disease transmitted to humans directly (via sexual or mother-to-child transmission) or indirectly (via vector *Aedes aegypti* mosquitoes, blood transfusion, or organ transplantation). In 2015, there was a sharp increase in infants born with microcephaly noted 6 months after detection of ZIKV. The first outbreak of ZIKV was noted in 2016 in the continental United States. ZIKV infection in adults presents as a rash and fever that is generally mild and self-limited. However, vertical transmission of ZIKV to the fetus can lead to a broad spectrum of neurological impairments, growth restriction, and fetal loss. This collective presentation is termed as **congenital Zika syndrome** (CZS). The fetuses and children diagnosed with CZS have been found to have microcephaly (a small head size), extra skin on the scalp, club feet, **arthrogryposis** (contractures of joints), increased muscle tone, spasticity, and hyperreflexia. Children with CZS are also noted to have atypical brain activity, seizures, and eye impairments leading to poor vision (da Silva Pone et al., 2018).

Follow-up studies of children with CZS show significantly delayed cognitive skills, motor skills, communication skills, and an increased incidence of cerebral palsy (Pessoa et al., 2018; Wheeler, 2018). The diagnosis of CZS is confirmed by blood or urine testing in the newborn period. Additional guidelines on evaluation and management of CZS are available through the CDC (Adebanjo et al., 2017). Currently, there is no vaccine available to prevent ZIKV infections. Management of a child with CZS involves an interdisciplinary and collaborative effort among obstetricians; neonatologists; pediatricians; neurologists; ophthalmologists; orthopedic surgeons; rehab specialists, including physical therapists, occupational therapists, and speech and language pathologists; early intervention services; social workers; and the educational system supporting the family of the child.

ENVIRONMENTAL TOXICANTS AND EPIGENETICS

Epigenetics is the study of heritable changes in gene expression that occur without changes in the DNA sequence (see Chapter 1). Epigenetic changes can be described as a mechanism by which genes can be switched on or off by chemical signals, similar to a dimmer switch on a light. These epigenetic changes can alter the ways in which genes produce proteins and signal other genes; they can last for months to years but are potentially reversible. Environmental toxins can induce phenotypic changes using several epigenetic mechanisms (e.g., DNA methylation, histone modifications, and microRNA [miRNA] expression) and can change genome function. When epigenetic changes occur in a developing fetus, they can alter cellular function (Javed, Chen, Lin, & Liang, 2016).

For instance, prenatal exposure to tobacco via maternal smoking has been associated with changes in DNA methylation patterns in several genes. This could lead to a decreased number of neurons in the fetus and alterations in neurodevelopment (Armstrong et al., 2016; Banik et al., 2017; Chatterton et al., 2017). Fetal exposure to alcohol also has been associated with alteration in genes via multiple mechanisms, including DNA methylation, histone modification, alterations in miRNA expression, and alterations in several genes impacting neurodevelopment (Banik et al., 2017). In regions with high levels of arsenic in the ground water (contaminated naturally or from mining or agriculture), adults have been noted to have dose-dependent DNA hypermethylation in their blood DNA (Chanda et al., 2006; Pilsner et al., 2007), and prenatal arsenic exposure has been associated with global methylation of cord blood DNA in a sex-specific manner (Pilsner et al., 2012). Endocrine disruptors are also increasingly recognized for their epigenetic influences on neurodevelopment, thyroid regulation, reproduction capacity, and other metabolic processes (Derghal, Djelloul, Trouslard, & Mounien, 2016; Stel & Legler, 2015; Walker & Gore, 2017).

THE SOCIETAL COST OF ENVIRONMENTAL TOXICANTS

It is very challenging to estimate the societal cost associated with environmental exposures. It is most commonly measured as disability adjusted life years and monetary burden to the economy. The global economic burden attributed to cognitive impairments caused by lead exposure in the United States was estimated to be $54 billion in the year 2010. For low- and middle-resource countries, the overall cost is estimated to be over $1 trillion (Grandjean & Bellanger, 2017). Cognitive impairments associated with methylmercury, organophosphates, and polybrominated diphenyl ethers have been estimated to have resulted in economic productivity losses in excess of $314 billion in the year 2010. These costs do not account for other neurodevelopmental disorders such as ADHD and autism. Fetal alcohol spectrum disorders are another segment of preventable developmental disorders, with estimated costs of $5.4 billion to the U.S. economy in the year 2003 (Popova, Stade, Bekmuradov, Lange, & Rehm, 2011).

PUBLIC POLICY IMPLICATIONS

The Toxic Substances Control Act (TSCA), passed in 1976 (PL 94-469), provided the EPA with the authority to require reporting, record keeping, testing requirements, and restrictions relating to chemical substances or mixtures. This law was amended and signed into law as the Frank R. Lautenberg Chemical Safety for the 21st Century Act (H.R.2576) in June 22, 2016. This new law prioritizes safety and risk evaluation of existing chemicals under the TSCA, and it requires affirmative findings on safety of any new chemical before it is introduced into the market (EPA, 2016). Although this is a step in the right direction, it will take some time for existing chemicals to be reviewed under the new law and for current guidelines to be updated reflecting available data on safety. It continues to be important to perform research and advocate for policy changes that are supportive of environmental chemical exposure prevention and management within the context of children's health and public health.

SUMMARY

- There are more than 1,000 chemicals identified as neurotoxicants based on human and animal studies.
- Chemical toxins have different effects on the human body depending on timing and dose exposure.
- Long-term neurodevelopmental adverse outcomes have been associated with *in utero* as well as postnatal exposure to multiple chemicals.
- Damage to the central nervous system (CNS) from environmental toxins can persist for years and is often irreversible.
- Mechanisms of action, such as epigenetic modifications, are being identified that can aid in the evaluation for safety of neurotoxicants.
- Because of the irreversible nature of damage observed in the CNS due to these environmental toxins, practitioners must focus on prevention of exposure.

ADDITIONAL RESOURCES

Agency for Toxic Substances & Disease Registry (ATSDR) Toxic Substances Portal: https://www.atsdr.cdc.gov/substances/index.asp

American Public Health Association (APHA): https://www.apha.org/topics-and-issues/environmental-health

American Association on Intellectual and Developmental Disabilities (AAIDD) Environmental Health Initiative: http://www.aaidd.org/ehi/index.cfm

Additional resources can be found online in Appendix D: Childhood Disabilities Resources, Services, and Organizations (see About the Online Companion Materials).

REFERENCES

Adebanjo, T., Godfred-Cato, S., Viens, L., Fischer, M., Staples, J. E., Kuhnert-Tallman, W., . . . Moore, C. A. (2017). Update: Interim guidance for the diagnosis, evaluation, and management of infants with possible congenital Zika virus infection—United States, October 2017. *MMWR: Morbidity and Mortality Weekly Report, 66*(41), 1089–1099. doi:10.15585/mmwr.mm6641a1

Alyea, R. A., & Watson, C. S. (2009). Differential regulation of dopamine transporter function and location by low concentrations of environmental estrogens and 17beta-estradiol. *Environmental Health Perspectives, 117*(5), 778–783. doi:10.1289/ehp.0800026

American Academy of Pediatrics. (2013). *Vaccine Safety: Examine the Evidence.* Retrieved from https://www.aap.org/en-us/Documents/immunization_vaccine_studies.pdf

Antunes dos Santos, A., Appel Hort, M., Culbreth, M., López-Granero, C., Farina, M., Rocha, J. B. T., & Aschner, M. (2016). Methylmercury and brain development: A review of recent literature. *Journal of Trace Elements in Medicine and Biology, 38*(Supplement C), 99–107. doi:https://doi.org/10.1016/j.jtemb.2016.03.001

Armstrong, D. A., Green, B. B., Blair, B. A., Guerin, D. J., Litzky, J. F., Chavan, N. R., . . . Marsit, C. J. (2016). Maternal smoking during pregnancy is associated with mitochondrial DNA methylation. *Environmental Epigenetics, 2*(3). 1–9. doi:10.1093/eep/dvw020

Atwood, D., & Paisley-Jones, C. (2017). *Pesticides industry sales and usage 2008–2012 market estimates.* Washington, DC: Environmental Protection Agency. Retrieved from https://www.epa.gov/sites/production/files/2017-01/documents/pesticides-industry-sales-usage-2016_0.pdf

Baghurst, P. A., McMichael, A. J., Wigg, N. R., Vimpani, G. V., Robertson, E. F., Roberts, R. J., & Tong, S. L. (1992). Environmental exposure to lead and children's intelligence at the age of seven years. The Port Pirie Cohort Study. *New England Journal of Medicine, 327*(18), 1279–1284. doi:10.1056/nejm199210293271805

Baker, T., Datta, P., Rewers-Felkins, K., Thompson, H., Kallem, R. R., & Hale, T. W. (2018). Transfer of inhaled cannabis into human breast milk. *Obstetrics and Gynecology, 131*(5), 783–788. doi:10.1097/aog.0000000000002575

Banderali, G., Martelli, A., Landi, M., Moretti, F., Betti, F., Radaelli, G., . . . Verduci, E. (2015). Short and long term health effects of parental tobacco smoking during pregnancy and lactation: A descriptive review. *Journal of Translational Medicine, 13*, 327. doi:10.1186/s12967-015-0690-y

Banik, A., Kandilya, D., Ramya, S., Stunkel, W., Chong, Y. S., & Dheen, S. T. (2017). Maternal factors that induce epigenetic changes contribute to neurological disorders in offspring. *Genes (Basel), 8*(6). doi:10.3390/genes8060150

Baranowska-Bosiacka, I., Falkowska, A., Gutowska, I., Gassowska, M., Kolasa-Wolosiuk, A., Tarnowski, M., . . . Chlubek, D. (2017). Glycogen metabolism in brain and neurons - Astrocytes metabolic cooperation can be altered by pre- and neonatal lead (Pb) exposure. *Toxicology, 390*, 146–158. doi:10.1016/j.tox.2017.09.007

Bellinger, D. C., Stiles, K. M., & Needleman, H. L. (1992). Low-level lead exposure, intelligence and academic achievement: a long-term follow-up study. *Pediatrics, 90*(6), 855–861.

Berghuis, S. A., Soechitram, S. D., Hitzert, M. M., Sauer, P. J., & Bos, A. F. (2013). Prenatal exposure to polychlorinated biphenyls and their hydroxylated metabolites is associated with motor development of three-month-old infants. *Neurotoxicology, 38*, 124–130. doi:10.1016/j.neuro.2013.07.003

Bouchard, M. F., Bellinger, D. C., Wright, R. O., & Weisskopf, M. G. (2010). Attention-deficit/hyperactivity disorder and urinary metabolites of organophosphate pesticides. *Pediatrics, 125*(6), e1270–1277. doi:10.1542/peds.2009-3058

Bouchard, M. F., Chevrier, J., Harley, K. G., Kogut, K., Vedar, M., Calderon, N., . . . Eskenazi, B. (2011). Prenatal exposure to organophosphate pesticides and IQ in 7-year-old children. *Environmental Health Perspectives, 119*(8), 1189–1195. doi:10.1289/ehp.1003185

Boucher, O., Jacobson, S. W., Plusquellec, P., Dewailly, E., Ayotte, P., Forget-Dubois, N., . . . Muckle, G. (2012). Prenatal methylmercury, postnatal lead exposure, and evidence of attention deficit/hyperactivity disorder among Inuit children in Arctic Quebec. *Environmental Health Perspectives, 120*(10), 1456–1461. doi:10.1289/ehp.1204976

Braun, J. M. (2017). Early-life exposure to EDCs: Role in childhood obesity and neurodevelopment. *Nature Reviews: Endocrinology, 13*(3), 161–173. doi:10.1038/nrendo.2016.186

Braun, J. M., Kahn, R. S., Froehlich, T., Auinger, P., & Lanphear, B. P. (2006). Exposures to environmental toxicants and attention deficit hyperactivity disorder in U.S. children. *Environmental Health Perspectives, 114*(12), 1904–1909.

Braun, J. M., Kalkbrenner, A. E., Just, A. C., Yolton, K., Calafat, A. M., Sjodin, A., . . . Lanphear, B. P. (2014). Gestational exposure to endocrine-disrupting chemicals and reciprocal social, repetitive, and stereotypic behaviors in 4- and 5-year-old children: The HOME study. *Environmental Health Perspectives, 122*(5), 513–520. doi:10.1289/ehp.1307261

Braun, J. M., Muckle, G., Arbuckle, T., Bouchard, M. F., Fraser, W. D., Ouellet, E., . . . Lanphear, B. P. (2017). Associations of prenatal urinary bisphenol A concentrations with child behaviors and cognitive abilities. *Environmental Health Perspectives, 125*(6), 067008. doi:10.1289/ehp984

Canfield, R. L., Henderson, C. R., Jr., Cory-Slechta, D. A., Cox, C., Jusko, T. A., & Lanphear, B. P. (2003). Intellectual impairment in children with blood lead concentrations below 10 microg per deciliter. *New England Journal of Medicine, 348*(16), 1517–1526. doi:10.1056/NEJMoa022848

Casas, M., Nieuwenhuijsen, M., Martinez, D., Ballester, F., Basagana, X., Basterrechea, M., . . . Bonde, J. P. (2015). Prenatal exposure to PCB-153, p,p'-DDE and birth outcomes in 9000 mother-child pairs: Exposure-response relationship and effect modifiers. *Environment International, 74*, 23–31. doi:10.1016/j.envint.2014.09.013

CBHSQ. (2015). *Behavioral health trends in the United States: Results from the 2014 national survey on drug use and health.* Rockville, MD: Center for Behavioral Health Statistics and Quality, Substance Abuse, and Mental Health Services Administration. Retrieved from http://www.samhsa.gov/data

Chanda, S., Dasgupta, U. B., Guhamazumder, D., Gupta, M., Chaudhuri, U., Lahiri, S., . . . Chatterjee, D. (2006). DNA hypermethylation of promoter of gene p53 and p16 in arsenic-exposed people with and without malignancy. *Toxicological Sciences, 89*(2), 431–437. doi:10.1093/toxsci/kfj030

Chatterton, Z., Hartley, B. J., Seok, M. H., Mendelev, N., Chen, S., Milekic, M., . . . Haghighi, F. (2017). In utero exposure to maternal smoking is associated with DNA methylation alterations and reduced neuronal content in the developing fetal brain. *Epigenetics Chromatin, 10*, 4. doi:10.1186/s13072-017-0111-y

Chen, M., Chang, C.-H., Tao, L., & Lu, C. (2015). Residential exposure to pesticide during childhood and childhood cancers: A meta-analysis. *Pediatrics, 136*(4), 719–729. doi:10.1542/peds.2015-0006

Clifford, A., Lang, L., & Chen, R. (2012). Effects of maternal cigarette smoking during pregnancy on cognitive parameters of children and young adults: A literature review. *Neurotoxicology and Teratology, 34*(6), 560–570. doi:10.1016/j.ntt.2012.09.004

Crume, T. L., Juhl, A. L., Brooks-Russell, A., Hall, K. E., Wymore, E., & Borgelt, L. M. (2018). Cannabis use during the perinatal period in a state with legalized recreational and medical marijuana: The association between maternal characteristics, breastfeeding patterns, and neonatal outcomes. *The Journal of Pediatrics, 197*, 90–96.

da Silva Pone, M. V., Moura Pone, S., Araujo Zin, A., Barros Mendes, P. H., Senra Aibe, M., Barroso de Aguiar, E., & de Oliveira Gomes da Silva, T. (2018). Zika virus infection in children: Epidemiology and clinical manifestations. *Child's Nervous System, 34*(1), 63–71. doi:10.1007/s00381-017-3635-3

Debes, F., Weihe, P., & Grandjean, P. (2016). Cognitive deficits at age 22 years associated with prenatal exposure to methylmercury. *Cortex, 74*, 358–369. doi:10.1016/j.cortex.2015.05.017

Delvaux, I., Van Cauwenberghe, J., Den Hond, E., Schoeters, G., Govarts, E., Nelen, V., . . . Sioen, I. (2014). Prenatal exposure to environmental contaminants and body composition at age 7–9 years. *Environmental Research, 132*, 24–32. doi:10.1016/j.envres.2014.03.019

Derauf, C., Kekatpure, M., Neyzi, N., Lester, B., & Kosofsky, B. (2009). Neuroimaging of children following prenatal drug exposure. *Seminars in Cell and Developmental Biology, 20*(4), 441–454. doi:10.1016/j.semcdb.2009.03.001

Derghal, A., Djelloul, M., Trouslard, J., & Mounien, L. (2016). An emerging role of micro-RNA in the effect of the endocrine disruptors. *Frontiers in Neuroscience, 10*, 318. doi:10.3389/fnins.2016.00318

Eiden, R. D., Schuetze, P., Shisler, S., & Huestis, M. A. (2018). Prenatal exposure to tobacco and cannabis: Effects on autonomic and emotion regulation. *Neurotoxicology and Teratology, 68*, 47–56. doi:10.1016/j.ntt.2018.04.007

Ejaredar, M., Nyanza, E. C., Ten Eycke, K., & Dewey, D. (2015). Phthalate exposure and children's neurodevelopment: A systematic review. *Environmental Research, 142,* 51–60. doi:10.1016/j.envres.2015.06.014

EPA. (2016). *Highlights of key provisions in Frank R. Lautenberg Chemical Safety for the 21st Century Act.* Washington, DC: Environmental Protection Agency. Retrieved from https://www.epa.gov/assessing-and-managing-chemicals-under-tsca/highlights-key-provisions-frank-r-lautenberg-chemical

Eskenazi, B., Kogut, K., Huen, K., Harley, K. G., Bouchard, M., Bradman, A., . . . Holland, N. (2014). Organophosphate pesticide exposure, PON1, and neurodevelopment in school-age children from the CHAMACOS study. *Environmental Research, 134,* 149–157. doi:10.1016/j.envres.2014.07.001

Eskenazi, B., Rosas, L. G., Marks, A. R., Bradman, A., Harley, K., Holland, N., . . . Barr, D. B. (2008). Pesticide toxicity and the developing brain. *Basic & Clinical Pharmacology & Toxicology, 102*(2), 228–236. doi:10.1111/j.1742-7843.2007.00171.x

Eubig, P. A., Aguiar, A., & Schantz, S. L. (2010). Lead and PCBs as risk factors for attention deficit/hyperactivity disorder. *Environmental Health Perspectives, 118*(12), 1654–1667. doi:10.1289/ehp.0901852

Evans, S. F., Kobrosly, R. W., Barrett, E. S., Thurston, S. W., Calafat, A. M., Weiss, B., . . . Swan, S. H. (2014). Prenatal bisphenol A exposure and maternally reported behavior in boys and girls. *Neurotoxicology, 45,* 91–99. doi:10.1016/j.neuro.2014.10.003

Evens, A., Hryhorczuk, D., Lanphear, B. P., Rankin, K. M., Lewis, D. A., Forst, L., & Rosenberg, D. (2015). The impact of low-level lead toxicity on school performance among children in the Chicago public schools: A population-based retrospective cohort study. *Environmental Health, 14*(1), 21. doi:10.1186/s12940-015-0008-9

Flak, A. L., Su, S., Bertrand, J., Denny, C. H., Kesmodel, U. S., & Cogswell, M. E. (2014). The association of mild, moderate, and binge prenatal alcohol exposure and child neuropsychological outcomes: A meta-analysis. *Alcoholism, Clinical and Experimental Research, 38*(1), 214–226. doi:10.1111/acer.12214

Froehlich, T. E., Lanphear, B. P., Auinger, P., Hornung, R., Epstein, J. N., Braun, J., & Kahn, R. S. (2009). Association of tobacco and lead exposures with attention-deficit/hyperactivity disorder. *Pediatrics, 124*(6), e1054–1063. doi:10.1542/peds.2009-0738

Gassowska, M., Baranowska-Bosiacka, I., Moczydlowska, J., Frontczak-Baniewicz, M., Gewartowska, M., Struzynska, L., . . . Adamczyk, A. (2016). Perinatal exposure to lead (Pb) induces ultrastructural and molecular alterations in synapses of rat offspring. *Toxicology, 373,* 13–29. doi:10.1016/j.tox.2016.10.014

Gibson, J. L. (2005). A plea for painted railings and painted walls of rooms as the source of lead poisoning amongst Queensland children. *Public Health Reports, 120*(3), 301–304.

Gilbert, S. G., & Weiss, B. (2006). A rationale for lowering the blood lead action level from 10 to 2 microg/dL. *Neurotoxicology, 27*(5), 693–701. doi:10.1016/j.neuro.2006.06.008

Glass, L., Moore, E. M., Akshoomoff, N., Jones, K. L., Riley, E. P., & Mattson, S. N. (2017). Academic difficulties in children with prenatal alcohol exposure: Presence, profile, and neural correlates. *Alcoholism, Clinical and Experimental Research, 41*(5), 1024–1034. doi:10.1111/acer.13366

Grandjean, P., & Bellanger, M. (2017). Calculation of the disease burden associated with environmental chemical exposures: Application of toxicological information in health economic estimation. *Environmental Health: A Global Access Science Source, 16*(1), 123. doi:10.1186/s12940-017-0340-3

Grandjean, P., Weihe, P., Debes, F., Choi, A. L., & Budtz-Jorgensen, E. (2014). Neurotoxicity from prenatal and postnatal exposure to methylmercury. *Neurotoxicology and Teratology, 43,* 39–44. doi:10.1016/j.ntt.2014.03.004

Grant, K. S., Petroff, R., Isoherranen, N., Stella, N., & Burbacher, T. M. (2018). Cannabis use during pregnancy: Pharmacokinetics and effects on child development. *Pharmacology and Therapeutics, 182,* 133–151. doi:10.1016/j.pharmthera.2017.08.014

Gross, L. A., Moore, E. M., Wozniak, J. R., Coles, C. D., Kable, J. A., Sowell, E. R., . . . Mattson, S. N. (2017). Neural correlates of verbal memory in youth with heavy prenatal alcohol exposure. *Brain Imaging and Behavior.* doi:10.1007/s11682-017-9739-2

Hadland, S. E., Knight, J. R., & Harris, S. K. (2015). Medical marijuana: Review of the science and implications for developmental behavioral pediatric practice. *Journal of Developmental and Behavioral Pediatrics: JDBP, 36*(2), 115–123. doi:10.1097/DBP.0000000000000129

Hagan, J. F., Balachova, T., Bertrand, J., Chasnoff, I., Dang, E., Fernandez-Baca, D., . . . Zubler, J. (2016). Neurobehavioral disorder associated with prenatal alcohol exposure. *Pediatrics, 138*(4). doi:10.1542/peds.2015-1553

Hanna-Attisha, M., LaChance, J., Sadler, R. C., & Champney Schnepp, A. (2015). Elevated blood lead levels in children associated with the Flint drinking water crisis: A spatial analysis of risk and public health response. *American Journal of Public Health, 106*(2), 283–290. doi:10.2105/AJPH.2015.303003

Harada, M. (1995). Minamata disease: Methylmercury poisoning in Japan caused by environmental pollution. *Critical Reviews in Toxicology, 25*(1), 1–24. doi:10.3109/10408449509089885

Hendrickson, T. J., Mueller, B. A., Sowell, E. R., Mattson, S. N., Coles, C. D., Kable, J. A., . . . Wozniak, J. R. (2017). Cortical gyrification is abnormal in children with prenatal alcohol exposure. *Neuroimage Clinical, 15,* 391–400. doi:10.1016/j.nicl.2017.05.015

Hoyme, H. E., Kalberg, W. O., Elliott, A. J., Blankenship, J., Buckley, D., Marais, A.-S., . . . May, P. A. (2016). Updated clinical guidelines for diagnosing fetal alcohol spectrum disorders. *Pediatrics, 138*(2). doi:10.1542/peds.2015-4256

Hughes, K., Bellis, M. A., Hardcastle, K. A., Sethi, D., Butchart, A., Mikton, C., . . . Dunne, M. P. (2017). The effect of multiple adverse childhood experiences on health: A systematic review and meta-analysis. *Lancet Public Health, 2*(8), e356–e366. doi:10.1016/s2468-2667(17)30118-4

Ino, T. (2010). Maternal smoking during pregnancy and offspring obesity: Meta-analysis. *Pediatrics International, 52*(1), 94–99. doi:10.1111/j.1442-200X.2009.02883.x

Ishido, M., Masuo, Y., Terasaki, M., & Morita, M. (2011). Rat hyperactivity by bisphenol A, but not by its derivatives, 3-hydroxybisphenol A or bisphenol A 3,4-quinone. *Toxicology Letters, 206*(3), 300–305. doi:10.1016/j.toxlet.2011.08.011

Jacobson, S. W., Jacobson, J. L., Molteno, C. D., Warton, C. M. R., Wintermark, P., Hoyme, H. E., . . . Meintjes, E. M. (2017). Heavy prenatal alcohol exposure is related to smaller corpus callosum in newborn MRI scans. *Alcoholism, Clinical and Experimental Research, 41*(5), 965–975. doi:10.1111/acer.13363

Jarmasz, J. S., Basalah, D. A., Chudley, A. E., & Del Bigio, M. R. (2017). Human brain abnormalities associated with prenatal alcohol exposure and fetal alcohol spectrum disorder. *Journal of Neuropathology and Experimental Neurology, 76*(9), 813–833. doi:10.1093/jnen/nlx064

Javed, R., Chen, W., Lin, F., & Liang, H. (2016). Infant's DNA methylation age at birth and epigenetic aging accelerators. *Biomed Research International, 2016*, 4515928. doi:10.1155/2016/4515928

Jusko, T. A., Henderson, C. R., Lanphear, B. P., Cory-Slechta, D. A., Parsons, P. J., & Canfield, R. L. (2008). Blood lead concentrations < 10 microg/dL and child intelligence at 6 years of age. *Environmental Health Perspectives, 116*(2), 243–248. doi:10.1289/ehp.10424

Kann, L., McManus, T., Harris, W., Shanklin, S., Flint, K., Hawkins, J., . . . Lowry, R. (2016). *Youth risk behavior surveillance-United States, 2015*. Washington, DC: Centers for Disease Control and Prevention.

Kidd, S. K., Anderson, D. W., & Schneider, J. S. (2008). Postnatal lead exposure alters expression of forebrain p75 and TrkA nerve growth factor receptors. *Brain Research, 1195*, 113–119. doi:10.1016/j.brainres.2007.12.012

Kim, Y., Cho, S.-C., Kim, B.-N., Hong, Y.-C., Shin, M.-S., Yoo, H.-J., . . . Bhang, S.-Y. (2010). Association between blood lead levels (<5μg/dL) and inattention-hyperactivity and neurocognitive profiles in school-aged Korean children. *Science of the Total Environment, 408*(23), 5737–5743. doi:https://doi.org/10.1016/j.scitotenv.2010.07.070

Lanphear, B. P., Hornung, R., Khoury, J., Yolton, K., Baghurst, P., Bellinger, D. C., . . . Roberts, R. (2005). Low-level environmental lead exposure and children's intellectual function: An international pooled analysis. *Environmental Health Perspectives, 113*(7), 894–899.

Lidsky, T. I., & Schneider, J. S. (2006). Adverse effects of childhood lead poisoning: The clinical neuropsychological perspective. *Environmental Research, 100*(2), 284–293. doi:10.1016/j.envres.2005.03.002

Mason, L. H., Harp, J. P., & Han, D. Y. (2014). Pb neurotoxicity: Neuropsychological effects of lead toxicity. *BioMed Research International, 2014*, 8. doi:10.1155/2014/840547

Masuo, Y., & Ishido, M. (2011). Neurotoxicity of endocrine disruptors: Possible involvement in brain development and neurodegeneration. *Journal of Toxicology and Environmental Health. Part B: Critical Reviews, 14*(5-7), 346–369. doi:10.1080/10937404.2011.578557

Mishra, P., Samarth, R., Pathak, N., Jain, S., Banerjee, S., & Maudar, K. (2009). Bhopal gas tragedy: Review of clinical and experimental findings after 25 years. *International Journal of Occupational Medicine and Environmental Health, 22*(3), 193–202.

Munoz-Quezada, M. T., Lucero, B. A., Barr, D. B., Steenland, K., Levy, K., Ryan, P. B., . . . Vega, C. (2013). Neurodevelopmental effects in children associated with exposure to organophosphate pesticides: A systematic review. *Neurotoxicology, 39*, 158–168. doi:10.1016/j.neuro.2013.09.003

Murch, S. (2004). A statement by Dr Simon Murch. Allegations concerning our 1998 study. *Lancet, 363*(9411), 821–822.

Neal, A. P., & Guilarte, T. R. (2010). Molecular neurobiology of lead (Pb(2+)): Effects on synaptic function. *Molecular Neurobiology, 42*(3), 151–160. doi:10.1007/s12035-010-8146-0

Neil, V. (2015). Thalidomide-induced teratogenesis: History and mechanisms. *Birth Defects Research Part C: Embryo Today: Reviews, 105*(2), 140–156. doi:doi:10.1002/bdrc.21096

Nygaard, E., Moe, V., Slinning, K., & Walhovd, K. B. (2015). Longitudinal cognitive development of children born to mothers with opioid and polysubstance use. *Pediatric Research, 78*(3), 330–335. doi:10.1038/pr.2015.95

Nygaard, E., Slinning, K., Moe, V., Due-Tonnessen, P., Fjell, A., & Walhovd, K. B. (2018). Neuroanatomical characteristics of youths with prenatal opioid and poly-drug exposure. *Neurotoxicology and Teratology, 68*, 13–26. doi:10.1016/j.ntt.2018.04.004

Nygaard, E., Slinning, K., Moe, V., & Walhovd, K. B. (2017). Cognitive function of youths born to mothers with opioid and poly-substance abuse problems during pregnancy. *Child Neuropsychology, 23*(2), 159–187. doi:10.1080/09297049.2015.1092509

Perera, F., Nolte, E. L., Wang, Y., Margolis, A. E., Calafat, A. M., Wang, S., . . . Herbstman, J. (2016). Bisphenol A exposure and symptoms of anxiety and depression among inner city children at 10–12 years of age. *Environmental Research, 151*, 195–202. doi:10.1016/j.envres.2016.07.028

Pessoa, A., van der Linden, V., Yeargin-Allsopp, M., Carvalho, M., Ribeiro, E. M., Van Naarden Braun, K., . . . Moore, C. A. (2018). Motor abnormalities and epilepsy in infants and children with evidence of congenital Zika virus infection. *Pediatrics, 141*(Suppl 2), S167–S179. doi:10.1542/peds.2017-2038F

Pilsner, J. R., Hall, M. N., Liu, X., Ilievski, V., Slavkovich, V., Levy, D., . . . Gamble, M. V. (2012). Influence of prenatal arsenic exposure and newborn sex on global methylation of cord blood DNA. *PloS One, 7*(5), e37147. doi:10.1371/journal.pone.0037147

Pilsner, J. R., Liu, X., Ahsan, H., Ilievski, V., Slavkovich, V., Levy, D., . . . Gamble, M. V. (2007). Genomic methylation of peripheral blood leukocyte DNA: Influences of arsenic and folate in Bangladeshi adults. *American Journal of Clinical Nutrition, 86*(4), 1179–1186.

Poole-Di Salvo, E., Liu, Y. H., Brenner, S., & Weitzman, M. (2010). Adult household smoking is associated with increased child emotional and behavioral problems. *Journal of Developmental and Behavioral Pediatrics, 31*(2), 107–115. doi:10.1097/DBP.0b013e3181cdaad6

Popova, S., Stade, B., Bekmuradov, D., Lange, S., & Rehm, J. (2011). What do we know about the economic impact of fetal alcohol spectrum disorder? A systematic literature review. *Alcohol and Alcoholism, 46*(4), 490–497. doi:10.1093/alcalc/agr029

Raanan, R., Harley, K. G., Balmes, J. R., Bradman, A., Lipsett, M., & Eskenazi, B. (2015). Early-life exposure to organophosphate pesticides and pediatric respiratory symptoms in the CHAMACOS cohort. *Environmental Health Perspectives, 123*(2), 179–185. doi:10.1289/ehp.1408235

Raciti, M., & Ceccatelli, S. (2017). Epigenetic mechanisms in developmental neurotoxicity. *Neurotoxicology and Teratology, 66*, 94–101. doi:10.1016/j.ntt.2017.12.002

Ramirez, G. B., Cruz, M. C., Pagulayan, O., Ostrea, E., & Dalisay, C. (2000). The Tagum study I: Analysis and clinical correlates of mercury in maternal and cord blood, breast milk, meconium, and infants' hair. *Pediatrics, 106*(4), 774–781.

Richardson, J. R., Taylor, M. M., Shalat, S. L., Guillot, T. S., 3rd, Caudle, W. M., Hossain, M. M., . . . Miller, G. W. (2015). Developmental pesticide exposure reproduces features of attention deficit hyperactivity disorder. *FASEB Journal, 29*(5), 1960–1972. doi:10.1096/fj.14-260901

Roozen, S., Peters, G. J., Kok, G., Townend, D., Nijhuis, J., & Curfs, L. (2016). Worldwide prevalence of fetal alcohol spectrum disorders: A systematic literature review including meta-analysis. *Alcoholism, Clinical and Experimental Research, 40*(1), 18–32. doi:10.1111/acer.12939

Rowe, C., Gunier, R., Bradman, A., Harley, K. G., Kogut, K., Parra, K., & Eskenazi, B. (2016). Residential proximity to organophosphate and carbamate pesticide use during pregnancy, poverty during childhood, and cognitive functioning in 10-year-old children. *Environmental Research, 150*, 128–137. doi:10.1016/j.envres.2016.05.048

Schneider, J. S., Anderson, D. W., Kidd, S. K., Sobolewski, M., & Cory-Slechta, D. A. (2016). Sex-dependent effects of lead and prenatal stress on post-translational histone modifications in frontal cortex and hippocampus in the early postnatal brain. *Neurotoxicology, 54*, 65–71. doi:10.1016/j.neuro.2016.03.016

Scott, J. C., Slomiak, S. T., Jones, J. D., Rosen, A. F. G., Moore, T. M., & Gur, R. C. (2018). Association of cannabis with cognitive functioning in adolescents and young adults: A systematic review and meta-analysis. *JAMA Psychiatry, 75*(6), 585–595. doi:10.1001/jamapsychiatry.2018.0335

Shelton, J. F., Geraghty, E. M., Tancredi, D. J., Delwiche, L. D., Schmidt, R. J., Ritz, B., . . . Hertz-Picciotto, I. (2014). Neurodevelopmental disorders and prenatal residential proximity to agricultural pesticides: The CHARGE study. *Environmental Health Perspectives, 122*(10), 1103–1109. doi:10.1289/ehp.1307044

Stein, L. J., Gunier, R. B., Harley, K., Kogut, K., Bradman, A., & Eskenazi, B. (2016). Early childhood adversity potentiates the adverse association between prenatal organophosphate pesticide exposure and child IQ: The CHAMACOS cohort. *Neurotoxicology, 56*, 180–187. doi:10.1016/j.neuro.2016.07.010

Stel, J., & Legler, J. (2015). The role of epigenetics in the latent effects of early life exposure to obesogenic endocrine disrupting chemicals. *Endocrinology, 156*(10), 3466–3472. doi:10.1210/en.2015-1434

Tan, C. H., Denny, C. H., Cheal, N. E., Sniezek, J. E., & Kanny, D. (2015). Alcohol use and binge drinking among women of childbearing age—United States, 2011–2013. *MMWR: Morbidity and Mortality Weekly Report, 64*(37), 1042–1046.

Tang-Peronard, J. L., Heitmann, B. L., Andersen, H. R., Steuerwald, U., Grandjean, P., Weihe, P., & Jensen, T. K. (2014). Association between prenatal polychlorinated biphenyl exposure and obesity development at ages 5 and 7 y: A prospective cohort study of 656 children from the Faroe Islands. *American Journal of Clinical Nutrition, 99*(1), 5–13. doi:10.3945/ajcn.113.066720

Tewar, S., Auinger, P., Braun, J. M., Lanphear, B., Yolton, K., Epstein, J. N., . . . Froehlich, T. E. (2016). Association of bisphenol A exposure and attention-deficit/hyperactivity disorder in a national sample of U.S. children. *Environmental Research, 150*, 112–118. doi:10.1016/j.envres.2016.05.040

Toscano, C. D., & Guilarte, T. R. (2005). Lead neurotoxicity: From exposure to molecular effects. *Brain Research: Brain Research Reviews, 49*(3), 529–554. doi:10.1016/j.brainresrev.2005.02.004

U.S. Food & Drug Administration. (2017a). *Eating fish: What pregnant women and parents should know* [Press release]. Retrieved from https://www.fda.gov/downloads/Food/FoodborneIllnessContaminants/Metals/UCM537120.pdf

U.S. Food & Drug Administration. (2017b). *Thimerosal and vaccines*. Retrieved from https://www.fda.gov/BiologicsBloodVaccines/SafetyAvailability/VaccineSafety/UCM096228#bib

Varma, D. R. (1987). Epidemiological and experimental studies on the effects of methyl isocyanate on the course of pregnancy. *Environmental Health Perspectives, 72*, 153–157.

Victor, B. G., Resko, S. M., Ryan, J. P., & Perron, B. E. (2018). Identification of domestic violence service needs among child welfare-involved parents with substance use disorders: A gender-stratified analysis. *Journal of Interpersonal Violence*. doi:10.1177/0886260518768569

Wagner-Schuman, M., Richardson, J. R., Auinger, P., Braun, J. M., Lanphear, B. P., Epstein, J. N., . . . Froehlich, T. E. (2015). Association of pyrethroid pesticide exposure with attention-deficit/hyperactivity disorder in a nationally representative sample of U.S. children. *Environmental Health: A Global Access Science Source, 14*, 44. doi:10.1186/s12940-015-0030-y

Walker, D. M., & Gore, A. C. (2017). Epigenetic impacts of endocrine disruptors in the brain. *Frontiers in Neuroendocrinology, 44*, 1–26. doi:10.1016/j.yfrne.2016.09.002

Weng, S. F., Redsell, S. A., Swift, J. A., Yang, M., & Glazebrook, C. P. (2012). Systematic review and meta-analyses of risk factors for childhood overweight identifiable during infancy. *Archives of Disease in Childhood, 97*(12), 1019–1026. doi:10.1136/archdischild-2012-302263

Wheeler, A. C. (2018). Development of infants with congenital Zika syndrome: What do we know and what can we expect? *Pediatrics, 141*(Suppl 2), S154–S160. doi:10.1542/peds.2017-2038D

Williams, J. F., & Smith, V. C. (2015). Fetal alcohol spectrum disorders. *Pediatrics*. doi:10.1542/peds.2015-3113

World Health Organization. (2006). *Statement on thiomersal*. Global Advisory Committee on Vaccine Safety. Retrieved from http://www.who.int/vaccine_safety/committee/topics/thiomersal/statement_jul2006/en/

Wozniak, J. R., Mueller, B. A., Mattson, S. N., Coles, C. D., Kable, J. A., Jones, K. L., . . . Sowell, E. R. (2017). Functional connectivity abnormalities and associated cognitive deficits in fetal alcohol spectrum disorders (FASD). *Brain Imaging and Behavior, 11*(5), 1432–1445. doi:10.1007/s11682-016-9624-4

Zhou, S., Rosenthal, D. G., Sherman, S., Zelikoff, J., Gordon, T., & Weitzman, M. (2014). Physical, behavioral, and cognitive effects of prenatal tobacco and postnatal secondhand smoke exposure. *Current Problems in Pediatric and Adolescent Health Care, 44*(8), 219–241. doi:10.1016/j.cppeds.2014.03.007

CHAPTER 3

Birth Defects and Prenatal Diagnosis

Rhonda L. Schonberg and Margaret B. Menzel

Upon completion of this chapter, the reader will

- Become familiar with the process of genetic counseling and the genetic screening/testing options available to couples prior to and during pregnancy
- Understand the uses and limitations of noninvasive prenatal maternal blood screening for genetic syndromes and birth defects
- Become knowledgeable regarding the indications for and limitations of first- and second-trimester evaluation of birth defects using the techniques of ultrasonography, fetal magnetic resonance imaging, and echocardiography
- Be aware of the techniques for and possible results from amniocentesis and chorionic villus sampling and be able to determine when these diagnostic tests may be indicated
- Understand the benefits of a multidisciplinary team in a comprehensive prenatal diagnosis center or fetal center for the counseling, evaluation, and management of fetal anomalies when they are identified
- Become familiar with alternative reproductive technology (ART), including *in vitro* fertilization with preimplantation genetic diagnosis, and understand under what circumstances couples might benefit from such technologies
- Understand the psychosocial issues and needs of families who are at increased risk for having children with genetic disorders or birth defects

The prenatal diagnosis of a child with a developmental disability or a genetic disorder has a major impact on parents, siblings, and extended family members. As parents come to terms with their child's disability or disorder, they may try to understand what happened and why. Although most infants in the United States are born without complications, 3% of all births, 1 in every 33 infants, is born with a birth defect or genetic disorder (Centers for Disease Control and Prevention, 2017). These events can affect any pregnant woman regardless of age, socioeconomic status, or ethnicity. Although medical professionals recognize certain circumstances that increase the risk of having a child with a birth defect (a number of which are discussed in this chapter), it must be acknowledged that most affected newborns will be born to couples who were unaware of any risk and had no family history of similarly affected children. When this occurs, genetic evaluation (discussed in Chapter 1) may help determine a diagnosis and mode of inheritance. Advances in prenatal screening and diagnosis have provided couples with the opportunity to gain detailed information about their fetus (e.g., the presence of, or increased risk for, a birth defect or genetic disorder) and examine a range of family planning options. This chapter discusses 1) genetic screening that is available prior to and during pregnancy, 2) diagnostic testing appropriate for fetuses who have been determined to be at an increased risk for a specific genetic disorder, and 3) alternative reproductive choices.

CASE STUDY

Jennifer, a 32-year-old experiencing her first pregnancy, opted for cell-free DNA noninvasive prenatal testing (DNA/NIPT) at 10 weeks' gestation because she had been told she could learn the gender of her fetus. The results were unexpected; instead of an XX (female) or XY (male) pattern, the fetus had findings consistent with a single sex chromosome XO (Turner syndrome, see Appendix B). Jennifer met with a genetic counselor who clarified that DNA/NIPT was a screening rather than a diagnostic test and had certain limitations to its accuracy, especially in detecting sex chromosome abnormalities. The genetic counselor reviewed further diagnostic testing options, including chorionic villus sampling (CVS) and amniocentesis. Jennifer declined further genetic testing at that time but agreed to have follow-up ultrasounds and fetal echocardiography given the increased risk for a congenital heart defect (CHD) in children with Turner syndrome. At her 12-week ultrasound, the **nuchal translucency measurement** (a measure of the collection of fluid under the skin at the back of the fetal neck) was increased, and a fetal echocardiogram at 20 weeks' gestation indicated a CHD—coarctation of the aorta. Both of these findings were consistent with a diagnosis of Turner syndrome. Jennifer then opted for amniocentesis, which confirmed the diagnosis.

This diagnosis allowed Jennifer and her husband time to prepare for the birth of a child with Turner syndrome. They met with a pediatric geneticist, and Jennifer was followed closely with fetal echocardiograms by a pediatric cardiologist as well. A plan for immediate postnatal evaluation of Jennifer's infant by cardiology/cardiovascular surgery and genetics personnel was put into place. She and her husband were connected with the Turner Syndrome Society and two other families who had come through the fetal medicine center and subsequently had children with Turner syndrome. Although learning about the diagnosis was initially difficult for Jennifer and her family, she felt empowered by the information she received and the plan she and her husband had in place for after the infant was born. Ultimately, Jennifer felt that learning about the diagnosis prenatally allowed her family time to digest the information and plan and prepare for the follow-up needed after delivery.

At birth, a cardiac evaluation determined that Jennifer's infant, Hope, had a critical CHD that required immediate surgery. The coarctation was successfully repaired by the cardiovascular surgeon and Hope, now 8 years old, is doing very well. She has typical features of Turner syndrome, such as being small and having a mild learning disability, but she is a happy and well-adjusted child. Hope will face other challenges as she gets older, but her mother has become an expert and advocate for Turner syndrome, and she is confident that Hope will have a happy and productive life.

Thought Questions:

How can the prenatal (versus postnatal) diagnosis of a birth defect or genetic syndrome be helpful for a family? Can you think of reasons why patient advocacy groups may be in favor of, or against, prenatal screening and diagnosis? Why might a fertile couple consider assisted reproductive technologies to have a child?

GENETIC ASSESSMENT AND CARRIER DETECTION

Assessing reproductive risk involves reviewing an individual's medical and pregnancy history and taking an extended family history. This includes obtaining information about the presence of birth defects, genetic disorders, unexplained infant deaths, and recurrent pregnancy losses. Information about maternal medication use and occupational or other exposures, including infections such as CMV, toxoplasmosis, or Zika virus, can also provide clues to possible reproductive risks (see Chapter 2).

As of 2017, more than 24,000 genetic disorders have been identified (National Center for Biotechnology Information, 2017). Specific genetic testing is clinically available for over 5,000 of these disorders, and the number continues to grow (National Center for Biotechnology Information, n.d.). Information about these genetic disorders is available to the lay public through 1) the Genetics Home Reference, a National Library of Medicine–supported database (http://ghr.nlm.nih.gov); 2) the Genetic Alliance, a clearinghouse for information and support groups for genetic disorders (http://www.geneticalliance.org); and 3) the National Organization for Rare Disorders (http://www.rarediseases.org).

Knowing an individual's ethnic background can be one of the initial steps in assessing reproductive risk. Individuals from certain ethnic backgrounds (e.g., Ashkenazi Jewish and Amish) have a higher risk of carrying specific gene mutations that are known to be associated with particular genetic disorders (see Table 3.1). In addition, the American College of Obstetrics and Gynecology (ACOG) recommends that all women who are pregnant or are considering pregnancy should have carrier screening for spinal muscular atrophy (SMA), Fragile X syndrome, hemoglobinopathies, and cystic fibrosis (ACOG, 2017a). SMA, most hemoglobinopathies, and cystic fibrosis are autosomal recessive disorders. Fragile X syndrome is X-linked. For recessive disorders, both parents must be carriers of a mutation in the same gene for there to be an increased risk of having an affected child (see Chapter 1). For Fragile X syndrome, the carrier state in the mother alone is sufficient to increase the risk to the fetus and can have health implications for the carrier mother as well (Wheeler et al., 2014). Advanced knowledge of risk provides couples with the opportunity to consider alternative reproductive options or to undergo prenatal diagnostic testing.

The cost of DNA analysis and sequencing has decreased precipitously since the mid-2000s. This, along with other advancing technologies, has prompted the development of expanded carrier screening wherein laboratories can offer screening panels of up to 100 or more conditions at a relatively low cost. Many obstetrics-gynecology and maternal fetal medicine practices are now offering this expanded carrier screening to couples of all ethnicities prior to or early in pregnancy. Although there are clear benefits of carrier screening, there are also limitations, such as different detection rates among disorders and residual risks based on an individual's ethnicity.

If an individual is found to be a carrier for a change in a gene associated with a particular condition, it is important that they meet with a genetic counselor. The woman can then learn about the clinical presentation of the disorder as well as the incidence, penetrance, and variability in expression so that she can decide whether to pursue additional testing in her partner and/or fetus (Grody et al., 2013).

A couple also may be at increased risk for having a child with a genetic disorder if a previous child or other close family member has been diagnosed with the disorder. In these situations, a detailed review of the family history, pregnancy history, and medical records is performed along with examination of the

Table 3.1. Disorders with increased carrier frequencies in particular ethnic groups

Ethnic group	Disorder at risk	Estimated carrier frequency
European and North American (Caucasian)	Cystic fibrosis	1 in 25
Ashkenazi Jewish (Eastern European Jewish)	Tay-Sachs disease	1 in 27
	Canavan disease	1 in 40
	Cystic fibrosis	1 in 25
	Gaucher disease (type 1)	1 in 15
	Bloom syndrome	1 in 100
	Niemann-Pick disease (type A)	1 in 90
	Fanconi anemia	1 in 90
	Glycogen storage disease (type 1A)	1 in 71
	Maple syrup urine disease (MSUD)	1 in 81
	Mucolipidosis IV (ML IV)	1 in 125
	Familial dysautonomia	1 in 36
African American or Western African	Sickle cell anemia	1 in 12
	Beta thalassemia	1 in 50
	Cystic fibrosis	1 in 61
Mediterranean	Beta thalassemia	1 in 15 to 1 in 20
Asian	Alpha thalassemia	1 in 8 to 1 in 20
French Canadian	Tay-Sachs disease	1 in 27
Southeast Asian	Beta thalassemia	1 in 4 to 1 in 150

This table was published in *Medical complications during pregnancy* (5th ed.), B.N. Burrow & T.P. Duffy, in the chapter Clinical Genetics, by Seashore, M.R., p. 216. Copyright W.B. Saunders, 1999; adapted by permission.

affected individual by a pediatric geneticist to verify or establish the diagnosis. This process is necessary in order to discuss reproductive risks and prenatal testing options for future pregnancies. See Box 3.1 to learn about the role of the genetic counselor in this process.

SCREENING TESTS DURING PREGNANCY

First- and second-trimester screening can modify the risk assessment for having a child with Down syndrome, trisomy 18, trisomy 13, a sex chromosome abnormality, and certain microdeletion syndromes. While the chance of having a child with a chromosomal abnormality increases with maternal age (Hook, 1981; Morris, Wald, Mutton, & Alberman, 2003; see Figure 3.1), the vast majority of pregnancies, and therefore most newborns with Down syndrome, are born to younger women. As a result, ACOG has recommended that prenatal screening and diagnostic testing be offered to all women, regardless of age (ACOG, 2017a); this is now considered the standard of care. The following sections describe the options for prenatal testing during the first and second trimesters.

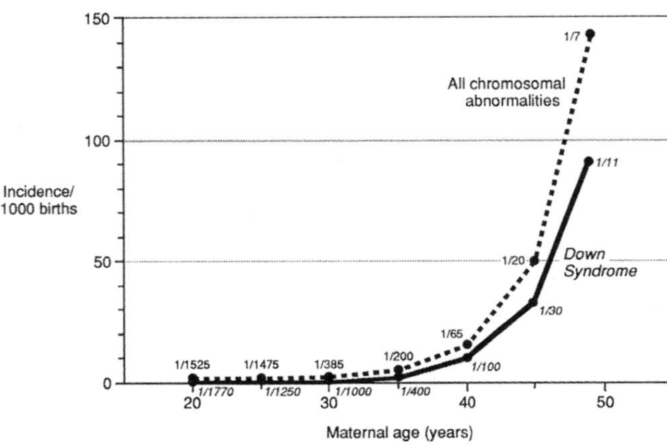

Figure 3.1. Risk of trisomy 21 and all chromosome abnormalities in pregnant women of various ages. Risk increases markedly after 35 years of age. (*Source:* Hook, 1981.)

First-Trimester Screening

Screening for **aneuploidy** (an abnormal number of chromosomes) and birth defects during the first trimester of pregnancy allows for earlier assessment, diagnosis, genetic counseling, and discussion of follow-up

BOX 3.1 INTERDISCIPLINARY CARE

The Genetic Counselor

Throughout the United States, many medical centers employ a genetic counselor (http://www.nsgc.org) to assist with this genetic assessment. The value of having a genetic counselor evaluate the patient and be a member of the multidisciplinary medical team is well documented (Lawrence, Menzel, & Bulas, 2016). With the rapid expansion of complex genetic screening and testing options, the importance of genetic counselors has only grown.

Genetic counselors are medical professionals with a master's degree in genetic counseling and board certification/eligibility through the American Board of Genetic Counseling (ABGC). They have specialized training and expertise in evaluating risks for genetic disease and communicating complex information to families and other health care providers in the prenatal, pediatric, oncology, or laboratory setting.

Meeting with a genetic counselor prior to or during pregnancy allows couples the time to review specific questions about their own pregnancy and family or medical history, as well as questions regarding prenatal screening and diagnostic options.

Genetic counselors can identify and provide resources such as support groups, counseling, patient-appropriate literature, and other family connections to patients. They help other members of a multidisciplinary prenatal team by sharing information with referring providers and communicating the following:

- Patient medical and family history
- The indication for referral
- Prior ultrasounds and genetic screening/testing results
- Guidance regarding patient expectations
- Follow-up on diagnoses

testing. Such screening includes ultrasonography, maternal serum (blood) screening, and DNA/NIPT. ACOG recommends that all women over 35 years old be offered both screening and diagnostic testing for chromosome abnormalities using **CVS** performed in the first trimester or **amniocentesis** performed in the second trimester (ACOG, 2016a; Wilson et al., 2013).

First-Trimester Ultrasound An early ultrasound can establish fetal viability, determine the number of fetuses (especially useful in cases involving assisted reproductive technology), suggest certain genetic/chromosomal disorders and birth defects (e.g., Down syndrome, CHDs, and meningomyelocele), and confirm gestational dating and placental positioning (Table 3.2). Fetal structural anomalies are found in up to 3% of all pregnancies, and approximately half of all major anomalies can be detected with a first-trimester ultrasound (Edwards & Hui, 2018). The highest detection rate with ultrasound at 11–14 weeks was for neck anomalies (92%), whereas limb (34%), face (34%), and genitourinary anomalies (34%) were associated with the lowest detection rate (Rossi & Perfumo, 2013). Increased nuchal translucency seen on an ultrasound, even in the absence of a chromosomal abnormality, is associated with adverse outcomes, including a greater incidence of CHD, other fetal anomalies, genetic syndromes (e.g., Turner syndrome), and fetal death (Sonek & Nicolaides, 2010). Given the association with CHD, a fetal echocardiogram is often recommended in these situations.

For women of advanced maternal age, early ultrasound can impact further testing strategies and clinical management. In one study, 16% of women over age 35 who had considered having cell-free fetal DNA screening altered their decision and care plan based on an abnormal first-trimester ultrasound finding. Some decided to have further diagnostic testing (i.e., amniocentesis or CVS) instead of screening, while others chose to end their pregnancy (Vora, Robinson, Hardesty, & Stamilo, 2017). First-trimester ultrasound is also most accurate for gestational dating. This is important for maternal serum screening for aneuploidy, which can be drawn as early as 9 weeks.

Table 3.2. Ultrasound findings in certain chromosomal abnormalities

Syndrome	Findings
Trisomy 13	Cleft lip and palate
	Congenital heart defect
	Cystic kidneys
	Polydactyly
	Midline facial defect
	Brain abnormalities (holoprosencephaly)
Trisomy 18	Clenched hands with overlapping fingers
	Congenital heart defect
	Polyhydramnios
	Growth retardation
	Rocker-bottom feet
	Omphalocele
Trisomy 21	Gastrointestinal malformations (duodenal atresia)
	Congenital heart defect
	Excess neck skin/increased nuchal translucency
	Absent nasal bone

Sources: D'Alton and DeCherney (1993); Nicolaides (2004); and Viora et al. (2005).

First-Trimester Maternal Serum Screening Testing of maternal serum-free **human chorionic gonadotropin (hCG)** and pregnancy-associated plasma protein A (PAPP-A) at 9–14 weeks' gestation, when used in combination with a first-trimester nuchal translucency ultrasound at 11–13 weeks, further contributes to the risk assessment. This combined screening has been found to correctly identify 90%–95% of fetuses with Down syndrome and trisomy 18 and 13, and it has less than a 5% false-positive rate (Anderson & Brown, 2009; Nicolaides, 2004). In addition to identifying these chromosomal abnormalities, levels of maternal, serum-free β-hCG or PAPP-A that are less than the 5th percentile or greater than the 95th percentile can indicate an adverse pregnancy outcome, specifically an increased risk for preeclampsia and/or intrauterine growth retardation, both of which warrant additional monitoring.

Fetal Echocardiogram A first-trimester fetal echocardiogram (ECHO) is useful for evaluating fetuses with an increased risk for congenital heart disease. Indications include 1) increased nuchal translucency, 2) a first-degree affected relative, 3) a known or suspected chromosome abnormality associated with CHD, 4) an extra cardiac abnormality, or 5) exposure to certain teratogens. Fetal ECHO permits the evaluation of the structure and function of the fetal heart and monitors fetal blood flow. Although it can be performed as early as 11 weeks' gestation in a high-risk fetus, the ECHO should be repeated at 18–20 weeks, when it is most accurate (Rayburn, Jolley, & Simpson, 2015). The presence of prenatally identified CHD can affect *in utero* management, delivery options, and neonatal intervention or follow up (Donofrio et al., 2014).

Cell-Free DNA/NIPT Screening Over the past decade, the landscape for prenatal screening has changed significantly with the advent of NIPT, also known as cell-free fetal DNA screening. During pregnancy, fetal DNA fragments from both the fetus and pregnant woman are present in the maternal bloodstream (Figure 3.2; Benn, Cuckle, & Pergament, 2013). Cell-free fetal DNA fragments, mostly of trophoblast origin, cross the placenta, enter the maternal circulation, and are cleared within hours. Fetal DNA detected during a pregnancy represents DNA from the current gestation. For women at increased risk for aneuploidy, the American College of Medical Genetics and Genomics (ACMG) suggests that maternal serum cell-free fetal DNA screening should be considered as a primary screening tool. NIPT is routinely available as a screen for trisomy 21, 18, and 13, with most laboratories quoting detection rates of 99% for trisomy 21 and 95% for trisomy 18 or 13. NIPT screening has recently expanded in scope, and many laboratories now include sex chromosome abnormalities and some microdeletion syndromes in their panels, although the **positive predictive value** (the proportion of positive results that correctly predicts the disorder being screened) is significantly lower.

Advantages of NIPT include 1) being done as early as 9 weeks in pregnancy and reliable throughout the remainder of pregnancy; 2) having a higher detection rate and lower false-positive rate than any of the other first- or second-trimester screens for Down syndrome, trisomy 18, and trisomy 13; and 3) being able to screen for other genetic abnormalities such as triploidy, sex chromosome abnormalities, and some micro deletion syndromes. It is important to remember, however, that NIPT is a screening, not a diagnostic tool like CVS or amniocentesis, and it has significant limitations. Approximately 0.5%–1% of women will receive an inconclusive test result due to an insufficient fetal fraction of free DNA, and mosaicism, partial trisomies, unbalanced translocations, and single-gene disorders cannot routinely be identified by NIPT (Cuckle, Benn, & Pergament, 2015). In addition, NIPT has not been validated in triplet or higher multiple pregnancies or in pregnancies conceived using egg donation. Also, unlike first- and second-trimester serum screening, NIPT does not detect maternal serum abnormalities that may indicate additional pregnancy or fetal complications, such as an increased risk for preeclampsia, intrauterine growth retardation, or other fetal abnormalities (Beulen et al., 2017).

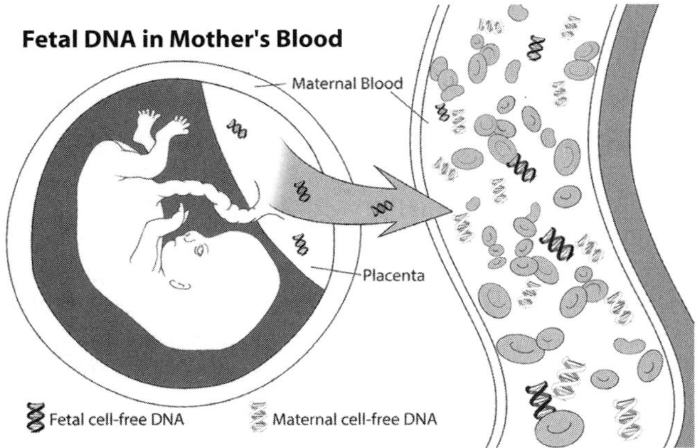

Figure 3.2. Cell-free fetal DNA enters maternal circulation through the placenta. Approximately 10% of DNA in maternal plasma is fetal. This allows testing for increased presence of DNA associated with certain chromosomes. It may also identify some microduplication or microdeletion syndromes in the fetus.

Although the sensitivity and specificity of NIPT in the low-risk population (women under 35 years of age at delivery) seems to be similar to that in the high-risk population, the positive predictive value is lower in the low-risk population given the lower prevalence of abnormalities (ACOG, 2015). Thus, the recommendation by ACOG continues to be that first-trimester maternal serum and ultrasound screening remains the first-line screen offered to the low-risk general obstetric population.

Chorionic Villus Sampling CVS involves obtaining a small biopsy of the **chorion,** the outermost membrane surrounding the embryo. Chorionic **villi,** consisting of rapidly dividing cells of fetal origin, can be analyzed directly or grown in culture prior to testing (Blakemore, 1988). CVS can be used for chromosome analysis, enzyme assay (for inborn errors of metabolism; see Chapter 16), molecular DNA analysis (identifying specific mutations that cause genetic diseases), and chromosome microarray analysis. It is not, however, diagnostic for neural tube defects, such as spina bifida, so a maternal serum α-fetoprotein (AFP) screen at 16+ weeks is recommended after a CVS.

CVS is performed at approximately 10–12 weeks' gestation, usually before a woman appears to be pregnant and prior to **quickening** (the detection of fetal movement by the mother). Using ultrasound guidance, a chorionic villus biopsy is performed either by suction through a small catheter passed into the cervix or by aspiration via a needle inserted through the abdominal wall and uterus (Figure 3.3). CVS is considered the safest invasive prenatal diagnostic procedure prior to the 14th week of gestation. There is a less than 1% risk of procedure-related pregnancy loss and, provided CVS is performed after 10 weeks' gestation, there is no increased risk of causing a fetal anomaly (Ogilvie & Akolekar, 2014).

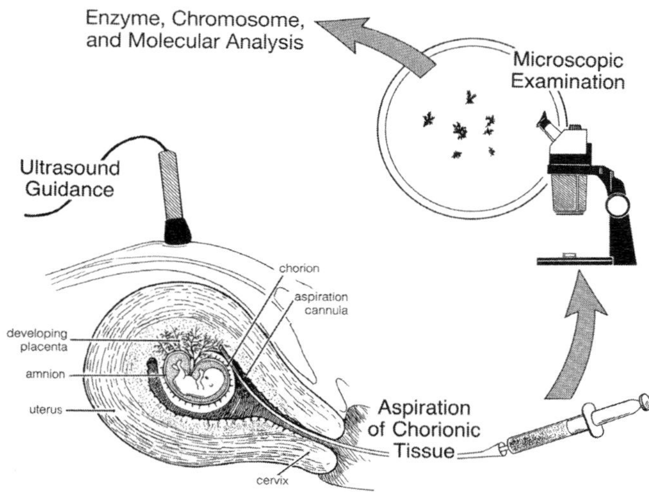

Figure 3.3. CVS is performed at 10–12 weeks' gestation. It can be transcervical or transabdominal. Guided by ultrasound, a catheter is inserted through the vagina and passed into the uterus, or a needle is inserted through the abdomen into the uterus. A small amount of chorionic tissue is removed by suction. The tissue is then examined under a microscope to make sure it is sufficient and sent to the lab. Karyotype, microarray, enzyme, and/or DNA analyses can be performed. Cell culture is needed for most analyses. Results are available in a few days in select situations; more often they are ready in 10–14 days.

Second-Trimester Screening

Maternal serum screening and ultrasonography are also offered in the second trimester. In addition, magnetic resonance imaging (MRI) and fetal echocardiography can add important information in select circumstances at this point in the pregnancy.

Second-Trimester Maternal Serum Screening

Because not all women present for prenatal care in the first trimester, second-trimester screening remains useful (Shamshirsaz, Benn, & Egan, 2010). Approximately 70% of pregnant women in the United States have a maternal serum screen and/or a detailed ultrasound study performed in the second trimester to screen for chromosome abnormalities, birth defects, or inadequate fetal growth.

For the quadruple (Quad) screen, a maternal blood specimen can be drawn at approximately 16 weeks' gestation and analyzed for 1) AFP, 2) β-hCG, 3) unconjugated serum estriol, and 4) inhibin A. In combination with first-trimester screening results, this screening can increase the detection rate for Down syndrome to about 95%, with a 5% false-positive rate (Anderson & Brown, 2009; Malone et al., 2005). These serum markers, combined with other indicators, including maternal age, weight, race, diabetes status, and number of fetuses, can also be used to assess the risk for neural tube defects (**spina bifida** and **anencephaly**), abdominal wall defects (**gastroschisis** and **omphalocele**), and trisomy 18 syndrome (see Appendix B). If the quad screen in the second trimester suggests an increased risk for a fetal abnormality, diagnostic testing by amniocentesis and a detailed ultrasound evaluation should be considered. It should be noted that correct gestational age assessment is essential for an accurate interpretation of all maternal serum screening results.

Second-Trimester Ultrasonography Approximately two-thirds of pregnant women undergo second-trimester **real-time ultrasonography**. Prenatal ultrasound studies at 18–22 weeks' gestation can identify more than 70% of major structural anomalies in fetuses. Once an abnormality is suspected, other imaging, such as a fetal echocardiogram or fetal MRI, may be suggested to further delineate the diagnosis and contribute to management (Edwards & Hui, 2018). Common anomalies detected by ultrasound imaging include neural tube defects, abdominal wall defects, facial clefts, renal anomalies, skeletal anomalies, brain anomalies, and CHD. Although the identification of structural abnormalities by ultrasound is improving, it does not replace definitive diagnostic testing for chromosomal abnormalities, micro duplication or deletion syndromes, genetic mutations, and biochemical analyses that are possible using amniocentesis or CVS. In most cases, ultrasound and other diagnostic testing complement each other in making a diagnosis.

Amniocentesis Amniocentesis is traditionally performed between 15 and 20 weeks' gestation, although it can be performed beyond 20 weeks in select situations. The procedure is done under ultrasound guidance in a sterile field. A needle is inserted just below the mother's umbilicus and through the abdominal and uterine walls. Once in the amniotic sac, 1 to 2 ounces of amniotic fluid are aspirated (Figure 3.4). Through natural processes, mostly fetal urination, the aspirated fluid is replenished within 24 hours. The risk of pregnancy loss following a genetic amniocentesis at 15+ weeks is approximately 0.5%. The specific loss risk is dependent on the provider performing the procedure and possible other maternal complications (Carlson & Vora, 2017; Ogilvie & Akolekar, 2014). Amniocentesis performed before 14 weeks' gestation has been associated with an increased risk of pregnancy loss, a higher incidence of musculoskeletal deformities (most often clubfoot), and a greater chance of amniotic fluid leakage. For this reason, CVS rather than amniocentesis continues to be the preferred procedure for first-trimester diagnosis (Wapner, 2005).

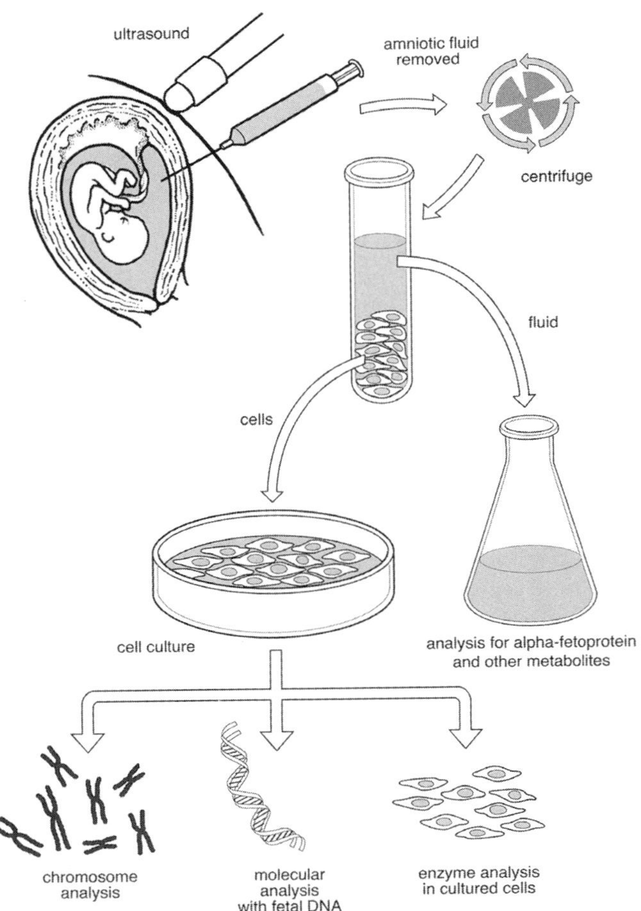

Figure 3.4. Amniocentesis. Approximately 1 to 2 ounces of amniotic fluid are removed at 16–20 weeks' gestation. The sample is spun in a centrifuge to separate the fluid from the fetal cells. The alpha-fetoprotein in the fluid is measured to screen for a neural tube or abdominal wall defect. The fluid can also be used to check for metabolites associated with inborn errors of metabolism when indicated. The cells are grown for a week, and then a karyotype, microarray, enzyme, or DNA analysis can be performed. Most results are available in 10–14 days. (*Source:* Rose & Mennuti, 1993.)

One advantage of amniocentesis over CVS or maternal serum screening is the ability to assay the amniotic fluid directly for abnormal levels of biochemical compounds, such as AFP for neural tube and some abdominal wall defects. Ultrasound evaluations cannot detect all cases of neural tube defects; however, when combined with an elevated amniotic fluid AFP level and a positive **acetylcholinesterase** test, an abnormal ultrasound identifies virtually all neural tube defects (Rose & Mennutti, 1993). The diagnosis of fetal infections such as CMV or toxoplasmosis is also most accurate using amniotic fluid rather than maternal serum.

MRI In selected instances, fetal MRI can add to the clinical understanding of an ultrasound variation when used at 17 weeks' gestation or later (Bulas, 2007; Reddy, Filly, & Copel, 2008). Because MRI uses ultrafast imaging sequences, neither the mother nor fetus requires sedation, and there are no other known maternal or fetal risks with its use. First-trimester evaluation of the fetus by MRI, however, is avoided because of limited resolution of fetal structures.

MRI is particularly useful in conjunction with ultrasound for evaluation of the fetal brain (Rossi & Perfumo, 2014). Among other structures, fetal brain MRI can demonstrate the presence (Figure 3.5A) or absence (Figure 3.5B) of the **corpus callosum** (the band of tissue connecting the two cerebral hemispheres), **Chiari malformations** (the downward displacement of the cerebellum through the opening at the base of the skull, seen most commonly in spina bifida), and **hydrocephalus** (significantly enlarged ventricles) (Glenn & Berkovich, 2006). MRI also is useful in the evaluation of the airway, for the identification of lung lesions, and complex abdominal pathology. It is particularly

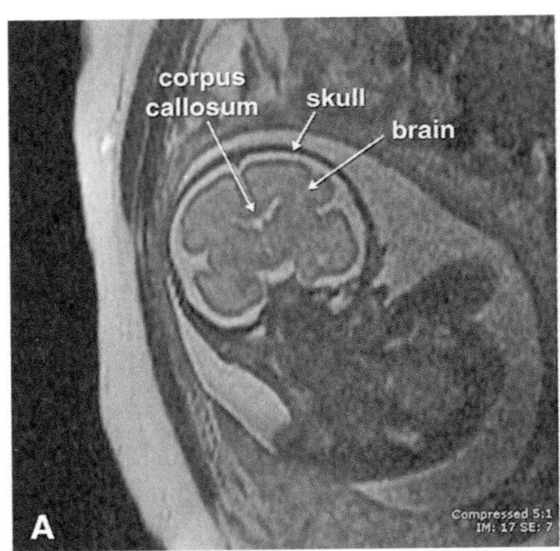

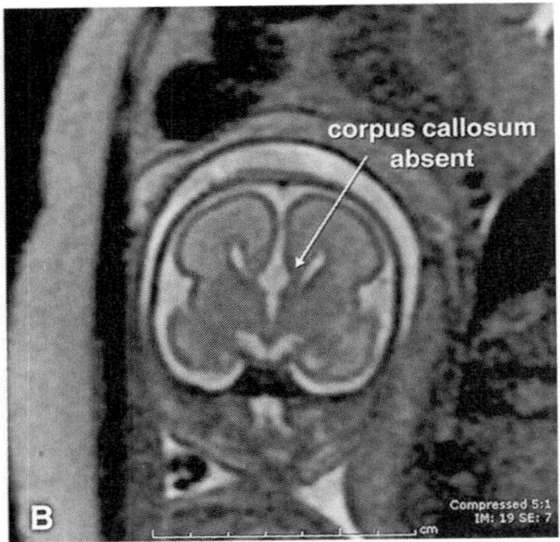

Figure 3.5. A) MRI images of a fetal brain with a corpus callosum. B) MRI images of a fetal brain with agenesis of the corpus callosum. (Courtesy of Dorothy I. Bulas, MD, Department of Diagnostic Imaging, Children's National Medical Center, Washington, DC)

beneficial when there is low or no amniotic fluid surrounding the fetus, as ultrasound imaging is limited in this situation.

Fetal Echocardiography The field of fetal cardiac medicine focuses on the diagnosis of CHD, assessment of cardiac function and the cardiovascular system, and evaluation of treatment options (Donofrio et al., 2014). CHD is the most common birth defect in children (occurring in 8.3 out of 1,000 children, or 0.8% of the population) and represents more than one-third of all deaths from birth defects (Marelli et al., 2014; Reddy et al., 2008). Fetal echocardiography is the best tool in the assessment of a fetus with CHD. This targeted ultrasound is ideally performed at 18–22 weeks' gestation, when the fetal heart is approximately the size of an adult's thumbnail. A family history of CHD, an increased nuchal translucency in the first trimester (Souka et al., 2005), maternal diabetes or lupus, a fetal diagnosis of Down syndrome or velocardiofacial syndrome (see Appendix B), or other birth defects noted by ultrasound all increase the likelihood that a CHD will be identified.

When a CHD is identified *in utero,* a detailed ultrasound study is indicated to screen for other malformations. Approximately 10%–15% of infants with CHD have an underlying chromosomal abnormality and will often have additional anomalies and intellectual disability (Table 3.2; Brown, 2000). Infants with isolated critical CHD are also at risk for developmental delay or cognitive impairments as a result of hypoxemia and morbidity from corrective cardiovascular surgery. When a fetus is identified with a CHD, genetic counseling and diagnostic testing via amniocentesis are warranted because the long-term outcome for a child with an isolated CHD can be much different than for a child with CHD as part of a chromosomal or genetic syndrome.

Because the fetal circulation differs from that of the newborn, not all CHDs can be identified prenatally; therefore, a careful cardiac evaluation should also be performed in the newborn period for infants known to be at increased risk. Early diagnosis and management is important in planning for prenatal or postnatal intervention and may play a role in improving the neurocognitive outcome. See Box 3.2 for more on genetic testing and fetal CHD.

Diagnostic Testing of Fetal Cells Both CVS and amniocentesis are well-established techniques for obtaining fetal cells. The most common testing requested is chromosomal analysis (karyotype) and/or microarray. When indicated, biochemical analysis for inborn errors of metabolism or DNA analysis for disorders such as fragile X syndrome or cystic fibrosis can also can be performed (Thompson, McInnes, & Willard, 2004). Indeed, any genetic disorder for which a familial DNA mutation has been identified can be assessed using DNA isolated from the fetal cells. Studies other than microarray and/or chromosome analysis are generally only considered when a pregnancy is thought to be at increased risk for a particular condition.

ACOG guidelines updated in 2016 recommend chromosomal microarray (CMA) as the first tier of

BOX 3.2 EVIDENCE-BASED PRACTICE

Genetic Testing and Fetal Congenital Heart Disease

Approximately 15% of fetuses with congenital heart disease (CHD) have a chromosome abnormality. Thus, all patients with a fetal diagnosis of CHD should be offered genetic counseling and prenatal diagnosis. The American College of Obstetrics and Gynecologists and Society for Maternal-Fetal Medicine now recommend offering chromosomal microarray analysis (versus karyotype alone) for those pursuing prenatal diagnosis when there are one or more structural abnormalities.

Regarding CHD specifically, the single nucleotide polymorphism microarray increases the likelihood of identifying clinically significant chromosomal differences that aren't detectable by karyotype. One study looking at the detection of microarray abnormalities in prenatal CHD found that 19.8% of fetuses with a CHD had an array abnormality (17.4% in isolated CHD and 25% in syndromic cases). When karyotype alone was performed, 14% of fetuses had a chromosomal abnormality (Turan et al., 2018; Mademont-Soler et al., 2013).

The take away message is the following:

- Genetic counseling is important for all patients with a prenatal diagnosis of CHD.
- Chromosomal microarray should be offered in lieu of, or in addition to, a normal karyotype for patients with a fetal diagnosis of CHD.

testing in the case of an ultrasound finding of a fetal structural anomaly, with the caveat that if the abnormality is strongly suggestive of a particular aneuploidy, a karyotype (chromosomal analysis) may be offered before CMA. In a prospective study by Wapner et al. (2012) evaluating fetuses with normal karyotype by amniocentesis or CVS, microarray analysis identified clinically relevant deletions or duplications in 6% of fetuses with a structural abnormality and 1.7% of those whose indication for prenatal diagnosis was advanced maternal age or abnormal screening results.

GENETIC COUNSELING AND DECISION MAKING

When a concern for a congenital abnormality is raised, prenatal testing offers parents the opportunity of learning more about the condition and making an informed decision on how to proceed. Some parents make the incredibly difficult and painful choice to terminate the pregnancy. For those who continue the pregnancy, there is time to learn more about the disorder prior to delivery, enabling the family to start preparing emotionally and logistically for the birth of a child who may require extensive supports. Prenatal testing ensures that if immediate postnatal surgical or other medical intervention is required, the family and medical team have time to develop a treatment plan. It may also provide the time to arrange for palliative care for a child who may not survive for very long after birth because of the severity of the anatomical abnormalities. Perinatal palliative care is a valuable option for families who choose to continue a pregnancy with a fetus where early postnatal death is likely. Clinicians specifically trained in palliative care can provide resources and support to help families make the most of the precious time they have with their child both inside and/or outside the womb. Resources for both patients and health care providers can be found at www.perinatalhospice.org.

Due to the complexity of prenatal testing and screening (see Figure 3.6), it is becoming more challenging for parents to process their options and make informed decisions; therefore, it is increasingly important for them to receive genetic counseling. As technology advances, the indications for prenatal diagnosis will continue to increase and detection will continue to improve; however, even the most sophisticated prenatal diagnostic technology cannot guarantee the birth of a "typical" child. Many of the disorders that cause developmental disabilities in the absence of structural malformations are not currently amenable to prenatal diagnosis unless there is a known familial genetic diagnosis.

DECREASING THE RISK OF A BIRTH DEFECT

Attention to certain environmental exposures during pregnancy can help decrease the risk for some birth defects. Recommendations include receiving early prenatal care, avoiding alcoholic beverages and tobacco, and minimizing unnecessary medications. In addition, pregnant women should try to avoid exposure to infection, excess vitamin A (e.g., Accutane for acne), and frequent consumption of fish that are known to have elevated mercury content (e.g., mackerel, marlin, orange roughy, swordfish, tilefish, and ahi tuna; ACOG, 2017b). Daily ingestion of 0.4 mg of folic acid (found in most multivitamins) by all women of childbearing age starting 3 months before attempted conception and continuing through the first trimester is recommended to reduce the risk of neural tube defects.

If not treated appropriately, a number of maternal conditions can also predispose an infant to birth defects or developmental delay. A woman with phenylketonuria is at risk of having a child with microcephaly and intellectual disability if she does not maintain a phenylalanine-restricted diet during pregnancy (see Chapter 16). If not under good control, chronic maternal disorders, including diabetes and lupus, increase the risk for congenital anomalies to the fetus. Certain medications taken to control illness, such as anti-epileptic drugs, can also increase the risk for birth defects. Ideally, the risks versus benefits of chronic medication use during pregnancy should be discussed by the patient and her care provider prior to conception.

ALTERNATIVE REPRODUCTIVE CHOICES

When a couple is at increased risk to have a child with a serious genetic disorder, reproductive options are available to minimize that risk utilizing **assisted reproductive technology** (ART). Given its complexities, genetic counseling is recommended prior to initiating ART.

Preimplantation Genetic Diagnosis

Preimplantation genetic diagnosis (PGD) is available for couples who 1) are at risk of having a child with a known genetic disorder, 2) wish to conceive an unaffected child that is biologically their own, and 3) want to avoid having to consider pregnancy termination. Originally introduced in 1990 for couples at risk of having a child with an X-linked disorder, PGD accuracy continues to improve with the use of next-generation sequencing (NGS) analysis to identify DNA sequence differences (i.e., single-gene mutations) (Dolan, Goldwaser, & Jindal, 2017; Stern, 2014).

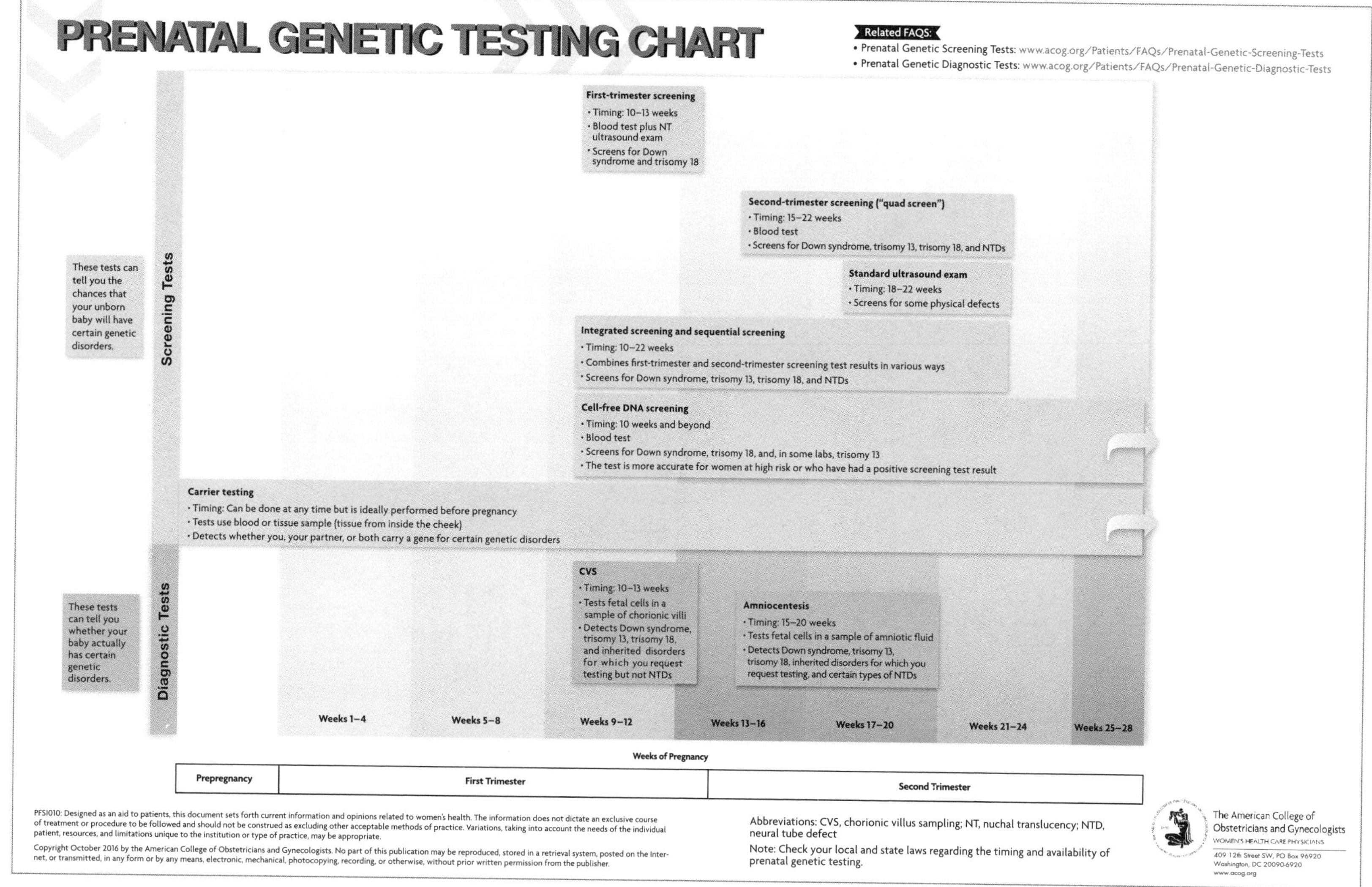

Figure 3.6. This American College of Obstetrics and Gynecology (ACOG) overview of prenatal testing includes the screening and diagnostic options available through pregnancy. (Reprinted with permission from American College of Obstetricians and Gynecologists. Prenatal genetic testing chart [infographic]. Washington, DC; American College of Obstetricians and Gynecologists; 2016. Available here: https://www.acog.org/Patients/FAQS/Prenatal-Genetic-Testing-Chart-Infographic. Retrieved December 12, 2017.)

There are two approaches to PGD, as illustrated in Figure 3.7. Both include the methods of ***in vitro* fertilization** (IVF). IVF is accomplished by harvesting a woman's egg cells and fertilizing them outside the womb with the father's sperm. The first involves **polar body testing** of the woman's eggs to establish the presence or absence of the mutation in question (e.g., looking for the Tay-Sachs gene mutations in a couple who are both carriers of this disorder). Only embryos from fertilized eggs determined to contain the normal gene(s) are then transferred to the mother's uterus to establish a pregnancy. The second approach is to perform IVF on harvested eggs (without testing the polar bodies) and allow them to develop in culture to the blastomere, or eight-cell stage. A single cell is then microdissected from each blastomere and analyzed for the presence of mutations or an abnormal chromosome number. Only unaffected embryos are subsequently transferred to the uterus. The greater the number of embryos created, the greater the likelihood of a genetically normal

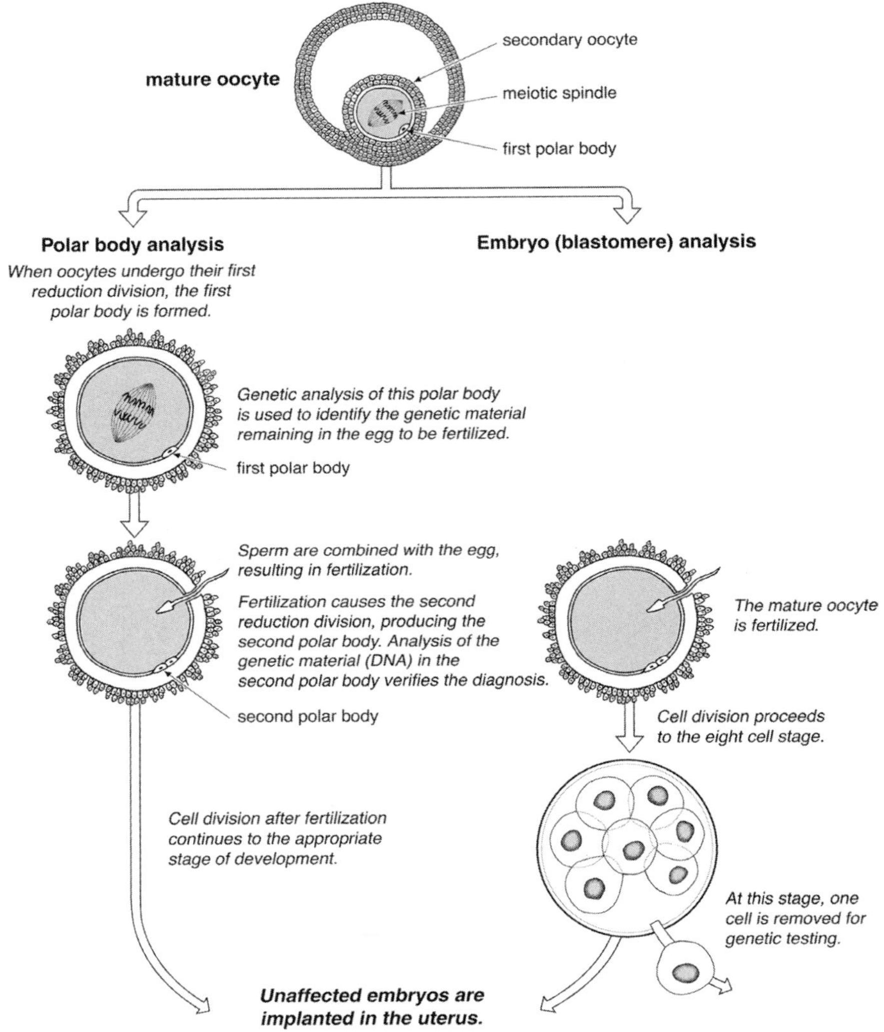
mature oocyte
secondary oocyte
meiotic spindle
first polar body
Polar body analysis
When oocytes undergo their first reduction division, the first polar body is formed.
Embryo (blastomere) analysis
Genetic analysis of this polar body is used to identify the genetic material remaining in the egg to be fertilized.
first polar body
Sperm are combined with the egg, resulting in fertilization.
Fertilization causes the second reduction division, producing the second polar body. Analysis of the genetic material (DNA) in the second polar body verifies the diagnosis.
second polar body
The mature oocyte is fertilized.
Cell division proceeds to the eight cell stage.
Cell division after fertilization continues to the appropriate stage of development.
At this stage, one cell is removed for genetic testing.
Unaffected embryos are implanted in the uterus.

Figure 3.7. Preimplantation genetic diagnosis (PGD). Individuals who undergo PGD begin the process as they would for *in vitro* fertilization. The ovary is stimulated to produce mature oocytes, which are then harvested for fertilization outside of the woman's body. These mature oocytes can be used for polar body analysis or fertilized and processed for a blastomere biopsy. This figure describes the path toward the preimplantation diagnosis using both methods. Polar body analysis is limited to those disorders or variations that would be present in the maternal genetic material whereas an embryo biopsy can analyze both maternal and paternal genetic contributions. As with *in vitro* fertilization, not all pregnancies will progress to term. Prenatal diagnosis at a later stage of gestation via CVS or amniocentesis is recommended to confirm an accurate diagnosis.

embryo. Approximately 30% of implanted embryos will survive to birth, but success is impacted by maternal age and other maternal factors. As diagnosis from a single cell remains a technical challenge and the risk of misdiagnosis cannot be eliminated (Wilton, Thornhill, Traeger-Synodinos, Sermon, & Harper, 2009), confirmatory prenatal diagnosis via CVS or amniocentesis is recommended after PGD.

As NGS and **whole-exome sequencing** become more accessible, care should be given to ethical considerations for the use of PGD outside of its original goals (Stern, 2014). PGD could theoretically be used to screen for or against particular traits rather than medical conditions, bringing us closer to the idea of "designer" infants. This would obviously be ethically suspect. It is important that regulating bodies, medical and legal organizations, patient advocacy groups, and government organizations stay engaged in the discussion of these issues.

Additional options within ART include artificial insemination or IVF with donor sperm or IVF using donor egg. Couples considering these options should assess 1) how donors are screened, 2) what carrier testing is performed to ensure that the donor and patient are not carriers for variations in genes for the same genetic disease, and 3) the donor's family history such as birth defects or known genetic conditions.

Another ART is intracytoplasmic sperm injection (ICSI), a technology available for men who have a low sperm count or poor sperm motility (Palermo et al., 1998). Sperm from the prospective father are harvested, and the cytoplasmic portions of the sperm are removed. The nucleus of the sperm is then introduced into a harvested egg by microinjection, and the developing blastocyst (early embryo) is subsequently transferred into the uterus. Single-embryo transfer is the most effective option to reduce the risk of multiple births (Tobias, Sharara, Rranasiak, Heiser, & Pickney-Clark, 2016). For approximately 1% of conceptions accomplished through ICSI, sex chromosome aneuploidy (e.g., an extra X or Y chromosome) has been reported. Although there had been concern about a 6.5% malformation rate secondary to the ART, recent data support other confounding factors that may be responsible for the increased identification of birth defects (Parazzinin et al., 2015).

All of these options are costly in terms of physical, emotional, and financial resources. At present these services are not always covered by health insurance plans. The risk of multiple gestations is also a concern, particularly if fetal reduction (i.e., abortion of one or more fetuses) is not an option the parents are willing to consider. Publications from Europe, the United States, and Australia have suggested an association between ART and imprinting (epigenetic) disorders such as Beckwith-Wiedemann syndrome (Chapter 1; Appendix B). However, because the absolute risk is small, routine screening for these imprinting disorders in children conceived by ART is not recommended at this time (Manipalviratn, DeCherney, & Segars, 2009).

When considering ART, couples should request detailed information regarding the techniques that are used, the risk of error in diagnosis, the risk of other anomalies or birth defects, the cost per attempt, the rate of successful pregnancies, and the risk of multiple gestations (e.g., twins or triplets; Stern, 2014; Wen et al., 2010). The American Society of Reproductive Medicine and the Society of Assisted Reproductive Technology are putting forth guidelines for using ART (http://www.asrm.org; http://www.sart.org). These sites have valuable information for patients and providers about the process and data from participating centers.

PSYCHOSOCIAL IMPLICATIONS OF PRENATAL TESTING

With prenatal screening and testing technology progressing rapidly, choices can be overwhelming for a family. Health care professionals and patients often avoid difficult preliminary discussions about how a couple would respond to the diagnosis of an abnormality or, if they already have a child with special needs, how they would respond to the recurrence of the disorder in a subsequent child. For some couples, having advanced knowledge allows for preparation prior to birth; for others, it may mean ending a pregnancy.

Many of these issues are best addressed prior to attempting a pregnancy to ensure that prenatal diagnostic techniques, genetic screening, and other specialized tests can be discussed in advance. Exploring each individual's reproductive choices and available options is time consuming, but necessary. It is imperative that health care professionals focus on the family's psychosocial needs along with the clinical information.

When a woman gives birth to a child with special needs or a child who does not survive long after birth, the experience can be devastating. Each family is unique, and assumptions by health care providers as to what a family should or should not do in a given situation must be avoided. Genetic counselors and medical geneticists who are trained in nondirective counseling can help families understand their options and choose a course of action that is consistent with the family's values and resources. Often, support groups or individual counseling can be beneficial.

Appropriate pretest genetic counseling should include information that is balanced (pros and cons), accurate, and up to date. It should be supported by materials that are easy to understand so pregnant women can be supported in their decision making and make an informed choice (Metcalfe, 2017). This is particularly true for couples who have an increased risk for conceiving a child with a specific genetic disorder or who have previously conceived a child with a birth defect, special needs, or genetic disorder. The array of screening and diagnostic tests can be both overwhelming and reassuring. Health care providers, working together with genetics professionals, are in a unique position to help families carefully consider and understand their reproductive options and the effects that prenatal diagnosis or genetic screening will have on them physically, emotionally, and financially.

SUMMARY

- Planning for a pregnancy allows time for the patient and health care provider to address maternal health issues; start prenatal vitamins, including 0.4 mg (or more) of folic acid daily; obtain genetic carrier testing; and review family history.
- Accurate dating leads to early prenatal care and access to early ultrasound and/or blood screening tests.
- Decisions about prenatal screening (i.e., cell-free fetal DNA) versus diagnostic studies (such as CVS or amniocentesis) are complex and ideally are addressed with an individual by a genetic counselor early in pregnancy.
- Imaging studies such as fetal echocardiogram and fetal MRI may be needed to further clarify abnormal prenatal findings noted on ultrasound or through abnormal NIPT or diagnostic test results.
- Earlier diagnosis of a fetal abnormality allows couples the opportunity to explore the appropriate options for ending a pregnancy and/or to creating a delivery and management plan.
- Assisted reproductive technology such as PGD or ICSI is an important option for some women/couples.
- Genetic counselors and centers specializing in fetal care are important resources for prenatal patients and families.
- Health care workers who understand the unique stress that prenatal patients and their families may experience are instrumental in getting families through trying times. This often includes referring patients for additional counseling.

ADDITIONAL RESOURCES

Genetic Alliance: http://www.geneticalliance.org

Genetics Home Reference: http://ghr.nlm.nih.gov

Genetic Testing Registry (GTR): https://www.ncbi.nlm.nih.gov/gtr/#genereviews

Additional resources can be found online in Appendix D: Childhood Disabilities Resources, Services, and Organizations (see About the Online Companion Materials).

REFERENCES

American College of Obstetrics and Gynecology. (2015). Cell-free DNA screening for fetal aneuploidy [Committee Opinion No. 640]. *Obstetrics & Gynecology, 126,* e31–e37.

American College of Obstetrics and Gynecology. (2016a). *ACOG issues new prenatal testing guidelines* [Practice Bulletin 163]. Washington, DC: Author.

American College of Obstetrics and Gynecology. [2016b]. *Prenatal genetic testing chart* [Infographic]. Retrieved from https://www.acog.org/Patients/FAQs/Prenatal-Genetic-Testing-Chart-Infographic

American College of Obstetrics and Gynecology. (2017a). *Counseling about genetic testing and communication of genetic test results* [Committee Opinion Number 693]. Washington, DC: Author.

American College of Obstetricians and Gynecologists. (2017b). *Reducing risks of birth defects.* Retrieved from http://www.acog.org/Patients/FAQs/Reducing-Risks-of-Birth-Defects

Anderson, D. L., & Brown, C. E. L. (2009). Fetal chromosome abnormalities: Antenatal screening and diagnosis. *American Family Physicians, 79*(2), 117–123.

Benn, P., Cuckle, H., & Pergament, E. (2013). Non-invasive prenatal testing for aneuploidy: Current status and future prospects. *Ultrasound in Obstetrics & Gynecology, 42*(1), 15–33.

Beulen, L., Faas, B. H. W., Feenstra, I., van Vugt, J. M. G., & Bekker, M. N. (2017). Clinical utility of non-invasive prenatal testing in pregnancies with ultrasound anomalies. *Ultrasound in Obstetrics & Gynecology, 49,* 721–728.

Blakemore, K. J. (1988). Prenatal diagnosis by chorionic villus sampling. *Obstetrics & Gynecology Clinics of North America, 15,* 179–213.

Brown, D. L. (2000). Family history of congenital heart disease. In C. B. Benson, P. H. Arger, & E. I. Bluth (Eds.), *Ultrasonography in obstetrics and gynecology: A practical approach* (pp. 155–166). New York, NY: Thieme Medical.

Bulas, D. (2007). Fetal magnetic resonance imaging as a complement to fetal ultrasonography. *Ultrasound, 23*(1), 3–22.

Carlson, L. M., & Vora, N. L. (2017). Prenatal diagnosis screening and diagnostic tools. *Obstetrics & Gynecology Clinics of North America, 44,* 245–256.

Centers for Disease Control and Prevention. (2017). *Birth defects.* Retrieved from https://www.cdc.gov/ncbddd/birthdefects

Cuckle, H., Benn, P., & Pergament, E. (2015). Cell-free DNA screening for fetal aneuploidy as a clinical service. *Clinical Biochemistry, 48*(15), 932–941. doi:10.1016/j.clinbiochem.2015.02.011

D'Alton, M. E., & DeCherney, A. H. (1993). Prenatal diagnosis. *The New England Journal of Medicine, 328,* 114–119.

Dolan, S. M., Goldwaser, T. H., & Jindal, S. K. (2017). Preimplantation genetic diagnosis for Mendelian conditions. *JAMA: The Journal of the American Medical Association, 318,* 859–860.

Donofrio, M. T., Moon-Grady, A. J., Hornberger, L. K., Copel, J. A., Sklansky, M. S., Abuhanad, A., . . . Rychik, J. (2014). Diagnosis and treatment of fetal cardiac disease. *Circulation, 129,* 2183–2242.

Edwards, L., & Hui, L. (2018). First and second trimester screening for fetal structural anomalies. *Seminars in Fetal & Neonatal Medicine, 23,* 102–111.

Glenn, O. A., & Barkovich, J. (2006). Magnetic resonance imaging of the fetal brain and spine: An increasingly important role in prenatal diagnosis: Part 2. *American Journal of Neuroradiology, 27,* 1807–1814.

Grody, W. W., Thompson, B. H., Gregg, A. R., Bean, L. H., Mohaghan, K. G., Schneider, A., & Lebo, R. V. (2013). ACMG position statement on prenatal/preconception expanded carrier screening. *Genetics in Medicine, 15,* 482–483.

Hook, E. B. (1981). Rates of chromosomal abnormalities at different maternal ages. *Obstetrics & Gynecology, 58,* 282–285.

Lawrence, A. K., Menzel, M. B., & Bulas, D. I. (2016). Prenatal counseling tools for the pediatric radiologist as part of a multidisciplinary team. *Pediatric Radiology, 46,* 172–176.

Mademont-Soler, I., Morales, C., Soler, A., Martínez-Crespo, J. M., Shen, Y., Margarit, E., . . . Sánchez, A. (2013). Prenatal diagnosis of chromosomal abnormalities in fetuses with abnormal cardiac ultrasound findings: Evaluation of chromosomal microarray-based analysis. *Ultrasound Obstetrics & Gynecology, 4,* 375–382.

Malone, F. D., Canick, J. A., Ball, R. H., Nyberg, D. A., Comstock, C. H., Bukowski, R., . . . and First- and Second-Trimester Evaluation of Risk (FASTER) Research Consortium. (2005). First-trimester or second-trimester screening, or both, for Down's syndrome. *The New England Journal of Medicine, 353*(19), 2001–2011.

Manipalviratn, S., DeCherney, A., & Segars, J. (2009). Imprinting disorders and assisted reproductive technology. *Fertility & Sterility, 91*(2), 305–315.

Marelli, A. J., Ionescu-Ittu, R., Mackie, A. S., Guo, L., Dendukuri, N., & Kaouache, M. (2014). Lifetime prevalence of congenital heart disease in the general population from 2000 to 2010. *Circulation, 130*(9), 749–756.

Metcalfe, S. A. (2017). Genetic counseling, patient education and informed decision making in the genomic era. *Seminars in Fetal & Neonatal Medicine, 23,* 142–149.

Morris, J. K., Wald, N. J., Mutton, D. E., & Alberman, E. (2003). Comparison models of maternal age-specific risk for Down syndrome live births. *Prenatal Diagnosis, 23,* 252–258.

National Center for Biotechnology Information. (n.d.). GTR: *Genetic Testing Registry.* Retrieved from https://www.ncbi.nlm.nih.gov/gtr/#genereviews

National Center for Biotechnology Information. (2017). *Online Mendelian Inheritance in Man.* Retrieved from http://www.ncbi.nlm.nih.gov/omim

Nicolaides, K. H. (2004). Nuchal translucency and other first-trimester sonographic markers of chromosomal abnormalities. *American Journal of Obstetrics & Gynecology, 191,* 45–67.

Ogilvie, C., & Akolekar, R. (2014). Pregnancy loss following amniocentesis or CVS sampling-time for a reassessment of risk. *Journal of Clinical Medicine, 3,* 741–746.

Palermo, G. D., Schlegel, P. N., Sills, E. S., Veeck, L. L, Zaninovic, N., Menendez, S., & Rosenwaks, Z. (1998). Births after intracytoplasmic injection of sperm obtained by testicular extraction from men with nonmosaic Klinefelter's syndrome. *The New England Journal of Medicine, 338,* 588–590.

Parazzinin, F., Cipriani, S., Bulfoni, G., Frigerio, A., Somigliana, E., & Mosca, F. (2015). The risk of birth defects after assisted reproduction. *Journal of Assisted Reproduction and Genetics 32*(3), 379–385.

Rayburn, W. F., Jolley, J. A., & Simpson, L. L. (2015). Advances in ultrasound imaging for congenital malformations during early gestation. *Birth Defects Research: Part A. Clinical & Molecular Teratology, 103*(4), 260–268.

Reddy, U. M., Filly, R. A., & Copel, J. A. (2008). Prenatal imaging: Ultrasonography and magnetic resonance imaging. *Obstetrics & Genecology, 112*(1), 145–157.

Rose, N. C., & Mennutti, M. T. (1993). Alpha-fetoprotein and neural tube defects. In J. J. Sciarra & P. V. Dilts, Jr. (Eds.), *Gynecology and obstetrics* (Rev. ed., pp. 1–14). New York, NY: HarperCollins.

Rossi, A. C., & Perfumo, F. (2014). Additional value of fetal magnetic resonance imaging in the prenatal diagnosis of central nervous system anomalies: A systematic review of the literature. *Ultrasound in Obstetrics & Gynecology, 44,* 388–393.

Rossi, A. C., & Perfumo, F. (2013). Accuracy of ultrasonography at 11-14 weeks of gestation for detection of fetal structural anomalies: A systematic review. *Obstetrics & Gynecology, 122,* 1160–1167.

Shamshirsaz, A. A., Benn, P., & Egan, J. F. (2010). The role of second-trimester screening in the post-first-trimester screening era. *Clinics in Laboratory Medicine, 30*(3), 667–676.

Sonek, J., & Nicolaides, K. (2010). Additional first-trimester ultrasound markers. *Clinics in Laboratory Medicine, 30*(3), 573–592.

Souka, A., von Kaisenberg, C., Hyett, J., Sonek, J. D., & Nicolaides, K. H. (2005). Increased nuchal translucency with normal karyotype. *American Journal of Obstetrics & Gynecology, 192*(4), 1005–1021.

Stern, H. J. (2014). Preimplantation genetic diagnosis: Prenatal testing for embryos finally achieving its potential. *Journal of Clinical Medicine, 3,* 280–309.

Thompson, M. W., McInnes, R. R., & Willard, H. F. (Eds.). (2004). *Thompson & Thompson genetics in medicine* (6th ed.). Philadelphia, PA: W.B. Saunders.

Tobias, T., Sharara, F. I., Rranasiak, J. M., Heiser, P. W., & Pickney-Clark, E. (2016). Promoting the use of elective single embryo transfer in clinical practice. *Fertility Research and Practice, 2*(1).

Turan, S., Asoglu, M. R., Benziv, R. G., Doyle, L., Harman, C., & Turan, O. M. (2018). Yield rate of chromosomal microarray analysis in fetuses with congenital heart defects. *European Journal of Obstetrics and Gynecology and Reproductive Biology, 221,* 172–176.

Viora, E., Errante, G., Sciarrone, A., Bastonero, S., Masturzo, G., Martiny, G., & Campogrande, M. (2005). Fetal nasal bone and trisomy 21 in the second trimester. *Prenatal Diagnosis, 25*(6), 511–515.

Vora, N. L., Robinson, S., Hardisty, E. E., & Stamilo, D. M. (2017). Utility or ultrasound examination at 10-14 weeks prior to cell-free DNA screening for fetal aneuploidy. *Ultrasound Obstetrics & Gynecology, 49,* 465–469.

Wapner, R. J. (2005) *Invasive prenatal diagnostic techniques. Seminars in Perinatology, 29*(6), 401–404.

Wapner, R. J., Martin, C. L., Levy, B., Ballif, B. C., Eng, C. M., Zachary, J. M., . . . Jackson, L. (2012). Chromosomal microarray versus karyotyping for prenatal diagnosis. *New England Journal of Medicine, 367,* 2175–2184.

Wen, S. W., Leader, A., White, R. R., Léveillé, M. C., Wilkie, V., Zhou, J., & Walker, M. C. (2010). A comprehensive assessment of outcomes in pregnancies conceived by in vitro fertilization/intracytoplasmic sperm injection. *European Journal of Obstetrics & Gynecology, 150*(2), 160–165.

Wheeler, A. C., Bailey, D. B. Jr., Berry-Kravis, E., Greenberg, J., Losh, M., Mailick, M., . . . Hagerman, R. (2014). Associated features in females with an FMR1 premutation. *Journal of Neurodevelopmental Disorders, 6*(1), 30. doi:10.1186/1866-1955-6-30

Wilson, K. L., Czerwinski, J. L., Hoskovee, S. J., Noblin, S. J., Sullivan, C. M., Harbison, A., . . . Singletary, C. N. (2013). NSGC practice guideline: Prenatal screening and diagnostic testing options for chromosome aneuploidy. *Journal of Genetic Counseling, 22*, 4–15.

Wilton, L., Thornhill, A., Traeger-Synodinos, J., Sermon, K. D., & Harper, J. C. (2009). The causes of misdiagnosis and adverse outcomes in PGD. *Human Reproduction, 24*(5), 1221–1228.

CHAPTER 4 Newborn Screening

Joan E. Pellegrino

Upon completion of the chapter, the reader will

- Understand the rationale for newborn screening
- Recognize the difference between a screening test and a diagnostic test
- Be familiar with the types of screening tests available
- Understand the limitations and pitfalls of screening

The birth of a new infant is a joyous time, but for some families a shadow is cast on their initial hopes by the worrisome results of a newborn screening test. The infant's mother will have undergone a number of screening procedures during the pregnancy (see Chapter 3), but she may be unaware that her newborn infant will also have several screening tests performed. This chapter describes the rationale for newborn screening, summarizes the types of disorders for which screening is conducted, and reviews the methods for ensuring proper follow-up on the results of newborn screening.

CASE STUDY

Denise, a 31-year-old healthy woman, was pregnant with her second child. The pregnancy was uncomplicated. She had a normal maternal serum screening test in the second trimester and normal prenatal ultrasounds. The delivery was uncomplicated, and she and her daughter, Ashley, were discharged home from the hospital when Ashley was 2 days of age. Ashley's parents were therefore upset and confused to receive a telephone call 4 days later, notifying them that Ashley had screened positive for medium chain acyl-CoA-dehydrogenase deficiency (MCAD), an inborn error of metabolism. They did not know what this disease was, and they did not understand why Ashley should screen positive for an "inherited" condition when they already had a healthy 2-year-old daughter at home. Denise did recall reading that her state had implemented expanded newborn screening, but she was unsure what this meant. Ashley was seen by her pediatrician and underwent diagnostic testing for MCAD. The diagnosis was confirmed, and Ashley was treated with a frequent, regular feeding schedule and remained asymptomatic (see Chapter 16).

Thought Question:

How often do we miss a genetic diagnosis as a cause of developmental disabilities, and could earlier diagnosis and treatment improve the outcome in many of these cases?

WHAT IS A SCREENING TEST?

A **screening test,** as the name implies, is a test designed to screen for, but not definitively diagnose, a particular condition. When applied to a group of individuals, a screening test separates those who are at increased risk for a condition from those who are at a lower risk. The ideal screening test would perform this operation with perfect accuracy, but in reality, all screening tests produce **false-positive results** that identify unaffected individuals as being at increased risk. Some screening tests also produce **false-negative results,** identifying affected individuals as not being at increased risk. As the goal of newborn screening is to identify *all* truly affected individuals, interpretive methods and screening algorithms are devised to decrease false-negative results while still trying to minimize false positives. In some cases, this is accomplished by setting a numerical cut-off for a test that favors the identification of truly affected individuals at the expense of over-identifying some unaffected individuals (Figure 4.1). Since any particular condition tested for by newborn screening is relatively rare, the number of individuals affected by that condition will be much smaller than the number of unaffected individuals. Depending on the technology used, this means that some positive screens may turn out to be false positives. For some conditions, retesting a child using the same or alternative screening tests will improve the screening process, but ultimately, a final group of individuals with positive screening results must undergo diagnostic testing. A **diagnostic test** is designed to more definitively confirm or exclude the presence of a disease or condition in a particular individual (i.e., to "make a diagnosis"). Diagnostic tests are meant to be done on individual patients and differ from population-based screening tests ("risk assessments").

WHY SCREEN NEWBORNS?

Of the hundreds of diseases and conditions that may potentially affect infants and young children, a limited number are appropriate for inclusion in a newborn screening program. In the United States, the number of conditions that are screened varies widely among the individual states. In 2005, the American College of Medical Genetics completed a report commissioned by the Health Resources and Services Administration that recommended universal screening for 29 specific core conditions and 25 secondary conditions (Newborn Screening Expert Group, 2005). The Advisory Committee on Heritable Disorders in Newborns and Children meets quarterly to review new conditions to add to the core screening panel (U.S. Department of Health and Human Services, 2018). As of September 2017, there are 34 disorders on the recommended uniform screening panel (Table 4.1) and another 26 secondary targets (Table 4.2). In general terms, the core conditions screened for must meet three criteria: They must be 1) serious (life threatening or life altering), 2) identifiable (a biomarker is available), and 3) treatable. In this context, being "treatable" does not necessarily mean that the condition is curable; it means that interventions should result in significant amelioration of the expected consequences of that condition. The types of diseases and disorders screened for generally fall into one of four categories: endocrine disorders, hemoglobinopathies, metabolic disorders, and other disorders (including immune disorders). While infectious

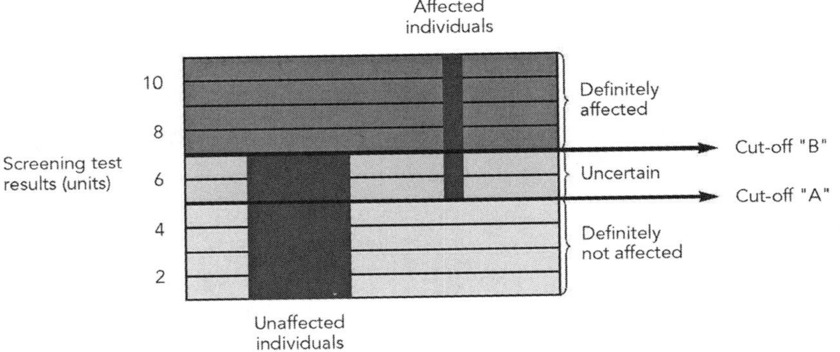

Figure 4.1. Setting a cut-off level for a screening test. In this example, a hypothetical screening test is applied with the ultimate goal of identifying individuals who are affected by a particular disease or condition. Individuals who ultimately prove to be unaffected show test results from 0 to 7 units; individuals who prove to be affected show test results ranging from 5 to 11 units. Individuals with test results above 7 or below 5 will be definitely identified by the screen as affected or unaffected; individuals testing between 5 and 7 may or may not be affected. If cut-off "A" is selected, all affected individuals will be correctly identified, but some unaffected individuals will be incorrectly identified as having disease (false positives). Because the number of unaffected individuals is so much larger than the number of individuals with disease, the majority of individuals testing positive will turn out to be unaffected. If cut-off "B" is selected, all unaffected individuals will be correctly identified, but some individuals with disease will be missed (false negatives). Selecting a cut-off level between "A" and "B" will result in a mix of false positives and false negatives.

Table 4.1. Recommended uniform screening panel—Core conditions

Type of disorder	Specific disorder
Amino acid disorders	
	Argininosuccinic aciduria (ASA)
	Citrullinemia type I
	Homocystinuria
	Maple syrup urine disease (MSUD)
	Phenylketonuria (PKU)
	Tyrosinemia type I
Organic acid disorders	
	3-hydroxy-3-methylglutaric aciduria (HMG)
	Glutaric acidemia type 1 (GA1)
	Isovaleric acidemia (IVA)
	3-methylcrotonyl-CoA carboxylase deficiency (3-MCC)
	Holocarboxylase synthetase deficiency
	Methylmalonic acidemia (cobalamin disorders)
	Methylmalonic acidemia (mutase deficiency)
	Beta-ketothiolase deficiency
	Propionic acidemia (PA)
Fatty acid oxidation disorders	
	Carnitine uptake defect/carnitine transport defects
	Long chain L-3 hydroxyacyl-CoA dehydrogenase deficiency (LCHAD)
	Medium chain acyl-CoA dehydrogenase deficiency (MCAD)
	Trifunctional protein deficiency (TFP)
	Very long chain acyl-CoA dehydrogenase deficiency (VLCAD)
Hemoglobinopathies	
	Hb S/S; Hb S/ßTh; Hb S/C
Endocrine disorders	
	Congenital adrenal hyperplasia
	Congenital hypothyroidism
Other	
	Biotinidase deficiency
	Cystic fibrosis
	Classical galactosemia
	Hearing loss
	Severe combined immune deficiency (SCID)
	Glycogen storage type 2 (Pompe)
	Mucopolysaccharidosis type 1 (Hurler)
	X-linked adrenoleukodystrophy
	Critical congenital heart disease

Sources: National Newborn Screening and Genetics Resource Center (2017) and U.S. Department of Health and Human Services (2018).

diseases are not part of the uniform panel, they are screened by some states and discussed below. In addition to disorders screened by blood, the panel has also recommended two disorders that are screened for by point-of-care studies performed in the nursery: hearing loss using a hearing screen (Choo & Meinzen-Derr, 2010; Wolff et al., 2010) and critical congenital heart disease (CHD) using the oxygen saturation measurement (Bruno & Havranek, 2015).

This chapter focuses on medical conditions that can be identified by newborn screening and that place the child at significant risk for developmental disabilities.

Table 4.2. Recommended uniform screening panel—Secondary targets

Type of disorder	Specific disorder
Amino acid disorders	
	Argininemia
	Citrullinemia II
	Defects of biopterin cofactor biosynthesis
	Defects of biopterin cofactor regeneration
	Hypermethioninemia
	Benign hyperphenylalaninemia
Organic acid disorders	
	2-methylbutyrylglycinuria (2MBG)
	2-methyl-3-hydroxybutyric aciduria (2M3HBA)
	3-methylglutaconic aciduria (3MGA)
	Isobutyrylglycinuria (IBG)
	Malonic acidemia (MAL)
	Methylmalonic academia with homocystinuria
	Tyrosinemia types II and III
Fatty acid oxidation disorders	
	2,4 dienoyl-CoA reductase deficiency (DE RED)
	Carnitine palmitoyltransferase I and II (CPT I and II)
	Carnitine acylcarnitine translocase deficiency (CACT)
	Medium-chain ketoacyl-CoA thiolase deficiency (MCKAT)
	Medium/short-chain L-3 hydroxyacyl-CoA dehydrogenase deficiency (M/SCHAD)
	Glutaric acidemia type II
	Short chain Acyl-CoA dehydrogenase deficiency (SCAD)
Other disorders	
	Galactokinase deficiency
	Galactose epimerase deficiency
	Other hemoglobinopathies
	T-cell–related lymphocyte deficiencies

It should be noted, however, that newborn screening is also conducted for additional conditions that carry significant medical and related emotional issues but do not place the infant at increased risk for developmental disabilities. These include congenital adrenal hyperplasia (White & Medscape, 2009), cystic fibrosis (Southern, Mérelle, Dankert-Roelse, & Nagelkerke, 2009), and sickle cell anemia/hemoglobinopathies (Benson & Therrell, 2010).

Hearing Loss

Infants are screened for hearing loss at the hospital where they are born. This is typically done at the bedside and is thus referred to as a point-of-care service. The incidence of severe to profound hearing loss is 1 out of 1,000, but it increases to 6 out of 1,000 when you include mild to moderate hearing loss. By 18 years of age, 17 out of 1,000 persons will be affected by some degree of permanent hearing loss (Grindle, 2014). In 2014, 97% of newborns were screened for hearing loss in the United States (current data are available at http://www.cdc.gov/ncbddd/hearingloss/data.html). The goals of screening for hearing loss are to 1) identify all children with a permanent loss by age 3 months, 2) initiate appropriate interventions by age 6 months, 3) establish a medical home for infants with permanent hearing loss, and 4) track data and quality metrics for public health initiatives. With the introduction of newborn hearing screening, the mean age of diagnosis of hearing loss has decreased from 2.5 years to 2 to 3 months of age. A detailed discussion of newborn hearing screening can be found in Chapter 7, and a discussion of the causes and interventions for hearing loss can be found in Chapter 26.

Critical Congenital Heart Disease

CHD is the most common congenital malformation, with an incidence of 8 to 12 per 1,000 live births. Critical

CHD (CCHD) occurs in about 1.5 per 1,000 newborns, accounting for 10%–15% of all heart defects. These are called critical defects as they require intervention in the first weeks of life or may cause significant morbidity (including developmental disabilities) or mortality (Frank, Bradshaw, Beckman, Mahle, & Martin, 2013). In one study, 50% of infants with previously undiagnosed CCHD died at home or in emergency departments (Chang, Gurvitz, & Rodriguez, 2008). Typically, these types of heart defects lead to low levels of oxygen in the newborn period and may be identified using **pulse oximetry screening** (a noninvasive method for monitoring oxygen saturation) at least 24 hours after birth. Some specific types of CCHDs are listed in Table 4.3. In September 2011, the U.S. Health and Human Services (HHS) Secretary added universal screening discharge pulse oximetry to the recommended universal screening panel in an effort to better identify asymptomatic infants with CCHD prior to discharge from the newborn nursery. Some states have been slow to recommend universal screening for these disorders due to problems with implementation (Studer, Smith, Lustik, & Carr, 2014). About 30 states have already implemented CCHD universal screening, and the remaining states either have some population screening or are working on implementation.

Endocrine Disorders

The endocrine system produces and regulates a variety of hormones that are critical to maintaining the body in a normal and balanced physiological state, called **homeostasis.** Several specific hormones are critical to the early growth and development of the central nervous system. Congenital hypothyroidism is a condition in which a newborn produces an inadequate amount of thyroid hormone. One in 3,000 infants is born with the condition, making it relatively common compared with many other disorders screened for in the newborn period. This is usually not due to a genetic defect. Early identification of this condition allows for early treatment with thyroid hormone replacement. Untreated infants have severe growth problems and atypical brain development, resulting in serious lifelong intellectual disability (Fingerhut & Olgemöller, 2009; Pass & Neto, 2009).

Table 4.3. Some specific critical congenital heart diseases

Coarctation of the aorta
Double-outlet right ventricle
d-Transposition of the great arteries
Ebstein anomaly
Hypoplastic left heart syndrome
Interrupted aortic arch
Pulmonary atresia (with intact septum)
Single ventricle
Total anomalous pulmonary venous return
Tetralogy of Fallot
Tricuspid atresia
Truncus arteriosus

Infectious Diseases

At the time of this writing, three states screen for human immunodeficiency virus (HIV), and another two states screen for ***Toxoplasmosis gondii.*** These are potentially serious infections in newborns. A positive screen for either of these organisms would require consultation with an infectious disease specialist for confirmation and treatment.

A positive HIV screen in the newborn indicates that the mother is infected and the newborn needs to be followed for the increased risk of disease. The goal of treatment for affected newborns with HIV is long-term suppression of viral replication with antiretroviral therapy (ARV) in order to prevent clinical symptoms of acquired immunodeficiency syndrome and to preserve the child's immune system. Guidelines for treatment are available via the HHS (see https://aidsinfo.nih.gov/). All pregnant women are offered HIV screening prenatally; this ensures that pregnant women who test positive can start ARV treatment and reduce the risk of "vertical" transmission to the fetus. As a result, there has been a more than a 70% reduction in the transmission of HIV from an infected mother to her newborn infant in the United States (Connor et al., 1994).

Untreated congenital toxoplasmosis results in multisystem disease, including seizures, visual impairments, and intellectual disability. The incidence of congenital toxoplasmosis ranges from 1 in 1,000 to 1 in 8,000 live births. Infants identified through newborn screening require treatment with pyrimethamine, sulfadiazine, and leucovorin over a year to reduce the incidence of the above sequelae (Röser, Nielsen, Petersen, Saugmann-Jensen, & Nørgaard-Pedersen, 2010).

Immune Disorders

Severe combined immunodeficiency (SCID) includes a group of disorders that leads to early childhood death as a result of severe infections (Puck, 2007). SCID is also known as the "bubble boy" or "bubble baby" disease because affected children used to be placed in a protected environment to reduce the risk of infection. Children receiving an early diagnosis via screening can benefit from hematologic stem cell transplantation (Lipstein et al., 2010). SCID was added to the recommended uniform screening panel in 2010 (see https://www.hrsa.gov/advisory-committees/heritable-disorders/index.html). As of 2018, it is being screened for in most states.

Metabolic Disorders

Metabolic disorders, also known as inborn errors of metabolism, represent a diverse group of genetic conditions that manifest as impairments of body chemistry at the cellular level (see Chapter 16). These conditions are often associated with the accumulation of atypical substances, or metabolites, in body fluids and tissues as a consequence of atypical functioning of proteins known as enzymes. Phenylketonuria (PKU) is a classic example of a screenable metabolic condition. In the United States, the incidence of PKU is 1 in 10,000, with an increased incidence in Caucasians of European decent. The disorder belongs to a group of metabolic conditions known as **amino acid disorders.** In PKU, a genetic mutation results in the deficiency of an enzyme needed to process phenylalanine, an amino acid common to most protein-laden foods, including meat and dairy products. Early identification of PKU by newborn screening allows implementation of a protein-restricted diet. In the absence of treatment, there is an accumulation of phenylalanine in blood and body tissues, with particularly severe consequences for the developing central nervous system.

Another relatively common metabolic disorder (with an incidence of 1 in 15,000) is MCAD, the disorder that Ashley has, as discussed in the opening case study. This disorder is the most common example of a group of metabolic conditions called **fatty acid oxidation disorders** (Kompare & Rizzo, 2008; Leonard & Dezateux, 2009). Normally, the body processes fat in order to release energy through oxidation. This is especially important during periods of fasting, when fat becomes the main source of energy for the body. Children with MCAD may become seriously ill after a period of fasting and may suffer permanent brain damage as a consequence of hypoglycemia. Careful monitoring and frequent feedings are essential, especially during infancy.

In addition to amino acid and fatty acid disorders, there are several other categories of metabolic diseases for which newborn screening is available. These include certain **urea cycle disorders, organic acidemias,** disorders of carbohydrate metabolism (e.g., **galactosemia**), and several miscellaneous enzyme deficiencies (e.g., **biotinidase deficiency**). These disorders are amenable to dietary intervention or to specific medical treatments. The newest group of disorders added to the uniform panel is storage disorders. These may be treatable with enzyme replacement therapy or stem cell transplant. **Pompe** (see Box 4.1) is a glycogen storage disorder that was added to the recommended universal screening panel in 2013. In 2015, both **mucopolysaccharidosis type 1** and **X-linked adrenoleukodystrophy** were added. As a group, the metabolic disorders now represent the largest number of potentially treatable conditions that can be identified through newborn screening and are the primary targets of the newest screening technologies.

HOW IS NEWBORN SCREENING DONE?

Most newborn screening tests rely on blood samples obtained during the first few days after birth (Fernhoff, 2009; Hiraki & Green, 2010; Levy, 2010). Testing begins by collecting a blood sample from a heel prick and blotting this onto a special filter-paper collection device. The sample is collected before the newborn is discharged from the birthing facility but after the infant has had an opportunity to feed, ideally at least 24 hours after birth. The infant must eat first because certain metabolic disorders cannot be detected until the body is challenged to metabolize the substances present in breast milk or formula. The filter paper is dried and sent to a newborn screening laboratory, usually a state Department of Health facility. The specimen is then divided into

BOX 4.1 EVIDENCE-BASED PRACTICE

Pompe's Addition to the Recommended Universal Screening Panel

Each disorder on the recommended uniform screening panel has an associated algorithm that helps clinicians decide what tests are needed in order to confirm or rule out a positive screen. When a new disorder is added to the newborn screening panel, then new algorithms and evidence-based treatment guidelines need to be devised. Pompe was approved in March 2015, and the Pompe Disease Newborn Screening Working Group recently published guidelines for the initial evaluation (algorithms) and management of confirmed positive patients (Burton et al., 2017).

multiple samples for use in a variety of tests screening for specific diseases. In the past, a different test was required for each disease. With the advent of tandem mass spectrometry, the number of tests that can be run on one sample has increased exponentially.

The mass spectrometer is a device that separates and quantifies ions based on their mass-to-charge ratio (American College of Medical Genetics & American Society of Human Genetics, 2000). The **tandem mass spectrometer (MS/MS)** consists of two of these devices separated by a reaction chamber such that accurate measurements of many different types of metabolites can be obtained at once (Chace, DiPerna, & Naylor, 1999). This is a very rapid and sensitive method for mass screening because a single sample can be screened in 1–2 minutes for numerous disorders (Chace, Kalas, & Naylor, 2003). This technology can improve the detection rate (lower the number of false positives) for diseases such as PKU (Marsden, Larson, & Levy, 2006). It is important to note that not all of the currently mandated disorders can be screened in this way, so other methods will continue to be needed.

Many states have second-tier testing if the initial biochemical test is found to be atypical. Second-tier testing is usually performed by the same laboratory that performed the initial screen and occurs automatically as part of the screening algorithm. Under this method, a sample is tested and flagged as atypical relative to an expected range for the test. The sample is then sent for a second-tier test that aids in the interpretation of the initial screening result. For example, a specimen might be atypical for immunoreactive trypsinogen (IRT), a test for cystic fibrosis. That sample may then be tested for at least some of the common DNA mutations associated with cystic fibrosis. If one or two mutations are found, the sample may be coded as positive. If no mutation is found then the sample may be coded as negative or positive depending on the level of IRT. Second-tier testing may involve genetic testing (testing of the DNA of the infant, see Chapter 1). By adding second-tier testing (such as DNA), the sensitivity of the test is increased. However, an increased number of carriers (false positives—individuals with a single copy of the mutated gene who actually do not have cystic fibrosis) are also identified (Baker et al., 2016).

WHAT SHOULD BE DONE WHEN A CHILD HAS A POSITIVE NEWBORN SCREEN?

In practice, each state decides how to handle positive screening results and how to follow up. In general, there should be prompt notification of the physician of record (usually the primary care pediatrician or family practitioner) and the infant's family. Definitive testing should confirm the diagnosis. If the diagnosis is confirmed, a treatment plan specific to that disorder should be initiated. The family is typically referred to a specialty consultant or program, and genetic counseling is offered. Some of the conditions screened for require urgent evaluation and onset of therapy, such as organic acidemias, carbohydrate and urea cycle disorders, and immune and endocrine diseases. All interventions require close collaboration among the medical specialist, primary care physician, public health department, and the family.

Even when the follow-up plan for a positive newborn screen operates efficiently and effectively, families experience significant stress related to the process. As previously discussed, many positive screens turn out to be false positives. In many conditions, for every 10 infants with a positive screen, only 1 will be found to actually have the disease. Even though these other 9 infants will ultimately prove to be unaffected, the process leading to this conclusion can be difficult for families. Mothers of false-positive infants have been found to have significantly increased stress level scores compared with mothers of screen-negative infants, and they score higher on measures of parent–child dysfunction. Having the child seen at a specialty center (e.g., a metabolic or genetic disorders clinic at an academic medical center) or communicating repeat screening results in person seems to improve this situation (Waisbren et al., 2003). While it is important for families to understand that a positive newborn screen does not automatically mean that their infant has a problem, it is equally important that appropriate follow-up is pursued in a timely fashion to allow identification of truly affected infants.

WHAT HAPPENS TO CHILDREN WITH CONFIRMED DISEASE?

Infants with a positive newborn screen are often referred to a center where they can be seen by a medical specialist who has expertise in the condition for which positive screening occurred (James & Levy, 2006). This may be a hematologist, a pulmonologist, an endocrinologist, an infectious disease specialist, or a geneticist. In some states, families may have access to multidisciplinary clinics that include nurses, genetic counselors, social workers, and nutritionists in addition to pediatrician specialists. The specialist conducts additional testing to confirm the specific diagnosis or to aid in genetic counseling. Once the diagnosis is established, the child will require ongoing (and often lifelong) care for that condition. The specific interventions employed will depend on the diagnosis (e.g., see Chapter 16). In general, the focus is to provide long-term therapy for the child and ongoing counseling to the family, with the ultimate goal of improving medical, neurodevelopmental, and psychosocial outcomes. Some disorders are relatively easy to manage with medications or supplements (e.g., thyroid hormone replacement therapy for congenital hypothyroidism or biotin therapy [a B vitamin] for biotinidase deficiency). Other disorders are more complex and may require a combination of medications, supplements, and dietary changes. For example, the treatment of PKU requires protein restriction and replacement of normal food items with synthetic, non-phenylalanine-containing substitutes and medication. This is usually achieved using special formulas (medical food) in infants and young children or supplemental nutrition bars in older children and adults. Although this sounds quite simple, for most individuals and families it is a very burdensome diet and is complicated by the fact that these specialized foods are costly and may not be covered by medical insurance. The cost of medication is a significant problem for individuals with storage disorders, as enzyme replacement therapy can cost hundreds of thousands of dollars each year (see Chapter 16).

As most of these disorders are inherited, genetic testing may be recommended to confirm the diagnosis or to provide additional prognostic information. Once a specific mutation is identified, prenatal diagnosis may be available for the next pregnancy if the family chooses to pursue this (see Chapter 3). The **recurrence risk** (risk that another child will be born with the same condition in the future) is an appropriate concern. Because most metabolic disorders are inherited as autosomal recessive traits (see Chapter 1), the statistical risk of recurrence is 25%.

WHAT IS THE RISK OF DEVELOPMENTAL DISABILITY IN CHILDREN WITH CONFIRMED DISEASE?

The neurodevelopmental and functional sequelae of a particular disorder identified through newborn screening is specific to that disorder. Unidentified and untreated these disorders invariably lead to significant morbidity. A few studies have addressed the issue of developmental outcomes in children who have an underlying metabolic disorder and were diagnosed by newborn screening. In one study (Waisbren et al., 2003), the children identified by newborn screening had fewer developmental and health problems and functioned better (as evidenced by developmental testing) compared with those children diagnosed at a later age based on clinical symptoms. The children identified through screening had fewer hospitalizations, shorter hospital stays, and 60% fewer medical problems, and they scored significantly higher on developmental testing. Despite this positive outlook, many of these diseases, especially the storage disorders, are still associated with severe developmental disabilities (Dhondt, 2010).

HOW CAN SCREENING FAIL?

There are a number of steps during which newborn screening can fail. First, the newborn may have been missed being screened at the hospital. Second, many states allow for exemptions from newborn screening based on religious or other reasons. Other possibilities are that the newborn may have been born at home, the newborn may have been transferred to another hospital, or the specimen could have been lost or misidentified. There are also reasons why an infant could screen negative but still have a disease (i.e., a false-negative result). For example, it is possible that the specimen was obtained too early. As previously noted, for some of the metabolic disorders, the infant needs to be at least 24 hours old and must have been fed an adequate amount of formula or breast milk before a screening test can be valid. If the infant has not eaten, then the metabolites for some of the diseases will not accumulate and the test will yield a false-negative result. For some disorders, the test is not accurate if the infant has had a blood transfusion. Things as simple as how much blood is collected, how long the sample is dried, how long it took to get to the state lab, and even the weather conditions during shipment can result in inaccurate test results. In addition, infants are sometimes "lost" to follow-up. It may be difficult to actually locate a specific infant due to a name change for the infant, family relocations, inadequate information provided with the sample (e.g., wrong address or telephone number), or a new physician of record.

Newborn screening can be particularly challenging in infants who are born prematurely or are critically ill in the neonatal intensive care unit. The false-positive rate increases with decreasing birth weight and gestation age and is significantly increased in very-low-birth-weight neonates (< 1,000 g) and infants with a gestational age of greater than 32 weeks. Strategies to decrease the false-positive rate include waiting for greater than 48 hours to obtain the first sample in infants with a gestational age of less than 32 weeks (Slaughter et al., 2010) and stopping nutrition 3 hours before sample collection (Morris et al., 2014).

The purpose of newborn screening is to identify affected infants, but as previously noted, a certain number of unaffected infants will be identified as being at risk. For some conditions, these false-positive cases turn out to represent individuals who are carriers for the condition. With the advent of DNA testing, an increasing number of carrier infants have been identified. These infants do not have the disease but are carrying one DNA mutation for the screened disease. In many cases, the families of these newborns will be referred to a specialty center for further testing and counseling. If it is determined that the infant is a carrier, then genetic counseling will be offered to the parents so that they can better understand the risk of recurrence for themselves, for their child (and his or her future children), and for the child's siblings (who may also be carriers for the condition).

THE PAST, PRESENT, AND FUTURE OF NEWBORN SCREENING

The first successful newborn screening program was started in Massachusetts in 1962 with screening for PKU (MacCready, 1963). Preventive screening was mandated by the state and subsequently adopted by other states over a period of several years. Expansion of newborn screening began in earnest in 1975, when a test was developed to screen for congenital hypothyroidism (Dussault et al., 1975; LaFranchi, 2010). The success of newborn screening for this disorder led to the addition of testing for an increasing number of disorders. Each year more than 4 million newborns are screened in the United States for a variety of disorders, and approximately 6,000 infants are diagnosed with a detectable and treatable disorder (National Newborn Screening and Genetics Resource Center, 2017; U.S. Department of Health and Human Services, 2018). Each state decides which disorders will be screened for, but the majority of states are providing universal screening for most of the 34 core conditions. Most states have mandatory screening (i.e., all newborns must be screened) with implied consent. Some states have a single designated laboratory that performs all screening testing; others contract with regional centers, university laboratories, or private laboratories. Each state must decide how the screening process is to be conducted, how to notify the parents and professionals of the results, and how to follow up on atypical results. Each state may make a different decision depending on a number of factors including its resources, population mix, and birth rate. However, with the passage of The Newborn Screening Saves Lives Act of 2008, most states have begun to follow a uniform practice for performing and following up on newborn screening (National Newborn Screening and Genetics Resource Center, 2017).

Further expansion of screening programs has been driven by consumer activism and new technologies (especially tandem mass spectroscopy). The HHS Secretary's Advisory Committee on Heritable Disorders in Newborns and Children has developed an evidence review process to consider additional conditions for universal screening. As of September 2017, they have evaluated 12 conditions and recommended the addition of 5 to the uniform panel. The advisory committee looks at the scientific evidence to make recommendations for inclusion in the screening panel by reviewing the condition, diagnosis, treatment, and screening methods. They consider the natural history of the disease, at how early and by what method the disease is diagnosed, and at the clinical variability and burden of disease. They also review information on the methods available for newborn screening, including the validity, sensitivity, positive-predictive value, cost, and whether or not it can be multiplexed (more than one disease identified from the same run). Then they review the diagnosis and treatment options to see if confirmation of the diagnosis is available and if early identification and treatment can improve the outcome (Calonge et al., 2010).

A state can also add diseases to their newborn screening panel through their own legislative acts. Therefore, some conditions that were not recommended by the advisory committee are, in fact, being tested for in a few specific states. The lysosomal storage disorders are a good example of this. These are a group of about 40 diseases in which there is progressive accumulation of a substance in the **lysosome** (a cellular organelle containing degradative enzymes) that is normally broken down. In lysosomal storage disorders, the substance is unable to be metabolized due to a defect in an enzyme. Some of these disorders are treatable by either enzyme replacement therapy or hematopoetic stem cell transplantation. However, in order to optimize treatment, it should begin as soon as possible, making early identification critical. Table 4.4 includes a variety of disorders, including lysosomal storage diseases, that are being screened for in at least one state. As new technologies are developed and therapeutic advances are made, the list of conditions recommended for newborn screening is likely to expand. As an example, with the completion of the Human Genome Project, the discovery of hundreds of mutations causing disorders being screened for opens the possibility of using expression microarray technology to screen for these mutations in the newborn period rather than to screen for metabolic impairments resulting from the mutations (the MS/

Table 4.4. Disorders screened in newborns by at least one state but not part of the recommended uniform screening panel

5-oxoprolinuria (pyroglutamic aciduria)
Carbamoylphosphate synthetase
Nonketotic hyperglycinemia
Prolinemia
Ethylmalonic encephalopathy
Glucose-6-phosphate dehydrogenase
Hyperammonemia/ornithinemia/citrullinemia (Ornithine transporter defect)
MPS-II mucopolysaccharidosis type II (Hunter syndrome)
Krabbe disease
Niemann-Pick disease
Gaucher disease
Fabry disease
Congenital human immunodeficiency virus
Congenital toxoplasmosis

Source: National Newborn Screening and Genetics Resource Center (2014).

MS method). Chromosomal microarray has become the first-tier test for individuals with developmental disabilities or congenital anomalies (Miller et al., 2010; also see Chapter 1). This technology could be used for newborn screening as well. Whole-genome sequencing studies have also been piloted for newborn screening (Bodian et al., 2016).

There is no doubt that newborn screening will expand in the future. The challenge will be to balance the legal, ethical, and social concerns that can be raised by expanded screening (DeLuca, 2017). As an example, there is clinical variation in many of the screenable diseases, making it difficult to know who to treat and when to institute therapy. Furthermore, DNA-based technology can detect carriers and also detect sequence variations and polymorphisms for which we have little information, making it difficult to know the clinical significance (Bodian et al., 2016). There may also be a paradigm shift from the newborn as the patient to the family as the patient. In this view, the family receives the information on carrier status and its implications for prenatal diagnoses in future pregnancies (McCabe & McCabe, 2008).

SUMMARY

- Screening tests are important tools used to help define increased risk for significant medical and genetic conditions.
- Screening tests can be used for mass screening of newborns, prenatal screening, and targeted screening of at-risk populations and ethnic groups.
- Newborn screening is an important and effective public health measure.
- Many infants have been identified by screening and have been successfully treated with improved outcomes though they may have lifelong complications.
- The number of disorders screened for has grown over time and will continue to increase.
- Parents have been the greatest advocates for expanding newborn screening and will continue to play a major role as we move forward (Lipstein et al., 2010).
- As more infants are identified with more disorders, future research will be aimed at developing innovative therapies to further improve outcomes.

ADDITIONAL RESOURCES

Baby's First Test: http://www.babysfirsttest.org/

Newborn Screening Portal, CDC: https://www.cdc.gov/newbornscreening/

MedlinePlus: https://medlineplus.gov/newbornscreening.html

Additional resources can be found online in Appendix D: Childhood Disabilities Resources, Services, and Organizations (see About the Online Companion Materials).

REFERENCES

American College of Medical Genetics & American Society of Human Genetics Test and Technology Transfer Committee. (2000). Tandem mass spectroscopy in newborn screening. *Genetics in Medicine, 2*, 267–269.

Baker, M. W., Atkins, A. E., Cordovado, S. K., Hendrix, M., Earley, M. C., & Farrell, P. M. (2016). Improving newborn screening for cystic fibrosis using next generation sequencing technology: A technical feasibility study. *Genetics in Medicine, 18*(3), 231–237.

Benson, J. M., & Therrell, B. L., Jr. (2010). History and current status of newborn screening for hemoglobinopathies. *Seminars in Perinatology, 34*(2), 134–144.

Bodian, D. L., Klein, E., Iyer, R. K., Wong, W. S. W., Kothiyal, P., Stauffer, D., . . . Solomon, B. D. (2016). Utility of whole-genome sequencing for detection of newborn screening disorders in a population cohort of 1,696 neonates. *Genetics in Medicine, 18*(3), 221–230.

Burton, B. K., Kronn, D. F., Hwu, W. L., & Kishnani, P. S. (2017, July). The initial evaluation of patients after positive newborn screening: Recommended algorithms leading to confirmed diagnosis of Pompe disease. *Pediatrics, 140*(Suppl. 1), S14–S23.

Bruno, C. J., & Havranek, T. (2015). Screening for critical congenital heart disease in newborns. *Advanced Pediatrics, 62*(1), 211–226. doi:10.1016/j.yapd.2015.04.002

Calonge, N., Green, N. S., Rinaldo, P., Llyod-Puryear, M., Dougherty, D., Boyle, C., . . . The Advisory Committee on Heritable Disorders in Newborns and Children. (2010). Committee report: Method for evaluating conditions nominated for population-based screening of newborns and children. *Genetics in Medicine, 12*(3), 153–159.

Chace, D. H., DiPerna, J. C., & Naylor, E. W. (1999). Laboratory integration and utilization of tandem mass spectroscopy in neonatal screening: A model for clinical mass spectroscopy in the next millennium. *Acta Paediatrica Supplement, 88,* 45–47.

Chace, D. H., Kalas, T. A., & Naylor, E. W. (2003). Use of tandem mass spectrometry for multianalyte screening of dried blood specimens from newborns. *Clinical Chemistry, 49,* 1797–1817.

Chang, R. K. R., Gurvitz, M., & Rodriguez, S. (2008). Missed diagnosis of critical congenital heart disease. *Archives of Pediatric and Adolescent Medicine, 162,* 969–974.

Choo, D., & Meinzen-Derr, J. (2010). Universal newborn hearing screening in 2010. *Current Opinions in Otolaryngology and Head and Neck Surgery, 18*(5), 399–404.

Connor, E. M., Sperling, R. S., Gelber, R., Kiselev, P., Scott, G., O'Sullivan, MJ, . . . Jacobson R. L. (1994). Reduction of maternal-infant transmission of human immunodeficiency virus type 1 with zidovudine treatment. Pediatric AIDS Clinical Trials Group Protocol 076 Study Group. *New England Journal of Medicine, 331*(18), 1173–1180. PMID:7935654

DeLuca, J. M. (2017, January–February). Public attitudes towards expanded newborn screening. *Journal of Pediatric Nursing,* e19–e23.

Dhondt, J. L. (2010). Expanded newborn screening: Social and ethical issues. *Journal of Inherited Metabolic Disease, 33*(Suppl. 2), S211–S217.

Dussault, J. H., Coulombe, P., Laberge, C., Letarte, J., Guyda, H., & Khoury, K. (1975). Preliminary report on a mass screening program for neonatal hypothyroidism. *Journal of Pediatrics, 86,* 670–674.

Fernhoff, P. M. (2009). Newborn screening for genetic disorders. *Pediatric Clinics of North America, 56*(3), 505–513.

Fingerhut, R., & Olgemöller, B. (2009). Newborn screening for inborn errors of metabolism and endocrinopathies: An update. *Analytical and Bioanalytical Chemistry, 393*(5), 1481–1497.

Frank, L. H., Bradshaw, E., Beckman, R., Mahle, W. T., & Martin, G. R. (2013). Critical congenital heart disease screening using pulse oximetry. *Journal of Pediatrics, 162*(3), 445–453.

Grindle, C. R. (2014). Pediatric hearing loss. *Pediatrics in Review, 35*(11), 456–464.

Hiraki, S., & Green, N. S. (2010). Newborn screening for treatable genetic conditions: Past, present, and future. *Obstetrics & Gynecology Clinics of North America, 37*(1), 11–21.

James, P. M., & Levy, H. L. (2006). The clinical aspects of newborn screening: Importance of newborn screening follow-up. *Mental Retardation and Developmental Disabilities Research Reviews, 12*(4), 246–254.

Kompare, M., & Rizzo, W. B. (2008). Mitochondrial fatty-acid oxidation disorders. *Seminars in Pediatric Neurology, 15*(3), 140–149.

LaFranchi, S. H. (2010). Newborn screening strategies for congenital hypothyroidism: An update. *Journal of Inherited Metabolic Disease, 33*(Suppl. 2), S225–S233.

Leonard, J. V., & Dezateux, C. (2009). Newborn screening for medium chain acyl CoA dehydrogenase deficiency. *Archives of Disease in Childhood, 94*(3), 235–238.

Levy, P. A. (2010). An overview of newborn screening. *Journal of Developmental & Behavioral Pediatrics, 31*(7), 622–631.

Lipstein, E. A., Vorono, S., Browning, M. F., Green, N. S., Kemper, A. R., Knapp, A. A., . . . Perrin, J. M. (2010). Systematic evidence review of newborn screening and treatment of severe combined immunodeficiency. *Pediatrics, 125*(5), e1226–1235.

MacCready, R. (1963). Phenylketonuria screening program. *The New England Journal of Medicine, 269,* 52–56.

Marsden, D., Larson, C., & Levy, H. L. (2006). Newborn screening for metabolic disorders. *Journal of Pediatrics, 148,* 577–584.

McCabe, L. L., & McCabe, E. R. B. (2008). Expanded newborn screening: Implications for genomic medicine. *Annual Review of Medicine, 59,* 163–175.

Miller, D. T., Adam, M. P., Aradhya, S., Biesecker, L. G., Brothman, A. R., Carter, N. P., . . . Ledbetter, D. H. (2010). Consensus statement: Chromosomal microarray is a first tier clinical diagnostic test for individuals with developmental disabilities or congenital anomalies. *The American Journal of Human Genetics, 86,* 749–764.

Morris, M., Fischer, K., Leydiker, K., Elliott, L., Newby, J., & Abdenur, J. (2014). Reduction in newborn screening metabolic false positive results following a new collection protocol. *Genetics in Medicine, 16,* 477–483.

National Newborn Screening and Genetics Resource Center. (2014). *Newborn screening status report.* Retrieved from http://genes-r-us.uthscsa.edu/sites/genes-r-us/files/nbsdisorders.pdf

National Newborn Screening and Genetics Resource Center. (2017). *National newborn screening status report.* Retrieved from http://genes-r-us.uthscsa.edu/

Newborn Screening Expert Group. (2005). Newborn screening: Towards a uniform screening panel and system. *Federal Register, 70,* 44. Retrieved from https://www.hrsa.gov/sites/default/files/hrsa/advisory-committees/heritable-disorders/newborn-uniform-screening-panel.pdf

Pass, K. A., & Neto, E. C. (2009). Update: Newborn screening for endocrinopathies. *Endocrinology Metabolism Clinics of North America, 38*(4), 827–737.

Puck, J. M. (2007). Neonatal screening for severe combined immune deficiency. *Current Opinion in Allergy and Clinical Immunology, 7*(6), 522–527.

Röser, D., Nielsen, H. V., Petersen, E., Saugmann-Jensen, P., & Nørgaard-Pedersen, P. B. (2010). Congenital toxoplasmosis: A report on the Danish neonatal screening programme 1999–2007. *Journal of Inherited Metabolic Disease, 33*(Suppl. 2), S241–S247.

Slaughter, J. L., Meinzen-Derr, J., Rose, S. R., Leslie, N. D., Chandraesekar, R., Linard, S. M., & Akinbi, H. T. (2010). The effects of gestational age and birth weight on false positive newborn screening rates. *Pediatrics, 126*(5), 910–916.

Southern, K. W., Mérelle, M. M., Dankert-Roelse, J. E., & Nagelkerke, A. D. (2009). Newborn screening for cystic fibrosis. *Cochrane Database Systematic Review, 21*(1), CD001402.

Studer, M. A., Smith, A. E., Lustik, M. B., & Carr, M. R. (2014). Newborn pulse oximetry screening detect critical congenital heart disease. *Journal of Pediatrics, 164,* 505–509.

U.S. Department of Health and Human Services. (2018). *Advisory Committee on Heritable Disorders in Newborns and Children.* Retrieved from https://www.hrsa.gov/advisory-committees/mchbadvisory/heritabledisorders/index.html

Waisbren, S. E., Albers, S., Amato, S., Ampola, M., Brewster, T. G., Demmer, L., & Levy, H. L. (2003). Effect of expanded newborn screening for biochemical genetic disorders on child outcomes and parental stress. *Journal of the American Medical Association, 290*(19), 2564–2572.

White, P. C., & Medscape. (2009). Neonatal screening for congenital adrenal hyperplasia. *Nature Reviews Endrocrinology, 5*(9), 490–498.

Wolff, R., Hommerich, J., Riemsma, R., Antes, G., Lange, S., & Kleijnen, J. (2010). Hearing screening in newborns: Systematic review of accuracy, effectiveness, and effects of interventions after screening. *Archives of Disease in Childhood, 95*(2), 130–135.

CHAPTER 5 Premature and Small-for-Dates Infants

Khodayar Rais-Bahrami and Billie Lou Short

Upon completion of this chapter, the reader will

- Recognize some of the causes of prematurity and reasons that infants may be small for their gestational age
- Be able to identify physical characteristics of the premature infant
- Understand the complications and illnesses associated with preterm birth
- Be aware of the methods used to care for low birth weight infants
- Know the results of outcome studies

The preterm infant is at an immediate disadvantage compared with the full-term infant. In addition to facing all of the usual challenges of making the transition from intrauterine to extrauterine life, the preterm infant must make these changes using organs that are not yet ready to perform the task. Almost every organ is immature (Hyman, Novoa, & Holzman, 2011). Decreased production of a substance called surfactant in the lungs can lead to respiratory distress syndrome (RDS); immaturity of the central nervous system places the preterm infant at increased risk for an **intraventricular hemorrhage** (IVH), **periventricular leukomalacia** (PVL), and **hydrocephalus;** and inadequate kidney function makes fluid and metabolic management difficult. An immature gastrointestinal tract impairs the infant's ability to digest and absorb certain nutrients and places the gut at risk for developing a life-threatening disorder called **necrotizing enterocolitis** (NEC) that results from inadequate blood supply to the small intestine. Finally, the preterm infant's eyes are more susceptible to the damaging effects of the oxygen that is used to treat respiratory distress. This may result in **retinopathy of prematurity** (ROP) and the potential for subsequent vision loss (see Chapter 7). Given all the risks, it is remarkable that most preterm infants overcome these acute problems with little residual effects. A minority, however, do sustain long-term medical and neurodevelopmental complications. A discussion of these complications and their prevention is the focus of this chapter.

CASE STUDY

Erin was born prematurely, at 23 weeks' gestation, weighing less than 500 grams (about 1 pound). During Erin's first day of life, she needed artificial ventilation and surfactant therapy to keep the air passages in her lungs open. By 2 months of age, she was doing well enough to receive a pressurized oxygen–air mixture through a high-flow **nasal cannula** (nose tube), but she had brief breathing arrests (**apnea**) associated with a slowed heart rate (**bradycardia**). These problems were treated successfully with caffeine and frequent physical stimulation. In addition, she developed NEC, leading to small bowel (intestine) perforation that required two major abdominal surgeries 10 weeks apart.

Meeting Erin's nutritional requirements was also a problem. Initially, she needed intravenous nutrition. Gradually, she was able to tolerate increasing amounts of elemental infant formula by a nasogastric (nose to stomach) tube, and by 3 months, she was strong enough to receive some of her feedings by bottle. At her 168th day of life (i.e., postconceptional age of 45 weeks), weighing 3,760 grams (8 pounds, 4½ ounces), Erin went home on oxygen and caffeine (to prevent apneic episodes) and was hooked up to an apnea monitor while taking all feedings by mouth. Her parents had been instructed how to administer oxygen therapy, how to use the monitor, and how to administer cardiopulmonary resuscitation (CPR) if she had a prolonged apneic episode. Although her overall prognosis is good, Erin will need continued medical and neurodevelopmental monitoring until she is school age.

Thought Question:

Define *SGA infants.* What are the maternal, placental, and fetal factors leading to SGA infants?

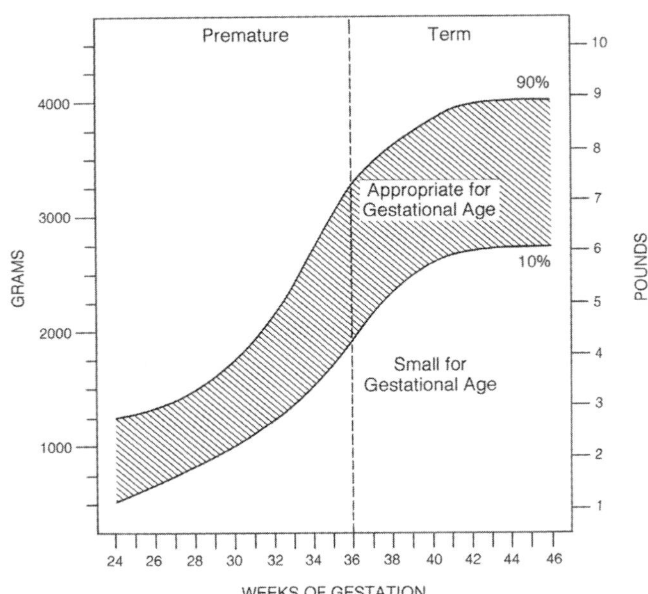

Figure 5.1. Newborn weight by gestational age. The shaded area between the 10th and 90th percentiles represents infants who are appropriate for gestational age. Weight below the 10th percentile makes an infant small for gestational age. Prematurity is defined as being born before 36 weeks' gestation. (From Lubchenco, L. O. [1976]. *The high risk infant*. Philadelphia, PA: W.B. Saunders; reprinted by permission.)

DEFINITIONS OF PREMATURITY AND LOW BIRTH WEIGHT

A preterm or premature infant is one born before or at 36 weeks' gestation. Although there is no universal system for birth weight classification, it is commonly accepted that an infant with a birth weight less than 2,500 grams (5½ pounds) is categorized as **low birth weight** (LBW), an infant born weighing less than 1,500 grams (3⅓ pounds) is **very low birth weight** (VLBW), and an infant with a birth weight lower than 1,000 grams (2¼ pounds) is **extremely low birth weight** (ELBW). An infant weighing less than 800 grams (1¾ pounds) is sometimes called a **micropreemie** (Dani, Poggi, Romangnoli, & Bertini, 2009). Assessment of gestational age is also important because LBW infants may represent prematurely born infants or those who have fetal growth restriction (see Chapter 6) and are **small for gestational age (SGA)**.

Small-for-Gestational-Age (SGA) Infants

SGA infants can be either full term or premature. In either case, they have a birth weight below the 10th percentile using a graph of population-specific birth weight verses gestational age (Figure 5.1). SGA infants are also referred to as dysmature, or small for dates. In addition to being small, these infants appear malnourished, usually because of **intrauterine or fetal growth restriction.** About one half of SGA births are attributable to maternal illness, smoking, or malnutrition (Grivell, Dodd, & Robinson, 2009). These infants tend to be underweight but have normal length and head circumference; they are said to have asymmetric SGA because of this discrepancy in growth pattern. The other half of SGA births are said to have symmetric SGA (equally deviant in length, weight, and head circumference). These infants may have been exposed *in utero* to alcohol or to infections such as cytomegalovirus (see Chapter 6). Infants with certain chromosomal and other genetic disorders also present as symmetrical SGA infants (Adams-Chapman et al., 2013). Even in uncomplicated pregnancies, SGA infants, as compared with **appropriate-for-gestational-age** newborns, have a significantly higher risk of neonatal morbidity and mortality and of being stillborn. The following morbidities are significantly more common among term SGA neonates when compared with appropriate-for-gestational-age neonates: An Apgar less than 4 at 5 minutes, respiratory distress syndrome, requirement for mechanical ventilation, NEC, grade 2 or 3 IVH, and neonatal sepsis. SGA infants, whether full term or preterm, are recognized as having an increased risk for many other complications in the newborn period (e.g., hypoxia, hypothermia, and hypoglycemia), increased perinatal and neonatal mortality, long-term growth impairments, and developmental disabilities (Argente, Mehls, & Barrios, 2010; de Bie, Oostrom, & Delemarre-van de Wall, 2010; Mendez-Figueroa, Truong, Pedroza, Khan, & Chauhan, 2016; Sinclair, Bottino, & Cowett, 2009).

Assessment of Gestational Age

Assessment of gestational age helps distinguish an appropriate-for-gestational-age infant from an SGA infant. In addition, it influences treatment approaches, neurodevelopmental assessment, and outcome. The gestational age is calculated from the projected birth date, or estimated date of confinement. This can be obtained using the Nägele rule: Add 7 days and subtract 3 months from the date of the last menstrual period. The accuracy of menstrual dating, however, is quite variable, especially in anticipated preterm deliveries. In most cases, uterine size is an accurate predictor of gestational age and can be measured by clinical and ultrasound examination. Another way of estimating gestational age is by noting when fetal activity first develops. **Quickening** is first felt by the mother at approximately 16–18 weeks' gestation. Fetal heart sounds can be first detected at approximately 10–12 weeks by ultrasound and at 20 weeks by fetoscope (similar to a stethoscope). Following birth, gestational age can be assessed using a clinical scoring system called the modified Dubowitz examination (discussed next). Another technique allows for estimating the degree of prematurity by examining the maturity of the lens of the eye in the first 24–48 hours of life (Nagpal, Kumar, & Ramji, 2004). Using a combination of these methods increases the accuracy of gestational age assessment.

Physical and Behavioral Characteristics of the Premature Infant

Several physical and developmental characteristics distinguish the premature infant from the full-term infant. Historically, the scoring system developed by Dubowitz, Dubowitz, and Goldberg (1970) and updated by Ballard and colleagues (1991) takes these characteristics into account and enables the physician to estimate the infant's gestational age with some accuracy (Figure 5.2). The limitation of this scoring system is the postnatal age of the infant. If the scoring is not performed within the first 24 hours of birth, neurological and some physical features (e.g., skin texture) can change, making the infant appear more mature. Also, any severely ill infant can be difficult to evaluate due to altered neurological status.

The main physical characteristics that distinguish a premature infant from a full-term infant are the presence of fine body hair (**lanugo**) and smooth, reddish skin, along with the absence of skin creases, ear cartilage, and breast buds (Figure 5.3). In addition to the physical appearance, premature infants display distinctive neurological and behavioral characteristics, including reduced muscle tone and activity and increased joint mobility (Constantine et al., 1987). Low muscle tone is particularly evident in the infant born before 28 weeks' gestation; it gradually improves with advancing gestational age, starting with the legs and moving up to the arms by 32 weeks gestational age. Thus, while the premature infant lies in a floppy, extended position, the full-term infant rests in a semi-flexed position. As flexion tone improves over the weeks after birth, increased joint mobility disappears. Finally, as compared with the full-term infant, the premature infant may appear behaviorally passive and have disorganized movements in the first weeks of life (Mandrich, Simons, Ritchie, Schmidt, & Mullet, 1994).

INCIDENCE OF PRETERM BIRTHS

The preterm birth rate in the United States declined for the seventh straight year in 2014 to 9.57%; the LBW rate was unchanged at 8.00%. The infant mortality rate decreased to a historic low of 5.82 infant deaths per 1,000 live births (Mathews & Driscoll, 2017). While preterm birth represents a minority of pregnancies, it is responsible for the majority of neonatal deaths and nearly one half of all cases of neonatal-onset neurodevelopmental disabilities, including cerebral palsy (Stavsky et al., 2017). The risk is highest in infants born before 32 weeks' gestation, representing 2% of all births. Preterm births occur twice as frequently in African Americans as in Caucasians. Of LBW infants weighing less than 2,500 grams, 70% are preterm and 30% are full-term infants who are SGA (Heron et al., 2010; Murphy, Mathews, Martin, Minkovitz, & Strobino, 2017).

CAUSES OF PREMATURE BIRTH

Preterm delivery is certainly a cause for concern and has been associated with a number of cofactors: obstetric interventions (e.g., cesarean sections); assisted reproduction techniques (e.g., *in vitro* fertilization); multiple-gestation births; substance abuse, low socioeconomic status, and low maternal educational level;

Neuromuscular Maturity

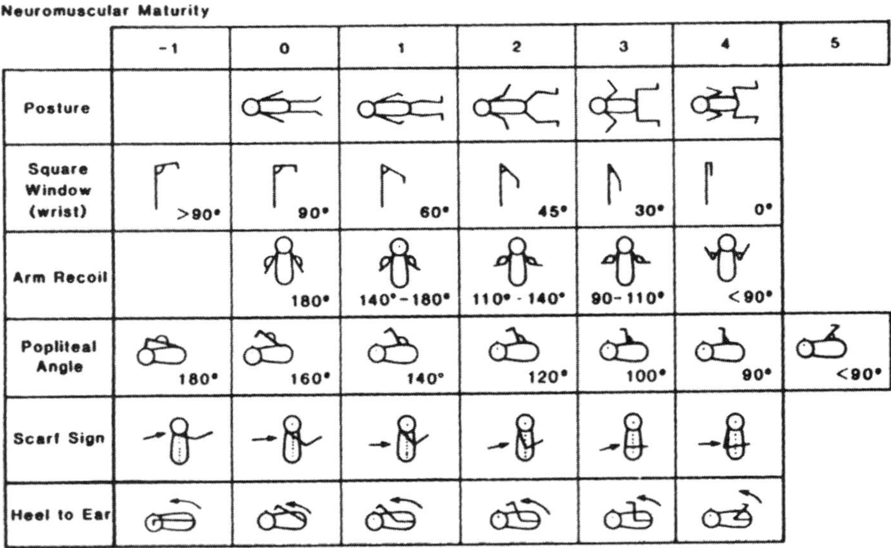

-1
0
1
2
3
4
5
Posture
Square Window (wrist)
>90°
90°
60°
45°
30°
0°
Arm Recoil
180°
140°-180°
110°-140°
90-110°
<90°
Popliteal Angle
180°
160°
140°
120°
100°
90°
<90°
Scarf Sign
Heel to Ear

Physical Maturity

Skin	sticky friable transparent	gelatinous red, translucent	smooth pink, visible veins	superficial peeling &/or rash. few veins	cracking pale areas rare veins	parchment deep cracking no vessels	leathery cracked wrinkled
Lanugo	none	sparse	abundant	thinning	bald areas	mostly bald	
Plantar Surface	heel-toe 40-50 mm: -1 <40 mm: -2	>50mm no crease	faint red marks	anterior transverse crease only	creases ant. 2/3	creases over entire sole	
Breast	imperceptible	barely perceptible	flat areola no bud	stippled areola 1-2mm bud	raised areola 3-4mm bud	full areola 5-10mm bud	
Eye/Ear	lids fused loosely: -1 tightly: -2	lids open pinna flat stays folded	sl. curved pinna; soft; slow recoil	well-curved pinna; soft but ready recoil	formed &firm instant recoil	thick cartilage ear stiff	
Genitals male	scrotum flat, smooth	scrotum empty faint rugae	testes in upper canal rare rugae	testes descending few rugae	testes down good rugae	testes pendulous deep rugae	
Genitals female	clitoris prominent labia flat	prominent clitoris small labia minora	prominent clitoris enlarging minora	majora & minora equally prominent	majora large minora small	majora cover clitoris & minora	

Maturity Rating

score	weeks
-10	20
-5	22
0	24
5	26
10	28
15	30
20	32
25	34
30	36
35	38
40	40
45	42
50	44

Figure 5.2. Scoring system to assess newborn infants. The scores for each of the neuromuscular and physical signs are added together to obtain a score called the "total maturity score." Gestational age is determined from this score. (This figure was published in *Journal of Pediatrics*, 119, 418, Ballard, J.L., Khoury, J.C., Wedig, K., et al. New Ballard score, expanded to include extremely premature infants, Copyright Elsevier, 1991; reprinted by permission.)

maternal infections; and adolescent pregnancies (Cantarutti, Franchi, Monzio Compagnoni, Merlino, & Corrao, 2017). Other risk factors include inadequate prenatal care, acute and chronic maternal illness, history of previous premature pregnancies, placental bleeding, preeclampsia, smoking, and substance abuse (see Box 5.1; Cantarutti et al., 2017). Congenital anomalies or injuries to the fetus may also lead to premature birth.

Although less than 3% of all pregnancies occur in adolescents, these pregnancies account for 14%–18% of all preterm births. A maternal age that is under 18 years is a major risk factor for complications in both mothers and neonates, especially in mothers aged younger than 15 years (Najati & Gojazadeh, 2010). Approximately half of preterm births are attributable to maternal infections, which are commonly undetected and untreated in low-income settings. In addition, up to 80% of early preterm births (births before 30 weeks' gestation) are associated with an intrauterine infection that precedes the rupture of membranes (Lee et al., 2015).

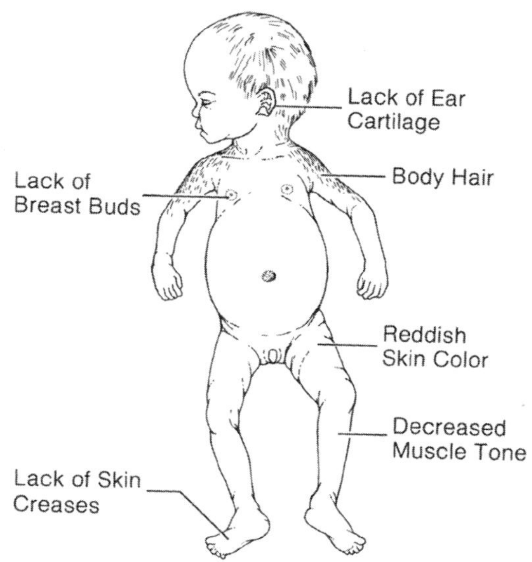

Figure 5.3. Typical physical features of a premature infant.

COMPLICATIONS OF PREMATURITY

The premature infant must undergo the same physiologic transitions to extrauterine life as the full-term infant. The preterm infant, however, must accomplish this difficult task using immature body organs. The result is a significant risk of complications in virtually every organ system, and this risk increases with the degree of prematurity.

Respiratory Problems

Respiratory problems are one of the most common and potentially life-threatening complications for premature infants born before 34 weeks. These problems result from the immaturity of the fetal lungs and the lack of production of **surfactant.** The section that follows discusses the acute respiratory issue of hyaline membrane disease (HMD) as well as the potential long-term consequences leading to bronchoplulmonary dysplasia (BPD).

Hyaline Membrane Disease HMD, also called RDS, is a disorder characterized by respiratory distress in the newborn period. The underlying impairment is decreased production of surfactant that normally keeps the **alveoli** (the terminal airway passages) open, permitting the exchange of oxygen and carbon dioxide (Figure 5.4). A chest x-ray can clinically confirm HMD, showing a "ground glass" appearance of the lungs. This results from the collapsed alveoli appearing dense and hazy in comparison with the air-filled lung of a typical full-term newborn, which appears translucent and black (Figure 5.5). The clinical course of HMD involves a peak severity between 24 and 48 hours after birth, followed by improvement over the next 24–48 hours. In uncomplicated cases, HMD will resolve within 72–96 hours after birth. This classical course of HMD has fortunately been modified by the administration of exogenous surfactant replacement therapy (Wirbelauer & Speer, 2009). Improvement in pulmonary function usually begins within minutes after the first dose of surfactant is injected through the trachea and into the lungs of the newborn; after one or two doses of surfactant, effective gas exchange can be achieved with a significantly lower level of oxygen and ventilatory support. Except in severe cases of HMD, it is unusual for an infant to require more than two doses of surfactant.

BOX 5.1 EVIDENCE-BASED PRACTICE

Risk Factors for Preterm Delivery

Preterm delivery is a significant concern that has been associated with a number of cofactors, such as obstetrical interventions (e.g., cesarean sections), assisted reproduction techniques (e.g., *in vitro* fertilization), multiple-gestation births, substance abuse, low socioeconomic status, low maternal educational level, maternal infections, and adolescent pregnancies (Cantarutti et al., 2017). Other risk factors include inadequate prenatal care, acute and chronic maternal illness, previous premature pregnancies, placental bleeding, preeclampsia, smoking, and substance abuse (Cantarutti et al., 2017). Congenital anomalies or injuries to the fetus may also lead to premature birth.

Although less than 3% of all pregnancies occur in adolescents, these account for 14%–18% of all preterm births. A maternal age of younger than 18 years is a major risk factor for complications in both mothers and neonates, especially in mothers younger than 15 years of age (Najati & Gojazadeh, 2010). Approximately half of preterm births are attributable to maternal infections, and up to 80% of early preterm births (births before 30 weeks' gestation) are associated with an intrauterine infection that precedes the rupture of membranes (Lee et al., 2015).

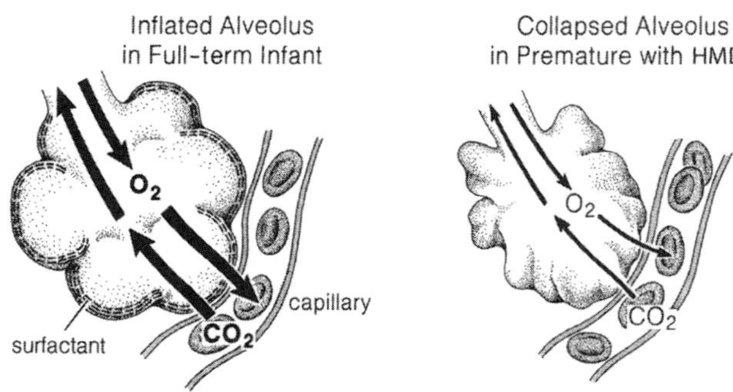

Figure 5.4. Schematic drawing of alveoli in a normal newborn and in a premature infant with respiratory distress syndrome. Note that the inflated alveolus is kept open by surfactant. Oxygen (O_2) moves from the alveolus to the red blood cells in the pulmonary capillary. Carbon dioxide (CO_2) moves in the opposite direction. This exchange is much less efficient when the alveolus is collapsed; the result is hypoxia.

Infants with mild HMD generally do well with supplemental oxygen alone or in combination with **continuous positive airway pressure** (CPAP). CPAP involves providing a mixture of oxygen and air under continuous pressure; this prevents the alveoli from collapsing between breaths. More severely affected infants may require the placement of an endotracheal tube for mechanical ventilatory support as well as administration of surfactant. Although surfactant therapy has significantly reduced mortality in ELBW premature infants, there has been no appreciable change in long-term pulmonary and neurodevelopmental complications in these infants (Patrianakos-Hoobler et al., 2010). Therefore, close follow-up to school entry is important.

A related approach to treating surfactant deficiency is to stimulate its production. There is evidence that administration of steroids to mothers 24–36 hours before preterm delivery stimulates surfactant production and pulmonary maturation in the fetus. This lessens the likelihood and/or severity of HMD. The effect of antenatal steroids is additive to postnatal surfactant replacement therapy in reducing respiratory distress and mortality. It is therefore recommended that steroids be given prior to birth for potential preterm delivery of fetuses between 24–36 weeks' gestational age (Roberts, Brown, Medley, & Dalziel, 2017).

Bronchopulmonary Dysplasia The improved survival of ELBW newborns has increased the number of infants at risk for various forms of long-term respiratory morbidity associated with mechanical ventilation, including **bronchopulmonary dysplasia (BPD)**. This term is generally used to describe infants who require supplemental oxygen and/or mechanical ventilation beyond 28 days postnatal age and/or corrected gestational age of 36 weeks with persistently atypical chest x-rays and respiratory examinations (e.g., rapid breathing or wheezing). BPD primarily occurs in infants who are born at less than 32 weeks' gestation and require mechanical ventilation during the first week of life for treatment of HMD. Although the frequency of BPD in VLBW neonates is high, in the majority of cases the disease is mild. Severe BPD is more common in neonates with associated comorbidities, such as late-onset sepsis or advanced **intraventricular hemorrhage (IVH)** (Kiciński, Kęsiak, Nowiczewski, & Gulczyńska, 2017).

The development of BPD has been attributed to lung injury from a combination of **barotrauma** (pressure damage from prolonged mechanical ventilation), oxygen toxicity, infection, and inflammation. The exact mechanism of BPD, however, remains poorly understood. Since the mid-2000s, newer methods of respiratory support, including high-frequency ventilation and surfactant therapy, have increased the survival rate of smaller and less mature infants, but the total number of infants who develop BPD has not decreased. BPD remains the most common chronic lung disease of infancy in the United States, with some 7,000 new cases being diagnosed each year. Long-term studies of pulmonary function in this population indicate that as these infants grow, there is clinical improvement.

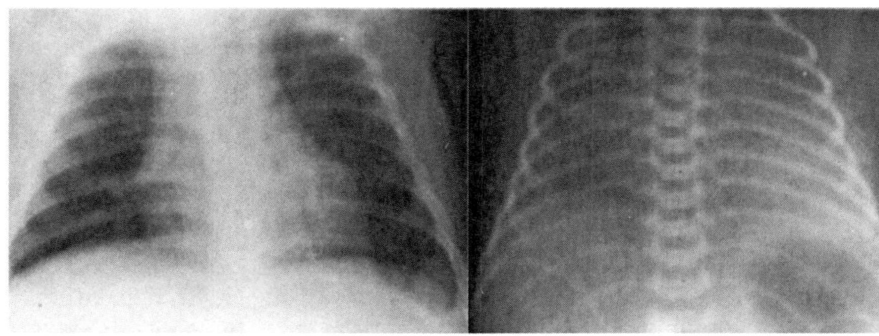

Figure 5.5. Chest x-rays of a normal newborn (left) and of a premature infant with respiratory distress syndrome (right), which shows a "white out" of the lungs due to surfactant deficiency.

Yet, children diagnosed with BPD are at increased risk for developing reactive airway disease or asthma in childhood and chronic obstructive pulmonary disease in adulthood (Vom Hove, Prenzel, Uhlig, & Robel-Tillig, 2014).

Approaches to postnatal prevention and treatment of BPD have included steroid therapy, supplemental vitamin A, high-frequency ventilation, use of bronchodilators (asthma medication), and administration of diuretics (to increase urinary excretion of excessive lung fluids). The use of postnatal steroids such as dexamethasone for prevention and treatment of BPD has been a matter of controversy. Although early postnatal corticosteroid treatment facilitates extubation (removal of the breathing tube) and reduces the risk of BPD, it can cause short-term adverse effects, including gastrointestinal bleeding, intestinal perforation, hyperglycemia (high blood sugar levels), hypertension, hypertrophic cardiomyopathy (inflammation of the heart), and growth failure. There is also the potential for steroids having long-term adverse effects on physical growth and neurodevelopment. It is not unusual for infants with BPD to require supplemental oxygen, diuretics, and bronchodilators after discharge from the hospital. Even with supportive care and treatment, infants with BPD may continue to have long-term problems, including limited tolerance of physical activity, feeding difficulties that contribute to poor physical growth, excessive caloric requirement, and an increased risk of cerebral palsy and other developmental disabilities (Abman et al., 2017; Kiciński et al., 2017).

Neurologic Problems

Premature infants are also at increased risk for neurologic problems that are often linked to their respiratory problems. These problems include **intraventricular hemorrhage (IVH)** (bleeding into the brain), **periventricular leukomalacia (PVL)** (damage to the white matter of the brain), **apnea** and **bradycardia** (brief periods of respiratory arrest and heart rates slowing), and damage to hearing from antibiotic use.

Intraventricular Hemorrhage IVH, defined as bleeding into the ventricular space within the brain hemispheres, is a significant neurological complication of extremely premature infants. The risk of IVH correlates directly with the degree of prematurity. Fortunately, its incidence appears to be declining. About half of IVH cases occur during the first day of life, and 90% by the third day of life (Brouwer, Groenendaal, Benders, & de Vries, 2014). Ultrasound of the head is the most reliable and safest technique for diagnosing IVH. The American Academy of Neurology Practice Parameter for "Neuroimaging of the Neonate" suggests that an initial screening ultrasound shortly after birth be performed on all preterm infants of less than 30 weeks' gestation to detect evidence of IVH. In addition, they recommend a follow-up ultrasound at 36–40 weeks postmenstrual age in order to detect CNS lesions, such as PVL and **ventriculomegaly** (enlargement of the ventricles), which will affect long-term outcomes (Brouwer et al., 2014). Magnetic resonance imaging (MRI) is better than ultrasound at detecting white matter abnormalities, hemorrhagic lesions, and cysts. Emerging data are providing evidence for the importance of this imaging modality at term-equivalent as a predictor of neurological outcome in VLBW preterm infants (El-Dib, Massaro, Bulas, & Aly, 2010).

IVH is commonly graded by four levels of severity (Volpe, 2008). Grade I is defined by bleeding into the germinal matrix, a network of blood vessels in the roof of the lateral ventricles. If the hemorrhage expands beyond the germinal matrix into the ventricular system, it is Grade II. Grades I and II account for the majority of IVH cases, and significant neurological impairment is fortunately rare with these types. About 20% of hemorrhages, however, are severe enough to dilate the ventricle (Grade III) or invade the brain substance (Grade IV). Grade IV is often called *periventricular hemorrhagic infarction.* These hemorrhages can lead to PVL, or damage of the white matter surrounding the ventricles (Volpe, 2008). The long-term neurological outcome for infants with IVH is related to the severity of the hemorrhage. Cerebral palsy (with or without intellectual disability) is seen in about 30% of patients with Grade III hemorrhages and in 75% of those with Grade IV hemorrhages (Pleacher, Vohr, Katz, Ment, & Allan, 2004; Sarkar, Bhagat, Dechert, Schumacher, & Donn, 2009).

Avoidance of hypoxic–ischemic events that lead to fluctuations in cerebral blood pressure, expert delivery room stabilization, effective resuscitation and ventilation, gentle handling, and use of muscle relaxants during mechanical ventilation have all been associated with a reduction in the incidence and severity of IVH (Volpe, 2008). A number of medications have been studied for preventing or treating IVH with varied results. These include antenatal use of steroids and postnatal use of phenobarbital, vitamin K, vitamin E, indomethacin, ethamsylate, ibuprofen, and recombinant activated factor VIIa (McCrea & Ment, 2008).

Periventricular Leukomalacia PVL is the most common form of cerebral white matter injury in preterm infants and results in cerebral palsy in 60%–100% of survivors (Huang et al., 2017). The periventricular white matter is the region of the brain closest to the ventricles. PVL occurs when this area sustains damage either due to low oxygen or low blood flow. This area is especially vulnerable to injury in the premature infant because the glial cells, a major constituent of white matter, undergo rapid growth by the end of the second trimester. During this period, they are more susceptible to injury caused by fluctuations in cerebral blood pressure. There is also evidence that **chorioamnionitis** (maternal infection involving the membranes surrounding the fetus) increases the risk of PVL (Huang et al., 2017).

PVL may occur in association with IVH or independently (Figure 5.6). The diagnosis of PVL is best made by serial cranial (head) ultrasounds that may show the development of cystic (cyst-like) lesions in the white matter. Serial cranial ultrasounds or an MRI at near-term gestation (or at term-equivalent gestation in VLBW neonates) also have been shown to be important predictors of the subsequent development of **spastic diplegia** (a form of cerebral palsy that impairs lower extremity function) and **hemiplegia** (a form of cerebral palsy that affects one side of the body (see Chapter 21). Large cysts (greater than 3 mm in diameter) place the neonate at increased risk of developing **spastic quadriplegia** (a form of cerebral palsy that affects all four limbs), visual impairment, intellectual disability, and seizures in early childhood (Huang et al., 2017).

Auditory Toxicity

ELBW infants are at increased risk for hearing loss because of multisystem illness and the frequent use of medications (such as aminoglycoside antibiotics and diuretics) and excessive environmental noise that can be toxic to the auditory system. Hearing loss is one of the most common health problems of infancy, affecting 1 in 700 to 1,000 newborns. The rate of hearing loss in preterm infants is between 2% and 15%, with the majority of the cases having no known cause (Zimmerman & Lahav, 2013). In 1995, the Joint Committee on Infant Hearing recommended that all VLBW infants undergo auditory screening. The committee further expanded this statement in 2000 to advocate testing for all newborns. The most commonly performed tests are brainstem auditory evoked response and **otoacoustic emission,** which are discussed in Chapter 7 (Ohl, Dornier, Czajka, Chobaut, & Tavernier, 2009).

Apnea and Bradycardia

Apnea is clinically defined as a respiratory pause lasting 15–20 seconds. It is usually associated with a decrease in heart rate to below 80 to 100 beats per minute (bradycardia) and systemic oxygen desaturations. It is the most common disorder of respiratory control found in the neonatal intensive care unit (NICU) and

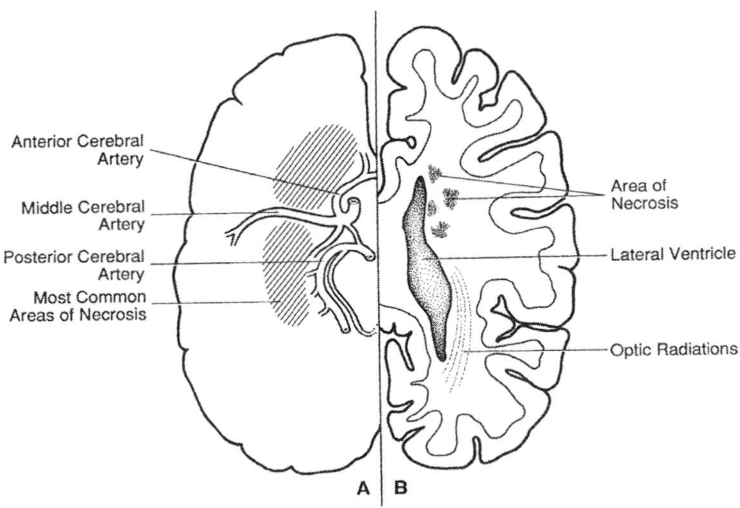

Figure 5.6. Periventricular leukomalacia. A) The blood vessel supply to the brain, and B) the brain structures. The area of the white matter surrounding the lateral ventricle (particularly the top part) is especially susceptible to hypoxic-ischemic damage because it is not well supplied by blood vessels. It lies in a watershed area between the anterior, middle, and posterior cerebral arteries. In premature infants, poor oxygenation and decreased blood flow associated with respiratory distress syndrome may lead to necrosis of this brain tissue, a condition termed *periventricular leukomalacia.* When the posterior portion is affected, the optic radiations may be damaged, resulting in cortical blindness.

can affect up to 85%–100% of premature newborns. It is related to immaturity of the central nervous system. (Goryniak, Szczęśniak, Śleboda, & Dołęgowska, 2017).

Apnea of prematurity (AOP) remains a major clinical problem and requires the neonatologist to make treatment choices that are sometimes difficult. AOP occurs in most infants of gestational age less than 33 weeks (Goryniak et al., 2017). It is a developmental disorder that usually reflects a physiological immaturity of brain control of respiration. However, neonatal diseases may be associated with AOP and play an additive role, resulting in an increased incidence of apnea. Careful screening should therefore be performed in order to make sure that no factor other than immaturity is involved in the occurrence of apnea. Short apnea (less than 10 seconds) without bradycardia and/or desaturation is not clinically significant. Prolonged apnea is defined as lasting for more than 15 to 20 seconds and/or is associated with bradycardia or oxygen desaturation. Prolonged apnea results in short-term disturbances of cerebral hemodynamics and oxygenation, which may negatively affect neurodevelopmental outcome. Treatment involves the administration of caffeine, which has been shown to reduce the incidence of apnea and decrease the risk of bronchopulmonary dysplasia, patent ductus arteriosus, and subsequent development of cerebral palsy (Goryniak et al., 2017).

Sudden Unexpected Infant Death Syndrome

The incidence of **sudden unexpected infant death (SUID)** syndrome fortunately decreased from 120 to 56 deaths per 100,000 live births between 1992 and 2001. While from 2001 to 2008 the rate remained constant, it then declined to 40 deaths per 100,000 live births in 2013. Although the rates have declined significantly, SUID remains the leading cause of post-neonatal (28 days to 1 year of age) mortality in the United States, with over 1,500 infants dying of the disorder in 2013. Ninety percent of SUID cases occur before an infant reaches the age of 6 months, peaking between 1 and 4 months of age (Moon, 2016). SUID occurs more frequently in premature infants than in full-term infants (Moon, 2016). Contrary to earlier beliefs, apnea of prematurity is not a major predisposing factor for SUID. However, because of the increased incidence of SUID among this population, extremely premature infants who are having significant apneic spells in the 2 weeks before discharge may be sent home with an apnea monitor (Committee on Fetus and Newborn, American Academy of Pediatrics, 2003). Although these monitors emit an alarm if the infant stops breathing and alerts the parents to intervene, studies on their use have not shown effectiveness in reducing the occurrence of SUID. The monitors do, however, provide reassurance to parents and physicians about the status of the infant. Parents of such high-risk infants should be trained in neonatal CPR prior to taking their infant home on an apnea monitor. The monitor is generally not required for more than a few months.

In 1992, in an effort to prevent SUID, the American Academy of Pediatrics' Task Force on Infant Position and SUID began recommending that infants be placed on their back for sleep. In addition, the Task Force recommended that fluffy blankets and toys not be placed in an infant's crib during sleep times and that the home environment be smoke free. These changes have resulted in a more than 50% reduction in the incidence of SUID as noted above (Moon, 2016).

Cardiovascular Problems

The most common cardiovascular problem in LBW infants is a **patent ductus arteriosus** (PDA). The ductus arteriosus is the fetal vessel that diverts blood flow from the lungs. It normally closes at birth, allowing blood to flow to the lungs and be oxygenated. About 30% of premature infants, and more than 50% of those born weighing less than 1,000 grams, will have a patent (open) ductus arteriosus diagnosed during the first few days of life (Hamrick & Hansmann, 2010). This is especially true in premature infants who have RDS. In these children, a PDA will divert blood from the lungs and further decrease oxygenation to the body and brain, increasing the work of the heart. This can lead to hypoxia, decreased blood flow to specific organs, and heart failure. The presence of a PDA can be detected by echocardiography, a form of ultrasound of the heart. Its management involves medical and supportive measures, including fluid restriction, diuresis (stimulation of urination), and the use of CPAP. If these measures fail, closure is possible using medications such as indomethacin or ibuprofen. In a small percentage of infants, surgical closure is required (Al Nemri, 2014; Noori, 2010).

Gastrointestinal Problems

Although premature infants may be born with a suck-and-swallow response, they are immature and poorly coordinated until approximately 32–34 weeks' gestation. Thus, most premature infants require **nasogastric** (nose to stomach) or **nasojejunal** (nose to small intestine) tube feedings until they can make the transition to oral feeding (Giannì et al., 2017). The nutritional needs of the premature infant are also different from those of the full-term infant and require the use of specialty formulas. In addition to physiological problems, premature infants are at increased risk for two major gastrointestinal disorders—**necrotizing enterocolitis (NEC)** and **gastroesophageal reflux disease (GERD)**—that can inhibit growth and be life-threatening.

Necrotizing Enterocolitis **NEC** is the most commonly acquired life-threatening intestinal disease in premature infants. It involves severe injury to a portion of the bowel wall. The exact cause of NEC is unknown, but prematurity appears to be the most common predisposing factor. Approximately 80% of infants with NEC are born at less than 38 weeks' gestation and weigh less than 2,500 grams at birth. Other predisposing factors include fetal distress, premature rupture of membranes, low Apgar scores, and exchange transfusion (where blood is gradually removed from the newborn and replaced with matched adult blood to treat Rh incompatibility). The incidence of NEC is 1 to 2 per 1,000 live births, occurring in 5%–10% of VLBW infants. Although the survival rate of extremely preterm infants has markedly increased, the number of deaths attributed to NEC has been increasing. Mortality rates from NEC range from 15%–30% (Samuels, van de Graaf, de Jonge, Reiss, & Vermeulen 2017).

Medical management of NEC involves withholding feedings, applying nasogastric suction to decrease pressure on the bowel wall, administering antibiotics to fight the suspected underlying infection, and providing intravenous fluids and nutrition to prevent dehydration and weight loss. Although medical treatment can be successful in many infants with NEC, approximately half require surgery to remove the diseased section of the bowel (Sheng et al., 2016). Survivors of NEC may experience a variety of postoperative complications related to the disease, the operation, or treatment measures. Surgery for NEC may involve removal of a large portion of the bowel, leading to decreased absorption of nutrients (Sheng et al., 2016). This is called short bowel syndrome and occurs in up to 11% of postsurgical NEC survivors. It results in chronic diarrhea, malabsorption, nutritional deficiencies, impaired growth, and the long-term need for intravenous nutrition (fats, carbohydrates, and amino acids provided intravenously through a central line).

Gastroesophageal Reflux Disease The immaturity of gastric sphincter muscular control and delayed stomach emptying in premature infants may result in GERD, a syndrome in which the contents of the stomach are regurgitated back into the **esophagus** (D'Agostino, Passarella, Martin, & Lorch, 2016). Infants with severe GERD are at increased risk for vomiting and **aspiration pneumonia** (a lung infection precipitated by the **aspiration** of food into the lung), which may be worsened by nasogastric tube feedings. Signs of GERD include refusal of oral feeding, apnea, irritability, and back arching. Treatment is targeted toward special positioning techniques and medications (see Chapter 10).

Retinopathy of Prematurity

Impairments in retinal vascular development after preterm birth lead to **retinopathy of prematurity (ROP),** formerly called *retrolental fibroplasia*. The highest risk infants are those born at less than 28 weeks gestational age and weighing less than 1 kilogram at birth (Chan-Ling, Gole, Quinn, Adamson & Darlow, 2017). A pediatric ophthalmologist should perform an examination for early detection of ROP at 4–6 weeks after birth or at 32–33 weeks' gestation (whichever comes first). Follow-up examinations should be done until retinal vascularization is complete, usually around term gestation (see Chapter 7). Preventive therapy with early human milk feeding and vitamins A and E supplements may decrease the severity of ROP in susceptible infants (Porcelli & Weaver, 2010). Severe ROP is treated by laser to prevent permanent retinal detachment.

Immunologic Problems

The premature infant is born with an immature immune system. As a result, the infant is at increased risk for infection in the first months of life (Wilińska, Warakomska, Głuszczak-Idziakowska, & Jackowska, 2016). Generalized bacterial and fungal infections, occurring in approximately 30% of extremely premature infants, are major life-threatening illnesses and can lead to a poor neurodevelopmental outcome (Wilińska et al., 2016). Premature infants who remain in the hospital for prolonged periods should receive routine immunizations based on their chronological age.

Other Physiologic Impairments

Premature infants are at increased risk for many of the same transient physiological impairments that occur in full-term infants. These include hyperbilirubinemia, anemia, hypoglycemia, hyperglycemia, hypocalcemia, and hypothermia. These problems place the premature infant at increased risk for brain damage.

Acidosis and hypoxia, resulting from inadequate respiration, can increase the permeability of the blood–brain barrier to bilirubin, making preterm infants more susceptible to **kernicterus.** In kernicterus, there is the deposition of bilirubin pigment in the brain, leading to athetoid cerebral palsy, hearing loss, vision problems, and/or intellectual disability. Thus, the bilirubin level that is used to determine whether phototherapy or an exchange transfusion should be performed is lower for the preterm infant than for the full-term infant (Maisels, Watchko, Bhutani, & Stevenson, 2012). **Glucose** and **electrolyte** instability are also common in premature infants, especially the ELBW infant.

Anemia usually is more of a problem for the premature infant than for the full-term infant because it decreases the oxygen-carrying capacity of the red blood cells and can lead to hypoxic–ischemic brain damage. Preterm infants, especially ELBW infants, are exposed to frequent blood draws as part of their routine care in the NICU, which lowers their red blood count. These infants develop anemia of prematurity due to inadequate production of erythropoietin, which normally stimulates the bone marrow to produce red blood cells. In severe cases, anemia of prematurity is corrected with blood transfusion and/or treatment with erythropoietin (Bishara & Ohls, 2009). In recent years, revised transfusion guidelines have significantly reduced the use of transfusions in the LBW premature infant and the need for erythropoietin in ELBW infants (Bishara & Ohls, 2009).

Finally, premature infants often have a transient deficiency of thyroid hormone production. In severe cases, this condition may be associated with neurodevelopmental impairments. However, in most cases, the hypothyroidism resolves without the need for thyroid hormone replacement therapy and does not negatively impact long-term outcomes (van Wassenaer-Leemhuis et al., 2014).

MEDICAL AND DEVELOPMENTAL CARE OF LOW BIRTH WEIGHT INFANTS

The best treatment for LBW infants is prevention of preterm births. This starts with identifying women at risk and providing them with education and prenatal health care. In addition, detecting preterm labor early and using labor-arresting agents and antenatal steroid therapy are very effective methods for preventing neonatal mortality and morbidity (Roberts et al., 2017). Prenatal care has improved appreciably since the 1970s, but the incidence of preterm delivery remains high. Preterm and SGA infants are best managed and cared for in high-risk obstetrical centers/children's hospitals with NICUs.

The increased survival rate of preterm infants has the potential for increasing the number of children with adverse neurodevelopmental outcome. Fortunately, since the year 2000 neurodevelopmental impairments have actually decreased among ELBW infants. A variety of perinatal and neonatal factors have been associated with this improved outcome, including increased antenatal steroid use and cesarean section delivery. These interventions have resulted in decreased risk of sepsis and less severe cranial ultrasound abnormalities. There has, however been no change in the rate of chronic lung disease despite the postnatal use of steroids to stimulate surfactant production (Pierrat et al., 2017).

As survival rates of preterm infants have improved, the focus of care is now on creating the optimal environment within the NICU for the premature infant to develop. Traditional NICU care has focused on medical protocols and procedures. A newer approach uses a more relationship-based, individualized, developmentally supportive model. This approach recognizes that the usual NICU setting is not optimal for the premature infant's developmental progress. Typical NICU care has involved the infant experiencing prolonged diffuse sleep states, unattended crying, a high ambient noise level, bright ambient light, a lack of opportunity for sucking, and poorly timed social and caregiving interactions.

The newer approach seeks to observe the infant's behavior and respond to it appropriately by providing individualized neurodevelopmental care and actively involving the parents in their infant's care (McAnulty et al., 2013). This involves documenting infant behavior, including breathing pattern, color fluctuations, startles, posture, and sleep state. Caregiving suggestions and environmental modifications are then based on these observations. One of the techniques involving the parent is termed **kangaroo care.** Once the premature infant has reached physiologic stability and does not require major respiratory support, he or she is placed on the parent's chest. Kangaroo care (parent–infant skin-to-skin contact) has been shown to improve preterm growth, decrease hospital-acquired infections, and possibly shorten hospital length of stay (Head, 2014). These developmental approaches have been associated with improved functioning of the neonate in the NICU, including the infant having a reduced number of apnea events, faster weight gain, improved oxygenation, motor maturity, and behavioral state organization. Research is ongoing to determine whether this approach carries long-term benefits.

In addition to environmental modifications that support development, early intervention services can be provided even before the child is discharged from the NICU. Once the infant is medically stable, a team consisting of a physical and/or occupational therapist, speech pathologist, developmental psychologist, and/or developmental pediatrician should evaluate the child. Care plans should be developed to provide parents with training regarding the ongoing developmental needs of the child after discharge (see Box 5.2). This may also include referral to an early intervention program in the community (see Chapter 31).

SURVIVAL OF LOW BIRTH WEIGHT INFANTS

Advances in medical technology in neonatal intensive care and their application to the premature infant have been very successful in reducing mortality. Since 1960, survival of LBW infants has increased from 50% to more than 90% (Table 5.1). This improvement has been even more remarkable in ELBW and micropreemie infants. ELBW infants who survive the first few days of extrauterine life have a far better chance of long-term survival. Although the overall survival for infants with a birth weight of less than 500 grams was only 8%, those who lived through the first 3 days of life had up to a 50% chance of survival. Infants in the 500- to 749-gram birth weight category had an overall survival rate of 50%. That increased to 70% if they survived through the third day and 80% by the end of the first week of life (Mohamed, Nada, & Aly, 2010). A more recent study has shown that infants who were born between 2005–2011 at 22 to 24 weeks' gestation had a significantly lower mortality compared with those born from 1998–2004 (42% versus 55%). Neurodevelopmental impairment among surviving infants also declined from 68% to 47% (Younge et al., 2016).

Table 5.1. Improvement in survival rates of premature infants

	Survival (%)		
Birth weight (g)	1960	1990	2004
500–750	10	30	50
750–1,000	20	70	85
1000–1,500	30	90	98
1500–2,000	50	90	> 98

Sources: Emsley et al. (1998); O'Shea et al. (1997); O'Shea et al. (1998); and Mohamed et al. (2010).

CARE AFTER DISCHARGE FROM THE HOSPITAL

The medical cost of the hospitalization and care of preterm infants who require prolonged NICU stays is extraordinarily high, often measured in hundreds of thousands of dollars. Length of stay is a major factor in this cost. As a result, many centers are developing care pathways that allow the medical team to consider earlier discharge than previously practiced for stable premature infants. This new approach needs to be monitored closely to ensure that earlier discharge does not compromise the health of infants and result in an increased risk of readmission to the hospital for treatment of medical complications.

Clinical criteria for discharging preterm LBW infants are based on the achievement of sufficient weight and maturity of body organ function to ensure medical stability and continued growth in a home environment. This generally involves the infant being

BOX 5.2 INTERDISCIPLINARY CARE

Specialty Services Required At or After Discharge

Many premature infants may still require specialty services at or after time of discharge to home, which may include some or all of the following services:

- Occupational therapy
- Physical therapy
- Speech therapy
- Ophthalmology follow-ups for retinopathy of prematurity
- Pulmonary follow-ups if discharged on home oxygen and with an apnea monitor
- Gastroenterology and nutritional follow-ups
- Neurodevelopmental follow-ups

able to feed well by mouth, continue to gain weight, maintain a stable body temperature outside of an isolette, and no longer experience episodes of apnea and bradycardia. Most preterm LBW infants meet these eligibility criteria at a postconceptional age of 35–37 weeks. For ELBW infants, discharge at a postconceptional age of 37–42 weeks is a more realistic goal (Jefferies, 2014). At the time of discharge, most infants weigh between 1,800 and 2,000 grams (4 to 4¼ pounds).

When premature infants are discharged, parents may be faced with the stress and difficulty of caring for an infant with many special needs. The prolonged duration of hospitalization and separation from parents also may have interfered with the usual parent–infant bonding. Premature infants may be more irritable, cry more often, and have poorer sleep–wake cycles compared with full-term infants. Because of an immature sucking pattern, they often require more frequent feedings. Specialized formula and/or breast milk supplementation with a human milk fortifier are now available to meet the caloric needs of premature infants post discharge.

As a result of these stresses, it is important to provide adequate support for the family after discharge, including close medical supervision and home-care visits by nursing and/or social work staff (Aydon, Hauck, Murdoch, Siu, & Sharp, 2017). Parental education regarding the needs of a growing preterm infant is extremely important. Ideally, the infant should be discharged to a home environment that is free of smoke and any other potential respiratory irritants such as kerosene heaters, fresh paint, and people with respiratory-related viral illness. Each of these factors plays a crucial role in causing subsequent respiratory illnesses or in exacerbating the underlying lung disease.

To prepare premature infants and their parents for the infant's discharge, most centers provide rooming-in services for the parents. This allows the parents to take over the care of their infant under the supervision of the NICU staff members who determine whether there are unforeseen problems. The parents also learn about the care of their infant, thereby reducing the stress and anxiety of taking a preterm infant home (Broedsgaard & Wagner, 2005).

EARLY INTERVENTION PROGRAMS

Early intervention programs have been shown to benefit the neurodevelopment of most premature infants through 3–5 years of age, although longer-term effects are still debated (Koldewijn et al., 2010; Spittle, Orton, Anderson, Boyd, & Doyle, 2015). In a study of children with birth weights less than 2 kilograms, there was no significant difference in Mental Developmental Index scores at 3 years of age (after adjustment for maternal education) between children who receive early intervention services and those who do not; however, there was a statistically significant benefit shown via full-scale IQ scores at 5 years. With respect to motor outcomes, there were no differences between the groups receiving services and those not receiving services (Nordhov et al., 2010).

These programs should start for many premature infants prior to discharge from the hospital and continue until the child reaches 3 years corrected age. Corrected age is calculated by first determining how premature the child was in weeks (subtract the child's gestational age at birth from 40 weeks); then that number is subtracted from the child's current chronological age. For example, a child born at 28 weeks was 12 weeks early. To obtain the corrected age, 12 weeks (i.e., 3 months) should be subtracted from the child's age. The corrected age for an 8 month old born at 28 weeks' gestation is therefore 5 months. This correction is generally done until 12–24 months chronological age.

The intervention strategy incorporates group meetings for parents, home visits, and after 24 months' chronological age, attendance at a multidisciplinary child development center with a low teacher-to-infant ratio (i.e., one teacher to three or four infants; see Chapter 31). It is important to recognize that even after completion of the early intervention program, many of these children continue to need special education services, including speech-language therapy, physical and/or occupational therapy, special education, behavior therapy, and treatment of emotional problems. If these children do not receive these services, the benefits of early intervention may be lost over time (Guralnick, 2012).

NEURODEVELOPMENTAL OUTCOME

Most infants born prematurely can be viewed during infancy as developing at a typical rate when their corrected or adjusted age is determined from their expected date of birth rather than from their actual birth date. There are, however, differences between full-term and preterm infants even when gestational age is taken into account. Although few premature infants develop cerebral palsy, in terms of motor skills, they often lack the smooth, rhythmic movement patterns of full-term infants. Devices such as walkers and jumpers should be avoided because they encourage the infant to stand on tiptoe and walk in an atypical pattern. In later infancy, visual-motor tasks that require the planned use of arms and hands are also more difficult. Coordinating reach and grasp, scooping with a spoon, managing a standard cup, copying block constructions, and completing crayon/paper tasks can be more difficult (Sripada et al., 2015).

By school age, the developmental status of preterm children who had birth weights above 1,500 grams is not very different from full-term infants. Late-preterm infants born at 34–36 weeks' gestational age who are otherwise healthy seem to have no real burdens regarding cognition, achievement, behavior, and socioemotional development throughout childhood (Gurka, LoCasale-Crouch, & Blackman, 2010). Children with birth weights below 1,500 grams and less than 32 weeks' gestation, however, have an increased risk for developmental disabilities. School-age children who were born very preterm or had ELBW are at greater risk of developing executive function deficits (seen in children with attention-deficit/hyperactivity disorder [ADHD], learning disabilities, and autism) and at greater risk of requiring ongoing neuropsychological follow-up through middle childhood (de Kieviet, van Elburg, Lafeber, & Oosterlaan, 2012; Eryigit Madzwamuse, Baumann, Jaekel, Bartmann, & Wolke, 2015; Hutchinson, De Luca, Doyle, Roberts, & Anderson 2013; Johnson et al., 2015; Joseph et al., 2017; Peralta-Carcelen et al., 2017).

In terms of behavior issues, children born prematurely are at risk for lower levels of social competence, and they are often less adaptable, less regular in their habits, less persistent, and more withdrawn. ADHD is also more common in this group (de Kieviet et al., 2012). Signs of ADHD may appear as early as 2 years of age, with hyperactivity and difficulty following verbal directions or listening to a story (see Chapter 19). In addition, there may be behavior differences such as sleep disturbances, feeding difficulties, tantrums, and/or resistance to limit setting (Johnson et al., 2015). Learning differences may be anticipated in children whose language is delayed and who demonstrate poor visual–motor coordination (Sripada et al., 2015; also see Chapter 20). Family factors have also been found to be strong predictors of future school performance (Garfield et al., 2017). Optimal school outcome has been significantly associated with increased parental education, child rearing by two parents, stability in family composition, socioeconomic status, and geographic residence.

Major developmental disabilities have been found in about one quarter of children with a birth weight less than 1,000 grams (i.e., ELBW infants and micropreemies). This includes cerebral palsy; hearing impairment; visual impairment; and, at 18–22 months' corrected age, a mean mental developmental index of less than 85 (Hintz, Newman, & Vohr, 2016). Although cerebral palsy, especially spastic diplegia, is not uncommon in children who were VLBW, many "outgrow" this diagnosis by school age and simply appear to be less coordinated or to have motor-associated learning difficulties.

In terms of predicting future neurodevelopmental disabilities, in one study, 30%–40% of ELBW infants with a normal cranial ultrasound were later found to have either cerebral palsy or intellectual disability (Hintz et al., 2016). A neonatal brain MRI at corrected term gestation and/or before discharge appears to be a better predictor of severe neurodevelopmental disorders (El-Dib et al., 2010; Hintz et al., 2016). In one study, sensorineural hearing impairments were correlated with neonatal sepsis and jaundice; neurological, developmental, neurosensory, and functional morbidities increased with a decreasing birth weight; and, overall, males were more at risk for disabilities than were females. In addition, infants born SGA are at increased risk for lower cognitive performance as young adults. However, this lower capacity is not considered sufficiently severe to affect their educational level or social adjustment (Yi, Yi, & Hwang, 2016).

SUMMARY

- When compared with full-term infants, LBW infants—in particular, VLBW infants/micropreemies—are at greater risk in the newborn period for many problems that may lead to long-term complications.
- Physiologic immaturity of organ systems often leads to RDS, hyperbilirubinemia, hypoglycemia, and hypocalcemia.
- Most of these infants recover from these transient complications without major long-term sequelae.
- Other problems, such as IVH, PVL, sepsis, and persistent apnea and bradycardia, are associated with poor neurodevelopmental outcome.
- With increased public awareness, improved prenatal care, advanced neonatal intensive care, increased parent involvement in the NICU, and access to early intervention services, the outcome of premature and SGA infants is likely to continue to improve.

ADDITIONAL RESOURCES

Mayo Clinic: Premature Birth: http://www.mayoclinic.com/health/prematurebirth/DS00137

Medline Plus: Premature Babies: http://www.nlm.nih.gov/medlineplus/prematurebabies.html

Premature Babies: Caring for Your Baby: http://familydoctor.org/handouts/283.html

Additional resources can be found online in Appendix D: Childhood Disabilities Resources, Services, and Organizations (see About the Online Companion Materials).

REFERENCES

Abman, S. H., Collaco, J. M., Shepherd, E. G., Keszler, M., Cuevas-Guaman, M., Welty, S. E., . . . Nelin, D. (2017). Interdisciplinary care of children with severe bronchopulmonary dysplasia. *Journal of Pediatrics, 181,* 12–28.

Adams-Chapman, I., Hansen, N. I., Shankaran, S., Bell, E. F., Boghossian, N. S., Murray, J. C., . . . Stoll, B. J. (2013). Ten-year review of major birth defects in VLBW infants. *Pediatrics, 132*(1), 49–61.

Al Nemri, A. M. H. (2014). Patent ductus arteriosus in preterm infant: Basic pathology and when to treat. *Sudanese Journal of Paediatrics, 14*(1), 25–30.

American Academy of Pediatrics Task Force on Infant Position and SIDS. (1992). Position and SIDS. *Pediatrics, 89,* 1120–1126.

Argente, J., Mehls, O., & Barrios, V. (2010). Growth and body composition in very young SGA children. *Pediatric Nephrology, 25*(4), 679–685.

Aydon, L., Hauck, Y., Murdoch, J., Siu, D., & Sharp, M. (2017). Transition from hospital to home: Parents' perception of their preparation and readiness for discharge with their preterm infant. *Journal of Clinical Nursing.* Advance online publication. doi:10.1111/jocn.13883

Ballard, J. L., Khoury, J. C., Wedig, K., Wang, L., Eilers-Walsman, B. L., & Lipp, R. (1991). New Ballard score, expanded to include extremely premature infants. *The Journal of Pediatrics, 119,* 417–423.

Bishara, N., & Ohls, R. K. (2009). Current controversies in the management of the anemia of prematurity. *Seminars in Perinatology, 33,* 29–34.

Broedsgaard, A., & Wagner, L. (2005). How to facilitate parents and their premature infant for the transition home. *International Nursing Review, 52,* 196–203.

Brouwer, A. J., Groenendaal, F., Benders, M. J., & de Vries, L. S. (2014). Early and late complications of germinal matrix-intraventricular haemorrhage in the preterm infant: What is new? *Neonatology, 106*(4), 296–303.

Cantarutti, A., Franchi, M., Monzio Compagnoni, M., Merlino, L., & Corrao, G. (2017). Mother's education and the risk of several neonatal outcomes: An evidence from an Italian population-based study. *BMC Pregnancy Childbirth, 17*(1), 221. doi:10.1186/s12884-017-1418-1

Chan-Ling, T., Gole, G. A., Quinn, G. E., Adamson, S. J., & Darlow, B. A. (2017). Pathophysiology, screening and treatment of ROP: A multi-disciplinary perspective. *Progress in Retinal and Eye Research.* Advance online publication. doi:10.1016/j.preteyeres.2017.09.002

Committee on Fetus and Newborn, American Academy of Pediatrics. (2003). Apnea, sudden infant death syndrome, and home monitoring. *Pediatrics, 111*(4), 914–917.

Constantine, N. A., Kraemer, H. C., Kendall-Tackett, K. A., Bennett, G. C., Tyson, J. E., & Gross, R. T. (1987). Use of physical and neurologic observations in assessment of gestational age in low-birth-weight infants. *The Journal of Pediatrics, 110,* 921–928.

D'Agostino, J. A., Passarella, M., Martin, A. E., & Lorch, S. A. (2016). Use of gastroesophageal reflux medications in premature infants after NICU discharge. *Pediatrics, 138*(6), pii: e20161977

Dani, C., Poggi, C., Romagnoli, C., & Bertini, G. (2009). Survival and major disability rate in infants born at 22–25 weeks of gestation. *Journal of Perinatal Medicine, 37*(6), 599–608. pii: e20161977

de Bie, H. M., Oostrom, K. J., & Delemarre-van de Waal, H. A. (2010). Brain development, intelligence and cognitive outcome in children born small for gestational age. *Hormone Research in Paediatrics, 73*(1), 6–14.

de Kieviet, J. F., van Elburg, R. M., Lafeber, H. N., & Oosterlaan, J. (2012). Attention problems of very preterm children compared with age-matched term controls at school-age. *Journal of Pediatrics, 161*(5), 824–829.

Dubowitz, L. M., Dubowitz, V., & Goldberg, C. (1970). Clinical assessment of gestational age in the newborn infant. *The Journal of Pediatrics, 77,* 1–10.

El-Dib, M., Massaro, A. N., Bulas, D., & Aly, H. (2010). Neuroimaging and neurodevelopmental outcome of premature infants. *American Journal of Perinatology, 27*(10), 803–818.

Emsley, H. C. A., Wardle, S. P., Sims, D. G., Chiswick, M. L., & D'Souza, S. W. (1998). Increased survival and deteriorating developmental outcome in 23 to 25 week old gestation infants, 1990–4 compared with 1984–9. *Archives of Disease in Childhood, Fetal and Neonatal Edition, 78,* F99–F104.

Eryigit Madzwamuse, S., Baumann, N, Jaekel, J., Bartmann, P., & Wolke, D. (2015). Neuro-cognitive performance of very preterm or very low birth weight adults at 26 years. *Journal of Child Psychology and Psychiatry, 56*(8), 857–864.

Garfield, C. F., Karbownik, K., Murthy, K., Falciglia, G., Guryan, J., Figlio, D. N., & Roth, J. (2017). Educational performance of children born prematurely. *JAMA Pediatrics, 171*(8), 764–770.

Giannì, M. L., Sannino, P., Bezze, E., Plevani, L., Esposito, C., Muscolo, S., et al. (2017). Usefulness of the Infant Driven Scale in the early identification of preterm infants at risk for delayed oral feeding independency. *Early Human Development, 23*(115), 18–22.

Goryniak, A., Szczęśniak, A., Śleboda, D., & Dołęgowska, B. (2017). Apnea of prematurity: Characteristic and treatment. *Postepy Biochemii, 63*(2), 151–154.

Grivell, R., Dodd, J., & Robinson, J. (2009). The prevention and treatment of intrauterine growth restriction. *Best Practice & Research Clinical Obstetrics and Gynaecology, 23*(6), 795–807.

Guralnick, M. J. (2012). Preventive interventions for preterm children: Effectiveness and developmental mechanisms. *Journal of Developmental and Behavioral Pediatrics, 33,* 352–364.

Gurka, M. J., LoCasale-Crouch, J., & Blackman, J. A. (2010). Long-term cognition, achievement, socioemotional, and behavioral development of healthy late-preterm infants. *Archives of Pediatrics and Adolescent Medicine, 164*(6), 525–532.

Hamrick, S. E., & Hansmann, G. (2010). Patent ductus arteriosus of the preterm infant. *Pediatrics, 125*(5), 1020–1030.

Head, L. M. (2014). The effect of kangaroo care on neurodevelopmental outcomes in preterm infants. *Journal of Perinatal and Neonatal Nursing, 28*(4), 290–299; quiz E3-4. doi:10.1097/JPN.0000000000000062

Heron, M., Sutton, P. D., Xu, J., Ventura, S. J., Strobino, D. M., & Guyer, B. (2010). Annual summary of vital statistics: 2007. *Pediatrics, 125*(1), 4–15. doi:10.1542/peds.2009-2416. Epub 2009 Dec 21.

Hintz, S. R., Newman, J. E., & Vohr, B. R. (2016). Changing definitions of long-term follow-up: Should "long term" be even longer? *Seminars in Perinatology, 40*(6), 398–409.

Huang, J., Zhang, L., Kang, B., Zhu, T., Li, Y., Zhao, F., . . . Mu, D. (2017). Association between perinatal hypoxic-ischemia and periventricular leukomalacia in preterm infants: A systematic review and meta-analysis. *PLoS One, 20;12*(9), e0184993. doi:10.1371/journal.pone.0184993

Hutchinson, E. A., De Luca, C. R., Doyle, L. W., Roberts, G., & Anderson, P. J. (2013). School-age outcomes of extremely preterm or extremely low birth weight children. *Pediatrics, 131*(4), e1053–1061.

Hyman, S. J., Novoa, Y., & Holzman, I. (2011). Perinatal endocrinology: Common endocrine disorders in the sick and premature newborn. *Pediatric Clinics of North America, 58*(5), 1083–1098.

Jefferies, A. L. (2014). Going home: Facilitating discharge of the preterm infant. *Paediatrics & Child Health, 19*(1), 31–42.

Johnson, S., Matthews, R., Draper, E. S., Field, D. J., Manktelow, B. N., Marlow, N., . . . Boyle, E. M. (2015). Early emergence of delayed social competence in infants born late and moderately preterm. *Journal of Developmental and Behavioral Pediatrics, 36*(9), 690–699.

Joint Committee on Infant Hearing. (1995). Joint Committee on Infant Hearing 1994 Position Statement. *Pediatrics, 95*(1), 152–156.

Joint Committee on Infant Hearing. (2000). Year 2000 position statement: Principles and guidelines for early hearing detection and intervention programs. *Pediatrics, 106*(4), 798–817.

Joseph, R. M., Korzeniewski, S. J., Allred, E. N., O'Shea, T. M., Heeren, T., Frazier, J. A., . . . & ELGAN Study Investigators. (2017). Extremely low gestational age and very low birthweight for gestational age are risk factors for autism spectrum disorder in a large cohort study of 10-year-old children born at 23-27 weeks' gestation. *American Journal of Obstetrics and Gynecology, 216*(3), 304.e1–304.e16.

Kiciński, P., Kęsiak, M., Nowiczewski, M., & Gulczyńska, E. (2017). Bronchopulmonary dysplasia in very and extremely low birth weight infants: Analysis of selected risk factors. *Polski Merkuriusz Lekarski, 20*(248), 71–75.

Koldewijn, K., van Wassenaer, A., Wolf, M. J., Meijssen, D., Houtzager, B., Beelen, A., . . . Nollet, F. (2010). A neurobehavioral intervention and assessment program in very low birth weight infants: Outcome at 24 months. *Journal of Pediatrics, 156*(3), 359–365.

Lee, A. C., Quaiyum, M. A., Mullany, L. C., Mitra, D. K., Labrique, A., Ahmed. P., . . . and Projahmo Study Group. (2015). Screening and treatment of maternal genitourinary tract infections in early pregnancy to prevent preterm birth in rural Sylhet, Bangladesh: a cluster randomized trial. *BMC Pregnancy Childbirth, 7*(15), 326. doi:10.1186/s12884-015-0724-8

Lubchenco, L. O. (1976). *The high risk infant*. Philadelphia, PA: Saunders.

Maisels, M. J., Watchko, J. F., Bhutani, V. K., & Stevenson, D. K. (2012). An approach to the management of hyperbilirubinemia in the preterm infant less than 35 weeks of gestation. *Journal of Perinatology, 32*(9), 660–664.

Mandrich, M., Simons, C. J., Ritchie, S., Schmidt, D., & Mullett, M. (1994). Motor development, infantile reactions and postural responses of preterm, at-risk infants. *Developmental Medicine and Child Neurology, 36,* 397–405.

Mathews, T. J., & Driscoll, A. K. (2017). Trends in infant mortality in the United States, 2005–2014. NCHS data brief, no. 279. Hyattsville, MD: National Center for Health Statistics.

McAnulty, G., Duffy, F. H., Kosta, S., Weisenfeld, N. I., Warfield, S. K., Butler, S. C., . . . Als, H. (2013). School-age effects of the newborn individualized developmental care and assessment program for preterm infants with intrauterine growth restriction: Preliminary findings. *BMC Pediatrics, 19*(13), 25. doi:10.1186/1471-2431-13-25

McCrea, H. J., & Ment, L. R. (2008). The diagnosis, management and postnatal prevention of intraventricular hemorrhage in the preterm neonate. *Clinics in Perinatology, 35,* 777.

Mendez-Figueroa, H., Truong, V. T., Pedroza, C., Khan, A. M., & Chauhan, S. P. (2016). Small-for-gestational-age infants among uncomplicated pregnancies at term: A secondary analysis of 9 Maternal-Fetal Medicine Units Network studies. *American Journal of Obstetrics and Gynecology, 215*(5), 628.e1–628.

Mohamed, M. A., Nada, A., & Aly, H. (2010). Day-by-day postnatal survival in very low birth weight infants. *Pediatrics, 126*(2), e360–e366.

Moon, R. Y. (2016). SIDS and other sleep-related infant deaths: Evidence base for 2016 updated recommendations for a safe infant sleeping environment. *Pediatrics, 138*(5), pii:e20162940.

Murphy, S. L., Mathews, T. J., Martin, J. A., Minkovitz, C. S., & Strobino, D. M. (2017). Annual summary of vital statistics: 2013-2014. *Pediatrics, 139*(6). pii: e20163239. doi:10.1542/peds.2016-3239

Nagpal, J., Kumar, A., & Ramji, S. (2004). Anterior lens capsule vascularity in evaluating gestation in small for gestation neonates. *Indian Pediatrics, 41,* 817–821.

Najati, N., & Gojazadeh, M. (2010). Maternal and neonatal complications in mothers aged under 18 years. *Journal of Patient Preference and Adherence, 4,* 219–222.

Noori, S. (2010). Patent ductus arteriosus in the preterm infant: To treat or not to treat? *Journal of Perinatology, 30,* S31–S37.

Nordhov, S. M., Rønning, J. A., Dahl, L. B., Ulvund, S. E., Tunby, J., & Kaaresen, P. I. (2010). Early intervention improves cognitive outcomes for preterm infants: Randomized controlled trial. *Pediatrics, 126*(5), e1088–e1094. Advance online publication. doi:10.1542/peds.2010-0778

Ohl, C., Dornier, L., Czajka, C., Chobaut, J. C., & Tavernier, L. (2009). Newborn hearing screening on infants at risk. *International Journal of Pediatrics Otorhinolaryngology, 73*(12), 1691–1695.

O'Shea, T. M., Klinepeter, K. L., Goldstein, D. J., Jackson, B. W., & Dillard, R. G. (1997). Survival and developmental disability in infants with birth weights of 501 to 800 grams, born between 1979 and 1994. *Pediatrics, 100*(6), 982–986.

O'Shea, T. M., Preisser, J. S., Klinepeter, K. L., & Dillard, R. G. (1998). Trends in mortality and cerebral palsy in a geographically based cohort of very low birth weight neonates born between 1982 and 1994. *Pediatrics, 101*(4), 642–647.

Patrianakos-Hoobler, A. I., Msall, M. E., Huo, D., Marks, J. D., Plesha-Troyke, S., & Schreiber, M. D. (2010). Predicting school readiness from neurodevelopmental assessments at age 2 years after respiratory distress syndrome in infants born preterm. *Developmental Medicine & Child Neurology, 52*(4), 379–385.

Peralta-Carcelen, M., Carlo W. A., Pappas, A., Vaucher, Y. E., Yeates, K. O., Phillips, V. A., . . . Bann, C. M. (2017). Behavioral problems and socioemotional competence at 18 to 22 months of extremely premature children. *Pediatrics, 139*(6). pii:e20161043. doi:10.1542/peds.2016-1043

Pierrat, V., Marchand-Martin, L., Arnaud, C., Kaminski, M., Resche-Rigon, M., Lebeaux, C., . . . Ancel, P. Y. (2017). Neurodevelopmental outcome at 2 years for preterm children born at 22 to 34 weeks' gestation in France in 2011: EPIPAGE-2 cohort study. *BMJ, 16*(358), j3448. doi:10.1136/bmj.j3448

Pleacher, M. D., Vohr, B. R., Katz, K. H., Ment, L. R., & Allan, W. C. (2004). An evidence-based approach to predicting low IQ in very preterm infants from the neurological examination: Outcome data from the Indomethacin intraventricular hemorrhage prevention trial. *Pediatrics, 113,* 416–419.

Porcelli, P. J., & Weaver, R. G., Jr. (2010). The influence of early postnatal nutrition on retinopathy of prematurity in extremely low birth weight infants. *Early Human Development, 86,* 391–396.

Roberts, D., Brown, J., Medley, N., & Dalziel, S. R. (2017). Antenatal corticosteroids for accelerating fetal lung maturation for women at risk of preterm birth. *Cochrane Database of Systematic Reviews, 21*(3), CD004454. doi:10.1002/14651858.CD004454.pub3

Samuels, N., van de Graaf, R. A., de Jonge, R. C. J., Reiss, I. K. M., & Vermeulen, M. J. (2017). Risk factors for necrotizing enterocolitis in neonates: A systematic review of prognostic studies. *BMC Pediatrics, 17*(1), 105. doi:10.1186/s12887-017-0847-3

Sarkar, S., Bhagat, I., Dechert, R., Schumacher, R. E., & Donn, S. M. (2009). Severe intraventricular hemorrhage in preterm infants: Comparison of risk factors and short-term neonatal morbidities between grade 3 and grade 4 intraventricular hemorrhage. *American Journal of Perinatology, 26*(6), 419–424.

Sheng, Q., Lv, Z., Xu, W., Liu, J., Wu, Y., Shi, J., & Xi, Z. (2016). Short-term surgical outcomes of preterm infants with necrotizing enterocolitis: A single-center experience. *Medicine (Baltimore), 95*(30), e4379. doi:10.1097/MD.0000000000004379

Sinclair, J. C., Bottino, M., & Cowett, R. M. (2009). Interventions for prevention of neonatal hyperglycemia in very low birth weight infants. *Cochrane Database of Systematic Reviews, 8*(3), CD007615.

Spittle, A., Orton, J., Anderson, P. J., Boyd, R., & Doyle, L. W. (2015). Early developmental intervention programmes provided post hospital discharge to prevent motor and cognitive impairment in preterm infants. *Cochrane Database of Systematic Reviews, 24*(11), CD005495.

Sripada, K., Løhaugen, G. C., Eikenes, L., Bjørlykke, K. M., Håberg, A. K., Skranes, J., & Rimol, L. M. (2015). Visual-motor deficits relate to altered gray and white matter in young adults born preterm with very low birth weight. *Neuroimage, 1*(109), 493–504.

Stavsky, M., Mor, O., Mastrolia, S. A., Greenbaum, S., Than, N. G., & Erez, O. (2017). Cerebral palsy—Trends in epidemiology and recent development in prenatal mechanisms of disease, treatment, and prevention. *Frontiers in Pediatrics, 13*(5), 21.

Van Wassenaer-Leemhuis, A., Ares, S., Golombek, S., Kok, J., Paneth, N., Kase, J., & LaGamma, E. F. (2014). Thyroid hormone supplementation in preterm infants born before 28 weeks gestational age and neurodevelopmental outcome at age 36 months. *Thyroid, 24*(7), 1162–1169.

Volpe, J. J. (2008). *Neurology of the newborn* (5th ed.). Philadelphia, PA: Saunders.

Vom Hove, M., Prenzel, F., Uhlig, H. H., & Robel-Tillig, E. (2014). Pulmonary outcome in former preterm, very low birth weight children with bronchopulmonary dysplasia: A case-control follow-up at school age. *Journal of Pediatrics, 164*(1), 40–45.

Wilińska, M., Warakomska, M., Głuszczak-Idziakowska, E., & Jackowska, T. (2016). Risk factors for adverse events after vaccinations performed during the initial hospitalization of infants born prematurely. *Developmental Period Medicine, 20*(4), 296–305.

Wirbelauer, J., & Speer, C. P. (2009). The role of surfactant treatment in preterm infants and term newborns with acute respiratory distress syndrome. *Journal of Perinatology, 29*(Suppl 2), S18–S22.

Yi, K. H., Yi, Y. Y., & Hwang, I. T. (2016). Behavioral and intelligence outcome in 8- to 16-year-old born small for gestational age. *Korean Journal of Pediatrics, 59*(10), 414–420.

Younge, N., Smith, P. B., Gustafson, K. E., Malcolm, W., Ashley, P., Cotton, C. M., . . . Goldstein, R. F. (2016). Improved survival and neurodevelopmental outcomes among extremely premature infants born near the limit of viability. *Early Human Development, 95,* 5–8. doi:10.1016/j.earlhumdev.2016.01.015

Zimmerman, E., & Lahav, A. (2013). Ototoxicity in preterm infants: Effects of genetics, aminoglycosides, and loud environmental noise. *Journal of Perinatology, 33*(1), 3–8.

PART II

The Child's Body
Physiology

CHAPTER 6 Fetal Development

Nickie N. Andescavage

Upon completion of this chapter, the reader will

- Explain the fundamental principles of fetal development from conception to term birth
- Describe the complex interplay of maternal-placental-fetal health during gestation
- Identify the various mechanisms that can disrupt normal fetal development

A single egg joins a single sperm cell, and 9 months later an infant is born. When all goes well, from those two cells will come 10 fingers and toes, one heart, two lungs, a brain, and other normally functioning body organs. Embryonic/fetal life allows for the protected development of the fertilized egg into a complex, multi-organ human through a highly structured pattern of development. However, deviations from normal development can have a significant and long-lasting impact. Early severe **anomalies** (congenital abnormalities) in the developmental sequence can result in a miscarriage, whereas more subtle anomalies may go undetected until after birth when functional impairment is noted.

This chapter provides an overview of normal human development. It describes the critical steps that take place in development as well as periods of vulnerability when body organs are particularly susceptible to long-lasting consequences if the normal developmental sequence is disrupted. It also explains the concept of the fetal origin of certain adult diseases, including heart disease, diabetes, cancer, and psychiatric-neurobehavioral disorders (Calkins & Devaskar, 2011; Fall & Osmond, 2013). Chapter 1 and Chapter 2 in this volume describe the genetic, biologic, and environmental influences that contribute to specific developmental disabilities; this chapter emphasizes how these and other factors influence fetal health and the long-term impact on neurodevelopment. It also provides an overview of the evaluation of fetal development, diagnostic considerations, and management strategies.

CASE STUDY

Jane is a 33-year-old woman pregnant with her first child and is currently in her second trimester. She is generally healthy, although she had significant nausea and vomiting during her first trimester that was treated with antiemetic medication. As the morning sickness has now subsided, her only current medication is a daily prenatal vitamin. Her family history is notable for hypertension (mother), type 2 diabetes (father), and a sister who had two miscarriages prior to the delivery of a healthy boy. Jane's work for an international nonprofit organization involves frequent travel to Central and South America. She is a nonsmoker and describes herself as a social drinker (1-2 glasses of wine per week). She immediately stopped drinking once she learned she was pregnant at 6 weeks' gestation. During a routine prenatal visit at 20 weeks' gestation, Jane's obstetrician noted that her uterus measured smaller than expected and arranged for a fetal imaging procedure to be performed. Fetal measurements on ultrasound revealed asymmetric (unequal in size/shape) fetal growth, and she was referred to a maternal-fetal medicine specialist for the further evaluation of her small-for-dates fetus.

Thought Questions:

What can affect the fetus and cause subsequent neurodevelopmental disabilities? What can be done to optimize fetal neurodevelopment?

OVERVIEW OF KEY ANATOMIC STRUCTURES

Early human development requires the close and interdependent interaction of the maternal-fetal-placental unit. By the end of the first trimester, the placenta is a mature, established organ that nourishes and protects the developing fetus through the close physical approximation of the maternal and fetal circulations (Figure 6.1). Blood from the maternal circulation reaches the placenta through the uterine arteries and **perfuses** (pushes blood to) the uterine wall. The mother's endometrial arteries then send the blood into the **intervillous space** (the space between the villi containing the vessels of the mother and embryo). The intervillous space surrounds and bathes the fetal vessels, promoting the transfer of gases (oxygen and carbon dioxide), nutrients, and waste between the fetus and mother.

The fetal circulation differs from the adult circulation in several important ways. The most nutrient-rich blood exits the placenta via the umbilical vein and returns to the fetus where two transient fetal structures (the **ductus venosus** and the **foramen ovale**) shunt this blood to the ascending aorta and thereby to the developing brain (Figure 6.2). These mechanisms allow for the most oxygenated and nutrient-dense blood to preferentially perfuse the developing brain. Any disruption in the maternal-placental-fetal circulation can have long-lasting consequences for the neurodevelopment of the fetus.

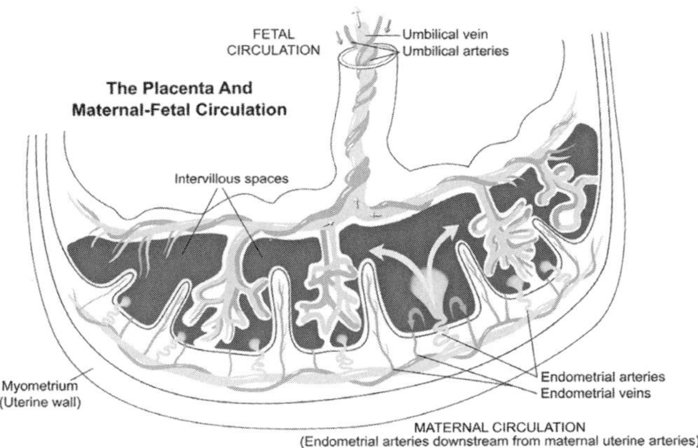

Figure 6.1. Placenta and maternal-fetal circulation. Blood from the maternal circulation reaches the placenta through the uterine arteries and perfuses the uterine wall. The endometrial arteries send blood into the intervillous space; the intervillous space, in turn, surrounds and bathes the fetal vessels, allowing for the transfer of gases, nutrients, and waste between the fetus and mother.

HUMAN DEVELOPMENT

Human development follows a highly ordered sequence of events and requires a consistent reference starting point. Embryologists use **postconceptional age** (PCA) as a metric for development. PCA dates the onset of human development from the presumed date of ovulation (when fertilization occurs). Within this context, intrauterine development is divided into two phases, the **embryotic period** (the first 8 postconceptional weeks) and the **fetal period** (from 9 weeks until birth).

Clinicians, on the other hand, use **gestational age** (GA) in weeks as a metric for embryonic-fetal

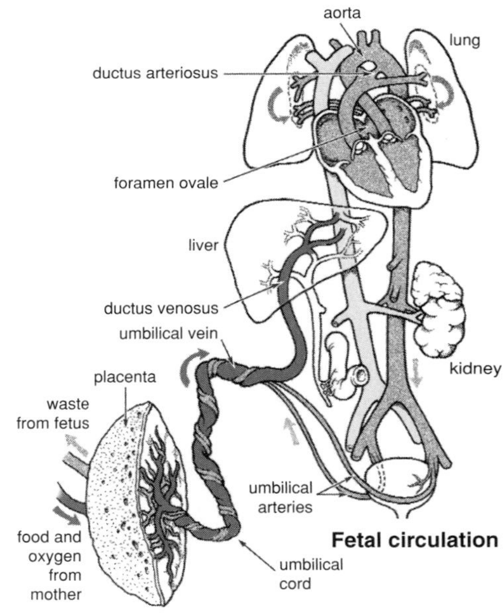

Figure 6.2. Fetal circulation: The foramen ovale and patent (open) ductus artesiosus allow the blood flow to bypass the unexpanded lungs.

development. The GA is measured from the first day of the last menstrual period, that is, 2 weeks earlier than PCA. Using GA, the intrauterine period is divided into trimesters. The first trimester extends to 12 weeks GA, the second from 13 to 28 weeks GA, and the third trimester from 29 weeks until term (40 weeks GA).

This section describes the timeline of typical human development during the embryonic and fetal periods (Figure 6.3). This information will lay the foundation to understand the next sections, which describe how deviations from developmental norms can contribute to neurodevelopmental disabilities.

The Embryonic Period

During the embryonic period, the individual body organs are formed. The heart is the first organ to develop, with a primitive heart tube and developing circulatory system beginning to function around 6 weeks GA. At this time, the **rostral** end of the neural tube (destined to become the fetal head) begins to differentiate into sections that will form the major components of the brain—the forebrain, midbrain, and hindbrain (Figure 6.4)—along with the basic components of the spinal cord.

The embryonic period is divided into three stages: germinal, gastrulation, and neurulation. Genetic and environmental induced defects during this period most commonly lead to miscarriage. However, some affected embryos survive and are born with disorders that can be associated with developmental disabilities. These disorders include chromosomal disorders (e.g., Down syndrome), single-gene disorders (e.g., neurofibromatosis), toxic exposures (e.g., fetal alcohol syndrome), and congenital malformations (e.g., neural tube defects).

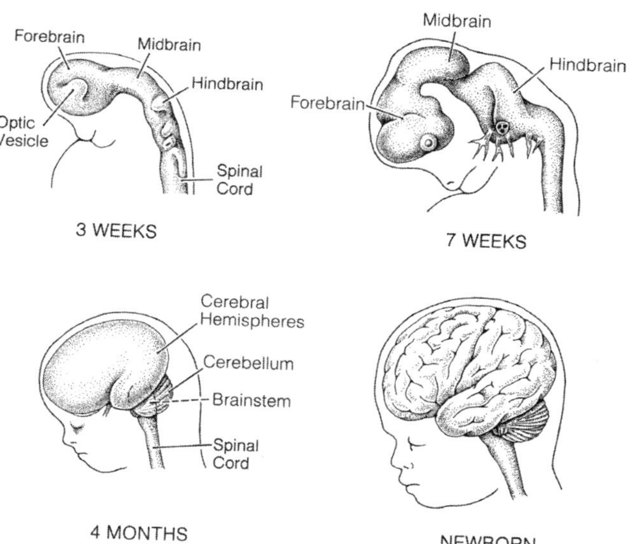

Figure 6.4. Development of the fetal brain. This is a side view illustrating the increasing complexity of the brain over time. The forebrain, or prosencephalon, develops into the cerebral hemispheres; the midbrain, or mesencephalon, develops into the brainstem; and the hindbrain, or rhombencephalon, develops into the cerebellum, pons, and medulla. Although all brain structures are formed by 4 months, the brain grows greatly in size and complexity during the final months of prenatal development.

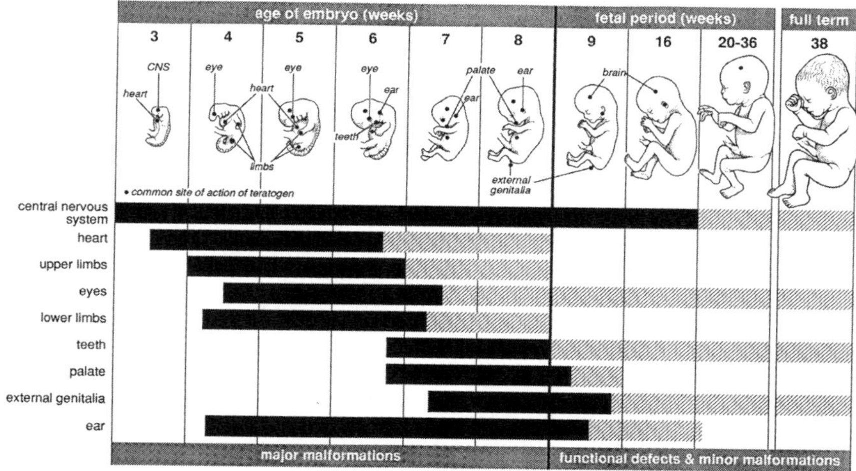

Figure 6.3. Embryogenesis and fetal development. (From Moore, K. L., & Persaud, T. V. N. [1993]. *Before we are born: Essentials of embryology and birth defects* [4th ed., inside back cover]. Philadelphia, PA: W. B. Saunders; adapted by permission.) The majority of major malformations results from deviations of normal embryonic development and coincide with the emergence of each major organ system. Insults to the developing fetus, after the basic structural elements of organ formation, typically result in functional defects or minor malformations.

Germinal Stage The **germinal stage** of human development occurs during the period between fertilization and implantation of the developing embryo (Figure 6.5). It begins with the fusion of the egg and sperm, resulting in a single-celled **zygote,** the fertilized egg cell. The zygote divides into two cells; then the two cells divide into four, four cells to eight, and so on. These dividing cells are known as **blastomeres** and create a spherical group of cells known as the **morula.** Within a few days of fertilization, these cells develop into two distinct cell types in a process known as cellular differentiation. The outer layer of cells becomes **trophoblast** cells, which will go on to develop the placenta; the inner mass cells or **embryoblasts** go on to form the human embryo.

Gastrulation Stage During the **gastrulation stage,** the developing embryo organizes into three layers of cells, with distinctive head-to-tail, front-to-back, and left-right differentiation. It is during this period that the forerunners of the structures and organs that make up an infant begin to develop. The outermost layer, or **ectoderm,** will give rise to the skin, nervous system, eyes, inner ear, and connective tissues. **Neural crest** cells are a transient group of cells that arise from the ectodermal layer and become the neurons, glia, and skin cells.

Abnormalities in the differentiation of neural crest cells are believed to underlie **neurocutaneous syndromes,** a collection of conditions that affect both skin and brain and lead to developmental disabilities. The most common of these disorders are neurofibromatosis, Sturge-Weber disease, and tuberous sclerosis. The middle layer, or **mesoderm,** will become the heart and circulatory system, bones, muscles, and kidneys. The inner layer, or **endoderm,** will develop into the lungs, intestine, thyroid, pancreas, and bladder.

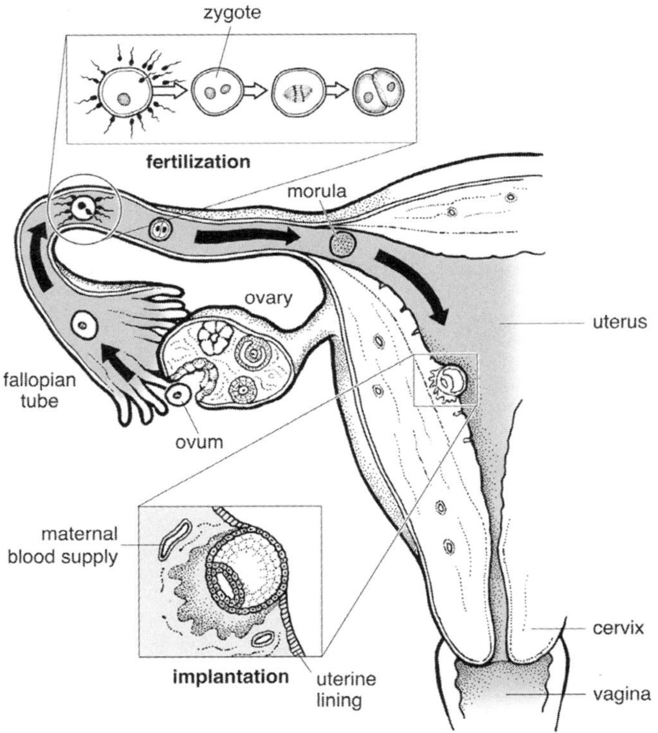

Figure 6.5. Germinal stage of fetal development. This figure shows the germinal stage of human development from fertilization to implantation of the blastocyst, or early embryo. The ovum (egg) is dropped from the ovary into the fallopian tube, where it is fertilized by a sperm. The fertilized egg begins dividing as it travels toward the uterus. Two distinct cell types begin to emerge—the outer layer (trophoblast) and inner cells (embryoblasts)—as it enters the uterine cavity and implants into the maternal wall.

Neurulation Stage In the **neurulation stage,** the disc-like structure of the developing embryo folds over to form the neural tube, which will eventually form the central nervous system, brain, and spinal cord (Figure 6.6). *Primary neurulation* is the process by which the flat neural plate develops a midline groove, the edges of which fold over, converge, and fuse. *Secondary neurulation* is a series of events that result in the creation of the neural tube by hollowing out its center.

Defects in primary neurulation result in congenital malformations known as neural tube defects, including spina bifida (**meningomyelocoele**) and **encephalocele.** Defects in secondary neurulation lead to the **caudal regression syndrome** that can result in major malformations of the lower vertebrae, pelvis, and spine.

The Fetal Period

Although all major organ systems have formed by the end of the embryonic period, they are not fully functional. For the remainder of gestation, termed the fetal

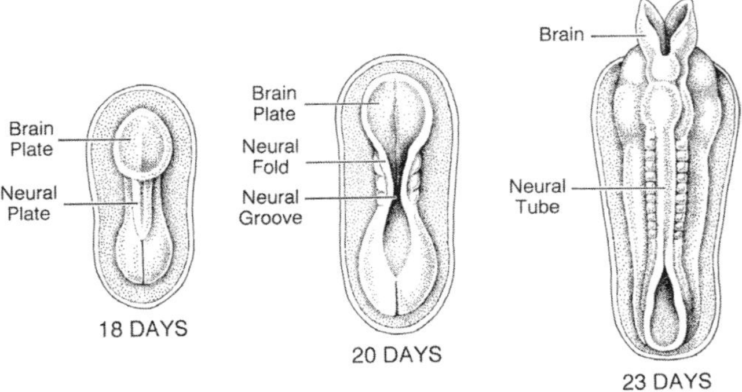

Figure 6.6. Neurulation. Development of the central nervous system during the first month of the embryonic period. This is a longitudinal view showing the gradual closure of the neural tube to form the spinal column and the rounding up of the head region to form the primitive brain.

period, the individual organs, organ systems, and body will grow and develop. As this text addresses neurodevelopmental disabilities, this section focuses on the structural development of the fetal brain and what can go wrong, particularly in the cerebrum and cerebellum. Cerebral development can be divided into four periods: 1) neural proliferation, 2) neuronal migration, 3) cortical organization and synapse formation, and 4) myelination.

Neural Proliferation Period **Neural proliferation** occurs during a sustained period of vigorous cellular division that peaks between 6 and 27 weeks GA. This period gives rise to precursors of the **neuronal** (grey matter) and **glial** (white matter) cell populations of the brain. There are two early populations of nerve cells: the dorsal neuroepithelium, which forms the neuronal population and pathways important for cognition, motivation, and memory, and the ventral neuroepithelium, which gives rise to the future interneuronal population that produces the neurotransmitter gamma aminobutyric acid (GABA). During early brain development, GABA exerts an excitatory function but later switches to become the principal inhibitory neurotransmitter. Maternal ingestion of antiepileptic medication (e.g., valproate) during this period can have teratogenic effects (causing anomalies) on the fetus through its impact on GABA.

The rapidly growing periventricular regions of the brain are particularly susceptible to injury during this time from viral infections (e.g., **cytomegalovirus [CMV]**) and exposure to radiation or alcohol (see Chapter 2). This can result in **microcephaly** (abnormally small head) and developmental disturbances of other body organs (Volpe, 2008).

Neuronal Migration Period After neuronal proliferation, the neurons start to migrate out toward the surface of the brain in successive waves beginning at 12 weeks GA and ending by 20 weeks GA. This results in the development of the folds (**gyri**) and grooves (**sulci**) that give the typically developed brain a walnut-like appearance and increase its surface area and complexity (see Figure 6.4).

Disturbances in cell signaling and neuronal migration can result in a variety of structural anomalies generally referred to as neuronal migration disorders, such as **lissencephaly** (a "smooth" brain with a lack of gyri and sulci) and **polymicrogyria** (too many small folds). In addition, disturbances in early neuronal migration may play a role in the subsequent development of complex partial seizures (see Chapter 22) and autism (see Chapter 18; Bystron, Blakemore, & Rakic, 2008; Zhao et al., 2006).

The **subplate zone,** just under the developing cortex, is a transient area that plays a critical role in the development of numerous cortical pathways and connections. These act as the relay zone and communication hub for higher cortical processing (Kostovic & Judas, 2010). Abnormalities in subplate development and function have been associated with several neuropsychiatric conditions including epilepsy (see Chapter 22), schizophrenia, and autism (see Chapter 18; Hoerder-Suabedissen & Molnár, 2015).

Cortical Organization and Synapse Formation
A **synapse** is the point at which an impulse passes from one neuron to another, resulting in neural activation or communication. Neural activation occurs early in development through gene activation and growth factor support, which lead to the formation of synapses. This can result in the major overproduction of synapses, requiring "pruning back" or reorganization during subsequent phases of brain development. This pruning activity does not occur properly in certain conditions such as Down syndrome and fragile X syndrome (see Chapter 15). Inadequate pruning has also been implicated in the development of attention-deficit/hyperactivity disorder (ADHD) and learning disabilities (see Chapters 19 and 20; Cellot & Cherubini, 2013; Naaijen et al., 2017).

The next phase of cortical organization involves the development and refinement of synapses. Synaptic communication allows for the establishment of the complex behavioral actions necessary in postnatal life. Rett syndrome and fragile X syndrome are genetic disorders that result from abnormalities in neuronal maturation and synaptic function and result in cognitive and behavioral disturbances (Banerjee, Castro, & Sur, 2012).

Myelination The efficacy of neural connectivity for both cognition and movement depends not only on the successful conduction of electrical impulses across synapses, but also on the speed and coordination of these transmissions. This process is facilitated and accelerated by axonal **myelination.** During myelination, **oligodendrocytes** (a type of neuronal support cell) attach and wrap myelin along the length of a neuronal axon. The sheath of myelin from the oligodendrocytes serves to insulate the neuron and facilitate the conduction of signals between cells.

During fetal development, myelination starts in the spinal cord and brainstem and proceeds upward toward the cerebrum. At 40 weeks' gestation (the time of a typical birth), myelination has only advanced into the brainstem, cerebellum, and **internal capsule** (white matter near the thalamus). Myelination of the cerebral white matter occurs relatively late, reaching its peak during the first year of postnatal life. Because of the prolonged period of myelination, early injury to oligodendrocytes and their progenitors may not result in clinical symptoms until well after birth. Oligodendrocytes and their progenitors are particularly vulnerable to infection, inflammation, and **hypoxia-ischemia** (lack of adequate oxygenation or blood circulation). Such events during the latter part of fetal life or in the premature neonate can permanently injure the developing oligodendrocytes and may be responsible for certain forms of cerebral palsy (see Chapter 21; Back et al., 2001).

The Developing Cerebellum Extensive cerebellar development during intrauterine life exposes it to a prolonged period of risk for injury and maldevelopment. In addition, cerebellar **hypoplasia** (undergrowth) has been associated with certain genetic disorders, including Dandy-Walker syndrome, Werdnig-Hoffman syndrome, and Walker-Warburg syndrome. Increasingly, injury or maldevelopment of the cerebellum is recognized as contributing to significant motor and nonmotor functions, including cognition, language, and behavioral regulation, especially in premature neonates (Limperopoulos et al., 2007).

PLACENTAL DEVELOPMENT AND FUNCTION

The human placenta is a temporary, yet critical organ necessary for human development. Connecting the fetus to the maternal uterine wall, the placenta allows for gas and nutrient exchange between the maternal and fetal circulations, as well as for the elimination of waste and toxins. It also performs critical immune and endocrine functions. Although the placenta allows for the close approximation of maternal and fetal circulations, the placental barrier maintains each as a distinct compartment (see Figure 6.1).

Nutrition and Excretion

One of the main functions of the placenta is the active and passive transfer of nutrients from the maternal to the fetal circulation. In return, the placenta allows for the excretion of toxins and waste from the fetal to the maternal circulation, where it can be further processed and excreted by the mother. Gases, including oxygen and carbon dioxide, can readily **diffuse** (passively move along a concentration gradient) across the placental barrier. Similarly, small molecules and electrolytes (like sodium and potassium) can cross the placental barrier via diffusion. Transporters on the placental membrane also allow for active diffusion against concentration gradients and for the engulfment and transport of larger proteins and nutrients (Walker et al., 2017).

Immunity

Immune cells from the placenta release **cytokines** (substances such as interferon, interleukin, and growth factors) into the maternal circulation that activate the maternal immune system. This activation increases antibody and immunoglobulin production in the mother. It also renders the fetus more immunocompetent and leads to the release of cytokines that promote placental implantation and growth. In addition, many maternal antibodies cross the placenta during the second half of pregnancy and provide passive immunity to the newborn for several months after birth. This helps protect the infant from developing infections and immunologic disorders (Malek, 2013). The placenta's immunologic features also protect the fetus from being physically rejected by the maternal immune system as would normally happen to a "foreign body."

Endocrine Function

The placenta is responsible for the production of numerous hormones throughout gestation that are necessary for normal maternal, fetal, and placental function. Immediately after implantation, the placenta produces human chorionic gonadotropin, progesterone, and estrogens—all of which facilitate normal implantation and development of the blastocyst. Hormones that increase later in gestation promote **angiogenesis** (growth of blood vessels) as well as general fetal and placental growth. In addition, the placenta produces many neurosteroids and neurosteroid precursors that are thought to be protective of the developing brain (Costa, 2016; Hirst, Palliser, Yates, Yawno, & Walker, 2008).

MATERNAL, FETAL, AND PLACENTAL ORIGINS OF DEVELOPMENTAL DISORDERS

As described previously, the steps necessary for a successful pregnancy and typical human development require a complex interplay of fetal, maternal, and placental factors. Beyond the genetic make-up of the fetus, it is now known that the early intrauterine environment greatly influences human development. Recognizing that there is significant overlap of maternal, placental, and fetal contributions to fetal health, this section describes general periods of vulnerability, focusing on the developing brain and the multifactorial mechanisms of disrupted brain development.

Preconception Period

In many ways, fetal vulnerability to developmental disabilities begins even prior to conception. These risks include parental age, health, and nutrition. Advanced maternal age is associated with impaired egg quality; rates of **aneuploidy** (the genetic mechanism responsible for trisomy 21, also called Down syndrome) increase up to 50% in older mothers (see Chapter 1). In addition, maternal age is believed to impact epigenetic modifications (where genes are turned on and off) that may further diminish egg quality. Advanced paternal age is also believed to impact sperm quality as well as increase the amount of DNA damage/mutation in sperm. In contrast to chromosomal anomalies associated with advanced maternal age, advanced paternal age is more commonly associated with single gene mutations resulting in autosomal dominant disorders (see Chapter 1). There have been some population-based cohort studies that suggest an association between advanced paternal age and the development of neuropsychiatric disease (e.g., schizophrenia and autism), presumably mediated by cumulative DNA damage to key genetic sites. Parental exposure to environmental toxins, such as mercury or lead, is an additional concern in the development of birth defects and low birth weight infants (Bray, Gunnell, & Davey Smith, 2006; Ge, Schatten, Zhang, & Sun, 2015; Sadler, 2015).

Optimizing maternal health is important during the period prior to conception as well as during pregnancy. Many chronic diseases that impact maternal cardiovascular function (e.g., diabetes mellitus, hypertension, and obesity) can compromise uterine blood flow and uterine-placental function. This placental dysfunction results in substandard nutrient transfer, chronic fetal hypoxia, fetal growth restriction, and premature birth. These conditions are well-described risk factors for brain injury and developmental disabilities. Maternal hyperglycemia due to poorly controlled diabetes mellitus can be teratogenic, particularly early in pregnancy. Using the preconception period to stabilize chronic maternal disease provides direct benefit by improving maternal cardiovascular status, glycemic index, and limiting or eliminating maternal medications that also may be teratogenic (Shannon, Alberg, Nacul, & Pashayan, 2014).

Preconception is also the time to improve maternal nutrition. Low pre-pregnancy weight is associated with premature birth, while folic acid and iron supplementation (if there is maternal iron-deficient anemia) are associated with improved fetal growth, decreasing the risk of fetal growth restriction, and low birth weight infants (De-Regil, Fernandez-Gaxiola, Dowswell, & Pena-Rosas, 2010; Dean, Lassi, Imam, & Bhutta, 2014; Hodgetts, Morris, Francis, Gardosi, & Ismail, 2015). Folic acid supplementation prior to conception and throughout pregnancy also has been estimated to reduce the risk for neural tube defects by 70% as well as congenital heart disease (Tur-Torres, Garrido-Gimenez, & Alijotas-Reig, 2017; Viswanathan et al., 2017). Multivitamin supplements help decrease other teratogenic risks.

Embryonic Period

Typically, deviations from normal development during the embryotic period result in major structural **malformations** (the complete or partial absence of a body structure or alteration of its normal configuration). It is estimated that up to one half of all conceptions result in miscarriage (often referred to as spontaneous abortions), with up to 80% occurring during the embryonic period. Of all miscarriages, approximately half occur because of genetic abnormalities, particularly chromosomal anomalies. The other half result from external factors affecting the mother, fetus, or placenta as discussed earlier (Petracchi, Colaci, Igarzabal, & Gadow, 2009).

The initial risk to the embryo is the implantation of the blastocyst during the germinal period. Antigen presentation from the developing embryo to the mother during implantation is the trigger to activate the maternal immune system and shift from a primarily cell-mediated to antibody-mediated immunity. If this shift does not occur, the embryo will be rejected, resulting in pregnancy loss. Another problem is if implantation occurs outside the uterus. This results in an ectopic pregnancy, which most commonly leads to embryonic death around the second month of gestation. Even the location of embryonic implantation within the uterus can become problematic. Optimal sites for implantation are along the **anterior** (front) or **posterior** (back) wall of the uterus. Implantation near the cervix can cause **placenta previa,** in which the placenta overlies the cervix and may result in bleeding or premature delivery.

Specific genetic mutations affecting formation of the cerebral hemispheres can result in **holoprosencephaly** (failure of forebrain development), which involves impaired cleavage of the cerebral hemispheres and associated facial malformations. Although this malformation is most commonly genetic in origin, similar disturbances in brain development can be seen after alcohol exposure (fetal alcohol syndrome) or retinoic acid exposure (high-dose vitamin A given for treatment of severe acne) during early embryonic development (Edison & Muenke, 2003).

High blood sugar levels, seen in mothers with uncontrolled diabetes, can act as a teratogen during embryogenesis, resulting in **caudal agenesis**—a condition in which there is **hypoplasia** (underdevelopment) and fusion of the lower limbs along with pelvic and **sacral** (base of the spine) anomalies (Sadler, 2015).

The emergence of **laterality** (dominance of right or left side) is also vulnerable to injury and maldevelopment during embryogenesis. The heart is the primary organ with significant laterality (left side dominant), and disruptions in the emergence of laterality leave the fetus particularly vulnerable to the development of critical congenital heart disease (e.g., hypoplastic left heart syndrome).

This period in development further coincides with neurulation, so that individuals with abnormal arrangements of body organs are also prone to "midline defects," including neural tube defects, cleft palate, and **omphaloceles** (a midline abdominal wall defect).

Fetal Period

Major structural malformations are less likely to occur in the fetal period, as most body organs have already formed. Rather, this period is marked by a vulnerability to disruptions in the typical growth and development of existing body organs. Environmental influences and toxins become increasingly important, as does the dose, duration, and developmental stage at the time of exposure (see Chapter 2). The fetal period marks the time for proliferation, organization, and refinement of the neuronal circuity of the brain that, if altered, can lead to the emergence of developmental disabilities. The next section of this chapter emphasizes the most common mechanisms of fetal injury, particularly brain injury, during the fetal period. These mechanisms include the following: 1) infection; 2) inflammation; 3) hypoxia, hypoperfusion, and ischemia; 4) polysubstance use and abuse; and 5) maternal stress, anxiety, and depression.

Infection The developing fetus is susceptible to injury from infections for a number of reasons. First, as previously discussed, alterations in the mother's immune system leave her vulnerable to infections. Maternal infections can spread to the fetus through multiple routes: transplacental, ascending, and perinatal transmission. **Transplacental transmission** refers to the passage of microbes from the maternal to fetal circulation via the placenta. **Ascending infections** refer to the transfer of microbes from the maternal genital tract through the cervix and across the amniotic membranes to the fetus. **Perinatal transmission** refers to the transfer of infection during the passage of the infant through the cervix during delivery.

Congenital infections affecting the fetus and newborn can occur at any time during pregnancy. The GA at exposure reflects different periods of fetal vulnerability and explains the wide spectrum of clinical symptoms that may be present at birth. Early exposures to infectious agents in pregnancy, particularly to certain viruses, can result in interruptions of cellular division and proliferation in addition to the direct viral effect of **cytotoxicity** (cellular toxicity) and cell death. As a result, it is not surprising that early exposure to many types of viruses can result in microcephaly and overall fetal growth restriction. The mother's immune status and pre-pregnancy exposures also impact the effect of viral infections on fetal development.

CMV is one of the most common congenital infections and can result in premature birth, growth restriction, microcephaly, seizures, and hearing loss. Up to 60% of women will have been exposed to CMV prior to pregnancy, so only 40% are susceptible to primary infection during pregnancy (Staras et al., 2006). There may be few or no symptoms of CMV infection in the mother. If symptoms do occur, they tend to be mild and include muscle aches, fatigue, and low-grade fever. For women who are susceptible to CMV infection, fortunately less than 10% will acquire the infection during pregnancy and expose their fetus to the virus (Hyde, Schmid, & Cannon, 2010).

Many infants with congenital CMV are asymptomatic at birth but present with neurodevelopmental delays later in life. Up to 15% of affected infants will manifest hearing loss, visual impairment, and intellectual disability within the first few years of life but without microcephaly (Fowler & Boppana, 2018). This group likely reflects later exposure during fetal life. As a result, early neuronal proliferation is preserved, resulting in a typical head size; however, disruption of neuronal migration and organization can lead to cognitive impairment (Silasi et al., 2015).

This contrasts with congenital herpes simplex virus (HSV), in that the vast majority of newborns contract HSV infection during delivery. For women with existing antibodies (up to 70% of the population), the risk of HSV transmission to the fetus is fortunately quite low. There is, however, nearly a 50% risk of transmission if the mother acquires her first HSV infection during pregnancy. For newborns who acquire perinatal HSV and develop **encephalitis** (brain infection) after birth, more than two thirds of survivors will manifest neurodevelopmental abnormalities even if they have received adequate antiviral therapy (James, Kimberlin, & Whitley, 2009; Shankar, Patil, & Skariyachan, 2017; Silasi et al., 2015).

The immature fetal immune system also contributes to the impact of congenital infections. **Congenital varicella syndrome (VZV)** occurs when the embryo or fetus is exposed to the varicella virus in the first 20 weeks of pregnancy and can result in microcephaly, intellectual disability, limb hypoplasia, and/or growth restriction. Although lifelong immunity is common after exposure to varicella as a child or adult, it is believed that congenital VZV results from reactivation of the virus transmitted by the mother to the fetus in the absence of a functioning fetal immune system (Lamont et al., 2011; Smith & Arvin, 2009).

The outbreak of **Zika virus** in Central and South America in 2015 identified this virus as a previously unrecognized teratogenic agent. Neuronal stem cells are particularly sensitive to the Zika virus, resulting in exaggerated cell death in the frontal and parietal lobes of the fetal brain. This can lead to microcephaly and intellectual disability that is more severe than in other congenital infections.

Although risks of fetal viral infection persist, advances in medicine have positively influenced the **vertical transmission** (passage from mother to infant during the period immediately before and after birth) of certain microbes. The prime examples are Rubella and human immunodeficiency virus (HIV). Rubella virus in pregnancy is associated with the development of cataracts, glaucoma, heart defects, intellectual disability, hearing loss, and dental anomalies in the progeny. However, the rates of congenital rubella have decreased dramatically since the 1970s as a result of the routine administration of the rubella vaccine to children, providing lifelong immunity (Silasi et al., 2015).

Advanced therapies for the treatment of HIV can reduce maternal viral counts to virtually undetectable levels and markedly decrease the risk of transmission of the virus from mother to child. However, elucidating the fetal impact of congenital HIV has been challenging, as the effects of the virus versus those of antiretroviral treatment are difficult to distinguish. The overall prevalence of birth defects in this population is estimated to be approximately 5%–7%, primarily affecting musculoskeletal and cardiovascular development (Williams et al., 2015).

Complicating the assessment of the impact of early infectious exposures on the developing fetus is evidence that **hyperthermia** (fever) associated with any infection can be teratogenic. Particularly in the embryonic period, elevated maternal temperature is associated with an increased risk of major malformations. Other viruses such as parvovirus B19 may not be teratogenic but can nonetheless cause significant fetal harm. Parvovirus has a predilection for destroying red blood cells, leading to fetal anemia, hypoxemia, and high-output cardiac failure. While not directly targeting the brain, cardiovascular collapse in the fetus can affect both survival and neurodevelopment (Ornoy & Ergaz, 2017; Sass et al., 2017).

Inflammation Acute and chronic inflammation, even in the absence of intrauterine infection, is associated with poor pregnancy outcome, including preterm birth, neonatal encephalopathy, and perinatal mortality. Chronic inflammation (most commonly **chorioamnionitis**) alone increases the chance of preterm delivery and potentially related brain injury. The severity of fetal inflammation at delivery has been associated with an increased risk of neurodevelopment disabilities, most prominently cerebral palsy. Placental inflammation has also been associated with fetal growth restriction, an independent risk factor for neurodevelopmental disabilities (Greer et al., 2012; Salas et al., 2013).

Hypoxia, Hypoperfusion, and Ischemia In critical congenital heart disease (CCHD), the normal patterns of blood circulation are disrupted, resulting in chronic **hypoxia** (lower than normal levels of circulating oxygen). Numerous neurodevelopmental abnormalities have been described in this population. Impaired brain growth and maturation is most impacted by hypoxia and hypoperfusion in the third trimester when there is a particularly high demand for nutrients because of rapid body growth (Clouchoux et al., 2013).

Chronic hypoxia is also seen when there is placental insufficiency. The result is fetal growth restriction and low birth weight. As with CCHD, many survivors of fetal growth restriction are at risk for lifelong motor, cognitive, and behavioral impairments (Malhotra et al., 2017).

As is true with chronic hypoxia, low perfusion states of the fetus can also result in neuro-developmental impairment (Ghi et al., 2004). In addition to parvovirus infection, conditions associated with fetal anemia (e.g., **Rh incompatibility,** in which maternal antibodies cross into the fetal circulation and destroy fetal red cells) can result in hypoperfusion and hypoxia.

Polysubstance Use and Abuse The maternal use of alcohol, cigarettes, marijuana, illicit drugs, and opioids during pregnancy can have a significant adverse impact on fetal health. Some of these substances have direct teratogenic effects on the fetus (see

Chapter 2), whereas others influence brain biochemistry through alterations in neurotransmitters. Some have direct toxic effects on the placenta, but all impact maternal behavior and health.

Alcohol exposure during pregnancy can result in a spectrum of disorders. The most severe form is fetal alcohol syndrome, a condition with profound physical, cognitive, and behavioral disabilities that likely results from early and high exposure to alcohol in the embryonic period. Alcohol also is toxic to the placenta, exacerbating placental disease and disrupting the normal hormonal functions of the fetal-placental unit.

Nicotine and smoking exposure throughout pregnancy is associated with fetal growth restriction and low birth weight as a result of decreased utero-placental and fetal umbilical vessel blood flow (Behnke, Smith, Committee on Substance Abuse, & Committee on Fetus and Newborn, 2013; Thakur et al., 2013). Nicotine also activates numerous brain pathways, including cholinergic, GABA, and glutamate receptors. These pathways are also activated by other compounds from cigarettes and smoke, including cyanide and cadmium. It is likely that these altered pathways play a role in the increased incidence of subsequent neurobehavioral and cognitive impairments (e.g., ADHD) in the child (Lin et al., 2017).

Cocaine and other stimulants increase dopamine and serotonin pathways, and opioids mimic natural endorphins and also activate those pathways. The increase in both legal (prescription opioid-containing pain medication) and illicit (heroin) opioid use during pregnancy in the United States has been so dramatic in recent years that it has reached epidemic proportions (Brown, Doshi, Pauly, & Talbert, 2016). Although the prescribed use of methadone and buprenorphine has helped individuals with heroin dependency and decreased the symptoms of neonatal abstinence syndrome, the long-term effects of these medications on fetal neurodevelopment is not well known (Jansson et al., 2017).

Maternal Stress, Anxiety, and Depression

Maternal stress has been known to influence the immune system of both mother and fetus and has been associated with deviations in neurodevelopment and neuropsychiatric conditions. Maternal stress hormones also are known to cross the placenta, stimulating the fetal stress axis and releasing fetal cortisol. Early fetal exposure to these stress hormones is associated with preterm delivery, long-term metabolic effects on the child (including obesity and hypertension), and altered behavioral and cognitive function.

Structurally, prenatal stress levels have been correlated with volumetric changes in the hippocampus and amygdala of the brain and in subsequent behavior in affected children, suggesting that early fetal exposures influence brain growth and development (Marques, Bjorke-Monsen, Teixeira, & Silverman, 2015). Advanced imaging of the brain that can identify and describe neuronal microstructure suggests that neural pathways in newborns exposed to maternal anxiety differ from healthy controls, particularly in regions of the brain controlling sensory and emotional processing (Rifkin-Graboi et al., 2015).

Maternal depression and depressive symptoms are common during pregnancy and the postpartum period. Maternal depression has been found to be associated with preterm delivery, decreased placental function, growth restriction, and increased neonatal complications. It also has been associated with subsequent developmental delays and behavior problems (increased anxiety and attention problems) in children born to these mothers.

Many women receive psychopharmacologic therapy during pregnancy. Selective serotonin reuptake inhibitors (SSRIs) are the most common medications prescribed for depression in pregnancy. Studies suggest SSRIs may increase the rates of miscarriage and preeclampsia, preterm birth, and fetal growth restriction (Andersen, Andersen, Horwitz, Poulsen, & Jimenez-Solem, 2014; Eke, Saccone, & Berghella, 2016), although it is unclear if these rates are higher in mothers with untreated depression compared with those with SSRI exposure. There are mixed reports of early SSRI exposure and congenital anomalies, although this risk seems small. Some studies suggest that prenatal SSRI exposure may impact neurodevelopmental outcome, although long-term studies on this relationship are lacking. Animal studies suggest that the type of antidepressants, the timing, and cumulative exposure can each influence fetal neurodevelopment (Olivier et al., 2013).

EVALUATION OF FETAL DEVELOPMENT

The primary tool for the evaluation of fetal development is a detailed medical history that elicits genetic and environmental risk factors (including dietary and lifestyle habits), as well as potential toxic and viral exposures. Routine screening for fetal maldevelopment involves obtaining maternal blood samples that measure pregnancy-specific biomarkers. Recent advances in genetic testing can now extract fetal DNA (cell-free DNA) from the maternal circulation (see Chapter 3). This process permits the prenatal diagnosis of chromosomal anomalies without the need for invasive procedures that carry risk to the developing fetus (i.e., amniocentesis and chorionic villus sampling). Fetal imaging, through ultrasound or magnetic resonance imaging, can also give significant insight into the developing fetus.

DIAGNOSTIC CONSIDERATIONS

Although the availability of cell-free DNA technology has transformed prenatal testing, there remain significant limitations. This technology has been best studied in the identification of chromosomal anomalies; the detection of nonchromosomal conditions is less reliable and currently not commercially available. For definitive genetic testing, the gold standard remains the evaluation of fetal tissue, either through chorionic villous sampling of the placenta or amniocentesis.

Similarly, advances in prenatal imaging have revolutionized the identification of major structural anomalies. However, structure and function are not synonymous, and clinicians are limited in predicting functional outcome from structural alterations alone. These limitations are most pronounced in the prognostication of neuropsychiatric and neurobehavioral conditions in which fairly normal structural evaluations of the brain are generally obtained.

OVERVIEW OF MANAGEMENT STRATEGIES

A significant challenge in the medical evaluation and care of the developing embryo/fetus is that severe malformations often occur before the mother is even aware she is pregnant. Therefore, many strategies to optimize pregnancy outcomes emphasize the initiation of care in the preconception period. Pre-pregnancy vaccinations and micronutrient supplementation are two interventions that have dramatically improved pregnancy outcomes.

Advances in obstetric and perinatalcare now allow for direct intervention of the fetus *in utero*—particularly for the early correction of major malformations. As one example, fetal surgery for the repair of neural tube defects may improve outcomes by preventing secondary injury to the developing spinal cord. Another example is fetal cardiac interventions, which may improve fetal circulation and ameliorate future neurodevelopmental impairment.

Other interventions are being developed to optimize utero-placental health through novel medications and nutritional supplements. Successful mammalian models of an artificial placenta present the possibility of having the human fetus grow outside of the uterus when the intrauterine environment will no longer sustain it (Partridge et al., 2017). These promising new therapies have the potential to transform fetal care, particularly in the setting of an adverse intrauterine environment, and revolutionize the way clinicians consider neuroprotection to prevent fetal derived developmental disabilities.

SUMMARY

- Fetal health involves a complex interplay of fetal-maternal-placental well-being. Specific adaptations of the fetal and placental circulations optimize nutrient transfer to the fetus, especially the fetal brain.
- Human development follows a highly structured pattern of development from conception through fetal development. The rapidly developing fetal brain results in varying periods of vulnerability throughout gestation, during which even the subtlest alteration can give rise to lifelong consequences.
- The placenta is a critical organ of fetal development that performs important nutritional, immunologic, and endocrine functions to support the developing fetus.
- Deviations from normal development can result from maternal, fetal, or placental disturbances. Such deviations may be genetic in origin or secondary to acquired illness, injury, or toxic exposure.
- A detailed medical history can identify a significant number of risk factors for developmental disorders in the fetus. Maternal serum testing and fetal testing through amniocentesis or chorionic villous sampling, along with structural evaluations of the fetus through ultrasound and magnetic resonance imaging, can aid in the diagnosis of many fetal conditions.
- Accurate fetal diagnostics will become increasingly important as novel fetal interventions become available.

ADDITIONAL RESOURCES

Baby Center: https://www.babycenter.com/fetal-development-week-by-week

MedlinePlus: https://medlineplus.gov/ency/article/002398.htm

Abnormal Fetal Development: https://embryology.med.unsw.edu.au/embryology/index.php/Abnormal_Development_-_Fetal_Growth_Restriction Technical description of influences on abnormal fetal development

Additional resources can be found online in Appendix D: Childhood Disabilities Resources, Services, and Organizations (see About the Online Companion Materials).

REFERENCES

Andersen, J. T., Andersen, N. L., Horwitz, H., Poulsen, H. E., & Jimenez-Solem, E. (2014). Exposure to selective serotonin reuptake inhibitors in early pregnancy and the risk of miscarriage. *Obstetrics & Gynecology, 124*(4), 655–661. doi:10.1097/AOG.0000000000000447

Back, S. A., Luo, N. L., Borenstein, N. S., Levine, J. M., Volpe, J. J., & Kinney, H. C. (2001). Late oligodendrocyte progenitors coincide with the developmental window of vulnerability for human perinatal white matter injury. *Journal of Neuroscience, 21*(4), 1302–1312.

Banerjee, A., Castro, J., & Sur, M. (2012). Rett syndrome: Genes, synapses, circuits, and therapeutics. *Frontiers in Psychiatry, 3*, 34. doi:10.3389/fpsyt.2012.00034

Behnke, M., Smith, V. C., Committee on Substance Abuse, & Committee on Fetus and Newborn. (2013). P renatal substance abuse: Short- and long-term effects on the exposed fetus. *Pediatrics, 131*(3), e1009–e1024. doi:10.1542/peds.2012-3931

Bray, I., Gunnell, D., & Davey Smith, G. (2006). Advanced paternal age: How old is too old? *Journal of Epidemiology and Community Health, 60*(10), 851–853. doi:10.1136/jech.2005.045179

Brown, J. D., Doshi, P. A., Pauly, N. J., & Talbert, J. C. (2016). Rates of neonatal abstinence syndrome amid efforts to combat the opioid abuse epidemic. *JAMA Pediatrics, 170*(11), 1110–1112. doi:10.1001/jamapediatrics.2016.2150

Bystron, I., Blakemore, C., & Rakic, P. (2008). Development of the human cerebral cortex: Boulder Committee revisited. *Nature Reviews Neuroscience, 9*(2), 110–122. doi:10.1038/nrn2252

Calkins, K., & Devaskar, S. U. (2011). Fetal origins of adult disease. *Current Problems in Pediatric and Adolescent Health Care, 41*(6), 158–176. doi:10.1016/j.cppeds.2011.01.001

Cellot, G., & Cherubini, E. (2013). Functional role of ambient GABA in refining neuronal circuits early in postnatal development. *Frontiers in Neural Circuits, 7*, 136. doi:10.3389/fncir.2013.00136

Clouchoux, C., du Plessis, A. J., Bouyssi-Kobar, M., Tworetzky, W., McElhinney, D. B., Brown, D. W., . . . Limperopoulos, C. (2013). Delayed cortical development in fetuses with complex congenital heart disease. *Cerebral Cortex, 23*(12), 2932–2943. doi:10.1093/cercor/bhs281

Costa, M. A. (2016). The endocrine function of human placenta: An overview. *Reproductive BioMedicine Online, 32*(1), 14–43. doi:10.1016/j.rbmo.2015.10.005

De-Regil, L. M., Fernandez-Gaxiola, A. C., Dowswell, T., & Pena-Rosas, J. P. (2010). Effects and safety of periconceptional folate supplementation for preventing birth defects. *Cochrane Database System Review*, 10, CD007950. doi:10.1002/14651858.CD007950.pub2

Dean, S. V., Lassi, Z. S., Imam, A. M., & Bhutta, Z. A. (2014). Preconception care: Nutritional risks and interventions. *Reproductive Health, 11*(Suppl. 3), S3. doi:10.1186/1742-4755-11-S3-S3

Edison, R., & Muenke, M. (2003). The interplay of genetic and environmental factors in craniofacial morphogenesis: Holoprosencephaly and the role of cholesterol. *Congenital Anomolies (Kyoto), 43*(1), 1–21.

Eke, A. C., Saccone, G., & Berghella, V. (2016). Selective serotonin reuptake inhibitor (SSRI) use during pregnancy and risk of preterm birth: A systematic review and meta-analysis. *BJOG, 123*(12), 1900–1907. doi:10.1111/1471-0528.14144

Fall, C., & Osmond, C. (2013). Commentary: The developmental origins of health and disease: An appreciation of the life and work of Professor David J. P. Barker, 1938–2013. *International Journal of Epidemiology, 42*(5), 1231–1232. doi:10.1093/ije/dyt207

Fowler, K. B., & Boppana, S. B. (2018). Congenital cytomegalovirus infection. *Seminars in Perinatology, 42*(3), 149–154. doi:10.1053/j.semperi.2018.02.002

Ge, Z. J., Schatten, H., Zhang, C. L., & Sun, Q. Y. (2015). Oocyte ageing and epigenetics. *Reproduction, 149*(3), R103–114. doi:10.1530/REP-14-0242

Ghi, T., Brondelli, L., Simonazzi, G., Valeri, B., Santini, D., Sandri, F., . . . Pilu, G. (2004). Sonographic demonstration of brain injury in fetuses with severe red blood cell alloimmunization undergoing intrauterine transfusions. *Ultrasound in Obstetrics & Gynecology, 23*(5), 428–431. doi:10.1002/uog.1035

Greer, L. G., Ziadie, M. S., Casey, B. M., Rogers, B. B., McIntire, D. D., & Leveno, K. J. (2012). An immunologic basis for placental insufficiency in fetal growth restriction. *American Journal of Perinatology, 29*(7), 533–538. doi:10.1055/s-0032-1310525

Hirst, J. J., Palliser, H. K., Yates, D. M., Yawno, T., & Walker, D. W. (2008). Neurosteroids in the fetus and neonate: Potential protective role in compromised pregnancies. *Neurochemistry International, 52*(4–5), 602–610. doi:10.1016/j.neuint.2007.07.018

Hodgetts, V. A., Morris, R. K., Francis, A., Gardosi, J., & Ismail, K. M. (2015). Effectiveness of folic acid supplementation in pregnancy on reducing the risk of small-for-gestational age neonates: A population study, systematic review and meta-analysis. *BJOG, 122*(4), 478–490. doi:10.1111/1471-0528.13202

Hoerder-Suabedissen, A., & Molnár, Z. (2015). Development, evolution and pathology of neocortical subplate neurons. *Nature Reviews Neuroscience, 16*, 133. doi:10.1038/nrn3915

Hyde, T. B., Schmid, D. S., & Cannon, M. J. (2010). Cytomegalovirus seroconversion rates and risk factors: Implications for congenital CMV. *Reviews in Medical Virology, 20*(5), 311–326. doi:10.1002/rmv.659

James, S. H., Kimberlin, D. W., & Whitley, R. J. (2009). Antiviral therapy for herpesvirus central nervous system infections: Neonatal herpes simplex virus infection, herpes simplex encephalitis, and congenital cytomegalovirus infection. *Antiviral Research, 83*(3), 207–213. doi:10.1016/j.antiviral.2009.04.010

Jansson, L. M., Velez, M., McConnell, K., Spencer, N., Tuten, M., Jones, H. E., . . . DiPietro, J. A. (2017). Maternal buprenorphine treatment and fetal neurobehavioral development. *American Journal of Obstetrics & Gynecology, 216*(5), e521–e528. doi:10.1016/j.ajog.2017.01.040

Kostovic, I., & Judas, M. (2010). The development of the subplate and thalamocortical connections in the human foetal brain. *Acta Paediatrica, 99*(8), 1119–1127. doi:10.1111/j.1651-2227.2010.01811.x

Lamont, R. F., Sobel, J. D., Carrington, D., Mazaki-Tovi, S., Kusanovic, J. P., Vaisbuch, E., & Romero, R. (2011). Varicella-zoster virus (chickenpox) infection in pregnancy. *BJOG, 118*(10), 1155–1162. doi:10.1111/j.1471-0528.2011.02983.x

Limperopoulos, C., Bassan, H., Gauvreau, K., Robertson, R. L., Jr., Sullivan, N. R., Benson, C. B., . . . duPlessis, A. J. (2007). Does cerebellar injury in premature infants contribute to the high prevalence of long-term cognitive, learning, and behavioral disability in survivors? *Pediatrics, 120*(3), 584–593. doi:10.1542/peds.2007-1041

Lin, Q., Hou, X. Y., Yin, X. N., Wen, G. M., Sun, D., Xian, D. X., . . . Chen, W. Q. (2017). Prenatal exposure to environmental tobacco smoke and hyperactivity behavior in chinese young children. *International Journal of Environmental Research and Public Health, 14*(10). doi:10.3390/ijerph14101132

Malek, A. (2013). Role of IgG antibodies in association with placental function and immunologic diseases in human pregnancy. *Expert Review of Clinical Immunol, 9*(3), 235–249. doi:10.1586/eci.12.99

Malhotra, A., Ditchfield, M., Fahey, M. C., Castillo-Melendez, M., Allison, B. J., Polglase, G. R., . . . Miller, S. L. (2017). Detection and assessment of brain injury in the growth-restricted fetus and neonate. *Pediatric Research, 82*(2), 184–193. doi:10.1038/pr.2017.37

Marques, A. H., Bjorke-Monsen, A. L., Teixeira, A. L., & Silverman, M. N. (2015). Maternal stress, nutrition and physical activity: Impact on immune function, CNS development and psychopathology. *Brain Research, 1617*, 28–46. doi:10.1016/j.brainres.2014.10.051

Naaijen, J., Bralten, J., Poelmans, G., Consortium, I., Glennon, J. C., Franke, B., & Buitelaar, J. K. (2017). Glutamatergic and GABAergic gene sets in attention-deficit/hyperactivity disorder: Association to overlapping traits in ADHD and autism. *Translational Psychiatry, 7*(1), e999. doi:10.1038/tp.2016.273

Olivier, J. D., Akerud, H., Kaihola, H., Pawluski, J. L., Skalkidou, A., Hogberg, U., & Sundstrom-Poromaa, I. (2013). The effects of maternal depression and maternal selective serotonin reuptake inhibitor exposure on offspring. *Frontiers in Cell Neuroscience, 7*, 73. doi:10.3389/fncel.2013.00073

Ornoy, A., & Ergaz, Z. (2017). Parvovirus B19 infection during pregnancy and risks to the fetus. *Birth Defects Research, 109*(5), 311–323. doi:10.1002/bdra.23588

Partridge, E. A., Davey, M. G., Hornick, M. A., McGovern, P. E., Mejaddam, A. Y., Vrecenak, J. D., . . . Flake, A. W. (2017). An extra-uterine system to physiologically support the extreme premature lamb. *Nature Communications, 8*, 15112. doi:10.1038/ncomms15112

Petracchi, F., Colaci, D. S., Igarzabal, L., & Gadow, E. (2009). Cytogenetic analysis of first trimester pregnancy loss. *International Journal of Gynecology & Obstetrics, 104*(3), 243–244. doi:10.1016/j.ijgo.2008.10.014

Rifkin-Graboi, A., Meaney, M. J., Chen, H., Bai, J., Hameed, W. B., Tint, M. T., . . . Qiu, A. (2015). Antenatal maternal anxiety predicts variations in neural structures implicated in anxiety disorders in newborns. *Journal of the American Academy of Child and Adolescent Psychiatry, 54*(4), 313–321, e312. doi:10.1016/j.jaac.2015.01.013

Sadler, T. W. (2015). *Langman's medical embryology* (13th ed.). Philadelphia, PA. Wolters Kluwer.

Salas, A. A., Faye-Petersen, O. M., Sims, B., Peralta-Carcelen, M., Reilly, S. D., McGwin, G., Jr., . . . Ambalavanan, N. (2013). Histological characteristics of the fetal inflammatory response associated with neurodevelopmental impairment and death in extremely preterm infants. *Journal of Pediatrics, 163*(3), 652–657, e651–e652. doi:10.1016/j.jpeds.2013.03.081

Sass, L., Urhoj, S. K., Kjaergaard, J., Dreier, J. W., Strandberg-Larsen, K., & Nybo Andersen, A. M. (2017). Fever in pregnancy and the risk of congenital malformations: A cohort study. *BMC Pregnancy Childbirth, 17*(1), 413. doi:10.1186/s12884-017-1585-0

Shankar, A., Patil, A. A., & Skariyachan, S. (2017). Recent perspectives on genome, transmission, clinical manifestation, diagnosis, therapeutic strategies, vaccine developments, and challenges of Zika virus research. *Frontiers in Microbiology, 8*, 1761. doi:10.3389/fmicb.2017.01761

Shannon, G. D., Alberg, C., Nacul, L., & Pashayan, N. (2014). Preconception healthcare and congenital disorders: systematic review of the effectiveness of preconception care programs in the prevention of congenital disorders. *Maternal and Child Health Journal, 18*(6), 1354–1379. doi:10.1007/s10995-013-1370-2

Silasi, M., Cardenas, I., Kwon, J. Y., Racicot, K., Aldo, P., & Mor, G. (2015). Viral infections during pregnancy. *American Journal of Reproductive Immunology, 73*(3), 199–213. doi:10.1111/aji.12355

Smith, C. K., & Arvin, A. M. (2009). Varicella in the fetus and newborn. *Seminars in Fetal Neonatal Medicine, 14*(4), 209–217. doi:10.1016/j.siny.2008.11.008

Staras, S. A., Dollard, S. C., Radford, K. W., Flanders, W. D., Pass, R. F., & Cannon, M. J. (2006). Seroprevalence of cytomegalovirus infection in the United States, 1988-1994. *Clinical Infectious Diseases, 43*(9), 1143–1151. doi:10.1086/508173

Thakur, G. A., Sengupta, S. M., Grizenko, N., Schmitz, N., Page, V., & Joober, R. (2013). Maternal smoking during pregnancy and ADHD: A comprehensive clinical and neurocognitive characterization. *Nicotine & Tobacco Research, 15*(1), 149–157. doi:10.1093/ntr/nts102

Tur-Torres, M. H., Garrido-Gimenez, C., & Alijotas-Reig, J. (2017). Genetics of recurrent miscarriage and fetal loss. *Best Practice & Research: Clinical Obstetrics & Gynaecology, 42*, 11–25. doi:10.1016/j.bpobgyn.2017.03.007

Viswanathan, M., Treiman, K. A., Kish-Doto, J., Middleton, J. C., Coker-Schwimmer, E. J., & Nicholson, W. K. (2017). Folic acid supplementation for the prevention of neural tube defects: An updated evidence report and systematic review for the US Preventive Services Task Force. *JAMA, 317*(2), 190–203. doi:10.1001/jama.2016.19193

Volpe, J. J. (2008). *Neurology of the newborn* (5th ed.). Philadelphia, PA: Saunders/Elsevier.

Walker, N., Filis, P., Soffientini, U., Bellingham, M., O'Shaughnessy, P. J., & Fowler, P. A. (2017). Placental transporter localization and expression in the human: The importance of species, sex, and gestational age differencesdagger. *Biology of Reproduction, 96*(4), 733–742. doi:10.1093/biolre/iox012

Williams, P. L., Crain, M. J., Yildirim, C., Hazra, R., Van Dyke, R. B., Rich, K., . . . Watts, D. H. (2015). Congenital anomalies and in utero antiretroviral exposure in human immunodeficiency virus-exposed uninfected infants. *JAMA Pediatrics, 169*(1), 48–55. doi:10.1001/jamapediatrics.2014.1889

Zhao, H., Wong, R. J., Nguyen, X., Kalish, F., Mizobuchi, M., Vreman, H. J., . . . Contag, C. H. (2006). Expression and regulation of heme oxygenase isozymes in the developing mouse cortex. *Pediatric Research, 60*(5), 518–523. doi:10.1203/01.PDR.0000242374.21415.f5

CHAPTER 7

The Senses *The World We See, Hear, and Feel*

Louis Pellegrino

Upon completion of this chapter, the reader will

- Explain the ways in which individuals use their senses to adapt to the world around and within them
- Describe the anatomy of vision and the development of the visual system
- Identify common methods of screening for vision problems
- Describe the anatomy of hearing and the development of the auditory system
- Identify common methods of screening for hearing problems
- Describe the components of the somatosensory system and their relationships to motor control and coordination

We often take for granted the great gift that we have in our senses. At every moment, our brains are awash with signals transmitted from myriad sensory receptors throughout our bodies, allowing us to sense the world around us and the world within us. The brain is, in fact, the primary sensory organ, and our eyes, ears, and other sensory organs serve to translate information in the environment and in our bodies into nerve impulses that the brain can use and understand.

The traditional "five senses" (vision, hearing, touch, smell, and taste) represent an oversimplification of the true complexity of the human sensory apparatus (Table 7.1). This chapter focuses on those systems of special relevance to developmental disabilities: the visual, auditory, and somatosensory systems. Emphasis is placed on the anatomy and development of these systems and on screening procedures used to identify vision, hearing, and sensory integration problems. Impairments of vision are discussed in detail in Chapter 25, impairments of hearing are discussed in Chapter 26, and sensory processing impairments as they relate to autism spectrum disorder are discussed in Chapter 18.

THE WORLD WE SEE

Humans are creatures of vision. More than any of the other senses, individuals rely on vision to keep track of the world around them. Even language is dominated by vision-related metaphors (e.g., "I *see* what you mean," "A good leader must have a *clear vision* for the future," "We need to *take a look at* that issue more closely," and "You don't have *the big picture*"). At some point in our lives, most individuals will experience challenges with vision that require professional attention, especially as they age. Yet, vision problems are also common in

Table 7.1. The human sensory apparatus

Name	Primary receptor(s)	Neurologic destination
The chemical senses (sensing chemical substances through direct contact with sensory organs)		
Taste	Taste receptors for salt, sweet, bitter, sour, and umami (savory) located in the taste buds of the tongue, palate, and pharynx	Gustatory cortex (part of the parietal cortex) via nuclei in the brainstem and thalamus
Smell (olfaction)	Olfactory cells located on the inner surfaces of the nasal cavity	Direct pathway from receptor cells to the primitive olfactory cortex; indirect pathways via the thalamus to the orbital frontal cortex
The remote senses (sensing energy sources from the external environment)		
Vision	Photoreceptors in the retina (rods and cones) transduce electromagnetic energy into nerve impulses	The visual cortex via the brainstem and thalamus
Hearing	Transduction of acoustic energy (pressure/sound waves) by hair cells in the cochlea into nerve impulses	The auditory cortex via the brainstem and thalamus
The internal senses (sensing changes inside the body and on body surfaces)		
Balance	The vestibular apparatus (of the inner ear) senses the position and movement of the head via movement of fluid within the semicircular canals, which is transduced by hair cells into nerve impulses	Output from the vestibular apparatus to multiple centers in the brain and spinal cord help regulate movement
Touch, pressure, pain, temperature	Mechanoreceptors (touch and pressure), nociceptors (pain), and thermoreceptors (temperature) in the skin	The somatosensory cortex via multiple pathways in the spinal cord, brainstem, and thalamus
"Body sense" (proprioception)	Stretch receptors (muscle spindles) and Golgi tendon organs sense active stretching and the state of tension in muscles and tendons; multiple receptor types sense movement and position of joints	Multiple pathways in the spinal cord and brainstem regulate motor output and movement, mostly at an unconscious level

children, especially those with developmental disabilities, and can have a significant impact on their lives.

The case study below illustrates the common issue of unidentified vision problems in children—especially younger children. In the United States, the prevalence of vision impairment in preschoolers aged 36 to 72 months is estimated to be 1.5%, which is equivalent to more than 174,000 children (Varma, Tarczy-Hornoch, & Jiang, 2017). Hispanic and African American children are at higher risk, and children with other developmental disabilities, such as cerebral palsy or intellectual disability, are at highest risk for visual problems. In fact, 75% of children with vision impairment have another developmental disability (Boyle et al., 2011).

CASE STUDY

Kayla is a smart, vivacious 7-year-old second grader who has been falling behind academically. She mastered her letters and numbers early in preschool and was reading first-grade material by the end of kindergarten. Her first-grade teacher described her as being one of her best students and a delight to have in the class. Her second-grade teacher saw a very different picture. Kayla seemed uncharacteristically distracted and didn't participate in classroom activities. She still enjoyed reading on her own, loved playing with her friends during recess, and seemed to learn well when her teacher worked with her one-on-one, but during group instruction she missed much of what was being taught. She wasn't being bullied and wasn't having problems at home.

Kayla's mother and teacher were both at a loss to explain the change in her demeanor. Early in the school year the school nurse performed vision screening on all of the students, and Kayla's mother and teacher were both surprised to learn that Kayla failed the screen. She was seen by an optometrist, who discovered that Kayla was near-sighted, or myopic, and had difficulty seeing distant objects. Once Kayla was fitted with glasses, she quickly recovered her enthusiasm for learning. Her teacher was amazed by the transformation and felt that she working with a different child. Her mother felt like she had her old Kayla back.

Thought Questions:

What measures could be taken to improve the identification of young children with vision problems? If a child has passed his or her newborn hearing screening test, is further testing ever necessary? If so, under what circumstances? How might an awareness of sensory processing problems in children influence the design of schools and classrooms?

Anatomy of the Visual System

The eye is the primary organ of vision (Figure 7.1). It is designed to transduce a portion of electromagnetic radiation, visible light, into nerve impulses that can be processed by the brain. Light first enters the eye through the **cornea,** a transparent tissue that is the primary refractive surface of the eye (Figure 7.2). The curved surface of the cornea bends (refracts) light so that it converges on the retina, the light-sensitive surface lining the back of the eye.

The amount of light that enters the eye is regulated by the contraction and relaxation of the donut-shaped **iris** (the colored part of the eye), which controls the size of the central **pupil.** The **lens** further focuses light through the central cavity of the eye (which is filled with a gelatinous fluid, the **vitreous humor**) onto the **retina.** The retina contains two types of photoreceptive cells, the **cones,** which respond to differences in color (related to the frequency of light waves), and the **rods,** which are sensitive to differences in brightness (related to the amplitude of light waves). There are three types of cones: 1) those that are most sensitive to low-frequency (red) light, 2) those most sensitive to mid-frequency (green) light, and 3) those most sensitive to high-frequency (blue) light. The cones are concentrated in the central area of the retina (the **fovea**) and subserve color vision for detail in bright daylight.

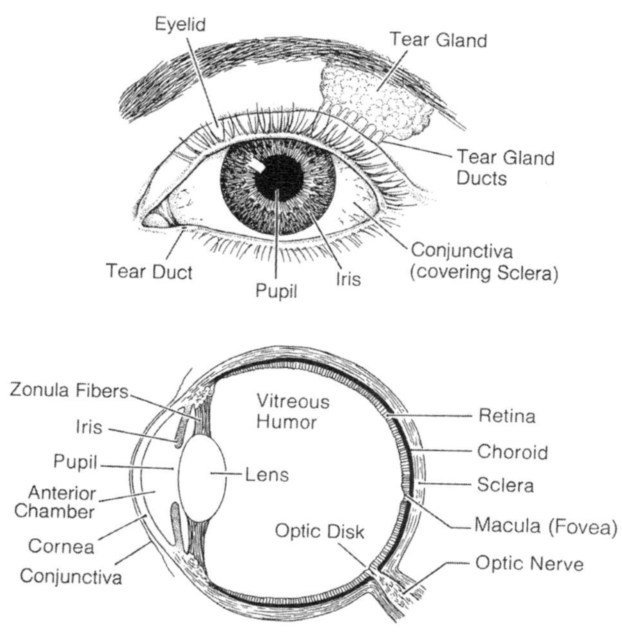

Figure 7.1. The anatomy of the eye. The eye is often likened to a camera. The pupil is like the shutter of a camera, which opens and closes to admit more or less light. Light is transmitted through the transparent tissues and fluids of the eye (the cornea, the fluid of the anterior chamber, the lens, and the vitreous humor) to the retina, where light energy is transduced into nerve impulses, which are then transmitted to the brain via the optic nerve.

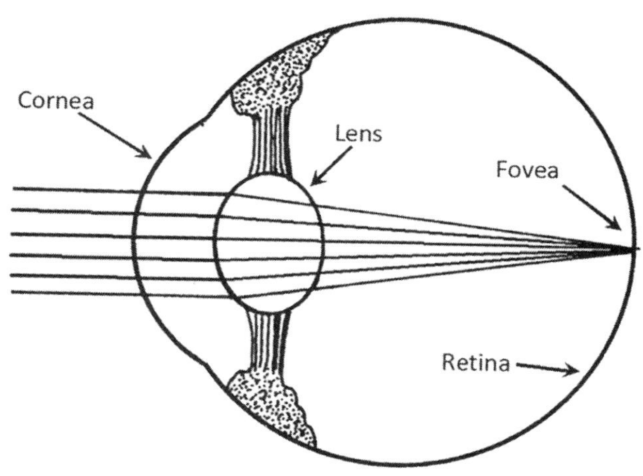

Figure 7.2. Refraction of light by the cornea and lens. The cornea, which is situated between the surrounding air and the fluid interior of the eye, is the primary refractive surface of the eye. Muscles attached to the lens change its shape, refining the focus of images falling on the fovea, the most sensitive center of vision on the retina.

Each cone is connected through intermediary cells to a single ganglion cell in the retina. Ganglion cells are the first in a series of nerve cells (neurons) that transmit information from the retina to the brain. This one-to-one arrangement of cones to ganglion cells ensures a high degree of accuracy in encoding detailed spatial information about the visual environment. Rods are far more numerous than cones, and they populate the periphery of the retina. They are most sensitive in low light conditions, and many rods tend to connect to individual ganglion cells, in effect amplifying their sensitivity in low light conditions. Because rods are not specifically responsive to particular colors, low light vision lends a grayish or dark blueish-green cast to the visual environment (Bear, Connors, & Paradiso, 2016).

Spatial information about the visual environment is "mapped" onto the retina, and that information is transmitted more or less intact throughout the nervous system. Fibers from the ganglion cells bundle together to form the right and left optic nerves, which meet at a crossroad in the visual system called the optic chiasm. At this point, nerve fibers carrying information about the left visual field *from both eyes* continue toward nerve centers on the right side of the brain, and fibers carrying information about the right visual field *from both eyes* continue toward nerve centers on the left side of the brain. In effect, the right brain sees the left side of the world, and the left brain sees the right side of the world.

Next, nerve fibers arrive at the "Grand Central Station" of vision in the brain, the lateral geniculate body of the thalamus. The thalamus is the major waystation in the brain for all types of sensory information, and visual information here "changes trains" and is transmitted to its final destination, the primary visual cortex.

The visual cortex, located in the back of the brain in the occipital lobe, has remarkable computational powers. Different modules within the cortex analyze different aspects of the visual environment, such as the shape and configuration of objects, color, and motion. Visual information is then processed further along two pathways in the cortex, the dorsal pathway and the ventral pathway (Figure 7.3). The dorsal pathway, sometimes referred to as the "where" or "action" stream, analyzes spatial information in the environment and is thought to aid the motor control system in planning movement. The ventral pathway, sometimes referred to as the "what" or "perception" stream, provides for object recognition and is thought to aid various higher-level cognitive processes involved in perception and memory (Goodale & Milner, 1992). A special area in the ventral pathway is dedicated to facial recognition, and damage to that area can result in a condition sometimes called "face blindness." Affected individuals have normal vision and object perception but cannot recognize people's faces, including close family members.

Development of Vision

In the human embryo, the eyes develop as a direct outgrowth of the embryonic brain (Figure 7.4). The first rudimentary precursors to the eyes appear at 4 weeks' gestation. By 7 weeks, the eyes have assumed their basic form, and by 15 weeks, they are fully formed.

In contrast to the auditory system, which receives significant stimulation prenatally, the visual system receives no input prior to birth. Infants are not born blind, however. Studies have demonstrated that they have at least a vague awareness of their visual environment, and quite early in infancy they demonstrate a preference for faces over other objects (Bremond-Gignac et al., 2011). Newborns have fewer cones in the retina than adults and so have limited color perception. They also have a lower density of connections in the thalamus and visual cortex compared with adults. Control of eye movements is also immature. Newborns can briefly fix their gaze on objects or faces, but their eyes often don't move together (this is called dysconjugate eye movements or gaze).

By 3 months of age, infants are able to fix on and follow objects with their eyes and the eyes consistently move together (conjugate gaze). By this age, infants also will blink in response to a visual threat (e.g., an object moving toward the face quickly), and they will attempt to coordinate vision with movement (e.g., reaching toward and batting at objects).

By 5 to 8 months of age, infants demonstrate evidence of improved color vision and depth perception, and from a neurologic perspective, they have achieved the highest synaptic density of connections within the visual system that they will ever have during their lifespan. These connections are gradually "pruned" as the visual system matures in a similar way to what happens in the brain. This high level of connectivity relates to the great plasticity of the visual system in infancy and early childhood. The immature nervous system in general, and the visual nervous system in particular, is better able to respond and adapt to visual and visual motor disturbances. For this reason,

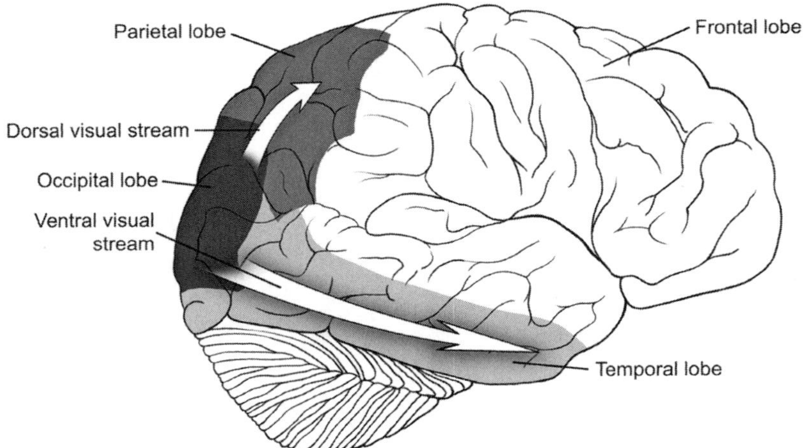

Figure 7.3. The ventral and dorsal visual pathways of the cortex. Visual data received by the primary visual cortex are further analyzed to provide visual context for movement (the "where" stream, located along the upper, or dorsal, surface of the brain) and to provide information for analysis of the details of the visual environment (the "what" stream, located along the lower, or ventral, surface of the brain).

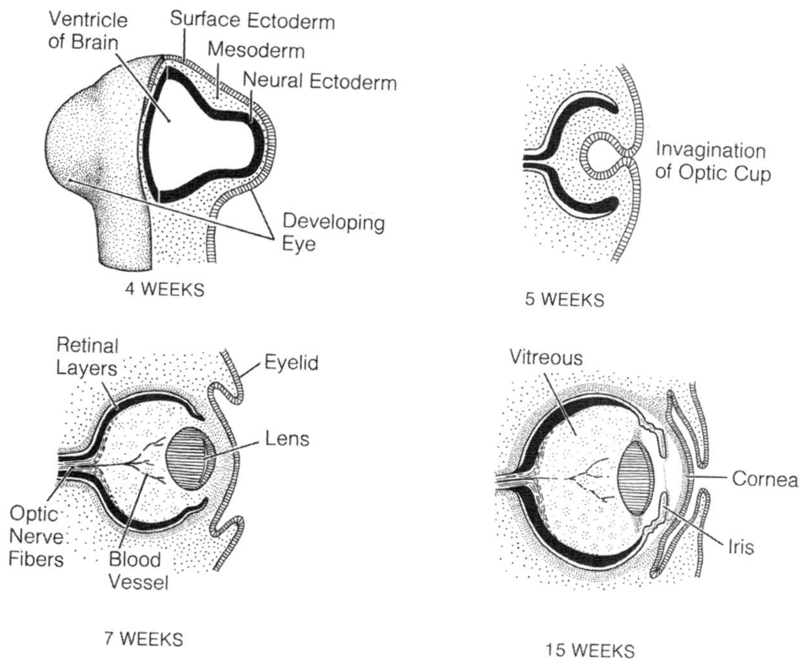

Figure 7.4. The embryonic development of the eye. The eyes first appear at 4 weeks' gestation as two spherical bulges, one on each side of the head. They indent in the next week to form the optic cups. By 7 weeks, the eyes have already assumed their basic form. The eye is completely formed by 15 weeks.

treatment of these problems earlier rather than later in childhood will result in more favorable outcomes for vision (see the discussion on amblyopia in Chapter 25). By 3 to 4 years of age, measures of visual acuity will generally average 20/40, and by 6 years of age, children achieve adult levels of visual acuity (fully mature vision), ideally 20/20.

Measuring Visual Acuity

When someone says, "I have 20/20 vision," it is understood that they have excellent vision and probably don't need glasses. The term *20/20* derives from how well an individual can see the lines on a standard eye chart. The first 20 in this ratio refers to the standard distance (20 feet) that a person would stand from the eye chart when being tested (for convenience, however, many charts are designed to be used at a distance of 10 feet). Vision is usually tested separately for each eye (the eye not being tested is covered). If the person being tested can see items on a chart that an adult with normal vision can see at 20 feet, that person is said to have 20/20 vision. If, on the other hand, the person being tested can only see items on the chart that adults with normal vision would be able to see at a distance of 40 feet, that person is said to have 20/40 vision. The larger the bottom number, the worse the vision. A person with 20/70 has a significant visual impairment and is said to have low vision; a person with 20/200 vision is said to be legally blind.

Different eye charts are used to test vision at different ages. The classic Snellen eye chart uses letters and should only be used in adults and older children who can read. Eye charts used for testing younger children include the HOTV chart, which uses various sizes of the capitalized letters *H, O, T,* and *V.* The child is asked to match the letter she sees to an example of the letters held close by the examiner (the child does not have to name the letters). Lea charts similarly use simple visual symbols (a circle, a square, and simplified drawings of a house and an apple) that a child is asked to match. Children as young as 2 to 3 years of age may be tested in this manner (American Academy of Ophthalmology, 2016; Rogers & Jordan, 2013).

Screening for Vision Problems

Whereas universal screening of newborns for hearing problems has become the norm (see discussion below), there is still a lack of consensus about how best to approach the issue of screening for visual deficits in young children. There is general agreement that vision problems should be identified as early as possible, that the process of surveillance for such problems should begin at birth, and that primary care providers (such as pediatricians and family practice physicians) have a particular responsibility to identify the risk factors for and the early signs of visual impairment (see Box 7.1 for a discussion of the role of schools and the school nurse in screening for vision problems). There is also agreement that children should have their vision screened using standard eye charts as early as possible (ideally beginning at 3 years of age).

Children who fail vision screening, have significant risk factors for visual impairment, or demonstrate abnormalities on examination of their eyes, including dysconjugate gaze, should be referred to a vision specialist for a comprehensive evaluation. Table 7.2 provides a summary of current recommendations for evaluation and referral. Recommendations have been made for all children to have a comprehensive assessment as early as 6 months of age (American Association for Pediatric Ophthalmology and Strabismus, 2017), but there are concerns that this would represent an inefficient use of resources. Likewise, attempts to provide universal screening outside of primary care settings have met with mixed results (Kemper, Fant, & Badgett, 2003; Rogers & Jordan, 2013).

Screening very young children (especially those less than 3 years old) represents a particularly difficult problem, but technology has provided answers. Instruments referred to as photoscreeners and autorefractors are available that allow testing of children as young as 1 year of age. These methods are noninvasive (for photoscreeners, the process is as simple as taking the equivalent of a snapshot of the child's eyes), require minimal cooperation from the child, and can be used in children who cannot be reliably screened using eye charts.

Instrument-based screening may actually be superior to eye charts for 3- to 6-year-olds (O'Hara, 2016). Limitations for their use include the initial cost of the instruments and lack of insurance coverage for the procedure. Despite these difficulties, the American Academy of Pediatrics and the American Academy of Ophthalmology have endorsed their use in recently published guidelines (Miller & Lessin, 2012).

THE WORLD WE HEAR

If vision is a window on the world, hearing is a gateway into the thoughts and feelings of others. Compared with vision, hearing is a more intrusive sense; individuals cannot stop hearing as easily as they can stop seeing by closing their eyes. Humans are constantly bathed in a sea of sound, and a primary task of the auditory system is to filter out the noise and allow individuals to focus on those things that are most important to hear. Very often, the things that are most necessary to hear are the words spoken by others.

In the course of early development, human beings are unique in their ability to become attuned to the discrete units of sounds (phonemes) of their native language (Jusczyk, 2002). Our capacity to speak and to understand others is critically dependent on this ability. Ensuring that children are born with intact hearing and thus have a clear path to learning to speak their native language is a high priority for parents and professionals alike.

The most common cause of temporary hearing loss in young children is otitis media with effusion (OME), an ear infection with middle ear fluid. By 1 year of age, 62% of children have had their first episode of

BOX 7.1 INTERDISCIPLINARY CARE

The School Nurse and Vision Screening

Because children typically have the most contact with their primary care providers (i.e., pediatricians, family practitioners, nurse practitioners, and physician assistants) through early childhood, these professionals have the greatest responsibility for identifying vision problems. Despite efforts to improve screening practices in these settings, shortfalls persist in this process (see text for discussion). The school nurse can serve as a crucial "safety net" in identifying children with vision problems who may have been previously missed. Vision problems may surface for the first time in elementary or middle school, and the school nurse is ideally situated to recognize these problems by providing in-school screening and by referring children for further assessment.

Guidelines exist for screening children through elementary school and beyond (Colorado Department of Education, 2017; National Association of School Nurses, 2017). School nurses are also well positioned, through their regular contact with students and teachers, to recognize children who may have "red flags" for vision problems (e.g., unexplained reading difficulties, unexplained deterioration in general academic performance).

Table 7.2. Vision screening recommendations

Age	Evaluation	Reasons for referral to vision specialist
Newborn–1 year	Examine eyes (external inspection) Assess vision (response to light younger than 3 months, fixation and following older than 3 months) Perform red reflex evaluation (looking for absent or asymmetric reflex)[a] Perform pupillary examination Review family history	Abnormal red reflex (urgent consultation) Family history of retinoblastoma in parent or sibling Refer any infant with poor tracking or eye misalignment in child younger than 3 months old
1–3 years	Obtain ocular history Examine eyes, lids, visual reactions, and eye alignment and motility with use of ophthalmoscope Perform pupillary examination Perform red reflex evaluation Use screening device (e.g., photoscreening, autorefraction), if available Perform visual acuity testing (HOTV, LEA symbols) in some 2- to 3-year-olds	Abnormal eye movements (strabismus) Chronic tearing or eye discharge Failed visual acuity testing Failed photoscreening
3–5 years	Obtain ocular history Examine eyes, lids, visual reactions, and eye alignment and motility Perform pupillary examinations Perform red reflex evaluation Perform visual acuity testing (HOTV, LEA symbols) Use a screening device, if available	Failed visual acuity test: 3–4 years: Cannot identify most items at 20/50 4–5 years: Cannot identify most items at 20/40 Two-line difference between eyes on visual acuity test Failed photoscreening
5 years and older	Perform ocular history Examine eyes, lids, visual reactions, and eye alignment and motility Perform pupillary examinations Perform red reflex evaluation Perform visual acuity testing (every 1–2 years)	Failed visual acuity test: Cannot identify most items at 20/30 Two-line difference between eyes on visual acuity test Trouble reading
At-risk children (any age)	Perform ocular history Examine eyes, lids, visual reactions, and eye alignment and motility Perform pupillary examinations Perform red reflex evaluation Perform visual acuity testing	Retinopathy of prematurity Family history of retinoblastoma, congenital glaucoma, congenital cataracts Other medical conditions associated with eye and vision problems Nystagmus (involuntary "jiggling" eye movements) Developmental delay, disability

Sources: American Association for Pediatric Ophthalmology and Strabismus (2017), Donahue and Baker (2016), and Rogers and Jordan (2013).

[a]*Red reflex evaluation:* Examine both eyes simultaneously from approximately 1 to 2 feet away, using an ophthalmoscope to view the red reflection (reflex) of the retina of each eye seen through a child's pupils (identical to the red-eye effect seen when taking a photograph). The red reflex should have a typical red appearance and should be the same brightness in each eye. If the appearance is abnormal (e.g., white or cloudy instead of red) or if the red reflex for one eye differs from the other, the child should be referred for a comprehensive vision assessment.

otitis media, and by 3 years of age, 83% of children have been affected (Rosa-Olivares, Porro, Rodriguez-Varela, Riefkohl, & Niroomand-Rad, 2015). Otitis media may develop during an upper respiratory infection, spontaneously as a result of eustachian tube dysfunction, or as a delayed sequelae of acute otitis media. Regardless of the etiology, if the middle ear infection is associated with effusion, it may cause a temporary conductive hearing loss that can impact language development if prolonged. Because OME is painless, it may escape diagnosis, but it should be carefully assessed for in children with delayed language development.

Current guidelines recommend tympanostomy tube placement for OME of 3 months or more duration (termed chronic) if it causes hearing loss (Rosenfeld et al., 2013). Tympanostomy tubes are surgically inserted, serve to aerate the middle ear, and help prevent future episodes of acute otitis media and OME. They typically extrude spontaneously within 1–2 years after insertion. Placement of tympanostomy tubes is the most common outpatient surgery performed in the United States. In fact, nearly 1 in 15 children will have tympanostomy tubes placed by 3 years of age (Rosenfeld et al., 2013).

Although the hearing loss associated with OME is most often a mild to moderate conductive hearing loss, moderate to profound persistent hearing loss from all causes occurs in about 4.5 out of every 1,000 children (Boyle et al., 2011). Significant hearing problems are especially common among children with other developmental disabilities, particularly trisomy 21 (discussed in detail in Chapter 26).

CASE STUDY

Henry is a 2-and-a-half-year-old boy with delayed speech and articulation errors. He passed his newborn hearing screen, but beginning in infancy he developed recurrent episodes of otitis media in one or both ears, as diagnosed by his pediatrician, Dr. Mendez. The acute inflammation always resolved with antibiotic treatment; however, Dr. Mendez has noted persistent fluid in the middle ear on several occasions. Henry has had three separate episodes of acute otitis media in the past year and persistent OME for the past 4 months. Henry's parents are concerned that these otologic problems may be affecting his speech and ask Dr. Mendez to test his hearing. She tells them that it would be best to have Henry tested by an audiologist. She also makes a referral to an otolaryngologist for consideration of placement of tympanostomy tubes. In the meantime, Henry has been evaluated by his county early intervention team, and he is receiving home-based speech therapy.

Anatomy of the Auditory System

The ear is designed to convert the mechanical energy of sound waves into nerve impulses that can be processed by the brain (Figure 7.5). The external ear and middle ear serve to transmit and amplify sound; the inner ear converts sound waves into nerve impulses, which are transmitted via central auditory pathways to the auditory cortex.

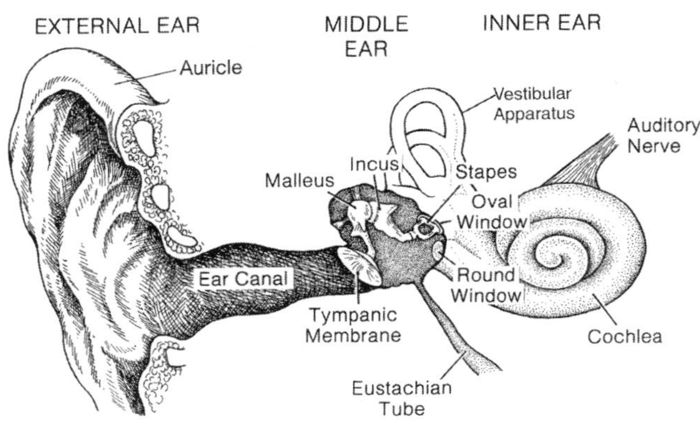

Figure 7.5. The anatomy of the ear. The external ear includes the auricle and the ear canal. The middle ear is composed of the tympanic membrane, or eardrum, and the three ear bones—the malleus, the incus, and the stapes. When the eustachian tube, which aerates the middle ear, is not functional, otitis media may develop. The stapes footplate lies on the oval window, the gateway to the inner ear. The inner ear contains the cochlea and the vestibular (balance) apparatus, collectively called the labyrinth.

The External and Middle Ear Sound waves are "collected," in a sense, by the external ear. The external ear is composed of the pinna or **auricle** (the part of the ear that can be seen when looking in the mirror) and the ear canal, which has glands in its wall that produce ear wax, or cerumen. The auricle is designed to funnel sound through the ear canal toward the ear drum, or **tympanic membrane** (TM), which lies at the end of the ear canal. The TM is made of thin, almost transparent tissue, and it vibrates readily in response to sound. It is attached to the **malleus** (Latin for "hammer"), which is the first in a series of tiny bones (called **ossicles**) that span the **middle ear** space. The malleus is rigidly connected to the **incus** (Latin for "anvil"), and the incus is flexibly connected to the **stapes** (Latin for "stirrup"). The flat face (footplate) of the stapes makes contact with a membrane covering the **oval window,** which is a part of the cochlea. This arrangement of TM-to-ossicles-to-oval window is designed to amplify the sounds that enter the ear. This is accomplished in two ways. The arrangement of the ossicles is such that they function as a lever, converting large but weak vibrations at the tympanic membrane into smaller but stronger vibrations at the oval window. The oval window also has a much smaller surface area than does the TM, which further serves to amplify the vibrations. Taken together, these two mechanisms amplify the sound pressure that reaches the oval window by a factor of 20 (Bear et al., 2016).

The Inner Ear The **cochlea** (Latin for "snail") and the **vestibular apparatus** (the organ of balance) constitute the **inner ear.** The cochlea is designed to convert the mechanical energy of the amplified vibrations presented at the oval window into nerve impulses that can be transmitted to the brain. If the spiral-shaped cochlea were unraveled and straightened, it would look like three fluid-filled tubes running parallel to each other (Figure 7.6). One tube, called the **scala vestibuli** (SV), originates at the oval window, and at its end encounters an opening (the helicotrema) that forms the origin of the **scala tympani** (ST). The ST runs back along the length of the cochlea to end at the round window. The SV and ST are filled with a sodium-rich fluid called perilymph. Because the SV and the ST are continuous with each other, vibrations at the oval window are transmitted through the perilymph to the round window. In between the SV and the ST lies the **scala media** (SM). In contrast to the SV and ST, the SM is filled with a potassium-rich fluid called endolymph.

The actual organ of hearing, the **organ of Corti,** runs along the base of the SM and rests on the **basilar**

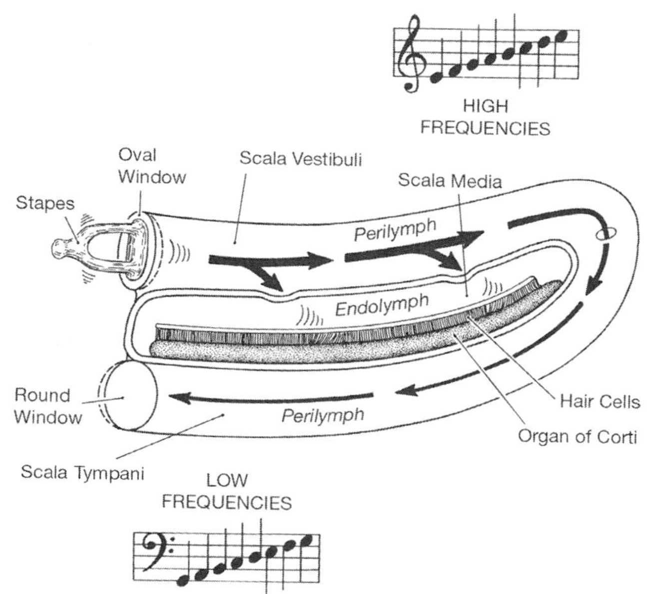

Figure 7.6. The anatomy of the cochlea. In this illustration, the cochlea has been "unfolded" for simplicity. Sound vibrations from the stapes are transmitted as waves in the perilymph, leading to displacement of the organ of Corti (see Figure 7.7). High-frequency sounds stimulate hair cells close to the oval window, whereas low-frequency sounds stimulate hair cells further along the cochlea.

membrane (Figure 7.7). The organ of Corti is covered by the **tectorial membrane.** Between the basilar and tectorial membranes are a single row of inner hair cells and three parallel rows of outer hair cells. The hair cells are anchored to the basilar membrane and have minuscule hair-like projections, called **stereocilia,** which project into the tectorial membrane. When pressure waves pass through the SV and ST, the basilar membrane is deformed and displaced, along with the attached hair cells, toward the tectorial membrane, causing the stereocilia to bend. When bent, tiny channels at the tips of the stereocilia open to allow an influx of potassium ions. This stimulates the release of an excitatory neurotransmitter, glutamate, which initiates nerve impulses in tiny tendrils projecting from the spiral ganglia of the auditory nerve. These impulses are then carried to the brain.

In summary,

1. Sound waves are funneled toward the tympanic membrane by the external ear.
2. The vibrations of the tympanic membrane are then transmitted and amplified by the ossicles, which create pressure waves in the fluid of the cochlea via the oval window.
3. These pressure waves displace the basilar membrane and with it the hair cells, causing a bending of the stereocilia that triggers (via the influx of potassium) the release of an excitatory neurotransmitter.
4. The release of glutamate initiates nerve impulses in the ganglion cells of the auditory nerve and completes the process of transduction of sound waves into nerve impulses.

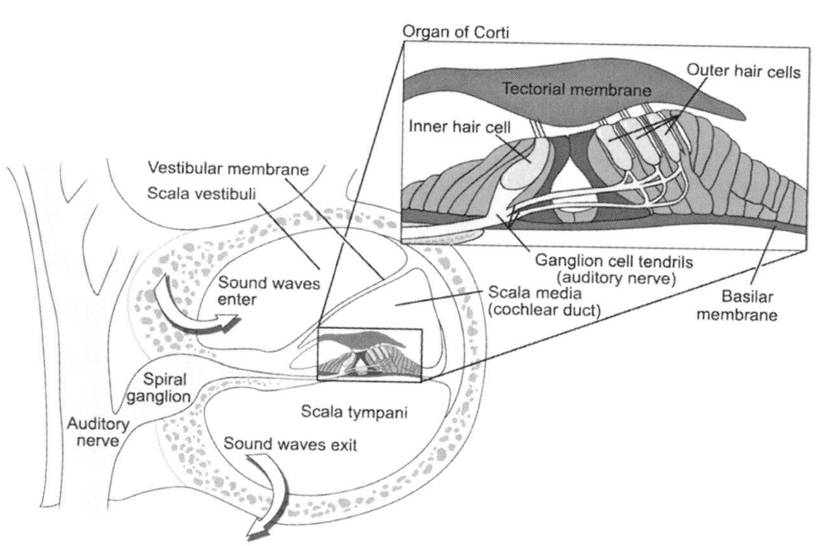

Figure 7.7. The cochlea and the organ of Corti. The organ of Corti, the true organ of hearing, is located on the basilar membrane in the scala media of the cochlea. The inner and outer hair cells attach to the basilar membrane, and their sterocilia reach the overlying tectorial membrane. Sound waves cause movement of the basilar membrane relative to the tectorial membrane, stimulating the inner hairs cells, which in turn synapse with ganglion cells of the auditory nerve, sending signals to the brain. The same movement stimulates the outer hairs to amplify the effect of sound on the cochlea.

Processing Sound Important details in this process relate to the nature of sound waves and the structural details of the middle and inner ears. Sound is, at its essence, a series of compression (pressure) waves transmitted through a medium, such as air. These pressure waves are usually depicted as sinusoidal waves, with peaks representing zones of compression and valleys representing zones of rarefaction (Figure 7.8). The waves are characterized by frequency (how close the waves are to each other, which relates to how many waves pass a given point in a given time interval) and intensity (the height of the waves). Frequency, which corresponds to **pitch** (whether a sound is high or low), is measured in Hertz (Hz, cycles per second), and intensity, which corresponds to loudness, is measured in decibels (dBs). Table 7.3 provides examples of decibel levels for representative environmental sounds.

The auditory system has a remarkable ability to modulate its response to both the intensity and frequency characteristics of sound. As sound waves are transmitted from the tympanic membrane to the ossicles of the middle ear, tiny muscles attached to the malleus and stapes contract or relax in response to the intensity (loudness) of the sound. Loud sounds cause contraction of the tensor tympani and the stapedius muscles to effectively reduce sound transmission through the malleus and stapes and protect the cochlea against sound injury.

When sound waves are transmitted into the cochlea via the oval window, the frequency (pitch) of the sounds is registered as a result of the special structural characteristics of the basilar membrane and the frequency-response characteristics of the hair cells. This membrane is narrower and stiffer at its origin near the oval window (the base) and wider and floppier at its terminus near the confluence of the scala vestibule and scala tympani. Because of this anatomy, more energetic, higher-frequency sounds are propagated shorter distances along the basilar membrane, and less energetic, lower-frequency sounds are propagated further along the basilar membrane. As a consequence, hair cells located near the base of the basilar membrane are situated to register higher-frequency sounds, and hair cells located near the apex of the basilar membrane are situated to register lower-frequency sounds. Because of this **tonotopic organization** of the cochlea, high-frequency and low-frequency sounds can be distinguished, and these distinctions can then be transmitted to the brain.

The phenomenon of **cochlear amplification** is another important factor in the process of sound transduction. As described above, sound waves are

Table 7.3. Volume of environmental sounds

dBA[a]	Example
0	Hearing threshold
10	Dropped pin
20	Rustling leaves
30	Whisper
40	Babbling brook
50	Refrigerator
60	Conversational speech
70	Shower
75	Vacuum cleaner
80	Alarm clock
85	**Threshold for hearing loss due to cumulative exposure**
90	Lawn mower
100	Motorcycle
110	Rock band
120	Thunderclap
130	Peak stadium crowd noise
140	Jet engine takeoff
150	Fighter jet launch
160	Shotgun
170	Airbag deploying
180	Rocket launch
194	**Sound waves become shock waves**

[a]dBA = Loudness in decibels adjusted for response of the human ear.
Adapted with permission from Noisehelp.com. See https://www.noisehelp.com/chart1.

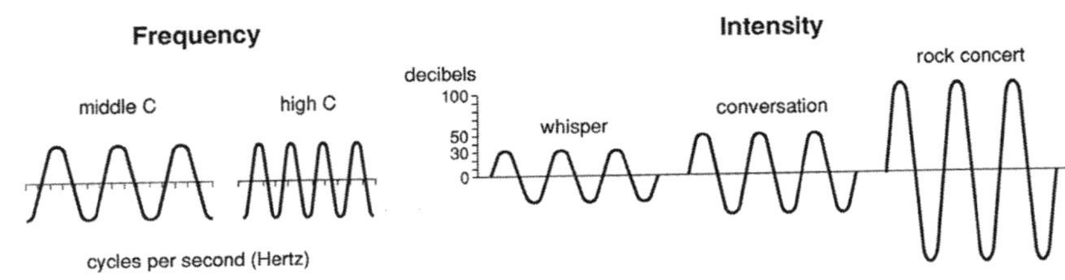

Figure 7.8. Frequency and intensity of sound waves. The frequency of a sound, or its pitch, is expressed as cycles per second, or hertz (Hz). Middle C is 261.6 Hz; one octave higher (high C) is 523.3 Hz. Intensity of sound is expressed as decibels (dB) and varies from a whisper at 30 dB to a rock concert at 100 dB or more.

mechanically amplified in the middle ear as they are transmitted from the tympanic membrane to the oval window. In the cochlea, the movement of the basilar membrane in response to sound is further amplified by the action of the outer hair cells. When the outer hair cells are stimulated by specific sound frequencies, they contract and relax in response to the bending of the stereocilia, enhancing the movement of the basilar membrane to which they are anchored. The response time for this is nearly instantaneous and is mediated by a special motor protein in the cell membranes of the outer hair cells called prestin, from the Italian word *presto*, for fast (Bear et al., 2016).

A curious side effect of cochlear amplification is a phenomenon known as otoacoustic emissions (OAEs). The contraction of the outer hair cells in response to sound causes the cochlea itself to vibrate, in effect generating its own sound, like a faint echo of the original sound stimulus. Humans typically cannot hear this sound, because it is drowned out by ambient sound, but the phenomenon of OAEs is used to screen for hearing problems in newborns (see below).

There are many similarities between the visual and auditory systems in how they transmit nerve impulses to the brain. When hair cells (especially inner hair cells) of the cochlea are excited by sound, they stimulate nerve impulses in ganglia cells of the auditory nerve (analogous ganglia cells are located in the retina in the visual system). Most of these impulses cross over to the opposite side of the brainstem and are transmitted through several way stations to the thalamus, the hub of sensory information, and arrive finally at the primary auditory cortex. Just as spatial information is retained in the transmission of visual information from the retina to the visual cortex, the frequency-specific (tonotopic) cochlear "sound map" of the world is faithfully reproduced at each level of the auditory nervous system.

Further processing of auditory information in the cortex is unique in humans because of the requirements of language. The human brain is especially effective at processing the subtle phonetic distinctions in speech, and the cortex is designed to support both the processing of phonemes (the basis of comprehension) and the encoding of phonemes (the basis of speech). As with processing in the visual cortex, there is a dorsal pathway, which subserves speech production, and a ventral pathway, which promotes language comprehension (Hickok, 2012; Hickok & Poeppel, 2007).

Development of Hearing

In the human embryo, the structures of the middle ear and cochlea are fully formed by 15 weeks' gestation (the beginning of the second trimester). By 20 weeks' gestation, these structures are individually capable of responding to sound in the intrauterine environment and have formed connections to the ganglion cells of the auditory nerve and to the nuclei in the brainstem. By 25 to 26 weeks' gestation, a loud noise *in utero* can produce changes in fetal heart rate and breathing patterns. By 28 to 30 weeks' gestation (the beginning of the third trimester) the entire auditory system comes "online." All of the neural connections from the cochlea to the temporal lobe of the cortex become active, and unborn infants begin to show behavioral responses to sound. It is at this stage that pregnant mothers may notice their infants moving in response to loud sounds in the external environment.

It is also at this stage (between 28 and 30 weeks' gestation) that exposure to sounds in the intrauterine environment allows the cochlea to begin fine-tuning its response to different frequencies of sound; this process is known as **tonotopic tuning.** This process allows individual hair cells (especially the inner hair cells) to become exquisitely sensitive to specific sound frequencies. By the end of this process, adjacent hair cells in the cochlea differ in their characteristic or prime frequency response by only 0.2% (or one-thirtieth of the difference between adjacent piano keys; Graven & Browne, 2008). Because the amniotic fluid that surrounds the unborn infant preferentially transmits lower frequency sounds, the cochlea becomes tonotopically attuned to lower frequency sounds first and to higher frequency sounds after the infant is born. After 32 weeks' gestation, unborn infants can recognize specific sounds, including and especially their mothers' voices, and also become aware of specific melodies, which they will show a preference for after they are born (Graven & Browne, 2008; Moon & Fifer, 2000).

In contrast to vision, which requires exposure to visual experiences and stimuli *after* birth for normal development, hearing requires exposure to sound, and to the right types of sound, *before* birth (beginning at 28 weeks' gestation). It is especially important for unborn infants to be exposed to environmental sounds (particularly voices and music) that allow them to develop an early sensitivity to phonemes. By contrast, very loud sounds, especially those above 60 dB, can be damaging to the delicate hairs cells of the developing cochlea. For this reason, placing headphones on a pregnant mother's abdomen to play music to an unborn infant is *not* advisable, as the loudness of this mode of sound delivery may easily be underestimated (Box 7.2).

Especially concerning is the potential impact of noise on children born prematurely. These children, some of whom are born as early as 23 weeks' gestational age, are exposed to a cacophony of sounds

BOX 7.2 EVIDENCE-BASED PRACTICE

Noise in the Newborn Intensive Care Unit

Based on years of research on the deleterious effects of exposure to loud noise to both the fetus and the premature infant, a multidisciplinary group of clinicians and researchers known as the Sound Study Group developed the following recommendations (Graven, 2000; Krueger, Horesh, & Crossland, 2012; Philbin, Robertson, & Hall, 2008).

Application to Practice

For the fetus:

- Women should avoid prolonged exposure to low-frequency sound (sound below 250 Hz) above 65 dB during pregnancy.
- Sound devices such as earphones should not be placed directly on a pregnant woman's abdomen.
- Special programs to supplement the fetal auditory experience (playing recorded music) are not recommended as the voice of the mother and normal sounds of the mother's body are sufficient for normal auditory development.

For the preterm infant:

- The hourly Leq (the equivalent steady noise level of an hour of sound, if noise levels were constant instead of varying) should not exceed 50 dB.
- The hourly L10 (the measured decibel level exceeded for 10% of an hour) should not exceed 55 dB.
- The 1-second Lmax (the highest decibel level exceeded for at least one-twentieth of a second in an hour) should not exceed 70 dB.
- Earphones and similar devices should not be placed on an infant's ears at any time.

Studies indicate that implementation of these recommendations in newborn intensive care units (NICUs) has been problematic. In one study, average noise levels measured in a NICU during the day and night ranged from 50 to 90 dB, with the highest measured Leq at 85.4 dB in a centrally located area of the unit (Matook, Sullivan, Salisbury, Miller, & Lester, 2010).

and loud noises in the acoustically challenging environment of the neonatal intensive care nursery. Recommendations have been developed for managing environmental noise in the classic multibed newborn intensive care unit (NICU), but significant concerns remain about implementation of these recommendations and about the long-term disabling effects of noise on former premature infants who already have many other risk factors for adverse developmental outcomes (see Chapter 5; Krueger et al., 2012). As a result, recently constructed NICUs have single-bed rooms where environmental noises can be better controlled.

The Auditory System and Language

The auditory system in humans is uniquely designed to support language processing and production. As mentioned previously, human infants are born with the ability to distinguish all of the phonemes represented by all languages (Jusczyk, 2002). This ability is promoted in part by the process of tonotopic tuning in the late prenatal and early postnatal periods, which makes the cochlea exquisitely sensitive to subtle differences in pitch, and by the unique organizational characteristics of the human cortex. Children 6 months of age typically show equal interest in and sensitivity to the sounds of all languages, but by 9 months, they begin to show a preference for the sounds, intonations, and rhythms of their native language. By 3 years of age, this preference is firmly entrenched. This is one of the reasons that developing fluency in a second language is much easier for a child exposed to the phonemic environment of that language prior to 3 years.

In a broader sense, early childhood represents a sensitive and critical period for language development. Children with a significant hearing loss are at a great risk for impairments of speech and language. Research shows that identifying and treating hearing problems as early as possible results in the best outcomes for language development. In particular, children who are born with significant hearing loss have the best language outcomes if interventions begin prior to 6 months of age (Centers for Disease Control and Prevention, 2017; Choo & Meinzen-Derr, 2010; Grindle, 2014; also see Chapter 17 for detailed information about speech and language disorders).

Types of Hearing Loss

There are several types of hearing loss (please see Chapter 26 for a detailed discussion). **Conductive hearing loss** (problems with the middle ear) is the most common type. It tends to be associated with minimal to moderate degrees of hearing loss and is often temporary. Because this type of hearing loss is often associated with otitis media, medical intervention (antibiotic therapy) or surgery (pressure equalizer tube placement) is often employed in its treatment.

By contrast, **sensorineural hearing loss** (resulting from abnormalities in the cochlea or auditory nerve) is often congenital. It may have a genetic origin and be progressive in nature. While less common than conductive hearing loss (occurring in about 1 out of 1,000 newborns), it is more often associated with severe to profound hearing loss. Interventions include the use of hearing aids; special education and targeted therapy; and, in some cases, cochlear implants. Although any degree of hearing loss can be associated with negative language outcomes, early identification of hearing loss is an especially high priority and is the primary target of screening programs in infants and young children (Centers for Disease Control and Prevention, 2017; Grindle, 2014).

Screening for Hearing Problems

Universal newborn hearing screening (UNHS) has now become the norm in the United States. This has revolutionized the identification of children with hearing loss, especially those with severe to profound sensorineural hearing loss. As of 2014, 97% of newborns in the United States were being screened for hearing loss (Centers for Disease Control and Prevention, 2017). Following the implementation of newborn screening, the mean age of identification for children with hearing loss has dropped from 2.5 years to 2 to 3 months (Harrison, Roush, & Wallace, 2003). The primary goals of UNHS are the following:

- Screen all infants by 1 month of age
- Identify all children with permanent hearing loss by 3 months of age
- Initiate appropriate interventions for hearing loss by 6 months of age
- Establish a medical home (see Chapter 30) for children with hearing loss
- Collect data and track progress with screening as a public health initiative

The Centers for Disease Control and Prevention provide an excellent resource for information related to hearing loss and newborn screening, including up-to-date statistics on the progress of UNHS at http://www.cdc.gov/ncbddd/hearingloss/data.html. Infants at increased risk of delayed onset of hearing loss (e.g., premature infants and those exposed to intrauterine infections) should be followed even if they pass newborn hearing testing.

Screening Methods

Currently two methods are used to screen hearing in newborns, **otoacoustic emission** (OAE) testing and **auditory brainstem response** (ABR) testing. OAE testing is based on the fact that the cochlea generates a subtle but detectible "echo" in response to an acoustic stimulus (based on the action of the cochlear amplification system; see previous discussion). The OAE device is inserted into the ear canal of the newborn and emits a continuous tone; a microphone picks up the cochlear response to this tone. An advantage of OAE testing is that it is easy to perform and can be done in a quiet, awake infant. It also requires less training to use. Disadvantages include difficulties in obtaining an accurate result in children with external or middle ear problems (e.g., earwax) and a fairly high rate of false-positive results (children having an abnormal test who actually have normal hearing). OAE is also based on the assumption that most causes of sensorineural loss (SNHL) are due to cochlear dysfunction, so it will miss those rarer instances when SNHL is due to auditory nerve dysfunction.

ABR testing is based on the fact that, when the auditory system is intact, acoustic stimuli presented to the ear will generate nerve impulses in the auditory nerve and brain that can be detected by electrodes placed on the scalp. There are both screening (automated) and full (nonautomated or diagnostic) versions of the test. The screening version is used for initial testing. A device is inserted into the ear canal that generates either high-frequency clicks or frequency-specific tones. Electrodes placed at strategic locations on the newborn's head pick up the signals generated as they progress through the nervous system. The advantages of the ABR are that it is less prone to interference from problems in the external or middle ears, has a lower false-positive rate than the OAE, and will detect SNHL due to both cochlear and auditory nerve abnormalities.

However, the ABR is more difficult to perform, requires more training to administer, and requires a quiet or sleeping infant (Grindle, 2014).

Most newborn screening programs for hearing loss employ a two-step process. Children who fail the initial screen (whether it is an OAE or an ABR) will typically be retested, often using a full ABR test. As mentioned previously, one of the goals of UNHS is to identity all children with congenital hearing loss by 3 months of age. As of 2014, although 97% of newborns were screened, of those who failed the initial screening, only 71% were identified as having or not having hearing loss by 3 months of age. This highlights the challenge of ensuring adequate follow-up for children with potential hearing loss (Centers for Disease Control and Prevention, 2017).

Congenital Cytomegalovirus Infection and Screening

Although the most common cause of congenital sensorineural hearing loss is genetic, the second most common cause is congenital cytomegalovirus (CMV) infection (see Chapter 26). CMV infection can be diagnosed by detection of the virus in saliva or urine, but because acquired infections are so common, it is imperative to test suspected infants in the newborn period to ensure an accurate diagnosis. Current recommendations include testing all children who have signs of CMV infection and all children who have failed newborn hearing screening. As of 2018, whether or not all newborns should be screened for congenital CMV is a point of active discussion since many cases that cause sensorineural hearing loss are asymptomatic. Identifying congenital CMV is especially important in light of reports that treatment with antiviral drugs may prevent SNHL and perhaps reverse the progression of SNHL in affected children (Choo & Meinzen-Derr, 2010; Oliver et al., 2009).

THE WORLD WE FEEL

When thinking about senses, the ones that tend to come to mind first are those that help individuals engage the world outside and around them; vision and hearing have particular primacy in this view of the senses. However, "below the hood" there exist myriad, inwardly directed sensory systems that help to sense and regulate the world. In many instances, these senses are not "sensed" in the usual meaning of the term. They do provide feedback about the internal state of an individual's body but often at an unconscious level. These internal sensors are especially critical to the regulation of movement and provide an awareness of the position of our bodies in space. These sensory systems are a critical part of the complex motor planning and control apparatus known as the **somatosensory system.**

The Somatosensory System

Taken together, the somatosensory system refers to all of the physiological systems that provide feedback about the internal states of the body to the central nervous system (CNS). The CNS is organized hierarchically: sensory data from the muscles, tendons, joints, and skin are fed back to the spinal cord and brainstem, where they are processed locally and provide direct feedback to reflex mechanisms that support rapid moment-by-moment motor control. Sensory data are further processed in the thalamus (the "Grand Central Station" of sensory processing at the heart of the brain, referred to in the previous discussions on vision and hearing) and ultimately arrive at the somatosensory cortex located in the parietal lobes of the brain (see Chapter 8).

Proprioception **Proprioception** refers to those components of the somatosensory system that provide feedback regarding the states of muscles, tendons, and joints. Proprioception, together with information from sensors in our skin (cutaneous sensation) and in our inner ear (vestibular sense or balance), provides individuals with "body awareness" and a sense of the position of the body in space.

Muscle Spindles Muscle spindles are special sensors located in all of the muscles of the body. They are also referred to as stretch receptors, because their primary function is to sense the state of stretch in muscles from moment to moment. Rapid stretching of muscles causes the muscle spindles to fire, and nerve impulses feed back to the spinal cord and trigger motor neurons that supply the same muscles to cause a compensatory muscular contraction. This is the basis of the familiar knee-jerk reflex (Bear et al., 2016; Shumway-Cook & Woollacott, 2017).

Golgi Tendon Organs Golgi tendon organs (GTOs) are located at the junction of muscles and their tendons; they are highly sensitive to changes in tension that result from muscle stretch or contraction. In contrast to muscles spindles (which are arranged in parallel with muscle fibers), GTOs (situated between muscles and the bones to which they are attached) are arranged in series with muscle fibers. Whereas muscle spindles provide feedback about muscle length, GTOs provide information about muscle tension. When a muscle tendon unit is under increased tension, GTOs send nerve impulses back to the spinal cord that result in inhibition of contraction of the same muscle. This allows for finely-graded movement and is thought to be especially important in the manipulation of fragile objects that must be held with steady, but not excessive pressure (Bear et al., 2016; Shumway-Cook & Woollacott, 2017).

Joint Receptors Several different sensor types are present in the joints of the body, some of which are similar to GTOs and others of which are similar to mechanoreceptors (pressure sensors) in the skin. Joint receptors are especially important in contributing to our awareness of joint angle, an important aspect of body awareness (Shumway-Cook & Woollacott, 2017).

Cutaneous Receptors The skin has an array of receptors that are sensitive to a wide variety of stimuli. Pain receptors (also called nociceptors) are sensitive to sources of mechanical and thermal energy that could cause tissue damage. Touch receptors (which include a variety of mechanoreceptors, or sensors that respond to mechanical changes in the skin) are sensitive to wide variations of pressure, vibration, rubbing, pinching, and pricking. High concentrations of particular types of touch receptors are present in our hands, especially in our fingertips, providing critical sensory feedback for fine motor control. Considered globally, cutaneous receptors throughout the body provide a crucial component of body awareness by furnishing the CNS with data regarding the state of our "interface" with the outside world (Bear et al., 2016).

The Vestibular System The **vestibular apparatus** (VA), located in the inner ear, assists our sense of balance (see Figure 7.7). The vestibular apparatus has two main components, the semicircular canals and the otolith organs. The **semicircular canals** consist of fluid-filled tubular structures that form three loops arranged at right angles to each other. The fluid moves in response to angular acceleration of the head (as when a child spins in circles) and provides the CNS with feedback regarding rotational movements of the head. The **otolith organs** (the utricle and the saccule) sit at the base of the vestibular apparatus near the convergence of the semicircular canals. These organs contain calcium carbonate crystals (called otoliths) that shift position with changes in head tilt. They are also sensitive to changes in linear acceleration (forward and backward movement) of the head. The main function of the otolith organs is to provide the CNS with feedback regarding the position of the head with respect to gravity (Bear et al., 2016; Shumway-Cook & Woollacott, 2017).

SENSORY INTEGRATION AND MOTOR CONTROL

Like the studio musician who cannot play his instrument without being able to hear feedback of his own performance, human beings cannot control their own movements and adaptive responses without constant feedback from every component of the sensory system. While the somatosensory system is especially important to motor control, our other senses (especially vision and hearing) also make an important contribution to the process. The idea of **sensory integration** arises from the recognition that the brain must perform an astonishing feat of computational analysis on a continuous stream of sensory and motor data to allow for even the simplest of movements.

CASE STUDY

Casey is a 10-year-old boy who was diagnosed with autism spectrum disorder (see Chapter 18) when he was 7 years old. Although his biggest challenges relate to his social skills and behavior, he has also struggled with "clumsiness," lack of coordination, and "sensory issues." The developmental pediatrician who diagnosed him with autism also diagnosed developmental coordination disorder and made reference to problems with "sensory integration" in her original diagnostic report.

In particular, Casey had severe aversions to loud noises, bright lights, strong odors, and an array of tactile sensations as a toddler and preschooler. He abhorred having his hair washed, would only take baths in lukewarm water, hated wearing socks, and preferred to be naked whenever that was allowed. Paradoxically, he seemed to be relatively insensitive to pain, and on one particular occasion, after a bad fall, he made no complaint of a badly swollen toe that was later found to be broken. As he got older, these "sensory issues" have improved, and he has learned to cope with the ones that have persisted. For example, he is allowed to wear headphones when his school has a fire drill, as sensitivity to loud noises is still a problem for him.

When a child like Casey is diagnosed with a developmental coordination disorder, clinicians must consider whether his physical awkwardness results from a primary problem with motor output or a problem with the integration of sensory data with the motor control system.

Dunn's Model of Sensory Processing

The concept of sensory integration recognizes that while sensory data are registered in multiple modalities (e.g., vision, hearing, touch, and balance; see Table 7.1), these divergent sources of information from the outside world and from within the body must be combined in order to provide for the possibility of a coherent and adaptive behavioral response. Theoretical approaches to sensory integration therefore take a unified, "trans-modal" approach to sensory data.

Dunn's Model of Sensory Processing (Dunn, 1997) has been particularly influential in this regard (Table 7.4). The model is based on a detailed analysis of the sensory profiles (see below) of typically developing children, and it characterizes individuals based on their sensitivity to sensory stimuli (or neurologic threshold for reacting to the stimuli) and their manner of responding to these stimuli. Children who have a *high sensory threshold* tend to have a low sensitivity (are hyposensitive) to sensory stimuli. For example, children with a high sensory threshold may seem unreactive to sounds that would gain the attention of most children. By contrast, children with *low sensory threshold* are overly sensitive (hypersensitive) to sensory stimuli. Sounds that might not be noticed by most children might be distracting or disturbing to these children.

Children also differ in their behavioral responses to stimuli. Those who are *passive responders* tend to be underreactive (hyporeactive) to sensory stimuli. Passive responders who are also hyposensitive (with a high sensory threshold) are said to have *low registration*. Children with low registration may seem insensitive to injury and may be surprisingly slow to respond to a cut or bruise that would elicit a dramatic response from most children. Passive responders who are hypersensitive (with a low sensory threshold) are said to be *sensory sensitive*. Sensory sensitive children might be bothered by being hugged but don't respond actively to their discomfort.

Children who are *active responders*, by contrast, tend to be overreactive (hyperreactive) to sensory stimuli. Active responders who are hyposensitive (with a high sensory threshold) are said to be *sensory seeking*. Sensory-seeking children may, for example, have a strong need for oral stimulation and will compulsively seek out things to chew, including nonfood items. Active responders who are hypersensitive (with a low sensory threshold) are said to be *sensory avoidant*. Sensory avoidant children will go out of their way to withdraw from situations that are overstimulating to them.

Screening and Assessment

In contrast to screening methods employed to identify problems with vision and hearing, which rely on specific, discrete screening methods and tools, screening and assessment of sensory processing involves a complex set of clinical processes that address all levels of sensory processing, from the registration of sensory data to adaptive behavioral responses in specific settings. These clinical processes are most often carried out by an occupational therapist (Box 7.3).

A number of specific screening tools are commonly employed in the evaluation of sensory processing. Two frequently used measures are the Sensory Profile-2 (Dunn, 2014) and the Sensory Processing Measure (Miller-Kuhaneck, Henry, Glennon, & Mu, 2007). The Sensory Profile-2 is keyed to Dunn's Model of Sensory Integration and provides a means of categorizing a child as being low registering, sensory sensitive, sensory seeking, or sensory avoidant. Several versions have been developed for different age groups for birth to adulthood. The Sensory Processing Measure (for ages 3 to 12 years) can assess sensory vulnerabilities in multiple settings and includes parent and teacher rating scales.

Table 7.4. Dunn's Model of Sensory Processing (Dunn, 1997)

		Continuum of behavioral response	
		Passive (hyporeactive)	**Active (hyperreactive)**
Continuum of neurologic/sensory registration	**High threshold (hypo-sensitive)**	*Low registration* • Less sensitive to sensory stimuli • Low level of reactivity manifests as slow or absent response to sensory stimuli	*Sensory seeking* • Less sensitive to sensory stimuli • High level of reactivity manifests as effort to access/experience (seek-out) sensory stimuli
	Low threshold (hyper-sensitive)	*Sensory sensitive* • More sensitive to sensory stimuli • Low level of reactivity manifests as distraction and discomfort	*Sensory avoidant* • More sensitive to sensory stimuli • High level of reactivity manifests as avoidance of offending stimuli

BOX 7.3 INTERDISCIPLINARY CARE

Sensory Integration and the Role of the Occupational Therapist

At its heart, occupational therapy is devoted to helping people adapt to and function optimally in their real-life settings. Occupational therapists (OTs) who work with children focus especially on helping them to develop functional independence with activities of daily living at home and to develop skills that support academic growth and classroom adaptation at school.

In these settings and in others, children with sensory challenges benefit from working with OTs in several ways. OTs provide an in-depth assessment of a child's profile of sensory sensitivities, needs, and responses, employing diagnostic tools and interpreting the results of these assessments in light of a child's specific circumstances. OTs often work with families and teachers to develop accommodations to the sensory features of the home and school environment. For example, a child with sensitivities to loud noise might be provided with noise cancelling headphones. OT-designed "sensory diets" offer a schedule of accommodations in specific settings (such as school) to help a child cope with the challenges of difficult sensory environments and complex schedules.

Direct interventions are also employed. These include sensory integration therapy (based on the work of Dr. A. Jane Ayres) and a variety of sensory based therapies that focus on providing children with coping strategies for dealing with an often unpredictable sensory environment. Some interventions use targeted sensory input (vestibular, proprioceptive, auditory, and tactile) by means of special techniques such as brushing, the application of "deep pressure," the use of weighted blankets and vests, and the use of swings (to provide vestibular input) in order to influence or modulate a child's pattern of sensory responsiveness. In each instance, the OT's therapy is tailored to a child's specific needs and circumstances, with the overall goal of improving functional adaptation and independence.

Occupation therapy researchers are working to clarify the efficacy of these various interventions. For example, a systematic review of research on the efficacy of sensory integration therapy in children found evidence of improvements in function and behavior across several domains but also recognized variability in the approaches employed in various studies and endorsed the need for further research (May-Benson & Koomar, 2010).

Sensory Processing Disorders

In the 1970s, A. Jean Ayres, PhD, proposed that some children may have abnormalities of these sensory integration processes that could lead not only to problems with motor control, but also to difficulties with other aspects of development, learning, and emotional regulation (Ayres, Robbins, & Pediatric Therapy Network, 2005). This led to the development of the concept of **sensory processing disorders.**

More recently, a classification system for sensory processing disorders has been proposed (Miller, Anzalone, Lane, Cermak, & Osten, 2007). Three types of sensory processing disorders are suggested:

- Sensory modulation disorder (subdivided into overresponsive, underresponsive, and sensory-seeking subtypes)
- Sensory discrimination disorder (difficult distinguishing among sensory stimuli)
- Sensory-based motor disability (subdivided into postural disorder and dyspraxia)

Although the therapeutic interventions for sensory processing disorders and the diagnosis itself have become widely employed, neither have been universally accepted. In the most recent edition of the *Diagnostic and Statistical Manual of Mental Disorders, Fifth Edition* (American Psychiatric Association, 2013), sensory disturbances have been recognized as a diagnostic component of autism spectrum disorder (see Chapter 18), but sensory processing disorders were not accepted as a separate diagnosis, pending further research (Zimmer & Desch, 2012).

SUMMARY

- The senses provide individuals with a means to adapt to the world around them and regulate their responses to that world.

- The visual system is designed to transduce electromagnetic energy into nerve impulses that can be interpreted by the brain.
- The visual system matures gradually after birth and requires appropriate visual input for typical development to occur.
- Vision screening can be accomplished in several ways and has as its goal the early identification of vision problems such as amblyopia.
- The hearing system is designed to transduce acoustic energy in the form of sound/pressure waves into nerve impulses that can be interpreted by the brain.
- The hearing system begins to mature before birth and requires appropriate auditory input for typical development to occur.
- Universal newborn hearing screening has become the norm, with the goal of identifying hearing loss (especially sensorineural hearing loss) prior to 3 months of age and implementing interventions for hearing loss by 6 months of age.
- The somatosensory system includes an array of internal sensors (receptors) that provide the basis for individuals' awareness of their own bodies and the position of their bodies in space.
- Integration of sensory data from multiple sources is needed for normal function of the motor control system and provides the basis for adaptive response to the environment.
- Therapeutic techniques targeting sensory integration are widely employed, and the concept of sensory processing disorders has been proposed, but universal acceptance awaits further research.

ADDITIONAL RESOURCES

American Association for Pediatric Ophthalmology and Strabismus: https://www.aapos.org/terms/conditions/131

The American Academy of Ophthalmology: Eye Screening: https://www.aao.org/eye-health/tips-prevention/children-eye-screening

Centers for Disease Control and Prevention: Newborn Hearing Screening: https://www.cdc.gov/ncbddd/hearingloss/parentsguide/understanding/newbornhearingscreening.html.

American Occupational Therapy Association, Inc.: Sensory Integration: https://www.aota.org/Practice/Children-Youth/SI.aspx

WebMD: Sensory Processing Disorder: https://www.webmd.com/children/sensory-processing-disorder#1

Kidhealth: Hearing Evaluation in Children: https://kidshealth.org/en/parents/hear.html

Additional resources can be found online in Appendix D: Childhood Disabilities Resources, Services, and Organizations (see About the Online Companion Materials).

REFERENCES

American Academy of Ophthalmology. (2016). Visual system assessment in infants, children, and young adults by pediatricians (Committee on Practice and Ambulatory Medicine, Section on Ophthalmology, American Association of Certified Orthoptists, American Association for Pediatric Ophthalmology and Strabismus, American Academy of Ophthalmology). *Pediatrics, 137*(1), 28–30.

American Association for Pediatric Ophthalmology and Strabismus. (2017). *Vision screening recommendations.* American Association for Pediatric Ophthalmology and Strabismus. Retrieved from https://www.aapos.org/terms/conditions/131

American Psychiatric Association. (2013). *Diagnostic and statistical manual of mental disorders* (5th ed.). Washington, DC: American Psychiatric Association.

Ayres, A. J., Robbins, J., & Pediatric Therapy Network. (2005). *Sensory integration and the child: Understanding hidden sensory challenges* (25th anniversary ed.). Los Angeles, CA: WPS.

Bear, M., Connors, B., & Paradiso, M. (2016). *Neuroscience: Exploring the brain.* Philadelphia, PA: Wolters Kluwer.

Boyle, C. A., Boulet, S., Schieve, L. A., Cohen, R. A., Blumberg, S. J., Yeargin-Allsopp, M., . . . Kogan, M. D. (2011). Trends in the prevalence of developmental disabilities in US children, 1997-2008. *Pediatrics, 127*(6), 1034–1042.

Bremond-Gignac, D., Copin, H., Lapillonne, A., Milazzo, S., & European Network of Study and Research in Eye Development (2011). Visual development in infants: Physiological and pathological mechanisms. *Current Opinion in Ophthalmology, 22* (Suppl.), S1–S8.

Centers for Disease Control and Prevention. (2017). *Hearing loss in children: Data and statistics.* Retrieved from http://www.cdc.gov/ncbddd/hearingloss/data.html

Choo, D., & Meinzen-Derr, J. (2010). Universal newborn hearing screening in 2010. *Current Opinions in Otolaryngology & Head and Neck Surgery, 18*(5), 399–404.

Colorado Department of Education. (2017). Guidelines for vision screening programs: Kindergarten through Grade 12. *School Nursing and Health—Health Services: Screening.* Retrieved from https://www.cde.state.co.us/healthandwellness/snh_healthservices

Donahue, S. P., & Baker, C. N. (2016). Procedures for the evaluation of the visual system by pediatricians (Committee on Practice Ambulatory Medicine, American Academy of Pediatrics Section on Ophthalmology, American Academy of Pediatrics, American Association of Certified Orthoptists, American Association for Pediatric Ophthalmology and Strabismus, American Academy of Ophthalmology). *Pediatrics, 137*(1).

Dunn, W. (1997). The impact of sensory processing abilities on the daily lives of young children and families: A conceptual model. *Infants & Young Children, 9*(4), 23–35.

Dunn, W. (2014). *Sensory Profile 2: User's manual.* San Antonio, TX: Psychological Corp.

Goodale, M. A., & Milner, A. D. (1992). Separate visual pathways for perception and action. *Trends in Neuroscience, 15*(1), 20–25.

Graven, S. N. (2000). Sound and the developing infant in the NICU: Conclusions and recommendations for care. *Journal of Perinatology, 20*(8 Pt 2), S88–S93.

Graven, S. N., & Browne, J. V. (2008). Auditory development of the fetus and infant. *Newborn & Infant Nursing Reviews, 8*(4), 187–193.

Grindle, C. R. (2014). Pediatric hearing loss. *Pediatrics in Review, 35*(11), 456–463; quiz 464. doi:10.1542/pir.35-11-456

Harrison, M., Roush, J., & Wallace, J. (2003). Trends in age of identification and intervention in infants with hearing loss. *Ear and Hearing, 24*(1), 89–95.

Hickok, G. (2012). The cortical organization of speech processing: Feedback control and predictive coding the context of a dual-stream model. *Journal of Communication Disorders, 45*(6), 393–402.

Hickok, G., & Poeppel, D. (2007). The cortical organization of speech processing. *Nature Reviews Neuroscience, 8*(5), 393–402.

Jusczyk, P. W. (2002). Some critical developments in acquiring native language sound organization during the first year. *Annals of Otology, Rhinology, & Laryngology—Supplement, 189*, 11–15.

Kemper, A. R., Fant, K. E., & Badgett, J. T. (2003). Preschool vision screening in primary care after a legislative mandate for diagnostic eye examinations. *Southern Medical Journal, 96*(9), 859–862.

Krueger, C., Horesh, E., & Crossland, B. A. (2012). Safe sound exposure in the fetus and preterm infant. *Journal of Obstetric, Gynecologic, & Neonatal Nursing, 41*(2), 166–170.

Matook, S. A., Sullivan, M. C., Salisbury, A., Miller, R. J., & Lester, B. M. (2010). Variations of NICU sound by location and time of day. *Neonatal Network—Journal of Neonatal Nursing, 29*(2), 87–95.

May-Benson, T. A., & Koomar, J. A. (2010). Systematic review of the research evidence examining the effectiveness of interventions using a sensory integrative approach for children. *American Journal of Occupational Therapy, 64*(3), 403–414.

Miller, L. J., Anzalone, M. E., Lane, S. J., Cermak, S. A., & Osten, E. T. (2007). Concept evolution in sensory integration: A proposed nosology for diagnosis. *American Journal of Occupational Therapy, 61*(2), 135–140.

Miller, J. M., & Lessin, H. R. (2012). Instrument-based pediatric vision screening policy statement. *Pediatrics, 130*(5), 983–986.

Miller-Kuhaneck, H., Henry, D. A., Glennon, T. J., & Mu, K. (2007). Development of the Sensory Processing Measure-School: Initial studies of reliability and validity. *American Journal of Occupational Therapy, 61*(2), 170–175.

Moon, C. M., & Fifer, W. P. (2000). Evidence of transnatal auditory learning. *Journal of Perinatology, 20*(8 Pt 2), S37–S44.

National Association of School Nurses. (2017). *Vision and eye health.* Retrieved from https://www.nasn.org/nasn-resources/practice-topics/vision-health

Noise Help. (2017). *Noise level chart.* Retrieved from http://www.noisehelp.com/noise-level-chart.html

O'Hara, M. A. (2016). Instrument-based pediatric vision screening. *Current Opinion in Ophthalmology, 27*(5), 398–401.

Oliver, S. E., Cloud, G. A., Sanchez, P. J., Demmler, G. J., Dankner, W., Shelton, M., . . . National Institute of Allergy (2009). Neurodevelopmental outcomes following ganciclovir therapy in symptomatic congenital cytomegalovirus infections involving the central nervous system. *Journal of Clinical Virology, 46*(Suppl. 4), S22–S26.

Philbin, M. K., Robertson, A., & Hall, J. W. (2008). Recommended permissible noise criteria for occupied, newly constructed or renovated hospital nurseries. *Advanced Neonatal Care, 8*(5, Suppl.), S11–S15.

Rogers, G. L., & Jordan, C. O. (2013). Pediatric vision screening. *Pediatrics in Review, 34*(3), 126–132.

Rosa-Olivares, J., Porro, A., Rodriguez-Varela, M., Riefkohl, G., & Niroomand-Rad, I. (2015). Otitis media: To treat, to refer, to do nothing: A review for the practitioner. *Pediatrics in Review, 36*(11), 480–486; quiz 487–488.

Rosenfeld, R. M., Schwartz, S. R., Pynnonen, M. A., Tunkel, D. E., Hussey, H. M., Fichera, J. S., . . . Schellhase, K. G. (2013). Clinical practice guideline: Tympanostomy tubes in children. *Otolaryngology—Head & Neck Surgery, 149*(1, Suppl.), S1–S35.

Shumway-Cook, A., & Woollacott, M. H. (2017). *Motor control: Translating research into clinical practice* (5th ed.). Philadelphia, PA: Wolters Kluwer.

Varma, R., Tarczy-Hornoch, K., & Jiang, X. (2017). Visual impairment in preschool children in the United States: Demographic and geographic variations from 2015 to 2060. *JAMA Ophthalmology, 135*(6), 610–616. doi:10.1001/jamaophthalmol.2017.1021

Zimmer, M., & Desch, L. (2012). Sensory integration therapies for children with developmental and behavioral disorders. *Pediatrics, 129*(6), 1186–1189. doi:10.1542/peds.2012-0876

CHAPTER 8

The Brain and Nervous System

Joseph Scafidi and Andrea Gropman

Upon completion of this chapter, the reader will

- Understand the anatomical structures of the brain and their purposes
- Know about the roles played by neurons, oligodendrocytes, and astrocytes in the function of the central nervous system
- Discover how neural stem cells develop into neurons and oligodendrocytes in the prenatal and postnatal brain
- Be able to explain the origin and function of cerebrospinal fluid and its associated blockage in hydrocephalus
- Understand current imaging technologies that help us evaluate the central nervous system

The **central nervous system** (CNS) is an incredibly complex system that is comprised of the brain and spinal cord. The CNS is responsible for receiving and processing sensory information, movement data, cognitive information, social behaviors, and other interactions with the surrounding world. An impairment of any part of this complex system reduces the ability of the individual to adapt to the environment, and it can lead to disorders as diverse as learning disabilities, **autism spectrum disorder** (ASD), **cerebral palsy**, and **epilepsy.** This chapter provides an overview of the interrelationships among the individual elements of the CNS and the peripheral nervous system (PNS). It also describes examples of CNS and PNS dysfunction and their effects on a child.

CASE STUDY

Thomas, born after a 41-week pregnancy, developed intermittent tonic-clonic activity of the right arm and leg at 18 hours of life. The duration of these events was between 1–3 minutes. In between, Thomas was noted to have less movement of the right arm and leg than the left. He was immediately transferred to the neonatal intensive care unit for suspicion of seizures, and neurology was consulted. A neurological exam revealed mild facial asymmetry, decreased motor strength of the right arm and legs, and **hyporeflexia** (decreased deep tendon reflexes) on the right side. Thomas was administered the medication phenobarbital to stop the seizures. An electroencephalogram (EEG) captured one of the events prior to phenobarbital administration and showed seizure activity emanating from the left central-temporal and parietal regions of the cortex. During periods when there were no seizure events, there was slowing of the EEG background activity in this region of the brain. Phenobarbital levels were adjusted to prevent further seizures. Magnetic resonance imaging (MRI) revealed a middle cerebral artery distribution acute stroke on the left affecting the frontal-parietal region (Figure 8.1). Thomas remained on phenobarbital for 1 week and then was weaned off of this medication.

A subsequent neurologic examination at 1 year of age revealed almost symmetric strength of his arm and leg but some **hyperreflexia** (increased deep tendon reflexes) on the right. It was noted that when reaching for objects or standing, Thomas favored using his left hand. It was also noted that age-appropriate fine motor skills were limited on the right compared with the left side. No delays were noted in his language, and no further seizures had been noted by the family. In summary, Thomas' diagnosis is neonatal seizures as a result of an acute left-sided stroke. Phenobarbital was administered to stop the seizures during the acute period and was stopped to prevent long-term side effects of medication. His outcome should be good, although he may retain subtle weakness on the right side of his body as a consequence of the stroke. At 2 years of age, Thomas will likely receive a diagnosis of right hemiplegic cerebral palsy.

Thought Questions:

What are the six main structures of the central nervous system? What are the major components of the peripheral nervous system and some disorders associated with it? What are the different diagnostic techniques for evaluating neurodevelopmental disorders? Compare and contrast the different diagnostic techniques for evaluating the central nervous system.

THE BRAIN AND SPINAL CORD

The brain and the spinal cord comprise the mature CNS and have six main structures: 1) the cerebral hemispheres, 2) basal ganglia, 3) thalamus, 4) brainstem, 5) cerebellum, and 6) spinal cord (Crossman & Neary, 2015).

The Cerebral Hemispheres

During embryonic development, the CNS develops from a layer of ectodermal cells that folds over and becomes the neural tube. In turn, the neural tube develops several swellings that eventually develop into the brain and spinal cord, and the cavity within the neural tube develops into the ventricles (see Chapter 6). The first bulge is the **prosencephalon**, which becomes the **telencephalon** and **diencephalon** (thalamus and hypothalamus). The telencephalon consists of the cerebral cortex, subcortical white matter (where the "wiring" of the brain is found), and deep masses of gray matter collectively called the **basal ganglia** (containing specialized groupings of neurons). Within each hemisphere, there is a fluid-filled cavity called the lateral **ventricle**. The main connection between the two hemispheres is a large band of axonal fibers called the **corpus callosum** that permits the exchange of information between the two hemispheres (Figure 8.2A and 8.2B). There are genetic and environmental factors that may interfere with the normal formation of the corpus callosum and, in the most severe cases, result in its complete lack of development (termed **agenesis** of the corpus callosum) (Palmer & Mowat, 2014). The importance of this exchange of information is highlighted by the results of a surgical procedure called a **corpus callosotomy.** In this operation, all or part of the corpus callosum is cut in an effort to control a severe seizure

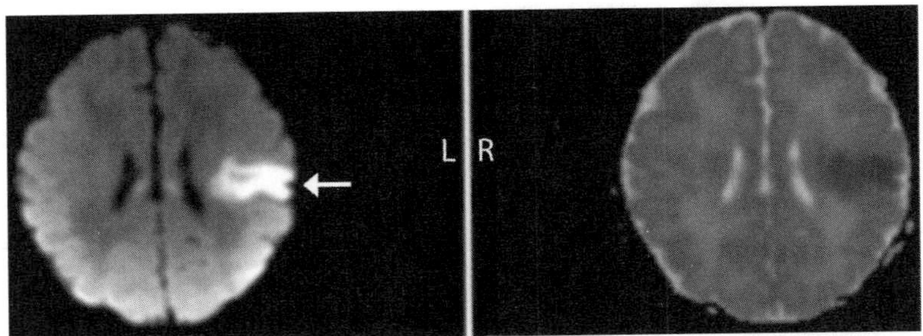

Figure 8.1. A full-term neonate that presented with neonatal seizures noted on the right side of the body. Magnetic resonance imaging on the third day of life revealed an acute left middle cerebral artery distribution stroke. The arrow on the left image points to the region where ischemia was present. Upon exam, the patient had evidence of right-sided body asymmetries.

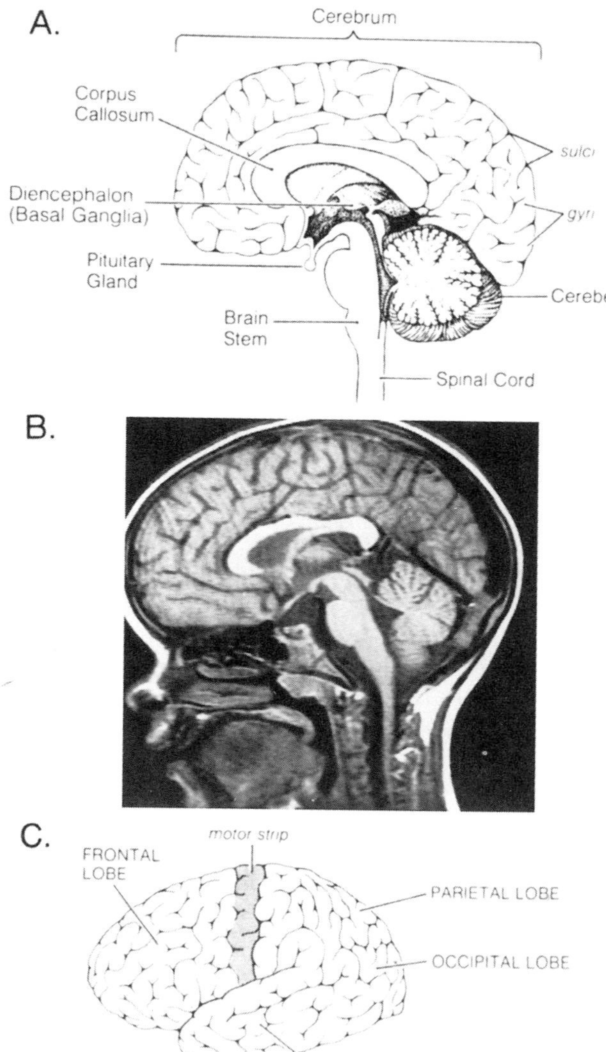

Figure 8.2. A) Sagittal view of the brain showing the component elements: cerebral hemispheres, diencephalon, cerebellum, brainstem, and spinal cord. B) Lateral view of brain by magnetic resonance imaging scan. Note the excellent reproduction of the structures of the brain. C) Side view of the left hemisphere. The cortex is divided into four lobes: frontal, parietal, temporal, and occipital. The motor strip, lying at the back of the frontal lobe, is highlighted. It initiates voluntary movement.

disorder (Graham et al., 2016). It has proven quite effective in decreasing the spread of seizure activity from one hemisphere to the other. In some adults, however, it has resulted in a disconnection syndrome and declines in language, visual-perceptual skills, and manual dexterity. This is the result of a decreased ability of the hemispheres to communicate with each other (Malmgren et al., 2015).

In early fetal life, the surface of the cerebral hemisphere is smooth. As the brain's complexity increases during the third trimester, involutions called **fissures** and **sulci** appear. Fissures, which are deeper than sulci, are first visible during fetal development and divide each hemisphere into four functional areas or lobes. The frontal lobe occupies the anterior third of the hemisphere; the parietal lobe sits in the middle-upper part of the hemisphere; the temporal lobe is in the middle-lower region; and the occipital lobe takes up the posterior quarter of each hemisphere (Figure 8.2C). The sulci are smaller involutions within each lobe, and the regions between the sulci are called convolutions or **gyri** (Figure 8.2A). Some gyri vary little in location and contour from one person to another, whereas others vary considerably. Sulci and gyri increase the surface area of the brain and permit additional growth within the limited space of the brain cavity.

The surface of the cerebral hemisphere, called the **cortex**, consists of gray matter. It is composed principally of **neurons** (nerve cell bodies) and **glia** (supporting cells). Below this gray matter lie the nerve fibers (**axons**) that are insulated and comprise the white matter. The function of the cerebral cortex is to initiate motion and thought processes, and to process sensory input. The cortex of each lobe is responsible for specific activities or functions, outlined in more detail below.

The Frontal Lobe

The frontal lobe controls voluntary motor activity and makes significant contributions to cognition and executive function (Burgess & Stuss, 2017; Nowrangi et al., 2014). It plays an important role in attention, impulse control, and emotion. Impaired frontal lobe function is responsible for conditions such as intellectual disability, attention-deficit/hyperactivity disorder (ADHD), and certain genetic disorders (e.g., autosomal dominant nocturnal frontal lobe epilepsy). The anterior cingulate cortex and fronto-insular cortex, in particular, are connected to process information across a variety of domains, including those related to attention, emotion, and effortful tasks (Craig, 2009; Engstrom, Karlsson, Landtblom, & Craig, 2015).

Within the frontal lobe the different regions of the body are represented topographically along a strip called the primary motor cortex (Brodmann area 4). The tongue and larynx, or voice box, are controlled from the lowest point followed in an upward sequence by the face, hand, arm, trunk, thigh, and foot (Figure 8.3). The tongue, larynx, and hand occupy a particularly large area along this strip because more neurons are necessary due to the complexity of speech and fine motor activity.

A nerve impulse initiated in the motor strip passes down the **pyramidal tract** (also called the **corticospinal pathway**) that connects the cortex with the spinal cord. Reaching the spinal cord, the impulse jumps across a

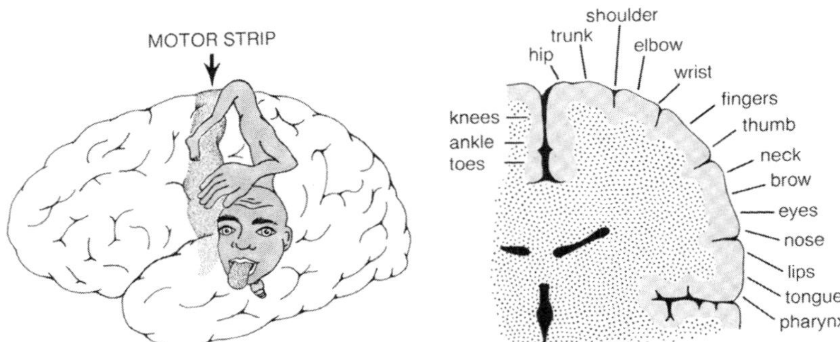

Figure 8.3. The motor strip. The cartoon figure represents body parts at various points on the strip. Note that the areas representing facial and hand muscles are very large. This is because of the intricate control necessary for speech and fine motor coordination. A cross-section of the motor strip is shown to the right.

synapse (junction between two nerve cells) to an anterior horn cell in the gray matter section of the spinal cord. This neuron relays the transmission via its axon to a peripheral nerve that connects to an appropriate muscle. The muscle subsequently contracts in response to the original signal from the motor strip in the cortex. In **spinal muscular atrophy** (Werdnig-Hoffman disease), the motor neuron dies during childhood, resulting in **hypotonia** (low muscle tone) and weakness (Shababi, Lorson, & Rudnik-Schoneborn, 2014; see Chapter 9).

Conversely, if the motor cortex or the pyramidal tract is damaged, increased tone in the form of spasticity results. In spasticity, the underlying involuntary muscle contractions controlled by the brainstem and spinal cord are no longer inhibited by pyramidal tract activity. As a result, voluntary movement becomes less fluid and muscle control is more difficult, as seen in cerebral palsy and other movement disorders (see Chapter 21). Therapeutic approaches to spasticity focus on manipulating neurotransmitters to reduce tone. For example, the drug baclofen, which decreases spasticity by increasing the activity of gamma-amino butyric acid (GABA), an inhibitory neurotransmitter, can be administered orally or into the spinal fluid using an implantable pump in individuals with cerebral palsy (Hasnat & Rice, 2015; He et al., 2014). Damage to the motor cortex can also lead to focal-onset seizures, as occurred with Thomas (see Chapter 22).

The frontal lobe is also important in abstract thinking. Via functional imaging techniques, the frontal lobe has been identified as the origin of executive function (Burgess & Stuss, 2017). This high-level abstract thinking is the planner and organizer for future activities. Children with autism, ADHD, and learning disabilities show deficiencies in executive function (Bos et al., 2017; Rubia et al., 2011; see Chapters 18–20).

Broca's area (Figure 8.4), the center for expressive language, typically resides in the left frontal lobe, anterior to the motor strip (see Chapter 17). The location can vary, particularly in children who are left-handed, have epilepsy, or have prior destructive lesions such as tumors or stroke (Avramescu-Murphy et al., 2017; Benjamin et al., 2017; Gaillard et al., 2011; Steinberg, Ratner, Gaillard, & Berl, 2013).

The Parietal Lobe Touch, pain, vibration, **proprioception** (the ability to sense the position, location, orientation, and movement of body parts), and temperature sensation are all processed within the parietal lobe. In addition, the parietal lobe contributes to the integration of stimuli from different regions, providing the ability to create a complete "picture." The primary sensory cortex (Brodmann area 3,1,2) is located in the postcentral gyrus of the brain and receives all sensory information in a **somatotopical** organization (point-for-point correspondence of an area of the body to a specific area in the brain) from the opposite side of the body. Information to the primary somatosensory cortex arrives from the **thalamus.** Injury to the thalamus

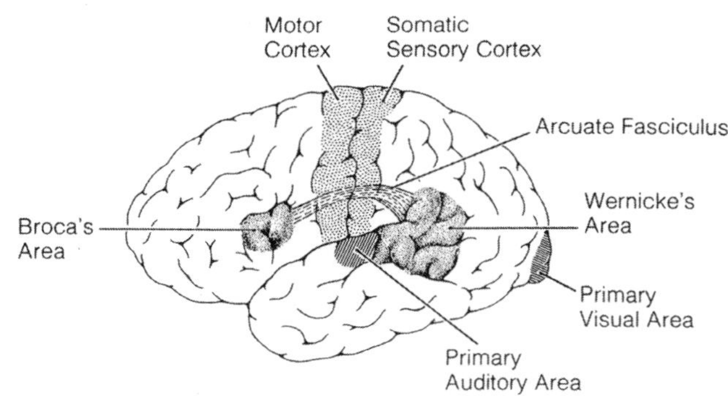

Figure 8.4. An adult neuropathological model of language. Sounds are received in Wernicke's area and passed on to Broca's area via nerve fibers of the arcuate fasciculus. Expressive language is formed here, and the motor cortex is then stimulated to produce speech.

(e.g., by a stroke) may produce **paresthesias** (numbness with a pins-and-needles sensation) on the opposite side of the body. A destructive lesion (e.g., a tumor or hemorrhage) in this area impairs sensation, including difficulty localizing painful stimuli or measuring their intensity. Although the primary visual cortex is in the occipital lobe, some higher levels of visual processing take place in the parietal lobe. There is evidence that the visual-perceptual problems experienced by children with learning disabilities and the difficulties in performing fine motor tasks found in children with ADHD may be related to parietal region abnormalities (Cubillo et al., 2010; Schulz et al., 2017).

The Temporal Lobe The temporal lobe is primarily involved in communication and sensation. The dominant hemisphere (the left side in more than 90% of people) is responsible for comprehending speech as well as contributing to the memory of auditory and visual experiences (Gaillard et al., 2011). It receives input from each ear, with somatotopical projection of the **cochlea** (the spiral-shaped cavity of the inner ear that resembles a snail shell and contains nerve endings essential for hearing) upon the acoustic area of the temporal lobe. Wernicke's area, the receptive language center, is found in the superior temporal gyrus. As with Broca's area, it is most commonly found on the left side, but its location can vary (Berl et al., 2014).

Within the base of each temporal lobe rests two structures, the **hippocampus** and **amygdala,** which serve special cognitive functions. The hippocampus plays an important role in memory and allows for learning of new information. The amygdala is involved in sensory processing and emotions and is part of the general-purpose "fight-or-flight" defense response control system.

Both the amygdala and hippocampus show structural abnormalities in autism, with the degree of abnormality being linked to the severity of impairment (Barnea-Goraly et al., 2014; Dziobek, Bahnemann, Convit, & Heekeren, 2010; Kleinhans et al., 2010). It is unclear if alterations in the hippocampus are a cause or an effect of the disorder's symptomatology. Studies in both animals and humans suggest that the hippocampus can undergo dynamic changes as a result of experience, behavior, and exercise (Insausti, Cebada-Sánchez, & Marcos, 2010; Korol, Gold, & Scavuzzo, 2013).

In humans, the amygdala is associated with emotional and social functions. Recent use of functional MRI (fMRI) has demonstrated that the human brain is equipped with specialized circuits for discriminating facial emotions. In particular, the crucial involvement of the amygdala in emotional face processing has been demonstrated by a large number of studies comparing patients with damaged amygdala and unaffected subjects (Damiano, Churches, Ring, & Baron-Cohen, 2011). Amygdala dysfunction has also been strongly implicated in the social deficits of autism as it is involved in the ability to read and relate to others' emotions.

Recent evidence suggests that several aspects of face processing are impaired in patients with autism (Damiano et al., 2011). The most reproducible features include atypical patterns of gaze processing, memory for facial identity, and recognition of the emotional content of facial expressions. Research studying face processing in autism focuses on impairments in a specific network of brain regions that are implicated in social cognition and face processing. These include the superior temporal sulcus (located in the temporal lobe), which plays a role in processing gaze and facial movements, and the fusiform face area (located on the ventral surface of the temporal lobe). It is not known how alterations in developmental processes and the role of experience interact during normal development and in autism to modify and influence this network.

Temporal lobe dysfunction can contribute to a number of disorders, the two most common being receptive **aphasia** and focal to bilateral seizures (Chatzikonstantinou, 2014; Mesulam et al., 2014). In receptive aphasia, the temporal lobe may have been damaged by a tumor, vascular insufficiency, or trauma. The individual is unable to understand spoken words but is able to speak, frequently in an unintelligible fashion. Individuals with focal seizures originating from the temporal lobe may initially experience a *déjà vu* or flashback phenomenon caused by stimulation of this brain area. The person may also have visual hallucinations, hear bizarre sounds, or smell unpleasant aromas, all of which emanate from the temporal lobe.

Treatment of refractory complex partial seizures may involve surgical removal of the seizure focus (Ravindra, Sweney, & Bollo, 2017). This surgery has been shown in adults to be superior to long-term antiepileptic drug use in terms of seizure control and quality of life (see Chapter 22). Although adults who undergo this neurosurgical procedure on the left side of the brain often sustain some language or memory loss, children appear less likely to experience this complication. This suggests that a child's brain is more flexible than an adult's, such that the nondominant hemisphere can take over some of the language functions of the damaged dominant area. In fact, children as old as 6 years have undergone total dominant **hemispherectomy** (removal of the left hemisphere for intractable generalized seizures with a left-sided focus) and have been able to recover speech function, presumably by incorporating other cortical locations in a new functional role (Bulteau et al., 2017; Johnston, 2009). This is a clear demonstration of the plasticity of the developing brain.

With hemispherectomy, the degree of language recovery varies according to the underlying cause of the seizure disorder (Bulteau et al., 2015; Ivanova et al., 2017).

In the temporal lobe, the primary auditory cortex receives input from both ears by way of the cochlear nerves via multiple synapses in the brainstem. Irritation of this cortex may cause a buzzing or roaring sensation in the ears. Because of the bilateral representation, unilateral damage does not result in deafness but may lead to a mild hearing loss. Bilateral lesions can result in a complete hearing loss.

The Occipital Lobe The primary visual receptive cortex is located in the occipital lobe. The right occipital lobe receives impulses from the right half of each **retina** (the nerve layer that lines the back of the eye, senses light, and creates impulses that travel through the optic nerve to the brain). This creates the left visual field, whereas the left visual cortex receives impulses from the left half of each retina (and creates the right visual field). The upper portion of this cortical area represents the upper half of each retina (the lower visual field), whereas the lower portion represents the lower half (the upper visual field). Irritation of the visual cortex can produce such visual hallucinations as flashes of light, rainbows, brilliant stars, or bright lines. Destructive lesions can cause defects in the visual fields on the opposite side without loss of central vision.

Visual stimuli are first interpreted in the visual-receptive area and then processed further in an adjacent part of the occipital lobe before being passed on to the temporal and parietal lobes (see Chapter 7). Here the identity of a viewed object and its location in space are further determined. In both the temporal and parietal lobes, the image is linked to what is heard and felt so that a proper interpretation can be made. Severe damage to the occipital region may cause **cortical visual impairment** (cortical blindness). In this condition, despite a normal visual apparatus and pathways leading toward the occipital lobe, the person is functionally blind.

Interconnections The white matter of the adult cerebral hemispheres contains nerve fibers of many sizes that are **myelinated** (sheathed by an insulating layer that increases the speed at which impulses are conducted). Some of these fibers serve to connect various regions of the brain. The most important of these interconnections is the corpus callosum, noted above (Figure 8.2A).

A second type of interconnection is formed by projection fibers that connect the cerebral cortex with lower portions of the brain or spinal cord. As an example, the **internal capsule** is a collection of fibers that projects from the cortex to the spinal cord; nerve impulses carried by these fibers control distant muscles. Destructive lesions such as tumors or strokes may compress or otherwise compromise the internal capsule and the pyramidal (motor) tract it contains. This will result in **hemiplegia** (spasticity and weakness on the opposite side of the body).

Finally, association fibers connect various cortical areas within the same hemisphere. There are short association fibers, or U fibers, that connect adjacent gyri, while long association fibers connect more widely separated gyri.

The Basal Ganglia and Thalamus

Deep beneath the cortical surface resides the **diencephalon** (Figure 8.2A), which consists of the thalamus and **hypothalamus.** Adjacent to the diencephalon are the **basal ganglia** and related structures. In humans, this primitive part of the brain modulates instructions from the motor cortex in directing voluntary movements. In lower vertebrates it directly controls motor activity. Anatomically, the basal ganglia include the **caudate nucleus** and the **putamen** (together called the **corpus striatum**), the **globus pallidus,** and the other gray matter areas at the base of the forebrain. Together, the putamen and the globus pallidus form the **lentiform nucleus.** The caudate nucleus is separated from the lentiform nucleus and thalamus by the **internal capsule.** Functionally, these collections of neurons, together with their connections and neurotransmitters, form an associated motor system.

Damage to the basal ganglia produces various movement disorders. Although voluntary movement is still possible, involuntary jerking or twisting, referred to as **choreoathetosis,** may also occur. Alternatively, individuals may experience rigidity or **dystonic** posturing (involuntary contraction of muscles, forcing limbs into abnormal, sometimes painful postures). Children with perinatal brain injury involving the basal ganglia may have **dyskinetic cerebral palsy** (Monbaliu et al., 2017).

In the center of the brain is a crucial structure called the thalamus. Nearly all sensory input from throughout the body must first pass through the thalamus prior to reaching the appropriate region of the cortex. The thalamus is often referred to as a major relay station responsible for transmission of information within the brain and across networks and pathways. It also is the seat of normal brain rhythms that are inhibitory and modulate control of movement.

The thalamus is comprised of multiple nuclei that have specific roles in what information is processed. Depending on the location of an injury, thalamic injury can present as movement disorders, cognitive dysfunction, language difficulty, problems with visual processing, and sleep-wake cycling difficulties. More diffuse injuries to the thalamocortical pathways (connecting the thalamus to the cortex) have also been found to result in abnormal excitation that may be related to a variety of neuropsychiatric and behavioral disorders. Neuroimaging studies have demonstrated that mild to moderate traumatic brain injury can result in disruption of thalamic resting state networks and that this injury correlates with reduced performance on neurocognitive testing (Han, Chapman, & Krawczyk, 2015). This continues to be an exciting area of research because of the contribution that the thalamic resting state network may have in autism and intellectual disability (Nair et al., 2015).

The Brainstem

In contrast to the cerebral hemispheres, which control voluntary actions, the brainstem controls more reflexive and involuntary activities. It is comprised of three distinct areas (midbrain, pons, and medulla) and connects the cerebral hemispheres to the spinal cord (Figure 8.5). Within it are the cranial nerves that control functions such as vision, hearing, swallowing, and articulation. These cranial nerves also affect facial expression, eye and tongue movement, salivation, and even breathing. In addition to the cranial nerve nuclei, the brainstem is composed of a vast array of fiber tracts relaying messages into and out of the brain. The corticospinal tract provides a passage of neural impulses from the cortex to the spinal cord. Conversely there are tracts that bring sensory information to the cortex via the thalamus. Therefore, any abnormality in this region affects function in distant locations. Children with cerebral palsy may have damage to the brainstem or to pathways that end in the brainstem. This damage might explain the high incidence of excessive salivation, swallowing problems, strabismus, and speech disorders in these children (see Chapter 21).

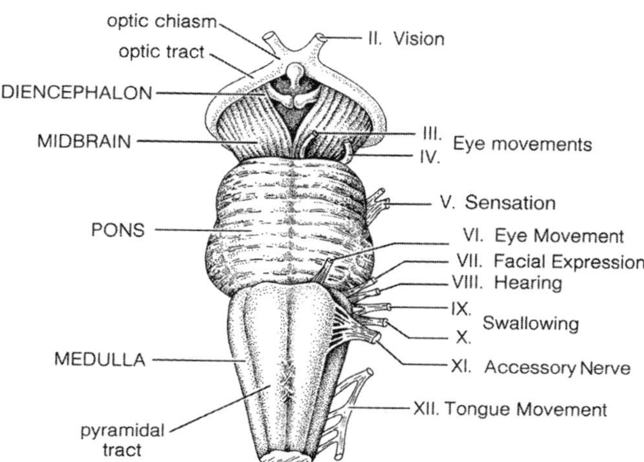

Figure 8.5. The three regions of the brainstem are shown: midbrain, pons, and medulla. The placement and function of 11 of the 12 cranial nerves are illustrated. (The first cranial nerve [smell] is not shown. It lies in front of the second cranial nerve, below the frontal lobe.) Note that the pyramidal tract runs from the cortex (not shown) into the brainstem. The pyramidal fibers cross over in the medulla. Thus, the right hemisphere controls left-side movement, and the left hemisphere controls right-side movement.

The Cerebellum

The **cerebellum** (Figure 8.2A and B) resides below the cerebral hemispheres and behind the brainstem. The importance of the cerebellum is increasingly being recognized for its contributions to coordination of voluntary motor activity, cognition, emotion, language, and learning. During the late fetal and early postnatal period, the cerebellum undergoes unparalleled rapid growth and development (Brossard-Racine & Limperopoulos, 2016). It helps coordinate voluntary motor activity by dampening skeletal muscular activity. This enables a smooth transition between activating **agonist** muscles (that work together) and inhibiting their counterpart antagonist muscles. Normal muscle coordination requires that cerebellar functions be integrated with those of the cerebral hemispheres and the basal ganglia. Although voluntary movement can occur without the cerebellum, such movements are **ataxic** (erratic and uncoordinated). An ataxic gait may be seen with cerebellar tumors, progressive neurological disorders (e.g., ataxia telangiectasia), cerebral palsy, certain genetic conditions, or as a side effect of certain medications.

Advanced imaging studies have revealed cortical-cerebellar connectivity during cognitive testing of memory and executive function (Koziol et al., 2014; Nguyen et al., 2017). Imaging using fMRI reveals cerebellar activation during a variety of cognitive tasks including those related to language, visual–spatial abilities, and executive function. Furthermore, resting-state functional connectivity data demonstrate that the cerebellum is part of cognitive networks that include the prefrontal and parietal association cortices (Koziol et al., 2014). The **clinical cerebellar cognitive affective syndrome,** occurring in patients with cerebellar lesions, provides further evidence of cerebellar involvement in cognitive functions. The syndrome causes deficits in spatial processing, working memory, language, and emotional labiality (Hoche, Guell, Vangel, Sherman, & Schmahmann, 2017).

A number of theories have been proposed regarding the specific contributions that the cerebellum makes to neural processes, including timing, sequencing, and learning associative relationships among elements (Baumann et al., 2015; Cheron, Marquez-Ruiz, & Dan, 2016; Freeman, 2014). This suggests that the cerebellum is important for extracting relevant information from the environment and optimizing motor output related to that information. These findings support the theory that the cerebellum is crucial to the formation of internal models, which may apply to both movement and cognitive functions.

The Spinal Cord

The spinal cord transmits motor and sensory messages between the brain and the rest of the body. In addition to permitting voluntary movement, the spinal cord acts to provide protective reflex arcs in both the upper and lower extremities, such as the deep tendon reflex elicited when the knee is tapped. The spinal cord is an elongated, cylindrical mass of nerve tissue that is continuous with the brainstem at its upper end and occupies the upper two thirds of the adult spinal canal within the vertebral column (Figure 8.6). It widens laterally in the neck and the lower back regions. These enlargements correspond to the origins of the nerves of the upper and lower extremities. The nerves of the **brachial plexus** originate at the **cervical** (neck) enlargement of the spinal cord and control arm movement; the nerves of the **lumbosacral plexus** arise from the **lumbar** (lower back) enlargement of the spinal cord and control leg movement. Injury to a newborn's brachial plexus most commonly occurs during a difficult vaginal delivery, resulting in weakness of the arm (Freeman, Goodyear, & Leith, 2017). Many patients with birth-related brachial plexus injuries recover enough motion and strength and do not need early surgery, but they do greatly benefit from occupational therapy.

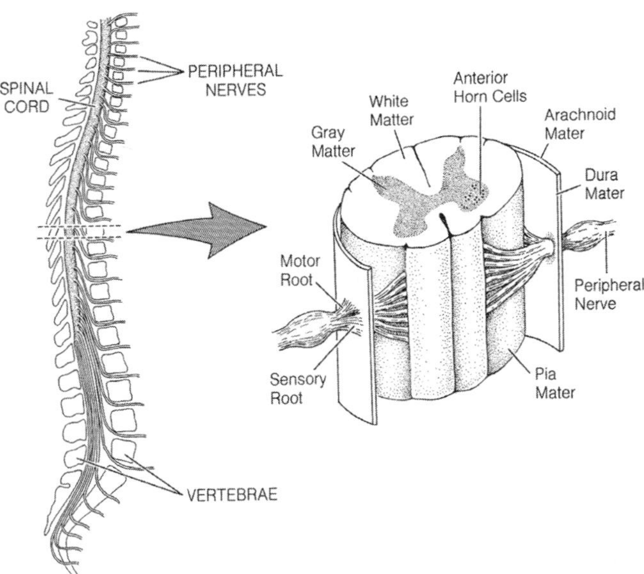

Figure 8.6. The spinal column. The spinal cord extends from the neck to the lower back. It is protected by the bony vertebrae that form the spinal column. The enlargement to the right shows a section of the cord taken from the upper back region. Note the meninges (the dura, arachnoid, and pia mater) surrounding the cord and the peripheral nerve on its way to a muscle. This nerve contains both motor and sensory components (roots). The spinal cord, like the brain, has both gray and white matter. The gray matter consists of various nerve cells, the most important of which are the anterior horn cells. These are destroyed in polio. The white matter contains nerve fibers wrapped in myelin, which gives the cord its glistening appearance.

The spinal cord is divided into approximately 30 segments—8 cervical, 12 thoracic (chest), 5 lumbar, 5 sacral (pelvic), and a few small coccygeal (tailbone) segments—that correspond to attachments of groups of nerve roots. Individual segments vary in length. They are about twice as long in the midthoracic region as in the cervical or upper lumbar area.

There are no sharp boundaries between segments within the cord itself. Each segment contributes four roots: a **ventral** (front) and **dorsal** (back) root arising from the left half and a similar pair of roots arising from the right half of the cord. Each root is made up of many individual rootlets. The dorsal nerve roots allow sensory input to ascend to the brainstem, whereas the ventral roots deliver motor input from the brainstem to the appropriate muscle.

If the spinal cord is damaged (e.g., due to trauma or a congenital malformation, such as a myelomeningocele), messages to and from the brain are short-circuited below the area of defect. The result is a loss (either partial or complete) of sensation and movement in the affected limbs. The paralysis, which is initially flaccid (hypotonic) but ultimately becomes spastic (hypertonic), may involve the legs (**paraplegia**) or all four extremities (**quadriplegia**) depending on the level of damage.

Cerebrospinal Fluid and the Hydrodynamic Balance

Cerebrospinal fluid (CSF) is now known to perform many functions. In addition to physically supporting the neural elements and serving to buffer the brain and spinal cord from excessive motion, CSF acts to provide nutritional support as well as remove excessive hormones and neurotransmitters. CSF may also serve as a "relief valve," adjusting its volume when there is an increase in intracranial pressure.

In adults approximately 600 to 700 milliliters of CSF is produced each day primarily by the **choroid plexus,** a collection of modified ependymal cells lining the ventricles of the brain. This fluid moves throughout the lateral and third ventricles and communicates with the fourth ventricle via the aqueduct of Sylvius (Figure 8.7). At the level of the fourth ventricle, the CSF exits to circulate over the surface of the brain as well as the spinal cord in the subarachnoid space. Absorption of CSF occurs at the **arachnoid granulations** over

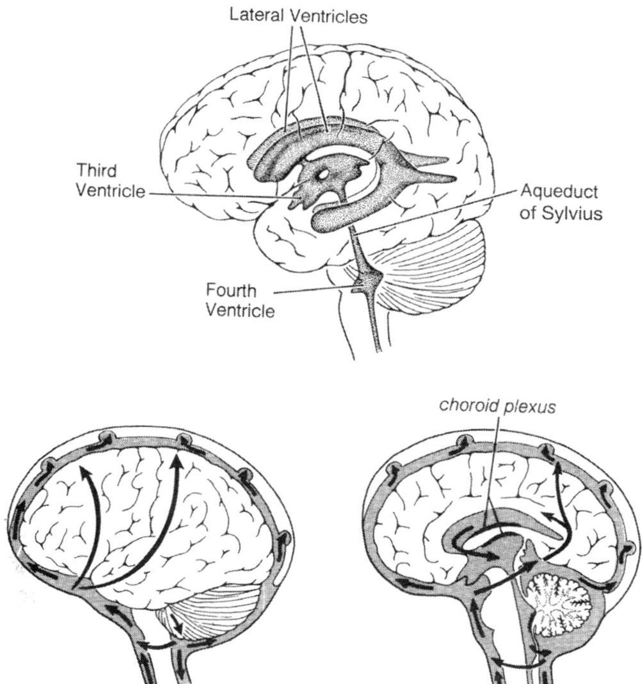

Figure 8.7. The ventricular system of the brain. The major parts of the ventricular system are shown (top). The flow of cerebrospinal fluid is shown (bottom). The fluid is produced by the choroid plexus in the roof of the lateral and third ventricles. Its primary route is through the aqueduct of Sylvius, into the fourth ventricle, and then into the spinal column, where it is absorbed. A secondary route is around the surface of the brain. A blockage, most commonly of the aqueduct of Sylvius, leads to hydrocephalus. (Lower illustrations from Milhorat, T.H. [1972]. *Hydrocephalus and the cerebrospinal fluid*. Philadelphia, PA: Lippincott Williams & Wilkins. http://www.lww.com. Copyright © 1972, The Williams & Wilkins Co., Baltimore, MD; adapted by permission.)

the superior surface of the brain. These granulations act as one-way valves to allow CSF to move into the blood stream.

Should an imbalance develop between CSF production and absorption, **hydrocephalus** may result (Figure 8.8). This usually congenital condition involves an abnormal accumulation of fluid in the cerebral ventricles, causing skull enlargement in the infant and brain compression. It can be caused by an obstruction of CSF flow within the ventricular system (frequently at the aqueduct of Sylvius) or at the exit of the ventricular system (at the foramina of Luschka and Magendie). This is known as a noncommunicating hydrocephalus. In contrast, a communicating hydrocephalus is caused by a malfunction at the level of the arachnoid granulations. In addition to inadequate absorption, overproduction of CSF can occur, as seen with tumors of the choroid plexus.

When fluid builds up inside the skull of an infant, the **sutures** (the joints connecting the bones of the skull) expand and dissipate the increased pressure at the expense of an increase in head circumference. This may

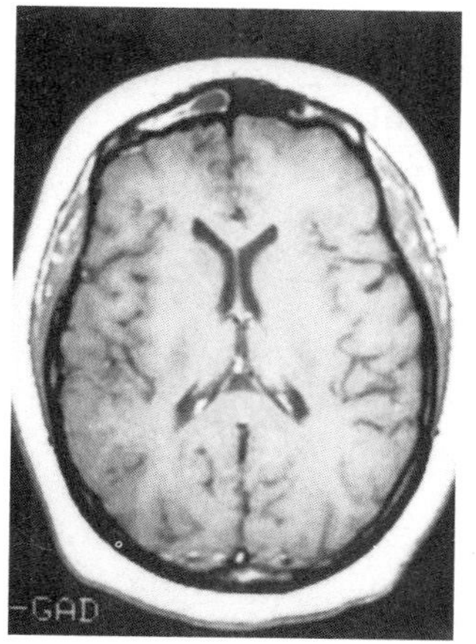

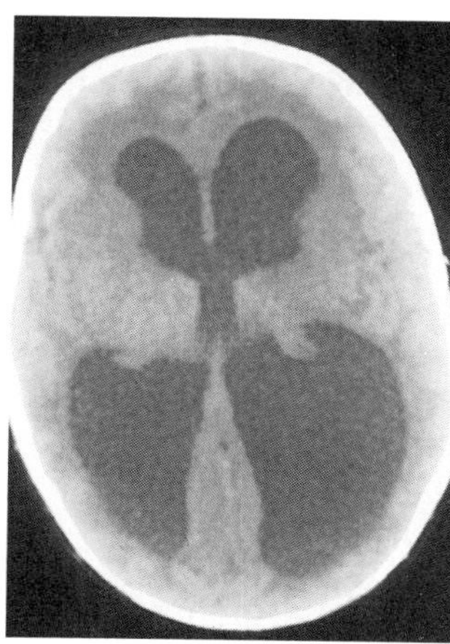

Figure 8.8. Normal magnetic resonance imaging scan (left) and computed tomography scan showing hydrocephalus (right). In the image to the right, note the rounded appearance of the frontal horns (top) as well as the differentially enlarged occipital horns (bottom). This is known as culpocephaly and is frequently seen in individuals with spina bifida.

present as a bulging **anterior fontanelle** ("soft spot"). The sutures generally close between 9–18 months, so hydrocephalus in a child older than 18 months may quickly lead to headache, vomiting, lethargy, and **focal** (localized) neurological changes. This buildup of fluid can be life-threatening at any age and is considered a medical emergency.

When hydrocephalus occurs, it is necessary to restore the balance between production and absorption of CSF, a treatment often accomplished via a shunting procedure that results in long-term drainage of CSF. The shunt's objective is to bypass the CSF obstruction, whether at the level of the arachnoid granulations or within the ventricular system. This usually involves diverting CSF from the head to another site, preferably the abdomen. The complication rate for this surgery is low, and the long-term outcome is reasonably good. Once in place, however, numerous obstacles remain in maintaining a working shunt and avoiding infection. Many children require shunt revisions as a result of infection or because obstructions develop within the shunt. Managing hydrocephalus, however, has been simplified and often allows for a near-typical lifestyle.

In children with noncommunicating hydrocephalus, either congenital (e.g., aqueductal stenosis) or acquired (e.g., secondary to a tumor), there is a surgical alternative to shunting. This procedure (endoscopic third ventriculostomy) involves perforating the floor of the third ventricle to create a new outflow route for the CSF, thus bypassing the obstruction completely. Endoscopic third ventriculostomy has the benefit of avoiding implants but is not feasible in all individuals with hydrocephalus (Lam, Harris, Rocque, & Ham, 2014).

In addition, there is a small but serious risk of injury to nearby vascular and neural structures (Robertson, Abd-El-Barr, Mukundan, & Gormley, 2017).

THE PERIPHERAL NERVOUS SYSTEM

The peripheral nerves allow neural impulses to move from the CNS (brain and spinal cord) to distant muscles and sensory organs. These nerves can have both motor and sensory fibers that run in opposite directions. Motor, or **efferent,** fibers transmit impulses from the brain to initiate movement, whereas sensory, or **afferent,** fibers carry signals from muscles, skin, and joints back to the brain. Sensory fibers convey information related to the position of a joint or the tone of a muscle following movement. Hyperexcitability of sensory neurons in the child with cerebral palsy contributes to spasticity. There are also a number of hereditary neuropathies that interfere with the peripheral nervous system (Stojkovic, 2016).

The regenerative capacity of the peripheral nervous system differs substantially from that of the CNS. Although the CNS is considered capable of limited regeneration, the peripheral nervous system can be repaired more easily. This ability to promote the regrowth of peripheral nerves is responsible for the success seen in surgical reconstruction for **brachial plexus** palsy sustained during vaginal delivery. The brachial plexus is a network of nerves that conducts signals from the spine to the shoulder, arm, and hand. Brachial plexus palsy is caused by damage to those nerves. Symptoms include a limp or paralyzed arm; lack of muscle control in the arm, hand, or wrist; and a lack of feeling or sensation in the arm or hand. Recovery of partial function is seen in 60%–90% of young children undergoing these procedures (Abid, 2016; Abzug & Kozin, 2010).

The **somatic** nervous system (SNS) is the part of the peripheral nervous system that is associated with the voluntary control of body movements via skeletal muscles and with the sensory reception of touch, hearing, and sight. The SNS consists of efferent nerves responsible for stimulating muscle contraction, including all the neurons connected with skeletal muscles, skin, and sense organs. Complex coordination between the motor and sensory system is necessary to ensure normal muscle tone. An imbalance can lead to either increased or decreased tone. Direct injury to the SNS will affect voluntary as well as reflex activities of the involved muscle and will cause flaccid weakness. This is in contrast to a CNS-presenting motor injury, which will present with increased tone in the form of spasticity.

Involuntary activities of the cardiovascular, digestive, endocrine, urinary, respiratory, and reproductive systems are controlled by the **autonomic nervous system.** This control begins in the diencephalon and terminates at the end organ (Figure 8.9). In contrast to the graded response of voluntary movements, the autonomic nervous system involves an on/off type of control. The best example of this is the fight-or-flight response. When a person feels threatened, physically or psychologically, several physiological changes take place simultaneously. Digestive system functions are suspended so that blood can be diverted to more important areas for actions involved in fight or flight, such as the brain and heart. Heart rate and blood pressure increase, and the air passages of the lungs expand in size. All of these changes prepare for a quick reaction to an emergency.

Although the autonomic nervous system works involuntarily in maintaining **homeostasis** (metabolic equilibrium of the body), voluntary adjustments come from the cerebral cortex to modulate these effects. The development of bowel and bladder control is the best example of this. In an infant, when the bladder or rectum fills, the outlet muscles release automatically and the infant urinates or defecates with no conscious control. Between the ages of 12 and 18 months, however, the child starts to be able to gain control over these functions. The cerebral cortex begins to send inhibitory signals to reduce the normal autonomic activity. As any parent knows only too well, this coordination requires months (or years) of fine-tuning to master consistent control. Individuals who have sustained damage to either the corticospinal tracts or the spinal cord

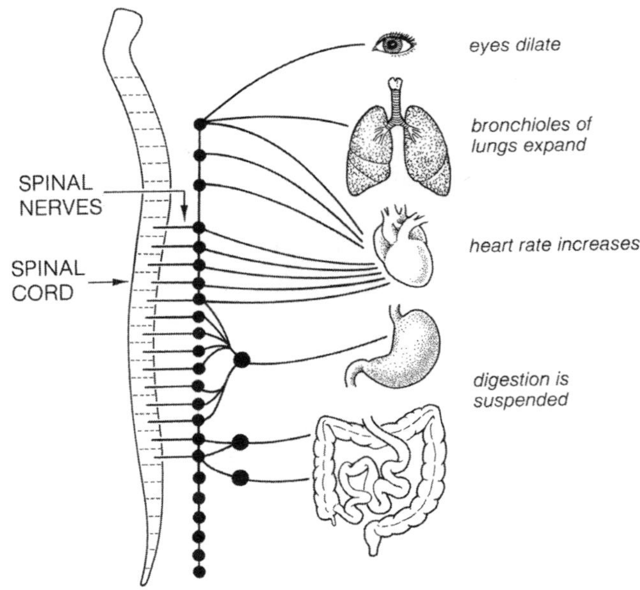

Figure 8.9. Autonomic nervous system. These nerves control such involuntary motor activities as breathing, heart rate, and digestion. This figure shows what occurs in fight-or-flight reactions (sympathetic).

are less able to inhibit the autonomic nervous system in this way. This explains the great difficulty that children with cerebral palsy, myelomeningocele, or traumatic brain injury may have in controlling bowel and bladder function.

THE MICROSCOPIC ARCHITECTURE OF THE BRAIN

The Neuron

Neurons are similar to other cells in that they have a cell body consisting of a nucleus and cytoplasm. Unlike other cells, however, they have a long process called an **axon,** which extends from the cell body, and many short jutting processes called **dendrites** (Figure 8.10). The axon carries impulses away from the nerve cell body, sometimes for a distance greater than a meter. Dendrites receive impulses from other neurons and carry them a short distance toward the cell body. The size and shape of dendrites may change with neuronal activity, suggesting that these changes may represent the anatomical basis for memory.

As the brain begins to organize by 5 weeks' gestation (a process that continues into early childhood), neurons develop from neural progenitor cells that first symmetrically proliferate (multiply) during the first 6 weeks of gestation and then shift to asymmetric cell division (Lui, Hansen, & Kriegstein, 2011). Most of the neural progenitor cells that eventually mature into postmitotic neurons are produced in the ventricular zone. They migrate radially to form the six-layered neocortex—with the sixth layer being formed first and the more superficial layers formed later by migrating cells (Lui et al., 2011). Once the neurons have migrated to their target region, they grow in size, differentiate, and develop neuronal processes (i.e., axons and dendrites). The major developmental features of this organizational period include 1) the establishment and differentiation of neurons; 2) the attainment of proper alignment, orientation, and layering of cortical neurons; 3) the elaboration of dendrites and axons; 4) the establishment of synaptic contacts; and 5) cell death and selective elimination of neuronal processes and synapses.

As the neurons develop, the growing axons are able to recognize various signaling molecules that are on the surface of other axons and cell bodies. They use these molecules as a means to navigate to their final destination. Based on these signaling cues, the axons move forward (sometimes rapidly), avoid obstacles, and stop when their target is reached. These guidance functions—sensory, motor, and integrative—are contained within the specialized tip of a growing axon, the growth cone (Tamariz & Varela-Echavarria, 2015).

Dendrites and Axons

As axons grow toward their respective dendritic targets, the dendrites respond by increasing the number of spines (projections) along their surface (Figure 8.11). The spines increase the surface area of the dendrites, permitting more elaborate communication between the neurons. In fact, increased dendritic outgrowth has been associated with enhanced memory, and deficient development of dendritic arborization has been observed in individuals with cognitive impairment, most notably in Down syndrome (Huttenlocher, 1991).

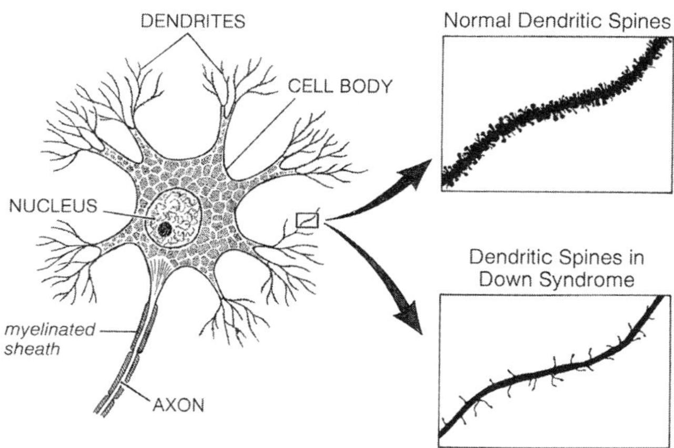

Figure 8.10. Illustration of a nerve cell (neuron) showing its component elements. The enlargements show the minute dendritic spines that increase the number of synapses or junctures among nerve cells. Note the diminished size and number of dendritic spines in a child with Down syndrome.

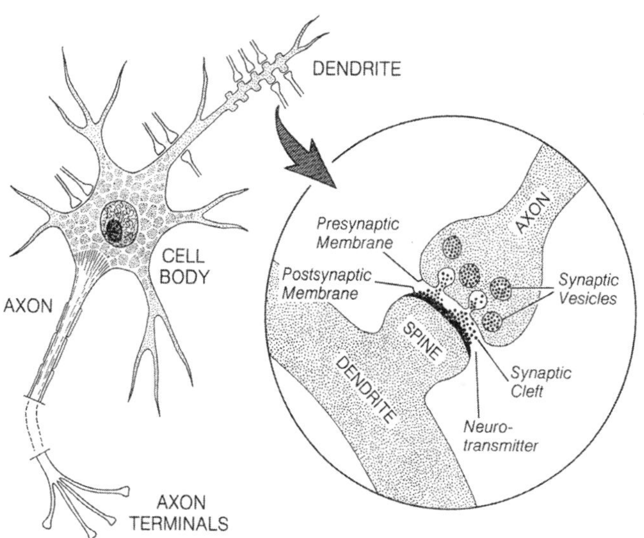

Figure 8.11. Central nervous system synapse. The enlargement shows the abutting of an axon against a dendritic spine. The space separating the two is the synaptic cleft. Neurotransmitter bundles are released into the cleft from vesicles in the presynaptic membrane. These permit transmission of an impulse across the juncture.

Synapses Proper function of the nervous system requires that two linkages form: 1) the needed communication between an axon from one neuron and the dendrite from a second neuron and 2) the communication between these two neurons once the connection is established. The point of contact between two neurons is called a **synapse** (Figure 8.11).

Synapses can be either chemical or electrical, with distinct characteristics for each type. In electrical synapses, there is a short distance between the two neurons, and there is a communication between the cytoplasm of the cells. Because of this, there is very little delay as an electric current passes from one neuron to the next, and the transmission is usually bidirectional.

In contrast, chemical synapses have a larger gap between the two neurons and no direct communication of the cytoplasm. Small **vesicles** (fluid-filled sacs within cells) containing specific neurotransmitters are released from the axon of one neuron and travel the distance between the cells to reach the receptors for that particular neurotransmitter on the dendrite of the second neuron. The effect on the postsynaptic cell can be either excitatory or inhibitory depending on the neurotransmitter and the cell type. Within a network of cells, electrical and chemical synapses work together to foster synchrony.

During early stages of brain development, there are initially an excess number of connections. This exuberant number of synapses throughout the brain gradually declines beginning during the early postnatal period and continuing throughout childhood and adolescence. This process of elimination of axons and dendrites is known as **synaptic pruning**. The purpose of this process is to remove redundancy and enhance connectivity between pertinent neural networks. During neuronal differentiation, the primitive neurons begin to express their distinctive physical and biochemical features. This process, called **arborization,** is much like the growth of a tree from a sapling. It even involves pruning, such that some new connections (synapses) remain established while others disappear. For example, in the visual cortex, synapses form most rapidly between 2 and 4 months after full-term birth, a critical time for the development of visual function. Maximum synaptic density is attained at 8 months of age, when the elimination of synapses begins. Synaptic strengthening and pruning continue through adolescence and into adulthood.

Glia

Glia account for more than half of the cells in the human brain. These macroglia cells—the oligodendrocytes and astrocytes—were originally thought to be simply support cells to the neurons. However, they are now known to play a crucial role as regulators of brain development, plasticity, and disease. They arise from neuroepithelial progenitor cells in the embryonic neural tube and prosencephalon. These neural progenitor cells during early embryonic development first give rise to the radial glia that generate neurons (described above). During the later stage of embryonic development, they begin to differentiate into astrocytes and oligodendrocytes.

Astrocytes are crucial for neuronal survival. They take up the nutrients from the vasculature in order to provide metabolic support to neurons. They also play an important role in a phenomena known as neurovascular coupling; they stimulate increased blood flow to the region where neurons are active in order to provide metabolic support for these regions (Mishra et al., 2016). Recent evidence supports the idea that astrocytes are responsible for regulating the flow of cerebral spinal fluid and its homeostasis (Brinker, Stopa, Morrison, & Klinge, 2014). At the synaptic level, they contribute to ionic balance and the removal and recycling of neurotransmitters.

Oligodendrocytes are the other CNS-specific glial cells and are responsible for myelination. Myelination of axons is important because it acts as an insulator, thus facilitating rapid signal transmission with minimal degradation. In the CNS, myelination begins during the third trimester of pregnancy. Oligodendrocyte progenitor cells differentiate and undergo complex morphological changes that result in the extension of their processes so that they can wrap around multiple axons. Due to the lipid content of myelin, its appearance is white. Effective **myelination** is necessary for the development of voluntary gross and fine motor movement and the suppression of **primitive reflexes** (see Chapters 9 and 21). While the majority of myelination occurs during the first 2 years of life, it continues to a lesser extent into early adulthood (Snaidero & Simons, 2014). Deficient myelin formation (hypomyelination) has been found using MRI in a number of conditions, including prematurity, congenital hypothyroidism, and malnutrition (Barkovich & Deon, 2016).

Outside of the CNS, the peripheral nervous system also requires rapid transmission of signals to and from the CNS. The glial cells that are responsible for myelin formation of the PNS are called **Schwann cells.** Unlike oligodendrocytes in the CNS, a single Schwann cell is responsible for wrapping a single axon; in fact, multiple Schwann cells may wrap a single axon. The embryonic origin of the glial cells that develop into Schwann cells are the neural crest cells.

Neurotransmitters

Neurotransmitters are chemicals that are released by one cell to cause an effect on a second cell. They differ from hormones in the scale of their action. While hormones are released into the bloodstream and can affect cells distant from the originating cell, neurotransmitters are released within the synapse and only affect cells that are in very close proximity. For a substance to be considered a neurotransmitter, it has to be synthesized within and released from the presynaptic neuron and has to exert a defined effect on the postsynaptic neuron.

In the case of chemical transmission at a synapse, the first step is the synthesis of the neurotransmitter within the presynaptic neuron. Many of these chemicals share a common precursor. For example, the neurotransmitters dopamine and norepinephrine are both synthesized from the amino acid tyrosine. Each neuron is specialized to use a specific neurotransmitter. After synthesis, the neurotransmitters are packaged and stored in vesicles within the axon to await release. When a **depolarizing current** (an electrical current causing a change in cell membrane voltage) passes through the axon, the vesicles spill their contents into the synapse. The neurotransmitters then travel the distance between the two neurons. The dendrite of the postsynaptic neuron has receptors that are specific for the released neurotransmitter. When the receptors are activated, there can be an excitatory or inhibitory response. The excess neurotransmitters within the synapse are then removed either by reuptake or by enzymatic breakdown. The function of the CNS can be altered by manipulating any of the steps in chemical transmission. Many commonly used medications for depression and anxiety belong to a group of prescription drugs known as **selective serotonin reuptake inhibitors.** Examples include fluoxetine (Prozac) and sertraline (Zoloft) (see Appendix C). These medications block the reuptake of serotonin after its release in the synaptic cleft, thereby increasing the availability and the duration of serotonin action in specific brain regions. Similarly, atomoxetine (Strattera) is a selective norepinephrine inhibitor and has been found to be effective in treating ADHD. Atomoxetine works differently from stimulant medications that directly stimulate levels of norepinephrine (see Chapter 19). Within the central, peripheral, and autonomic nervous system there are a variety of identified neurotransmitters. Table 8.1 provides a simplified summary of the characteristics of some of the major neurotransmitters.

Table 8.1. Characteristics of some of the major neurotransmitters

Neurotransmitter	Location	Function	Associated disorder
Acetylcholine	Nucleus basalis Neuromuscular junction Autonomic nervous system	Stimulates muscle contraction at the neuromuscular junction	Myasthenia gravis (loss of receptors) Botulism (impaired release)
Dopamine	Substantia nigra	Initiates and controls movement	Parkinson's disease (deficiency) Schizophrenia (excess)
Norepinephrine	Locus ceruleus Sympathetic nervous system	Maintains vigilance and responsiveness	Alzheimer's disease
Serotonin	Raphe nuclei	Involved in the sleep–wake cycle, emotions, food intake, thermoregulation, and sexual behavior	Depression (deficiency)
Histamine	Hypothalamus	Regulates hormones	
GABA	Inhibitory interneurons throughout the brain and spinal cord	Principal inhibitory neurotransmitter	Epilepsy (deficiency)
Glycine	Inhibitory interneurons in the spinal cord	Inhibits antagonist muscles	Nonketotic hyperglycinemia (excess)
Glutamate	Excitatory neurons throughout the brain and spinal cord	Principal excitatory neurotransmitter	Huntington disease (excess) Acute brain injury (excess)

Source: Kandel, Schwartz, and Jessell (2000).
Key: GABA, gamma-aminobutyric acid.

TECHNIQUES FOR EVALUATING THE CENTRAL NERVOUS SYSTEM

Computed Tomography

High-speed computed tomography (CT) scans, which are produced from multiple thin-cut x-rays, are a routine part of evaluating a child with hydrocephalus, trauma, craniofacial disorders, new-onset seizures, or brain and skull tumors. The CT provides excellent bone definition and allows the physician to discern whether acute brain pathology is present including hemorrhage, edema (swelling), or tumor. Three-dimensional CT scans also can provide sophisticated reconstruction of complex skull-base disorders, while CT angiography offers good resolution of blood vessels and flow abnormalities. CT scans can often be obtained quickly, so they may not require sedation in young children, as opposed to MRI scans, which take longer to acquire, making sedation necessary.

CT can be supplemented with intravenous (IV) contrast, which helps define areas of blood-brain barrier breakdown. The addition of IV contrast is especially helpful in cases of infection or a suspected tumor. Most infections and many (but not all) tumors will appear bright with the addition of contrast, aiding in visualization of these lesions. Conversely, IV contrast typically does not help in certain clinical scenarios such as a closed head injury or hydrocephalus.

While CT is a powerful diagnostic tool, the associated radiation exposure is greater than that from a typical chest x-ray. Not only are children more sensitive to radiation and thus at an increased risk from exposure, but they also will have a longer lifetime than adults for any negative effects from exposure to manifest (Antonucci et al., 2017; Bulas, Goske, Applegate, & Wood, 2009). In addition to the risk to the individual, one must consider the potential population risk of increased cancer rates as use of CT has become more common (Pearce et al., 2012). While CT remains a mainstay in evaluating the child's nervous system in the acute setting (e.g., traumatic brain injury), decreased radiation or alternative methods of imaging, such as MRI, are becoming the mainstay in most diagnostic situations.

Magnetic Resonance Imagining

MRI scanning has surpassed all other imaging modalities for evaluating brain structure. It is particularly useful in investigating developmental abnormalities of the brain, in assessing the causes of epilepsy, in identifying chronic hemorrhage, and in visualizing brain tumors.

Over the last decade, improvements in MRI technology and science have allowed physicians to collect information not only about alterations in structure, but also alterations in function, brain metabolism, and microscopic damage to the brain's gray and white matter. This is done by using special MRI software in the routine MRI scanner. These new sequences have been used clinically as well as part of research studies to learn more about brain networks that underlie cognition and how different developmental disorders may be similar or different in terms of brain function.

Children with intellectual disability may have a structural cause for the underlying deficit. It may be qualitative or quantitative and therefore can be measured by MRI. Some findings may be nonspecific but nonetheless may be helpful in identifying a physiologic process (e.g., whether it involves the gray matter or white matter), determining the timing of the insult (e.g., an old neonatal stroke versus a recent stroke in a child with sickle cell disease), assessing the potential for reversibility, or following up to see if a condition is static or progressive. Other findings on MRI may be so specific that they help to identify the definitive cause of a child's intellectual disability. An example would be the diagnosis of a major structural brain anomaly such as holoprosencephaly, lissencephaly, or a malformation of the cerebellum (see Chapter 3). Applying the newer modalities of MRI that probe function, microstructure, and metabolism can assess brain injury at its earliest onset as well as provide a basis for following the course of the disease or gauging the effects of interventions.

New discoveries and applications over the past decades include 1) fluid-attenuated inversion recovery imaging, which allows much better analysis of disorders that affect the white matter (see Figure 8.12); 2) fMRI, which enables one to visualize brain activation patterns while a patient performs a cognitive or motor task in the scanner (see Figure 8.13); 3) diffusion weighted imaging and diffusion tensor imaging to look at microscopic damage in white matter; and 4) magnetic resonance spectroscopy (MRS), which enables a noninvasive biochemical examination of the brain (Figure 8.14). A systematic approach based on pattern recognition of brain involvement is particularly useful

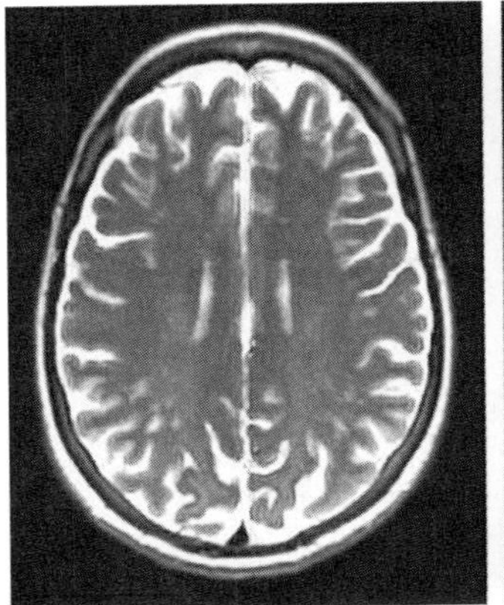
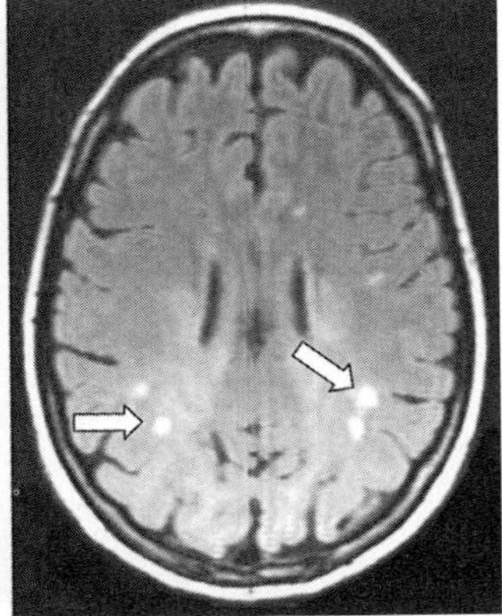

Figure 8.12. On routine T2 imaging (left), white matter lesions may be difficult to visualize. However, on the fluid-attenuated inversion recovery imaging (right) sequence the white matter lesions are clearly evident. (*Source:* Kandel, Schwartz, & Jessell, 2000.)

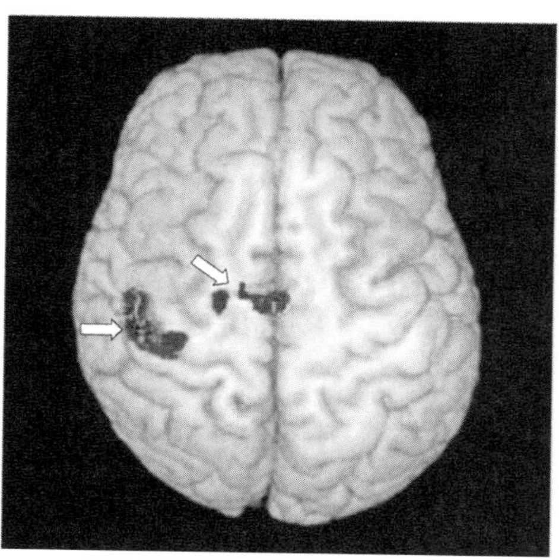

Figure 8.13. Activation map typical of an fMRI. In this figure, the left motor strip is being activated in the area indicated by the arrows. A task that elicits motor response would be expected to produce such a motor response. In an individual who has motor impairment, this area may show less activation and other areas may activate in a compensatory response.

in the analysis of brain MRI scans in patients with inborn errors of metabolism (see Chapter 16).

Since the mid-2000s, fMRI has emerged as a valuable tool for imaging the time course of activity associated with neurocognitive processes in the brain (Gaillard & Berl, 2012). This technology has wide-ranging applications for both basic research into brain function and for clinical research into the neurophysiology of neurological and psychiatric illness. fMRI detects minute changes in regional blood flow and metabolism and can be useful in localizing brain regions involved in such activities as reading, speaking, listening, and moving. Differences have been found in individuals with dyslexia versus standard-achievement-level readers (Krafnick, Flowers, Luetje, Napoliello, & Eden, 2014). In epilepsy, fMRI is useful in localizing language and memory function, as well as seizure foci, and it may one day replace more invasive testing of these functions (Gaillard & Berl, 2012).

MRS is a versatile noninvasive technique capable of producing information on a large number of brain metabolites. This technology is readily available and often performed in the same session as conventional MRI. MRS techniques complement conventional and advanced imaging and are proving useful in diagnosing, treating, and predicting progression. To date there are no clear guidelines for the use of MRS in childhood neurological diseases. However, many studies demonstrate that MRS can serve as a useful tool to predict outcome after perinatal brain injury, facilitate the diagnosis of metabolic disorders or mass (tumor) lesions, and provide additive information in the workup of children with epilepsy (Gropman, 2010; Rincon et al., 2016).

The most commonly used spectroscopy in clinical practice is hydrogen (1H)-MRS. The following neurometabolites can be assessed by MRS: 1) N-acetyl aspartate, a mitochondrial-derived metabolite made in neurons that is a marker of neuronal integrity, neuronal number, and during white matter development

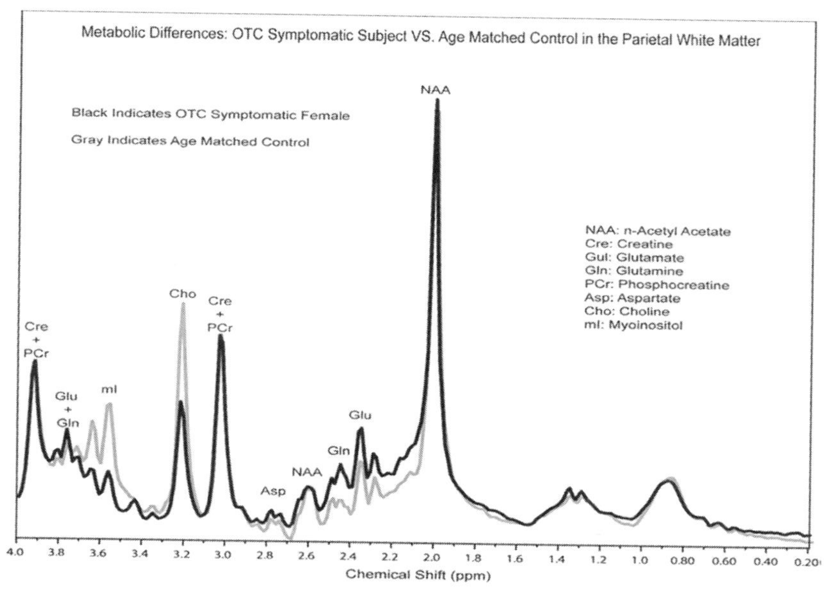

Figure 8.14. 1H-MRS comparing a normal subject (gray) with a subject with OTC deficiency (black). A peak difference can be seen, specifically, higher Gln in OTC deficiency, lower Cho in OTC deficiency, and ml in OTC deficiency. (*Key:* 1H-MRS, hydrogen magnetic resonance spectroscopy; OTC, ornithine transcarbamylase)

is responsible for contributing to myelin lipids; 2) creatine, an energy marker; 3) choline, a cell membrane component; 4) myoinositol, a small sugar that is involved in intracellular signaling, cell volume, and osmoregulation; and 5) lactate, a marker elevated in conditions where energy metabolism is compromised. With special software and more specific acquisition protocols, the neurotransmitters glutamate, glutamine, and GABA can also be measured. Figure 8.14 demonstrates an MRS comparing a normal subject with one of the inborn errors of metabolism, ornithine transcarbamylase.

Single Photon Emission Computer Tomography and Positron Emission Tomography

Like fMRI, single photon emission computer tomography (SPECT) and positron emission tomography (PET) are techniques that demonstrate metabolically active regions in the brain. A radioactive-labeled compound, most commonly glucose, is injected into the bloodstream, and SPECT or PET is then used to assess the compound's selective uptake in various brain regions. Both techniques have been used in the past to diagnose strokes, tumors, and brain injury following head trauma. SPECT and PET have also been employed to evaluate seizure disorders prior to surgery (Kumar & Chugani, 2017). Table 8.2 summarizes the advantages and disadvantages of each of these different imaging techniques. As with CT, there is radiation exposure associated with SPECT and PET scans that must be factored in when weighing the risks and benefits of these diagnostic studies in children.

Electroencephalography

Whereas CT and MRI show the structure of the brain and SPECT, PET, and fMRI show its metabolic activity, there are additional tests that can be useful in assessing the function of the brain. An electroencephalogram (EEG) utilizes scalp electrodes to measure intracranial electrical activity (see Chapter 22). This is a noninvasive test that detects the summation of neuronal discharges in the superficial layers of the cerebral cortex. In epilepsy, an EEG can show a pattern that is indicative of epileptiform ("seizure-like") activity. Coupled with continuous video monitoring, EEG becomes a powerful tool to match seizure type with the location of the seizure focus in the brain. It can detect seizures that may not be evident clinically and can show the effects of various treatments, both medical and surgical, on seizure activity. EEG is also useful in evaluating mental status changes associated with diffuse neurological dysfunction (as might occur in encephalitis or infection of the brain). The background EEG is important because the frequency (Hertz) of the waveforms is a key characteristic used to define normal or abnormal EEG rhythms. In certain situations, EEG waveforms of a certain frequency for age and/or state of alertness may be viewed as abnormal because they demonstrate irregularities in amplitude or rhythmicity. While the EEG is a useful diagnostic tool, a routine EEG is not completely sensitive or specific. A normal EEG does not rule out the possibility that the patient has seizures or epilepsy. Alternatively, an abnormal EEG does not signify that the patient is having seizures or has epilepsy. Repeated EEG studies as well as careful history taking will increase the yield of diagnosing seizures in patients.

Electromyography and Nerve Conduction Studies

Up to this point, the discussion of techniques for evaluating the nervous system has focused on evaluating the CNS. Although there is limited imaging to assess the peripheral nervous system (e.g., MRI to evaluate the brachial plexus), functional testing is readily

Table 8.2. Advantages and disadvantages of each neuroimaging technique

Imaging technique	Advantages	Disadvantages
Computed tomography (CT)	High resolution of bony anatomy; quick and readily available; usually does not require sedation	Lower resolution of brain structures compared to MRI
Magnetic resonance imaging (MRI)	Extremely high resolution of brain structures; images obtained in multiple planes; no radiation exposure	Takes longer to acquire images compared with CT; often requires sedation
Positron emission tomography (PET)/single photon emission computed tomography (SPECT)	Shows brain function in addition to structure by tracking the uptake of radioactive glucose	Limited availability at many centers
Functional MRI (fMRI)	Shows function by detecting variation in regional blood flow; lends better structural resolution than PET/SPECT	Requires significant patient cooperation; not feasible for individuals who are very young or who have severe intellectual disability

available in the form of **electromyography** (EMG) and **nerve conduction studies** (NCS). These studies involve placement of needle electrodes at various points on the body to test motor and sensory function of the peripheral nerves. EMG and NCS can be used to define traumatic injury or peripheral neuropathy. In addition, these studies can be a helpful aid in surgical cases that involve dissection near either sensory or motor pathways.

SUMMARY

- The nervous system is composed of central and peripheral elements.
- The CNS (the brain and spinal cord) is complex in both its structure and function.
- Various techniques allow better assessment of the brain for diagnosis of a broad range of clinical pathology.
- There are multiple modalities to assess structure and function of the central and peripheral nervous system.
- As the field's understanding of both normal and abnormal neurological function improves, better therapeutic avenues will be forthcoming.

ADDITIONAL RESOURCES

Neuropsychological Review: The basics of brain development: https://www.ncbi.nlm.nih.gov/pmc/articles/PMC2989000/

Urban Child Institute: http://www.urbanchildinstitute.org/why-0-3/baby-and-brain

MedlinePlus: Brain malformations: https://medlineplus.gov/brainmalformations.html

Additional resources can be found online in Appendix D: Childhood Disabilities Resources, Services, and Organizations (see About the Online Companion Materials).

REFERENCES

Abid, A. (2016). Brachial plexus birth palsy: Management during the first year of life. *Orthopedics & Traumatology: Surgery & Research, 102,* S125–S132.

Abzug, J. M., Kozin, S.H. (2010). Current concepts: Neonatal brachial plexus palsy. *Orthopedics, 33,* 430–435.

Antonucci, M. C., Zuckerbraun, N. S., Tyler-Kabara, E. C., Furtado, A. D., Murphy, M. E., & Marin, J. R. (2017). The burden of ionizing radiation studies in children with ventricular shunts. *Journal of Pediatrics, 182,* 210–216.

Avramescu-Murphy, M., Hattigen, E., Forster, M. T., Oszvald, A., Anti, S., Frisch, S., . . . Jurcoane, A. (2017). Post-surgical language reorganization occurs in tumors of the dominant and non-dominant hemisphere. *Clinical Neuroradiology, 27,* 299–309.

Barkovich, A. J., & Deon, S. (2016). Hypomyelinating disorders: An MRI approach. *Neurobiology of Disease, 87,* 50–58.

Barnea-Goraly, N., Frazier, T. W., Piacenza, L., Minshew, N. J., Keshavan, M. S., Reiss, A. L., & Hardan, A. Y. (2014). A preliminary longitudinal volumetric MRI study of amygdala and hippocampal volumes in autism. *Progress in Neuro-Psychopharmacology and Biological Psychiatry, 48,* 124–128.

Baumann, O., Borra, R. J., Bower, J. M., Cullen, K. E., Habas, C., Ivry, R. B., . . . Sokolov, A. A. (2015). Consensus paper: The role of the cerebellum in perceptual processes. *Cerebellum, 14,* 197–220.

Benjamin, C. F., Walshaw, P. D., Hale, K., Gaillard, W. D., Baxter, L. C., Berl, M. M., . . . Brookheimer, S. Y. (2017). Presurgical language fMRI: Mapping of six critical regions. *Human Brain Mapping, 38,* 4239–4255.

Berl, M. M., Zimmaro, L. A., Khan, O. I., Dustin, I., Ritzl, E., Duke, E. S., . . . Gaillard, W. D. (2014). Characterization of atypical language activation patterns in focal epilepsy. *Annals of Neurology, 75,* 33–42.

Bos, D. J., Oranje, B., Achterberg, M., Vlaskamp, C., Ambrosino, S., de Reus, M. A., . . . Durston, S. (2017). Structural and functional connectivity in children and adolescents with and without attention deficit/hyperactivity disorder. *The Journal of Child Psychology and Psychiatry, 58,* 810–818.

Brinker, T., Stopa, E., Morrison, J., & Klinge, P. (2014). A new look at cerebrospinal fluid circulation. *Fluid Barriers CNS, 11,* eCollection.

Brossard-Racine, M., & Limperopoulos, C. (2016). Normal cerebellar development by qualitative and quantitative MR imaging: From the fetus to the adolescent. *Neuroimaging Clinics of North America, 26,* 331–339.

Bulas, D. I., Goske, M. J., Applegate, K. E., & Wood, B. P. (2009). Image gently: Why we should talk to parents about CT in children. *American Journal of Roentgenology, 192,* 1176–1178.

Bulteau, C., Grosmaitre, C., Save-Pedebos, J., Leunen, D., Delalande, O., Dorfmuller, G., . . . Jambaque, I. (2015). Language recovery after left hemispherectomy for Rasmussen encephalitis. *Epilepsy & Behavior, 53,* 51–57.

Bulteau, C., Jambaque, I., Chiron, C., Rodrigo, S., Dorfmuller, G., Dulac, O., . . . Noulhiane, M. (2017). Language plasticity after hemispherectomy of the dominant hemisphere in 3 patients: Implications of non-linguistic networks. *Epilepsy & Behavior, 69,* 86–94.

Burgess, P. W., & Stuss, D. T. (2017). Fifty years of prefrontal cortex research: Impact on assessment. *Journal of the International Neuropsychological Society, 23,* 755–767.

Chatzikonstantinou, A. (2014). Epilepsy and the hippocampus. *Frontiers of Neurology and Neuroscience, 34,* 121–142.

Cheron, G., Marquez-Ruiz, J., & Dan, B. (2016). Oscillations, timing, plasticity, and learning in the cerebellum. *Cerebellum, 15,* 122–138.

Craig, A. D. (2009). How do you feel — now? The anterior insula and human awareness. *Nature Reviews Neuroscience, 10,* 59–70.

Crossman, A. R., & Neary, D. (2015). *Neuroanatomy: An illustrated colour text* (5th ed.). Philadelphia, PA: Churchill Livingstone.

Cubillo, A., Halari, R., Ecker, C., Giampietro, V., Taylor, E., & Rubia, K. (2010). Reduced activation and inter-regional functional connectivity of fronto-striatal networks in adults with childhood attention-deficit/hyperactivity disorder (ADHD) and persisting symptoms during tasks of motor inhibition and cognitive switching. *Journal of Psychiatric Research, 44*(10), 629–639.

Damiano, C., Churches, O., Ring, H., & Baron-Cohen, S. (2011). The development of perceptual expertise for faces and objects in autism spectrum conditions. *Autism Research, 4*(4), 297–301.

Dziobek, I., Bahnemann, M., Convit, A., & Heekeren, H. R. (2010). The role of the fusiform–amygdala system in the pathophysiology of autism. *Archives of General Psychiatry, 67*(4), 397–405.

Engstrom, M., Karlsson, T., Landtblom, A. M., & Craig, A. D. (2015) Evidence of conjoint activation of the anterior insular and cingulate cortices during effortful tasks. *Frontiers in Human Neuroscience, 8*, 1071.

Freeman, J. H. (2014). The ontogeny of associative cerebellar learning. *International Review of Neurobiology, 117*, 53–72.

Freeman, M. D., Goodyear, S. M., & Leith, W. M. (2017). A multistate population-based analysis of linked maternal and neonatal discharge records to identify risk factors for neonatal brachial plexus injury. *International Journal of Gynecology & Obstetrics, 136*, 331–336.

Gaillard, W. D., Berl, M. M., Duke, E. S., Ritzl, E., Miranda, S., Liew, C., . . . Theodore, W. H. (2011). fMRI language dominance and FDG–PET hypometabolism. *Neurology, 76*(15), 1322–1329.

Gaillard, W. D., & Berl, M. M. (2012). Chapter 24–Functional magnetic resonance imaging: Functional mapping. *Handbook of Clinical Neurology, 107*, 387–398.

Graham, D., Tisdall, M. M., & Gill, D. (2016). Corpus callosotomy outcomes in pediatric patients: A systemic review. *Epilepsia, 57*, 1053–1068.

Gropman, A. (2010). Brain imaging in urea cycle disorders. *Molecular Genetics and Metabolism, 100*, S20–S30.

Han, K., Chapman, S. B., & Krawczyk, D. C. (2015). Altered amygdala connectivity in individuals with chronic traumatic brain injury and comorbid depressive symptoms. *Frontiers in Neurology, 6*, eCollection.

Hasnat, M. J., & Rice, J. E. (2015). Intrathecal baclofen for treating spasticity in children with cerebral palsy. *Cochrane Database of Systematic Reviews, 11*, CD004552.

He, Y., Brunstrom-Hernandez, J. E., Thio, L. L., Lackey, S., Gaebler-Spira, D., Kuroda, M. M., . . . Jusko, W. J. (2014). Population pharmacokinetics of oral baclofen in pediatric patients with cerebral palsy. *The Journal of Pediatrics, 164*, 1181–1188.

Hoche, F., Guell, X., Vangel, M. G., Sherman, J. C., & Schmahmann, J. D. (2017). The cerebellar cognitive affective/Schmahmann syndrome scale. *Brain, 141*, 248–270.

Huttenlocher, P. R. (1991). Dendritic and synaptic pathology in mental retardation. *Pediatric Neurology, 7*, 79–85.

Insausti, R., Cebada-Sánchez, S., & Marcos, P. (2010). Postnatal development of the human hippocampal formation. *Advances in Anatomy, Embryology, and Cell Biology, 206*, 1–86.

Ivanova, A., Zaidel, E., Salamon, N., Bookheimer, S., Uddin, L. Q., & de Bode, S. (2017). Intrinsic functional organization of putative language networks in the brain following hemispherectomy. *Brain Structure and Function, 222*, 3795–3805.

Johnston, M. V. (2009). Plasticity in the developing brain: Implications for rehabilitation. *Developmental Disabilities Research Review, 15*(2), 94–101.

Kleinhans, N. M., Richards, T., Weaver, K., Johnson, L. C., Greenson, J., Dawson, G., & Aylward, E. (2010). Association between amygdala response to emotional faces and social anxiety in autism spectrum disorders. *Neuropsychologia, 48*(12), 3665–3670.

Korol, D. L., Gold, P. E., & Scavuzzo, C. J. (2013). Use it and boost it with physical and mental activity. *Hippocampus, 23*, 1125–1135.

Koziol, L. F., Budding, D., Andreasen, N., D'Arrigo, S., Bulgheroni, S., Imamizu, H., . . . Yamazaki, T. (2014). Consensus paper: The cerebellum's role in movement in cognition. *Cerebellum, 13*, 151–177.

Krafnick, A. J., Flowers, D. L., Luetje, M. M., Napoliello, E. M., & Eden, G. F. (2014). An investigation into the origin of anatomical differences in dyslexia. *Journal of Neuroscience, 34*(3), 901–908. doi:10.1523/JNEUROSCI.2092-13.2013. PMID:24431448

Kumar, A., & Chugani, H. T. (2017). The role of radionuclide imaging in epilepsy, Part 1: Sporadic temporal and extratemporal lobe epilepsy. *Journal of Nuclear Medicine Technology, 45*, 14–21.

Lam, S., Harris, D., Rocque, B. G., & Ham, S. A. (2014). Pediatric endoscopic third ventriculostomy: A population-based study. *Journal Neurosurgery: Pediatrics, 14*, 455–464.

Lui, J. H., Hansen, D. V., & Kriegstein, A. R. (2011). Development and evolution of the human neocortex. *Cell, 146*, 18–36.

Malmgren, K., Rydenhag, B., & Hallbook, T. (2015). Reappraisal of corpus callosotomy. *Current Opinion in Neurology, 28*, 175–181.

Mesulam, M. M., Rogalski, E. J., Wieneke, C., Hurley, R. S., Geula, C., Bigio, E. H., . . . Weintraub, S. (2014). Primary progressive aphasia and the evolving neurology of the language network. *Nature Reviews Neurology, 10*, 554–569.

Mishra, A., Reynolds, J. P., Chen, Y., Gourine, A. V., Rusakov, D. A., & Attwell, D. (2016). Astrocytes mediate neurovascular signaling to capillary pericytes but not to arterioles. *Nature Neuroscience, 19*, 1619–1627.

Monbaliu, E., Himmelmann, K., Lin, J. P., Ortibus, E., Bonouvrie, L., Feys, H., . . . Dan, B. (2017). Clinical presentation and management of dyskinetic cerebral palsy. *Lancet Neurology, 16*, 741–749.

Nair, A., Carper, R. A., Abbott, A. E., Chen, C. P., Solders, S., Nakutin, S. . . . Muller, R. A. (2015). Regional specificity of aberrant thalamocortical connectivity in autism. *Human Brain Mapping, 36*, 4497–4511.

Nguyen, V. T., Sonkusare, S., Stadler, J., Hu, X., Breakspear, M., & Guo, C. C. (2017). Distinct cerebellar contributions to cognitive-perceptual dynamics during natural viewing. *Cerebral Cortex, 27*, 5652–5662.

Nowrangi, M. A., Lyketsos, C., Rao, V., & Munro, C. A. (2014). Systematic review of neuroimaging correlates of executive functioning: Converging evidence from different clinical populations. *The Journal of Neuropsychiatry and Clinical Neurosciences, 26*, 114–125.

Palmer, E. E., & Mowat, D. (2014). Agenesis of the corpus callosum: A clinical approach to diagnosis. *American Journal of Medical Genetics Part C (Seminars in Medical Genetics), 166C*, 184–197.

Pearce, M. S., Salotti, J. A., Little, M. P., McHugh, K., Lee, C., Kim, K. P., . . . Berrington de Gonzalez, A. (2012). Radiation exposure from CT scans in childhood and subsequent risk of leukaemia and brain tumors: A retrospective cohort study. *Lancet, 380*, 499–505.

Ravindra, V. M., Sweney, M. T., & Bollo, R. J. (2017). Recent developments in the surgical management of paediatric epilepsy. *Archives of Disease in Childhood, 102*, 760–766.

Rincon, S. P., Blitstein, M. B., Caruso, P. A., Gonzalez, R. G., Thibert, R. L., & Ratai, E. M. (2016). The use of magnetic resonance spectroscopy in the evaluation of pediatric patients with seizures. *Pediatric Neurology, 58*, 57–66.

Robertson, F. C., Abd-El-Barr, M. M., Mukundan, S., & Gormley, W. B. (2017). Ventriculostomy-associated hemorrhage: A risk assessment by radiographic simulation. *Journal of Neurosurgery, 127*, 532–536.

Rubia, K., Halari, R., Cubillo, A., Smith, A. B., Mohammad, A. M., Brammer, M., & Taylor, E. (2011). Methylphenidate normalizes fronto-striatal underactivation during interference inhibition in medication-naïve boys with attention-deficit/hyperactivity disorder. *Neuropsychopharmacology, 36*, 1575–1586.

Shababi, M., Lorson, C. L., & Rudnik-Schoneborn, S. S. (2014). Spinal muscular atrophy: A motor neuron disorder or multi-organ disease? *Journal of Anatomy, 224*, 15–28.

Schulz, K. P., Li, X., Clerkin, S. M., Fan, J., Berwid, O. G., Newcorn, J. H., & Halperin, J. M. (2017). Prefrontal and parietal correlates of cognitive control related to the adult outcome of attention-deficit/hyperactivity disorder diagnosed in childhood. *Cortex, 90*, 1–11.

Snaidero, N., & Simons, M. (2014). Myelination at a glance. *Journal of Cell Science, 127*, 2999–3004.

Steinberg, M. E., Ratner, N. B., Gaillard, W., & Berl, M. (2013). Fluency patterns in narratives from children with localization related epilepsy. *Journal of Fluency Disorders, 38*, 193–205.

Stojkovic, T. (2016). Hereditary neuropathies: An update. *Revue Neurologique, 172*, 775–778.

Tamariz, E., & Varela-Echavarria, A. (2015). The discovery of the growth cone and its influence on the study of axon guidance. *Frontiers in Neuroanatomy, 9*, eCollection.

CHAPTER 9

Muscles, Bones, and Nerves

Peter B. Kang

Upon completion of this chapter, the reader will

- Describe how the neuromuscular and musculoskeletal systems function and are integrated
- Recognize the common signs and symptoms of neuromuscular and musculoskeletal disorders
- Learn the utility, appropriate use, and interpretation of standard diagnostic tests for neuromuscular and musculoskeletal disorders
- Identify the most common neuromuscular and musculoskeletal diseases of childhood and their treatments, including recently developed molecular therapies

Together, the neuromuscular and musculoskeletal systems are responsible for the ability to sit, stand, and move; impairments of these systems are major causes of developmental disability in childhood. This chapter provides a general overview of key anatomical structures, identifies the signs and symptoms of neuromuscular and musculoskeletal disorders, describes common disorders of the neuromuscular and musculoskeletal systems, and reviews evaluation and management methods and principles. Importantly, it explains how an integrated health care and school system can improve the lives of children affected by such disorders.

CASE STUDY

Praya is a 4-month-old female infant brought to the pediatrician's office for evaluation and treatment for concerns of floppiness and poor weight gain. She was born full term after an uncomplicated gestation, but her parents report that she feeds poorly and that milk sometimes pools in her mouth. During the examination, she has a weak cry and has trouble lifting her head from the exam table. Her muscle tone seems diminished when she is picked up, both in vertical and prone positions. She has limited antigravity movements of her arms and legs.

Thought Questions:

What should be the overall assessment of this case? Does this infant appear to have a central nervous system or peripheral nervous system disease, and—if so—what features of the clinical presentation would help with the diagnostic evaluation?

OVERVIEW OF THE NEUROMUSCULAR AND MUSCULOSKELETAL SYSTEMS

The neuromuscular system is the neurological network that connects the brain and spinal cord to the musculoskeletal system. Its major components are 1) the **anterior horn cells** (lower motor neurons) in the spinal cord, 2) the peripheral nerves in the extremities, 3) the neuromuscular junction, which joins the nerves and muscles, and 4) the skeletal muscles (Figure 9.1). The musculoskeletal system consists of the skeletal muscles, tendons, bones, joints, and ligaments.

In order for a muscle to produce voluntary movement across a joint, an electrical signal originates in the cortex of the brain (within an upper motor neuron) and then passes through the spinal cord to an anterior horn cell; there, an axon extends down a peripheral nerve until it ends at a neuromuscular junction (Figure 9.1). The electrical impulse triggers the release of the neurotransmitter acetylcholine, which jumps across the synapse, or gap, at this junction. The acetylcholine binds

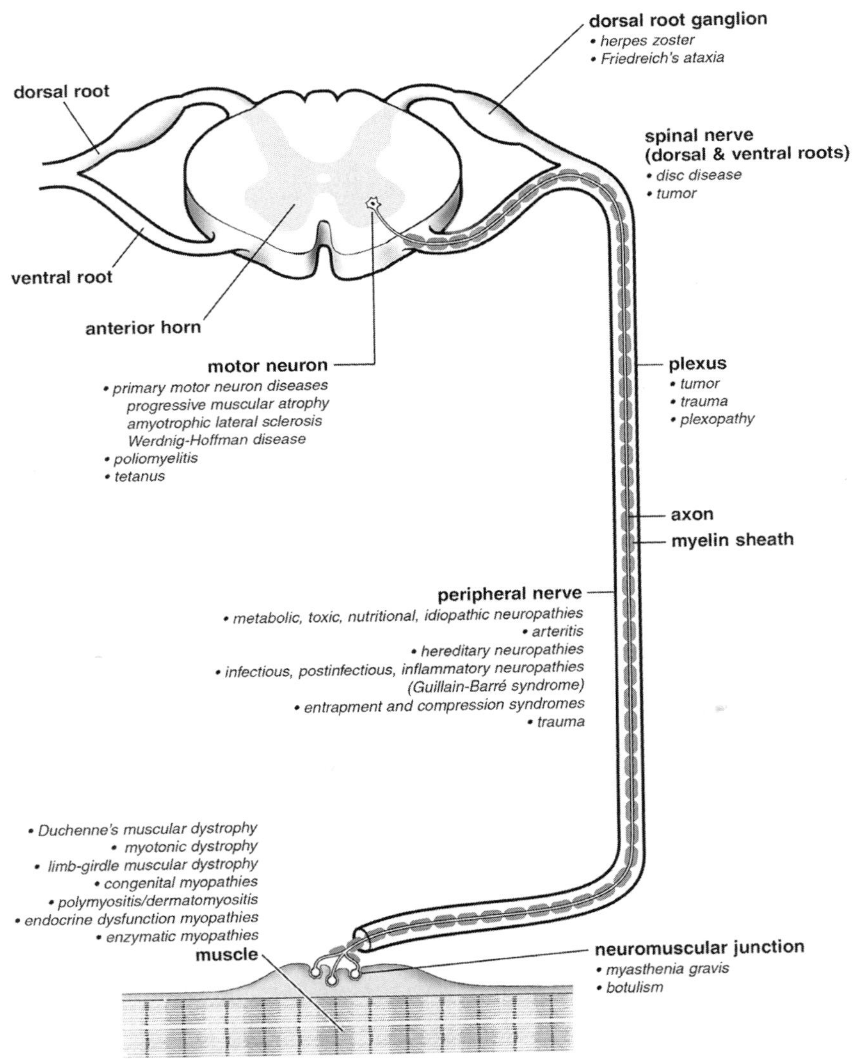

Figure 9.1. The neuromuscular system. The central components of the nervous system include the brain and spinal cord. Descending corticospinal pathways carry signals from the brain through the spinal cord to motor neurons in the anterior horns of the spinal cord. The motor neurons are generally regarded as being the first segment of the peripheral nervous system. Signals are transmitted from the motor neurons down the peripheral nerves, then across the neuromuscular junction to skeletal muscle. These signals initiate muscle contraction, leading to movement of the musculoskeletal system. Sensory signals are transmitted from the sensory nerves to the spinal cord, and then to the brain, which continuously integrates this information to monitor the state of the environment and the neuromuscular and musculoskeletal systems.

to receptors in the muscle fiber; and these receptors generate a new electrical signal that propagates through the muscle fiber and stimulates muscle contraction.

The **sarcomere** is the basic contractile unit in the muscle fiber; it is composed of a number of proteins that bind to each other in a dynamic manner. To help organize, modulate, and coordinate motor activities, signals are sent to the brain through the sensory system, providing information about the body's position in space.

The main function of skeletal muscle is to contract by shortening, thereby moving limbs, with joints used as fulcrums. **Agonist** muscles reinforce each other's movements, while **antagonist** muscles oppose one another. For example, when you flex your arm at the elbow, the biceps contracts, as does the brachialis; the triceps, however, relax. If all these muscles contracted simultaneously, your arm would be held stiffly in an **isometric contraction** (i.e., muscular contraction against resistance in which the length of the muscle remains the same). Therefore, to move your arm, the brain sends signals that generate contraction of some muscles and relaxation of others in that arm.

The bones of the skeleton form the body's internal scaffolding. They range in size from the auditory ossicles (inner ear bones) that measure less than a half inch each at the long axis to the femur (thigh bone), which is roughly 18 inches long in adults. As growth takes place and the bone is subject to different forces, the bone responds by changing its shape, a process referred to as remodeling. These changes usually increase the tensile strength and stability of the bone, making it less susceptible to fracture. On average, a given portion of a child's bone turns over approximately once a year. In an adult, the reshaping continues even though growth has stopped. The average bone segment of an adult turns over approximately every 7 years.

SYMPTOMS AND SIGNS OF NEUROMUSCULAR AND MUSCULOSKELETAL DISORDERS

Neuromuscular and musculoskeletal disorders classically present with motor impairments as cardinal symptoms, with weakness and other findings such as gait abnormalities identified on examination. It is important to note that in some cases, respiratory, cardiac, and sensory symptoms may be initial or dominant components of the clinical presentation. Spine abnormalities such as scoliosis, kyphosis, and lordosis, along with contractures, may in some cases be **idiopathic** (cause unknown), especially scoliosis, but in other cases they may provide a diagnostic clue to the presence of these disorders.

Respiratory and Cardiac Issues

In most cases, respiratory and cardiac issues do not arise from neuromuscular or musculoskeletal disorders. However, they constitute frequent complications of these disorders, especially respiratory issues. In addition, in rare instances, they may constitute early manifestations of such conditions. Examples include late-onset **Pompe disease** (a genetic lysosomal storage disorder), in which respiratory distress may be an early symptom, and Becker muscular dystrophy, in which cardiomyopathy is sometimes the first sign of disease. Some neuromuscular disorders affect the respiratory muscles, resulting in an abnormal sleep pattern or **sleep apnea** (brief periods of respiratory arrest). These children may suffer from daytime somnolence and often appear fatigued or easily distractible at school.

Muscle Bulk, Tone, and Strength

Pseudohypertrophy (apparent muscle enlargement due to overgrowth of connective tissue), especially of the calves and in conjunction with weakness, may be a sign of **Duchenne muscular dystrophy (DMD)** and Becker muscular dystrophy; less frequently it accompanies other muscular dystrophies. In contrast, muscle atrophy is found in neuropathies such as **Charcot-Marie-Tooth disease (CMT)** but may also be seen in some myopathies and muscular dystrophies.

It is important to differentiate between tone abnormalities and strength abnormalities. Tone is the muscle's passive ability to respond to stretch, whereas strength represents the force that the muscle exerts actively. Children can have **hypertonia** (high tone and an overreactive response to a normal stimulus) or **hypotonia** (low tone, with a lesser response to a stimulus). Many neuromuscular or musculoskeletal disorders are linked to disturbances in tone. Hypertonia and spasticity are seen primarily in central nervous system (CNS) disorders that affect the upper motor neuron or its axons in the brain and spine, whereas hypotonia can be seen not only in lesions of the CNS (upper motor neuron), but also in peripheral nervous system (lower motor neuron) involvement. In infants, preserved strength in the setting of hypotonia is usually associated with a central nervous system process, whereas weakness in conjunction with hypotonia is usually associated with a peripheral nervous system process.

Muscle weakness can be **proximal** (involving muscles or body segments closer to the center of the body) or **distal** (involving muscles or body segments farther from the center of the body). Proximal muscle weakness affects the shoulder and hip girdle muscles (often seen in **myopathies,** which are primary disorders of muscle). Children with weak shoulder and hip girdle muscles have difficulty rising from a floor or chair, reaching objects on a high shelf, climbing jungle gyms, and/or doing push-ups. Testing the ability of the child to grasp and manipulate objects demonstrates selective control, a skill necessary to operate hand controls. Children with distal muscle weakness may thus have trouble holding a pen or pencil, finishing long writing activities on time, and/or using scissors. Proximal or distal lower extremity weakness often causes gait abnormalities (see the following sections).

Sensation

Sensory symptoms such as numbness, **paresthesias** (abnormal skin sensations, such as burning, prickling, itching, and tingling) and pain may result from disorders of the peripheral sensory nerves (e.g., peripheral neuropathies) or from CNS disorders. Sensory nerve fibers tell the brain where the body is in space, so affected children may have a clumsy gait or feel unsteady in the dark, requiring visual input for balance.

Scoliosis, Kyphosis, and Lordosis

Scoliosis is a **lateral** (sideways) curvature of the spinal column, **kyphosis** is an excessive **anterior** (forward) curvature of the spine, and **lordosis** is an excessive **posterior** (backward) curvature. Isolated scoliosis in an otherwise healthy child or adolescent is usually not associated with a neuromuscular or musculoskeletal condition. Idiopathic scoliosis occurs frequently during the adolescent growth spurt, especially in young women. However, scoliosis, kyphosis, lordosis, or a combination of these may be complications of numerous neuromuscular and musculoskeletal disorders. The appearance of these vertebral abnormalities in a younger child or of one of them in conjunction with other concerning findings should prompt careful evaluation.

Because spinal curves are best managed before they become severe, the spine of a child at greater risk (e.g., a child with meningomyelocele or muscular dystrophy) should be examined regularly. Early clues suggesting scoliosis are unequal heights of the shoulders or a slanting of the waist. Also, as the ribs attach to the thoracic (chest level) spine, they may follow the curve of the vertebrae, causing a rib rise or "rib hump" when the child bends forward. School screening examinations for scoliosis are designed to look for these physical findings in order to detect scoliosis as early as possible.

Contractures and Gait Abnormalities

When a neuromuscular or musculoskeletal disorder prevents full range of motion around a joint for a prolonged period of time, a joint **contracture** (shortening of the tendons around a joint) can develop, resulting in a fixed loss of joint motion. In an ankle joint contracture, the Achilles tendon shortens and the child walks on his or her toes. Toe-walking, limping, walking with a wide-based gait, and other gait abnormalities should prompt a medical evaluation.

In an ambulatory child, observing the gait pattern is a valuable part of the physical examination. During normal gait, the head and trunk should be level, with minimal sway from side to side. The child should be able to maintain balance while standing on one leg and swinging the opposite leg through. The leg that is swinging should clear the ground, and the foot should not drag.

Strong pelvic muscles are needed for a child to rise from a seated position and to climb stairs. Children with hip girdle weakness often need to pull on a handrail to walk up steps or to push off with their hands in order to rise from a chair. To get up from the floor, such children often use a Gowers maneuver: First, they turn to face the floor; then they use their hands on the floor to support part of their weight as they straighten their knees; and, finally, they push their hands on their thighs to achieve an erect posture.

Distal muscle weakness (often seen in neuropathies) affects the hands and feet; children may trip and fall frequently because they cannot lift their feet or toes when walking. They also may not be able to walk on their heels and may "slap" their feet while walking (a condition called *foot drop*). Orthotic devices may stabilize distal leg weakness and lessen the frequency and severity of falls.

Joint Abnormalities

Joint abnormalities can be identified with range-of-motion testing. Range of motion is a passive assessment, meaning the patient should be relaxed while the examiner moves the extremities. The upper extremities should be examined for range of motion of the shoulders, elbows, and hands. The examiner should be able to lift the child's arms above the head. The elbows should straighten fully, often even a few degrees beyond full extension (known as hyperextension). All fingers should be able to be straightened and brought out of the palm.

The hip exam, like the spine exam, should be performed often, as early treatment of hip problems leads to the best outcomes. The examiner should be able to

abduct (spread apart) the hips easily and symmetrically. Loss of hip abduction may indicate a hip dislocation or **subluxation** (partial dislocation). Another means of assessing whether the hip is dislocated is to look for discrepancies in knee heights with the hips and knees flexed and the ankles together, while the patient is **supine** (lying on their back).

The knee must be straight for standing, but it must flex to 90 degrees for comfortable sitting and flex even farther for easy stair climbing. Contractures of the hamstrings can limit knee movement and impair the ability to stand.

The ankle should be examined for **plantarflexion** (downward motion of the foot) and **dorsiflexion** (upward movement of the foot). The ability to dorsiflex beyond a neutral position is important for both walking and sitting and should be tested with the knee both extended and flexed. A child should be able to maintain the feet in a **plantargrade** (flat on the floor) position while walking and maintain as much flexibility in the feet as possible. Heel cord contractures, which may lead to balance problems and toe-walking, are commonly seen in a range of neuromuscular disorders, including muscular dystrophies.

LABORATORY TESTING AND RADIOGRAPHY

There is an ever-expanding array of diagnostic options available for neuromuscular and musculoskeletal disorders, most prominently genetic testing and advanced imaging modalities such as ultrasound and extremity MRI studies. However, it is important to remember the ongoing importance of more traditional test modalities, such as basic serum muscle enzyme measurements, electrophysiology, and muscle and nerve biopsies.

Serum Testing

Measurements of muscle enzyme levels in **serum** (the protein-rich liquid that separates out when blood coagulates) are useful as initial screening laboratory tests in the evaluation of potential neuromuscular disorders, especially due to their low costs. The most well-known of these is the creatine phosphokinase (CPK), also known as the creatine kinase level. Aldolase is also useful as an adjunctive muscle enzyme marker. Significant elevations in muscle enzyme levels suggest the presence of a muscle disease. Mild to moderate elevations may be difficult to interpret, as they may be normal variants, signs of muscle disease, or sometimes signs of a neurogenic disease such as spinal muscular atrophy.

Genetic Testing

Genetic testing for mutations (see Chapter 1) has been a boon to diagnosing inherited diseases, including neuromuscular and musculoskeletal disorders, and it can spare an increasing number of patients from invasive and painful diagnostic procedures such as electromyography and biopsies. However, genetic test results are not always definitive and must be interpreted with care. Close coordination with a geneticist or another physician who is experienced in diagnosing and treating the disease in question will increase the likelihood of accurate application to clinical practice. Thus, traditional diagnostic tests for neuromuscular disease remain relevant and useful for many of these patients for the foreseeable future.

Electrophysiology

Nerve conduction studies and **electromyography** (EMG), a recording of electric potentials found in muscle fibers, are useful in diagnosing a variety of neuromuscular disorders, including anterior horn cell disease, neuropathies, neuromuscular junction disorders, and some myopathies. Advances in genetic testing and immunohistochemistry of biopsy specimens have changed referral patterns for pediatric patients with suspected neuromuscular disorders (Karakis, Liew, Darras, Jones, & Kang, 2014). In particular, Duchenne and Becker muscular dystrophies are now primarily diagnosed with genetic testing and these patients are rarely referred to the EMG laboratory. Spinal muscular atrophy is usually diagnosed with genetic testing as well, although in cases in which the diagnosis must be confirmed rapidly, EMG is still important prior to genetic confirmation. EMG continues to play an important role in the initial evaluation of Charcot-Marie-Tooth disease, as many children present with subtle signs that raise the possibility of this diagnosis but end up not having a neuropathy (Karakis, Gregas, Darras, Kang, & Jones, 2013). EMG is technically demanding and should be performed only by an electromyographer experienced in performing these studies in children. This is important both for diagnostic accuracy and for the comfort of the child, as the procedure involves electrical stimulations during the nerve conduction studies, followed by needle examination of the muscle. EMG remains useful for a range of diagnostic neuromuscular questions in children (Karakis et al., 2014).

Biopsy

Muscle, nerve, and skin biopsies have traditionally been essential to the diagnosis of many neuromuscular and musculoskeletal disorders. Genetic testing, however, has changed the profile of patients who are referred for these tests; patients with Duchenne and Becker muscular dystrophies rarely need muscle biopsies, as they can usually be diagnosed by identification of mutations from blood samples. Genetic testing has also begun to supplant muscle biopsy in suspected cases of limb-girdle muscular dystrophy, although a higher proportion of these patients will need biopsies at some point during their evaluations. When biopsies are needed, advances in genetics and biochemistry have enhanced the sophistication of their interpretation, as immunohistochemistry of biopsy sections can detect protein deficiencies that may indicate a specific genetic defect.

Radiography

Abnormal musculoskeletal exam findings can be illuminated by plain x-rays of the involved areas, which can help detect movement limitations caused by bony deformity. X-rays are helpful in detecting the shapes of bones but are a poor gauge of the quality of bone because bone loss will not be apparent until at least one third of the bone is gone. Bone density is best measured by a bone density scan.

Ultrasonography and magnetic resonance imaging (MRI) have only recently been applied to the evaluation of possible muscle disorders, but certain myopathies show distinct patterns of muscle involvement that may be detected by such methods (Wattjes, Kley, & Fischer, 2010). These tests have the potential to spare some children from undergoing invasive diagnostic procedures such as muscle biopsy, or to assist in the selection of a muscle for biopsy that may have an optimal diagnostic yield.

DISORDERS OF THE NEUROMUSCULAR SYSTEM

Within the traditional anatomical categories of neuromuscular disorders (anterior horn cell disease, neuropathy, disorders of the neuromuscular junction, and muscle disease), knowledge of various genetic and immune etiologies has expanded knowledge to a remarkable degree in the past several decades.

Anterior Horn Cells: Spinal Muscular Atrophy

The nerve cells (neurons) in the spinal column that control movement are called anterior horn cells. In the past, the most well-known disease associated with damage to the anterior horn cell was paralytic poliomyelitis. Thanks to the polio vaccine, this viral illness is no longer endemic in the United States. Currently, the most common disorder affecting the anterior horn cell in children is **spinal muscular atrophy** (SMA; Darras & Kang, 2007).

SMA is characterized by degeneration of alpha-motor neurons in the brainstem and spinal cord. There is a subsequent involvement of motor nerves, leading to progressive weakness that is nearly always predominantly proximal and symmetrical, with diffuse weakness in more severe cases and at later stages of disease. Intelligence is preserved (von Gontard et al., 2002). Most cases are associated with homozygous deletions in the *SMN1* gene, making this an autosomal recessive disorder (Lefebvre et al., 1995; Melki et al., 1994). SMA was historically the most common inherited cause of death in infancy, with an estimated incidence of 10 to 16.7 per 100,000 live births (Merlini, Stagni, Marri, & Granata, 1992; Pearn, 1973; Pearn, 1978); these estimates have more recently been adjusted to 8.5 to 10.3 per 100,000 live births (Arkblad, Tulinius, Kroksmark, Henricsson, & Darin, 2009; Jedrzejowska et al., 2010; Lally et al., 2017; Prior et al., 2010; Sugarman et al., 2012). SMA has traditionally been divided into three clinical variants based primarily on the milestones attained: SMA I, SMA II, and SMA III.

SMA I Children with SMA I (previously known as Werdnig-Hoffman disease) have onset typically before 6 months of age and are never able to sit or walk. Infants with SMA I develop diffuse hypotonia and weakness with **areflexia** (lack of deep tendon reflexes). Swallowing and breathing difficulties are serious, life-threatening complications that may occur at any time. Without interventions, affected children rarely survive beyond 2 years of age and often die much earlier. This prognosis, however, has changed dramatically with recent therapeutic developments. Placement of gastrostomy feeding tubes and respiratory interventions, including both noninvasive and invasive options, can extend these children's life expectancies, sometimes for years. If a gastrostomy tube is to be placed, it should be done as early as possible. Lung interventions may include pulmonary hygiene (used to clear mucus and secretions from the airways), noninvasive pressure support ventilation (delivery of mechanical ventilation without the need for artificial airway), and tracheostomy with full mechanical ventilation. Families and physicians should decide collaboratively on a treatment plan based on their ethical judgment about the quality of life they feel is best.

SMA II In SMA II, patients sit at some point during childhood, but never walk. Onset is usually between 6 and 18 months. Infants and toddlers with SMA II typically present with hypotonia, areflexia, and delayed motor milestones. They are also susceptible to difficulties swallowing and breathing, but these complications tend to occur later and progress more slowly than in SMA I. Nutritional and respiratory therapies are similar to those used in SMA I. Scoliosis is a frequent and disabling complication in these children, for which spine surgery is often helpful. Depending on the severity of the individual case and the level of intervention, life expectancy has traditionally ranged from late childhood through early adulthood. More recent advances in ventilatory approaches to these patients, and novel molecular therapies have dramatically improved this prognosis.

SMA III Patients with SMA III are able to sit and walk, and they usually have onset of motor difficulties after 18 months of age but before adulthood. Children with SMA III often present with gait difficulties, proximal weakness, and areflexia, sometimes severe enough to cause delayed motor milestones. The weakness is almost always symmetrical, though some exceptions have been described (Kang, Krishnamoorthy, Jones, Shapiro, & Darras, 2006). Hypotonia, while present, is not as prominent a feature. Difficulties swallowing and breathing are rare, and life expectancy is usually not affected.

Therapy Until recently, therapy for SMA was primarily supportive. However, a novel antisense oligonucleotide drug (nusinersen) has been developed that has shown efficacy and safety in symptomatic infants with SMA I and II and was approved by the U.S. Food and Drug Administration (FDA) in 2016 (Finkel et al., 2016; Finkel et al., 2017; Mercuri et al., 2018a) (see Box 9.1). The therapy must be administered **intrathecally** (into the spinal canal) and at this time requires ongoing dosing indefinitely. Further studies are ongoing regarding the use of gene therapy approaches as well (Mendell et al., 2017).

Disorders of the Peripheral Nerves: Charcot-Marie-Tooth Disease (CMT)

Neuropathy and *peripheral neuropathy* are general terms that imply that some damage has occurred to the nerve. Neuropathies can be motor, sensory, or sensorimotor (a combination of the two). The term *mononeuropathy* implies that only a single nerve is damaged, whereas *polyneuropathy* refers to a generalized process that affects all or most nerves, albeit with varying degrees of severity. The acute autoimmune neuropathy, Guillain-Barré syndrome, usually does not lead to significant prolonged disability, with the exception of some cases that involve prominent axonal loss; it will not be discussed in detail here.

BOX 9.1 EVIDENCE-BASED PRACTICE

Effect of Treatment with Nusinersen on Outcome in Spinal Muscular Atrophy

Spinal muscular atrophy is an autosomal recessive neuromuscular disorder that is caused by an insufficient level of survival motor neuron (SMN) protein. Nusinersen is an antisense oligonucleotide drug that modifies pre–messenger RNA splicing of the *SMN2* gene and thus promotes increased production of full-length SMN protein, correcting the defect. The authors conducted a randomized, double-blind, sham-controlled, phase 3 efficacy and safety trial of nusinersen in infants with spinal muscular atrophy (SMA I and II). The primary treatment goals were improved motor-milestones and prolonged survival of this usually rapidly fatal disease. In the study a significantly higher percentage of infants in the nusinersen group than in the control group had improved motor milestones (37 of 73 infants [51%] vs. 0 of 37 [0%]). Furthermore, the likelihood of survival was higher in the nusinersen group than in the control (untreated) group. Infants identified and treated earlier were more likely than those with a longer duration disease to benefit from nusinersen. In summary, among infants with spinal muscular atrophy, those who received nusinersen were more likely to be alive and have improvements in motor function than those in the control group. Early treatment may be necessary to maximize the benefit of the drug.

From Finkel, R. S., Mercuri, E., Darras, B. T., Connolly, A. M., Kuntz, N. L., Kirschner, J., . . . Endear Study Group. (2017). Nusinersen versus sham control in infantile-onset spinal muscular atrophy. *New England Journal of Medicine, 377*(18), 1723–1732; reprinted by permission.

CMT disease is the most common inherited polyneuropathy; in an epidemiologic study from Norway it was found to affect 1 in 1,214 individuals (Braathen, 2012). An alternative term for this disorder, *hereditary motor and sensory neuropathy,* is also used. CMT is classified based on the inheritance pattern (autosomal dominant or recessive) and physiology (demyelinating or axonal). *Demyelination* refers to a disease process in which the myelin insulation surrounding nerve axons is stripped off, whereas axonal loss refers to a process in which the axons themselves degenerate.

The major categories of polyneuropathies are CMT1 (dominant, demyelinating), CMT2 (dominant, axonal), CMTX (X-linked, axonal and/or demyelinating), and CMT4 (recessive, axonal and/or demyelinating). Déjerine-Sottas disease was previously known as CMT3 and is a rare, early-onset form of CMT that may be associated with more significant long-term motor disabilities than the classic phenotype of CMT. There is genetic and phenotypic overlap with congenital hypomyelinating neuropathy. The most common form of CMT is CMT1A, which is caused by a duplication in the *PMP22* gene (Lupski et al., 1991). Hereditary neuropathy with liability to pressure palsies (HNPP) is a related disorder in which patients are susceptible to compression neuropathies after minor trauma. HNPP is typically caused by a deletion of the *PMP22* gene rather than a duplication.

Onset of CMT depends on the specific type and may occur at birth or not until adulthood, but many cases are diagnosed in the first 2 decades of life. Patients with CMT typically present with weakness and wasting of the foot and lower leg muscles, which may result in foot drop and a high-steppage gait with frequent tripping and falling. Foot deformities, such as **pes cavus** (high arches) and hammertoes (a condition in which the ends of the toes curl downward), result from weakness of the intrinsic foot muscles (Laura et al., 2018). Some children can present with **pes planus** (flat feet) and need arch supports. The degeneration of myelin, axons, or both results in muscle weakness and atrophy in the extremities, and the degeneration of sensory nerves results in a reduced ability to feel heat, cold, and pain. Because of the muscle weakness, contractures develop over time, especially at the heel cords, and sometimes curvature of the spine occurs (Shy, 2004).

In general, CMT is slowly progressive, and people with most forms of CMT have a normal life expectancy. There is currently no cure, but physical therapy, occupational therapy, braces and other orthopedic devices, and orthopedic surgery (see Box 9.2) can help individuals with CMT finish school, work, and live functional lives despite the disabling symptoms of the disease (Bertorini, Narayanaswami, & Rashed, 2004; McDonald, 2001; Shy, 2004). Vitamin C therapy has been investigated for the treatment of CMT, but clinical trials in adults (Micallef et al., 2009; Verhamme et al., 2009) and children (Burns et al., 2009) showed no clear benefit.

Diseases of the Neuromuscular Junction: Myasthenia Gravis

The peripheral nerves end at the neuromuscular junction. For a nerve impulse to cross the synapse separating the nerve and muscle, the chemical neurotransmitter acetylcholine must be released from the nerve terminal, cross the space between the nerve and muscle, bind to its receptor on the muscle membrane (much like a key fitting into a keyhole), and generate the muscle membrane impulse that will transmit the signal to the contractile structures within the muscle cell. Impairment of any of the mechanisms that allow a nerve impulse to transmit signals to stimulate muscle movement can result in a myasthenic disorder (from *myo* meaning muscle and *asthenia* meaning fatigability). In rare instances, myasthenic syndromes are genetic

BOX 9.2 INTERDISCIPLINARY CARE

Orthopedic Surgery

Orthopedic surgery, or orthopedics, is the branch of surgery concerned with conditions involving the musculoskeletal system. In the pediatrics age group orthopedic surgeons use both surgical and nonsurgical means to treat musculoskeletal disorders and other developmental disabilities as well as acute injuries such as broken bones. Pediatric orthopedic surgeons train as residents and fellows for at least 6 years following medical school. For children with developmental disabilities, they may perform surgery to correct hip dislocation, spinal curvatures, and/or spasticity. They also work as part of a rehabilitative team (see Chapter 32) to design orthoptic supports, wheelchair assistance, and physical and occupational therapy.

in origin (called congenital myasthenic syndrome), but they are most often acquired as autoimmune disorders. In children and adolescents, acquired autoimmune myasthenia is typically referred to as juvenile myasthenia gravis. The most common symptoms are **diplopia** (double vision), **ptosis** (drooping eyelid), **dysphagia** (difficulty swallowing), **dysarthria** (changes in voice quality), and extremity weakness. These symptoms result from cranial nerve involvement, which is almost always present. The symptoms tend to worsen with activity and toward the end of the day. In the most severe cases, breathing and swallowing may be impaired (Chiang, Darras, & Kang, 2009).

Treatment of juvenile myasthenia gravis generally targets improving neuromuscular transmission and increasing muscle strength while suppressing the production of abnormal antibodies. Pyridostigmine is a drug that is a common first-line therapy. It is an acetylcholinesterase inhibitor, which means that it prevents the neurotransmitter acetylcholine from being metabolized at the neuromuscular junction, raising its effective levels. At high doses, pyridostigmine can cause cholinergic side effects (including excessive secretions and sometimes worsening of myasthenia symptoms), but in general it is well tolerated. Its main drawback is that it is a relatively weak therapy, and often patients will need immunomodulatory therapy as well.

There are three standard immunomodulatory therapies available for myasthenia gravis: plasmapheresis, intravenous immunoglobulin, and steroids (Liew et al., 2014). Plasmapheresis requires central venous access (a surgically placed central line into a large central vein) in younger children and others with small-caliber peripheral veins. In older children and adolescents with large-caliber veins, the treatments can be performed through a peripheral vein (standard intravenous therapy). Intravenous immunoglobulin has also been used in some cases. Steroid therapy may be the most traditional approach, but it is associated with significant side effects when used on a long-term basis, especially in children and adolescents. When a child needs additional therapy beyond the traditional immunomodulatory therapies, steroid-sparing immunomodulatory agents may be used. Due to the significant side effect profile of chronic corticosteroid use, steroid-sparing agents are likely to be used before steroids in the future.

Thymectomy is a surgical procedure that removes the thymus, a gland in the chest that plays a key role in regulating immune responses. This procedure appears to induce partial or complete remission in some cases of juvenile myasthenia gravis (Kogut, Bufo, Rothenberg, & Lobe, 2000; Tracy, McRae, & Millichap, 2009).

Disorders of Muscle: Muscular Dystrophies and Myopathies

The two major categories of inherited muscle disease in childhood are muscular dystrophies and congenital myopathies. Muscular dystrophies are characterized by the progressive destruction of muscle tissue, whereas congenital myopathies typically involve either the abnormal accumulation of certain proteins or other developmental abnormalities in the muscle fibers. These findings can be observed on microscopic examination of skeletal muscle tissue obtained at biopsy.

Muscular dystrophies tend to be progressive, whereas the clinical course in congenital myopathies varies. There is a vast array of muscular dystrophies, including limb-girdle muscular dystrophies, congenital muscular dystrophies, facioscapulohumeral muscular dystrophy, and Emery-Dreifuss muscular dystrophy. Genetic etiologies have been defined for each of these categories of disease.

Duchenne Muscular Dystrophy DMD is the most common form of muscular dystrophy in childhood. It is a progressive skeletal muscle disorder caused by mutations in the X-linked DMD gene, resulting in the absence of dystrophin, a major muscle protein (Hoffman, Brown, & Kunkel, 1987; Monaco et al., 1986). The incidence of Duchenne muscular dystrophy is approximately 1 in 3,300 male births (Jeppesen, Green, Steffensen, & Rahbek, 2003). This disorder is associated with a high spontaneous mutation rate (Van Essen, Busch, te Meerman, & ten Kate, 1992), so a significant number of boys with Duchenne muscular dystrophy have no family history of the disease.

The disease manifests in early childhood, although abnormal muscle CPK levels and microscopic signs of muscle damage may be observed at birth. Delayed walking and frequent falls are characteristic initial symptoms. Boys with Duchenne muscular dystrophy often walk on their tiptoes. Manifestations of proximal hip girdle muscle weakness become apparent by 3–5 years of age when the child starts having difficulties climbing in the playground, getting up from the floor, climbing stairs, and running. Weakness in the quadriceps and gluteus maximus muscles makes it difficult for the child to rise from the floor to a standing position, and affected boys use the Gowers maneuver (described earlier) to compensate. Weakness in the gluteus medius muscles leads to a waddling gait. **Pseudohypertrophy** (enlargement that is due primarily to fibrosis and fatty infiltration of muscle, rather than a true increase in muscle fiber diameter or numbers) of various muscles occurs, most commonly at the calves (Figure 9.2).

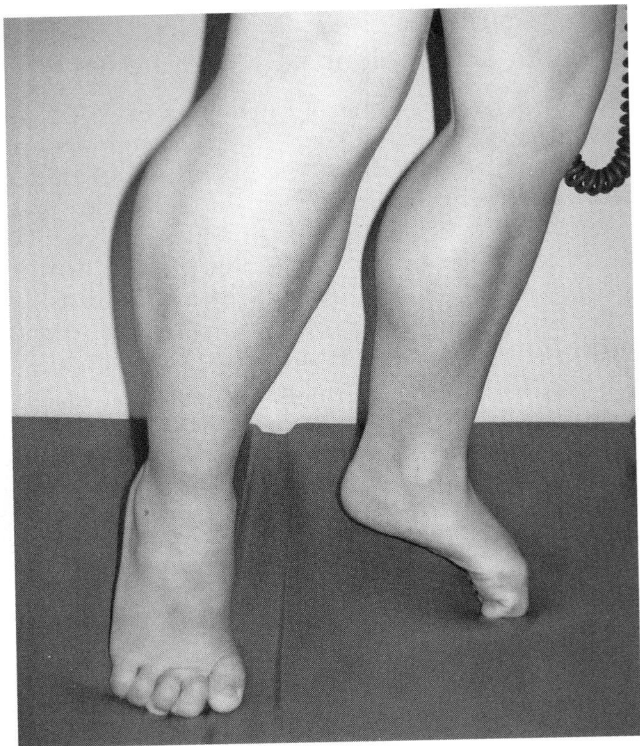

Figure 9.2. Pseudohypertrophy of the calf muscles in a 5-year-old boy with Duchenne muscular dystrophy, characterized by a deletion in exon 45 in *DMD*, the dystrophin gene. (Courtesy of Peter B. Kang, M.D.)

Accelerated deterioration in strength and balance often results from intercurrent disease or surgically induced immobilization. If tendon releases are performed, mobilization in a walking splint or cast is needed as soon as possible to prevent a decrease in muscle strength from disuse. When ambulation is no longer possible, typically by the ages of 10–12 years, contractures in the lower extremities become more pronounced and may involve the shoulders. Daily physical therapy and occupational therapy services at school and daily stretching exercises at home are imperative.

Corticosteroid treatment of Duchenne muscular dystrophy has become a standard component of clinical care, although the optimal age for initiation of this therapy remains controversial (Birnkrant et al., 2018b). Oral prednisone (a steroid medication) stabilizes or improves strength and, in many cases, prolongs the ambulatory phase of the disease by 1–3 years (Griggs et al., 1993). The synthetic steroid deflazacort was approved by the FDA in 2017 due to evidence suggesting that it may have a milder side effect profile compared with prednisone, especially with respect to weight gain (Griggs et al., 2016). One exception to the finding of a lower side effect profile is the formation of asymptomatic cataracts, which tends to be more common with deflazacort (Biggar, Gingras, Fehlings, Harris, & Steele, 2001; Campbell & Jacob, 2003; Moxley et al., 2005). At this time, the differences in side effect profiles are relatively modest so that either corticosteroid is a viable option (Griggs et al., 2016). Dietary supplements have generally not been found to improve outcome (Escolar et al., 2005).

Kyphoscoliosis (abnormal curvature of the vertebral column in two planes, a combination of kyphosis and scoliosis) can develop at any time but typically accelerates after ambulation is lost. This complication not only causes pain and postural problems, but also exacerbates pulmonary issues due to loss of effective lung volume. Baseline spine x-ray images should be obtained for comparison with future studies to monitor the development of scoliosis. Both manual and power wheelchairs are useful. When the kyphoscoliosis is severe enough, usually at 30 to 50 degrees of curvature, spinal fusion surgery with rod placement may be warranted to help preserve lung function and improve posture (Brook, Kennedy, Stern, Sutherland, & Foster, 1996). The optimal time for surgical intervention is while lung and cardiac functioning is satisfactory (Finder et al., 2004).

Cardiac and respiratory abnormalities are almost universal in the later stages of the disease, and one or the other of these complications constitutes the immediate cause of death in most cases. Cardiac manifestations include cardiomyopathy and cardiac arrhythmias. The progression of cardiomyopathy (inflammation of the heart muscle impairing its function) may be slowed by the use of certain drugs. Progressive respiratory failure occurs from a combination of decreased lung capacity and function. Noninvasive ventilatory support, in combination with interventions to promote appropriate secretion clearance and coughing, is now commonly recommended to counteract this decline.

Lower-than-average IQ scores have been reported in individuals with Duchenne muscular dystrophy, although results have not been consistent and many children have typical cognition (Felisari et al., 2000). Certain cognitive areas such as verbal memory, digit span, and auditory comprehension are more affected than others (Hinton, De Vivo, Nereo, Goldstein, & Stern, 2000). Deletions localized in a specific part of the dystrophin gene are preferentially associated with cognitive impairment (Giliberto, Ferreiro, Dalamon, & Szijan, 2004). The incidence of neurobehavioral issues, ranging from attention-deficit/hyperactivity disorder to autism spectrum disorder, seem to be increased as well in boys with Duchenne muscular dystrophy (Hendriksen & Vles, 2008; Wu, Kuban, Allred, Shapiro, & Darras, 2005).

The life expectancy for patients with Duchenne muscular dystrophy without significant interventions was previously less than 2 decades. The supportive and medical therapies, including spinal fusion surgery, steroids, cardiac medications, and noninvasive ventilatory support, have together helped lengthen the life expectancy in many cases to the fourth decade and in some cases to the fifth decade. Treatment by a multidisciplinary neuromuscular team is critical to implementing such a care plan.

The only treatment that has had an effect on the primary muscle weakness in Duchenne muscular dystrophy has been corticosteroids, as previously noted. In 2016, however, an antisense oligonucleotide therapy (eteplirsen), given by intravenous injection weekly, was approved by the FDA to restore the reading frame of the dystrophin gene in certain boys with Duchenne muscular dystrophy. This approach, referred to as exon skipping, appears to have the potential to partially restore the reading frame of the gene in patients with mutations amenable to skipping of exon 51 in dystrophin, representing about 13% of affected boys (Mendell et al., 2016). More treatments that take advantage of exon skipping are expected to follow in the years to come.

Congenital Myopathies Congenital myopathies usually present in infancy with marked hypotonia and weakness, feeding difficulties, and respiratory insufficiency. Within each type of congenital myopathy, there is a spectrum of severity, and later onset variants have been identified for several subtypes due to advances in genetic diagnosis (Dubowitz & Fardeau, 1995; Ryan et al., 2003). In contrast to muscular dystrophies, congenital myopathies are more likely to be associated with cranial nerve involvement (facial weakness, eye movement abnormalities, or both) and early respiratory complications.

The classic congenital myopathies include centronuclear myopathy (including X-linked myotubular myopathy), nemaline myopathy, central core disease, and congenital fiber type disproportion (Riggs, Bodensteiner, & Schochet, 2003). These diseases are listed in order of decreasing overall severity, although there is overlap among these subtypes.

Causative mutations in various genes that encode structural muscle proteins, often localizing to the sarcomere, have been linked with each type of congenital myopathy. Mutations in the *MTM1* gene cause myotubular myopathy (Laporte et al., 1996), and centronuclear myopathy has been associated with several genes to date: *DNM2* (Bitoun et al., 2005), *BIN1* (Nicot et al., 2007), and *RYR1* (Wilmshurst et al., 2010). Nemaline myopathy has been associated with mutations in an ever-increasing number of genes, including *ACTA1* (Nowak et al., 1999), *CFL2* (Agrawal et al., 2007), *NEB* (Pelin et al., 1999), *TNNT1* (Johnston et al., 2000), *TPM2* (Donner et al., 2002), and *TPM3* (Laing et al., 1995). Central core disease and isolated malignant hyperthermia have been associated with mutations in the *RYR1* gene (Quane et al., 1993; Zhang et al., 1993). The clinical spectrum of *RYR1* myopathies continues to expand.

Caring for a child with a congenital myopathy will depend on specific complications. Respiratory interventions include invasive (i.e., tracheostomy and mechanical ventilation) and noninvasive supports depending on the individual case. A range of orthotic devices and orthopedic procedures may be helpful at various stages of the disease. Nutritional support may also be needed. No pharmacological treatment currently exists for any form of the disorders, though recent research has shown promising results for gene therapy in animal models of myotubular myopathy (Daniele et al., 2018; Elverman et al., 2017; Tasfaout et al., 2018), and a human clinical trial is thus underway. These children generally have typical cognitive development, so education should be provided at the appropriate age and grade level. However, some children may have difficulty speaking due to facial and tongue weakness and sometimes due to a tracheostomy, so an augmentative/alternative communication evaluation is essential (see Chapter 36). Rehabilitation focuses on improving daily living skills (see Chapter 32).

DISORDERS OF THE MUSCULOSKELETAL SYSTEM

Musculoskeletal disorders may involve abnormalities of just one limb or joint or the entire skeleton. This section discusses the different types of musculoskeletal disorders, providing an example of each. These include joint disorders, such as arthrogryposis; skeletal dysplasias, such as achondroplasia; and connective tissue disorders, such as osteogenesis imperfecta.

Joint Disorders: Arthrogryposis

The term **arthrogryposis** refers to congenital joint contractures. Arthrogryposis multiplex congenita is a syndrome in which arthrogryposis is present in at least two major joints, with an incidence estimated to range from 1 in 3,000 to 1 in 12,000 live births (Darin, Kimber, Kroksmark, & Tulinius, 2002). The final common pathway for the development of the characteristic contractures is significant prolonged fetal immobility (Gordon, 1998). More than 150 distinct causes of arthrogryposis multiplex congenita have been identified (Hall, 1997). The etiologies can be divided into endogenous (having an internal cause or origin) and exogenous (having an external cause or origin) categories. Endogenous causes are often genetic in nature and include multiorgan system genetic syndromes, connective tissue diseases, and central and peripheral nervous system disorders. Exogenous causes are typically maternal and include structural uterine problems, placental insufficiency, maternal myasthenia gravis, and maternal multiple sclerosis (Livingstone & Sack, 1984). When a neuromuscular cause of arthrogryposis multiplex congenita is suspected, electrophysiological testing and muscle biopsy are complementary and should both be pursued when possible (Kang et al., 2003).

Although spinal deformity at birth is uncommon for infants with arthrogryposis, 35% of patients will develop scoliosis or lordosis by adulthood (Nouraei, Sawatzky, MacGillivray, & Hall, 2017). Most curves are resistant to bracing. Physical therapy and occupational therapy, however, are helpful in maintaining joint motion and maximizing functional development. In cases of arthrogryposis associated with other congenital anomalies, the child may have additional medical problems that must be addressed.

Long-term orthopedic management is directed at maximizing function. Because arthrogryposis can be caused by many disorders, there is no single management plan. The common goals are independent ambulation or wheelchair mobility, self-care, and the ability to be employed and live independently. The initial treatment of any contracture involves gentle stretching and range-of-motion exercises. Once the joint is in a proper position, a lightweight splint may help prevent recurrence. If a joint's range of motion is not functional, casting or surgical soft-tissue release followed by casting may improve it. The limitations of surgical interventions should be kept in mind in this patient population (Lahoti & Bell, 2005).

Skeletal Dysplasias: Achondroplasia

The skeletal dysplasias are a large, genetically diverse group of conditions characterized by abnormalities in the development, growth, and maintenance of the skeleton. Many of these disorders result in disproportionate short stature (Savarirayan & Rimoin, 2002). There are approximately 175 different skeletal dysplasias (OMIM, 2011; Orioli, Castilla, & Barbosa-Neto, 1986; Stoll, Dott, Roth, & Alembik, 1989).

Achondroplasia is the most common form of short stature associated with disproportionately shortened limbs. The incidence has been estimated to be 3.6 to 6.0 in every 100,000 live births in the United States (Waller et al., 2008). It has been found to result from a point mutation in the gene coding for fibroblast growth factor receptor 3 (Matsui et al., 1998). The condition is inherited as an autosomal dominant trait, and most individuals have the same genetic mutation, so the condition's physical manifestations tend to be similar across individuals (Bellus et al., 1995). It is important to monitor affected children for potentially serious complications such as hydrocephalus, craniocervical junction compression (a decrease in the space between the lower brainstem and cervical cord that can lead to spinal cord compression), upper airway obstruction, and kyphosis (Trotter & Hall, 2005).

Thoracolumbar kyphosis (curvature of the mid-lower spine in the front to back plane) is present to some degree in most infants with achondroplasia as a result of their enlarged heads, hypotonia, and ligamentous laxity (double jointedness). The kyphosis typically improves spontaneously once the child begins to walk, but 10%–15% of children require bracing or surgical correction of the curvature (Ain & Browne, 2004; Ain & Shirley, 2004). Careful monitoring is essential, and support for the back, particularly in the very young child, may be helpful.

The major impairments of the extremities include short limbs, limited elbow and hip extension, and knee and leg deformities that can impede ambulation. **Genu verum** (bowed legs) occurs in 40% of individuals with achondroplasia, but only 25% will experience a clinically significant deformity that requires surgical correction (Beals & Stanley, 2005). Significant advances have been made in surgical limb-lengthening procedures, but it still takes about 3 years to achieve the desired lengthening. Growth hormone therapy has achieved only limited success in people with achondroplasia (Hagenas & Hertel, 2003), and impacts on final adult heights are modest (Harada et al., 2017), so it is not regarded as standard of care.

Connective Tissue Disorders: Osteogenesis Imperfecta

Connective tissue disorders are caused by the mechanical failure of collagen (the main structural protein found in skin and other connective tissues), which results in joint hypermobility. Examples of connective tissue disorders include Ehlers-Danlos syndrome and Marfan syndrome.

Osteogenesis imperfecta (OI) is caused by a failure of formation of type I collagen, the scaffolding on which bone mineral is laid down. Bone deformities and frequent fractures are typical complications of this disease. Blue **sclera** (the part of the eye that is normally white) is a classic physical finding in this disease, but a true blue color is typically only seen in type I, whereas bluish-gray sclera or normal sclera are more typical in other subtypes. Poor dentition is seen in more severe cases. Traditionally, the clinical diagnosis of OI has been supported by a skin biopsy to test for the underlying genetic defect (Minch & Kruse, 1998), but genetic testing of blood leukocytes is now the standard diagnostic approach (Van Dijk & Sillence, 2014). OI has been estimated to have a prevalence of 9.5 in 100,000 births (Lindahl et al., 2015). Causative mutations are most commonly found in *COL1A1* (on chromosome 17) and *COL1A2* (on chromosome 7) (Lindahl et al., 2015), though numerous other associated genes have been identified.

Orthopedic care has been the mainstay in managing OI and involves measures to prevent fractures, treat acute fractures, and correct bony deformities. People with OI are particularly susceptible to disuse osteoporosis (bone weakness); therefore, promoting mobility in both daily life and after an injury is essential. Placing rods inside the bones for support at the time of a fracture or in conjunction with **osteotomies** (surgical cuts through the bone to correct deformities) can improve the bone alignment, shorten rehabilitation time, and help prevent future fractures. Scoliosis occurs in 39%–80% of individuals with OI (Wallace, Kruse, & Shah, 2017). Because thoracic curves can decrease lung capacity (Widmann et al., 1999), orthopedic consultation is recommended for monitoring curve progression, with spine fusion surgery performed if necessary (Engelbert, Pruijs, Beemer, & Helders, 1998).

The bone fragility seen in OI is due to disturbed organization of bone tissue, decreased bone mass, and altered bone geometry. Children with OI do not form as much bone compared with unaffected children, and children with moderate to severe OI form essentially the same amount of bone as they resorb. This imbalance informs the rationale for treating affected children with bisphosphonates (e.g., alendronate, typically used to treat osteoporosis in postmenopausal women), and these are now commonly prescribed for this disorder. Bisphosphonate therapy has been shown to increase bone mineral density, but it is not certain yet whether these treatments reduce the incidence of fractures and other clinical complications, and it is not clear what regimen of bisphosphonate therapy is optimal, including the question of the relative merits of oral versus intravenous administration (Dwan, Phillipi, Steiner, & Basel, 2016).

MANAGEMENT PRINCIPLES

Recommended standards of care have been published for Duchenne muscular dystrophy (Birnkrant et al., 2018a, Birnkrant et al., 2018b, Birnkrant et al., 2018c; Bushby et al., 2010a; Bushby et al., 2010b) and spinal muscular atrophy (Finkel et al., 2018; Mercuri et al., 2018b), and these standards provide greater detail regarding the care of such disorders. While they are by no means the last word on the subject, they summarize what is currently known about caring for children with these conditions and what gaps in knowledge persist.

General management principles for the care of children with neuromuscular and musculoskeletal disorders involve medical care, rehabilitation management, preventing contractures promoting bone health, and providing educational services; these approaches are described below.

Medical Care

The autoimmune neuromuscular disorders, including chronic inflammatory demyelinating polyradiculoneuropathy (CIDP) and myasthenia gravis, typically respond to immunomodulatory therapies including plasmapheresis, intravenous immunoglobulin, and steroids. Guillain-Barré syndrome (closely related to CIDP) responds to immunomodulatory therapies and intravenous immunoglobulin.

Two important precautions apply to patients with primary muscle diseases:

1. **Rhabdomyolysis** (breakdown of muscle tissue) and **myoglobinuria** (the resulting spillage of myoglobin, a heme pigment, into the urine) may occur in isolation or as part of certain muscle diseases (Mathews et al., 2011). These complications occur especially in the context of strenuous exercise, dehydration, or both. Whenever this reaction occurs, the individual should be taken to the nearest emergency department immediately, as the myoglobinuria aspect of the reaction has the potential to cause permanent kidney damage. Intravenous fluids will avert renal injury in most cases.
2. **Malignant hyperthermia** (a life-threatening elevation of body temperature associated with the administration of an anesthetic agent) can occur in patients with *RYR1* mutations (MacLennan et al., 1990; McCarthy et al., 1990) or in the setting of muscle diseases, including muscular dystrophies and congenital myopathies such as *RYR1*-associated central core disease (Quane et al., 1993; Zhang et al., 1993).

Medical therapies for inherited neuromuscular disorders are often limited, but there are important medications for certain disorders. Albuterol (an asthma medication) appeared to increase patients' strength in two studies involving patients with SMA II (Kinali et al., 2002; Pane et al., 2008), and some clinicians now prescribe this for certain SMA patients. Its efficacy, however, has not been proven in a randomized controlled trial. Steroids have been shown to improve the motor outcome in Duchenne muscular dystrophy, as discussed earlier. Also, specific subtypes of congenital myasthenic syndrome respond to various medications. It is important to note that new molecular therapies are being developed, and a handful have been recently approved for spinal muscular atrophy and Duchenne muscular dystrophy, as described earlier.

It is important for children with neuromuscular disease to have routine immunizations as recommended by the American Academy of Pediatrics (2010), especially when there is a high risk of pulmonary complications. They should also receive the pneumococcal and annual influenza (flu) vaccine. Certain immunizations may need to be deferred for some patients, such as those with active or recent episodes of Guillain-Barré syndrome and patients with active cases of CIDP. Parents of such patients should discuss the advisability of having certain vaccinations with the child's physicians.

Children with myopathies and muscular dystrophies are at increased risk for sleep apnea. Symptoms may be noticeable during daytime and often involve fatigue, falling asleep during class, or morning headaches. A **polysomnogram** (sleep study) with continuous carbon dioxide monitoring is the best way to assess the need for ventilatory support. Provision of noninvasive nocturnal ventilation can significantly increase the quality of life and lengthen life expectancy (Baydur et al., 2000).

Rehabilitation Management

Physical therapy and rehabilitation play an important role in maximizing functional status and tone, and they may even slow the progression of some diseases, although this effect is subtle and difficult to prove. Some evidence suggests that such interventions may have a beneficial impact on outcomes for these diseases (Cup et al., 2007), but it is clear that further data are needed to draw definitive conclusions (Dunaway et al., 2016).

In muscular dystrophies there is a consensus that high-resistance exercises, especially those involving eccentric contractions (i.e., weight lifting and abdominal crunches), are damaging to the muscle cell membrane and should be avoided (Ansved, 2003). However, the impact of a sedentary life is equally negative (McDonald, 2002). Therefore, active, nonresistive exercises are encouraged, such as swimming (with the proper safeguards). An active lifestyle will also prevent excessive weight gain, especially if the child is receiving steroids. Daily walks help maintain strength and slow contracture formation (see Chapter 32).

Both the nature and quantity of activity should be modified so that fatigue does not remain after a night's sleep. Wheelchair games can be played when ambulation is lost. Children with neuromuscular disorders who are confined to bed because of the disease, injury, or surgery require physical therapy, including range-of-motion exercises, with prompt progression to more active exercise, including walking when possible. In the event of leg fractures, walking casts should be used as soon as possible (Siegel, 1977), and every effort should be made to limit the amount of time the child spends in a cast.

For those children who develop difficulty with activities of daily living, occupational therapy evaluation at school is essential to assess self-feeding, self-care, torso positioning within the classroom, and writing. A keyboard should be provided to complete school tasks, and an assistive technology evaluation should be performed. A voice recorder is useful for taking notes, or a note-taker can be appointed. Some students may require a classroom aide in order to participate fully in the academic environment and safely navigate the school building, and this should be built into their individualized education program (see Chapter 33).

Preventing Contractures

Stretching exercises, nighttime splinting, or both should be recommended as soon as tightness of the heel cords is noticed in order to prevent contractures (Hyde et al., 2000). A standing board tilted at an appropriate angle may be used for limited periods during the day to help stretch the Achilles tendon in children who do not ambulate. If stretching and **orthoses** (bracing) are not effective, surgical release of tight heel cords may be beneficial (Goertzen, Baltzer, & Voit, 1995). Temporary bracing after tendon surgery is necessary for optimal results. Further details on orthoses may be found in Chapter 32.

Promoting Bone Health

In children with neuromuscular and musculoskeletal disorders, a fracture can occur with little or no trauma (e.g., from gentle range-of-motion exercises during physical therapy). Such fractures are called pathologic fractures and may result from bone fragility (especially in osteogenesis imperfecta), as a secondary effect of a medication (e.g., steroids or antiepileptic drugs), or as weakness from disuse (Sambrook & Jones, 1995). Children may manifest pathological fractures as swelling and increased warmth of the fractured extremity. Weight-bearing activities are important for maintaining bone density as bones have internal receptors that recognize weight-bearing activity and send signals to make bones stronger in response. Similarly, it is essential that these children be given diets rich in calcium and vitamin D, with supplementation of vitamin D recommended in many cases depending on the specific disease and the stage of illness.

Educational Services

Children with acute neuromuscular disorders including myasthenia gravis, inflammatory myopathies, and inflammatory neuropathies may require prolonged admissions to the hospital, which can entail extended absences from school. Some children require homebound instruction during convalescence. Once the child returns to school, supportive measures such as physical therapy and occupational therapy may be very helpful (Table 9.1). Children with fluctuating disorders such as myasthenia gravis may require access to elevators, modified physical education programs, additional rest periods during the day, or a shortened school day. Children with chronic disorders such as congenital and hereditary progressive myopathies, as well as chronic polyneuropathies, may require specialized rehabilitation care.

Table 9.1. School accommodations for children with neuromuscular and musculoskeletal disorders

Physical and occupational therapy
Stretching
Range-of-motion exercises
Muscle cramp massage
Safety training (on stairs and playground)
Hallway safety
Accommodating activities of daily living to changing physical needs (e.g., toileting, lunchtime/cafeteria safety)
Adapted or modified physical education and sports for individuals with disabilities
Consultation for body positioning, seating, and gross- and fine-motor function
Assistive technology
Specialized accommodations
Provision of an additional set of textbooks to avoid having to transport books from one classroom to another
Access to an elevator
Consideration of students' physical needs when designing class schedule
Preferential seating in the classroom
Consideration of students' physical needs when developing a school emergency evacuation plan
Consideration of students' needs when planning field trips and school events

Steroids are used in neuromuscular diseases such as Duchenne muscular dystrophy, chronic inflammatory demyelinating polyradiculoneuropathy, and myasthenia gravis. Two side effects, behavior problems and weight gain, may occur shortly after starting the medication and may persist. Changes in behavior related to the chronic treatment could impact school performance and interpersonal relationships. Steroids can cause depression, hyperactivity, and behavioral changes, including, in rare instances, psychosis. Sometimes adjusting the dose can improve these symptoms, but in other cases the side effects are severe enough that the medication needs to be discontinued.

A child receiving steroids also tends to have increased appetite and weight gain, as well as slowing of linear growth and bone demineralization. Unwanted weight gain can be especially detrimental in children with a neuromuscular disease, including those with muscular dystrophies. The increased body weight burdens the already weak muscles, and this can obscure the benefits of steroid treatment. This problem can sometimes be avoided or mitigated, however, if the child follows a healthy diet. Children on steroids should bring lunch to school whenever possible in order to follow their diet, and they should avoid snacks between meals.

SUMMARY

- The neuromuscular and musculoskeletal systems support the physical structure of the body and help carry out essential movements.
- Diseases affecting these systems have a significant impact on a child's functional capacity and independence.
- Classic signs and symptoms of these diseases may in some cases be straightforward, but in other cases they may be subtle or involve other organ systems and thus be difficult to recognize.
- Genetic advances over the past several decades have facilitated detailed descriptions of genetic subtypes of numerous disorders.
- The child's care team should include family members; primary care physicians; and medical

specialists such as child neurologists, orthopaedic surgeons, therapists, and rehabilitative specialists.

- The goals of therapy are to gain or retain function, conserve energy, prolong life expectancy when possible, and improve quality of life.
- Therapy may involve a combination of medical and nonmedical approaches, including medications; bracing; physical therapy; occupational therapy; seating systems; adaptive equipment; and, when necessary, surgery.
- Historically, cures have been elusive, but this has begun to change as highly sophisticated disease-modifying therapies are beginning to win approval from the FDA for some of these disorders.
- These disorders are under active investigation, with the goal of developing new treatment approaches, including the repair of genetic material, more effective medications, and improved surgical techniques.

ADDITIONAL RESOURCES

Muscular Dystrophy Association: http://www.mdausa.org

Spinal Muscular Atrophy Foundation (SMA Foundation): http://www.smafoundation.org/

Gillette Children's Hospital: https://www.gillettechildrens.org/conditions-care/neuromuscular-disorders

Additional resources can be found online in Appendix D: Childhood Disabilities Resources, Services, and Organizations (see About the Online Companion Materials).

REFERENCES

Agrawal, P. B., Greenleaf, R. S., Tomczak, K. K., Lehtokari, V. L., Wallgren-Pettersson, C., Wallefeld, W., . . . Beggs, A. H. (2007). Nemaline myopathy with minicores caused by mutation of the CFL2 gene encoding the skeletal muscle actin-binding protein, cofilin-2. *American Journal of Human Genetics, 80,* 162–167.

Ain, M. C., & Browne, J. A. (2004). Spinal arthrodesis with instrumentation for thoracolumbar kyphosis in pediatric achondroplasia. *Spine, 29,* 2075–2080.

Ain, M. C., & Shirley, E. D. (2004). Spinal fusion for kyphosis in achondroplasia. *Journal of Pediatric Orthopedics, 24,* 541–545.

American Academy of Pediatrics. (2010). Policy statement—Recommended childhood and adolescent immunization schedules—United States, 2010. *Pediatrics, 125,* 195–196.

Ansved, T. (2003). Muscular dystrophies, influence of physical conditioning on the disease evolution. *Current Opinion in Clinical Nutrition and Metabolic Care, 6,* 435–439.

Arkblad, E., Tulinius, M., Kroksmark, A. K., Henricsson, M., & Darin, N. (2009). A population-based study of genotypic and phenotypic variability in children with spinal muscular atrophy. *Acta Paediatrica, 98*(5), 865–872.

Baydur, A., Layne, E., Aral, H., Krishnareddy, N., Topacio, R., Frederick, G., & Bodden, W. (2000). Long term non-invasive ventilation in the community for patients with musculoskeletal disorders, 46 year experience and review. *Thorax, 55,* 4–11.

Beals, R. K., & Stanley, G. (2005). Surgical correction of bowlegs in achondroplasia. *Journal of Pediatric Orthopedics, B14,* 245–249.

Bellus, G. A., Hefferon, T. W., Ortiz de Luna, R. I., Hecht, J. T., Horton, W. A., Machado, M., . . . Francomano, C. A. (1995). Achondroplasia is defined by recurrent G380R mutations of FGFR3. *American Journal of Human Genetics, 56,* 368–373.

Bertorini, T., Narayanaswami, P., & Rashed, H. (2004). Charcot–Marie–Tooth disease (hereditary motor sensory neuropathies) and hereditary sensory and autonomic neuropathies. *Neurologist, 10,* 327–337.

Biggar, W. D., Gingras, M., Fehlings, D. L., Harris, V. A., & Steele, C. A. (2001). Deflazacort treatment of Duchenne muscular dystrophy. *Journal of Pediatrics, 138,* 45–50.

Birnkrant, D. J., Bushby, K., Bann, C. M., Alman, B. A., Apkon, S. D., Blackwell, A., . . . DMD Care Considerations Working Group. (2018a). Diagnosis and management of Duchenne muscular dystrophy, part 2: Respiratory, cardiac, bone health, and orthopaedic management. *Lancet Neurology, 17*(4), 347–361.

Birnkrant, D. J., Bushby, K., Bann, C. M., Apkon, S. D., Blackwell, A., Brumbaugh, D., . . . DMD Care Considerations Working Group. (2018b). Diagnosis and management of Duchenne muscular dystrophy, part 1: Diagnosis, and neuromuscular, rehabilitation, endocrine, and gastrointestinal and nutritional management. *Lancet Neurology, 17*(3), 251–267.

Birnkrant, D. J., Bushby, K., Bann, C. M., Apkon, S. D., Blackwell, A., Colvin, M. K., . . . DMD Care Considerations Working Group. (2018c). Diagnosis and management of Duchenne muscular dystrophy, part 3: Primary care, emergency management, psychosocial care, and transitions of care across the lifespan. *Lancet Neurology, 17*(5), 445–455.

Bitoun, M., Maugenre, S., Jeannet, P.Y., Lacène, E., Ferrer, X., Laforêt, P., . . . Guichenev, P. (2005). Mutations in dynamin 2 cause dominant centronuclear myopathy. *Nature Genetics, 37,* 1207–1209.

Braathen, G. J. (2012). Genetic epidemiology of Charcot-Marie-Tooth disease. *Acta Neurologica Scandinavia Supplementum, 193,* iv–22.

Brook, P. D., Kennedy, J. D., Stern, L. M., Sutherland A. D., & Foster, B. K. (1996). Spinal fusion in Duchenne's muscular dystrophy. *Journal of Pediatric Orthopedics, 16,* 324–331.

Burns, J., Ouvrier, R. A., Yiu, E. M., Joseph, P. D., Kornberg, A. J., Fahey, M. C., & Ryan, M. M. (2009). Ascorbic acid for Charcot-Marie-Tooth disease type 1A in children: A randomised, double-blind, placebo-controlled, safety and efficacy trial. *Lancet Neurology, 8*(6), 537–544.

Bushby, K., Finkel, R., Birnkrant, D. J., Case, L. E., Clemens, P. R, Cripe, L., . . . DMD Care Considerations Working Group. (2010a). Diagnosis and management of Duchenne muscular dystrophy, part 1, diagnosis, and pharmacological and psychosocial management. *Lancet Neurology, 9,* 77–93.

Bushby, K., Finkel, R., Birnkrant, D. J., Case, L. E., Clemens, P. R, Cripe, L., . . . DMD Care Considerations Working Group. (2010b). Diagnosis and management of Duchenne muscular dystrophy, part 2, implementation of multidisciplinary care. *Lancet Neurology, 9,* 177–189.

Campbell, C., & Jacob, P. (2003). Deflazacort for the treatment of Duchenne dystrophy, a systematic review. *BMC Neurology, 3,* 7.

Chiang, L. M., Darras, B. T., & Kang, P. B. (2009). Juvenile myasthenia gravis. *Muscle & Nerve, 39,* 423–431.

Cup, E. H., Pieterse, A. J., Ten Broek-Pastoor, J. M., Munneke, M., van Engelen, B. G., Hendricks, H. T., . . . Osstendorp, R. Al. (2007). Exercise therapy and other types of physical therapy for patients with neuromuscular diseases: A systematic review. *Archives of Physical Medicine and Rehabilitation, 88*(11), 1452–1464.

Daniele, N., Moal, C., Julien, L., Marinello, M., Jamet, T., Martin, S., . . . Buj-Bello, A. (2018). Intravenous administration of a MTMR2-encoding AAV vector ameliorates the phenotype of myotubular myopathy in mice. *Journal of Neuropathology & Experimental Neurology, 77*(4), 282–295.

Darin, N., Kimber, E., Kroksmark, A.K., & Tulinius, M. (2002). Multiple congenital contractures, birth prevalence, etiology, and outcome. *Journal of Pediatrics, 140,* 61–67.

Darras, B. T., & Jones, H. R. (2000). Diagnosis of pediatric neuromuscular disorders in the era of DNA analysis. *Pediatric Neurology, 23,* 289–300.

Darras, B. T., & Kang, P. B. (2007). Clinical trials in spinal muscular atrophy. *Current Opinions in Pediatrics, 19,* 675–679.

Donner, K., Ollikainen, M., Ridanpaa, M., Christen, H.J., Goebel, H.H., de Visser, M., . . . Wallgren-Pettersson, C. (2002). Mutations in the beta–tropomyosin (TPM2) gene—A rare cause of nemaline myopathy. *Neuromuscular Disorders, 12,* 151–158.

Dubowitz, V., & Fardeau, M. (1995). Proceedings of the 27th ENMC sponsored workshop on congenital muscular dystrophy. 22–24 April 1994, The Netherlands. *Neuromuscular Disorders, 5,* 253–258.

Dubowitz, V., Kinali, M., Main, M., Mercuri, E., & Muntoni, F. (2002). Remission of clinical signs in early Duchenne muscular dystrophy on intermittent low-dosage prednisolone therapy. *European Journal of Paediatric Neurology, 6,* 153–159.

Dunaway, S., Montes, J., McDermott, M. P., Martens, W., Neisen, A., Glanzman, A. M., . . . Pandya, S. (2016). Physical therapy services received by individuals with spinal muscular atrophy (SMA). *Journal of Pediatric Rehabilitation Medicine, 9*(1), 35–44.

Dwan, K., Phillipi, C. A., Steiner, R. D., & Basel, D. (2016). Bisphosphonate therapy for osteogenesis imperfecta. *Cochrane Database System Review, 10,* CD005088.

Elverman, M., Goddard, M. A., Mack, D., Snyder, J. M., Lawlor, M. W., Meng, H., . . . Childers, M. K. (2017). Long-term effects of systemic gene therapy in a canine model of myotubular myopathy. *Muscle Nerve, 56*(5), 943–953.

Engelbert, R. H., Pruijs, H. E., Beemer, F. A., & Helders, P. J. (1998). Osteogenesis imperfecta in childhood, treatment strategies. *Archives of Physical Medicine and Rehabilitation, 79,* 1590–1594.

Escolar, D. M., Buyse, G., Henricson, E., Leshner, R., Florence, J., Mayhew, J., . . . CINRG Group. (2005). CINRG randomized controlled trial of creatine and glutamine in Duchenne muscular dystrophy. *Annals of Neurology, 58,* 151–155.

Felisari, G., Martinelli Boneschi, F., Bardoni, A., Sironi, M., Comi, G. P., Robotti, M., . . . Bresolin, N. (2000). Loss of Dp140 dystrophin isoform and intellectual impairment in Duchenne dystrophy. *Neurology, 55,* 559–564.

Finder, J. D., Birnkrant, D., Carl, J., Farber, H. J., Gozal, D., Iannoccone, S. T., . . . American Thoracic Society. (2004). Respiratory care of the patient with Duchenne muscular dystrophy, ATS consensus statement. *American Journal of Respiratory and Critical Care Medicine, 170,* 456–465.

Finkel, R. S., Chiriboga, C. A., Vajsar, J., Day, J. W., Montes, J., De Vivo, D. C., . . . Bishop, K. M. (2016). Treatment of infantile-onset spinal muscular atrophy with nusinersen: A phase 2, open-label, dose-escalation study. *Lancet, 388,* 3017–3026.

Finkel, R. S., Mercuri, E., Darras, B. T., Connolly, A. M., Kuntz, N. L., Kirschner, J., . . . Endear Study Group. (2017). Nusinersen versus sham control in infantile-onset spinal muscular atrophy. *New England Journal of Medicine, 377*(18), 1723–1732.

Finkel, R. S., Mercuri, E., Meyer, O. H., Simonds, A. K., Schroth, M. K., Graham, R. J., . . . S. M. A. Care Group. (2018). Diagnosis and management of spinal muscular atrophy: Part 2: Pulmonary and acute care; medications, supplements and immunizations; other organ systems; and ethics. *Neuromuscular Disorders, 28*(3), 197–207.

Giliberto, F., Ferreiro, V., Dalamon, V., & Szijan, I. (2004). Dystrophin deletions and cognitive impairment in Duchenne/Becker muscular dystrophy. *Neurological Research, 26,* 83–87.

Goertzen, M., Baltzer, A., & Voit, T. (1995). Clinical results of early orthopaedic management in Duchenne muscular dystrophy. *Neuropediatrics, 26,* 257–259.

Gordon, N. (1998). Arthrogryposis multiplex congenita. *Brain & Development, 20,* 507–511.

Griggs, R. C., Moxley, R. T., 3rd, Mendell, J. R., Fenichel, G. M., Brooke, M. H., Pestronk, A., . . . Pandya, S. (1993). Duchenne dystrophy, randomized, controlled trial of prednisone (18 months) and azathioprine (12 months). *Neurology, 43,* 520–527.

Griggs, R. C., Miller, J. P., Greenberg, C. R., Fehlings, D. L., Pestronk, A., Mendell, J. R., . . . Meyer, J. M. (2016). Efficacy and safety of deflazacort vs prednisone and placebo for Duchenne muscular dystrophy. *Neurology, 87,* 2123–2131.

Hagenas, L., & Hertel, T. (2003). Skeletal dysplasia, growth hormone treatment and body proportion, comparison with other syndromic and non-syndromic short children. *Hormone Research, 60*(3), 65–70.

Hall, J. G. (1997). Arthrogryposis multiplex congenita, etiology, genetics, classification, diagnostic approach, and general aspects. *Journal of Pediatric Orthopedics, 6,* 159–166.

Harada, D., Namba, N., Hanioka, Y., Ueyama, K., Sakamoto, N., Nakano, Y., . . . Seino, Y. (2017). Final adult height in long-term growth hormone-treated achondroplasia patients. *European Journal of Paediatrics, 176*(7), 873–879.

Hendriksen, J. G., & Vles, J. S. (2008). Neuropsychiatric disorders in males with Duchenne muscular dystrophy, frequency rate of attention–deficit/hyperactivity disorder (ADHD), autism spectrum disorder, and obsessive-compulsive disorder. *Journal of Child Neurology, 23,* 477–481.

Hinton, V. J., De Vivo, D. C., Nereo, N. E., Goldstein, E., & Stern, Y. (2000). Poor verbal working memory across intellectual level in boys with Duchenne dystrophy. *Neurology, 54,* 2127–2132.

Hoffman, E. P., Brown, R. H., Jr., & Kunkel, L. M. (1987). Dystrophin, the protein product of the Duchenne muscular dystrophy locus. *Cell, 51,* 919–928.

Hyde, S. A., FlŁytrup, I., Glent, S., Kroksmark, A. K., Salling, B., Steffensen, B. F., . . . Erlandsen, M. (2000). A randomized comparative study of two methods for controlling Tendo

Achilles contracture in Duchenne muscular dystrophy. *Neuromuscular Disorders, 10,* 257–263.

Jedrzejowska, M., Milewski, M., Zimowski, J., Zagozdzon, P., Kostera-Pruszczyk, A., Borkowska, J., . . . Hausmanowa-Petrusewicz, I. (2010). Incidence of spinal muscular atrophy in Poland—more frequent than predicted? *Neuroepidemiology, 34*(3), 152–157.

Jeppesen, J., Green, A., Steffensen, B. F., & Rahbek, J. (2003). The Duchenne muscular dystrophy population in Denmark, 1977–2001, prevalence, incidence and survival in relation to the introduction of ventilator use. *Neuromuscular Disorders, 13,* 804–812.

Johnston, J. J., Kelley, R. I., Crawford, T. O., Morton, D. H., Agarwala, R., Koch, T., . . . Biesecker, L. G. (2000). A novel nemaline myopathy in the Amish caused by a mutation in troponin T1. *American Journal of Human Genetics, 67,* 814–821.

Jungbluth, H., Davis, M. R., Muller, C., Counsell, S., Allsop, J., Chattopadhyay, A., . . . Muntoni, F. (2004). Magnetic resonance imaging of muscle in congenital myopathies associated with RYR1 mutations. *Neuromuscular Disorders, 14,* 785–790.

Kang, P. B., Lidov, H. G., David, W. S., Torres, A., Anthony, D. C., Jones, H. R., & Darras, B. T. (2003). Diagnostic value of electromyography and muscle biopsy in arthrogryposis multiplex congenita. *Annals of Neurology, 54,* 790–795.

Kang, P. B., Krishnamoorthy, K. S., Jones, R. M., Shapiro, F. D., & Darras, B. T. (2006). Atypical presentations of spinal muscular atrophy type III (Kugelberg-Welander disease). *Neuromuscular Disorders, 16,* 492–494.

Karakis, I., Gregas, M., Darras, B. T., Kang, P. B., & Jones, H. R. (2013). Clinical correlates of Charcot-Marie-Tooth disease in patients with pes cavus deformities. *Muscle Nerve, 47*(4), 488–492.

Karakis, I., Liew, W., Darras, B. T., Jones, H. R., & Kang, P. B. (2014). Referral and diagnostic trends in pediatric electromyography in the molecular era. *Muscle Nerve, 50*(2), 244–249.

Kinali, M., Mercuri, E., Main, M., De Biasia, F., Karatza, A., Higgins, R., . . . Muntoni, F. (2002). Pilot trial of albuterol in spinal muscular atrophy. *Neurology, 59,* 609–610.

Kogut, K. A., Bufo, A. J., Rothenberg, S. S., & Lobe, T. E. (2000). Thoracoscopic thymectomy for myasthenia gravis in children. *Journal of Pediatric Surgery, 35,* 1576–1577.

Lahoti, O., & Bell, M. J. (2005). Transfer of pectoralis major in arthrogryposis to restore elbow flexion, deteriorating results in the long term. *Journal of Bone and Joint Surgery, British Volume, 87,* 858–860.

Lally, C., Jones, C., Farwell, W., Reyna, S. P., Cook, S. F., & Flanders, W. D. (2017). Indirect estimation of the prevalence of spinal muscular atrophy type I, II, and III in the United States. *Orphanet Journal of Rare Diseases, 12*(1), 175.

Laing, N. G., Wilton, S. D., Akkari, P. A., Dorosz, S., Boundy, K., Blumbergs, P., . . . Love, D. R. (1995). A mutation in the alpha tropomyosin gene TPM3 associated with autosomal dominant nemaline myopathy. *Nature Genetics, 9,* 75–79.

Laporte, J., Hu, L. J., Kretz, C., Mandel, J. L., Kioschis, P., Coy, J. F., . . . Dahl, N. (1996). A gene mutated in X-linked myotubular myopathy defines a new putative tyrosine phosphatase family conserved in yeast. *Nature Genetics, 13,* 175–182.

Laura, M., Singh, D., Ramdharry, G., Morrow, J., Skorupinska, M., Pareyson, D., . . . Inherited Neuropathies Consortium. (2018). Prevalence and orthopedic management of foot and ankle deformities in Charcot-Marie-Tooth disease. *Muscle Nerve, 57*(2), 255–259.

Lefebvre, S., Burglen, L., Reboullet, S., Clermont, O., Burlet, P., Viollet, L., . . . Zeviani, M. (1995). Identification and characterization of a spinal muscular atrophy–determining gene. *Cell, 180,* 155–165.

Liew, W. K. M., Powell, C. A., Sloan, S. R., Shamberger, R. C., Weldon, C. B., Darras, B. T., & Kang, P. B. (2014). Comparison of plasmapheresis and intravenous immunoglobulin as maintenance therapies for juvenile myasthenia gravis. *JAMA Neurology, 71,* 575–580.

Lindahl, K., Astrom, E., Rubin, C. J., Grigelioniene, G., Malmgren, B., Ljunggren, O., & Kindmark, A. (2015). Genetic epidemiology, prevalence, and genotype-phenotype correlations in the Swedish population with osteogenesis imperfecta. *European Journal of Human Genetics, 23*(8), 1042–1050.

Livingstone, I. R., & Sack, G. H., Jr. (1984). Arthrogryposis multiplex congenita occurring with maternal multiple sclerosis. *Archives of Neurology, 41,* 1216–1217.

Lupski, J. R., de Oca–Luna, R. M., Slaugenhaupt, S., Pentao, L., Guzzetta, V., Trask, B. J., . . . Patel, P. I. (1991). DNA duplication associated with Charcot–Marie–Tooth disease type 1A. *Cell, 66,* 219–232.

MacLennan, D. H., Duff, C., Zorzato, F., Fujii, J., Phillips, M., Korneluk, R.G., . . . Worton, R. G. (1990). Ryanodine receptor gene is a candidate for predisposition to malignant hyperthermia. *Nature, 343,* 559–561.

Mathews, K. D., Stephan, C. M., Laubenthal, K., Winder, T. L., Michele, D. E., Moore, S. A., & Campbell, K. P. (2011). Myoglobinuria and muscle pain are common in patients with limb-girdle muscular dystrophy 2I. *Neurology, 76,* 194–195.

Matsui, Y., Yasui, N., Kimura, T., Tsumaki, N., Kawabata, H., & Ochi, T. (1998). Genotype phenotype correlation in achondroplasia and hypochondroplasia. *Journal of Bone and Joint Surgery, British Volume 80,* 1052–1056.

McCarthy, T. V., Healy, J. M., Heffron, J. J., Lehane, M., Deufel, T., Lehmann-Horn, F., . . . Johnson, K. (1990). Localization of the malignant hyperthermia susceptibility locus to human chromosome 19q12–13.2. *Nature, 343,* 562–564.

McDonald, C. M. (2001). Peripheral neuropathies of childhood. *Physical Medicine and Rehabilitation Clinics of North America, 12,* 473–490.

McDonald, C. M. (2002). Physical activity, health impairments, and disability in neuromuscular disease. *American Journal of Physical Medicine and Rehabilitation, 81,* S108–S120.

McMillan, H. J., Darras, B. T., Kang, P. B., Saleh, F., & Jones, H. R. (2009). Pediatric monomelic amyotrophy, evidence for poliomyelitis in vulnerable populations. *Muscle & Nerve, 40,* 860–863.

Melki, J., Lefebvre, S., Burglen, L., Burlet, P., Clermont, O., Millasseau, P., . . . Le Paslier, D. (1994). De novo and inherited deletions of the 5q13 region in spinal muscular atrophies. *Science, 264,* 1474–1477.

Mendell, J. R., Goemans, N., Lowes, L. P., Alfano, L. N., Berry, K., Shao, J., . . . Eteplirsen Study Group and Telethon Foundation DMD Italian Network. (2016). Longitudinal effect of eteplirsen versus historical control on ambulation in Duchenne muscular dystrophy. *Annals of Neurology, 79,* 257–271.

Mendell, J. R., Al-Zaidy, S., Shell, R., Arnold, W. D., Rodino-Klapac, L. R., Prior, T. W., . . . Kaspar, B. K. (2017). Single-dose gene-replacement therapy for spinal muscular atrophy. *New England Journal of Medicine, 377*(18), 1713–1722.

Mercuri, E., Darras, B. T., Chiriboga, C. A., Day, J. W., Campbell, C., Connolly, A. M., . . . Cherish Study Group. (2018a). Nusinersen versus sham control in later-onset spinal muscular atrophy. *New England Journal of Medicine, 378*(7), 625–635.

Mercuri, E., Finkel, R. S., Muntoni, F., Wirth, B., Montes, J., Main, M., . . . S. M. A. Care Group. (2018b). Diagnosis and management of spinal muscular atrophy: Part 1: Recommendations for diagnosis, rehabilitation, orthopedic and nutritional care. *Neuromuscular Disorders, 28*(2), 103–115.

Merlini, L., Stagni, S. B., Marri, E., & Granata, C. (1992). Epidemiology of neuromuscular disorders in the under-20 population in Bologna Province, Italy. *Neuromuscular Disorders, 2,* 197–200.

Micallef, J., Attarian, S., Dubourg, O., Gonnaud, P. M., Hogrel, J. Y., Stojkovic, T., . . . Blin, O. (2009). Effect of ascorbic acid in patients with Charcot-Marie-Tooth disease type 1A: A multicentre, randomised, double-blind, placebo-controlled trial. *Lancet Neurology, 8*(12), 1103–1110.

Minch, C. M., & Kruse, R. W. (1998). Osteogenesis imperfecta, a review of basic science and diagnosis. *Orthopedics, 21,* 558–567; quiz 568–569.

Monaco, A. P., Neve, R. L., Colletti-Feener, C., Bertelsen, C. J., Kurnit, D. M., & Kunkel, L. M. (1986). Isolation of candidate cDNAs for portions of the Duchenne muscular dystrophy gene. *Nature, 323,* 646–650.

Moxley, R. T., 3rd, Ashwal, S., Pandya, S., Connolly, A., Florence, J., Mathews, K., . . . Wade, C. (2005). Practice parameter, corticosteroid treatment of Duchenne dystrophy, report of the Quality Standards Subcommittee of the American Academy of Neurology and the Practice Committee of the Child Neurology Society. *Neurology, 64,* 13–20.

Nicot, A. S., Toussaint, A., Tosch, V., Kretz, C., Wallgren-Petterson, C., Iwarsson, E., . . . Laporte, J. (2007). Mutations in amphiphysin 2 (BIN1) disrupt interaction with dynamin 2 and cause autosomal recessive centronuclear myopathy. *Nature Genetics, 39,* 1134–1139.

Nouraei, H., Sawatzky, B., MacGillivray, M., & Hall, J. (2017). Long-term functional and mobility outcomes for individuals with arthrogryposis multiplex congenita. *American Journal of Medical Genetics Part A, 173*(5), 1270–1278.

Nowak, K. J., Wattanasirichaigoon, D., Goebel, H. H., Wilce, M., Pelin, K., Donner, K., . . . Laing, N. G. (1999). Mutations in the skeletal muscle alpha–actin gene in patients with actin myopathy and nemaline myopathy. *Nature Genetics, 23,* 208–212.

OMIM. (2011). *Online Mendelian Inheritance in Man*. McKusick-Nathans Institute of Genetic Medicine, Johns Hopkins University, Baltimore, MD. Retrieved from http://omim.org/

Orioli, I. M., Castilla, E. E., & Barbosa-Neto, J. G. (1986). The birth prevalence rates for the skeletal dysplasias. *Journal of Medical Genetics, 23,* 328–332.

Pane, M., Staccioli, S., Messina, S., D'Amico, A., Pelliccioni, M., Mazzone, E.S., . . . Mercuri, E. (2008). Daily salbutamol in young patients with SMA type II. *Neuromuscular Disorders, 18,* 536–540.

Pearn, J. (1978). Incidence, prevalence, and gene frequency studies of chronic childhood spinal muscular atrophy. *Journal of Medical Genetics, 15,* 409–413.

Pearn, J. H. (1973). The gene frequency of acute Werdnig–Hoffmann disease (SMA type 1). A total population survey in North-East England. *Journal of Medical Genetics, 10,* 260–265.

Pelin, K., Hilpela, P., Donner, K., Sewry, C., Akkari, P.A., Wilton, S. D., . . . Wallgren-Pettersson, C. (1999). Mutations in the nebulin gene associated with autosomal recessive nemaline myopathy. *Proceedings of the National Academy of Sciences of the USA, 96,* 2305–2310.

Prior, T. W, Snyder, P. J., Rink, B. D., Pearl, D. K., Pyatt, R. E., Mihal, D. C., . . . Garner, S. (2010). Newborn and carrier screening for spinal muscular atrophy. *American Journal of Medical Genetics Part A, 152A*(7), 1608–1616.

Quane, K. A., Healy, J. M., Keating, K. E., Manning, M. B., Couch, F. J., Palmucci, L. M., . . . McCarthy, V. (1993). Mutations in the ryanodine receptor gene in central core disease and malignant hyperthermia. *Nature Genetics, 5,* 51–55.

Riggs, J. E., Bodensteiner, J. B., & Schochet, S. S., Jr. (2003). Congenital myopathies/dystrophies. *Neurological Clinics, 21,* 779–794; v–vi.

Ryan, M. M., Ilkovski, B., Strickland, C. D., Schnell, C., Sanoudou, D., Midgett, C., . . . Beggs, A. H. (2003). Clinical course correlates poorly with muscle pathology in nemaline myopathy. *Neurology, 60,* 665–673.

Sambrook, P. N., & Jones, G. (1995). Corticosteroid osteoporosis. *British Journal of Rheumatology, 34,* 8–12.

Savarirayan, R., & Rimoin, D. L. (2002). The skeletal dysplasias. *Best Practice & Research of Clinical Endocrinology & Metabolism, 16,* 547–560.

Shy, M. E. (2004). Charcot–Marie–Tooth disease, an update. *Current Opinion in Neurology, 17,* 579–585.

Siegel, I. M. (1977). Fractures of long bones in Duchenne muscular dystrophy. *Journal of Trauma, 17,* 219–222.

Stoll, C., Dott, B., Roth, M. P., & Alembik, Y. (1989). Birth prevalence rates of skeletal dysplasias. *Clinical Genetics, 35,* 88–92.

Sugarman, E. A., Nagan, N., Zhu, H., Akmaev, V. R., Zhou, Z., Rohlfs, E. M., . . . Allitto, B. A. (2012). Pan-ethnic carrier screening and prenatal diagnosis for spinal muscular atrophy: Clinical laboratory analysis of >72,400 specimens. *European Journal of Human Genetics, 20*(1), 27–32.

Tasfaout, H., Lionello, V. M., Kretz, C., Koebel, P., Messaddeq, N., Bitz, D., Cowling, B. S. (2018). Single intramuscular injection of AAV-shRNA reduces DNM2 and prevents myotubular myopathy in mice. *Molecular Therapy, 26*(4), 1082–1092.

Tracy, M. M., McRae, W., & Millichap, J. G. (2009). Graded response to thymectomy in children with myasthenia gravis. *Journal of Child Neurology, 24,* 454–459.

Trotter, T. L., & Hall, J. G. (2005). Health supervision for children with achondroplasia. *Pediatrics, 116,* 771–783.

Van Dijk, F. S., & Sillence, D. O. (2014). Osteogenesis imperfecta: clinical diagnosis, nomenclature and severity assessment. *American Journal of Medical Genetics Part A, 164A*(6), 1470–1481.

Van Essen, A. J., Busch, H. F., te Meerman, G. J., & ten Kate, L. P. (1992). Birth and population prevalence of Duchenne muscular dystrophy in The Netherlands. *Human Genetics, 88,* 258–266.

Verhamme, C., de Haan, R. J., Vermeulen, M., Baas, F., de Visser, M., & van Schaik, I. N. (2009). Oral high dose ascorbic acid treatment for one year in young CMT1A patients: A randomised, double-blind, placebo-controlled phase II trial. *BMC Medicine, 7,* 70.

von Gontard, A., Zerres, K., Backes, M., Laufersweiler-Plass, C., Wendland, C., Melchers, P., . . . Rudnik- Schöneborn, S. (2002). Intelligence and cognitive function in children and adolescents with spinal muscular atrophy. *Neuromuscular Disorders, 12,* 130–136.

Wallace, M. J., Kruse, R. W., & Shah, S. A. (2017). The spine in patients with osteogenesis imperfecta. *Journal of the American Academy of Orthopaedic Surgeons, 25*(2), 100–109.

Waller, D. K., Correa, A., Vo, T. M., Wang, Y., Hobbs, C., Langlois, P. H., . . . Hecht, J. T. (2008). The population-based prevalence of achondroplasia and thanatophoric dysplasia in selected regions of the US. *American Journal of Medical Genetics Part A, 146A*(18), 2385–2389.

Wang, C. H., Finkel, R. S., Bertini, E. S., Schroth, M., Simonds, A., Wong, B., . . . Trela, A. (2007). Consensus statement for standard of care in spinal muscular atrophy. *Journal of Child Neurology, 22,* 1027–1049.

Wattjes, M. P., Kley, R. A., & Fischer, D. (2010). Neuromuscular imaging in inherited muscle diseases. *European Radiology, 20*(10), 2447–2460.

Widmann, R. F., Bitan, F. D., Laplaza, F. J., Burke, S. W., DiMaio, M. F., & Schneider, R. (1999). Spinal deformity, pulmonary compromise, and quality of life in osteogenesis imperfecta. *Spine, 24,* 1673–1678.

Wilmshurst, J. M., Lillis, S., Zhou, H., Pillay, K., Henderson, H., Kress W, . . . Jungbluth, H. (2010). RYR1 mutations are a common cause of congenital myopathies with central nuclei. *Annals of Neurology, 68,* 717–726.

Wu, J. Y., Kuban, K. C., Allred, E., Shapiro, F., & Darras, B. T. (2005). Association of Duchenne muscular dystrophy with autism spectrum disorder. *Journal of Child Neurology, 20,* 790–795.

Zhang, Y., Chen, H. S., Khanna, V. K., De Leon, S., Phillips, M. S., Schappert, K., . . . MacLennan, D. H. (1993). A mutation in the human ryanodine receptor gene associated with central core disease. *Nature Genetics, 5,* 46–50.

CHAPTER 10 Nutrition

Lina Diaz-Calderon, Virginia Gebus, and Laurie S. Conklin

Upon completion of this chapter, the reader will

- Understand nutritional requirements and their assessment in children
- Identify how developmental disabilities modify nutritional requirements
- Recognize the fundamental role of nutrition in the growth and development of children
- Be aware of how nutritional interventions are included in a child's care plan
- Understand the importance of working with a multidisciplinary team to tailor a specific approach to nutrition support based on the child and family's needs

Food selection and preparation are major cultural characteristics of all societies, and within the context of home and family, providing and preparing meals for children expresses parental love and concern. Nutrition is the study of foods, their nutrients, and other components of the diet that affect biological processes and health (Brown, 2014). Human requirements for protein, fats, carbohydrates, vitamins, and minerals vary with age, activity level, medical diagnosis, genetic heritage, and physiological state (Institute of Medicine, 2005). For many children, a regular diet prepared by the family provides all of the nutrients, minerals, and vitamins needed for typical growth and development. In children with developmental disabilities, however, a typical diet may present challenges. For instance, as a result of motor impairments a child with cerebral palsy (CP) may have difficulty ingesting sufficient food (see Chapter 21). A child with autism spectrum disorder (ASD) may have food selectivity that results in nutritional deficiencies (see Chapter 18). Conversely, a child with Prader-Willi syndrome often engages in **hyperphagia** (pathological overeating), and a child with **meningomyelocoele** may become obese through inactivity.

The impact of nutrition is greatest during infancy and childhood, when the body is actively growing; optimizing growth and nutrition in this period can improve cognitive outcomes (Harding, Cormack, Alexander, Alsweiler, & Bloomfield, 2017). For children with developmental disabilities, however, the need for medical nutritional therapy (MNT) may be lifelong. MNT is defined as the manipulation of nutrients and dietary components to affect a disease or condition (American Dietetic Association, 2010). This therapy also takes into account the psychosocial environment in which the child lives. This chapter focuses on the nutritional needs of children with developmental disabilities and emphasizes MNT as part of a comprehensive care plan.

CASE STUDY

Abraham is a 12-year-old boy, born at 34 weeks' gestational age, who has spastic quadriplegia and chronic lung disease. He has been hospitalized several times for pneumonia. His weight plots at a *z*-score of -2.6 and height at a *z*-score of -2.7, but his BMI percentile is normal. Over time, his *z*-scores have become further from the normal range. On a cerebral palsy (CP) growth chart, stratified for age, degree of motor involvement, and tube feeding status, his weight-for-age plots less than the 20th percentile in the "zone of concern," where increased morbidity and mortality may result because of impaired nutritional status (Rempel, 2015). Abraham's parents report an intake of over 2,000 calories daily, but when observed eating a meal, Abraham has significant losses due to oropharyngeal incoordination, poor bolus formation, and inadequate control of bolus propulsion. He is noted to have gastroesophageal reflux and coughing while feeding, and meals take well over 45 minutes to complete. Abraham had a modified barium swallow study with a speech therapist, which demonstrated laryngeal penetration with thin and thickened liquids, but not with pureed consistency. A meeting to allow shared decision making was held, which included the family, physician, and registered dietician. At this meeting Abraham's risk of aspiration and effects of malnutrition on his health were discussed (Adams, Elias, & Council on Children with Disabilities, 2014), as well as the benefits of MNT. As a result, a nasogastric tube was placed for administration of supplemental feedings overnight and boluses during the day (Kuperminc et al., 2013). Abraham continues to consume and enjoy pureed foods in smaller amounts. Water was added to his feeding regimen in order to meet his full fluid needs daily. The management of constipation with this increase in fluids and the addition of a stool softener has improved his tolerance of feedings. Abraham continues to see his dietician for regular guidance regarding his trajectory of weight gain and adjustments to his feeding regimen to suit the family's daily schedule.

Thought Questions:

Who are the team members that contribute to nutritional evaluation and support for children with disabilities, and what roles do they play? What are some of the most common nutritional issues for children with developmental disabilities? What are some ways to provide proper nutrition to a child who is unable to ingest food and drink in a typical way?

TYPICAL GROWTH DURING CHILDHOOD

Nutritional requirements for infants and children are determined by what is needed to produce optimal growth and development. The average full-term infant weighs 3.4 kilograms (about 7.5 pounds) at birth and gains 20 to 30 grams (about 1 ounce) each day for several months. By 4–6 months of age, the infant's birth weight has doubled, and by 12 months, it has tripled (National Center for Health Statistics, 2000, 2008a; Weintraub, 2011). As the child becomes more active, weight gain slows to about 2.5 kilograms per year until approximately 9–10 years of age, when the adolescent growth spurt begins. Length advances at a slower pace than weight, increasing by 50% during the first year of life (from an average of 50 centimeters or about 19.5 inches at birth), doubling by 4 years of age, and tripling by 13 years of age. Age-based reference ranges for height velocity in U.S. children have been described (Kelly et al., 2014). Another measure of growth, increase in head circumference, parallels brain growth. Head circumference increases by approximately 1 centimeter per month during the first year of life. Brain weight doubles by 1 year of age and quadruples by 3 years of age (Dekaban, 1978; National Center for Health Statistics, 2000, 2008a).

In addition to the basic measures of growth (i.e., weight, length, and head circumference), a number of useful growth indices have been developed to provide a more nuanced and clinically relevant way of measuring a child's nutritional status. Among these, the formula used most often is the **body mass index** (BMI), a measure of the relationship between weight and stature (length) for children older than 2 years of age that was developed by the Centers for Disease Control and Prevention (CDC; National Center for Health Statistics, 2010; see Table 10.1). By placing weight into the context of a child's overall size and body habitus, the BMI can be a useful screening tool to assess whether a child is overweight or underweight (NCD Risk Factor Collaboration, 2017). The measurements of weight and stature can be plotted on the World Health Organization (WHO) growth charts for infants and children from 0 to 2 years of age (https://www.cdc.gov/growthcharts/who_charts.htm), the CDC growth charts for children and adolescents from 2 to 20 years of age (https://www.cdc.gov/growthcharts/clinical_charts.htm), or the CP growth charts that include children up to 20 years of age and separates them using the Gross Motor Function Class System. The CP growth chart allows children to be plotted based on a population with similar functional disabilities. When using these charts, weight between the 20th and 95th percentile is acceptable (Brooks, Day, Shavelle, & Strauss, 2011). However, some children may

Table 10.1. Growth parameters and nutrition assessment[a]

Growth parameter	Utility in nutrition assessment
Weight for age *z*-score	Key parameter for monitoring short- and long-term changes in nutritional status
Length for age *z*-score	Key measure of linear growth and assessment of long-term nutritional status
Head circumference for age (inches or centimeters)	Key proxy for brain growth
Weight-to-height proportionality *z*-score	Provides a rough estimate of nutritional status by relating weight to stature; birth to 24 months of age (WHO growth charts)
Body mass index *z*-score (BMI = weight in pounds × 703 / height in inches × height in inches)	Provides an estimate of body fat relative to weight and height; > 2 years of age (CDC growth charts)
Rate of weight and length accretion (change in weight or length over a given time interval)	Precise method of tracking patterns and rates of growth
Body fat indices	Direct measures of body fat using reliable, specialized equipment and techniques

[a]May apply specialty (disease-specific) growth charts for growth assessment.

have an altered body composition that can skew these measurements and interpretations; for instance, a child with CP may have microcephaly or contractures. In these situations, triceps skinfold thickness and mid-upper arm circumference are used as a proxy for body composition (i.e., lean and fat mass; Addo & Himes, 2010; Addo, Himes, & Zemel, 2017; Mramba et al., 2017). A triceps skinfold measurement is a screen for depleted fat stores. A mid-arm circumference assesses a child's muscle mass, bone, and fat reserves and can be measured in a reproducible way (Rempel, 2015). While these measurements require specialized equipment and techniques that are not as widely available, they do offer an even more accurate way of assessing this critical aspect of a child's nutritional status.

NUTRITIONAL GUIDELINES

Research-based nutrition guidelines published by the National Academies of Sciences estimate daily intake of specific vitamins and minerals based on age and gender (Institute of Medicine, 1997, 2001, 2005, 2010). Energy and protein intake recommendations were updated in 2006 (Institute of Medicine of the National Academies, 2006) and have been incorporated into the nutrients included in food labels. They are also reflected in the standard growth charts commonly used by health care professionals (National Centers for Health Statistics, 2000; WHO Multicentre Growth Reference Study Group, 2006). The concept of a "balanced diet" derives from these standard nutritional guidelines and is based on the notion that typical children will require specific amounts and proportions of certain nutrients. Although these guidelines are a good starting point for determining the nutritional requirements for children with disabilities, adjustments are often required. In some cases, an apparently "unbalanced" diet is appropriate for a child with a specific condition. An all-liquid diet or a diet of only a few different foods may be recommended for a child with limited oral-motor skills. For a child with a special metabolic condition for example, it may be critically important that certain elements of the diet be reduced, eliminated, or enhanced to avoid the buildup of toxic metabolites. Table 10.2 provides other examples of how specific dietary components and calorie content can be manipulated to address the special needs of specific medical conditions and disabilities (Isaacs & Zand, 2007).

NUTRITIONAL ISSUES IN CHILDREN WITH DEVELOPMENTAL DISABILITIES

Children with developmental disabilities have many of the same nutrition issues as typically developing children. These include being overweight or underweight, refusing to eat or drink a variety of foods and beverages, and fighting for control with parents at mealtimes. However, children with neurological impairments are at risk for multiple nutrition-related problems including poor linear growth, micronutrient deficiencies, and low bone mineral density (Romano et al., 2017). They are also prone to more serious and varied problems that are especially related to impaired oral motor skills (e.g., swallowing incoordination among children with cerebral palsy), medical problems (e.g., chronic gastroesophageal reflux among children with hypotonia or a history of prematurity; see Box 10.1), delayed gastric emptying, and food refusal (e.g., dislike of certain food textures among children with ASD; Bandini et al., 2010; Romano et al., 2017). As a result, common nutritional

Table 10.2. Dietary adjustments for specific medical conditions and disabilities

Dietary element	Condition	Specific adjustment required
Fats	Smith-Lemli-Opitz syndrome	Cholesterol (purified form) increased
	Long-chain fatty acid oxidation disorders	Fat decreased, greater than 75% of nutrition from fat-free foods
	Uncontrollable seizures	Ketogenic diet, fat increased
Proteins	Phenylketonuria, maple syrup urine disease	Natural protein decreased by more than 80%, addition of protein substitutes, vitamins, and minerals
Carbohydrates	Glycogen storage disease type 1	Specific types of sugar (e.g., sucrose, fructose, galactose, lactose) decreased
	Galactosemia, lactose intolerance	Specific types of sugar (e.g., galactose, lactose) decreased
	Hereditary fructose intolerance	Specific types of sugar (e.g., fructose) decreased
Vitamins and minerals	Vitamin B_{12} disorders	Vitamin B12 increased, often protein content decreased
	Iron-deficiency anemia	Foods rich in iron increased or supplemental iron added
	Rickets	Foods rich in calcium and vitamin D increased or supplements added
Energy (calorie)	Obesity and overweight	Calories decreased 10%–30% (fats, proteins, carbohydrates), activity level increased
	Hypotonia in Down syndrome or Prader-Willi syndrome (if obese)	Calories decreased 30%–40% (fats, proteins, carbohydrates)

advice for typically developing children may not be appropriate for children with developmental disabilities (see Table 10.3). Instead, diets may need to be targeted to specific conditions and/or developmental disabilities, as illustrated in Table 10.2.

Undernutrition

Pediatric malnutrition (undernutrition) is defined as an imbalance between nutrient requirement and intake resulting in cumulative deficits of energy, protein, or micronutrients that may negatively affect growth, development, or other relevant outcomes (Mehta et al., 2013). Recognizing undernutrition and malnutrition in children with disabilities may be difficult because nutrient needs and activity levels may be higher or lower than typical, as noted above (Penagini et al., 2015). For example, short stature is usually not a sign of limited nutrition in children with Turner syndrome (Cohen et al., 2008). Thin appearance is common in spastic quadriplegia (a severe form of cerebral palsy; Motil, 2010; see Chapter 21). However, concern about the adequacy of energy intake is more common in children with disabilities than in typically developing children. Needs for increased energy and protein are commonly observed in children with such conditions as prematurity (Harding et al., 2017), cystic fibrosis (Sullivan & Mascarenhas, 2017), and Rett syndrome (Leonard et al., 2013). In these cases, the goal of MNT is to provide extra calories and protein (as food or nutritional supplements) to achieve adequate weight gain and linear growth.

Poor Linear Growth and Low Bone Mineral Density

Typically, an important measure of sufficient nutrition in children is adequate linear growth. Yet, many developmental disabilities are associated with atypical growth patterns. As a result, it may be difficult to determine whether a child with a developmental disability who has apparent inadequate growth is truly undernourished (Marchand, Motil, & NASPGHAN Committee on Nutrition, 2006). Extra calories and nutrients may not normalize linear growth in certain medical conditions that are known to be associated with short stature, such as translocation chromosomal disorders, Turner syndrome, Down syndrome, Williams syndrome, chromosome 22q11 microdeletion syndromes (i.e., velocardiofacial syndrome and DiGeorge syndrome), meningomyelocoele (Liusuwan, Widman, Abresch, Styne, & McDonald, 2007), chronic kidney disease (Rodig et al., 2014), and fetal alcohol syndrome (Del Campo & Jones, 2017). These syndromes are described in Appendix B. Diagnosis-specific growth charts are based on smaller population groups than the standard growth charts for typically developing children, yet they help set realistic expectations for growth after a diagnosis has been made (Arvay et al., 2005).

If a child is consistently plotted below the 3rd percentile, it can be difficult to make comparisons over time. Growth charts that allow comparison of units of standard deviation from norms for reference age groups (*z*-score comparisons) are recommended when assessing growth and nutritional status in these children.

BOX 10.1 EVIDENCE-BASED PRACTICE

Gastroesophageal Reflux Disease

Gastroesophageal reflux disease (GERD) is commonly seen in children with neurological impairment, with an incidence as high as 70% (Bayram et al., 2016). Gastroesophageal reflux (GER) involves the passage of gastric contents into the esophagus with or without regurgitation and vomiting. GERD occurs when GER leads to troublesome symptoms, which vary with age and degree of neurological impairment, and/or complications such as esophagitis, Barrett metaplasia, or esophageal stenosis (Rosen et al., 2018).

The diagnosis of GERD is based primarily on clinical suspicion, which can be strengthened by additional diagnostic investigations that aim to quantify and qualify GERD. A detailed history and physical exam should be obtained to assess "red flag" symptoms and signs that suggest an alternative underlying disease other than GERD that needs to be addressed and treated appropriately (Rosen et al., 2018). Objective testing for the diagnosis of GERD in children, such as esophageal pH or pH/multichannel intraluminal impedance monitoring, are useful to

1. Correlate persistent troublesome symptoms with acid and non-acid gastroesophageal reflux events
2. Clarify the role of acid and non-acid reflux in the etiology of esophagitis and other signs of symptoms suggestive of GERD
3. Determine the efficacy of acid suppression therapy

However, these tests can be difficult to perform in certain children with neurological impairment, and treatment for GERD may be started based on clinical suspicion.

Treatment for GERD involves nonpharmacological, pharmacological, and surgical options. Feeding modifications, including formula or food thickeners, reduced feeding volumes or more frequent feedings, and hydrolyzed or amino-acid based formulas, may improve some symptoms of GERD (Rosen et al., 2018). Feeding modifications should be carefully implemented based on the child's neurological impairment, oral-motor skills, and feeding route. A 4- to 8-week trial of histamine-2 receptor antagonists or proton pump inhibitors with careful clinical follow up is also acceptable management in patients with neurological impairment (Romano et al., 2017). Laparoscopic antireflux surgery, mainly Nissen fundoplication, is currently accepted as the gold standard surgical procedure for children with severe, medically refractory GERD (Fukahori et al., 2016).

Points to Remember

1. Diagnosis of GERD is based on clinical suspicion. A detailed history and physical exam should be obtained to rule out alternative diseases that may present in a similar manner.
2. Nonpharmacological, pharmacological, and surgical treatments should be tailored according to patient's symptoms, neurological impairment, and GERD-associated complications.

Table 10.3. Common nutrition advice that may not apply to children with disabilities

Common nutrition advice	How this advice may not apply to children with disabilities
"If she won't eat now, don't worry; she will eat when she is hungry."	The child may not respond to hunger cues.
	Hunger may be masked by fatigue, medications, or specific medical conditions.
"Don't worry. Others in the family are small."	Genetic and hereditary factors are important to identify, but many "small" children with disabilities are often undernourished due to lack of sufficient intake.
"He's just picky."	Behaviorally based feeding problems are common in children with disabilities.
	Some food refusals are key symptoms of an underlying medical problem.
"He's failing to thrive."	Many disabilities are associated with atypical growth patterns (disability-specific growth charts allow for more accurate interpretation of growth patterns).
"He eats the same foods all the time. He should eat a variety of foods."	Monotonous self-restricted eating patterns are common in children with developmental disabilities, especially those who have autism spectrum disorder.
	Some medical conditions (especially metabolic disorders) require a limited range of food types to prevent complications.

A *z*-score allows for quantification and longitudinal follow up of measurements that consistently fall above or below the upper limits of measurement on a growth chart (Becker et al., 2015). Total calorie deficit may not be the only cause for poor growth; protein and specific micronutrient deficiencies may also contribute to this problem (i.e., zinc, vitamin B_{12}, vitamin D, and iron).

Low bone mineral density is prevalent in neurologically impaired children, and it may affect linear growth (Romano et al., 2017). Limited ambulation, long-term administration of anti-epileptic drugs, reduced sun exposure, and poor nutrient intake are all factors that contribute to low bone mineral density. It is important to evaluate and optimize the child's bone health by providing an adequate intake of calcium, vitamin D, and phosphorus and promoting physical activity with the aid of a therapist (Golden, Abrams, & Committee on Nutrition, 2014). Children at risk for low bone mineral density should be evaluated using dual-energy radiograph absorptiometry (DXA) (Bianchi et al., & Clinical Society for Clinical Densitometry, 2013). Scans of the lateral distal femur are valuable for children with immobilization disorders or contractures who cannot be positioned for a spine or whole-body DXA (Bachrach, Gordon, & AAP Section on Endocrinology, 2016). Serum levels of 25-OH vitamin D, calcium, phosphorous, and parathyroid hormone also should be monitored.

Obesity

Children are also considered malnourished if they consume too much energy. Obesity is caused by excessive energy intake relative to energy expenditure and is typically defined, using the CDC growth chart, by a BMI greater than the 95th percentile for age. Notably, BMI includes assumptions about stature and body composition that may not be appropriate for certain children with disabilities. For example, **scoliosis** may interfere with accurate height measurements, which, in turn, can affect the calculation of the BMI. The American Academy of Pediatrics (Barlow & Expert Committee, 2007) provides guidelines for prevention, assessment, and treatment of overweight and obese children. Yet, some of these recommendations may not apply to children with neurological impairments who have varied levels of activity and different comorbidities that may affect food intake. Therefore, it is crucial to have serial monitoring of weight gain and screening for obesity-related complications including dyslipidemia, diabetes, hypertension, and nonalcoholic fatty liver disease in these children and adjust their nutritional care plan to prevent overweight and obesity. More research is needed to better understand unique risk factors and interventions necessary to maintain a healthy body weight in children with developmental disabilities (Curtin, Must, Phillips, & Bandini, 2017). It is important to remember that cultural beliefs and practices may influence parental perceptions of their children's health status and feeding behaviors, and parents may have different definitions of what they consider to be "healthy." Assessing the family's knowledge and perceptions about health, social supports and networks, hunger cues, and healthful diets may assist health care providers in communicating health issues more sensitively and respectfully (Pena et al., 2012).

When Developmental Disabilities Limit Eating

Children with developmental disabilities may lack an appetite or have physical difficulties in eating. In these situations, mealtime, rather than being a pleasure, becomes an aversive experience for both the child and parents. It is thus imperative to identify the root causes of the eating problem and to design an appropriate therapy program. A child unable to eat because of fatigue and weakness resulting from a neuromuscular disability merits a different approach than a child who refuses to eat as a consequence of behavioral or cognitive issues. Children with dyskinetic cerebral palsy for instance may have such severe difficulty chewing and swallowing that they may risk aspiration pneumonia as well as undernutrition. In this case, nutritional therapy might be directed at providing alternative routes for nutrition, such as **gastrostomy** tube formula feedings (Romano et al., 2017). The child's risk of aspiration and degree of oral motor dysfunction can be studied by video-fluoroscopic assessment of chewing and swallowing function using different food and beverage textures and various feeding positions (Romano et al., 2017). A multidisciplinary team should perform careful assessment of feeding difficulties in children with developmental disabilities (Kerzner et al., 2015; see Chapter 29). Speech and language therapy and occupational therapy are often an important part of treating feeding problems.

Children with ASD may have severe and persistent restricted food preferences. However, a study by Edmond, Emmet, Steer, and Golding in 2010 showed that while children with ASD may have decreased variability in their diets, adequate energy intake is maintained, resulting in typical growth. Behavior management techniques may be utilized to gradually add new food items to the menu of the child with ASD (see Chapter 18). Such techniques may involve offering rewards for trying new foods or encouraging the child to participate in food preparation.

MEDICAL NUTRITIONAL THERAPY

The overall goal of MNT is to achieve the child's growth potential and maintain adequate nutritional status. It is crucial to have a multidisciplinary team (physician, registered dietitians, nurse, social worker, and occupational and speech therapists) that works with the family to assess the child's underlying medical condition and nutritional status and develops an individualized plan for nutritional interventions that optimizes the child's health.

Nutritional Assessment and Care Plan

The tools of MNT are the nutritional assessment and care plan that is customized to the needs of each child. A nutritional assessment usually answers the following questions:

1. Is the child being fed a diet that meets his or her nutritional requirements?
2. Is the child growing as expected for his or her age, gender, and condition?
3. Is there a feeding or eating problem interfering with growth or with meeting nutritional requirements?
4. Does the child require alternative means of nutritional support? (Riddick-Grisham, 2004, p. 328)

The nutritional assessment is the first step in the process of documenting a child's status. This involves the steps outlined in Table 10.4; the measurement and interpretation of growth parameters are defined in Table 10.1. If a child's nutritional status is not optimal, recommendations are made to improve the diet and feeding or eating practices.

Table 10.4. Elements of a nutrition assessment

Review the child's medical history (including diagnosis, laboratory findings, medications used, and developmental levels).
Assess and interpret the child's growth parameters (see Table 10.1).
Obtain the child's dietary history from caregivers (including intake patterns for food and drink, portion sizes, meal duration, and use of supplements).
Analyze and interpret the dietary intake information, based on the child's age and gender, for macronutrients (protein, fats, and carbohydrates), micronutrients (vitamins and minerals), fluids, and other dietary components (e.g., dietary fiber); computer dietary analysis programs can be used.
Summarize impressions of the child's nutritional status and the adequacy of his or her diet; make recommendations and referrals.

The nutrition care plan articulates recommendations and spells out monitoring and follow-up needs. Table 10.5 shows common interventions found in a nutrition care plan. In addition to offering general dietary and feeding recommendations, a well-developed nutrition care plan addresses the role of food in the family life and in its culture, taking into consideration their meal and snack patterns, food choices, and food preparation. When estimating daily energy requirements, it should also take into account that parents may overestimate or overreport a child's caloric intake. For children with cerebral palsy, their nutrition care plan should account for calorie losses due to gastroesophageal reflux or retained exaggerated infant reflexes like tonic bite, tongue, or jaw thrust. Furthermore, plans should factor in a child's degree of neurological disability, mobility, feeding difficulties, mode of nutritional support, and the need for weight gain or weight loss (Shaikhkhalil & Meyers, 2015). Decreased activity may lead to overnutrition, especially in children who are fed by feeding tube. Lower calorie formulas with adequate protein and micronutrients should be used instead of diluting the formula. If obesity is a family problem, the weight loss plan should involve changing the entire family's eating patterns. If the family culture involves ingesting fatty and fried foods, a plan should be developed with the family to incorporate different cooking patterns. When providing food is equated by the parents to providing love, emotional needs may

Table 10.5. Sample interventions found in a nutrition care plan

Analyze and interpret home intake diet record.
Recommend meal and snack schedules or timing.
Counter side effects from medications (e.g., increased appetite, effect on taste).
Prevent overweight or underweight.
Monitor planned weight gain, weight loss, or catch-up growth.
Modify diets for specific nutrients, such as low protein, high calorie, or low fat.
Reinforce breast feeding, infant formula, or formula preparation steps.
Select foods to address food texture problems or avoid choking.
Manage food refusals, food jags, or other food behaviors.
Demonstrate how to determine portion sizes and measure foods.
Order special formulas or supplements.
Reinforce signs of hunger, fullness, and right pace of eating or feeding.
Document food insecurity and refer the family to community nutrition programs.
Coordinate with other health care providers and educators.
Complete referrals for the Special Supplemental Nutrition Program for Women, Infants, and Children (WIC) as well as for early intervention services or other providers.

be interfering with appropriate nutritional intake. If food is used as a behavioral reinforcer, another equally effective non-food reinforcer (e.g., attention) may need to be identified and implemented.

Methods of Nutritional Support

Oral food is the preferred method of feeding children. However, some children may require enteral nutritional support. Enteral tube feeding is necessary in children who 1) cannot meet their energy, fluid, or nutrient needs orally; 2) are at risk for aspiration; 3) have oral motor feeding difficulties; or 4) have difficulties with medication administration (Monczka, 2015; see Box 10.2 for more examples). The most common developmental disabilities that require nutritional support include cerebral palsy (e.g., spastic quadriplegia), progressive neurologic disorders (e.g., Tay-Sachs disease), poorly controlled seizure disorders (e.g., Lennox-Gastaut syndrome), and certain inborn errors of metabolism (e.g., urea cycle disorders) (Monczka, 2015). Current clinical and nutritional status of the child, length of time enteral feedings are likely to be required, and the type of feeding regimen that may best fit the needs of the child and family should be considered when determining the type of enteral access (Shaikhkhalil & Meyers, 2015). Nasogastric tube feeding is used for short-term nutritional support (less than 12 weeks) or in children who are awaiting gastrostomy tube placement. A gastrostomy tube can be placed surgically or endoscopically; it allows direct access to the stomach through the anterior wall and direct enteral administration of feedings (Abdelhadi, Rahe, & Lyman, 2016). Gastrostomy tube feeding can help bypass some eating difficulties and decrease the family's psychological stress around nutritional issues. Children at high risk for aspiration due to neurologic or swallowing dysfunction, anatomical abnormalities, or gastrointestinal dysmotility may benefit from tube feedings that bypass the stomach (i.e., gastrojejunal, also called GJ-tubes). It is crucial to provide detailed education to the child's family and other caregivers about feeding tubes and site care (Table 10.6; Abdelhadi, Rahe, & Lyman, 2016).

Establishing a feeding regimen to optimize a child's nutritional status requires assessment of 1) the child's medical condition, 2) the goal of growth rate, 3) the previous history of feeding tolerance, and 4) the family's daily schedule. Multiple bolus feedings (a set amount of nutrition given via nasogastric or gastrostomy tube over a short period of time) throughout the day is the preferred enteral feeding regimen as opposed to continuous feedings. This simulates the physiological response to feeding and allows for a convenient and flexible schedule for caregivers. For some children with bolus feeding intolerance (marked by abdominal distention or discomfort, vomiting, or frequent regurgitation) resulting from delayed gastric emptying or for children at high risk for aspiration, continuous postpyloric feedings or jejunal feedings may be required (Abdelhadi, Rahe, & Lyman, 2016; Shaikhkhalil & Meyers, 2015).

BOX 10.2 INTERDISCIPLINARY CARE

The Multidisciplinary Care Team of a Child Receiving Enteral Tube Feedings: Role of the Nurse

A multidisciplinary team approach is critical when managing the care of a child who receives feedings delivered by enteral tube, typically including involvement by a physician, nurse, occupational therapist, speech therapist, physical therapist, registered dietician, and pharmacist. The nurse plays a particularly important role in this team and provides the following care:

- Teaches home and school caregivers how to prepare and administer enteral formula
- Provides emotional support for caregivers, identifying family stressors and anxiety associated with tube feeding
- Provides coordination and technical support while teaching about enteral access device placement, management, and troubleshooting if problems arise
- Assesses the health literacy of the caregiver and comprehension of information, adjusting the delivery of information if needed
- Works with caregivers to understand and use formula delivery methods like enteral pumps
- Works to balance calories consumed orally with those delivered enterally, especially when a child is transitioning off enteral feedings
- Communicates with home caregivers regarding changes in the feeding plan

Table 10.6. Feeding tubes care and troubleshooting issues

Feeding tube	Site care	When to be concerned
Nasogastric	Secure the tube to the child's face with hypoallergenic adhesion products. Fix excess tubing to the back of the child to keep out of sight and prevent accidental dislodgement.	1. Vomiting with feedings. 2. Increase in abdominal distention. 3. Respiratory distress during feedings. 4. Yellow drainage from the nostril (move the tube to the opposite nostril and assess for sinusitis).
Gastrostomy	Wash skin with soap and water. Keep area dry and clean. Rotate tube once or twice daily. Replace with a new tube every 12 weeks after health provider has done first tube change.	1. Dislodgement: Management is based on the time from placement. 2. Pain with feeds could indicate an infection or misplaced tube. 3. Erosion, erythema, and induration of the surrounding skin. 4. Increase in abdominal distention—may vent the gastric port to allow air to come out to alleviate distention. 5. Respiratory distress during feedings.
Gastrojejunostomy	Wash skin with soap and water. Keep area dry and clean. Never rotate. Provide continuous formula drip only via jejunal port.	1. Same as above. 2. Vomiting formula could indicate jejunal port has migrated back to the stomach.

Table 10.7 provides a sample dietary intake for a child with spastic quadriplegia who receives a combination of oral, bolus, and continuous feedings via a gastrostomy tube.

Nutrition Support Formulas

A wide range of formulas are available as food replacements, food supplements, and nutrition support as described in Table 10.8. These differ from infant formulas in terms of energy content, **osmolarity** (concentration of a solution), and the level of supplemented vitamins and minerals. Nutrition support formulas differ from one another in specific nutrients, caloric density, intended use, and mode of administration. Children older than 1 year of age who require nutritional supplementation may be transitioned to pediatric formulas (intended for children up to 10 years old) that provide 30 calories per fluid ounce as compared with regular infant formulas that provide 20 calories per fluid ounce. Children older than age 10 may use a formula intended for adults (Joeckel & Phillips, 2009). Protein-free or carbohydrate-free formulas employed in inborn errors of metabolism entail additional arrangements (see Chapter 16). They cannot be used alone as they create a nutritional deficiency; they need to be mixed with other formulas or foods (Isaacs & Zand, 2007).

Table 10.7. Sample intake and feeding schedule for a child with a limited ability to eat by mouth and supplemented feedings via gastrostomy tube

6:30 a.m.	Stop night feeding pump
9:30 a.m.	Oral snack at school: milk in a cup and spoon-fed applesauce
11:45 a.m.	School lunch: modified soft texture, 30% self-feeding
1:00 p.m.	Gastrostomy feeding of 8 fluid ounces of complete nutritional supplement
3:30 p.m.	After-school snack at home: self-fed cookie and milk in a cup
6:00 p.m.	Supper with family: mashed potato with gravy on a spoon and juice in a cup
8:30 p.m.	Start night feeding of 50 milliliters per hour complete nutritional supplement, providing 40% of daily calories and 60% of daily protein intake

SPECIAL NUTRITIONAL CONCERNS IN CHILDREN WITH DISABILITIES

Children with developmental disabilities may require specialized diets to address nutritional concerns associated with their disability. Common nutritional concerns associated with specific developmental disabilities are listed in Table 10.9. In most cases, families of children with specialized diets benefit from the involvement of a registered dietitian who can help monitor the diets and provide consultative support to schools and other agencies. A multidisciplinary team, which should include a nurse, dietician, and pharmacist, among other professionals, will ensure appropriate implementation of dietary recommendations.

Therapeutic Diets

Low-protein diets, used for certain inborn errors of metabolism, and the **ketogenic diet**, used in some children with intractable epilepsy, provide examples of customized diets that differ in composition and goals.

Table 10.8. Selected formulas for children with disabilities

Formulas and their components	Use based on diagnosis or condition
Standard infant formulas; 20 calories per fluid ounce[a]	Full-term newborns up to 1 year
Premature transitional formula; 22 calories per fluid ounce[a]	Discharge formula for infants with birth weight of < 1,800 grams, on limited volume intake or a history of osteoporosis or poor growth
Complete nutritional supplements; 30 calories per fluid ounce[a]	Meal or snack substitutes
	Increase calories
	Ensure intake of specific nutrients (e.g., protein)
Formulas modified in the balance of nutrients; these are not used alone	Protein free: protein-restricted diets
	Carbohydrate restricted: ketogenic diet
	Fat altered: diets for gastrointestinal disorders or long-chain fatty acid oxidation disorders
	Specific amino acids removed: phenylketonuria

[a]Calories per fluid ounce can be adjusted based on a child's needs.

Table 10.9. Common nutrition concerns of particular developmental disabilities

Prematurity-related nutrition problems, likely in the first 3 years	Formula changes to accommodate medical problems
	Delayed self-feeding and oral-motor dysfunction
	Rate of growth corrected for preterm birth
	Difficulty with setting feeding schedules
	Variable appetite, especially with illness
	Gastrointestinal problems (constipation, gastroesophageal reflux, reduced appetite, milk protein allergy)
Neuromuscular disorders (e.g., spinal muscular atrophy)	Difficulty gaining weight, particularly with frequent illness
	Excessive weight gain due to immobility and high calorie intake
	Underweight with low muscle mass
	Short stature
	Gastrointestinal issues (constipation, gastroesophageal reflux, gastroparesis)
	Feeding difficulties or oral-motor dysfunction limiting food types
	Need to consider supplementation or gastrostomy tube placement
	Unusual growth patterns
Developmental delays/intellectual disability (e.g., Down syndrome, Prader-Willi syndrome)	Underweight or overweight
	Unusual level of activity, either higher or lower
	Delayed self-feeding skills
	Self-restricted diet
	Difficulty identifying hunger and fullness
	Constipation, which may or may not be alleviated with dietary fiber
Attention-deficit/hyperactivity disorder	Distractibility interfering with eating and sitting during meal times
	Lack of structured meal and snack patterns
	Possible decreased appetite as a medication side effect
Epilepsy	Difficulty with socializing at meals
	A growth plateau is likely, even if eating well
	Possible changes in appetite as medication side effect
	A post-seizure state is likely to interfere with meals and energy intake
	Unusual growth patterns in children with poorly controlled seizures

Both types of diet are similar in that they require close monitoring and may cause behavior problems around food at home, in school, and at restaurants. Table 10.10 shows a sample daily nutritional intake for a 10-year old with phenylketonuria (PKU) who is complying well with a low-protein diet.

As a result of the effectiveness of early dietary treatment for PKU, the list of inborn errors of metabolism treated early in life through diet has increased markedly (Evans, Truby, & Boneh, 2017; Frazier et al., 2014; Singh et al., 2013). As newborn screening and knowledge of dietary interventions expands, the focus has shifted toward developing evidence- and consensus-based guidelines for nutritional management of inherited metabolic disorders, with a goal of optimizing longer-term outcomes for patients (Singh, Rohr, & Splett, 2013; Osara et al., 2015).

Another example of medical treatment through dietary modification is shown in Table 10.11, which presents a sample dietary intake for an older child on a ketogenic diet. A ketogenic diet is deliberately designed to be very high in fat content and very low in carbohydrates, while providing adequate calories and protein for growth. This diet results in the accumulation of ketones in the body; ketones are thought to be the mechanism of improved seizure control (see Chapter 22). The sample diet shown is for an older child who eats regular foods; however, some children on the ketogenic diet are not able to consume food by mouth and rely on specific fat-modified formulas that are administered through a gastrostomy tube (Zupec-Kania & Spellman, 2008).

Table 10.10. Sample diet for a 10 year old with phenylketonuria (PKU)

Breakfast	1/2 cup cereal
	6 fluid ounces rice milk
	1 low-protein blueberry muffin
	8 fluid ounces PKU formula
Lunch	Medium garden salad with 2 tablespoons of ranch dressing
	Small order of french fries
	12 fluid ounces non-diet soft drink
After-school snack	Baked apple slices with brown sugar and cinnamon
	8 fluid ounces PKU formula
Dinner	Hot dog bun with 1 slice low-protein cheese, mustard, ketchup, and pickles
	Pear
	8 fluid ounces PKU formula

Table 10.11. Sample ketogenic diet: Intake for an older child on a 4-to-1 (fat-to-protein plus carbohydrate) ratio

Breakfast	Omelet made with 35 grams egg, 35 grams butter, 20 grams mushroom
Lunch	55 grams beef bologna
	15 grams black olives
	30 grams mayonnaise
	20 grams tomato
After-school snack	Carbohydrate-free multivitamin and mineral pill
	20 grams strawberries
	55 grams heavy whipping cream
Dinner	25 grams chicken breast cooked in 25 grams butter
	25 grams avocado
	25 grams green beans cooked in 20 grams butter
Snack	50 grams carrot sticks
	25 grams mayonnaise

Food Allergies

While there is not a clear linkage of food allergies to developmental disabilities, food allergies are common in the general population, and, as such, are also prevalent in children with disabilities. A food allergy is an adverse reaction to food caused by an immune response. The most common food allergens in the United States are milk, soy, egg, wheat, peanut, tree nut, fish, and seafood. Poor nutritional outcomes may occur in children with food allergies as a consequence of diet restrictions that may severely impact nutrient intake. Nutrition education should focus on foods to be avoided. Nutritionally complete hypoallergenic formulas are available to supplement a child's intake and ensure adequate growth (Meyer et al., 2016). Eosinophilic esophagitis (EoE) is a specific type of allergy in which inflammation of the esophagus may lead to feeding aversion or picky eating. EoE is one of the most common conditions diagnosed during the assessment of feeding problems in children (Furuta & Katzka, 2015).

Constipation

Gastrointestinal dysfunction is a frequent concern for children with developmental disabilities. Immobility, low enteral fluid intake, and medication side effects are all factors that contribute to constipation, especially in children and adults with cerebral palsy. Increasing dietary fiber by substituting whole wheat bread for white bread and fresh unpeeled apples for apple juice, are often suggested to families dealing with children with disabilities who are fed by mouth. For tube-fed children, providing a fiber-containing formula and additional fluid in the form of free water via gastrostomy or jejunostomy tube may alleviate constipation. Constipation that is refractory to increasing fiber in the diet can be treated using stool softeners or stimulant laxatives (lactulose, polyethylene glycol or milk of magnesia, bisacodyl, or senna; Tabbers et al., 2014).

Celiac Disease

Celiac disease may present with symptoms of diarrhea, abdominal pain, anemia, constipation, or poor growth. Celiac disease involves a permanent sensitivity to gluten, the protein portion of wheat and rye. Some children with celiac disease also have to avoid oats. Children with Down syndrome, Turner syndrome, and Williams syndrome have a higher incidence of celiac disease than children in the typically developing population (Hill et al., 2016). In affected children, a gluten-free diet has to be followed strictly, even when children are asymptomatic. The North American Society for Pediatric Gastroenterology, Hepatology, and Nutrition (Hill et al., 2016) provides detailed guidelines for the evaluation and chronic management of children with celiac disease. Many processed foods from both grocery stores and restaurants must be avoided because they contain wheat and other flours for fillers and binding agents. Potato-, soy-, and rice-based products can be used as substitutes for regular breads and pastas, although these specialized foods may be prohibitively expensive for many families.

Dietary Self-Restriction

Dietary self-restriction is a common problem in children with developmental disabilities, manifesting as food refusal, selectivity by type of food or food texture, oral-motor delay, and **dysphagia** (see Chapter 29). As noted previously, ASD is particularly associated with a selective eating pattern (Hyman et al., 2012; Kerzner et al., 2015). Sensitivities to food colors, textures, and temperature are often reported as leading to food refusal. When not given preferred foods, the child completely refuses to eat and may have temper tantrums. The child may also prefer to drink rather than to eat foods, and so a high proportion of total calories may come from one type of drink. Interventions to improve the child's diet may include providing a complete vitamin and mineral supplement and adding new foods one at a time, offering them many times (15 to 20 times) over 1–2 months paired with positive reinforcers (i.e., foods the child likes; see Chapter 34). Usually children with ASD have typical growth and caloric intake despite their unusual eating habits.

NUTRITION WITHIN COMPLEMENTARY HEALTH APPROACHES

In response to the large number of children with developmental disabilities, many products, treatments, and medicines have been created to improve nutrition. Products claiming to boost energy or correct nutritional deficiencies are especially attractive to parents. Data from the 2007 National Health Interview Survey show that one in nine children used **complementary health approaches (CHA)** in 2006 (National Center for Health Statistics, 2008b; see Chapter 39). Most parents who use CHA for their children do not spontaneously share that information with their care provider. It is important that providers inquire about the use of CHA and be aware of potential interactions of various supplements with medications or other aspects of care (Shaikhkhalil & Meyers, 2015). In the developmental disability population, the use of CHA is most commonly associated with attention-deficit/hyperactivity disorder, ASD, and cerebral palsy. CHA approaches that are promoted to improve nutrition include **megavitamin therapy,** amino acid and mineral supplements, and herbal remedies. Although CHA approaches are often presumed to be harmless, the safety of these approaches has not been well documented, and no CHA nutritional therapy has been proven effective by scientific methods (Kemper, Vohra, Walls, & the Task Force of Complementary and Alternative Medicine and the Provisional Section on Complementary, Holistic, and Integrative Medicine, 2008). CHA in the form of nutritional supplements can lead to an increased risk for or new side effects of medication received to control the underlying disability (e.g., antiepileptic drugs). Thus, a child's medical and nutrition history should include a comprehensive list of supplements (Kemper et al., 2008).

SUMMARY

- Underweight, overweight, constipation, food allergies, feeding difficulties, and other gastrointestinal disturbances that interfere with appetite are more common in children with developmental disabilities than in typically developing children.
- Typical dietary guidelines for Americans (U.S. Department of Agriculture, 2010) and the MyPlate plan (U.S. Department of Agriculture, n.d.) are not sufficient resources for customizing nutrition recommendations for many children with developmental disabilities.

- Medical nutritional therapy that includes a nutritional assessment and care plan should be part of the comprehensive care for children with developmental disabilities.

ADDITIONAL RESOURCES

Dietary reference intake for healthy children from the U.S. Department of Agriculture: https://www.nal.usda.gov/fnic/dri-tables-and-application-reports

Growth charts:

- WHO charts for infants and children from 0 to 2 years of age: https://www.cdc.gov/growthcharts/who_charts.htm
- CDC charts for children and adolescents from 2 to 20 years of age: https://www.cdc.gov/growthcharts/clinical_charts.htm
- CP growth charts: http://www.lifeexpectancy.org/articles/GrowthCharts.shtml

Additional resources can be found online in Appendix D: Childhood Disabilities Resources, Services, and Organizations (see About the Online Companion Materials).

REFERENCES

Adams, R. C., Elias, E. R., & Council on Children with Disabilities. (2014). Nonoral feeding for children and youth with developmental or acquired disabilities. *Pediatrics, 134*, e1745–e1762.

Abdelhadi, R. A., Rahe, K., & Lyman, B. (2016). Pediatric enteral access device management. *Nutrition in Clinical Practice*, 31(6), 748–761.

Addo, O. Y., Himes, J. H., & Zemel, B. S. (2017). Reference ranges for midupper arm circumference, upper arm muscle area, and upper arm fat area in US children and adolescents aged 1-20y. *American Journal of Clinical Nutrition, 105*(1), 111–120.

Addo, O. Y., & Himes, J. H. (2010). Reference curves for triceps and subscapular skinfold thicknesses in US children and adolescents. *American Journal of Clinical Nutrition, 91*, 635–642.

American Dietetic Association. (2010). Position of the American Dietetic Association: Integration of medical nutrition therapy and pharmacotherapy. *Journal of the American Dietetic Association, 110*, 950–956.

Arvay, J., Zemel, B. S., Gallagher, P. R., Rovner A. J., Mulberg, A. E., Stallings, V. A., . . . Haber, B. A. (2005). Body composition of children aged 1 to 12 years with biliary atresia or Alagille syndrome. *Journal of Pediatric Gastroenterology and Nutrition, 40*, 146–150.

Bachrach, L. K., Gordon, C. M., & AAP Section on Endocrinology. (2016). Bone densitometry in children and adolescents. *Pediatrics, 138*, e20162398.

Bandini, L. G., Anderson, S. E., Curtin, C., Cermak, S., Evans, E. W., Scampini, R., . . . Must, A. (2010). Food selectivity in children with autism spectrum disorders and typically developing children. *Pediatrics, 157*, 259–264.

Bandini, L. G., Curtin, C., Hamad, C., Tybor, D. J., & Must, A. (2005). Prevalence of overweight in children with developmental disorders in the continuous national health and nutrition examination survey (NHANES) 1999–2002. *Pediatrics, 146*(6), 738–743.

Barlow, S., & Expert Committee. (2007). Expert committee recommendations regarding prevention, assessment, and treatment of child and adolescent overweight and obesity: Summary report. *Pediatrics, 120*(4), S164–S192.

Bayram, A. K., Canpolat, M., Karacabey, N., Gumus, H., Kumandas, S., Doğanay, S., . . . Per, H. (2016). Misdiagnosis of gastroesophaeal reflux disease as epileptic seizures in children. *Brain & Development, 38*, 274–279.

Becker, P., Carney, L. N., Corkins, M. R., Monczka, J., Smith, E., Smith, S. E., . . . White, J.V.; Academy of Nutrition and Dietetics; American Society for Parenteral and Enteral Nutrition (2015). Consensus statement of the Academy of Nutrition and Dietetics/American Society for Parenteral and Enteral Nutrition: Indicators recommended for the identification and documentation of pediatric malnutrition (undernutrition). *Nutrition in Clinical Practice*, 30, 147-161.

Bianchi, M. L., Leonard, M. B., Bechtold, S., Hogler, W., Mughal, M. Z., Schonau, E., . . . Ward, L. M.; International Society for Clinical Densitometry (2013). Bone health in children and adolescents with chronic diseases that may affect the skeleton: The 2013 ISCD pediatric official positions. *Journal of Clinical Densitometry, 17*, 281–294.

Brooks, J., Day, S., Shavelle, R., & Strauss, D. (2011). Low weight, morbidity, and mortality in children with cerebral palsy: New clinical growth charts. *Pediatrics, 128*, e299–e307.

Brown, J. E. (Ed.). (2014). *Nutrition through the life cycle* (6th ed.). Boston, MA: Cengage Learning.

Cohen, P., Rogol, A. D., Deal, C. L., Saenger, P., Reiter, E. O., Ross, J. L., . . . Wit, J. M.; 2007 ISS Consensus Workshop participants (2008). Consensus statement on the diagnosis and treatment of children with idiopathic short stature: A summary of the growth hormone research society, the Lawson Wilkins Pediatric Endocrine Society, and the European Society for Paediatric Endocrinology Workshop. *The Journal of Clinical Endocrinology and Metabolism, 93*, 4210–4217.

Curtin, C., Must, A., Phillips, S., & Bandini, L. (2017). The healthy weight research network: A research agenda to promote healthy weight among youth with autism spectrum disorder and other developmental disabilities. *Pediatric Obesity, 12*, e6–e9.

Dekaban, A. S. (1978). Changes in brain weights during the span of human life: Relation of brain weights to body heights and body weights. *Annals of Neurology, 4*(4), 345–356.

Del Campo, M., & Jones, K. L. (2017). A review of the physical features of the fetal alcohol spectrum disorders. *European Journal of Medical Genetics, 60*(1), 55–64.

Edmond, A., Emmett, P., Steer, C., & Golding, J. (2010). Feeding symptoms, dietary patterns, and growth in young children with autism spectrum disorders. *Pediatrics*, 126, e337.

Evans, M., Truby, H., & Boneh, A. (2017). The relationship between dietary intake, growth, and body composition in inborn errors of intermediary protein metabolism. *Journal of Pediatrics, 188*, 163–172.

Frazier, D. M., Allgeier, C., Homer, C., Marriage, B. J., Ogata, B., Rohr, F., . . . Singh, R. H. (2014). Nutrition management guideline for maple syrup urine disease: An evidence- and consensus-based approach. *Molecular Genetics and Metabolism, 112*(3), 210–217.

Fukahori, S., Yagi, M., Ishii, S., Asagiri, K., Saikusa, N., Hashizume, N., . . . Tanaka, Y.(2016). Laparoscopic Nissen fundoplication mainly reduces the volume of acid reflux and potentially improves mucosal integrity up to the middle esophagus in neurologically impaired children detected by esophageal combined pH-multichannel intraluminal impedance measurements. *Journal of Pediatric Surgery, 51,* 1283–1287.

Furuta, G. T., & Katzka, D. A. (2015). Eosinophilic esophagitis. *New England Journal of Medicine, 373,* 1640–1648.

Golden, N. H., Abrams, S. A., & Committee on Nutrition. (2014). Optimizing bone health in children and adolescents. *Pediatrics, 134,* e1229–e1243.

Harding, J. E., Cormack, B. E., Alexander, T., Alsweiler, J. M., & Bloomfield, F. H. (2017). Advances in nutrition of the newborn infant. *Lancet, 389*(10079), 1660–1668.

Hill, I. D., Fasano, A., Guandalini, S., Hoffenberg, E., Levy, J., Reilly, N., & Verma, R. (2016). NASPGHAN Clinical report on the diagnosis and treatment of gluten-related disorders. *Journal of Pediatric Gastroenterology and Nutrition, 63,* 156–165.

Hyman, S. L., Stewart, P. A., Schmidt, B., Cain, U., Lemcke, N., Foley, J. T., . . . Ng, P. K. (2012). Nutrient intake from food in children with autism. *Pediatrics, 130*(Suppl. 2), S145–S153.

Institute of Medicine, Food and Nutrition Board. (1997). *Dietary reference intakes for calcium, phosphorus, magnesium, vitamin D, and fluoride.* Washington, DC: National Academies Press.

Institute of Medicine, Food and Nutrition Board. (2001). *Dietary reference intakes for vitamin A, vitamin K, arsenic, boron, chromium, copper, iodine, iron, molybdenum, nickel, silicon, vanadium, and zinc.* Washington, DC: National Academies Press.

Institute of Medicine, Food and Nutrition Board. (2005). *Dietary reference intakes for energy, carbohydrate, fiber, fat, fatty acids, cholesterol, protein, and amino acids.* Washington, DC: National Academies Press.

Institute of Medicine, Food and Nutrition Board. (2010). *Dietary reference intakes for vitamin D and calcium.* Washington, DC: The National Academies Press.

Institute of Medicine of the National Academies. (2006). *Dietary reference intakes. The essential guide to nutrient requirements.* Washington, DC: The National Academies Press.

Isaacs, J. S., & Zand, D. J. (2007). Single-gene autosomal recessive disorders and Prader-Willi syndrome: An update for food and nutrition professionals. *Journal of the American Dietetic Association, 107,* 466–478.

Joeckel, R. J., & Phillips, S. K. (2009). Overview of infant and pediatric formulas. *Nutrition in Clinical Practice, 24,* 356–362.

Kelly, A., Winer, K. K., Kalkwarf, H., Oberfield, S. E., Lappe, J., Gilsanz, V., . . . Zemel, B. S. (2014). Age-based reference ranges for annual height velocity in US children. *Journal of Clinical Endocrinology and Metabolism, 99*(6), 2104–2112.

Kemper, K. J., Vohra, S., Walls, R., & the Task Force of Complementary and Alternative Medicine and the Provisional Section on Complementary, Holistic, and Integrative Medicine. (2008). The use of complementary and alternative medicine in pediatrics. *Pediatrics, 122,* 1374–1386.

Kerzner, B., Milano, K., MacLean, W. C., Jr., Berall, G., Stuart, S., & Chatoor, I. (2015). A practical approach to classifying and managing feeding difficulties. *Pediatrics, 135*(2), 344–353.

Kuperminc, M. N., Gottrand, F., Samson-Fang, L., Arvedson, J., Bell, K., Craig, G. M., . . . Sullivan, P. B. (2013). Nutritional management of children with cerebral palsy: A practical guide. *European Journal of Clinical Nutrition, 67,* S21–S23.

Leonard, H., Ravikumara, M., Baikie, G., Naseem, N., Ellaway, C., Percy, A., . . . Downs, J.; Telethon Institute for Child Health Research (2013). Assessment and management of nutrition and growth in Rett syndrome. *Journal of Pediatric Gastroenterology Nutrition, 57*(4), 451–460.

Liusuwan, R. A., Widman, L. M., Abresch, R. T., Styne, D. M., & McDonald, C. M. (2007). Body composition and resting energy expenditure in patients aged 11 to 21 years with spinal cord dysfunction compared to controls: Comparisons and relationships among groups. *The Journal of Spinal Cord Medicine, 30,* S105–S111.

Marchand, V., Motil, K. J. & NASPGHAN Committee on Nutrition (2006). Nutrition support for neurologically impaired children: A clinical report of the North American Society for Pediatric Gastroenterology, Hepatology, and Nutrition. *Journal of Pediatric Gastroenterology and Nutrition, 43*(1), 123–135.

Mehta, N. M., Corkins, M. R., Lyman, B., Malone, A., Goday, P. S., Carney, L. N., . . . Schwenk, W. F.; American Society for Parenteral and Enteral Nutrition Board of Directors. (2013). Defining pediatric malnutrition: a paradigm shift toward etiology-related definitions. *Journal of Parenteral and Enteral Nutrition, 37,* 460–481.

Meyer, R., DeKoker, C., Dziubak, R., Godwin, H., Dominguez-Ortega, G., Chebar Lozinsky, A., . . . Shah, N. (2016). The impact of the elimination diet on growth and nutrient intake in children with food protein induced gastrointestinal allergies. *Clinical and Translational Allergy, 14*(6), 25.

Monczka, J. (2015). Parenteral and enteral nutrition support: Determining the best way to feed. In M. Corkins (Ed.), *The A.S.P.E.N. pediatric nutrition support core curriculum.* Silver Springs, MD: American Society for Parenteral and Enteral Nutrition.

Motil, K. J. (2010). Developmental delay. In M. Corkins (Ed.), *The A.S.P.E.N. pediatric nutrition support core curriculum.* Silver Springs, MD: American Society for Parenteral and Enteral Nutrition.

Mramba, L., Ngari, M., Mwangome, M., Muchai, L., Bauni, E., Walker, A. S., . . . Berkley, J. A. (2017). A growth reference for mid upper arm circumference for age among school age children and adolescents, and validation for mortality: Growth curve construction and longitudinal cohort study. *BMJ, 358,* j3423. doi:10.1136/bmj.j3423

National Center for Health Statistics. (2000). *NCHS growth curves for children 0–19 years.* Washington, DC: U.S. Government Printing Office.

National Center for Health Statistics. (2008a). *Anthropometric reference data for children and adults: United States, 2003–2006.* Washington, DC: U.S. Government Printing Office.

National Center for Health Statistics. (2010). *Changes in terminology for childhood overweight and obesity.* Washington, DC: U.S. Government Printing Office.

NCD Risk Factor Collaboration. (2017). Worldwide trends in body-mass index, underweight, overweight, and obesity from 1975-2016: A pooled analysis of 2416 population-based measurement studies in 128.9 million children, adolescents, and adults. *Lancet, 390*(10113), 2627–2642.

Osara, Y., Coakley, K., Aisthorpe, A., Stembridge, A., Quirk, M., Splett, P. L., . . . Singh, R. H. (2015). The role of evidence analysts in creating nutrition management guidelines for inherited metabolic disorders. *Journal of Evaluation in Clinical Practice 21*(6), 1235–1243.

Pena, M., Dixon, B., & Taveras, E. M. (2012). Are you talking to ME? The importance of ethnicity and culture in childhood obesity prevention and management. *Childhood Obesity, 8*(1), 23–27.

Penagini, F., Mameli, C., Fabiano, V., Brunetti, D., Dilillo, D., & Zuccotti, G. V. (2015). Dietary intakes and nutritional issues in neurologically impaired children. *Nutrients, 7*(11), 9400–9415.

Rempel, G. (2015). The importance of good nutrition in children with cerebral palsy. *Physical Medicine and Rehabilitation Clinics of North America, 26*, 39–56.

Riddick-Grisham, S. (Ed.). (2004). *Pediatric life care planning and case management.* Boca Raton, FL: CRC Press.

Rodig, N. M., McDermott, K. C., Schneider, M. F., Hotchkiss, H. M., Yadin, O., Seikaly, M. G., . . . Warady, B.A. (2014). Growth in children with chronic kidney disease: A report from the Chronic Kidney Disease in Children Study. *Pediatric Nephrology, 29*, 1987–1995.

Romano, C., van Wynckel, M., Hulst, J., Broekaert, I., Bronsky, J., Dall'Oglio, L., . . . Gottrand, F. (2017). European Society for Paediatric Gastroenterology, Hepatology, and Nutrition guidelines for the evaluation and treatment of gastrointestinal and nutritional complications in children with neurological impairment. *Journal of Pediatric Gastroenterology and Nutrition, 65*(2), 242–264.

Rosen, R., Vandeplas, Y., Singendonk, M., Cabana, M., DiLorenzo, C., Gottrand, F., . . . Tabbers, M. (2018). Pediatric gastroesophageal reflux clinical practice guidelines: Joint recommendations of the North American Society for Pediatric Gastroenterology, Hepatology, and Nutrition and the European Society for Pediatric Gastroenterology, Hepatology, and Nutrition. *Journal of Pediatric Gastroenterology and Nutrition, 66*, 516–554.

Shaikhkhalil, A. K., & Meyers, R. (2015). Neurological impairment. In M. Corkins (Ed.), *The A.S.P.E.N. pediatric nutrition support core curriculum.* Silver Spring, MD: American Society for Parenteral and Enteral Nutrition.

Singh, R. H., Rohr, F., & Splett, P. L. (2013). Bridging evidence and consensus methodology for inherited metabolic disorders: creating nutrition guidelines. *Journal of Evaluation in Clinical Practice, 19*(4), 584–590.

Singh, R. H., Cunningham, A. C., Mofidi, S., Douglas, T. D., Frazier, D. M., Hook, D. G., & Rohr, F. (2015). Updated, web-based nutrition management guideline for PKU: An evidence and consensus based approach. *Molecular Genetics and Metabolism, 118*(2), 72–83.

Sullivan, J. S., & Mascarenhas, M. R. (2017). Nutrition: Prevention and management of nutritional failure in cystic fibrosis. *Journal of Cystic Fibrosis, 16*(Suppl 2), S87–S93.

Tabbers, M. M., DiLorenzo, C., Berger, M. Y., Faure, C., Langendam, M. W., Nurko, S., . . . Benninga, M. A. (2014). Evaluation and treatment of functional constipation in infants and children: Evidence-based recommendations from ESPGHAN and NASPGHAN. *Journal of Pediatric Gastroenterology and Nutrition, 58*, 258–274.

U.S. Department of Agriculture. (n.d.). *ChooseMyPlate.* Retrieved from http://www.choosemyplate.gov

U.S. Department of Agriculture. (2010). *Dietary guidelines for Americans.* Retrieved from http://www.cnpp.usda.gov/DGAs2010-DGACReport.htm

Weintraub, B. (2011). Growth. *Pediatrics in Review, 32*(9), 404–406.

WHO Multicentre Growth Reference Study Group. (2006). WHO Child Growth Standards based on length/height, weight and age. *Acta Paediatrica (Suppl. 450)*, 76–85.

Williams, R. A., Mamotte, C. D., & Burnett, J. R. (2008). Phenylketonuria: An inborn error of phenylalanine metabolism. *Clinical Biochemical Review, 29*, 31–41.

World Health Organization. (2006). WHO Child Growth Standards: Length/Height-for-Age, Weight-for-Age, Weight- for-Length, Weight-for-Height and Body Mass Index-for-Age: Methods and Development. Geneva, Switzerland: World Health Organization.

Zupec-Kania, B. A., & Spellman, E. (2008). An overview of the ketogenic diet for pediatric epilepsy. *Nutrition in Clinical Practice, 23*, 589–596.

PART III

Developmental Assessment

CHAPTER 11 Child Development

Louis Pellegrino

Upon completion of this chapter, the reader will

- Define *child development* and key terms related to this concept
- Describe the various theoretical perspectives on child development
- Explain the uses and potential misuses of developmental milestones
- Discuss trends in child development with reference to the concept of human adaptability
- Distinguish between typical and atypical development
- Explain the importance and uses of developmental surveillance and developmental screening

Most people are familiar with the concept of child development, at least in a general sense. They know that dramatic changes in appearance, behavior, and ability characterize childhood, and many have at least a vague memory of having gone through these processes. It can be more difficult to define development in precise terms and especially problematic to clarify what is meant by terms such as *typical* or *normal* with reference to the processes of development.

This chapter addresses these issues and provides a basis for the discussions on diagnosing developmental disabilities in subsequent chapters.

CASE STUDY

Isabella is a 2-year-old girl from a bilingual family; both Spanish and English are spoken in her home. She is seen 1 week after her second birthday for a well-child visit. Her pediatrician, who is also bilingual, asks Isabella's mother if she has any concerns. Isabella's mother feels that her daughter is growing well, has been healthy, and has a cheerful disposition, but she is concerned that her daughter is not talking yet. Isabella seems to understand most of what is said to her (in Spanish and English) and is surprisingly adept at making her needs and wants known through the use of pointing, vocalizing (especially grunting), eye gaze, eye contact, and "body language." Although she doesn't use recognizable words, she speaks a kind of "gibberish" that occasionally sounds vaguely like real words. She recognizes and responds to her name, can identify a few body parts and pictures in books by pointing, and can respond to simple instructions, such as "go get your coat." She walks and runs well, is learning how to jump, can use a spoon and a fork, pretends to feed her stuffed animals, and has developed an independent streak, with occasional tantrums when she doesn't get what she wants.

Isabella's pediatrician decides to administer a developmental screening test, which consists of a series of simple questions answered by Isabella's mother. The screen reveals that Isabella "passes" in all areas, except language development. Although her mother is sure that Isabella hears well, the pediatrician recommends that Isabella have her hearing tested by an audiologist. She also refers Isabella to the local early intervention team to further assess her development and determine if she is eligible for home-based speech therapy.

Isabella's mother wonders if speaking two languages at home might be confusing to Isabella; relatives have told her that she should only speak to Isabella in English. The pediatrician reassures her that living in a bilingual home does not cause language delays and that, in the long run, being bilingual confers significant developmental and cognitive advantages.

Thought Questions:

How might some developmental milestones be more useful in some clinical situations more than others? How can atypical development be distinguished from variations in typical development?

DEFINING CHILD DEVELOPMENT

Development in a generic sense can refer to anything that changes over time (e.g., a photographic negative develops), but it most often describes an organic process of change. For the purposes of this book, the term *development* is used with reference to changes in human thought, behavior, and function. Development is distinguished from the term *growth*, which refers more specifically to physical increases in height, weight, head size, and sexual maturation. Although the concepts of growth and development are obviously connected, the techniques used to measure and describe them tend to be separate.

As applied to the individual human being, the term *development* can possess different meanings. On the one hand, a person changes in response to a specific set of life circumstances and experiences. In this sense, every human being has a unique developmental history that can never be replicated. On the other hand, individuals experience changes in cognition, emotion, and specific abilities that likely indicate a common "blueprint" that transcends individual life histories or cultures. For example, walking is begun and mastered at about the same age and seems to follow a fairly consistent sequence across cultures. Similarly, children universally and spontaneously learn to speak their native languages and do so in a predictable sequence of steps without any explicit instruction in vocabulary or grammar.

Additional general changes in behavior and social-emotional responses also occur on a predictable timeline and in predictable ways. Typically, infants begin to exhibit "stranger anxiety" at about 6 or 7 months of age, toddlers demonstrate limit-testing behavior as part of increasing autonomy, school-age children become enamored of rules and enjoy a sense of industrious accomplishment, and preteens and teens experience a sense of independence and identity in the context of intensified peer relations.

Human development is wonderfully varied but reasonably predictable and, for the purposes of this discussion, may be defined as follows: *Development* refers to the characteristic, predictable ways in which behavior changes during the human life cycle. At its most basic level, *behavior* refers to any action that a person can perform and another can observe. Moving a leg, sneezing, saying a word, and composing a symphony are all forms of human behavior. Behavior can be characterized as simple (moving an arm) or complex (playing a concerto). Some forms of behavior are inherently more meaningful than others (e.g., talking versus coughing). With regard to the definition of development, behavior that is most directly relevant to real-life situations tends to be of greatest interest (e.g., identifying pictures in a book, using a spoon, or riding a bike). Behavior is also used as a proxy for aspects of cognition and emotion that are critically important to development but that cannot be observed directly (for example, using shape drawing as a proxy for one aspect of nonverbal cognition). Observing and interpreting behavior is, in fact, the primary focus of developmental assessment.

In everyday speech, the word *normal* usually describes something that is usual or expected. For example, "The weather is normal for this time of year," means that the temperature, humidity, and presence or absence of precipitation is close to average or to be expected based on previous experience. Saying the weather is normal doesn't necessarily convey a value judgement. People speak of "bad weather" with regard to a damaging thunderstorm, but such a storm might be normal for the peak of summer in a particular area.

When referring to human development and behavior as normal or abnormal, the message does tend to carry good or bad connotations. For example, when a parent scolds a child for misbehaving, and asks, "Why can't you act *normal*?," the parent is really saying that the behavior is not only different from what is expected but that it is also bad. Saying that a child's speech development is abnormal also implies, perhaps more subtly, that there is something bad or wrong with that child's speech.

In discussions of behavior and development, it is therefore preferable to use the term *typical* to express the idea of usual, expected, or average and *atypical* to convey that which is unusual, unexpected, or significantly different from average. Although these terms are also less than perfect in avoiding value judgment (in particular, the word *atypical* does have at least a mildly negative connation to most ears), they are still preferable to *normal* and *abnormal* and seem to be the best options, especially when attempting to emphasize a child's abilities rather than disabilities.

THEORETICAL PERSPECTIVES ON DEVELOPMENT

Several theoretical perspectives help practitioners and families understand child development, including those concerning the brain (biology, maturation, and cognition), the environment, and social context. Key theories are summarized in Table 11.1.

A common theme of all developmental theories is the idea of adaptation. Each theory in its own way considers development to be an adaptive response of the human organism to its environment. The dynamic systems theory (Thelen & Smith, 1994) is a striking example of this. This theory draws on mathematical concepts of dynamic systems and considers behavioral change as an emergent property of an organism in a specific environmental context. Developmental sequences, rather than being rigidly predetermined, are seen as processes of dynamic change of a specific organism to a specific set of circumstances organized around a specific task. For example, a child with specific physical characteristics who tries to pull herself up to a standing position using the edge of a coffee table is exhibiting an adaptive response.

The Brain

Development is dependent on the brain, and the predictable behavioral changes that characterize development occur in parallel with the maturation of the central nervous system. Functional and structural changes in the human nervous system are most dramatically evident during fetal life and early childhood but continue into adulthood (see Chapters 6 and 8). These processes promote and are intimately connected to developmental change. For example, myelination of key **corticospinal pathways** (pathways from the cortex of the brain to the spinal cord that orchestrate movement) during the first year of life is one of the main determinants of early gross motor development, such as rolling over, sitting, and crawling (Volpe, 2018). Critical changes in the brain's functional organization occur toward the end of the second year of life that create an opportunity for explosive language development that typically occurs between 18 and 24 months of age (Redcay, Haist, & Courchesne, 2008).

Changing nervous system **plasticity** (the ability of the nervous system to change or adapt) over the course of the human life cycle also creates opportunities and constraints on development. One example of this phenomenon is the well-known observation that young children much more easily attain fluency in a foreign language than do adults or older children (i.e., beyond 8 or 9 years of age). Indeed, there appears to be a sensitive period for language acquisition during these early years, and children who miss this opportunity will most likely never develop fluency in any language (Werker & Hensch, 2015). The good news for adults is that although there is decreased brain plasticity with age, learning continues unabated through the entire life cycle. The brain works by creating a rich network of functional connections within and across many cortical and subcortical domains, and these networks are continually enhanced and elaborated throughout the life span.

Biology, Maturation, and Cognition

A number of developmental theories have emerged during the 19th and 20th centuries in an attempt to provide an explanatory framework for the processes of developmental change. Of these, Sigmund Freud's theory of psychosexual development is one of the best known and perhaps most notorious (Freud & Strachey, 2000). Freud viewed the conflict between in-born biological drives and external societal restrictions as being the engine of developmental and behavioral change. Although most of the specifics of his theories are no longer accepted, his idea of development as occurring in a series of stages, each dependent on the one before, has had a lasting influence.

Erik Erikson's psychosocial stage theory (Erikson & Coles, 2000) has given us a model for development through the life span that describes a series of existential crises that must each be successfully overcome. The most famous of these is the identity crisis of adolescence, and the idea of a "midlife crisis" in popular usage also stems from Erikson's ideas.

Other development theories have focused on the biological underpinnings of developmental change. Attachment theory, for example, emphasizes the critical importance of the infant–caregiver bond and describes early infancy as a critical period within which such

Table 11.1. Developmental theories in a nutshell

Theory	Focus	Key components
Theories emphasizing biological and maturational factors		
Gesell: Maturational theory of development (Shaffer & Kipp, 2014)	Genetically determined blueprint for development unfolds in specific sequences	Definitions of specific sequences of development and recognizable, testable milestones form the basis of subsequent screening/testing
Freud: Psychosexual stage theory (Freud & Strachey, 2000)	Conflict between biological drives and societal restrictions generates developmental change	The psyche is classified into domains (id, ego, superego) and stages of personality development are defined (oral, anal, phallic, latent, genital) based on interactions and conflicts among the domains
Erikson: Psychosocial stage theory (Erikson & Coles, 2000)	A series of psychosocial crises drives development (also has a maturational/psychosexual orientation as an offshoot of Freud's theory)	Eight stages are defined (trust, autonomy, initiative, industry, identity, intimacy, generativity, integration) in relation to their opposites; at each stage a crisis (e.g., identity crisis in adolescence) is faced, allowing the person to advance to the next stage
Bolby: Attachment theory (Bowlby, 2005)	Infants are born with an innate need to form attachments with caregivers to ensure survival	Child–parent interactions yield different patterns of attachment (secure, insecure, anxious) that result in different developmental and behavior outcomes
Ethology and evolutionary psychology (Shaffer & Kipp, 2014)	Behavior and development are explained in terms of evolutionary adaptation	Behavioral analogies to other animal species (especially primates) in conjunction with information from paleontology and anthropology inform theories regarding current human development and behavior
Theories emphasizing cognitive factors		
Piaget: Cognitive development stage theory (Wadsworth, 2004)	Cognitive processes and ways of thinking are constructed through interactions with the environment	Stages are defined (sensorimotor, pre-operational, concrete operational, formal operational) based on the manner of thought that characterizes each stage, starting with basic motoric responses to sensory stimuli and ending with abstract thought
Information processing theory (Shaffer & Kipp, 2014)	Model based on analogy to computer processing	Cognition develops through modifications to the information-processing machinery of the brain
Theories emphasizing environmental factors		
Behavioral theories of child development (Shaffer & Kipp, 2014)	The child is a blank slate that is shaped through behavioral conditioning	Environment determines behavior and development through association, conditioning, and reinforcement (e.g., behaviors associated with rewards are reinforced)
Bandura: Social learning theory (Bandura, 1977)	The social context is critical to learning	Conditioning and reinforcement alone cannot explain behavior; social observation and modeling lead to learning and the acquisition of new skills
Theories emphasizing social and cultural factors		
Vygotsky: Sociocultural theory (Vygotsky & Cole, 1978)	Learning is inherently a social process	Development occurs through active, hands-on engagement in activities of increasing difficulty and complexity with family and peers facilitating (scaffolding) the process
Bronfenbrenner: Ecological theory (Bronfenbrenner, 1979)	The cultural context drives development	Nested developmental settings starting from those closed to the individuals (e.g., home, school) and extending to broader societal settings (the culture with its laws, history and traditions) determine the roles, activities, and relationships that drive developmental change
Theories emphasizing processes of adaptation		
Dynamic systems theory (Thelen & Smith, 1994)	Mathematical concepts of dynamic systems applied to developmental change	Behavioral change and development are emergent properties of complex systems that include the individual, the environment, and multiple particular elements of each that are in constant flux

bonds must form (Bowlby, 2005). Arnold Gesell saw genetics and neurology as providing a blueprint for developmental change and focused on mapping these changes by identifying easily observable and testable milestones. His work has had a lasting influence on developmental screening and testing procedures. Ethological theories have taken an evolutionary perspective on development and behavior and have drawn on observations of other primate species for analogies to human behavior (Shaffer & Kipp, 2014).

One of the most influential developmental theories is Piaget's cognitive development stage theory (Wadsworth, 2004). Piaget proposed that our interactions with the environment are governed by the construction of cognitive processes during childhood, which he called schemas. These schemas arise through processes of adaptation to the environment, which he referred to as assimilation (processing information using existing schemas) and accommodation (creating new schemas to process new types of information). The first stage (sensorimotor) provides the foundation by connecting sensory perceptions to motor responses via the construction of cognitive intermediaries. Subsequent stages (pre-operational, concrete operational, and formal operational) elaborate on these cognitive structures to provide an increasingly complex and abstract means of responding to the world around us.

Selma Fraiberg drew on Piaget's description of the pre-operational stage of development to describe the charming idiosyncrasies and "magical thinking" of the preschool years in her influential work, *The Magic Years* (Fraiberg, 2015). The interest of school-aged children in rules and in understanding how things work through the use of basic logic is explained in Piaget's theory as manifestations of the concrete operational stage of development. The turbulence of the adolescent mind as it struggles to grapple with existential realities and abstract ideas is explained in Piaget's theory as a manifestation of the formal operational stage of development.

In recent years, information processing theory, a concept of cognitive psychology, has emerged to reemphasize the importance of cognitive processes in development and behavior. The theory draws heavily on analogies to computer processing to create a modular scheme of human cognition with a strong emphasis on the basic mechanisms of attention, memory, and learning (Shaffer & Kipp, 2014).

The Environment and Social Context

Other developmental theories (see Table 11.1) have emerged to emphasize the importance of the environment in developmental change. Behavioral theories of development have emphasized the importance of environmental contingencies in reinforcing some behaviors preferentially, especially through the association of preferred behaviors with rewards (e.g., receiving parental praise for good behavior). The most radical behavioral model, B. F. Skinner's operant conditioning theory, considers a child to be a "blank slate" whose behavioral responses are entirely governed by these environmental contingencies (Skinner, 1966). Although this form of the theory has not stood the test of time, behavioral principles have had a lasting impact in clinical practice, where they have provided the basis for a variety of therapies such as applied behavioral analysis to address maladaptive behaviors (see Chapter 34).

Other theories have emphasized the social and cultural context of learning and development. Social learning theory (Bandura, 1977) emphasizes the importance of social modeling and imitation in learning. Vygotsky's sociocultural theory (Vygotsky & Cole, 1978) emphasizes the importance of family, teachers, and peers in facilitating hands-on learning. He introduced the concept of the **zone of proximal development,** which represents the space between what learners can do on their own and what they are not ready to do at all; it is the place where or circumstances within which children are able to learn new, difficult things with the help and support of others. Because of its clarity and utility, Vygotsky's theory has had a lasting influence on educational practices and teacher training. Bronfenbrenner's ecology theory (Bronfenbrenner, 1979) emphasizes the cultural context and the roles, activities, and relationships engendered by that context that determine individual behavior to a greater or lesser degree.

DEVELOPMENTAL MILESTONES

Developmental theory can offer a framework for thinking about developmental processes, but it is necessary to find a way to operationalize the discussion of typical development by invoking the concept of the developmental milestone. Simply defined, a **developmental milestone** is a behavior, ability, or skill that emerges at a particular age in most children and which can easily be observed and described. For example, most children take their first independent steps at approximately 12 months of age (Figure 11.1). Of course, some children start a bit earlier than this and others a bit later. About 90% of children have started taking independent steps by about 14 months of age, and so children who start walking after this age are considered "delayed" for this milestone (Piper & Darrah, 1994).

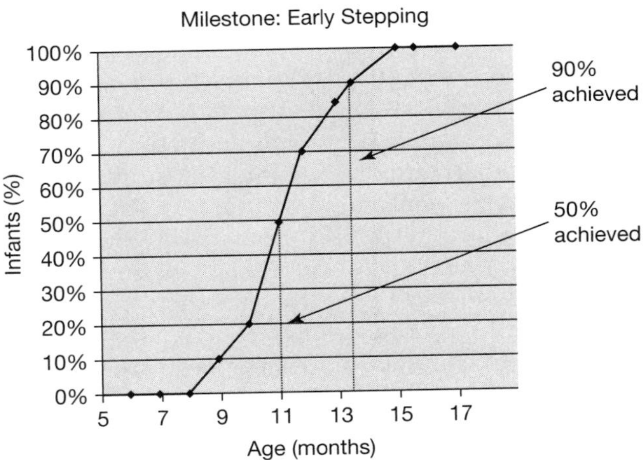

Figure 11.1. Milestone: early stepping. 50% of children take their first independent steps by 11 months; 90% have achieved this milestone by 13.5 months. (Adapted with permission from Piper, M.C., & Darrah, J. [1994]. Motor assessment of the developing infant [p. 165]. Philadelphia, PA: W.B. Saunders; Copyright © 1994 Elsevier.)

Milestones are characterized as belonging to several specific functional domains/streams, which usually include the following:

- Gross motor (skills involving the movement of the body or limbs as a whole)
- Fine motor (skills involving the manipulation of objects with the hands)
- Language and communication
- Cognitive and problem-solving
- Self-care (adaptive)
- Play
- Social

Each of these domains may be combined or subdivided in different ways to suit the clinical or scientific purpose for which they are being used (this is sometimes referred to informally as "lumping" or splitting"). For example, language, communication, and social domains are often combined ("lumped") into a larger communication/socialization domain for the purposes of emphasizing the broad range of skills important to social interactions (this is done to characterize one of the two large domains of dysfunction associated with autism spectrum disorder [ASD]; see Chapter 18). By contrast, language milestones may be subdivided ("split") into expressive skills (spoken language), receptive skills (comprehension), and pragmatic skills (social/functional communication) for the purposes of carrying out a detailed analysis of a child's language abilities. The way that specific domains are combined or subdivided is determined by the purpose for which they are being used (examples of various clinical uses of milestones are shown in Table 11.2).

Clinical Usefulness

Developmental milestones are a necessary part of every aspect of clinical practice involving the assessment and management of children with potential or actual developmental challenges. But not all developmental milestones are weighted equally. Thousands of milestones have been described by a multitude of observers, but they vary significantly in practical utility. In general, the most useful milestones have the following characteristics:

1. They emerge in most children within a reasonably narrow and predicable range of ages.
2. They are easy to observe and describe.
3. They don't vary tremendously in appearance from person to person.
4. They are functionally relevant.

Some milestones, such as a child taking her first independent steps, have all of these characteristics, whereas many others only have some of them. For example, in the fine-motor/adaptive domain of a well-known developmental screening test, a milestone referred to as the "thumb wiggle" is described (Frankenburg, Dodds, Archer, Shapiro, & Bresnick, 1992). A child is simply asked to wiggle her thumb after demonstration. Approximately 50% of children are able to do this by 39 months of age, and 90% are able to do it by 45 months of age. As a milestone, it emerges within a predicable range of ages, is easily observed and described, and is consistent in appearance. However, it could be argued that the

Table 11.2. Clinical uses of developmental milestones

Type of assessment	Purpose
Developmental surveillance	Monitoring and tracking of developmental progress
Developmental screening (with standardized screening instruments)	Identifying at-risk children for further evaluation
Diagnostic interview	Reviewing the history of developmental progress to establish the diagnosis of a developmental disability
Norm-referenced testing (with standardized instruments)	Comparing a child's scores to reference populations (e.g., IQ, academic achievement tests)
Criteria-referenced testing (with standardized instruments)	Comparing a child's progress against predetermined standards of performance (e.g., tests assessing reading progress based on established standards for grade level)

thumb wiggle has much less functional relevance than other motor milestones, such walking and running.

By contrast, a milestone such as crawling, which has clear functional relevance, is notoriously variable in its presentation. Most children do some type of crawling toward the end of their first year, but the style of crawling can vary considerably, from belly (commando) crawling to crawling on hands and knees to "bear" crawling (walking on all fours). The emergence of these various forms of crawling occurs with considerable variability with respect to other, more predictable early motor milestones; in fact, some children skip crawling altogether. So, although crawling is considered an important early motor milestone, it has limited utility in determining whether a particular child has delayed motor development.

In clinical practice, developmental milestones also vary considerably in how they are observed and recorded. In many instances, caregivers (usually parents) are simply asked to report whether they have observed a behavior (milestone) at home—in other words, caregivers are used as proxy observers by the clinician. Milestones for language, social skills, and self-care skills are often elicited in this way. Other milestones are directly observed by the clinician, either passively or actively. For example, noting that a child walks into a room constitutes a passive observation of that skill. Other milestones are actively elicited, either by means of imitation (e.g., asking a child to hop on one foot after a clinician shows him how) or by providing a model (e.g., showing a child a picture of a circle and asking her to copy it). It is important to note that the method of observation may influence whether a child can demonstrate a particular skill. For example, a 2-year-old who may not be able to copy a circle from a picture may be able to imitate an adult drawing a circle.

Limitations and Misuses

In the hands of an experienced clinician, developmental milestones are essential tools that, when used correctly, yield critical information about a child's developmental well-being. However, as with any tool, the characteristics and limitations of milestones must be understood to avoid being misused. In particular, milestones vary considerably in their level of precision. Developmental milestones are typically presented in the form of tables (see Table 11.3) demonstrating what skills emerge at what ages for different domains of development. These tables are typically derived from multiple sources, and the quality of evidence with regard to the precision of these milestones varies considerably (Dosman, Andrews, & Goulden, 2012).

In general, motor milestones and milestones for self-care skills tend to be more precisely defined and have a higher quality of evidence to support them than do milestones for language, social-emotional, and cognitive development. This is not to say that motor and self-care milestones are more important than other types of milestones; indeed, depending on the clinical circumstance, the other domains may and often do take precedence. It is therefore incumbent upon clinicians and early childhood educators to understand how and why they are using milestones and, in particular, what they are trying to accomplish when they encounter a child who may have a developmental concern.

DEVELOPMENT AND ADAPTATION: TRENDS AND KEY MILESTONES

Tables of developmental milestones (see Table 11.3) are necessary and useful, but in and of themselves they are not very effective at conveying a sense of the dynamism of the developmental process and its relation to real-world challenges. At its most basic level, development is fundamentally a process of adaptation, and developmental trajectories can best be understood with reference to the question, "What makes it possible for a child to develop into a fully functional adult?" To answer this question, one must consider how a child gradually adapts to both his/her physical and sociocultural environments.

Human beings are expert at adapting to change. This adaptability is a consequence of our evolutionary inheritance of bipedal locomotion (walking), tool use and advanced adaptive behaviors (problem-solving skills, especially those involving highly advanced fine-motor capabilities), our propensity for hypersocial behavior, and our capacity for symbolic thought and language.

It is useful to think of the processes of development as a kind of recapitulation of these evolutionary adaptations, and trends in development can be described accordingly in four broad categories: mobility (bipedalism), adaptive skills (tool use; manipulating the environment), hypersociality and theory of mind, and symbolic thought and language (Tuttle, 2017).

Mobility

Mobility refers to the ability of an organism to move in and successfully navigate a particular physical environment. The key developmental milestone for mobility in humans is independent walking, which first emerges for most children by 12 months of age. Early

Table 11.3. Developmental milestones*

Number of months/years	Domain						
	Gross motor	Fine motor	Self-help	Problem-solving	Social/emotional	Receptive language	Expressive language
Birth–1 month	Chin up in prone Turns head in supine Primitive reflexes evident	Hands fisted near face **Palmar grasp reflex dominant**	**Sucks well**	Follows face	**Discriminates mother's voice** Cries out in distress	Startles to voice/sound	Throaty noises
2 months	Chest up in prone Head bobs in sitting	Hands unfisted 50% Holds hands together Retains rattle placed in hand	Opens mouth at sight of breast or bottle	Reacts to visual threat Recognizes mother Follows large, high-contrast objects	**Reciprocal smile** **Responds to adult voice and smile**	Alerts to voice/sound	Coos **Social smile (6 weeks)** **Vowel-like noises**
4 months	Sits with trunk support **No head lag when pulled to sit** Props on wrists in prone Rolls front to back	**Hands mostly open** Reaches for objects Plays with rattle Clutches at clothes	Brings hands to mouth Briefly holds onto breast or bottle	**Reaches for face, ring, rattle** Follows object in circle Regards toys Mouths objects Shakes rattle Stares at new face longer	Expresses disgust Visually follows person across room Smiles at pleasurable sight/sound Stops crying to parent voice **Reciprocal vocalizations**	Regards speaker Orients toward voice Stops crying to soothing voice	**Laughs out loud** Vocalizes when talked to and when alone
6 months	Sits momentarily propped on hands Pivots in prone Bears weight on 1 hand in prone **Rolls both ways** Primitive reflexes minimally evident	**Palmar grasp of cube (voluntary)** **Transfers objects between hands** Rakes at small objects **Reaches and grasps**	**Eats pureed baby food** Feeds self crackers Places hands on bottle	Turns head to look for dropped spoon Regards small objects Touches reflection and vocalizes Removes cloth from face Bangs and shakes toys	Recognizes caregiver visually Forms attachment relationship with caregiver **Stranger anxiety**	Responds to name Stops to "no" Gestures for "up"	Says "ah-goo"; razzes, squeals (5 months) **Reduplicative babbling with consonants ("bababa")** Reciprocal vocalizations with caregiver Smiles/vocalizes to mirror
7 months	**Sits steadily without support** Puts arms out to sides for balance Bounces on feet when held	**Radial-palmar grasp** (thumb-side of hand used for grasping)	Refuses excess food	Explores different aspects of toys Observes cube in each hand Finds partially hidden object	**Looks from object to parent and back when wanting help**	Looks toward familiar object when named Attends to music	Increasing variety of syllables

9 months	**Pulls to stand** Bear walks (on all fours)	**Radial-digital (thumb-finger) grasp** Bangs two cubes together Removes cube from cup, peg from pegboard	**Holds own bottle** Finger foods (bits of cereal) Bites, chews cookie	**Seeks object after it falls silently to the floor** Inspects, rings bell Pulls string attached to ring to obtain ring	Lets parents know when happy, upset **Gaze monitoring (follows adult glance)** Uses sounds to get attention **Separation anxiety** **Follows a point** ("Oh, look at . . .") Recognizes familiar people	Responds to "Come here" Looks for named family members **Orients to name well** Orients to bell	**Says "dada" and "mama" (nonspecific)** Nonreduplicative babbling ("dagaba") Imitates sounds Shakes head "no"
10 months	**Cruises around furniture** Creeps (crawls on hands and knees) Walks with 2 hands held	**Isolates index finger and pokes**	Drinks from cup held by caregiver	**Uncovers a toy under cloth** Pokes at pellet in bottle Tries to put cube in cup, but may not be able to let go	Experiences fear Looks preferentially when name is called	Enjoys peek-a-boo Waves "bye-bye" back	**Says "dada" specific** Waves "bye-bye"
12 months	**Independent steps**	**Fine pincer (thumb-index finger) grasp** Holds crayon, scribbles after demo Attempts 2-cube tower Stirs with spoon Throws objects	**Finger feeds well** Cooperates with dressing	Rattles spoon in cup Lifts box lid to find toy	**Shows objects to parent to share interest** Point to desired objects	Stops activity when told "no" Bounces to music Follows one-step command with gesture Looks toward 2 named objects	**Says first words** (other than "mama" or "dada") **Points to desired objects** Vocalizes to songs; uses gestures with vocalizations (e.g., waving, reaching)
15 months	Stoops to pick up toy; walks carrying toy Runs stiffly Climbs on furniture	**Builds 3-cube tower** Places 10 cubes in cup Imitates back-and-forth scribble Places round peg in pegboard	Uses spoons with some spilling Chews well Removes socks/shoes Attempts to brush hair	Dangles ring by string Reaches around clear barrier to obtain object Unwraps toy in cloth Dumps pellet out of bottle after demonstration **Turns pages in book** Places circle in single-shaped puzzle	Shows desire to please caregiver Solitary play Functional play; purposeful exploration of toys (trial and error) **Points to objects to express interest** **Shows empathy** Hugs back when hugged	Responds to 1-step commands without gesture Points to 1 body part Gets named object from another room on command Points out 1 named object out of 3	Uses 3–5 words **Points to objects to express interest** Vowel-like noises Jargon ("jibber-jabber") mixed with real words

(*continued*)

Table 11.3. *(continued)*

Number of months/years	Domain						
	Gross motor	Fine motor	Self-help	Problem-solving	Social/emotional	Receptive language	Expressive language
18 months	**Runs well** Throws ball Walks backward Creeps up and down stairs	Builds 4-cube tower Scribbles spontaneously Imitates vertical line (crudely)	Picks up and drinks from cup Removes some clothes Gets into adult chair Moves about house without adult	Dumps pellet from bottle spontaneously Places circle in a form board of 3 shapes Finds toy seen hidden under several layers Matches pairs of objects	Kisses touching lips to skin Periodically visually relocates caregiver Shows embarrassment, shame Shows possessiveness **Pretend play with others (e.g., tea party)**	Points to 2 of 3 named pictures; 2/3 objects Points to 3 body parts Points to self, understands "mine" Points to familiar people when named	Uses 10–25 words Uses "giant" words ("all gone," "gimme") Copies animal sounds **Begins pointing to, naming pictures**
24 months	Walks up and down stairs, both feet on each step, holding rail **Kicks a ball** **Throws overhand**	Builds single-line "train" of cubes **Imitates vertical and horizontal line and circle** Completes pegboard of round pegs	**Uses spoon well; drinks well from cup;** sucks through straw **Gets undressed (no buttons); unzips; tries to put on shoes**	Deduces location of familiar object **Completes form board of 3 shapes (circle, square [20 months], triangle)** Sorts objects Matches objects to pictures Shows use of familiar objects	Expresses thoughts about feelings Tea party with stuffed animals Kisses with pucker Watches other children intently; **parallel play** Shows defiance Begins to mask emotions for social etiquette	Points to 5–10 pictures; 5–6 body parts; 4 pieces of clothing Follows 2-step commands Understands me/you	**Use 50+ words** **Two-word phrases** (noun + verb) **50% intelligible** Refers to self by name Can name several pictures
30 months	**Jumps in place** Walks up stairs, alternating feet, with rail	**Builds 8-cube tower** Builds "train" of cubes with stack Turns pages crudely Unscrews jar lid	Pulls pants up with help Verbalizes need for toilet Washes hands Brushes teeth with help	Matches shapes and colors Points to small details in pictures Replaces circle in reversed form board	Reduced separation anxiety **Imitates adult activities** (e.g., sweeping, talking on the phone)	Understands "just one" Follows 2 prepositional commands ("put block in/on box") Understands action words ("playing," "washing")	**Uses 1st and 2nd person pronouns** ("me," "I," "mine," "you"), **phrases, partial sentences** Names objects by use

3 years	Walks swinging arms opposite legs (synchronous gait) **Walks up stairs, alternating feet, no rail** Walks forward heel to toe Balances on 1 foot for 3 seconds Catches ball stiffly **Pedals a tricycle**	**Copies circle** Imitates 3-cube bridge Imitates cross-cuts with scissor crudely	**Independent eating** Puts on coat, shoes (no laces); unbuttons **Toilet trained** Pours liquids from one container to another	**Draws 2- to 3-part person** Understands long/short, big/small, more/less **Knows own gender and age** Matches letters, numbers	Some sharing Fears imaginary things **Imaginative play** Says what another person is thinking	Understands 3 prepositional commands Understands dirty, wet Points to objects by use Points to parts of pictures Understands negatives Groups objects (foods, toys)	Uses 200+ words **Uses simple, grammatical sentences** Uses pronouns correctly (including 3rd person) Gives first and last name Counts to 3 Begins to use past tense Uses plurals **75% intelligible** Asks to be read to
4 years	**Standing broad jump, 1 to 2 feet** Gallops **Catches bounced ball (4½ years)** Balances on 1 foot for 4–8 seconds; hops on 1 foot 2 to 3 times	**Copies square** Imitates 3-cube gate Writes first part of name Ties a single knot	**Uses fork well** Goes to toilet alone; wipes after bowel movement **Washes face and hands** **Brushes teeth alone** **Buttons**	Draws 4- to 6-part person Can give amounts < 5 correctly Simple analogies (e.g., dad/boy: mom/?); ice/cold: fire/?; ceiling/up: floor/?) Points to letters/numbers when named Counts to 4 Recognizes common signs	**Tells fibs**, tries to trick others Has a preferred friend Labels happiness, sadness, fear, and anger in self Group play	Follows 3-step commands Points to things that are same vs. different Names things based on description (e.g., "You read it" -> book) Understands adjectives	Uses 300–1,000 words **Tells stories, jokes** Uses "feeling" words **Uses past tense well** Uses words about time **100% intelligible** **Can engage in back and forth conversation**
5 years	**Walks down stairs, alternating feet, with rail** **Skips** Jumps backwards Balances on 1 foot for > 8 seconds; hops on 1 foot 15 times Running broad jump, 2–3 feet Walks backward heel to toe	**Copies a triangle** **Cuts with scissors well** **Writes first name** Builds stairs with cubes from model Puts paper clip on paper	**Spreads with knife** **Independent dressing** **Bathes independently**	Draws 8- to 10-part person Gives amounts < 10 Identifies coins **Knows 10 colors** **Counts to 10** **Knows letters and numbers well** **Knows sounds of consonants and short vowels by the end of kindergarten; reads 25 words**	Has group of friends Apologizes Responds verbally to the good fortune of others	Knows right and left on self Points to different one in series Understands "er" endings (e.g., skater) Enjoys rhyming and alliteration Points correctly to side, middle, corner	Uses 2,000 words **Retells stories with clear beginning, middle, and end** **Responds to "why" questions** Repeats 6- to 8-word sentence Knows telephone number Defines simple words

(*continued*)

Table 11.3. *(continued)*

Number of months/years	Domain						
	Gross motor	Fine motor	Self-help	Problem-solving	Social/emotional	Receptive language	Expressive language
6 years	Tandem walks	**Copies a diamond; flag** Cuts with scissors well **Writes first and last name;** forms letters with downgoing and counterclockwise strokes Builds stairs with cubes from memory	Ties shoes Combs hair **Looks both ways at street** Remembers to bring belongings	Draws 12- to 14-part person Number concepts to 20 Simple addition/subtraction Understands seasons **Sounds out regularly spelled words** **Reads 250 words by the end of first grade**	**Has best friend of same sex** **Plays board games** Distinguishes fantasy from reality Wants to be like friends, please them Enjoys school	Asks what unfamiliar words mean Can tell which words do not belong in a group	**Uses 10,000 words** Describes events in order Knows days of the week Repeats 8- to 10-word sentence **Uses future tense**

Sources: Gerber, Wilks, and Erdie-Lalena (2010, 2011) and Wilks, Gerber, and Erdie-Lalena (2010).

*Items in bold are key milestones referred to in the text.

OUR EVOLUTIONARY HERITAGE

Bipedal locomotion (upright walking) first emerged about 3 to 6 million years ago when prehuman hominins (human-like apes) branched off from the ancestral line that produced chimpanzees. The most famous example is the Australopithecine "Lucy," who was essentially a bipedal chimpanzee adapted for life on the African savannah (away from the forest). She had a small body and a small brain but could walk on two legs.

The genus *Homo* (early humans) branched off from other hominins about 2.8 million years ago and developed more complex cooperative social structures and tool use to allow for a greater reliance on hunting and cooking. This allowed a change in gut anatomy and physiology (shorter intestines) and increased the caloric density of the diet to support larger bodies and, most importantly, larger brains. The rudiments of culture and language were likely present. *Homo erectus* was the first hominin to migrate extensively from Africa to Eurasia. Neanderthals evolved from a subgroup of these in Europe, and Devonians evolved in central Asia.

Homo sapiens (modern humans) emerged in Africa about 200,000 to 300,000 years ago during a period of significant climate change, which pushed our species toward increased adaptability. Modern humans evolved to be experts at adapting to change by becoming hypersocial beings who could anticipate thoughts and intentions of others (theory of mind) and who could think symbolically (a primary manifestation being the emergence of language; Tuttle, 2017).

gross motor development subserves the emergence of this key ability.

At birth, movement patterns are dominated by **primitive reflexes** (Accardo, 2008). These are "programmed" motor responses that are present at birth, such as the ability to orient toward and suckle a nipple. They gradually fade during the first year and are replaced by voluntary motor responses, except in children with cerebral palsy, in which case the pathological persistence of primitive reflexes may be observed (see Chapter 21).

By 7 months of age, most children have developed enough head and trunk control that they are able to maintain a sitting position on their own. They have also developed a number of **automatic movement reactions,** or protective responses, such as propping their arms forward or to the side to catch themselves if they begin to tip over. A parallel development during these early months is the emergence of floor mobility skills, such as belly ("commando") crawling and rolling over, which culminate in creeping (crawling on knees and extended arms) by the end of the first year. The trend toward floor, or "horizontal," mobility is quickly overcome in most children by an increasing emphasis on "vertical" mobility. By 9 months of age, most children can pull up to a standing position while holding on to furniture, and by 10 months they can walk holding on to furniture (also called "cruising"). Most children take their first independent steps by about 12 months of age.

The further development of mobility-related skills during the toddler and preschool years can be characterized as an elaboration of skills in five categories: standing and balancing, walking, running and jumping, climbing, and general coordination (Gerber, Wilks, & Erdie-Lalena, 2010).

Standing and Balancing

By about 14 months of age, most children can stand up without holding on to anything, and by 15 months, they can stoop down to pick up a toy. By their second birthday, most children can easily squat down and stand back up at will, and they usually do so multiple times in a typical day. By 30 months of age, they can stand on a balance beam without falling off. By 3 years of age, most children can balance on one foot for 3 seconds or more, and by their fourth birthday they can hop on one foot two or three times. By 5 years of age, they can typically balance on one foot for more than 8 seconds and can hop on one foot 15 times.

Walking

When children start walking at 12 months of age, they are of course a bit unsteady, but most children are walking well by 15 months of age and can also carry a toy while they walk. Most children can walk backwards by 18 months of age. Between 2½ and 3 years of age, most children develop the adult pattern of walking with their arms swinging opposite of their legs, referred to as **synchronous gait.** By 3 years of age, most children can walk heal-to-toe forward, and by 5 years of age, they can do this backward.

Running and Jumping

Some children seem to start running as soon as they have learned to walk, but most can at least run stiffly by 15 months of age and can run well by 18 months. Most children can jump in place by 30 months of age and can make a standing broad jump 1 to 2 feet by 4 years of age. By 4 years of age most children can also "gallop," which is an honest but awkward attempt at skipping, and they can actually skip (as well as make a running broad jump) by 5 years of age.

Climbing By 15 months of age, most children can climb on furniture, and by 18 months they can crawl (creep) up and down stairs. By 24 months, they can usually walk up and down stairs, stopping with both feet on each step, while holding onto a rail. By 3 years, most children can walk upstairs using alternating feet, and they can even do this without holding onto a rail; by 5 years they can descend the stairs with alternating feet, but it may still take a few years before they can do so without holding on to a rail.

General Coordination General coordination refers to gross motor skills that especially involve coordination of the legs and arms together and require complex motor planning, timing, and balance. This discussion will focus on ball-handling skills and learning to ride a bicycle. Most children can first throw objects with clear intent by about 12 months of age and can first throw a ball stiffly by 18 months of age. By 24 months most children can throw a ball overhand and kick a ball. Most children can catch a ball with their arms stiffly extended by 3 years of age, can catch a bounced ball by 4½ years of age, and many children can play at least a rudimentary game of catch by 5 to 6 years of age.

Most children can pedal a tricycle by 3 years of age (the motion of pedaling is similar to the motion of climbing stairs with alternating feet, which also emerges at this age). Ages at which children learn to ride a bicycle tend to be extremely variable, and for that reason are often not included in charts of developmental milestones. In general, many children can learn to ride a bike with training wheels by kindergarten, but it can take years before a child can ride a bike without training wheels, although many have accomplished this by the time they have entered second grade.

Adaptive Skills

For the purposes of this discussion, **adaptive skills** refer to the broad range of abilities that allow human beings to manipulate their environment. This includes the literal manipulation of the environment with the hands through the application of fine-motor skills and the abstract manipulation of the environment by means of a variety of cognitive and problem-solving abilities (Gerber et al., 2010; Wilks, Gerber, & Erdie-Lalena, 2010).

Early Fine Motor Skills The first year of life is marked by the development of basic fine motor skills, and a key milestone is the development of the **pincer grasp** (the ability to pick up a small object between the tips of the thumb and index finder) by 12 months of age. At birth, the hands are dominated by a primitive reflex called the **palmar grasp reflex.** Newborns automatically grab any object that comes into contact with the palm of the hand. By 4 months, this reflex has faded, and the child begins to grasp objects voluntarily. By 6 months, most infants can use a palmar grasp (using the fingers and thumb as a unit, like a mitten) to reach for and pick up objects like a 1-inch cube, but they have trouble picking up smaller objects, like a bit of cereal. At this age children can also transfer objects between hands. By 7 months of age, most infants tend to use the thumb and first few fingers of the hand (**radial-palmar grasp**) to pick up objects rather than using the whole hand. By 9 months, the fingers are able to operate independent of each other (like a glove), such that an object can be grasped between the thumb and the side of the first finger (**radial-digital grasp**). The grasp pattern matures into the **pincer grasp** described above by the first birthday.

Later Fine Motor Skills As early as 9 months of age, infants begin to experiment with the properties of objects that they have learned to grasp (for example, banging two cubes together). By 12 months, infants usually begin to use objects as a means to an end (trying to scribble with a crayon or trying to stack one block on another); in other words, shortly after 1 year of age, most children have learned how to use objects as tools. Although any object that comes within a young child's reach is subject to experimentation, it is customary to describe the progression of skills with representative and commonly available objects: cubes and cups, crayons, pegboards, puzzles, and scissors.

Cubes and Cups, Pegboards, and Puzzles Most infants can retrieve a cube from a cup by 8 months of age, but they cannot usually release a cube into a cup voluntarily until after 10 months. By 15 months, they can fill a cup with cubes and drop things on the floor from a highchair; in fact, many 1-year-olds make this into a game, and they relish enticing their caregivers to repeatedly retrieve the dropped objects, only to be dropped again (this game is sometimes called casting).

Once a child can control the release of an object more precisely, he can then move on to more advanced skills, such as stacking. By 15 months of age, most children can build a two- to three-cube tower; they can also release a small pellet into a bottle. Between 2½ and 3 years of age, children generally have developed sufficient dexterity to be able to construct a tower of 10 cubes. During the preschool years children develop increasing sophistication in their ability to create more complex forms with blocks that reflect increasing dexterity and problem-solving abilities (Figure 11.2).

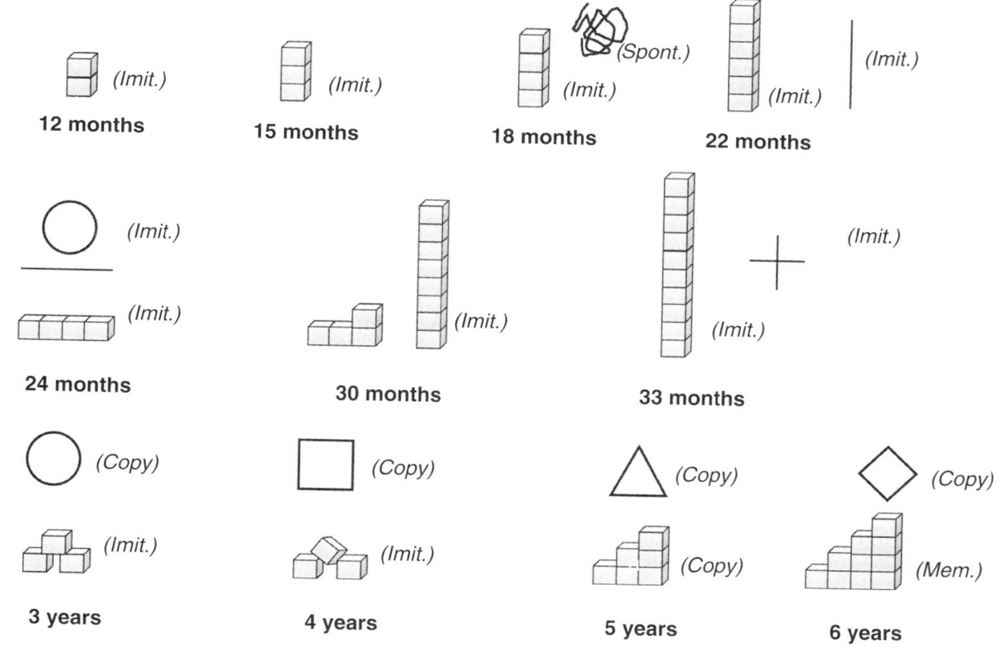

Figure 11.2. Fine motor skills: cubes and shapes. Figures illustrate the progression of fine motor skills as demonstrated by the ability of a child to construct with cubes and drawings. (*Key: Spont.*, produced spontaneously; *Imit.*, produced by imitation after demonstration by an adult; *Copy*, copied from a model; *Mem.*, produced from memory of a model; data from Gerber et al., 2010.)

Pegboards are often used in developmental testing and are a relatively pure measure of dexterity in contrast to other fine motor tasks that make greater cognitive demands. Infants can first remove a round peg from a pegboard at the same age that they can first remove a cube from a cup (8 months). By 15 months, they can place a single round peg in a pegboard and complete a pegboard with round pegs well before their second birthday.

Compared with pegboards, puzzles make relatively greater demands on visual-spatial reasoning and cognition. Most 18 month olds can place a circle shape into a puzzle consisting of a circle, square, and triangle, and they can usually complete the puzzle by 24 months (although 2-year-olds get confused if you flip the puzzle over so the shapes change position).

Crayons and Scissors Children start experimenting with crayons by making marks or scribbles on paper (or walls, if paper is not available) as early as 12 to 15 months. By 24 months, they can imitate producing vertical and horizontal lines and approximations of circles after demonstration. By 3 years of age, most children can draw a circle from a copy without needing its production demonstrated, and the ability to produce more difficult shapes follows (see Figure 11.2). By this age, most children are also able to draw a person with two or three parts. By 6 years of age, most children can draw a much more detailed picture of a person with more than a dozen parts.

The ability to use scissors along with the ability to draw simple shapes are among the skills often included in lists of kindergarten readiness. Most children are first able to operate scissors awkwardly by 3 years of age, but they can usually use them well by their fifth birthday.

Problem-Solving: Memory and Object Permanence Relatively few fine motor skills are pure manifestations of motor dexterity; most require cognitive and problem-solving abilities to a greater or lesser extent. Indeed, the ability to manipulate the environment mentally far exceeds the limits of human physical dexterity and pervades every aspect of adult functioning.

Fundamental to these cognitive abilities is the capacity to remember, register, record, and retain mental traces or images of the world. Humans are not born with this ability fully formed. Prior to 6 months of age, infants seem to live purely "in the moment." If something (or someone) is not immediately available to their senses, they no longer exist as far as the infant is concerned (this is the ultimate example of the expression "out of sight, out of mind"). It is thought that very young infants lack the ability to form a stable mental image of the things in their world.

Their ability changes as early as 7 months of age, when infants begin to look for objects that are partially hidden, suggesting that they are forming a mental image of something that is only partially visible. By 11 months, they are able to retrieve objects completely hidden under a cloth or cup as they have retained the image. This early ability to create and sustain a stable mental image of objects is called **object permanence.** This is fundamental to memory and is necessary to the development of all subsequent cognitive skills. It is also critical to one's emotional and social life. It is no coincidence that **stranger anxiety** (unease in the presence of strangers) emerging at 6 months and **separation anxiety** (fear at losing sight of a caregiver) emerging at 9 months arise at the same time as object permanence. Both milestones rely on the child's ability to form a stable mental image of the caregiver to draw on when faced with a stranger or the absence of that caregiver. Object permanence is also necessary to the development of the **theory of mind,** a critical aspect of social cognition (see below).

Problem-Solving: Self-Care Skills A prominent and practical manifestation of burgeoning problem-solving skills in early childhood is the acquisition of self-care skills. Skills in this domain also draw heavily on other functional domains, including basic fine and gross motor function, and occur in specific social contexts. Whether a child learns to eat with a spoon or with chopsticks, what types of clothes a child will wear, and expectations for hygiene and toileting are culturally determined.

Drinking and Eating As early as 6 months of age, most infants are able to feed themselves easy-to-grasp finger foods, such as crackers, and by 12 months of age, they are starting to be able to drink from a cup. By 12 to 15 months, a mature chewing pattern has also emerged such that children are safely able to manage a wider variety of food textures. By 15 months, most children can use a spoon awkwardly to feed themselves, and by their second birthday, can use both a spoon and a cup well; most children are also able to drink through a straw at this stage. By 3 years of age, most children can feed themselves an entire meal. By 4 years of age, most children can use a fork well, and by 5 years they can spread with a butter knife.

Dressing Between 6 and 12 months, infants learn to cooperate with getting dressed, and by 15 months, most have figured out how to remove their shoes and socks. By 18 months, they can typically take off other clothing items, and by 24 months most can get undressed on their own (unless buttons slow them down; they can usually unzip zippers, though). By 3 years, they can get dressed with help, and by 4 years they can manage buttons on their own. By 5 years of age, most children can completely dress themselves except for tying their shoes, which in an age of Velcro and slip-on shoes is often learned much later.

Hygiene and Toileting Children are typically dependent on caregivers for hygiene and toileting needs until their second birthday, although many will experiment with combs and brushes and fuss when they need a diaper change by 18 months of age. By 30 months most children can wash their hands and brush their own teeth with assistance. Most will have started the process of toilet training, although the onset and completion of this task is extremely variable. By 4 years of age, most children are toilet trained, can go to the toilet on their own, and can wipe themselves after a bowel movement. At this age, most children can also wash their face and hands and brush their teeth without help. By 5 years of age, most children can dress and bath independently, and by 6 years, most can comb and brush their own hair without help.

Problem-Solving: Preacademic Skills For the purposes of this discussion, preacademic skills refer to knowledge about colors, shapes, letters, numbers, books, and words that provide the foundation for kindergarten (i.e., kindergarten-readiness skills). The ability to match and sort objects and to recognize and categorize pictures forms the basis for these skills. As previously discussed, by 12 months of age most children have begun to use objects with a purpose in mind, and it is also at this age that children begin to show an interest in looking at pictures in books.

By 15 months, children begin to play with shape puzzles, and they become familiar with how to turn the pages of a book. By 18 months, children can typically match pairs of objects, and by 24 months they can sort objects and match objects to pictures. By 30 months, these matching skills have been extended to colors and shapes, as well as to letters and numbers by 3 years of age. By 4 years of age, most children have learned to identify common colors and shapes by pointing to them and can also point out some letters and numbers. Most can count to four by rote and are beginning to be able to identify quantities.

By 5 years of age, most children can name all of the letters and numbers, can name 10 colors, have learned the sounds of the consonants and short vowels, and may recognize a few words. They can count to 10 by rote and identify amounts up to 10 as well. By 5 years most children can also write their first name. By the end of kindergarten, most children can read 25 words, and by the end of first grade, most children can sound out words well, read 250 words, write their first and last names, and perform simple addition and subtraction.

Hypersociality and Theory of Mind

Humans are intensely social beings, and, along with language use, this hypersociality is a hallmark of our species. The social brain hypothesis (Dunbar, 2009) proposes that the cognitive requirements of functioning in large social groups was the crucial factor in driving the evolution of larger brains, greater intelligence, and the emergence of symbolic thought and language in our species. Stated differently, the ability of human beings to anticipate the thoughts and intentions of others and to grapple with the complexities of interpersonal relationships made our species smarter and made it possible for us to survive in and adapt to an unpredictable world.

The ability to understand something about the thoughts and intentions of others—to perceive the world from their perspective—is referred to as **theory of mind** (von dem Hagen, Stoyanova, Rowe, Baron-Cohen, & Calder, 2014). Theory of mind is fundamental to social cognition and human social interactions and, when lacking, results in one of the most significant developmental disabilities, ASD (see Chapter 18).

Some of the rudiments of theory of mind are evident even in early infancy. Infants are born recognizing their mothers' voices, and by 2 months of age they can recognize familiar faces and demonstrate a reciprocal social smile. By 4 months, this reciprocity extends to back-and-forth vocalizations, and by 6 months a clear attachment to the primary caregiver is evident. With the advent of object permanence (see previous discussion), 6 month olds can also maintain a stable mental image of their primary caregiver, and this, along with the attachment that has formed, leads to the emergence of stranger and separation anxiety (Gerber, Wilks, & Erdie-Lalena, 2011).

By 8 months of age, children demonstrate **gaze monitoring.** A child notices that her mother is looking at something across the room, and she follows her mother's glance to see what she is looking at. This simple act suggests something profound—that the child is seeing that room from her mother's perspective. In other words, the child is exhibiting **perspective-taking,** a fundamental component of theory of mind. By 9 months, children can similarly track where someone is pointing, and by 12 months children begin to use pointing themselves as a means of indicating wants and needs (this is referred to as **proto-imperative pointing**). Children typically engage their parents with eye contact, look toward the desired object, point to the desired object, and then look back at the parent while continuing to point. This suggests reciprocity in perspective-taking; the child perceives his/her parent's point of view and then uses pointing, eye contact, and vocalizations to influence the parent to see things from the child's perspective and respond accordingly. By 15 months of age, the child will also point to objects simply to express interest or share an experience, as if to say, "See what I'm looking at, I want you to look, too." This is referred to as **proto-declarative pointing.**

By 18 months of age, children demonstrate embarrassment and shame, as well as empathy, all of which presuppose an awareness of the perceptions and emotional states of others in the social environment. It is also at this age that the capacity for **pretend play** (e.g., having a "tea party") emerges. Pretend play, even when done alone, has at its heart the idea of intentionality and agency (acting to produce a particular result) learned through social interaction and applied to the world of things. When a child plays with a stuffed animal or doll, he is imputing the qualities of mind, feeling, and agency to that toy.

Between 18 and 24 months, children develop an increasing sense of autonomy, and they begin to exhibit defiant behavior in an attempt to establish the priority of their own intentions and desires above those of their caregivers. Two-year-olds exhibit the ability to **parallel play** (playing in the company of other children); by 3 years, they are able to engage in **cooperative play** (involving sharing, turn taking, and common goals). Three-year-olds have a vivid imagination, and they are able to engage in true **imaginative play,** which includes the ability to imagine that a thing is something other than itself (e.g., that a stick is a magic wand). It is also at this age that children develop fears of imaginary creatures. Four-year-olds are able to use this capacity to imagine things being "other than they actually are," to tell fibs, or to try to "trick" others by saying something they know to be untrue in order to get a reaction.

Four-year-olds are also able to pass the "ultimate" test of theory of mind, the false belief test (Bauminger-Zviely, 2013). This is also called the **Sally-Ann Test,** after the original version of the test (Baron-Cohen, Leslie, & Frith, 1985). The child being tested is presented with the follow scenario:

> Sally and Ann are together in a room; Sally has a basket. Ann has a box. Sally puts a marble in the basket and leaves the room. While Sally is gone, Ann moves the marble to the box. When Sally comes back, where will she look for her marble?

A 3-year-old presented with this puzzle believes that Sally will look in the box because the 3-year-old knows it's there, but a typical 4-year-old will realize that, from Sally's perspective, the marble should still be where she left it.

The continued development of theory of mind and the nuances of perspective-taking are at the basis of ongoing emotional development throughout the life span. It provides the foundation for friendship and also serves as the basis for the development of a mature morality based on an appreciation of the interests and needs of others (Killen & Smetana, 2013). It also helps to explain people's interest in gossip and the contemporary obsession with social media; this propensity seems to be built into one's DNA and hardwired into the brain.

Symbolic Thought and Language

Since the advent of the Internet, humans are inundated with words and language in its myriad forms and are liable to think of its written manifestations when we hear the word "language." But written language is a relatively recent invention, and language is fundamentally a social and verbal phenomenon with a biological origin. The fact that language has a basis in biology is supported by the observation that children seem to be "programmed" for language learning and typically become fluent in their native language through simple social exposure to its use without any formal instruction. Infants also show a sensitive period in early infancy, during which time their auditory system is able to process any phoneme of any language. After about 9 months of age, children become preferentially sensitive to the phonemes of their native language. And as noted previously, language has a firm basis in our hypersocial nature. Through reciprocal gestures, facial expressions, and vocalizations, infants establish the basis for communication well before their first birthday and well before they can use spoken language.

When children do begin to speak, their first words are usually "mama" and "dada" (if the spoken language is English). They begin to use other words by 12 months of age, but it is clear that they can understand words such as "no" and the names of family members well before they can speak. Between 12 and 18 months of age, children gradually acquire the ability to use other single words and can typically say about 10 to 25 words by 18 months. Up to this point, children tend to enjoy using words to label objects and pictures, and to a limited degree they use words to indicate wants and needs. They, however, are still reliant on gestures, facial expressions, and nonspecific vocalizations to make their needs known.

Typically beginning between 18 and 24 months, children undergo a radical expansion and transformation of their language skills. By 24 months, children are using a minimum of 50 words. More importantly, they are beginning to combine words into phrases, and eventually sentences, using the grammar of their native language. Initially phrases are dominated by simple nouns and verbs, but by 30 months other parts of speech, such as pronouns, come into use. By 3 years of age, most children can use complete, grammatical sentences that are intelligible most of the time, and they can say more than 200 individual words. By 4 years of age, children are using as many as 1,000 words, and they can tell simple stories and jokes, use the past tense, and engage in reciprocal (back-and-forth) conversation. By 5 years of age children can use the future tense, complex sentence forms, and can retell complicated stories with a clear beginning, middle, and end (see Chapter 17 for a detailed discussion of speech, language, and communication).

DISTINGUISHING TYPICAL AND ATYPICAL DEVELOPMENT

Isabella, the 2-year-old described in the case study at the beginning of this chapter, presented with a very common developmental concern, a delay in the development of her speech and language skills. The term "delay" figures prominently in discussions of developmental problems, and in this case recognizes that Isabella is not doing something (talking) that we would expect a child her age would do. **Developmental delays** may refer to the late emergence of a particular skill or milestone or the general slowing of development within or across broader domains of development. Development that is more delayed in some domains than others is referred to as a **dissociated** pattern of delay. Development that is significantly delayed across all domains is referred to as a **global developmental delay.**

Development can also deviate or diverge from typical patterns of development. Whereas a child with delays exhibits typical milestones at later-than-expected ages, a child with divergent traits exhibits qualitatively different skills or behaviors that are not usually seen in most children at any point during their development. For example, children with ASD (see Chapter 18) exhibit a variety of divergent behaviors such as echolalia (randomly repeating bits of favorite TV shows or conversation) or unusual, repetitive body movements, such as hand flapping. Depending on the nature of the developmental problem, children will exhibit variable degrees of delay and divergence, and it is the task of the developmental practitioner to recognize, identify, and characterize the nature of these changes (Accardo, 2008; Voigt, 2018; see Chapter 12 for a detailed discussion of the use of these concepts in the diagnostic process).

Recognizing Problems: Developmental Surveillance

Isabella's speech difficulties first came to light when her pediatrician asked her mother about developmental milestones as part of a well-child visit. Her pediatrician was knowledgeable about typical development and routinely inquired about specific milestones at each well-child visit. As part of her training, she learned to use charts and tables of developmental milestones as references for typical development, and she incorporated this information into the questions that she asked parents about their children.

The process of review of developmental progress over time is known as **developmental surveillance.** Primary care providers, including pediatricians, family practitioners, nurse practitioners, and physician assistants, are uniquely positioned to provide such surveillance due to their frequent contact with young children throughout the critical early stages of their development. Optimizing the parent–practitioner partnership is critical to ensuring the success of developmental surveillance as parents are the primary source of the information that forms the basis for surveillance (see Box 11.1).

Developmental surveillance provides the foundation and context for all other processes of developmental assessment, but it has its pitfalls. Clinicians vary considerably with regard to their level of experience and expertise in identifying developmental differences. Variability also exists in the degree to which individual clinicians prioritize developmental issues relative to the many other concerns that are addressed during a typical well-child visit. Some clinicians utilize up-to-date developmental references and surveillance tools, whereas others may rely on their memory of potentially out-of-date information from early in their training. Studies indicate that as a consequence of this variability, many children with potentially significant developmental concerns may not be identified for early intervention services (Thomas, Cotton, Pan, & Ratliff-Schaub, 2012). Surveillance is therefore considered a necessary, but not entirely sufficient, part of the process of identifying delayed and divergent development.

Recognizing Problems: Developmental Screening

In addition to asking Isabella's mother about her development, her pediatrician also administered a standardized screening test. In 2006, the American Academy of Pediatrics (AAP), recognizing the limitations of developmental surveillance, published guidelines recommending that all children routinely undergo developmental screening using a standardized screening tool (test) at 9, 18, and 30 months of age (see Box 11.2). In addition, the screening tool should be used at any visit when surveillance suggests a developmental problem (Council on Children with Disabilities, 2006).

Several commonly used developmental screening tests are described in Table 11.4. The original recommendations were subsequently modified to allow screening at 24 months as an alternative to 30-month testing, mainly because most primary care offices do not see children for well-child visits at 30 months (visits are keyed to vaccination schedules; Marks & LaRosa, 2012).

Isabella's pediatrician decided to administer a screening test both because of the child's age and because of concerns about speech identified through surveillance. **Screening tests** are primarily designed to distinguish children who are at risk for developmental problems from those who are not, and, as such, they usually yield a "pass" or "fail" result. Depending on

BOX 11.1 INTERDISCIPLINARY CARE

The Parent–Practitioner Partnership in Recognizing Development Delay

Because they have regular contact with children during the early, critical stages of development, medical practitioners (pediatricians, family practice physicians, pediatric nurse practitioners, and physician assistants) have a mandate to identify developmental problems and refer children for early intervention. This goal can only be accomplished in close partnership with parents and other primary care givers, whose knowledge of and concerns about their children form the basis for developmental surveillance and screening. Indeed, it is typically parents who first recognize problems in their children, and the wise practitioner will take these concerns seriously and act promptly. A "wait-and-see" approach to development delay is almost never advisable.

BOX 11.2 EVIDENCE-BASED PRACTICE

Implementing Recommendations for Developmental Screening

The American Academy of Pediatrics (AAP)'s 2006 guidelines for developmental screening and surveillance recommended automatic administration of a validated screening tool for all children at ages 9, 18, and 24 or 30 months (Council on Children with Disabilities, 2006). A survey of pediatricians completed in 2009 revealed that although the recommendations did result in a significant increase in screening, more than one half of practitioners were still not following the AAP guidelines (Radecki, Sand-Loud, O'Connor, Sharp, & Olson, 2011).

In response to this, the New Mexico Developmental Screening Initiative was created (Malik, Booker, Brown, McClain, & McGrath, 2014). Seven large practices in a large urban area were involved in an intensive quality improvement project to improve rates of developmental screening. After 1 year, rates of screening in these practices improved from 27% to 92%.

the test, a "fail" result should prompt either follow-up screening procedures or referral for diagnostic assessment and potential services.

Many screening tests utilize specific developmental milestones in the assessment process, but the limitations of individual milestones are overcome by incorporation of multiple milestones into the process of standardization of the test as a whole. Other screening tests, such as the one that Isabella's pediatrician used, rely instead on caregiver report of concern about

Table 11.4. Commonly used developmental screening tools

Screening tool	Characteristics	Administration and uses	Interpretation
Ages and Stages Questionnaires®, Third Edition (ASQ®-3; Squires, Bricker, & Potter, 2009)	0–60 months Sensitivity 70%–90%; Specificity 76%–91% Based on specific milestones by age	Self-administered (parent) with or without clinician assistance 30 items 10–15 minutes Used as first-line screening tool for general developmental concerns and to aid surveillance	Yields pass or fail results for domains and recommendations for referral
Modified Checklist for Autism in Toddlers, Revised (M-CHAT-R; Robins et al., 2014)	16–30 months Based on specific questions regarding communication and socialization skills	Self-administered (parent) 20 items 5–10 minutes	Yields scores: high risk (8–20; referral for EI), medium risk (3–7; rescreen with M-CHAT-R/F), low risk (0–2; reassurance)
Modified Checklist for Autism in Toddlers, Revised with Follow-up (M-CHAT-R/F; Robins et al., 2014)	16–30 months Based on specific questions regarding communication and socialization skills	Interview by clinician 5–10 minutes Used to rescreen medium risk scores from M-CHAT-R	Scores 2 or greater indicated referral; other rescreen at future visits
Parents' Evaluation of Developmental Status (PEDS; Glascoe, 2007)	0–9 years Sensitivity 74%–79%; Specificity 70%–80% Based on parental concern Available in 14 languages	0–9 years Sensitivity 74%–79%; Specificity 70%–80% Based on parental concern Available in 14 languages	Scores fall into categories (decision pathways) (high risk = referral; moderate risk = further screening or referral; low risk = education and reassurance)
Parents' Evaluation of Developmental Status—Developmental Milestones (PEDS-DM; Brothers, Glascoe, & Robertshaw, 2008)	0–8 years Sensitivity 70% or greater; Specificity 77%–93% Based on specific milestones by age	Administered by clinician 6–8 items 4–10 minutes Used to supplement PEDS, to rescreen moderate risk PEDS, and to aid surveillance	Yields pass or fail results Interpretation made in conjunction with other screening tools (such as the PEDS)

Sensitivity refers to the percentage of children with true delays correctly identified. *Specificity* refers to the percentage of children without delays correctly identified. Developmental screening tests should have sensitivities and specificities > 70%.

development, and they are based on research recognizing that parents/caregivers reliably identify developmental problems in their children (Glascoe & Marks, 2011). An effective screening test is simple and fast to administer, and it can identify children with developmental problems (the test has good sensitivity) as well as children who do *not* have developmental problems (the test has good specificity).

Because of increasing concerns about identifying children with ASD, the AAP has also recommended that autism-specific screening tests be administered to all children at 18 and 24 months of age (Zwaigenbaum et al., 2015).

Early Intervention

The primary purpose of developmental surveillance and screening is to identify children for referral to early intervention. Multiple studies have identified the importance of providing early intervention in optimizing long-term developmental outcomes in children at risk for or manifesting developmental disabilities (Wallander et al., 2014). **Early intervention** refers to a specific, federally mandated program for children from birth to 3 years of age (see Chapter 31), but it more broadly refers to a variety of special education services and therapeutic interventions that are employed throughout early childhood.

Developmental Diagnosis

Developmental surveillance and screening are critical to identifying children with atypical development, but they do not, in and of themselves, diagnose the nature of these problems. The diagnostic process, which involves a complex consideration of a child's developmental history combined with the results of screening and testing procedures, is discussed in detail in Chapter 12.

SUMMARY

- The term *development* refers to the characteristic, predictable ways that behavior changes during the human life cycle and can be characterized in terms of specific functional domains.
- The term *typical* is preferred to the term *normal* when describing developmental change as experienced by most children.
- A variety of developmental theories have been developed in an attempt to describe and explain the complexities of child development.
- Developmental milestones are used to map the processes of developmental change, and while they are indispensable in clinical practice, they must be understood and used carefully to avoid misuse and misinterpretation.
- It is useful to think of the processes of development as a kind of recapitulation of the evolutionary adaptations of our species.
- Trends in development can be described in four broad categories: mobility (bipedalism), adaptive skills (tool use; manipulating the environment), theory of mind (hypersociality), and language (symbolic thought).
- Atypical development occurs when a child exhibits delays or otherwise diverges from expected developmental trajectories, either in some domains more than others (dissociated development) or across all domains of function (globally impaired development).
- Clinicians, and primary care providers in particular, have a mandate to identify children with atypical development through the processes of developmental surveillance and screening.
- The use of standardized screening tools is recommended at 9, 18, and 24 or 30 months or when concerns arise about a child's development at any age.

ADDITIONAL RESOURCES

Ages and Stages: Birth to 12 months: http://www.extension.iastate.edu/Publications/PM1530A.pdf

American Academy of Pediatrics: Bright Futures:

https://brightfutures.aap.org/families/Pages/Resources-for-Families.aspx

Centers for Disease Control: Developmental Monitoring and Screening:

https://www.cdc.gov/ncbddd/childdevelopment/screening.html

Additional resources can be found online in Appendix D: Childhood Disabilities Resources, Services, and Organizations (see About the Online Companion Materials).

REFERENCES

Accardo, P. J. (Ed.). (2008). *Capute & Accardo's neurodevelopmental disabilities in infancy and childhood* (3rd ed.). Baltimore, MD: Paul H. Brookes Publishing Co.

Bandura, A. (1977). *Social learning theory*. Englewood Cliffs, NJ: Prentice Hall.
Baron-Cohen, S., Leslie, A. M., & Frith, U. (1985). Does the autistic child have a "theory of mind"? *Cognition, 21*(1), 37–46.
Bauminger-Zviely, N. (2013). False-belief task. In F. R. Volkmar (Ed.), *Encyclopedia of autism spectrum disorders*. Retrieved from https://link.springer.com/referenceworkentry/10.1007%2F978-1-4419-1698-3_91
Brothers, K. B., Glascoe, F. P., & Robertshaw, N. S. (2008). PEDS: Developmental milestones—An accurate brief tool for surveillance and screening. *Clinical Pediatrics, 47*(3), 271–279.
Bowlby, J. (2005). *The making and breaking of affectional bonds*. London, England; New York, NY: Routledge.
Bronfenbrenner, U. (1979). *The ecology of human development: Experiments by nature and design*. Cambridge, MA: Harvard University Press.
Council on Children with Disabilities. (2006). Identifying infants and young children with developmental disorders in the medical home: An algorithm for developmental surveillance and screening. *Pediatrics, 118*(1), 405–420.
Dosman, C. F., Andrews, D., & Goulden, K. J. (2012). Evidence-based milestone ages as a framework for developmental surveillance. *Paediatrics & Child Health, 17*(10), 561–568.
Dunbar, R. I. (2009). The social brain hypothesis and its implications for social evolution. *Annals of Human Biology, 36*(5), 562–572.
Erikson, E. H., & Coles, R. (2000). *The Erik Erikson reader* (1st ed.). New York, NY: W.W. Norton.
Fraiberg, S. H. (2015). *The magic years: Understanding and handling the problems of early childhood*. New York, NY: Scribner.
Frankenburg, W. K., Dodds, J., Archer, P., Shapiro, H., & Bresnick, B. (1992). The Denver II: A major revision and restandardization of the Denver Developmental Screening Test. *Pediatrics, 89*(1), 91–97.
Freud, S., & Strachey, J. (2000). *Three essays on the theory of sexuality*. New York, NY: Basic Books.
Gerber, R. J., Wilks, T., & Erdie-Lalena, C. (2010). Developmental milestones: Motor development. *Pediatrics in Review, 31*(7), 267–276.
Gerber, R. J., Wilks, T., & Erdie-Lalena, C. (2011). Developmental milestones 3: Social-emotional development. *Pediatrics in Review, 32*(12), 533–536.
Glascoe, F. P. (2007). *Parents' evaluation of developmental status:An evidence-based approach to developmental-behavioral screening and surveillance*. Nashville, TN: Ellsworth & Vandermeer Press.
Glascoe, F. P., & Marks, K. P. (2011). Detecting children with developmental-behavioral problems: The value of collaborating with parents. *Psychological Test and Assessment Modeling, 53*(2), 258–279.
Killen, M., & Smetana, J. (Eds.). (2013). *Handbook of moral development* (2nd ed.). New York, NY: Psychological Press.
Malik, F., Booker, J. M., Brown, S., McClain, C., & McGrath, J. (2014). Improving developmental screening among pediatricians in New Mexico: Findings from the developmental screening initiative. *Clinical Pediatrics, 53*(6), 531–538.
Marks, K. P., & LaRosa, A. C. (2012). Understanding developmental-behavioral screening measures. *Pediatrics in Review, 33*(10), 448–457; quiz 457–448. doi:10.1542/pir.33-10-448
Piper, M. C., & Darrah, J. (1994). *Motor assessment of the developing infant*. Philadelphia, PA: Saunders.
Radecki, L., Sand-Loud, N., O'Connor, K. G., Sharp, S., & Olson, L. M. (2011). Trends in the use of standardized tools for developmental screening in early childhood: 2002–2009. *Pediatrics, 128*(1), 14–19.
Redcay, E., Haist, F., & Courchesne, E. (2008). Functional neuroimaging of speech perception during a pivotal period in language acquisition. *Developmental Science, 11*(2), 237–252.
Robins, D. L., Casagrande, K., Barton, M., Chen, C. M., Dumont-Mathieu, T., & Fein, D. (2014). Validation of the Modified Checklist for Autism in Toddlers, Revised with Follow-up (M-CHAT-R/F). *Pediatrics, 133*(1), 37–45.
Shaffer, D. R., & Kipp, K. (2014). *Developmental psychology: Childhood and adolescence* (9th ed.). Belmont, CA: Wadsworth Cengage Learning.
Skinner, B. F. (1966). *Contingencies of reinforcement*. New York, NY: Appleton-Century-Crofts. Reprinted 2013, B. F. Skinner Foundation.
Squires, J., Bricker, D., & Potter, L. (2009). *Ages & Stages Questionnaires®, third edition (ASQ®-3) user's guide*. Baltimore, MD: Paul H. Brookes Publishing Co.
Thelen, E., & Smith, L. B. (1994). *A dynamic systems approach to the development of cognition and action*. Cambridge, MA: MIT Press.
Thomas, S. A., Cotton, W., Pan, X., & Ratliff-Schaub, K. (2012). Comparison of systematic developmental surveillance with standardized developmental screening in primary care. *Clinical Pediatrics, 51*(2), 154–159.
Tuttle, R. H. (2017). Human evolution. *Britannica*. Retrieved from https://www.britannica.com/science/human-evolution
Voigt, R. G. (2018) Making developmental-behavioral diagnoses. In R. G. Voigt, M. M. Macias, S. M. Myers, & D. D. Tapia (Eds.), *American Academy of Pediatrics developmental and behavioral pediatrics* (2nd ed.; pp. 187–221). Itasca, IL: American Academy of Pediatrics.
Volpe, J. J. (2018). *Volpe's neurology of the newborn* (6th ed.). Philadelphia, PA: Elsevier.
von dem Hagen, E. A., Stoyanova, R. S., Rowe, J. B., Baron-Cohen, S., & Calder, A. J. (2014). Direct gaze elicits atypical activation of the theory-of-mind network in autism spectrum conditions. *Cerebral Cortex, 24*(6), 1485–1492.
Vygotsky, L. S., & Cole, M. (1978). *Mind in society: The development of higher psychological processes*. Cambridge, MA: Harvard University Press.
Wadsworth, B. J. (2004). *Piaget's theory of cognitive and affective development* (Classic ed.). Boston, MA: Pearson/A and B.
Wallander, J. L., Biasini, F. J., Thorsten, V., Dhaded, S. M., de Jong, D. M., Chomba, E., . . . Carlo, W. A. (2014). Dose of early intervention treatment during children's first 36 months of life is associated with developmental outcomes: An observational cohort study in three low/low-middle income countries. *BMC Pediatrics, 14*, 281.
Werker, J. F., & Hensch, T. K. (2015). Critical periods in speech perception: New directions. *Annual Review of Psychology, 66*, 173–196. doi:10.1146/annurev-psych-010814-015104
Wilks, T., Gerber, R. J., & Erdie-Lalena, C. (2010). Developmental milestones: Cognitive development. *Pediatrics in Review, 31*(9), 364–367.
Zwaigenbaum, L., Bauman, M. L., Fein, D., Pierce, K., Buie, T., Davis, P. A., . . . Wagner, S. (2015). Early screening of autism spectrum disorder: Recommendations for practice and research. *Pediatrics, 136(Suppl. 1)*, S41–S59.

CHAPTER 12

Diagnosing Developmental Disabilities

Scott M. Myers

Upon completion of this chapter, the reader will

- Recognize the major streams/domains of development and their role in defining the spectrum and continuum of developmental disabilities
- Understand atypical patterns of development including delay, dissociation, deviance, and regression and their role in developmental diagnosis
- Discover the components of the developmental diagnostic evaluation and how they contribute to the diagnostic formulation

Children typically present for developmental diagnostic evaluation because of concerns about not attaining cognitive, motor, or social/adaptive milestones or about the presence of aberrant behaviors. These issues may be raised spontaneously by parents or other caregivers or teachers, or they may be elicited by health care providers through developmental surveillance and screening (American Academy of Pediatrics et al., 2006; Bellman, Byrne, & Sege, 2013). The diagnostic process enables the clinician to begin to answer the four fundamental questions that most parents have when they seek evaluation:

1. What is wrong with my child? (Diagnosis)
2. What is going to happen to my child over time? (Natural history/prognosis)
3. What can be done to improve my child's condition? (Treatment)
4. What caused my child's condition? (Etiology)

In this chapter, general principles and processes involved in diagnosis of developmental disabilities are reviewed. Details about each of the specific disabilities and procedures, such as developmental or psychological testing, are available in other chapters in this volume (Chapters 11 and 13) and in other current textbooks in the field (e.g., Accardo, 2008; Augustyn, Zuckerman, & Caronna, 2011; Carey, Crocker, Coleman, Elias, & Feldman, 2009; Sonksen, 2016; Voigt, Macias, Myers, & Tapia, 2018; Wolraich, Drotar, Dworkin, & Perrin, 2008). The focus is on developmental disabilities caused by brain dysfunction rather than those caused by sensory deficits (e.g., blindness or deafness); orthopedic impairments; or disorders of the spinal cord, peripheral nervous system, or muscle.

CASE STUDY

At her 18-month routine health supervision visit, Julia's parents raised concerns about delays in her attainment of developmental milestones and lack of intelligible speech. These concerns were validated by a parent-completed general developmental screening measure, and her pediatrician confirmed the concerns and noted that her head circumference measurement was at the 98th percentile for age. She was referred to the local early intervention program for evaluation, which confirmed delays in cognitive, communication, social-emotional, adaptive, and physical development. Speech-language therapy, occupational therapy, and physical therapy were initiated. Audiological assessment was completed, and her hearing was found to be normal. Because of the macrocephaly (large head size) and developmental delays, magnetic resonance imaging of Julia's brain was completed. The results were normal.

Speech development progressed more slowly than other aspects of development, and Julia developed some repetitive behaviors and other features that raised concerns about the possibility of autism, prompting referral for additional evaluation. Neurodevelopmental assessment at age 3.5 years revealed global developmental delay (GDD), including delays of approximately 35% in receptive language and nonverbal problem-solving abilities and approximately 60% in expressive language. General adaptive functioning was also significantly subaverage. Speech intelligibility was very poor, and she had difficulty imitating words. However, although she exhibited some features commonly associated with autism, Julia did not meet criteria for autism spectrum disorder (ASD). Her height and weight were both at approximately the 40th percentile, her body mass index was just above the 50th percentile, and her head circumference was at the 98th percentile. No dysmorphic features or structural anomalies were noted. Neurologic examination was notable for mild neuromotor abnormalities, including mild hypotonia; mixed or unclear hand dominance; and qualitatively immature coordination. Chromosomal microarray analysis (CMA; see Chapter 1) was recommended to try to determine the etiology of Julia's GDD, superimposed expressive language disorder (suspected to be a motor speech disorder), macrocephaly, and mild neuromotor abnormalities; she was referred to a pediatric speech-language pathologist with expertise in the diagnosis and treatment of motor speech disorders in young children.

The speech-language pathologist determined that Julia met criteria for childhood apraxia of speech. As such, he increased the intensity of therapy, focusing on improving functional communication through the use of sign language and gestures, while building on sounds in her phonemic repertoire to increase verbal output. Chromosomal microarray analysis revealed an almost 600-kb deletion on the short arm of chromosome 16 at 16p11.2, consistent with a molecular diagnosis of 16p11.2 recurrent deletion syndrome, which explained her developmental diagnoses. The test results and implications were explained to her parents with the help of a genetic counselor, and they were relieved to learn that neither of them had the deletion, meaning that this was a *de novo* (new) deletion in Julia; as such, the chance that their subsequent children would have 16p11.2 recurrent deletion syndrome was estimated to be less than 1%. Radiographs of the spine ruled out vertebral anomalies and scoliosis, which occur in about 20% of individuals with this deletion, and her parents were counseled about the increased risk of obesity and, less commonly, seizures. Her family became active in a support group and found it very helpful to meet other children and families affected by 16p11.2 recurrent deletion syndrome. When Julia was 5 years old, the diagnosis of GDD was replaced by the diagnosis of mild intellectual disability (ID), based on the results of psychological testing.

Thought Questions:

How might different meanings of the term *diagnosis* convey different information and treatment implications? What is the value of conceptualizing neurodevelopmental disorders as clinical manifestations of a common denominator, namely developmental brain dysfunction?

DEVELOPMENTAL PRINCIPLES

Development is an end product of neural function that unfolds over time as a result of 1) innate factors determined by the DNA sequence and heritable epigenetic modifications that make up an individual's biological endowment and 2) experiential influences that either affect neurodevelopment beneficially (e.g., environmental enrichment) or deleteriously (e.g., traumatic or hypoxic-ischemic brain insults or toxic stress) during sensitive periods of neuromaturation (Wang, 2018). The complex, dynamic processes that make up child development can be described clinically by quantifiable milestones and qualitative features and can be divided into three primary "streams" (also referred to as "domains") of development: motor, cognitive, and neurobehavioral. Each of the primary streams can be broken down into narrower streams of development, which can be assessed independently (Table 12.1). The motor stream includes gross and fine motor skills as well as oral motor function (e.g., chewing, swallowing, and motor aspects of speech). The cognitive, or central processing, stream includes receptive and expressive language abilities and nonverbal problem-solving/perceptual reasoning.

Table 12.1. Streams of development

Motor
Gross motor
Fine motor
Oral motor
Cognitive (or central processing)
Language
Receptive
Expressive
Nonverbal problem-solving/perceptual reasoning
Neurobehavioral
Social behavior
Adaptive emotional behavior, self-regulation, and mental status

The neurobehavioral stream includes fundamental aspects of social and emotional behavior, self-regulation, and mental status. These include the development of reciprocal social interaction, impulse control, attention, the development of an appropriately varied repertoire of interests and activities, and the development of adaptive regulation of mood and anxiety.

ATYPICAL PATTERNS OF DEVELOPMENT

Based on careful study of the development of thousands of infants and children, Gesell observed that typical development is methodical, orderly (sequential), timed, and therefore largely predictable (Gesell, Halvorsen, & Amatruda, 1940; Gesell & Amatruda, 1947). This principle is the basis for using developmental milestones and tests as markers of neuromaturation. Independent assessment of skills within each stream of development facilitates recognition of patterns of atypical development. The terms *delay, dissociation,* and *deviance* describe variations in the attainment of developmental milestones as manifestations of underlying brain dysfunction, and analysis of these three types of variation is helpful in distinguishing among diagnostic possibilities (Accardo, Accardo, & Capute, 2008; Capute & Palmer, 1980; Voigt, 2018; also see Chapter 11).

Developmental delay refers to a significant lag in the attainment of milestones in one or more areas of development; milestones are attained in the typical sequence but at a slower rate. Traditionally, a delay of 22.5%–25% or greater in the rate of development, or performance that is 1.5 to 2 standard deviations or more below the norm, has been considered to be significant. The developmental quotient (DQ) is a useful means of quantifying development within a stream as a percentage of normal. The DQ is therefore a ratio; that is, the child's developmental age (DA) in a particular area of development divided by his or her chronological age (CA) and multiplied by 100 to yield a percentage ($DQ = DA / CA \times 100$). For example, a 20-month-old child who is found to have gross motor skills at the level expected of a typically developing 12 month old has a DQ in the gross motor stream of $12 / 20 \times 100 = 60$. This child can thus be said to be exhibiting a 40% delay in gross motor development or to be progressing at 60% of the typical rate within the gross motor stream. The functional DA equivalent is determined based on comparison to typical milestones in a particular area of development using tables of normal milestones that are available in textbooks (e.g., Accardo, 2008; Sonksen, 2016) and review articles (Scharf, Scharf, & Stroustrup, 2016) or assessment instruments that yield age equivalents in different streams of development, such as the Capute Scales (Cognitive Adaptive Test/Clinical Linguistic and Auditory Milestone Scale [CAT/CLAMS]; Accardo & Capute, 2005), the Parents' Evaluation of Developmental Status: Developmental Milestones (PEDS:DM; Brothers, Glascoe, & Robertshaw, 2008), and the Child Development Inventory (CDI; Ireton, 1992).

Developmental dissociation refers to a significant difference in developmental rates between two of the major areas of development: gross motor, fine motor, problem-solving, expressive language, receptive language, and social/adaptive. Typical sequences of development are maintained, but there is asynchrony, resulting in one or more areas of development being significantly out of phase with other areas. By convention, a DQ or rate discrepancy of greater than 15 percentage points between two major areas of development is typically considered to represent dissociation in infants or young children. In older children, a difference in standard scores of more than 1 to 1.5 standard deviations on standardized measures traditionally defines a significant discrepancy between academic achievement and intellectual ability (Peterson & Pennington, 2015; Shaywitz, Morris, & Shaywitz, 2008).

Developmental deviance refers to nonsequential unevenness in the achievement of milestones within one or more streams of development (e.g., within-task scatter). This phenomenon is typically described qualitatively, rather than as a rate, quotient, or standard score, although some investigators have attempted to quantify deviance in the form of intrasubtest scatter (inconsistent or unusual response patterns to test items within a single scale on a standardized test; Godber, Anderson, & Bell, 2000; VanMeter, Fein, Morris, Waterhouse, & Allen, 1997). Typical developmental sequences are not maintained, and deviance is intrinsically abnormal.

Whereas children exhibiting delay and dissociation attain milestones in a manner that would be expected for a younger typically developing child, deviance is not typical for any age.

GDD has often been defined in the literature as significant delays in two or more of the following domains: gross motor/fine motor, speech/language, cognition, social/personal, and adaptive functioning (i.e., activities of daily living; Moeschler & Shevell, 2014; Riou, Ghosh, Francoeur, & Shevell, 2009). According to this definition, a child with spastic diplegic cerebral palsy (CP) causing isolated motor delay and secondary adaptive deficits and an infant exhibiting 25% delays in expressive language and gross motor skills (with average receptive language and problem-solving abilities) would both be considered to have GDD. The assumption that having delays in any two domains is equivalent to having general intellectual delay is inherently problematic; for example, Riou and colleagues (2009) demonstrated that among preschoolers with a diagnosis of GDD, 73% had an IQ greater than 70 and 20% had average intelligence.

The alternate definition of GDD restricts its use to young children with significant delays in both language and nonlanguage cognition (problem-solving) accompanied by deficits in adaptive behavior (activities of daily living). This definition more closely approximates applying the concept of ID to children who may be too young to obtain a valid and reliable IQ measurement. In these children, continued development at the same trajectory would predict functioning within the ID range. Of course, this does not mean that all children with GDD will ultimately have ID because developmental trajectories may change, but the greater the degree of GDD, the higher the predictive validity of an early childhood diagnosis (Elbaum & Celimi-Aksoy, 2017; VanderVeer & Schweid, 1974). Consistent with the latter approach, in 2013 the fifth edition of the *Diagnostic and Statistical Manual of Mental Disorders* (*DSM-5*) introduced GDD as a diagnostic classification to describe children under the age of 5 years who exhibit developmental delays "in several areas of intellectual functioning," and categorized this diagnosis within the intellectual disabilities subgroup of neurodevelopmental disorders (American Psychiatric Association, 2013).

Once specific areas of delay have been identified, the concept of dissociation becomes particularly important in defining and distinguishing among the various developmental disability diagnoses. Mixed receptive and expressive language disorders, for example, are defined by language development that is delayed and dissociated from other streams of development, especially nonlanguage cognition/problem-solving. In the case of expressive language disorders, there is dissociation between the expressive and receptive components of the language stream; expressive language development is delayed, but receptive language and nonlanguage cognition are intact. Specific learning disabilities are also determined by dissociation, or discrepancy; academic underachievement in a specific area (e.g., reading, mathematics, or written expression) is unexpected because the child appears to have all of the factors (i.e., intact sensory abilities, adequate intelligence and motivation, and exposure to reasonable instruction) needed to achieve but continues to struggle (Fletcher & Miciak, 2017; Peterson & Pennington, 2015; Shaywitz et al., 2008). In the past, discrepancy between academic achievement and intellectual ability (as measured by IQ) was used as the primary indicator of the presence of a specific learning disability. However, the weight of the evidence suggests that there is little difference between IQ-discrepant and nondiscrepant low-achieving children in achievement, behavior, cognitive processes (e.g., phonological awareness), prognosis, response to treatment, or neuroimaging markers of brain function (Fletcher & Miciak, 2017; Peterson & Pennington, 2015). Current approaches emphasize the discrepancy between actual and expected response to quality instruction, and IQ tests are not required for diagnosis of a specific learning disability (see Chapter 20; Fletcher & Miciak, 2017; Peterson & Pennington, 2015). Important components of a learning disability evaluation include assessment of academic achievement using well-validated standardized measures, instructional response, and contextual factors that interfere with achievement, such as other disorders (e.g., attention-deficit/hyperactivity disorder [ADHD]) or toxic stress (Fletcher & Miciak, 2017). Absolute developmental delay relative to age does not have to be present for dissociation to be significant, since, for example, a child with an IQ of 130 and standard scores of approximately 100 on measures of reading achievement may have a specific reading disability based on poorer-than-expected reading performance despite quality instruction (Gilman et al., 2013).

Developmental deviance may present in young children as failure to accomplish simple tasks or skills in a given developmental sequence while unexpectedly performing tasks that are more complex. For example, a 2-year-old child who can use single words to label more than 50 different objects or pictures and correctly identify colors and shapes, yet does not use words to make requests, does not say "mama" or "dada," and still engages in immature jargoning is exhibiting significantly deviant language development. Strong rote memory skills accompanied by weak comprehension and pragmatic (social) language skills may contribute to this deviant profile and may suggest the presence of ASD (Boucher, 2012; Myers & Challman, 2018). Most individually administered standardized psychometric tests include items that are arranged hierarchically, so in order to be able to administer only the appropriate portion of the test to a particular child, a "basal" and a "ceiling" must be established. Typically, this means that the child must answer a certain number of consecutive items correctly to establish a basal, and the test is stopped when the child answers a certain number of consecutive items incorrectly (ceiling). Developmental deviance, especially in older children with learning disorders, may be suggested by a much-wider-than-average number of items between the basal and the ceiling on a particular test or subtest because of tending to pass more advanced items in the hierarchy while failing easier items (Accardo et al., 2008; Godber et al., 2000). Deviance in motor development may occur in children with CP due to abnormal muscle tone and control. For example, a child with spastic diplegia may be able to stand holding on and cruise along furniture before being able to sit independently.

Another phenomenon that may be detected by history or upon serial assessment is **developmental regression,** which is the loss of previously attained milestones. A child who has truly regressed developmentally is no longer capable of performing previously mastered skills. Regression may occur following a period of typical development or may be superimposed on preexisting atypical development (Baird et al., 2008; Meilleur & Fombonne, 2009). According to population-based studies, approximately 20% of children with ASD lose previously established language and/or social interaction skills at a mean age of 21–24 months (Barger, Campbell, & McDonough, 2013). The reported rate of regression is higher (35%–40%) in clinic-based samples and survey studies (Barger et al., 2013). However, the true prevalence of meaningful regression may be lower because these studies are plagued by problems with case definition and reliance on parent-reported skill loss without verification by rigorous clinical information gathering (Barbaresi, 2016). In addition, very few cases of frank regression have been reported in prospective studies of high-risk infants (Jones, Gliga, Bedford, Charman, & Johnson, 2014). Although unexplained developmental regression is not unique to ASD, the available evidence suggests that it is more frequent in children with ASD than in those with other diagnoses such as GDD and specific language impairment (Baird et al., 2008; Pickles et al., 2009). However, the rate of developmental regression, including language regression, is also high (22%) in children with severe or profound congenital visual impairment (Dale & Sonksen, 2002). Landau-Kleffner syndrome, or acquired epileptic aphasia, is a rare epilepsy syndrome that affects otherwise typically developing children between 3 and 7 years of age and involves loss of the ability to understand and use spoken language (Shbarou & Mikati, 2016). Most affected children also have clinical seizures (see Chapter 22). Global regression involving language, motor, and cognitive skills may indicate the presence of an inborn error of metabolism or neurodegenerative disorder, brain tumor, or subclinical seizures, and it therefore always warrants investigation (Greene, 2013; Kelley, 2008).

Specific types of isolated regression in motor skills, such as deterioration in gait in someone with a known disability, may be explained by the history and physical exam and warrant further evaluation and/or treatment. For example, deterioration in gait in a child or adolescent with spastic diplegia may be due to the mechanics of linear growth and weight gain in the setting of abnormal tone and the development of contractures requiring medical or surgical intervention. Similar deterioration in gait accompanied by increasing spasticity in the legs, change in bowel and bladder function, and progressive scoliosis in an individual with spina bifida would prompt evaluation for tethering or syrinx of the spinal cord.

Spectrum and Continuum of Developmental Disabilities

The various developmental disorders that result from neurologically based abnormalities in cognitive, motor, and neurobehavioral function have been referred to as the *spectrum* of developmental disabilities (Accardo et al., 2008; Voigt, 2018). Within each group of disorders, there also exists a spectrum of severity and prevalence. These conditions range from high-prevalence, low-severity conditions such as dyslexia/specific reading disability, developmental coordination disorder (DCD), and ADHD to low-prevalence, high-severity conditions such as ID and CP (Accardo et al., 2008; Boyle et al., 2011; Voigt, 2018). Severity is determined by the degree of developmental delay, dissociation, and/or deviance, and, as with most other pathologies, the milder forms are more common than the most severe forms.

In contrast to focal neurologic deficits that occur in the mature nervous system as a result of insults such as cerebrovascular accidents, developmental brain dysfunction tends to be diffuse, resulting in observable manifestations in cognitive, motor, and neurobehavioral functioning (Figure 12.1). Clinical developmental disability syndromes may be primarily cognitive (e.g., ID, a language disorder, or a specific learning disability), motor (e.g., CP or DCD), or neurobehavioral (e.g., ASD or ADHD) conditions, but careful examination typically reveals additional impairments in the other streams of development. In fact, the presence of

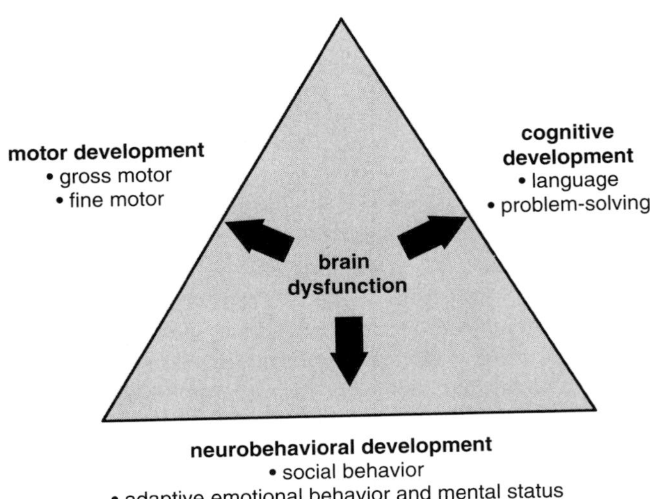

Figure 12.1. Adaptation of Capute's triangle: Developmental brain dysfunction impacts all three major streams of development. (*Source:* Capute, 1991)

additional impairments or coexisting disorders is the rule rather than the exception. This concept is referred to as the *continuum* of developmental disabilities.

The epidemiology of developmental disabilities supports the concept of a continuum across streams of development, as essentially all developmental disorders co-occur with other developmental disorders much more frequently than expected by chance. For example, data from population-based epidemiologic studies suggest that 31%–65% of children with CP also have an IQ less than 70 (Pakula, Van Naarden Braun, & Yeargin-Alsopp, 2009; Türkoğlu, Türkoğlu, Çelik, & Uçan, 2017; Yin Foo et al., 2013). Even among those individuals with CP but without ID, the prevalence of below-average IQ, learning disabilities, speech and language disorders, and ADHD is high (Odding, Roebroeck, & Stam, 2006). ASD has been reported to occur in 6.9%–8.7% of children with CP (Christensen et al., 2014; Delobel-Ayoub, Klapouszczak et al., 2017). Insults causing brain dysfunction severe enough to result in CP also increase the risk of other neurological and sensory dysfunction; also increased in this population are rates of epilepsy (20%–46%), visual impairment (2%–19%), and hearing impairment (2%–6%) (Pakula et al., 2009). In addition, the neuromotor impairment associated with CP often leads to secondary associated conditions, such as orthopedic deformities, chronic constipation, gastroesophageal reflux, malnutrition, poor growth, osteopenia, and skin breakdown (see Chapter 21).

The developmental profile can be conceptualized as an iceberg, with one or more visible tips representing the defining features of the primary diagnoses, and the submerged portion representing the larger continuum of manifestations of underlying brain dysfunction (Accardo et al., 2008). For example, a child with ADHD, by definition, exhibits symptoms of inattention and/or hyperactivity/impulsivity that are inappropriate for age and developmental level and that interfere significantly with functioning. However, the ADHD symptoms (tip of the iceberg) are usually accompanied by other signs and symptoms below the surface, such as motor coordination deficits, tics, neurologic "subtle" or "soft" signs upon examination, learning deficits, pragmatic language impairment, social skills deficits, sleep problems, obsessive thoughts, compulsive behaviors, anxiety, depressed or irritable mood, and disruptive behaviors. These are manifestations of the underlying brain dysfunction and its interaction with environmental influences and experiences. Often, some of these symptoms of neurological dysfunction are prominent enough to meet diagnostic criteria for one or more other disorders, such as a specific learning disability, DCD, Tourette syndrome, obsessive-compulsive disorder, or oppositional-defiant disorder (additional visible tips of the iceberg). Other symptoms may remain subthreshold in terms of additional diagnoses but may still be important to address when planning treatment.

Comorbidity among developmental disorders is primarily due to the diffuse nature of the underlying brain dysfunction, which is often genetic in origin, although environment and experience may be important modifiers of this effect. For example, studies of twins have shown that reading disorder (RD), math disorder (MD), and ADHD are familial and heritable and that the etiology of the comorbidity between RD and MD (28%–64%), RD and ADHD (10%–40%), and MD and ADHD (12%–36%) is primarily explained by common genetic influences (Willcutt et al., 2010). A genetic abnormality may result in different phenotypes due to incomplete penetrance, variable expressivity, or interactions between genes and the environment. A gene/environment (G × E) interaction is said to occur if environmental circumstances modify the expression of an individual's genetic background, either strengthening or weakening the phenotype. Significant G × E interactions have been described in psychiatric conditions such as conduct disorder and depression and are being explored in developmental disabilities such as ADHD and ASD (Willcutt et al., 2010).

DIAGNOSTIC CLASSIFICATION

Diagnostic labels, whether *disease* names that imply a known etiology or pathophysiology or *disorder* names that are defined by clusters of attributes or symptoms less closely related to a single cause, are the usual means by which clinicians access the relevant medical literature to guide management decisions and communicate about conditions with patients, families, and colleagues (Clark, Cuthbert, Lewis-Fernández, Narrow, & Reed, 2017). Diagnostic classification is important for treatment planning, prognostication, and other aspects of clinical care for specific individuals as well as for etiologic and outcomes research and societal allocation of resources (Table 12.2).

In most branches of medicine, systematic classification systems based on etiology and pathophysiology predominate; conditions are differentiated first by cause (e.g., infectious, genetic, neoplastic, autoimmune, or traumatic) and second by how these processes disturb organ structure and function (e.g., pneumonia, skeletal dysplasia, leukemia, hepatitis, or brain injury). In developmental medicine and psychiatry, however, conditions are described primarily phenomenologically as disorders or symptom-cluster syndromes rather than as diseases with known causes (Clark et al., 2017; Hyman, 2010). Although categorization based on phenomenology is useful for establishing a common language that can be applied with reasonably good interrater reliability, limitations of this approach for capturing clinical and biological realities are apparent based on the within-disorder etiologic heterogeneity (multiple causality), high rates of comorbidity among disorders, shared risk factors and etiologies across disorders, scientifically arbitrary nature of diagnostic thresholds, and large numbers of individuals who have substantial impairment but do not quite fulfill the diagnostic criteria (Clark et al., 2017; Hyman, 2010; Lilienfeld & Treadway, 2016; Moreno-De-Luca et al., 2013).

While a definitive etiologic diagnosis can be made in a subset of individuals with any developmental disorder, there is not a one-to-one correspondence between a developmental disorder diagnosis and etiologic diagnosis. Chromosomal microarray analysis and next-generation sequencing studies have made it clear that there is substantial genetic overlap between and among neurodevelopmental disorders; for example, the same pathogenic copy number variants and single nucleotide variants have been detected in individuals with ASD, ID, epilepsy, schizophrenia, and other clinical presentations (Coe, Girirajan, & Eichler, 2012; Gonzalez-Mantilla, Moreno-De-Luca, Ledbetter, & Martin, 2016; Moreno-De-Luca et al., 2013). Neurodevelopmental disorders, which share overlapping symptoms and risk factors and frequently co-occur, can be conceptualized as clinical manifestations of a common denominator, "developmental brain dysfunction," rather than causally and pathophysiologically distinct entities (see Box 12.1; Gonzalez-Mantilla et al., 2016; Moreno-De-Luca et al., 2013).

Table 12.2. Importance of diagnostic classification

Clinical care
Parent/caregiver education
Treatment planning
Etiologic investigation
Identification of associated deficits
Genetic counseling
Prognostication
Reimbursement
Research
Epidemiology
Etiology
Natural history
Treatment efficacy/outcomes
Societal resource allocation
Planning, funding, and distribution of services and supports
Identification and correction of gaps in knowledge and service delivery
Training of health care and other professionals
Education and prevention efforts
Research funding

Levels of Diagnosis

Disorders of development and behavior can be described at three different levels, each of which has clinical significance (see Figure 12.2; Table 12.3). This conceptualization is shown in Figure 12.2 as an inverted triangle, with the broad first level (specific impairments) at the top, narrower second level (categorical diagnoses) in the middle, and very narrow third level (etiologic diagnosis) at the bottom. An individual may have many specific impairments or symptoms that identify a smaller number of categorical disorders or symptom-cluster syndromes that are due to one underlying etiology or a very small number of distinct etiologies.

Specific Impairments The first level of diagnosis, which is descriptive and may not be traditionally thought of as representing a diagnosis at all, is the level of identifying and labeling pertinent signs and symptoms as specific impairments or deficits. A prerequisite for formulating categorical diagnoses (disorders or symptom-cluster syndromes), delineation of functionally impairing symptoms is essential for treatment planning, since educational, behavioral, and psychopharmacologic interventions most often address these specific impairments rather than the categorical diagnostic classification or etiologic diagnosis

BOX 12.1 EVIDENCE-BASED PRACTICE

The Research Domain Criteria Initiative

Significant challenges to the validity of current diagnostic classification systems include the high rates of comorbidity among disorders, the scientifically arbitrary nature of diagnostic thresholds, the large number of patients who have substantial impairment but are subthreshold for diagnosis, and the imprecise relationships between etiologies and diagnoses (Clark et al., 2017; Hyman, 2010; Lilienfeld & Treadway, 2016). In recent years, advances in genetic testing and the application of the new technologies to well-characterized patient cohorts have resulted in increasing recognition that often a clinical disorder can have multiple different genetic causes (etiologic heterogeneity) and that a particular genetic variant can cause multiple different clinically distinct disorders (variable expressivity; Moreno-De-Luca et al., 2013; Stessman, Turner, & Eichler, 2016).

In response to these issues, the National Institute of Mental Health launched the Research Domain Criteria (RDoC) initiative to develop for research purposes new ways of classifying developmental and psychiatric disorders based on dimensions of observable behavior and neurobiological measures (Cuthbert, 2015; Insel et al., 2010). The RDoC approach employs a dimensional rather than categorical framework, is transdiagnostic in seeking markers of neural dysfunction, and is translational in emphasis (Clark et al., 2017; Cuthbert, 2015; Cuthbert & Insel, 2013; Insel et al., 2010; Lilienfeld & Treadway, 2016). The goal is to identify brain mechanisms that explain the etiology and pathophysiology of these disorders, leading to earlier and more accurate diagnosis; prediction of treatment responses and outcomes; and, ultimately, development of more effective treatments that are based on neurobiology rather than symptoms (Insel et al., 2010). The RDoC initiative neither replaces nor excludes other classification systems; it is a paradigm designed to promote research that facilitates application of neuroscience to diagnostic classification, providing scaffolding for a large-scale research program that may ultimately yield an alternative to the *Diagnostic and Statistical Manual of Mental Disorders* and the *International Classification of Diseases* (Cuthbert, 2015; Lilienfeld & Treadway, 2016).

(Myers & Challman, 2018; Myers, Johnson, & Council on Children with Disabilities, 2007).

It is the specific deficits that are addressed, for example, by educational and habilitative interventions, with the goal of building developmentally appropriate skills and increasing functional independence. Challenging behaviors and symptoms associated with developmental disabilities (e.g., aggression, self-injurious behavior,

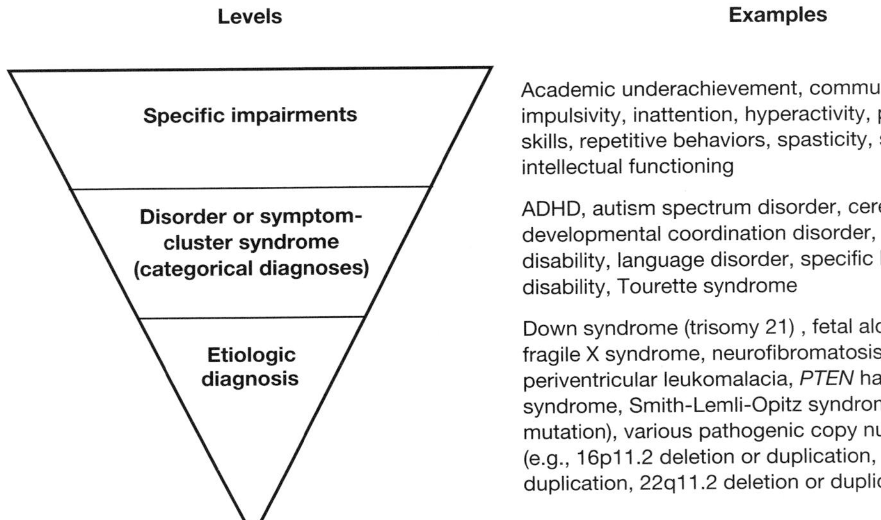

Figure 12.2. Levels of diagnosis. (*Key:* ADHD, attention-deficit/hyperactivity disorder.)

Table 12.3 Significance of each level of diagnosis

Level of Diagnosis	Importance					
	Treatment					
	Behavioral, educational	Psychopharmacologic	Genetic counseling	Identification of associated medical problems	Prognostication	Resource allocation
Specific impairments	++	++	–	–/+	+/++	+
Categorical diagnoses	+	+	+	+	++	++
Etiologic diagnosis	–	–/+*	++	++	+	–/+

Key: –, minimal or no importance; +, important; ++, very important; *emerging importance (may become very important with future advances).

property destruction, elopement, compulsions, and others) may interfere with functioning and contribute substantially to the burden on families. In most cases, problem-focused behavioral interventions informed by functional behavior assessment are an important and effective component of treatment (Hanley, Iwata, & McCord, 2003; Harvey et al. 2009; McGuire et al., 2016; see Chapter 34). These interventions address the specific observable behaviors, not the diagnostic classification.

Even psychopharmacologic treatments are often determined more by the specific impairments or target symptoms than by categorical or etiologic diagnoses. The traditional psychiatric model of psychopharmacologic decision making involves first making the diagnosis of a specific disorder, such as ADHD or depression, and then choosing a medication based on that diagnosis. However, because symptoms exist on a continuum and occur across different disorders, and modifications of diagnostic criteria are necessary in order to apply many psychiatric diagnoses to individuals with more severe disabilities, the value of categorical distinctions in selecting pharmacologic treatment is often unclear. Therefore, a target-symptom approach is often the most appropriate treatment strategy (Accordino et al., 2016; Bostic & Rho, 2006; Myers, 2007; see Chapter 28).

In addition to considering impairments that are intrinsic to the individual, it is important to also consider the child's abilities and the practical impact of environmental, early experiential, and societal factors. The International Classification of Functioning, Disability, and Health for Children and Youth classification system focuses on impairment and enablement in body structures and functions, activities, and participation/involvement, as well as the influences of environmental and personal factors, that would be described at this level of diagnosis (Msall & Msall, 2008; Wolraich and Drotar, 2008).

Categorical Diagnoses: Disorders, Symptom-Cluster Syndromes The second level of diagnosis involves recognizing patterns of specific impairments as disorders or clusters of symptoms that represent clinical syndromes (e.g., ADHD, ASD, ID, and mixed receptive-expressive language disorder) and categorizing them as such. This is the primary way that developmental disability diagnoses are classified using the *International Classification of Diseases* (ICD-10; World Health Organization, 1992) and *DSM-5* (American Psychiatric Association, 2013) diagnostic classification systems. Although there are significant weaknesses, as described previously, categorical diagnoses are reasonably reliable and very useful for communication. Identification of the categorical diagnoses is important for guiding and attempting to standardize treatment; identifying associated problems that meet threshold for a diagnostic label; providing a prognosis; and communicating information to patients, families, and treatment providers, including educators, habilitative therapists, psychologists, and health care providers. Epidemiologic information is also most often collected at this level of diagnosis, and this information can be used to guide resource allocation.

Etiologic Diagnosis The third level of diagnosis, the etiologic diagnosis, involves identifying the specific underlying cause of the developmental disorder, which may be genetic, metabolic, teratogenic, infectious, hypoxic-ischemic, traumatic, a combination of more than one of these, or unknown/idiopathic. This etiologic level of diagnosis is commonly determined in individuals with disorders of the spinal cord, peripheral nervous system, or sensory deficits (such as blindness or deafness); this level of diagnosis currently can be determined in only a minority of individuals with brain-based developmental disabilities. In general, the more severe the brain-based developmental disability, the more likely a specific etiologic diagnosis can be identified. For example, among individuals with ID, a specific etiology is much more likely to be determined if the cognitive impairment is severe (defined as an IQ less than 50) than if it is mild (an IQ between 50 and 70) (D'Arrigo et al., 2016; Yeargin-Allsopp et al., 1997). With the development of chromosomal microarray analysis and next-generation sequencing, the diagnostic yield of genetic testing has increased to 55%–70% for severe ID (Vissers, Gilissen, & Veltman, 2016).

The etiologic diagnosis is important, especially in the case of genetic disorders for which accurate counseling regarding recurrence risk can be provided and, in some cases, associated medical problems can be identified, treated, and perhaps prevented as a result of their known association with the genetic abnormality. For example, a child who is found to have a 22q11.2 deletion (see Appendix B) as the cause of his or her ID or ASD is at increased risk for cardiac, palatal, immune, and renal anomalies, as well as psychiatric disorders, and there is a 6%–10% chance that one of the parents has the deletion (McDonald-McGinn & Sullivan, 2011). If a parent is affected, he or she has a 50% chance of passing the deletion to each of his or her children. In addition, individuals with the 17q12 recurrent deletion are at risk for structural and functional renal disease and maturity-onset diabetes of the young, type 5, and require monitoring (Mitchel et al., 2016), and in the case of certain genetic epilepsies, knowing the etiologic molecular diagnosis allows important refinement of antiepileptic therapy decisions (Poduri, 2017).

The value of determining an etiologic diagnosis is not limited to genetic disorders that directly affect neurological function, and genetic tests are not the only valuable studies. For example, brain imaging may reveal an **infarction** as the cause of a young child's hemiplegia. This would prompt further evaluation that might identify a constitutional **coagulopathy** (clotting disorder) for which additional treatment, stroke recurrence risk counseling, and family genetic counseling are available. An infant with congenital cytomegalovirus infection requires serial assessments for hearing loss, which may be delayed in onset and/or progressive, and in the case of certain inborn errors of metabolism, neuroprotective or even curative treatment can be provided if the diagnosis is made early (see Chapter 16).

All of these important aspects of medical management are more closely linked to etiologic diagnosis than to categorical (level 2) diagnoses or specific impairments (Table 12.3). Discoveries about the neurobiology of genetic neurodevelopmental disorders have led to pharmacological interventions to improve cognitive function in animal models of various disorders, and with human clinical trials for single-gene disorders, such as tuberous sclerosis complex, fragile X syndrome, and Rett syndrome, we have entered the era of neuroscience-driven pharmacotherapy that depends on the etiologic diagnosis rather than the disorder- or symptom-level diagnosis (Jeong & Wong, 2016; van Karnebeek, Bowden, & Berry-Kravis, 2016).

THE DIAGNOSTIC PROCESS

Similar to other areas of medicine, the diagnostic process in developmental medicine consists of taking a history, completing a physical examination, generating a differential diagnosis, planning tests and investigations, formulating a provisional or definitive diagnosis, and developing a management plan. However, in developmental medicine, the examination includes developmental and/or psychoeducational testing as an extension of the neurologic exam. In addition, there are essentially two levels of differential diagnosis: one addressing the categorical diagnosis (e.g., ID or ASD) and the other addressing the etiologic diagnosis (e.g., 22q11.2 deletion syndrome or fragile X syndrome). Laboratory tests and other investigations such as neuroimaging and neurophysiologic studies primarily address the etiologic differential diagnosis or medical conditions that may be associated with the categorical diagnosis.

The diagnostic evaluation format will vary depending on the availability of local resources and clinician preferences. One approach involves employing an interdisciplinary or multidisciplinary team specializing in developmental disabilities. This includes individuals from a variety of disciplines including psychology, speech-language pathology, occupational therapy, physical therapy, special education, social work, audiology, and various medical subspecialties. Alternatively, the diagnostic evaluation may be conducted by an individual clinician-specialist who is capable of interpreting and integrating information from various disciplines and comfortable with making developmental diagnoses, even if there is not an interdisciplinary team that meets in person. Most often, this is a neurodevelopmental pediatrician, developmental-behavioral pediatrician, child psychologist, neuropsychologist, child and adolescent psychiatrist, or pediatric neurologist.

The diagnostic evaluation should incorporate the following elements (Davie, 2012; Huerta & Lord, 2012; Myers & Challman, 2018; Steiner, Goldsmith, Snow, & Chawarska, 2012):

1. *Caregiver interview*, including a thorough medical history and review of systems, a developmental and behavioral history (past milestone attainment

and current abilities), a social history, and a three-generation family history. Standardized rating scales completed by parents/caregivers and teachers or other professionals are commonly used to quantify symptoms and compare them to normative populations.

2. *Review of pertinent medical and educational records,* including any available standardized testing done by early intervention evaluators, psychologists, speech-language pathologists, occupational therapists, physical therapists, and special educators. Although not necessary for categorical diagnosis, it is helpful to note the results of any previous etiologic investigations and other pertinent tests that have been completed (e.g., genetic testing, audiometry, and central nervous system [CNS] imaging).
3. *Direct clinical assessment,* including a physical examination (with an emphasis on the neurologic examination and evaluation for **dysmorphology**), developmental/psychological testing (appropriate for age and level of ability), and neurobehavioral observation/elicitation. In the case of team evaluations, the developmental or psychoeducational testing is often completed by someone other than the physician. In some cases, even a physician diagnostician who is working independently will review and interpret the results of current standardized testing performed by professionals in other disciplines in lieu of directly administering tests herself/himself.
4. *Integration of information and determination of categorical diagnoses,* most often using current criteria from the *DSM-5* (American Psychiatric Association, 2013) or the *ICD-10* (World Health Organization, 1992), although the diagnostician is not limited to these classification systems. Clinical judgment is informed by the information gathered in steps 1 to 3.
5. *Consideration of etiologic possibilities* and determination of appropriate investigations to evaluate for etiologic diagnoses and/or associated medical conditions.

Many clinicians choose to gather some historical information in advance by having parents complete medical, developmental, and family history questionnaires, which allows consultation time to be used for more focused questioning (Davie, 2012; Horridge, 2011). This process may also increase the accuracy of historical information because it gives families the opportunity to reflect on the questions without pressure or time constraints, to review milestones in baby books or journals, and to ask relatives about family history. In some practice models, the diagnostic process involves more than one office visit.

Chief Complaint and Age of Presentation

In all branches of medicine, the physician starts the diagnostic process by asking about the presenting symptoms and concerns, or the "chief complaint." In the field of developmental disabilities, the age of presentation/referral to the developmental specialist is closely tied to the nature of the chief complaint and developmental diagnosis (Lock, Shapiro, Ross, & Capute, 1986; Shapiro & Gwynn, 2008; Shevell, Majnemer, Rosenbaum, & Abrahamowicz, 2001). Although caregivers may detect severe hearing or vision impairment in infants at 3–6 months of age based on a lack of appropriate response to sounds or visual tracking, concerns arising in the first 6 months of life are usually based not on developmental delays, but rather on medical risk factors. These include major congenital anomalies; obvious dysmorphic features; failed newborn hearing screening; or known central nervous system insults, such as severe intraventricular hemorrhage or hypoxic-ischemic encephalopathy. Physiologic instability resulting from frequent seizures, feeding dysfunction, or poor weight gain may also trigger concerns about development in early infancy. Concerns presenting at 6–18 months of age are most often related to delayed attainment of gross motor milestones, and common diagnoses include CP and other types of neuromotor dysfunction, including central hypotonia and neuromuscular disorders (Crawford, 1996; Ehrmann Feldman et al., 2005; Lock et al., 1986; Shevell et al., 2001).

Children with delayed language development tend to present at 18–36 months of age, and common diagnoses among this group include language disorders, GDD/ID, and ASD. Toddlers with both delayed language and problem-solving skills (GDD) tend to present for diagnostic evaluation slightly earlier than those with primary language disorders (median ages 27 months and 32 months, respectively; Lock et al., 1986). One study found that among 17- to 36-month-old children with ASD receiving early intervention services in Louisiana, the most common first concern reported by parents was delayed communication (74%), followed by challenging behaviors (24%) and social skills deficits (12%) (Kozlowski, Matson, Horovitz, Worley, & Neal, 2011). However, communication impairment was also the most frequent initial concern reported by parents of toddlers with other developmental disorders (81%), and no single area of concern distinguished ASDs from other developmental disorders.

Disruptive behaviors, including tantrums, oppositional and defiant behaviors, impulsivity, hyperactivity, and aggressive or destructive behavior, can present over a wide range of ages, from 24 months to school age and beyond. These behaviors are associated with a variety of developmental and behavioral diagnoses. Whereas the hyperactivity and impulsivity of ADHD, combined presentation (ADHD-C) may prompt referral in the preschool period, children with predominantly inattentive presentation ADHD (ADHD-I) typically are not recognized until inattention, distractibility, and poor organizational skills interfere with academic functioning in elementary school or later (see Chapter 19). Individuals with ADHD-I tend to manifest impairment later (after age 7 in 43%), have primarily academic problems, and exhibit fewer social and behavioral problems than those with ADHD-C (Applegate et al., 1997). Concerns about academic achievement or school performance may present as early as age 3–5 years in these children, but these issues more commonly arise as problems in the elementary school years or later. As a result, learning disorders or disabilities are primarily diagnosed in school-age children or adolescents with ADHD.

Information Gathering

The Medical History A careful prenatal and perinatal history may identify risk factors, such as toxic or teratogenic exposure, premature birth, or maternal complications (e.g., infection, gestational diabetes mellitus, pregnancy-induced hypertension, hypothyroidism, or other significant illness; Bellman et al., 2013; Horridge, 2011; Whitaker & Palmer, 2008). In addition to eliciting any potential history of perinatal hypoxic-ischemic insult, the clinician may identify markers of fetal abnormality, such as hypoactive or hyperactive fetal movements, evidence of distress noted on fetal monitoring, breech presentation, or abnormal brain/body growth (i.e., microcephaly, macrocephaly, and small for gestational age status). The neonatal history is focused on identifying pertinent complications and treatments, especially in infants who were born prematurely and/or had medical or surgical problems requiring intensive care, and eliciting evidence of nonspecific neurobehavioral or neuromotor abnormalities that may provide insight into the integrity of the CNS. Examples of the latter include excessive quietness, irritability, persistent colic, altered sleep–wake cycle, feeding problems, jitteriness, floppiness, and stiffness. Complications such as intraventricular or **parenchymal** CNS hemorrhage, **periventricular leukomalacia,** neonatal seizures, severe hyperbilirubinemia, chronic lung disease associated with prematurity (especially with early postnatal steroid treatment), and retinopathy of prematurity should be noted (see Chapters 5 and 25).

The medical history beyond the neonatal period is also helpful in establishing risk and providing clues to the etiology of developmental problems (Bellman et al., 2013; Whitaker & Palmer, 2008). Pertinent findings include past acute medical conditions (e.g., meningitis, encephalitis, and traumatic brain injury), chronic illnesses that have the potential to impact development and behavior (e.g., malnutrition, recurrent infections, cancer, sickle-cell anemia, and chronic renal disease; see Chapter 24), and environmental exposures (e.g., lead; see Chapter 2). The medical history may also provide clues suggesting the possibility of a metabolic disorder (e.g., episodic neurological dysfunction, unusual prostration with illness, or intolerance of fasting) or genetic syndrome (e.g., congenital anomalies such as congenital heart defects, cleft palate, or **hypospadias**). Specific prompts are often required to elicit all of the pertinent issues from parents; important medical problems may be omitted by parents unless there is a specific review of systems and inquiry about hospitalizations or other medical consultants who have participated in the child's care. It is especially important to inquire whether the child has had formal hearing and vision screening. Sometimes anomalies that were surgically corrected are not mentioned by parents until the clinician inquires specifically about previous surgical procedures.

Developmental and Behavioral History A thorough and accurate developmental and behavioral history requires substantial skill, experience, and time to complete, but it is usually the most informative aspect of the neurodevelopmental diagnostic assessment (Davie, 2012; Horridge, 2011; Leppert, 2011; Montgomery, 2008; Whitaker & Palmer, 2008). The components of the developmental and behavioral history are outlined in Table 12.4. Developmental milestones (see Chapter 11) are the cornerstones of the developmental and behavioral history; they provide the information necessary to identify developmental delays and atypical patterns of development, including dissociation, deviance, and regression, as described previously.

Useful milestones must have precise definitions, occur within a narrow normative time frame, be clinically observable and useful to the child, and have predictive validity (Accardo et al., 2008; Bellman et al., 2013; Shapiro & Gwynn, 2008). Questions about current abilities should seek more detail than those on past milestones, which should focus on more notable milestones that are easier to recall by parents. When eliciting a current history of babbling in an infant, for example, the clinician must first define for the parent

Table 12.4 Developmental and behavioral history

Age of developmental milestone attainment and current functioning	
Gross motor skills	Academic achievement (strengths, weaknesses)
Fine motor skills	Social skills
Communication/language skills (receptive, expressive, pragmatic)	Adaptive skills (self-care, activities of daily living)
Problem-solving skills/nonlanguage cognition	Play/leisure skills and interests
Identification of atypical developmental patterns	
Delay, dissociation, deviance	
Regression	
Adaptive and maladaptive emotional behavior, self-regulation, and mental status	
Challenging behaviors	*Sensory modulation issues (tactile, auditory, visual, olfactory, vestibular)*
Inattention, distractibility	Overresponsivity
Disorganization	Underresponsivity
Hyperactivity	Sensation-seeking, unusual sensory exploration
Impulsivity	*Food- or meal-related problems, pica*
Noncompliance, oppositional and defiant behavior	*Sleep problems*
Tantrums, emotional outbursts	Difficulty falling asleep, bedtime resistance
Aggression	Nightwakings
Self-injurious behavior	Early morning awakening
Repetitive behaviors	Snoring, gasping, apnea
Stereotypy	Excessive sleep
Obsessions	*Anxiety*
Compulsions	*Mood problems*
Perseveration	Depression, mania, irritability, lability
Rituals, nonfunctional routines	*Conduct problems*
Tics	Lying, stealing, truancy, vandalism, cruelty to animals, fire setting
	Enuresis, encopresis

that babbling is consonant-vowel combinations. Then they can explore where the child is in the hierarchy of babbling, which typically progresses from single syllables ("da") to reduplicative strings ("dadada") of varying length. This is followed by an increased repertoire of reduplicative strings ("dadada," "bababa," or "gagaga") and then nonreduplicative strings ("badabagaba"). If the child were a 3 year old who is speaking in phrases, the clinician would not go into this level of detail about babbling while eliciting the expressive language history because this is not something that parents would be likely to recall. The clinician would instead focus on milestones such as when the first meaningful words were spoken and when the child began to use novel two-word combinations. More detailed questions are reserved for current abilities (e.g., vocabulary, length and content of phrases and sentences, use of pronouns, use of plurals, and intelligibility).

The experienced diagnostician not only has a thorough knowledge of the average age of attainment of milestones in all areas of development, but is also able to improve parent recall of developmental achievements by linking them to important family events. This might include asking about function during past holidays, birthdays, or summer vacations (e.g., "How was your child moving around on her first birthday? Was she crawling, pulling up to a standing position, cruising along furniture, or walking independently?"). Each area of development is reviewed chronologically to ascertain the age at which specific important milestones were attained as well as the current level of functioning (Leppert, 2011; Whitaker & Palmer, 2008).

This approach allows retrospective analysis of developmental rate in each stream and recognition of changes in trajectory over time, such as improving trajectory ("catch-up"), plateau, or regression. This is analogous to obtaining past growth measurements and plotting them on appropriate growth curves to facilitate recognition of important patterns, such as crossing percentiles due to a plateau in linear or head circumference growth or loss of weight.

It is also important to thoroughly explore whether there are challenging or maladaptive behaviors and, if so, to obtain specific descriptions of the challenging behaviors (Table 12.4). Standardized rating scales may be helpful in eliciting and quantifying various aspects of behavior from different sources, including parents and teachers, but they are not independently diagnostic and should not replace the clinician interview (American Academy of Pediatrics, Task Force on Mental Health, 2010). If the child exhibits challenging disruptive behaviors such as tantrums or aggressive outbursts, for example, it is important to specifically describe 1) the specific behaviors (e.g., screaming, crying, throwing things, hitting, kicking, and dropping to the floor and flailing arms and legs); 2) their frequency, intensity, and duration; 3) exacerbating factors/triggers (e.g., time, setting/location, demand situations, denials, and transitions); 4) ameliorating factors and response to behavioral interventions; 5) time trends (increasing, decreasing, or stable); and 6) degree of interference with functioning. In this way, it is often possible to formulate working hypotheses about the functions of the behaviors and what aspects of the environment are maintaining these behaviors through inadvertent reinforcement (see Chapters 27 and 34). A published practice pathway for the evaluation and management of irritability-related challenging behavior in ASD includes a stepwise approach to collecting this type of information and a detailed checklist that can be applied to other diagnoses and behavioral symptoms (McGuire et al., 2016). Ultimately, after the child's developmental functioning in all major streams has been assessed, it is possible to judge whether the behaviors that concern the parent are inappropriate for the child's developmental level or whether they are actually typical behaviors once understood in the context of the child's developmental level of functioning or "developmental age." For example, parents who express concern and frustration about their 6-year-old child's inattention, impulsivity, tantrums in response to denials, and nocturnal enuresis may begin to understand the behaviors and approach them more appropriately when they are put in the context of the child's developmental age of 3 years.

Family History The primary goal of the family history, which should include at least three generations, is to identify genetic risk and clues to specific genetic etiology, including pattern of inheritance (Pyeritz, 2012; Saal & Chen, 2013). Parental ages at conception, history of prior fetal losses, educational levels, early educational difficulties, and major medical problems should be queried. Family history should include known genetic conditions; malformation syndromes; structural birth defects; and developmental and neurological disorders such as ID, ASD, CP, muscular dystrophies, ADHD, learning disorders, language disorders, developmental delays, epilepsy, tic disorders, hearing loss, and blindness (Hoyme, 2013; Saal & Chen, 2013). It is also often helpful to ask about whether any past family members were slow learners, required special education services or any extra help in school, needed a wheelchair for mobility, or were unable to live independently as adults. Psychiatric conditions, such as schizophrenia, depression, bipolar disorder, anxiety disorders, obsessive-compulsive disorder, and substance abuse, should also be explored.

The pattern of individuals with ID in a family, for example, may suggest autosomal dominant, autosomal recessive, X-linked, or mitochondrial inheritance (see Chapter 1). Even in the absence of any other family members with major developmental disabilities, the presence of other conditions may point to a specific genetic etiology. For example, a history of anxiety and difficulty with math in the mother and an undiagnosed tremor and ataxia syndrome in the maternal grandfather of a boy with GDD, hyperactivity, and gaze avoidance raises the possibility of fragile X syndrome (see Chapter 15). Factors such as ethnicity; consanguinity; and a history of multiple fetal losses, infant deaths, progressive or neurodegenerative disorders, or conditions associated with abnormal energy metabolism (e.g., myopathy, myoclonic epilepsy, cardiomyopathy, retinitis pigmentosa, ophthalmoplegia, sensorineural deafness, or peripheral neuropathy) may suggest an increased risk of metabolic disease (Greene, 2013; Kelley, 2008).

Social History Potential protective and deleterious psychosocial and socioeconomic factors should be explored. Parental education, cultural beliefs, family support systems, and previous experience with people with disabilities may impact the ability and willingness of parents or grandparents and extended family members to accept the diagnosis and treatment recommendations (see Chapter 37). A history of abuse or neglect of the child may be particularly relevant to the interpretation of the child's behavior, attachment, and social functioning; previous involvement with child protective service agencies or foster care should be queried. Psychosocial stressors, such as recent crises or transitions, financial or marital difficulties, and mental health or substance abuse issues, may impact the child's development and behavior and the ability of the family to access resources and comply with treatment recommendations. If there are behavioral concerns about the child, it is important to determine the parents' expectations and behavior management strategies.

The child's educational/habilitative intervention history is also important. This includes utilization of early intervention services, preschool programs (including Head Start), and special education services. Any history of grade retention should be noted. Details of the current educational program should always be explored because a significant mismatch between educational expectations or demands and the child's current abilities is likely to result in poor progress and often behavioral or emotional problems, especially in school-age children. The timing and types of concerns voiced by the teachers and other school staff should be noted, along with previous disciplinary actions, such as frequent loss of recess or other privileges, afterschool detention, or suspension from school.

Physical Examination The diagnostic evaluation should include a complete general physical and neurological examination. Particularly important aspects of the general physical examination include assessment for abnormal growth, dysmorphic features, evidence of visceral storage such as **hepatomegaly** (enlarged liver) and **splenomegaly** (enlarged spleen), and skin manifestations of neurocutaneous disorders or other genetic syndromes (Greene, 2013; Hoyme, 2013).

Aberrations in growth such as short stature, tall stature, obesity, microcephaly, and macrocephaly may provide important clues to the etiology of the developmental disability (Hoyme, 2013). For some underlying causes, such as hypothyroidism, effective treatment is available. Important alterations in the trajectory or velocity of growth may be exposed by plotting serial measurements on normal population growth curves, revealing crossing of multiple percentile lines. For example, an infant with a rapidly increasing head circumference may have hydrocephalus and require surgical intervention. A plateau in head growth after 6 months of age resulting in acquired microcephaly in a female infant in the second year of life may be a manifestation of Rett syndrome. The visible change over time on the growth curve is much more informative than just a single measurement at the time of evaluation.

The child also should be examined for congenital anomalies, which can be classified as major or minor. Major anomalies usually require medical or surgical intervention, whereas minor anomalies generally do not require intervention but may be of cosmetic concern and diagnostic significance (Toriello, 2008). Major and minor anomalies occur much more commonly in children with developmental disabilities than in typically developing children. In individuals with three or more minor anomalies, the chance of having a major anomaly, a dysmorphic syndrome, or both increases greatly (Hoyme, 2013; Toriello, 2008). Measurements should be recorded and compared with normative values in order to confirm or refute clinical impressions of abnormal size, proportions, or spacing of body parts (Gripp, Slavotinek, Hall, & Allanson, 2013). A clinical impression of **hypotelorism** (eyes close together), for example, should be confirmed by measurements because it is a strong indicator of abnormal brain development. Findings such as a **submucosal** cleft palate are important not only because of the treatable impact on speech, feeding, and conductive hearing loss, but also as a clue to an underlying genetic syndrome such as 22q11.2 deletion syndrome. Documentation of detailed descriptions of anomalies is useful for later searching the literature and online databases for potential diagnoses, which can in turn lead to a reasonable approach to laboratory testing (Greene, 2013; Hoyme, 2013; Toriello, 2008).

Coarse facial features, a large tongue, corneal clouding, hepatomegaly, and splenomegaly may be due to a lysosomal storage disease (e.g., mucopolysaccharidoses or Gaucher disease) (Greene, 2013; Kelley, 2008; see Chapter 16 and Appendix B). In all children, the skin should be carefully examined, along with the other accessible ectodermal derivatives (hair, teeth, and nails). Hyperpigmented or hypopigmented lesions, vascular anomalies, and other lesions such as various types of fibromas and hamartomas are prominent aspects of neurocutaneous syndromes such as neurofibromatosis, tuberous sclerosis, Sturge-Weber syndrome, ataxia-telangiectasia, and incontinentia pigmenti (Korf & Bebin, 2017; Ruggieri & Praticò, 2015; see Appendix B). Linear streaks or whorls of hypopigmentation, sometimes referred to as hypomelanosis of Ito, are often associated with mosaicism for a variety of chromosomal abnormalities (Ruggieri & Praticò, 2015; see Chapter 1).

The neurologic examination of children with developmental disabilities includes standard evaluation of cranial nerve function, posture/station, muscle strength, muscle tone, deep tendon reflexes, cerebellar function, gait, coordination, and sensation. Abnormalities such as unusual movements; pathological reflexes; and significant asymmetry of function, strength, tone, or deep tendon reflexes are recorded. In infants and young children, markers of neuromotor maturation, such as primitive reflexes and postural reactions, should be examined (Blasco, 1992). Older children are assessed for markers of neuromaturation and neurodysfunction, such as upper extremity posturing during stressed gait maneuvers and finger-tapping tasks (Larson et al., 2007; Martins et al., 2013; Montgomery, 2008). Neurologic "subtle" or "soft" signs such as dysrhythmia and overflow movements, which are unintentional and unnecessary movements that accompany voluntary activity, are often detected. Mirror overflow, for example, includes movements that occur on the opposite side of the body during tasks such as sequential finger-tapping (Cole, Mostofsky, Gidley Larson, Denckla, & Mahone, 2008; Mostofsky, Newschaffer, & Denckla, 2003). Although most basic motor skills are mastered by age 6 or 7, some subtle signs may persist in typically developing children until about age 10 (Larson et al., 2007). However, prominent persistence into late childhood or adolescence may indicate atypical neurological development. These subtle signs are more common in children and adolescents with developmental disabilities, including ADHD, learning disorders, high-functioning ASD, obsessive-compulsive disorder, and Tourette syndrome, and are related to decreased inhibitory control (Cole et al., 2008; Martins et al., 2013; Mostofsky et al., 2003).

Developmental Testing and Neurobehavioral Status Exam In addition to assessing each stream of development by history, the diagnostician evaluates each child by direct observation and elicitation (Davie, 2012; Leppert, 2011; Montgomery, 2008; Stein & Lukasik, 2009). Formal testing is either completed by the clinician or the results of current testing done by professionals in other disciplines are reviewed or both. Language and nonlanguage/problem-solving aspects of cognition are measured directly. Age-appropriate quantifiable visual-motor measures, such as those that assess figure copying, drawing, and written output, and those that do not require pencil and paper (e.g., block design tasks) are included, and the qualitative aspects of the child's performance (e.g., pencil grasp, tremor or overflow movements, and qualitative features of the final product) are carefully observed and recorded. In older preschoolers and school-age children, academic achievement is also typically measured using standardized instruments.

Reviews of many of the specific developmental and psychoeducational tests available for assessing children and adolescents are included in Chapter 13 of this volume and elsewhere (Feldman & Messick, 2008; Kral, 2018; Montgomery, 2008; Stein & Lukasik, 2009). In general, physicians who perform independent evaluations tend to use tests that are relatively brief to administer, such as the Capute Scales (CAT/CLAMS; Accardo & Capute, 2005), the Battelle Developmental Inventory (BDI–2; Newborg, 2005), the Mullen Scales of Early Learning (MSEL; Mullen, 1995), the Stanford-Binet Intelligence Scales for Early Childhood (Early SB5; Roid, 2005), the Young Children's Achievement Test (YCAT; Hresko, Peak, Herron, & Bridges, 2000), the Peabody Picture Vocabulary Test, Fourth Edition (PPVT-4; Dunn & Dunn, 2007), the Kaufman Brief Intelligence Test (KBIT-2; Kaufman & Kaufman, 2004), Raven's Coloured Progressive Matrices (Raven, Court, & Raven, 1995), and the Wide Range Achievement Test (WRAT-4; Wilkinson & Robertson, 2006). They also use portions or subtests of various measures, such as the Gesell Developmental Schedules (Gesell & Amatruda, 1947; Gesell et al., 1940) and others, to assess different domains of development.

Adaptive functioning is usually quantified using standardized interviews such as the Vineland Adaptive Behavior Scales, Third Edition (Vineland-3; Sparrow, Cicchetti, & Saulnier, 2016) or caregiver-completed rating scales such as the Adaptive Behavior Assessment System (ABAS-3; Harrison & Oakland, 2015), but these may be supplemented by direct observation and elicitation. Criterion-referenced functional measures such as the broad-based Functional Independence Measure for Children (WeeFIM; Msall et al., 1994) and the motor domain-specific Gross Motor Function Classification System (Palisano et al., 2007) are useful for determining an individual's current ability to perform the tasks of daily living and to fulfill expected social roles. These evaluations can often be used as meaningful outcome measures and to suggest supports necessary for successful progress (Msall & Msall, 2008).

Social behavior is often quantified as part of a broad adaptive measure such as the Vineland-3 or the ABAS-3 but must be directly assessed as well. Appropriate toys should be available to the child so that spontaneous independent play can be observed (often while the clinician is conducting the parent interview) and interactive play can be elicited by the examiner or spontaneously initiated by the child. Eye contact, including referential gaze shifts; response to joint attention bids; and initiation of social communicative interactions, such as bringing/showing toys to the parents to share interest and positive affect, and commenting should be assessed. Direct assessment measures specific to certain disorders are often utilized when needed to further evaluate clinical suspicion or narrow the differential diagnosis. For example, the appropriate module of the Autism Diagnostic Observation Schedule (Lord et al., 2012) or the standard or high-functioning version of the Childhood Autism Rating Scale (CARS2-ST or CARS2-HF; Schopler, Van Bourgondien, Wellman, & Love, 2010) may be administered (see Chapter 18).

Maladaptive behavior is also typically quantified using standardized rating scales completed by parents or teachers to supplement the history obtained by interview and review of records. The American Academy of Pediatrics Task Force on Mental Health (2010) has published a comprehensive review of available informal tools and standardized instruments, including broad measures (some of which include adaptive behaviors as well) and narrow measures targeting specific disorders or types of symptoms (e.g., ADHD, depression, and conduct problems). Important information can also be gained from qualitative assessment of anxiety, attention, distractibility, impulse control, activity level, compliance, and atypical repetitive behaviors or resistance to change during the interview, testing, and physical examination. Deviations from the norm may be readily apparent upon observation of the child's behavior during the various aspects of the evaluation. It is common, however, not to witness challenging behaviors such as tantrums, self-injury, aggression, and irritability during the evaluation, and even a child with significant ADHD may exhibit few overt symptoms. This does not negate the history provided by the parents, especially when verified by documentation from teachers, therapists, or other family members such as grandparents, since many children are able to temporarily modify their behavior for a few hours, especially in a one-on-one or very small group setting. In contrast, the history is suspect if the child clearly exhibits skills such as appropriate imaginative play and reciprocal social interaction during the evaluation despite parental report that the child never exhibits these behaviors at home or in other settings.

Diagnostic Formulation

Ultimately, the diagnostic process is an exercise in the reduction of uncertainty through information gathering, serial hypothesis generation and testing, and deductive reasoning. The developmental evaluation should culminate in a diagnostic formulation, which in turn guides etiologic investigation and management recommendations. All of the information gathering in the form of the history-taking, record review, and direct clinical assessment provides the input that the clinician then must compare to existing scientific knowledge of typical and atypical development and behavior to identify the pertinent problems and develop hypotheses to explain these problems in a list called a differential diagnosis.

For over a century, the Oslerian paradigm of formulating a differential diagnosis has been pivotal to best-practice medicine (Pearn, 2011). The differential diagnosis is defined as a list of conditions consistent with the individual's history and observed signs arranged in ranked order of decreasing likelihood. It is constantly modified throughout the evaluation process as additional information becomes available, with potential diagnoses being added, eliminated, and moved up or down on the list. The quality of differential diagnosis depends on clinician history-taking and examination skills, ability to assign relative weights of importance to specific symptoms and signs, and knowledge of disorders of development and behavior and their causes (Pearn, 2011).

The clinician actually formulates and modifies the differential diagnosis throughout the history-taking process. This is further refined by considering the direct clinical assessment; it may be helpful to tabulate the data obtained from the developmental testing, physical examination, and neurobehavioral status examination (Figure 12.3) to facilitate identifying the pertinent problems and narrowing the differential diagnosis through pattern recognition (such as discrepancies suggesting developmental dissociation).

Because developmental disabilities result from diffuse brain dysfunction, the set of problems identified through the thorough evaluation process is likely to include cognitive, motor, and neurobehavioral manifestations and sometimes CNS morphologic anomalies (e.g., microcephaly or structural malformation on brain imaging) or neurophysiologic abnormalities (e.g., seizures, abnormal EEG). This may lead to the tendency to arrive at a long list of diagnoses that is essentially the same list of concerns that the parents had expressed except that it has been translated into medical terminology. Such an approach is not very helpful or very satisfying to parents. Almost 50 years ago, McKusick (1969) used the terms *lumping* and *splitting* to describe two positions on the origin of genetic diseases and emphasized that both had an important place: lumping in connection with pleiotropism ("many from one"—multiple phenotypic features arising from one etiologic factor) and splitting in connection with heterogeneity ("one from many"—the same or almost the same phenotype arising from several different etiologic factors). In developmental disabilities, although splitting is

Domain	Test(s)	Age level	SS or DQ	Grade level	Pertinent qualitative information
Language, verbal IQ					
Problem-solving, nonverbal IQ					
Working memory, processing speed, other					
Visual-motor, fine motor					
Gross motor					
Reading					
Decoding					
Fluency					
Comprehension					
Mathematics					
Writing					
Other academic or pre-academic achievement					
Adaptive behavior					
Social-emotional behavior					
Maladaptive behavior (rating scales)					
General physical exam					
Neurologic exam					
Neurobehavioral status exam					

Figure 12.3. Sample format for tabulating neurodevelopmental assessment data. (*Key:* DQ, developmental quotient; SS, standard score.)

emphasized in the information-gathering process, etiologic diagnosis, and identification of specific impairments to be addressed in treatment, lumping is the key to parsimonious diagnostic classification at the disorder or syndrome level. The diagnostician must emphasize the importance of the forest over the trees.

For example, a particular child may exhibit deficits in language and nonlanguage cognition, self-help skills/activities of daily living, phonology, semantic and pragmatic aspects of language, socialization with peers, reading comprehension, math computation, written output, and motor coordination. The child may also have challenging behaviors including inattention, impulsivity, hyperactivity, tantrums, noncompliance, preference for structure and routine, and perseveration on certain topics or questions. All of these findings can be explained by the single diagnosis of moderate ID rather than a list of diagnoses including moderate ID, ASD, ADHD, GDD, phonological disorder, DCD, and oppositional defiant disorder. Alternatively, the child may be appropriately and meaningfully diagnosed with several categorical disorders (e.g., moderate ID, ASD, and disruptive behavior [e.g., *DSM-5: unspecified disruptive, impulse control,* and *conduct disorder*]), yet there is likely a single underlying etiology that may or may not be identified through laboratory investigations. Even when a relatively long list of diagnoses is appropriate, it is important to emphasize that the child has one problem, brain dysfunction, and that these diagnoses represent the most parsimonious description of the manifestations of that brain dysfunction.

Once the diagnostic evaluation has been completed, the diagnoses and recommendations for treatment and further evaluation are presented to the family. Often, referrals are made to specialists in other disciplines, such as special education, speech-language therapy, occupational therapy, or physical therapy (usually within the early intervention or education systems) in order to develop and implement specific treatment plans. In some cases, further evaluation is required to delineate the diagnoses, and referral to a neuropsychologist, clinical psychologist, or speech-language pathologist for additional testing may be necessary.

When explaining the developmental profile and diagnostic formulation to parents, one can start with writing *brain dysfunction* in the center of a blank piece of paper, followed by listing beneath it the child's pertinent problems (impairments), divided into the three categories—*cognitive, neuromotor,* and *neurobehavioral*—and sometimes a fourth category, *anatomic/physiologic* (used when there are CNS-related anomalies, such as microcephaly or macrocephaly, or known neurophysiologic abnormalities, such as seizures or an abnormal EEG). Below the three or four parallel columns of impairments, the categorical diagnoses are listed while explaining the meaning of each. Next, one can go back to the top of the paper and diagram the various causes of brain dysfunction, followed by crossing out those that do not pertain to the child and arriving at those that should be further investigated. This leads to a discussion of recommendations for laboratory tests, imaging studies, and/or other additional evaluations (or brief discussion of why further investigation is not necessary). The potential influence of environmental and experiential influences fits well into the discussion at this point. All of this leads to a piece of paper looking like something similar to Figure 12.4 but specific to the individual. The diagnosis list and profile of impairments can also be referred to during discussion of treatment recommendations.

Etiologic Evaluation

Decision making regarding genetic etiologic evaluation in children with developmental disabilities is informed by a rapidly expanding literature base. Expert recommendations regarding etiologic investigations depend on the specific diagnoses (especially the presence or absence of GDD, ID, or ASD), physical examination findings, neurobehavioral profile, and family history. Less-severe disabilities, such as language disorders, specific learning disabilities, and ADHD, usually do not require etiologic investigation, such as laboratory or imaging studies, unless the history and/or physical examination suggest the possibility of a specific etiology that requires further evaluation (e.g., vision or hearing impairment, obstructive sleep apnea, thyroid dysfunction, lead toxicity, or physical stigmata of a genetic syndrome). Guidelines pertaining to individuals with GDD, ID, ASD, and CP have been published by organizations including the American College of Medical Genetics and Genomics, the American Academy of Pediatrics, the American Academy of Neurology and Child Neurology Society, the American Academy of Child and Adolescent Psychiatry, the International Standard Cytogenomic Array Consortium (now part of the NIH-funded Clinical Genome Resource [ClinGen]), and others (Ashwal et al., 2004; Manning & Hudgins, 2010; Michelson et al., 2011; Miller et al., 2010; Mithyantha et al., 2017; Moeschler & Shevell, 2014; Muhle et al., 2017; Schaefer, Mendelsohn, & Professional Practice and Guidelines Committee, 2013). Unfortunately, the specific test recommendations tend to become rapidly outdated due to the development of new technology, and the publication of new guidelines may lag several years behind state-of-the-art care.

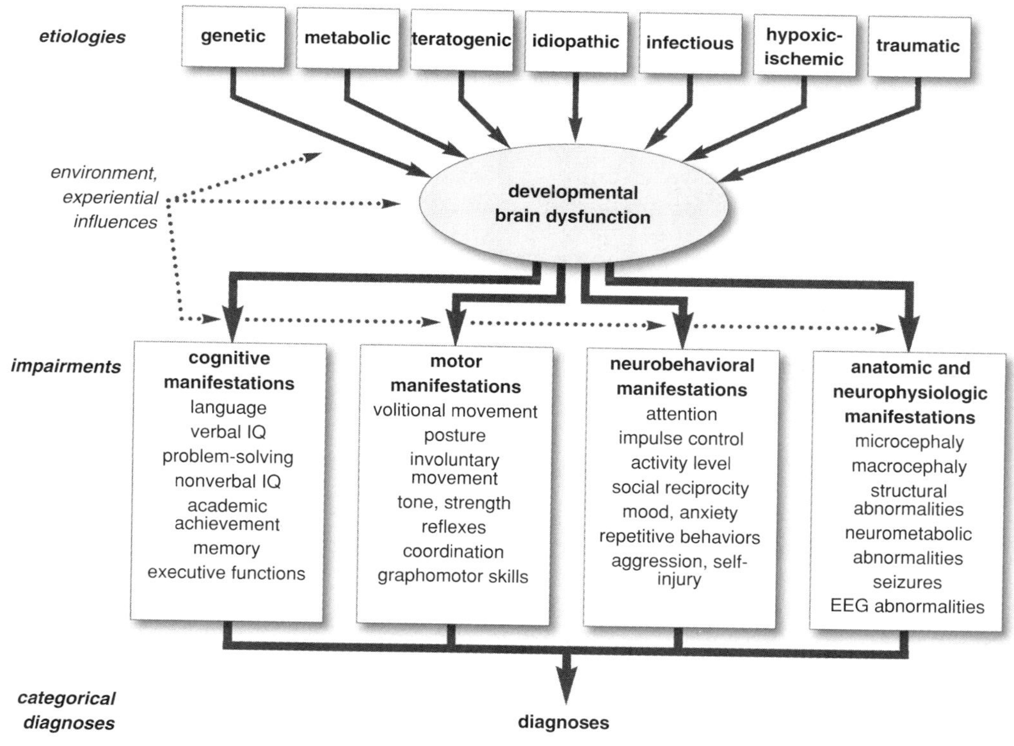

Figure 12.4. Diagnostic formulation diagram.

BOX 12.2 INTERDISCIPLINARY CARE

The Role of the Genetic Counselor

As professionals who have advanced training in medical genetics and counseling, genetic counselors are an increasingly important part of the interdisciplinary care team for children with developmental disabilities and their families. Traditional roles of genetic counselors include the following (National Society of Genetic Counselors' Definition Task Force, 2006):

- Interpreting family and medical histories to assess the chance of disease occurrence or recurrence
- Educating families, other health care professionals, and the general public about inheritance; genetic testing; management of specific genetic conditions; prevention; research opportunities; and resources for information, advocacy, and support
- Providing counseling to facilitate informed choices and adaptation to a diagnosis or health risk and providing psychosocial support to individuals and families
- Serving as patient advocates, including referring individuals and families to community or state support services

There is consensus that a genetic evaluation should be offered to every person with ID, GDD, and ASD (Muhle et al., 2017), and advances such as the development of chromosomal microarray and next-generation sequencing technologies have led to a substantial increase in the likelihood of obtaining a causal molecular diagnosis (Finucane & Myers, 2016; Retterer et al., 2016; Stessman, Turner, & Eichler, 2016; Vissers et al., 2016). An outcome of more widespread genetic testing and higher diagnostic yield is that there are more individuals and families who would benefit from counseling and education about the implications of their new molecular diagnoses.

As the availability and complexity of genetic tests has increased, pretest counseling and consenting, interpretation of test results, and explanation of the findings (including variants of uncertain significance) to families have become much more complicated. In addition, test results often require reinterpretation over time, including comparison to large genomic data resources because the status of some variants changes as more information becomes available. The expertise of genetic counselors allows them to fulfill these roles, making them invaluable members of the developmental disabilities health care team.

When a specific syndrome or metabolic disorder is suspected based on the history, physical examination, and record review, the next step is to proceed with the appropriate targeted testing or referral to a medical geneticist. In the case of a child presenting with GDD, ID, or ASD, if there is no strong suspicion of a particular diagnosis or testing for suspected diagnoses is negative, a reasonable approach is to pursue CMA and, in most cases, fragile X DNA analysis. If these are unrevealing, whole-exome sequencing (see Chapter 1) should be considered (Muhle et al., 2017; Myers & Challman, 2018). These tests must be explained to families so that they understand the potential benefits and risks as well as the range of potential results (including finding variants of uncertain significance and secondary findings), and involvement of a genetic counselor is highly desirable (see Box 12.2). Some families decline etiologic investigation for various reasons, including concerns about cost or insurance coverage, potential assignment of responsibility or "guilt" to one parent, issues of future insurability of the child, lack of curative treatment based on etiology, and not wanting to put the child through any discomfort or risk associated with tests. However, most families are interested and find the information to be helpful (Lingen et al., 2016; Reiff et al., 2015).

SUMMARY

- Developmental brain dysfunction, whether genetic or due to other pathology, varies in severity and is manifested as a spectrum/continuum of disorders ranging from high-prevalence, low-severity conditions such as ADHD, learning disabilities, and DCD to low-prevalence, high-severity conditions such as ID and CP.
- Most developmental disorders can have many different causes, and most etiologic diagnoses can result in a variety of different clinical disorders.
- The process of developmental diagnosis includes not only assigning categorical diagnoses, but also

delineating associated deficits, which are typically the primary targets of intervention, quantifying severity, and searching for an underlying etiology.

- The developmental profile compiled during diagnostic evaluation is vital for determining prognosis and guiding treatment planning.

ADDITIONAL RESOURCES

The American Society of Human Genetics (ASHG): http://www.ashg.org/press/healthprofessional.shtml#1

MedlinePlus: https://medlineplus.gov/developmentaldisabilities.html

Centers for Diseases Control and Prevention: https://www.cdc.gov/ncbddd/developmentaldisabilities/facts.html

Additional resources can be found online in Appendix D: Childhood Disabilities Resources, Services, and Organizations (see About the Online Companion Materials).

REFERENCES

Accardo, P. J. (2008). *Capute & Accardo's neurodevelopmental disabilities in infancy and childhood. Vol. I: Neurodevelopmental diagnosis and treatment* (3rd ed.). Baltimore, MD: Paul H. Brookes Publishing Co.

Accardo, P. J., & Capute, A. J. (2005). *The Capute Scales: Cognitive Adaptive Test/Clinical Linguistic & Auditory Milestone Scale (CAT/CLAMS).* Baltimore, MD: Paul H. Brookes Publishing Co.

Accardo, P. J., Accardo, J. A., & Capute, A. J. (2008). A neurodevelopmental perspective on the continuum of developmental disabilities. In P. J. Accardo (Ed.), *Capute & Accardo's neurodevelopmental disabilities in infancy and childhood: Vol. I: Neurodevelopmental diagnosis and treatment* (3rd ed., pp. 3–25). Baltimore, MD: Paul H. Brookes Publishing Co.

Accordino, R. E., Kidd, C., Politte, L. C., Henry, C. A., & McDougle, C. J. (2016). Psychopharmacological interventions in autism spectrum disorder. *Expert Opinion on Pharmacotherapy, 17,* 937–952.

American Academy of Pediatrics, Council on Children With Disabilities, Section on Developmental Behavioral Pediatrics, Bright Futures Steering Committee, & Medical Home Initiatives for Children With Special Needs Project Advisory Committee. (2006). Identifying infants and young children with developmental disorders in the medical home: An algorithm for developmental surveillance and screening. *Pediatrics, 118,* 405–420.

American Academy of Pediatrics, Task Force on Mental Health. (2010). Supplemental appendix S12: Mental health screening and assessment tools for primary care. *Pediatrics, 125,* S173–S192.

American Psychiatric Association. (2013). *Diagnostic and statistical manual of mental disorders* (5th ed.). Arlington, VA: American Psychiatric Publishing

Applegate, B., Lahey, B. B., Hart, E. L., Biederman, J., Hynd, G. W., Barkley, R. A., . . . Shaffer, D. (1997). Validity of the age-of-onset criterion for ADHD. A report from the DSM-IV field trials. *Journal of the American Academy of Child & Adolescent Psychiatry, 36,* 1211–1221.

Ashwal, S., Russman, B. S., Blasco, P. A., Miller, G., Sandler, A., Shevell, M., & Stevenson, R. (2004). Practice parameter: Diagnostic assessment of the child with cerebral palsy: Report of the Quality Standards Subcommittee of the American Academy of Neurology and the Practice Committee of the Child Neurology Society. *Neurology, 62,* 851–863.

Augustyn, M., Zuckerman, B., & Caronna, E. B. (2011). *The Zuckerman Parker handbook of developmental and behavioral pediatrics for primary care* (3rd ed.). Philadelphia, PA: Lippincott Williams & Wilkins.

Baird, G., Charman, T., Pickles, A., Chandler, S., Loucas, T., Meldrum, D., . . . Simonoff, E. (2008). Regression, developmental trajectory, and associated problems in disorders in the autism spectrum: The SNAP study. *Journal of Autism and Developmental Disorders, 38,* 1827–1836.

Barbaresi, W. J. (2016). The meaning of "regression" in children with autism spectrum disorder: Why does it matter? *Journal of Developmental and Behavioral Pediatrics, 37,* 506–507.

Barger, B. D., Campbell, J. M., & McDonough, J. D. (2013). Prevalence and onset of regression within autism spectrum disorders: A meta-analytic review. *Journal of Autism and Developmental Disorders, 43,* 817–828.

Bellman, M., Byrne, O., & Sege, R. (2013). Developmental assessment of children. *BMJ, 346,* e8687. doi:10.1136/bmj.e8687

Blasco, P. A. (1992). Normal and abnormal motor development. *Pediatric Rounds, 1,* 1–6.

Bostic, J. Q., & Rho, Y. (2006). Target-symptom psychopharmacology: Between the forest and the trees. *Child and Adolescent Psychiatric Clinics of North America, 15,* 289–302.

Boucher, J. (2012). Research review: Structural language in autistic spectrum disorder—characteristics and causes. *Journal of Child Psychology and Psychiatry and Allied Disciplines, 53,* 219–233.

Boyle, C. A., Boulet, S., Schieve, L. A., Cohen, R. A., Blumberg, S. J., Yeargin-Allsopp, M., . . . Kogan, M. D. (2011). Trends in the prevalence of developmental disabilities in US children, 1997-2008. *Pediatrics, 127,* 1034–1042.

Brothers, K. B., Glascoe, F. P., & Robertshaw, N. S. (2008). PEDS: Developmental Milestones—an accurate brief tool for surveillance and screening. *Clinical Pediatrics, 47,* 271–279.

Capute, A. (1991). The expanded Strauss syndrome: MBD revisited. In P. J. Accardo, T. A. Blondis, & B. Y. Whitman (Eds.), *Attention deficit disorders and hyperactivity in children* (pp. 27–36). New York, NY: Marcel Dekker.

Capute, A. J., & Palmer, F. B. (1980). A pediatric overview of the spectrum of developmental disabilities. *Journal of Developmental and Behavioral Pediatrics, 1,* 66–69.

Carey, W. B., Crocker, A. C., Coleman, W. L., Elias, E. R., & Feldman, H. M. (2009). *Developmental-behavioral pediatrics* (4th ed.). Philadelphia, PA: Saunders.

Christensen, D., Van Naarden Braun, K., Doernberg, N. S., Maenner, M. J., Arneson, C. L., Durkin, M. S., . . . Yeargin-Allsopp, M. (2014). Prevalence of cerebral palsy, co-occurring autism spectrum disorders, and motor functioning: Autism and Developmental Disabilities Monitoring Network, USA, 2008. *Developmental Medicine & Child Neurology, 56,* 59–65.

Clark, L. A., Cuthbert, B., Lewis-Fernández, R., Narrow, W. E., & Reed, G. M. (2017). Three approaches to understanding and classifying mental disorder: ICD-11, DSM-5, and the National Institute of Mental Health's Research Domain Criteria (RDoC). *Psychological Science in the Public Interest, 8,* 72–145.

Coe, B. P., Girirajan, S., & Eichler, E. E. (2012). The genetic variability and commonality of neurodevelopmental disease. *American Journal of Medical Genetics Part C: Seminars in Medical Genetics, 160C,* 118–129.

Cole, W. R., Mostofsky, S. H., Gidley Larson, J. C., Denckla, M. B., & Mahone, E. M. (2008). Age-related changes in motor subtle signs among girls and boys with ADHD. *Neurology, 71,* 1514–1520.

Crawford, T. O. (1996). Neuromuscular disorders. In A. J. Capute & P. A. Accardo (Eds.), *Developmental disabilities in infancy and childhood: Vol. II: The spectrum of developmental disabilities* (2nd ed., pp. 151–162). Baltimore, MD: Paul H. Brookes Publishing Co.

Cuthbert, B. N. (2015). Research domain criteria: Toward future psychiatric nosologies. *Dialogues in Clinical Neuroscience, 17,* 89–97.

Cuthbert, B. N., & Insel, T. R. (2013). Toward the future of psychiatric diagnosis: The seven pillars of RDoC. *BMC Medicine, 11,* 126. doi:10.1186/1741-7015-11-126

Dale, N., & Sonksen, P. (2002). Developmental outcome, including setback, in young children with severe visual impairment. *Developmental Medicine & Child Neurology, 44,* 613–622.

D'Arrigo, S., Gavazzi, F., Alfei, E., Zuffardi, O., Montomoli, C., Corso, B., . . . Pantaleoni, C. (2016). The diagnostic yield of array comparative genomic hybridization is high regardless of severity of intellectual disability/developmental delay in children. *Journal of Child Neurology, 31,* 691–699.

Davie, M. (2012). Developmental assessment in the over 5s. *Archives of Disease in Childhood, Education and Practice Edition,97,* 2–8.

Delobel-Ayoub, M., Klapouszczak, D., van Bakel, M. M. E., Horridge, K., Sigurdardottir, S., Himmelmann, K., & Arnaud, C. (2017). Prevalence and characteristics of autism spectrum disorders in children with cerebral palsy. *Developmental Medicine & Child Neurology, 59,* 738–742.

Dunn, L. M., & Dunn, D. M. (2007). *Peabody Picture Vocabulary Test, Fourth Edition, manual.* Minneapolis, MN: NCS Pearson.

Ehrmann Feldman, D., Couture, M., Grilli, L., Simard, M. N., Azoulay, L., & Gosselin, J. (2005). When and by whom is concern first expressed for children with neuromotor problems? *Archives of Pediatric and Adolescent Medicine, 159,* 882–886.

Elbaum, B., & Celimli-Aksoy, S. (2017). Empirically identified subgroups of children served in Part C early intervention programs. *Journal of Developmental and Behavioral Pediatrics, 38,* 510–520.

Feldman, H. M., & Messick, C. (2008). Assessment of speech and language. In M. L. Wolraich, D. D. Drotar, P. H. Dworkin, & E. C. Perrin (Eds.), *Developmental-behavioral pediatrics: Evidence and practice* (pp. 177–190). Philadelphia, PA: Mosby.

Finucane, B., & Myers, S. M. (2016). Genetic counseling for autism spectrum disorder in an evolving theoretical landscape. *Current Genetic Medicine Reports, 4,* 147–153. doi:10.1007/s40142-016-0099-9

Fletcher, J. M., & Miciak, J. (2017). Comprehensive cognitive assessments are not necessary for the identification and treatment of learning disabilities. *Archives of Clinical Neuropsychology, 32,* 2–7.

Gesell, A., & Amatruda, C. S. (1947). *Developmental diagnosis: Normal and abnormal child development, clinical methods and pediatric applications* (2nd ed.). New York, NY: Paul B. Hoeber.

Gesell, A. L., Halverson, H. M., & Amatruda, C. S. (1940). *The first five years of life: A guide to the study of the preschool child.* New York, NY: Harper.

Gilman, B. J., Lovecky, D. V., Kearney, K., Peters, D. B., Wasserman, J. D., . . . Rimm, S. B. (2013). Critical issues in the identification of gifted students with co-existing disabilities: The twice-exceptional. *SAGE Open, 3,* 1–16. doi:10.1177/2158244013505855

Godber, T., Anderson, V., & Bell, R. (2000). The measurement and diagnostic utility of intrasubtest scatter in pediatric neuropsychology. *Journal of Clinical Psychology, 56,* 101–112.

Gonzalez-Mantilla, A. J., Moreno-De-Luca, A., Ledbetter, D. H., & Martin, C. L. (2016). A cross-disorder method to identify novel candidate genes for developmental brain disorders. *JAMA Psychiatry, 73,* 275–283.

Greene, C. L. (2013). Recognizing inborn errors of metabolism. In R. A. Saul (Ed.), *Medical genetics in pediatric practice* (pp. 111–133). Itasca, IL: American Academy of Pediatrics.

Gripp, K. W., Slavotinek, A. M., Hall, J. G., & Allanson, J. E. (Eds.). (2013). *Handbook of physical measurements* (3rd ed.). New York, NY: Oxford University Press.

Hanley, G. P., Iwata, B. A., & McCord, B. E. (2003). Functional analysis of problem behavior: A review. *Journal of Applied Behavior Analysis, 36,* 147–185.

Harrison, P. L., & Oakland, T. (2015). *Adaptive Behavior Assessment System* (3rd ed.). Torrance, CA: Western Psychological Services.

Harvey, S. T., Boer, D., Meyer, L. H., & Evans, I. M. (2009). Updating a meta-analysis of intervention research with challenging behaviour: treatment validity and standards of practice. *Journal of Intellectual and Developmental Disabilities, 34,* 67–80.

Horridge, K. A. (2011). Assessment and investigation of the child with disordered development. *Archives of Disease in Childhood, Education and Practice Edition, 96,* 9–20.

Hoyme, H. E. (2013). Assessing dysmorphology in primary care. In R. A. Saul (Ed.), *Medical genetics in pediatric practice* (pp. 135–174). Itasca, IL: American Academy of Pediatrics.

Hresko, W. P., Peak, P. K., Herron, S. R., & Bridges, D. L. (2000). *Young Children's Achievement Test.* Austin, TX: PRO-ED.

Huerta, M., & Lord, C. (2012). Diagnostic evaluation of autism spectrum disorders. *Pediatric Clinics of North America,* 12(59), 103–111.

Hyman, S. E. (2010). The diagnosis of mental disorders: The problem of reification. *Annual Review of Clinical Psychology, 6,* 155–179.

Individuals with Disabilities Education Improvement Act, PL 108–446, 20 U.S. §1400 et seq. (2004).

Insel, T., Cuthbert, B., Garvey, M., Heinssen, R., Kozak, M., Pine, D. S., . . . Wang, P. (2010). Research Domain Criteria (RDoC): Toward a new classification framework for research on mental disorders. *American Journal of Psychiatry, 167,* 748–751.

Ireton, H. (1992). *Child Development Inventory manual.* Minneapolis, MN: Behavior Science Systems.

Jeong, A., & Wong, M. (2016). mTOR inhibitors in children: Current indications and future directions in neurology. *Current Neurology and Neuroscience Reports, 16,* 102.

Johnson, C. P., Myers, S. M., & Council on Children with Disabilities. (2007). Identification and evaluation of children with autism spectrum disorders. *Pediatrics, 120,* 1183–1215.

Jones, E. J., Gliga, T., Bedford, R., Charman, T., & Johnson, M. H. (2014). Developmental pathways to autism: A review of prospective studies of infants at risk. *Neuroscience Biobehavioral Reviews, 39,* 1–33.

Kaufman, A. S., & Kaufman, N. L. (2004). *Kaufman Brief Intelligence Test, Second Edition manual.* Minneapolis, MN: NCS Pearson.

Kelley, R. I. (2008). Metabolic diseases and developmental disabilities. In P. J. Accardo (Ed.), *Capute & Accardo's neurodevelopmental disabilities in infancy and childhood: Vol. I: Neurodevelopmental diagnosis and treatment* (3rd ed., pp. 115–145). Baltimore, MD: Paul H. Brookes Publishing Co.

Korf, B. R., & Bebin, E. M. (2017). Neurocutaneous disorders in children. *Pediatrics in Review, 38,* 119–128.

Kozlowski, A. M., Matson, J. L., Horovitz, M., Worley, J. A., & Neal, D. (2011). Parents' first concerns of their child's development in toddlers with autism spectrum disorders. *Developmental Neurorehabilitation, 14,* 72–78.

Kral, M. C. (2018). Interpreting psychoeducational testing reports, individualized family service plans (IFSP), and individualized education program (IEP) plans. In R. G. Voigt, M. M. Macias, S. M. Myers, & D. D. Tapia (Eds.), *American Academy of Pediatrics developmental and behavioral pediatrics* (2nd ed., pp. 477–493). Itasca, IL: American Academy of Pediatrics.

Larson, J., Mostofsky, S. H., Goldberg, M. C., Cutting, L. E., Denckla, M. B., & Mahone, E. M. (2007). Effects of gender and age on motor exam in developing children. *Developmental Neuropsychology, 32,* 543–562.

Leppert, M. L. (2011). Neurodevelopmental assessment and medical evaluation. In R. G. Voigt, M. M. Macias, & S. M. Myers (Eds.), *AAP developmental and behavioral pediatrics* (pp. 93–119). Elk Grove Village, IL: American Academy of Pediatrics.

Lilienfeld, S. O., & Treadway, M. T. (2016). Clashing diagnostic approaches: DSM-ICD versus RDoC. *Annual Review of Clinical Psychology, 12,* 435–463.

Lingen, M., Albers, L., Borchers, M., Haass, S., Gärtner, J., Schröder, S., . . . Zirn, B. (2016). Obtaining a genetic diagnosis in a child with disability: Impact on parental quality of life. *Clinical Genetics, 89,* 258–266.

Lock, T. M., Shapiro, B. K., Ross, A., & Capute, A. J. (1986). Age of presentation in developmental disability. *Journal of Developmental and Behavioral Pediatrics, 7,* 340–345.

Lord, C., Rutter, M., DiLavore, P. S., Risi, S., Gotham, K., & Bishop, S. L. (2012). *Autism Diagnostic Observation Schedule, Second Edition (ADOS-2) manual (Part 1): Modules 1-4.* Torrence, CA: Western Psychological Services.

Manning, M., & Hudgins, L. (2010). Array-based technology and recommendations for utilization in medical genetics practice for detection of chromosomal abnormalities. *Genetics in Medicine, 12,* 742–745.

Martins, I. P., Lauterbach, M., Luís, H., Amaral, H., Rosenbaum, G., Slade, P. D., & Townes, B. D. (2013). Neurological subtle signs and cognitive development: A study in late childhood and adolescence. *Child Neuropsychology, 19,* 466–478.

McDonald-McGinn, D. M., & Sullivan, K. E. (2011). Chromosome 22q11.2 deletion syndrome (DiGeorge syndrome/velocardiofacial syndrome). *Medicine, 90,* 1–18.

McGuire, K., Fung, L. K., Hagopian, L., Vasa, R. A., Mahajan, R., Bernal, P., . . . Whitaker, A. H. (2016). Irritability and problem behavior in autism spectrum disorder: A practice pathway for pediatric primary care. *Pediatrics, 137*(Suppl. 2), S136–S148.

McKusick, V. A. (1969). On lumpers and splitters, or the nosology of genetic disease. *Perspectives in Biology and Medicine, 12,* 298–312.

Meilleur, A.-A. S., & Fombonne, E. (2009). Regression of language and non-language skills in pervasive developmental disorders. *Journal of Intellectual Disability Research, 53,* 115–124.

Michelson, D. J., Shevell, M. I., Sherr, E. H., Moeschler, J. B., Gropman, A. L., & Ashwal, S. (2011). Evidence report: Genetic and metabolic testing on children with global developmental delay: Report of the Quality Standards Subcommittee of the American Academy of Neurology and the Practice Committee of the Child Neurology Society. *Neurology, 77,* 1629–1635.

Miller, D. T., Adam, M. A., Aradhya, S., Biesecker, L. G., Brothman, A. R., Carter, N. P., . . . Ledbetter, D. H. (2010). Consensus statement: Chromosomal microarray is a first-tier clinical diagnostic test for individuals with developmental disabilities or congenital anomalies. *American Journal of Human Genetics, 86,* 749–764.

Mitchel, M. W., Moreno-De-Luca, D., Myers, S. M., Finucane, B., Ledbetter, D. H., & Martin, C. L. (2016). 17q12 recurrent deletion syndrome. In M. P. Adam, H. H. Ardinger, R. A. Pagon, & S. E. Wallace (Eds.), *GeneReviews®* [Internet]. Seattle, WA: University of Washington, Seattle. Retrieved from https://www.ncbi.nlm.nih.gov/books/NBK401562/

Mithyantha, R., Kneen, R., McCann, E., & Gladstone, M. (2017). Current evidence-based recommendations on investigating children with global developmental delay. *Archives of Disease in Childhood, 102,* 1071–1076.

Moeschler, J. B., & Shevell, M. (2014). Committee on Genetics. Comprehensive evaluation of the child with intellectual disability or global developmental delays. *Pediatrics, 134,* e903–e918.

Montgomery, T. (2008). Neurodevelopmental assessment of school-age children. In P. J. Accardo (Ed.), *Capute & Accardo's neurodevelopmental disabilities in infancy and childhood: Vol. I: Neurodevelopmental diagnosis and treatment* (3rd ed., pp. 405–417). Baltimore, MD: Paul H. Brookes Publishing Co.

Moreno-De-Luca, A., Myers, S. M., Challman, T. D., Moreno-De-Luca, D., Evans, D. W., & Ledbetter, D. H. (2013). Developmental brain dysfunction: Revival and expansion of old concepts based on new genetic evidence. *Lancet Neurology, 12,* 406–414.

Mostofsky, S. H., Newschaffer, C. J., & Denckla, M. B. (2003). Overflow movements predict impaired response inhibition in children with ADHD. *Perceptual & Motor Skills, 97,* 1315–1331.

Msall, M. E., DiGuadio, K., Rogers, B. T., LaForest, S., Lyon, N., Campbell, J., . . . Duffy, L. C. (1994). The Functional Independence Measure for Children (WeeFIM): Conceptual basis and pilot use in children with developmental disabilities. *Clinical Pediatrics, 33,* 421–430.

Msall, M. E., & Msall, E. R. (2008). Functional assessment in neurodevelopmental disorders. In P. J. Accardo (Ed.), *Capute & Accardo's neurodevelopmental disabilities in infancy and childhood: Vol. I: Neurodevelopmental diagnosis and treatment* (3rd ed., pp. 419–444). Baltimore, MD: Paul H. Brookes Publishing Co.

Muhle, R. A., Reed, H. E., Vo, L. C., Mehta, S., McGuire, K., Veenstra-VanderWeele, J., & Pedapati, E. (2017). Clinical diagnostic genetic testing for individuals with developmental disorders. *Journal of the American Academy of Child & Adolescent Psychiatry, 56,* 910–913.

Mullen, E. M. (1995). *Mullen Scales of Early Learning manual.* Circle Pines, MN: American Guidance Service.

Myers, S. M. (2007). The status of pharmacotherapy for autism spectrum disorders. *Expert Opinion on Pharmacotherapy, 8,* 1579–1603.

Myers, S. M., & Challman, T. D. (2018). Autism spectrum disorder. In R. G. Voigt, M. M. Macias, S. M. Myers, & D. D. Tapia (Eds.), *American Academy of Pediatrics developmental and behavioral pediatrics* (2nd ed., pp. 407–475). Itasca, IL: American Academy of Pediatrics.

Myers, S. M., Johnson, C. P., & Council on Children with Disabilities. (2007). Management of children with autism spectrum disorders. *Pediatrics, 120,* 1162–1182.

National Society of Genetic Counselors' Definition Task Force, Resta, R., Biesecker, B. B., Bennett, R. L., Blum, S., Estabrooks Hahn, S., . . . Williams, J. L. (2006). A new definition of genetic counseling: National society of genetic counselors' task force report. *Journal of Genetic Counseling, 15*(2), 77–83.

Newborg, J. (2005). *Battelle Developmental Inventory* (2nd ed.). Itasca, IL: Riverside Publishing.

Odding, E., Roebroeck, M. E., & Stam, H. J. (2006). The epidemiology of cerebral palsy: Incidence, impairments and risk factors. *Disability & Rehabilitation, 28,* 183–191.

Pakula, A. T., Van Naarden Braun, K., & Yeargin-Alsopp, M. (2009). Cerebral palsy: Classification and epidemiology. *Physical Medicine & Rehabilitation Clinics of North America, 20,* 425–452.

Palisano, R., Rosenbaum, P., Bartlett, D. J., & Livingston, M. (2007). *Gross Motor Function Classification System: Expanded and revised* (GMFCS-E&R). Retrieved from https://canchild.ca/system/tenon/assets/attachments/000/000/058/original/GMFCS-ER_English.pdf

Pearn, J. (2011). Differentiating diseases: The centrum of differential diagnosis in the evolution of Oslerian medicine. *Fetal and Pediatric Pathology, 30,* 1–15.

Peterson, R. L., & Pennington, B. F. (2015). Developmental dyslexia. *Annual Review of Clinical Psychology, 11,* 283–307.

Pickles, A., Simonoff, E., Conti-Ramsden, G., Falcaro, M., Simkin, Z., Charman, T., . . . Baird, G. (2009). Loss of language in early development of autism and specific language impairment. *Journal of Child Psychology and Psychiatry, 50,* 843–852.

Poduri, A. (2017). When should genetic testing be performed in epilepsy patients? *Epilepsy Currents, 17,* 16–22.

Pyeritz, R. E. (2012). The family history: the first genetic test, and still useful after all those years? *Genetics in Medicine, 14,* 3–9.

Raven, J. C., Court, J. H., & Raven, J. (1995). *Manual for Raven's Progressive Matrices and Vocabulary Scales: Section 2: Coloured Progressive Matrices.* Oxford, United Kingdom: Oxford Psychologists Press.

Reiff, M., Giarelli, E., Bernhardt, B. A., Easley, E., Spinner, N. B., Sankar, P. L., & Mulchandani, S. (2015). Parents' perceptions of the usefulness of chromosomal microarray analysis for children with autism spectrum disorders. *Journal of Autism and Developmental Disorders, 45,* 3262–3275.

Retterer, K., Juusola, J., Cho, M. T., Vitakaza, P., Millan, F., Gibellini, F., . . . Bale, S. (2016). Clinical application of whole-exome sequencing across clinical indications. *Genetics in Medicine, 18,* 696–704.

Riou, E. M., Ghosh, S., Francoeur, E., & Shevell, M. I. (2009). Global developmental delay and its relationship to cognitive skills. *Developmental Medicine & Child Neurology, 51,* 600–606.

Rogers, S. J. (2004). Developmental regression in autism spectrum disorders. *Mental Retardation and Developmental Disabilities Research Reviews, 10,* 139–143.

Roid, G. (2005). *Stanford-Binet Intelligence Scales for Early Childhood.* Itasca, IL: Riverside Publishing.

Ruggieri, M., & Praticò, A. D. (2015). Mosaic neurocutaneous disorders and their causes. *Seminars in Pediatric Neurology, 22,* 207–233.

Saal, H. M., & Chen, E. (2013). Family history and pedigree construction. In R. A. Saul (Ed.), *Medical genetics in pediatric practice* (pp. 73–109). Itasca, IL: American Academy of Pediatrics.

Schaefer, G. B., Mendelsohn, N. J., & Professional Practice and Guidelines Committee. (2013). Clinical genetics evaluation in identifying the etiology of autism spectrum disorders: 2013 guideline revisions. *Genetics in Medicine, 15,* 399–407.

Scharf, R. J., Scharf, G. J., & Stroustrup, A. (2016). Developmental milestones. *Pediatrics in Review, 37,* 25–37.

Schopler, E., Van Bourgondien, M. E., Wellman, G. J., & Love, S. R. (2010). *Childhood Autism Rating Scale, Second Edition manual.* Los Angeles, CA: Western Psychological Services.

Shapiro, B. K., & Gwynn, H. (2008). Neurodevelopmental assessment of infants and young children. In P. J. Accardo (Ed.), *Capute & Accardo's neurodevelopmental disabilities in infancy and childhood: Vol. I: Neurodevelopmental diagnosis and treatment* (3rd ed., pp. 367–382). Baltimore, MD: Paul H. Brookes Publishing Co.

Shaywitz, S. E., Morris, R., & Shaywitz, B. A. (2008). The education of dyslexic children from childhood to young adulthood. *Annual Review of Psychology, 59,* 451–475.

Shbarou, R., & Mikati, M.A. (2016). The expanding clinical spectrum of genetic pediatric epileptic encephalopathies. *Seminars in Pediatric Neurology, 23,* 134–142.

Shevell, M. I., Majnemer, A., Rosenbaum, P., & Abrahamowicz, M. (2001). Profile of referrals for early childhood developmental delay to ambulatory subspecialty clinics. *Journal of Child Neurology, 16,* 645–650.

Sonksen, P. M. (2016). *Developmental assessment: Theory, practice and application to neurodisability. A practical guide from Mac Keith Press.* London, United Kingdom: Mac Keith Press.

Sparrow, S. S., Cicchetti, D. V., & Saulnier, C. A. (2016). *Vineland Adaptive Behavior Scales, Third Edition (Vineland-3).* Bloomington, MN: Pearson.

Stein, M. T., & Lukasik, M. K. (2009). Developmental screening and assessment: Infants, toddlers, and preschoolers. In W. B. Carey, A. C. Crocker, W. L. Coleman, E. R. Elias, & H. M. Feldman (Eds.), *Developmental-behavioral pediatrics* (4th ed., pp. 785–796). Philadelphia, PA: Saunders.

Steiner, A. M., Goldsmith, T. R., Snow, A. V., & Chawarska, K. (2012). Practitioner's guide to assessment of autism spectrum disorders in infants and toddlers. *Journal of Autism and Developmental Disorders, 42,* 1183–1196.

Stessman, H. A., Turner, T. N., & Eichler, E. E. (2016). Molecular subtyping and improved treatment of neurodevelopmental disease. *Genome Medicine, 8,* 22. doi:10.1186/s13073-016-0278-z

Toriello, H. V. (2008). Role of the dysmorphologic evaluation in the child with developmental delay. *Pediatric Clinics of North America, 55,* 1085–1098.

Türkoğlu, G., Türkoğlu, S., Çelik, C., & Uçan, H. (2017). Intelligence, functioning, and related factors in children with cerebral palsy. *Archives of Neuropsychiatry, 54,* 33–37.

van Karnebeek, C. D., Bowden, K., & Berry-Kravis, E. (2016). Treatment of neurogenetic developmental conditions: From 2016 into the future. *Pediatric Neurology, 65,* 1–13.

VanderVeer, B., & Schweid, E. (1974). Infant assessment: Stability of mental functioning in young retarded children. *American Journal of Mental Deficiency, 79,* 1–4.

VanMeter, L., Fein, D., Morris, R., Waterhouse, L., & Allen, D. (1997). Delay versus deviance in autistic social behavior. *Journal of Autism and Developmental Disorders, 27,* 557–569.

Vissers, L. E., Gilissen, C., & Veltman, J. A. (2016). Genetic studies in intellectual disability and related disorders. *Nature Reviews Genetics, 17,* 9–18.

Voigt, R. G. (2018). Making developmental-behavioral diagnoses. In R. G. Voigt, M. M. Macias, S. M. Myers, & D. D. Tapia (Eds.), *American Academy of Pediatrics developmental and behavioral pediatrics* (2nd ed., pp. 187–221). Itasca, IL: American Academy of Pediatrics.

Voigt, R. G., Macias, M. M., Myers, S. M., & Tapia, D. D. (Eds.). (2018). *American Academy of Pediatrics developmental and behavioral pediatrics* (2nd ed.). Itasca, IL: American Academy of Pediatrics.

Wang, P. P. (2018). Nature, nurture, and their interactions in child development and behavior. In R. G. Voigt, M. M. Macias, S. M. Myers, & D. D. Tapia (Eds.), *American Academy of Pediatrics developmental and behavioral pediatrics* (2nd ed., pp. 5–20). Itasca, IL: American Academy of Pediatrics.

Whitaker, T. M., & Palmer, F. B. (2008). The developmental history. In P. J. Accardo (Ed.), *Capute & Accardo's neurodevelopmental disabilities in infancy and childhood. Vol. I: Neurodevelopmental diagnosis and treatment* (3rd ed., pp. 297–310). Baltimore, MD: Paul H. Brookes Publishing Co.

Wilkinson, G. S., & Robertson, G. J. (2006). *Wide Range Achievement Test, Fourth Edition manual.* Lutz, FL: Psychological Assessment Resources.

Willcutt, E. G., Pennington, B. F., Duncan, L., Smith, S. D., Keenan, J. M., Wadsworth, S., . . . Olson, R. K. (2010). Understanding the complex etiologies of developmental disorders: Behavioral and molecular genetic approaches. *Journal of Developmental and Behavioral Pediatrics, 31,* 533–544.

Wolraich, M. L., & Drotar, D. D. (2008). Diagnostic classification systems. In M. L. Wolraich, D. D. Drotar, P. H. Dworkin, & E. C. Perrin (Eds.), *Developmental-behavioral pediatrics: Evidence and practice* (pp. 109–122). Philadelphia, PA: Mosby.

Wolraich, M. L., Drotar, D. D., Dworkin, P. H., & Perrin, E. C. (2008). *Developmental-behavioral pediatrics: Evidence and practice.* Philadelphia, PA: Mosby.

World Health Organization. (1992). *The ICD-10 Classification of Mental and Behavioral Disorders.* Geneva, Switzerland: World Health Organization.

Yeargin-Allsopp, M., Murphy, C. C., Cordero, J. F., Decoufle, P., & Hollowell, J. G. (1997). Reported biomedical causes and associated medical conditions for mental retardation among 10-year-old children, Metropolitan Atlanta, 1985 to 1987. *Developmental Medicine & Child Neurology, 39,* 142–149.

Yin Foo, R., Guppy, M., & Johnston, L. M. (2013). Intelligence assessments for children with cerebral palsy: A systematic review. *Developmental Medicine & Child Neurology, 55,* 911–918.

CHAPTER 13 Neuropsychological Assessment

Lauren Kenworthy and Laura Gutermuth Anthony

Upon completion of this chapter, the reader will

- Understand the purpose of neuropsychological assessment
- Be able to describe a model of neuropsychological assessment that incorporates development, brain, and context
- Be familiar with the domains of functioning that neuropsychological assessments address
- Understand how to formulate referral questions and interpret testing results in order to inform treatment
- Know how to maximize the impact of an assessment through effective dissemination of findings and recommendations
- Be able to apply these concepts to a specific case

This chapter focuses on general principles and practical aspects of neuropsychological and cognitive assessment. In order to ensure that the application of this topic is clear, this chapter refers to a specific case about a boy named John throughout (see Case Study, Parts 1–10) to illustrate key points.

CASE STUDY, PART 1

John is an 8-year-old boy in the second grade who was referred for a neuropsychological evaluation following difficulties with socialization and schoolwork. He had previously been diagnosed with a sensory integration disorder, motor delay, and anxiety. As a result of this new neuropsychological evaluation, he received a diagnosis of autism spectrum disorder (ASD). John is a boy with many strengths, including precocious math and science abilities. His parents also report that he has a good sense of humor, likes to learn, and is devoted to a few important people in his life. But he is described as socially isolated, "rude" to his teacher, and inflexible. John also has difficulty producing satisfactory written work.

Thought Questions:

When would standard psychoeducational testing be sufficient, and when would neuropsychological testing be indicated? How might the results of neuropsychological testing be translated into a comprehensive treatment plan, including recommendations for home, school, and therapy?

THE PURPOSE OF NEUROPSYCHOLOGICAL ASSESSMENT

The **neuropsychological assessment** is a valuable tool for determining diagnosis, prognosis, and functional abilities in children (Kaufman, Boxer, & Bilder, 2013). It is particularly important for children with complex environmental, medical, psychiatric, and cognitive factors affecting behavior and learning. Neuropsychological assessment's unique contribution is its ability to provide an integrated understanding of emotional, cognitive, and other factors in an individual child for the purposes of building an effective treatment plan (Braun et al., 2011). See Box 13.1 for a description of the roles of different types of psychologists for children with neurodevelopmental disabilities.

There are currently no medical treatments for the core symptoms of many neurodevelopmental disabilities. For example, primary interventions for intellectual and learning disabilities (ID/LD) and ASD are linguistic, behavioral, and cognitive. In the case of attention-deficit/hyperactivity disorder (ADHD), there are potent medications that target core symptoms, but they are most effective in children when used in combination with behavioral and cognitive interventions (Hinshaw, Arnold, & MTA Cooperative Group, 2015). Because most children with neurodevelopmental disabilities receive school-based services, intervention recommendations that coordinate school, home, and therapeutic settings are a fundamental step to a comprehensive treatment plan (Wolraich & DuPaul, 2010). In addition, there is a great deal of variability within the cognitive profiles of children with neurodevelopmental disabilities. For these two reasons, a neuropsychological evaluation that delineates cognitive strengths and weaknesses and makes specific recommendations regarding classroom placement, accommodations, special education, and therapy can serve as the cornerstone of an effective treatment plan for a child with a neurodevelopmental disability.

Since the 1990s, **neuropsychology** has evolved to better meet the needs of children with neurodevelopmental disabilities. The advent of brain imaging and other sophisticated diagnostic techniques has shifted neuropsychology's role from diagnosis and lesion location to the determination of functional capacities and needs in real-world settings, such as home and school (Burgess et al., 2006; Kenworthy, Yerys, Anthony, & Wallace, 2008; Hardy et al., 2017). Matarazzo (1990) documented this shift in his seminal paper distinguishing *psychological testing,* which is focused on producing test scores, from *psychological assessment,* which incorporates test scores into a broad-based assessment of a person's abilities and environment. Bernstein (2000) elaborated on this in the context of pediatric neuropsychology, saying "The primary goal of a comprehensive clinical assessment [of a child] is . . . to produce a comfortable, competent 25-year-old" (p. 408), which requires an assessment designed to promote optimum fit between an individual child's cognitive, social, and behavioral profile and the environments in which that child learns and develops (Baron, 2004). This is typically what parents most want from an assessment; however, when evaluations are geared toward the presentation of "test results" or performance on specific criterion-based testing, as within school settings, it is easy for this goal to become lost.

A MODEL FOR DEVELOPMENTAL NEUROPSYCHOLOGICAL ASSESSMENT

The developmental neuropsychological assessment model described by Bernstein (2000) is ideally suited to the needs of children with neurodevelopmental disabilities because it emphasizes identification of diagnostic behavioral clusters or domains, which pose specific risks to the developing child in specific contexts (e.g., elementary school). Bernstein's model of assessment has three key interacting variables: 1) development, 2) brain, and 3) context.

Development is the first key variable. An understanding of development in typical children and in the specific child being assessed is a hallmark of a good assessment. This means knowing that reversing letters when writing is typical in 5 year olds and not expected in 8 year olds, for example. Professionals engaged in assessment must also understand an individual child's developmental trajectory and how a neurodevelopmental disorder may alter brain functions that in turn change the way a child learns and develops other abilities. Piaget (1952) first provided this understanding of children as constructing knowledge through experience. A child's development occurs in the context of his or her own specific brain and environment interacting together. **Joint attention** is a good example of a neurocognitive ability that influences how a child benefits from his or her environment. Joint attention, or the ability to share attention between another person and an object, plays an early developing "self-organizing role" in helping children learn from their social environment (Mundy & Newell, 2007). Impairments in joint attention, as occur in autism, have downstream effects on language, intelligence, and social abilities (Mundy, 2018). Assessment of a developing brain also requires an appreciation of plasticity and consideration of possible brain reorganization following injury. An understanding of the typical course of development, the timing of the insult or injury and its potential effects on brain structure, and the ability to benefit from context are all important (Hunter, Hinkle, & Edidin, 2012; see Case Study, Part 2).

CASE STUDY, PART 2

Developmental variables are key to understanding John's neuropsychological profile. The development of his pre-academic skills was precocious. For example, he could recite the alphabet at 18 months of age, demonstrating a facility for memorizing discrete units of information. At 5 years of age, he demonstrated very strong expressive and receptive language skills, and he achieved a superior verbal IQ score. But now, at 8 years of age, John is expected to formulate multiple sentences on a topic of his teacher's choosing, and his precocious vocabulary and verbal memorization skills do not support him on this higher-order academic language task. They do, however, allow him to tell his teacher in very sophisticated language what is wrong with her assignments.

The *brain* is Bernstein's second key variable for assessment. Assessment of a child with a neurodevelopmental disability occurs in the context of an understanding of the neural substrate, or brain structure/function, expected for that disability and observed in the individual child being assessed. It can be very powerful for parents and the treatment team to understand which components of a child's behavior are related to brain-based differences in processing, understanding, and producing information, as opposed to behaviors that may be learned, or even willful, on the child's part. Distinguishing between these two sources of behavior is what helps parents distinguish when a child "can't"—as opposed to "won't"—do what they expect (Kenworthy et al., 2014). In the case of "can't," parents and treatment teams can clearly understand that changes in the demand or context will be needed (see Case Study, Part 3). For example, most children with ADHD and ASD struggle with executive dysfunction, especially disorganization. Many of them cannot sit down on their own initiative at home to begin homework, but if the context is altered to be more supportive, through the provision of a written schedule, checklist, breaks, and rewards, they are successful.

CASE STUDY, PART 3

By learning about John's brain-based deficits in executive function, in particular his disorganization and inflexibility, his teacher was able to understand that this bright boy with an oversized vocabulary really *couldn't* organize words into written responses on specific topics of her choosing *unless* he was taught a highly structured writing rubric. Like many of us, until instructed otherwise, she assumed that a boy with John's core language abilities and considerable intelligence must be *choosing* not to write.

This leads directly to the final key variable in assessment, the *context* within which the child develops (see Figure 13.1) and is performing. Context is defined by Bernstein to include all aspects of a child's environment, and it is important for many reasons. It is essential to understand how a child's context and history may affect his or her performance during an assessment. For example, impaired vocabulary in a 7-year-old child who comes from a home in which books are read to him daily raises concerns regarding possible abnormalities in left frontal-temporal brain networks and suggests the need for specialized therapy. The same vocabulary in a child whose family speaks a language different from that in which the assessment was administered may simply indicate a familial and cultural basis for the vocabulary deficit and the need for increased exposure to English. The context of the assessment itself is vital as well. The 7-year-old child with impaired vocabulary may be reacting poorly to the assessment setting. Perhaps the examiner was unable to develop adequate rapport with the child, who became very anxious and provided only minimal responses. Many children behave differently in school, home, and clinical settings, and thus information must be gathered about performance in each setting to create a complete picture. Finally, an understanding of future contexts is important for an assessment to effectively predict risk and make recommendations. For example, a 4-year-old child with impaired phonological awareness and poor ability to break words down into individual sounds may be thriving in a nonacademic preschool but is at great

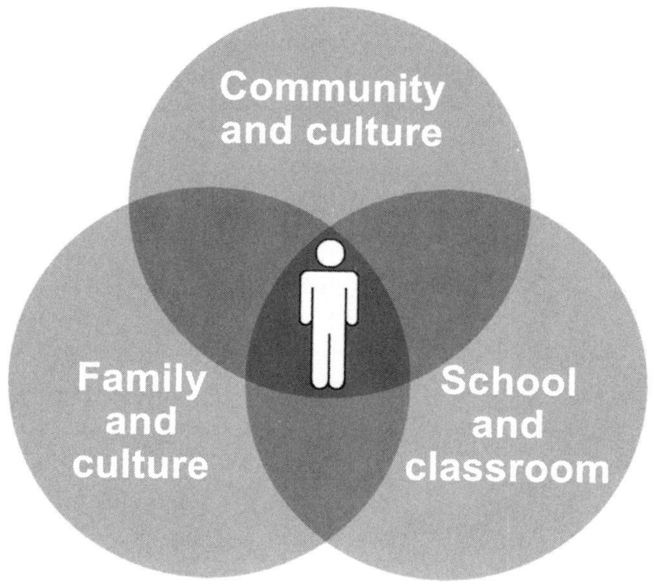

Figure 13.1. Viewing the child in context.

risk of failure in a kindergarten setting where reading skills are emphasized. Likewise, a very bright but disorganized fifth grader is at great risk for increased difficulties when he or she makes the transition to middle school with its demands for managing multiple subjects, teachers, and longer assignments. Delineation of risks is what drives practical recommendations for intervention. Development, and successful recommendations for enhancing development, do not exist in a vacuum. They occur within specific settings that can affect the course and prognosis of a child's difficulties, the way these difficulties are expressed, and the success of treatment. For this reason, *tests should not be used or interpreted in isolation* (see Case Study, Part 4).

CASE STUDY, PART 4

In John's case, consideration of context was important for many reasons. For example, although his parents were concerned about his lack of social skills, John had a close friend his age who did not have any neurodevelopmental disabilities. He saw his friend frequently, and his ability to sustain this friendship raised questions about whether he had greater social interaction abilities than his parents gave him credit for. Review of the context revealed, however, that this friend was a member of a family that socialized with John's whole family on a regular basis, and so John was not sustaining the friendship independently, but rather benefitted from a highly supported social context.

Assessment requires the integration of 1) test performance, behavioral observations, and contextual information provided by parents, teachers, and treatment team; 2) principles of development; and 3) knowledge of brain function. This information is integrated across the span of the child's development and across the settings the child inhabits. Baron (2004) terms this process *convergence profile analysis,* highlighting the fact that one test score or reported behavior is insufficient to generate an accurate cognitive profile. For example, take an assessment designed to answer whether or not a child has an attention deficit. All of the following questions must be answered before a determination can be made:

1. Is there a history of problems paying attention, or is it a new problem?
2. Is the child inattentive to all types of stimuli (people, words, and pictures) or just some types?
3. Is the child inattentive at home, at school, and in the clinician's office, or just in some settings?
4. What are the demands being placed on the child to pay attention, and what attention demands will he or she confront in the future?
5. What other cognitive, emotional, or contextual factors are affecting the child's ability to pay attention?
6. Have medical sources of attention problems, such as sleep disturbance and thyroid abnormalities, been ruled out?

A comprehensive neuropsychological assessment should provide a thorough investigation of each of the domains of functioning that are described in the next section of this chapter. The goal is to delineate a pattern of cognitive and behavioral strengths and weaknesses, to identify the risks posed by a child's profile in the contexts he or she inhabits, and to generate recommendations to ameliorate those risks through accommodations, special education, and therapy (see Case Study, Part 5).

CASE STUDY, PART 5

Convergence profile analyses were essential for interpreting John's attention data. His parents reported that John had considerable difficulty maintaining focused attention at home, but he performed well on a computerized attention task during the assessment. His attention to the examiner's spoken directions was somewhat less consistent, but he usually knew exactly what to do before she had finished giving directions anyway. He was least attentive in the assessment when the examiner tried to chat with him about her own interests and experiences. His teacher reported that John had problems attending to instructions, to class discussion, and to tasks that he found boring, but she also reported that he had excellent focus once he was engaged in independent work on a task that interested him. John also experienced problems with generalized anxiety, which contributed to difficulty falling asleep. Integrating these data across contexts and tasks suggests that John does not have a pervasive problem with attention, but rather has increasing difficulty attending as the context becomes less structured and predictable, as the demands on executive function increase (home versus school), and as the social content of the material increases (e.g., having good attention to a computerized task or in independent work but poor attention when people are talking to him). This points to executive and social deficits as the primary problem, not attention. John's remarkable intelligence is another key factor affecting attention, as he typically understands information very quickly and thus is more easily bored. Finally, his sleep problems and anxiety may contribute to John's attention problems, a finding that has important implications for treatment strategies.

BOX 13.1 INTERDISCIPLINARY CARE

The Varieties of Psychology

What are the differences among a neuropsychologist, a clinical child psychologist, and a school psychologist? The American Psychological Association (2012) defines the three specialties this way:

1. Clinical neuropsychology is a specialty in professional psychology that applies principles of assessment and intervention based upon the scientific study of human behavior as it relates to normal and abnormal functioning of the central nervous system. The specialty is dedicated to enhancing the understanding of brain–behavior relationships and the application of such knowledge to human problems. A pediatric neuropsychologist is a specialist within clinical neuropsychology who addresses these considerations in infants, children, adolescents, and emerging adults.
2. Clinical child psychology is a specialty in professional psychology that develops and applies scientific knowledge to the delivery of psychological services to infants, toddlers, children, and adolescents within their social context. Of particular importance to the specialty of clinical child psychology is an understanding of developmental models and their relationships with the basic psychological needs of children and adolescents, as well as how the family and other social contexts influence the socioemotional adjustment, cognitive development, behavioral adaptation, and health status of children and adolescents.
3. School psychology is a health service provider specialty within professional psychology that is concerned with the science and practice of psychology with children, youth, and families; learners of all ages; and the schooling process. The basic education and training of school psychologists prepare them to provide a range of psychological diagnosis, assessment, intervention, prevention, health promotion, and program development and evaluation services with a special focus on the developmental processes of children and youth within the context of schools and other educational systems.

Practically speaking, there is a fair amount of overlap, and most neuropsychologists are trained in either clinical or school psychology programs with specialized coursework and training. It could happen that a child like John could see all three types of psychologists, either at the same time as part of a multidisciplinary team or consecutively as new or different assessment questions emerge. For example, John's neuropsychologist might evaluate how his developmental brain differences impact his everyday functioning; John's clinical psychologist could assess for other mental health issues, such as his anxiety or sleep problems, or lead his treatment team after diagnosis; and John's school psychologist could be instrumental in setting up a successful program of adaptations and interventions in school to help him be a successful student. Alternatively, John could be assessed and treated by only one of these professional subspecialties.

Adapted from the American Psychological Association. Recognized Specialties and Proficiencies in Professional Psychology. http://www.apa.org/ed/graduate/specialize/recognized.aspx

DOMAINS OF FUNCTIONING ASSESSED IN NEUROPSYCHOLOGICAL EVALUATIONS

A comprehensive neuropsychological assessment includes a description of strengths and weaknesses. For each neuropsychological domain, the assessment should provide a clear summary statement describing the child's abilities and an integration of data from multiple sources. A full assessment includes multiple methods—for example, parent and child clinical interviews and/or structured standardized interviews such as the Autism Diagnostic Observation Schedule, Second Edition (ADOS-2; Lord, Rutter, DiLavore, & Risi, 2012) and the Autism Diagnostic Interview, Revised (ADI-R; Rutter, Le Couteur & Lord, 2003); norm-referenced rating scales from the parent, teacher, and child (self-report); behavioral observations; standardized, norm-referenced tests in relevant domains; and sometimes supplemental subjective measures (see Box 13.2). Although the specific neuropsychological domains and their labels can vary somewhat depending on the examiner, the most commonly referenced domains of functioning are defined below. Table 13.1 also lists these domains, indicates neurodevelopmental disabilities that may be associated with deficits in each domain, and gives examples of relevant data sources regarding each domain. There is also a table listing many common tests associated with each of these domains in the appendix at the end of this chapter (see Appendix 13.1).

BOX 13.2 EVIDENCE-BASED PRACTICE

Focused Models of Assessment

- In the field of pediatric neuropsychology, the norm had been to conduct a comprehensive, 1–2 day evaluation that sampled all domains of functioning; however, many professionals now are emphasizing the importance of a focused battery. Youngstrom (2013) argues that an evidence-based assessment is targeted and parsimonious: Specific, clinically relevant questions are addressed with the briefest, most focused evaluation possible. Thus, if a child has a specific problem or a simple diagnostic question (e.g., whether he or she has attention-deficit/hyperactivity disorder) a comprehensive neuropsychological assessment may be an inefficient use of time and money. Conversely, a child who is having trouble making friends and struggles with anxiety, emotional outbursts, and writing and reading at school may need a comprehensive evaluation in order to inform differential diagnoses and investigate possible weaknesses across many domains of functioning.
- One downside of comprehensive evaluations is the time required to produce and read the reports they generate. A recent survey of neuropsychologists and their referral sources revealed that many neuropsychologists do not believe that the reports they write are read in their entirety and that 73% of referral sources feel that slow turnaround time of reports negatively affects their patients' care. The components of neuropsychological reports that they found most helpful are the diagnosis, impression, and recommendations sections (Postal et al., 2018).
- Models for triaging assessment referrals and customizing assessment protocols and reports are increasingly important to make sure that the referral questions are answered efficiently. Hardy and colleagues (2017) have elaborated a graduated system of evaluation with three tiers of assessment for children with medical conditions affecting the central nervous system:
    1. Universal monitoring by the medical treatment team (with brief questionnaires or computerized tasks)
    2. Targeted screening by the neuropsychologist for those children with greatest risk or who are identified to be at risk through monitoring
    3. Comprehensive evaluation for those for whom screening is inadequate to address concerns

General Intelligence

General intelligence is commonly discussed in neuropsychological assessments and is often considered the benchmark against which other cognitive abilities are measured. For example, a child with an overall IQ score that is in the intellectually deficient range would not be identified as having a specific visual processing deficit unless difficulties in that domain were greater than what would be expected based on his or her IQ. Yet, it is important to recognize that general intelligence scores have narrower implications for a child's ability to become a successful and happy 25 year old than is often assumed by parents. Intelligence testing originated in early 20th-century France as a method to predict which children would succeed in school. Its development in 20th-century America included the delineation of separate factors in intelligence with a strong emphasis on verbal knowledge and spatial performance as key factors in determining overall intellectual abilities. **Crystallized intelligence** (using knowledge and experience) versus **fluid intelligence** (solving novel problems) is another common dichotomy. Processing speed has played an increasing role in our understanding of performance on IQ tests, particularly in children with congenital or acquired brain abnormalities (see Donders & Strong, 2015). In any case, Gardner's (1983) seminal book on multiple intelligences serves as an important reminder that IQ scores capture only a fraction of the many abilities that govern a person's performance in the real world. Other caveats regarding measures of general intelligence are that 1) crystallized and verbal knowledge measures are affected by the home and school environment, 2) IQ scores are unstable in young children and are not necessarily predictive of later performance on intelligence tests, and 3) the causes of poor performance have been oversimplified. For example, Wechsler Processing Speed Index scores are heavily reliant on fast processing but also on fast motor output, a demand that is not recognized by their name.

Table 13.1 Common neurocognitive domains and associated neurodevelopmental disorders

Domain	Examples of associated neurodevelopmental disorders	Examples of key data sources
General intelligence	Intellectual disability	Standardized IQ tests
Attention	Attention-deficit disorder Emotional disorders (anxiety, depression, trauma) Traumatic brain injury Epilepsy	Parent and teacher rating scales and qualitative report Observations during assessment Standardized tests
Executive function	Attention-deficit disorder Autism Reading disability Prematurity Nonverbal learning disability Traumatic brain injury	Parent and teacher rating scales and qualitative report Observations during assessment Standardized tests
Language	Language-based learning disabilities (reading, writing) Developmental language disorders Autism Hearing impairment	Observations during assessment Standardized tests School work Qualitative parent and teacher report
Visual perceptual	Nonverbal learning disability Prematurity Visual impairment	Standardized tests Observations during assessment
Learning/memory	Autism Attention-deficit disorder Learning disabilities Developmental language disorders Nonverbal learning disability Traumatic brain injury Intellectual disability Epilepsy	Standardized tests Observations during assessment Qualitative parent and teacher report
Social cognition	Autism Nonverbal learning disability	Parent and teacher rating scales and qualitative report Structured interview observations Standardized tasks
Motor/sensory	Cerebral palsy Attention-deficit/hyperactivity disorder Autism Nonverbal learning disability	Standardized tests Observations during assessment Work samples
Emotional adjustment	Depression Anxiety disorder Trauma Adjustment problems Bipolar disorder Attention-deficit disorder Medical disorders	Parent and teacher rating scales and qualitative report Observations and self-report during assessment Projective measures
Adaptive/academic	All	Parent and teacher qualitative report and report on standardized adaptive behavior interviews Standardized academic tests/tasks Work samples

The Wechsler Arithmetic subtest requires listening to a word problem and then performing arithmetic operations without paper to produce an answer. As a result, the task includes auditory processing (listening to the question), verbal processing (identifying the quantities and operations required), working memory (maintaining the key elements in working memory and performing operations on them), and exposure to arithmetic.

Attention

Attention is closely associated with, and sometimes even subsumed under, executive function. Common subdomains within the concept of attention include orienting, focusing, shifting, and sustaining attention. Attention relies on complex distributed networks in the brain (Mesulam, 2000; Posner, 2016). Attention is affected by a diverse array of factors including anxiety, arousal (most sleepy people are inattentive), difficulty of the task (e.g., dyslexic children are inattentive specifically on reading-related tasks), motivation (e.g., interest level in the material), and the novelty, as well as the type, of the situation. A finding of impaired attention should be based on data showing difficulty paying attention in several different contexts (home and school), on a variety of tasks, and in the absence of other interfering mental states.

Executive Function

Executive function is an umbrella term that captures a set of cognitive abilities that governs behavior regulation and goal-oriented activity. These cognitive processes include working memory, inhibition, flexibility, monitoring, planning, and generativity (Rogers & Bennetto, 2000). Executive functions rely on complex interconnected brain networks emphasizing frontal and subcortical nodes (Hunter et al., 2012; Stuss & Benson, 1984). Executive functions are notoriously difficult to capture in the standard test-based assessment, as the assessments are usually conducted in a quiet room with one highly supportive adult examiner prompting performance. In this structured environment, the examiner 1) provides the plan, 2) organizes the activities, 3) gives explicit instructions and cues regarding performance, 4) probes for elaboration, 5) presents tasks one at a time, and 6) generally supports executive control (Gioia, Isquith, Guy, & Kenworthy, 2015). Such support makes it difficult to reveal deficits in this area and, in fact, is the approach a teacher takes to assist a child with executive function deficits. Therefore, intact performance on an executive function test should not be considered adequate evidence of intact executive function. Often some subdomains of executive function are intact while others are impaired in a child with a neurodevelopmental disability. By school age, delineation of performance in specific subdomains (e.g., inhibition/impulse control versus planning or self-monitoring) is informative for targeting specific interventions (e.g., interventions to support and improve weak working memory are quite different than those targeting impulse control or flexibility; see Case Study, Part 6).

CASE STUDY, PART 6

John, like many children with high-functioning ASD, had specific executive function deficits affecting his ability to organize, integrate, and plan using complex information or multistep tasks, which affected his ability to write essays at school. He required targeted interventions to help him learn to use a specific writing rubric that provided familiarity and structure to this otherwise open-ended, overwhelming task. John also struggled with cognitive inflexibility and needed to learn routines and scripts to help him be more flexible. On the other hand, John's ability to manipulate numbers in working memory was remarkable, and he generally had adequate impulse control.

Language

This domain addresses the ability to understand language, use language to express needs and wants, establish social relationships, and make the sounds of speech (see Chapter 17). Often subsumed under the language domain are a full range of communicative abilities, including motor speech capacities and pragmatic nonverbal communications such as gestures. At its core, the language domain involves the phonological, semantic, syntactic, and formulation abilities that enable us to distinguish and combine sounds, build a vocabulary, and combine words into sentences and longer utterances. Language abilities rely heavily on frontotemporal brain networks, typically in the left hemisphere (Bear & Connors, 2016). Language skills are often divided between receptive or comprehension abilities and expressive abilities, which can be divergent. Although most neurocognitive evaluations screen basic language abilities and can be helpful in differentiating the unique contributions of attention, executive function, social cognition, and language difficulties to a problem in the child's functioning, a significant concern regarding language abilities typically also merits a full speech and language assessment (see Case Study, Part 7).

CASE STUDY, PART 7

John's basic language abilities related to phonology, semantics, and syntax were very strong and supported fluent reading, decoding, excellent vocabulary, and a sophisticated use and understanding of words and sentence syntax. His communication deteriorated, however, as executive demands to organize and integrate information into paragraphs or as pragmatic language demands to use gestures and eye contact increased. Finally, inflexibility drove him to be overly precise in his use of language and interfered with his ability to maintain a conversation about topics that were not intrinsically interesting to him.

Visual Processing

The brain supports a variety of visual processing abilities, including perception and spatial location. Right hemisphere posterior brain structures are frequently involved, although the neural underpinnings of visual processing are complex (see Baron, 2004, for review). Visual processing is closely associated with visual construction skills, which also require motor output; perception of visual gestalts; and visual pattern recognition, often associated with visual reasoning. All of these skills rely on intact or corrected vision. Isolated deficits in this domain are not common in neurodevelopmental disabilities, and it is important to recognize that a significantly lower Wechsler Performance IQ score than Verbal IQ score cannot be interpreted in isolation to indicate a perceptual deficit (see Case Study, Part 8). Such a discrepancy can result from many different conditions, including executive dysfunction and highly enriched verbal teaching at home and at school. A true deficit in this domain should be confirmed with performance data other than IQ scores, such as scores on tests of visual learning and memory.

CASE STUDY, PART 8

John's IQ scores showed a significant discrepancy between very superior Verbal IQ and average Performance IQ. Yet, he is a gifted math student and has strong visual learning abilities. Observation of John's approach to the tasks that constitute the Performance IQ revealed that his inflexibility and tendency to focus on details slowed his performance and reduced his score, implicating executive dysfunction, not a perceptual deficit.

Learning and Memory

Although true memory impairments are relatively rare in children with neurodevelopmental disabilities, learning deficits are common. Learning can be impaired for visual or verbal information in the context of core deficits in language or visual processing. Executive dysfunction also typically interferes with effective information retrieval in response to open-ended queries (e.g., "How was your day?") and with learning large amounts of information but not with information retrieval in structured conditions (e.g., multiple choice) or when learning simpler data. A neuropsychological evaluation should provide specific insights into how a child learns best and in which learning conditions the child will require extra support (e.g., only during lectures, written responses, or independent reading). Optimizing learning is a key intervention for all children since their major academic task is to learn new information (see Case Study, Part 9).

CASE STUDY, PART 9

In John's case, it was useful to delineate the difference between his prodigious learning and memory abilities for small chunks of information such as words, facts, and mathematic operations and his much greater difficulty with learning and retrieving large chunks of information from memory. In the assessment, he struggled with learning and remembering a large, complex abstract figure; in his daily life, he struggled to learn from his experiences.

Social Cognition

Social perception and cognition rely on fronto-temporal brain networks that support a person's ability to perceive social stimuli such as faces, facial expressions, voice intonation, and body language. The brain also "reasons" using social information, such as understanding human relationships and having a theory of mind; this social reasoning ability is commonly referred to as social cognition (for reviews, see Frith & Frith, 2010). However, our ability to measure social cognition with standardized tools is still quite limited. With the exception of basic social perception tasks (such as learning and remembering faces and recognizing facial expressions), measuring social cognition largely relies on parent and teacher report, observation, and responses in structured interviews. For planning successful interventions, it is essential to have an understanding of whether a child with a neurodevelopmental disability can accurately perceive and express social cues, have a theory of mind, and reason with social information.

Motor/Sensory

The motor and sensory domains encompass a broad range of gross and fine motor abilities as well as sensory perception. Standardized motor tasks eliciting speed, strength, and dexterity, such as quickly placing pegs in a board, tracing a curvy line, or imitating a gait or hand movement, can provide information about the subtle motor impairments often seen in neurodevelopmental disabilities. These impairments can profoundly affect a child's ability to produce written work at school, to carry out key activities of daily living, or to simply sit up straight in his or her chair. A complex or pervasive motor difficulty often merits a physical or occupational therapy evaluation. Sensory information regarding visual, auditory, and tactile perception can also be collected with standardized assessments and can be particularly important for children with focal brain damage. Oversensitivity and undersensitivity to sensory stimuli are included in the diagnostic criteria for autism (American Psychiatric Association, 2013) and are best assessed by observation and parent or teacher report.

Emotional Adjustment

Emotional adjustment should be evaluated in any comprehensive assessment because it has a major impact on a child's overall functioning level, the intervention plan, and specific neurocognitive functions. Mood, anxiety, and any other emotional difficulties interfering with a child's functioning and ability to regulate mood and behavior should all be assessed. These data may inform diagnosis of comorbid psychiatric disorders. They may also indicate alternative explanations for cognitive impairments. For example, working memory can be impaired by anxiety (Ferreri, Lapp & Peretti, 2011); depression slows down motor response and generally impairs performance on tasks requiring cognitive effort (Buyukdura, McClintock, & Croarkin, 2011); and even hallucinations occur in a small number of children, which certainly interfere with attention (Castaneda et al., 2008). Parent, teacher, and child reports on standardized measures, as well as a qualitative report of symptoms and concerns, are useful. In addition to an interview with the child, which can be play based for younger children, the child's response to projective measures is often informative. Projective measures present incomplete or ambiguous stimuli (such as drawings, sentence beginnings, or inkblots) and are designed to elicit information about the child's internal state.

Adaptive/Academic

Adaptive and academic skills are best thought of as outcomes of the pattern of strengths and weaknesses in a child's core cognitive domains, combined with the full range of contextual factors described above. They reflect how successfully the child is coping with the demands of daily living (e.g., showing age-appropriate toileting, dressing, grooming, communication, and social skills) and accumulating academic knowledge and skills.

ENSURING THAT ASSESSMENT INFORMS MANAGEMENT

Useful Assessments Are Driven by Appropriate Referral Questions

Neuropsychological assessment can answer or provide input on a wide range of questions, but there are at least as many questions that it cannot, or should not, answer. A comprehensive neuropsychological assessment can often provide input in the following areas: 1) diagnostic clarification, 2) the child's level of developmental or cognitive functioning, 3) patterns of strengths and weaknesses, 4) school placement or program eligibility determinations, 5) progress or deterioration over time, 6) forensic issues, and 7) suggestions for treatment. Assessment can rarely definitively answer questions such as "What caused this to happen?"

A good referral request asks a clear, answerable question. Some examples of appropriate questions would be whether a child has ASD, whether a child's difficulties are due to language or attention problems, or whether a child is receiving appropriate services and making the expected level of progress. Providing the evaluator with information about the strengths and weaknesses of the child, the family system, and the current educational plan will increase the utility of the assessment. Specifying which exact tests should be given is not useful. There may be very good reasons for not giving a certain test, such as any of the threats to validity described below.

An Understanding of the Purpose and Limits of Psychometric Data Informs Effective Use of Assessment Results

When selected, administered, and scored appropriately, standardized test instruments provide important normative benchmarks against which to compare performance. They complement nonstandardized data and provide key information about how a child's abilities compare with same-age typically developing children. One study (Meyer et al., 2001) compared psychological tests with medical tests like magnetic resonance imaging, Pap smears, and electrocardiograms and found that psychological tests generally predict outcomes just as well as medical tests do.

The term *psychometrics* refers to the branch of psychology addressing the design, administration, and interpretation of quantitative (numerical) tests that measure psychological factors such as intelligence, aptitude, and personality traits (Upton & Cook, 2008). Psychometric approaches have proven to be extraordinarily useful over time but have been criticized for being overly reductionistic (tending to oversimplify complex phenomena by breaking them down into constituent parts). Because of the inherent limitations of the psychometric approach, professionals are often required to meet standards for training and experience in order to be able to purchase psychological tests and to be licensed to administer and interpret those tests (American Educational Research Association, American Psychological Association, National Council of Measurements in Education, & Joint Committee on Standards for Educational and Psychological Testing, 2014). This sets a very high standard for the appropriate interpretation of any test score and should caution unqualified people against attempting to interpret scores.

Psychometric measures should be interpreted with caution for many reasons. Psychometrics do not model the neural substrate (e.g., a test score does not map neatly onto brain regions or functions) or place behavior in context. Further, psychological tests are rarely pure (e.g., they do not measure only the domain they are supposed to measure), are not completely objective (e.g., variability in examiners or cultural factors can have a significant impact on scores), and are not always reliable and even less often valid. The results of any psychometric measure are only as good as the measure itself. The largest factors that contribute to score accuracy include 1) the use of standardized procedures; 2) the reliability of the test; 3) the validity of the test; and 4) the quality, size, recency, and diversity of the normative sample. Described below are some of the most important psychometric factors a neuropsychologist considers.

What Does It Mean for a Test to Be Standardized? A test is standardized if 1) it has exact procedures for administration, including the qualifications of the administrator; 2) it has instructions and questions that must be repeated in exactly the same way every time (i.e., the administrator must "stick to the script"), 3) the exact same materials are used every time; and 4) rules for scoring are specifically defined and are not subjective (Sattler, 2018).

What Does It Mean for a Test to Be Reliable? Reliability is a measure of how consistent a score is over time (test-retest reliability), between examiners (interrater reliability), across different forms of the test (alternate forms reliability), and within the items of the test (internal consistency). Reliability can be affected by the length of the test, variability in the normative sample, the difficulty range of the items (it is important that items are neither too difficult nor too easy), and how well the administration and scoring procedures are described.

Reliable change refers to the extent to which the change in an individual's scores fall beyond the range that could be attributed to the measurement variability of the instrument or the effects of practice. Many new standardized assessment tools often provide Reliable Change Index scores.

What Does It Mean for a Test to Be Valid (and What About Bilingualism, Culture, Race, Ethnicity, and Income Levels)? A test is valid if it accurately measures what it is supposed to measure. A well-standardized test has undergone many different types of checks for validity under controlled situations. However, most tests are used outside of these controlled situations, and therefore the evaluator should tell the reader of the report how valid he or she believes a child's assessment to be and how predictive the assessment is likely to be of that child's functioning. For instance, most individually administered tests (such as IQ tests) are not valid if repeated within 6–12 months because practicing the tasks improves performance on those tasks. Child-specific factors can also reduce the validity of a test result. Was the child hungry, tired, ill, or distracted? Was the child taking any medication that could affect results? Cultural factors should always be considered as a potential threat to validity; a test's questions may contain content and assume knowledge that are foreign to the child's environment. For example, a child from Taiwan may not be able to correctly categorize the fruits we typically eat in the United States. Poor performance in this case relates to the child's culture, not to her categorization or abstract thinking ability. But we also know that no test is without biases, which may be more subtle and may disproportionally identify children from "nondominant" cultures for some categories of special education services or contribute to the underidentification of children for gifted services (Voulgarides, Fergus, & Thorius, 2017). In the United States this is a particular problem with testing of African American and Hispanic populations and contributes to educational disparities (see Chapter 42).

Sometimes a certain child will need accommodations during testing or will need to be given special tests, and the report should acknowledge these factors and how they affect validity. A child with cerebral palsy (CP) or other physical disabilities may need to be given motor-free tests, and even verbal tests should not be timed. When a child with a language disorder is assessed in other domains, nonverbal tests should be given (such as the Leiter or the Comprehensive Test of Non-Verbal Intelligence). A child who speaks a different language should either receive culturally appropriate nonverbal tests or a test that has been carefully translated, adapted, and standardized in the child's native language and culture; bilingual children should receive some testing in both of their languages (Sanchez et al., 2013). Some testing accommodations are less dramatic, such as allowing the child to stand or move around the room, instituting reward systems, and breaking the testing up into several sessions. But these accommodations should be noted in the report, as the validity of the findings may be tied to them. This can also be helpful in alerting teachers and parents to specific accommodations that are likely to improve performance at home and at school.

The validity of tests can also be challenged by intentional efforts on the part of the person being assessed to make mistakes or "malinger." A formal assessment of effort, using embedded or standalone "symptom validity" tests, is an important component of evidence-based practice in neuropsychological assessment (Greve, Durtis, & Bianchini, 2013). Effort testing should be included in most assessments. Performance on these tasks should be noted in a section of the neuropsychological report that addresses the validity of the assessment.

Why Is It Important for a Test to Be Norm-Referenced? A test is norm-referenced if it has been given to a large number of people (the sample) who are representative of the population of interest. An individual child's performance is measured against the performance of all children of the same age in the normative sample in order to generate a standard score. The larger and more diverse the normative sample is, the more useful this standard score is. Cultural, linguistic, and physical factors that the child does not share with the normative sample will reduce its utility. The normative sample also must be recent, as children's scores in the population change over time. For example, cognitive intelligence scores have been shown to increase by about three standard score points per decade (Trahan, Stuebing, Hiscock, & Fletcher, 2014).

What Is a Standardized Score? Standardized scores are statistically derived from the normative sample during test development. All standardized scores assume that the scores range according to a normal distribution (see Figure 13.2). There are several types of standardized scores. Test scores can be expressed as follows:

1. *Age or grade equivalents.* Performance is typical of a specific age group or grade level in the normative sample. While age and grade equivalents are the most intuitive of the standardized scores and are the most easily understood by parents and teachers, they should not be used for making diagnostic or placement decisions because of their low reliability and validity (American Educational Research Association et al., 2014).

2. *Percentiles.* This ranks the child's relative position in the normative sample. For example, a child's score at the 80th percentile means that the child performed better than 80% of children in the sample.

3. *Deviation scores.* The child's performance is assessed in relation to the distance from the mean in terms of standard deviations (SD). The SD of a score is a

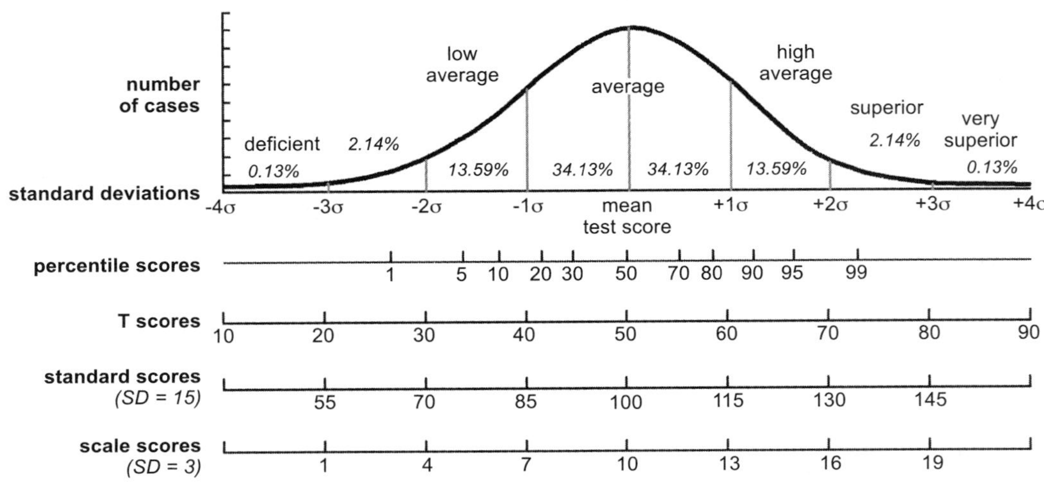

Figure 13.2. The normal curve.

measure of how much variability there is in scores in terms of distance from the mean (average). Standard scores, scale scores, *t*-scores, and *z*-scores are all deviation scores. Standard scores typically have a mean of 100 and an SD of 15. Scale scores typically have a mean of 10 and an SD of 3. *T*-scores have a mean of 50 and an SD of 10, and *z*-scores have a mean of 0 and an SD of 1.

Most children (about 68%) obtain scores within 1 SD of the mean. These scores are considered "average." The further a score is away from the mean, the fewer children obtain that score. Figure 13.2 represents what is commonly referred to as the "Bell curve" or the normal distribution of scores in a group of individuals. The area under the curve represents the number of children obtaining that score. If Figure 13.2 represents a total of 1,000 children, then 680 children would obtain scores in the area of the curve representing the "average range." However, only one child would obtain a score in the small area under the curve in the "very superior range," which is the area of the curve 4 SDs above the mean. The general labels used to describe scores are depicted in Figure 13.2, but each test may also use its own descriptive labels depending on what the test is measuring. For example, a child who scores very low on an anxiety measure, such as a *t*-score of 20, is not said to be "deficient" of anxiety symptoms. Instead, a *t*-score of 70 on the anxiety measure may be described as "clinically significant," meaning that the score indicates noteworthy anxiety symptoms.

Interpreting the clinical significance of variability between scores often requires more than simply understanding the standardized score itself. It is important to recognize, for example, that intra-individual variability in standardized scores on different tests is expected, especially in children (Schretlen & Sullivan, 2013). A good assessment takes into account expected variability and only reports "strengths" and "weaknesses" on tasks with scores that are more discrepant than is typical for that measure.

Effective Feedback and Dissemination of Findings

A meta-analysis (Poston & Hanson, 2010) showed that when psychological assessment and the sharing of assessment results is done in a collaborative fashion with the child and his/her family and the feedback is offered in a sensitive, clinically meaningful manner, the assessment process itself functions as a therapeutic intervention. Effective communication of assessment results is essential for optimizing the power of an assessment as an intervention tool. When a child is referred for a medical specialist's consultation, the professional making the referral wants the specialist's interpretation and integration of information to answer the referral question and to suggest avenues of treatment, if needed. The same is true of referrals for neuropsychological assessments. Presentation of cognitive strengths and weaknesses, appropriate diagnoses, primary risks, and recommendations should all be communicated in a collaborative conversation and in language that both the referring professional and the parents can understand. One important way to make sure that test results are clear is to describe all test scores in a consistent, clearly explained manner. Increased standardization in the reporting of test data with standardized qualitative descriptors for normalized test scores (e.g., "average" or "superior") is an evidence-based practice (Schoenberg & Rum, 2017). Many reports describe test performance in multiple ways, which is needlessly confusing.

An assessment's value is determined by its usefulness and intelligibility to the family and education/treatment team of the child being assessed. Standards of care include offering in-person feedback regarding the findings of an evaluation, providing recommendations for an effective treatment plan, and writing a report that serves as a document that parents and referral sources can share with schools, members of the treatment team, and others who may intervene on behalf of the child. It is essential that the written report is completed in a timely manner and that the diagnostic formulation, impression, and recommendation sections of the report are clearly written and accessible to the reader, as these are the most commonly read portions of neuropsychological reports (Postal et al., 2018).

Often the most important intervention resulting from an assessment is simply to see the child's behavior in a new light. For example, a child who is described by his teacher as unmotivated can now be seen as a child with short-term memory problems, an attention disorder, or depression. This reframing of the problem can lead teachers, parents, and other adults to change their intervention strategies and to modify their interactions with and expectations of the child. This in turn can lead to a difference in how the child sees himself/herself. The first step in this reframing process is to confirm that the parents understand the assessment results. Follow-up questions regarding what was communicated during the assessment feedback session are important because misunderstandings are common. Provision of resources that will help the family move toward a greater understanding of their child's strengths, weaknesses, risks, needed interventions and accommodations, and prognosis may enable parents to be their child's best advocate.

Implementation of Recommendations

The next step is to make sure that a plan is in place so that all necessary recommendations can be implemented. This can be an overwhelming process for parents, particularly if their child needs multiple types of interventions and accommodations. It is important to help parents recognize that many assessments provide recommendations meant to be implemented over a period of several years. Prioritizing among recommendations and identifying key initial targets for intervention can be helpful. Referral sources often assist families in this process; they report that the diagnosis, impression, and recommendations sections of neuropsychological reports are especially valuable in supporting their efforts to help families (Postal et al., 2018). Very often, recommendations will call for changes in both school-based and home/outpatient-based services (see Case Study, Part 10).

CASE STUDY, PART 10

John's assessment report led to several significant changes. Perhaps most important, his parents and teachers became better able to distinguish his "can'ts" from his "won'ts." He was provided with some social coaching to help him read social cues and understand how his behavior can seem rude to others. An individualized education program (IEP) was established in school, which allowed him to use extra supports for writing assignments and provided specialized speech and language therapy targeting language pragmatic and formulation skills and special education services targeting executive functions and writing. In addition, he got help from a peer buddy on the playground to ensure inclusion in games and activities. John's school services were supplemented by outpatient services in social skills training and anxiety reduction techniques by a skilled therapist. His parents also received coaching in how to organize John's day and to set up a comprehensive reward system.

School-Based Recommendations School-based services in private schools are up to the discretion of the school. Some private schools offer specialized services to students, but they are not required to do so and may charge an additional fee. There are three options for services in public schools: 1) informal supports and accommodations negotiated with the child's teacher or the student support team, 2) a 504 plan to provide formalized accommodations that will allow a student with a disability to access the general curriculum, or 3) an IEP to formulate specific and measurable goals. In order to make progress toward meeting those goals, formalized services must usually be provided to the student (e.g., special education or speech-language therapy), and those services may be provided in a mainstream classroom, resource room, special classroom, or special school depending on the student's needs. Every student has a right to an appropriate education in the least restrictive environment possible (see Chapter 33). School-based services are generally well coordinated across disciplines. The quality of school-based services varies widely, however, from county to county and sometimes even from one school to another within a county. Having an outside professional review the services a child is receiving and monitor the progress the child is making is helpful for many families. If the family needs extra help navigating the school-based meetings, they may want to hire an educational specialist/advocate, a professional who knows the laws and the local schools, or a special education attorney if the family is heading toward mediation or a due process hearing. The free-access web site http://www.wrightslaw.com has more information on advocating for special education services.

Home/Outpatient-Based Services Getting services through a disconnected service system, as most out-of-school systems are, requires active advocacy skills from parents. Parents often find themselves filling multiple roles, including case manager and treatment coordinator, as well as having to obtain insurance authorizations, schedule and transport their child, and act as a treatment provider at home. Many parents need help in the identification and coordination of treatment team members. All treatment providers and key school personnel should see the assessment report. Communication among team members is vital. If the child's needs are complicated, a short conference call is useful to make sure that everyone has the same information and that there is consistency across settings. Over time, it is useful to review recommendations and discuss suggestions that have not yet been tried or next steps to consider. Risk factors identified in the report should also be monitored. Too often, an evaluation is reviewed once and then ignored when in fact it contains data relevant to the treatment plan for a schoolchild for several years after the assessment. The final step of effective implementation of an assessment is following up at the appropriate time for recommended reevaluations.

SUMMARY

- The primary purpose of neuropsychological assessment is to educate the child, his or her family, and the treatment and educational team about the child's profile of cognitive strengths and weaknesses and emotional and behavioral functioning.

- This profile is used to identify where the child is at risk of difficulty and to develop a plan for making environmental accommodations or for teaching the child missing skills so that those risks can be mitigated.
- A successful model of neuropsychological assessment requires the integration of understanding brain structure and function, development, and context. Understanding the neural substrate available to a child at his or her stage of development, as well as the demands placed by the contexts the child inhabits, informs the description of the child's neuropsychological profile and treatment plan.
- The neuropsychological profile typically addresses multiple domains of functioning, including general intelligence, attention, executive, language, visual, learning and memory, social cognition, sensory, motor, emotional, adaptive, and academic performance.
- Appropriate referral questions, followed by thorough assessment and effective dissemination of findings and recommendations to families and treatment teams, maximizes the impact of neuropsychological assessment on children's lives.

ADDITIONAL RESOURCES

American Psychological Association: http://www.apa.org/topics/testing/index.aspx

National Council on Measurement in Education: http://www.ncme.org

The Standards for Educational and Psychological Testing: http://www.apa.org/science/programs/testing/standards.aspx

Additional resources can be found online in Appendix D: Childhood Disabilities Resources, Services, and Organizations (see About the Online Companion Materials).

REFERENCES

Achenbach, T. M., & Rescorla, L. A. (2001). *Manual for the ASEBA school-age forms & profiles*. Burlington, VT: University of Vermont.

Aman, M. G., & Singh, N. N. (1986). *Aberrant behavior checklist*. East Aurora, NY: Slosson Educational Publications.

American Educational Research Association, American Psychological Association, National Council of Measurement in Education & Joint Committee on Standards for Educational and Psychological Testing (2014). *Standards for educational and psychological testing*. Washington, DC: American Educational Research Association.

American Psychological Association. (2012). *Education and training guidelines: A taxonomy for education and training in professional psychology health service specialties*. Retrieved from http://www.apa.org/ed/graduate/specialize/taxonomy.pdf

American Psychiatric Association. (2013). *Diagnostic and statistical manual of mental disorders* (5th ed.). Washington, DC: Author.

Baron, I. (2004). *Neuropsychological evaluation of the child*. New York, NY: Oxford University Press.

Bayley, N. (2006). *Bayley Scales of Infant and Toddler Development: Technical manual*. San Antonio, TX: Harcourt Brace and Company.

Bear, M. F., & Connors, B. W. (2016). *Neuroscience: Exploring the brain* (4th ed.). Philadelphia PA: Wolters Kluwer.

Beery, K. E., & Beery, N. A. (2004). *The Beery-Buktenica Developmental Test of Visual-Motor Integration, Sixth Edition*. Minneapolis, MN: NCS Pearson.

Bernstein, J. (2000). Developmental neuropsychological assessment. In K. O. Yeates, M. D. Ris, & H. G. Taylor (Eds.), *Pediatric neuropsychology: Research, theory, and practice* (pp. 405–438). New York, NY: Guilford Press.

Bowers, L., Huisingh, R., & LoGiudice, C. (2005). *Test of Problem Solving 3: Elementary*. East Moline, IL: LinguiSystems.

Brandon, A. D., & Bennett, T. L. (1989). *Digital Finger Tapping Test*. Los Angeles, CA: Western Psychological Services.

Braun, M., Tupper, D., Kaufmann, P, McCrea, M., Postal, K., Westerveld, M., . . . Deer, T. (2011). Neuropsychological assessment: A valuable tool in the diagnosis and management of neurological, neurodevelopmental, medical, and psychiatric disorders. *Cognitive Behavioral Neurology, 24*, 107–114.

Briggs Gowan, M. J., & Carter, A. S. (2006). *ITSEA/BITSEA: Infant-Toddler and Brief Infant-Toddler Social and Emotional Assessment*. San Antonio, TX: The Psychological Corporation.

Burgess, P., Alderman, N., Forbes, C., Costello, A., Coates, L., Dawson, D., . . . Channon, S. (2006). The case for the development and use of 'ecologically valid' measures of executive function in experimental and clinical neuropsychology. *Journal of the International Neuropsychological Society, 12*(2), 194–209. doi:10.1017/S1355617706060310

Buyukdura, J. S., McClintock, S. M., & Croarkin, P. E. (2011). Psychomotor retardation in depression: Biological underpinnings, measurement, and treatment, *Progress in Neuro-Psychopharmacology & Biological Psychiatry, 35*(2), 395–409. doi:10.1016/j.pnpbp.2010.10.019

Castaneda, A., Tuulio-Henriksson, A., Marttunen, M., Suvisaari, J., & Lönnqvist, J. (2008). A review on cognitive impairments in depressive and anxiety disorders with a focus on young adults. *Journal of Affective Disorders, 106*(1–2), 1–27. doi:10.1016/j.jad.2007.06.006

Conners, C. K. (2008). *Conners' Continuous Performance Test* (3rd ed.). North Tonawanda, NY: Multi-Health Systems.

Conners, C. K., & MHS Staff. (2004). *Conners' Continuous Performance Test (CPT II)*. North Tonawanda, NY: Multi-Health Systems.

Constantino, J. N., & Gruber, C. P. (2012). *Social Responsiveness Scale, Second Edition (SRS-2)*. Torrance, CA: Western Psychological Services.

Delis, D. C., Kramer, J. H., Kaplan, E., & Ober, B. A. (1994). *California Verbal Learning Test—Children's Version*. San Antonio, TX: Harcourt Brace and Company.

Donders, J., & Strong, C. A. H. (2015). Clinical utility of the Wechsler Adult Intelligence Scale-Fourth Edition after traumatic brain injury. *Assessment, 22*(1), 17–22. doi:10.1177/1073191114530776

Elliott, C. D. (2007). *Differential Ability Scales-Second Edition, administration & scoring manual*. San Antonio, TX: PsychCorp.

Ferreri, F., Lapp, L. K., & Peretti, C. S. (2011). Current research on cognitive aspects of anxiety disorders. *Current Opinion in Psychiatry, 24*(1), 49–54.

Folio, M. R., & Fewell, R. R. (2000). *Peabody Developmental Motor Scales—Second Edition*. Austin, TX: PRO-ED.

Frith, U., & Frith, C. D. (2010). The social brain: Allowing humans to boldly go where no other species has been. *Philosophical Transactions of the Royal Society B: Biological Sciences, 365*(1537), 165–176.

Gardner, H. (1983). *Frames of mind: The theory of multiple intelligences*. New York, NY: Basic Books.

Gioia, G. A., & Isquith, P. K. (2004). Ecological assessment of executive function in traumatic brain injury. *Developmental Neuropsychology, 25*(1), 135–158. doi:10.1207/s15326942dn2501&2_8

Gioia, G. A., Isquith, P. K., Guy, S. C., & Kenworthy, L. (2000). *Behavior Rating Inventory of Executive Function, Second Edition*. Lutz, FL: PAR.

Gioia, G. A., Isquith, P. K., Guy, S. C., & Kenworthy, L. (2015). *Behavior Rating Inventory of Executive Function, Second Edition (BRIEF-2)*. Odessa, FL: Psychological Assessment Resources.

Goldman, R., & Fristoe, M. (2015). *Goldman-Fristoe Test of Articulation, Third Edition (GFTA-3)*. Circle Pines, MN: American Guidance Service, Inc.

Greve, K. W., Durtis, K. L., & Bianchini, K. J. (2013). Symptom validity testing: A summary of recent research. *Neuropsychology science and practice I* (pp. 61–94). New York, NY: Oxford University Press.

Hammill, D. D., Pearson, N. A., & Wiederholt, J. L. (2009). *Comprehensive Test of Nonverbal Intelligence—Second Edition*. Austin, TX: PRO-ED.

Hardy, K. K., Olson, K., Cox, S. M., Kennedy, T., & Walsh, K. S. (2017). Systematic review: A prevention-based model of neuropsychological assessment for children with medical illness. *Journal of Pediatric Psychology, 42*(8), 815–882. doi:10.1093/jpepsy/jsx060

Harrison, P. L., & Oakland, T. (2015). *Adaptive Behavior Assessment System, Third Edition manual*. Torrance, CA: Western Psychological Services.

Heaton, R. K., Chelune, G. J., Talley, J. L., Kay, J. H., & Curtiss, G. (1993). *Wisconsin Card Sorting Test Manual*. Odessa, FL: Psychological Assessment Resources.

Hinshaw, S. P., Arnold, L. E., & MTA Cooperative Group. (2015). Attention-deficit hyperactivity disorder, multimodal treatment, and longitudinal outcome: evidence, paradox, and challenge. *WIREs Cognitive Science, 6*, 39–52. doi:10.1002/wcs.1324

Hunter, S. J., Hinkle, C. D., & Edidin, J. P. (2012). The neurobiology of executive functions. In S. J. Hunter & E. P. Sparrow (Eds.), *Executive function and dysfunction* (pp. 37–64). New York, NY: Cambridge University Press.

Kaufman, D. A. S., Boxer, O., and Bilder, R. M. (2013). Evidence-based science and practice in neuropsychology: A review. In S. Koffler, J. Morgan, I. S. Baron, & M.F. Greiffenstein (Eds.), *Neuropsychology science and practice I* (pp. 1–38). New York, NY: Oxford University Press.

Kenworthy, L., Anthony, L. G., Alexander, K. C., Werner, M. A., Cannon, L., & Greenman, L. (2014). *Solving executive functioning challenges: Simple ways to get kids with autism unstuck and on target*. Baltimore, MD: Brookes Publishing Co.

Kenworthy, L., Yerys, B., Anthony, L., & Wallace, G. (2008). Understanding executive control in autism spectrum disorders in the lab and in the real world. *Neuropsychology Review, 18*(4), 320–338. doi:10.1007/s11065-008-9077-7

Lord, C., Rutter, M., DiLavore, P. C., & Risi, S. (2012). *The Autism Diagnostic Observation Schedule, Second Edition (ADOS-2)*. Torrance, CA: Western Psychological Services.

Matarazzo, J. (1990). Psychological assessment versus psychological testing: Validation from Binet to the school, clinic, and courtroom. *American Psychologist, 45*(9), 999–1017. doi:10.1037/0003-066X.45.9.999

Mesulam, M. M. (2000). *Principles of behavioral and cognitive neurology*. New York, NY: Oxford University Press.

Meyer, G., Finn, S., Eyde, L., Kay, G., Moreland, K., Dies, R., . . . Reed, G. M. (2001). Psychological testing and psychological assessment: A review of evidence and issues. *American Psychologist, 56*(2), 128–165. doi:10.1037/0003-066X.56.2.128

Meyers, J. E., & Meyers, K. R. (1996). *Rey Complex Figure Test and Recognition Trial*. Odessa, FL: Psychological Assessment Resources.

Mullen, E. M. (1995). *Mullen Scales of Early Learning*. Circle Pines, MN: American Guidance Service.

Mundy, P. (2018). A review of joint attention and social-cognitive brain systems in typical development and autism spectrum disorder. *European Journal of Neuroscience, 47*(6), 497–514. doi:10.1111/ejn.13720

Mundy, P., & Newell, L. (2007). Attention, joint attention, and social cognition. *Current Directions in Psychological Science, 16*(5), 269–274. doi:10.1111/j.1467–8721.2007.00518.x

Piaget, J. (1952). *The origins of intelligence in children*. New York, NY: International Universities Press.

Posner, M. I. (2016). Orienting of attention: Then and now. *The Quarterly Journal of Experimental Psychology (Hove), 69*(10), 1864–1875. doi:10.1080/17470218.2014.937446

Postal, K., Chow, C., Jung, S., Erickson-Moreo, K., Geier, F., & Lanca, M. (2018). The stakeholders' project in neuropsychological report writing: A survey of neuropsychologists' and referral sources' views of neuropsychological reports, *The Clinical Neuropsychologist, 32*(3), 326–344. doi:10.1080/13854046.2017.1373859

Poston, J. M., & Hanson, W. E. (2010). Meta-analysis of psychological assessment as a therapeutic intervention. *Psychological Assessment, 22*(2), 203–212. doi:10.1037/a0018679

Reitan, R. M. (1979). *Halstead-Reitan Neuropsychological Test Battery*. Tucson, AZ: Reitan Neuropsychology Laboratory/Press.

Rogers, S. J., & Bennetto, L. (2000). Intersubjectivity in autism: The roles of imitation and executive function. In A. P. Wetherby & B. Prizant (Eds.), *Autism spectrum disorders: A transactional developmental perspective* (pp. 79–107). Baltimore, MD: Paul H. Brookes Publishing Co.

Roid, G. H., Miller, L. J., Pomplun, M., & Koch, C. (2013). *Leiter International Performance Scale, Third Edition*. Wood Dale, IL: Stoelting Co.

Rutter, M., Le Couteur, A., & Lord, C. (2003). *Autism Diagnostic Interview, Revised (ADI-R)*. Los Angeles, CA: Western Psychological Services.

Sanchez, S. V., Rodriguez, B. J., Soto-Huerta, M. E., Villarreal, F. C., Guerra, N. S., & Flores, B. B. (2013). A case for multidimensional bilingual assessment. *Language Assessment Quarterly, 10*(2), 160–177.

Sattler, J. M. (2018) *Assessment of Children: Cognitive Foundations and Applications, Sixth Edition*. La Mesa, CA: Jerome M. Sattler, Publisher, Inc.

Schoenberg, M. R., & Rum, R. S. (2017). Towards reporting standards for neuropsychological study results: A proposal to minimize communication errors with standardized qualitative descriptors for normalized test scores. *Clinical Neurology and Neurosurgery, 162,* 72–79.

Schrank, F. A., McGrew, K. S., & Mather, N. (2014). *Woodcock-Johnson IV.* Rolling Meadows, IL: Riverside Publishing Company.

Schretlen, D. J., & Sullivan, C. (2013). Intraindividual variability in cognitive test performance. In S. Koffler, J. Morgan, I. S. Baron, & M.F. Greiffenstein (Eds.), *Neuropsychology science and practice I* (pp. 39–60). New York, NY. Oxford University Press.

Sheslow, D., & Adams, W. (2003). *Wide Range Assessment of Memory and Learning, Second Edition.* Lutz, FL: PAR.

Sparrow, S., Cicchetti, D., & Saulnier, C. A. (2005). *Vineland Adaptive Behavior Scales, Third Edition: Manual.* Bloomington, MN: Pearson.

Stuss, D. T., & Benson, D. F. (1984). Neuropsychological studies of the frontal lobes. *Psychological Bulletin, 95*(1), 3–28. doi:10.1037/0033-2909.95.1.3

Trahan, L., Stuebing, K. K., Hiscock, M. K., & Fletcher, J. M. (2014). The Flynn effect: A meta-analysis. *Psychological Bulletin, 140*(5), 1332–1360. http://doi.org/10.1037/a0037173

Upton, G., & Cook, I. (2008). *A dictionary of statistics* (2nd ed.) New York, NY: Oxford University Press.

Voulgarides, C. K., Fergus, E., & Thorius, K. A. K. (2017). Pursuing equity: Disproportionality in special education and the reframing of technical solutions to address systemic inequities. *Review of Research in Education, 41,* 61–87. doi:10.3102/0091732X16686947

Wechsler, D. (2008). *Wechsler Adult Intelligence Scale–Fourth Edition.* San Antonio, TX: Pearson.

Wechsler, D. (2011). *Wechsler Abbreviated Scale of Intelligence, Second Edition.* Bloomington, MN: Pearson.

Wechsler, D. (2014). *Wechsler Intelligence Scale for Children—Fifth Edition: Technical and interpretive manual.* Bloomington, MN: Pearson.

Wiig, E., Semel, E., & Secord, W. A. (2013). *Clinical evaluation of language fundamentals* (5th ed.). Bloomington, MN: Pearson.

Wilkinson, G. S., & Robertson, G. J. (2006). *Wide Range Achievement Test 4 (WRAT4).* Lutz, FL: PAR.

Wolraich, M. L., & DuPaul, G. J. (2010). *ADHD diagnosis and management: A practical guide for the clinic and the classroom.* Baltimore, MD: Paul H. Brookes Publishing Co.

Youngstrom, E. A. (2013). Future directions in psychological assessment: Combining evidence based medicine innovations with psychology's historical strengths to enhance utility. *Journal of Clinical Child & Adolescent Psychology, 42,* 139–159.

Youngstrom, E., LaKind, J. S., Kenworthy, L., Lipkin, P. H., Goodman, M., Squibb, K., . . . Anthony, L. G. (2010). Advancing the selection of neurodevelopmental measures in epidemiological studies of environmental chemical exposure and health effects. *International Journal of Environmental Research and Public Health, 7,* 229–268.

Zimmerman, I. L., Steiner, V. G., & Pond, R. E. (2011). *Preschool Language Scale, Fifth Edition.* San Antonio, TX: Harcourt Brace Jovanovich.

Appendix 13.1 Examples of Widely Used Neurodevelopmental Measures Organized by Functional Domain

Measure	Scale name	Age range	Admin. time	Advantages	Disadvantages	References
General intelligence						
Bayley Scales of Infant Development, Third Edition (Bayley-III)	Adaptive behavior, cognitive, language composite, motor composite	1–42 months	50–90 min.	One of the only instruments available in the age range, recently restandardized, extended floors and ceilings, improved evidence of reliability and validity	Difficult to administer and confounded by significant language demands	Bayley (2006)
Mullen Scales of Early Learning (AGS Edition)	Early learning composite Gross motor; visual reception; fine motor; receptive language; expressive language	Birth–68 months	~15 min. (for 1 year olds) to 60 min. (for 5 year olds)	Limited language demands	Old normative data	Mullen (1995)
Wechsler Intelligence Scales for Children—Fifth Edition (WISC-V)	Full scale, verbal comprehension, visual spatial, working memory, fluid reasoning, processing speed	6–16 years	60–90 min.	Most widely used test of cognitive ability in children and adolescents; excellent norms; familiar; stronger measurement of working memory than previous	Not tied to strong theory of intelligence; relatively weak assessment of processing speed	Wechsler (2014)
Wechsler Adult Intelligence Scales (WAIS-IV)	Full scale, verbal comprehension, perceptual reasoning, working memory, processing speed, general ability	16–90 years	60–90 min.	Reliable, good norms, commonly administered	Not tied to strong theory of intelligence; relatively weak assessment of processing speed and working memory	Wechsler (2008)
Wechsler Abbreviated Scale of Intelligence (WASI-II)	Full scale, verbal comprehension, perceptual reasoning	6–90 years	30 min.	Validated as a brief measure of verbal, nonverbal, and general cognitive ability; very precise scores; Matrix Reasoning can be administered nonverbally	No coverage of processing speed, working memory, or other aspects of cognitive ability	Wechsler (2011)
Comprehensive Test of Nonverbal Intelligence (CTONI-2)	Pictorial analogies, geometric analogies, pictorial categories, geometric categories, pictorial sequences, geometric sequences	6 years–89 years, 11 months	60 min.	Minimizes cultural bias, good for children with language disorders	Less predictive of some aspects of functioning than verbally loaded scales	Hammill, Pearson, and Wiederholt (2009)
Leiter International Performance Scale, Third Edition	Cognitive; attention & memory	3–75 years	20–45 min.	Covers wide age range; minimal bias across cultures; strong theoretical model guiding revision	Special training may be needed for good standardization, though the reduction from 20 subtests to 10 subtests in the third edition helps.	Roid, Miller, Pomplun, and Koch (2013)
Differential Abilities Scale–II (DAS-II)	General Cognitive Ability, Verbal Ability, Nonverbal Ability, Spatial Ability	2.5 years–17 years, 11 months	60 min.	Good norms, conceptual model, strong psychometrics, nonverbal subtests can be administered without language	No working memory or processing speed	Elliott (2007)

Attention						
Conners' Continuous Performance Test (3rd ed.)	Total score (also a short form, a *DSM* form, and a global form)	6–18 years	5–20 min.	Parent, teacher, and youth forms; includes *DSM-IV* content; extensive research base; includes validity scales	Cumbersome to score without computer software; short forms validated in embedded version (not separate administration)	Conners (2008)
Continuous Performance Test–II (CPT)	Sustained attention, omissions, commissions, variability, standard error	3+ years	15–20 min.	Standardized task that measures multiple performance facets of attention	Relatively small number of minorities included in the norm sample; overall mild correlations between CPT and ADHD rating scales	Conners and MHS Staff (2004)
Executive functioning						
Behavior Rating Inventory of Executive Functioning (BRIEF-2)	Global executive composite	5–18 years	10–15 min.	Parent and teacher forms; inexpensive; collateral source of information about executive functioning Comprehensive coverage of subdomains of executive functioning; ecologically valid measure; used extensively in research with good sensitivity; easy to administer and complete	Informant ratings are susceptible to bias; report of everyday executive function does not necessarily accurately parse subdomains of executive function.	Gioia, Isquith, Guy, and Kenworthy (2000)
Rey Complex Figure Test	Copy strategy	6–89 years	45 min., including 30-min. delayed interval	New manual (1996) improves scoring criteria and guidelines, as well as norms Developmental scoring norms capture problem-solving strategy (as opposed to outcome score), which is a key correlate of executive functions that is often not addressed	Wide developmental variation and limited normative sample compromise sensitivity Scoring system is complex and prone to error; requires specific training for adequate accuracy	Meyers and Meyers (1996)
Wisconsin Card Sorting Test (WCST)	Perseverative errors	6.5 years–89 years, 11 months	20–30 min.	Relevant construct for neurotoxicity	Difficult to reliably score if not using computer administration; not representative norms; complex relationship between scales and executive function	Heaton, Chelune, Talley, Kay, and Curtiss (1993)
Language						
Goldman-Fristoe Test of Articulation-3	Sounds in words, sounds in sentences, stimulability	2–21 years	15 min.	Strong standardization sample; good norm-referenced scores	Technical information based on administrations by speech pathologists; unclear how results would vary with less trained raters; use with caution with speakers of nonstandard English	Goldman and Fristoe (2015)

(*continued*)

Appendix 13.1 *(continued)*

Measure	Scale name	Age range	Admin. time	Advantages	Disadvantages	References
Preschool Language Scale, Fifth Edition (PLS)	Auditory comprehension, expressive communication	Birth–7 years, 11 months	45–60 min.	Spanish version available, with dual-language administration and scoring Spanish norms developed with both monolingual and bilingual children	Potential for variability in administration and scoring means that a high degree of training is needed for consistency	Zimmerman, Steiner, and Pond (2011)
Clinical Evaluation of Language Fundamentals (Fifth Edition) (CELF-5)	Core language, receptive language, expressive language, language content, language memory, pragmatics	5–21 years (preschool version also available)	30–45 min.	Easy to learn; computer-assisted scoring; focuses on specific skills and areas of functioning (versus achievement) Telepractice option available (Q-Global)		Wiig, Semel, and Secord (2013)
California Verbal Learning Test, Children's Version (CVLT-C)	Verbal learning, memory	5–16 years	15–20 min.	Widely used test of verbal learning and memory, short, measures recognition and recall		Delis, Kramer, Kaplan, and Ober (1994)
Test of Problem Solving Child and Adolescent (TOPS 3 Elementary)	Pragmatic language	6 years–12 years, 11 months	35 min.	Assesses language-based critical-thinking skills	Lengthy to administer	Bowers, Huisingh, and LoGiudice (2005)
Visual perceptual						
Beery-Buktenica Developmental Test of Visual Motor Integration (6th Edition)	Visual motor integration, visual perception, motor coordination	2–99 years for full form	10–15 min.	Culture-free, easy to administer, used in many countries, can be administered in groups	Scoring somewhat difficult	Beery and Beery (2004)
Performance subtests from IQ measures (e.g., WISC, DAS)	Block design, digit cancellation, copy, etc.	Various	Various	Well-normed; clear scoring; readily available	Not validated as stand-alone tests; scores on single scale driven by multiple factors	Elliott (2007); Wechsler (2014)
Learning/memory						
Wide Range Assessment of Memory and Learning (WRAML-2)	Visual memory index, verbal memory index, attention/concentration, general memory index, screening memory index	5 years –84 years, 11 months	60 min. for all core subtests	Wide age range; new norms; stronger factor structure than earlier version	Lengthy administration time; often only specific subtests are used	Sheslow and Adams (2003)

Social cognition						
Social Responsiveness Scale, Second Edition (SRS-2) Parent and teacher forms	Total, social cognition, social communication, social awareness, social motivation, restricted interests, and repetitive behavior	2.5–18 years	15–20 min.	Exceptional evidence of construct validity; inexpensive to administer; gender normed	No age norms	Constantino and Gruber (2012)
Autism Diagnostic Observation Schedule, Second Edition (ADOS-2)	Social affect, restricted and repetitive behavior, overall total, comparison score	12 months–adult	40–60 min.	Modules chosen based on language skill, good validity, play- and interview-based assessment	Difficult to administer and score reliably, extensive training needed	Lord, Rutter, DiLavore, and Risi (2012)
Autism Diagnostic Interview, Revised (ADI-R)	Communication, social, repetitive interests/behaviors	4 years–adult	1.5–2.5 hours	Comfortable for parents, thorough	Retrospective parent report, difficult to administer and score reliably, extensive training needed, lengthy	Rutter, Le Couteur, and Lord (2003)
Motor/sensory						
Peabody Developmental Motor Scales	Fine motor quotient, gross motor quotient, plus 9 subtest scores	Birth–72 months	2–3 hours (20–30 min. per subtest)	Minimal training needed because of clear instructions and objective scoring; easy to administer	Limited data on children with special needs; kit does not include all materials needed for administration; small objects are a choke hazard and need cleaning if mouthed	Folio and Fewell (2000)
Digital Finger Tapping	Digital finger tapping	Various norms; college student for digital version	10 min. with scoring	Easy to administer; electronic counter enhances accuracy	Poor norms; limited psychometric data; primarily suited to research use with comparison groups	Brandon and Bennett (1989)
Finger Tapping (Halstead-Reitan)	Finger tapping	15–64 years	10 min. with scoring	Easy to administer; widely recognized test	Small and dated norms	Reitan (1979)
Finger Tapping (Findeis and Weight Meta-Norms)	Finger tapping	5–14 years	10 min. with scoring	Easy to administer	Pools data from 20 different studies to create "norms"	Baron (2004)
Emotional adjustment						
Achenbach Child Behavior Checklist	Total problems, externalizing, internalizing, attention problems	1.5 years–young adult	10–15 min.	Multiple versions, multiple informants, forms and norms for multiple age ranges, large research and clinical literature with wide variety of medical conditions	Omits some content likely to be relevant, including theory of mind, mania scale; Scales do not map directly onto psychiatric diagnoses	Achenbach and Rescorla (2001)
Aberrant Behavior Checklist (ABC)	Irritability, lethargy, stereotypy, hyperactivity, inappropriate speech	5–51+ years	~5 min. for a rater familiar with subject's behavior	Good content coverage; sensitive to treatment effects	Manual provides incomplete psychometric information; although often used as parent or teacher rating, less validation of these formats	Aman and Singh (1986)

(continued)

Appendix 13.1 *(continued)*

Measure	Scale name	Age range	Admin. time	Advantages	Disadvantages	References
Infant-Toddler Social and Emotional Assessment (ITSEA)	Problem total; competence total; also externalizing, internalizing, dysregulation, competence, and maladaptive item clusters	12–35 months	20–30 min.	Parent form, parent interview form, and childcare provider form; Spanish translation available; brief screening version (BITSEA)	Little technical information about childcare provider or Spanish forms	Briggs Gowan and Carter (2006)
Adaptive/academic						
Adaptive Behavior Assessment System, Third Edition (ABAS-3)	Parent form, general adaptive, composite	Birth–89 years	15–20 min.	Multiple versions for different ages and parents and daycare providers; extensive construct validity	Like any parent checklist, ABAS is susceptible to misinterpretation and bias	Harrison and Oakland (2015)
Vineland Adaptive Behavior Scale, Third Edition (Vineland-3)	Adaptive behavior composite, communication, daily living skills, socialization, motor skills (optional), maladaptive behavior (optional)	Birth–90 years	20–60 min. 15–20 min.	Well-validated in multiple clinical groups Interview and informant-report versions; multiple versions for different ages and parents and daycare providers; extensive construct validity	Time and expertise intensive measure for the interview version; can take more than 1 hour to complete Administration of interview version requires expertise gained through graduate-level training programs in psychology or social work	Sparrow, Cicchetti, and Saulnier (2005)
Wide Range Achievement Test 4 (WRAT-4)	Word reading, sentence comprehension, reading composite, spelling, math computation	5 years–94 years, 11 months	15–25 min. for ages 5 to 7 for whole test; 30–45 min. for over age 7 for whole test	Short, alternative forms allows retesting, part can be administered in group format	Captures basic learning difficulties with reading decoding, and math computation, but is not sensitive to learning disabilities associated with executive function, processing speed, motor output, reading comprehension, or written expression	Wilkinson and Robertson (2006)
Woodcock-Johnson–IV	Cognitive abilities, achievement, and oral language	2–90+ years	Variable, ~5 min. per test	Relatively easy to administer; sensitive to the effects of processing speed and motor output deficits on academics		Schrank, McGrew, and Mather (2014)

Adapted and updated from Youngstrom, E., LaKind, J.S., Kenworthy, L., Lipkin, P.H., Goodman, M., Squibb, K., . . . Anthony, L.G. (2010). Advancing the selection of neurodevelopmental measures in epidemiological studies of associations between environmental chemical exposure and adverse health effects. *International Journal of Environmental Research and Public Health, 7,* 229–268. doi:10.3390/ijerph7010229.

PART IV

Developmental Disabilities

CHAPTER 14 Intellectual Disability

Bruce K. Shapiro and Mark L. Batshaw

Upon completion of this chapter, the reader will

- Understand the definition of the term *developmental delay* and the implications of the terms *mental retardation* and *intellectual disability*
- Be aware of the various causes of intellectual disability
- Recognize the various interventions in intellectual disability
- Be aware of the different levels of functioning and independence that individuals with intellectual disability can achieve

Intellectual disability refers to a heterogeneous group of disorders that have significant deficits in reasoning that impairs the individual's ability to function in day to day life. People with intellectual disability have the capacity to learn, but they have difficulty adapting that knowledge to novel situations. There are many different causes of intellectual disability. Consequently, the range of the cognitive impairment seen in intellectual disability is wide and comorbid disorders are the rule. A multimodal, individualized approach to management can optimize the individual's ability to participate in everyday life.

CASE STUDY

Daniel's mother, Marina, noticed many signs in his early development that indicated atypical development. (In the following paragraphs, the typical ages for these developmental milestones are indicated in parentheses after the age at which Daniel achieved them).

As an infant, Daniel showed little interest in his environment and was not very alert. Although Marina tried to breastfeed him, his suck was weak, and he frequently regurgitated his formula. He was floppy and had poor head control. His cry was high pitched, and he was difficult to comfort. He would sit in an infant seat for hours without complaint.

In social and motor development, Daniel was delayed. With regard to his social development, Daniel smiled at 5 months (2 months) but was not very responsive to his parents' attention. He did not start babbling until 13 months (6 months). With regard to gross motor development, Daniel could hold his head up at 4 months (1 month), roll over at 8 months (5 months), and sit up at 14 months (6 months). He transferred objects from one hand to the other at 14 months (5 months).

When evaluated with the Bayley Scales of Infant Development–Third Edition (BSID-III; Bayley, 2006) at 16 months of age, Daniel's mental age was found to be 7 months and he received a mental developmental index (similar to an intelligence quotient [IQ] score) of less than 50. He progressed from an early intervention program to a special preschool program. Prior to school entry at age 6, Daniel was retested on the Stanford-Binet

Intelligence Scales, Fifth Edition (SB5; Roid, 2003). His score indicated a mental age of 2 years and 8 months and an IQ score of 40. Concomitant impairments in adaptive behavior were demonstrated by the Vineland Adaptive Behavior Scales, Third Edition (Vineland-3; Sparrow, Chrichetti, & Saulnier, 2016), which revealed communicative, self-care, and social skill challenges.

Thought Question:

How early can you determine that a child has intellectual disability, and why does it matter?

DEFINING INTELLECTUAL DISABILITY

The term *intellectual disability* (ID) has replaced the older term *mental retardation*. This change was codified in federal legislation in 2010, when Rosa's Law (Pub. L. 111-256) was enacted, which changed the term used in federal legislation from *mental retardation* to *intellectual disability*. The federal definition of the term itself did not change and comes from the Individuals with Disabilities Education Improvement Act (IDEA) of 2004 (PL 108–446), which defines intellectual disability as "significantly sub-average general intellectual functioning, existing concurrently with deficits in adaptive behavior and manifested during the developmental period that adversely affects a child's educational performance." Two other authoritative groups, the American Psychiatric Association (APA, 2013) and the American Association on Intellectual and Developmental Disabilities (AAIDD; Schalock et al., 2009) maintain the same three criteria of adaptive behavior deficits, subaverage intellectual function, and onset during the developmental period. Yet, their definitions shift the focus from IQ to adaptive behavior deficits. It is likely that the term *intellectual disability* will be replaced by the term *intellectual developmental disorder*. The latter has been proposed by the World Health Organization's *International Classification of Diseases* (ICD-11) nomenclature as a health condition and is defined as "a group of developmental conditions characterized by a significant impairment of cognitive functions which are associated with limitations of learning, adaptive behavior and skills" (Bertelli, Munir, Harris, & Salvador-Carulla, 2016).

Adaptive Impairments

Individuals fulfilling the diagnosis of intellectual disability must demonstrate adaptive deficits that impair their ability to adapt to or function in daily life when compared with peers of similar age or culture. Indeed, it is the deficits in adaptive function that bring children to our attention. These impairments limit or restrict an individual's participation and performance in one or more aspects of daily life activities, such as communication, social participation, function at school or work, or personal independence at home or in community settings. The limitations result in the need for ongoing support at home, school, work, or independent life. Typically, adaptive behavior is measured using individualized, standardized, culturally appropriate, and psychometrically sound tests (APA, 2013).

The AAIDD (Schalock et al., 2009) divides adaptive function into three domains: conceptual, practical, and socialization. Conceptual skills include such things as language and literacy, money, time, number concepts, and self-direction. Practical skills include the activities of daily living, occupational skills, health care, travel/transportation, schedules/routines, safety, use of money, and use of the telephone. Social skills encompass interpersonal skills, social responsibility, self-esteem, gullibility, naïveté, social problem-solving, and the ability to follow rules/obey laws and to avoid being victimized. The AAIDD definition of intellectual disability requires deficits to exist in one of the three domains of adaptive behavior.

Intellectual Functioning

There is general agreement that the definition of intellectual disability requires that a person must have significantly subaverage intellectual functioning and impairments in adaptive abilities with onset during the developmental period; however, disagreements over operationalizing this definition have arisen for both biological and philosophical reasons. The first controversial issue is that the definition involves the assessment of intellectual functioning. The average level of intellectual functioning in a population corresponds to the apex of a bell-shaped curve (Figure 14.1). Two standard deviations on either side of the mean encompass 95% of a population sample and approximately defines the range of typical intellectual functioning. By definition, the average IQ score is 100, and the standard deviation (a statistical measure of dispersion from the mean) of most IQ tests is 15 points. Historically, a person scoring more than 2 standard deviations below the mean, or below an IQ of 70, has been considered to have intellectual disability.

Statisticians, however, point out that there is a measurement variance of approximately 5 points in assessing IQ by most psychometric tests. In other words, repeated testing of the same individual will produce scores that vary by as much as 5 points (American Psychiatric Association, 2000). Using this schema, intellectual disability would be diagnosed in an individual with

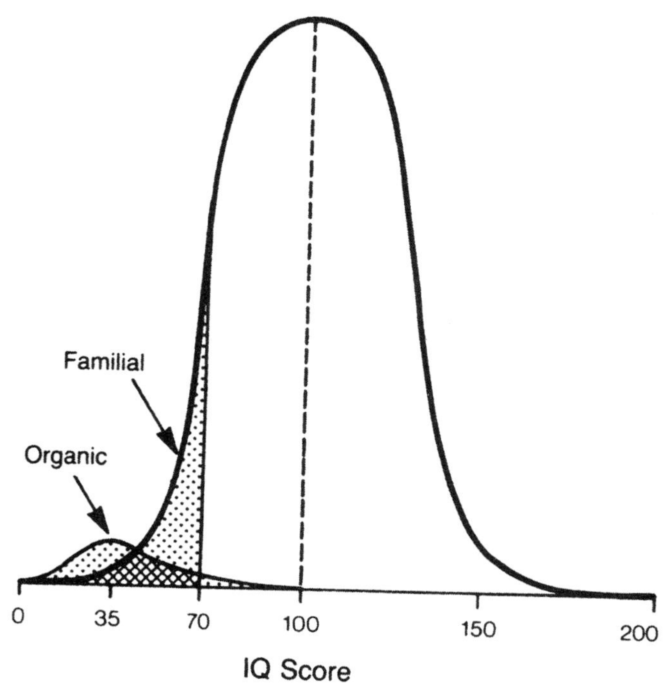

Figure 14.1. Bimodal distribution of intelligence. The mean IQ score is 100. An IQ score of less than 70, or 2 standard deviations below the mean, can indicate intellectual disability. The second, smaller curve takes into account individuals who have intellectual disability because of birth trauma, infection, inborn errors, or other organic causes. This explains why more individuals have severe to profound intellectual disability than are predicted by the familial curve alone. (From Zigler, E. [1967]. Familial mental retardation: A continuing dilemma. *Science, 155*, 292–298. http://www.aaas.org. Reprinted with permission from AAAS.)

an IQ score between 70 and 75 who exhibits significant impairments in adaptive behavior, whereas it would not be diagnosed in an individual with an IQ of 65 to 70 who demonstrates adaptive skills in the typical range.

Measured IQ may not be stable over time. Children may grow into or out of intellectual disability. Some young children may evidence a decelerating trajectory of intellectual growth and move into the diagnosis as adolescents. Alternatively, children may have an intellectual growth rate that accelerates over time and grow out of the diagnosis. Others develop sufficient adaptive behavior to no longer meet the criteria for intellectual disability.

In addition to changes in the individual, there appears to be a change in performance on IQ measures in a population. This phenomenon, known as the Flynn effect, holds that there is a relationship between the length of time that an instrument is in use and the individual's score on that instrument. This is based on the observation that the mean IQ increased on every restandardization sample in a population for major intelligence tests (Schalock et al., 2009).

Cognitive functioning is not always uniform across all neurodevelopmental domains. An example is found in a study by Wang and Bellugi (1993), who compared neuropsychological testing results in children with Down syndrome and Williams syndrome. Although the full-scale IQ scores in both groups were similar, the pattern of cognitive strengths and weaknesses was very different. The individuals with Williams syndrome had much stronger skills in language but much poorer visual-perceptual abilities than did the children with Down syndrome. When volumetric analysis of magnetic resonance imaging (MRI) scans was performed, the cortical areas involved in language acquisition were much more developed in individuals with Williams syndrome; conversely, the basal ganglia area that is involved in visual-perception was more developed in individuals with Down syndrome.

Beyond any measurement variability, a more fundamental concern of some theorists is the underlying value of an IQ score. Gardner (1983) challenged the dichotomous (verbal-vs.-performance) structure of intelligence assessed by many IQ tests. He proposed that intelligence comprises a wider range of abilities, not only the traditional linguistic and logical-mathematical skills, but also musical, spatial, bodily-kinesthetic, and interpersonal characteristics. However, this approach has not gained wide acceptance as it does not have a clear neuropsychological or neuroanatomical basis. Although it is acknowledged that a single IQ score averages a person's cognitive abilities and may not capture all forms of intelligence, there is evidence that a significantly subnormal IQ score is a meaningful predictor of future cognitive function.

Finally, there are the concerns over predictive validity and cultural bias. Infant psychological tests are notoriously poor predictors of adult IQ scores, although they clearly differentiate severe impairments from typical functioning. In addition, cultural bias has been suggested as one explanation for differences in IQ scores found among individuals from various racial, ethnic, and socioeconomic groups.

CLASSIFICATION OF INTELLECTUAL DISABILITY

Intellectual disability is comprised of a group of conditions that arise from many different causes and that have many different expressions. Although the diagnosis of intellectual disability is important, the classification of intellectual disability is equally important. Etiologic evaluation, neurobiological mechanisms, management, planning, and prognosis are all predicated on the ability to classify the disorder. There are many methods for classification, but this chapter focuses on five: 1) degree of intellectual impairment, 2) adaptive behavior, 3) required supports, 4) domains of disability, and 5) etiology.

Degree of Intellectual Impairment

There is controversy about classifying the levels of intellectual disability. In the fourth edition of the *Diagnostic and Statistical Manual of Mental Disorders* published by the APA (*DSM-IV*), an individual was classified as having mild intellectual disability if his or her IQ level was 50 to approximately 70, moderate intellectual disability if his or her IQ level was 35 to approximately 50, severe intellectual disability if his or her IQ level was 20 to approximately 35, and profound intellectual disability if his or her IQ level was below 20 to 25 (APA, 2000). While this classification has been met with widespread acceptance in the medical community, it should be noted that classification solely on the basis of IQ is incomplete and does not capture all of an individual's adaptive abilities. *DSM-5* abandoned specific IQ scores as a diagnostic criterion, although it retained the general notion of functioning two or more standard deviations below the general population.

It has also been suggested that intellectual disability should be simply dichotomized into mild (an IQ score of 50 to approximately 70) and severe (an IQ score below 50). This suggestion is based on the discrete biological division between mild intellectual disability and the more severe forms, with different etiologies and outcomes. This dichotomy has not been widely accepted for clinical purposes because the medical, educational, and habilitative needs are quite different between individuals with moderate impairments and those with profound impairments.

Adaptive Behavior

In the *DSM-5*, the APA has advocated for classifying intellectual disability by adaptive behavior (APA, 2013). This classification is addressed below in the section on outcomes. While this classification may be a more complete view of a person's everyday function in conceptual, social, and practical domains than classification by degree of intellectual impairment, it is most useful when dealing with adults. This system is less useful in developing children and when encountering discordance in the domains of adaptive behavior.

Required Supports

The AAIDD takes a different approach in defining the degree of severity of intellectual disability, relying not on IQ scores, but rather on the patterns and intensity of needed support (i.e., intermittent, limited, extensive, or pervasive support). This definition marks a philosophical shift from an emphasis on degree of impairment to a focus on the abilities of individuals to function in an inclusive environment. This shift is controversial because it assumes that adaptive behaviors can be independent of cognition, and it does not provide clear guidelines for establishing diagnostic eligibility of children with IQ scores in the upper limits of the range connoting intellectual disability. This chapter (and other chapters throughout this book) uses the *DSM-IV* categories in discussing medical issues and the AAIDD's categories in discussing educational and other interventions, emphasizing the capabilities rather than the impairments of individuals with intellectual disability.

Domains of Disability

Another way to classify intellectual disability is to use the terminology developed by the National Center for Medical Rehabilitation Research (Msall, 2005). This model defines five domains: pathophysiology, impairment, functional limitation, disability, and societal limitation (Table 14.1). Pathophysiology focuses on the cellular, structural, or functional events resulting from injury, disease, or genetic abnormality that underlie the developmental disability. Impairment refers to the losses that result from the pathophysiological event. Functional limitation describes the restriction or lack of ability to perform a normal function. Disability is the inability to perform activities or limitation in the performance of activities. Societal limitations focus on barriers to full participation in society. Table 14.1 illustrates how this system can be applied to children with Prader-Willi syndrome, fetal alcohol spectrum disorder, and Down syndrome. The advantage of this approach is that it leads directly from diagnosis to treatment and that it focuses on how to overcome limitations. The approach also acknowledges the change in emphasis in the diagnosis of intellectual disability from impairment and functional limitations to disability and societal limitations. This is consistent with the move from focusing on the intensity of the disability (e.g., severe) to the support needed to function in society (e.g., requiring extensive support). This approach is also in keeping with the process for developing an individualized education program (IEP) for a school-age child (see Chapter 33).

Etiology

Classification of intellectual disability by cause (etiology) has increased as the ability to identify genetic

Table 14.1. Relationship between disability domains and treatments in Prader-Willi syndrome, fetal alcohol spectrum disorder, and Down syndrome

Pathophysiology	Impairment/ Disorder	Functional limitation	Disability	Societal limitation	Treatment
Deletion in chromosome 15	Prader-Willi syndrome	Intellectual disability Feeding disorder	Learning and adaptive skills below age level Obesity	Noninclusive school settings Stereotyping because of obesity and intellectual disability Underestimating abilities	Education Activities to promote weight loss
In utero alcohol exposure	Fetal alcohol spectrum disorder	Intellectual disability Behavioral disturbances	Learning and adaptive skills below age level but variable Severe hyperactivity common	Noninclusive school settings Stigma because of etiology Overestimating abilities because of variable cognitive profile	Education Mental health Interventions as required
Trisomy 21	Down syndrome	Intellectual disability	Learning and adaptive skills below age level	Noninclusive school settings Stereotyping because of intellectual disability Underestimating abilities	Education programs to raise societal awareness

Source: Msall et al. (2003).
Note: Even though each child may have similar degrees of intellectual disability, the pattern of disability and type of treatments may vary widely.

causes of intellectual disability has advanced. It has also led to the establishment of family support and advocacy groups for specific disorders (e.g., Down syndrome, fragile X syndrome, and Williams syndrome). In one study, the etiology of intellectual disability was able to be divided into five classification groups at 4 years of age: environmental (44.4%), genetic (20.5%), idiopathic (12.6%), neonatal sequelae (13.2%), and other diseases (9.3%) (Karam et al., 2016). Grouping by etiology provides greater biologic homogeneity and facilitates neurobiologic research that elucidates the brain mechanisms of intellectual disability and the potential for prevention, amelioration, or cure. The decreasing cost and increased availability of genetic testing have enhanced our ability to diagnose etiologies of many individuals with moderate-profound intellectual disability, and it is now part of the diagnostic regimen for these individuals (see Chapter 12).

PREVALENCE OF INTELLECTUAL DISABILITY

The epidemiology of intellectual disability suggests that there are two distinct populations: Mild intellectual disability is more likely to be associated with social disadvantage and familial factors (Reichenberg et al., 2016), whereas severe intellectual disability is more typically linked to a biological/genetic origin (Karam et al., 2015). There is often, however, an interaction between nature and nurture. Postnatal environmental influences mediate biological processes through mechanisms that may be indirect (e.g., epigenetics; see Chapter 1) and are not fully understood at the present. In addition, postnatal environmental factors may affect the expression of neurodevelopmental dysfunction. For example, a child may have an initial biological insult (e.g., intrauterine growth restriction [IUGR]) that can be compounded by postnatal environmental variables, such as poor nutrition, social disadvantage, or physical abuse). Mothers who never finished high school are four times more likely to have children with mild intellectual disability than are women who completed high school (Mendola, Selevan, Gutter, & Rice, 2002). The explanation for this is unclear, but it may involve a genetic component (i.e., inheritance of a cognitive impairment) and socioeconomic factors (e.g., poverty and poor nutrition). The application of early intervention services to high-risk infants who are also at socioeconomic risk has resulted in improved cognitive outcomes (see Chapter 31).

The prevalence of intellectual disability depends on the definition used, the method of ascertainment, and the population studied. In various studies it has ranged between 6.7 (Boyle et al., 2011) and 10.37 (Van Naarden Braun et al., 2015) per 1,000. Males are more likely to manifest intellectual disability than females with a ratio of approximately two to one.

The variability in the prevalence of intellectual disability seems to be related to mild intellectual disability. The prevalence of severe intellectual disability is relatively constant across countries and across time, accounting for 0.3%–0.5% of the population. By contrast, the prevalence of mild intellectual disability shows significant variability.

According to statistics of IQ tests, 2.5% of the population could be predicted to have intellectual disability, and another 2.5% could be predicted to have superior intelligence (Figure 14.1). The IQ scores of 85% of individuals with intellectual disability (about 2.1% of the population) should fall in the range of mild intellectual disability (2 to 3 standard deviations below the mean). If, however, individuals who score low on IQ tests because of social disadvantage are excluded from the count, the prevalence of mild intellectual disability is only about half these predictions, somewhere between 0.8% and 1.2% (Heikura et al., 2003). Other factors that impact the prevalence of mild intellectual disability are 1) diagnostic overshadowing (e.g., providing a primary diagnosis of learning disability, language disorder, autism, developmental delay, or a mental health disorder rather than intellectual disability), 2) improved evaluation instruments, 3) professional disinclination to use this diagnosis in children, and 4) the inappropriate use of the term *developmental delay* in older children. Diagnostic substitution of autism spectrum disorder (ASD) as a primary diagnosis instead of intellectual disability has had an especially important impact on the prevalence of intellectual disability (see Chapter 18). Finally, it is possible that the prevalence of mild intellectual disability is decreasing because of public welfare (improved nutrition), health (anticipatory guidance), and education (early intervention) measures that have been implemented.

Whatever the prevalence, the diagnosis of intellectual disability appears to peak at 10–14 years of age, acknowledging that, as expected, children with mild impairments are identified significantly later than those with more severe impairments.

Etiology

The specific origins of mild intellectual disability are identifiable in less than half of affected individuals (Moeschler, Shevell, & American Academy of Pediatrics Committee on Genetics, 2006). The most common biological causes are certain genetic/chromosomal syndromes—for example, velocardiofacial syndrome; fetal deprivation (e.g., IUGR); perinatal complications (e.g., encephalopathy or infection); and intrauterine exposure to drugs of abuse, especially alcohol (Hoyme et al., 2016). Although definite genetic causes are less common (5% in mild intellectual disability versus 47% in severe intellectual disability), familial clustering of mild intellectual disability is common. In children with severe intellectual disability, a biological origin can be identified in about three quarters of cases. The most common identifiable causes are Down syndrome, fragile X syndrome, and fetal alcohol spectrum disorders, which together account for almost one third of all currently detectable cases of severe intellectual disability (Hoyme et al., 2016).

One way of dividing the biological origins of intellectual disability is by their timing in the developmental sequence; in general, the earlier the problem, the more severe its consequences. This is consistent with finding a prenatal cause in about three quarters of individuals with an identifiable cause of severe intellectual disability (Gropman & Batshaw, 2010).

Chromosomal disorders (e.g., Down syndrome and Prader-Willi syndrome,), certain single-gene defects (e.g., Rubinstein-Taybi syndrome, Hurler syndrome, and Kabuki syndrome), abnormalities of brain development that affect early embryogenesis (e.g., holoprosencephaly), and inborn errors of metabolism (see Chapter 16) are the most common and severe examples of biologic origin of intellectual disability. Together, these groups of genetically based causes of severe intellectual disability account for more than two thirds of identifiable causes and encompass more than 700 disorders (see http://www.ncbi.nlm.nih.gov/omim for more information).

Insults in the first and second trimesters as a result of substance abuse (e.g., fetal alcohol spectrum disorders), infections (e.g., cytomegalovirus), and other pregnancy problems (e.g., IUGR) occur in 10% of cases. Fetal deprivation in the third trimester due to placental damage, preeclampsia, or hemorrhage (see Chapter 6) and problems in the perinatal period (see Chapter 5) now account for less than 10% of identifiable causes of severe intellectual disability. Five percent are the result of postnatal brain damage, most commonly meningitis/encephalitis and traumatic brain injury (see Chapter 23). Overall, the recurrence risk in families with one child who has severe intellectual disability of unknown origin is 3%–9% (De Souza, Halliday, Chan, Bower, & Morris, 2009). Recurrence risk for intellectual disability of known origin, however, varies according to the cause. A family whose child has intellectual disability following neonatal meningitis does not have a significantly increased risk of having future affected children, whereas a woman who has had one child with a fetal alcohol spectrum disorder has a 30%–50% risk of having other affected children if she continues to abuse alcohol during pregnancy. The risk of recurrent Down syndrome ranges from less than 1% for trisomy 21 to more than 10% for a balanced translocation (De Souza et al., 2009). If the cause of intellectual disability is a Mendelian disorder (see Chapter 1), such as neurofibromatosis (an autosomal dominant trait), Hurler syndrome (an autosomal recessive trait), or fragile X syndrome (an X-linked trait), the recurrence risk ranges from 0%–50% depending on the inheritance pattern of the specific disorder.

DIAGNOSIS AND CLINICAL MANIFESTATIONS

Parents usually seek an evaluation for developmental delay when their child fails to meet specific developmental milestones (Table 14.2). In early infancy, these include a lack of responsiveness, unusual muscle tone or posture, and feeding difficulties. Between 6 and 15 months of age, motor delay is the most common concern. Language and behavior problems are the most common concerns after 18 months. If there is evidence of a significant developmental lag over time, the child should be sent for a comprehensive evaluation. Ideally, this evaluation should include an examination by a physician (pediatrician, neurodevelopmental pediatrician, developmental-behavioral pediatrician, child psychiatrist, geneticist, or pediatric neurologist) experienced in early childhood development and developmental disabilities, preferably in tandem with a clinical/educational psychologist and a social worker. Depending on the child's age and impairments, he or she also may need to be seen for early intervention assessment by an early childhood educator, advanced practice nurse, speech-language pathologist, or audiologist. If the child displays motor impairments, a physical therapist, an occupational therapist, and possibly a physiatrist should also be involved. Following the assessment, an individual family service plan (IFSP) is developed in the context of an early intervention program (see Chapter 31).

The term *global developmental delay* is most commonly used as a temporary diagnosis in young children who are at risk for developmental disabilities (Moeschler, Shevell, & American Academy of Pediatrics Committee on Genetics, 2014). Global developmental delay is applied to children younger than 5 years of age who show a significant delay in achieving age-appropriate neurodevelopmental milestones in two or more of the major areas of child development: cognition, language, motor, self-help, and social-emotional development. It is often, although not always, predictive of a future diagnosis of intellectual disability (Riou, Ghosh, Francoeur, & Shevell, 2009).

Global developmental delay is recognized by the failure of the child to meet age-appropriate expectations based on the typical sequence of development. In the first months of life, delayed development can be manifested by a lack of visual or auditory response, an inadequate suck, and/or floppy or spastic muscle tone. Later in the first year, lack of language and motor delays in sitting and walking may suggest developmental delay (see Box 14.1). When a child continues to show significant delays in all developmental areas, intellectual disability is the most likely diagnosis.

Global developmental delay should be distinguished from the less specific developmental delay. Unfortunately, some medical practitioners continue to use the term *global developmental delay* long after the more specific diagnosis of intellectual disability can be made. Developmental delay, as an educational term, is defined by each state and may be used as a category of disability for children younger than age 9 years (IDEA, 2004).

Although developmental delay is the most common presenting concern in children who turn out to have intellectual disability, sensory impairment, ASD, or cerebral palsy, it does not always indicate a developmental disability. Isolated mild delays in expressive language (particularly in boys) or in gross motor abilities often resolve over time. These mild early delays, however, often signal an increased risk of the child developing academic or behavioral difficulties by school age.

Table 14.2. Presentations of intellectual disability by age

Age	Area of concern
Newborn	Dysmorphisms (structural abnormalities) Major physiologic dysfunction (e.g., eating, breathing)
2–4 months	Failure to interact with the environment (e.g., parent suspects child is deaf or has a visual impairment)
6–18 months	Gross motor delay (e.g., sitting, crawling, walking)
18 months–3 years	Language
3–5 years	Language Behavior (including play) Fine motor (e.g., cutting, coloring)
5+ years	Academic achievement Behavior (e.g., attention, anxiety, mood, conduct)

Source: Shapiro and Batshaw (2002).

BOX 14.1 EVIDENCE-BASED PRACTICE

How Early Is Early?

The Eden Cohort is a prospective longitudinal study that seeks to identify prenatal and early postnatal nutritional, environmental, and social determinants associated with children's health and typical or atypical development. This study comprised 1,100 infants who were recruited during their pregnancy and were followed through 5–6 years of age. Developmental milestones were collected in a standard fashion at 4, 8, 12, and 24 months. Questionnaires were derived from Brunet-Lezine Psychomotor Development Scale, a scale that is widely used in France. The MacArthur-Bates Communicative Development Inventories, short French version, a listing of 100 common words that a young child uses, was given at 24 months to quantify expressive vocabulary. The Wechsler Preschool and Primary Inventory was administered at 5–6 years. Data were grouped as gross motor, fine motor, socialization, and language domains (at 4 months groupings were motor and socialization/communication). Using multivariate analysis, the authors found that 1) a substantial amount of the later IQ variance was predicted by the 24-month evaluation; 2) early language skills more strongly predicted later IQ than other cognitive domains; and 3) several cognitive domains, but particularly language skills from the age of 8 months, predicted disabled children (IQ < 70) at 5–6 years. This study supports the contention that language is the best predictor of cognitive development and that developmental monitoring, even at very young ages, can detect children at risk for later intellectual disability (Peyre, Charkaluk, Forhan, Heude, & Ramus, 2017).

MEDICAL DIAGNOSTIC TESTING

No single method exists for detecting all causes of intellectual disability (Moeschler et al., 2014). As a result, diagnostic testing should be based on the medical history and a physical examination. For example, a child with an unusual facial appearance, a history of other affected family members, or multiple congenital anomalies should be referred to a geneticist. With the increased ability to identify genetic disorders, even minor anomalies may be worth pursuing (see Chapter 1). A male with unusual physical features or a family history of intellectual disability or ASD should probably have molecular studies for fragile X syndrome. A child with a progressive neurological disorder will need extensive metabolic investigation (see Chapter 16), and a child with seizure-like episodes should have an electroencephalogram (see Chapter 22). Finally, an MRI scan may be warranted in children with abnormal head growth or asymmetrical neurological findings (e.g., one side of the body weaker than the other). These tests, however, should not be seen as screening tools to be used in all children with intellectual disability because their yield of useful results is low unless there is a specific reason for performing the study and their cost is high.

Although these are the most common reasons for performing diagnostic tests, it now seems clear that some children with subtle physical or neurological findings also may have determinable biological origins of their intellectual disability. It has been shown that a significant percentage of unexplained intellectual disability can be accounted for by genomic copy number variants (see Chapter 1). Chromosome microarrays and next-generation sequencing have revolutionized gene discovery in intellectual disability (Mefford, Batshaw, & Hoffman, 2012). Chromosome microarray analysis, which is recommended as a first-line test in the genetic workup of children with intellectual disability, developmental delays, autism, and congenital anomalies, provides a molecular diagnosis in 15%–20% of cases. Exome sequencing and whole-genome sequencing have moved rapidly into the diagnostic laboratory to identify specific genetic mutations (Rump et al., 2016; Zahir et al., 2017). It is important to mention that whole-genome sequencing is not clinically available yet but will be in the near future and will detect mutations that whole exome has not been able to identify. In addition, MRI scans have been found to document a significant number of subtle markers of cerebral malformations in about 10% of children with intellectual disability (Barkovich & Raybaud, 2004).

The extent to which one should investigate the cause of a child's intellectual disability is based on a number of factors. First, what is the degree of intellectual disability? One is less likely to find a biological cause in a child with mild intellectual disability than in a child with a severe disability. Second, is there a specific diagnostic path to follow? If there is a medical history, a family history, or physical findings pointing to a specific cause, a diagnosis is more likely to be made. Conversely, in the absence of these indicators, it is difficult to choose specific tests to perform. Third, are the parents planning to have additional children? If so, clinicians are more likely to intensively seek disorders for which prenatal diagnosis or a specific early treatment option is available (e.g., inborn errors of metabolism). Finally, and most importantly, what are the parents' wishes? Different families have different levels of investment in searching for the cause of the intellectual disability. Some focus exclusively on treatment, while others are so directed at obtaining a diagnosis that they have difficulty accepting intervention until a specific cause has been determined. Both extremes and every perspective in between must be respected, and supportive anticipatory guidance should be provided in the context of parent education for the "here and now" as well as for the future.

PSYCHOLOGICAL TESTING

The routine evaluation for intellectual disability should include an individual intelligence test (see Chapter 13). The most commonly used tests in children are the BSID-III (Bayley, 2006), the SB5 (Roid, 2003), and the Wechsler scales: the Wechsler Preschool and Primary Scale of Intelligence–Fourth Edition (WPPSI-IV; Wechsler, 2012) and the Wechsler Intelligence Scale for Children–Fifth Edition (WISC-V; Wechsler et al., 2015).

As noted in the APA definition of intellectual disability, in addition to testing intelligence, adaptive skills (including social functioning) also should be measured. The most commonly used test of adaptive behavior is the Vineland-3 (Sparrow et al., 2016). Other tests of adaptive behavior that are used commonly include the Scales of Independent Behavior—Revised (Bruininks, Woodcock, Weatherman, & Hill, 1996) and the Adaptive Behavior Assessment System–Third Edition (ABAS-3; Harrison & Oakland, 2015).

Interpretation of Test Results

In infants and young children with typical development, there is substantial variability in IQ scores on repeated cognitive testing and consequently poor predictive validity until around 10 years of age. Accuracy is enhanced if repeated testing confirms a stable rate of cognitive development. The predictive value of infant tests is further limited because such tests are primarily dependent on nonlanguage items, whereas language skills remain the best predictors of future IQ scores. These tests do permit the differentiation of infants with severe intellectual disability from typically developing infants, but they are less helpful in distinguishing between a typically developing child and one with a mild intellectual disability. In general, however, there is less variability seen with cognitive growth in children with intellectual disability, and so predictive validity is enhanced compared with children with typical development.

Although children with intellectual disability usually score below average on all subscale scores, they may score in the typical range in one or more performance areas in the Wechsler scales. Overall, these scales are quite accurate in predicting adult IQ scores when administered to school-age children. The evaluator, however, must ensure that conditions that may contribute to falsely low IQ scores do not confound the test performance. These include motor impairments, communication disorders, sensory impairments, speaking a language other than English, extremely low birth weight, or insufficient schooling; such conditions may invalidate certain intelligence tests and require modification of others. The presence of such conditions always requires caution with regard to interpretation.

There is usually, but not always, a good correlation between scores on intelligence tests and adaptive scales (Bloom & Zelko, 1994). Adaptive abilities, however, are more responsive to intervention efforts than are the cognitive abilities measured by IQ. Adaptive abilities are also more variable, which may relate to the underlying condition. For example, individuals with Prader-Willi syndrome have stable adaptive skills through adulthood, while individuals with fragile X syndrome may have increasing impairments over time (Jacquemont et al., 2004; Klaiman et al., 2014).

COMORBID/ASSOCIATED CONDITIONS

Intellectual disability is often accompanied by other impairments called comorbid conditions or associated deficits. Although a mild intellectual disability is frequently an isolated disorder, moderate-profound intellectual disability is often paired with medical, motor, behavioral, and communication disorders that affect the child's developmental outcome. The prevalence of these associated impairments correlates with the severity of the disability (Barnhill, Cooper, & Fletcher, 2017; Crocker, Prokic, Morin, & Reyes, 2014; Oeseburg, Jansen, Dijkstra, Groothoff, & Reijneveld, 2010a; Oeseburg, Jansen, Groothoff, Dijkstra, & Reijneveld, 2010b; Oliver & Richards, 2015; Robertson, Hatton, Emerson, & Baines, 2015). Comorbid conditions include cerebral palsy, seizure disorders, communication disorders, sensory impairments (hearing and/or visual deficits), and psychological/behavioral disorders (e.g., mood disorders, ASD, attention-deficit/hyperactivity disorder [ADHD], self-injury, aggression, and conduct disorders; Table 14.3).

Approximately 20% of children with severe intellectual disability have cerebral palsy, which may also be associated with feeding problems and failure to thrive. Seizure disorders also occur in about 20% of children with intellectual disability. Communication deficits (speech-language impairments) beyond those related to the cognitive impairment also are frequent. Finally, psychological and behavior disorders occur in up to half of children with intellectual disability (Cooper & van der Speck, 2009). In considering intervention strategies, identifying these comorbid conditions and working toward their treatment is essential in order to obtain an optimal outcome.

Associated deficits may make it difficult to distinguish intellectual disability from other developmental disabilities. Certain distinguishing features, however, frequently exist. In isolated intellectual disability, language and nonverbal reasoning skills are significantly delayed, whereas gross motor skills tend to be less affected. Conversely, in cerebral palsy, motor impairments are often more prominent than cognitive impairments. In communication disorders, expressive and/or receptive language skills are more delayed than nonverbal reasoning skills. In ASD, social skills impairments and atypical behaviors are superimposed on cognitive (especially communication) impairments. In some instances, repeated assessments may be necessary to determine the primary developmental disability.

Table 14.3. Percentage of children with intellectual disability who have associated chronic health conditions

Epilepsy	22%
Cerebral palsy	19.8%
Hearing problems	4.5%
Vision problems	2.2%–26.8%
Down syndrome	11.0%
Fragile X	1.9%
Autism spectrum disorder	17.2%
ADHD/hyperkinetic disorder	9.5%
Conduct disorder	5.1%
Oppositional defiant disorder	12.4%
Anxiety disorder	17.1%

Source: Osesburg, Dijkstra, Groothoff, Reijneveld, and Jansen (2011).

Key: ADHD, attention-deficit/hyperactivity disorder.

TREATMENT, MANAGEMENT, AND INTERVENTIONS

The most useful treatment approach for children with intellectual disability consists of multimodal efforts directed at many aspects of the child's life—education, social and recreational activities, behavior problems, and associated impairments (Shapiro & Batshaw, 2016; Wehmeyer et al, 2017). Support for parents, siblings, and other caregivers (both family members and unrelated caregivers) is also important (see textbox titled Cultural Competence and Intellectual Disability, along with Chapter 37).

Educational Services

Education is the single most important discipline involved in intervention for children with intellectual disability and their families (see Chapters 31 and 33). The achievement of good outcomes in an educational program is dependent on the interaction between the student and teacher. Educational programs must be relevant to the child's needs and address the child's

CULTURAL COMPETENCE AND INTELLECTUAL DISABILITY

In caring for individuals with intellectual disability, it is important to be sensitive to cultural issues that can affect care. It can be generally assumed that parents love their children and want what is best for them. However, as professionals, we cannot assume that all families will attempt to achieve an optimal outcome for their child in the same way, and the culture they live in may present challenges. In some cultures, the visible presence of a child with a disability may adversely impact the marriage prospects of other children in the family. The family may thus want to homeschool the child or have him or her in a segregated school. In other cultures, traditional rather than modern medicine may be practiced, which may affect the use of needed medication or surgery. The practitioner who does not understand and respect the culture that defines the family may lose the opportunity to continue caring for the child. Therefore, it is essential to understand and respect the cultural background that may define the families with whom you work. It is often possible to work within these confines and still provide excellent and respectful care.

BOX 14.2 INTERDISCIPLINARY CARE

The Special Education Teacher

Perhaps the most important discipline in caring for a child with intellectual disability is special education. The special education teacher is essential in designing and then carrying out the individualized family service plan (IFSP; for early intervention) or individual education program (IEP; for primary and secondary school). The teacher is the hub of care for the child with intellectual disability, bringing in other disciplines as needed to assist in developing an effective learning environment. The teacher is trained in both pedagogical techniques and behavior management for children with special education needs and is also tasked with assessing the progress of the child educationally and revising the curriculum as needed to optimally serve the student.

individual strengths and challenges. The child's developmental level and his or her requirements for support and goals for independence provide a basis for establishing an IFSP in early intervention programs and an IEP in school programs (see Box 14.2).

It should also be remembered that learning begins at home in the context of a child's family. Early intervention for infants and toddlers (birth to 3 years) usually takes place in the home as well. The home continues to be the primary educational setting for 3 to 4 year olds, although many children attend out-of-home center-based or preschool programs. At age 5, most children enter kindergarten for half- or full-day sessions and are introduced to a more formal learning environment. Formal special education services are provided in the school setting thereafter.

Leisure and Recreational Needs

In addition to education, the child's physical, social, and recreational needs should be addressed (Andrews, Falkmer, & Girdler, 2015; Patel & Greydanus, 2010; Verdonschot, de Witte, Reichrath, Buntinx, & Curfs, 2009; Wehmeyer et al., 2017). Peer socialization in play and recreational activities constitutes an important part of social-emotional development and builds resilience. As such, socialization competencies and experiences (e.g., dealing with social conflict, managing anger, making needs known, and expressing affection or unhappiness) can exert a significant influence upon developmental outcomes and school readiness and participation and can eventually influence future success in adult life. In the ideal world, children with intellectual disability would participate as equals in all recreation and leisure activities. Although young children with intellectual disability are not usually excluded from play activities, parents still may have a difficult time finding age- and skill-appropriate adaptive play equipment (cost can be a significant factor) or socially oriented play groups (transportation costs and availability of inclusive programs are additional compromising factors). Furthermore, adolescents with intellectual disability are often not included by their typically developing peers in extracurricular sports and social activities. Yet, participation in sports or related exercise regimens should be encouraged with all children, as functionally appropriate, because it offers many immediate and long-term benefits, including weight management, development of physical coordination, maintenance of cardiovascular fitness, and improvement of self-image. For some individuals, these needs can be met through the Special Olympics.

Social activities are equally important to the social and emotional development of youth with intellectual disabilities. Such activities should include those with adolescents of the opposite gender and with typically developing youth. These activities, however, need to be based on the youth's functionally adaptive and age-appropriate behaviors. Examples of normalizing activities include participation in summer camps; school dances; school or family trips; dating or socialization in youth groups or school clubs; visits to movies, restaurants, and other socializing establishments; and other typical recreational events. These activities should also include opportunities for increasing social-emotional independence away from direct parental oversight. They should additionally involve exposure to novel experiences in which the individual has the opportunity to test, grapple with, and practice his or her overall adaptive competencies (see Chapter 40). While parental oversight may diminish during this period, sufficient supports are needed to ensure that the adolescent with intellectual disability is not targeted, bullied, or taken advantage of in these settings.

Behavior Therapy

Although most children with intellectual disability do not have behavior disorders, behavior problems do occur with a greater frequency in this population than among children with typical development (Munir, 2016). To facilitate the child's socialization and to avoid limiting academic opportunities, significant behavior problems must be addressed (see Chapter 34). Behavior problems may result from associated neurodevelopmental disorders (e.g., ADHD or sensory disorders); primary or secondary psychiatric disorders (e.g., mood disorders); unrealistic parental expectations; family, financial, or social difficulties; and school-related adjustment difficulties (Deutsch, Dube, & McIlvane, 2008). Many behavior problems result from a mismatch between the demands of the situation and the child's abilities. Often, behavior problems represent attempts by the child to communicate, gain attention, or avoid performing a task. In assessing problematic behavior, one must first consider whether a behavior is appropriate for the child's "cognitive" age rather than for his or her chronological age. The child's chronological age, however, needs to be considered when addressing behavioral challenges in real-life settings. An environmental change, such as a more appropriate classroom, may improve behavior problems for some children; for others, behavior management techniques (see Chapter 34) or the use of psychotropic medication may be appropriate.

Treatment of Comorbid Conditions

Comorbid conditions must be addressed to achieve an optimal outcome for the individual with intellectual disability. Comorbid conditions include, for example, cerebral palsy; sensory impairments; seizure disorders; speech disorders; ADHD; anxiety disorders; depression; ASD; and other disorders of language, behavior, or perception. Treatment of comorbid conditions may require ongoing physical therapy, occupational therapy, speech-language therapy, behavioral therapy, adaptive equipment, eyeglasses, hearing aids, medication, and so forth. Failure to adequately identify and treat these problems may negatively influence functional outcomes and result in difficulties in the home, school, or neighborhood environment.

Use of Medication

Medication is not useful in treating the core symptoms of intellectual disability; no drug has been found to improve cognitive function in these individuals. Medication may be helpful, however, in treating comorbid behavioral and emotional disorders (McQuire, Hassiotis, Harrison, & Pilling, 2015; Risen, Accardo, & Shapiro, 2010). These drugs are generally directed at specific symptom complexes, including ADHD (e.g., stimulants and alpha-2-adrenergic agonists), self-injurious behavior or aggression (e.g., mood stabilizers and neuroleptics), and mood or obsessive-compulsive disorders (e.g., selective serotonin reuptake inhibitors). The properties of these psychopharmaceutical drugs are outlined in Chapter 38. Before long-term therapy with any drug is initiated, a short trial should be conducted. Even if a medication proves successful, its use should be reevaluated at least yearly to assess the need for continued treatment.

Family Counseling

All families benefit from anticipatory guidance regarding their child's health and development, and this is especially true for those families who have children with intellectual disability (Coren, Hutchfield, Thomae, & Gustafsson, 2010). Many families adapt well, but some have significant emotional challenges. Among the factors that have been associated with family coping skills are the severity of the child's disability, number of siblings, stability of the parents' relationship, parental age, mental and physical health of the family, financial stability, expectations and acceptance of the child's diagnosis, supportiveness of the extended family, and availability of community resources and respite care services. In families in which the emotional demands of having a child with intellectual disability are great, family counseling and sibling support groups should be an integral part of the treatment plan (Crnic, Neece, McIntyre, Blacher, & Baker, 2017; see Chapter 37).

Periodic Reevaluation

Since the needs of children and their families change over time, a child's health, learning, and adaptive and behavioral goals must be reassessed periodically, and management programs must be adjusted accordingly. A periodic review should include information about the child's health status as well as his or her functioning at home, at school, and in other social contexts. Other evaluations, such as formal **psychoeducational** testing, may be needed (see Chapter 13). Reevaluation should be undertaken at transition points, at any time the child is not meeting expectations, and when he or she is moving from one service provision system to another. Reevaluations are needed during early childhood and preschool years to ensure that the program remains appropriate as the child matures.

Children with intellectual disability and their families experience many transitions. Among the predictable transition points are 1) from recognition to identification, 2) from identification to diagnosis, 3) from diagnosis to intervention, 4) from intervention to primary education, 5) from early elementary school to later elementary school, 6) from elementary to middle school, 7) from middle school to high school, and 8) from high school to post high school (including specialized college program for individuals with ID).

Transition programs for typical adolescents center on the move from pediatric to adult health services. For adolescents with intellectual disability (and other developmental disabilities), this transition is more complex. IDEA (2004) requires that all students with an individualized education program begin transition planning before the student is 16 years old and that the plan is based on the student's individual needs, strengths, skills, and interests (see Chapter 33). Among the domains that should be addressed in a complete transition plan are 1) self-determination and decision making, 2) transition of health care (including needed therapies), 3) transition of mental health services, 4) home living, 5) community living, 6) continuing education, 7) employment, 8) leisure and socialization, 9) protection from exploitation, and 10) legal (including parental wills, estate planning, and trusts) services (Neece, Kraemer, & Blacher, 2009; Seo, Shogren, Wehmeyer, Little, & Palmer 2017).

Additional factors that complicate transition into adulthood for individuals with intellectual disability are the termination of the entitlement to education and related services afforded by IDEA and a lack of availability of case management services that help coordinate across therapeutic domains.

OUTCOME

Except for individuals with severe-profound intellectual disability, IQ scores alone are not good predictors of outcome. Outcome instead depends on the interplay of many factors including 1) the underlying cause of the intellectual disability; 2) the degree of functional disability; 3) the presence of comorbid conditions (such as epilepsy) and behavior problems; 4) the capabilities of the family; and 5) the supports, community services, and training provided to the child and family (Patel, Greydanus, Calles, & Pratt, 2010).

As adults, many people with mild intellectual disability are able to gain functional literacy and some economic and social independence and only require intermittent supports (Seltzer et al., 2009). Adults with mild intellectual disability show impairments in abstract thinking, executive function, short-term memory, and functional academics. Communication, conversation, language, and social judgement may be more immature than expected for age, and limited understanding of risk in social situations is common (APA, 2013). Support for health care decisions and legal matters is often required. Such adults may need periodic assistance, especially when under social or economic stress. Some marry and live successfully in the community, either independently or in supervised settings (Felce et al., 2008). Life expectancy usually is not adversely affected.

For individuals with moderate intellectual disability, the goals of education are to enhance adaptive abilities, functional academics, and vocational skills to ensure that these individuals are better able to live in the adult world (Totsika, Felce, Kerr, & Hastings, 2010). Academic skill development is typically at an elementary school level. Social and communicative behavior is markedly different from typical peers, but enduring friendships may be established. Personal care and household tasks require instruction, and reminders may be needed. Contemporary gains, including supported employment, have benefited these individuals the most. Supported employment challenges the view that prerequisite skills must be taught before there can be successful vocational adaptation. Instead, individuals are trained by a coach to do a specific job in

ETHICAL CONSIDERATIONS

The rights of an individual with intellectual disability have not always been considered in our society, and this was an ethical failure. Individuals with intellectual disability were segregated in schools for the "retarded"; they were deprived of advanced medical care (such as transplants), experimented on without their consent, and their civil rights were not respected (sterilization). Fortunately, the civil rights movement in the 1960s also benefited people with disabilities. There was the integration of children with disabilities into typical classes, the requirement of consent by the individual (or primary caregiver) for medical or research procedures, and the provision of other basic rights that all citizens should have.

the setting in which the person works. This approach bypasses the need for extended time mastering "prerequisite skills" and has resulted in successful work adaptation in the community for many people with intellectual disability. Outcome studies have documented the benefits and effectiveness of this approach (Stephens, Collins, & Dodder, 2005). People with intellectual disability requiring limited support (e.g., individuals with Down syndrome) generally live at home or in a supervised setting in the community.

As adults, people with severe to profound intellectual disability require extensive to pervasive support in activities of daily living, decision making, and communication. They may, however, perform simple tasks in supervised settings. These individuals often have comorbid conditions such as cerebral palsy, seizure disorders, and sensory impairments that further limit their adaptive functioning, yet most people with this level of intellectual disability are able to live in the community with supportive adaptations in their environment and with supervisory oversight. Family-based, community-supported care is preferable to institutional care for these individuals, but it is often difficult to achieve for a variety of reasons (e.g., parents' advanced ages, lack of financial support, familial or community resistance, and comorbid conditions). As a result, some of these individuals with severe medical problems, major behavioral disturbances, or disrupted families require out-of-home living in such settings as foster homes, alternative living units, group homes, nursing homes, or residential schools. People who require extensive or pervasive supports have increased utilization of medical and behavioral health care and often have a shortened life span (Kilgour, Starr, & Whalley, 2010).

SUMMARY

- Development is an ordered process that is linked to the maturation of the central nervous system.
- With intellectual disability, development is altered so that intellectual and adaptive skills are impaired.
- In most cases of mild intellectual disability, the underlying cause is unclear and may be tied to environmental effects.
- In individuals with severe intellectual disability there is usually a definable biologic, often genetic, cause.
- Most people with intellectual disability have a mild degree of impairment, require only intermittent support, and are often able to achieve some degree of economic and social independence.
- The early identification of a global developmental delay is important to ensure appropriate treatment and to enable the child to develop and use all of his or her capabilities.
- Treatment should be multimodal, supporting the education, mental and physical health, adaptive behavior, and communication skills of individuals with intellectual disability.

ADDITIONAL RESOURCES

American Association on Intellectual and Developmental Disabilities: http://aaidd.org/

The Arc of the United States: http://thearc.org

President's Committee for People with Intellectual Disabilities: http://www.acf.hhs.gov/programs/pcpid/index.html

Additional resources can be found online in Appendix D: Childhood Disabilities Resources, Services, and Organizations (see About the Online Companion Materials).

REFERENCES

American Psychiatric Association. (2000). *Diagnostic and statistical manual of mental disorders* (4th ed.) Washington, DC: Author.

American Psychiatric Association. (2013). *Diagnostic and statistical manual of mental disorders* (5th ed.) Washington, DC: Author.

Andrews, J., Falkmer, M., & Girdler, S. (2015). Community participation interventions for children and adolescents with a neurodevelopmental intellectual disability: A systematic review. *Disability and Rehabilitation, 37*(10), 825–833. doi:10.3109/09638288.2014.944625

Barkovich, A. J., & Raybaud, C. A. (2004). Malformations of cortical development. *Neuroimaging Clinics of North America, 14*(3), 401–423.

Barnhill, J., Cooper, S.-A., & Fletcher, R. J. (2017). *Diagnostic Manual-Intellectual Disability 2 (DM-ID): A textbook of diagnosis of mental disorders in persons with intellectual disability* (2nd ed.). Kingston, NY: NADD Press.

Bayley, N. (2006). *Bayley Scales of Infant Development: Third edition manual.* San Antonio, TX: Harcourt Assessment.

Bertelli, M. O., Munir, K., Harris, J., & Salvador-Carulla, L. (2016). "Intellectual developmental disorders": Reflections on the international consensus document for redefining "mental retardation-intellectual disability" in ICD-11. *Advances in Mental Health and Intellectual Disabilities, 10*(1), 36–58. doi:10.1108/AMHID-10-2015-0050

Bloom, A. S., & Zelko, F. A. (1994). Variability in adaptive behavior in children with developmental delay. *Journal of Clinical Psychology, 50,* 261–265.

Bourke, J., de Klerk, N., Smith, T., & Leonard, H. (2016). Population-based prevalence of intellectual disability and autism spectrum disorders in Western Australia:

A comparison with previous estimates. *Medicine, 95*(21), e3737. doi:10.1097/MD.0000000000003737

Boyle, C. A., Boulet, S., Schieve, L. A., Cohen, R. A., Blumberg, S. J., Yeargin-Allsopp, M., . . . Kogan, M. D. (2011). Trends in the prevalence of developmental disabilities in US children, 1997–2008. *Pediatrics, 127*(6), 1034–1042.

Bruininks, R. H., Woodcock, R. W., Weatherman, R. F., & Hill, B. K. (1996). *Scales of Independent Behavior–Revised (SIB-R).* Chicago, IL: Riverside Publishing.

Canadian Task Force on Preventive Health Care. (2016). Recommendations on screening for developmental delay. *Canadian Medical Association Journal, 188*(8), 579–587. doi:10.1503/cmaj.151437

Centers for Disease Control and Prevention. (1996). State-specific rates of mental retardation—United States, 1993. *Morbidity and Mortality Weekly Report, 45*(3), 61–65.

Cooper, S. A., & van der Speck, R. (2009). Epidemiology of mental ill health in adults with intellectual disabilities. *Current Opinion in Psychiatry, 22*(5), 431–436. doi:10.1097/YCO.0b013e32832e2a1e.

Coren, E., Hutchfield, J., Thomae, M., & Gustafsson, C. (2010). Parent training support for intellectually disabled parents. *Cochrane Database of Systematic Reviews, 16*(6), CD007987.

Crnic, K. A., Neece, C. L., McIntyre, L. L., Blacher, J., & Baker, B. L. (2017). Intellectual disability and developmental risk: Promoting intervention to improve child and family well-being. *Child Development, 88*(2), 436–445. doi:10.1111/cdev.12740

Crocker, A. G., Prokić, A., Morin, D., & Reyes, A. (2014). Intellectual disability and co-occurring mental health and physical disorders in aggressive behaviour. *Journal of Intellectual Disability Research, 58*(11), 1032–1044. doi:10.1111/jir.12080. PMID: 23952483

De Souza, E., Halliday, J., Chan, A., Bower, C., & Morris, J. K. (2009). Recurrence risks for trisomies 13, 18, and 21. *American Journal of Medical Genetics Part A, 149A*(12), 2716–2722.

Deutsch, C. K., Dube, W. V., & McIlvane, W. J. (2008). Attention deficits, attention-deficit/hyperactivity disorder, and intellectual disabilities. *Developmental Disabilities Research Reviews, 14*(4), 285–292.

Felce, D., Perry, J., Romeo, R., Robertson, J., Meek, A., Emerson, E., & Knapp, M. (2008). Outcomes and costs of community living: Semi-independent living and fully staffed group homes. *American Journal of Mental Retardation, 113*(2), 87–101.

Fletcher, R., Loschen, E., Stavrakaki, C., & First, M. (2007). *Diagnostic Manual-Intellectual disability (DM-ID): A clinical guide for diagnosis of mental disorders in persons with intellectual disability.* Kingston, NY: NADD Press.

Gardner, H. (1983). *Frames of mind: The theory of multiple intelligences.* New York, NY: Basic Books.

Gropman, A. L., & Batshaw, M. L. (2010). Epigenetics, copy number variation, and other molecular mechanisms underlying neurodevelopmental disabilities: New insights and diagnostic approaches. *Journal of Developmental and Behavioral Pediatrics, 31*(7), 582–591.

Harrison, P. L., & Oakland, T. (2015). *Adaptive Behavior Assessment System-3.* San Antonio, TX: Pearson.

Heikura, U., Taanila, A., Olsen, P., Hartikainen, A. L., von Wendt, L., & Järvelin, M. R. (2003). Temporal changes in incidence and prevalence of intellectual disability between two birth cohorts in Northern Finland. *American Journal of Mental Retardation, 108*(1), 19–31.

Hoyme, H. E., Kalberg, W. O., Elliott, A. J., Blankenship, J., Buckley, D., Marais, A. S., . . . May, P. A. (2016). Updated clinical guidelines for diagnosing fetal alcohol spectrum disorders. *Pediatrics, 138*(2), e20154256. doi:10.1542/peds.2015-4256.

Individuals with Disabilities Education Improvement Act of 2004, PL 108–446, 20 U.S. §1400 *et seq.*

Jacquemont, S., Farzin, F., Hall, D., Leehey, M., Tassone, F., Gane., L., . . . Hagerman, R. J. (2004). Aging in individuals with the FMR1 mutation. *American Journal on Mental Retardation, 109*(2), 154–164.

Karam, S. M., Barros, A. J. D., Matijasevich, A., Dos Santos, I. S., Anselmi, L., Barros, F., . . . Black, M. M. (2016). Intellectual disability in a birth cohort: Prevalence, etiology, and determinants at the age of 4 years. *Public Health Genomics, 19*(5), 290–297. doi:10.1159/000448912

Karam, S. M., Riegel, M., Segal, S. L., et al. (2015). Genetic causes of intellectual disability in a birth cohort: A population-based study. *American Journal of Medical Genetics Part A, 167*(6), 1204–1214. doi:10.1002/ajmg.a.37011

Kilgour, A. H., Starr, J. M., & Whalley, L. J. (2010). Associations between childhood intelligence (IQ), adult morbidity and mortality. *Maturitas, 65*(2), 98–105.

Klaiman, C., Quintin, E.-M., Jo, B., Lightbody, A. A., Hazlett, H. C., Piven, J., . . . Reiss, A. L. (2014). Longitudinal profiles of adaptive behavior in fragile X syndrome. *Pediatrics, 134*(2), 315–324. doi:10.1542/peds.2013-3990

McQuire, C., Hassiotis, A., Harrison, B., & Pilling, S. (2015). Pharmacological interventions for challenging behaviour in children with intellectual disabilities: A systematic review and meta-analysis. *BMC Psychiatry, 15,* 303. doi:10.1186/s12888-015-0688-2. PMID:26611280. PMCID:PMC4662033

Mefford, H. C., Batshaw, M. L., & Hoffman, E. P. (2012). Genomics, intellectual disability, and autism. *The New England Journal of Medicine, 366*(8), 733–743. doi:10.1056/NEJMra1114194

Mendola, P., Selevan, S. G., Gutter, S., & Rice, D. (2002). Environmental factors associated with a spectrum of neurodevelopmental deficits. *Mental Retardation and Developmental Disabilities Research Reviews, 8*(3), 188–197.

Moeschler, J. B., Shevell, M., & American Academy of Pediatrics Committee on Genetics. (2006). Clinical genetic evaluation of the child with mental retardation or developmental delays. *Pediatrics, 117,* 2304–2316.

Moeschler, J. B., Shevell, M., & American Academy of Pediatrics Committee on Genetics. (2014). Comprehensive evaluation of the child with intellectual disability or global developmental delay. *Pediatrics, 134*(3), e903–e918. doi:10.1542/peds.2014-1839

Msall, M. E. (2005). Measuring functional skills in preschool children at risk for neurodevelopmental disabilities. *Mental Retardation and Developmental Disability Research Reviews, 11*(3), 263–273.

Msall, M. E., Avery, R. C., Tremont, M. R., Lima, J. C., Rogers, M. L., & Hogan, D. P. (2003). Functional disability and school activity limitations in 41,300 school-age children: Relationship to medical impairments. *Pediatrics, 111*(3), 548–53. PMID: 12612235

Munir, K. M. (2016). The co-occurrence of mental disorders in children and adolescents with intellectual disability/intellectual developmental disorder. *Current Opinion in Psychiatry, 29*(2), 95–102. doi:10.1097/YCO.0000000000000236

Neece, C. L., Kraemer, B. R., & Blacher, J. (2009). Transition satisfaction and family well being among parents of young adults with severe intellectual disability. *Intellectual and Developmental Disabilities, 47*(1), 31–43.

Oeseburg, B., Jansen, D. E., Dijkstra, G. J., Groothoff, J. W., & Reijneveld, S. A. (2010a). Prevalence of chronic diseases in adolescents with intellectual disability. *Research in Developmental Disabilities, 31*(3), 698–704. doi:10.1016/j.ridd.2010.01.011. PMID: 20188511

Oeseburg, B., Jansen, D. E., Groothoff, J. W., Dijkstra, G. J., & Reijneveld, S. A. (2010b). Emotional and behavioural problems in adolescents with intellectual disability with and without chronic diseases. *Journal of Intellectual Disabilities Research, 54*(1), 81–89. doi:10.1111/j.1365-2788.2009.01231.x. PMID: 20122098

Oeseburg, B., Dijkstra, G. J., Groothoff, J. W., Reijneveld, S. A., & Jansen, D. E. (2011). Prevalence of chronic health conditions in children with intellectual disability: A systematic literature review. *Intellectual and Developmental Disabilities, 49*(2), 59–85.

Oliver, C, & Richards, C. (2015). Practitioner review: Self-injurious behaviour in children with developmental delay. *Journal of Child Psychology and Psychiatry, 56*(10), 1042–1054. doi:10.1111/jcpp.12425. PMID: 25916173

Patel, D. R., & Greydanus, D. E. (2010). Sport participation by physically and cognitively challenged young athletes. *Pediatric Clinics of North America, 57*(3), 795–817.

Patel, D. R., Greydanus, D. E., Calles, J. L., Jr., & Pratt, H. D. (2010). Developmental disabilities across the lifespan. *Disease-a-Month, 56*(6), 304–397.

Peyre, H., Charkaluk, M. L., Forhan, A., Heude, B., & Ramus, F. (2017). EDEN Mother–Child Cohort Study Group. Do developmental milestones at 4, 8, 12 and 24 months predict IQ at 5-6 years old? Results of the EDEN mother-child cohort. *European Journal of Paediatric Neurology, 21*(2), 272–279. doi:10.1016/j.ejpn.2016.11.001

Reichenberg, A., Cederlöf, M., McMillan, A., Trzaskowski, M., Kapra, O., Fruchter, E., . . Lichenstein, P. (2016). Discontinuity in the genetic and environmental causes of the intellectual disability spectrum. *Proceedings of the National Academy of Sciences of the United States of America, 113*(4), 1098–1103. doi:10.1073/pnas.1508093112

Riou, E. M., Ghosh, S., Francoeur, E., & Shevell, M. I. (2009). Global developmental delay and its relationship to cognitive skills. *Developmental Medicine and Child Neurology, 5*(8), 600–606.

Risen, S., Accardo, P. J., & Shapiro, B. K. (2010). A clinical approach to the pharmacological management of behavioral disturbance in intellectual disability. In B. K. Shapiro & P. J. Accardo (Eds.), *Neurogenetic syndromes: Behavioral issues and their treatment* (pp.185–216). Baltimore, MD: Paul H. Brookes Publishing Co.

Robertson, J., Hatton, C., Emerson, E., & Baines, S. (2015). Prevalence of epilepsy among people with intellectual disabilities: A systematic review. *Seizure, 29*, 46–62. doi:10.1016/j.seizure.2015.03.016. PMID:26076844

Roid, G. (2003). *Stanford-Binet Intelligence Scales, Fifth Edition (SB5).* Chicago, IL: Riverside Publishing.

Rump, P., Jazayeri, O., van Dijk-Bos, K. K., Johansson, L. F., van Essen, A. J., Verheij, J. B., . . . Sikkema-Raddatz, B. (2016). Whole-exome sequencing is a powerful approach for establishing the etiological diagnosis in patients with intellectual disability and microcephaly. *BMC Medical Genomics, 9*, 7. doi:10.1186/s12920-016-0167-8

Schalock, R., Borthwick-Duffy, S. A., Buntinx, W. H. E., Coulter, D. L., & Ellis, M. C. (2009). *Intellectual disability: Definition, classification, and systems of support* (11th ed.). Washington, DC: American Association on Intellectual and Developmental Disabilities.

Seltzer, M. M., Floyd, F. J., Greenberg, J. S., Hong, J., Taylor, J. L., & Doescher, H. (2009). Factors predictive of midlife occupational attainment and psychological functioning in adults with mild intellectual deficits. *American Journal of Intellectual and Developmental Disability, 114*(2), 128–143.

Seo, H., Shogren, K. A., Wehmeyer, M. L., Little, T. D., & Palmer, S. B. (2017). The impact of medical/behavioral support needs on the supports needed by adolescents with intellectual disability to participate in community life. *American Journal on Intellectual and Developmental Disabilities, 122*, 173–191. doi:10.1352/1944-7558-122.2.173

Shapiro, B., & Batshaw, M. (2016). Intellectual disability. In R. Kliegman, B. Stanton, J. W. St. Geme, N. F. Schor, & R. E. Behrman (Eds.), *Nelson textbook of pediatrics* (20th ed.; pp. 216–222). Philadelphia, PA: Elsevier.

Shapiro, B. K., & Batshaw, M. L. (2002). Mental retardation. In F. D. Burg, J. R. Ingelfinger, R. A. Polin, & A. A. Gershon (Eds.), *Gellis and Kagan's current pediatric therapy* (17th ed.) (pp. 309–402). Philadelphia, PA: W.B. Saunders.

Sparrow, S. S., Crichetti, D. V., & Saulner, C. A. (2016). *Vineland Adaptive Behavior Scales, Third Edition (Vineland-3).* San Antonio, TX: Pearson.

Stephens, D. L., Collins, M. D., & Dodder, R. A. (2005). A longitudinal study of employment and skill acquisition among individuals with developmental disabilities. *Research in Developmental Disabilities, 26*(5), 469–486.

Totsika, V., Felce, D., Kerr, M., & Hastings, R. P. (2010). Behavior problems, psychiatric symptoms, and quality of life for older adults with intellectual disability with and without autism. *Journal of Autism and Developmental Disorders, 40*(10), 1171–1178.

Van Naarden Braun, K., Christensen, D., Doernberg, N., Schieve, L., Rice, C., Wiggins, L., ... Yeargin-Allsopp, M. (2015). Trends in the prevalence of autism spectrum disorder, cerebral palsy, hearing loss, intellectual disability, and vision impairment, Metropolitan Atlanta, 1991–2010. *PLoS ONE, 10*(4), e0124120. doi:10.1371/journal.pone.0124120

Verdonschot, M. M., de Witte, L. P., Reichrath, E., Buntinx, W. H., & Curfs, L. M. (2009). Community participation of people with an intellectual disability: A review of empirical findings. *Journal of Intellectual Disability Research, 53*(4), 303–318.

Wang, P. P., & Bellugi, U. (1993). Williams syndrome, Down syndrome, and cognitive neuroscience. *American Journal of Diseases of Childhood, 147*, 1246–1251.

Wechsler, D. (2012). *Wechsler Preschool and Primary Scale of Intelligence–Fourth Eedition.* San Antonio, TX: The Psychological Corporation.

Wechsler, D. (2015). *Wechsler Intelligence Scale for Children–Fifth Edition.* San Antonio, TX: NCS Pearson.

Wehmeyer, M. L., Brown, I., Percy, M., Shogren, K. A., & Lung, W-L. A. (2017). *A comprehensive guide to intellectual & developmental disabilities* (2nd ed.). Baltimore, MD: Paul H. Brookes Publishing Co.

Zahir, F. R., Mwenifumbo, J. C., Chun, H.-J. E., Lim, E. L., Van Karnebeekk C. D. M., Couse, M., . . . Marra, M. A. (2017). Comprehensive whole genome sequence analyses yields novel genetic and structural insights for intellectual disability. *BMC Genomics, 18*, 403. doi:10.1186/s12864-017-3671-0

CHAPTER **15**

Down Syndrome and Fragile X Syndrome

Elizabeth Berry-Kravis, Katherine Myers, and Nancy J. Roizen

After completion of this chapter, the reader will

- Recognize the physical characteristics of Down syndrome
- Be aware of the substantial increase in life expectancy in individuals with Down syndrome
- Identify the health issues that are common in children with Down syndrome
- Appreciate the increased incidence of autism in children with Down syndrome
- Know the clinical differences between a premutation and full mutation for fragile X syndrome
- Be alert to the physical findings of fragile X syndrome
- Be able to identify the clinical presentation of fragile X syndrome
- Have an approach to treating the medical and behavioral problems found in fragile X syndrome

Down syndrome (DS) is the most common chromosomal **etiology** (cause) of intellectual disability, while fragile X syndrome (FXS) is the most common inherited form of intellectual disability (ID). In this chapter, DS and FSX are discussed in depth because they are associated with multiple medical problems, as well as behavior challenges that require identification and intervention.

DS was one of the first symptom complexes associated with ID to be identified as a syndrome. In 1866, Dr. John Langdon Down, for whom the syndrome is named, published the first compete physical description of DS, which included a similarity of facial features among affected individuals (Down, 1866). Nearly 100 years later, in 1959, researchers identified the underlying chromosomal abnormality—an additional chromosome 21—that causes DS (Lejeune, Gautier, & Turpin, 1959). More recently, in 2000, an international collaborative group of scientists completed the genomic sequence of HSA21q (the long arm of chromosome 21, which accounts for the findings of the syndrome) (Hattori et al., 2000).

FXS is the most common cause of X-linked ID (Lubs, Stevenson, & Schwartz, 2012). It was initially identified in 1943, when Martin and Bell described a family with 11 males across two generations with an X-linked form of ID, which came to be known as Martin-Bell syndrome (Martin & Bell, 1943). In 1969, researchers developed a cytogenetic (chromosome) test that identified a break or constriction of a region of the X chromosome, which was initially referred to a "marker X" and was later referred to a "fragile X" (Lubs, 1969). In 1991, a gene associated with multiple CGG nucleotide repeats was identified that coincided with the fragile X site. It was named the *fragile X mental retardation 1* [*FMR1*] gene and became the basis of a new, more accurate test for FXS (Verkerk et al., 1991). In 2001, a fragile X–associated tremor/ataxia syndrome was discovered (FXTAS; Hagerman et al., 2001).

CASE STUDY

Jerome is a 13-year-old boy with DS. He experiences complex behavioral problems as well as bilateral mild to moderate hearing loss, obesity, sleep apnea, enuresis (lack of urinary control), refractive errors, and mild gastroesophageal reflux disease (*GERD*). On psychoeducational testing at 6 years of age, he had a full-scale intelligence quotient (IQ) of 50. ADHD was diagnosed and he began stimulant medication, which helped with inattention and impulsivity. By 8 years of age, all observers reported anxiety with transitions, panic attacks, and melt downs with aggression at school, which improved with a selective serotonin reuptake inhibitor (SSRI). However, by 10 years of age he was not functioning well at school, and his family moved him to a state-developed homeschool program. He is functioning well with counseling, medication, as well as careful management of social opportunities. Now, at 14 years of age, there are issues with medical treatment. Fortunately, his hearing loss has not progressed, but Jerome refuses to wear his hearing aids. His obesity has increased. Sleep apnea improved with tonsillectomy and adenoidectomy. His enuresis (urinary incontinence) was treated with medication and has resolved. He wears glasses. His GERD has also resolved.

CASE STUDY

James is a 20-year-old young man who had an uneventful birth, delayed early motor development, and a mild strabismus (weak eye muscles) noted in the first year of life that was managed with patching and glasses. He walked at 15 months; was able to say only a few words by age 2; and had recurrent ear infections, which were initially thought to be the cause of his language delay. The delay persisted after myringotomy tube placement (see Chapter 26), however, and he did not talk in phrases until age 4. He was treated with speech and occupational therapy and evaluated for developmental delay by a specialist, who noted him to have flat feet but otherwise unremarkable physical features. Subsequent testing of cognitive and adaptive skills confirmed that James had moderate ID. Genetic testing revealed an *FMR1* full mutation consistent with a diagnosis of FXS. Behavior became very hyperactive around age 3, and he was hypersensitive to sounds and had tactile defensiveness. His attention ability was limiting at school, and so at age 5 he was started on stimulant medication, which improved his ability to stay at his seat and be on task. He performed at about half his age level at school, with particular problems with writing and math, but he had better, though still delayed, visual memory and reading skills. He had a special education program with partial inclusion through high school. He was better able to control hyperactive behavior as he became older, but by high school age, he was anxious about performing school work, resisted going out to do new things, did not like crowds, and seemed to be more reclusive. He would sometimes become upset and aggressive when things did not go his way. His anxiety and aggression were improved with treatment with an SSRI (see Chapter 27), which also allowed better ability to participate in his vocational training at job sites.

Thought Questions:

How do children with DS compare to those with FXS in factors of genetics, behavioral issues, and ID? How are medical complications similar for children with DS and FXS?

DOWN SYNDROME

Prevalence

DS is the most common chromosomal abnormality diagnosed in the United States. With increased births to older mothers and elective terminations of pregnancies, the overall birth prevalence has been steady at about 1 in 700 births. With advances in medical care, the median life expectancy has increased from 4 years in 1950 to 58 years in 2010 (de Graaf, Buckley, & Skotko, 2015).

Physical Characteristics

The distinct physical features of DS include 1) low muscle tone (infants appear "floppy"); 2) flat facial features with a small nose; 3) an upward slant to the eyes; 4) small skin folds on the inner corner of the eyes; 5) small, atypically shaped ears; and 6) a single deep crease across the center of the palm (Jones, Jones, & del Campo, 2013). Medical complications affect almost every body organ system and are described in greater detail below (Bull & American Academy of Pediatrics Committee on Genetics, 2011). They include congenital heart defects; endocrine abnormalities; sensory impairments; growth and obesity problems; dental concerns; gastrointestinal (GI), renal, and urinary tract abnormalities; epilepsy; hematologic disorders; and skin conditions. In addition, there are cognitive deficits, including mild to moderate ID and a later risk of Alzheimer disease, and neurobehavioral issues.

Chromosomal Findings

DS occurs due to chromosomal abnormalities in chromosome 21. Specifically, three types of abnormalities result in extra copies of the DS area of chromosome 21: Trisomy of chromosome 21 accounts for approximately 94% of the cases, translocation for 4.3%, and mosaicism for 2.1% (Jones et al., 2013; see Chapter 1).

Medical complications occur with similar frequency in the three types of the chromosomal abnormalities. Studies indicate that children with translocation DS do not differ cognitively from those with trisomy 21. By contrast, children with mosaic DS, perhaps because not all cells are affected, on average score higher on IQ tests than those with trisomy 21 or translocation DS (Fischler & Koch, 1991).

Early Identification

The American College of Obstetricians and Gynecologists recommends that all pregnant women should be offered screening before 20 weeks' gestation and diagnostic testing for DS if desired (Carmichael et al., 2017; Gill, Quezada, Revello, Akolekar, & Nicolaides, 2015; see Chapter 3). After birth, if there are signs of DS, diagnosis can be evaluated by chromosome analysis (karyotype) of the blood. Common signs in more than 75% of newborns include oblique (slanted) palpebral fissures (eye openings), a wide space between the first and second toes, increased neck tissue, hypotonia (low muscle tone), and a flat facial profile (Jones et al., 2013).

Medical Problems

Children with DS have an increased risk of abnormalities in almost every organ system (Bull & American Academy of Pediatrics Committee on Genetics, 2011). Knowledge of these possible medical complications enables the health care provider to evaluate the child for the more common conditions (e.g., congenital heart malformation, hearing problems, vision problems, and obstructive sleep apnea). Health care providers should also monitor, (e.g., thyroid problems, hemoglobin, and growth), prevent (e.g., gingivitis and obesity), and be vigilant for symptoms of other medical problems (e.g., diabetes and urological abnormalities). There is a risk for **diagnostic overshadowing** (presuming that symptoms are simply a consequence of the DS) that can lead to postponing or missing a diagnosis. DS clinics with physicians and other professionals involved in the care of children and adults with DS can help evaluate concerns and problems, taking into consideration the contribution of medical, behavioral, and developmental factors (Box 15.1).

Obstructive Sleep Apnea and Airway Concerns

Obstructive sleep apnea is when breathing intermittently stops when the airway is blocked. Symptoms include snoring, apnea, restless sleep, daytime sleepiness, frequent night awakenings, and behavior problems. Although pneumonia and other airway problems are not usually considered in the system review in children with DS, they are the most common reason for children with DS to be admitted to the hospital and the leading cause of excess mortality (McDowell & Craven, 2011).

Hearing Problems As many as 26% of newborns with DS fail their newborn hearing screen, and after diagnostic evaluation the prevalence of congenital hearing loss is estimated at 15%–20% in newborns (Tedeschi et al., 2015). In addition, children with DS who pass their newborn hearing screen can still develop conductive, sensorineural, and mixed hearing loss (see Chapter 26).

BOX 15.1 INTERDISCIPLINARY CARE

The Clinic Coordinator

For a Down syndrome clinic, the clinic coordinator, often a social worker or a nurse, is the person who helps parents keep track of the needed evaluations, monitoring, their outcomes, and follow-ups so that the parents are supported in their pursuit of optimal care for their child.

In school-age children, 22%–30% experience transient hearing loss with frequent **otitis media** (OM) and 24.9% have a permanent hearing loss, most frequently bilateral (75.4%) and conductive (33.3%) (Nightengale, Yoon, Wolter-Warmerdam, Daniels, & Hickey, 2017).

Vision Problems Deficits in **visual acuity** (nearsightedness or farsightedness) occur in 30%–62% of DS cases, with **amblyopia** (loss of vision with brain suppressing vision) occurring in 3%–20% of cases of DS. Other eye conditions like **strabismus** (crossed eyes; 20%–60%) and **nystagmus** (jiggling of the eyes; 10%–20%), as well as cataracts, are also found more frequently than in the general population (Creavin & Brown, 2009; Roizen, Mets, & Blondis, 1994).

Congenital Heart Defects In children with DS, 44% have congenital heart defects, the most common being **endocardial cushion defect** (resulting in connection between the two upper chambers, or atria, of the heart and the two lower chambers, or ventricles, of the heart; 30%), followed by **atrial septal defect** (connection between the two upper chambers; 25%), and **ventricular septal defect** (a connection between the two lower chambers; 22%) (Stoll, Dott, Alembik, & Roth, 2015).

Dental Problems The most serious dental problem common among children with DS is early-onset **periodontal disease** (disease of tissue surrounding the gums), which involves **gingivitis** (gum inflammation) and regression of the bone that anchors the teeth. In addition, children with DS are more likely than their healthy peers to have delayed eruption and **malocclusions** (abnormal contact of opposing teeth). Many individuals with DS have dental anomalies (e.g., fused teeth; **microdontia,** or small teeth; and missing teeth) and **bruxism** (teeth grinding). Interestingly, children with DS are less affected by dental **caries** (cavities) than are typically developing children (58% versus 78%; Dieguez-Perez, de Nova-Garcia, Mourelle-Martinez, & Bartolome-Villar, 2016).

Thyroid Disease Newborns with DS have an increased prevalence of congenital hypothyroidism (in-born deficiency of thyroid hormone production) resulting from impaired development of the thyroid gland. Hypothyroidism needing supplemental thyroid therapy has been identified in 17.5% of newborns (Purdy, Singh, Brown, Vangala, & Devaskar, 2014). The incidence increases with age, with perhaps 24% having a thyroid disorder by 10 years of age and 50% by adulthood (Iughetti et al., 2014; Pierce, Fanchi, & Pinter, 2017). Although hypothyroidism predominates, hyperthyroidism (excess thyroid hormone production) associated with Hashimoto's thyroiditis (an inflammatory condition of the thyroid gland) is also found.

Seizures and Neurological Problems Children with DS are at risk for a variety of neurologic problems, including seizures and strokes. A survey of more than 350 children and adolescents with DS revealed epileptic seizures in 8%, of which 47% were partial seizures, 32% were infantile spasms, and 21% were generalized tonic-clonic seizures (Goldberg-Stern et al., 2001; see Chapter 22). Moyamoya disease (blocked arteries at the base of the brain) is a rare progressive disorder that is associated with strokes. Of children less than 15 years of age admitted to the hospital with moyamoya, 9.5% have DS (Kainth, Chaudhry, Kainth, Suri, & Qureshi, 2013).

Celiac Disease and Gastrointestinal Problems GI problems are increased in DS and include celiac disease, constipation, congenital GI malformations, and gastroesophageal reflux. **Celiac disease,** sensitivity to wheat and other grains, is reported in at least 5% of children with DS (Szaflarska-Popolawska et al., 2016). Congenital GI malformations are found in 6% of children with DS, most frequently presenting in the newborn period with poor feeding, vomiting, or aspiration pneumonia. The most common malformations are **duodenal** (first section of the intestine) stenosis (narrowing) or **atresia** (blockage) (67%); imperforate (closed) anus (14%); and Hirschsprung disease (lack of innervation of the colon; 14%) (Stoll et al., 2015).

Obesity and Growth Although children with DS are proportional at birth, they frequently become lighter for their height initially and then gain proportionally more weight compared with height. Eventually 47.8% develop obesity (defined as a body mass index [BMI] greater than 95%) compared with 12.1% in a community sample (Basil et al., 2016). There can also be problems with poor gain in weight and/or height related to medical conditions like congenital heart failure or celiac disease.

Leukemias and Anemia Leukemias are the most common cancer in children with DS and account for 97% of all malignancy in children with DS 15 years of age or younger. Individuals with DS have a 10- to 20-fold higher relative risk than the general population, with a cumulative risk of 2% by 5 years of age (Rabin & Whitlock, 2009). Children with DS have low dietary intake of iron (Luke, Sutton, Schoeller, & Roizen, 1996). Iron deficiency or iron deficiency anemia are found in 10% of this population (Dixon et al., 2010).

Orthopedic Problems Orthopedic problems can be painful and interfere with function. Problems include hip subluxation (instability and dislocation of the hip joint), **patellar** (knee cap) and other joint instability, and **pes planus** (flat feet). The most perplexing and potentially serious problem is **atlantoaxial instability** (partial subluxation of the upper spine; Figure 15.1), which occurs in 10%–30% of individuals with DS as a result of atlanto-occipital and atlantoaxial hypermobility; about 2% of these are symptomatic (Bull & American Academy of Pediatrics Committee on Genetics, 2011).

Other Frequent Medical Problems Children with DS also may experience type I diabetes, rheumatoid arthritis, alopecia (hair loss), vitiligo (loss of pigment in skin), testicular cancer, and urologic and renal disorders. In children with DS, type I diabetes has a 4.2-fold increased prevalence compared with the general population (Bergholdt, Eising, Nerup, & Pociot, 2006; Whooten, Schmitt, & Schwartz, 2017). Juvenile idiopathic arthritis is six times higher than in the general pediatric population and is associated with joint subluxation in half of the cases. The average delay from symptom onset to diagnosis is 2 years (Juj & Emery, 2009); this is a good example of diagnostic overshadowing. Testicular cancer is the only solid tumor in DS with an increased incidence (Hasle, Friedman, Olsen, & Rasmussen, 2016). The spectrum of renal and urologic malformations occurs in 3.2% of the DS population, with an odds ratio of 4.5 compared with the general population (Kupferman, Cruschel, & Kupchik, 2009).

Evaluation and Treatment of Medical Complications

Since children with DS may have increased risk for medical problems, as discussed above, medical providers must ensure that they are engaging in evaluation, screening, and prevention for common conditions. They must remain vigilant for symptoms of these or other medical complications throughout their work with children with DS. Recommendations for preventive health care for children and adolescents with DS are outlined below and summarized in Figure 15.2.

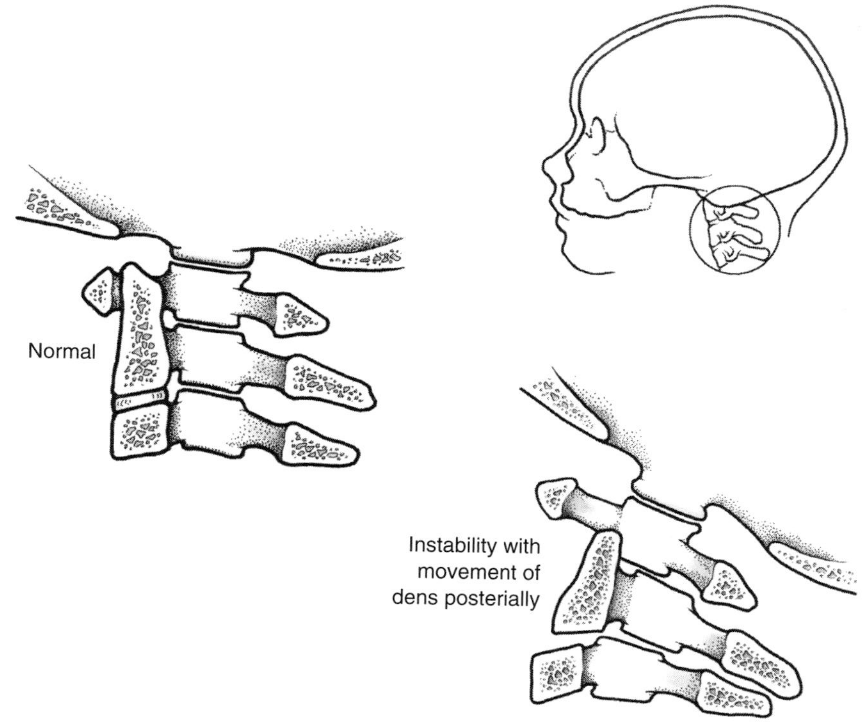

Figure 15.1. Children with DS are at risk of developing subluxation (partial dislocation) of the atlantoaxial or atlanto-occipital joint, as shown in this illustration (right side). A typical neck region is shown for comparison (left side). This subluxation predisposes these children to spinal injury with trauma. This abnormality can be detected by X-ray or an MRI scan of the neck.

	Birth to 1 month	Infancy months						Early childhood years					Late childhood years									
		2	4	6	8	10	12	1	2	3	4	5	5	7	9	11	13	13	15	17	19	21
Karyotype	•																					
Echocardiogram	•																					
Hearing screen and follow-up	•																					
Audiological[1]				•				Every 6 months														
Ear specific audiogram[1]													Annually									
Eye exam for cataracts[2]	•																					
Ophthalmology referral		Once in 1st 6 mo						Annually					Every 2 years					Every 3 years				
TSH (Thyroid Stimulating Hormone)	•			•			•	Annually														
CBC[3] (complete blood count) and differential	•																					
Hb[4] (hemoglobin)								Annually														
Hb only																		Annually				
Radiographic swallowing assessment[5]	If symptomatic																					
Lateral neck x ray in neutral position[6]	If symptomatic																					
Tissue transglutaminase IgA and quantitative IgA[7]								If symptomatic														
Echocardiogram[8]																		If symptomatic				

1. If normal hearing established, do behavioral audiogram and tympanometry until bilateral ear specific testing possible. Refer child with abnormal hearing to otolaryngologist.
2. Referral to ophthalmologist who has experience with Down syndrome to assess for strabismus, cataracts, and nystagmus.
3. To rule out transient myeloproliferative disorder; polycythemia.
4. Hb annually; CRP (c-reactive protein) and ferritin or CHr (reticulocyte hemoglobin content) if possible risk of iron deficiency or Hb < 11 g.
5. If marked hypotonia, slow feeding, choking with feeds, recurrent or persistent respiratory symptoms, failure to thrive.
6. If myelopathic symptoms: obtain neutral position spine films and, if normal, obtain flexion and extension films and refer to pediatric neurosurgeon or orthopedic surgeon with expertise in evaluation and treating atlanto-axial instability.
7. If symptoms of celiac disease are present.
8. If symptoms of acquired mitral or aortic valve disease such as increased fatigue, shortness of breath, or exertional dyspnea or abnormal physical examination findings such as a new murmur or gallop.

Figure 15.2. Recommendations for preventive health care for children and adolescents with Down syndrome. (*Source:* Bull & American Academy of Pediatrics Committee on Genetics, 2011.)

Obstructive Sleep Apnea: Evaluation and Symptomatic Vigilance In light of the high incidence of sleep apnea, the American Academy of Pediatrics (AAP) recommends a sleep study for all children with DS by 4 years of age regardless of whether they have symptoms of sleep apnea. First-line treatment is usually tonsillectomy with and without an adenoidectomy, which decreases symptoms in 50% of individuals but has a low cure rate (17%–20%; Nation & Brigger, 2017). Continuous positive airway pressure with a mask is sometimes possible and effective, but it is uncomfortable. Newer interventions include tongue reduction and other surgery at the base of the tongue. Hypoglossal nerve stimulator implantation is presently in a multicenter trial (Bassett & Musso, 2017; Diercks et al., 2018). Obstructive sleep apnea is associated with lower IQ and behavior problems and eventually can lead to heart failure (Lott & Dierssen, 2010). See Box 15.2 for more information on obstructive sleep apnea and DS.

Hearing Problems: Evaluation After newborn screening for hearing loss (see Chapter 7), the AAP health supervision guidelines recommends hearing screening starting at 6 months of age and every 6 months to 5 years of age and then annually (Bull & American Academy of Pediatrics Committee on Genetics, 2011). Treatment for hearing loss commonly includes surgical placement of pressure equalization tubes (PET; Bernardi, Pires, Oliveria, & Nisihara, 2017; Manickam, Shott, Heithaus, & Shott, 2016) and less frequently hearing aid use (Yaneza, Hunter, Irwin, & Kubba, 2016) and cochlear implants (Phelan, Henderson, Green, & Bruce, 2016). Of school-age children, 23% used hearing aids or had them recommended in a treatment plan (Nightengale et al., 2017). In a 15-year longitudinal study from infancy of 57 children with DS who were consistently monitored for hearing loss, PET placement occurred in 88.8%, normal hearing was present in 38%–44%, and tympanic membrane perforations were present in 17% of ears (Manickam et al., 2016).

Vision Problems: Evaluation The AAP recommendation is for infants with DS to be evaluated by an ophthalmologist experienced with children by 6 months of age, or sooner if there are any concerns. Unless more frequent visits are indicated, follow-up evaluations are recommended to occur annually from 1 to 5 years of age, then every 2 years from 5 to 19 years of age, and then every 3 years from 13 to 21 years of age.

Cardiac: Evaluation An echocardiogram is recommended for the newborn with DS, even if there has been a prior fetal echocardiogram (Bull & American Academy of Pediatrics Committee on Genetics, 2011). Data indicate that children with DS have a similar rate of mortality as do other children with the same heart defect (Fudge et al., 2010). Since the early 2000s, there has been a trend toward increased use of invasive therapy, including corrective or palliative cardiac surgery and therapeutic catheterization, in children less than 12 months of age (Dias et al., 2016). In a cross-sectional study of children with DS, the parents of children with congenital heart disease reported that 55% needed cardiac surgery at a mean age of 9.6 months (Roizen et al., 2014).

Dental: Monitoring Children with DS need early and regular dental care to prevent and limit the development of gingivitis, which eventually can lead to loss of teeth. Arguably, all children with DS need orthodontic treatment for their malocclusion (Andersson, Axelsson, & Katsaris, 2016), but not all can tolerate the discomfort.

Thyroid: Monitoring As with all newborns, infants with DS are routinely screened for thyroid dysfunction. The initial screen should include a thyroid-stimulating hormone (TSH). Follow-up TSH screening should occur at 6 and 12 months of age and then continued annually (Bull & American Academy of Pediatrics Committee on Genetics, 2011; Whooten et al., 2017). More frequent

BOX 15.2 EVIDENCE-BASED PRACTICE

Obstructive Sleep Apnea and Down Syndrome

In a study of 3-year-olds with Down syndrome (DS) chosen for having normal hearing and followed from infancy, at least 57% had evidence of obstructive sleep apnea when evaluated by **polysomnograms** (i.e., a sleep study). Of the 69% of parents who reported no sleep problems in their child with DS, 54% of their children were found to have abnormal sleep study results (Shott et al., 2006). This study increased awareness of the frequency of obstructed sleep apnea in preschoolers with DS and the need to identify it and develop interventions that work.

TSHs are indicated if the child displays plateauing height, behavior problems, or an unexpected lack of cognitive progress (Lott & Dierssen, 2010). If there is clinical and laboratory evidence of thyroid disease, treatment is indicated.

Seizures and Other Neurological Problems: Vigilance

When comparing children with and without DS who develop infantile spasms (see Chapter 22), the median age of diagnosis (6–7 months) and time from diagnosis to treatment (1.0 day) does not differ, nor is there a difference in treatment timelines. Compared with other children with **idiopathic** (no-identified-cause) infantile spasms, children with DS appear to be more responsive to treatment (Beatty, Wrede, & Blume, 2017). Children with infantile spasms and associated neurological insults are more likely to progress to epilepsy.

Celiac and GI Problems: Symptomatic Vigilance

Presenting symptoms of celiac disease can include abdominal pain, constipation, diarrhea, failure to thrive, reflux, vomiting, short stature, and fatigue (Khatib, Baker, Ly, Kozielski, & Baker, 2016). The AAP recommended health supervision for children with DS who have symptoms of celiac disease is screening with blood tissue transglutaminase immunoglobulin A (IgA) and quantitative IgA (Bull & American Academy of Pediatrics Committee on Genetics, 2011). Medical evaluation and treatment are recommended for constipation unresponsive to dietary intervention, signs of a bowel obstruction, or GE reflux.

Obesity and Growth: Monitoring and Prevention

Several factors contribute to the development of obesity in DS, including a lower resting metabolic rate (Luke, Roizen, Sutton, & Schoeller, 1994), decreased activity level, and preferring indoor activities compared with siblings. In 2015, updated growth charts for children and adolescents with DS were published for monitoring growth (Zemel et al., 2015). The recommendation is that for children with DS who are 10 years of age or older, the Centers for Disease Control (CDC) BMI growth chart 85th percentile is a better indicator of excess adiposity (100% sensitivity) than the new DS-specific BMI charts, which have low sensitivity (62.3%; Hatch-Stein et al., 2016; Whooten et al., 2017).

Leukemias: Vigilance

Signs of leukemia include bruising due to low platelets, fatigue due to anemia, and frequent or unusual infections, and these should be evaluated given the increased risk of leukemia in DS. With the newest treatment trials, myeloid leukemia in DS has an 89.9% 5-year event-free survival rate and an overall survival rate of 93% for the majority of children, but for less than 10%, the leukemia is refractory and relapses, with a 5-year overall survival rate of 34.4% (Taub et al., 2017). For acute lymphoblastic leukemia, on contemporary protocols, the outcomes for children with DS continue to be poorer than for children without DS, with a 5-year event-free survival rate of 65.6% for children with DS compared with 87.7% for children without DS and an overall survival rate of 70% for children with DS compared with 92.2% for children without DS (Patrick et al., 2014).

Orthopedic Problems: Vigilance

Symptoms of atlantoaxial instability include new neck pain, torticollis (stiff neck), loss of motor skills such as limping, loss of bowel or bladder control, having new difficulty climbing stairs, or any neurological changes. Parents should be advised to have their child seen urgently by a physician the day that the symptoms are first noticed. The child needs plain lateral cervical spine radiography (a side-view neck x-ray) in the neutral position. If there are any abnormalities, the child should be immediately referred to a pediatric neurosurgeon or orthopedic surgeon experienced in the evaluation and treatment of atlantoaxial instability (Bull & American Academy of Pediatrics Committee on Genetics, 2011).

Development and Behavior

Intellectual disability (see Chapter 14) is found almost universally in children with DS. In general, in the first 24 months of life, children pass developmental milestones at twice the age of typically developing children. Mental developmental quotients on the Bayley Scales of Infant Development from 6 to 24 months are in the 50s and 60s, while the motor developmental quotients are in the 40s and 50s. At 10 years of age, average developmental quotients are 39.9 (standard deviation: 9.4) with age-equivalent functioning at 51.2 (plus or minus 12.10) months. In adaptive function at 10 years of age, the total age-equivalent level of functioning is 54.4 months, with strength in socialization and weakness in daily living (communication = 45, daily living = 39.7, socialization = 50, combined = 41). Early developmental outcomes at 12 and 24 months correlate with outcomes at 10.7 years (Marchal et al., 2016).

Children with DS are stereotyped as being amiable and happy. Temperament studies, however, have shown them to have behavioral profiles comparable to typically developing children (Chapman & Husketh, 2000). Compared with the general population, individuals with DS are at increased risk for experiencing behavioral, emotional, and psychiatric problems (18%–23%). But compared with other children with IDs who are at 30%–40% risk, children with DS are at decreased risk. Children and youth with DS have been found to have high rates of provocative behaviors and low-level aggressive behaviors (e.g., 73% disobedient, 65% argumentative, and 50% demanding attention). In addition, 6%–8% of children with DS are diagnosed with ADHD, like Jerome in our case study (Dykens, 2007). The prevalence of psychotropic medication use in children and adolescents with DS is higher than in the general population (25% versus 17%). Nervous system stimulants are most frequently prescribed for children from 5 to 11 years, with declining use thereafter. By contrast, the use of SSRI for the treatment of anxiety and depression increases into adolescence and young adulthood (Downes, Anixt, Esbensen, Wiley, & Meinzen-Derr, 2015). There are some reports of psychosis or depression with psychotic features in adolescents and young adults, with marked motoric slowing in daily activities and in expressive language (Dykens et al., 2015).

The reported prevalence of autism spectrum disorder (ASD) in DS is between 7% and 16%. (Dykens, 2007; Richards, Jones, Groves, Moss, & Oliver, 2015). In those who have regression with the development of autism, the loss of language is reported to occur later than in non-DS autism development (61.8 months versus 19.7 months; Castillo et al., 2008). In addition, children with DS who have autism have poorer development in all areas, and seizures are more likely.

DS disintegrative disorder is a rare phenomenon of acute or semi-acute cognitive and functional decline that can have features of autism or depression; it generally occurs in the preteen or teen years. Extensive evaluations may identify dysfunctional sleep or thyroid dysfunction. Most are treated with SSRIs, and generally upon follow-up months to years later, 50% are somewhat better (Mircher et al., 2017; Worley et al., 2015).

It appears that virtually all individuals with DS have the characteristic neuropathology of Alzheimer's disease by 45 years of age, although not all individuals have clinical signs. They have increased concentrations of brain amyloid, which is associated with neurofibrillary tangles. A number of genes on chromosome 21 have been implicated in Alzheimer's disease (Lott & Dierssen, 2010).

Intervention: Educational and Services

Parents of a newborn with DS should be provided with a balanced view of the possible outcomes and information on intervention and support. They should be given current materials on infants with DS and contact information for the point of entry for the early intervention system (see Chapter 31). In addition, information regarding local and national parent support /advocacy programs such as the National Down Syndrome Society (www.ndss.org, which focuses on advocacy), the National Down Syndrome Congress (www.ndsccenter.org, which focuses on the needs of families and offers an annual meeting), and Gigi's Playhouse (www.gigisplayhouse.org, which provides an array of programs and support) should be offered. Information on respite care and supplemental security income (SSI) is also helpful (see Chapter 37).

The educational program of the child with DS needs to provide the optimal environment for learning. A balance of inclusion in learning environments with typically developing children and the provision of specialized therapeutic interventions needs to be planned to meet each child's needs (Chapter 33). Most frequently, children with DS have strengths in visual-motor skills, and so a visual approach to teaching that uses aids such as written instructions, visual organizers, and schedules capitalizes on this strength. Data indicate that an inclusive educational setting supports academic development, especially in the areas of language and literacy (de Graaf & van Hove, 2015).

In their role as advocates for their child with DS, most parents consider using alternative and complementary therapies for improvement in cognitive function (Prussing, Sobo, Walker, & Kurtin, 2005). Eighty-seven percent of these parents do at some time treat their child with an alternative therapy, most commonly combination nutritional therapy (e.g., Nutrivene; Ellis et al., 2008; Prussing et al., 2005; Vacca & Valenti, 2015; see Chapter 39). Although there are many studies of alternative therapies in individuals with DS, few meet even the minimal methodology criteria of scientific studies (Roizen, 2005). The efforts to improve the health and lives of individuals with DS have resulted in the development of the Down Syndrome Medical Interest Group, which includes a network of Down syndrome clinics (Box 15.1; www.dsmig-usa.org) and also has resulted in the formation of organizations within the research community (including the National Institutes of Health) with the purpose of developing a data collection site that parents can populate with information on their child (www.dsconnect.nih.gov) as well as the development of the Trisomy 21 Research Society (Delabar et al., 2016).

Outcomes

Since the 1970s, the prognosis for a productive and positive life experience for individuals with DS and their families has continued to improve, with the credit going to the efforts of parents' advocacy. But significant barriers remain. The most difficult challenges include medical complications, bullying or ostracism, disappointments regarding the achievement of certain adult milestones (e.g., obtaining a driver's license), and a lack of adequate services and supports in adulthood (Hanson, 2003). However, there is increased interest in adults with DS and increased efforts to review the limited data on adults (Steingass, Chicoine, McGuire, & Roizen, 2011) and develop health care guidelines (Capone et al., 2018).

With the introduction in the 1980s of **supported employment** (in which individuals with disabilities have a job coach), adults with DS are able to hold jobs with improved pay, improved benefits, and better working conditions. In a survey about employment completed by parents regarding their adult children with DS, 50% were employed in some capacity, with 3% of those in competitive employment (Kumin & Schoenbrodt, 2015). Most frequently for individuals with special needs like those with DS, employment is in food services, landscaping, filing, factories, and environmental services.

FRAGILE X SYNDROME

Prevalence

FXS is the most common known single-gene cause of ID and ASD, with an estimated frequency of about 1 to 4,000 to 5,000 (Coffee et al., 2009). Prevalence varies somewhat between different populations, but the disorder affects all ethnic groups worldwide.

Genetics

FXS is one of a set of disorders, termed fragile X–associated disorders (FXD), which are caused by mutations of the *FMR1* gene on the X chromosome (see Chapter 1). These mutations involve the expansion of a trinucleotide repeat (CGG) sequence in the promotor region of the *FMR1* gene. The **promotor region** of a gene controls the transcription of that gene into mRNA, which is then translated into a functional protein—in this case, the fragile X mental retardation protein (FMRP). Normally, the promotor region of the *FMR1* gene has 5 to 44 CGG repeats, which allows for normal transcription and translation of the gene. Some individuals have 55 to 200 CGG repeats; they are said to have a **premutation.** The prevalence of premutation is estimated to be about 1 in 151 to 1 in 209 females and 1 in 430 to 1 in 468 males in the United States. The premutation is associated with two well-defined adult-onset diseases: FXTAS (a late-onset progressive neurological disorder) and fragile X–associated primary ovarian insufficiency (FXPOI). These individuals are still able to produce FMRP, the gene product of the *FMR1* gene, so they *do not* have FXS (although individuals with more than 150 repeats may have some characteristics of FXS due to a mild reduction in FMRP; Willemsen, Levenga, & Oostra, 2011).

For most female premutation carriers, there is an increased risk for passing on the *FMR1* gene as a **full mutation** (more than 200 CGG repeats); male premutation carriers (and, surprisingly, even males with the full mutation) can only pass the premutation to their offspring (Yrigollen et al., 2014). The full mutation results in silencing of the *FMR1* gene so little or no *FMR1* mRNA is made, and thus most males with the full mutation make little or no FMRP. The substantial reduction or lack of FMRP is what causes these individuals to have FXS. Because the *FMR1* gene is located on the X chromosome, girls who receive the full mutation from their mothers will have a normal *FMR1* gene on the X chromosome that they receive from their fathers. They would therefore have at least some production of FMRP and tend to have milder manifestations of the symptoms of FXS (Loesch, Huggins, & Hagerman, 2004). By contrast, boys who receive the full mutation from their mothers receive no counterbalancing normal *FMR1* gene from their fathers and so have the typical features of FXS (with some variability in severity depending on differences in FMRP production and variation in the amount of gene inactivation in different cells in the body [mosaicism]; Willemsen et al., 2011). Because *FMR1* expansions tend to increase in size as they are passed from generation to generation, FXDs affect families in multiple generations.

Physical Features, Typical Presentations, Diagnostic Testing, and Early Identification

Physical features of FXS include macro-orchidism (large testes) in virtually all adult males with FXS. A characteristic pattern of facial features is seen in a percentage of individuals with FXS, including prominent ears, macrocephaly (large head), long face, prominent jaw and forehead, midfacial hypoplasia (reduced dimensions of the midfacial area), and high arched palate. Connective tissue laxity, leading to hyperextensible joints, flat feet, and soft skin, is common in FXS but not present in all individuals (Hagerman & Hagerman, 2002). Physical features are sufficiently variable that they cannot be used as indicators of which individuals to screen for the presence of FXS.

Developmental delays are the first sign of FXS. Motor development is often only mildly delayed; the most common presentation leading to an FXS diagnosis is speech delay, which is seen in most boys with FXS and a significant proportion of girls. Some higher functioning boys and many girls present at school age with behavioral difficulties, ADHD, anxiety, or academic delay.

The average age of diagnosis of FXS is about 3 years (Bailey, Raspa, Bishop, & Holiday, 2009), although developmental delays can be identified in most boys by age 9–12 months (Box 15.3). There has been a recent collaborative initiative (CDC & AAP, 2016) of the AAP, CDC, and FXS community to bring the age of diagnosis down to 2 years or less, to obtain earlier intervention, and earlier family counseling regarding genetic risks and reproductive options to allow for prenatal testing or preimplantation genetic diagnosis. Pilot newborn screening studies for FXS have been conducted (Bailey et al., 2017) and are ongoing, but additional work is needed for FXS to be considered for mandatory screening.

Medical Complications

Medical problems more prevalent in FXS than in the general population based on recent data from nine FXS clinics in the Fragile X Clinical and Research Consortium (FXCRC; see Box 15.4) include frequent OM (males 55%, females 46%), strabismus (males 17%, females 13%), seizures (males 12%, females 3%, usually in childhood), sleep disorders (males/females 27%), gastroesophageal reflux (males/females 11%), sleep apnea (males/females 7%), and loose stools (males 12%, females 7%) (Kidd et al., 2014; see Figure 15.3). Treatment of medical problems is important as these problems can impact development and behavior. Primary care physicians should look for and ask about symptoms that might be related to these problems at routine yearly well-child visits and should refer to specialists for further evaluation and management if needed. The type and timing of follow up for these problems will depend on severity and whether medication intervention is implemented.

Treatment of Medical Problems

Since children with FXS have expressive language delays and recurrent OM that may lead to conductive hearing loss and further language and articulation issues, it is important that all OM and any other ear-related issues be treated promptly and appropriately. Hearing should be monitored carefully, and there should be a relatively low threshold for early pressure equalization tube placement in children with FXS and recurrent OM (Bennett & Haggard, 1999). If chronically infected adenoids and tonsils become a problem, adenoidectomy and/or tonsillectomy may be performed at the same time as the PE tubes are inserted.

Children with FXS should have vision screening yearly or every other year during childhood to ensure that any acuity issues are being addressed so these do not compound problems with reading and academics. When present, strabismus should be managed with eye patching, vision therapy, or surgery to avoid amblyopia and aggravation of visual processing problems.

For concerns about episodes that might be seizures, an electroencephalogram (EEG) should be obtained (see Chapter 22). The EEG can be used to distinguish behavioral spells from seizures. Typically, individuals would be treated after two documented seizures with anticonvulsants that are least likely to cause sedation (Berry-Kravis et al., 2010), with a plan to discontinue treatment after an individual with FXS is seizure-free for 2 years.

Monitoring and managing obstructive sleep apnea and other sleep problems are of particular importance in FXS due to their relationship to decrements in daytime performance and behavior (Goodlin-Jones, Tang, & Anders, 2009; Kronk et al., 2010). Sleep problems may require behavioral or medical treatment. When symptoms of obstructive sleep apnea are clearly present, management with tonsillectomy/adenoidectomy is indicated.

Individuals with FXS have increased risk for being overweight and for somewhat diminished height in adulthood. It is important to encourage healthy diet, calorie restriction when necessary, and exercise programs for 30–40 minutes four to five times a week to minimize problems associated with increased weight.

When GE reflux is present, antacids should be used when needed to prevent pain and esophagitis. As individuals with FXS are not always able to describe heartburn, the only sign of GE reflux may be behavioral

BOX 15.3 EVIDENCE-BASED PRACTICE

Testing for Fragile X Syndrome

Diagnostic testing for fragile X syndrome (FXS) is recommended for all children who have intellectual disability or developmental disabilities of undetermined etiology. Children with FXS have developmental delay identified by 9–12 months, but the average age of diagnosis is 3 years. Bailey and colleagues (2017) are conducting a pilot newborn screening study that could enable early identification and targeted intervention.

BOX 15.4 INTERDISCIPLINARY CARE

The Fragile X Clinical and Research Consortium

The Fragile X Clinical and Research Consortium (FXCRC; https://fragilex.org/research/) was created in association with the National Fragile X Foundation in 2006 to establish standards of care for fragile X syndrome (FXS) with optimized care delivery at sites geographically more available to families relative to the prior few clinics specializing in FXS. The FXCRC has grown from 11 to 27 clinics, has published on medical problems, and has created consensus documents regarding the management of issues important for those with FXD. These documents are published on the NFXF web site and are updated at regular intervals (https://fragilex.org/2017/treatment-and-intervention/consensus-fragile-x-clinical-research-consortium-clinical-practices/). The majority of clinics that have joined the FXCRC feel that the organization has been helpful for improving clinical care, providing more services, and increasing the ability of the clinic to participate in clinical trials (Liu et al., 2016). It also appears that when individuals are seen at an FXCRC specialty clinic, unmanaged issues are identified and can be treated (Visootsak et al., 2016).

The FXCRC also serves as a research network to allow recruitment of cohorts across multiple sites to better study the FXS population without the biases of small studies. Most of the FXCRC clinics participate in and contribute data to the FORWARD (Fragile X Online Registry with Accessible Research Database) longitudinal natural history study of FXS, which is funded by the CDC (Sherman et al., 2017). This study is expected to produce extensive information about the life trajectory of FXS in terms of medical, educational, functional/adaptive, behavioral, vocational, and social issues.

outbursts occurring in patterns during the day in relation to meals or sleep dysfunction with frequent night awakenings.

Some individuals with FXS benefit from orthotics or shoe inserts for foot pronation and flat feet to help with motor development when young and to avoid leg pain and reduce gait problems when older.

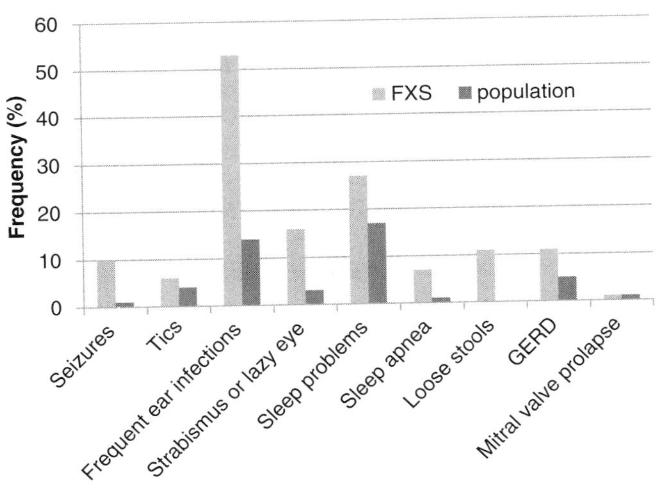

Figure 15.3. Frequency of medical conditions in FXS in the United States relative to control populations of typically developing children. (*Sources:* Fragile X Clinical and Research Consortium: www.fragilex.org; Kidd et al., 2014). (*Key:* FXS, fragile X syndrome; GERD, gastroesophageal reflux disease.)

Neurodevelopment, Cognitive Profile, and Behavioral Issues

The majority of males with FXS will meet criteria for mild to severe ID (Kaufmann, Abrams, Chen, & Reiss, 1999). Average IQ in adult males with FXS is 40–50, with a mental age of about of 5–6 years. Females with FXS are often less affected than males, with about 25% having cognitive impairment and others frequently being diagnosed with learning disabilities (de Vries et al., 1996). Average IQ in females is about 80, with a range from severe impairment to normal or even superior ability. There is a relatively consistent pattern of intellectual weaknesses and strengths distinct to both males and females with FXS, generally milder in severity in females (Freund, Reiss, & Abrams, 1993). Relative weaknesses include visuospatial skills, working memory, processing of sequential information, and attention (Dykens, Hodapp, & Leckman, 1987) while there are relative strengths in visual memory, simultaneous processing, and long-term memory (see Chapters 13 and 20). These patterns are important to recognize to optimize education programming.

The full-scale IQ score decreases with age as children with FXS become older (Dykens et al., 1987; Fisch et al., 1996; Fisch et al., 1999). Standard scores on the Vineland Adaptive Behavior Scale for overall adaptive behavior as well as subdomains decline with age during childhood, in males more so than in females with FXS (Klaiman et al., 2014). Decline in standard scores for intelligence and adaptive function does not reflect regression but rather failure to keep pace with the normal rate of intellectual development. These scores are stable in adulthood.

The behavioral phenotype in males with FXS covers a wide spectrum. Most common broad categories of behavioral dysfunction seen in FXS are attention/hyperactivity, hyperarousal, anxiety, and aggression. Females with FXS have the same spectrum of behavioral difficulties but with milder symptomology.

Attention disorders, including impulsivity, hyperactivity, and inattention, are extremely common in FXS and result in a comorbid ADHD diagnosis in as many as 73% of males (Baumgardner, Reiss, Freund, & Abrams, 1995; Hagerman & Falkenstein, 1987; Turk, 1998) and 30%–63% of females (Freund et al., 1993; Hagerman et al., 1992; Mazzocco, Pennington, & Hagerman, 1993). Anxiety disorders, including generalized anxiety and particularly specific phobias and social anxiety (Cordeiro, Ballinger, Haberman, & Hessl, 2011; Freund et al., 1993; Hagerman et al., 1992), have been reported in 86.2% of males with FXS and 76.9% of females with FXS (Cordeiro et al., 2011).

Hyperarousal, an overreaction to sensory input, can be triggered in FXS by a wide range of situations, including noises, new environments, crowds, interpersonal distance, eye contact, and new people (Cohen, 1995). The effects of this hyperarousal are widespread and include high levels of motor activity (e.g., running and jumping), stereotypic motor movements (e.g., hand flapping), gaze aversion, and perseverative behaviors (Bailey et al., 1998; Belser & Subhaler, 2001; Cohen, 1995).

Aggression and self-injurious behavior (SIB) are often linked to hyperarousal or anxiety and are especially detrimental to family functioning, quality of life (Bailey et al., 2012), and participation in daily activities. SIB typically begins at 1 to 3 years of age (Symons, Byiers, Raspa, Bishop, & Bailey, 2010). Aggression typically occurs later, frequently during the pubescent and postpubescent periods (Bailey et al., 2012).

Language development is significantly delayed for most individuals with FXS. In general, individuals with FXS have stronger receptive than expressive language skills (McDuffie, Kover, Abbeduto, Lewis, & Brown, 2012), with particular strengths in receptive vocabulary. Pragmatic language (see Chapter 17) is also delayed, and young children with FXS have been shown to have difficulties with joint attention, reciprocating positive facial expressions, eye gaze, and turn-taking (Murphy & Abbeduto, 2005; Roberts, Mirrett, Anderson, Burchinal, & Neebe, 2002). Males with FXS demonstrate high rates of perseverative language, tangential (off-topic) language, overly literal interpretation of language, and decreased topic initiation and maintenance (Bailey et al., 1998; Sudhalter, Cohen, Silverman, & Wolf-Schein, 1994).

About one half to two thirds of males and about 20% of females with FXS meet the criteria for ASD (Wang, Berry-Kravis, & Hagerman, 2010; see Chapter 18). These two disorders share multiple behaviors, including pragmatic deficits, language delays, reduced eye contact, difficulty with regulation of attention and activity level, SIB, and aggression. Characteristics that tend to differ between FXS and idiopathic ASD include a higher rate of ID, more severe motor coordination deficits, worse expressive than receptive language, generally higher interest in socialization (although limited by anxiety), and better imitation skills in FXS relative to idiopathic ASD. Children with FXS and a codiagnosis of ASD are at higher risk of seizures and chronic sleep disorders, more severe behavioral issues in all areas except anxiety, and higher use of antipsychotics and alpha-agonists to target aggressive behavior relative to those with FXS without ASD (Kaufmann et al., 2017).

Supportive Interventions for Educational and Behavioral Problems

Current treatment of FXS includes therapy, educational strategies that take into account cognitive and behavioral strengths and weaknesses in FXS, treatment of medical problems, behavioral modification, and psychopharmacology for behaviors creating dysfunction (Berry-Kravis, Sumis, Hervey, & Mathur, 2012).

Occupational therapy, physical therapy, and speech therapy should be included as part of a comprehensive intervention program based on the specific needs of the individual child with FXS. Therapy techniques that have been validated for autism are often helpful for FXS, but they must be modified based on what is known about the FXS phenotype. Individuals with FXS have been shown to display better behavioral and adaptive functioning when their environment and supportive programming are well matched to their needs (Hessl et al., 2001), and therefore a highly individualized behavioral, therapeutic, and educational intervention plan is needed both for home and school or work environments.

The use of medications such as stimulants for attention and hyperactivity, SSRIs for anxiety, alpha-agonists for hyperactivity and overarousal, and antipsychotics for irritable and aggressive behaviors appears to be helpful by assessment in a clinical setting in approximately 50%–70% of patients (Berry-Kravis et al., 2012; see Chapter 27). Response is not complete, however, and data from a national survey on FXS showed that approximately 10%–20% of respondents thought that medication was not helpful at all for behavior problems, while only approximately 40% felt the medication was helping a lot (Bailey et al., 2012). Thus, there is a clear unmet need in FXS for better treatments for behavior and for any treatments that target cognitive deficits. Treatments that modify the underlying disorder would be an extremely important advance (see Box 15.4 for more information on FXCRC).

Progress Toward Targeted Treatment

Recent studies of the neurobiology and synaptic mechanisms resulting from absence of the FMRP in FXS have become an important window on future targeted treatments for FXS, ASD, and related neurodevelopmental disorders (Wang et al., 2010; Yu & Berry-Kravis, 2014). FMRP is an mRNA binding protein that regulates the expression of proteins at synapses in neurons and thus is involved in adjusting synaptic strength and plasticity in response to activation of a particular neuron (Berry-Kravis, 2014; Huber, Gallagher, Warren, & Bear, 2002). An animal model of FXS, known as the *Fmr1* knockout mouse, makes no functional FMRP. It has been a critical resource in understanding the role of FMRP in neurons, identifying cellular targets for treatment, and exploring the effects of potential disease-modifying agents. Successful preclinical testing of disease-targeted treatments in mice, rats, and flies has demonstrated reversal of disease phenotypes (particular features of neurons and behaviors seen in the FXS animal models), leading to a number of early-phase and several larger clinical trials in humans (Berry-Kravis et al., 2016; Berry-Kravis et al., 2017; Gross, Hoffman, Bassell, & Berry-Kravis, 2015; Youssef et al., 2018). These studies have been plagued by uncertainties about how to optimally demonstrate treatment effects and disease modification in a clinical trial setting for a population of individuals with developmental disabilities (Berry-Kravis et al., 2016; Berry-Kravis et al., 2017; Erickson et al., 2017; Gross et al., 2015; Youssef et al., 2018). Major trial design issues include variable dosing windows; the timing (age) and length of treatment necessary; the need for cognitive/behavioral interventions to assess drug effects on learning; large placebo effects; and the lack of validated, sensitive biomarkers and functional outcome measures in FXS (Berry-Kravis et al., 2013; Budimirovic et al., 2017; Erickson et al., 2017). Work is ongoing to resolve these issues so that in the future, treatment to reverse the underlying disorder will eventually replace or complement supportive treatment.

There is significant overlap in molecular and cellular pathways involving FMRP, and FMRP binds to and regulates many key autism gene products (Iossifov et al., 2012; Steinberg & Webber, 2013; Waltes et al., 2014). Thus, progress in development of targeted treatments for FXS may result in targeted treatments to reverse CNS defects and clinical manifestations of ASD, other neurodevelopmental disabilities, and ID.

SUMMARY

- DS is associated with a variety of medical conditions and complications in nearly all organ systems.
- There is a risk for **diagnostic overshadowing,** which can lead to postponing or missing a diagnosis. Therefore, it is important for health care providers to closely evaluate individuals with DS for medical concerns and be vigilant with their medical care.
- An appropriate educational program for a child with DS should provide a balance of inclusion in learning environments with typical children and therapeutic interventions for each child's needs.
- Treatment of medical problems in both DS and FXS is important as they can impact development and behavior.
- Early identification of FXS enables early intervention.
- FXCRC is seeking to develop targeted treatments of FXS to improve development and behavior.

ADDITIONAL RESOURCES

National Down Syndrome Congress (NDSC): http://ndsccenter.org

National Down Syndrome Society (NDSS): http://www.ndss.org

Down Syndrome Connect: https://www.dsconnect.nih.gov

FRAXA Research Foundation: http://www.fraxa.org

The National Fragile X Foundation: http://www.FragileX.org

CDC Fragile X Syndrome information webpage: https://www.cdc.gov/ncbddd/fxs/index.

Additional resources can be found online in Appendix D: Childhood Disabilities Resources, Services, and Organizations (see About the Online Companion Materials).

REFERENCES

Andersson, E. M., Axelsson, S., & Katsaris, K. P. (2016). Malocclusion and the need for orthodontic treatment in 8-year-old children with Down syndrome: A cross-sectional population-based study. *Special Care Dentistry, 36*(4), 194–200.

Bailey, D. B., Berry-Kravis, E., Gane, L. W., Guarda, S., Hagerman, R., Powell, C. M., . . . Wheeler, A. (2017). Fragile X newborn screening: Lessons learned from a multisite screening study. *Pediatrics, 139*(Suppl. 3), S216–S225. PMID:28814542

Bailey, D. J., Mesibov, G. B., Hatton, D. D., Clark, R. D., Roberts, J. E., & Mayhew, L. (1998). Autistic behavior in young boys with fragile X syndrome. *Journal of Autism and Developmental Disorders, 28*(6), 499.

Bailey, D. B., Raspa, M., Bishop, E., & Holiday, D. (2009). No change in the age of diagnosis for fragile X syndrome: Findings from a national parent survey. *Pediatrics, 124,* 527–533.

Bailey, D. B., Raspa, M., Bishop, E., Mitra, D., Martin, S., Wheeler, A., . . . Sacco, P. (2012). Health and economic consequences of fragile X syndrome for caregivers. *Journal of Developmental & Behavioral Pediatrics, 33*(9), 705–712.

Bailey, D. B., Raspa, M., Bishop, E., Olmsted, M., Mallya, U. G., & Berry-Kravis, E. (2012). Medication utilization for targeted symptoms in children and adults with fragile X syndrome: US survey. *Journal of Developmental-Behavioral Pediatrics, 33*(1), 62–69.

Basil, J. S., Santoro, S. L., Martin, L. J., Healy, K. W., Chini, B. A., & Saal, H. M. (2016). Retrospective study of obesity in children with Down syndrome. *Journal of Pediatrics, 173,* 143–148.

Bassett, E. C., & Musso, M. F. (2017). Otolaryngologic management of Down syndrome patients what is new? *Current Opinion in Otolaryngology Head and Neck Surgery, 25*(6), 493–497.

Baumgardner, T. L., Reiss, A. L., Freund, L. S., & Abrams, M. T. (1995). Specification of the neurobehavioral phenotype in males with fragile X syndrome. *Pediatrics, 95*(5), 744.

Beatty, C. Q., Wrede, J. E., & Blume, H. K. (2017). Diagnosis, treatment, and outcomes of infantile spasms in trisomy 21 population. *Seizure: European Journal of Epilepsy, 45,* 184–188.

Belser, R. C., & Sudhalter, V. (2001). Conversational characteristics of children with fragile X syndrome: Repetitive speech. *American Journal of Mental Retardation, 106*(1), 28–38.

Bennett, K. E., & Haggard, M. P. (1999). Behavior and cognitive outcomes from middle ear disease. *Archives of Disease in Childhood, 80*(1), 28–35.

Bergholdt, R., Eising, S., Nerup, J., & Pociot, F. (2006). Increased prevalence of Down's syndrome in individuals with type 1 diabetes in Denmark: A nationwide population-based study. *Diabetologia, 49,* 1179–1182.

Bernardi, G. G., Pires, C. T. F., Oliverira, N. P., & Nisihara, R. (2017). Prevalence of pressure equalization tube placement and hearing loss in children with Down syndrome. *International Journal of Pediatric Otorhinolaryngology, 98,* 48–52.

Berry-Kravis, E. (2014). Mechanism-based treatments in neurodevelopmental disorders: Fragile X syndrome. *Pediatric Neurology, 50*(4), 297–302.

Berry-Kravis, E., Des Portes, V., Hagerman, R., Jacquemont, S., Charles, P., Visootsak, J., . . . von Raison, F. (2016). Mavoglurant in adults and adolescents with fragile X syndrome: Results of randomized, double-blind, placebo-controlled trials. *Science Translational Medicine, 8,* 321ra5.

Berry-Kravis, E., Hagerman, R., Visootsak, J., Budimirovic, D., Kaufmann, W. E., Walton-Bowen, K., . . . Carpenter, R. L. (2017). Arbaclofen in fragile X syndrome: Results of phase 3 trials. *Journal of Neurodevelopmental Disorders, 9,* 3. PMID:28616094

Berry-Kravis, E., Hessl, D., Abbeduto, L., Reiss, A., Beckel-Michener, A., Urv, T., & Outcome Measures Working Groups. (2013). Outcome measures for fragile X syndrome clinical trials: Consensus Statement from the NIH Fragile X Coordinating Group. *Journal of Developmental-Behavioral Pediatrics, 34,* 508–522.

Berry-Kravis, E., Raspa, M., Loggin-Hester, L., Bishop, E., Holiday, D., & Bailey, D. (2010). Seizures in fragile X syndrome: Characteristics and co-morbid diagnoses. *American Journal of Intellectual and Developmental Disabilities, 115,* 461–472.

Berry-Kravis, E., Sumis, A., Hervey, C., & Mathur, S. (2012). Clinic-based retrospective analysis of psychopharmacology for behavior in fragile X syndrome. *International Journal of Pediatrics,* Article ID 843016, doi:10.1155/2012/843016

Budimirovic, D. B., Berry-Kravis, E., Erickson, C. A., Hall, S. S., Hessl, D., Reiss, A. L., . . . Kaufmann, W. E. (2017). Updated report on tools to measure outcomes of clinical trials in fragile X syndrome. *Journal of Neurodevelopmental Disorders, 9,* 14.

Bull, M. J., & American Academy of Pediatrics Committee on Genetics. (2011). Clinical report: Health supervision for children with Down syndrome. *Pediatrics, 128,* 393–404.

Capone, G. T., Chicoine, B., Bulova, P., Stephens, M., Hart, S., Crissman, B., . . . Down Syndrome Medical Interest Group DSMIG-USA Adult Health Care Workgroup. (2018). Co-occurring medical conditions in adults with Down syndrome: A systematic review toward the development of health care guidelines. *American Journal of Medical Genetics, 176A,* 116–133.

Carmichael, J. B., Liu, H. P., Janik, D., Hallahan T.W., Nicolaides, K. H., & Krantz, D. A. (2017). Expanded conventional first trimester screening. *Prenatal Diagnosis, 37,* 802–807.

Castillo, H., Patterson, B., Hickey, F., Kinsman, A., Howard, J. M., Mitchell, T., . . . Molloy, C. A. (2008). Difference in age at regression in children with autism with and without Down syndrome. *Journal of Developmental & Behavioral Pediatrics, 29,* 89–93.

Centers for Disease Control and Prevention & American Academy of Pediatrics. (2016). *CDC and AAP bust fragile X myths.* Retrieved from https://www.cdc.gov/features/fragile-x-myths/index.html

Chapman, R. S., & Hesketh, L. J. (2000). Behavioral phenotype of individuals with Down syndrome. *Mental Retardation and Developmental Disabilities Research Reviews, 6,* 84–95.

Coffee, B., Keith, K., Albizua, I., Malone, T., Mowrey, J., Sherman, S. L., . . . Warren, S. T. (2009). Incidence of fragile X syndrome by newborn screening for methylated FMR1 DNA. *American Journal of Human Genetics, 85,* 503–514.

Cohen, I. L. (1995). A theoretical analysis of the role of hyperarousal in the learning and behavior of fragile X males. *Mental Retardation and Developmental Disabilities Research Reviews,* 1(4), 286–291.

Cordeiro, L., Ballinger, E., Hagerman, R., & Hessl, D. (2011). Clinical assessment of DSM-IV anxiety disorders in fragile X syndrome: Prevalence and characterization. *Journal of Neurodevelopment Disorders,* 3(1), 57–67.

Creavin, A. L., & Brown, R. D. (2009). Ophthalmic abnormalities in children with Down syndrome. *Journal of Pediatric Ophthalmology and Strabismus, 46,* 76–82.

de Graaf, G., Buckley, F., & Skotko, B. G. (2015). Estimates of the live births, natural losses, and elective terminations with Down syndrome in the United States. *American Journal of Medical Genetics Part A, 167A,* 756–767.

de Graaf, G., & van Hove, G. (2015). Learning to read in regular and special schools: A follow-up study of students with Down syndrome. *Life Span and Disability, 18*(1), 7–39.

Delabar, J. -M., Allinquant, B., Bianchi, D., Blumenthal, T., Dekker, A., Edgin, J., . . . Busciglio, J. (2016). Changing paradigms, in Down syndrome: The first international conference of Trisomy 21 Research Society. *Molecular Syndromology, 7*, 251–261.

de Vries, B. B., Wiegers, A. M., Smits, A. P., Mohkamsing, S., Duivenvoorden, H. J., Fryns, J. P., . . . Niermeijer, M. F. (1996). Mental status of females with an FMR1 gene full mutation. *American Journal of Medical Genetics, 58*(5), 1025.

Dias, F. M., Cordeiro, S., Menezes, I., Nogueira, G., Teixeira, A., Marques, M., . . . Anjos, R. (2016). Congenital heart disease in children with Down syndrome: What has changed in the last three decades? *Acta Medica Portuguesa, 29*, 613–620.

Dieguez-Perez, M., de Nova-Garcia, M. -Q., Mourelle-Martinez, M. R., & Bartolome-Villar, B. (2016). Oral health in children with physical (cerebral palsy) and intellectual (Down syndrome) disabilities: Systematic review 1. *Journal of Clinical Experimental Dentistry, 8*(3), e337–e343.

Diercks, G. R., Wentland, C., Keamy, D., Kinane, T. B., Skotko, B., de Guzman, V., . . . Hartnick, C. J. (2018). Hypoglossal nerve stimulation in adolescents with Down syndrome and obstructive sleep apnea. *JAMA Otolaryngology—Head & Neck Surgery, 144*(1), 37–42. doi:10.1001/jamaoto.2017.1871

Dixon, N. E., Crissman, B. G., Smith, P. B., Zimmerman, S. A., Worley, G., & Kishnani, P. S. (2010). Prevalence of iron deficiency in children with Down syndrome. *Journal of Pediatrics, 157*, 967–971.

Down, J. L. H. (1866). Observations on an ethnic classification of idiots. *Clinical Lecture Reports, London Hospital, 3*, 559.

Downes, A., Anixt, J. S., Esbensen, A. J., Wiley, S., & Meinzen-Derr, J. (2015). Psychotropic medication use in children and adolescents with Down syndrome. *Journal of Developmental & Behavioral Pediatrics, 36*, 613–619.

Dykens, E. M. (2007). Psychiatric and behavioral disorders in persons with Down syndrome. *Mental Retardation and Developmental Disabilities Research Reviews, 13*, 272–278.

Dykens, E. M., Hodapp, R. M., & Leckman, J. F. (1987). Strengths and weaknesses in the intellectual functioning of males with fragile X syndrome. *American Journal of Mental Deficiency, 92*(2), 234.

Dykens, E. M., Shah, B., Davis, B., Baker, C., Fife, T., & Fitzpatrick, J. (2015). Psychiatric disorders in adolescents and young adults with Down syndrome and other intellectual disabilities. *Journal of Neurodevelopmental Disorders, 7*(1), 9–20.

Ellis, J. M., Tan, H. K., Gilbert, R. E., Muller, D. P. R., Henley, W., Moy, R., . . . Logan, S. (2008). Supplementation with antioxidants and folinic acid for children with Down's syndrome: Randomized controlled trial. *British Medical Journal, 336*, 594.

Erickson, C. A., Davenport, M. H., Schaefer, T. L., Wink, L. K., Pedapati, E. V., & Sweeney, J. A. (2017). Fragile X targeted pharmacotherapy: Lessons learned and future directions. *Journal of Neurodevelopmental Disorders, 9*, 7.

Fisch, G. S., Carpenter, N., Holden, J. J. A., Howard-Peebles, P. N., Maddalena, A., Borghgraef, M., . . . Fryns, J. P. (1999). Longitudinal changes in cognitive and adaptive behavior in fragile X females: A prospective multicenter analysis. *American Journal of Medical Genetics, 83*(4), 308.

Fisch, G. S., Simensen, R., Tarleton, J., Chalifoux, M., Holden, J. J. A., Carpenter, N., et al. (1996). Longitudinal study of cognitive abilities and adaptive behavior levels in fragile X males: A prospective multicenter analysis. *American Journal of Medical Genetics, 64*(2), 356.

Fishler, K., & Koch, R. (1991). Mental development in Down syndrome mosaicism. *American Journal of Mental Retardation, 96*, 345–351.

Freund, L. S., Reiss, A. L., & Abrams, M. T. (1993). Psychiatric disorders associated with fragile X in the young female. *Pediatrics, 91*(2), 321.

Fudge, J. C., Jr., Li, S., Jaggers, J., O'Brien, S. M., Peterson, E. D., Jacobs, J. P., . . . Pasquali, S. K. (2010). Congenital heart surgery outcomes in Down syndrome: Analysis of a national clinical data base. *Pediatrics, 126*, 314–322.

Gill, M. M., Quezada, M. S., Revello, R., Akolekar, R., & Nicolaides, K. H. (2015). Analysis of cell free DNA in maternal blood in screening for fetal aneuploidies: Update meta-analysis. *Ultrasound Oster Gynecology, 45*, 249.

Goldberg-Stern, H., Strawsburg, R. H., Paterson, B., Hickey, F., Bae, M., Godoth, N., . . . Degrauw, T. J. (2001). Seizure frequency and characteristics in children with Down syndrome. *Brain Development, 23*, 375–378.

Goodlin-Jones, B., Tang, K., Liu, J., & Anders, T. F. (2009). Sleep problems, sleepiness and daytime behavior in preschool-age children. *Journal of Child Psychology & Psychiatry, 50*(12), 1532–1540.

Gross, C., Hoffmann, A., Bassell, G. J., & Berry-Kravis, E. M. (2015). Therapeutic strategies in fragile X syndrome: From bench to bedside and back. *Neurotherapeutics, 12*, 584–608.

Hagerman, R. J., & Falkenstein, A. R. (1987). An association between recurrent otitis media in infancy and later hyperactivity. *Clinical Pediatrics, 26*(5), 253–257.

Hagerman, R. J., & Hagerman, H. P. (2002). *Fragile X syndrome diagnosis, treatment, and research* (3rd ed.). Baltimore, MD: John Hopkins University Press.

Hagerman, R. J., Jackson, C., Amiri, K., O'Connor, R., Sobesky, W., & Silverman, A. C. (1992). Girls with fragile X syndrome: Physical and neurocognitive status and outcome. *Pediatrics, 89*(3), 395–400.

Hagerman, R. J., Leehey, M., Heinrichs, W., Tassone, F., Wilson, R., Hills, J., . . . Hagerman, P. J. (2001). Intention tremor, parkinsonism, and generalized brain atrophy in male carriers of fragile X. *Neurology, 57*, 127–130.

Hanson, M. (2003). Twenty-five years after early intervention: A follow-up of children with Down syndrome and their families. *Infants and Young Children, 16*, 354–365.

Hasle, H., Friedman, J. M., Olsen, J. H., & Rasmssen, S. A. (2016). Low risk of solid tumors in persons with Down syndrome. *Genetic Medicine, 18*(11), 1151–1157.

Hatch-Stein, J. A., Zemel, B. S., Prasad, D., Kalkwarf, H. J., Pipan, M., Magge, S. N., . . . Kelly, A. (2016). Body composition and BMI growth charts in children with Down syndrome. *Pediatrics, 138*, 1–8.

Hattori, M., Fujiyama, A., Taylor, T. D., Watanabe, H., Yada, T, Part, H. -S., . . . Yaspo, M. (2000). The DNA sequence of human chromosome 21. *Nature, 405*, 311–319.

Hessl, D., Dyer-Friedman, J., Glaser, B., Wisbeck, J., Barajas, R. G., Taylor, A., . . . Reiss, A. L. (2001). The influence of environmental and genetic factors on behavior problems and autistic symptoms in boys and girls with fragile X syndrome. *Pediatrics, 108*(5), 1–9.

Huber, K. M., Gallagher, S. M., Warren, S. T., & Bear, M. R. (2002). Altered synaptic plasticity in a mouse model of fragile X mental retardation. *Proceedings of the National Academy of Sciences of the United States of America, 99*, 7746–7750.

Iliff, A. J., Renoux, A. J, Krans, A., Usdin, K., Sutton, M. A., & Todd, P. K (2013). Impaired activity-dependent FMRP translation and enhanced mGluR-dependent LTD in Fragile X premutation mice. *Human Molecular Genetics, 22,* 1180–1192.

Iossifov, I., Ronemus, M., Levy, D., Wang, Z., Hakker, I., Rosenbaum, J., . . . Wigler, M. (2012). De novo gene disruptions in children on the autistic spectrum. *Neuron, 74,* 285–299.

Iughetti, L., Predieri, B., Bruzzi, P., Predieri, F., Vellani, G., Madeo, S. F., . . . Wigler, M. (2014). Ten-year longitudinal study of thyroid function in children with Down's syndrome. *Hormonal Research Paediatrics, 82*(2), 113–121.

Jones, K. L., Jones, M. C., & Campo, M. D. (2013). *Smith's recognizable patterns of human malformation* (7th ed.). Philadelphia, PA: Elsevier Saunders.

Juj, H., & Emery, H. (2009). The arthropathy of Down syndrome: An underdiagnosed and under-recognized condition. *The Journal of Pediatrics, 154*(2), 234–238.

Kainth, D. S., Chaudhry, S. A., Kainth, H. S., Suri, F. K., & Qureshi, A. (2013). Prevalence and characteristic of concurrent Down syndrome in patients with moyamoya disease. *Neurosurgery, 72,* 210–215.

Kaufmann, W. E., Abrams, M. T., Chen, W., & Reiss, A. L. (1999). Genotype, molecular phenotype, and cognitive phenotype: Correlations in fragile X syndrome. *American Journal of Medical Genetics, 83*(4), 286.

Kaufmann, W. E., Kidd, S. A., Andrews, H., Budimirovic, D. B, Esler, A., Haas-Givler, B., . . . Berry-Kravis, E. (2017). Autism spectrum disorder in fragile X syndrome: Characterization using FORWARD. *Pediatrics, 139*(Suppl. 3), S194–S206. PMID:28814540

Khatib, M., Baker, R. D., Ly, E. K., Kozielski, R., & Baker, S. S. (2016). Presenting pattern of pediatric celiac disease. *Journal of Pediatric Gastroenterology and Nutrition, 62,* 60–63.

Kidd, S. A., Lachiewicz, A., Barbouth, D., Blitz, R. K., Delahunty, C., McBrien, D., . . . Berry-Kravis, E. (2014). Fragile X syndrome: A review of associated medical problems. *Pediatrics, 134*(5), 995–1005.

Klaiman, C., Quintin, E. -M., Lightbody, A. A., Hazlett, H. C., Piven, J., . . . Reiss, A. L. (2014). Longitudinal profiles of adaptive behavior in fragile X syndrome. *Pediatrics, 134*(2), 315–324.

Kronk, R., Bishop, E. E., Raspa, M., Bickel, J. O., Mandel, D. A., & Bailey, D. B. (2010). Prevalence, nature, and correlates of sleep problems among children with fragile X syndrome based on a large scale parent survey. *Sleep, 33*(5), 679–687.

Kumin, L., & Schoenbrodt, L. (2015). Employment in adults with Down syndrome in the United States: Results from a national survey. *Journal of Applied Research in Intellectual Disabilities, 29*(4), 330–345. doi:10.1111/jar.12182

Kupferman, J. C., Cruschel, C. M., & Kupchik, G. S. (2009). Increased prevalence of renal and urinary tract anomalies in children with Down syndrome. *Pediatrics, 124,* e615–e621.

Lejeune, J., Gautier, M., & Turpin, R. (1959). Etudes des chromosomes somatiques de neufenfants mongoliens [Study of somatic chromosomes of new children with mongolism]. *Comptes Rendus de l'Académie des Sciences, 248,* 1721–1722.

Liu, J. A, Hagerman, R. J., Miller, R. M., Craft, L. T., Finucane, B., Tartaglia, N., . . . Cohen, J., (2016). Clinicians' experiences with the Fragile X Clinical and Research Consortium. *American Journal of Medical Genetics, 9999A,* 1–6. PMID:27604509

Loesch, D. Z., Huggins, R. M., & Hagerman, R. J. (2004). Phenotypic variation and FMRP levels in fragile X. *Mental Retardation and Developmental Disabilities Research Reviews, 10,* 31–41.

Lott, I. T., & Dierssen, M. (2010). Cognitive deficits and associated neurological complications in individuals with Down's syndrome. *The Lancet Neurology, 9,* 623–633.

Lubs, H. A. (1969). A marker X chromosome. *American Journal of Human Genetics, 21*(3), 231–244.

Lubs, H. A., Stevenson, R. E., & Schwartz, C. E. (2012). Fragile X and X-linked intellectual disability: Four decades of discovery. *American Journal of Human Genetics, 90*(4), 579–590. doi:10.1016/j.ajhg.2012.02.018

Luke, A., Roizen, N. J., Sutton, M., & Schoeller, D. A. (1994). Energy expenditure in children with Down syndrome correcting metabolic rate for movement. *Journal of Pediatrics, 125,* 825–839.

Luke, A., Sutton, M., Schoeller, D., & Roizen, N. (1996). Nutrient intake and obesity in prepubescent children with Down syndrome. *Journal of the American Dietetic Association, 96,* 1262–1267.

Manickam, V., Shott, G. S., Heithaus, D., & Shott, S. R. (2016). Hearing loss in Down syndrome revisited—15 years later. *International Journal of Pediatric Otorhinolaryngology, 88,* 203–207.

Marchal, J. P., Maurice-Stamer, H., Houtzager, B. A., von Rozenburg-Marres, S. L. R., Oostrom, K. J., Grootenhuis, M. A., . . . van Trotsenburg, A. S. P. (2016). Growing up with Down syndrome: Development from 6 months to 10.7 years. *Research in Developmental Disabilities, 59,* 437–450.

Martin, J. P., & Bell, J. (1943). A pedigree of mental defect showing sex-linkage. *Journal of Neurology and Psychiatry, 6*(3-4), 154–157.

Mazzocco, M. M., Pennington, B. F., & Hagerman, R. J. (1993). The neurocognitive phenotype of female carriers of fragile X: Additional evidence for specificity. *Journal of Developmental & Behavioral Pediatrics, 14*(5), 328–335.

McDowell, K. M., & Craven, D. I. (2011). Pulmonary complications of Down syndrome during childhood. *Journal of Pediatrics, 158*(2), 319–324.

McDuffie, A., Kover, S., Abbeduto, L., Lewis, P., & Brown, T. (2012). Profiles of receptive and expressive language abilities in boys with comorbid fragile X syndrome and autism. *American Journal of Intellectual and Developmental Disabilities, 117*(1), 18.

Mircher, D., Cieuta-Walti, C., Marey, I., Rebillat, A-S, Cretu, L., Milenko, E., . . . Ravel, A. (2017). Acute regression in young people with Down syndrome. *Brain Science, 7*(6), 57.

Murphy, M. M., & Abbeduto, L. (2005). Indirect genetic effects and the early language development of children with genetic mental retardation syndromes: The role of joint attention. *Infants & Young Children, 18*(1), 47–59.

Nation, J., & Brigger, M. (2017). The efficacy of adenoidectomy for obstructive sleep apnea in children with Down syndrome: A systematic review. *Otolaryngology—Head and Neck Surgery, 157,* 401–408.

Nightengale, E., Yoon, P., Wolter-Warmerdam, K., Daniels, D., & Hickey, F. (2017). Understanding hearing and hearing loss in children with Down syndrome. *American Journal of Audiology, 26,* 301–308.

Patrick, K., Wade, R., Goulden, N., Rowntree, C., Hough, R., Moorman, A. V., . . . Mitchell, C. D. (2014). Outcome of Down syndrome associated acute lymphoblastic leukaemia treated on a contemporary protocol. *British Journal of Haematology, 165,* 552–555.

Phelan, E., Pal, R., Henderson, L., Green, K. M., & Bruce, I. A. (2016). The management of children with Down syndrome and profound hearing loss. *Cochlear Implants International, 17*(1), 52–57.

Pierce, M. J., Fanchi, S. H., & Pinter, J. D. (2017). Characterization of thyroid abnormalities in a large cohort of children with Down syndrome. *Hormone Research in Paediatrics, 87*, 170–178.

Prussing, E., Sobo, E. J., Walker, E., & Kurtin, P. S. (2005). Between desperation and disability right: A narrative analysis of complementary/alternative medicine use by parents for children with Down syndrome. *Social Science & Medicine, 60*, 587–598.

Purdy, I. B., Singh, N., Brown, W. L., Vangala, S., & Devaskar, U. P. (2014). Revising early hypothyroidism screening in infants with Down syndrome. *Journal of Perinatology, 34*, 936–940.

Rabin, K. R., & Whitlock, J. A. (2009). Malignancy in children with trisomy 21. *The Oncologist, 14*, 164–173.

Richards, C., Jones, C., Groves, L., Moss, J., & Oliver, C. (2015). Prevalence of autism spectrum disorder phenomenology in genetic disorders: a systematic review and meta-analysis. *Lancet Psychiatry, 2*, 909–916.

Roberts, J. E., Mirrett, P., Anderson, K., Burchinal, M., & Neebe, E. (2002). Early communication, symbolic behavior, and social profiles of young males with fragile X syndrome. *American Journal of Speech Language Pathology, 11*(3), 295–304.

Roizen, N. J. (2005). Complementary and alternative medicine in Down syndrome. *Mental Retardation and Developmental Disabilities Research Reviews, 11*, 149–155.

Roizen, N. J. (2010). Overview of health issues in Down syndrome. *International Review of Research in Mental Retardation, 39*, 3–33.

Roizen, N. J., Magyar, C. I., Kuschner, E. S., Sulkes, S. B., Druschel, C., van Wijngaarden, E., . . . Hyman, S. L. (2014). A community cross-sectional survey of medical problems in 440 children with Down syndrome in New York State. *Journal of Pediatrics, 164*, 871–875.

Roizen, N. J., Mets, M. B., & Blondis, T. A. (1994). Ophthalmic disorders in children with Down syndrome. *Developmental Medicine and Child Neurology, 36*, 594–600.

Seltzer, M. M., Baker, M. W., Hong, J., Maenner, M., Greenberg, J., & Mandel, D. (2012). Prevalence of CGG expansions of the FMR1 gene in a US population-based sample. *American Journal of Medical Genetics Part B, Neuropsychiatric Genetics, 159B*, 589–597.

Sherman, S. L., Kidd, S. A., Berry-Kravis, E., Andrews, H., Lincoln, S., Swanson, M., . . . Brown, W. T. (2017). Fragile X Online Registry With Accessible Research Database (FORWARD): Experience from the Fragile X Clinical and Research Consortium to study the natural history of fragile X syndrome. *Pediatrics, 139*(Suppl. 3), S183–S193. PMID:28814539

Shott, S. R., Amin, R., Chini, B., Heubi, C., Hotze, S., & Akers, R. (2006). Obstructive sleep apnea: Should all children with Down syndrome be tested? *Archives of Otolaryngology, Head, and Neck Surgery, 132*, 432–436.

Steinberg, J., & Webber, C. (2013). The roles of FMRP-regulated genes in autism spectrum disorder: Single- and multiple-hit genetic etiologies. *The American Journal of Human Genetics, 93*, 825–839.

Steingass, K. J., Chicoine, B., McGuire, D., & Roizen, N. J. (2011). Developmental disabilities grown up: Down syndrome. *Journal of Developmental & Behavioral Pediatrics, 32*(7), 548–558.

Stoll, C., Dott, B., Alembik, Y., & Roth, M. P. (2015). Associated congenital anomalies among cases with Down syndrome. *European Journal of Medical Genetics, 58*, 674–680.

Sudhalter, V., Cohen, I. L., Silverman, W., & Wolf-Schein, E. G. (1994). Conversational analyses of males with fragile X, Down syndrome, and autism: Comparison of the emergence of deviant language. *American Journal of Mental Retardation, 94*(4), 431–441.

Symons, F. J., Byiers, B. J., Raspa, M., Bishop, E., & Bailey, D. B. (2010). Self-injurious behavior and fragile X syndrome: findings from the national fragile X survey. *American Journal of Intellectual and Developmental Disabilities, 115*(6), 473–481.

Szaflarska-Popolawska, A., Soroczynska-Wrzyszcz, N., Barg, E., Jozefczuk, J., Grzybowska-Chiebowszyk, B. K. U., Wiecek, S., . . . Cukrowska, B. (2016). Assessment of coeliac disease prevalence in patients with Down syndrome in Poland—A multi-centre study. *Przeglad Gastroenterologiczny, 11*(1), 41–46.

Tassone, F., Long, K. P., Tong, T. -H., Lo, J., Gane, L. W., Berry-Kravis, E., . . . Hagerman, R. J. (2012). FMR1 CGG allele size and prevalence ascertained through newborn screening in the United States. *Genome Medicine, 4*, 100.

Taub, J. W., Berman, J. N., Hitzler, J. K., Sorrell, A. D., Lacayo, N. J., Mast, K., . . . Gamis, A. S. (2017). Improved outcomes for myeloid leukemia of Down syndrome: A report from the Children's Oncology Group AAML0431 trial. *Blood, 129*(25), 3304–3313.

Tedeschi, A. S., Roizen, N. J., Taylor, H. G., Murray, G., Curtis, C. A., & Parikh, A. S. (2015). The prevalence of congenital hearing loss in neonates with Down syndrome. *Journal of Pediatrics, 166*(1), 168–171.

Turk, J. (1998). Fragile X syndrome and attentional deficits. *Journal of Applied Research in Intellectual Disabilities, 11*(3), 175.

Vacca, R. A., & Valenti, D. (2015). Green tea ECCG plus fish oil omega-3 dietary supplements rescue mitochondrial dysfunctions and are safe in the Down's syndrome child. *Clinical Nutrition, 34*, 783–784.

Verkerk, A. J., Pieretti, M., Sutcliffe, J. S., Fu, Y. H., Kuhl, D. P., Pizzuti, A., . . . Zhang, F. P. (1991). Identification of a gene (FMR-1) containing a CGG repeat coincident with a breakpoint cluster region exhibiting length variation in fragile X syndrome. *Cell, 65*(5), 905–914.

Visootsak, J., Kidd, S., Anderson, T., Bassell, J. L., Sherman, S., & Berry-Kravis, E. (2016). Importance of a specialty clinic for individuals with genetic conditions: Fragile X syndrome as a model. *American Journal of Medical Genetics, 170*, 3144–3149. PMID:27649377

Waltes, R., Duketis, E., Knapp, M., Anney, R. J., Huguet, G., Schilitt, S., . . . Chiocchetti, A. G. (2014). Common variants in genes of the postsynaptic FMRP signaling pathway are risk factors for autism spectrum disorders. *Human Genetics, 133*, 781–792.

Wang, L. W., Berry-Kravis, E., & Hagerman, R. J. (2010). Fragile X: Leading the way for targeted treatments in autism. *Neurotherapeutics, 7*(3), 264–274.

Willemsen, R., Levenga, J., & Oostra, B. A. (2011). CGG repeat in the FMR1 gene: Size matters. *Clinical Genetics, 80*, 214–225.

Whooten, R., Schmitt, J., & Schwartz, A. (2017). Endocrine manifestations of Down syndrome. *Current Opinion in Endocrinology Diabetes, and Obesity, 25*, 61–66. oi:10.1097/MED.0000000000000382

Worley, G., Crissman, B. G., Cadogan, E., Milleson, C., Adkins, D. W., & Kishnani, P. S. (2015). Down syndrome disintegrative disorder: New-onset autistic regression, dementia, and insomnia in older children and adolescents with Down syndrome. *Journal of Child Neurology, 30*(9), 1147–1152.

Yaneza, M. M., Hunter, K., Irwin, S., & Kubba, H. (2016). Hearing in school-aged children with trisomy 21—results of a longitudinal cohort study in children identified at birth. *Clinical Otolaryngology, 41*(6), 711–717.

Youssef, E. A., Berry-Kravis, E., Czech, C., Hagerman, R. J., Hessl, D., Wong, C. Y., . . . FragXis Study Group. (2018). Effect of the mGluR5-NAM Basimglurant on behavior in adolescents and adults with fragile X syndrome in a randomized, double-blind, placebo-controlled trial: FragXis phase 2 results. *Neuropsychopharmacology, 43*(3), 503–512.

Yrigollen, C. M., Martorell, L., Durbin-Johnson, B. D., Naudo, M., Genoves, J., Murgia, A., . . . Tassone, F. (2014). AGG interruptions and age affect *FMR1* allele stability during transmission. *Journal of Neurodevelopmental Disorders, 6*, 24.

Yu, T. W., & Berry-Kravis, E. (2014). Autism and fragile X syndrome. *Seminars in Neurology, 34*, 258–265.

Zemel, B. S., Pipan, M., Stallings, V.A., Hall, W., Schadt, K., Freedman, D. A., . . . Thorpe, P. (2015). Growth charts for children with Down syndrome in the United States. *Pediatrics, 136*(5), e1204–e12011.

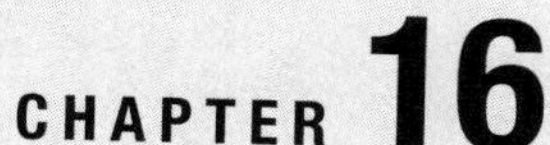

CHAPTER 16 Inborn Errors of Metabolism

Nicholas Ah Mew, Erin MacLeod, and Mark L. Batshaw

Upon completion of this chapter, the reader will

- Understand the term *inborn error of metabolism*
- Know the differences among a number of these inborn errors, including amino acid disorders, organic acidemias, fatty acid oxidation defects, mitochondrial disorders, peroxisomal disorders, and lysosomal storage diseases
- Identify the characteristic clinical symptoms and diagnostic tests for these disorders
- Know which of these disorders have newborn screening tests available
- Recognize different approaches to treatment
- Understand the outcome and range of developmental disabilities associated with inborn errors of metabolism

The food we eat contains fats, proteins, and carbohydrates that must be broken down into smaller components and then metabolized by thousands of enzymes that maintain body functions. Approximately 1 in 2,500 children are born with a deficiency in one of the enzymes that normally catalyzes an important biochemical reaction in the cells (OMIM, 2018). These children are said to have an inborn error of metabolism. Such an enzyme deficiency can result in the accumulation of a toxic chemical compound behind the enzyme block or lead to a deficiency of a product normally produced by the deficient enzyme (Figure 16.1). The result may be organ damage or dysfunction (often the brain), varying degrees of disability, or even death. For example, children with phenylketonuria (PKU) have a deficiency in the enzyme that normally converts one amino acid (phenylalanine) to another (tyrosine). An inherited deficiency of this enzyme (phenylalanine hydroxylase) leads to the accumulation of phenylalanine, which at high levels is toxic to the brain (Figure 16.1; Jahja et al., 2017; Singh et al., 2014; Vockley et al., 2014). If PKU is not recognized and treated soon after birth, severe intellectual disability ensues. In contrast, in children with congenital adrenal hypoplasia, an inherited enzyme deficiency leads to decreased production of certain steroid hormones (e.g., cortisol) that are essential for typical body function. Females with this deficiency may be born with ambiguous genitalia because they produce abnormal amounts of the male steroid sex hormone (testosterone) *in utero* (Auchus, 2015; Turcu & Auchus, 2015). Fortunately, for these disorders and others, newborn screening tests and early treatment have

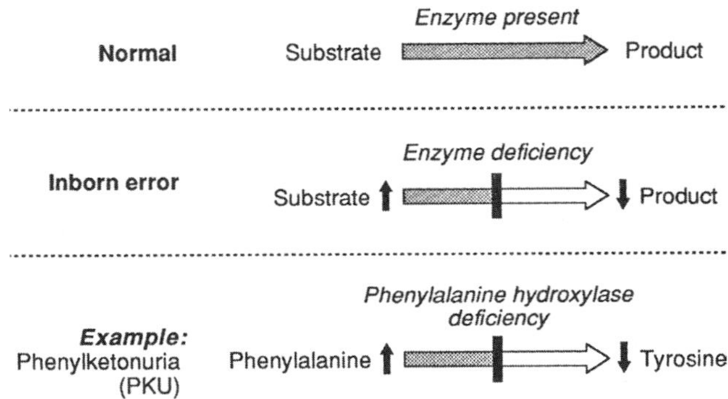

Figure 16.1. Inborn errors of metabolism are genetic disorders involving an enzyme deficiency. This enzyme block leads to the accumulation of a toxic substrate and/or the deficient synthesis of a product needed for normal body function. In PKU, there is a toxic accumulation of phenylalanine behind the deficient enzyme, phenylalanine hydroxylase.

permitted children who are affected to grow up with typical intelligence and normal physiological functioning. Not all inborn errors of metabolism can be as effectively treated, however, because of delays in diagnosis or lack of an effective intervention. This chapter provides examples from a range of inborn errors of metabolism to explain diagnostic and therapeutic advances that are improving the outcome of people with these disorders.

CASE STUDY

Lisa was discharged from the hospital at 3 days of age. Her parents were surprised and upset when they were called back a week later after doctors reported that she had abnormal results for her screening test for PKU. Amino acid studies confirmed the diagnosis of PKU, and Lisa was placed on a formula that was free of phenylalanine. She was also allowed to breastfeed a small amount. As Lisa grew, her parents could hardly believe there was a problem because Lisa looked and acted like a typically developing child and achieved her developmental milestones on time, sometimes making PKU seem like a "silent disorder." The visits to the metabolism clinic were focused on educating her parents and Lisa about her special diet. Though Lisa struggled to find independence, her providers would remind her of the importance of "diet for life." As a result of dietary indiscretions, Lisa had poor metabolic control that began to impact her academic performance. She was unfortunately found to be a nonresponder to the pharmaceutical interventions available, requiring her to continue her strict dietary regimen. She eventually graduated from college, got married, and recognized the importance of returning to her special diet in order to have a healthy infant and avoid the manifestations of uncontrolled maternal PKU, which include microcephaly, intellectual disability, and heart defects in her baby.

CASE STUDY

Darnel babbled at 6 months and sat without support shortly thereafter. His parents became concerned, however, when at 1 year of age he had made no further progress. If anything, he seemed less steady in sitting and was uninvolved with his surroundings. His pediatrician worried that Darnel might have an autism spectrum disorder. By 18 months, there were graver concerns. Darnel was no longer able to roll over; he was very floppy and did not appear to respond to light or sound. His pediatrician referred Darnel to a genetics clinic, where an extensive workup eventually diagnosed him as having Tay-Sachs disease, a genetic disorder affecting lipid metabolism in the brain. Over the next 3 years, Darnel slipped into an unresponsive condition and required tube feeding. He finally succumbed to aspiration pneumonia. As a result of the diagnosis, his parents decided to undergo prenatal diagnosis in subsequent pregnancies. They now have two healthy children, and his mother underwent one termination of a fetus that was affected.

Thought Questions:

As a metaphor for inborn errors of metabolism, imagine that the human body is an efficiently run city and that each road represents a chemical reaction catalyzed by a unique enzyme. What happens to car traffic in the city if one of the roads is blocked? How would this differ if it were a major highway that was blocked versus a small road? How about if only two lanes of the highway were obstructed rather than the whole highway? What if the only road to the only electric power plant is permanently blocked? What would happen to the parking lot of the car manufacturing plant if its exit were obstructed?

TYPES OF INBORN ERRORS OF METABOLISM

Inborn errors of metabolism were first described approximately 100 years ago (Garrod, 1908). Since then, a number of new metabolic disorders have been described each year. In fact, over 300 additional disorders have been identified in the last decade alone (Saudubray et al., 2016). The majority of these enzyme deficiencies are inherited as autosomal recessive traits, in which both parents carry a genetic change on one of their two copies of the gene (see Chapter 1). These carriers are healthy and develop typically due to the normal second copy of the gene. Individuals who are affected usually inherit two abnormal genes and have no normal version. A few metabolic disorders are transmitted as X-linked disorders or through mitochondrial inheritance (see Chapter 1). Prenatal diagnosis is available for most of these disorders (see Chapter 4). See Table 16.1 for further classifications of metabolic disorders.

Although there are many different ways of categorizing these disorders, inborn errors of metabolism are often divided into 1) those that are clinically "silent" for a relatively long period before being recognized, 2) those that produce acute metabolic crises, and 3) those that cause progressive organ damage or dysfunction (Table 16.2).

Among the silent disorders are certain abnormalities involving amino acids or organic acids (e.g., PKU) or metals (e.g., Wilson disease). Disorders producing acute toxicity include certain inborn errors in the metabolism of small molecules, including ammonia, amino acids, organic acids, fatty acids, lactic acid, and simple sugars (Levy, 2009a, 2009b; Vernon, 2015). Inborn errors of metabolism causing progressive disorders include most **glycogen** storage and peroxisomal and lysosomal storage disorders. The specific names of the disorders are often derived from their deficient enzyme (e.g., **ornithine transcarbamylase [OTC] deficiency,** a urea cycle disorder [UCD]).

Silent disorders, such as PKU, do not manifest as life-threatening crises, but if left untreated, they lead to irreversible brain damage and developmental disabilities. These disorders contrast with inborn errors that cause episodic symptoms, such as OTC deficiency, that may be acutely life-threatening with each decompensation, typically starting in early infancy. In both cases, an infant who is affected is generally protected in the womb because the maternal circulation can remove the toxic chemical or provide the missing product. After birth, however, the infant must rely on his or her own metabolic pathways, and if they are abnormal, toxicity occurs rapidly or over time, depending on the severity of the defect. In progressive disorders, there is a gradual accumulation of large molecules. These molecules are stored in the cells of various body organs, including the brain, where they ultimately cause damage, leading to physical or neurological deterioration. Many of the small-molecular disorders, both those that are silent and those with acute symptoms, are treatable with fairly good outcome if treatment is started early. The large-molecular disorders, with a few notable exceptions, have been far more difficult to treat, and their outcome generally remains poor.

Clinical Manifestations

The clinical manifestations of the various inborn errors of metabolism fall along a spectrum, from lack of overt symptoms to life-threatening episodes.

The silent disorders like PKU do not manifest symptoms such as lethargy, coma, or regression of skills. Instead, children who are untreated develop at a slower-than-expected rate and are usually not identified as having intellectual disability until later in childhood.

Table 16.1. Categorical classification of metabolic disorders*

Protein-related metabolic disorders	Proteins are large molecules (macromolecules) composed of chains of amino acids (AAs) Proteins are the main structural components of the cells and tissues of the body Special proteins called enzymes catalyze (speed up or facilitate) chemical reactions in the body Protein in food (a macronutrient) is present in meat, fish, dairy, and eggs in large amounts, and in plants (especially beans and legumes) in smaller amounts	
Disorder	Metabolic defect	Examples
Aminoacidopathies	Proteins are broken down into AAs Defects in the early steps of the breakdown of AAs lead to accumulation of specific AAs that are toxic in high amounts Abnormal quantities of AAs are found in the blood (abnormal quantitative plasma AAs)	*Phenylketonuria* (excess AA phenylalanine)** *Maple syrup urine disease* (excess branched-chain AAs: leucine, isoleucine, valine) Homocystinuria (excess AA homocysteine and methionine) *Tyrosinemia* (excess AA tyrosine)
Organic acidemias	AAs are broken down into organic acids (OA) and ammonia (NH3) Defects in later steps in the breakdown of AAs lead to an accumulation of OAs, NH3, and other metabolic by-products (e.g., acyl carnitine) in the blood OAs acidify the blood, causing metabolic acidosis OAs and other metabolic byproducts accumulate in the urine (abnormal quantitative urine OAs)	*Propionic acidemia* *Methylmalonic acidemia* *Glutaric acidemia type I* Isovaleric acidemia

(continued)

Table 16.1. *(continued)*

Disorder	Metabolic defect	Examples
Urea cycle disorders	AAs are broken down into OA and NH3 Ammonia is toxic and must be converted into urea and excreted by the kidneys Defects in the synthesis of urea from ammonia result in accumulation of ammonia in the blood (hyperammonemia), abnormalities of plasma AAs, and the presence of orotic acid in the urine	*Ornithine transcarbamylase deficiency* Citrullinemia Arginosuccinic aciduria
Fat-related metabolic disorders	Fats are large molecules (macromolecules) composed of long fatty acid (FA) chains held together by a small molecule (glycerol) Fats are the main energy storage molecules of the cells and tissues of the body Fats in food (a macronutrient) are present in meat, fish, dairy, and eggs as animal fats and in plants as oils	
Disorder	Metabolic defect	Examples
Fatty acid oxidation disorders	Fats are broken down into FAs Defects in the breakdown of FAs lead to accumulation of FA byproducts called acyl carnitines (abnormal acyl carnitine profile) Defects in the breakdown of FAs lead to decreased production of glucose, resulting in low blood sugar, especially after fasting (hypoglycemia)	Medium-chain acyl CoA dehydrogenase deficiency Long-chain 3-hydroxy acyl CoA dehydrogenase deficiency Very long-chain acyl CoA dehydrogenase deficiency Primary carnitine deficiency
Carbohydrate-related metabolic disorders	Carbohydrates are large molecules (macromolecules) composed of chains of simple sugars Carbohydrates are a major energy source for the body and are stored as glycogen in the liver and in muscles Carbohydrates in food (a macronutrient) are present in fruits, vegetables, and grains; the sugar lactose is present in milk, and other sugars, such as fructose, are present in fruit	
Disorder	Metabolic defect	Examples
Disorders of carbohydrate/sugar metabolism	Carbohydrates are broken down into sugars Defects in the breakdown of sugars leads to an accumulation of toxic amounts of the sugar and metabolic products in the body (abnormal plasma sugar levels) Untreated infants develop jaundice, liver dysfunction, blood clotting abnormalities, and severe infections	*Galactosemia* Hereditary fructose intolerance
Disorders of carbohydrate degradation	Carbohydrates are stored in the liver and in muscles as the macromolecule glycogen The liver utilizes glycogen to later provide a slow release of glucose to the rest of the body and maintain blood glucose levels In contrast, each muscle (including the heart) stores carbohydrates as glycogen for its own future use Defects in the breakdown of glycogen result in accumulation of toxic quantities of glycogen in the liver or muscles or both A defect in liver glycogen breakdown may result in hypoglycemia and liver failure A defect in muscle glycogen breakdown may result in muscle pain, fatigue, and heart failure (cardiomyopathy) One disorder of carbohydrate degradation (Pompe disease) is also classified as a lysosomal disorder because the deficient enzyme is located in lysosomes	Hepatic *glycogen storage diseases* (e.g., type I, III, IV, VI) Muscle glycogen storage diseases (e.g., type II, V)
Lysosomal disorders	Lysosomes are spherical organelles found in the cytoplasm of cells throughout the body Lysosomes contain enzymes that "digest" large, complex molecules (macromolecules) including mucopolysaccharides (made of complex chains of sugars, also known as glycosaminoglycans [GAGs]) and sphingolipids (specially modified lipid molecules)	

Disorder	Metabolic defect	Examples
Mucopolysaccharidoses (MPSs)	Lysosomes are deficient in enzymes that break down MPSs/GAGs MPS molecules accumulate in tissues Urine GAG analysis is used as a screening test for MPSs	*MPS I (Hurler syndrome)* MPS II (Hunter syndrome) *MPS III (Sanfilippo syndrome)* MPS IVa (Morquio syndrome) MPS VI (Maroteaux-Lamy syndrome) MPS VII (Sly syndrome)
Sphingolipidoses	Lysosomes are deficient in enzymes that break down sphingolipids Sphingolipids are present to varying degrees in different tissues of the body, many of which are important in the nervous system Types of sphingolipids include sphingomyelin, globosides, and gangliosides	*Tay-Sachs disease* *Niemann-Pick disease type A and B* *Fabry disease* *Krabbe disease* *Metachromatic leukodystrophy* *Gaucher disease*
Other lysosomal disorders	Other lysosomal disorders include oligosacchridoses, lipidoses, and lysosomal transport diseases	Neuronal ceroid lipofuscinoses Sialuria (Salla disease)
Peroxisomal disorders	Peroxisomes are organelles found in the cytoplasm of cells throughout the body Peroxisomes are important in the breakdown (oxidation) of very long-chain FAs (VLCFAs) and branched-chain FAs	
Disorder	Metabolic defect	Examples
Deficiency of peroxisomal oxidation	Peroxisomes are unable to breakdown VLCFAs or branched-chain FAs Individuals present with neurologic deterioration and developmental regression during childhood	X-linked *adrenoleukodystrophy*
Severe depletion or absence of peroxisomes (peroxisomal biogenesis disorders)	Peroxisomes are deficient or absent Infants are born with multiple physical anomalies and neurologic and sensory deficits Usually fatal in infancy	*Zellweger syndrome*
Mitochondrial disorders	Mitochondria are complex, double-membraned organelles found in the cytoplasm of cells throughout the body Mitochondria are critical to the production of energy from the breakdown products of proteins, carbohydrates, and fats Mitochondria are inherited exclusively from the mother and have their own DNA, but most mitochondrial functions rely on the products of nuclear ("regular") genes that are inherited from both parents (see Chapter 1)	
Disorder	Metabolic defect	Examples
Mutations of mitochondrial DNA	Mitochondria are critical to energy production through the body but are especially important in tissues that have high energy demands The brain, muscles, heart, and eyes are especially affected by mitochondrial dysfunction Individuals affected have a wide range of symptoms, including stroke-like episodes, diabetes, hearing loss, heart and visual abnormalities, and accumulation of lactic acid in the blood (lactic acidosis)	*MELAS (mitochondrial encephalomyopathy, lactic acid, and stroke-like episodes)* Kearns-Sayre syndrome
Mutations of nuclear DNA affecting mitochondrial function	Multiple energy-dependent tissues and organs are affected Affected individuals can present in infancy with severe developmental delays, seizures, muscle weakness, and lactic acidosis and liver dysfunction	Leigh syndrome Mitochondrial depletion syndromes

*Adapted with permission from Rice, G. M., & Steiner, R. D. (2016). Inborn Errors of Metabolism (Metabolic Disorders). *Pediatrics in Review, 37*(1), 3–15.

**Examples of metabolic disorders discussed in the main chapter text are *italicized*. See Appendix B for descriptions of the individual disorders.

Table 16.2. Examples of inborn errors of metabolism

Type I: Silent disorders
Phenylketonuria (PKU)
Type II: Disorders presenting in acute metabolic crisis
Urea cycle disorders (ornithine transcarbamylase [OTC] deficiency)
Organic acidemias (propionic acidemia)
Fatty acid oxidation disorders (very long-chain Acyl-CoA dehydrogenase [VLCAD] deficiency)
Type III: Disorders with progressive neurological deterioration
Lysosomal storage disorders (Gaucher disease, Pompe disease, Fabry disease, mucopolysaccharidoses, Tay-Sachs disease, metachromatic leukodystrophy)
Peroxisomal storage disorders (X-linked adrenoleukodystrophy, Zellweger disease)
Mitochondrial disorders (mitochondrial encephalomyopathy, lactic acidosis, and stroke-like episodes [MELAS])

Life-threatening crises characterize the second group of inborn errors of metabolism. Affected individuals with these disorders appear to be unaffected at birth. Severely affected infants will present by a few days of age with vomiting, respiratory distress, and lethargy before slipping into coma. These symptoms, however, mimic those observed in other severe newborn illnesses such as sepsis (blood-borne infection), brain hemorrhage, heart and lung malformations, and gastrointestinal obstruction, so that making the correct diagnosis is difficult. If specific metabolic testing of the blood and urine is not performed, the disease will go undetected. Undiagnosed and untreated, virtually all children who are affected will die quickly. One study reported that 60% of children with newborn onset inborn errors of the **urea** cycle (causing elevated ammonia level) had at least one sibling who died before the disorder was correctly diagnosed in a subsequent child (Batshaw et al., 1982). Even with "heroic" treatment, which may include **dialysis** to "wash out" the toxin (ammonia), many infants do not survive, and severe developmental disabilities may occur in those who do (Bilgin, Unal, Gunduz, Uncu, & Tiryaki, 2014; Posset et al., 2016).

In children with neonatal-onset disease, DNA analysis typically shows mutations that cause the absence of the enzyme or the formation of a completely nonfunctional enzyme. Enzyme activity levels are generally undetectable (see Chapter 1). By contrast, some children with the same inborn error of metabolism have less severe mutations that result in reduced (rather than absent) amount of enzymes or that result in enzymes that are only partially dysfunctional. These children typically have later onset of clinical signs and more variable or subtle symptoms. For instance, some individuals with fatty acid oxidation disorders do not present in infancy but instead present when illness or exercise results in severe muscle weakness and breakdown of muscle tissue (Hisahara et al., 2015). In the case of children with milder urea cycle disorders, symptoms of behavioral change, cyclical vomiting, and lethargy are often provoked by excessive protein intake or intercurrent infections such as a gastrointestinal virus or a cold (Lichter-Konecki et al., 2016; Posset et al., 2016). Although these children generally have a better outcome than those with neonatal-onset disease, they remain at risk for life-threatening metabolic crises throughout life. In addition, although their developmental disabilities may be less severe than those in children with neonatal-onset disease, children with later onset disease rarely escape without some residual cognitive impairment, ranging from attention-deficit/hyperactivity disorder (ADHD) and learning disabilities to intellectual disability.

The third clinical presentation of inborn errors of metabolism is in the form of slowly progressive disorders. These often result from the accumulation of a large molecule in a cellular compartment, such as the lysosome or the peroxisome, eventually interfering with cellular processes. Over 50 lysosomal storage disorders (Beck, 2018; Rastall & Amalfitano, 2017) and over 15 peroxisomal disorders (Braverman, D'Agostino, & MacLean, 2013; Wanders et al., 2017) have been described to date.

In the most severe of these disorders, the deleterious effects may begin prenatally, resulting in clinical features at birth that worsen with age. Such is the case with Zellweger syndrome, which may already present at birth with hypotonia, seizures, liver failure, and renal cysts. In other disorders, infants appear unaffected at birth, but they gradually develop progressive loss of motor and cognitive skills beginning in later infancy or early childhood that, if left untreated, commonly leads to death in childhood. In the case of Tay-Sachs disease, Darnel's disorder in the case study, the child who is affected appears to develop typically until 3–12 months of age, at which point skill development halts. For the next 1–2 years, the child gradually loses all skills, begins having seizures, and exhibits decreases in muscle tone, vision, hearing, and cognition. Death usually results from malnutrition or aspiration pneumonia. Unfortunately, no effective treatment currently exists for this disorder.

Enzyme replacement therapy, however, has been successful in treating several lysosomal disorders (Gaucher disease, Fabry disease, Pompe disease, and mucopolysaccharidoses) in which target organs other than the brain are accessible to a recombinant (genetically engineered) enzyme (Dornelles et al., 2017; El Dib et al., 2017; Kishnani & Beckemeyer, 2014; Stirnemann et al., 2017). However, the synthetic enzyme does not cross the blood–brain barrier (the network of blood vessels and cells around the brain that acts as a filter for blood flowing to the central nervous system), and so it does not halt or reverse the cognitive effects of these disorders. Some clinical studies have explored injecting synthetic enzyme intrathecally (into the spinal canal so that it reaches the cerebrospinal fluid) as a treatment for disorders in which the brain is a target organ. Medications that reduce production of the toxic metabolite (i.e., substrate reduction therapies) have also been a successful therapeutic avenue and have been used in conjunction with enzyme replacement therapies (Stirnemann et al., 2017). Stem cell and bone marrow transplantation have also been somewhat effective in certain mucopolysaccharidoses and leukodystrophies (Boelens & van Hasselt, 2016; Chiesa, Wynn, & Veys, 2016).

MECHANISM OF BRAIN DAMAGE

The causes of brain damage in the various inborn errors of metabolism are not completely understood. Research is starting to provide some clues that may eventually lead to improved treatment.

Neurotoxins appear to play a role in certain metabolic disorders. For example, in nonketotic hyperglycinemia, an inborn error of amino acid metabolism, there is an accumulation of **glycine,** leading to uncontrolled seizures (Van Hove, Coughlin, & Scharer, 2013). Glycine appears to produce excitotoxicity at a neurotransmitter receptor, leading to the influx of calcium ions and water into the neuron. This causes swelling and, eventually, cell death.

In some disorders, more than one neurotoxin may be involved. Scientists believe that in inborn errors of the urea cycle, the accumulating toxins, both ammonia and glutamine, directly cause nerve cells to swell and indirectly cause excitotoxic damage to the brain (Braissant et al., 2013). If children are rescued from the ammonia-induced coma within a day or two, the neurotoxic effect can subside and outcome can be fairly good (Bilgin et al., 2014). If the coma is prolonged, however, irreversible brain damage occurs.

ASSOCIATED DISABILITIES

The toxic accumulation of metabolic compounds or the deficient synthesis of essential products results in a range of developmental disabilities in children with inborn errors of metabolism. The most common are intellectual disability and cerebral palsy. However, in certain inborn errors, there are also rather specific impairments. These are sometimes associated with distinctive pathological features in the brain, which may eventually permit a better understanding of brain development and function. For example, children with glutaric acidemia type I, other organic acidemias, and mitochondrial disorders can have dyskinetic cerebral palsy associated with calcifications of the basal ganglia (deep-brain structures important in the control of movement; Falk, 2010; Gitiaux et al., 2008; Gouider-Khouja, Kraoua, Benrhouma, Fraj, & Rouissi, 2010). In Zellweger syndrome, a disorder of **peroxisome** formation, children exhibit multiple malformations that are more commonly associated with chromosomal abnormalities, including an atypical facial appearance, kidney cysts, and congenital heart defects (Braverman et al., 2013). This indicates an embryonic origin of the abnormalities, unlike the other disorders described above, where abnormalities occur as a result of an accumulation of a toxin or lack of a needed product after birth. Prior to birth, the placenta typically acts like a dialyzing system to remove these toxins produced by the fetus.

DIAGNOSTIC TESTING

A genetics evaluation should be considered for all children with significant intellectual or physical disabilities of unknown origin. As a part of that evaluation, particular attention will be paid to potential metabolic disorders if a child displays any of the following signs or symptoms: cyclical behavioral changes, vomiting and lethargy, enlargement of the liver or spleen, cardiomyopathy, evidence of neurological deterioration or regression, or a family history suggestive of an inherited disorder (Kamboj, 2008). An increasing number of clinically available biochemical and molecular tests can lead to a specific diagnosis. In some disorders, early diagnosis leads to therapy with an improved outcome. Even in currently untreatable disorders, a specific diagnosis may permit effective genetic counseling.

A metabolic evaluation is not required, however, for all children with developmental disabilities. It is expensive, and the diagnostic yield is quite low.

Diagnosis of an inborn error of amino acid or organic acid metabolism relies primarily on blood and urine tests to detect toxins or specific biochemical markers. The most common blood tests are for blood ammonia, lactic acid, acylcarnitines, and amino acids; urine is principally tested for organic acids. Metabolic evaluations are individualized based on the specific biochemical pathway that is suspected to be involved. Brain degenerative conditions such as lysosomal storage disorders are typically diagnosed by measuring the suspected deficient enzyme activity in blood or cultured skin cells (Martins et al., 2009). Mutation analysis is increasingly being utilized as a first-line test, as the simultaneous DNA sequencing of numerous suspected genes may more rapidly lead to the diagnosis. Imaging studies (e.g., magnetic resonance imaging, magnetic resonance spectroscopy, computed tomography scan, and electroencephalogram), and other neurological measures (e.g., nerve conduction velocity and electromyography) may also prove helpful in diagnosing these disorders. In many disorders, alterations in brain structure or function are evident on imaging prior to the onset of clinical symptoms.

NEWBORN SCREENING

Because individual inborn errors of metabolism are rare (typically occurring in fewer than 1 in 10,000 births) and the diagnosis is easily missed, efforts have been directed at developing newborn mass screening methods for the detection of the more common and treatable disorders (Weismiller, 2017). In these disorders, rapid diagnosis and treatment are often essential in achieving a favorable outcome; therefore, screening efforts have focused on newborn infants. The first newborn screening test for PKU was developed in 1959, and it was successful in detecting more than 90% of infants who were affected. Subsequently, methods have been established for screening over 30 inborn errors of metabolism as well as other disorders (see Newborn Screening, Chapter 4). This expanded screening, now employing tandem mass spectrometry and other techniques in state-run screening laboratories, is offered to families in newborn nurseries. In the United States, the specific inborn errors of metabolism screened varies between states based on local legislation, which is typically guided by conditions on the recommended uniform screening panel (see Chapter 4). State-specific information is provided by the Health Resources and Services Administration of the U.S. Department of Health and Human Services (www.babysfirsttest.org).

Although these tests have proved to be remarkably effective, parents should be reminded that a positive test only indicates a higher than normal likelihood of a genetic disorder that needs to be confirmed or ruled out by additional confirmatory testing in the specialized clinic. In addition, the tests detect only a fraction of inborn errors of metabolism, whereas parents might incorrectly assume that these tests are diagnostic for all disorders causing severe developmental disabilities.

THERAPEUTIC APPROACHES

Figure 16.2 illustrates the varying approaches to treating inborn errors of metabolism. These methods include 1) substrate deprivation (limiting the influx of a potentially toxic compound normally metabolized by the defective enzyme); 2) externally supplying the deficient product; 3) stimulating an alternative pathway around the enzyme block; 4) providing a cofactor to stimulate the deficient enzyme; and 5) boosting or restoring enzyme activity by supplying the deficient enzyme, transplanting an organ that has normal enzyme activity, or using gene therapy to correct the genetic defect or to insert a normal copy of the gene. Each of these approaches is illustrated by specific disorders in Table 16.3.

Substrate Deprivation

Most inborn errors of metabolism involve a failure to metabolize to completion one of the three primary macronutrients: carbohydrates, fats, or amino acids. As a result, there occurs a toxic accumulation of an intermediate of the deficient metabolic pathway. Therefore, the mainstay of treatment is dietary restriction of the precursor (carbohydrate, fat, or amino acid) to the potential toxin. For example, children with PKU are placed on a phenylalanine-restricted diet in order to prevent the phenylalanine accumulation that is associated with brain damage (Figure 16.1; Singh et al., 2014). This involves a diet consisting of a special phenylalanine-restricted formula combined with low-protein foods. It is important to note that the diet for individuals with PKU cannot be completely free of phenylalanine. Phenylalanine is an essential amino acid, and a small amount is necessary for normal growth and development. Although simple in concept, these diets are extremely hard to follow. Someone like Lisa, introduced in the first case study, may only be allowed 6 grams of natural protein a day, the same amount as

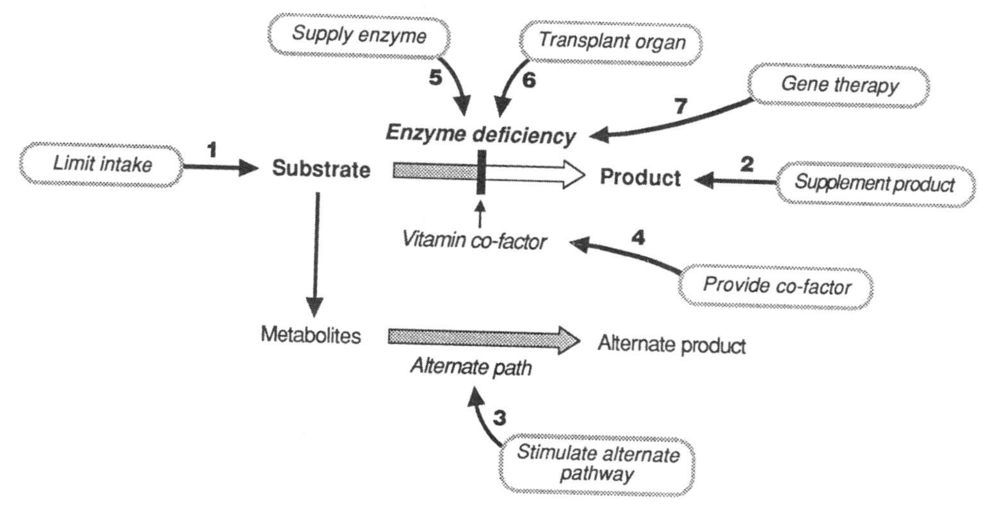

Figure 16.2. Approaches to treatment of inborn errors of metabolism. Treatment can be directed at 1) substrate deprivation, limiting the influx of a potentially toxic compound; 2) supplementing the deficient product; 3) stimulating an alternate metabolic pathway; 4) providing a cofactor to activate residual enzyme activity; or 5) increasing enzyme activity by supplying the deficient enzyme, transplanting an organ with intact enzyme, or gene therapy to correct the genetic defect or to insert a normal copy of the gene.

in three fourths of a cup of pasta. The average adult female takes in 50 to 70 grams of protein a day.

Fortunately, phenylalanine-restricted diets are quite effective for individuals with PKU. A classic study showed that the IQ scores of children who began this treatment within the first month of life were around 100, whereas the scores of those initially treated later in childhood were 20 to 50 points lower (Hanley, Linsao, & Netley, 1971). A low-phenylalanine diet was initially thought to be essential only through early childhood to prevent IQ decline (Michals, Azen, Acosta, Koch, & Matalon, 1988; Waisbren, Mahon, Schnell, & Levy,

Table 16.3. Examples of treatment approaches for inborn errors of metabolism

Approaches	Disorder	Specific treatment
Substrate deprivation	Phenylketonuria (PKU)	Phenylalanine restriction
	Maple syrup urine disease	Branch chain amino acid restriction
	Galactosemia	Galactose restriction
	Tyrosinemia	NTBC/nitisinone (Orfadin)
	Gaucher disease	Miglustat (Zavesca), eliglustat (Cerdelga)
Externally supplementing the deficient product	Glycogen storage disease	Cornstarch
	Ornithine transcarbamylase deficiency	Citrulline
	Phenylketonuria	Tyrosine
Stimulating an alternative pathway	Urea cycle disorders	Phenylbutyrate (Buphenyl, Ravicti)
	Organic acidemias	Carnitine (Carnitor)
	Isovaleric acidemia	Glycine
Providing a cofactor	Biotinidase deficiency	Biotin (vitamin B_7)
	Homocystinuria	Pyridoxine (vitamin B_6)
	PKU	Tetrahydrobiopterin (BH4, sapropterin, KUVAN)
Replacing an enzyme	Fabry disease	Agalsidase beta (Fabrazyme)
	Gaucher disease	Imiglucerase (Cerezyme)
	Morquio disease	Elosulfase alfa (Vimizim)
Transplanting an organ	X-linked adrenoleukodystrophy	Bone marrow transplant
	Ornithine transcarbamylase deficiency	Liver transplant
	Methylmalonic acidemia	Liver and kidney transplant

For entries with parenthetical text, text with initial capitalization indicates a brand name.

1987). However, "diet for life" is now the accepted approach among metabolic specialists in order to optimize cognitive outcomes, avoid executive functioning challenges, and prevent changes in brain white matter (Hood, Rutlin, Shimony, Grange, & White, 2017; van Spronsen et al., 2017; Vockley et al., 2014). See Box 16.1 for more information on metabolic specialists.

In addition to learning about the neurological risks of PKU, individuals with PKU should understand the importance of good metabolic control before conception. An elevated maternal phenylalanine level poses a serious threat for the fetus of a woman with PKU who is without dietary control (Prick, Hop, & Duvekot, 2012). Prick and colleagues' synthesis of case reports and case series on maternal PKU showed that before newborn screening and effective treatment were available, men and women with PKU had severe intellectual disability and women did not often bear children. Their analysis showed that since effective treatment has become available, most women with PKU have been able to become mothers. Many of the women in the cohort of this study had stopped following the phenylalanine-restricted diet during childhood. Unexpectedly, almost all of the children born to these women were found to have congenital abnormalities, including microcephaly, congenital heart disease, cleft lip and palate, and gastrointestinal and urinary tract abnormalities, and they were later found to have intellectual disability. These children, however, did not have PKU; they were only carriers. Instead, the intellectual disability and other abnormalities were caused by the **teratogenic** effect (interfering with normal embryonic development) of the mother's high phenylalanine levels on the developing fetus (Prick et al., 2012). Studies have also shown that lowering the phenylalanine levels in pregnant mothers with PKU significantly improves the chances for typical development of offspring. As a result, it is now advised that women with PKU continue life-long dietary restriction (Vockley et al., 2014) and that tight phenylalanine control be achieved for at least 3 months prior to conception (American College of Obstetricians and Gynecologists Committee on Genetics, 2015).

Galactosemia is another disorder where substrate deprivation is used to prevent the accumulation of toxins. Infants with galactosemia develop liver failure in the first few days of life due to consumption of breast milk or lactose-containing formula. When lactose is removed from the diet, these life-threatening complications improve and infants grow as expected (Berry, 2017). However, even with adequate dietary restriction, individuals with galactosemia can exhibit speech delay, developmental delay, and premature ovarian failure (Coss et al., 2013; Frederick, Cutler, & Fridovich-Keil, 2017; van Calcar et al., 2014).

There are also nondietary approaches to substrate deprivation. One example is the inhibition of a pathway upstream to prevent the formation of toxic products behind the enzymatic block. In hereditary tyrosinemia type I, the drug NTBC, an herbicide derivative, has been found to inhibit tyrosine degradation in children who are affected, preventing the downstream formation of a toxic compound that causes liver and kidney disease and liver cancer (Chinsky et al., 2017; Das, 2017). Similarly, several substrate reduction therapies have been developed for lysosomal storage disorders, including eliglustat for Gaucher disease and miglustat for both Gaucher and Niemann-Pick C1 disease. These medications inhibit the formation of glucosylcermide,

BOX 16.1 INTERDISCIPLINARY CARE

Role of the Metabolic Dietitian

Metabolic dietitians are essential members of the care team for individuals with inborn errors of metabolism. With a sound understanding of biochemistry, these registered dietitians translate the scientific necessity of the special diets required to prevent the toxic buildup of metabolites to families, while also ensuring adequate growth and nutrition. For the majority of inborn errors of metabolism, if the toxic metabolite (e.g., phenylalanine in phenylketonuria, fat in fatty acid oxidation disorders) were completely eliminated from the diet, the individual would fail to grow appropriately and may develop overt nutritional deficiencies. Metabolic dietitians are able to individualize diet plans that prevent deficiency and promote growth while still being practical and attainable. Food is the cornerstone of many cultures. Metabolic dietitians must therefore incorporate the importance of following an extremely restrictive diet into the individual cultural beliefs and habits of families. For many families their metabolic dietitian is their first contact for any challenge related to their rare disorder. In addition to providing nutrition knowledge, metabolic dietitians often serve as insurance advocates, professional resources for school meetings, and coordinators of care related to these rare diseases.

reducing the accumulated substrate load and improving clinical outcome (Coutinho et al., 2016; Stirnemann et al., 2017). Current clinical trials are also investigating the use of genistein as a substrate reduction therapy in mucopolysaccharidosis type III, also known as Sanfilippo syndrome (de Ruijter et al., 2012).

Externally Supplementing the Deficient Product

Some children with inborn errors of metabolism are given replacements for the enzyme product they are missing. For example, the medical formulas for the treatment of PKU are enhanced in tyrosine, the product of the deficient enzyme. Tyrosine is an important precursor for a number of neurotransmitters. The goals of PKU management include both controlling phenylalanine elevations and ensuring adequate tyrosine intake (Singh et al., 2014). Similarly, the primary treatment for a group of disorders called glycogen storage diseases is uncooked cornstarch. In these disorders, individuals are unable to utilize the glycogen in their liver for energy (glucose), and cornstarch is given to provide a slow release source of glucose and prevent recurrent hypoglycemia (Kishnani et al., 2014).

Stimulating an Alternative Pathway

It is now possible to treat some metabolic disorders by stimulating an alternative pathway that detours around the enzymatic block. For example, children with inborn errors of the urea cycle cannot convert toxic ammonia to nontoxic urea. Treatment by dietary protein restriction alone has proven unsuccessful because the degree of restriction required to prevent an accumulation of ammonia does not allow a sufficient diet to permit sustained growth or prolonged survival (Shih, 1976). A different approach is to use the drug glycerol phenylbutyrate to stimulate an alternate pathway for ammonia excretion. By providing a detour around the enzymatic block and converting the ammonia to an alternate nontoxic product, phenylacetylglutamine, instead of urea, this drug allows the majority of children with urea cycle disorders to survive, although many have developmental disabilities (Rüegger et al., 2014).

Providing a Cofactor

For certain individuals with metabolic diseases, providing a large dose of a vitamin cofactor results in amplification of residual enzyme activity or enhanced enzyme stability and clinical improvement. This approach has been used most effectively in treating children with an organic acidemia called biotinidase deficiency (Wolf, 2016). These children, who develop symptoms of acidosis and coma because of a defect in the enzyme biotinidase, show remarkable improvement if the vitamin biotin is provided at a very high (but nontoxic) dosage. The primary defect in biotinidase deficiency is the inability of the body to recycle the vitamin biotin. Biotin is an essential cofactor for a number of critical enzymes in multiple metabolic pathways. By giving these children large doses of biotin, these enzymes are normalized. In other disorders, the mutation may affect the binding site for enzyme cofactors. In some of these cases, providing large quantities of a vitamin cofactor may stabilize and even normalize enzyme activity. This type of vitamin therapy can minimize symptoms and improve outcomes for children with certain forms of another organic acidemia called methylmalonic acidemia (using vitamin B_{12}; Manoli, Sloan, & Venditti, 2005) and an amino acid disorder called homocystinuria (using vitamin B_6; Morris et al., 2017). Certain individuals with PKU respond well to tetrahydrobiopterin, the cofactor for the phenylalanine hydroxylase enzyme. Although tetrahydrobiopterin does not completely eliminate the need for a special diet in PKU, it does allow for some dietary liberalization and improved plasma phenylalanine levels (Singh et al., 2014; Vockley et al., 2014). In some disorders, providing a cofactor for treatment is so effective it eliminates all signs of disease. This can become challenging for families who culturally are suspicious of traditional medicine or question a diagnosis in their child who appears "normal." Continuously reviewing the basis of the diagnosis and the risks of not treating may be needed to ensure that families remain compliant with treatment recommendations.

Replacing an Enzyme

The previously discussed methods of therapy use indirect approaches to improve the child's condition. Supplying the missing enzyme is a direct approach to correct the inborn error. Intravenous injections of a synthetic enzyme first proved successful in treating the lysosomal storage disorder Gaucher disease, which is associated with the accumulation of glucocerebroside in cells of the liver, spleen, and bone marrow. With severe infantile Gaucher disease, the glucocerebroside accumulates in the brain as well. Individuals who receive biweekly injections of the deficient enzyme show marked improvements, including significant shrinkage of the liver and spleen (Stirnemann et al., 2017). This enzyme, however, cannot cross the blood–brain barrier, making replacement therapy ineffective for those children with severe infantile Gaucher disease. As of 2017, specific enzyme replacement therapy has been approved for Fabry disease; Gaucher disease; glycogen storage disease type II (Pompe disease); lysosomal acid lipase disease (Wolman); and mucopolysaccharidoses type I, II, IV, and VI (Hurler, Hunter, Morquio, and Maroteau-Lamy disease). Enzyme replacement therapy continues to be investigated as a therapy for other lysosomal storage diseases (see Box 16.2).

Another strategy that has been employed is the administration of a substitute enzyme, rather than replacement of the enzyme that is deficient. An example of this type of enzyme substitution that has shown promise is phenylalanine ammonia lyase (an enzyme produced by plants and fungi but not by humans) in the treatment of PKU. In clinical trials, intermittent subcutaneous injections of phenylalanine ammonia lyase appears to reduce the phenylalanine load and allow less severe dietary restriction (Bell et al., 2017; Sarkissian et al., 2008).

Although replacement therapy seems ideal, it is not without shortcomings. These synthetic enzymes are some of the most expensive drugs in the world. In addition, the enzyme must be injected at frequent intervals throughout the individual's life, and antibodies can develop against the foreign protein just as antibodies against insulin develop in some individuals with diabetes. Many individuals experience hypersensitivity reactions to their infusions, ranging from mild flushing and nausea to severe, life-threatening anaphylactic (allergic) reactions.

Transplanting an Organ

Some deficient enzymes can be replaced by transplanting a body organ that contains the enzyme. For example, bone marrow, umbilical cord blood, and stem cell transplantation have been performed in individuals with certain lysosomal and peroxisomal storage disorders, including juvenile metachromatic leukodystrophy, adrenoleukodystrophy, and Hurler syndrome. These disorders, marked by neurological and physical deterioration and early death, are caused by the deficiency of enzymes found in many body organs, including bone marrow cells. In a number of studies, transplantation, by providing the deficient enzyme, has resulted in improvement in symptoms and, in some cases, arrest of disease progression. It is questionable, however, whether it has an effect on brain function (Beckmann, Miller, Dietrich, & Orchard, 2017; Boelens & van Hasselt, 2016; Chiesa et al., 2016; Parini et al., 2017; Saute et al., 2016).

Liver transplantation has been associated with biochemical correction and improvement in symptoms of certain inborn errors of amino acid metabolism, most notably urea cycle disorders and maple syrup urine disease (MSUD; Diaz et al., 2014; Lichter-Konecki et al,, 2016; Yu, Rayhill, Hsu, & Landis, 2015). Liver transplantation has also been used to treat severe cases of propionic acidemia (PA) and has been associated with an improvement in metabolic control, reversal of cardiomyopathy, and possible improvement in neurologic function (Nagao et al., 2013; Shchelochkov, Carrillo, &

BOX 16.2 EVIDENCE-BASED PRACTICE

Novel Therapies

Inborn errors of metabolism are very rare. Therefore, the standard treatment for most disorders is based on limited clinical studies, case reports, or expert opinion (Häberle et al., 2012; Morris et al., 2017; van Wegberg et al., 2017). Although treatments continue to be developed for inborn errors of metabolism, there are fewer therapies than are available for more common disorders. Thus novel therapies that show promise frequently are employed and can become part of standard care even before robust evidence of their efficacy is available.

Since the mid-2000s, a growing number of clinical studies in some lysosomal disorders have demonstrated the benefit of infused enzyme replacement (e.g., Gaucher disease, Pompe disease, Fabry disease, and mucopolysaccharidoses) and hematopoietic stem cell transplant (e.g., X-linked adrenoleukodystrophy [X-ALD], mucopolysaccharidoses). Notably, both Pompe disease and X-ALD had previously been nominated to be considered for addition to the Secretary of Health and Human Services Recommended Uniform Screening Panel (RUSP), in 2008 and 2012, respectively, but they were rejected at the time due to insufficient evidence. However, in 2015, based on new evidence, Pompe disease was the first lysosomal disorder to be added to the RUSP, and it was quickly followed in 2016 by the addition of X-ALD and MPS-1. Long-term outcome data of enzyme replacement or stem cell transplant in these disorders are still very limited. Even so, the addition of these three disorders to the RUSP greatly changes the paradigm of newborn screening; additional disorders will likely be added in the coming years.

Venditti, 2016). However, unlike those with a urea cycle disorder or maple syrup urine disease, individuals with propionic acidemia must continue a modified protein diet post transplant, as the risk of metabolic decompensation is not eliminated (Fraser & Venditti, 2016). Liver transplantation has also been used to treat tyrosinemia when there is liver damage and the risk for liver cancer. In some cases of methylmalonic acidemia, liver transplantation in conjunction with kidney transplantation has been effective (Niemi et al., 2015). Organ transplantation carries a risk of mortality as high as 10%–20% (Cuenca, Kim, & Vakili, 2017) and an even higher risk of morbidity. In addition, transplant recipients require immunosuppression drugs for life, and the long-range outcomes for transplant recipients is still uncertain.

Using Gene Therapy

In theory, an ideal treatment for an inborn error of metabolism would involve the insertion of a normal gene to compensate for a defective one, or correction (editing) of the defective gene. This would allow for the production of a normal enzyme, thereby permanently correcting or curing the disorder. However, in clinical research studies, progress has been slow (Hanna, Rémuzat, Auquier, & Toumi, 2017), and some trials have been associated with severe adverse events, including a death in an early trial in urea cycle disorders (Cavazzana-Calvo, Lagresle, Hacein-Bey-Abina, & Fischer, 2005; Raper et al., 2003). As of 2017, gene therapy trials have been successful in treating only a few nonmetabolic disorders, such as blood cancers (Locke et al., 2017; Maude et al., 2014), hemophilia, and hereditary blindness (Le Meur et al., 2017).

For brain-based disorders, there is the problem of getting across the blood–brain barrier. There is the potential for therapeutic application of hematopoietic stem cell gene therapy with intracerebral gene transfer (brain gene therapy) in individuals with metachromatic leukodystrophy and adrenoleukodystrophy (Eichler et al., 2017; Sevin, Cartier-Lacave, & Aubourg, 2009). Intrathecal delivery of gene therapy is also being explored (Hinderer et al., 2017).

OUTCOME

The range of outcomes in inborn errors of metabolism varies enormously. In most disorders that can be detected by newborn screening, such as PKU, children who are affected have usually done well. Their IQ generally falls within the average range, if somewhat lower than that of their parents. They are, however, at increased risk for having learning disabilities and ADHD (Jahja et al., 2017; Palermo et al., 2017; Singh et al., 2014; van Spronsen et al., 2017; Vockley et al., 2014). Less favorable outcomes occur in other inborn errors of amino acid and organic acid metabolism. Although these children are surviving longer, many manifest developmental disabilities. Among children with metabolic disorders associated with progressive neurological disorders, such as certain lysosomal storage diseases, there has been only limited improvement in mortality and morbidity.

SUMMARY

- Although inborn errors of metabolism are rare, their consequences are often devastating.
- Therapy is effective for a number of these disorders.
- Children who are affected often must continue treatment for the rest of their lives, which may prove difficult.
- For therapy to succeed, it must be started early.
- The expansion in the number of disorders that are tested by newborn screening bodes well for early identification and treatment with the possibility of improved outcome.

ADDITIONAL RESOURCES

The National Organization for Rare Disorders (NORD): http://www.rarediseases.org

GeneReviews: https://www.ncbi.nlm.nih.gov/books/NBK1116/

The American College of Medical Genetics and Genomics: https://www.acmg.net/

Additional resources can be found online in Appendix D: Childhood Disabilities Resources, Services, and Organizations (see About the Online Companion Materials).

REFERENCES

American College of Obstetricians and Gynecologists Committee on Genetics (2015). ACOG committee opinion no. 636. *Obstetrics & Gynecology, 125*, 1548–1550.

Auchus, R. J. (2015). The classic and nonclassic congenital adrenal hyperplasias. *Endocrine Practice, 21*(4), 383–389.

Batshaw, M. L., Brusilow, S., Waber, L., Blom, W., Brubakk, A. M., Burton, B.K., . . . Schafer, I. A. (1982). Treatment of inborn errors of urea synthesis: Activation of alternative pathways of waste nitrogen synthesis and excretion. *The New England Journal of Medicine, 306*(23), 1387–1392.

Beck, M. (2018). Treatment strategies for lysosomal storage disorders. *Developmental Medicine and Child Neurology, 60*(1), 13–18.

Beckmann, N. B., Miller, W. P., Dietrich, M. S., & Orchard, P. J. (2017). Quality of life among boys with adrenoleukodystrophy following hematopoietic stem cell transplant. *Child Neuropsychology, 24*(7), 1–13.

Bell, S. M., Wendt, D. J., Zhang, Y., Taylor, T. W., Long, S., Tsuruda, L., . . . Fitzpatrick, P. A. (2017). Formulation and PEGylation optimization of the therapeutic PEGylated phenylalanine ammonia lyase for the treatment of phenylketonuria. *PLoS One, 12*(3), e0173269. doi:10.1371/journal.pone.0173269

Berry, G. T. (2017). Classic galactosemia and clinical variant galactosemia. In M. P. Adam, H. H. Ardinger, R. A. Pagon, S. E. Wallace, L. J. H. Bean, H. C. Mefford, . . . N. Ledbetter (Eds.), *GeneReviews* [Internet]. Seattle, WA: University of Washington, Seattle. Retrieved from https://www.ncbi.nlm.nih.gov/books/NBK1518/

Bilgin, L., Unal, S., Gunduz, M., Uncu, N., & Tiryaki, T. (2014). Utility of peritoneal dialysis in neonates affected by inborn errors of metabolism. *Journal of Peadiatrics and Child Health, 50*(7), 531–535.

Boelens, J. J., & van Hasselt, P. M. (2016). Neurodevelopmental outcome after hematopoietic cell transplantation in inborn errors of metabolism: Current considerations and future perspectives. *Neuropediatrics, 47*(5), 285–292. doi:10.1055/s-0036-1584602

Braissant, O., McLin, V. A., & Cudalbu, C. J. (2013). Ammonia toxicity to the brain. *Journal of Inherited Metabolic Disease, 36*, 595. doi:10.1007/s10545-012-9546-2

Braverman, N. E., D'Agostino, M. D., & MacLean, G. E. (2013). Peroxisome biogenesis disorders: Biological, clinical and pathophysiological perspectives. *Developmental Disabililities Research Reviews, 17*, 187–196. doi:10.1002/ddrr.1113

Cavazzana-Calvo, M., Lagresle, C., Hacein-Bey-Abina, S., & Fischer, A. (2005). Gene therapy for severe combined immunodeficiency. *Annual Review of Medicine, 56*, 585–602.

Chiesa, R., Wynn, R. F., & Veys, P. (2016). Haematopoietic stem cell transplantation in inborn errors of metabolism. *Current Opinion in Hematology, 23*(6), 530–535.

Chinsky, J. M., Singh, R., Ficicioglu, C., van Karnebeek, C. D. M., Grompe, M., Mitchell, G., . . . Scott, C. R. (2017). Diagnosis and treatment of tyrosinemia type I: A US and Canadian consensus group review and recommendations. *Genetics in Medicine, 19*(12), 1–16. doi:10.1038/gim.2017.101

Coss, K. P., Doran, P. P., Owoeye, C., Codd, M. B., Hamid, N., Mayne, P. D., . . . Treacy, E. P. (2013). Classical galactosaemia in Ireland: Incidence, complications and outcomes of treatment. *Journal of Inherited Metabolic Disease, 36*(1), 21–27.

Coutinho, M. F., Santos, J. I., Matos, L., & Alves, S. (2016). Genetic substrate reduction therapy: A promising approach for lysosomal storage disorders. *Diseases, 4*(4), pii:E33. doi:10.3390/diseases4040033

Cuenca, A. G., Kim, H. B., & Vakili, K. (2017). Pediatric liver transplantation. *Seminars in Pediatric Surgery, 26*(4), 217–223. doi:10.1053/j.sempedsurg.2017.07.014

Das, A. M. (2017). Clinical utility of nitisinone for the treatment of hereditary tyrosinemia type-1 (HT-1). *The Application of Clinical Genetics, 10*, 43–48. doi:10.2147/TACG.S113310

de Ruijter, J., Valstar, M. J., Narajczyk, M., Wegrzyn, G., Kulik, W., Ijlst, L., . . . Wijburg, F. A. (2012). Genistein in Sanfilippo disease: A randomized controlled crossover trial. *Annals of Neurology, 71*(1), 110–120. doi:10.1002/ana.22643

Diaz, V. M., Camarena, C., de la Vega, A., Martinez-Pardo, M., Diaz, C., Lopez, M., . . . Jara, P. (2014). Liver transplantation for classical maple syrup urine disease: Long-term follow-up. *Journal of Pediatric Gastroenterology and Nutrition, 59*(5), 636–639.

Dornelles, A. D., Artigalás, O., da Silva, A. A., Ardila, D. L. V., Alegra, T., Pereira, T. V., . . . Schwartz, I. V. D. (2017). Efficacy and safety of intravenous laronidase for mucopolysaccharidosis type I: A systematic review and meta-analysis. *PLoS ONE, 12*(8), e0184065. doi:10.1371/journal.pone.0184065

Eichler, F., Duncan, C., Musolino, P. L., Orchard, P. J., De Oliveira, S., Thrasher, A. J., . . . Williams, D. A. (2017). Hematopoietic stem-cell gene therapy for cerebral adrenoleukodystrophy. *New England Journal of Medicine, 377*(17), 1630–1638. doi:10.1056/NEJMoa1700554

El Dib, R., Gomaa, H., Ortiz, A., Politei, J., Kapoor, A., & Barreto, F. (2017). Enzyme replacement therapy for Anderson-Fabry disease: A complementary overview of a Cochrane publication through a linear regression and a pooled analysis of proportions from cohort studies. *PLoS ONE, 12*(3), e0173358. doi:10.1371/journal.pone.0173358

Falk, M. J. (2010). Neurodevelopmental manifestations of mitochondrial disease. *Journal of Developmental and Behavioral Pediatrics, 31*(7), 610–621.

Folling, A. (1934). Excretion of phenylalanine in urine: An inborn error of metabolism associated with intellectual disability. *Hoppe-Seyler's Zeitschrift fur Physiologische Chemie, 227*, 169–176.

Fraser, J. L., & Venditti, C. P. (2016). Methylmalonic and propionic acidemias: Clinical management update. *Current Opinion in Pediatrics, 28*(6), 682–693.

Frederick, A. B., Cutler, D. J., & Fridovich-Keil, J. L. (2017). Rigor of non-dairy galactose restriction in early childhood, measured by retrospective survey, does not associate with severity of five long-term outcomes quantified in 231 children and adults with classic galactosemia. *Journal of Inherited Metabolic Disease*, Advance online publication. doi:10.1007/s10545-017-0067-x

Garrod, A. E. (1908). The Croonian Lectures on inborn errors of metabolism: Delivered before the Royal College of Physicians of London. *The Lancet*(172), 4429, 142–148

Gitiaux, C., Roze, E., Kinugawa, K., Flamand-Rouvière, C., Boddaert, N., Apartis, E., . . . Bahi-Buisson, N. (2008). Spectrum of movement disorders associated with glutaric aciduria type 1: A study of 16 patients. *Movement Disorders, 23*(16), 2392–2397.

Gouider-Khouja, N., Kraoua, I., Benrhouma, H., Fraj, N., & Rouissi, A. (2010). Movement disorders in neuro-metabolic diseases. *European Journal of Paediatric Neurology, 14*(4), 304–307.

Häberle, J., Boddaert, N., Burlina, A., Chakrapani, A., Dixon, M., Huemer, M., . . . Dionisi-Vici, C. (2012). Suggested guidelines for the diagnosis and management of urea cycle disorders. *Orphanet Journal of Rare Diseases, 7*, 32. doi:10.1186/1750-1172-7-32

Hanley, W. B., Linsao, L. S., & Netley, C. (1971). The efficacy of dietary therapy for phenylketonuria. *Canadian Medical Association Journal, 104*(12), 1089–1091.

Hanna, E., Rémuzat, C., Auquier, P., & Toumi, M. (2017). Gene therapies development: Slow progress and promising prospect. *Journal of Market Access & Health Policy, 5*(1), 1265293. doi:10.1080/20016689.2017.1265293

Hinderer, C., Bell, P., Katz, N., Vite, C. H., Louboutin, J. P., Bote, E., . . . Wilson, J. M. (2017). Evaluation of intrathecal routes of administration for adeno-associated viral vectors in large animals. *Human Gene Therapy*, Advance online publication. doi:10.1089/hum.2017.026

Hisahara, S., Matsushita, T., Furuyama, H., Tajima, G., Shigemastsu, Y., Imai, T., & Shimohama, S. (2015). A heterozygous missense mutation in adolescent-onset very long-chain acyl-CoA dehydrogenase deficiency with exercise-induced rhabdomyolysis. *The Tohoku Journal of Experimental Medicine, 235*(4), 305–310.

Hood, A., Rutlin, J., Shimony, J. S., Grange, D. K., & White, D. A. (2017). Brain white matter integrity mediates the relationship between phenylalanine control and executive abilities in children with phenylketonuria. *Journal of Inherited Metabolic Disease, 33,* 41–47.

Jahja, R., van Spronsen, F. J., de Sonneville, L. M. J., van der Meere, J. J., Bosch, A. M., Hollak, C. E. M., . . . Huijbregts, S. C. J. (2017). Long-term follow up of cognition and mental health in adult phenylketonuria: A PKU-COBESO study. *Behavior Genetics, 47*(5), 486–497 doi:10.1007/s10519-017-9863-1

Jakóbkiewicz-Banecka, J., Wegrzyn, A., & Wegrzyn, G. (2007). Substrate deprivation therapy: A new hope for patients suffering from neuronopathic forms of inherited lysosomal storage diseases. *Journal of Applied Genetics, 48*(4), 383–388.

Kamboj, M. (2008). Clinical approach to the diagnoses of inborn errors of metabolism. *Pediatric Clinics of North America, 55*(5), 1113–1127, viii.

Kishnani, P. S, Austin, S. L., Abdenur, J. E., Arn, P., Bali, D. S., Boney, A., Chung, W. K., . . . American College of Medical Genetics and Genomics. (2014). Diagnosis and management of glycogen storage disease type 1: A practice guideline of the American College of Medical Genetics and Genomic. *Genetics in Medicine, 16*(11), e1.

Kishnani, P., & Beckemeyer, A. (2014). New therapeutic approaches for Pompe disease: Enzyme replacement therapy and beyond. *Pediatric Endocrinology Reviews, 12*(Suppl. 1), 114–124.

Le Meur, G., Lebranchu, P., Billaud, F., Adjali, O., Schmitt, S., Bézieau, S., . . . Weber, M. (2017). Safety and long-term efficacy of AAV4 gene therapy in patients with RPE65 Leber congenital amaurosis. *Molecular Therapy, 26*(1), 256–268. doi:10.1016/j.ymthe.2017.09.014

Levy, P. A. (2009a). Inborn errors of metabolism: Part 1: Overview. *Pediatrics in Review, 30*(4), 131–137.

Levy, P. A. (2009b). Inborn errors of metabolism: Part 2: Specific disorders. *Pediatrics in Review, 30*(4), e22–e28.

Lichter-Konecki, U., Caldovic, L., Morizono, H., & Simpson, K. (2016). Ornithine transcarbamylase deficiency. In M. P. Adam, H. H. Ardinger, R. A. Pagon, S. E. Wallace, L. J. H. Bean, H. C. Mefford, . . . N. Ledbetter (Eds.), *GeneReviews®* [Internet]. Seattle, WA: University of Washington, Seattle. Retrieved from https://www.ncbi.nlm.nih.gov/books/NBK154378/#otc-def.Diagnosis

Locke, F. L., Neelapu, S. S., Bartlett, N. L., Siddiqi, T., Chavez, J. C., Hosing, C. M., Ghobadi, A., . . . Go, W. Y. (2017). Phase 1 results of ZUMA-1: A multicenter study of KTE-C19 anti-CD19 CAR T cell therapy in refractory aggressive lymphoma. *Molecular Therapy, 25*(1), 285–295. doi10.1016/j.ymthe.2016.10.020

Manoli, I., Sloan, J. L., & Venditti, C. P. (2005). Isolated methylmalonic acidemia. In M. P. Adam, H. H. Ardinger, R. A. Pagon, S. E. Wallace, L. J. H. Bean, H. C. Mefford, . . . N. Ledbetter (Eds.), *GeneReviews®* [Internet]. Seattle, WA: University of Washington, Seattle. Retrieved from https://www.ncbi.nlm.nih.gov/books/NBK1231/

Martins, A. M., Valadares, E. R., Porta, G., Coelho, J., Semionato, F. J. Pianovski, M. A. Kerstenetzky, M. S., . . . Brazilian Study Group on Gaucher Disease and other Lysosomal Storage Diseases. (2009). Recommendations on diagnosis, treatment, and monitoring for Gaucher disease. *The Journal of Pediatrics, 155*(4, Suppl.) S10–S18. doi:10.1016/j.jpeds.2009.07.004

Maude, S. L., Frey, N., Shaw, P. A., Aplenc, R., Barrett, D. M., Bunin, N. J., . . . Grupp, S. A. (2014). Chimeric antigen receptor T cells for sustained remissions in leukemia. *New England Journal of Medicine, 371*(16), 1507–1517. doi:10.1056/NEJMoa1407222

Michals, K., Azen, C., Acosta, P., Koch, R., & Matalon, R. (1988). Blood phenylalanine levels and intelligence of 10-year-old children with PKU in the National Collaborative Study. *Journal of the American Diabetic Association, 88*(10), 1226–1229.

Morris, A. A., Kožich, V., Santra, S., Andria, G., Ben-Omran, T. I., Chakrapani, A. B., . . . Chapman, K. A. (2017). Guidelines for the diagnosis and management of cystathionine beta-synthase deficiency. *Journal of Inherited Metabolic Disease, 40*(1), 49–74. doi:10.1007/s10545-016-9979-0

OMIM. (2018). *Online Mendelian Inheritance in Man.* McKusick-Nathans Institute of Genetic Medicine, Johns Hopkins University (Baltimore, MD). Retrieved from https://omim.org/

Nagao, M., Tanaka, T., Morii, M., Wakai, S., Horikawa, R., & Kasahara, M. (2013). Improved neurologic prognosis for a patient with propionic acidemia who received early living donor liver transplantation. *Molecular Genetics and Metabolism, 108*(1), 25–29.

Niemi, A. K., Kim, I. K., Krueger, C. E., Cowan, T. M., Baugh, N., Ferrell, R., . . . Enns, G. M. (2015). Treatment of methylmalonic acidemia by liver or combined liver-kidney transplantation. *Journal of Pediatrics, 166*(6), 1455–1461, e1.

Palermo, L., Geberhiwot, T., MacDonald, A., Limback, E., Hall, S. K., & Romani, C. (2017). Cognitive outcomes in early-treated adults with phenylketonuria (PKU): A comprehensive picture across domains. *Neuropsychology, 31*(3), 255–267. doi:10.1037/neu0000337

Parini, R., Deodato, F., Di Rocco, M., Lanino, E., Locatelli, F., Messina, C., Rovelli, A., & Scarpa, M. (2017). Open issues in mucopolysaccharidosis type 1–Hurler. *Orphanet Journal of Rare Diseases, 12*(1), 112.

Posset, R., Garcia-Cazorla, A., Valayannopoulos, V., Teles, E. L., Dionisi-Vici, C., Brassier, A., . . . Additional individual contributors of the E-IMD consortium. (2016). Age at disease onset and peak ammonium level rather than interventional variables predict the neurological outcome in urea cycle disorders. *Journal of Inherited Metabolic Disease, 39*(5), 661–672.

Prick, B. W., Hop, W. C., & Duvekot, J. J. (2012). Maternal phenylketonuria and hyperphenylalaninemia in pregnancy: Pregnancy complications and neonatal sequelae in untreated and treated pregnancies. *American Journal of Clinical Nutrition, 95*(2), 374–382. doi:10.3945/ajcn.110.009456

Raper, S. E., Chirmule, N., Lee, F. S., Wivel, N. A., Bagg, A., Guang-ping, G., . . . Batshaw, M. L. (2003). Fatal systemic inflammatory response syndrome in an ornithine transcarbamylase deficient patient following adenoviral gene transfer. *Molecular Genetics and Metabolism, 80*(1–2), 148–158.

Rastall, D. P. W., & Amalfitano, A. (2017). Current and future treatments for lysosomal storage disorders. *Current Treatment Options in Neurology, 19,* 45. doi:10.1007/s11940-017-0481-2

Rice, G. M., & Steiner, R. D. (2016). Inborn errors of metabolism (metabolic disorders). *Pediatrics in Review, 37*(1), 3–15.

Rüegger, C. M., Lindner, M., Ballhausen, D., Baumgartner M.R., Beblo S., Das A., Gautschi, M., . . . Häberle, J. (2014).

Cross-sectional observational study of 208 patients with non-classical urea cycle disorders. *Journal of Inherited Metabolic Disease, 37*, 21. doi:10.1007/s10545-013-9624-0

Sarkissian, C. N., Gámez, A., Wang, L., Charbonneau, M., Fitzpatrick, P., Lemontt, J. F., . . . Scriver, C. R. (2008). Preclinical evaluation of multiple species of PEGylated recombinant phenylalanine ammonia lyase for the treatment of phenylketonuria. *Proceedings of the National Academy of Sciences of the United States of America, 105*(52), 20894–20899.

Saudubray, J. M. (2016). *Inborn metabolic diseases: Diagnosis and treatment* (6th ed.). New York, NY: Springer Berlin Heidelberg.

Saute, J. A., Souza, C. F., Poswar, F. O., Donis, K. C., Campos, L. G., Deyl, A. V., . . . Jardim, L. B. (2016). Neurological outcomes after hematopoietic stem cell transplantation for cerebral X-linked adrenoleukodystrophy, late onset metachromatic leukodystrophy and Hurler syndrome. *Arquivos de Neuro-Psiquiatria, 74*(12), 953–966.

Sevin, C., Cartier-Lacave, N., & Aubourg, P. (2009). Gene therapy in metachromatic leukodystrophy. *International Journal of Clinical Pharmacology and Therapeutics, 47*(Suppl. 1), S128–131.

Shapiro, B. E., Pastores, G. M., Gianutsos, J., Luzy, C., & Kolodny, E. H. (2009). Miglustat in late-onset Tay-Sachs disease: A 12-month, randomized, controlled clinical study with 24 months of extended treatment. *Genetics in Medicine, 11*(6), 425–433.

Shchelochkov, O. A., Carrillo, N., & Venditti, C. (2016). Propionic acidemia. In M. P. Adam, H. H. Ardinger, R. A. Pagon, S. E. Wallace, L. J. H. Bean, H. C. Mefford, . . . N. Ledbetter (Eds.), *GeneReviews®* [Internet]. Seattle, WA: University of Washington, Seattle. Retrieved from https://www.ncbi.nlm.nih.gov/books/NBK92946/

Shih, V. E. (1976). Hereditary urea-cycle disorders. In S. Grisolia, R. Baguena, & E. Mayor (Eds.), *The urea cycle* (pp. 367–414). Hoboken, NY: John Wiley & Sons.

Singh, R. H., Rohr, F., Frazier, D., Cunningham, A., Mofidi, S., Ogata, B., . . . van Calcar, S. C. (2014). Recommendations for the nutrition management of phenylalanine hydroxylase deficiency. *Genetics in Medicine, 16*(2), 121–131.

Stirnemann, J., Belmatoug, N., Camou, F., Serratrice, C., Froissart, R., Caillaud, C., . . . Berger, M. G. (2017). A review of Gaucher disease pathophysiology, clinical presentation and treatments. *International Journal of Molecular Sciences, 18*(2), 441. doi:10.3390/ijms18020441

Turcu, A. F., & Auchus, R. J. (2015). The next 150 years of congenital adrenal hyperplasia. *The Journal of Steroid Biochemistry and Molecular Biology, 153*, 63–71.

van Calcar, S. C., Bernstein, L. E., Rohr, F. J., Scaman, C. H., Yannicelli, S., & Berry, G. T. (2014). A re-evaluation of life-long severe galactose restriction for the nutrition management of classic galactosemia. *Molecular Genetics Metabolism, 112*(3), 191–197.

Van Hove, J., Coughlin, II, C., & Scharer, G. (2002). Glycine encephalopathy. In M. P. Adam, H. H. Ardinger, R. A. Pagon, S. E. Wallace, L. J. H. Bean, H. C. Mefford, . . . N. Ledbetter (Eds.), *GeneReviews®* [Internet]. Seattle, WA: University of Washington, Seattle. Retrieved from https://www.ncbi.nlm.nih.gov/books/NBK1357/

van Spronsen, F. J., van Wegberg, A. M. J., Ahring, K., Belanger-Quintana, A., Blau, N., Bosch, A. M., . . . MacDonald, A. (2017). Key European guidelines for the diagnosis and management of patients with phenylketonuria. *Lancet Diabetes & Endocrinology, 5*(9), 743–756.

van Wegberg, A. M. J, MacDonald, A., Ahring, K., Bélanger-Quintana, A., Blau, N., Bosch, A., . . . van Spronsen, F. J. (2017). The complete European guidelines on phenylketonuria: Diagnosis and treatment. *Orphanet Journal of Rare Diseases, 12*, 162.

Vernon, H. J. (2015). Inborn errors of metabolism: Advances in diagnosis and therapy. *JAMA Pediatrics, 169*(8), 778–782. doi:10.1001/jamapediatrics.2015.0754

Vockley, J., Andersson, H. C., Antshel, K. M., Braverman, N. E., Burton, B. K., Frazier, D. M., . . . Berry, S. A. (2014). American College of Medical Genetics and Genomics Therapeutics Committee. Phenylalanine hydroxylase deficiency: Diagnosis and management guideline. *Genetics in Medicine, 16*(2), 188–200. doi:10.1038/gim.2013.157

Waisbren, S. E., Mahon, B. E., Schnell, R. R., & Levy, H. L. (1987). Predictors of intelligence quotient and intelligence quotient change in persons treated for phenylketonuria early in life. *Pediatrics, 79*(3), 351–355.

Wanders, R. J. A., Klouwer, F. C. C., Ferdinandusse, S., Waterham, H. R., & Poll-Thé, B. T. (2017). Clinical and laboratory diagnosis of peroxisomal disorders. In M. Schrader (Ed.), *Peroxisomes. Methods and protocols* (pp. 329–342). New York, NY: Humana Press.

Weismiller, D. G. (2017). Expanded newborn screening: Information and resources for the family physician. *American Family Physician, 95*(11), 703–709.

Wolf, B. (2016). Biotinidase deficiency. In M. P. Adam, H. H. Ardinger, R. A. Pagon, S. E. Wallace, L. J. H. Bean, H. C. Mefford, . . . N. Ledbetter (Eds.), *GeneReviews®* [Internet]. Seattle, WA: University of Washington, Seattle. Retrieved from https://www.ncbi.nlm.nih.gov/books/NBK1322/

Yu, L., Rayhill, S. C., Hsu, E. K., & Landis, C. S. (2015). Liver transplantation for urea cycle disorders: Analysis of the United Network for Organ Sharing Database. *Transplantation Proceedings, 47*(8), 2413–2418.

CHAPTER 17

Speech and Language Disorders

Barbara L. Ekelman and Barbara A. Lewis

Upon completion of this chapter, the reader will

- Differentiate among children with various speech sound disorders, namely articulation, phonology, and apraxia
- Differentiate among children with various language disorders, namely receptive and expressive language disorders involving phonological awareness, morphology, syntax, semantics, and pragmatics
- Identify the possible etiological bases for speech and language disorders, their prevalence, and common comorbid conditions
- Employ evidence-based practices for the treatment and remediation of speech and language disorders
- Discuss prognostic indicators for outcomes and variables associated with persistent speech and language disorders

For most children, the basics of speech and language emerge effortlessly over the first 3 years of life, progressing from babbling to first words to simple sentences, with further complexities of language developing well into later childhood. Yet for other children, developmental milestones for speech and language are delayed and not achieved according to age expectations. Some of these children go on to have significant speech, language, and learning disabilities that require intervention and can have lifelong social-emotional, academic, and occupational consequences. These individuals present with various profiles of speech, language, and learning impairments. This chapter will review the diagnosis and treatment of these disorders, applying evidence-based practices.

CASE STUDY

Steve's parents were concerned that his speech development was delayed. He was late to talk, and his first words contained mostly vowel sounds, in particular the "uh" sound. When Steve was 2½ years old, he attended a preschool setting for 2 days each week and played appropriately with his peers. However, although Steve made frequent attempts to communicate, his speech remained unintelligible, especially to unfamiliar listeners. The preschool teacher encouraged his parents to have him tested, so the parents spoke to Steve's pediatrician about their concerns, and the pediatrician referred the family to the local early intervention program (see Chapter 31) through which Steve received a speech-language evaluation. The pediatrician also recommended an audiological evaluation. The audiologist and speech-language pathologist (SLP) evaluated Steve when he was 2 years, 10 months of age. The audiologist ruled out hearing loss as the basis for Steve's speech-language delays (see Box 17.1 for a discussion of the roles of the multidisciplinary team in Steve's care).

The SLP administered the Preschool Language Scale–Fifth Edition (PLS-5; Zimmerman, Steiner, & Pond, 2011), the Goldman-Fristoe Test of Articulation–Third Edition (GFTA-3; Goldman & Fristoe, 2015), and the Clinical Assessment of Articulation and Phonology–Second Edition (CAAP-2; Secord & Donohue, 2014). Steve scored above the mean in the average range on the PLS-5 (suggesting well-developed general language skills), but he scored 2 standard deviations (SDs) below the mean on the GFTA-3 and CAAP-2 (suggesting specific impairments of articulation). Steve's mother completed the Vineland Adaptive Behavior Scales–Third Edition, Parent Interview (Vineland-3; Sparrow, Cicchetti, & Saulnier, 2016). The test results confirmed a speech sound disorder (SSD; an articulation and phonological disorder) and a spoken language disorder (SLD). Interestingly, Steve's socialization score on the Vineland-3 was high. Steve's SLD qualified him for preschool early intervention services through his public school (see Chapter 33).

Steve received speech services one time per week from age 2 years, 10 months to 4 years, 2 months. The intervention focused on correcting multiple speech sound errors, including omissions, syllable reductions, substitutions, cluster reductions, and fronting of back sounds. Both articulation and phonological approaches were implemented for therapy.

Thought Questions:

When a child has a significant speech delay, how can professionals best develop an "action plan" for characterizing the nature and possible causes of the delay, and what bearing does this have on designing a plan for evaluation and treatment? For children diagnosed with a speech or language disorder in preschool, what sort of problems may develop as they get older, and what can professionals do to monitor for these problems?

DEFINITIONS, DESCRIPTIONS, AND CLASSIFICATIONS

Speech and language disorders can be classified as speech sound disorders and spoken language disorders, both of which are described in this section. Diagnostic criteria of communication disorders according to the American Psychiatric Association's *Diagnostic*

BOX 17.1 INTERDISCIPLINARY CARE

Multidisciplinary Team Members Involved in Steve's Care

Pediatrician: The pediatrician follows the child's health and development over time. The pediatrician agrees that Steve's spoken language disorder warrants a speech-language evaluation at this time. He also refers Steve to an audiologist to rule out hearing loss (either sensorineural or conductive; see Chapter 26) as the cause for his speech-language delays.

Audiologist: The audiologist tests hearing acuity. The audiologist wants to determine whether Steve has a sensorineural hearing loss or a conductive hearing loss due to fluid build-up in his middle ear. Steve's air and bone conduction thresholds and tympanometry test results show excellent hearing.

SLP: The SLP works to improve Steve's speech and language skills (listening, speaking, reading comprehension, and written expression), memory, retrieval, and residual speech sound errors.

Occupational Therapist: The occupational therapist's goals for Steve are to improve pencil grip and letter formation (place, manner, spacing, and sizing).

Learning Specialist: The learning specialist works to improve Steve's reading (decoding, fluency, and comprehension) and writing (spelling and written expression) skills.

Psychiatrist: The child psychiatrist will determine if Steve has an attention deficit and will rule out other psychological factors such as depression and anxiety. A psychiatrist's treatment may be focused on medication management of ADHD.

Psychologist: The psychologist will assess Steve's cognitive abilities and learning skills. He will help Steve succeed academically, behaviorally, and socially in school.

and Statistical Manual of Mental Disorders–Fifth Edition (*DSM-5*; APA, 2013) are also briefly addressed.

Speech Sound Disorders

Some children have difficulty learning and producing speech sounds. Although there is great variability in the typical rate at which children learn speech sounds, some children lag significantly behind their peers in producing intelligible speech. These children are said to have a **speech sound disorder (SSD)**. Children with an SSD may not be intelligible to family members or friends.

Children may have difficulty with speech sounds for different reasons. Some children have difficulty learning the sound system of their language and the rules for combining sounds. These children have a **phonological disorder.** Other children have difficulty producing the speech sounds. They may substitute one sound for another, omit a sound altogether, or distort a sound. These children have an **articulation disorder.** Many children, such as Steve in the case study, have a combination of a phonological disorder and an articulation disorder.

There is a developmental sequence of speech sound acquisition, with sounds that are more easily produced and more frequently used in the language mastered first. Early sounds are /m/, /b/, /y/, /n/, /w/, /d/, /p/, /d/, and /h/. Next, /t/, /ng/, /k/, /g/, /f/, /v/, /ch/, and /j/ are learned. Later developing sounds are /sh/, /th/, /s/, /z/, /l/, and /r/. Consonant clusters (/sp/, /st/, /sk/, /br/, /bl/, /spr/, /str/, and /skr/) are also typically mastered later. By 8 years of age, most children employ the adult speech sound system with few or no sound errors in conversation. Common speech sound errors are described with examples in Table 17.1.

Sometimes the cause for an SSD is readily identifiable. Children with hearing loss, cleft palate, cerebral palsy, and other medical conditions typically present with SSDs because of their sensory impairments or because of physical limitations that affect their ability to generate accurate speech sounds. However, for the majority of children with SSDs, the cause of the speech difficulty is unknown. Professionals have speculated as to possible reasons for SSDs. For example, some children may have difficulty discriminating and processing different speech sounds and therefore do not learn the sounds correctly (**phonological processing deficits**). Other children may not form accurate representations of the sounds in the brain or may have trouble storing them in memory (weak phonological representations). Another group of children may have difficulty with planning and executing a motor program for producing the speech sounds (**childhood apraxia of speech** [CAS]), and still another group may have motor incoordination or weakness of the muscles needed to articulate intelligible speech (**developmental dysarthria**). It is important for every child with speech sound difficulties to have a comprehensive evaluation performed by a licensed and certified SLP to determine the specific problems that the child has and to develop an appropriate therapy plan to remediate these difficulties.

Table 17.1. Examples of speech sound errors

Error	Description	Examples
Omissions	Deletion of a sound within a word	"**tr**uck" to "-uck"
Substitutions	Substituting one sound in a word for another	"**t**ar" to "**k**ar"
Distortions	Substituting a typical sound for an atypical/idiosyncratic sound	Pronouncing the "s" sound around the side of the tongue rather than over the top of the tongue
Additions	Adding extra sounds to words	"dog" to "dog**ga**"
Fronting of back sounds	Sounds typically produced in the back of the mouth are moved to the front	"**g**oat" to "**d**oat"
Backing of front sounds	Sounds typically produced in the front of the mouth are moved to the back (less common than fronting)	"**d**og" to "**g**og"
Final consonant deletion	Final consonant sounds are dropped in multiple words	"fee**t**" to "fee-"
Initial consonant deletion	Initial consonant sounds are dropped in multiple words	"**d**ig" to "-ig"
Cluster reductions	Reduction of two adjacent consonant sounds to one	"**sn**ake" to "-**n**ake"
Syllable reductions	Syllables dropped from words	"**ba**nana" to "-nana"
Gliding	Liquid sounds (L & R) are changed to glides (Y & W)	"ye**ll**ow" to "ye**y**o" "**l**eg" to "**w**eg"
Metathesis	Order of sounds in a word are changed (with or without sound substitutions)	"**spagh**etti" to "**pask**etti"

As defined by the American Speech, Language, and Hearing Association (ASHA), CAS is a neurological childhood (pediatric) SSD in which the precision and consistency of movements underlying speech are impaired in the absence of neuromuscular deficits. CAS may occur as the result of known neurological impairment, in association with complex neurobehavioral disorders of known or unknown etiology, or as an idiopathic neurogenic SSD. The core impairment in motor planning the spatiotemporal parameters of movement sequences results in errors in speech sound production and **prosody** (the melody, flow, and rhythm of speech). Children with CAS may have difficulty moving from one articulatory configuration to another (Strand, 2017). Comorbid spoken language disorders and specific reading disabilities are often observed in children with CAS (ASHA, 2007). CAS is rare with prevalence estimates between 0.125% (Shriberg, Aram, & Kwiatkowski, 1997) and 1.0% (Yoss & Darley, 1974).

Children with CAS often present with early developmental difficulties that may be indicative of suspected CAS. These include problems with feeding as an infant, little vocal play or babbling, little imitation in infancy, a family history of speech disorders, delayed onset of language, and gross and fine motor incoordination. The diagnostic criteria for CAS are controversial, and often a course of therapy is required before a diagnosis is made. Exclusionary criteria include sensory disorders, cognitive impairment, receptive language deficit, emotional /pragmatic disorder, and poor muscle tone. Hallmark characteristics include groping movements of the articulators and trial-and-error behaviors to produce speech sounds, deviant speech development, receptive abilities better than expressive abilities, inconsistent errors, prosody disturbances, and slow progress in therapy. Speech characteristics include unusual errors not found in children with other types of SSD, a large percentage of omission errors, difficulty producing and maintaining appropriate voicing (switching a consonant sound that engages the vocal cords for one that does not, or vice versa; e.g., /b/ for /p/), vowel and diphthong errors, difficulty sequencing speech sounds and syllables, difficulty with nasality and nasal emission, groping behaviors and silent posturing, prosodic impairments, and difficulty identifying rhymes and syllables (Murray, McCabe, Heard, & Ballard, 2015).

It is important for every child with speech sound difficulties to have a comprehensive evaluation performed by a licensed and certified SLP to determine the specific problem(s) that the child has and to develop an appropriate therapy plan to remediate these difficulties.

Spoken Language Disorders

ASHA defines a **spoken language disorder (SLD)** as "a significant impairment in the acquisition and use of language across modalities (e.g., speech, sign language, or both) due to deficits in comprehension and/or production across any of the five language domains (i.e., phonology, morphology, syntax, semantics, pragmatics)" (https://www.asha.org/Practice-Portal/Clinical-Topics/Spoken-Language-Disorders/ pg1). An SLD may occur in isolation or in combination with other developmental disorders such as autism spectrum disorder (ASD), Down syndrome, intellectual disabilities, and many other neurodevelopmental disorders. Some SLDs are acquired as in the case of traumatic brain injury. A child with SLD may present with **receptive language** (comprehension) delays and/or **expressive language** (production) delays.

Children with SLD are heterogeneous and often exhibit different profiles of language skills across the domains of **semantics** (meaning), **syntax** (structure), morphology (smallest units of meaning), **pragmatics** (rules and conventions), and **phonology** (sound system) (see Table 17.2 for detailed definitions). An assessment by an SLP will determine if language skills are delayed but following a typical developmental course or if they are deviant (disordered) and presenting with an unusual pattern of language errors. For example, some children with an SLD present with specific problems with syntax and phonology while semantics and pragmatic language skills remain intact. Other children have a severe communication deficit that includes nonverbal as well as verbal communication. See Box 17.2 for more information on comorbid language disorders.

Diagnostic Criteria

The *DSM-5* provides diagnostic criteria and features for a broad range of developmental disorders that may involve speech and language disorders such as autism spectrum disorder (ASD). It includes information on differential diagnosis, comorbid disorders, and risk factors.

The specific diagnostic category of communication disorders includes language disorder, SSD, childhood-onset fluency disorder, social communication disorder, and unspecified communication disorder. The unspecified communication disorder is assigned when symptoms are present but do not meet a sufficient number of the diagnostic criteria to warrant a more specific diagnosis.

The *DSM-5* has made several controversial changes to the diagnosis of communication disorders, including

Table 17.2. Speech and language definitions, descriptions, and classifications

Phonology	The sound system of a language and the rules that govern the sound combinations
Phonological awareness	Metalinguistic awareness of all levels of the speech sound system, including word boundaries, stress patterns, syllables, onset-rime units, and phonemes; a more encompassing term than phoneme awareness, which is the explicit understanding that words are composed of phonemes (i.e., segments of sound smaller than a syllable) plus the knowledge that each of these phonemes has distinctive features (Moats, 2010; Moore-Brown & Montgomery, 2001)
Phonological working memory	Temporary storage of speech codes in memory that allows the meaning of language to be extracted and stored in longer term memory (Moats, 2010).
Phonological retrieval	Retrieval of the phonological form of a word from long-term memory; refers to the mental act of formulating and pronouncing the word (Moats, 2010).
Prosody	The melody, flow, and rhythm of spoken language; melodic changes in syllable stress, pitch, loudness, and duration (Plante & Beeson, 2004)
Morphology	The study of morphemes, the smallest units of language that have meaning; free morphemes (cat, dog, me, etc.) can stand alone to convey meaning and cannot be reduced any further without losing meaning; bound morphemes (-ing, -s, -er, etc.) cannot stand alone and must be attached to a free morpheme to convey meaning (Shipley & McAfee, 1998)
Syntax	The rule system governing sentence formation; the study of sentence structure (Moats, 2010)
Semantics	The study of the meaning of language, including meaning at the word, sentence, and conversational levels; also known as content (Shipley & McAfee, 1998)
Pragmatics	The system of rules and conventions for using language and related gestures in social contexts; the study of that rule system (Moats 2010)
Discourse	The organization of sentences into larger cohesive communication units and the ability to process and formulate these units (Moats, 2010)
Metalinguistics	The ability to think about and analyze language in a critical manner, including the ability to understand humor, multiple meanings, inferences, and figurative language (Vinson, 2012)
Receptive language	The individual's ability to understand and process language (Kaderavek, 2011)
Expressive language	The language a person produces spontaneously, without imitating another person's verbalizations (Pence Turnbull & Justice, 2017)

BOX 17.2 EVIDENCE-BASED PRACTICE

Comorbid Language Disorders Associated with Speech Sound Disorders

About 50% of preschool children with speech sound disorders (SSDs) have comorbid language impairment. That is, in addition to speech sound deficits, these children may have problems with vocabulary, grammar, morphology, and/or social language. Language impairments may be limited to expressive language or may involve both receptive and expressive language. Children with early speech and language deficits are at risk for reading, spelling, and written language difficulties at school age and adolescence. Spoken language skills lay the foundation for reading and written language.

Lewis and colleagues (2015) followed 140 children with SSDs identified during early childhood through adolescence. Individuals with an SSD and comorbid language impairment had poorer literacy skills than those with SSD only or no history of SSD. Risk factors for language and literacy problems in adolescence included persistent SSD, history of early language impairment, and lower nonverbal cognitive ability.

- These results underscore the importance of completing a comprehensive evaluation by kindergarten with at-risk children who have already been identified as toddlers as having speech language delays/disorders.
- These results underscore the dangers of a "wait and see" approach to servicing children with suspected speech language delay.

the addition of social communication disorder and the elimination of specific language impairment (Rice, 2016). Individuals who present with other disorders described in the *DSM-5* such as ASD, specific learning disability, attention-deficit/hyperactivity disorder (ADHD), and intellectual disability may also meet the criteria for a communication disorder and should be assessed by an SLP (Paul, 2013).

CASE STUDY

Steve was discharged from speech-language therapy when he was 4 years, 2 months of age because his speech sound production skills were age appropriate. His classmates could understand his speech, and his social communication and play skills were excellent. When Steve was 5 years old and entering kindergarten, his mother expressed concerns about his language development (vocabulary and syntax) and the impact his early SSD would have on literacy development. His mother also noted that Steve's speech had a "stuttering" quality because he had trouble finding the right words, repeated words and partial phrases, and often revised his verbal output. Telling a story seemed to be a laborious process for him.

The school SLP administered three subtests (Sentence Structure, Word Structure, and Expressive Vocabulary) from the Clinical Evaluation of Language Fundamentals Preschool–Second Edition (CELF-P2; Semel, Wiig, & Secord, 2004) and collected a brief speech sample. The school SLP provided no specific information for receptive versus expressive language, syntax, semantics, or early literacy skills. Based on the analysis of the speech sample, the SLP ruled out the diagnosis of stuttering (see Box 17.3 for a discussion comparing normal dysfluency and persistent stuttering). Steve's CELF-P2 Core Language score of 98 placed him within the average range. The special service team did not qualify him for continued support services in kindergarten.

Steve's first-grade teacher contacted special services mid-year because she was concerned about Steve's language and learning development. In the area of listening, she noted Steve had trouble following spoken directions and remembering what was said and that he often asked for clarifications. In the area of speaking,

BOX 17.3 EVIDENCE-BASED PRACTICE

Normal Dysfluency or Persistent Stuttering?

Speech-language pathologists (SLPs) and pediatricians are often confronted with the dilemma of determining if a young preschool child (usually between 2 and 4 years of age) is presenting with early signs of stuttering or if the child is exhibiting normal dysfluencies typical of young children who are acquiring language. A common practice is to "wait and see" as normal dysfluencies generally disappear between 6 and 12 months from onset. However, this policy may delay intervention for children who will become persistent stutterers. Some speech characteristics of normal dysfluencies that may assist in distinguishing these from true stuttering behaviors include whole phrase repetition (instead of syllable repetitions), lack of tension, prolongations and blocking (inability to produce a word; i.e., getting "stuck"), and a negative family history for stuttering (Coleman, 2013).

Recent research also suggests that language characteristics may indicate risk for true stuttering. In one study, children with more rapid growth rates of productive syntax recovered more often than children with slower rates (Leech, Ratner, Brown, & Weber, 2017). Another study of children between 28 and 43 months of age demonstrated that as grammatical abilities increased, dysfluencies decreased (Hollister, Van Horne, & Zebrowski, 2017). Smith and Weber (2017) have proposed a multifactorial dynamic pathway theory of the development of stuttering that incorporates motor, linguistic, emotional, and genetic/epigenetic factors.

- These findings suggest that a "wait and see" policy to differentiate normal dysfluencies from persistent stuttering in young children is not appropriate.
- SLPs should consider characteristics of the dysfluencies as well as other factors, such as language development, family history of stuttering, gender of the child, and level of parent concern when determining whether to intervene.
- Recent studies suggest that early persistent stuttering may be related to slower language growth. Children with dysfluencies should be monitored for language delays that may impact later academic performance.

she indicated difficulties with asking and answering questions, use of vocabulary, describing and expressing thoughts, use of appropriate grammar and sentence structure, and difficulty articulating sounds. In the area of reading, she reported that Steve had trouble with sound play (rhyming, letter names, and letter sounds), sounding out words, understanding and explaining what was read, and remembering details. In the area of writing, she noted Steve did not have a proper pencil grip and that his handwriting was below grade-level expectations.

A multifactored evaluation was completed at his school and an evaluation team report (ETR) was written. In sum, the results of testing indicated multiple areas of weakness: expressive language (produced language or speech), **phonological processing** (including phonological awareness, memory, and retrieval; see Table 17.2), auditory processing, reading, writing, and speech sound production.

The school occupational therapist administered the Beery-Buktenica Developmental Test of Visual-Motor Integration–Sixth Edition (VMI-6; Beery, Buktenica, & Beery, 2010). Steve's scores for visual-motor integration and motor coordination fell in the below-average range. His score for visual perception fell in the above-average range. The special education team developed an individualized education program (IEP) (see Chapter 33) for Steve that described the services he needed in order to access the curriculum. He was scheduled to work with the SLP, learning specialist, and occupational therapist both within and outside the general education classroom.

PREVALENCE AND EPIDEMIOLOGY

Speech and language disorders are highly prevalent in young children. The National Center for Health Statistics reported that in 2012, 7.7% of children 3–17 years of age had a communication disorder based on interviews of parents and caregivers (Black, Vahratian, & Hoffman, 2015). Speech problems were the most common (5%), followed by language problems (3.3%). One third of the children 3–10 years of age and one fourth of the children 11–17 years of age had comorbid disorders. Communication disorders were more prevalent in young children (11% at 3–6 years of age) than older children (9.3% at 7–10 years and 4.9% at 11–17 years) and more common in boys (9.6%) than girls (5.7%).

Speech Sound Disorders

SSDs are one of the most common types of communication disorders in children, with prevalence rates of 15.6% at 3 years of age (Campbell et al., 2003), 3.4% at 4 years of age (Eadie et al., 2015), and 3.8% at 6 years of age (Shriberg, Tomblin, & McSweeny, 1999). At 6 years of age, 25% of children with early SSD continue to present with SSD. For most individuals, the SSD resolves by early grade school (approximately 8 years of age), but for others speech sound errors persist into adolescence and beyond (persistent SSD). More than one half of children with early SSD, as well as the majority of those with persistent SSD, encounter later academic difficulties in language, reading, and spelling (Lewis et al., 2015). Rates of persistent SSD vary based on age of assessment, criteria for persistent SSD, and whether the sample is clinically based or population based. One population-based estimate of persistent SSD is 3.6% of children at 8 years of age (Wren, Miller, Peter, Emond, & Roulstone, 2016).

Spoken Language Disorder

A large population-based study (Tomblin et al., 1997) examined 7,218 kindergarten children and reported a 7.4% overall prevalence rate of SLDs (8% in boys and 6% in girls). Another study reported that 7.58% of 4–5 year olds entering school have a clinically significant language disorder of unknown cause that adversely impacts learning (Norbury et al., 2016). Children whose SLD persists to the age of literacy acquisition are more likely to have difficulty learning to read (Snowling, Duff, Nash, & Hulme, 2016). The comorbidity of SSD and SLD has been reported in 1.3% of children (Shriberg et al., 1999). In children with SSD and SLD, 6% to 21% have been found to have receptive language disorders, and 38%–62% have been found to have expressive language disorders (Shriberg & Austin, 1998). Rates are higher for children with persistent disorders. For example, 11%–15% of children with persistent SSD have SLD, and 5%–8% of children with persisting SLD have SSD.

Comorbid Disorders

Other disorders such as specific reading disability (SRD; see Chapter 20) and ADHD (see Chapter 19) are often comorbid with speech and language disorders (Figure 17.1 illustrates the relationship between spoken and written language). The prevalence of SRD is estimated at 7% when defined as 1.5 SD below the mean on a test of reading achievement and 9% in a clinically ascertained population (Pennington & Bishop, 2009; Peterson & Pennington, 2012). Approximately one half of individuals with SLD meet the criteria for SRD (Catts, Fey, Tomblin, & Zhang, 2002; Snowling, Bishop, & Stothard, 2000), while fewer children with SSDs meet the criteria for SRD. Children with combined SSD and SLD are more likely to have SRD than those children

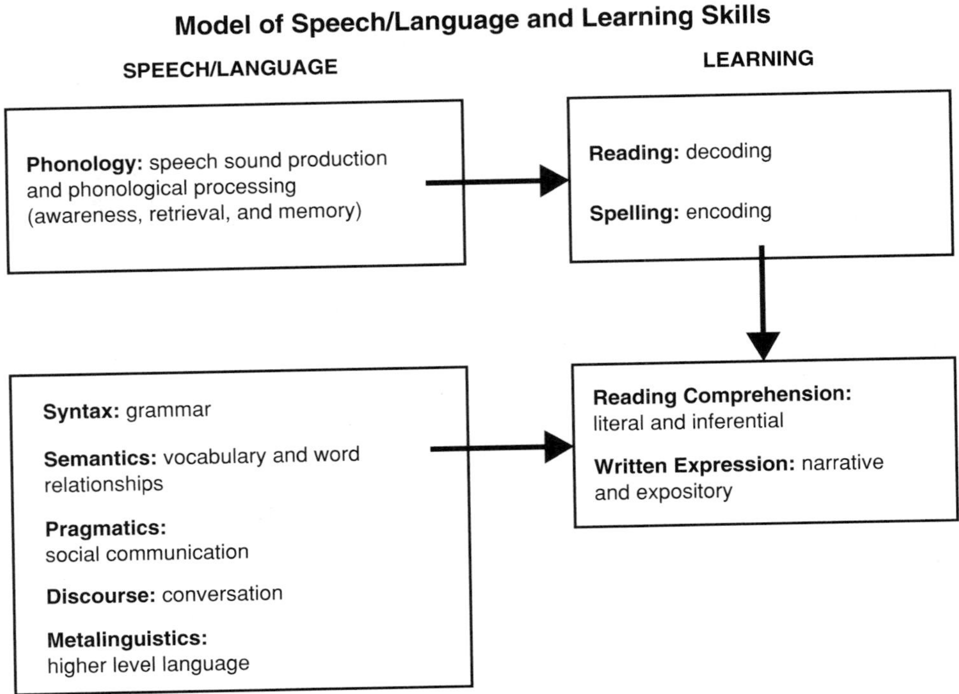

Figure 17.1. Model of speech/language and learning skills, which depicts the relationship between spoken and written language. The phonology of spoken language is related to reading decoding and spelling, and spoken language skills (syntax, semantics, pragmatics, discourse, and metalinguistics) contribute to reading comprehension skills and written expression. Also shown is the relationship between reading decoding and spelling and reading comprehension and written expression.

with SSD alone (Lewis et al., 2015). The high rates of comorbidity of SSD, SLD, and SRD are not surprising as they all involve components of language, especially phonology (see Box 17.4).

ADHD is often comorbid with SSD, spoken language disorder (SLD), and specific reading disability (SRD). Clinical studies have found that the comorbidity of SLD and ADHD ranges from 16% to 24% (Mueller & Tomblin, 2012). This rate drops to 3.3% of adolescents with persistent SLD (Snowling et al., 2006). Approximately 30% of children with SRD also have ADHD (International Dyslexia Association, 2008), and

BOX 17.4 EVIDENCE-BASED PRACTICE

Phonological Awareness and Reading Disorders

Individuals with speech sound disorders with and without an additional language impairment perform more poorly than controls on phonological awareness measures (Skebo et al., 2013). Children with more atypical or nondevelopmental speech sound errors (e.g., deletion of initial consonants) have more difficulty with phonological awareness tasks than children with typical errors (developmental /s/, /z/, /l/, and /r/; Preston & Edwards, 2010). Deficits in phonological awareness have been identified as one of the strongest early predictors of reading disorders (Wagner, Torgesen, Rashotte, & Pearson, 2013). Phonological awareness is the ability to manipulate phonemes in spoken words as well as the awareness of the sound structure of language.

- These results suggest that phonological awareness skills should be evaluated in kindergarten to identify children at risk for reading difficulties.
- These results indicate that developing phonological awareness skills should be part of the kindergarten curriculum.

language impairment is highly correlated with ADHD, with rates greater than 40% of children with combined SRD and ADHD (Helland, Posserud, Helland, Heimann, & Lundervold, 2016).

CASE STUDY

In fourth grade, Steve had no residual speech sound errors. His phonological awareness, phonics skills, and spelling skills were adequate. He wrote neatly with a proper pencil grip. However, Steve's reading vocabulary was limited, and he had difficulty understanding what he read and expressing himself in writing. Although Steve used simpler sentences to express himself, his social communication skills were excellent. Steve had an excellent work ethic, and he always turned his homework in on time even though he had to spend many more hours than his classmates to complete assignments. Because of Steve's working memory and processing limitations, his teacher was concerned he might have a comorbid ADHD (see Chapter 19 for a discussion of ADHD and comorbid language disorder). A child psychiatrist specializing in ADHD assessed Steve and ruled out an attention deficit. Based on Steve's latest ETR, he continues to qualify for an IEP to receive services from the SLP. The intervention is focused on written expression, vocabulary development, and reading comprehension.

ETIOLOGY

The etiology of speech and language disorders is complex due to the many neurobiological, anatomical, genetic, environmental, and cognitive factors that impact speech and language development. Some children have medical conditions that disrupt the acquisition of speech and language such as cleft lip and palate, hearing impairment (see Box 17.5 for a discussion of the impact of chronic otitis media on speech and language development), cerebral palsy, and syndromes with associated intellectual disabilities and cranial facial abnormalities. However, for many children with speech and language disorders, no known etiology for the disorder is identified; these cases are sometimes referred to as idiopathic. Table 17.3 presents risk factors associated with speech and language disorders.

Neurological Foundations of Speech and Language

Advances in neuroimaging techniques have provided new noninvasive methods to study speech and language processing in the brain (see Chapter 8). Studies utilizing these technologies have identified differences in brain structures as well as differences in language processing in children with speech and language

BOX 17.5 EVIDENCE-BASED PRACTICE

Middle Ear Infections and Speech-Language Development

There is a substantial body of research on the impact of otitis media with effusion (OME) on speech and language development (Casby, 2001). Approximately 66% of young children by 3 years of age and 80% of children by 4 years of age experience OM. OME results in a temporary mild to moderate hearing loss at an age when language skills are emerging. Since the hearing loss is fluctuating with normal hearing between OME episodes, the child may be exposed to inconsistent models of speech and language that result in a failure to encode clear phonological representations.

Longitudinal studies have demonstrated early speech and language delays in children with chronic OME around 2 years of age, but these delays are no longer apparent at 7 years of age (Zumach, Gerrits, Chenault, & Anteunis, 2010). However, recent studies have demonstrated a relationship between OME and literacy, presumably due to poor phonological awareness skills (Carroll & Breadmore, 2018). A study of Australian indigenous school children indicated that OME may be one factor affecting literacy skills (Timms, Williams, Stokes, & Kane, 2014).

- Children's hearing should be screened routinely until 7 years of age, and hearing should be tested at any age when speech, language, or learning problems are identified.
- Although early OME has not been demonstrated to impact school-age language skills, it is important to monitor early hearing and provide preschool therapy for children with delays to ensure kindergarten readiness.
- OME may be related to poorer literacy skills in at-risk populations.
- Articulation therapy is highly effective after the OM has resolved and hearing acuity returns.

Table 17.3. Risk factors associated with speech and language disorders

Examples	
Prenatal	Infections of amniotic fluid or membrane, maternal drug or alcohol use, maternal kidney infection, multiple gestation, placental bleeding, excessive or insufficient amniotic fluid, and maternal preeclampsia (hypertension, proteinuria, edema) (see Chapter 3)
Perinatal	Long labor, uncontrolled delivery, abnormal presentation of the infant, cesarean section, fetal distress, placental abnormalities, any perinatal condition that causes brain injury (see Chapter 3)
Neonatal	Low or unusually high birth weight, prematurity, hyperbilirubinemia, poor feeding, any kind of infection, physical anomalies (see Chapter 5)
Medical and genetic	Prolonged hospitalizations, syndromes such as Down syndrome, fragile X, Prader-Willi, neurological abnormalities (see Chapters 1, 3, and 15)
Environmental factors	Family environment, maternal education (affects mother's interaction with the child), low SES, toxins such as lead (see Chapter 2)
Cognitive factors	Inefficient auditory processing, poor verbal memory, learning disabilities, intellectual disability (see Chapters 14 and 20)
Sensory deficits	Congenital or acquired hearing impairments including sensory neural hearing loss, conductive hearing loss including chronic otitis media with effusion (see Chapter 26)

disorders. Structural differences include asymmetry of brain structures, differing amounts of white matter in the brain, and additional gyri in the frontal and temporal lobes. Language-processing differences identified include an increase in the number of brain structures activated, atypical bilateral brain activation patterns, hypo-activation in the frontal and parietal lobes, and neural differences in response to auditory stimuli (Hickok, 2009; Price, 2010; Tkach et al., 2011).

Although these technologies promise exciting new developments in the understanding of the neurological bases of speech and language, some limitations should be noted. For example, it is not known whether these brain differences cause the speech and language disorder or whether having a speech and language disorder results in these observed differences. In addition, other developmental disorders present with similar brain differences, and therefore these neurological differences are not unique to speech and language disorders. Finally, other family members may share these brain differences but do not report a history of speech and language disorders suggesting that other factors, such as genetics, may contribute to language skills (Paul & Norbury, 2012).

Genetic Bases of Speech and Language Disorders

Some children with speech and language disorders have been diagnosed with genetic syndromes. However, most children who are referred to SLPs have no known genetic basis for their disorder, although case histories often indicate other family members with speech, language, and reading difficulties. Since the mid-1990s, advances in genetic technology have allowed for genome-wide studies of speech and language disorders. These studies have identified some candidate genes for speech and language disorders as well as conditions that are often comorbid such as reading disorders and ADHD (Lewis et al., 2006; Worthey et al., 2013).

One such gene, the *FOXP2* gene, which is located on chromosome 7q13, was discovered in a large British family referred to as the "KE family" (Lai, Fisher, Hurst, Vargha-Khadem, & Monaco, 2001; Morgan, Fisher, Scheffer, & Hildebrand, 2017). Affected family members, spanning three generations, presented with orofacial apraxia, persistent SSDs, impairments in IQ, language disorders, and reading difficulties. Neuroimaging studies confirmed that the *FOXP2* gene influenced neurodevelopment in multiple areas of the brain that support speech and language. However, mutations in *FOXP2* are rare (Morgan et al., 2017; Reuter et al., 2017; Vargha-Khadem, Gadian, Copp, & Mishkin, 2005).

Other candidate genes were subsequently identified (*KIAA0319, TTRAP, DCDC2 BDNF, DRD2, AVPR1, CYP19A1,* and *CNTNAP2*, among others) that are also known to influence neurodevelopment and are associated with multiple developmental disorders, including speech, language, reading, and ADHD (Newbury & Monaco, 2010). There is no single gene responsible for the majority of cases of speech and language disorders. Heterogeneous effects of risk genes may act alone or together to give rise to multiple profiles of speech and language skills that may culminate in the same diagnosis and general impairment on the surface. The nature and severity of the disorder might vary at different developmental stages as genes may be turned on and off during the life span. The environment may act in concert with genes to give rise to cognitive skills (endophenotypes) such as phonological awareness skills, memory, vocabulary, and cognitive abilities. These endophenotypes contribute to multiple disorders such as SSDs, SLD, or SRD. Environmental factors such as early intervention or speech-language therapy might modify the resulting phenotype.

The SLP is often the first professional to treat a child with a developmental delay. A working knowledge of genetics may assist the SLP in making referrals to geneticists and genetic counselors when indicated. Knowledge of the features of genetic conditions may result in accurate prognosis, targeted interventions, and appropriate educational plans for the child.

ASSESSMENT AND DIAGNOSIS

The assessment, diagnosis, and remediation of speech and language disorders is a multimodal process. It involves evaluating speech sound and language skills in the contexts of speaking, listening, reading, and writing. The diagnostic process is not conducted in isolation; rather, information from parents, pediatricians, teachers, psychologists, and special educators, as available, is considered during part of the diagnostic process. Pediatricians are responsible for following and documenting a child's developmental history and managing medical needs. Psychologists and psychiatrists provide information about a child's intelligence, attention, and socioemotional development. Learning specialists and teachers provide information about a child's in-class reading and writing history in relation to same-age peers. There are several models for how the assessment team functions together (see Chapter 30).

Test battery selection depends on the age of the child being tested, the time allotted for testing, and the areas of concern. Specialists working in hospitals or schools often carry heavy case loads and do not have the luxury of time; therefore, it is sometimes necessary to shorten the test protocol. In these instances, it is important to get a sampling across skill areas to identify discrepancies.

Screening tools are often used to identify children who need further assessment and what specific areas are of greatest concern. The percentage of children who fail a screening test varies greatly depending on the age of the child who is screened and the screening tool employed. Before choosing a screening measure, the sensitivity (the degree to which a measure identifies a child as having a problem) and the specificity (the degree to which a measure accurately identifies a child as not having a problem) should be addressed. There are informal screening measures and formal, standardized screening tests. Informal measures may include collecting a language sample through conversation with the child; asking the child to perform simple tasks, such as counting to ten or writing his name; or asking the child to answer simple questions, such as his age or the name of his teacher. Formal screenings evaluate single word articulation, phonology, and other levels of receptive and expressive language, comparing the child's test performance with a normative sample or criterion. Examples of early childhood screenings include the CELF-5 Screening Test (Wiig, Semel, & Secord, 2013b) and the Fluharty-2 (Fluharty, 2001).

In the case study, Steve was administered a comprehensive battery in Grades 1, 4, and 11. Tests were selected and administered to assess cognition (Wechsler Intelligence Scale for Children–Fifth Edition [WISC-V]; Wechsler, 2014); receptive and expressive foundational language at the phonological, syntactic, and semantics levels (CELF-5; Wiig & Secord, 2013a; Peabody Picture Vocabulary Test–Fourth Edition [PPVT-4]; Dunn & Dunn, 2007; Expressive Vocabulary Test–Second Edition [EVT-2]; Williams, 2007; Test of Auditory Processing Skills–Third Edition [TAPS-3]; Martin & Brownell, 2005; Comprehensive Test of Phonological Processing–Second Edition [CTOPP-2]; Wagner, Torgesen, Rashotte, & Pearson, 2013); higher-level language at the pragmatic and semantic levels (CELF-5 Metalinguistics; Wiig & Secord, 2014); and learning (Woodcock-Johnson IV Tests of Achievement [WJ IV ACH]; Schrank, Mather, & McGrew, 2014).

Steve's full-scale IQ on the WISC-V fell in the average range across time periods. In first grade, Steve's expressive language, auditory processing, phonological awareness, and memory skills fell well below his full-scale IQ. His speech sound deficit interfered with the development of adequate phonological awareness skills, which, in turn, negatively impacted his basic reading and spelling development. In addition to compromised phoneme-grapheme (sound-letter) knowledge, Steve's lower reading comprehension score was also negatively impacted by memory and auditory processing limitations.

By fourth grade, Steve's phonological awareness and phoneme-grapheme knowledge skills had improved, and his reading of nonsense words and spelling scores fell within the normal limits. However, his reading vocabulary, reading comprehension, and written expression scores fell in the below-average range because of persistent language deficits. Steve's performance on the CELF-5 Metalinguistic Test indicated adequate meta-pragmatic skills (social communication skills) and below-average meta-semantic skills (understanding multiple meanings and abstract idioms), suggesting that Steve had good social communication skills but was missing deeper meanings that are being conveyed in conversation.

By 11th grade, Steve's language scores fell within normal limits, with the exception of the TAPS-3 auditory comprehension, auditory reasoning, and memory scores. Steve's foundational language skills were average, and his higher-level language skills fell in the above-average range. Steve continues to have reading comprehension concerns.

CASE STUDY

As an 11th grader, Steve's exceptional strengths include his work ethic, determination, desire to be a good student, positivity, and great sense of humor. Beyond being a hard worker in school and a talented athlete, he is very socially aware. He picks up on social cues and nuances. He instinctively gets a sense of those around him and goes out of his way to make sure people feel comfortable. Steve's strong social skills are especially impressive given his longstanding history of speech-language and learning difficulties.

Steve is performing well in school, although reading comprehension continues to be an area of weakness for him, especially if he is not given the opportunity to re-read information to glean deep meaning. Steve continues to struggle with working memory and listening skills; however, he compensates for these limitations by following up with his teachers or friends when he has missed information. His higher-level language skills are excellent. Steve feels confident with his school performance because he is given extended time on tests and in-class assignments. With the accommodation of extended time, he does well on in-class tests. The school psychologist is requesting that Steve be given extended time on standardized tests (e.g., the SAT and ACT) because of his longstanding history of language-based learning difficulties.

TREATMENT, MANAGEMENT, AND INTERVENTION

The identification and support of students with speech and language disorders is a goal of response to intervention (RTI), which is explained in the following section. This is followed by descriptions of evidence-based practice interventions for SSDs and SLDs.

Response to Intervention

An **RTI** is a multi-tiered approach to the early identification and support of students with learning and behavior needs. It also considers how well children respond to intervention for a variety of disabilities that impact their school performance (see Chapter 20). Speech and language disorders may impede learning due to impairments in both spoken and written language. Components of RTI include universal screening, high-quality instruction, interventions matched to student need, frequent monitoring of progress, and use of a data-based approach to making educational decisions (see Chapter 33). SLPs assist in the implementation of RTI through direct screening, assessment and treatment, collaboration with team members, and consultation with classroom teachers to provide support for children with communication disorders.

The SLP may function in a consultant role to parents, classroom teachers, and speech-language pathology assistants. In this role, the SLP conducts the assessment, designs the intervention, and supervises its implementation. The SLP may conduct individual or group therapy outside of the classroom or choose direct intervention within the classroom setting creating a more natural and functional communication environment. In other models, the SLP works collaboratively with other therapists such as occupational and physical therapists to optimize communication in daily living. Therapy should actively involve the child, follow the child's lead when possible, and take into account the culture of the child's family.

Intervention for Speech Sound Disorders

Children with SSDs may require a motor-based intervention approach if the disorder is thought to be articulatory based or a linguistic phonological approach if the disorder is hypothesized to result from inadequate knowledge of the sound system. Often a combination of both approaches is employed. In a motor-based approach to intervention, the child is first taught to discriminate and contrast the sounds in error. For example, if a child has the /k/ sound in error, pictures of a cat and bat may be presented. The child is asked to point to the picture that starts with the /k/ sound. Next, the target sounds are taught in isolation followed by single syllables, words, phrases, and sentences. The ultimate goal is to produce target sounds correctly in conversational speech. In a phonological-based approach, the goal is to teach phonological rules, sound contrasts, and phonological patterns of the language. For example, if a child deletes the final consonant sounds in words, he or she is presented with the syllable /ka/ and is asked to add the /t/ on the end of the word. Other sounds such as /p/, /b/, and /n/ may be added to the end of /ka/ to produce the words *cap, cab,* and *can.* In the phonological approach, the goal is to generalize the final consonant rule across multiple words.

A child with a more severe SSD, such as CAS, requires intensive and early intervention. A motor programming–based approach is essential because the core feature of CAS is difficulty with the motor planning aspects of speech production (Strand, 2017). Motor programming approaches utilize motor-learning principles, including the need for many repetitions of speech movements to help the child acquire skills and to accurately, consistently, and automatically make sounds and sequences of sounds. Remediation of CAS should progress systematically through hierarchies of task difficulty.

Other important recommendations for therapy for SSD include 1) stressing sequences of movements, 2) using repetitions of drill-oriented sessions, 3) considering auditory discrimination training, 4) emphasizing self-monitoring, 5) providing multiple modality input, 6) manipulating prosodic features, 7) employing compensatory strategies, and 8) providing successful experiences (Strand, McCauley, Wiegand, Stoekel, & Baas, 2013).

Intervention for Spoken Language Disorders

Children with SLDs may require intervention for social language skills, vocabulary, and grammar. Children with social language deficits, such as ASD, may demonstrate limitations in their use of language. They may lack a variety of pragmatic language skills, including presupposition (social knowledge of the listener's perspective, also known as theory of mind; see Chapter 18), referential skills (identifying for the listener what content the speaker is referring to), staying on topic, taking conversational turns, and recognizing and repairing conversational breakdowns. Therapists often use social stories that describe a situation that the child encounters in daily living to model appropriate social language skills.

Children with SLD may exhibit deficits in vocabulary, which may also impact written language, as proficient readers have strong vocabularies. Vocabulary should be taught employing a developmental sequence. For example, early quantitative words are *one, many, much, some,* and *more.* Later acquired quantitative words are *few, couple, nearly,* and *almost.* Qualitative words should be taught in pairs such as *big/little, tall/short, hot/cold,* and *wide/narrow.* Spatial and temporal terms may include *in, on, at, by, in front, behind, before, after, first,* and *last.* Early conjunctions are *and, but, because, when, or, if, although,* and *unless.*

Older students with SLD may have difficulty with multiple meanings for words, idioms, and figurative language such as metaphors and similes. Some children may present with word-retrieval difficulties and word-finding difficulties due to a lack of established representation in the child's **lexicon** (vocabulary) or poor word retrieval. Intervention should focus on organization of the child's lexicon and generalization to everyday use. Games can be used to teach categorization of common items such as food or animals.

Many children with SLD have difficulty with morphology and syntax. Intervention for these deficits should follow a developmental sequence. Morphological interventions seek to establish awareness of syllables and sounds, identify roots and affixes, and understand relationships with other words. Syntactic interventions may focus on pronouns, plurals, and verb tenses. In older children and adolescents, therapy includes increasing the complexity of the individual's spoken and often written language by elaboration of noun phrases, adverbial phrases, and embedded sentences.

OUTCOMES

Children with early childhood histories of SSD and SLD present with differing longitudinal trajectories of speech, language, literacy, and academic skills. Previous studies have identified risk factors for poor outcomes for individuals with SSD, including male gender, comorbid disorders, persistent speech sound errors, lower nonverbal cognitive abilities, motor impairment, maternal education, and social disadvantage (Harrison & McLeod, 2010; Lewis et al., 2015; Wren et al., 2016). A family history of speech, language, and learning disorders confers additional risk for poor outcomes. Children whose SSD and SLD resolve before adolescence tend to have better outcomes than those whose disorders persist into school age and adolescence.

SLDs may persist into adolescence and adulthood. For many children, their SLDs may resolve by early elementary school; however, the individual may continue to experience difficulty with written language (see Chapter 20). The development of written language relies on the language base established with the acquisition of spoken language, and draws on phonological awareness skills, vocabulary, morphology, and syntax shared with spoken language (See Figure 17.1). Children with SLD are at risk for literacy difficulties due to poor oral language and narrative abilities, phonological awareness, and vocabulary. They demonstrate difficulty with alphabetic knowledge, phoneme-grapheme correspondences, spelling and orthographic knowledge, and word awareness (see Chapter 20).

Although spoken language lays the foundation for written language, they differ in significant ways. For example, literacy is more formal and must be explicitly taught to children, whereas spoken language emerges effortlessly for most children. Literacy utilizes different perceptual and cognitive processes. In written language, vocabulary and sentence construction is more explicit to allow for complex connections among ideas, and the focus is on a central topic with a predictable organization of ideas. Children with early childhood SLDs should be monitored for literacy development. The interaction among the severity of the disorder, comorbid conditions, and early and appropriate interventions impacts the long-term educational, occupational, and social-emotional outcomes for the individual.

SUMMARY

- Children with speech and language disorders comprise a heterogeneous group with different profiles of deficits.
- The SLP's scope of practice includes screening, assessment, diagnosis, and treatment of speech, language, and learning disorders.
- The etiological basis for a disorder is critical in identifying profiles of deficits and strengths.
- Tailored interventions should be designed for specific speech, language, and learning profiles.
- Comorbid conditions may impact long-term outcomes for children with speech, language, or learning disorders.

ADDITIONAL RESOURCES

American Academy of Pediatrics on Speech Development: http://www.parenting.com/article/aap-speech-delay

American Speech and Hearing Association (ASHA): https://www.asha.org/

National Institute of Deafness and Other Communication Disorders: https://www.nidcd.nih.gov/health/specific-language-impairment

Additional resources can be found online in Appendix D: Childhood Disabilities Resources, Services, and Organizations (see About the Online Companion Materials).

REFERENCES

American Psychiatric Association. (2013). *Diagnostic and statistical manual of mental disorders* (5th ed.). Washington, DC: Author.

American Speech-Language-Heading Association. (2007). *Childhood apraxia of speech (technical report).* Retrieved from https:/www.asha.org/policy/tr2007-00278/

American Speech-Language-Heading Association. (n.d.). *Spoken language disorders (practice portal).* Retrieved from http://www.asha.org/Practice-Portal/Clinical-Topics/Spoken-Language-Disorders/

Beery, K., Buktenica, N., & Beery, N. (2010). *Beery VMI: Development Test of Visual-Motor Integration* (6th ed.). Bloomington, MN: Pearson/PsychCorp.

Black, L. I., Vahratian, A., & Hoffman, H. J. (2015). Communication disorders and use of intervention services among children aged 3–17 years: United States, 2012. Retrieved from https://www.cdc.gov/nchs/data/databriefs/db205.pdf

Campbell, T. F., Dollaghan, C. A., Rockette, H. E., Paradise, J. L., Feldman, H. M., Shriberg, L. D., . . . Kurs-Lasky, M. (2003). Risk factors for speech delay of unknown origin in 3-year-old children, *Child Development, 74*, 346–357.

Carroll, J. M., & Breadmore, H. L. (2018). Not all phonological awareness deficits are created equal: evidence from a comparison between children with otitis media and poor readers. *Developmental Science, 21*(3):e12588. doi:10.1111/desc.12588

Casby, M. W. (2001). Otitis media and language development: A meta-analysis. *American Journal of Speech Language Pathology, 10*, 65–80.

Catts, H. W., Fey, M. E., Tomblin, J. B., & Zhang, X. (2002). A longitudinal investigation of reading outcomes in children with language impairments. *Journal of Speech and Hearing Research, 45*, 1142–1147.

Coleman, C. (September 26, 2013). How can you tell if childhood stuttering is the real deal? *ASHA Leader Blog.* Retrieved from https://blog.asha.org/2013/09/26/how-can-you-tell-if-childhood-stuttering-is-the-real-deal/

Dunn, L. M., & Dunn, D. M. (2007). *Peabody Picture Vocabulary Test* (4th ed.). Bloomington, MN: Pearson/PsychCorp.

Eadie, P., Morgan, A., Ukoumunne, O. C., EEcen, K. T., Wake, M., & Reilly, S. (2015). Speech sound disorder at 4 years: Prevalence, comorbidities, and predictors in a community cohort of children. *Developmental Medicine and Child Neurology, 57*, 578–584.

Fluharty, N. B. (2001). *Fluharty 2: Fluharty Preschool Speech and Language Screening Test.* Austin, TX: PRO-ED.

Goldman, R., & Fristoe, M. (2015). *Goldman-Fristoe Test of Articulation* (3rd ed.). Bloomington, MN: Pearson/PsychCorp.

Harrison, L. J., & McLeod, S. (2010). Risk and protective factors associated with speech and language impairment in a nationally representative sample of 4- to 5-year-old children. *Journal of Speech, Language, and Hearing Research, 53*, 508–529.

Helland, W. A., Posserud, M., Helland, T., Heimann, M., & Lundervold, A. (2016). Language impairments in children with ADHD and in children with reading disorder. *Journal of Attention Disorders, 20*, 581–589.

Hickok, G. (2009). The functional neuroanatomy of language. *Physics of Life Reviews, 6*, 121–143.

Hollister, J., Van Horne, A. O., & Zebrowski, P. (2017). The relationship between grammatical development and disfluencies in preschool children who stutter and those who recover. *American Journal of Speech Language Pathology, 26,* 44–56.

International Dyslexia Association. (2008). *Fact sheet.* Retrieved from http://www.interdys.org

Kaderavek, J. N. (2011). *Language disorders in children: Fundamental concepts of assessment and intervention.* Upper Saddle, NJ: Pearson.

Lai, C. S., Fisher, S. E., Hurst, J. A., Vargha-Khadem, F., & Monaco, A. P. (2001). A forkhead-domain gene is mutated in a severe speech and language disorder. *Nature, 413,* 519–523.

Leech, K. A., Ratner, N. B., Brown, B., & Weber, C. M. (2017). Preliminary evidence that growth in productive language differentiates childhood stuttering persistence and recovery. *Journal of Speech, Language, and Hearing Research, 60,* 3097–3109.

Lewis, B. A., Shriberg, L. D., Freebairn, L. A., Hansen, A. J., Stein, C. M., Taylor, H. G., . . . Iyengar, S. K. (2006). The genetic bases of speech sound disorders: Evidence from spoken and written language. *Journal of Speech, Language, and Hearing Research, 49,* 1294–1312.

Lewis, B. A., Freebairn, L., Tag, J., Ciesla, A. A., Iyengar, S. K., Stein, C. M., . . . Taylor, H. G. (2015). Adolescent outcomes of children with early speech sound disorders with and without language impairment. *American Journal of Speech-Language Pathology, 24*(2), 150–163.

Martin, N., & Brownell, R. (2005). *Test of Auditory Processing Skills* (3rd ed.). Novato, CA: Academic Therapy Publications.

Moats, L. C. (2010). *Speech to print: Language essentials for teachers* (2nd ed.). Baltimore, MD: Paul H. Brookes Publishing Co.

Moore-Brown, B. J., & Montgomery, J. K. (2001). *Making a difference for America's children: Speech-language pathologists in public schools.* Eau Claire, WI: Thinking Publications.

Morgan, A., Fisher, S. E., Scheffer, I., & Hildebrand, M. (2017). FOXP-2 related speech and language disorders. In M. P. Adam, H. H. Ardinger, R. A. Pagon, S. E. Wallace, L. J. H. Bean, H. C. Mefford, . . . N. Ledbetter (Eds.), *GeneReviews* [Internet]. Seattle, WA: University of Washington, Seattle.

Mueller, K. L., & Tomblin, J. B. (2012). Examining the comorbidity of language impairment and attention-deficit/hyperactivity disorder. *Topics in Language Disorders, 32*(3), 207–227.

Murray, E., McCabe, P., Heard, R., & Ballard, K. J. (2015). Differential diagnosis of children with suspected apraxia of speech. *Journal of Speech, Language and Hearing Research, 58,* 43–60.

Newbury, D. F., & Monaco, A. P. (2010). Genetic advances in the study of speech and language disorders. *Neuron, 68,* 309–320.

Norbury, C. F., Gooch, D., Wray, C., Baird, G., Charman, T., Simonoff, E., . . . Pickles, A. (2016). The impact of nonverbal ability on the prevalence and clinical presentation of language disorder: Evidence from a population study. *Journal of Child Psychology and Psychiatry, 57,* 1247–1257.

Paul, D. (2013). A quick guide to the DSM-5. *The ASHA Leader, 18,* 52–54.

Paul, R., & Norbury, C. F. (2012). *Language disorders from infancy through adolescence* (4th ed.). St. Louis, MO: Elsevier.

Pennington, B., & Bishop, D. (2009). Relations among speech, language, and reading disorders. *Annual Review of Psychology, 60,* 283–306.

Peterson, R., & Pennington, B. (2012). Developmental dyslexia. *Lancet, 379,* 1997–2007.

Pence Turnbull, K. L., & Justice, L. M. (2017). *Language development from theory to practice* (3rd ed.). Upper Saddle, NJ: Pearson.

Plante, E., & Beeson, P. M. (2004). *Communication and communication disorders* (2nd ed.). Boston, MA: Pearson.

Preston, J., & Edwards, M. L. (2010). Phonological awareness and types of sound errors in preschoolers with speech sound disorders. *Journal of Speech, Language, and Hearing Research, 53,* 44–60.

Price, C. (2010). The anatomy of language: A review of 100 fMRI studies published in 2009. *Annals of the New York Academy of Sciences, 1191,* 62–88.

Reuter, M. S., Riess, A., Moog, U. Briggs, T. A., Chandler, K. E., Rauch, A., . . . Zweier, C. (2017). FOXP2 variants in 14 individuals with developmental speech and language disorders broaden the mutational and clinical spectrum. *Journal of Medical Genetics, 54,* 64–72.

Rice, M. L. (2016). Specific language impairment, nonverbal IQ, attention-deficit/hyperactivity disorder, cochlear implants, bilingualism, and dialectal variants: Defining boundaries, clarifying clinical conditions, and sorting out cases. *Journal of Speech, Language, and Hearing Research, 59,* 122–132.

Schrank, F. A., Mather, N., & McGrew, K. S. (2014). *Woodcock-Johnson IV Tests of Achievement.* Rolling Meadows, IL: Riverside.

Secord, W., & Donohue, J. S. (2014). *Clinical Assessment of Articulation and Phonology* (2nd ed.). Greenville, SC: Super Duper Publications.

Semel, E., Wiig, E., & Secord, W. (2004). *Clinical Evaluation of Language Fundamentals – Preschool-2.* Bloomington, MN: Pearson/PsychCorp.

Shipley, K. G., & McAfee, J. G. (1998). *Assessment in speech-language pathology* (2nd ed.). San Diego, CA: Singular Publishing Group.

Shriberg, L. D., Aram, D. M., & Kwiatkowski, J. (1997). Developmental apraxia of speech: I. Descriptive perspectives. *Journal of Speech, Language, and Hearing Research, 40,* 273–285.

Shriberg, L. D., & Austin, D. (1998). Comorbidity of speech-language disorders: Implications for a phenotype marker for speech delay. In R. Paul (Ed.), *Exploring the speech language connection* (pp. 73–117). Baltimore, MD: Paul H. Brookes Publishing Co.

Shriberg, L. D., Tomblin, J. B., & McSweeny, J. L. (1999). Prevalence of speech delay in 6-year-old children and comorbidity with language impairment. *Journal of Speech, Language, and Hearing Research, 42,* 1461–1481.

Skebo, C., Lewis, B. A., Freebairn, L., Tag, J., Avrich, A., & Stein, C. M. (2013). Predictors of reading skills at elementary, middle and high school for children with and without speech sound disorders. *Language, Speech, and Hearing Services in Schools, 40,* 360–373.

Smith, A., & Weber, C. (2017). How stuttering develops: The multifactorial dynamic pathways theory. *Journal of Speech, Language, and Hearing Research, 60,* 2483–2505.

Snowling, M., Bishop, D. V. M., & Stothard, S. E. (2000). Is preschool language impairment a risk factor for dyslexia in adolescence? *Journal of Child Psychology and Psychiatry, 41,* 587–600.

Snowling, M. J., Bishop, D. V. M., Stothard, S. E., Chipchase, B., & Kaplan, C. (2006). Psychosocial outcomes at 15 years of children with a preschool history of speech-language impairment. *Journal of Child Psychology and Psychiatry, 47,* 759–765.

Snowling, M. J., Duff, F. J., Nash, H. M., & Hulme, C. (2016). Language profiles and literacy outcomes of children with resolving, emerging or persisting language impairments. *Journal of Child Psychology and Psychiatry, 57*(12), 1360–1369.

Sparrow, S. S., Cicchetti, D. V., & Saulnier, C. A. (2016). *Vineland Adaptive Behavior Scales* (3rd ed.). Bloomington, MN: Pearson/PsychCorp.

Strand, E. (2017). Appraising apraxia: When a speech sound disorder is severe, how do you know if its apraxia of speech? *ASHA Leader, 22,* 50–58.

Strand, E., McCauley, R. J., Weigand, S. D., Stoekel, R. E., & Baas, B. S. (2013). A motor speech assessment for children with severe speech disorders: Reliability and validity evidence. *Journal of Speech, Language, and Hearing Research, 56,* 505–520.

Timms, L., Williams, C., Stokes, S. F., & Kane, R. (2014). Literacy skills of Australian Indigenous school children with and without otitis media and hearing loss. *International Journal of Speech and Language Pathology, 16,* 327–334.

Tkach, J. A., Chen, X., Freebairn, L. A., Schmithorst, V. J., Holland, S. K., & Lewis, B. A. (2011). Neural correlates of phonological processing in speech sound disorder: A functional magnetic resonance imaging study. *Brain and Language, 119,* 42–49.

Tomblin, J. B., Records, N., Buckwalter, P., Zhang, X., Smith, E., & O'Brien, M. (1997). Prevalence of specific language impairment in kindergarten children. *Journal of Speech, Language, and Hearing Research, 40,* 1245–1260.

Vargha-Khadem, F., Gadian, D. G., Copp, A., & Mishkin, M. (2005). *FOXP2* and the neuroanatomy of speech and language. *Nature Reviews Neuroscience, 6,* 131–138.

Vinson, B. P. (2012). *Preschool and School-Age Language Disorders* (1st ed.). Clifton Park, NY: Delmar Cengage Learning.

Wagner, R. K., Torgesen, J. K., Rashotte, C. A., & Pearson, N. A. (2013). *Comprehensive Test of Phonological Processing* (2nd ed.). Austin, TX: PRO-ED.

Wechsler, D. (2014). *Wechsler Intelligence Scale for Children* (5th ed.). Bloomington, MN: Pearson/PsychCorp.

Wiig, E. H., Semel, E. M., & Secord, W. (2013a). *Clinical Evaluation of Language Fundamentals* (5th ed.). Bloomington, MN: Pearson/PsychCorp.

Wiig, E. H., Semel, E. M., & Secord, W. (2013b). *Clinical Evaluation of Language Fundamentals: Screening Test* (5th ed.). Bloomington, MN: Pearson/PsychCorp.

Wiig, E. H., & Secord, W.A. (2014). *Clinical Evaluation of Language Fundamentals–Fifth Edition: Metalinguistics.* Bloomington, MN: Pearson/PsychCorp.

Williams, K. T. (2007). *Expressive Vocabulary Test* (2nd ed.). Bloomington, MN: Pearson/PsychCorp.

Worthey, E. A., Raca, G., Laffin, J. J., Wilk, B. M., Harris, J. M., Jakielski, K. J., . . . Shriberg, L. D. (2013). Whole-exome sequencing supports genetic heterogeneity in childhood apraxia of speech. *Journal of Neurodevelopmental Disorders, 5,* 5–29.

Wren, Y., Miller, L. L., Peter, T. J., Emond, A., & Roulstone, S. (2016). Prevalence and predictors of persistent speech sound disorder at eight years old: Findings from a population cohort study. *Journal of Speech, Language, and Hearing Research, 59,* 647–673.

Yoss, K. A., & Darley, F. L. (1974). Developmental apraxia of speech in children with defective articulation. *Journal of Speech and Hearing Research, 17,* 399–416.

Zimmerman, I., Steiner, V., & Pond, R. (2011). *Preschool Language Scale* (5th ed.). Bloomington, MN: Pearson/PsychCorp.

Zumach, A., Gerrits, E., Chenault, M., & Anteunis, L. (2010). Long-term effects of early-life otitis media on language development. *Journal of Speech, Language, and Hearing Research, 53,* 34–43.

CHAPTER 18 Autism Spectrum Disorder

Deborah Potvin and Allison B. Ratto

Upon completion of this chapter, the reader will

- Be familiar with the core features of autism spectrum disorder
- Understand the importance and process of screening, early identification, and intervention for autism
- Be able to identify the conditions associated with autism spectrum disorder
- Be familiar with the developmental course and outcomes

Autism spectrum disorder (ASD) is a neurodevelopmental disorder characterized by persistent impairments in reciprocal social communication and social interactions and restricted, repetitive patterns of behavior, interest, or activities. These core diagnostic features are present from an early age and significantly impact daily functioning; however, the manifestation of these symptoms and their impact vary based on the nature and severity of the autistic features; chronological age; temperament; and the individual's level of intellectual, language, and adaptive functioning.

This heterogeneity complicates the diagnosis and treatment of individuals with autism. In addition, autism is often seen in the context of comorbid medical and behavioral conditions, which can cloud diagnosis and change prognosis and treatment needs. Despite these challenges, evidence of the effectiveness of early and intensive intervention in improving adaptive, intellectual, and language function in young children with autism (Hampton & Kaiser, 2016; Reichow, 2012) lends urgency to the need for effective diagnosis. See the textbox titled A Note about Language for a brief discussion of the language used in this chapter.

CASE STUDY

Diego is a 4-year-old boy with a history of language delay who is having behavioral difficulties at home and school. As an infant, he was irritable and difficult to soothe. He started speaking some Spanish words at around 12 months of age, but by 24 months, he still spoke only a few single words and no phrases. Although his parents were told this was because he was learning two languages, Diego's older sister did not have this same problem. His parents sought out early intervention services for him, and Diego was identified as having a language delay. With speech therapy, he began making progress and now, at age 4, is speaking in short sentences, primarily in English. His language tends to be somewhat repetitive, and he often uses phrases out of context that he has heard on television. He has learned all of his letters and numbers, and he often surprises his

A NOTE ABOUT LANGUAGE

There is debate about the value of person-first versus identity-first language among professionals, self-advocates, and families in the world of autism. Person-first language (i.e., "person with autism spectrum disorder") is considered standard practice among most professionals, and families often prefer this language as well, arguing that this emphasizes the humanity and dignity of the individual. Self-advocates often prefer identify-first language (i.e., "autistic person"), arguing that a person cannot be separated from his/her autism and that "autistic" should be used in the same way as terms describing culture (e.g., "Muslim woman," "African American boy"). This chapter utilizes person-first language for consistency with common professional practice and other sections of this text. However, the reader is encouraged to read the Autistic Self-Advocacy Network's statement on identity-first language for additional perspective (www.autisticadvocacy.org). The terms *autism* and *ASD* are used interchangeably in this chapter as they are in clinical practice.

teachers by reading words aloud. Diego is a friendly, outgoing boy. He often walks up to adults and other children and touches them or tries to hand them a toy even if he has never met them before. He and his younger brother like to play with cars and sometimes act out their favorite movies together. Diego often follows other children around on the playground at school, but he struggles to play cooperatively with them. If other children do not want to play "his way," Diego often becomes upset and has a tantrum. He gets very upset when he has to have his hair or nails cut, and he covers his ears and hides whenever his mother uses the vacuum cleaner. He sometimes flaps his hands when he is excited or stressed. Diego is rarely able to sit still for more than a few minutes and struggles to pay attention at school. His parents tried giving him a stimulant medication that his pediatrician prescribed, but they stopped the medication after he became very anxious and agitated. His parents and teachers are proud of his early academic skills, but they are worried about his problems participating in classroom activities and getting along with other children.

CASE STUDY

Michael was born at term following an unproblematic pregnancy and delivery. His parents became concerned around the age of 9 months, when he was not babbling like other children his age. He was seen for his first assessment at 12 months, with findings of appropriate gross and fine motor skills and delays in both expressive and receptive language. Following this initial assessment, Michael began receiving early intervention services, including intensive speech and language therapy. At follow-up assessments at 18, 24, and 30 months, Michael showed slow but steady progress with language and, by the age of 2½, was using a few consistent signs. The question of a possible ASD diagnosis was raised by the parents, but Michael's therapists described him as a happy and social little boy and pointed out that he showed no clear repetitive behaviors. However, at his 36-month assessment, Michael showed subtle regression in his language skills and had stopped using his signs. Although quite pleasant and calm, he did not engage with the assessment tasks and spent most of the time in repetitive play, including opening and closing the doors and watching toys as he dropped them to the floor. At that time, Michael was diagnosed with an ASD and began intensive **applied behavior analysis (ABA)** therapy. Through therapy, he continued to make gains in adaptive skills (e.g., toileting and classroom routines). He showed little progress with language, and his family decided to introduce an augmentative/alternative communication device at the age of 5. The use of this device was initially focused on allowing Michael to request preferred activities and foods, but, as Michael became more comfortable, it evolved to include everyday routines. At the age of 6, Michael entered first grade in a primary autism classroom, which allowed for ABA-based instruction as well as opportunities to interact with typically developing children in the context of a buddies program.

CASE STUDY

Kay was born prematurely, at 31 weeks' gestational age, weighing 3 pounds, 5 ounces. Despite her early arrival, she had a fairly uneventful stay in the neonatal intensive care unit and was able to go home after 6 weeks, breathing and eating on her own. Her parents were very aware of the risks for early developmental delays in children born prematurely and monitored Kay's development carefully. To their delight, she appeared to meet all of her developmental milestones on time.

As a preschooler, however, Kay's teacher began to express concerns about some of her behaviors. She had a hard time adjusting to any changes in the routine, often becoming upset and quickly spiraling into a full meltdown when there was a minor change to the schedule. She was also a bit slow with some fine motor skills, including cutting and drawing. In addition, around this time, Kay's parents noted that her play seemed different from the other children. Although she enjoyed pretend play with her dolls and toy ponies, she tended to repeat the same scenes over and over. She was happy to have her parents play with her if they would stick with the script, but she got upset if other children tried to join her. Because of these concerns, Kay started participating in play therapy and occupational therapy.

As she progressed through elementary school, Kay was eager to make friends and have play dates. However, when other children came over, she typically greeted them enthusiastically but then went off to play on her own. Although the other girls in her class had moved on to different types of play, Kay still preferred to act out scenes with her toy ponies and had expanded that interest to reading every book she could find about horses. Kay was also struggling in school. The meltdowns continued to occur on a regular basis at school and at home had become more intense. In particular, when doing homework Kay needed to have everything "just so" and would become distraught and unable to continue if there was a single mistake or problem that seemed too hard. Although she seemed to have a strong vocabulary and learned to read easily, she had difficulty paying attention during group lessons and had a hard time answering questions about what she had read.

With these ongoing difficulties interfering with her school work and creating a stressful home environment, Kay was referred for a speech and language assessment. Although her core language skills were age appropriate, the speech-language therapist was concerned about her pragmatic or social language and recommended a more comprehensive, neuropsychological assessment. Following this assessment, Kay was finally diagnosed with ASD at the age of 10. In addition to changes in her school program and the introduction of an individualized education program (IEP), Kay began participating in cognitive behavioral therapy (CBT) with a practitioner experienced in working with girls with autism and joined a social skills group, which included cognitive flexibility training.

Thought Questions:

How can medical providers facilitate early diagnosis of ASD? Once a diagnosis is established, what recommendations should families receive about further evaluation and intervention? How can providers prepare families for some of the changes and struggles that occur as children with autism develop? How does autism's presentation change in the presence of comorbid neurodevelopmental or medical conditions, and how do these comorbid conditions affect diagnosis, intervention, and developmental trajectory? What are the advantages and disadvantages of different educational settings for children with ASD? What measures can be taken to successfully include a child with ASD in a general education setting? When might a more specialized setting be appropriate?

DEFINITIONS, DESCRIPTION, AND CLASSIFICATIONS

There is significant heterogeneity among individuals with ASD. Still, they all share two core domains of symptoms: impairments in social communication and restricted/repetitive patterns of behavior and interest (see diagnostic criteria in Table 18.1).

Persistent Deficits in Social Communication and Interaction

Impairments in social communication and interaction skills are critical to the diagnosis of ASD. The American Psychiatric Association's *Diagnostic and Statistical Manual of Mental Disorders, Fifth Edition* (*DSM-5*) criteria for ASD require that individuals show evidence of core difficulties in three areas: 1) nonverbal communication, 2) social-emotional reciprocity, and 3) social relationships (APA, 2013). There must be evidence that these difficulties began in early development, though the *DSM-5* acknowledges that some individuals, particularly those with higher cognitive and intellectual abilities, may not show functional impairment from these challenges until later ages, as social demands increase and become more subtle and complex (see the Previous Diagnostic Categories textbox).

Impairments in **nonverbal communication** are among those most classically associated with ASD. Individuals with ASD commonly have difficulty in making eye contact and fluidly coordinating eye gaze with other communicative behaviors. Impaired eye gaze is one of the earliest and most consistent signs of ASD, emerging as early as the first year of life (Baranek, 1999; Clifford et al., 2007). Eye-tracking studies have found that individuals with ASD spend less time looking at people's eyes and more time focused on objects and, when looking to faces, more time fixated on the mouth (Chawarska, Macari, & Shic, 2012; Klin, Jones, Schultz, Volkmar, & Cohen, 2002). Impairments in other aspects of nonverbal communication are also common in ASD, including a reduced range of facial expressions, reduced use of gestures, and markedly flat or unusual vocal intonation or **prosody** (patterns of stress and intonation in speech) (Rapin & Dunn, 2003).

Along with problems using nonverbal communication behaviors, individuals with ASD also have difficulty understanding nonverbal communication from others, including problems with accurately interpreting facial expressions, tone of voice, and body language (Dawson, Webb, & McPartland, 2005; Silverman, Bennetto, Campana, & Tanenhaus, 2010). Several studies have also found that attending to faces, which engenders positive emotions in typically developing

Table 18.1. Diagnostic criteria for autism spectrum disorder

A. Persistent deficits in social communication and social interaction across multiple contexts, as manifested by the following, currently or by history (examples are illustrative, not exhaustive; see text):
   1. Deficits in social-emotional reciprocity, ranging, for example, from abnormal social approach and failure of normal back-and-forth conversation; to reduced sharing of interests, emotions, or affect; to failure to initiate or respond to social interactions.
   2. Deficits in nonverbal communicative behaviors used for social interaction, ranging, for example, from poorly integrated verbal and nonverbal communication; to abnormalities in eye contact and body language or deficits in understanding and use of gestures; to a total lack of facial expressions and nonverbal communication.
   3. Deficits in developing, maintaining, and understanding relationships, ranging, for example, from difficulties adjusting behavior to suit various social contexts; to difficulties in sharing imaginative play or in making friends; to absence of interest in peers.

Specify current severity:

Severity is based on social communication impairments and restricted, repetitive patterns of behavior.

B. Restricted, repetitive patterns of behavior, interests, or activities, as manifested by at least two of the following, currently or by history (examples are illustrative, not exhaustive; see text):
   1. Stereotyped or repetitive motor movements, use of objects, or speech (e.g., simple motor stereotypes, lining up toys or flipping objects, echolalia, idiosyncratic phrases).
   2. Insistence on sameness, inflexible adherence to routines, or ritualized patterns of verbal or nonverbal behavior (e.g., extreme distress at small changes, difficulties with transitions, rigid thinking patterns, greeting rituals, need to take same route or eat same food every day).
   3. Highly restricted, fixated interests that are abnormal in intensity or focus (e.g., strong attachment to or preoccupation with unusual objects, excessively circumscribed or perseverative interests).
   4. Hyper- or hyporeactivity to sensory input or unusual interest in sensory aspects of the environment (e.g. apparent indifference to pain/temperature, adverse response to specific sounds or textures, excessive smelling or touching of objects, visual fascination with lights or movement).

Specify current severity:

Severity is based on social communication impairments and restricted, repetitive patterns of behavior.

C. Symptoms must be present in the early developmental period (but may not become fully manifest until social demands exceed limited capacities, or may be masked by learned strategies in later life).

D. Symptoms cause clinically significant impairment in social, occupational, or other important areas of current functioning.

E. These disturbances are not better explained by intellectual disability (intellectual developmental disorder) or global developmental delay. Intellectual disability and autism spectrum disorder frequently co-occur; to make comorbid diagnoses of autism spectrum disorder and intellectual disability, social communication should be below that expected for general developmental level.

Note: Individuals with a well-established DSM-IV diagnosis of autistic disorder, Asperger's disorder, or pervasive developmental disorder not otherwise specified should be given the diagnosis of autism spectrum disorder. Individuals who have marked deficits in social communication, but whose symptoms do not otherwise meet criteria for autism spectrum disorder, should be evaluated for social (pragmatic) communication disorder.

Specify if:

With or without accompanying intellectual impairment
With or without accompanying language impairment
Associated with a known medical or genetic condition or environmental factor
(**Coding note**: Use additional code to identify the associated medical or genetic condition.)
Associated with another neurodevelopmental, mental, or behavioral disorder
(**Coding note**: Use additional code[s] to identify the associated neurodevelopmental, mental, or behavioral disorder[s].
With catatonia (refer to the criteria for catatonia associated with another mental disorder)
(**Coding note**: Use additional code 293.89 catatonia associated with autism spectrum disorder to indicate the presence of the comorbid catatonia.)

individuals, tends to activate the amygdala and feelings of fear and anxiety in those with ASD.

Although impairments in verbal communication (i.e., language skills) are not required for the diagnosis of ASD, they are nonetheless a common feature of the disorder. Language delay is the most frequent first concern for parents of children later diagnosed with ASD (Chawarska et al., 2007). Although language delay from infancy is the most common presentation, in about 25%–30% of children with ASD early language development is typical but subsequently plateaus or regresses between 18 and 24 months (Parr et al., 2011; Rogers, 2004). Impairments in core language may persist throughout the lifespan, with an estimated 30% of individuals with autism classified as minimally verbal in adulthood (Tager-Flusberg & Kasari, 2013). These

PREVIOUS DIAGNOSTIC CATEGORIES

In the *DSM-IV-TR* (APA, 2000), ASD was captured under the category of Pervasive Developmental Disorders and individuals could be diagnosed with Autistic Disorder, Asperger's Disorder, or Pervasive Developmental Disorder–Not Otherwise Specified. Studies of differential diagnosis and long-term outcomes did not support distinctions between these diagnoses (particularly between Autistic Disorder and Asperger's Disorder) and found that even when using gold-standard diagnostic procedures, diagnostic categorization was not reliable across sites (Lord et al., 2012a; Witwer & Lecavalier, 2008). These findings drove the decision to move to the single category of Autism Spectrum Disorder in the *DSM-5,* which includes the provision that anyone diagnosed under *DSM-IV-TR* retains his or her diagnosis under *DSM-5*. Providers may still encounter families and individuals who refer to their *DSM-IV-TR* diagnosis. This is particularly true for individuals diagnosed with Asperger syndrome, who often identify more strongly with this label due in part to its more positive associations with intelligence and savant-like skills in the media and society at large.

individuals often communicate through augmentative/alternative communication (AAC) supports, discussed in more detail below.

Among those with intact core language skills, impairments in higher-order language, such as language organization, verbal reasoning, and pragmatic skills, are common (Boucher, 2012). Individuals with ASD may have an impressive vocabulary and strong cognitive abilities but still struggle with understanding idioms, metaphors, sarcasm, and other subtle, nonconcrete features of language. See the Social Communication Disorder textbox for a brief discussion of a new clinical diagnosis introduced in the *DSM-5*.

Impairments in both verbal and nonverbal communication skills contribute to broader difficulties in **social-emotional reciprocity** (i.e., difficulties relating to others). In early childhood, these deficits often manifest through reduced **joint attention,** which is the ability to share a common point of reference, such as a child pointing to an airplane flying overhead and saying "Look!" while pointing and using eye gaze (Mundy & Newell, 2007). Young children with ASD are less likely to initiate joint attention with others and often struggle to respond to others' joint attention bids. Young children with ASD are also less likely to spontaneously give and show objects to others and often prefer to play alone (Zwaigenbaum, Bryson, & Garon, 2013). As children age, deficits in social-emotional reciprocity are evident through more complex difficulties and as social cognition deficits.

Children and adults on the spectrum commonly struggle to initiate and maintain reciprocal conversations with others (Paul, Orlovski, Marcino, & Volkmar, 2009). They often have difficulty demonstrating interest in others' ideas and experiences and have trouble picking up on subtle conversational cues. Individuals with ASD also commonly struggle with **theory of mind,** which is the ability to intuit and understand others' thoughts, emotions, and perspectives, particularly when they differ from one's own experience (Yirmiya, Erel, Sheked, & Solmonica-Levi, 1998). They may assume that others' experiences are the same as their own or simply be unable to guess what another person is thinking or feeling.

Reduced social-emotional reciprocity in turn leads to difficulties in initiating and maintaining relationships with others, particularly with peers (Travis, Sigman, & Ruskin, 2001). While children with autism

SOCIAL COMMUNICATION DISORDER

The *DSM-5* introduced the new, clinical diagnosis of Social (Pragmatic) Communication Disorder, characterized by "persistent difficulties in the social use of verbal and nonverbal communication" (APA, 2013, p. 47) in children who do not meet diagnostic criteria for ASD. Deficits in social communication are present across a range of neurodevelopmental disabilities and have been shown to be present in children who do not show the restricted, repetitive patterns of behavior, interest, or activities associated with ASD (Bishop & Norbury, 2002), though the variable presentation of restricted, repetitive behaviors between individuals and across the lifespan raises concerns about accurately distinguishing between the two disorders. In addition, further research is needed to understand appropriate assessment techniques and treatments for this new diagnosis (Norbury, 2014).

were historically thought of as being unable to develop attachments to others, including their parents, more recent research has shown that while attachment behaviors may differ, these children generally develop very close bonds with their parents and other individuals important to them (Rutgers, Bakermans-Kranenburg, van Ijzendoorn, & van Berckelaer-Onnes, 2004).

Most consistently, children and adults with ASD struggle with peer relationships (Bauminger & Kasari, 2000; Orsmond, Krauss, & Seltzer, 2004). Some may prefer to be alone and actively avoid playing with peers, while others are highly socially motivated but struggle to make and keep friends due to their social skill deficits. In early and middle childhood, deficits in play skills contribute to difficulty developing peer relationships (Jordan, 2003).

Children with ASD often struggle to develop functional play (using toys as intended) and pretend play (using objects representationally and engaging in "make believe"), and they have trouble playing cooperatively with others (Kasari, Freeman, & Papparella, 2006). Some children learn to engage in pretend play but do so in a highly "scripted" manner, following the same routine each time or being unable to incorporate others' ideas into play.

As these children age and move into adolescence and adulthood, the overwhelming majority express an interest in dating and sexual activity but are less likely than their non-autistic counterparts to develop romantic relationships, particularly long-term relationships (Byers, Nichols, & Voyer, 2013; Strunz et al., 2017). Of note, rates of same-sex attraction, attraction to both sexes, and gender nonconforming feelings are significantly higher in adults with ASD, and this may further complicate their romantic relationships (Dewinter, De Graaf, & Begeer, 2017).

Restricted/Repetitive Patterns of Behavior, Interest, and Activities

Although differences in social "give and take" are considered central to the diagnosis of autism, **restricted/repetitive behaviors and interests** (RRBIs) are often the most visible symptoms (Leekam, Prior, & Uljarevic, 2011). Strict adherence to routines is common among people with ASD. This can extend to food selectivity, rituals related to daily routines, and difficulties with transitions and changes in their usual environments. For example, having a substitute teacher for the day or needing to take a different route to school may be extremely distressing for a child with ASD. Repetitive motor mannerisms, such as hand flapping or intense spinning, may also be observed, as well as repetitive use of objects, such as lining things up or becoming intensely focused on the parts of an object (e.g., repetitively spinning wheels on a toy car). Young children with autism may have attachments to unusual items rather than to soft or cuddly toys.

Repetitive, stereotyped, and idiosyncratic language is also a common feature of ASD. Individuals may engage in immediate **echolalia** (repeating others' speech) or use delayed echolalia or "scripting," in which they parrot previously heard phrases or sentences (Rapin & Dunn, 2003). Individuals with ASD may also speak in an overly formal manner, with younger children sometimes described as speaking like "little professors."

Unusual responses to sensory input are commonly reported as well (Marco, Hinkley, Hill, & Nagarajan, 2011). These may include insensitivity to some inputs, such as pain or temperature, or overreactions to other inputs, such as noises, touch, or odors. For example, a child may cover his or her ears and scream in response to certain sounds, such as a vacuum cleaner or blender, or refuse to have his or her nails cut or hair trimmed. The same child may also actively seek out other sensory experiences by staring out of the corners of their eyes, sniffing objects without a clear scent, or stroking surfaces or textures.

Restricted interests are also a common feature of autism. Individuals may develop intense interests in and knowledge of highly specific topics. These topics may be unusual (e.g., vacuum cleaners or road signs), or they may be common interests that are pursued with uncommon intensity (e.g., trains or *Star Wars*). Restricted/repetitive behaviors and interests often change in their presentation, focus, and intensity over the lifespan. These symptoms can significantly impair an individual's daily functioning and impede social interactions, but they do not necessarily do so. Behaviors that are present but not impairing (e.g., hand-flapping or intense interest in flags) do not need to be directly targeted for treatment. It is also worth noting that many self-advocates with ASD have pointed out the potential benefits of restricted/repetitive behaviors and interests. For example, an intense interest may help an individual to identify a career path or develop friendships around shared interests. Likewise, although strict adherence to routines may interfere with functioning, it may also reduce anxiety by ensuring that an individual knows what to expect.

Specifiers and Severity Levels

In recognition of the removal of separate diagnostic categories and use of the single label "ASD" for all individuals, the *DSM-5* provides a number of specifiers for clinicians to use; clinicians should identify whether or not the individual has a co-occurring intellectual

Table 18.2. Severity levels for autism spectrum disorder

Severity level	Social communication	Restricted, repetitive behaviors
Level 3 "Requiring very substantial support"	Severe deficits in verbal and nonverbal social communication skills cause severe impairments in functioning, very limited initiation of social interactions, and minimal response to social overtures from others. For example, a person with few words of intelligible speech who rarely initiates interaction and, when he or she does, makes unusual approaches to meet needs only and responds to only very direct social approaches.	Inflexibility of behavior, extreme difficulty coping with change, or other restricted/repetitive behaviors markedly interfere with functioning in all spheres. Great distress/difficulty changing focus or action.
Level 2 "Requiring substantial support"	Marked deficits in verbal and nonverbal social communication skills; social impairments apparent even with supports in place; limited initiation of social interactions; and reduced or abnormal responses to social overtures from others. For example, a person who speaks simple sentences, whose interaction is limited to narrow special interests, and who has markedly odd nonverbal communication.	Inflexibility of behavior, difficulty coping with change, or other restricted/repetitive behaviors appear frequently enough to be obvious to the casual observer and interfere with functioning in a variety of contexts. Distress and/or difficulty changing focus or action.
Level 1 "Requiring support"	Without supports in place, deficits in social communication cause noticeable impairments. Difficulty initiating social interactions and clear examples of atypical or unsuccessful responses to social overtures of others. May appear to have decreased interest in social interactions. For example, a person who is able to speak in full sentences and engages in communication but whose to-and-fro conversation with others fails and whose attempts to make friends are odd and typically unsuccessful.	Inflexibility of behavior causes significant interference with functioning in one or more contexts. Difficulty switching between activities. Problems of organization and planning hamper independence.

impairment, language impairment, or catatonia and whether the ASD is conceptualized as occurring secondary to a known medical, genetic, or environmental factor or to another neurodevelopmental, mental health, or behavioral condition. Clinicians are also encouraged to specify the severity of the condition using one of three severity levels (Table 18.2), which are determined based on the level of impairment in social communication and restricted/repetitive behaviors. There has been very limited research on these severity levels. Thus far, findings have emphasized that there is a considerable degree of heterogeneity in ASD severity and that impairments in social communication, restricted/repetitive behaviors, adaptive behavior, and intellectual ability are often discrepant with one another within individuals (Mehling & Tassé, 2016; Weitlauf, Gotham, Vehorn, & Warren, 2014). Research on the stability of the *DSM-5* severity levels over time has not yet been performed; however, given the variability of developmental trajectories in ASD, it is expected severity levels may change over the lifespan.

Strengths of the Autism Spectrum

In addition to the challenges experienced by individuals with autism, it should also be noted that there are several strengths associated with this condition. Individuals with ASD may have an exceptional memory, an excellent eye for detail, advanced visual-spatial skills, and strong abilities for logical and hierarchical reasoning (De Martino, Harrison, Knafo, Bird, & Dolan, 2008; Happé & Frith, 2006; Narzisi, Muratori, Calderoni, Fabbro, & Urgesi, 2013). For this reason, autistic traits have been commonly found in professionals working in math, computer science, and other sciences; adults on the spectrum may be particularly likely to excel in these fields (Baron-Cohen, Wheelwright, Skinner, Martin, & Clubley, 2001).

DEVELOPMENTAL COURSE OF AUTISM SPECTRUM DISORDER

As a neurodevelopmental disorder, autism is a condition that grows and changes with the child (see Table 18.3). Some symptoms may begin to emerge in the first year of life, though these are not commonly noted other than in severe cases or by parents with a family history (e.g., an older child) with ASD. Parents may describe an infant as being very difficult to soothe or as being quite content to be left alone. They may begin to notice that the infant is less likely to make eye contact or babbles less frequently than other children of the same age.

Symptoms of ASD are most often first observed in the second year of life (between 12–24 months of age). By far, the most common symptom parents report as their initial concern is a delay in language skills,

Table 18.3. Prominent symptoms and challenges by age

Birth–12 Months	12–24 Months	2–5 Years	Middle Childhood	Adolescence	Adulthood
Reduced eye contact and gaze to faces Lack of social smile Reduced babbling and vocalizations Unusual sensory responses Impaired motor coordination	Language delays Lack of gestures Poor joint attention Repetitive play and behaviors No response to name Possible developmental regression	Reduced peer interactions Unusual or stereotyped language Deficits in pretend play Unusual and restricted interests Insistence on sameness	Deficits in reciprocal conversation Poor friendship quality Problems with attention and learning	Problems with executive functioning Poor understanding of social cues Poor hygiene and self-care Social isolation and bullying	Under-employment Housing challenges Difficulties with activities of daily living Few and poor quality relationships

including acquisition of first words and phrases. Many children with ASD do not point or wave hello or goodbye. Children may be described as preferring to play alone and often do not try to engage their parents' interest (for example, by bringing items to them), in contrast to typically developing children who frequently seek parental attention. Parents may also notice unusual play at this age, such as spending a significant amount of time lining up or banging objects and failing to engage in early functional and symbolic play (e.g., pretending to talk on a toy phone or feeding or rocking a baby doll).

In the preschool period, problems playing with other children often become central—they may actively resist playing with peers or may only be willing to play with others if they play according to the child's rules. They may engage in very little pretend play or only do so by carefully reenacting favorite movies or television shows. Children at this age may be easily overwhelmed by transitions and upset by changes in routine or new experiences. Preschool teachers often describe a child who has frequent tantrums, struggles to participate in group activities, and has strong preferences for repeating the same activities over and over.

Most children with ASD are diagnosed by the time they exit the preschool period (CDC, 2018). Some children, however, particularly those who have strong intellectual and language abilities or who have known medical or genetic conditions (e.g., epilepsy) may be diagnosed later (Clarke et al., 2005). During the middle childhood years (elementary and early middle school), problems with attention and academic skills may be most prominent. Difficulties with writing and reading comprehension are common, given the demands for language and executive functioning involved in these tasks. Children who were able to play with peers in the preschool period may begin to struggle more with friendships at this age as the social interactions become more complex. They may be teased or bullied by other children for their social differences. Children who continue to have meltdowns or tantrums may need well-structured behavioral supports in place, particularly in the school setting.

As children enter puberty and adolescence, the risk for developing comorbid conditions, such as anxiety and depression, increases as they become more aware of their differences and feel increasingly separate from their peers. Problems navigating romantic relationships and sexual feelings may also emerge. Very intelligent children who performed well on the more rote academics of elementary school may have more difficulties in middle and high school. The transition to adulthood is often difficult. Individuals may struggle to be successful in postsecondary education or in work settings, often due to problems with social skills and executive functioning rather than an inability to perform the key tasks. Underachievement and underemployment, a lack of daytime activities, and reduced ability to live independently are common.

PREVALENCE AND EPIDEMIOLOGY

The Centers for Disease Control and Prevention (CDC)'s most recent study—from 2018—reported the prevalence of ASD as approximately 1 in 59 children in the United States. Other countries have reported similar rates, with some variations by ascertainment method and local awareness of autism (Baron-Cohen et al., 2009; Elsabbagh et al., 2012; Kim et al., 2011). There has been a consistent and significant increase in diagnostic rates over time throughout the world. Although researchers are still investigating the factors contributing to this increase, there is mounting evidence that the observed change in prevalence is due largely to increasing awareness of ASD and changes in diagnostic practices over time, such that many children, particularly those from minority populations, who would have previously gone undiagnosed or been diagnosed with another condition (e.g., attention-deficit/hyperactivity disorder, intellectual disability) are now being identified as having ASD (Coo et al., 2008; Hertz-Picciotto & Delwiche, 2009). The autism spectrum has also expanded over time to include an increasing number of individuals without co-occurring intellectual disability. Fifteen to twenty years ago, approximately 70% of children with autism were classified as intellectually disabled (Fombonne, 2003); more recent studies have found that only 31% of children with ASD also have intellectual disability (CDC, 2018).

Prevalence rates of ASD are affected by a number of demographic factors, including gender, race/ethnicity, and family income. Autism has always been identified in females at a substantially lower rate than in males, with most epidemiological studies reporting an approximately male-to-female ratio of 4 to 1 (Fombonne, 2009). However, a recent meta-analysis of epidemiological studies found that the true ratio is likely closer to 3 to 1, with findings suggesting that females with ASD are more likely to be undiagnosed (Loomes, Hull, & Mandy, 2017). It is also well established that the sex imbalance in prevalence varies with cognitive ability; among individuals with co-occurring intellectual disability, a smaller male-to-female ratio of approximately 2 to 1 exists, while a much larger ratio of as much as 6 to 1 occurs among those with average to above average IQ (Fombonne, 2009; Kirkovski, Enticott, & Fitzgerald, 2013).

Many in the field have described a female protective effect (e.g., Robinson, Lichtenstein, Anckarsater, Happé, & Ronald, 2013), by which female sex directly reduces the risk of autism, and there is evidence that there may be a higher genetic threshold for autism in females (Gilman et al., 2011; Jacquemont et al., 2014; Robinson et al., 2013). However, it has also been hypothesized that ASD may be "camouflaged" in females and that current diagnostic procedures may be biased against females, particularly those without co-occurring intellectual disability (Kirkovski et al., 2013; Lai et al., 2016).

Females have been found to have significant delays in receiving an autism diagnosis relative to males (Begeer et al., 2013; Shattuck et al., 2009; Siklos & Kerns, 2007). This may be due in part to relative social strengths among females on the spectrum, who may show more developmentally appropriate vocabulary and core language skills (Halladay et al., 2015; Hiller et al., 2016), more intact play and imitation skills (Knickmeyer, Wheelwright, & Baron-Cohen, 2008), and greater concerns with being liked by peers (Hiller et al., 2016; Kirkovski et al., 2013). In addition, some authors have noted that the lower rate of restricted/repetitive behaviors and interests among females relative to males on the spectrum (Mandy et al., 2012; Van Wijngaarden-Cremers et al., 2014) may actually be driven in part by clinician bias, as females may have restricted interests in more "normative" content areas (e.g., books, celebrities, and animals; Halladay et al., 2015; Kirkovski et al., 2013).

Of note, gender identity also likely plays an important role in the manifestations of ASD. Individuals with ASD are significantly more likely to endorse gender nonconforming feelings and behaviors (Strang et al., 2014). Rates of ASD and autistic traits are also significantly elevated among individuals presenting for treatment of gender dysphoria (de Vries, Noens, Cohen-Kettenis, van Berckelaer-Onnes, & Doreleijers, 2010; Edwards-Leeper & Spack, 2012).

Prevalence rates also vary by race/ethnicity. Data from the CDC prevalence studies have consistently found lower rates of diagnosis among Black, Latino, and Asian American children (CDC, 2007, 2012, 2016, 2018). Ethnic minority children also tend to be diagnosed later than their white peers (Liptak et al., 2008; Mandell, Novak, & Zubritsky, 2005; Pedersen et al., 2012). Perhaps due in part to these delays in diagnosis, ethnic minority children have also been reported to have more severe forms of ASD and higher rates of co-occurring intellectual disability than white children (Jarquin, Wiggins, Schieve, & Naarden-Braun, 2011; Liptak et al., 2008), even within samples controlled for socioeconomic status (Mandell et al., 2005; Tek & Landa, 2012).

Economic disparities continue to have a significant effect on access to care among families in the United States (Mandell et al., 2009; see Chapter 42). ASD was initially conceptualized as a disorder of the wealthy; it was believed that highly educated, wealthy parents were more likely to engage in "cold" parenting styles that engendered autistic symptoms in their children as opposed to the warmer, more nurturing parenting styles of low- to middle-income parents (Bettelheim, 1967; Sanua, 1984). Subsequent studies demonstrated that differences in diagnostic rates could be accounted for by biased recruitment in research samples (Schopler, Andrews, & Strupp, 1979; Wing, 1980). However, more recent studies continue to find that low-income children in the United States are less likely to be diagnosed with ASD and tend to be diagnosed significantly later than their middle-income and high-income peers (Durkin et al., 2010; Liptak et al., 2008; Mandell et al., 2005). Although the reasons for this discrepancy are not fully understood, it is suspected to be largely driven by disparities in access to health care and educational supports and knowledge of developmental milestones and disorders.

ETIOLOGY: CAUSES OF AUTISM SPECTRUM DISORDER

ASD has multiple etiologies, with the weight of research pointing to a strong genetic component, while ongoing studies continue to investigate the influence of environmental factors. However, even as our understanding of the etiology of autism expands, for most individuals the cause of an autism diagnosis remains unknown. What is fairly clear is that, with the exception of a minority of children with a perinatal or neonatal neurodevelopmental insult (Lindquest, Carlsson, Persson, & Uvebrant, 2006), ASD is a condition that is present from birth, with infants who go on to develop ASD showing subtle motor delays within the first year of life, well before the emergence of early language and social differences (Bhat, Galloway, & Landa, 2012).

The Genetics of Autism

Research shows strong evidence for a genetic etiology in ASD. The risk of autism in a younger sibling of a child with autism has been found to be as high as 18.7% (Ozonoff et al., 2011), lending weight to the importance of parent education of children with autism and careful monitoring of their younger siblings. Likewise, twin studies have shown a strong concordance (e.g., both twins having ASD) for identical twins (76%), with lower rates for same-sex fraternal twins (34%; Frazier et al., 2014). Although some of these studies point to the interplay between genetics and a shared intrauterine environment in the development of ASD (Hallmayer et al., 2011), others suggest linear inheritance with very little environmental influence (Sandin et al., 2017; Tick, Bolton, Happe, Rutter, & Rijsdijk, 2016).

Despite strong evidence for the role of genetics in ASD, there is not yet a clear genetic pathway to explain ASD, with most research pointing to multiple pathways. A minority of ASD cases are associated with genetic disorders that have known etiologies (see Table 18.4). Historically, several genetic disorders, including Prader-Willi syndrome, Angelman syndrome, tuberous sclerosis complex, and fragile X syndrome (see Appendix B, Chapter 1, and Chapter 15), have been associated with higher rates of autism, although even in these syndromes the majority of affected individuals do not meet criteria for autism.

With the increasing prevalence of genetic testing through chromosomal microarray (CMA; see Chapter 1), knowledge of the breadth of genetic syndromes associated with autism has expanded. Recent large-scales studies suggest that between 5%–9% of individuals with autism who complete chromosomal microarray analysis have clinically significant or pathogenic findings (Ho et al., 2016; McGrew, Peters, Crittendon, & Veenstra-VanderWeele, 2012; Tammimies et al., 2015). In addition, approximately 25% of individuals are found to have gene variants of uncertain significance (Ho et al., 2016). However, these findings still reflect the lack of a clear genetic etiology in many individuals with autism, supporting the importance of research on the role of polygenic inheritance, copy number variants, and high numbers of common genetic variants in the genetics of autism (see Chapter 1).

Environmental Factors

It may be that environmental factors interact with genes to cause the symptoms of ASD. The sections that follow describe the evidence, or lack thereof, for associations of obstetric complications, neurodevelopmental insults, intrauterine exposure, prenatal infections, and toxic environmental exposure with ASD.

Obstetric Complications Neither large epidemiological studies nor meta-analyses have strongly associated particular prenatal, perinatal, or neonatal complications with the development of ASD. However, obstetric optimality scores, which reflect the overall health of the pregnancy, delivery, and newborn period, are lower in children subsequently diagnosed with ASD (Dodds et al., 2011; Lyall et al., 2012), and meta-analyses show higher rates of complications during pregnancies of children born with ASD (Gardener, Spiegelman, & Buka, 2009). The causal direction of these findings is unclear, including whether factors that predispose a child to ASD also compromise fetal well-being or whether subtle compromises in fetal well-being increase susceptibility to ASD.

Neurodevelopmental Insults Researchers and clinicians are increasingly recognizing the elevated risk of autism in medically complex children whose medical history is linked with early neurodevelopmental insults. Studies have consistently linked premature birth with an increased risk for ASD. More focused investigations have shown a strong association between extreme prematurity (< 26 weeks' gestation) and ASD, with some estimates indicating that up to 8% of children with a history of extreme prematurity meet criteria for ASD (Johnson et al., 2010). Clinically, children born prematurely may present with a subtle and qualitatively different presentation of autism characteristics than seen in other children with ASD.

Clinicians are also becoming more aware of an increased risk of ASD in children with other medical conditions associated with early neurodevelopmental

Table 18.4. Genetic disorders associated with autism

Genetic disorder	Genetic defect	Primary features	Prevalence of autism
Rett's syndrome	Mutations in the *MeCP2* gene	Global regression following 6-18 months of typical development; intellectual disability; loss of purposeful hand movements	61%[a]
Cohen's syndrome	Mutations in *COH1* gene on 8q22	Developmental delay; intellectual disability; microcephaly; hypotonia	54%
Cornelia de Lange syndrome	Mutations in *NIPBL, SMC1A, HDAC8, RAD21*, and/ or *SMC3* gene	Slow growth; moderate to severe intellectual disability; bone abnormalities	43%
Tuberous Sclerosis complex	Mutations in *TSC1* or *TSC2* gene	Numerous benign tumors; intellectual disability; behavioral difficulties; seizures	36%
Angelman syndrome	Mutation in *UBE3A* gene	Developmental delay; intellectual disability; severe speech impairment; ataxia; seizures; microcephaly	34%
CHARGE syndrome	Mutation in CHD7 gene	Multiple physical and neurological abnormalities; delays in motor development	30%
Fragile X syndrome	Mutation in the *FMR1* gene on the X chromosome	Mild to moderate intellectual disability in males, with higher intellectual functioning in females; behaviors difficulties; seizures	30%[b]; 22%[c]
Neurofibromatosis type 1 (NF1)	Mutations in the *NF1* gene	Skin discoloration and tumors along nerves in skin, brain, and other areas; typical intellectual functioning; ADHD; learning disabilities	18%
Down syndrome	Trisomy 21	Mild to moderate intellectual disability; hypotonia; characteristic facial features	16%
Noonan's syndrome	Mutations in *PTPN11, SOS1*, or *RIT1* gene	Characteristic facial features; slow growth; heart defects, bleeding problems; range of intellectual functioning	15%
William's syndrome	Deletion of material from chromosome 7	Characteristic facial features; heart defects; mild to moderate intellectual disability; hypersocial personality	12%
22q11.2 deletion syndrome	Deletion on 22q11.2, with implications for *COMT* and *TBX1* genes	Characteristic facial features; heart defects; cleft palate; risk for developing schizophrenia and bipolar disorder; developmental delays; ADHD; learning disabilities	11%

Sources: For syndrome information: National Library of Medicine (2017); for prevalence information: Richards, Jones, Groves, Moss, and Oliver. (2015).
[a]females only; [b]males only; [c]mixed sex

insults. For instance, children with hydrocephalus and cerebral palsy (Lindquest et al., 2006) and congenital heart disease (reviewed in Cassidy et al., 2017) have been found to be at higher risk for ASD. Although the interplay between the neurological insults related to these disorders and the possible underlying genetic factors remains unclear, these findings highlight the need for consistent developmental screenings for these children, with a caution against attributing or "writing off" early developmental concerns to a child's medical history and not pursuing appropriate interventions.

Intrauterine Exposure Substances that result in an increased risk of birth defects in the developing fetus are termed teratogens (see Chapter 6). These include maternal medications, drugs of abuse, chemicals, and radiation. Past investigations of teratogens tended to focus on substances associated with an increased risk of congenital malformations and perinatal complications; however, increasing recognition is now being given to the neurobehavioral effects of these substances (Gentile, 2010). For example, thalidomide, a medication used to treat nausea in pregnant women in the early 1960s, was associated with limb deformities in the exposed fetuses. Many years later, adults who had been exposed to thalidomide *in utero* were also found to have higher rates of ASD (Strömland, Nordin, Miller, Akerström, & Gillberg, 1994). More recently, increased rates of ASD have been found in children exposed in utero to valproic acid, an anti-seizure medication (Christensen et al., 2013). Findings on prenatal exposure to antidepressants have been mixed, with more recent studies suggesting that previously found associations might be better explained by the underlying maternal mood disorder (Brown et al., 2017).

Prenatal Infections Prenatal infection with rubella increases the risk for cerebral palsy, intellectual disability, visual impairments, and ASD depending on the timing of the infection (Chess, 1971). Fortunately, the measles, mumps, and rubella (MMR) vaccination-based immunity in women has all but eliminated this cause of ASD in the United States. Although not as pronounced, an increased risk for autism has also been associated with children with congenital cytomegalovirus. Other viruses and bacteria that commonly infect pregnant women are not specifically associated with a higher risk of ASD in their children. However, a mother's own immune response to infections might cause subtle brain differences in the fetus that could predispose a child to ASD. Large epidemiological studies have found a slightly increased risk of ASD in children whose mother had an infection during pregnancy, particularly if the infection was diagnosed during an inpatient stay—and thus was suspected to be more severe (Jiang et al., 2016; Zerbo et al., 2015).

Toxic Environmental Exposure No known environmental or chemical exposures have been associated with an increased risk for ASD. Toxic exposure has been investigated through studies of air quality, heavy metal exposure, and exposure to endocrine-disrupting chemicals (e.g., PCBs, see Chapter 2). However, much of this research has been hampered by poor or limited designs (Modabbernia, Velthorst, & Reichenberg, 2017). The effect of exposure to mothers and infants, as well as the effect on brain development, needs to be explored in a more systematic way.

Vaccines

Extensive research has found no evidence of a causal link between vaccines and ASD. However, despite the weight of this research, concerns about vaccines and ASD continue to contribute to lower vaccination rates, particularly among younger siblings of children with ASD (Glickman, Harrison, & Dobkins, 2017). Thus, in light of these continued concerns and recent outbreaks of illness that may be prevented by vaccines, therapists and providers should be able to discuss this topic clearly with families.

Since the initial allegation of an association of the MMR vaccine with developmental regression and ASD, a large body of evidence has been published that has refuted the connection. The journal that published the article retracted the publication because of improper scientific practices (The Editors of The Lancet, 2010). Population-based studies, in fact, do not demonstrate an increase in the rate of ASD diagnosis with the introduction of the MMR vaccination (Demicheli, Jefferson, Rivetti, & Price, 2005). Madsen et al. (2002) compared the rate of autism in more than 400,000 children in Denmark who received the MMR vaccine with about 100,000 children who did not get the vaccine. There was no difference in the rate of autism. Likewise, there is no evidence that the body's immune reaction to the vaccines raises the risk of developing ASD (DeStefano, Price, & Weintraub, 2013). Despite this evidence against a connection between vaccination and ASD, there continues to be a decreased rate of immunization by parents concerned about a possible association (Glickman et al., 2017; Leask, Booy, & McIntyre, 2010). Families should be reassured that the immunization schedule advocated by the American Academy of Pediatrics (AAP) is not associated with the development of ASD.

A second hypothesis relates the ethylmercury-based preservative thimerosal (used as a preservative in pediatric vaccines prior to 2001) to symptoms of ASD in genetically susceptible children (Bernard, Enayati, Redwood, Roger, & Binstock, 2001). After removal of thimerosal from vaccines in Denmark, the rate of diagnosis of ASD actually increased (Madsen et al., 2003), although this could be attributed to the broadened diagnostic criteria and increased awareness of ASD in families and providers.

Brain Development and Neural Circuitry

Differences in the neuroanatomy of children with ASD are present from early in development and subtly affect a number of different regions of the brain, suggesting that autistic brains do look and work differently. However, research is still in the process of defining and quantifying that difference.

Development The early overgrowth theory is one of the most prominent theories explaining the dynamic relationship between neurodevelopment and the emergence of ASD symptoms. This theory hypothesizes that genetic predisposition and/or environmental factors contribute to increased cellular proliferation, migration, and differentiation in the developing brain of a young child with autism (Dinstein, Haar, Atsmon, & Schtaerman, 2017). These factors lead to hyperexpansion of the cortical surface between the ages of 6–12 months, followed by a period of overgrowth in total brain volume, between the ages of 12–24 months (Hazlett et al., 2017). The location of early cortical hyperexpansion within the sensory areas and the correspondence of the timing of these neurological changes with the timing of the emergence of early sensory symptoms and characteristic social deficits raise further questions about the interplay between these neurological changes and the symptoms of ASD. Interestingly, the overgrowth theory has also been traditionally linked with evidence of **macrocephaly** (large heads) and accelerated head growth in children with ASD (Elder, Dawson, Toth, Fein, & Munson, 2008). However, more recent studies have found no difference in head circumference in children with and without ASD (Dinstein et al., 2017; Zwaigenbaum et al., 2014).

Neural Circuitry The heterogeneity of the behavioral presentation of ASD has complicated research into neuroanatomical differences associated with the disorder. Although there is some agreement as to the brain regions involved in the key features of ASD, including social-communication deficits, repetitive behaviors, and executive functioning weaknesses, research into how these brain regions differ in individuals with ASD has led to inconsistent and sometimes contradictory findings. In general, the neural systems associated with autism are thought to include the 1) fronto-temporal and frontal parietal regions, 2) limbic brain regions, 3) fronto-striatal circuitry, and (4) cerebellum (Duerden, Mak-Fan, Taylor, & Roberts, 2012; reviewed in Ecker, 2017; see Chapter 8 for a discussion of brain anatomy). In addition, individuals with autism show reduced connectivity in the neural circuitry associated with these regions, including the social circuitry of the fronto-temporal regions (Pelphrey, Shultz, Hudac, & Vander Wyk, 2011), the circuitry of the fronto-parietal regions (Solomon et al., 2009), and the fronto-striatal circuitry (Shafritz, Dichter, Baranek, & Belger, 2008). The correlation between reduced connectivity within these neural circuits and performance on measures of social cognition, cognitive control, and repetitive behaviors, respectively, supports the development of a neurobiological model of autism.

DIAGNOSIS AND ASSESSMENT

A diagnosis of ASD is most often the result of an extended process that begins with concerns from parents, teachers, pediatricians, or others in the child's life. As noted above, concerns usually begin within the first few years of life but may not emerge until later for children with more intact core cognitive skills. In young children, the first step in this process is screening, most often performed by the child's pediatrician. Delays in language or social engagement or the presence of repetitive behaviors may raise initial concerns. Formal screening tools are often utilized as part of this process; the most commonly used of these is the Modified Checklist for Autism in Toddlers (M-CHAT; Pandey et al., 2008; Robins, Fein, Barton, & Green, 2001). The M-CHAT is a brief parent questionnaire suitable for screening toddlers in a pediatrician's office. Although sensitive to symptoms of ASD, it is not specific unless the items endorsed by the family are examined further by interview. The M-CHAT authors have subsequently developed an interview used to confirm the screening questionnaire (Pandey et al., 2008). A revised version was recently published, the Modified Checklist for Autism in Toddlers, Revised with Follow-up (M-CHAT-R/F) with improved positive predictive values (Robins et al., 2014). The M-CHAT is made freely available on the authors' web site with both online and hand scoring (see Additional Resources) and has been translated into several languages. Other well-validated screening tools include the First Year Inventory and the Screening Tool for Toddlers and Young Children (Reznick, Baranek, Reavis, Watson, & Crais, 2007; Stone, Coonrod, Turner, & Pozdol, 2004). See Box 18.1 for more on early diagnosis.

Once a child has "failed" an initial screening, he or she is referred to early intervention services, school-based assessment teams, and/or developmental specialists. ASD is most often diagnosed by physicians and psychologists, especially those with specialized training in this diagnosis, such as developmental pediatricians, pediatric neurologists and psychiatrics, clinical psychologists and neuropsychologists, and speech-language pathologists working as part of a multidisciplinary team. Many other professionals who work with these children (including speech-language pathologists, occupational therapists, behavioral analysts, educators, and social workers) make key contributions to the diagnostic process through their insights, observations, and experience. A thorough medical examination should be conducted to rule out underlying medical conditions; this often includes a referral to an audiologist to rule out hearing impairment. The physical examination should also include an examination of the skin, as children with neurocutaneous syndromes (e.g., tuberous sclerosis) are at higher risk for autism.

At minimum, making a diagnosis of ASD requires gathering information from parents and other caregivers about current symptoms and a thorough developmental, medical, and psychiatric history, along with direct observation and evaluation of the child's social communication skills and behavior. The Autism Diagnostic Interview-Revised (Rutter, LeCouteur, & Lord, 2003) is a structured interview that specifically evaluates current and historical symptoms of ASD; however, it is quite lengthy and is most commonly utilized in research. In clinical practice, providers often utilize

BOX 18.1 EVIDENCE-BASED PRACTICE

The Stability of Early Diagnosis

Evidence of the effectiveness of early and intensive intervention in improving outcomes for young children with autism lends urgency to the need for effective, early diagnosis. However, the intensity and expense of early intervention also comes with concerns about the accuracy of early diagnosis of autism in children under the age of 3. Ozonoff and associates (2015) studied the stability of early diagnosis in a group of children at high risk for developing autism, comparing early diagnosis at 18 or 24 months with a final diagnosis at 36 months. With diagnosis based on 1) Autism Diagnostic Observation Schedule assessment, 2) use of *DSM-IV* clinical criteria, and 3) diagnosis by a licensed clinician, they found a high degree of stability, 93% at 18 months and 82% at 24 months. Most strikingly, early diagnosis was highly specific (99% at 18 months and 95.5% at 24 months), with the majority of children who were diagnosed with autism at 18 or 24 months retaining that diagnosis at 36 months. However, many children who eventually received an autism diagnosis at 36 months were not diagnosed at either 18 or 24 months, suggesting that some children have a period of early development during which autism features slowly emerge.

- Clinical diagnosis of autism can be accurately made before the age of 3 and can allow for implementation of appropriate early intervention.
- Not all children with autism can be diagnosed before the age of 3, reflecting the importance of periodic screening and follow-up for children at risk for autism or with early developmental delays who do not initially meet criteria for an autism diagnosis.

unstructured interviews, along with parent questionnaires, such as the Social Communication Questionnaire (Rutter, Bailey, & Lord, 2003) or the Social Responsiveness Scale–2 (Constantino & Gruber, 2012). Clinicians should observe the child in the office in play interactions and conversation.

The use of the Autism Diagnostic Observation Schedule–2 (ADOS-2; Lord et al., 2012b) has become widespread in both research and clinical practice for direct observation of ASD symptoms. The ADOS-2 is a semistructured assessment of social communication skills that consists of a series of activities adapted based on the child's language and developmental level. It is primarily play based for younger children and is increasingly driven by conversation skills for older children and adolescents/adults.

Although the ADOS-2 is a very valuable tool, it is important to recognize that its results should not be used in isolation to make diagnostic determinations. In addition to parent report and direct evaluation of the child's social communication skills, best practice for the evaluation of ASD includes formal assessment of cognitive abilities, language skills, motor skills, and other psychiatric symptoms, as well as the input of teachers and others familiar with the child. Neuropsychological evaluation can be critical to understanding the profile of many children with autism and making appropriate recommendations (see Chapter 13). The diagnostic assessment of a child with possible ASD is often best accomplished in the context of a comprehensive, multidisciplinary evaluation of the child's strengths and weaknesses. A team approach to assessment yields not only a diagnosis, but also critical recommendations based on a global view of the child's abilities and challenges. See Box 18.2 for further discussion on the interdisciplinary team that supports evaluation.

Following the diagnosis of ASD, the AAP recommends that all children be referred for genetic testing, including a chromosome microarray (AAP, 2010). Ongoing management and continuing care should occur with a developmental pediatrician, pediatric psychiatrist, pediatric neurologist, or primary care pediatrician who is well versed in the management of children with ASD. The physician can guide families in determining when additional evaluations are needed, accessing treatments, prescribing medications to help with managing co-occurring symptoms, and coordinating with other medical providers and systems of care. Children who show signs of possible seizures or other neurological abnormalities should also be referred to a neurologist. Although additional medical and biological evaluations are often pursued by families, there is no scientific evidence to support measurement of heavy metal levels in hair, blood, or urine; immunologic parameters in blood; stool flora; urine peptides; or yeast metabolites in the urine in children with ASD (Levy & Hyman, 2005). Periodic assessment

BOX 18.2 INTERDISCIPLINARY CARE

The Role of the Psychologist

A clinical psychologist is a doctoral-level clinician with extensive training and experience in providing comprehensive mental health and behavioral assessment and care for individuals and families. A neuropsychologist is a psychologist with specialized training in the applied science of brain-behavior relationships. In practice, both psychologists and neuropsychologists work extensively with children with autism. Though their roles are often interchangeable, a psychologist may be more likely to provide ongoing treatment/care while a neuropsychologist may be more involved with extensive, periodic assessments, particularly for children with complex medical histories or comorbid diagnoses that impact neurological functioning.

The diagnostic assessment of a child with autism is best accomplished within a multidisciplinary team, and the psychologist or neuropsychologist plays an important role on that team, helping to ensure that the assessment yields both an accurate diagnosis and recommendations for appropriate treatment within the home and school settings. Following the initial diagnosis, the psychologist or neuropsychologist will also play a role in ongoing care and care management. Often families will meet with the psychologist on a regular basis to check in about their children's progress and to discuss any shift or changes that need to be made to the school or therapy programs. Periodic, psychological assessments of cognitive abilities, language skills, motor skills, and other psychiatric symptoms help to monitor a child's progress and guide treatment recommendations, while an extensive neuropsychological assessment, which adds evaluation of attention, learning and memory, and executive functioning, can provide important information for understanding the complex profile of children with autism and guiding educational programming and intervention.

of the child's cognitive, language, motor, and educational skills is strongly recommended throughout the lifespan to evaluate progress, provide updated treatment recommendations, and assist the family in long-term planning and preparation for the transition to adulthood (see Chapter 40).

ASSOCIATED CONDITIONS

Children with ASD often present with a number of comorbid or co-occurring conditions. These comorbid conditions can shape the presentation and functioning of children on the autism spectrum, with specific behavioral phenotypes associated with specific genetic syndromes (Moss & Howlin, 2009). Likewise, the level of adaptive functioning and the number and type of comorbid psychiatric conditions also strongly influence the presentation of ASD in particular individuals (Kraper, Kenworthy, Popal, Martin, & Wallace, 2017). A number of these associated conditions are described below.

Neurodevelopmental Conditions

Neurodevelopmental conditions often co-occur with ASD. The sections that follow discuss the evidence base for the co-occurrence of intellectual disability, attention-deficit/hyperactivity disorder (ADHD), and tic disorder.

Intellectual Disability As noted previously, although older studies found that the majority of individuals with ASD also had an intellectual disability (Yeargin-Allsopp et al., 2003), more recent research suggests that only about 30% of children with ASD have a co-occurring intellectual disability. This decrease in the prevalence of intellectual disability corresponds with the expansion of the autism spectrum to include individuals with higher-functioning forms of autism and relatively intact cognition (CDC, 2016). Conversely, among individuals with intellectual disability, ASD is one of the most commonly co-occurring conditions, with one study finding that approximately one fifth (18%) of children with intellectual disability also had a diagnosis of autism (Tonnsen et al., 2016). In individuals with ASD, a co-occurring intellectual disability is associated with lower adaptive functioning and increased levels of repetitive and self-injurious behaviors (Matson & Shoemaker, 2009).

Attention-Deficit/Hyperactivity Disorder The *DSM-IV-TR* dictated that ADHD could not be diagnosed in a child with ASD. The *DSM-5,* published in 2013, now recognizes the disorders as two distinct, yet frequently co-occurring, conditions. The rate of co-occurrence remains less than clear, with estimates ranging from 16%–50% (Hanson et al., 2013; Rao & Landa, 2014; Sinzig, Walter, & Doepfner, 2009). Children with ASD and co-occurring ADHD present with lower cognitive functioning, more severe social deficits, and lower adaptive functioning than children with ASD alone (Rao & Landa, 2014). They also demonstrate lower performance on measures of verbal working memory and delayed recall (Andersen, Hovik, Skogli, Egeland, & Oie, 2013). Investigators analyzing the often overlapping symptoms of the two disorders have attempted to explain the relationship between the core symptoms of inattention and impulsivity/hyperactivity in ADHD on the one hand and the social deficits and repetitive behaviors in ASD on the other (Sokolova et al., 2017). However, the clinical manifestation of ADHD and ASD as comorbid disorders tends to vary in different children. While some individuals show clear symptoms of inattention and hyperactivity/impulsivity, others show reduced sustained attention that could be attributed either to ADHD or to decreased social awareness or interest.

Tic Disorder Tic disorders, including persistent motor tic disorder, persistent vocal tic disorder, and Tourette disorder, are commonly associated with ADHD, obsessive-compulsive disorder, and disruptive behavior disorder (Scahill, Specht, & Page, 2014). In addition, up to 22% of children with ASD have a co-occurring tic disorder. ASD-associated tic disorders most often occur in children with comorbid intellectual disability, and there is a clear correlation between the level of intellectual disability and the prevalence of tic disorders (Canitano & Vivanti, 2007). It is important, but sometimes difficult, to distinguish between tics due to a tic disorder, compulsive behaviors due to obsessive compulsive disorder, and repetitive and stereotyped behaviors associated with ASD.

Psychiatric Conditions

Additional psychiatric disorders commonly co-occur in children with ASD. Until recently, the rates of co-occurrence were poorly understood due to both the difficulty of diagnosing psychiatric disorders, which may have symptoms that overlap those of ASD, and to the phenomenon of diagnostic overshadowing—the tendency to attribute the symptoms of a comorbid psychiatric condition to the primary developmental disability. Recent research has documented a very high rate of psychiatric comorbidity among children and adolescents with ASD. Studies show that 56%–95% of youth with autism meet criteria for a comorbid psychiatric disorder and the majority meets criteria for more than one psychiatric disorder (Joshi et al., 2010; Salazar et al., 2015; van Steensel, Bogels, & de Bruin, 2013). Although the association between IQ and level of psychiatric comorbidity is unclear, findings of higher rates of psychiatric disorders in youth with ASD who *do not* have intellectual disability (Salazar et al., 2015; Selten, Lundberg, Rai, & Magnusson, 2015) suggests that these individuals may experience higher levels of anxiety or may simply be better able to verbalize their psychiatric symptoms. Although anxiety is the most common psychiatric comorbidity (Salazar et al., 2015), youth with ASD also show high rates of obsessive compulsive disorder (Griffiths, Farrell, Waters, & White, 2017), depression (McPheeters, Davis, Navarre, & Scott, 2011), bipolar disorder, and psychotic disorders (Selten et al., 2015).

Treatment of the comorbid psychiatric conditions in ASD has generally followed from the treatments used in youth without ASD, sometimes with and sometimes without clear evidence of the efficacy of these interventions in the ASD population. For example, CBT has been modified to meet the needs of individuals with ASD with the inclusion of social stories and visual supports as well as the use of well-structured workbooks. This modified approach to CBT has been found to be effective in addressing anxiety and obsessive compulsive disorder (Iniesta-Sepulveda et al., 2017; Ung, Selles, Small, & Storch, 2015). By contrast, medications such as selective serotonin reuptake inhibitors (SSRIs; see Chapter 38), which are widely used in people with ASD for the treatment of anxiety and obsessive-compulsive symptoms, have a less well-established evidence base (Vasa et al., 2016).

Genetic Disorders

ASD occurs with greater frequency in children with known genetic disorders. As discussed previously, approximately 5%–9% of individuals with autism who complete genetic testing (i.e., CMA) have clinically significant findings, with links to known genetic syndromes (Ho et al., 2016; McGrew et al., 2012; Tammimies et al., 2015). Overall, approximately 10% of individuals with autism have an associated genetic condition. Syndrome-associated autism may differ from idiopathic autism (autism due to unknown causes) with regard to physical, behavioral, and developmental characteristics (Moss & Howlin, 2009). In part, this difference may be due to the known correlation between the severity of intellectual disability and autism symptomology (Matson & Shoemaker, 2009; Skuse, 2007); in other words, genetic disorders with an increased risk for intellectual disability also show an increased risk for ASD. However, across groups, the degree of intellectual disability associated with particular genetic disorders does not always account vfor the prevalence of ASD (Richards, Jones, Groves, Moss, & Oliver, 2015). In addition, as genetic testing becomes more sensitive and accessible, the number of known genetic disorders with links to ASD may increase, while the line between syndromic and idiopathic autism becomes less clear.

A recent meta-analysis identified 12 known genetic syndromes with increased prevalence of autism phenomenology, with the highest prevalence of autism phenomenology found in females with Rett syndrome, a genetic disorder previously included under the classification of Pervasive Developmental Disorders in *DSM-IV-TR*. Information on these genetic disorders, their symptomology, and the prevalence of autism phenomenology is provided below. In addition, increased rates of autism have been linked to an ever-growing, though less-studied, list of genetic disorders including 2q37 deletion syndrome, 22q13 deletion syndrome, Duchenne and Becker's muscular dystrophy, hyopmelanosis of Ito syndrome, Joubert syndrome, Klinefelter syndrome, Lujan-Fryns syndrome, phenylketonuria syndrome, Potocki Lupski syndrome, PTEN mutations, Smith-Lemli-Opitz syndrome, Smith-Magenis syndrome, Sotos syndrome, Timothy syndrome, and Turner syndrome (Zafeiriou, Ververi, Dafoulis, Kalyva, & Vargiami, 2013). A number of these disorders are described in Appendix B.

Epilepsy

The co-occurrence of epilepsy in individuals with ASD has been well established (see Chapter 22). However, the rate of co-occurrence remains poorly defined, with higher rates in clinical samples (28%; Valvo et al., 2013) and lower rates in population studies (8.6%; Thomas, Hovinga, Rai, & Lee, 2017). In children with ASD, epilepsy is more common in females and in children with intellectual disability (Thomas et al., 2017) and is associated with increased deficits in social skills, even when compared with other children with autism and similar intellectual functioning (Ho et al., 2016). In addition, individuals with ASD are more likely to have abnormal EEG findings, even in the absence of clinical seizures (Valvo et al., 2013).

Associated Impairments

Children with ASD often have trouble with sleeping, feeding, and toileting. These impairments can cause significant functional limitations and are a source of stress for the child and the family. Management of children with autism should include assessment of these areas of functioning and help with accessing appropriate interventions and supports. In addition to the more formal interventions described below, Autism Speaks (www.autismspeaks.org) provides toolkits to help families and providers apply evidence-based strategies for addressing these difficulties.

Sleep Disorders Children with ASD are nearly twice as likely as typical peers to be diagnosed with a sleep disorder (Elrod & Hood, 2015; see Chapter 28). Overall, children with ASD have shorter than expected overall sleep times and more difficulty falling asleep, with sleep difficulties being more apparent in children with comorbid intellectual disability (Elrod et al., 2016). Disordered sleep is associated with behavioral dysregulation, including aggression, irritability, hyperactivity, and inattention (Mazurek & Sohl, 2016). Evidence supports the use of behavioral approaches, including individual counseling and parent-training programs (Malow et al., 2014). Melatonin, a naturally occurring substance that is sold as a supplement, may also be helpful for those children who do not respond to behavioral supports alone (Wright et al., 2011).

Feeding Disorders Although "picky" eating is quite common among young children, the prevalence of selective eating is much higher in children with ASD (Sharp et al., 2013). Children with autism will often reject foods based on textures, color, smell, brand, packaging, food group, or temperature (Marshall, Hill, Ziviani, & Dodrill, 2014), leading to diets that may be restricted to only one or two preferred foods and that may cause considerable stress for families. Beyond this selectivity, which appears to be associated with the characteristic behavioral/cognitive rigidity and sensory sensitivities of ASD, children with ASD may also struggle with the oral motor skills necessary for feeding (Marshall et al., 2014). Treatment for feeding disorders general falls into one of three categories: behavioral approaches (e.g., approaches using ABA-based techniques to introduce and reward eating new foods); sensory-based approaches (e.g., approaches such as the sequential oral sensory [SOS] approach, which uses systematic desensitization across a hierarchy of textures, within a play-based environment), and cognitive behavioral approaches (e.g., approaches combining exposure therapy with building strategies to cope with anxiety around food). See Chapters 10 and 29 on nutrition and feeding disorders for more information.

Gastrointestinal Symptoms and Toileting Difficulties Gastrointestinal symptoms are often reported in children with ASD, including a higher rate of constipation, diarrhea, and abdominal pain (McElhanon, McCracken, Karpen, & Sharp, 2014). In addition, symptoms are associated with higher levels of social impairment and lower levels of social awareness (Gorrindo et al., 2012), reflecting the need for careful evaluation of children who may not be able to describe pain or discomfort. Associated with these gastrointestinal symptoms, children with ASD generally take longer to toilet train and show higher rates of daytime and nighttime wetting and fecal incontinence (von Gontard, Pirrung, Niemczyk, & Equit, 2015). While it found insufficient evidence for specific treatment guidelines, a current consensus opinion recommended that children with ASD and gastrointestinal symptoms be worked up with the same care as children without ASD, with the additional caveats that these children may present with behavioral changes indicating pain or discomfort and may be best served by treatment incorporating both behavioral and medical care (Buie et al., 2010).

TREATMENT, MANAGEMENT, AND INTERVENTIONS

Early intervention has long been the mantra of ASD treatment. While there are no treatments that can cure autism, early and intensive intervention has been shown to positively impact both core impairments associated with autism and associated behavioral difficulties. Appropriate treatment differs according to a child's presentation and needs and typically changes over the course of development. Comprehensive treatment typically includes direct behavioral therapy and interventions to build communication, social, and adaptive skills and the provision of school-based services, as well as treatment by allied health professionals (e.g., speech-language pathologists) and treatment and monitoring by relevant medical disciplines (e.g., developmental pediatrics, neurology, and psychiatry). It should be noted that treatment of ASD is complicated by core difficulties with generalizing skills across different settings (Plaisted, 2001). For instance, individuals with ASD may demonstrate gains in targeted skills within the context of treatment or while treatment is occurring, but they often struggle to demonstrate skills outside of the immediate treatment context and may also have trouble maintaining these gains over time. Thus, many of the treatments described below as being *efficacious* may be limited in their *effectiveness*. Continual reinforcement of new skills is strongly recommended for individuals with ASD to support the maintenance of treatment gains.

Applied Behavior Analysis

The strongest evidence-based treatment for applied behavior analysis (ABA). ABA combines principles of learning and motivation with an understanding that consequences of behavior (whether positive or negative) reinforce or extinguish subsequent behavior (Granpeesheh & Tarbox, 2009). The behavioral principles of operant learning (see Chapter 34) were initially used in a program for preschool children with autism developed by Dr. Ivar Lovaas (1987). His studies demonstrated that intensive early intervention that specifically teaches the component skills necessary for development was associated with subsequent typical classroom performance in almost half of the 20 children with autism studied (McEachin, Smith, & Lovaas, 1993). This model initially tested a 40-hour-per-week program that was based on individual therapy using discrete trial teaching, prompting, and reinforcement. Later studies reported qualitative improvement even in children who do not have the dramatic response to behavioral treatment as a result of comorbid intellectual disability (Smith, Eikeseth, Klevstran, & Lovaas, 1997). Generalization of skills to the home and classroom are an important component of the treatment plan (Foxx, 2008).

ABA may target a range of areas affected in autism, including communication, play skills, social interactions, activities of daily living (e.g., toileting, brushing teeth), and maladaptive behaviors (e.g., self-injury, aggression). It is specifically designed to be provided in the child's natural setting, which includes their home, school, and community. An ABA program is often highly intensive (e.g., as much as 30 hours per week), and consistency across settings is thought to be critical to the generalization of skills. The program is most often designed by a Board Certified Behavioral Analyst (BCBA; see Box 18.3) and implemented by a team of therapists. School programs may also be built on ABA principles. ABA includes a range of techniques and approaches, which vary in their primary goals and evidence for efficacy (Vismara & Rogers, 2010). There is strong and growing evidence of efficacy for some specific ABA programs for autism, including the Early Start Denver Model (Dawson et al., 2010), Pivotal Response Treatment (Koegel, Koegel, & Brookman, 2003), the Early Social Interaction Project (Wetherby et al., 2014), and the Joint Attention Symbolic Play Engagement and Regulation (JASPER) intervention (Kasari et al., 2006). There is also growing evidence that early intensive behavioral intervention, defined as 20–40 hours weekly of ABA and individualized instruction for children with autism under the age of 4, usually lasting for 2–3 years, may result in large developmental gains and a reduced need for long-term services (Odom et al., 2010; Reichow, Barton, Boyd, & Hume, 2014).

Speech-Language Therapy

Speech-language therapy is one of the most widely used treatments for autism. Speech therapy may target core language skills, such as following multi-step directions or speaking in grammatically correct sentences.

BOX 18.3 INTERDISCIPLINARY CARE

The Role of the BCBA

Board Certified Behavioral Analysts (BCBAs) are individuals with extensive training and experience in applied behavioral analysis (ABA). For children with autism who receive ABA, BCBAs often take a leading role in designing and implementing the therapeutic program. Typically, a BCBA's work will begin with assessment of the child and their needs. This assessment can range from informal observation and discussion with the family about their concerns or goals to formal assessment, such as the Verbal Behavior Milestones Assessment and Placement Program. Once a BCBA has a solid understanding of a child's current level of functioning and behavioral needs, they will create a therapeutic program designed to build target skills and reduce problematic behaviors. The ABA program will include clear behavioral goals as well as a plan for charting behavior and assessing progress. Although some BCBAs provide direct therapy, many supervise behavior therapists who provide the direct therapy or train parents and teachers. Regardless of the model, the BCBA is continuously involved in assessing the child's progress and modifying the therapeutic program appropriately. In addition, for children with complex therapeutic needs, the BCBA may work as part of an interdisciplinary team, coordinating with occupational therapists, speech therapists, teachers, and special educators.

For young children with language delays or those who are minimally verbal, speech therapists may introduce AAC supports. AAC can be relatively "low-tech," such as the use of the Picture Exchange Communication System (PECS; Bondy & Frost, 2001; Charlop-Christy, Carpente, Le, LeBlanc, & Kellet, 2002), in which children are taught to give pictures of desired items to others to communicate and to gradually sequence pictures into phrases or sentences. Spoken language is always paired with the PECS symbols, and children who use these approaches have been found to make greater gains in spoken language than those who do not. AAC can also be more "high-tech" for children who have long-term difficulties with spoken language, such as through the use of a voice-output device (VOD), in which the child touches a symbol or types words into a tablet or similar device that then "speaks" aloud for the child. Speech therapists are also well equipped to target pragmatic language and social difficulties, such as skills for greeting, conversations, and understanding and using nonverbal communication.

Social Skills Training

Social skills programs, particularly in group formats, are commonly offered for children and adolescents with autism, although research has not consistently supported the efficacy of all of these interventions (Reichow, Steiner, & Volkmar, 2012; White, Koenig, & Scahill, 2007). Peer-mediated approaches, particularly for young children, are among those with the best evidence of efficacy (Watkins et al., 2015; Wong et al., 2015). In these programs, typically developing children are taught to model appropriate behaviors and support children with autism in playing with their peers. Social skills groups are popular and generally try to improve social skills by providing children and adolescents with direct instruction in interpreting and accurately responding to social cues, along with opportunities for practice with direct feedback on their performance. Among these, one of the best established is the Program for the Education and Enrichment of Relational Skills (Laugeson, Frankel, Gantman, Dillon, & Mogil, 2012), which teaches real-world social behaviors and utilizes instruction and feedback from both peers and adults. Social Stories (Gray, 2000) are also widely used by families, teachers, and professionals. These are simple stories with visual supports, adapted to a child's individual needs, that break down social situations for children to help them understand how they are expected to behave.

Occupational Therapy

At its core, the goal of occupational therapy is to help individuals to develop independence with everyday activities. This often includes a strong focus on addressing fine motor deficits that may interfere with daily functioning, such as difficulties fastening buttons or writing with a pencil. Fine motor skills are the area most commonly targeted by school-based occupational therapists. Increasingly, occupational therapists have begun to offer additional interventions to children with autism to address their other needs. Sensory integration therapy and related techniques used to address the sensory processing problems in autism are common; however, it is important to note that there has been minimal research on these approaches and the research that has been conducted has been of poor quality; thus, sensory integration is not considered an evidence-based practice at this time (Lang et al., 2012). Some occupational therapists may also target social skills or executive functioning abilities, although these interventions are more often offered by other professionals (e.g., psychologists, speech-language pathologists, BCBAs, educators) who generally have more focused training and experience in the design and implementation of these interventions.

Medications

There are no medications that have been shown to treat the core impairments associated with autism (i.e., social communication deficits, rigid thinking, and repetitive behaviors). Medications can, however, play a role in addressing behavioral difficulties associated with autism and can help with comorbid conditions such as ADHD, anxiety, and depression (see Chapter 38). Risperidone (brand name: Risperdal) and aripiprazole (brand name: Abilify) are the only FDA-approved medications for treating the irritability commonly associated with autism, and both have a well-established evidence basis for this use (Hirsch & Pringsheim, 2016; Siegel & Beaulieu, 2012). Likewise, methylphenidate (common brand name: Ritalin) has been shown to be efficacious in addressing ADHD symptoms in children with autism, with emerging evidence as to the efficacy of nonstimulant medications, including the class of alpha-2 agonists (generic names: clonidine and guanfacine) and atomoxetine (brand name: Strattera), although with lower effect sizes than seen in studies of children with uncomplicated ADHD (Reichow, Volkmar, & Bloch, 2013). Evidence is less clear on the efficacy of SSRIs in treating repetitive behaviors or anxiety associated with autism (Carrasco, Volkmar, & Bloch, 2012; Vasa et al., 2016). In considering medication, it is important to understand that, relative to their neurotypical peers, children with autism have elevated rates of adverse effects and can experience adverse effects that are different than those seen in children without autism, including increased social withdrawal (Reichow et al., 2013).

School-Based Services

An appropriate educational program is an important aspect of treatment for children with autism. Many children with autism, particularly if they present with early language delays, will begin receiving educational and therapeutic services through an individualized family service plan (see Chapter 31). These services are provided for children from 0–3 years under the Individuals with Disabilities Education Improvement Act of 2004 (IDEA; PL 108-446) and are geared toward providing early intervention services and parent training within the context of the home environment, often before any formal diagnosis.

From the ages of 3 to 21, most children with autism receive special education services through an individualized education program (IEP), which lays out specific goals for each child, as well as the services that will be provided to help them reach those goals (see Chapter 33). Eligibility for special education is determined not only by the presence of a disability, but also by the educational impact of that disability and the need for special education services. Thus, while many children with autism will qualify under the classification of Autism, others may qualify for additional classifications of Specific Learning Disability or Other Health Impairment for attention difficulties. In addition, for children with strong core cognitive and academic skills, the educational impact of their autism may not be apparent in their academic work, yet they will require special education instruction in social and communication skills to allow them to participate and learn within the social and verbal environment of the classroom. Regardless of the eligibility classification, it is important that the IEP for a child with autism go beyond academic difficulties to address broader difficulties with organization, social skills, communication, behavioral regulation, and adaptive skills.

The IDEA Act provides for a free appropriate public education that allows the child to make adequate yearly progress within the least-restrictive environment. Children with autism may be served in a variety of educational settings from mainstream classrooms to inclusion classrooms, self-contained classrooms or programs, and placement in nonpublic schools dedicated to serving children with autism. In deciding on an appropriate placement for a child with autism, there is often an attempt to balance the intensity of intervention needs against the benefits of integration with typical peers. Although the benefit of placement in the least-restrictive environment is an underlying principle of IDEA and of the special education field more broadly, the benefit of inclusive placement has not been fully studied for children with autism, with some studies showing gains in adaptive and cognitive functioning and others showing slower than expected progress (Ferraioli & Harris, 2011).

Although the inclusive environment may allow children with autism to learn how to participate in the community and to have models of appropriate behavior, children with more intense social-communication deficits and highly self-directed attention may not benefit from this environment. These children may need the more highly structured environment provided by a self-contained placement, which can allow for instruction using highly specialized techniques (e.g., visually based learning, ABA-based teaching strategies) and can accommodate needs for low sensory and social stimulation in order to reduce stress.

In addition to outlining the primary placement, the IEP can also specify appropriate related services, which are necessary to allow children to gain the skills needed to benefit from classroom instruction. As with interventions outside of school, schools may offer a wide range of related services, including speech therapy, occupational therapy, physical therapy, behavior support services, social skills training, and counseling.

As a student nears graduation, his or her IEP must also include a transition plan, which lays out postgraduation goals for living, education, and employment and the steps needed to accomplish those goals, from participating in vocational classes to meeting with social service agencies and taking advanced classes (Chapter 33). Given the low rates of full employment among individuals with ASD, this transition plan is an essential part of school programming for young adults with autism. In the years leading up to graduation, the school programming should have a joint focus on academic skills and on the functional and vocational skills that will help the student maximize his/her independence as an adult. Even for the student with strong cognitive and academic skills, transition planning is necessary to ensure that the individual has the organizational and social skills needed in college and career settings.

Decisions about a child's special education program are made by the IEP team, of which the parents are an essential part. Therefore, it is important that parents understand the special education process and are able to bring their understanding of and priorities for their child to the educational team.

Complementary Health Approaches

Complementary health approaches (CHA) form a group of practices and products generally thought to be outside of conventional medical approaches, although often used in conjunction with more traditional treatments (Chapter 39). These practices are widely used in autism, with approximately one fourth of families reporting that they used at least one alternative treatment (Perrin et al., 2012). Many of these treatments have a basis in anecdotal evidence or in studies without a clear control group or without clearly controlled, randomized trials. Reviews of the use of CHA in autism have largely noted limited findings and the need for more systematic research. Given the lack of a "cure" for ASD, families of these children may be particularly susceptible to these practices. The Association for Science in Autism Treatment (www.asatonline.org) and the National Standards Project (www.nationalautismcenter.org/national-standards-project/) provide up-to-date information about the evidence base for popular autism treatments. Providers are often most effective when they speak to families supportively and provide information about risks and benefits of various treatments. Families should be educated about and strongly advised against the use of CHA treatments known to be dangerous to children.

Dietary treatments are one of the most commonly used CHA treatments, most notably the gluten-free, casein-free (GFCF) diet, although concerns have been raised about the nutritional effects of these restricted diets. A recent, small double-blind study of the GFCF diet found no evidence of its effectiveness in addressing core symptoms of autism or behavior problems (Hyman et al., 2016). Similarly, reviews on the use of high levels of supplements, including B6 and omega-3 fatty acids, have noted limited research studies with inconclusive findings (James, Montgomery, & Williams, 2011; Nye & Brice, 2005). A newer approach, which involves the use of cord blood to treat autism symptoms, also has little research basis, although a recent study found that the treatment was well tolerated, paving the path for more robust clinical trials (Dawson et al., 2017). Likewise, although small in scale, trials with intranasal oxytocin show some promising, but inconsistent, results in addressing the core social deficits associated with autism (Anagnostou et al., 2012; Guastella et al., 2015).

In addition to these generally safe, alternative treatments, two widely used treatments have been found to be both lacking in evidence of effectiveness and potentially harmful: 1) chelation therapy, which aims to remove heavy metals from the blood, but can lead to serious kidney damage (James, Stevenson, Silove, & Williams, 2015), and 2) hyperbaric oxygen therapy, which can lead to damage to the ear (Xiong, Chen, Luo, & Mu, 2016).

OUTCOMES

The heterogeneity among individuals with ASD ensures that outcomes likewise vary significantly. The sections that follow briefly trace the variability of outcomes from identification to adulthood.

Developmental Trajectories Children with autism show a great deal of variability in their developmental trajectories, although much of that variability appears to be set fairly early in development. With regard to the initial presentation of autism, children generally fall into one of two groups: those with early onset of symptoms, exhibiting early and widespread developmental disruption, and those with later onset of symptoms, who have a period of apparent typical development followed by slower development or regression. However, regardless of the age of onset, symptoms and presentations are often similar by 2 years of age (Landa, Gross, Stuart, & Faherty, 2013). Once diagnosed, for many children, their trajectories are consistent with their initial presentation (Lord, Bishop, & Anderson, 2015). While children who present with lower nonverbal skills and more severe autistic symptoms show slower development of core language, intellectual, and social skills, children who initially present with higher nonverbal skills show strong progress, with clear improvement in language and intellectual skills, sometimes to the point of "catching up" with their typically developing peers (Fountain, Winter, & Bearman, 2012; Pickles, Anderson, & Lord, 2014). Although a small group of "late bloomers" show rapid rates of developmental progress between the ages of 3 and 5, much of the difference between trajectories is evident between the ages of 2 and 3. Likewise, although language continues to develop, there is little change in language trajectory after the age of 6. In terms of long-term trajectories, the majority of individuals with autism continue to show a decline in symptom severity as they progress through childhood and adolescence (Howlin & Magiati, 2017), and approximately 70% achieve functional language on at least a 5-year-old level (Pickles et al., 2014).

Optimal Outcomes Although autism is generally considered a lifelong disability, approximately 10% of individuals who initially and accurately were diagnosed with autism at a young age will lose their autism diagnosis later in life (Anderson, Liang, & Lord, 2014). In early development these children are more likely to have received treatment at a young age and are characterized by higher verbal IQ, lessening of repetitive behaviors between the ages of 2 and 3, and a trend toward improved social skills during that same period (Anderson et al., 2014). For these individuals, social and communication skills continue to improve through childhood and early adolescence. As adults, these individuals, previously diagnosed with autism, appear to have social, communication, and language skills comparable to typically developing peers (Fein et al., 2013), although they do have higher rates of ADHD and anxiety (Orinstein et al., 2015).

Adults with Autism Outcomes among adults with autism are quite variable. While some individuals are able to live fully independent lives with a long-term partner or spouse, many adults with autism continue to need assistance in many domains. Intellectual functioning and language skills are the strongest predictors of outcomes for adults with autism. Few individuals with intellectual disability, or who lack functional language, are able to live on their own or achieve independent employment. However, even individuals with average or above-average intellectual functioning show low rates of employment, low levels of independent living, and few social contacts, although studies show variability in the prevalence of these difficulties (Farley et al., 2009; Howlin & Magiati, 2017).

Unfortunately, these outcome measures for individuals with autism but without intellectual disability do not appear to have shown significant improvement over the past decade despite the increase in available services for young children with autism and higher rates of individuals achieving advanced, post–high school education (Howlin & Magiati, 2017). In addition, as a whole, individuals with autism show high rates of psychiatric comorbidity (Gadke, McKinney, & Oliveros, 2016) and higher levels of mortality, with a lower age of death and a death rate that is nearly double that of the typically developing population (Howlin & Magiati, 2017). These mortality statistics reflect both the comorbidities associated with autism and the difficulties that individuals with autism may have in accessing medical care. In many ways, the outcomes of adults with autism reflect the essential gap between intellectual functioning and adaptive skills, with even individuals with average to above-average IQ showing global adaptive deficits (Kenworthy, Case, Harms, Martin, & Wallace, 2010). However, these outcomes also highlight the dearth of services or interventions geared toward adults with autism and toward improving everyday functioning in this population.

SUMMARY

- ASD is a neurodevelopmental disorder characterized by impairment in core social-communication abilities, along with the presence of restricted, repetitive patterns of behavior, interest, and activity.
- Although ASD is present from birth, first concerns are typically not apparent until between the ages of 1 and 2. For children with stronger language and core cognitive skills, concerns may not become apparent until much later, when social demands outpace their abilities.

- The majority of children with ASD have comorbid neurodevelopmental or psychiatric conditions that impact their functioning. Intellectual disability and ADHD are two of the most common, co-occurring conditions.
- Early diagnosis and treatment of ASD have been shown to improve many areas of functioning and to decrease the need for later services. Comprehensive treatment often includes intensive behavioral intervention as well as treatments to build social and communication skills.

ADDITIONAL RESOURCES

Autism Society of America: http://www.autism-society.org

Autism Speaks: http://www.autismspeaks.org

National Center on Birth Defects and Developmental Disabilities (NCBDDD): Autism Information Center: http://www.cdc.gov/ncbddd/autism/index.htm

Autistic Self-Advocacy Network: www.autisticadvocacy.org

Additional resources can be found online in Appendix D: Childhood Disabilities Resources, Services, and Organizations (see About the Online Companion Materials).

REFERENCES

American Academy of Pediatrics. (2010). Clinical genetic testing for patients with autism spectrum disorders. *Pediatrics, 125,* e727–2735. doi:10.1542/peds.2009-1684

American Psychiatric Association. (2000). *Diagnostic and statistical manual of mental disorders* (4th ed., text rev.). Washington, DC: Author.

American Psychiatric Association. (2013). *Diagnostic and statistical manual of mental disorders* (5th ed.). Washington, DC: Author.

Anagnostou, E., Soorya, L., Bartz, J., Halpern, D., Wasserman, S., Wang, A. T., . . . Hollander, E. (2012). Intranasal oxytocin versus placebo in the treatment of adults with autism spectrum disorders: A randomized controlled trial. *Molecular Autism, 3*(1), 16. doi:10.1186/2040-2392-16

Andersen, P. N., Hovik, K. T., Skogli, E. W., Egeland, J., & Oie, M. (2013). Symptoms of ADHD in children with high-functioning autism are related to impaired verbal working memory and verbal delayed recall. *PLoS ONE, 8,* e64842. doi:10.1371/journal.pone.0064842

Anderson, D. K., Liang, J. W., & Lord, C. (2014). Predicting young adult outcome among more and less cognitively able individuals with autism spectrum disorders. *Journal of Child Psychology and Psychiatry, 55*(5), 485–494.

Baranek, G. T. (1999). Autism during infancy: A retrospective video analysis of sensory-motor and social behaviors at 9-12 months of age. *Journal of Autism and Developmental Disorders, 29*(3), 213–224. Retrieved from http://www.ncbi.nlm.nih.gov/pubmed/10425584

Baron-Cohen, S., Scott, F. J., Allison, C., Williams, J., Bolton, P., Matthews, F. E., & Brayne, C. (2009). Prevalence of autism-spectrum conditions: UK school-based population study. *The British Journal of Psychiatry, 194,* 500–509. doi:10.1192/bjp.bp.108.059345

Baron-Cohen, S., Wheelwright, S., Skinner, R., Martin, J., & Clubley, E. (2001). The autism-spectrum quotient (AQ): Evidence from Asperger syndrome/high-functioning autism, males and females, scientists and mathematicians. *Journal of Autism and Developmental Disorders, 31,* 5–17. doi:10.1023/A:1005653411471

Bauminger, N., & Kasari, C. (2000). Loneliness and friendship in high-functioning children with autism. *Child Development, 71,* 447–456. doi:10.1111/1467-8624.00156

Begeer, S., Mandell, D., Wijnker-Holmes, B., Venderbosch, S., Rem, D., Stekelenburg, F., & Koot, H. M. (2013). Sex differences in the timing of identification among children and adults with autism spectrum disorders. *Journal of Autism and Developmental Disorders, 43*(5), 1151–1156. doi:10.1007/s10803-012-1656-z

Bernard, S. A., Enayati, A., Redwood, L., Roger, H., & Binstock, T. (2001). Autism: A novel form of mercury poisoning. *Medical Hypotheses, 56*(4), 462–471. doi:10.1054/mehy.2000.1281

Bettelheim, B. (1967). *The empty fortress: Infantile autism and the birth of self.* New York, NY: Free Press.

Bhat, A., Galloway, J., & Landa, R. J. (2012). Relationship between early motor delay and later communication delay in infants at risk for autism. *Infant Behavior and Development, 35(4),* 838–846.

Bishop, D. V., & Norbury, C. F. (2002). Exploring the borderlands of autistic disorder and specific language impairment: a study using standardised diagnostic instruments. *Journal of Child Psychology and Psychiatry, 43*(7), 917–929.

Bondy, A. S., & Frost, L. A. (2001). The Picture Exchange Communication System. *Behavior Modification, 25*(5), 725–744. doi:10.1177/0145445501255004

Boucher, J. (2012). Research review: Structural language in autistic spectrum disorder—characteristic and causes. *Journal of Child Psychology and Psychiatry, 53,* 219–233. doi:10.1111/j.1469-7610.2011.02508.x

Brown, H. K., Ray, J. G., Wilton, A. S., Lunsky, Y., Gomes, T., & Vigod, S. N. (2017). Association between serotonergic antidepressant use during pregnancy and autism spectrum disorder in children. *JAMA, 317*(15), 1544–1552. doi:10.1001/jama.2017.3415

Buie, T., Campbell, D. B., Fuchs, III, G. J., Furuta, G. T., Levy, J., VandeWater, J., . . . Winter, H. (2010). Evaluation, diagnosis, and treatment of gastrointestinal disorders in individuals with ASDs: A consensus report. *Pediatrics, 125*(Supplement 1), S1–S18. doi:10.1542/peds.2009-1878C

Byers, E. S., Nichols, S., & Voyer, S. D. (2013). Challenging stereotypes: Sexual functioning of single adults with high functioning autism spectrum disorder. *Journal of Autism and Developmental Disorders, 43,* 2617–2627. doi:10.1007/s10803-013-1813-z

Canitano, R., & Vivanti, G. (2007). Tics and Tourette syndrome in autism spectrum disorders. *Autism: The International Journal of Research & Practice, 11*(1), 19–28.

Carrasco, M., Volkmar, F. R., & Bloch, M. H. (2012). Pharmacologic treatment of repetitive behaviors in autism spectrum disorders: Evidence of publication bias. *Pediatrics, 129*(5), E1301–E1310.

Cassidy, A. R., Ilardi, D., Bowen, S. R., Hampton, L. E., Heinrich, K. P., Loman, M. M., . . . Wolfe, K. R. (2017): Congenital heart disease: A primer for the pediatric neuropsychologist, *Child Neuropsychology, 24*(7), 859–902. doi:10.1080/09297049.2017.1373758

Centers for Disease Control and Prevention. (2007). Prevalence of autism spectrum disorders—Autism and Developmental Disabilities Monitoring Network, United States, 2006. *Morbidity and Mortality Weekly Report, 58,* 1–20.

Centers for Disease Control and Prevention. (2012). Prevalence of autism spectrum disorders: Autism and Developmental Disabilities Monitoring Network, 14 Sites, United States, 2008. *Morbidity and Mortality Weekly Report. Surveillance Summaries, 61*(3), 1–19.

Centers for Disease Control and Prevention. (2016). Prevalence and characteristics of autism spectrum disorder among children aged 8 years—Autism and Developmental Disabilities Monitoring Network, 11 sites, United States, 2012. *Morbidity and Mortality Weekly Report Surveillance Summaries, 65*(3), 1–23. doi:10.15585/mmwr.ss6503a1

Centers for Disease Control and Prevention. (2018). Prevalence of autism spectrum disorder among children aged 8 years—Autism and Developmental Disabilities Monitoring Network, 11 sites, United States, 2014. *Morbidity and Mortality Weekly Report Surveillance Summaries, 67*(6), 1–23. doi:10.15585/mmwr.ss6706a1.

Charlop-Christy, M. H., Carpenter, M., Le, L., LeBlanc, L. A., & Kellet, K. (2002). Using the Picture Exchange Communication System (PECS) with children with autism: Assessment of PECS acquisition, speech, social-communicative behavior, and problem behavior. *Journal of Applied Behavior Analysis, 35*(3), 213–231. doi:10.1901/jaba.2002.35-213

Chawarska, K., Macari, S., & Shic, F. (2012). Context modulates attention to social scenes in toddlers with autism. *Journal of Child Psychology and Psychiatry, 53,* 903–913. doi:10.1111/j.1469-7610.2012.02538.x

Chawarska, K., Paul, R., Klin, A., Hannigen, S., Dichtel, L., & Volkmar, F. (2007). Parental recognition of developmental problems in toddlers with autism spectrum disorders. *Journal of Autism and Developmental Disorders, 37(1),* 62–72. doi:10.1007/s10803-006-0330-8

Chess, S. (1971). Autism in children with congenital rubella. *Journal of Autism and Child Schizophrenia, 1*(1), 33–47.

Christensen, J., Grønborg, T. K., Sørensen, M. J., Schendel, D., Parner, E. T., Pedersen, L. H., & Vestergaard, M. (2013). Prenatal valproate exposure and risk of autism spectrum disorders and childhood autism. *JAMA, 309*(16), 1696–1703. doi:10.1001/jama.2013.2270

Clarke, D. F., Roberts, W., Daraksan, M., Dupuis, A., McCabe, J., Wood, H., . . . Weiss, S. K. (2005). The prevalence of autistic spectrum disorder in children surveyed in a tertiary care epilepsy clinic. *Epilepsia, 46,* 1970–1977. doi:10.1111/j.1528-1167.2005.00343.x

Clifford, S., Dissanayake, C., Bui, Q. M., Huggins, R., Taylor, A. K., & Loesch, D. Z. (2007). Autism spectrum phenotype in males and females with fragile X full mutation and premutation. *Journal of Autism and Developmental Disorders, 37*(4), 738–747. doi:10.1007/s10803-006-0205-z

Constantino, J. N., & Gruber, C. (2012). *The Social Responsiveness Scale Manual, Second Edition (SRS-2).* Los Angeles, CA: Western Psychological Services.

Coo, H., Oulette-Kuntz, H., Lloyd, J. E. V., Kasmara, L., Holden, J. J. A., & Lewis, M. E. S. (2008). Trends in autism prevalence: Diagnostic substitution revisited. *Journal of Autism and Developmental Disorders, 38,* 1036–1046. doi:10.1007/s10803-007-0478-x

Dawson, G., Rogers, S., Munson, J., Smith, M., Winter, J., Greenson, J., . . . Varley, J. (2010). Randomized, controlled trial of an intervention for toddlers with autism: The Early Start Denver model. *Pediatrics, 125*(1), e17–e23. doi:10.1542/peds.2009-0958

Dawson, G., Sun, J. M., Davlantis, K. S., Murias, M., Franz, L., Troy, J., . . . Kurtzberg, J. (2017). Autologous cord blood infusions are safe and feasible in young children with autism spectrum disorder: Results of a single-center Phase I open-label trial. *Stem Cells Translational Medicine, 6*(5), 1332–1339. doi:10.1002/sctm.16-0474

Dawson, G., Webb, S. J., & McPartland, J. (2005). Understanding the nature of face processing impairment in autism: Insights from behavioral and electrophysiological studies. *Developmental Neuropsychology, 27*(3), 403–424. doi:10.1207/s15326942dn2703_6de

De Martino, B., Harrison, N. A., Knafo, S., Bird, G., & Dolan, R. J. (2008). Explaining enhanced logical consistency during decision making in autism. *Journal of Neuroscience, 28,* 10746–10750. doi:10.1523/JNEUROSCI.2895-08.2008

de Vries, A. L. C., Noens, I. L. J., Cohen-Kettenis, P. T., van Berckelaer-Onnes, I. A., & Doreleijers, T. A. (2010). Autism spectrum disorders in gender dysphoric children and adolescents. *Journal of Autism and Developmental Disorders, 40,* 930–936. doi:10.1007/s10803-010-0935-9

Demicheli, V., Jefferson, T., Rivetti, A., & Price, D. (2005). Vaccines for measles, mumps and rubella in children. *Cochrane Database of Systematic Reviews, 19*(4), CD004407. doi:10.1002/14651858.CD004407.pub2

DeStefano, F., Price, C. S., & Weintraub, E. S. (2013). Increasing exposure to antibody-stimulating proteins and polysaccharides in vaccines is not associated with risk of autism. *Journal of Pediatrics, 163*(2), 561–567. doi:10.1016/j.jpeds.2013.02.001

Dewinter, J., De Graaf, H., & Begeer, S. (2017). Sexual orientation, gender identity, and romantic relationships in adolescents and adults with autism spectrum disorder. *Journal of Autism and Developmental Disorders, 47,* 2927–2934. doi:10.1007/s10803-017-3199-9

Dinstein, I., Haar, S., Atsmon, S., & Schtaerman, H. (2017). No evidence of early head circumference enlargements in children later diagnosed with autism in Israel. *Molecular Autism, 8,* 1–9. doi:10.1186/s13229-017-0129-9

Dodds, L., Fell, D., Shea, S., Armson, B., Allen, A., & Bryson, S. (2011). The role of prenatal, obstetric and neonatal factors in the development of autism. *Journal of Autism and Developmental Disorders, 41*(7), 891–902. doi:10.1007/s10803-010-1114-8

Duerden, E. G., Mak-Fan, K. M., Taylor, M. J., & Roberts, S. W. (2012). Regional differences in grey and white matter in children and adolescents with autism spectrum disorders: An activation likelihood estimate (ALE) meta-analysis. *Autism Research, 5,* 49–66.

Durkin, M. S., Maenner, M. J., Meaney, F. J., Levy, S. E., DiGiuseppi, C., Nicholas, J. S., . . . Schieve, L. A. (2010). Socioeconomic inequality in the prevalence of autism spectrum disorder: Evidence from a U.S. cross-sectional study. *PLoS One, 5*(7), e11551. doi:10.1371/journal.pone.0011551

Ecker, C. (2017). The neuroanatomy of autism spectrum disorder: An overview of structural neuroimaging findings and their translatability to the clinical setting. *Autism, 21(1),* 18–28. doi:10.1177/1362361315627136

The Editors of The Lancet. (2010). Retraction—Ileal-lymphoid-nodular hyperplasia, non-specific colitis, and pervasive developmental disorder in children. *The Lancet, 375*(9713), 445–445. doi:10.1016/S0140-6736(10)60175-4

Edwards-Leeper, L., & Spack, N. (2012). Psychological evaluation and medical treatment of transgender youth in an interdisciplinary "Gender Management Service" (GeMS) in a major pediatric center. *Journal of Homosexuality, 59*, 321–336. doi:10.1080/00918369.2012.653302

Elder, L. M., Dawson, G., Toth, K., Fein, D., & Munson, J. (2008). Head circumference as an early predictor of autism symptoms in younger siblings of children with autism spectrum disorder. *Journal of Autism and Developmental Disorders, 38*(6), 1104–1111. doi:10.1007/s10803-007-0495-9

Elrod, M. G., & Hood, B. S. (2015). Sleep differences among children with autism spectrum disorders and typically developing peers: A meta-analysis. *Journal of Developmental and Behavioral Pediatrics, 36*(3), 166–177. doi:10.1097/DBP.0000000000000140

Elrod, M. G., Nylund, C. M., Susi, A. L., Gorman, G. H., Hisle-Gorman, E., Rogers, D. J., & Erdie-Lalena, C. (2016). Prevalence of diagnosed sleep disorders and related diagnostic and surgical procedures in children with autism spectrum disorders. *Journal of Developmental and Behavioral Pediatrics, 37*(5), 377–384. doi:10.1097/DBP.0000000000000248

Elsabbagh, M., Divan, G., Kohn, Y. -J., Kim, Y. S., Kauchali, S., Marcín, C., . . . Fombonne, E. (2012). Global prevalence of autism and other pervasive developmental disorders. *Autism Research, 5*, 160–179. doi:10.1002/aur.239

Farley, M. A., McMahon, W. M., Fombonne, E., Jenson, W. R., Miller, J., Gardner, M., . . . Coon, H. (2009). Twenty-year outcome for individuals with autism and average or near average cognitive abilities. *Autism Research, 2*(2), 109–118. doi:10.1002/aur.69

Fein, D., Barton, M., Eigsti, I., Kelley, E., Naigles, L., Schultz, R. T., . . . Tyson, K. (2013). Optimal outcome in individuals with a history of autism. *Journal of Child Psychology and Psychiatry, 54*(2), 195–205.

Ferraioli, S. J., & Harris, S. L. (2011). Effective educational inclusion of students on the autism spectrum. *Journal of Contemporary Psychotherapy, 41*(1), 19–28. doi:10.1007/s10879-010-9156-y

Fombonne, E. (2003). Epidemiological surveys of autism and other pervasive developmental disorders: An update. *Journal of Autism and Developmental Disorders, 33*(4), 365–382.

Fombonne, E. (2009). Epidemiology of pervasive developmental disorders. *Pediatric Research, 65*, 591–598. doi:10.1203/PDR.0b013e31819e7203

Fountain, C., Winter, A. S., & Bearman, P. S. (2012). Six developmental trajectories characterize children with autism. *Pediatrics, 129*(5), e1112–e1120. doi:10.1542/peds.2011-1601

Foxx, R. M. (2008). Applied behavior analysis treatment of autism: The state of the art. *Child and Adolescent Psychiatric Clinics of North America, 17*(4), 821–834. doi:10.1016/j.chc.2008.06.007

Frazier, T. W., Thompson, L., Youngstrom, E. A., Law, P., Hardan, A. Y., Eng, C., & Morris, N. (2014). A twin study of heritable and shared environmental contributions to autism. *Journal of Autism and Developmental Disorders, 44*(8), 2013–2025. doi:10.1007/s10803-014-2081-2

Gadke, D. L., McKinney, C., & Oliveros, A. (2016). Autism spectrum disorder symptoms and comorbidity in emerging adults. *Child Psychiatry and Human Development, 47*(2), 194–201. doi:10.1007/s10578-015-0556-9

Gardener, H., Spiegelman, D., & Buka, S. L. (2009). Prenatal risk factors for autism: Comprehensive meta-analysis. *The British Journal of Psychiatry, 195*(1), 7–14. doi:10.1192/bjp.bp.108.051672

Gardener, H., Spiegelman, D., & Buka, S. L. (2011). Perinatal and neonatal risk factors for autism: A comprehensive meta-analysis. *Pediatrics, 128*(2), 344–355. doi:10.1542/peds.2010-1036

Gentile, S. (2010). Neurodevelopmental effects of prenatal exposure to psychotropic medications. *Depression and Anxiety, 27*, 675–686.

Gilman, S. R., Iossifov, I., Levy, D., Ronemus, M., Wigler, M., & Vitkup, D. (2011). Rare de novo variants associated with autism implicate a large functional network of genes involved in formation and function of synapses. *Neuron, 70*(5), 898–907. doi:10.1016/j.neuron.2011.05.021

Glickman, G., Harrison, E., & Dobkins, K. (2017). Vaccinations rates among younger siblings of children with autism. *New England Journal of Medicine, 377*, 1099-1101. doi:10.1056/NEJMc1708223

Gorrindo, P., Williams, K. C., Lee, E. B., Walker, L. S., McGrew, S. G., & Levitt, P. (2012). Gastrointestinal dysfunction in autism: Parental report, clinical evaluation, and associated factors. *Autism Research, 5*(2), 101–108. doi:10.1002/aur.237

Granpeesheh, D., & Tarbox, J. (2009). Applied behavior analytic interventions for children with autism: A description and review of treatment research. *Annals of Clinical Psychiatry, 21*(3), 162–173.

Gray, C. (2000). *The new Social Story book*. Arlington, TX: Future Horizons.

Griffiths, D. L., Farrell, L. J., Waters, A. M., & White, S. W. (2017). Clinical correlates of obsessive compulsive disorder and comorbid autism spectrum disorder in youth. *Journal of Obsessive-Compulsive and Related Disorders, 14*, 90–98. doi:10.1016/j.jocrd.2017.06.006

Guastella, A. J., Gray, K. M., Rinehart, N. J., Alvares, G. A., Tonge, B. J., Hickie, I. B., . . . Einfeld, S. L. (2015). The effects of a course of intranasal oxytocin on social behaviors in youth diagnosed with autism spectrum disorders: A randomized controlled trial. *Journal of Child Psychology and Psychiatry, 56*(4), 444–452. doi:10.1111/jcpp.12305

Halladay, A. K., Bishop, S., Constantino, J. N., Daniels, A. M., Koenig, K., Palmer, K., . . . Szatmari, P. (2015). Sex and gender differences in autism spectrum disorder: summarizing evidence gaps and identifying emerging areas of priority. *Molecular Autism, 6*(36). doi:10.1186/s13229-015-0019-y

Hallmayer, J., Cleveland, S., Torres, A., Phillips, J., Cohen, B., Torigoe, T., . . . Risch, N. (2011). Genetic heritability and shared environmental factors among twin pairs with autism. *Archives of General Psychiatry, 68*(11), 1095–1102. doi:10.1001/archgenpsychiatry.2011.76

Hampton, L. H., & Kaiser, A. P. (2016). Intervention effects on spoken-language outcomes for children with autism: A systematic review and meta-analysis. *Journal of Intellectual Disability Research, 60*(5), 444-463.

Hanson, E., Cerban, B., Slater, C., Caccamo, L., Bacic, J., & Chan, E. (2013). Brief report: Prevalence of attention deficit/hyperactivity disorder among individuals with an autism spectrum disorder. *Journal of Autism and Developmental Disorders, 43*(6), 1459–1464.

Happé, F., & Frith, U. (2006). The weak coherence account: Detail-focused cognitive style in autism spectrum disorders. *Journal of Autism and Developmental Disorders, 36*, 5–25. doi:10.1007/s10803-005-0039-0

Hazlett, H. C., Gu, H., Munsell, B. C., Kim, S. H., Styner, M., Wolff, J. J., . . . Piven, J. (2017). Early brain development in infants at high risk for autism spectrum disorder. *Nature, 542*(7641), 348.

Hertz-Picciotto, I., & Delwiche, L. (2009). The rise in autism and the role in age at diagnosis. *Epidemiology, 20,* 84-90. doi:10.1097%2FEDE.0b013e3181902d15

Hiller, R. M., Young, R. L., & Weber, N. (2016). Sex differences in pre-diagnosis concerns for children later diagnosed with autism spectrum disorder. *Autism, 20*(1), 75–84. doi:10.1177/1362361314568899

Hirsch, L. E., & Pringsheim, T. (2016). Aripiprazole for autism spectrum disorders (ASD). *The Cochrane Database of Systematic Reviews,* 6, CD009043. doi:10.1002/14651858.CD009043.pub3

Ho, K. S., Twede, H., Vanzo, R., Harward, E., Hensel, C. H., Martin, M. M., Page, S., . . . Wassman, R. (2016). Clinical performance of an ultrahigh resolution chromosomal microarray optimized for neurodevelopmental disorders. *BioMed Research International, 2016*(7). doi:10.1155/2016/3284534

Howlin, P., & Magiati, I. (2017). Autism spectrum disorder: outcomes in adulthood. *Current Opinion in Psychiatry, 30*(2), 69–76. doi:10.1097/YCO.0000000000000308

Hyman, S., Stewart, P., Foley, J., Cain, U., Peck, R., Morris, D., . . . Smith, T. (2016). The gluten-free/casein free diet: A double-blind challenge trial in children with autism. *Journal of Autism and Developmental Disorders, 46*(1), 205–220. doi:10.1007/s10803-015-2564-9

Iniesta-Sepulveda, M., Nadeau, J., Ramos, A., Kay, B., Riemann, B., & Storch, E. (2017). An initial case series of intensive cognitive-behavioral therapy for obsessive-compulsive disorder in adolescents with autism spectrum disorder. *Child Psychiatry and Human Development, 49*(1), 9–19. doi:10.1007/s10578-017-0724-1

Jacquemont, S., Coe, B. P., Hersch, M., Duyzend, M. H., Krumm, N., Bergmann, S., . . . Eichler, E. E. (2014). A higher mutational burden in females supports a "female protective model" in neurodevelopmental disorders. *American Journal of Human Genetics, 94*(3), 415–425. doi:10.1016/j.ajhg.2014.02.001

James, S., Montgomery, P., & Williams, K. (2011). Omega-3 fatty acids supplementation for autism spectrum disorders (ASD). *The Cochrane Database of Systematic Reviews, 11,* CD007992. doi:10.1002/14651858.CD007992.pub2

James, S., Stevenson, S. W., Silove, N., & Williams, K. (2015). Chelation for autism spectrum disorder (ASD). *The Cochrane Database of Systematic Reviews, 5,* CD010766.

Jarquin, V. G., Wiggins, L. D., Schieve, L. A., & Naarden-Braun, K. V. (2011). Racial disparities in community identification of autism spectrum disorders over time; Metropolitan Atlanta, Georgia, 2000-2006. *Journal of Developmental & Behavioral Pediatrics, 32*(3), 179–187. doi:10.1097/DBP.0b013e31820b4260

Jiang, H., Xu, L., Shao, L., Xia, R., Yu, Z., Ling, Z., . . . Ruan, B. (2016). Maternal infection during pregnancy and risk of autism spectrum disorders: A systematic review and meta-analysis. *Brain Behavior and Immunity, 58,* 165–172. doi:10.1016/j.bbi.2016.06.005

Johnson, S., Hollis, C., Kochhar, P., Hennessy, E., Wolke, D., & Marlow, N. (2010). Autism spectrum disorders in extremely preterm children. *Journal of Pediatrics, 156*(4), 525–531. doi:10.1016/j.jpeds.2009.10.041

Jordan, R. (2003). Social play and autistic spectrum disorders: A perspective on theory, implications and educational approaches. *Autism, 7,* 347–360. doi:10.1177/1362361303007004002

Joshi, G., Petty, C., Wozniak, J., Henin, A., Fried, R., Galdo, M., . . . Biederman, J. (2010). The heavy burden of psychiatric comorbidity in youth with autism spectrum disorders: A large comparative study of a psychiatrically referred population. *Journal of Autism and Developmental Disorders, 40*(11), 1361–1370. doi:10.1007/s10803-010-0996-9

Kasari, C., Freeman, S., & Papparella, T. (2006). Joint attention and symbolic play in young children with autism: A randomized controlled intervention study. *Journal of Child Psychology and Psychiatry, 47,* 611–620. doi:10.1111/j.1469-7610.2005.01567.x

Kenworthy, L., Case, L., Harms, M., Martin, A., & Wallace, G. (2010). Adaptive behavior ratings correlate with symptomatology and IQ among individuals with high-functioning autism spectrum disorders. *Journal of Autism and Developmental Disorders, 40*(4), 416–423. doi:10.1007/s10803-009-0911-4

Kim, Y. S., Levanthal, B. L., Koh, Y.-J., Fombonne, E., Laska, E., Lim, E. -C., . . . Grinker, R. R. (2011). Prevalence of autism spectrum disorders in a total population sample. *American Journal of Psychiatry, 168,* 904–912. doi:10.1176/appi.ajp.2011.10101532

Kirkovski, M., Enticott, P. G., & Fitzgerald, P. B. (2013). A review of the role of female gender in autism spectrum disorders. *Journal of Autism and Developmental Disorders, 43*(11), 2584–2603. doi:10.1007/s10803-013-1811-1

Klin, A., Jones, W., Schultz, R., Volkmar, F., & Cohen, D. (2002). Visual fixation patterns during viewing of naturalistic social situations as predictors of social competence in individuals with autism. *Archives of General Psychiatry, 59*(9), 809–816. doi:10.1001/archpsyc.59.9.809

Knickmeyer, R. C., Wheelwright, S., & Baron-Cohen, S. B. (2008). Sex-typical play: Masculinization/defeminization in girls with an autism spectrum condition. *Journal of Autism and Developmental Disorders, 38*(6), 1028–1035. doi:10.1007/s10803-007-0475-0

Koegel, R. L., Koegel, L. K., & Brookman, L. I. (2003). Empirically supported pivotal response interventions for children with autism. In A. E. Kazdin, Yale University School of Medicine, & Child Study Centers (Eds.), *Evidence-based psychotherapies for children and adolescents* (pp. 341–357). New York, NY: Guilford Press.

Kraper, C., Kenworthy, L., Popal, H., Martin, A., & Wallace, G. (2017). The gap between adaptive behavior and intelligence in autism persists into young adulthood and is linked to psychiatric co-morbidities. *Journal of Autism and Developmental Disorders, 47*(10), 3007–3017. doi:10.1007/s10803-017-3213-2

Lai, M.-C., Lombardo, M. V., Ruigrok, A. N., Chakrabarti, B., Auyeung, B., Szatmari, P., . . . MRC AIMS Consortium. (2016). Quantifying and exploring camouflaging in men and women with autism. *Autism, 21*(6), 690–702. doi:10.1177/1362361316671012

Landa, R. J., Gross, A. L., Stuart, E. A., & Faherty, A. (2013). Developmental trajectories in children with and without autism spectrum disorders: The first 3 years. *Child Development, 84*(2), 429–442.

Lang, R., O'Reilly, M., Healy, O., Rispoli, M., Lydon, H., Streusand, W., . . . Didden, R. (2012). Sensory integration therapy for autism spectrum disorders: A systematic review. *Research in Autism Spectrum Disorders, 6*(3), 1004–1018.

Laugeson, E. A., Frankel, F., Gantman, A., Dillon, A. R., & Mogil, C. (2012). Evidence-based social skills training for adolescents with autism spectrum disorders: The UCLA PEERS program. *Journal of Autism and Developmental Disorders, 42*(6), 1025–1036.

Leask, J., Booy, R., & McIntyre, P. B. (2010). MMR, Wakefield, and The Lancet: What can we learn? *The Medical Journal of Australia, 193*(1), 5–7.

Leekam, S. R., Prior, M. R., & Uljarevic, M. (2011). Restricted and repetitive behaviors in autism spectrum disorders: A review of research in the last decade. *Psychological Bulletin, 137*, 562–593. doi:10.1037/a0023341

Levy, S. E., & Hyman, S. L. (2005). Novel treatments for autistic spectrum disorders. *Mental Retardation and Developmental Disabilities Research Reviews, 11*(2), 131–142. doi:10.1002/mrdd.20062

Lindquest, B., Carlsson, G., Persson, E. -K., & Uvebrant, P. (2006). Behavioral problems and autism in children with hydrocephalus. *European Child and Adolescent Psychiatry, 15*, 214–219. doi:10.1007/s00787-006-0525-8

Liptak, G. S., Benzoni, L. B., Mruzek, D. W., Nolan, K. W., Thingvoll, M. A., Wade, C. M., & Fryer, G. E. (2008). Disparities in diagnosis and access to health services for children with autism: Data from the National Survey of Children's Health. *Journal of Developmental & Behavioral Pediatrics, 29*(3), 152–160.

Loomes, R., Hull, L., & Mandy, W. P. L. (2017). What is the male-to-female ratio in autism spectrum disorder? A systematic review and meta-analysis. *Journal of the American Academy of Child & Adolescent Psychiatry, 56*, 466–474. doi:10.1016/j.jaac.2017.03.013

Lord, C., Bishop, S., & Anderson, D. (2015). Developmental trajectories as autism phenotypes. *American Journal of Medical Genetics. Part C, Seminars in Medical Genetics, 169*(2), 198–208. doi:101002/ajmg.c.31440

Lord, C., Petkova, E., Hus, V., Gan, W., Lu, F., Martin, D. M., . . . Algermissen, M. (2012a). A multisite study of the clinical diagnosis of different autism spectrum disorders. *Archives of general psychiatry, 69*(3), 306–313.

Lord, C., Risi, S., Lambrecht, L., Cook, E. H. Jr., Leventhal, B. L., DiLavore, P. C., . . . Rutter, M. (2000). The Autism Diagnostic Observation Schedule–Generic: A standard measure of social and communication deficits associated with the spectrum of autism. *Journal of Autism and Developmental Disorders, 30*(3), 205–223.

Lord, C., Rutter, M., DiLavore, P. C., Risi, S., Gotham, K., & Bishop, S. (2012b). *Autism Diagnostic Observation Schedule: ADOS-2*. Los Angeles, CA: Western Psychological Services.

Lovaas, O. (1987). Behavioral treatment and normal educational and intellectual functioning in young autistic children. *Journal of Consulting and Clinical Psychology, 55*(1), 3–9. doi:10.1037//0022-006X.55.1.3

Lyall, K., Pauls, D., Spiegelman, D., Ascherio, A., & Santangelo, S. (2012). Pregnancy complications and obstetric suboptimality in association with autism spectrum disorders in children of the Nurses' Health Study II. *Autism Research, 5*(1), 21–30. doi:10.1002/aur.228

Madsen, K. M., Hviid, A., Vestergaard, M., Schendel, D., Wohlfahrt, J., Thorsen, P., . . . Melbye, M. (2002). A population-based study of measles, mumps, and rubella vaccination and autism. *New England Journal of Medicine, 347*(19), 1477–1482.

Madsen, K. M., Lauritsen, M. B., Pedersen, C. B., Thorsen, P., Plesner, A. M., Andersen, P. H., & Mortensen, P. B. (2003). Thimerosal and the occurrence of autism: Negative ecological evidence from Danish population-based data. *Pediatrics, 112*(3, Pt 1), 604–606.

Malow, B. A., Adkins, K., Reynolds, A., Weiss, S., Loh, A., Fawkes, D., . . . Clemons, T. (2014). Parent-based sleep education for children with autism spectrum disorders. *Journal of Autism and Developmental Disorders, 44*(1), 216–228. doi:10.1007/s10803-013-1866-z

Mandell, D. S., Novak, M. M., & Zubritsky, C. D. (2005). Factors associated with age of diagnosis among children with autism spectrum disorders. *Pediatrics, 116*(6), 1480–1486. doi:10.1542/peds.2005-0185

Mandell, D. S., Wiggins, L. D., Carpenter, L. A., Daniels, J., DiGuiseppi, C., Durkin, M. S., . . . Kirby, R. S. (2009). Racial/ethnic disparities in the identification of children with autism spectrum disorders. *American Journal of Public Health, 99*(3), 493–498. doi:10.2105/AJPH.2007.131243

Mandy, W., Chilvers, R., Chowdhury, U., Salter, G., Seigal, A., & Skuse, D. (2012). Sex differences in autism spectrum disorder: Evidence from a large sample of children and adolescents. *Journal of Autism and Developmental Disorders, 42*(7), 1304–1313. doi:10.1007/s10803-011-1356-0

Marco, E. J., Hinkley, L. B. N., Hill, S. S., & Nagarajan, S. S. (2011). Sensory processing in autism: A review of neurophysiologic findings. *Neuropsychiatric Disorders and Pediatric Psychiatry, 69*, 48R–54R. doi:10.1203/PDR.0b013e3182130c54

Marshall, J., Hill, R. J., Ziviani, J., & Dodrill, P. (2014). Features of feeding difficulty in children with autism spectrum disorder. *International Journal of Speech-Language Pathology, 16*(2), 151–158. doi:10.3109/17549507.2013.808700

Matson, J. L., & Shoemaker, M. (2009). Intellectual disability and its relationship to autism spectrum disorders. *Research in Developmental Disabilities, 30*, 1107–1114. doi.org/10.1016/j.ridd.2009.06.003

Mazurek, M. O., & Sohl, K. (2016). Sleep and behavioral problems in children with autism spectrum disorder. *Journal of Autism and Developmental Disorders, 46*(6), 1906.

McEachin, J. J., Smith, T., & Lovaas, O. I. (1993). Long-term outcome for children with autism who received early intensive behavioral treatment. *American Journal on Mental Retardation, 97*(4), 359–372.

McElhanon, B. O., McCracken, C., Karpen, S., & Sharp, W. G. (2014). Gastrointestinal symptoms in autism spectrum disorder: A meta-analysis. *Pediatrics, 133*(5), 872–883. doi:10.1542/peds.2013-3995

McGrew, S. G., Peters, B. R., Crittendon, J. A., & Veenstra-VanderWeele, J. (2012). Diagnostic yield of chromosomal microarray analysis in an autism primary care practice: Which guidelines to implement? *Journal of Autism and Developmental Disorders, 42*(8), 1582–1591. doi:10.1007/s10803-011-1398-3

McPheeters, M. L., Davis, A., Navarre, J. R., & Scott, T. A. (2011). Family report of ASD concomitant with depression or anxiety among US children. *Journal of Autism and Developmental Disorders, 41*, 646–653. doi:10.1007/s10803-010-1085-9

Mehling, M. H., & Tassé, M. J. (2016). Severity of autism spectrum disorders: Current conceptualization, and transition to DSM-5. *Journal of Autism and Developmental Disorders, 46*, 2000–2016. doi:10.1007/s10803-016-2731-7

Modabbernia, A., Velthorst, E., & Reichenberg, A. (2017). Environmental risk factors for autism: an evidence-based review of systematic reviews and meta-analyses. *Molecular Autism, 8*, 1–16. doi:10.1186/s13229-017-0121-4

Moss, J., & Howlin, P. (2009). Autism spectrum disorders in genetic syndromes: Implications for diagnosis, intervention and understanding the wider autism spectrum disorder population. *Journal of Intellectual Disability Research, 53*(10), 852–873. doi:10.1111/j.1365-2788.2009.01197.x

Mundy, P., & Newell, L. (2007). Attention, joint attention and social cognition. *Current Directions in Psychological Science, 16*(5), 269–274. doi:10.1111/j.1467-8721.2007.00518.x

Narzisi, A., Muratori, F., Calderoni, S., Fabbro, F., & Urgesi, C. (2013). Neuropsychological profile in high-functioning autism spectrum disorders. *Journal of Autism and Developmental Disorders, 43*, 1895–1909. doi:10.1007/s10803-012-1736-0

National Library of Medicine. (2017). *Genetics home reference* [Internet]. Retrieved from https://ghr.nlm.nih.gov/

Norbury, C. F. (2014). Practitioner review: Social (pragmatic) communication disorder conceptualization, evidence, and clinical implications. *Journal of Child Psychology and Psychiatry, 55*, 204–216. doi:10.1111/jcpp.12154

Nye, C., & Brice, A. (2005). Combined vitamin B6-magnesium treatment in autism spectrum disorders. *Cochrane Database of Systematic Reviews, 19*(4), CD003497.

Odom, S. L., Collet-Kilnenberg, L., Rogers, S. J., & Hatton, D. D. (2010). Evidence-based practices in interventions for children and youth with autism spectrum disorders. *Preschool School Failure, 54*, 275–282. doi:10.1080/10459881003785506

Orinstein, A., Tyson, K., Suh, J., Troyb, E., Helt, M., Rosenthal, M., . . . Fein, D. (2015). Psychiatric symptoms in youth with a history of autism and optimal outcome. *Journal of Autism and Developmental Disorders, 45*(11), 3703–3714. doi:10.1007/s10803-015-2520-8

Orsmond, G. I., Krauss, M. W., & Seltzer, M. M. (2004). Peer relationships and social and recreational activities among adolescents and adults with autism. *Journal of Autism and Developmental Disorders, 34*, 245–256. doi:10.1023/B:JADD.0000029547.96610.df

Ozonoff, S., Young, G. S., Carter, A., Messinger, D., Yirmiya, N., Zwaigenbaum, L., . . . Stone, W. L. (2011). Recurrence risk for autism spectrum disorders: A baby siblings research consortium study. *Pediatrics, 128*(3), 2010–2825. doi:10.1542/peds.2010-2825

Ozonoff, S., Young, G. S., Landa, R. J., Brian, J., Bryson, S., Charman, T., . . . Iosif, A. (2015). Diagnostic stability in young children at risk for autism spectrum disorder: A baby siblings research consortium study. *Journal of Child Psychology and Psychiatry and Allied Disciplines, 56*(9), 988–998. doi:10.1111/jcpp.12421

Pandey, J., Verbalis, A., Robins, D. L., Boorstein, H., Klin, A., Babitz, T., . . . Fein, D. (2008). Screening for autism in older and younger toddlers with the Modified Checklist for Autism in Toddlers. *Autism, 12*(5), 513–535. doi:10.1177/1362361308094503

Parr, J., LeCouteur, A., Baird, G., Rutter, M., Pickles, A., Fombonne, E., & Bailey, A. J. (2011). Early developmental regression in autism spectrum disorder: Evidence from an international multiplex sample. *Journal of Autism and Developmental Disorders, 41*(3), 332–340.

Paul, R., Orlovski, S. M., Marcino, H. C., & Volkmar, F. (2009). Conversational behaviors in youth with high-functioning ASD and Asperger syndrome. *Journal of Autism and Developmental Disorders, 39*, 115–125. doi:10.1007/s10803-008-0607-1

Pedersen, A., Pettygrove, S., Meaney, F. J., Mancilla, K., Kessler, D. B., Grebe, T. A., & Cunniff, C. (2012). Prevalence of autism spectrum disorders in Hispanic and non-Hispanic white children. *Pediatrics, 129*(3), e629–e635. doi:10.1542/peds.2011-1145

Pelphrey, K. A., Shultz, S., Hudac, C. M., & Vander Wyk, B. C. (2011). Research review: Constraining heterogeneity: The social brain and its development in autism spectrum disorder. *Journal of Child Psychology and Psychiatry, 52*(6), 631–644. doi:10.1111/j.1469-7610.2010.02349.x

Perrin, J. M., Coury, D. L., Hyman, S. L., Cole, L., Reynolds, A. M., & Clemons, T. (2012). Complementary and alternative medicine use in a large pediatric autism sample. *Pediatrics, 130*(Suppl. 2), S77–S82. doi:10.1542/peds.2012-0900E

Pickles, A., Anderson, D. K., & Lord, C. (2014). Heterogeneity and plasticity in the development of language: A 17 year follow-up of children referred early for possible autism. *Journal of Child Psychology and Psychiatry, and Allied Disciplines, 55*(12), 1354–1362. doi:10.1111/jcpp.12269

Plaisted, K. C. (2001). Reduced generalization in autism: An alternative to weak central coherence. In J. A. Burack & T. Charman (Eds.), *The development of autism: Perspectives from theory and research* (pp. 149–169). Mahwah, NJ: Erlbaum.

Rao, P. A., & Landa, R. J. (2014). Association between severity of behavioral phenotype and comorbid attention deficit hyperactivity disorder symptoms in children with autism spectrum disorders. *Autism, 18*(3), 272–280. doi:10.1177/1362361312470494

Rapin, I., & Dunn, M. (2003). Update on the language disorders of individuals on the autistic spectrum. *Brain and Development, 25*(3), 166–172. doi:10.1016/S0387-7604(02)00191-2

Reichow, B. (2012). Overview of meta-analysis on early intensive behavioral intervention for young children with autism spectrum disorders. *Journal of Autism and Developmental Disorders, 45*, 512–520.

Reichow, B., Steiner, A., & Volkmar, F. (2012). Social skills groups for people aged 6 to 21 with autism spectrum disorders (ASD). *Cochrane Developmental, Psychosocial and Learning Problems Group, 2012*(7), *8(2)*, 266–315. doi:10.1002/14651858.CD008511.pub2

Reichow, B., Volkmar, F. R., & Bloch, M. H. (2013). Systematic review and meta-analysis of pharmacological treatment of the symptoms of attention-deficit/hyperactivity disorder in children with pervasive developmental disorders. *Journal of Autism and Developmental Disorders, 43*(10), 2435–2441.

Reichow, B., Barton, E. E., Boyd, B. A., & Hume, K. (2014). Early intensive behavioral intervention (EIBI) for youth children with autism spectrum disorders (ASD): A systematic review. *Campbell Systematic Reviews, 23*(6), 616–620. doi:10.4073/csr.2014.9

Reznick, J. S., Baranek, G. T., Reavis, S., Watson, L. R., & Crais, E. R. (2007). A parent-report instrument for identifying one-year-olds at risk for an eventual diagnosis of autism: The first year inventory. *Journal of Autism and Developmental Disorders, 37*(9), 1691–1710. doi:10.1007/s10803-006-0303-y

Richards, C., Jones, C., Groves, L., Moss, J., & Oliver, C. (2015). Prevalence of autism spectrum disorder phenomenology in genetic disorders: A systematic review and meta analysis. *The Lancet Psychiatry, 2*(10), 2909–2916. doi:10.1016/S2215-0366(15)00376-4

Robins, D. L., Casagrande, K., Barton, M., Chen, C. M. A., Dumont-Mathieu, T., & Fein, D. (2014). Validation of the modified checklist for autism in toddlers, revised with follow-up (M-CHAT-R/F). *Pediatrics, 133*(1), 37–45.

Robins, D. L., Fein, D., Barton, M. L., & Green, J. A. (2001). The Modified Checklist for Autism in Toddlers: An initial study investigating the early detection of autism and pervasive developmental disorders. *Journal of Autism and Developmental Disorders, 31*(2), 131–144.

Robinson, E. B., Lichtenstein, P., Anckarsater, H., Happe, F., & Ronald, A. (2013). Examining and interpreting the female protective effect against autistic behavior. *Proceedings of the National Academy of Sciences, 110*(13), 5258–5262. doi:10.1073/pnas.1211070110

Rogers, S. J. (2004). Developmental regression in autism spectrum disorders. *Mental Retardation and Developmental Disabilities Research Reviews, 10*(2), 139–143. doi:10.1002/mrdd.20027

Rutgers, A. H., Bakermans-Kranenburg, M. J., van Ijzendoorn, M. H., & van Berckelaer-Onnes, I. A. (2004). Autism and attachment: A meta-analytic review. *Journal of Child Psychology and Psychiatry, 45,* 1123–1134. doi:10.1111/j.1469-7610.2004.t01-1-00305.x

Rutter, M., Bailey, A., & Lord, C. (2003). *Social Communication Questionnaire.* Torrance, CA: Western Psychological Services.

Rutter, M., LeCouteur, A., & Lord, C. (2003). *Autism Diagnostic Interview–Revised.* Torrance, CA: Western Psychological Services.

Salazar, F., Baird, G., Chandler, S., Tseng, E., O'Sullivan, T., Howlin, P., . . . Simonoff, E. (2015). Co-occurring psychiatric disorders in preschool and elementary school-aged children with autism spectrum disorder. *Journal of Autism and Developmental Disorders, 45*(8), 2283–2294. doi:10.1007/s10803-015-2361-5

Sandin, S., Lichtenstein, P., Kuja-Halkola, R., Hultman, C., Larsson, H., & Reichenberg, A. (2017). The heritability of autism spectrum disorder. *JAMA, 318*(12), 1182–1184. doi:10.1001/jama.2017.12141

Sanua, V. D. (1984). Is infantile autism a universal phenomenon? An open question. *International Journal of Social Psychiatry, 30*(3), 163–177. doi:10.1177/002076408403000301

Scahill, L., Specht, M., & Page, C. (2014). The prevalence of tic disorders and clinical characteristics in children. *Journal of Obsessive-Compulsive and Related Disorders, 3*(4), 3394–3400. doi:10.1016/j.jocrd.2014.06.002

Schopler, E., Andrews, C., & Strupp, K. (1979). Do autistic children come from upper-middle class parents? *Journal of Autism and Developmental Disorders, 9*(2), 139–152.

Selten, J., Lundberg, M., Rai, D., & Magnusson, C. (2015). Risks for nonaffective psychotic disorder and bipolar disorder in young people with autism spectrum disorder: A population-based study. *JAMA Psychiatry, 72*(5), 483–489. doi:10.1001/jamapsychiatry.2014.3059

Shafritz, K. M., Dichter, G. S., Baranek, G. T., & Belger, A. (2008). The neural circuitry mediating shifts in behavioral response and cognitive set in autism. *Biological Psychiatry, 63,* 974-980. doi:10.1016/j.biopsych.2007.06.028

Sharp, W. G., Berry, R. C., McCracken, C., Nuhu, N. N., Marvel, E., Saulnier, C. A., . . . Jaquess, D. L. (2013). Feeding problems and nutrient intake in children with autism spectrum disorders: A meta-analysis and comprehensive review of the literature. *Journal of Autism and Developmental Disorders, 43*(9), 2159–2173.

Shattuck, P. T., Durkin, M., Maenner, M., Newschaffer, C., Mandell, D. S., Wiggins, L., . . . Cuniff, C. (2009). Timing of identification among children with an autism spectrum disorder: Findings from a population-based surveillance study. *Journal of the American Academy of Child & Adolescent Psychiatry, 48*(5), 474–483. https://doi.org/10.1097/CHI.0b013e31819b3848

Siegel, M., & Beaulieu, A. (2012). Psychotropic medications in children with autism spectrum disorders: A systematic review and synthesis for evidence-based practice. *Journal of Autism and Developmental Disorders, 42*(8), 1592–1605. doi:10.1007/s10803-011-1399-2

Siklos, S., & Kerns, K. A. (2007). Assessing the diagnostic experiences of a small sample of parents of children with autism spectrum disorders. *Research in Developmental Disabilities, 28*(1), 9–22. doi:10.1016/j.ridd.2005.09.003

Skuse, D. H. (2007). Rethinking the nature of genetic vulnerability to autistic spectrum disorders. *Trends in Genetics, 23,* 387–395. doi: 0.1016/j.tig.2007.06.003

Silverman, L. B., Bennetto, L., Campana, E., & Tanenhaus, M. K. (2010). Speech-and-gesture integration in high functioning autism. *Cognition, 115*(3), 380–393. doi:10.1016/j.cognition.2010.01.002

Sinzig, J., Walter, D., & Doepfner, M. (2009). Attention deficit/hyperactivity disorder in children and adolescents with autism spectrum disorder: Symptom or syndrome? *Journal of Attention Disorders, 13*(2), 117–126.

Smith, T., Eikeseth, S., Klevstran, M., & Lovaas, O. I. (1997). Intensive behavioral treatment for preschoolers with severe mental retardation and pervasive developmental disorder. *American Journal on Mental Retardation, 102*(3), 238–249. doi:10.1352/0895-8017(1997)102[[0238:IBTFPW]]2.0.CO;2

Sokolova, E., Oerlemans, A. M., Rommelse, N. N., Groot, P., Hartman, C. A., Glennon, J. C., . . . Buitelaar, J. K. (2017). A causal and mediation analysis of the comorbidity between attention deficit hyperactivity disorder (ADHD) and autism spectrum disorder (ASD). *Journal of Autism and Developmental Disorders, 47*(6), 1595–1604.

Solomon, M., Ozonoff, S. J., Ursu, S., Ravizza, S., Cummings, N., Ly, S., & Carter, C. S. (2009). The neural substrates of cognitive control deficits in autism spectrum disorders. *Neuropsychologia, 47,* 2515–2526. doi:10.1016/j.neuropsychologia.2009.04.019

Strang, J. F., Kenworthy, L., Dominska, A., Sokoloff, J., Kenealy, L. E., Berl, M., . . . Wallace, G. L. (2014). Increased gender variance in autism spectrum disorders and attention deficit hyperactivity disorder. *Archives of Sexual Behavior, 43*(8), 1525–1533. doi:10.1007/s10508-014-0285-3

Stone, W. L., Coonrod, E. E., Turner, L. M., & Pozdol, S. L. (2004). Psychometric properties of the STAT for early autism screening. *Journal of Autism and Developmental Disorders, 34*(6), 691–701.

Strömland, K., Nordin, V., Miller, M., Akerström, B., & Gillberg, C. (1994). Autism in thalidomide embryopathy: A population study. *Developmental Medicine and Child Neurology, 36*(4), 351–356.

Strunz, S., Schermuck, C., Ballerstein, S., Ahlers, C. J., Dziobek, I., & Roepke, S. (2017). Romantic relationships and relationship satisfaction among adults with Asperger syndrome and high-functioning autism. *Journal of Clinical Psychology, 73,* 113:125. doi:10.1002/jclp.22319

Tager-Flusberg, H., & Kasari, C. (2013). Minimally verbal school-aged children with autism spectrum disorder: The neglected end of the spectrum. *Autism Research, 6,* 468–478. doi:10.1002/aur.1329

Tammimies, K., Marshall, C. R., Walker, S., Kaur, G., Thiruvahindrapuram, B., Lionel, A. C., . . . Fernandez, B. A. (2015). Molecular diagnostic yield of chromosomal microarray analysis and whole-exome sequencing in children with autism spectrum disorder. *JAMA, 314*(9), 895–903. doi:10.1001/jama.2015.10078

Tek, S., & Landa, R. J. (2012). Differences in autism symptoms between minority and non-minority toddlers. *Journal of Autism and Developmental Disorders. 42(9),* 1967–1973. doi:10.1007/s10803-012-1445-8

Thomas, S., Hovinga, M. E., Rai, D., & Lee, B. K. (2017). Brief report: Prevalence of co-occurring epilepsy and autism spectrum disorder: The U.S. National Survey of Children's Health 2011-2012. *Journal of Autism and Developmental Disorders, 47*(1), 224–229. doi:10.1007/s10803-016-2938-7

Tick, B., Bolton, P., Happe, F., Rutter, M., & Rijsdijk, F. (2016). Heritability of autism spectrum disorders: A meta-analysis of twin studies. *Journal of Child Psychology and Psychiatry, 57*(5), 585–595.

Tonnsen, B. L., Boan, A. D., Bradley, C. C., Charlest, J., Cohen, A., & Carpenter, L. A. (2016). Prevalence of autism spectrum disorders among children with intellectual disability. *American Journal on Intellectual and Developmental Disabilities, 121*(6), 487–500.

Travis, L., Sigman, M., & Ruskin, E. (2001). Links between social understanding and social behavior in verbally able children with autism. *Journal of Autism and Developmental Disorders, 31*(2), 119–130.

Ung, D., Selles, R., Small, B. J., & Storch, E. A. (2015). A systematic review and meta analysis of cognitive behavioral therapy for anxiety in youth with high-functioning autism spectrum disorders. *Child Psychiatry and Human Development, 46*(4), 533–547. doi:10.1007/s10578-014-0494-y

Valvo, G., Baldini, S., Brachini, F., Apicella, F., Cosenza, A., Ferrari, A. R., . . . Sicca, F. (2013). Somatic overgrowth predisposes to seizures in autism spectrum disorders. *PLoS One, 8*(9), e75015. doi:10.1371/journal.pone.0075015.

van Steensel, F. A., Bogels, S. M., & de Bruin, E. I. (2013). Psychiatric comorbidity in children with autism spectrum disorders: A comparison with children with ADHD. *Journal of Child and Family Studies, 22*(3), 368–376.

Van Wijngaarden-Cremers, P. J. M., van Eeten, E., Groen, W. B., Van Deurzen, P. A., Oosterling, I. J., & Van der Gaag, R. J. (2014). Gender and age differences in the core triad of impairments in autism spectrum disorders: A systematic review and meta-analysis. *Journal of Autism and Developmental Disorders, 44*(3), 627–635. doi:10.1007/s10803-013-1913-9

Vasa, R. A., Mazurek, M. O., Mahajan, R., Bennett, A. E., Bernal, M. P., Nozzolillo, A. A., . . . Coury, D. L. (2016). Assessment and treatment of anxiety in youth with autism spectrum disorders. *Pediatrics, 137*(Suppl. 2), S115–S123. doi:10.1542/peds.2015-2851J

Vismara, L. A., & Rogers, S. J. (2010). Behavioral treatments in autism spectrum disorder: What do we know? *Annual Review of Clinical Psychology, 6*(1), 447–468. doi:10.1146/annurev.clinpsy.121208.131151

von Gontard, A., Pirrung, M., Niemczyk, J., & Equit, M. (2015). Incontinence in children with autism spectrum disorder. *Journal of Pediatric Urology, 11*(5), 264.e1. doi:10.1016/j.jpurol.2015.04.015

Watkins, L., O'Reilly, M., Kuhn, M., Gevarter, C., Lancioni, G.E., Sigafoos, J., & Lang, R. (2015). A review of peer-mediated social interaction interventions for students with autism in inclusive settings. *Journal of Autism and Developmental Disorders, 45*, 1070–1083. doi:10.1007/s10803-014-2264-x

Wechsler, D. (2003). *The Wechsler Intelligence Scale for Children—Fourth Edition*. London, United Kingdom: Pearson.

Weitlauf, A. S., Gotham, K. O., Vehorn, A. C., & Warren, Z. E. (2014). Brief report: DSM-5 "levels of support": A comment on discrepant conceptualizations of severity in ASD. *Journal of Autism and Developmental Disorders, 44*, 471–476. doi:10.1007/s10803-013-1882-z

Wetherby, A. M., Guthrie, W., Woods, J., Schatschneider, C., Holland, R. D., Morgan, L., & Lord, C. (2014). Parent-implemented social intervention for toddlers with autism: An RCT. *Pediatrics, 134*(6), 1084–1093.

White, S. W., Keonig, K., & Scahill, L. (2007). Social skills development in children with autism spectrum disorders: A review of the intervention research. *Journal of Autism and Developmental Disorders, 37*, 1858–1868.

Wing, L. (1980). Childhood autism and social class: A question of selection? *British Journal of Psychiatry, 137*, 410–417.

Witwer, A. N., & Lecavalier, L. (2008). Examining the validity of autism spectrum disorder subtypes. *Journal of Autism and Developmental Disorders, 38*(9), 1611–1624.

Wong, D., Odom, S. L., Hume, K. A., Cox, A. W., Fettig, A., Kucharczyk, S., . . . Schultz, T. R. (2015). Evidence-based practices for children, youth, and young adults with autism spectrum disorder: A comprehensive review. *Journal of Autism and Developmental Disorders, 45*, 1951–1966. doi:10.1007/s10803-014-2351-z

Wright, B., Sima, D., Smart, S., Alwazeer, A., Alderson-Day, B., Allgar, V., . . . Miles, J. (2011). Melatonin versus placebo in children with autism spectrum conditions and severe sleep problems not amenable to behaviour management strategies: A randomized controlled crossover trial. *Journal of Autism and Developmental Disorders, 2*, 175. doi:10.1007/s10803-010-1036-5

Xiong, T., Chen, H., Luo, R., & Mu, D. (2016). Hyperbaric oxygen therapy for people with autism spectrum disorder (ASD). *The Cochrane Database of Systematic Reviews, 10*, CD010922.

Yeargin-Allsopp, M., Rice, C., Karapurkar, T., Doernberg, N., Boyle, C., & Murphy, C. (2003). Prevalence of autism in a US metropolitan area. *Journal of American Medical Association, 289*(1), 49–55. doi:10.1001/jama.289.1.49

Yirmiya, N., Erel, O., Shaked, M., & Solomonica-Levi, D. (1998). Meta-analyses comparing theory of mind abilities of individuals with autism, individuals with mental retardation, and normally developing individuals. *Psychological Bulletin, 124*, 283–307.

Zafeiriou, D. I., Ververi, A., Dafoulis, V., Kalyva, E., & Vargiami, E. (2013). Autism spectrum disorders: The quest for genetic syndromes. *American Journal of Medical Genetics, Part B: Neuropsychiatric Genetics, 162*(4), 327366. doi:10.1002/ajmg.b.32152

Zerbo, O., Qian, Y., Yoshida, C., Grether, J., Water, J., & Croen, L. (2015). Maternal infection during pregnancy and autism spectrum disorders. *Journal of Autism & Developmental Disorders, 45*(12), 4015–4025. doi:10.1007/s10803-013-2016-3

Zwaigenbaum, L., Bryson, S., & Garon, N. (2013). Early identification of autism spectrum disorders. *Behavioural Brain Research, 251*, 133–146. doi:10.1016/j.bbr.2013.04.004

Zwaigenbaum, L., Young, G. S., Stone, W. L., Dobkins, K., Ozonoff, S., Brian, J., . . . Messinger, D. (2014). Early head growth in infants at risk of autism: A baby siblings research consortium study. *Journal of the American Academy of Child and Adolescent Psychiatry, 53*(10), 1053–1062. doi:10.1016/j.jaac.2014.07.007

CHAPTER 19 Attention-Deficit/ Hyperactivity Disorder

Marianne Glanzman and Neelam Kharod Sell

Upon completion of this chapter, the reader will

- Be familiar with the diagnostic criteria for attention-deficit/hyperactivity disorder
- Be aware of some of the causes of inattention and hyperactivity
- Understand the components of the diagnostic process
- Be aware of commonly associated symptoms and conditions
- Know the different approaches to management
- Understand the natural history and outcomes for this disorder

Attention-deficit/hyperactivity disorder (ADHD) is one of the most prevalent neurodevelopmental/mental health conditions in childhood. It is characterized by developmentally inappropriate levels of inattention and distractibility and/or hyperactivity and impulsivity that cause impairment in adaptive functioning at home, school, and in social situations. ADHD often persists into adolescence and adulthood. Treatment, including educational and psychosocial interventions, medication, and lifestyle modifications, can substantially improve short-term behavioral, academic, and social functioning. Optimal outcomes, however, have not been achieved, in part because sustained multimodal treatment is not widely accessible. Our understanding of the brain and genetic bases for the symptoms of ADHD has progressed rapidly over the past 30 years and may ultimately provide new insights into prevention and treatment.

CASE STUDY

Ricky, age 7, is in second grade. His teacher reports that he is having great difficulty learning to read. He also is quite disruptive in class, frequently not listening to directions, getting out of his seat, making tangential comments, and talking out of turn. His first-grade teacher reported similar problems, but these difficulties were attributed to him having to adjust to the new school, as he had attended a Montessori kindergarten previously. His parents and soccer coach have also noticed problems with his ability to follow directions and pay attention. Ricky was adopted shortly after birth, so there is no family history available. He has, however, always had a "difficult" temperament. He was a colicky infant with poor sleep patterns. As a preschooler, he was demanding and inflexible, and he would exhaust all those around him with his need to negotiate when he was asked to comply with a directive.

His parents and teachers feel that he is still quite immature and demanding, as he requires much more attention than other children his age in order to accomplish even routine daily activities.

A comprehensive evaluation revealed that Ricky has ADHD, combined presentation (ADHD-C) and a learning disability in reading, though he is intellectually gifted. Ricky was considered to be at significant risk for both academic and behavior difficulties; as such, his interdisciplinary team decided to put a multimodal treatment plan into place. Stimulant medication was started, and it proved dramatically helpful at school, as well as on weekends and school vacations, in improving functioning in social situations and activities of daily living. Counseling was also begun, focusing on the development of a consistent behavior management plan at home and school, as well as social skill instruction. At school, Ricky received resource room assistance for reading and language arts, enrichment programming in math, and weekly meetings with the school counselor for a social skills group.

Thought Questions:

How might a parent, teacher, or doctor of a school-age child distinguish inattention related to ADHD from inattention related to other causes? How might professionals counsel the parents of a child newly diagnosed with ADHD regarding treatment options? When the parents of a newly diagnosed child ask, "What does the future hold for our child with ADHD?", how should a professional respond to convey both hopefulness and realism?

DIAGNOSIS AND ADHD PRESENTATIONS

ADHD is a neurobehavioral syndrome; as of 2018, there are no available medical or psychological tests to definitively make the diagnosis. Instead, the diagnosis depends on "ruling in" symptoms of ADHD and "ruling out" other causes of the symptoms through the use of interviews and rating scales to systematically collect information from parents, teachers, and (older) children (which will be discussed in a section that follows titled "The Evaluation Process") (American Academy of Pediatrics [AAP], 2011).

The current diagnostic criteria consist of two major clusters of symptoms: inattention and hyperactivity/impulsivity. These criteria, outlined in the *Diagnostic and Statistical Manual* of *Mental Disorders, Fifth Edition* (*DSM-5*), of the American Psychiatric Association (APA, 2013), are shown in Table 19.1. In order to meet criteria for the diagnosis, children must have six of the nine symptoms in either or both categories. Those 17 years of age and older are only required to have five symptoms. Additional requirements for all presentations include 1) evidence of several symptoms before age 12 that have persisted for at least 6 months; 2) occurrence of several symptoms across multiple settings (i.e., school and home); 3) functional impairment as a result of symptoms in academic, social, or adaptive/occupational activities; and 4) symptoms cannot be better accounted for by another disorder such as a psychotic, mood, personality, or substance use disorder (APA, 2013).

Two additional diagnostic categories may be used when full criteria are not met. Other Specified ADHD is used when some, but not all, required symptoms are present. In addition, 1) the symptoms must be causing functional impairment, 2) the individual must not meet criteria for another neurodevelopmental disorder, and 3) the clinician must be able to articulate what is missing from the full criteria. For example, a 12-year-old child without another neurodevelopmental diagnosis who has five rather than six of the required symptoms and declining academic performance attributable to inattentive symptoms would receive this diagnosis. Unspecified ADHD is used when symptoms characteristic of ADHD are present and cause functional impairment and there is no other neurodevelopmental diagnosis but the clinician does not choose to specify what requirements are missing. This diagnosis is most often used when insufficient information is available to determine whether or not full criteria are met.

Changes in the diagnostic formulation from the *Diagnostic and Statistical Manual, Fourth Edition, Text Revision* (*DSM-IV-TR*; APA, 2000), to the current *DSM-5* (APA, 2013) include further specifying examples of symptoms to improve relevance to adolescents and adults, increasing the required age at which symptoms are first noted to be impairing from 7 to 12, and reducing the number of required symptoms from 6 to 5 in older adolescents and adults (Dalsgaard, 2013).

ADHD Combined Presentation is the most commonly diagnosed presentation in clinical samples and the most studied presentation of ADHD. It is associated with social impairment, increased prevalence of coexisting internalizing (anxiety and mood) and externalizing (oppositional defiant and conduct) disorders, and academic underachievement (Baeyens, Roeyers, & Walle, 2006; Spencer, Biederman, & Mick, 2007).

ADHD Inattentive Presentation is the most common presentation in broad epidemiologic samples (excluding preschoolers; Willcutt, 2012). It refers to individuals who do not display significant levels of hyperactivity but have significant problems in maintaining attention. The ratio of girls to boys with this

Table 19.1. Diagnostic criteria for attention-deficit/hyperactivity disorder

A. A persistent pattern of inattention and/or hyperactivity-impulsivity that interferes with functioning or development, characterized by (1) and/or (2):

1. Inattention/distractibility: Six (or more) of the following symptoms that have persisted for at least 6 months to a degree that is inconsistent with developmental level and that negatively impacts directly on social and academic/occupational activities:

   Note: The symptoms are not solely manifestations of oppositional behavior, defiance, hostility, or failure to understand tasks or instructions. For older adolescents and adults (those ages 17 or older), five symptoms are required.

   a. Often fails to give close attention to details or makes careless mistakes in schoolwork, work, or other activities (e.g., overlooks or misses details, work is inaccurate).

   b. Often has difficulty sustaining attention in tasks or play activities (e.g., has difficulty remaining focused during lectures, conversations, or lengthy reading).

   c. Often does not seem to listen when spoken to directly (e.g., mind seems elsewhere, even in the absence of any obvious distraction).

   d. Often does not follow through on instructions and fails to finish schoolwork, chores, or duties in the workplace (e.g., starts tasks but quickly loses focus and is easily sidetracked)

   e. Often has difficulty organizing tasks and activities (e.g., difficulty managing sequential tasks; difficulty keeping materials and belongings in order; has messy, disorganized work; has poor time management; fails to meet deadlines).

   f. Often avoids, dislikes, or is reluctant to engage in tasks that require sustained mental effort (e.g., schoolwork or homework; for older adolescents and adults, preparing reports, completing forms, reviewing lengthy papers).

   g. Often loses things necessary for tasks or activities (e.g., school materials, pencils, books, tools, wallets, keys, paperwork, eyeglasses, mobile telephones).

   h. Is often easily distracted by extraneous stimuli (for older adolescents and adults, may include unrelated thoughts).

   i. Is often forgetful in daily activities (e.g., doing chores, running errands; for older adolescents and adults, returning calls, paying bills, keeping appointments).

2. Hyperactivity and impulsivity: Six (or more) of the following symptoms that have persisted for at least 6 months to a degree that is inconsistent with developmental level and that negatively impacts directly on social and academic/occupational activities:

   Note: The symptoms are not solely manifestations of oppositional behavior, defiance, hostility, or failure to understand tasks or instructions. For older adolescents and adults (those ages 17 or older), five symptoms are required.

   a. Often fidgets with hands or feet or squirms in seat.

   b. Often leaves seat in classroom or in other situations in which remaining seated is expected (e.g., leaves his or her place in the classroom, in the office or other workplace, or in other situations that require remaining in place).

   c. Often runs about or climbs excessively in situations in which it is inappropriate (**Note:** In adolescents or adults, may be limited to feeling restless).

   d. Often unable to play or engage in leisure activities quietly.

   e. Is often "on the go," acting as if "driven by a motor" (e.g., is unable to be or uncomfortable being still for extended time, as in restaurants, meetings; may be experienced by others as being restless or difficult to keep up with).

   f. Often talks excessively.

   g. Often blurts out answers before a question has been completed (e.g., completes people's sentences; cannot wait for turn in conversation).

   h. Often has difficulty waiting his or her turn (e.g., while waiting in line).

   i. Often interrupts or intrudes on others (e.g., butts into conversations, games, or activities; may start using other people's things without asking or receiving permission; for adolescents or adults, may intrude into or take over what others are doing).

B. Several inattentive or hyperactive-impulsive symptoms were present prior to age 12 years.

C. Several inattentive or hyperactive-impulsive symptoms are present in two or more settings (e.g., home, school, or work; with friends or relatives; in other activities).

D. There is clear evidence that the symptoms interfere with, or reduce the quality of, social, academic, or occupational functioning.

E. The symptoms do not occur exclusively during the course of schizophrenia or another psychotic disorder and are not better explained by another mental disorder (e.g., mood disorder, anxiety disorder, dissociative disorder, personality disorder, substance intoxication or withdrawal).

Specify whether:

314.01(F90.2) Combined presentation: If both Criterion A1 (inattention) and Criterion A2 (hyperactivity-impulsivity) are met for the past 6 months.

314.00 (F90.0) Predominantly inattentive presentation: If Criterion A1 (inattention) is met but Criterion A2 (hyperactivity-impulsivity) is not met for the past 6 months

314.01 (F90.1) Predominantly hyperactive-impulsive presentation: If Criterion A2 (hyperactivity-impulsivity) is met and Criterion A1 (inattention) is not met for the past 6 months.

Specify if:

In partial remission: When full criteria were previously met, fewer than the full criteria have been met for the past 6 months, and the symptoms still result in impairment in social, academic, or occupational functioning.

Specify current severity:

Mild: Few, if any, symptoms in excess of those required to make the diagnosis are present, and if symptoms result in no more than minor impairments in social or occupational functioning.

Moderate: Symptoms or functional impairment between "mild" and "severe" are present

Severe: Many symptoms in excess of those required to make the diagnosis, or several symptoms that are particularly severe, are present, or the symptoms result in marked impairment in social or occupational functioning.

presentation is slightly higher than for the other presentations, and it is usually identified at a later age. The pattern of psychiatric comorbidity also differs from that of the combined presentation with fewer oppositional disorders or conduct disorders, but with more anxiety and mood disorders. Educational impairments are the most prominent difficulty experienced by this group (Baeyens et al., 2006; Barkley, 1998; Stefanatos & Baron, 2007). There is some evidence to suggest that the specific nature of inattention in this presentation may differ from the inattention shown by those with the combined presentation. A "slow" cognitive tempo is characteristic of some individuals with the inattentive presentation, and their inattention may be characterized by slow processing speed rather than distractibility (Becker et al., 2016).

ADHD Hyperactive/Impulsive Presentation was first identified in the *DSM-IV* (APA, 1994) and refers to children who do not display significant levels of attention problems in the presence of hyperactivity and impulsivity. The specific presentations of ADHD are not necessarily stable over time (Lahey, Pelham, Loney, Lee, & Willcutt, 2005). In particular, the hyperactive/impulsive presentation is most often diagnosed in preschool age boys and may change over time to the combined presentation as young children may have not yet reached an age at which attention problems are impairing (Greenhill, Posner, Vaughan, & Kratochvil, 2008). There is ongoing research regarding the two major symptom domains of ADHD. Some research suggests that the inattentive and hyperactive/impulsive presentations have different genetic influences, although both are highly heritable (Nikolas & Burt, 2010).

While there is general agreement on the conceptualization of ADHD as a disorder with specific core features and a desire to specify and quantify symptoms as much as possible, there is also agreement that a clear dividing line between presence and absence of the disorder does not exist. ADHD is increasingly recognized as the severe end of a symptom continuum, with a wide range in the degree of subthreshold symptom severity (Balázs & Keresztény, 2014; McLennan, 2016). The concept of a continuum is supported by genetic studies that show that genetic differences conferring risk for ADHD are more commonly present, not only in those with the diagnosis, but also in those with some symptoms (Middeldorp et al., 2016; Stergiakouli et al., 2015). There are also developmental studies that show that the youngest children in a specific grade are more likely to be diagnosed with ADHD than the oldest children in that grade (Sayal, Chudal, Hinkka-Yli-Salomäki, Joelsson & Sourander, 2017).

PREVALENCE AND EPIDEMIOLOGY

Prevalence is the proportion of a population who have a specific characteristic, or in this case, diagnosis, in a given time period. Point prevalence refers to the presence of the diagnosis at the time of the study, whereas lifetime prevalence, more commonly used in adults, refers to a history of ever having had the diagnosis. The prevalence of ADHD varies based on the population studied and the methods used. Studies based on endorsement of symptoms on questionnaires typically result in higher prevalence rates than studies that include a diagnostic interview to assess for other possible causes of symptoms and for a significant level of functional impairment (Polanczyk, Salum, Sugaya, Caye, & Rhode, 2015). Studies that use community, or population-based, samples also show higher rates, as a substantial group may have been previously undiagnosed (Rowland et al., 2015). Finally, the use of *DSM-5* rather than *DSM-IV* criteria increases prevalence rates due to the later age of onset allowed and a reduced number of symptoms required in older adolescents and adults (Vande Voort, He, Jameson, & Merikangas, 2014).

In the previous edition of this text, the estimated prevalence of ADHD in school-age children in the United States was 7%–10%. Newer studies suggest a rate of 8%–15% (McKeown et al., 2015; Rowland et al., 2015; Wolraich et al., 2014). It remains controversial as to whether this increase is due to the change in diagnostic criteria described above or whether there is a true increase in prevalence. A recent meta-analysis of world-wide studies (Polanczyk, Willcutt, Salum, Kieling, & Rohde, 2014) suggests that when methodological characteristics of the studies are taken into account, there has not been a true increase in the rate of ADHD. World-wide studies suggest a pooled prevalence of 3%–7% (Polanzyck et al., 2015; Thomas, Sanders, Doust, Beller, & Glasziou, 2015).

There continues to be significant variation in the rate of identification of ADHD in different populations. The rate of clinical identification is somewhat lower in the United States in Hispanic and African American children than for Caucasian children for reasons that likely include differences in cultural attitudes and ascertainment as well as differences in access to care, although prevalence rates of symptoms are similar (Alvarado & Modesto-Lowe, 2017; APA, 2013; Pastor, Reuben, Duran, & Hawkins, 2015). Identification rates of ADHD have consistently been lower in the United Kingdom (1.4%–3%) than in the United States, where different diagnostic criteria are used and underidentification has been hypothesized (Taylor, 2017; Thapar & Cooper, 2016). Studies in other European countries suggest intermediate rates between the United Kingdom and the United States (Taylor, 2017).

Prevalence rates in preschoolers and adults are derived from fewer studies. In preschoolers, prevalence estimates using *DSM-III* (APA, 1980) or *DSM-IV-TR* criteria range from 2%–5.7% (Egger & Angold, 2006) with slightly lower rates (1.9%) in a Scandinavian sample (Wichstrøm et al., 2012). In adults, pooled prevalence estimates are approximately 5% (Willcutt, 2012). These studies were done using *DSM-IV* criteria, and changes to *DSM-5* are likely to result in an increase in prevalence in older adolescents and adults (Dalsgaard, 2013).

In clinic-referred samples, the ratio of boys to girls diagnosed with ADHD ranges from 6 to 1 to 12 to 1, although in community samples that ratio is closer to 2 to 1 in children and 1.6 to 1 in adults (APA, 2013; Biederman et al., 2005). It is presumed that boys are referred more often than girls due to a higher rate of co-occurring aggressive behavior and oppositional and conduct disorders. Girls, on the other hand, may be more likely than boys to be referred because of the inattentive presentation and associated learning and internalizing disorders (mood and anxiety disorders), as well as disordered eating (Quinn, 2008; Rucklidge, 2010).

ADHD is estimated to persist from preschool into childhood, from childhood into adolescence, and from adolescence into adulthood in the majority of cases. The diagnosis is estimated to persist into adulthood in 2%–5% of the population in the United States (Barkley, 2010).

CLINICAL PRESENTATION

The presenting symptoms of ADHD tend to differ with age. During the preschool years, excessive activity level and impulsivity are typically the most prominent symptoms. This is often accompanied by cognitive inflexibility and emotional dysregulation. In combination, these symptoms may lead to impulsive aggression. Given the high activity level and short attention span of the typical preschooler, only children severely affected with ADHD will differ sufficiently from the developmental norm to fully meet the criteria for the disorder. Children in this age group who meet diagnostic criteria for ADHD have a greater rate of developmental delay, intellectual disability, coordination disorder, language disorders, autism spectrum disorder (ASD), and comorbid internalizing and externalizing disorders (Chacko, Wakschlag, Hill, Danis, & Espy, 2009; Smith et al., 2017; Tandon & Pergjika, 2017). In order to make an accurate diagnosis, children who present in the preschool period should be carefully assessed for hearing and vision deficits and the developmental disorders mentioned above, all of which have some similarities in presentation to ADHD (Daley, Jones, Hutchings, & Thompson, 2008). The majority of preschoolers diagnosed with ADHD will continue to meet criteria for the disorder in elementary school (Faraone, Biederman, & Mick, 2006; Lahey et al., 2004; Riddle et al., 2013). Symptom severity, cognitive ability, and family factors are key predictors of persistence into school age (Caye et al., 2016; Cherkasova, Sulla, Dalena, Ponde, & Hechtman, 2013).

Upon entering elementary school, problems with listening and compliance, task completion, work accuracy, and social interactions are common concerns of parents and teachers. Determining whether learning problems are caused by ADHD, coexist with ADHD, or are causing ADHD symptoms is an important component of making the diagnosis and developing a treatment plan in school-age children. While no "foolproof" formula for doing so exists, a careful history about timing and setting of symptoms and response to interventions can help clinicians develop a working hypothesis.

In adolescence, observable hyperactivity may decline significantly (Faraone et al., 2006; Lahey et al., 2005; Riddle et al., 2013). Concerns often focus around work completion, organization, and following rules. Approximately 65% of children with ADHD diagnosed early in childhood continue to meet the criteria for the disorder in adolescence, while an additional group will meet criteria for other specified ADHD or unspecified ADHD because of a reduced number of symptoms. The same factors that predict persistence from preschool into childhood continue to predict persistence into adolescence, with the addition of comorbid externalizing disorders predicting both persistence of ADHD symptoms and degree of impairment (Caye et al., 2016; Cherkasova et al., 2013).

Occasionally, individuals are not diagnosed with ADHD until adolescence, although they must have had symptoms by history that were impairing in childhood in order to meet current diagnostic criteria. Children who were able to cope during the early grades—typically because of low levels of hyperactivity/impulsivity; strong intellectual, social, athletic, or other strengths; and supportive families and school personnel—may present in adolescence. Their attentional/executive systems may finally be overwhelmed by the demands for processing increased volumes of reading and writing as well as the complex social, time management, organizational, and higher-order thinking and language processing skills required of them in high school.

Recent birth cohort studies using questionnaires suggest that a substantial percentage of older adolescents and adults who were not diagnosed with ADHD in childhood had significant symptoms of ADHD at the time of the study, suggesting that there might be an adult-onset form of the disorder (Agnew-Blais et al., 2016; Caye et al., 2016; Moffitt et al., 2015). However, prospective direct evaluation follow-up of a community sample of children without ADHD showed that up to 95% of those who met symptom criteria of ADHD in late adolescence/early adulthood by questionnaire in the absence of a childhood diagnosis had either fluctuations in cognitive symptoms or another disorder that could account for the symptoms, the most common being substance use disorder. Adolescent late-onset cases were often transient and limited to adolescence (Sibley et al., 2018).

Across all age groups, the most common factors predicting persistence into the subsequent age group are severe symptoms of ADHD; treatment for ADHD (which may be a marker of severity); the presence of disruptive behavior, oppositional defiant disorder, conduct disorder, or depression; and a family history of persistent ADHD (Caye et al., 2016; Riddle et al., 2013).

COMMON COEXISTING CONDITIONS

There are several conditions that occur more frequently in individuals with ADHD than in individuals without it, typically referred to as "comorbid" or "coexisting" conditions. Less frequently, another condition mimics ADHD and is the primary cause of inattentive or hyperactive symptoms rather than coexisting with ADHD (see later section in this chapter on the evaluation process). Coexisting conditions are important to identify during an evaluation because 1) they will often require additional or different treatment and, 2) unless treated, they may prevent adequate treatment of ADHD.

More than half of children and adolescents with ADHD presenting to a specialty clinic will have a coexisting disorder, including externalizing disorders (oppositional and conduct disorders), internalizing disorders (mood and anxiety disorders), learning disorders, and tic disorders (Pliszka, 2000; Singer, 2005). Approximately 25% will have more than one coexisting disorder (Jensen & Steinhausen, 2015). In clinical samples, most will have an externalizing behavior disorder, such as oppositional defiant disorder (approximately 60%; characterized by noncompliance and defiance of authority) or conduct disorder (approximately 20%; characterized by more serious antisocial behaviors) (Conner, Steeber, & McBurnett, 2010; Jensen & Steinhausen, 2015). There is an association between hyperactive/impulsive symptoms and oppositionality (Wood, Rijsdijk, Asherson, & Kuntsi, 2009). Estimates of internalizing disorders (anxiety and depression) in ADHD vary considerably from study to study, ranging from 14%–83%. Anxiety disorders occur in approximately 15%–35% of children with ADHD and may include separation anxiety, generalized anxiety, phobic, or obsessive compulsive disorder (OCD; Schatz & Rostain, 2006). Comorbid anxiety and ADHD may lead to increased school problems and functional impairment as compared with either disorder alone (Hammerness et al., 2009a). Depression is relatively common in the general population, with rates of approximately 2% in childhood and increasing to up to as high as 24% in some studies in adolescence. There appears to be an increased risk for unipolar depression in individuals with ADHD, but this varies widely with study design. What is consistent is an increasing risk in adolescence and young adulthood and in those with a family history of depression (Meinzer, Pettit, & Viswesvaran, 2014). Childhood bipolar disorder is difficult to diagnose due to a gradual and less distinct onset of symptoms compared with the symptoms described for adults in the *DSM-5*. Children are likely to have episodic irritability or atypical mood, intermittent explosiveness, psychomotor agitation characterized by talkativeness or motor restlessness, and signs of disordered thinking (Galanter & Leibenluft, 2008). There is evidence that juvenile onset of depression and subthreshold symptoms of depression and mania may be predictors of bipolar disorder in children (Faedda et al., 2015). Bipolar disorder has a lifetime prevalence of approximately 2% in adults, with most reporting onset of symptoms before the age of 18 years (Marangoni, De Chiara, & Faedda, 2015). It is particularly difficult to distinguish from ADHD due to an overlap in several symptoms, especially when internalizing and externalizing disorders coexist with ADHD.

Three main learning disabilities have been studied in relation to ADHD-specific disorders of reading, mathematics, and written language. Disorders of reading (including dyslexia, a disorder of reading at the word reading level) are the most common—and most studied—learning disability. The prevalence of a specific reading disability (RD) among students with ADHD ranges from 25%–48%. Reading disorders and ADHD have both distinct and shared neuropsychological factors that impact the rapid retrieval of linguistic information that is critical for fluent reading. While weak phonological processing and rapid naming are specific to reading disorder, and inattention and poor response inhibition are specific to ADHD, both share features of slow processing speed and weak verbal working memory. Approximately 11%–30% of children with ADHD have comorbid specific mathematics disorders, which may manifest as difficulty with calculation, problem-solving, or both. Math disorders may be related to weak visuospatial working memory in particular.

Approximately 55%–64% of children with ADHD have disorders of written language. In addition to inattention, the higher rates of weakness in visual-motor coordination, fine motor coordination, working memory, organization, and planning seen in ADHD likely contribute to the high rate of comorbidity (Pham & Riviere, 2015).

Tic disorders, including transient, chronic motor, or vocal tic disorder, or Tourette syndrome occur in as many as 20% of school-age children at some point in time, with transient tics being the most common and Tourette syndrome being the least common (Scahill, Specht, & Page, 2014). Tics occur at higher rates in children with ADHD, with about a 20% current (point) prevalence (Schlander, Schwarz, Rothenberger, & Roessner, 2011; Yoshimasu et al., 2012). Conversely, approximately 50% of children with tic disorders have ADHD (Cooke & So, 2016). Tics can occur on a spectrum from mild (which may not even be reported by parents) to the more severe (in which tics have important physical, emotional, and social impact). Group data show no increase in rates of tic disorders in children with ADHD on psychostimulant medications, but these medications may increase tics in specific individuals (Erenberg, 2006). In children with ADHD and Tourette syndrome, ADHD often appears first, and ADHD typically causes greater functional impairment than does the tic disorder (Cooke & So, 2016; Denckla, 2006; Singer, 2005). Persistent tics are often associated with externalizing and internalizing disorders, including obsessive-compulsive disorder as well as ADHD (Kraft et al., 2012; Pollak et al., 2009; Scahill et al., 2014).

In prior editions of the *DSM*, the presence of ASD was an exclusionary criterion for diagnosing ADHD; thus, the two diagnoses could not co-exist. The current edition allows both diagnoses when criteria are met for both. Given the overlap in social deficits and poorly regulated behavior, determining whether ASD is present instead of, or in addition to, ADHD can be difficult; this is discussed further in the later section on evaluation in this chapter. ASD is estimated to be present in 20%–65% of children with ADHD, and ADHD is estimated to be present in 30%–80% of children with ASD (Sokolova et al., 2017; van der Meer et al., 2012). Both genetic and neuropsychological factors (such as inattention, executive dysfunction, motor speed and variability, emotion recognition, and detail-focused processing) likely underlie the high rates of coexistence. It has even been hypothesized that ASD is the severe end of a single diagnostic continuum that includes ADHD, since within a population sample ADHD subgroups with and without ASD symptoms exist but all ASD subgroups have ADHD symptoms (van der Meer et al., 2012).

More severe ADHD symptoms and the male gender are associated with a higher risk of ASD (Green et al., 2015); attention dysfunction (especially maintaining and switching focus) is a particularly important common factor in ADHD and ASD (Sokolova et al., 2017; Visser, Rommelse, Greven, & Buitelaar, 2016). In children with both diagnoses, those diagnosed with ADHD as young children are diagnosed with ASD 3 years later on average, and they are more than 30 times more likely to be diagnosed after age 6 (Miodovnick, Harstad, Sideridis & Huntington, 2015). The highest rate of coexistence occurs in adolescence, likely due to a significant increase in the demands for social adaptability and executive skills during the transition process to independence (Hartman, Geurts, Franke, Buitelaar, & Rommelse, 2016).

Developmental coordination disorder (DCD), defined as a significant impairment in the acquisition and execution of coordinated motor skills leading to impairment in daily activities, is one of the more frequent conditions coexisting with ADHD. Impaired motor coordination can have a significant effect on the acquisition of adaptive, athletic, and writing skills, further impairing daily, social, and academic functioning. Although it is thought to occur in 5%–20% of the childhood population, it is seen in 30%–50% of children with ADHD (Cairney, Veldhuizen, & Szatmari, 2010). Boys are diagnosed two to seven times more often than girls. Core ADHD symptoms such as high activity level, impulsivity, and distractibility, as well as symptoms associated with ADHD, such as variable reaction time, weak working memory, and slow processing speed, can also contribute to difficulties with motor performance. Distinguishing the two etiologies of motor impairments in children with ADHD (secondary versus coexisting DCD) is a subject of ongoing research (Goulardins, Marques, & De Oliveira, 2017).

ASSOCIATED IMPAIRMENTS

Individuals with ADHD often have associated impairments. These may include symptoms that are not related to the core symptoms of ADHD or symptoms of coexisting disorders that do not meet full criteria for a diagnosis. Nonetheless, they can be significantly impairing and may require additional interventions. These include impairments in executive, language, social, academic, and adaptive functions; emotional regulation; and sleep.

Executive functions (EFs; see Chapter 13) include sustaining and shifting attention, being able to hold and manipulate information in order to complete a task (working memory), organizing and prioritizing incoming information, planning ahead, self-monitoring, and inhibiting responses (Martinussen, Hayden, Hogg-Johnson & Tannock, 2005). While ADHD is defined and diagnosed based on the presence of observed behavior, neuropsychological investigations suggest that impairments in executive function based in the frontal/prefrontal cortex may in part underlie the impairments seen in the majority of children with ADHD. Not all children with ADHD have executive dysfunction based on neuropsychological tests, and executive function impairments are not specific to ADHD as they also occur with ASD, learning disability, and depression (Diamond, 2013; Duff & Sulla, 2015; Vilgis, Silk, & Vance, 2015; Weyandt, 2005; Willcutt, Doyle, Nigg, Faraone, & Pennington, 2005). Other neurocognitive characteristics often seen in individuals with ADHD, such as slow processing speed and variability in reaction time, are also associated with symptoms and impairment (Jacobson et al., 2011; Pievsky & McGrath, 2017). Executive functions develop throughout childhood and adolescence, and their rapid development in adolescence may underlie improvements in ADHD in this age group (Satterthwaite et al., 2013).

Language impairments also commonly occur in children with ADHD (Sciberras et al., 2014), although rates vary widely from study to study (Redmond, 2016). Some children have deficits in the structural language components that are commonly tested when language concerns are suspected, such as vocabulary, phonology, semantics, and syntax. Pragmatic language deficits, however, which may not be routinely tested, are even more common and may exist when structural language is in the normal range for age (Green, Johnson, & Bretherton, 2014). Pragmatic deficits may underlie the social difficulties common in children and adolescents with ADHD (Leonard, Milich, & Lorch, 2011) and may include excessive talking, poor conversational turn-taking, and reduced organization of expressive language (i.e., starting in the middle of a narrative, not recognizing the background needed by the listener, poor sequencing of content, and excessive tangential explanation). Difficulty with verbal memory, listening comprehension, and organization of verbal output also occur in children with ADHD, even in the absence of specific language impairments (McInnes, Humphries, Hogg-Johnson, & Tannock, 2003). Impairments in auditory processing can also occur with symptoms of ADHD and contribute to academic underachievement (Dawes & Bishop, 2009).

Academic underachievement is a concern of many parents of school-age children with ADHD, even in the absence of criteria for a learning disability. Inattention, not hyperactivity/impulsivity, is predictive of poorer performance on academic measures (Semrud-Clikeman, 2012). Difficulty reading (most often in the form of problems with fluency, comprehension, or engagement with—and retention of—written material) often occurs in students with ADHD (Friedman, Rapport, Raiker, Orban, & Eckrich, 2017b), even in the absence of a diagnosed reading disability (Ghelani, Sidhu, Jain, & Tannock, 2004; Willcutt, Pennington, Olson, Chabildas, & Hulslander, 2005). Other academic problems commonly seen in children with ADHD include math calculation and applied problem-solving and written expression (Friedman, Rapport, Orban, Eckrich, & Calub, 2017b; Molitor, Langberg, & Evans, 2016).

Problems with writing are especially common in children with ADHD; they are likely due to a combination of difficulties with fine motor control, visual motor integration, inefficiencies in working memory, and impairments of organization and planning. In a study of ADHD and written-language disorder (WLD), the cumulative incidence of written-language disorder in children with ADHD was 64.5% for boys and 57% for girls, compared with 16.5% for boys and 9.4% for girls without ADHD. For both boys and girls with ADHD, the risk of written-language disorder in the absence of a comorbid RD was similar, but interestingly, the risk for written-language disorder was increased for girls with ADHD and reading disability compared with boys with ADHD and reading disability (Yoshimasu et al., 2011).

Executive function impairments, particularly weak working memory, contribute independently from ADHD symptoms to academic difficulties. In fact, weak working memory is emerging as the primary factor related to academic impairment in children and adolescents with ADHD (Friedman et al., 2017b; Jacobson et al., 2011; Kasper, Alderson, & Hudec, 2012; Simone, Marks, Bedard, & Halperin, 2018). It is predictive of academic function, symptom persistence, and degree of impairment (Karalunas et al., 2017; Simone et al., 2018; Sjowall, Bohlin, Rydell, & Thorell, 2017; van Lieshout et al., 2017). Slow processing speed also contributes to academic deficits, best documented for reading skills, but it also has an impact on adaptive skills, anxiety, and social competence (Cook, Braaten, & Surman, 2017).

Many children with ADHD have social difficulties and face peer rejection, an important risk factor for later negative outcomes. Social skill deficits include disruptive and inappropriate social behaviors, deficient social cognition and social problem-solving, and poor emotional regulation (Gardner & Gerdes, 2015). They have difficulty "reading" the nuances of social behavior or inhibiting impulsive responses. They may react excessively or overly negatively to the behavior of others. Some children with ADHD have difficulty initiating or sustaining verbal turn-taking or other reciprocal aspects of peer relations, and they may find themselves passively or actively ignored and without the deeper friendships that older school children begin to develop. They may be inflexible or perfectionistic, leading to "bossiness" with peers. Many children with ADHD tend to overestimate their social competency and don't recognize and adjust their maladaptive behavior (Owens, Goldfine, Evangelista, Hoza, & Kaiser, 2007). As a result, their peers appear to recognize their differences and reject them within a very short time (Sibley, Evans, & Serpell, 2010). Other children with ADHD are acutely aware of their social differences, and their self-esteem suffers as a result. Peer difficulties persist even after reduction in symptoms of ADHD with stimulants or behavioral intervention (Gardner & Gerdes, 2015; Hoza, 2007; Nijmeijer et al., 2007). Peer difficulties are equally problematic in girls with ADHD (Kok, Groen, Fuermaier, & Tucha, 2016), even though they may not have the same rates of externalizing behavior symptoms. Peer rejection persists into adolescence and can lead to further negative outcomes (Mrug et al., 2012).

Sleep problems as well as specific sleep disorders are more common in children and adolescents with ADHD than in their peers (25%–55%; Bioulac, Micoulaud-Franchi, & Philip, 2015). These include behaviorally based insomnia, circadian rhythm disorders, sleep-disordered breathing, and sleep-related movement disorders, including restless leg syndrome/periodic limb movement disorder (Cortese et al., 2013; Tsai, Hsu, & Huang, 2016; see Chapter 28). Parents report more bedtime resistance, sleep-onset difficulty, night awakenings, difficulty with morning awakenings, and daytime sleepiness (Cortese, Faraone, Konofal, & Lecendreux, 2009). Objectively, polysomnograms and actigraphs show increased latency to sleep onset, decreased sleep efficiency, more sleep-stage shifts per hour, and a higher apnea-hypopnea index (Cortese et al., 2009) but not alterations in sleep architecture or REM sleep (Baglioni et al., 2016). Co-existing internalizing conditions, such as anxiety or depression, further increase the risk for sleep problems (Accardo et al., 2012). The relationship between sleep and ADHD is bidirectional—ADHD symptoms can worsen sleep quality and quantity, while reduced sleep quality and quantity can cause or exacerbate ADHD symptoms. The propensity for sleep problems in ADHD may be based on shared genetic and anatomical underpinnings. Genes related to catecholaminergic and circadian rhythms and the dorsolateral and ventrolateral prefrontal and dorsal anterior cingulate cortices have been implicated in both (Cortese et al., 2013). ADHD may contribute to sleep problems via an increased risk for poor sleep hygiene (i.e., difficulty with bedtime routines, use of electronics before bed, difficulty slowing down thoughts or body, and insomnia-related side effects of several medications for ADHD; Cortese et al., 2013). Medications for ADHD have been shown to cause longer sleep latency, worse sleep efficiency, and shorter sleep duration (Kidwell, Van Dyk, Lundahl, & Nelson, 2015). Sleep disorders contribute to or cause ADHD symptoms via excessive daytime sleepiness, while treatment of sleep-disordered breathing with adeno-tonsillectomy may improve ADHD symptoms (Bioulac et al., 2015; Vélez-Galarraga, Guillén-Grima, Crespo-Eguílaz, & Sánchez-Carpintero, 2016).

Children with ADHD also have an increased incidence of problems with motor coordination, which may impair written work in school and social participation in athletic activities (Martin, Piek, & Hay, 2006). Half of children with ADHD will also meet criteria for developmental coordination disorder (DCD), characterized by poor motor performance to a degree that causes functional impairment. Impairments in visual-spatial organization and cerebellar function are thought to be common underlying mechanisms for these two disorders (Piek & Dyck, 2004).

CAUSES OF ADHD

Genetics

The most common etiological factor in the development of ADHD is heredity. Siblings of children with ADHD are between five and seven times more likely to be diagnosed with ADHD than children from unaffected families. Each child of a parent with ADHD has a 25% chance of having ADHD (Faraone et al., 2005; Sharp, McQuillin, & Gurling, 2009). Between 55%–92% of identical twins will be concordant for ADHD, and heritability is estimated at 76% (Faraone et al., 2005). Genetic changes may be as small as single substitutions of one nucleotide in the coding or noncoding region of the DNA for a gene (single nucleotide polymorphisms [SNPs]) or somewhat larger copy number variants (CNVs), which are increased or decreased numbers of copies of a gene or part of a gene (see Chapter 1). Large duplications or deletions of genetic material that inactivate the protein product of a gene are referred to as mutations. A large number of single nucleotide polymorphisms and a small number of copy number variants have been associated with ADHD symptoms. Large mutations do not appear to cause ADHD in isolation, but they do cause genetic syndromes that may include ADHD symptoms as part of a larger clinical phenotype (i.e., fragile X syndrome or 22q deletion syndrome; see Chapters 1 and 15 and Appendix B).

Initially, the search for genetic causes of ADHD focused on specific genes that might be suspected to play a role based on their involvement in the dopamine and norepinephrine neurotransmitter systems.

Dopamine-related genes are candidate genes for investigating the basis for ADHD because evidence from multiple sources indicates that dopamine is involved in the modulation of attention and behavioral regulation in the frontal cortex and its connections, particularly the striatum (see Chapter 8). Norepinephrine is another neurotransmitter that plays an important role in orienting attention and regulating alertness in the frontal cortex and in other areas of the cortex and lower brain. Medications that are effective in ameliorating ADHD symptoms have consistently been shown to affect one or both of these neurotransmitters (Banaschewski, Becker, Scherag, Franke, & Coghill, 2010; Kieling, Goncalves, Tannock, & Castellanos, 2008). In molecular genetic studies of families (linkage analysis), specific **alleles** (common variants of a gene found in a given population) of particular candidate genes have been found to occur at higher frequencies in individuals who have ADHD than can be explained by chance alone. Different alleles tend to be present in those individuals within the family who do not have ADHD. This suggests that specific alleles of these genes may confer susceptibility to ADHD and can be used to identify genes that confer susceptibility to ADHD. More recently, genome-wide association studies (GWAS) have allowed detection of genetic changes associated with ADHD in locations throughout the entire genome, even when the gene at that location is not suspected or when the function of the particular gene in that location is unknown.

Multiple candidate genes, a large number of single nucleotide polymorphisms, and a small number of copy number variants have been associated with susceptibility to ADHD, including genes related to the dopamine, norepinephrine, serotonin, acetylcholine, gamma aminobutyric acid, and glutamate neurotransmitter systems, as well as genes associated with neuronal migration and plasticity, cell adhesion, neurotransmitter release and cell signaling, cell division, and neuroimmunology (Akutagava-Martins, Rhode, & Hutz, 2016; Banaschewski et al., 2010), but none explain a substantial proportion of the risk for ADHD in all but a small number of families. Thus, researchers have begun to explore polygenic risk (the effect of having multiple susceptibility alleles) and pathway analysis (the effect of having multiple susceptibility alleles in a specific functional pathway in the brain). These studies are preliminary, but they support the concept that multiple genes are together involved in one or more of the processes listed above and therefore confer susceptibility to ADHD (Lima et al., 2016; Middeldorp et al., 2016; Mooney et al., 2016).

It has also been shown that there is overlap in the susceptibility genes based on single nucleotide polymorphism analysis across different neuropsychiatric and developmental disorders, with ADHD having a statistically significant overlap with major depressive disorder (Cross-Disorder Group of the Psychiatric Genomics Consortium et al., 2013) and educational underattainment (Shadrin et al., 2018). Having a higher number of susceptibility genes has also been shown to increase the risk for the presence of co-existing conditions and persistence of ADHD symptoms over time (Riglin et al., 2016). In addition, **epigenetic** changes (see Chapter 1), such as increased methylation in genes related to the neurotransmitter systems, can influence the expression of ADHD symptoms. For example, in studies of identical (monozygotic) twins discordant for ADHD, increased methylation of the D4 subtype of the dopamine receptor, rather than single nucleotide polymorphisms or copy number variants, predicted ADHD symptoms (Chen et al., 2018; Dadds, Schollar-Root, Lenroot, & Moul, 2016).

Other Etiologic Factors

Although the most common etiology of ADHD is genetic, other conditions known to affect brain development may result in ADHD symptoms or increase the risk of those genetically at risk for the disorder. These can be grouped into five general categories: 1) specific genetic syndromes, 2) prenatal exposure to toxins, 3) prenatal exposure to maternal metabolic conditions, 4) hypoxia- ischemia, and 5) medical conditions. Rather than directly "causing" ADHD, these risk factors are likely to affect the neuropsychological processes such as memory, temporal processing, response variability, and executive function skills that lead to symptoms of this diagnosis (Seo et al., 2015; Wiggs, Elmore, Nigg, & Nikolas, 2016). These factors increase the risk for other developmental disorders as well, such as autism and decreased IQ. Most studies typically indicate an "association" rather than prove a "cause," and most do not control for all possible associated factors. For example, prematurity may be associated with a higher risk for ADHD via an increased risk for hypoxia-ischemia rather than from the prematurity itself (Sciberras, Mulraney, Silva, & Coghill, 2017).

Genetic syndromes in which ADHD is more common than in the general population include sex chromosome abnormalities (Klinefelter syndrome, Turner syndrome, and fragile X syndrome) and other syndromes that may be inherited or genetic (e.g., neurofibromatosis type 1, Williams syndrome, and the 22q11 deletion syndrome; see Appendix B; reviewed by Lo-Castro, D'Agati, & Curatolo, 2010). Toxins linked to ADHD include prenatal exposures to cigarette smoking, lead (even at low levels; Ha et al., 2009; Nicolescu et al., 2010; Seo et al., 2015; see Chapter 2), alcohol, cocaine, antidepressants (Figueroa, 2010), long-term exposure to acetaminophen (Ystrom et al., 2017), and pesticides (reviewed in Mostafalou & Abdollahi, 2017). Maternal metabolic conditions that are associated with higher rates of ADHD include maternal thyroid disease (reviewed in Fetene, Betts, & Alati, 2017) and possibly maternal high fat diet/obesity (reviewed in Sullivan, Nousen, & Chamiou, 2014). In children with ADHD who do not have a family history, there is an increased incidence of complications during labor, delivery, and infancy (Sprich-Buckminster, Biederman, Milberger, Faraone, & Lehman, 1993). Pregnancy, labor, delivery and perinatal complications, prematurity, and low birth weight have been associated with an increased risk for ADHD in some studies, likely via the shared factor of prenatal or perinatal hypoxia-ischemia (Sciberras et al., 2017; Smith, Schmidt-Kastner, McGeary, Kaczorowski, & Knopik, 2016). Children who undergo surgery for congenital heart disease have alterations in cerebral blood flow, both prenatally and in association with the surgical intervention, and they have a higher risk for subsequent attention problems (Shillingford et al., 2009). Medical conditions associated with a higher risk for ADHD include prenatal and perinatal infection; traumatic brain injury (Chapman et al., 2010; Yeates et al., 2005); nutrient deficiencies such as iron, magnesium, zinc, and vitamin D (Villagomez & Ramtekkar, 2014; reviewed in Wang, Huang, Zhang, Qu, & Mu, 2017); and atopic (allergic) disease (Schans, Cicek, de Vries, Hak, & Hoekstra, 2017).

Structural and Functional Differences in the Brain

Multiple lines of evidence suggest that structural and functional differences exist in the brains of individuals with ADHD. The original study showing widespread differences in brain function, particularly in the prefrontal cortex, was done in adults with childhood-onset ADHD using positron emission tomography (PET) scanning (Zametkin et al., 1990; see Chapter 8). PET scans require the systemic injection of radioactive tracers to label neuronal activity and thus are difficult to justify for routine or repeated use in children. In contrast, magnetic resonance imaging (MRI), which uses a magnetic field and radiowaves to delineate brain structure, is considered safe and noninvasive; many studies of ADHD have used this technology. Volumetric MRI scans have shown important differences in the shape, thickness, and volume of specific brain areas compared with controls in many studies. Six regions have shown consistent differences: 1) the frontal lobes (including the dorsolateral prefrontal cortex and dorsal anterior cingulate cortex), 2) the inferior parietal cortex, 3) the basal ganglia (particularly the right striatum), 4) the corpus callosum (particularly anteriorly), 5) the cerebellum, and 6) the parieto-temporal regions (reviewed in Friedman & Rapoport, 2015; Frodl & Skokauskas, 2012; Mahone et al., 2011; Wyciszkiewicz, Pawlak, & Krawiec, 2017). Studies of the amygdala and hippocampus, part of the limbic system, have also shown anomalies in shape and volume in children with ADHD (Hoogman et al., 2017). Networks in the frontal cortex serve as the "executive center," processing incoming stimuli; connecting to other structures; and coordinating appropriate cognitive, emotional, and motor responses. The cerebellum and basal ganglia are thought to be involved because these areas are critical to motor planning, behavioral inhibition, and motivation. The hippocampus is involved in memory and the amygdala in facial and emotional processing. When compared with controls, these regions are 3%–4% smaller in subjects with ADHD and involve both gray and white matter, and these differences are present early in childhood (Shaw & Rabin, 2009). Longitudinal studies have shown delays in cortical maturation patterns in children with ADHD, resulting in reduced cortical thickness for age (particularly in the prefrontal cortex). Typically, after reaching maximal thickness at 10–14 years of age, a normal process of cortical thinning occurs into young adulthood (Giedd, Raznahan, Alexander-Bloch, Schmitt, Gotay, & Rapoport, 2015). In individuals with remitting ADHD, cortical thinning is reduced, ultimately resulting in cortical thickness similar to controls. Individuals in whom ADHD persists do not show a reduction in the degree of cortical thinning, resulting in a thinner cortex in adulthood (Shaw et al., 2013). Similar longitudinal developmental differences are found in the basal ganglia of children with ADHD (Shaw et al., 2014).

Functional MRI (fMRI) is a noninvasive MRI technique that measures variations in regional oxygen uptake in the brain, which correlates with cellular activity. fMRI studies indicate that subjects with ADHD have hypoactivation of the prefrontal cortex, parietal cortex, cerebellum, and caudate nucleus and that stimulant medication can increase activation in these areas (Casey, Nigg, & Durston, 2007). fMRI also allows detection of networks of brain regions that are activated simultaneously, either at rest or during performance of a task. The default mode network is a group of connected brain regions that become active or inactive simultaneously. This network includes the medial prefrontal, posterior cingulate/precuneus, and temporoparietal cortical areas. The default mode network is active when the brain is "at rest" and must be suppressed in order to initiate a cognitively demanding task. The cognitive control or executive network (including dorsolateral prefrontal, anterior cingulate, anterior insular, supplementary motor, and posterior parietal cortical areas) is activated for demanding cognitive tasks such as using working memory, inhibiting behavior, and cognitive shifting (see Chapter 8 for further information regarding the anatomy and structural organization of the brain). Studies suggest that the default mode network is more strongly connected in children and adults with ADHD, which may make it more difficult to suppress in order to initiate cognitively demanding tasks (Metin et al., 2015; Mohan et al., 2016).

Diffusion-weighted (DW) MRI uses the diffusion of water molecules to illuminate tissue microarchitecture. A specific type of DW-MRI called diffusion tensor imaging is particularly useful for mapping white matter tracts in the brain (see Chapter 8). Studies in children, adolescents, and adults with ADHD have shown differences in white matter tracts connecting fronto-stratial-cerebellar regions, posterior brain regions, and right and left hemispheres (Chen et al., 2016; Tamm, Barnea-Goraly, & Reiss, 2012; Yoncheva et al., 2016). This technique also suggests that ADHD combined and inattentive presentations may have different white matter connectivity characteristics (Ercan et al., 2016; Svatkova et al., 2016). As with volumetric findings, those with persistent ADHD have been shown to have more prominent white matter tract anomalies (Friedman & Rapoport, 2015). Furthermore, differences in white matter microarchitecture have been shown to be inherited (Sudre et al., 2017), providing a link among symptoms, genetics, and brain structure.

Structural and functional imaging scans show convergent findings about the networks of brain regions that function differently in individuals with ADHD across the age spectrum. While they are not yet sufficiently specific to be used diagnostically, this can be anticipated in the not-too-distant future.

THE EVALUATION PROCESS

Evaluating a child for ADHD requires assessment of 1) symptoms of ADHD; 2) different conditions that might cause the same symptoms; 3) coexisting conditions; and 4) any associated medical, psychosocial, or learning issues that may not reach the threshold for a specific diagnosis but may nonetheless influence the treatment plan. In order to cover these four areas, a comprehensive history, physical/neurological examination, and academic assessment must be completed. Findings in these examinations may prompt additional investigations, including consultation from specialists.

The history, generally taken from the parents, with the child's participation depending on age, includes current status and concerns, previous treatments and their effects, prenatal and perinatal events, medical history, developmental, psychiatric and behavioral history, educational course, social and family circumstances, and biological family history for ADHD symptoms and associated disorders. The main pediatric and child psychiatric professional organizations—the American Academy of Pediatrics (AAP) and the American Academy of Child and Adolescent Psychiatry (AACAP)—provide guidelines for the assessment of ADHD, and they both emphasize the importance of adhering to the *DSM* diagnostic criteria. Information from teachers, typically in the form of standardized rating scales, should be included to document impairment in the school setting (AACAP, 2007; AAP, 2011). The medical examination should focus on growth parameters and physical signs of sensory, genetic, chronic medical, and neurologic disorders, as well as mental status, informal communicative ability and insight, and motor skills.

Educational testing (including intellectual, achievement, and processing measures) will be necessary for many children, and it should focus on the careful assessment for learning disabilities, memory and processing problems, and areas of academic weakness that may not meet criteria for a learning disability (see Chapters 13 and 20). Additional support may allow the child to make better academic progress rather than falling further behind. This should include assessments of reading mechanics and comprehension, spelling, mathematical concepts and computation, and writing. Tests of verbal and visual memory and processing efficiency can be useful in identifying reasons for intellectual achievement discrepancies and can inform choices about educational remediation strategies.

Standardized interview formats and rating scales for parents and teachers collect information about symptoms of ADHD and related conditions, comparing the level of symptoms to age- and gender-matched peers, and they assess the level of functional impairment. In addition, rating scales designed for teachers allow the required collection of information from more than one setting. Commonly used rating scales to assess *DSM* ADHD symptoms include the ADHD Rating Scale-5 for Children and Adolescents (DuPaul, Power, Anastopoulos, & Reid, 2016), the Conners-3 Rating Scales (Conners, 2008), the Swanson, Nolan and Pelham (SNAP) rating scale (Swanson et al., 2012), and the Vanderbilt Rating Scale (Collett, Ohan, & Myers, 2003; Pelham et al., 2005; Wolraich et al., 2003).

Structured diagnostic interviews are quite time-consuming and require training for standardized administration; therefore, they are most often used in psychiatric and research settings. Commonly used structured diagnostic interviews include the Diagnostic Interview Schedule for Children (Shaffer Fisher, Lucas, Dulcan, & Schwab-Stone, 2000) and the Kiddie

Schedule for Affective Disorders and Schizophrenia (K-SADS; Kaufman et al., 1997). These allow the exploration of other diagnoses that may be the cause of the child's symptoms or may co-exist with ADHD (Leffler, Riebel, & Hughes, 2015). Broad rating scales, such as the Child Behavior Checklist and Teacher Report Form (Achenbach & Rescorla, 2001) or the Behavior Assessment System for Children (Reynolds & Kamphaus, 2015), may also be used for this purpose (Collett et al., 2003; Pelham et al., 2005).

Because comprehensive information is required, several professionals are typically involved (e.g., physician, psychologist, and teacher). The primary person responsible for formulating the diagnosis and communicating the findings and recommendations to the family must be experienced with the range of coexisting conditions and associated impairments. This person is typically a physician (pediatrician, neurodevelopmental or developmental-behavioral pediatrician, or a neurologist or psychiatrist) or psychologist. Additional professionals, such as speech-language pathologists, occupational therapists, and learning specialists, may be asked to provide input (see Box 19.1). While such a complex evaluation can be coordinated through a primary care setting, there are also a number of barriers related to knowledge, time, resources, and medical/mental health insurance coverage that limit access to a thorough evaluation for many children (Rushton, Fant, & Clark, 2004).

TREATMENT OF ADHD

Most treatment plans for ADHD will include education about the disorder and one or more of the following interventions: behavioral and family counseling, educational interventions, and medication. Often a combination of treatments is used because of the chronicity and multiple types of impairment caused by ADHD (AAP, 2011).

Education About ADHD and Emotional Support for Families

Parents and older children need to learn as much as possible about ADHD to allow them to be effective decision makers and advocates. The clinician can provide some information directly but should also guide the family toward resources such as national support and advocacy organizations, books and online resources, and parent support groups. Growing up with or parenting a child with ADHD can be a significant challenge. Parents and children will need emotional support to perform the difficult work needed to address the symptoms and consequences of ADHD.

BOX 19.1 INTERDISCIPLINARY CARE

The ADHD Team

Physician evaluators of children with attention-deficit/hyperactivity disorder (ADHD) may be primary pediatricians, developmental and behavioral pediatricians, pediatric neurologists, or child and adolescent psychiatrists. Psychologists may also evaluate, diagnose, and make treatment recommendations for children with ADHD. Additional team members who provide invaluable input for diagnosis and treatment include the following:

- The school psychologist is the school team leader who may perform a comprehensive psychoeducational evaluation to determine a student's eligibility for special education services, develop an individualized education program (IEP) if needed, or serve as team leader in developing a Chapter 15/Section 504 accommodation plan if needed in the absence of an IEP.
- The student's teacher is the school team member who will have direct experience with the student's strengths and weaknesses and who may be the first to recognize a student's need for additional intervention in the academic environment. The teacher may have implemented modifications informally and will have knowledge of what has and has not been helpful.
- The speech-language pathologist, occupational therapist, and physical therapist may be involved in the evaluation and treatment of children with language, speech, and fine and gross motor difficulties, respectively, in order to reduce the chance that these impairments will further affect a child's ability to attend to, and complete, tasks that require these skills in school and community settings.
- The behavior specialist may work with other team members to develop a positively oriented behavior support plan.

Behavioral Counseling and Social Skill Intervention

Behavior therapy is the type of counseling intervention with the best documented efficacy in preschoolers (Greenhill et al., 2008; Murray, 2010) and school-age children (DuPaul, Gormley, & Laracy, 2014) with ADHD, especially if there are additional disruptive behaviors (Coates, Taylor, & Sayal, 2015; Eyberg, Nelson, & Boggs, 2008). It involves training parents and teachers in the principles of behavior management that are adapted for a particular child in a particular setting. Behavior therapy changes behavior by altering the antecedents to, or consequences of, the behavior in such a way that it increases the chances that the child will successfully engage in the desired behaviors and reduces the chances that the child will engage in unwanted behaviors (see Chapter 34). Studies also suggest efficacy of behavior therapy in adolescents with ADHD, though there are limited data, and additional psychosocial interventions are more often necessary in this age group (Robin, 2008; Young & Amarasinghe, 2010). Parent/teacher training can also improve parenting skills and the adult–child relationship as well as decrease subsequent child conduct problems (Daley et al., 2014; Williford & Shelton, 2014).

Behavior therapy can be done in individual or group sessions and forms the basis for most parent training and classroom management programs for children with ADHD. Studies have consistently found that these interventions result in at least short-term improvements in the behavior (Pelham & Fabiano, 2008; Young & Amarasinghe, 2010) and homework problems (Langberg et al., 2010) of children with ADHD. A study of a very intensive behavioral intervention that also included social skill building and emotional support found some persistent benefit from this intervention 15 months after the intervention ended (MTA Cooperative Group, 2004a); however, this level of treatment intensity is unlikely to be widely available (Young & Amarasinghe, 2010). Factors that may interfere with successful parent training in behavior management include parental depression or ADHD, high levels of marital discord (Chronis, Chacko, Fabiano, Wymbs, & Pelham, 2004), low maternal parental self-efficacy, and multiple coexisting conditions in the child (van den Hoofdakker et al., 2010). Behavior therapy is the first line of treatment in preschoolers with ADHD, whereas medication treatment with behavior therapy is generally recommended in school-age children (AAP, 2011; Council on Early Childhood, Committee on Psychosocial Aspects of Child and Family Health, and Section on Developmental and Behavioral Pediatrics, 2016).

There is insufficient evidence to recommend family therapy as a specific treatment for core ADHD symptoms (Bjornstad & Montgomery, 2005); however, disruptive behavior can lead to increasingly negative and coercive patterns of parent–child interaction (Deault, 2010). There is some evidence for its effectiveness for families with a defiant adolescent (Robin, 2014). Family therapy can help to mitigate the effects of parenting a child with ADHD on the marital relationship and sibling interactions. It also may be necessary when parents cannot agree on an intervention plan or other family stressors interfere with implementation of a treatment plan.

Cognitive behavioral therapy (CBT) changes behavior by helping individuals to change self-defeating thought and behavior patterns. It is a well-documented treatment for depression and anxiety and has recently been shown to be effective in the treatment of ADHD in adults (Safren et al., 2010; Solanto et al., 2010; Young & Amarasinghe, 2010) and adolescents (Modesto-Lowe, Charbonneau, & Farahmand, 2017). Preliminary evidence in adults with ADHD suggests that CBT may actually enhance white matter connectivity in fronto-parietal and cerebellar networks (Wang et al., 2016). Individual psychotherapy or play therapy may be helpful for children with coexisting mood, anxiety, or self-esteem problems but is not effective in treating the core symptoms of ADHD (Barkley, 2004).

Coaching is an emerging approach to improve the daily functioning of (typically) older teens and adults with ADHD, but there is little empiric research support at this time (Prevatt, 2016). It involves regular meetings between the individual with ADHD and his or her coach to identify executive function impairments leading to problems in daily functioning and to develop systems and strategies to address them. Coaching is most likely to be successful when the individual recognizes the problems and wishes to address them but cannot seem to do it without help. It does not address core symptoms of ADHD, coexisting conditions, or motivational or emotional problems. Coaches are typically psychologists, educators, social workers, or successful adults with ADHD. A positive step in the field has been the development of professional standards and certification procedures (Murphy, Ratey, Maynard, Sussman, & Wright, 2010). Coaching is often done online, allowing access to individuals who may not live near a coach.

Interpersonal difficulties, such as peer victimization (bullying) and social isolation, are common in individuals with ADHD (Hoza, 2007; Nijmeijer et al., 2007) and may result, in part, from the social skill deficits described earlier in this chapter; thus, social skill interventions may be recommended as part of a comprehensive treatment plan. Social skill groups are often conducted in school or other group settings and teach by modeling, practicing, and reinforcing prosocial behaviors. When social skills interventions for children with ADHD are evaluated as a single intervention, however, the results have generally been disappointing (Abikoff et al., 2004; Barkley, 2004; Storebø et al., 2011). It seems that children "know" or can be taught appropriate skills but then do not apply them when needed. The social skills interventions that seem to be the most effective are intensive, sustained, and conducted in naturalistic settings (i.e., at a camp or school, rather than in a clinic) and are combined with parent training in behavior reinforcement (Mikami, Jia, & Jiwon, 2014; Pelham & Fabiano, 2008). See Box 19.2 for more information on the efficacy of behavioral interventions.

Educational Treatment

Behavioral treatments, such as token reinforcement systems, differential teacher attention, daily behavior report cards, and environmental modifications (e.g., preferential seating), are important in the school setting for supporting students with ADHD. However, it has become apparent that these students are at risk for underachievement even when attention is managed with medication or behavior therapy. Interventions aimed at improving study skills, organization, planning, memory and use of memory strategies, and homework completion are often needed, whether provided in a tutoring setting or as part of a school-based educational program (DuPaul, Gormley, & Laracy, 2014). These interventions are particularly relevant in middle school and high school, as the increased demand for executive and study skills can be overwhelming for students with deficits in these areas. While typical students may develop these skills spontaneously as work demands increase, the student with ADHD typically requires both explicit teaching of the skills and behavioral reinforcement for implementing them over extended periods of time (Evans, Langberg, Egan, & Molitor, 2014).

Appropriate school programs are extremely important for children with ADHD, many of whom have coexisting learning disabilities. When children with ADHD are in need of more assistance than is typically provided in the classroom, they may qualify for modification within their general education classes or in special education settings under either Section 504 of the Rehabilitation Act of 1973 (PL 93-112, Section 504) or the Individuals with Disabilities Education Improvement Act of 2004 (IDEA, 2004; PL 108-446); Chapter 33).

A child with ADHD who needs modification of curricular materials, demands, or teaching methods should have an individualized education program (IEP; see sites.ed.gov/idea/). Although ADHD is not one of the disabilities specifically included under IDEA, some children with ADHD will have an IEP under a coexisting condition such as specific learning disability, speech-language impairment, or emotional disturbance. Others will be provided an IEP under the IDEA category of "Other Health Impaired." When a learning disability is present, specific intervention for the learning disability as well as intervention for ADHD are recommended, and this will require an IEP.

A child with ADHD who is less educationally impaired by his or her symptoms may still be eligible

BOX 19.2 EVIDENCE-BASED PRACTICE

Sequencing Medication and Behavioral Interventions for ADHD

In a study of 146 children with attention-deficit/hyperactivity disorder (ADHD), subjects (ages 5–12, 76% male) were randomized to receive a "low dose" of behavioral intervention or extended-release medication. After a minimum of 8 weeks of treatment, insufficient responders were randomized to either a "higher dose" of the same treatment or the other treatment. They were treated and assessed for 1 school year. Those who analyzed the results were blinded. Parents, teachers, and those who provided the treatment and collected data were not. The primary outcome measure was classroom rule violations; secondary outcomes included out-of-class disciplinary events and parent and teacher ratings of disruptive and social behavior. Although a higher percentage of children beginning with behavioral treatment required medication than the reverse (67% vs. 47%), behavioral treatment first resulted in better primary and secondary outcome scores and lower medication dose at the end of the study, as well as better parent attendance at the behavior treatment sessions (Pelham et al., 2016).

for accommodations through a "Section 504 Plan" (www2.ed.gov/about/offices/list/ocr/504faq.html). Accommodations allow the child with ADHD to successfully "access" the regular education environment. These may include (but are not limited to) 1) regular home–school communication; 2) a behavior program to support desired behaviors; 3) a plan to ensure that the student understands and is following through on instructions; 4) modifications of testing time, format, or environment; 5) visual supports for verbal information; 6) an extra set of materials at home; and 7) technological assistance, such as the use of recording devices, recorded books, and a laptop for typing and speech-to-print applications.

Pharmacological Treatment

Stimulant medications are the most effective and commonly prescribed medications for ADHD. Atomoxetine, sustained-release guanfacine, and sustained-release clonidine are the only nonstimulant medications approved by the U.S. Food and Drug Administration (FDA) for the treatment of ADHD. Non–FDA-approved medications that have been used to treat ADHD include antidepressants (bupropion and tricyclics) and immediate-release or short-acting guanfacine and clonidine. There is emerging evidence that combination therapy with extended-release guanfacine and stimulant medication can be helpful in children with suboptimal response to monotherapy (Childress, 2012; McCracken et al., 2016). See Chapter 38 and Appendix C for information on medication formulations, dosages, and side effects.

Stimulant Medication Stimulant medications, including methylphenidate and amphetamine (see Table 19.2), have been used for the treatment of children with disruptive behaviors for over 70 years and have been more frequently used and more thoroughly studied than any other psychopharmacologic treatment in children. According to data collected from the National Survey on Children's Health in the United States, approximately 70% of children diagnosed with ADHD take medication, with 3.5 million children being treated overall (Visser et al., 2015). Stimulants are statistically more effective than nonstimulant options (Coghill et al., 2017) and appear to work equally well regardless of gender or *DSM* subtype, with treatment initiated more in boys and for combined or hyperactive/impulsive subtypes (Barbaresi et al., 2014). Preschoolers appear to have a somewhat less beneficial-effect/side-effect ratio than older children (see later section titled Stimulants in Preschoolers). There is some evidence that pharmacogenomics may aid in treatment decision making as studies show that dose response of stimulants (Stein et al., 2014) as well as side effects are linked to neuroreceptor genotype (Levy, Wimalaweera, Moul, Brennan, & Dadds, 2013). Various pharmacogenetic testing kits are available, but there is limited evidence for their clinical value.

Beneficial Effects Stimulant medications significantly reduce symptoms in 70%–90% of children and adolescents correctly diagnosed with ADHD (Wigal, 2009). They result in a rapid and often dramatic improvement in attention and distractibility and a decrease in impulsivity and hyperactivity. In addition, they improve academic productivity and accuracy, improve parent–child interactions, and decrease aggression. Teacher ratings of behavior, as well as the child's quality of life, improve with stimulant treatment (Punja et al., 2016; Storebø et al., 2015), and stimulants improve driving performance in adolescents and young adults with ADHD (Gobbo & Louzã, 2014). Stimulants may also have positive effects on academic achievement (Lu et al., 2017), although these are modest compared with their effects on behavior, indicating that additional interventions are needed in these areas (Jitendra, DuPaul, Someki, & Tresco, 2008; MTA Cooperative Group, 2004a, 2004b; Raggi & Chronis, 2006). The positive effects of stimulants on executive function appear to be in the areas of attention and response inhibition (Pauls et al., 2012) as well as working memory, reaction time, and variability (Coghill et al., 2014). Children with more severe executive function impairments show an increased response to stimulant treatment of ADHD symptoms (Hale et al., 2011; Kubas, Backenson, Wilcox, Piercy & Hale, 2012). Stimulants have "normalizing" effects on biological parameters that differentiate individuals with ADHD from their peers including activation patterns in the frontal cortex using fMRI (Rubia, Alegria, & Brinson, 2014), cortical-striatal-cerebellar attentional networks, basal ganglia surface morphology, and event-related brain (electrical) potentials (Bush et al., 2008; Ozdag, Yorbik, Ulas, Hamamcioglu, & Vural, 2004; Rubia et al., 2011; Sobel et al., 2010).

However, although beneficial effects on behavior have been very clearly demonstrated in short- to intermediate-term studies, long-term studies show no significant long-term reduction in symptoms (Swanson et al., 2017). It should also be noted that response to stimulant treatment is not diagnostic of ADHD, since individuals with other psychiatric or developmental disorders, and even individuals with typical development and mental health, display similar effects when given stimulant medication (Rapaport et al., 1978).

Table 19.2. Stimulant medications commonly used to treat attention-deficit/hyperactivity disorder

Brand name	Generic name of active medication	Usual duration of action (hours)	Dosages available (milligrams)	Other
Ritalin	D,L-methylphenidate	3–4	Tablets–5, 10, 20	
Focalin	D-methylphenidate	3–4	Tablets–2.5, 5, 10	Contains only the active isomer of methylphenidate; typical dose is half that of D,L-methylphenidate
Focalin XR	D-methylphenidate	8–12 (12 for 20-mg dose)	Capsules–5, 10, 20, 30	Capsule can be opened and sprinkled
Methylin	D,L-methylphenidate	3–4	Tablets–2.5, 5, 10 Suspension–5 mg/5 ml and 10 mg/5 ml	Tablets are grape flavored and chewable
Metadate CD	D,L-methylphenidate	6–8	Capsules–10, 20, 30, 40, 50, 60	Capsule can be opened and sprinkled; 30% of dose immediately released
Ritalin LA	D,L-methylphenidate	6–8	Capsules–10, 20, 30, 40, 50, 60	Capsule can be opened and sprinkled; 50% of dose immediately released
Concerta	D,L-methylphenidate	10–12	Capsule–18, 27, 36, 54	Must be swallowed whole; 22% of dose immediately released
Daytrana	D,L-methylphenidate	Up to 12	Patch–10, 15, 20, 30	Duration depends on timing of removal
Aptensio XR	D,L-methylphenidate	8–10	Capsule – 10, 15, 20, 30, 40, 50, 60	40% released immediately; capsule can be opened and sprinkled
Quillivant XR	D,L-methylphendiate	10–12	Oral suspension–25 mg/5 mL	20% immediate release
Quillichew ER	D,L-methylphendiate	6–8	chewable tablet–20, 30, 40	20% immediate release
Cotempla XR	D,L-methylphenidate	8–10	Orally disintegrating tablet–8.6, 17.3, 25.9	25% immediate release
Dexedrine	Dextroamphetamine	3–6	Tablet–5	
Dexedrine Spansules	Dextroamphetamine	6–8	Capsule–5, 10, 15	
Adderall	Mixed salts of amphetamine	3–6	Tablets–5, 7.5, 10, 12.5, 15, 20, 30	
Adderall XR	Mixed salts of amphetamine	8–10	Capsule–5, 10, 15, 20, 25, 30	Capsule can be opened and sprinkled; 50% of dose immediately released
Vyvanse	Lisdexamfetamine	12	Capsule–20, 30, 40, 50, 60, 70	Inactive until lysine cleaved from amphetamine in the gastrointestinal tract
Dynavel XR	D,L-amphetamine	10–12	Oral suspension–2.5-mg amphetamine base/mL	Each mL is the equivalent of 4 mg amphetamine salt
Procentra	Dextroamphetamine sulfate	4–6	Oral solution 5 mg/5 mL	Immediate release, bubble gum flavoring
Zenzedi	Dextroamphetamine sulfate	3–6	Tablet–2.5, 5, 7.5, 10, 15, 20, 30	Immediate release
Evekeo	D,L-amphetamine	4–6	Tablet–5, 10	BID dosing; immediate release
Adzensys XR	D,L-amphetamine	6-8	Tablet–3.1, 6.3, 9.4, 12.5, 15.7, 18.8	Orally disintegrating tablet; 50% immediate release and 50% extended release
Mydayis	Mixed salts of amphetamine	12–16	Capsule–12.5, 25, 37.5, 50	Extended release; approved for age 13 and older only

Formulations Methylphenidate and amphetamine come in a variety of formulations (see Table 19.2). The beneficial effects and side effects of these two types of stimulants are nearly identical, although 30%–40% of children may respond better to one medication than the other (May & Kratochvil, 2010). A few meta-analyses indicate that amphetamine may improve symptoms to a slightly greater degree than methylphenidate, but these studies did not take tolerability into account (Faraone & Buitelaar, 2010; Stuhec, Munda, Svab, & Locatelli, 2015). Amphetamine-based stimulants are typically given at one half to two thirds the dose of the methylphenidate-based stimulants to account for differences in the potency of the two medications. Likewise, dex-methylphenidate, the isolated, more effective d-isomer, has approximately twice the potency of d,l-methylphenidate and is given at approximately half the dose. Lisdexamfetamine is the only prodrug formulation, requiring cleavage of the attached lysine by gastrointestinal enzymes for activation.

The onset of action of immediate-release forms of methylphenidate and amphetamine is usually within 30 minutes of taking the dose. Based on the technology used to extend the duration of release, different formulations vary in how much of the medication is released immediately and time to onset, how the remainder is released (in a later bolus versus continuously), and duration of effect. Although Table 19.2 gives the typical duration of effect for the various formulations, there is significant variation among individuals. The methylphenidate patch is the only formulation that gives individuals the capacity to vary the duration of action on a daily basis (up to 10 hours) based on the timing of patch removal (Noven Therapeutics, LLC—http://www.daytrana.com/). There have been studies looking at the comparative efficacy of stimulants; however, the methods used for direct comparison of these studies have been inconsistent. The efficacy of stimulants varies based on pharmacokinetics and desired timing of positive effects; therefore, the formulation should be based on the needs of the individual (Coghill et al., 2013). For example, stimulants that release 50% of medication immediately (e.g., Ritalin LA, Focalin XR) seem to be more effective in the first four hours of treatment than OROS methylphenidate (e.g., Concerta), which is 33% immediate release.

Side Effects The most common adverse effects of stimulants are decreased appetite, headaches, stomachaches, growth, and sleep problems (Clavenna & Bonati, 2017; May & Kratochvil, 2010). As headaches, stomachaches, and sleep problems are common in untreated children with ADHD, it is important to determine the nature and frequency of these symptoms prior to starting the medication. The relationship of ADHD with sleep disturbances is explored in detail earlier in this chapter. There is an association with long-acting methylphenidate and sleep problems (Kidwell et al., 2015) with mixed results, as preexisting sleep problems show some improvement on higher doses (Becker, Froehlich, & Epstein, 2016).

Decreased appetite, weight loss, and abdominal pain are the most commonly reported gastrointestinal adverse effects in children (Holmskov et al., 2017). Decreased appetite is the most common adverse effect, but it is typically limited to lunchtime hours, with compensation at breakfast and dinner. Fewer children have more extensive appetite suppression and weight loss. These children may benefit from caloric and nutrient supplementation to prevent weight loss and maintain adequate nutrition, or they may be able to eat in between doses of shorter-acting formulations. Appetite suppression and abdominal pain will prevent some children from tolerating stimulants; however, this common adverse effect may be relieved by adjusting the dose or changing stimulant type (Wolraich, McGuinn, & Doffing, 2007). It may be that the minority of children who experience abdominal discomfort have an underlying gastrointestinal condition that renders them prone to related side effects, such as gastroesophageal reflux, gastritis, or other inflammatory conditions. Treatment of the underlying condition may then allow such children to tolerate pharmacologic treatment for ADHD.

Less common, but potentially more problematic side effects include "rebound" effects, tics, and social withdrawal. *Rebound* refers to a temporary worsening of symptoms, including irritability, increased activity, or mood swings, when the medication wears off. Although it is estimated that 30% of school-age children experience some rebound effects, they are significant enough to require altering the medication regimen in only about 10% of cases (Carlson & Kelly, 2003). Preliminary results suggest that some young adults may have increased driving errors during rebound (Cox et al., 2008). Some children do become withdrawn on stimulant medication. This may improve with dose adjustment or switching to another medication. The best ways to mitigate medication side effects is an area that has not been systematically researched and is typically based on common clinical experience rather than scientific evidence.

Tics have been reported to occur in approximately 10% of children treated with stimulants (Lipkin, Goldstein, & Adesman, 1994), but they have also been reported in a similar percentage of community control samples (22% of preschoolers, 8% of elementary school children, and 3.4% of adolescents; Gadow & Sverd, 2006). Early reports suggested that stimulants induced or exacerbated tics (Gadow & Sverd, 2006; Palumbo, Spencer, Lynch, CoChien, & Faraone, 2004), but recent meta-analyses indicate that this is less common than originally thought (Cohen et al., 2015; Pringsheim & Steeves, 2011). In addition, tics that appear to be stimulant induced or exacerbated usually subside with time, after the dose is reduced, or when treatment is discontinued. In rare cases, tics that appear to have been induced by stimulants do not resolve or may even worsen over time. Given that tics and ADHD commonly co-occur (Denckla, 2006; Gadow & Sverd, 2006), it is possible that those individuals whose tics appear to be induced by stimulants have a biological predisposition to develop tics. Clonidine, guanfacine, and atomoxetine (discussed below) can be alternative treatments in this population (Pringsheim & Steeves, 2011; Rizzo, Gulisano, Cali, & Curatolo, 2013).

Growth velocity slows by approximately 1.2 centimeters per year on average in prepubertal children during at least the first 2 years of continuous treatment with stimulants (MTA Cooperative Group, 2004b). In one study by Swanson and colleagues (2006), in preschoolers growth was 20% less and weight gain 55% less than expected over the first year of treatment. However, when school-age children were followed for up to 3 years, the slowed growth rates tended to stabilize, although growth rebound did not occur (Swanson et al., 2007).

Adult research suggests that stimulants can trigger activation of mania or psychosis in individuals with comorbid bipolar disorder if untreated (Viktorin et al., 2017). Research on children is limited in this area. Cardiovascular side effects secondary to sympathomimetic effects are more commonly part of anticipatory guidance with medication treatment of ADHD in pediatric use. Recent studies show no significant difference in QTc interval (an increased QTc interval on an electrocardiogram has been associated with increased risk of cardiac arrhythmias; Lamberti et al., 2015) with stimulant use, although an increase in pulse (heart rate) and blood pressure is still significant (Hennissen et al., 2017; Vitiello et al., 2012). In children without underlying cardiac abnormalities, recent research is conflicting, with some studies suggesting that cardiac adverse effects are rare and not associated with stimulant use (Olfson et al., 2012; Shin, Roughead, Park, & Pratt, 2016), while others suggesting an increase in adverse effects with stimulant use (Dalsgaard, Primdal Kvist, Leckman, Skyt Nielson, & Simonsen, 2014). Significant adverse effects are so rare that they should prompt an investigation for underlying medical causes that may be exacerbated by the medication. The FDA and Health Canada have recommended that stimulants not be used in individuals with known heart disease, including structural heart problems, rhythm abnormalities, and hypertension. Relevant professional organizations in pediatrics, psychiatry, and cardiology are in agreement about the importance of a careful personal and family history for risk factors for sudden death. These include palpitations, syncope or near-syncope, the presence of congenital structural abnormalities, hypertrophic cardiomyopathy, Marfan syndrome, long QT syndrome, and Wolff-Parkinson-White syndrome. During treatment, there should be regular monitoring of interim cardiovascular history, including concomitantly used medications with cardiovascular effects and pulse and blood pressure checks (Vetter et al., 2008; Warren et al., 2009). In the absence of risk factors or symptoms, the value of additional screening and cardiac assessment or monitoring is unclear and controversial at this time.

Potential for Substance Abuse and Diversion

Stimulants are classified as controlled substances by the Drug Enforcement Agency (DEA). There is increased monitoring of controlled substances due to recent increases in abuse and diversion of both stimulants and opioids. Most states have implemented prescription monitoring programs to limit diversion of medications while supporting access for appropriate medical use (www.deadiversion.usdoj.gov/faq/rx_monitor.htm).

When injected or taken intranasally, stimulants can produce a "high." However, when taken as directed, oral stimulants for ADHD do not induce euphoria or dependence due to their relatively slow uptake into the brain (Volkow & Swanson, 2003). The use of slow-release forms, in which the medication is mixed with other substances and released slowly, makes abuse even less likely to occur (Faraone & Upadhyaya, 2007). Lisdexamfetamine is also less likely to be abused as it is a prodrug, which requires processing in the GI tract, and is unable to be inhaled or used intravenously.

While prescribed stimulants are relatively ineffective for producing euphoria, diversion of stimulants for staying awake for prolonged periods of study or other activities is much more common in both college and high school students (Clemow & Walker, 2014). Approximately 17% of college students report using stimulants that are not prescribed to them for ADHD in this manner (Benson, Flory, Humphreys, & Lee, 2015). Coaching adolescents about managing their medication before they go to college and providing anticipatory guidance about how they will manage requests from peers to share their medication are important aspects of clinical practice for prescribing physicians. Use of medication contracts to encourage appropriate use of stimulants and deter diversion is another option for prevention (Colaneri, Keim, & Adesman, 2017).

In adolescents, a clinical diagnosis of ADHD is correlated with higher rate of substance abuse and substance use disorders (Charach, Yeung, Climans, & Lillie, 2011; Lee, Humphreys, Flory, Liu, & Glass, 2011), particularly with comorbid conduct disorder (Harty, Ivanov, Newcorn, & Halperin, 2011). However, treatment with stimulant medication does not increase this risk (Molina et al., 2013), and it may lower the long-term risk of substance use (Quinn et al., 2017).

Given the high rate of comorbidity of ADHD and substance abuse, physicians need to consider how to best treat such individuals. Current recommendations include psychosocial treatments for both ADHD and substance abuse, careful monitoring, and pharmacological treatment of ADHD with a nonstimulant. However, when nonstimulants are ineffective, the use of a long-acting stimulant, which is less likely to be abused, can be considered (Harstadt, Levy, & Committee on Substance Abuse, 2014).

Initiating and Monitoring Therapy Medication should be only one part of a comprehensive treatment plan that may include behavior therapy and parent training (AAP, 2011). Considerations regarding medication include duration of coverage needed, specific targets for improvement, and any previous treatment experience. In most circumstances, a stimulant is used as a first-line agent (AAP, 2011). School day (8–9 hours) or 12-hour coverage options exist in both stimulant categories. Immediate-release products lasting 3–5 hours may be helpful in several circumstances. They can be used when 12-hour coverage isn't required (for example, on weekends). They may be given after school on certain days to extend the duration of effect (especially to help with after school activities such as homework or sports). They are also sometimes used in the morning to take advantage of their rapid onset when the long-acting formulation being used reaches an effective level too slowly to be effective for the beginning of the school day.

Optimal dose is determined by the effectiveness and side effects profile and is best determined by a dose titration protocol so that a variety of dosage levels can be evaluated. During a dose titration protocol, it is important for parents, students, and teachers to have sufficient opportunity to observe for effects and side effects and to provide feedback. This may be difficult in preschoolers if they do not have a teacher or other outside care provider or with adolescents as they may have multiple teachers during the day (AAP, 2011). Typically, a new medication or dose will be started on the weekend so that parents can monitor their child before sending him or her to school, and then each dose will be monitored for a week. Standardized rating scales should be obtained before starting and at the end of the week on each dose. Most standardized rating scales focus on the core symptoms of ADHD or *DSM-5* criteria. It is also helpful to obtain feedback about functional changes in the areas of completion of activities of daily living, quality of social interaction, and academic accuracy and productivity. When parent and teacher rating scale results do not agree, it is important to consider reasons for this. It may signal additional diagnoses or symptoms and the need for additional interventions such as parent training or specialized instruction. If a child does not respond or has significant side effects on one stimulant, it is reasonable to try a stimulant from the other class (methylphenidate versus amphetamine; AACAP, 2007). Sometimes a child will show a better response to one formulation or release pattern over another, even within the same stimulant category, and some children who do not tolerate or respond to either stimulant category may respond to a nonstimulant such as atomoxetine or guanfacine (see discussion below). Certain side effects, such as prominent tics, significant anxiety, and persistent irritability, may lead to consideration of a nonstimulant trial or medication combination. Lack of response to a series of rationally considered trials should prompt a reevaluation of the diagnosis, evaluation for coexisting conditions, and an assessment of compliance and other medical or psychosocial factors that may interfere with effective treatment.

School achievement, behavior, relationships, mood, vital signs, and growth velocity should be monitored at baseline, after medication or dose adjustments, and at regular intervals (typically every 3–6 months) to ensure continued beneficial responses and the absence of significant adverse effects. No specific laboratory tests are indicated as part of the monitoring. Clinical history and exam may lead a clinician to order tests to rule out abnormalities that may coexist, exacerbate symptoms, limit effectiveness of medication treatment, or relate to observed side effects. These include ferritin (an iron-binding protein to rule-out iron deficiency anemia) and thyroid hormone levels, a celiac panel, sleep study, electroencephalography (EEG), and bone age x-ray. During childhood it is important to periodically assess whether medication is still effective. Since most children will continue to benefit throughout their school years, it is important to consider with parents and teachers how to best do such an assessment without substantially compromising the student's functioning.

As children become adolescents and young adults, additional targets for medication management become important that make a longer duration of coverage relevant. These include more hours spent doing homework and extracurricular activities, after-school jobs, the requirement for social decision making with increasingly serious implications, and the need for consistent concentration while driving. Driving performance (but not knowledge) has been shown to be impaired in individuals with ADHD, and effective medication treatment has been shown to improve performance (Gobbo & Louzã, 2014).

Stimulants in Preschoolers Stimulants have been used increasingly in children 3–5 years of age, although rates of medication use have stabilized since guidelines for treatment of ADHD in preschoolers were released by the AAP in 2011 (Fiks et al., 2016). Current guidelines recommend behavioral therapy as the first-line treatment for preschool ADHD, although only a small percentage of families enrolled in one large multisite study of ADHD treatment in more severely affected preschoolers felt that it was sufficient (Greenhill et al., 2006). Dextroamphetamine is the only FDA-approved stimulant for children in this age range. Although methylphenidate has been studied more frequently than dextroamphetamine or mixed salts of amphetamine in preschool children with ADHD, methylphenidate is not FDA approved for children under 6 years of age. The range of effective doses in mg/kg is similar to that found in school-age children, but the percentage of preschool children with a beneficial response may be slightly lower than in elementary school-age children, and side effects, particularly adverse emotional reactivity and growth rate reductions, may be more common (Kratochvil, Greenhill, March, Burke, & Vaughn, 2004; Swanson et al., 2006; Wigal et al., 2006). In a study by Vitiello and colleagues (2007), effectiveness was maintained over 10 months of follow up, but an almost 50% dose increase was required.

Typically, immediate-release methylphenidate up to three times daily has been the treatment regimen used in most studies; there is little information about the use of long-acting formulations in preschoolers. Preliminary open-label studies suggest effectiveness for a longer-acting beaded methylphenidate formulation (Maayan et al., 2009), but further research has been limited. There are few studies on the use of nonstimulants in this age range.

Nonstimulant Medications for ADHD Between 10%–30% of children with ADHD will not benefit from stimulants or will have adverse side effects that preclude their use. Nonstimulant medications may be helpful in this group. These medications fall into three categories: norepinephrine reuptake inhibitors, antidepressants, and alpha-2-adrenergic agonists.

Norepinephrine Reuptake Inhibitors Atomoxetine (e.g., Strattera) is the only norepinephrine reuptake inhibitor that is FDA approved for the treatment of ADHD (in individuals 6 years of age and over). It is effective in reducing ADHD symptoms compared with placebo and is not inferior to stimulant medications (Gayleard & Mychailyszyn, 2017; Shang, Pan, Lin, Huang, & Gau, 2015). A comprehensive review of atomoxetine trials in children, teens, and adults has demonstrated that atomoxetine improves parent and teacher ratings of attention and decreases their ratings of hyperactivity and impulsivity at doses of 1.2–1.4 mg/kg/day (Bushe & Savill, 2014; Savill et al., 2015; Schwartz & Correll, 2014). There is no clear benefit to increased-dose or twice-daily dosing in children with ADHD only (Waxmonsky, Waschbusch, Akinnusi, & Pelham, 2011), but benefits persist in the absence of serious adverse effects for 2–4 years (the longest duration thus far reported) without development of tolerance or progressive ineffectiveness over time (Donnelly et al., 2009; Garnock-Jones & Keating, 2009; Kratochvil et al., 2006). It is effective for ADHD in children and adolescents with a variety of coexisting conditions and does not worsen (or may improve) coexisting symptoms, including tics and anxiety (Garnock-Jones & Keating, 2009) and oppositional defiant disorder (Dittman et al., 2011). Nonetheless, it does not appear to be more effective in children with internalizing disorders than those without internalizing disorders (Scott, Ripperger-Suhler, Rajab, & Kjar, 2010). Preliminary evidence suggests that the benefits of atomoxetine may exceed effects on core ADHD symptoms to include improvements in reading and executive function skills (Adler, Clemow, Williams, & Durell, 2014; Maziade et al., 2009; Wehmeier et al., 2012). There are some studies that have suggested improvement in endorsement of core ADHD symptoms in preschool-age children (Ghuman et al., 2009a), but functional and clinical improvement were less apparent (Kratochvil et al., 2011).

Atomoxetine may take a few days before one begins to see effects and several weeks to reach the maximum effect. Similarly, beneficial effects may dissipate gradually when it is discontinued, and some children remain improved over baseline (Buitelaar et al., 2007); there is no adverse effect of abrupt discontinuation (Wernicke et al., 2004). It is generally given once daily in the morning but can be given twice daily to extend coverage into the evening. Fatigue and gastrointestinal upset are relatively common side effects, but atomoxetine is unlikely to cause sleep disturbance.

Gastrointestinal upset is typically prevented by giving the medication with food; foods containing protein or fat are particularly effective for this purpose. Some children experience weight loss during the first few months of treatment, but the average reduction in height and weight percentiles is generally maximal after 18 months of continued use. The loss is about 2% at 2 years and is resolved by 5 years in all except the largest children (Spencer et al., 2007). Growth effects can occur with atomoxetine but do not appear to be clinically significant over longer time periods. In a 5-year prospective study, maximal growth decrements occurred in the second year of treatment. Weight was 9.9 percentile points below that expected at 15 months of treatment, and height was 6.6 percentile points below expectations at 18 months. At 5 years, average height and weight percentiles were similar to the starting values for the majority of children. Some children who were above the mean for weight or height initially remained at lower percentiles at 5 years (Spencer et al., 2007).

Other side effects include dizziness, irritability, somnolence, and allergic reactions. Increases in pulse and blood pressure do occur, but these are typically not clinically significant. Other, more significant cardiovascular events have not been reported. Prescribing information includes a black box warning about the increased risk of suicidal ideation; thus, monitoring for depression, mood instability, and behavioral activation is critical.

Atomoxetine is metabolized by cytochrome P450 (CYP2D6), a system of liver enzymes important in the metabolism of many drugs, and levels may be affected in individuals who are rapid or slow metabolizers and by other medications that inhibit CYP2D6. Although genotyping for these variants is not currently a routine practice, dose reduction should be considered in those with prominent early side effects (ter Laak et al., 2010) or those taking another medication that is a CYP2D6 inhibitor, such as a selective serotonin reuptake inhibitor (SSRI; Sauer, Ring, & Witcher, 2005). A recent review of safety reported that incidents of hepatotoxicity are rare in children and adolescents treated with atomoxetine (Reed et al., 2016).

Antidepressants Several types of antidepressants have been found to be effective in children with ADHD, although they are not FDA approved for this purpose. A recent *Cochrane Review* of tricyclic antidepressants (TCAs) in children (including desipramine and nortriptyline) reported that the TCAs improve ADHD symptoms in children compared with a placebo, although they were not as effective as stimulants for most children (Otasowie, Castells, Ehimare, & Smith, 2014). Using a TCA may also be indicated when there are significant side effects from other medications or when there is an increased risk for substance abuse/diversion.

Compared with stimulants, TCAs have advantages that are like those of atomoxetine. They have a longer duration of action, low abuse potential, and tend not to exacerbate tics. However, they have many more potentially problematic cardiovascular, neurologic (tingling, incoordination, tremors) and anticholinergic (blurred vision, dry mouth) side effects that limit their use. Drug levels should be checked, as there can be large individual differences in metabolism of these medications (Banaschewski et al., 2004). Electrocardiograms must be obtained at baseline and monitored for cardiovascular changes. Overdoses can be lethal, and a few cases of sudden death, presumably from cardiac arrhythmias, have occurred in children taking appropriate doses of desipramine, although causality could not be clearly established (Popper, 2000).

Bupropion is a chemically distinct antidepressant whose precise mechanism of action in ADHD treatment remains unknown. It is a weak dopamine and norepinephrine reuptake inhibitor; this may explain its benefit. It has been shown to improve ADHD symptoms in both children and adults. Beneficial effects may be detected as early as 3 days after initiation of treatment, but maximum effects may not be seen until 4 weeks of treatment (Conners et al., 1996). On average, the magnitude of the effects is similar to or slightly less than those of stimulants (Jafarinia et al., 2012; Maneeton, Maneeton, Srisurapanont, & Woottliluk, 2011), but side effects are more commonly reported with methylphenidate (Mohammedi, Hafezi, Galeiha, Hajiaghaee, & Akhondzadeh, 2013). Gastrointestinal complaints, drowsiness, and rashes are the most common side effects with bupropion; insomnia can also occur. Bupropion treatment is associated with a slightly increased risk of drug-induced seizures (about 4 per 1,000 individuals). The use of high doses, a previous history of seizures, and the presence of an eating disorder seem to increase the risk for seizures. Bupropion also may exacerbate tic disorders. Both sustained- and extended-release formulations have been shown to provide extended symptom control throughout the day in adults (Maneeten, Maneeten, Srisurapanont, & Martin, 2014; Wilens et al., 2005).

Alpha-2-Adrenergic Agonists The alpha-2-adrenergic agents clonidine and guanfacine have been used for the treatment of ADHD since the 1980s. Clonidine has also been used for aggression and insomnia (Banaschewski et al., 2004). Short-acting guanfacine and clonidine are not FDA approved as treatment for ADHD but have been used off-label. However, in 2009, the FDA approved a long-acting form of guanfacine (Intuniv) for the treatment of ADHD in children and adolescents. Recent Phase 3 trials have shown extended-release guanfacine to be effective in reducing ADHD symptoms (Hervas et al., 2014; Wilens et al., 2015). This is true both as monotherapy and as adjunctive therapy with stimulants. There is no difference between morning and evening administration of extended-release guanfacine (Newcorn et al., 2013). As with other medications that affect primarily the noradrenergic system, clonidine and guanfacine do not tend to exacerbate tics and may reduce them (Bloch, Panza, Landeros-Weisenberger, & Leckman, 2009). Disadvantages of the immediate-release forms of these medications include 1) sedation and dry mouth, 2) rapid peaking of levels, and 3) decreased compliance as a result of the need for frequent dosing (reviewed in Sallee, 2010). The most common side effects are somnolence, headache, and fatigue, but they tend to subside over time (Faraone & Glatt, 2010; Hervas et al., 2014; Wilens et al., 2015). Cardiovascular changes have been noted to be mild and not clinically significant. Open-label continuation of treatment has demonstrated safety and effectiveness for up to 2 years (Biederman et al., 2008; Sallee et al., 2009). Although there is a theoretical concern about rebound hypertension with abrupt discontinuation, this was not found in a study of abrupt discontinuation in healthy young adults (Kisicki, Fiske, & Lyne, 2007). A clonidine patch changed weekly has been available since 1984, although it is not FDA approved for the treatment of ADHD. In 2010, a twice-daily, extended-release clonidine tablet (Kapvay; Shionogi, Inc.) was approved for use in children and adolescents ages 6 to 17. Clinical trials support the safety and efficacy of extended-release clonidine for the treatment of ADHD symptoms as both monotherapy (Jain, Segal, Kollins, & Khayrallah, 2011) and adjunctive therapy with stimulants (Kollins et al., 2011).

TREATMENT WITH COEXISTING CONDITIONS

Treatment of Children with ADHD and Intellectual Disability

ADHD can be diagnosed in the presence of intellectual disability when inattention or hyperactivity and impulsivity exceed expectations for the child's delayed developmental level and cause additional functional impairment. Studies suggest that methylphenidate can be effective for ADHD symptoms and cognitive task performance in preschoolers and school-age children with intellectual disability; however, they have a lower response rate (around 50%) and an increased risk for side effects, such as stereotypic behavior and emotional lability (Deutsch, Dube, & McIlvane, 2008; Ghuman et al., 2009b; Handen & Gilchrist, 2006). The likelihood of a positive response does not appear to be related to IQ or autistic features (Simonoff et al., 2013). Young children with an intellectual disability are more likely to be prescribed a nonstimulant (Osunsanmi & Turk, 2016). Atomoxetine does have positive effects on ADHD symptoms based on a recent review (Aman et al., 2014), but lower IQ may decrease efficacy of treatment (Mazzone, Reale, Mannino, Cocuzza, & Vitiello, 2011). An initial double-blind, placebo-controlled study of guanfacine in a small number of children with intellectual disability, autism, or both who previously failed methylphenidate treatment showed improvements in hyperactivity and aberrant behavior but not in attention (Handen, Sahl, & Hardan, 2008). Atypical antipsychotics, particularly risperidone (Risperdal), may also be helpful for hyperactivity and disruptive behaviors in children with intellectual disability (Filho et al., 2005; Handen & Gilchrist, 2006; Olfson, Crystal, Huang, & Gerhard, 2010); however, there are few studies using double-blind, placebo-controlled methods (Thompson, Maltezos, Paliokosta, & Xenitidis, 2009). An open-label study in children and adolescents showed continued effectiveness for up to 2 years (Reyes, Croonenberghs, Augustyns, & Eerdekends, 2006). The development of metabolic syndrome (the combination of obesity, hypertension, high cholesterol, and high blood sugar levels) is a significant risk with the use of atypical antipsychotics (Weiss et al., 2009; see Chapter 38).

Treatment of ADHD and Autism Spectrum Disorder

Older studies of children with autism suggested that the benefit to side effects ratio of stimulants (primarily methylphenidate) was not sufficient to warrant their use in this population; however, newer studies show positive effects (Abanilla, Hannahs, Wechsler, & Silva, 2005). Since a higher IQ is associated with better response, more recent inclusion of individuals with milder autism spectrum symptoms and higher IQ may have shifted the results.

In one study, extended-release methylphenidate was shown to improve hyperactivity, impulsivity, and inattention in children with ASD compared with a placebo, with both parents and teachers noting positive effects that were highly concordant (Pearson et al., 2013). Positive effects have also been reported on attention to social interaction and self-regulation (Jahromi et al., 2009). However, methylphenidate does not appear to help rigidity or stereotypic behavior, and an increased susceptibility to side effects has been noted compared with the rates seen in children with ADHD in the absence of ASD or intellectual disability (Handen, Johnson, & Lubetsky, 2000).

A randomized, controlled trial (RCT) showed modest improvements in ADHD symptoms with atomoxetine in 6–17 year olds with ASD, with no serious adverse effects (Harfterkamp et al., 2012). Extended-release guanfacine was found to be effective for treating ADHD symptoms in children with ASD, with minor side effects on pulse and blood pressure noted during one RCT (Scahill et al., 2015). Earlier studies showed similar modest effects with clonidine for ADHD target symptoms with ASD (Jaselskis, Cook, Fletcher, & Leventhal, 1992), but more recent studies in this population are limited. If using these medications, clinicians must be vigilant for both positive and negative changes in behavior, as well as physical side effects.

Atypical antipsychotics such as risperidone and apriprazole have been shown to improve irritability, aggression, and stereotyped behavior in children with autism (Arnold et al., 2010; Marcus et al., 2011; McDougle et al., 2005). Risperidone may improve hyperactivity (Posey, Stigler, Erickson, & McDougle, 2008) and impulsivity as well (Lemmon, Gregas, & Jeste, 2011). Positive behavioral effects were noted in long-term studies as well (Kent, Hough, Singh, Karcher, & Pandina, 2013). There is less evidence for effectiveness of antidepressants, anxiolytics, and mood stabilizers (Aman, Farmer, Hollway, & Arnold, 2008).

Treatment of ADHD and Externalizing Disorders (Oppositional Defiant Disorder and Conduct Disorder)

Individuals with ADHD and conduct disorder are at much higher risk of developing substance abuse or antisocial personality disorder and of being involved in criminal activity than individuals with ADHD alone (Turgay, 2009). Oppositional defiant disorder and conduct disorder are difficult to treat (see Chapter 27), but they typically respond best to comprehensive approaches involving both behavioral interventions and medication (Reale et al., 2017). About 60% of individuals with oppositional defiant disorder will develop conduct disorder (Turgay, 2009).

Pharmacologic studies may evaluate individuals with oppositional defiant disorder and conduct disorder separately or as one experimental group. Furthermore, some studies identify the characteristic of aggression rather than a specific diagnosis as the independent variable. The term *externalizing disorders* will be used hereafter to refer to all of these conditions collectively.

Individuals with ADHD and externalizing disorders respond well to stimulants for their ADHD symptoms. In addition, the externalizing symptoms are likely to improve, so stimulants should be considered the first-line pharmacologic treatment for externalizing disorders with ADHD (Pringsheim, Hirsch, Gardner, et al., 2015). When children with aggression appear to be stimulant nonresponders, a systematic, carefully monitored titration protocol to identify the optimal dose—in combination with behavior therapy—may show sufficient improvement up to 50% of the time to support continued stimulant monotherapy (Blader, Pliszka, Jensen, Schooler, & Kafantaris, 2010). Atomoxetine has been shown to be equally efficacious for ADHD symptoms with or without additional externalizing disorders (Dell'Agnello et al., 2009), and recent comparison studies show that it is as effective as stimulants for the treatment of comorbid externalizing symptoms (Garg, Arun, & Chavan, 2015). Both stimulants and atomoxetine have a small but finite risk of exacerbating depression, mood lability, or aggression, so these symptoms should be monitored with regular follow-up visits. Extended-release guanfacine has also been shown to be effective for treating ADHD and reducing externalizing symptoms (Connor, Steeber, & McBurnett, 2010; Wilens et al., 2015), with less evidence demonstrated for clonidine monotherapy (Connor et al., 2010; Ming, Mulvey, Mohanty, & Patel, 2011). Additional medications that demonstrate effectiveness for some individuals with externalizing disorders include mood stabilizers (such as lithium or divalproex sodium), SSRIs, and atypical antipsychotics (Loy, Merry, Hetrick, & Stasiak, 2017; Nevels, Dehon, Alexander, & Gontkovsky, 2010; Pliszka et al., 2006). Medication combinations may eventually prove to be most useful for this group of children, but they require further study before they can be FDA approved (McBurnett & Pfiffner, 2009; Spencer, 2009).

Treatment of ADHD and Internalizing Disorders

The treatment of children with ADHD and anxiety can be challenging because the ADHD core symptoms may not respond as well to methylphenidate (Ter-Stepanian, Grizenko, Zappitelli, & Joober, 2010) or because anxiety may be exacerbated by stimulants. Recent studies have found a reduction in social phobia and separation anxiety in children with comorbid ADHD that are treated with stimulants (Golubchik, Golubchik, Sever, & Weizman, 2014; Golubchik, Sever, & Weizman, 2014). Although anxiety may inhibit impulsivity, it also may make working memory impairments worse (Schatz & Rostain, 2006). Psychosocial intervention such as CBT has been shown to be particularly efficacious in children with coexisting anxiety disorders and may be a critical component of treatment in this group of children (Houghton, Alsalmi, Tan, Taylor, & Durkin, 2017; MTA Cooperative Group, 1999b). One algorithm derived by expert consensus (The Texas Children's Medication Algorithm) recommends initiating treatment with a stimulant and then adding an SSRI if anxiety does not improve sufficiently when the ADHD symptoms are treated effectively (Pliszka et al., 2006). Atomoxetine has been shown to be effective in children with ADHD and comorbid anxiety (Hutchison, Ghuman, Ghuman, Karpov, & Schuster, 2016) and may allow some children to be treated with one rather than two medications. When symptoms of depression are present, the more severe disorder should be treated first, with an SSRI being used for depression and a stimulant for ADHD (Pliska et al., 2006). Other antidepressants that also treat ADHD symptoms (TCAs and bupropion) are options if a stimulant is not tolerated or is not effective. The finding that SSRIs and other antidepressants can increase suicidal ideation in individuals with depression underscores the need for close monitoring even with newer agents (Hetrick, McKenzie, Cox, Simmons, & Merry, 2012).

Treatment of ADHD with Tic Disorders

Although the presence of tics or a personal or family history of Tourette syndrome are listed as contraindications to stimulant use by the pharmaceutical companies that manufacture these medications, this stance appears to be unnecessarily restrictive (see Side Effects). ADHD symptoms may cause much more functional impairment than do tics and thus be the priority for treatment (Denckla, 2006; Pringsheim & Steeves, 2011). Most children do not have significant tic exacerbations in response to therapeutic stimulant doses (Cohen et al., 2015). Nonstimulant medications (atomoxetine, guanfacine, and clonidine) can be tried first and may improve existent tics (Bloch et al., 2009). TCAs may also treat ADHD without inducing or exacerbating tics, but their safety profile is a limitation. If stimulants are the only effective medication and do exacerbate tics, the addition of guanfacine or clonidine is recommended (AACAP, 2007). If these are not effective, risperidone or pimozide may be used for tic suppression (Pliszka et al., 2006), along with newer atypical antipsychotics, such as aripiprazole, which have shown improved efficacy with fewer side effects. The antiepileptic medication topiramate may also be an effective tic suppressant, though further study is needed (Yang et al., 2016).

Treatment of ADHD with Medication Combinations

As described previously, it is common for individuals with ADHD to have one or more coexisting conditions. Medications approved for the treatment of ADHD do not typically address the coexisting symptoms, with some exceptions—atomoxetine may have positive effects on anxiety (Kratochvil et al., 2005; Spencer, 2009) and oppositional defiant disorder (Dittman et al., 2011), and alpha-adrenergic agonists may improve aggression (Connor et al., 2010; Sallee, 2010) and tics (Bloch et al., 2009; Pliszka et al., 2006).

Combinations of methylphenidate with alpha-adrenergic agonists (Kollins et al., 2011; Wilens et al., 2012), SSRIs, (Spencer, 2009), atomoxetine (Kratochvil et al., 2005; Wilens et al., 2008), and atypical antipsychotics have all shown some benefit for individuals with ADHD and coexisting conditions (Sallee, 2010; Spencer, 2009). However, there are limited data on combination pharmacological treatments in children with ADHD (Catalá-López et al., 2017). Preliminary investigation indicates that atomoxetine with fluoxetine is a safe and effective combination for ADHD with coexisting anxiety or depressive symptoms. The safety information is important given that both medications are substrates for P450–CY2D6 liver metabolism (Kratochvil et al., 2005). In addition, there is evidence for a combined efficacy of atomoxetine and stimulants (Ozbaran, Kose, Yuzuguldu, Atar, & Aydin, 2015), but larger studies are needed as adverse effects can be more common (Hammerness et al., 2009b). Despite increasing evidence for effectiveness and the widespread need for optimal management of ADHD with coexisting conditions, there are only two recent FDA-approved medication combinations for ADHD or ADHD with coexisting conditions, sustained-release clonidine (Kapvay; Shionogi, Inc.) and sustained-release guanfacine (Intuniv; Shire, Inc.) with a stimulant.

ALTERNATIVE THERAPIES

Elimination diets, nutrient supplementation, and brain training techniques are the most frequently studied alternative treatments for ADHD. Recently, benefits of aerobic exercise and mindfulness meditation have also been reported. Dietary treatments include three different approaches: the elimination of certain foods or additives, nutrient supplementation, and the provision of a "high-quality," whole-foods diet that decreases additives and increase nutrients. The two most commonly identified additive-free diets are the Feingold Program (elimination of artificial colors and flavors; the preservatives BHA, BHT, and TBHQ; and naturally occurring salicylates found in some fruits and vegetables), and a British version (elimination of artificial colors and the preservative sodium benzoate). There are, in fact, no accurately designed studies of the Feingold diet. Studies in the early 1970s, which purported to test this hypothesis, contained methodological flaws that would have minimized positive results. Nonetheless, 10%–20% of children were noted to respond, and preschoolers were noted to have a much higher response rate (Bateman et al., 2004; Kaplan, McNichol, Conte, & Moghadam, 1989). Studies focusing on the role of artificial colors and sodium benzoate in the general population of children in the United Kingdom (not selecting for those identified as having ADHD-related symptoms) have revealed small, but significant detrimental effects of these substances on the behavior of 3-year-old and 8- to 9-year-old children (Bateman et al., 2004; McCann et al., 2007). The adverse effect of additives in a subgroup of children in this study was moderated by polymorphisms in histamine degradation genes, suggesting that histamine response may play a role in the effects of additives on behavior (Stevenson et al., 2010). Meta-analyses of double-blind, placebo-controlled elimination diet trials have found positive effects, though with relatively small effect sizes (Nigg, Lewis, Edinger, & Falk, 2012; Pelsser, Frankena, Toorman, & Pereira, 2017; Schab & Trinh, 2004; Sonuga-Barke et al., 2013), likely due to significant response in a relatively small subgroup of subjects. In the future, it will be important to elucidate the factors that predict response as well as underlying mechanisms (Nigg & Holton, 2014).

The elimination of specific foods may also improve ADHD-related symptoms. Commonly allergenic foods are typically most often implicated, and in past studies the children who reacted to these foods also reacted to artificial colors (Carter et al., 1993; Egger, Carter, Graham, Gumley, & Soothill, 1985; Schmidt et al., 1997). A recent controlled, though not blinded, study of this approach in young children with ADHD resulted in an approximately 50% improvement on parent and teacher ADHD rating scales (Pelsser et al., 2009). The mechanism for this observation is unknown, but case reports documented improvement in ADHD symptoms when IgG-mediated food reactions were eliminated (Ritz & Lord, 2005). However, there are no well-controlled studies at this time. The elimination of sugar has not been found to be an effective intervention (Wolraich, Wilson, & White, 1995). It is important to note that elimination of high salicylate fruits and vegetables (in the Feingold Program) or allergenic foods (in an oligoantigenic diet) are not meant to be long-term practices, but rather following a 2- to 6-week full elimination, individual foods are added back singly to identify specific triggers. Most children do not need to eliminate all of the potential triggers. These diets can be nutritionally adequate for children who eat a variety of foods, but children who eliminate multiple foods for extended periods might benefit from consultation with a knowledgeable dietitian to ensure that appropriate substitutes are chosen to ensure adequate long-term nutrient intake.

Children with ADHD have been shown to be relatively deficient in iron, zinc, magnesium, and vitamin D (Bener, Kamal, Bener, & Bhugra, 2014; Sharif, Madani, Tabatabaei, & Tabatabaee, 2015; Wang, Huang, Zhang, Qu, & Mu, 2017), but treatment studies have shown limited effects (Hariri & Azadbakht, 2015; Lange et al., 2017). Studies of multinutrient supplementation, however, have shown positive effects under randomized, blinded, placebo-controlled conditions in both adults (Rucklidge, Frampton, Gorman, & Boggis, 2014) and children (Rucklidge, Eggleston, Johnstone, Darling, & Frampton, 2017) with ADHD. In children, attention, emotional regulation, aggression, and overall function improved, but hyperactive-impulsive symptoms did not. "Megadoses" of vitamins or minerals can have toxic effects and are not recommended.

Levels of polyunsaturated fatty acids (PUFAs), including the omega 3s, docohexanoic acid (DHA) and ecosapentanoic acid (EPA) and the omega 6s, arachidonic acid (AA), and gamma-linoleic acid (GLA), are lower in children with ADHD than controls (Montgomery, Burton, Sewell, Spreckelsen, & Richardson, 2013). Omega-3s are important components of neuronal cell membranes, and omega-6s are important in cell-to-cell signaling in the brain and periphery. Supplementation has shown positive effects, with small effect sizes, when a combination of the three anti-inflammatory PUFAs (EPA, DHA, and GLA) have been used in adequate doses for a sufficient length of time (reviewed in Cooper, Tye, Kuntsi, Vassos, & Asherson, 2016; Derbyshire, 2017; Gillies, Sinn, Lad, Leach, & Ross, 2013; Hawkey & Nigg, 2014). While adding PUFAs to effective methylphenidate treatment does not appear to provide additional benefit, one study indicates that children who do not have a good response to methylphenidate may respond to PUFAs (Perera, Jeewandara, Seneviratne, & Guruge, 2012). Recently, the FDA approved a combined omega-3–phosphatidylserine product as a medical food (Vayarin; Vaya Pharmaceuticals), which has been found to be effectively incorporated into brain cell membranes (Vaisman et al., 2008). It has shown positive effects in children with ADHD, but only in a subgroup; thus, overall effect sizes are small. This and other studies suggest that oppositional and emotional dysregulation symptoms may respond more so than core ADHD symptoms (Cooper et al., 2016; Manor et al., 2012). Since children with ADHD appear to be deficient due to altered metabolism of PUFAs rather than decreased intake (Colter, Cutler, & Meckling, 2008), initial measurement of PUFA levels, followed by individualized treatment, may be a more appropriate way to assess the effects of supplementation. For example, a recent study in which EPA treatment alone did show positive effects also found higher levels of arachidonic acid (an omega-6 EFA) among responders (Gustafsson et al., 2010).

There is an association between unhealthy diets and more symptoms related to ADHD (and other childhood disorders) when children are exposed prenatally and during early childhood (Jacka et al., 2013) and a two-fold risk for diagnosis of ADHD in adolescence when children follow a diet that is higher in fat, saturated fat, and sugar than recommended (Howard et al., 2011). Similarly, the risk for ADHD correlates inversely with adherence to the Mediterranean diet (low in processed foods and sugars and high in fruits, vegetables, fish and olive oil; Ríos-Hernández, Alda, Farran-Codina, Ferreira-García, & Izquierdo-Pulido, 2017). While these studies demonstrate an association between these differing diets and risk for ADHD, it is possible that dietary differences may be a consequence of, rather than cause of, ADHD symptoms. Further research is needed to establish a causative role of these diets in the genesis of ADHD symptoms. Overall, science is moving in the direction that supports a "clean," whole-foods based diet with adequate nutrients and healthy fats for ADHD as well as for other mental health conditions.

Several techniques that "train" brain activity with the goal of improving attention and working memory are under investigation. EEG biofeedback is the treatment that has been studied most extensively. Quantitative EEG studies indicate that subjects with ADHD have a lower level of alpha and beta brain waves, which are associated with alert, thinking states, and a higher level of theta and delta waves, which are associated with drowsiness. EEG biofeedback uses computer technology to train the individual to produce more of the brain wave patterns associated with concentration and to suppress those associated with overarousal or underarousal (Monastra, 2008). There is some evidence for effectiveness in improving ADHD symptoms and computerized measures of attentional control, but this tends to be stronger when control subjects have no treatment (rather than sham treatment) and are therefore not blinded (Holtmann, Sonuga-Barke, Cortese, & Brandeis, 2014). Persistence of treatment effects at 6 months is inconsistent (Geladé et al., 2017; Gevensleben et al., 2010) as is generalization of improved EEG measures to improved task performance (Janssen et al., 2016). Some recent randomized controlled trials found positive effects in combination with medication (González-Castro, Cueli, Rodríguez, García, & Álvarez, 2016; Lee & Jung, 2017), which require further investigation. It has been proposed that differences in specific training, duration of treatment, and outcome measures may contribute to inconsistent results. It has also been proposed that combining future neurofeedback studies with functional MRI may help to clarify the impact of neurofeedback training on brain activity in specific regions during task performance, which may provide insight into variable results (Sitaram et al., 2017).

Computerized working memory training is the next most frequently studied brain training approach. Studies of this approach also show somewhat inconsistent results, with some showing significant positive effects on a range of outcomes including memory, executive skills, and behavior (Farias et al., 2017), while others show modest effects (Kirk, Gray, Ellis, Taffe, & Cornish, 2017) or no significant effects at all (Hitchcock & Westwell, 2017). Reviews indicate that improvements are stronger for the specific trained skill (working memory) than for more applied skills (academic achievement and ADHD symptom control), and effects are smaller when treatment and control groups are blinded to the intervention (Rapport, Orban, Kofler, & Friedman, 2013; Robinson, Kaizar, Catroppa, Godfrey, & Yeates, 2014; Sonuga-Barke, Brandeis, Holtmann, & Cortese, 2014). Studies show task-dependent enhancement of brain activation in expected regions after training, and, as with neurofeedback, these neurophysiologic measures may be used in future studies to help clarify inconsistencies in outcome among current studies (Hoekzema et al., 2010; Stevens, Gaynor, Bessette, & Pearlson, 2016). While brain training approaches may be beneficial for some students, the current consistency and quality of evidence does not allow for a uniform recommendation for these treatments, which can be time-intensive and costly.

Aerobic exercise appears to provide benefits, not only for core symptoms of ADHD, but also for social, emotional, and behavioral outcomes as well as some cognitive/executive function and motor skills. The quality and consistency of studies does not allow the development of a specific exercise prescription at this time, however, and it should be considered an adjunctive intervention (Cerrillo-Urbina et al., 2015; Hoza, Martin, Pirog, & Shoulberg, 2016; Kamp, Sprlich, & Holmberg, 2014; Tan, Pooley, & Speelman, 2016). Mindfulness meditation can strengthen attentional control, and there is preliminary evidence for benefits for individuals with ADHD (Cassone, 2015).

OUTCOME

Symptoms of ADHD decline over time, and rates of persistence vary widely depending on methodology, with about 30%–50% showing persistence of the disorder and over 60% showing persistence of some symptoms (Caye et al., 2016). Unfortunately, even with a reduction in core symptoms, longitudinal follow-up studies indicate that functional impairments persist (Lee, Sibley, & Epstein, 2016).

Compared with their peers, young adults with ADHD have lower educational and employment performance and attainment; fewer friendships and more social problems; poorer driving records; and a higher chance of sexually transmitted disease, unplanned pregnancy, injuries, and even mortality (Dalsgaard, Ostergaard, Leckman, Mortensen, & Pedersen, 2015; Fischer, Barkley, Smallish, & Fletcher, 2007; Loe & Feldman, 2007; Wehmeier, Schacht, & Barkley, 2010). Youth with ADHD are also at higher risk for emerging coexisting conditions in their young adult years, including antisocial behavior, substance abuse, mood, anxiety, and eating disorders (Groenman, Janssen, & Oosterlaan, 2017; Klein et al., 2012; Nazar et al., 2016; Yilmaz et al., 2017). Inattention predicts poor academic outcome, but hyperactivity tends to predict the antisocial behavior and other adverse outcomes (Sasser, Kalvin, & Bierman, 2016). The presence of conduct disorder predicts some of the most severe outcome risks, including failure to graduate from high school, early sexual activity and parenthood, antisocial behavior, and substance use (Barkley et al., 2006; Caye et al., 2016).

Understanding the factors that result in the suboptimal outcomes faced by youth with ADHD is hampered by the difficulty in performing well-controlled, prospective, long-term studies. The heterogeneity in ADHD symptoms and trajectories also hamper outcome studies. For example, studies show that there are subsets of children with low levels of symptoms that remain stable, symptoms that decline or even resolve over time, and high levels of symptoms that remain high (Sasser et al., 2016). Childhood predictors of persistent symptoms into adulthood include the severity of symptoms in childhood (Caye et al., 2016) as well as several factors that predict poorer outcomes for all children, including lower IQ, the presence of other mental health conditions, limited family resources, marital problems, and decreased parental monitoring/involvement (Roy et al., 2017). Biological factors associated with persistence and severity of ADHD in population studies include the **polygenic risk score** and pattern of cortical development. A large number of gene variants confer risk for ADHD, and having a larger number of these (i.e., a higher polygeneic risk score) is correlated with baseline symptom severity, symptom persistence, and more comorbid diagnoses (Riglin et al., 2016). Different sets of genes are related to baseline severity and persistence (Pingault et al., 2015). Longitudinal imaging studies suggest that atypical cortical development is evident in those individuals with persistent or worsening trajectories, while a pattern of cortical development that is more similar to controls was seen in those with declining/remitting symptoms (Shaw et al., 2013).

When children receive evidence-based treatment, including medication and psychosocial interventions, there are also different response trajectories. The MTA study has been the largest clinical trial of ADHD treatments to date (MTA Cooperative Group, 1999a). It was a prospective multisite treatment study of 576 children with ADHD combined presentation (ADHD-C) between the ages of 7 and 9 years. Children were randomized into one of four treatment groups: medication management, intensive behavioral treatment, medication and intensive behavioral treatment, and standard community care. After 14 months of treatment, they returned to community treatment; the participants were then followed prospectively for 16 years (Hechtman et al., 2016).

In this study, there were three patterns of initial response to treatment: 1) About 34% of the subjects showed an initial mild improvement that gradually increased over time, 2) about 52% showed an initial substantial improvement that was maintained over time, and 3) about 14% had an initial substantial improvement and then deteriorated over time. Long-term outcomes paralleled initial treatment responses regardless of the specific treatment (Hechtman et al., 2016). The second group had the most favorable outcome. They were less impaired at baseline, had less psychosocial adversity, and were more frequently in the medication or combined treatment groups. The third group had the poorest outcome. They had increased severity at baseline, lower IQs, decreased social skills, more coexisting conditions, and more psychosocial risk factors.

Across studies, subgroups with a trajectory of resolving or declining symptoms have a lower level of negative outcomes than those with persistent symptoms. Those with resolving symptoms may not differ from controls in terms of mood and anxiety disorders and substance use (Hechtman et al., 2016), but they still have poorer educational and employment outcomes (Barkley, 2016).

Unfortunately, treatment with the evidence-based interventions of medication and behavior therapy, while showing robust short-term benefit, does not consistently translate into improved long-term outcomes. The initial benefit of medication treatment in the MTA study did not appear to hold up over time, even in those who remained on medication (Swanson et al., 2017). It must be noted, however, that there is a very limited number of studies of long-term medication or psychosocial treatments. It must also be acknowledged that, in the MTA study, those who remained on medication or continued to receive psychosocial treatment in the community most likely had the severest symptoms. There is, however, evidence for a positive impact of medication treatment on academic achievement when children, adolescents, and young adults are actively taking medication (Lu et al., 2017; Scheffler et al., 2009). There is also a positive impact on driving safety (Chang et al., 2017), injuries (Man et al., 2017), and hospital contacts (Dalsgaard, Nielson, & Simonsen, 2014), as well as a likely reduction in substance abuse (Quinn et al., 2017) and criminality (Dalsgaard et al., 2014).

Improvements in social, educational, employment, and mental health outcomes are not as well documented, and they are also harder to measure. Some studies do show positive outcomes that last beyond short-term treatment. The MTA study showed positive effects of combined psychosocial and medication treatment in children with coexisting disorders, especially anxiety disorders, and improved outcomes with treatment for children with the most psychosocial disadvantage (Swanson et al., 2008). There also appears to be a benefit from pharmacologic, nonpharmacologic, and combined treatment on measures of self-esteem and some measures of social function (Harpin, Mazzone, Raynaud, Kahle, & Hodgkins, 2016).

It has been theorized that current evidence-based treatments may not sufficiently sustain, generalize, or affect key areas of functional impairment because they do not fully target the neurocognitive and functional skills deficits associated with ADHD (Chacko, Kofler, & Jarrett, 2014). There is some evidence for improved functional outcomes with skill-based training for children and adolescents. This includes organizational and study skills in combination with parent training in the provision of reinforcements for using learned skills (Abikoff et al., 2013; DuPaul et al., 2014; Evans et al., 2014) as well as for cognitive behavior therapy in young adults (Weiss et al., 2012). These approaches are only beginning to be widely used, and, unfortunately, sustained treatment is not widely accessible. It remains to be determined whether the combination of skill-based, sustained, and intensive psycho-social-educational treatments with medication and biological optimization (nutrition and sleep and stress management) can improve long-term outcomes for children with ADHD.

SUMMARY

- ADHD is a prevalent neurodevelopmental condition that has a significant impact on the lives of affected children, their families, and the educational and medical/mental health systems.
- The core features of ADHD (difficulty sustaining mental effort, hyperactivity, and impulsivity) lead to impairment in academic, occupational, social, and adaptive functions without effective intervention.
- Coping with ADHD is made more complicated by commonly coexisting conditions, including learning disorders, oppositional defiant disorder, and anxiety disorders.
- ADHD is highly genetic, but adverse conditions in the prenatal and perinatal period can contribute to symptoms. Multiple lines of evidence suggest a biological basis involving frontal cortical, basal ganglia, and cerebellar pathways and biogenic amine neurotransmitters, particularly dopamine and norepinephrine.
- Treatments for ADHD include counseling, with a particularly focus on behavior management, accommodations in the classroom, addressing coexisting conditions, and medication.
- Additional treatments, including dietary modifications, exercise and meditation, training in study/organizational and executive function skills, and cognitive therapy, in adults warrant further investigation.
- Our increasing recognition of the complexity and uniqueness of each child with ADHD, as well as increasing options for treatment, offer children growing up with ADHD the opportunity to experience success.

ADDITIONAL RESOURCES

A.D.D. WareHouse: http://www.addwarehouse.com

Attention Deficit Disorder Association: http://www.add.org

CHADD (Children and Adults with ADHD): http://www.chadd.org

Additional resources can be found online in Appendix D: Childhood Disabilities Resources, Services, and Organizations (see About the Online Companion Materials).

REFERENCES

Abanilla, P. K., Hannahs, G. A., Wechsler, R., & Silva, R. R. (2005). The use of psychostimulants in pervasive developmental disorders. *Psychiatric Quarterly, 76,* 271–281. doi:10.1007/s11126-005-2980-7

Abikoff, H., Gallagher, R., Wells, K. C., Murray, D. W., Huang, L., Lu, F., & Petkova, E. (2013). Remediating organizational functioning in children with ADHD: Immediate and long-term effects from a randomized controlled trial. *Journal of Consulting and Clinical Psychology, 81*(1), 113–128. doi:10.1037/a0029648

Abikoff, H., Hechtman, L., Klein, R. G., Gallagher, R., Fleiss, K., Etcovitch, J., & Pollack, S. (2004). Social functioning in children with ADHD treated with long-term methylphenidate and multimodal psychosocial treatment. *Journal of the American Academy of Child & Adolescent Psychiatry, 43,* 820–829. doi:10.1097/01.chi.0000128797.91601.1a

Accardo, J. A., Marcus, C. L., Leonard, M. B., Shults, J., Meltzer, L. J., & Elia, J. (2012). Associations between psychiatric comorbidities and sleep disturbances in children with attention-deficit/hyperactivity disorder. *Journal of Developmental and Behavioral Pediatrics, 33,* 97–105.

Achenbach, T. M., & Rescorla, L. A. (2001). *Manual for the ASEBA School-Age Forms & Profiles*. Burlington: University of Vermont.

Adler, L. A., Clemow, D. B., Williams, D. W., & Durell, T. M. (2014). Atomoxetine effects on executive function as measured by the BRIEF-A in young adults with ADHD: A randomized, double-blind, placebo-controlled study. *PLoS One, 9*(8), e104175. doi:10.1371/journal.pone.0104175

Agnew-Blais, J. C., Polanczyk, G. V., Danese, A., Wertz, J., Moffitt, T. E., & Arseneault, L. (2016). Evaluation of the persistence, remission, and emergence of attention-deficit/hyperactivity disorder in young adulthood. *JAMA Psychiatry, 73*(7), 713–720. doi:10.1001/jamapsychiatry.2016.0465

Akutagava-Martins, G. C., Rohde, L. A., & Hutz, M. H. (2016). Genetics of attention-deficit/hyperactivity disorder: An update. *Expert Review of Neurotherapeutics, 16,* 145–156. doi:10.1586/14737175.2016.1130626

Alvarado, C., & Modesto-Lowe, V. (2017). Improving treatment in minority children with attention/deficit hyperactivity disorder. *Clinical Pediatrics, 56,* 171–176. doi:10.1177/0009922816645517

Aman, M. G., Farmer, C. A., Hollway, J., & Arnold, L. E. (2008). Treatment of inattention, overactivity, and impulsiveness in autism spectrum disorders. *Child & Adolescent Psychiatric Clinics of North America, 17,* 713–738. doi:10.1016/j.chc.2008.06.009

Aman, M. G., Smith, T., Arnold, L. E., Corbett-Dick, P., Tumuluru, R., Hollway, J. A., . . . Handen, B. (2014). A review of atomoxetine effects in young people with developmental disabilities. *Research in Developmental Disabilities, 35*(6), 1412–1424. http://doi.org/10.1016/j.ridd.2014.03.006

American Academy of Pediatrics. (2011). Clinical practice guideline: ADHD: Clinical practice guideline for the diagnosis, evaluation, and treatment of attention-deficit/hyperactivity disorder in children and adolescents. *Pediatrics, 128,* 1–16.

American Academy of Child and Adolescent Psychiatry. (2007). Practice parameter for the use of stimulant medications in the treatment of children, adolescents, and adults. *Journal of the American Academy of Child and Adolescent Psychiatry, 46,* 894–921.

American Psychiatric Association. (1980). *Diagnostic and statistical manual of mental disorders* (3rd ed.) Wahsington, DC: Author.

American Psychiatric Association. (1994). *Diagnostic and statistical manual of mental disorders* (4th ed.) Wahsington, DC: Author.

American Psychiatric Association. (2000). *Diagnostic and statistical manual of mental disorders* (4th ed., text rev). Washington, DC: Author.

American Psychiatric Association. (2013). *Diagnostic and statistical manual of mental disorders* (5th ed.). Washington, DC: Author.

Arnold, L. E., Farmer, C., Kraemer, H. C., Davies, M., Witwer, A., Chuang, S., . . . Swiezy, N. B. (2010). Moderators, mediators, and other predictors of risperidone response in children with autistic disorder and irritability. *Journal of Child & Adolescent Psychopharmacology, 20,* 83–93. doi:10.1089/cap.2009.0022

Baeyens, D., Roeyers, H., & Walle, J. V. (2006). Subtypes of attention-deficit/hyperactivity disorder (ADHD): Distinct or related disorders across measurement levels? *Child Psychiatry & Human Development, 36,* 403–417. doi:10.1007/s10578-006-0011-z

Baglioni, C., Nanovska, S., Regen, W., Spiegelhalder, K., Feige, B., Nissen, C., . . . Riemann, D. (2016). Sleep and mental disorders: A meta-analysis of polysomnographic research. *Psychological Bulletin, 142*(9), 969–990. doi:10.1037/bul0000053

Balázs, J., & Keresztény, Á. (2014). Subthreshold attention deficit hyperactivity in children and adolescents: A systematic review. *European Child and Adolescent Psychiatry, 23,* 393–408.

Banaschewski, T., Becker, K., Scherag, S., Franke, B., & Coghill, D. (2010). Molecular genetics of attention-deficit/hyperactivity disorder: An overview. *European Child & Adolescent Psychiatry, 19,* 237–257. doi:10.1007/s00787-010-0090-z

Banaschewski, T., Roessner, V., Dittman, R. W., Santosh, P. J., & Rothenberger, A. (2004). Non-stimulant medications in the treatment of ADHD. *European Child & Adolescent Psychiatry, 13*(Supp. 1), 102–116. doi:10.1007/s00787-004-1010-x

Barbaresi, W. J., Katusic, S. K., Colligan, R. C., Weaver, A. L., Leibson, C. L., & Jacobsen, S. J. (2014). Long-term stimulant medication treatment of attention-deficit/hyperactivity disorder: results from a population-based study. *Journal of Developmental and Behavioral Pediatrics, 35*(7), 448–457.

Barkley, R. A. (1998). Attention-deficit hyperactivity disorder. *Scientific American, 279,* 66–71. doi:10.1038/scientificamerican0998-66

Barkley, R. A. (2004). Adolescents with attention-deficit/hyperactivity disorder: An overview of empirically-based treatments. *Journal of Psychiatric Practice, 10,* 39–56. doi:10.1097/00131746-200401000-00005

Barkley, R. A. (2010). Against the status quo: Revising the diagnostic criteria for ADHD. *Journal of the American Academy of Child & Adolescent Psychiatry, 49,* 205–207. doi:10.1016/j.jaac.2009.12.005

Barkley, R. A. (2016). Recent longitudinal studies of childhood attention-deficit/hyperactivity disorder: Important themes and questions for future research. *Journal of Abnormal Psychology, 125,* 248–255. doi:10.1037/abn0000125

Barkley, R. A., Fischer, M., Smallish, L., & Fletcher, K. (2006). Young adult outcome of hyperactive children: Adaptive functioning in major life activities. *Journal of the American Academy of Child & Adolescent Psychiatry, 45,* 192–202. doi:10.1097/01.chi.0000189134.97436.e2

Bateman, B., Warner, J. O., Hutchinson, E., Dean, T., Rowlandson, P., Gant, C., . . . Stevenson, J. (2004). The effects of a double-blind, placebo controlled, artificial food colorings and benzoate preservative challenge on hyperactivity in a general population sample of preschool children. *Archives of Diseases in Children, 89,* 506–511. doi:10.1136/adc.2003.031435

Becker, S. P., Leopold, D. R., Burns, G. L., Jarrett, M. A., Langberg, J. M., Marshall, S. A., . . . Willcutt, E. G. (2016). The internal, external, and diagnostic validity of sluggish cognitive tempo: A meta-analysis and critical review. *Journal of the American Academy of Child and Adolescent Psychiatry, 55*(3), 163–178. doi:10.1016/j.jaac.2015.12.006

Becker, S. P., Froehlich, T. E., & Epstein, J. N. (2016). Effects of methylphenidate on sleep functioning in children with attention-deficit/hyperactivity disorder. *Journal of Developmental and Behavioral Pediatrics, 37*(5), 395–404. doi:10.1097/DBP.0000000000000285

Bener, A., Kamal, M., Bener, H., & Bhugra, D. (2014). Higher prevalence of iron deficiency as strong predictor of attention deficit hyperactivity disorder in children. *Annals of Medical & Health Sciences Research, 4*(Suppl. 3), S291–S297. doi:10.4103/2141-9248.141974

Benson, K., Flory, K., Humphreys, K. L., & Lee, S. S. (2015). Misuse of stimulant medication among college students: A comprehensive review and meta-analysis. *Clinical Child and Family Psychology Review, 18*(1), 50–76. doi:10.1007/s10567-014-0177-z

Biederman, J., Kwon, A., Aleardi, M., Chouinard, V. A., Marino, T., Cole, H., . . . Faraone, S. V. (2005). Absence of gender effects on attention deficit hyperactivity disorder: Findings in non-referred subjects. *American Journal of Psychiatry, 162,* 1083–1089.

Biederman, J., Melmed, R. D., Patel, A., McBurnett, K., Donahue, J., & Lyne, A. (2008). Long-term, open-label extension study of guanfacine extended release in children and adolescents with ADHD. *CNS Spectrums, 13,* 1047–1055.

Bioulac, S., Micoulaud-Franchi, J. -A., & Philip, P. (2015). Excessive daytime sleepiness in patients with ADHD—Diagnostic and management strategies. *Current Psychiatry Reports, 17,* 69. doi:10.1007/s11920-015-0608-7

Bjornstad, G., & Montgomery, P. (2005). Family therapy for attention-deficit disorder or attention-deficit/hyperactivity disorder in children and adolescents. *Cochrane Database of Systematic Reviews, 2,* CD005042. doi:10.1002/14651858.CD005042.pub2

Blader, J. C., Pliszka, S. R., Jensen, P. S., Schooler, N. R., & Kafantaris, V. (2010). Stimulant-responsive and stimulant-refractory aggressive behavior among children with ADHD. *Pediatrics, 126,* e796–e806. doi:10.1542/peds.2010-0086

Bloch, M. H., Panza, K. E., Landeros-Weisenberger, A., & Leckman, J. F. (2009). Meta-analysis: Treatment of attention-deficit/hyperactivity disorder in children with comorbid tic disorders. *Journal of the American Academy of Child & Adolescent Psychiatry, 48,* 884–893. doi:10.1097/CHI.0b013e3181b26e9f

Buitelaar, J. K., Michelson, D., Danckaerts, M., Gillberg, C., Spencer, T. J., Zuddas, A., . . . Biederman, J. (2007). A randomized, double-blind study of continuation treatment for attention-deficit/hyperactivity disorder after 1 year. *Biological Psychiatry, 61,* 694–699. doi:10.1016/j.biopsych.2006.03.066

Bush, G., Spencer, T., Holmes, J., Shin, L. M., Valera, E. M., Seidman, L. J., . . . Biederman, J. (2008). Functional magnetic resonance imaging of methylphenidate and placebo in attention-deficit/hyperactivity disorder during the multi-source interference task. *Archives of General Psychiatry, 65,* 102–114. doi:10.1001/archgenpsychiatry.2007.16

Bushe, C. J., & Savill, N. C. (2014). Systematic review of atomoxetine data in childhood and adolescent attention-deficit hyperactivity disorder 2009-2011: Focus on clinical efficacy and safety. *Journal of Psychopharmacology, 28*(3), 204–211. doi:10.1177/0269881113478475

Cairney, J., Veldhuizen, S., & Szatmari, P. (2010). Motor coordination and emotional-behavioral problems in children. *Current Opinion in Psychiatry, 23,* 324–329. doi:10.1097/YCO.0b013e32833aa0aa

Carlson, G. A., & Kelly, K. L. (2003). Stimulant rebound: How common is it and what does it mean? *Journal of Child and Adolescent Psychopharmacology, 13,* 137–142. doi:10.1089/104454603322163853

Carter, C. M., Urbanowicz, M., Hemsley, R., Mantilla, L., Storbel, S., Graham, P. J., & Taylor, E. (1993). Effects of a few foods diet in attention deficit disorder. *Archives of Diseases in Childhood, 69,* 564–568. doi:10.1136/adc.69.5.564

Casey, B. J., Nigg, J. T., & Durston, S. (2007). New potential leads in the biology and treatment of attention deficit-hyperactivity disorder. *Current Opinions in Neurology, 20,* 119–124. doi:10.1097/WCO.0b013e3280a02f78

Cassone, A. R. (2015). Mindfulness training as an adjunct to evidence-based treatment for ADHD within families. *Journal of Attention Disorders, 19,* 147–157. doi:10.1177/1087054713488438

Catalá-López, F., Hutton, B., Núñez-Beltrán, A., Page, M. J., Ridao, M., Macías Saint-Gerons, D., . . . Moher, D. (2017). The pharmacological and non-pharmacological treatment of attention deficit hyperactivity disorder in children and adolescents: A systematic review with network meta-analyses of randomised trials. *PLoS One,* 12(7), e0180355. doi:10.1371/journal.pone.0180355

Caye, A., Swanson, J., Thapar, A., Sibley, M., Arseneault, L., Hechtman, L., . . . Rohde, L. A. (2016). Life span studies of ADHD—Conceptual challenges and predictors of persistence and outcome. *Current Psychiatry Reports, 18*(12), 111. doi:10.1007/s11920-016-0750-x

Cerrillo-Urbina, A. J., García-Hermoso, A., Sánchez-López, M., Pardo-Guijarro, M. J., Santos Gómez, J. L., & Martinez-Vizcaíno, V. (2015). The effects of physical exercise in children with attention deficit hyperactivity disorder: A systematic review and meta-analysis of randomized control trials. *Child: Care, Health, and Development, 41,* 779–788. doi:10.1111/cch.12255

Chacko, A., Kofler, M., & Jarrett, M. (2014). Improving outcomes for youth with ADHD: A conceptual framework for combined neurocognitive and skill-based treatment approaches. *Clinical Child & Family Psychology Review, 17,* 368–384. doi:10.1007/s10567-014-0171-5

Chacko, A., Wakschlag, L., Hill, C., Danis, B., & Espy, K. A. (2009). Viewing preschool disruptive behavior disorders and attention-deficit/hyperactivity disorder through a developmental lens: What we know and what we need to know. *Child & Adolescent Psychiatric Clinics of North America, 18,* 627–643. doi:10.1016/j.chc.2009.02.003

Chang, Z., Quinn, P. D., Hur, K., Gibbons, R. D., Sjolander, A., Larsson, H., & D'Onofrio, B. M. (2017). Association between medication use for attention-deficit/hyperactivity disorder and risk of motor vehicle crashes. *JAMA Psychiatry, 74,* 597–603. doi:10.1001/jamapsychiatry.2017.0659

Chapman, L. A., Wade, S. L., Walz, N. C., Taylor, H. G., Stancin, T., & Yeates, K. O. (2010). Clinically significant behavior problems during the 18 months following early childhood traumatic brain injury. *Rehabilitation Psychology, 55,* 48–57. doi:10.1037/a0018418

Charach, A., Yeung, E., Climans, T., & Lillie, E. (2011). Childhood attention-deficit/hyperactivity disorder and future substance use disorders: Comparative meta-analyses. *Journal of the American Academy of Child and Adolescent Psychiatry, 50*(1), 9–21. doi:10.1016/j.jaac.2010.09.019

Chen, L., Hu, X., Ouyang, L., He, N., Liao, Y., Liu, Q., . . . Gong, Q. (2016). A systematic review and meta-analysis of tract-based spatial statistics studies regarding attention-deficit/hyperactivity disorder. *Neuroscience & Biobehavoral Reviews, 68,* 838–847. doi:10.1016/j.neubiorev.2016.07.022

Chen, Y. C., Sudre, G., Sharp, W., Donovan, F., Chandrasekharappa, S. C., Hansen, N., . . . Shaw, P. (2018). Neuroanatomic, epigenetic and genetic differences in monozygotic twins discordant for attention deficit hyperactivity disorder. *Molecular Psychiatry, 23*(3), 683–690. doi:10.1038/mp.2017.45

Cherkasova, M., Sulla, E. M., Dalena, K. L., Pondé, M. P., & Hechtman, L. (2013). Developmental course of attention deficit hyperactivity disorder and its predictors. *Journal of the Canadian Academy of Child & Adolescent Psychiatry, 22*, 47–54.

Childress, A. C. (2012). Guanfacine extended release as adjunctive therapy to psychostimulants in children and adolescents with attention deficit/hyperactivity disorder. *Advances in Therapy, 29*(5), 385–400. doi:10.1007/s12325-012-0020-1

Chronis, A. M., Chacko, A., Fabiano, G. A., Wymbs, B. T., & Pelham, W. E., Jr. (2004). Enhancements to the behavioral parent training paradigm for families of children with ADHD: Review and future directions. *Clinical Child & Family Psychology Review, 7*, 1–27. doi:10.1023/B:CCFP.0000020190.60808.a4

Clavenna, A., & Bonati, M. (2017). Pediatric pharmacoepidemiology—Safety and effectiveness of medicines for ADHD. *Expert Opinion on Drug Safety, 16*(12), 1335–1345. doi:10.1080/14740338.2017.1389894

Clemow, D. B., & Walker, D. J. (2014). The potential for misuse and abuse of medications in ADHD: A review. *Postgraduate Medical Review, 126*(5), 64–81. doi:10.3810/pgm.2014.09.2801

Coates, J., Taylor, J. A., & Sayal, K. (2015). Parenting interventions for ADHD: A systematic literature review and meta-analysis. *Journal of Attention Disorders, 19*, 8310843. doi:10.1177/1087054714535952

Coghill, D., Banaschewski, T., Zuddas, A., Pelaz, A., Gagliano, A., & Doepfner, M. (2013). Long-acting methylphenidate formulations in the treatment of attention-deficit/hyperactivity disorder: A systematic review of head-to-head studies. *BMC Psychiatry, 13*, 237. doi:10.1186/1471-244X-13-237

Coghill, D. R., Seth, S., Pedroso, S., Usala, T., Currie, J., & Gagliano, A. (2014). Effects of methylphenidate on cognitive functions in children and adolescents with attention-deficit/hyperactivity disorder: Evidence from a systematic review and a meta-analysis. *Biological Psychiatry, 76*(8), 603–615. doi:10.1016/j.biopsych.2013.10.005

Coghill, D. R., Banaschewski, T., Soutullo, C., Cottingham, M. G., & Zuddas, A. (2017). Systematic review of quality of life and functional outcomes in randomized placebo-controlled studies of medications for attention-deficit/hyperactivity disorder. *European Child and Adolescent Psychiatry, 26*(11), 1283–1307. doi:10.1007/s00787-017-0986-y

Cohen, S. C., Mulqueen, J. M., Ferracioli-Oda, E., Stuckelman, Z. D., Coughlin, C. G., Leckman, J. F., & Bloch, M. H. (2015). Meta-analysis: Risk of tics associated with psychostimulant use in randomized, placebo-controlled trials. *Journal of the American Academy of Child & Adolescent Psychiatry, 54*(9): 728–736. doi:10.1016/j.jaac.2015.06.011.

Colaneri, N., Keim, S., & Adesman, A. (2017). Physician practices to prevent ADHD stimulant diversion and misuse. *Journal of Substance Abuse Treatment, 74*, 26–34. doi:10.1016/j.jsat.2016.12.003

Collett, B. R., Ohan, J. L., & Myers, K. M. (2003). Ten-year review of rating scales. V. Scales assessing attention-deficit/hyperactivity disorder. *Journal of the American Academy of Child & Adolescent Psychiatry, 42*, 1015–1037. doi:10.1097/00004583-200310000-00006

Colter, A. L., Cutler, C., & Meckling, K. A. (2008). Fatty acid status and behavioral symptoms of attention deficit hyperactivity disorder in adolescents: A case-control study. *Nutrition Journal, 7*, 8. doi:10.1186/1475-2891-7-8

Conners, C. K. (2008). Conners-3 Rating Scales (manual). *Multihealth Systems*. Retrieved from www.mhs.com

Conners, C. K., Casat, C. D., Gualtieri, C. T., Weller, E., Reader, M., Reiss, A., . . . Ascher, J. (1996). Bupropion hydrochloride in attention deficit disorder with hyperactivity. *Journal of the American Academy of Child and Adolescent Psychiatry, 35*, 1314–1321. doi:10.1097/00004583-199610000-00018

Connor, D. F., Steeber, J., & McBurnett, K. (2010). A review of attention-deficit/hyperactivity disorder complicated by symptoms of oppositional defiant disorder or conduct disorder. *Journal of Developmental & Behavioral Pediatrics, 31*, 427–440. doi:10.1097/DBP.0b013e3181e121bd

Cook, N. E., Braaten, E. B., & Surman, C. B. H. (2017). Clinical and functional correlates of processing speed in pediatric attention-deficit/hyperactivity disorder: A systemic review and meta-analysis. *Child Neuropsychology, 27*, 1–19. doi:10.1080/09297049.2017.1307952

Cooke, T., & So, T. -Y. (2016). Attention deficit hyperactivity disorder and occurrence of tic disorders in children and adolescents—What is the verdict. *Current Pediatric Reviews, 12*, 230–238. doi:10.2174/1573396312666160728113443

Cooper, R. E., Tye, C., Kuntsi, J., Vassos, E., & Asherson, P. (2016). The effect of omega-3 polyunsaturated fatty acid supplementation on emotional dysregulation, oppositional behavior and conduct problems in ADHD: A systematic review and meta-analysis. *Journal of Affective Disorders, 190*, 474–482. doi:10.106/j.jad.2015.09.053

Cortese, S., Brown, T. E., Corkum, P., Gruber, R., O'Brien, L. M., Stein, M., . . . Owens, J. (2013). Assessment and management of sleep problems in youths with attention-deficit/hyperactivity disorder. *Journal of the American Academy of Child & Adolescent Psychiatry, 52*(8), 784–796. doi:10.1016/j.jaac.2013.06.001

Cortese, S., Faraone, S. V., Konofal, E., & Lecendreux, M. (2009). Sleep in children with attention-deficit/hyperactivity disorder: Meta-analysis of subjective and objective studies. *Journal of the American Academy of Child & Adolescent Psychiatry, 48*, 894–908.

Council on Early Childhood, Committee on Psychosocial Aspects of Child and Family Health, and Section on Developmental and Behavioral Pediatrics. (2016). Addressing early childhood emotional and behavioral problems. *Pediatrics, 138*, 1. doi:10.1542/peds.2016-3023.

Cox, D. J., Moore, M., Burket, R., Merkel, L. R., Mikami, A. L., & Kovatchev, B. (2008). Rebound effects with long-acting amphetamine or methylphenidate stimulant medication preparations among adolescent male drivers with attention-deficit/hyperactivity disorder. *Journal of Child & Adolescent Psychopharmacology, 18*, 1–10. doi:10.1089/cap.2006.0141

Cross-Disorder Group of the Psychiatric Genomics, C., Lee, S. H., Ripke, S., Neale, B. M., Faraone, S. V., Purcell, S. M., . . . International Inflammatory Bowel Disease Genetics Consoritum. (2013). Genetic relationship between five psychiatric disorders estimated from genome-wide SNPs. *Nature Genetics, 45*(9), 984–994. doi:10.1038/ng.2711

Dadds, M. R., Schollar-Root, O., Lenroot, R., & Moul, C. (2016). Epigenetic regulation of the DRD4 gene and dimensions of attentiondeficit/hyperactivity disorder in children. *European Journal of Child & Adolescent Psychiatry, 25*, 1081–1089. doi:10.1007/s00787-016-0828-3

Daley, D., Jones, K., Hutchings, J., & Thompson, M. (2008). Attention deficit hyperactivity disorder in pre-school children: Current findings, recommended interventions and future directions. *Child: Care, Health and Development, 35*, 754–766. doi:10.1111/j.1365-2214.2009.00938.x

Daley, D., van der Oord, S., Ferrin, M., Danckaerts, M., Doepfner, M., Cortese, S., . . . European ADHD Guidelines Group. (2014). Behavioral interventions in attention-deficit/

hyperactivity disorder: A meta-analysis of randomized controlled trials across multiple outcome domains. *Journal of the American Academy of Child & Adolescent Psychiatry, 53*(8), 835–847, doi:10.1016/j.jaac.2014.05.013

Dalsgaard, S. (2013). Attention-deficit/hyperactivity disorder (ADHD). *European Child and Adolescent Psychiatry, 22*(Suppl. 1), S43–S48.

Dalsgaard, S., Nielson, H. S., & Simonsen, M. (2014). Consequences of ADHD medication use for children's outcomes. *Journal of Health Economics, 37,* 137–151. doi:10.1016/j.jhealeco.2014.05.05

Dalsgaard, S., Ostergaard, S. D., Leckman, J. F., Mortensen, P. B., & Pedersen, M. G. (2015). Mortality in children, adolescents, and adults with attention deficit hyperactivity disorder: A nationwide cohort study. *Lancet, 385,* 2190–2196. doi:10.106/S0140-6736(14)61684-6

Dalsgaard, S., Primdal Kvist, A., Leckman, J. F., Skyt Nielsen, H., & Simonsen, M. (2014). Cardiovascular safety of stimulants in children with attention-deficit/hyperactivity disorder: A nationwide prospective cohort study. *Journal of Child and Adolescent Psychopharmacology, 24*(6), 302–310. doi:10.1089/cap.2014.0020

Dawes, P., & Bishop, D. (2009). Auditory processing disorder in relation to developmental disorders of language, communication and attention: A review and critique. *International Journal of Language & Communication Disorders, 44,* 440–465. doi:10.1080/13682820902929073

Deault, L. C. (2010). A systematic review of parenting in relation to the development of comorbidities and functional impairments in children with attention-deficit/hyperactivity disorder (ADHD). *Child Psychiatry and Human Development, 41,* 168–192. doi:10.1007/s10578-009-0159-4

Dell'Agnello, G., Zuddas, A., Masi, G., Curatolo, P., Besana, D., & Rossi, A. (2009). Use of atomoxetine in patients with attention-deficit hyperactivity disorder and co-morbid conditions. *CNS Drugs, 23,* 739–753. doi:10.2165/11314350-000000000-00000

Denckla, M. B. (2006). Attention deficit hyperactivity disorder: The childhood comorbidity that most influences the burden of disability. In J. T. Walkup, J. W. Mink, & P. J. Hollenbeck (Eds.), *Advances in neurology: Volume 99: Tourette syndrome* (pp. 17–21). Philadelphia, PA: Lippincott Williams & Wilkins.

Derbyshire, E. (2017). Do omega-3/6 fatty acids have a therapeutic role in children and young people with ADHD? *Journal of Lipids.* Advance online publication. doi:10.1155/2017/6285218

Deutsch, C. K., Dube, W. V., & McIlvane, W. J. (2008). Attention deficits, attention-deficit hyperactivity disorder, and intellectual disabilities. *Developmental Disabilities Research Reviews, 14,* 285–292. doi:10.1002/ddrr.42

Diamond, A. (2013). Executive functions. *Annual Review of Psychology, 64,* 135–168. doi:10.1146/annrev-psych-113011-143750

Dittmann, R. W., Schacht, A., Helsberg, K., Schneider-Fresenius, C., Lehmann, M., Lehmkuhl, G., & Wehmeier, P. M. (2011). Atomoxetine versus placebo in children and adolescents with attention-deficit/hyperactivity disorder and comorbid oppositional defiant disorder: A double-blind, randomized, multicenter trial in Germany. *Journal of Child & Adolescent Psychopharmacology, 21*(2), 97–110. doi:10.1089/cap.2009.0111

Donnelly, C., Bangs, M., Trzepacz, P., Jin, L., Zhang, S., Witte, M. M., . . . Spencer, T. J. (2009). Safety and tolerability of atomoxetine over 3 to 4 years in children and adolescents with ADHD. *Journal of the American Academy of Child & Adolescent Psychiatry, 48,* 176–185. doi:10.1097/CHI.0b013e318193060e

Duff, C. T., & Sulla, E. M. (2015). Measuring executive function in the differential diagnosis of attention-deficit/hyperactivity disorder: Does it really tell us anything? *Applied Neuropsychology: Child, 4,* 188–196. doi:10.1080/21622965.2013.848329

DuPaul, G. J., Gormley, M. J., & Laracy, S. D. (2014). School-based interventions for elementary school students with ADHD. *Child & Adolescent Psychiatric Clinics of North America, 23,* 687–697. doi:10.1016/j.chc.2014.05.003

DuPaul, G. J., Power, T. J., Anastopoulos, A. D., & Reid, R. (2016). *ADHD Rating Scale-5 for Children and Adolescents.* New York, NY: Guilford Press.

Education for All Handicapped Children Act of 1975, PL 94-142, 20 U.S.C. §§ 1400 *et seq.*

Egger, H. L., & Angold, A. (2006). Common emotional and behavioral disorders in preschool children: Presentation, nosology, and epidemiology. *Journal of Child Psychology and Psychiatry, 47,* 313–337. doi:10.1111/j.1469-7610.2006.01618.x

Egger, J., Carter, C. M., Graham, P. J., Gumley, D., & Soothill, J. F. (1985). Controlled trial of oligoantigenic treatment in the hyperkinetic syndrome. *The Lancet, 325*(8428), 540–546. doi:10.1016/S0140-6736(85)91206-1

Ercan, E. S., Suren, S., Bacanli, A., Yazici, K. U., Calli, C., Ardic, U. A., . . . Rohde, L. A. (2016). Altered structural connectivity is related to attention deficit/hyperactivity subtypes: A DTI study. *Psychiatry Research: Neuroimaging, 256,* 57–64. doi:10.1016/j.pscychresns.2016.04.002

Erenberg, G. (2006). The relationship between Tourette syndrome, attention-deficit hyperactivity disorder, and stimulant medication: A critical review. *Seminars in Pediatric Neurology, 12,* 217–221. doi:10.1016/j.spen.2005.12.003

Evans, S. W., Langberg, J. M., Egan, T., & Molitor, S. J. (2014). Middle school-based and high school-based interventions for adolescents with ADHD. *Child & Adolescent Psychiatric Clinics of North America, 23,* 699–715. doi:10.1016/j.chc.2014.05.004

Eyberg, S. M., Nelson, M. M., & Boggs, S. R. (2008). Evidence-based psychosocial treatments for children and adolescents with disruptive behavior. *Journal of Clinical Child & Adolescent Psychology, 37,* 215–237. doi:10.1080/15374410701820117

Faedda, G. L., Marangoni, C., Serra, G., Salvatore, P., Sani, G., Vazquez, G. H., . . . Koukopoulos, A. (2015). Precursors of bipolar disorders: A systematic literature review of prospective studies. *Journal of Clinical Psychiatry, 76*(5), 614–624. doi:10.4088/JCP.13r08900

Faraone, S. V., Biederman, J., & Mick, E. (2006). The age-dependent decline of attention deficit hyperactivity disorder: A meta-analysis of follow-up studies. *Psychological Medicine, 36,* 159–165. doi:10.1017/S003329170500471X

Faraone, S. V., & Buitelaar, J. (2010). Comparing the efficacy of stimulants for ADHD in children and adolescents using meta-analysis. *European Child & Adolescent Psychiatry, 19,* 353–364. doi:10.1007/s00787-009-0054-3

Faraone, S. V., & Glatt, S. J. (2010). Effects of extended-release guanfacine on ADHD symptoms and sedation-related adverse events in children with ADHD. *Journal of Attention Disorders, 13,* 532–538. doi:10.1177/1087054709332472

Faraone, S. V., Perlis, R. H., Doyle, A. E., Smoller, J. W., Goralinick, J. J., Holmgren, M. A., & Sklar, P. (2005). Molecular genetics of attention-deficit/hyperactivity disorder. *Biological Psychiatry, 57,* 1313–1323. doi:10.1016/j.biopsych.2004.11.024

Faraone, S. V., & Upadhyaya, H. P. (2007). The effect of stimulant treatment for ADHD on later substance abuse and the potential for medication misuse, abuse, and diversion. *Journal of Clinical Psychiatry, 68,* e28. doi:10.4088/JCP.1107e28

Farias, A. C., Cordeiro, M. L., Felden, E. P., Bara, T. S., Benko, C. R., Coutinho, D., . . . McCracken, J. T. (2017). Attention-memory training yields behavioral and academic improvements in children diagnosed with attention-deficit hyperactivity disorder comorbid with a learning disorder. *Neuropsychiatric Disease and Treatment, 13,* 1761–1769. doi:10.2147/NDT.S136663

Fetene, D. M., Betts, K. S., & Alati, R. (2017). Maternal thyroid dysfunction during pregnancy and behavioral and psychiatric disorders of children: A systematic review. *European Journal of Endocrinology, 177,* R261–R273. doi:10.1530/EJE-16-0860

Figueroa, R. (2010). Use of antidepressants during pregnancy and risk of attention-deficit/hyperactivity disorder in the offspring. *Journal of Developmental Behavioral Pediatrics, 31,* 1–8.

Fiks, A. G., Ross, M. E., Mayne, S. L., Song, L., Liu, W., Steffes, J., . . . Wasserman, R. (2016). Preschool ADHD diagnosis and stimulant use before and after the 2011 AAP Practice Guideline. *Pediatrics, 138*(6). pii:e20162025

Filho, A. G. C., Bodanese, R., Silva, T. L., Alvares, J. P., Aman, M., & Rohde, L. A. (2005). Comparison of risperidone and methylphenidate for reducing ADHD symptoms in children and adolescents with moderate mental retardation. *Journal of the American Academy of Child & Adolescent Psychiatry, 44,* 748–755.

Fischer, M., Barkley, R. A., Smallish, L., & Fletcher, K. (2007). Hyperactive children as young adults: Driving abilities, safe driving behavior, and adverse driving outcomes. *Accident Analysis & Prevention, 39,* 94–105. doi:10.1016/j.aap.2006.06.008

Friedman, L. A., & Rapoport, J. L. (2015). Brain development in ADHD. *Current Opinion in Neurobiology, 30,* 106–111. doi:10.1016/j.conb.2014.11.007

Friedman, L. M., Rapport, M. D., Orban, S. A., Eckrich, S. J., & Calub, C. A. (2017a). Applied problem-solving in children with ADHD: The mediating roles of working memory and mathematical calculation. *Journal of Abnormal Child Psychology, 45*(2). Advance online publication. doi:10.1007/s10802-017-0312-7

Friedman, L. M., Rapport, M. D., Raiker, J. S., Orban, S. A., & Eckrich, S. J. (2017b). Reading comprehension in boys with ADHD: The mediating roles of working memory and orthographic conversion. *Journal of Abnormal Child Psychology, 45,* 273–287. doi:10.1007/s10802-016-0171-7

Frodl, T., & Skokauskas, N. (2012). Meta-analysis of structural MRI studies in children and adults with attention deficit hyperactivity disorder indicates treatment effects. *Acta Psychiatrica Scandinavica, 125,* 114–126. doi:10.1111/j.1600-0447.2011.01786.x

Gadow, K. D., & Sverd, J. (2006). Attention-deficit/hyperactivity disorder, chronic tic disorder, and methylphenidate. In J. T. Walkup, J. W. Mink, & P. J. Hollenbeck (Eds.), *Advances in neurology: Vol. 99: Tourette syndrome* (pp. 197–207). Philadelphia, PA: Lippincott Williams & Wilkins.

Galanter, C. A., & Leibenluft, E. (2008). Frontiers between attention deficit hyperactivity disorder and bipolar disorder. *Child & Adolescent Psychiatric Clinics of North America, 17,* 325–346. doi:10.1016/j.chc.2007.11.001

Gardner, D. M., & Gerdes, A. C. (2015). A review of peer relationships and friendships in youth with ADHD. *Journal of Attention Disorders, 19,* 844–855. doi:10.1177/108705413501552

Garg, J., Arun, P., & Chavan, B. S. (2015). Comparative efficacy of methylphenidate and atomoxetine in oppositional defiant disorder comorbid with attention deficit hyperactivity disorder. *International Journal of Applied and Basic Medical Research, 5*(2), 114–118. doi:10.4103/2229-516X.157162

Garnock-Jones, K. P., & Keating, G. M. (2009). Atomoxetine: A review of its use in attention-deficit hyperactivity disorder in children and adolescents. *Pediatric Drugs, 11,* 203–226.

Gayleard, J. L., & Mychailyszyn, M. P. (2017). Atomoxetine treatment for children and adolescents with attention-deficit/hyperactivity disorder (ADHD): A comprehensive meta-analysis of outcomes on parent-rated core symptomatology. *Attention Deficit Hyperactivity Disorders, 9*(3), 149–160. doi:10.1007/s12402-017-0216-y

Gelade, K., Janssen, T. W. P., Bink, M., Twisk, J. W. R., van Mourik, R., Maras, A., & Oosterlaan, J. (2018). A 6-month follow-up of an RCT on behavioral and neurocognitive effects of neurofeedback in children with ADHD. *European Child & Adolescent Psychiatry, 27*(5), 581–593. doi:10.1007/s00787-017-1072-1

Gevensleben, H., Holl, B., Albrecht, B., Schlamp, D., Kratz, O., Studer, P., & Heinrich, H. (2010). Neurofeedback training in children with ADHD: 6-month follow-up of a randomized controlled trial. *European Journal of Child & Adolescent Psychiatry, 19,* 715–724. doi:10.1007/s00787-010-0109-5

Ghelani, K., Sidhu, R., Jain, U., & Tannock, R. (2004). Reading comprehension and reading related abilities in adolescents with reading disabilities and attention-deficit/hyperactivity disorder. *Dyslexia: The Journal of the British Dyslexia Association, 10,* 364–384. doi:10.1002/dys.285

Ghuman, J. K., Aman, M. G., Ghuman, H. S., Reichenbacher, T., Gelenberg, A., Wright, R., . . . Fort, C. (2009a). Prospective, naturalistic, pilot study of open-label atomoxetine treatment in preschool children with attention-deficit/hyperactivity disorder. *Journal of Child & Adolescent Psychopharmacology, 19,* 155–166. doi:10.1089/cap.2008.054

Ghuman, J. K., Aman, M. G., Lecavalier, L., Riddle, M. A., Gelenberg, A., Wright, R., & Fort, C. (2009b). Randomized, placebo-controlled, crossover study of methylphenidate for attention-deficit/hyperactivity disorder symptoms in preschoolers with developmental disorders. *Journal of Child & Adolescent Psychopharmacology, 19,* 329–339. doi:10.1089/cap.2008.0137

Giedd, J. N., Raznahan, A., Alexander-Bloch, A., Schmitt, E., Gotay, N., & Rapoport, J. L. (2105). Child Psychiatry Branch of the National Institute of Mental Health Longitudinal Structural Magnetic Resonance Imaging Study of Human Brain Development. *Neuropsychopharmacology Reviews, 40,* 43–49. doi:10.1038/npp.2014.236

Gillies, D., Sinn, J. K., Lad, S. S., Leach, M. J., & Ross, M. J. (2013). Polyunsaturated fatty acids (PUFA) for attention deficit hyperactivity disorder (ADHD) in children and adolescents. *Cochrane Database of Systematic Reviews, 7,* CD007986. doi:10.1002/14651858.CD007986.pub2

Gobbo, M. A., & Louzã, M. R. (2014). Influence of stimulant and non-stimulant drug treatment on driving performance in patients with attention deficit hyperactivity disorder: A systematic review. *European Neuropsychopharmacology, 24*(9), 1425–1443. doi:10.1016/j.neuro.2014.06.006

Golubchik, P., Golubchik, L., Sever, J. M., & Weizman, A. (2014). The beneficial effect of methylphenidate in ADHD with comorbid separation anxiety. *International Clinical Psychopharmacology, 29*(5), 274–278. doi:10.1097/YIC.0000000000000034

Golubchik, P., Sever, J., & Weizman, A. (2014). Methylphenidate treatment in children with attention deficit hyperactivity disorder and comorbid social phobia. *International Clinical Psychopharmacology, 29*(4), 212–215. doi:10.1097/YIC.0000000000000029

González-Castro, P., Cueli, M., Rodríguez, C., García, T., & Álvarez, L. (2016). Efficacy of neurofeedback versus pharmacological support in subjects with ADHD. *Applied Psychophysiology & Neurofeedback, 41*, 17–25. doi:10.1007/s10484-015-9299-4

Goulardins, J. B., Marques, J. C. B., & De Oliveira, J. A. (2017). Attention deficit hyperactivity disorder and motor impairment: A critical review. *Perceptual and Motor Skills, 124*, 425–440. doi:10.1177/0031512517690607

Green, J. L., Rinehart, N., Anderson, V., Nicholson, J. M., Jongeling, B. & Sciberras, E. (2015). Autism spectrum disorder symptoms in children with ADHD: A community-based study. *Research in Developmental Disabilities, 47*, 175–184. doi:10.1016/j.ridd.2015.09.016

Green, B. C., Johnson, K. A., & Bretherton, L. (2014). Pragmatic language difficulties in children with hyperactivity and attention problems: An integrated review. *International Journal of Language & Communication Disorders, 49*, 15–29. doi:10.1111/1460-6984.12056

Greenhill, L. L., Kollins, S., Abikoff, H., McCracken, J., Riddle, M., Swanson, J., . . . Cooper, T. (2006). Efficacy and safety of immediate-release methylphenidate treatment for preschoolers with ADHD. *Journal of the American Academy of Child & Adolescent Psychiatry, 45*, 1284–1293. doi:10.1097/01.chi.0000235077.32661.61

Greenhill, L. L., Posner, K., Vaughan, B. S., & Kratochvil, C. J. (2008). Attention-deficit/hyperactivity disorder in preschool children. *Child and Adolescent Psychiatric Clinics of North America, 17*, 347–366. doi:10.1016/j.chc.2007.11.004

Groenman, A. P., Janssen, T. W. P., & Oosterlaan, J. (2017). Childhood psychiatric disorders as risk factor for subsequent substance abuse: A meta-analysis. *Journal of the American Academy of Child & Adolescent Psychiatry, 56*, 556–569. doi:10.1016/j.jaac.2017.05.004

Gustafsson, P. A., Birberg-Thronberg, U., Duchen, K., Landgren, M., Malmberg, K., Pelling, H., & Karlsson, T. (2010). EPA supplementation improves teacher-rated behavior and oppositional symptoms in children with ADHD. *Acta Paediatrica, 99*, 1540–1549. doi:10.1111/j.1651-2227.2010.01871.x

Ha, M., Kwon, H. J., Lim, M. H., Jee, Y. K., Hong, Y. C., Leem, J. H., . . . Jo, S. -J. (2009). Low blood levels of lead and mercury and symptoms of attention deficit hyperactivity in children: A report of the children's health and environment research (CHEER). *Neurotoxicology, 30*, 31–36. doi:10.1016/j.neuro.2008.11.011

Hale, J. B., Reddy, L. A., Semrud-Clikeman, M., Hain, L. A., Whitaker, J., Morley, J., . . . Jones, N. (2011). Executive impairment determines ADHD medication response: Implications for academic achievement. *Journal of Learning Disabilities, 44*(2), 196–212. doi:10.1177/0022219410391191

Hammerness, P., Geller, D., Petty, C., Lamb, A., Bristol, E., & Biederman, J. (2009a). Does ADHD moderate the manifestation of anxiety disorders in children? *European Child & Adolescent Psychiatry, 19*, 107–112. doi:10.1007/s00787-009-0041-8

Hammerness, P., Georgiopoulos, A., Doyle, R. L., Utzinger, L., Schillinger, M., Martelon, M., . . . Wilens, T. E. (2009b). An open study of adjunct OROS-methylpheniate in children who are atomoxetine partial responders: II. Tolerability and pharmacokinetics. *Journal of Child & Adolescent Psychopharmacology, 19*, 493–499. doi:10.1089/cap.2008.0126

Handen, B. L., & Gilchrist, R. (2006). Practitioner review: Psychopharmacology in children and adolescents with mental retardation. *Journal of Child Psychology & Psychiatry, 47*, 871–882. doi:10.1111/j.1469-7610.2006.01588.x

Handen, B. L., Johnson, C. R., & Lubetsky, M. (2000). Efficacy of methylphenidate among children with autism and symptoms of attention-deficit hyperactivity disorder. *Journal of Autism & Developmental Disorders, 30*, 245–255.

Handen, B. L., Sahl, R., & Hardan, A. Y. (2008). Guanfacine in children with autism and/or intellectual disabilities. *Journal of Developmental & Behavioral Pediatrics, 29*, 303–308. doi:10.1097/DBP.0b013e3181739b9d

Harfterkamp, M., van de Loo-Neus, G., Minderaa, R. B., van der Gaag, R. J., Escobar, R., Schacht, A., . . . Hoekstra, P. J. (2012). A randomized double-blind study of atomoxetine versus placebo for attention-deficit/hyperactivity disorder symptoms in children with autism spectrum disorder. *Journal of the American Academy of Child & Adolescent Psychiatry, 51*(7), 733–741. doi:10.1016/j.jaac.2012.04.011

Hariri, M., & Azadbakht, L. (2015). Magnesium, iron, and zinc supplementation for the treatment of attention deficit hyperactivity disorder: A systematic review on the recent literature. *International Journal of Preventative Medicine, 6*, 83. doi:10.4103/2008-7802.164313

Harpin, V., Mazzone, L., Raynaud, J. P., Kahle, J., & Hodgkins, P. (2016). Long-term outcomes of ADHD: A systematic review of self-esteem and social function. *Journal of Attention Disorders, 20*, 295–305. doi:10.1177/1087054713486516

Harstad, E., Levy, S., & Committee on Substance Abuse. (2014). Attention-deficit/hyperactivity disorder and substance abuse. *Pediatrics, 134*(1), e293–e301. doi:10.1542/peds.2014-0992

Hartman, C. A., Geurts, H. M., Frabke, B., Buitelaar, J. K., & Rommelse, N. N. J. (2016). Changing ASD-ADHD symptom co-occurrence across the lifespan with adolescence as a crucial time window: Illustrating the need to go beyond childhood. *Neuroscience and Biobehavioral Reviews, 71*, 529–541. doi:10.1016/j.neubiorev.2016.09.003

Harty, S. C., Ivanov, I., Newcorn, J. H., & Halperin, J. M. (2011). The impact of conduct disorder and stimulant medication on later substance use in an ethnically diverse sample of individuals with attention-deficit/hyperactivity disorder in childhood. *Journal of Child & Adolescent Psychopharmacology, 21*(4), 331–339. doi:10.1089/cap.2010.0074

Hawkey, E. & Nigg, J. T. (2014). Omega-3 fatty acid and ADHD: Blood level analysis and meta-analytic extension of supplementation trials. *Clinical Psychology Review, 34*, 496–505. doi:10.1016/j.cpr.2014.05.005

Hechtman, L., Swanson, J. M., Sibley, M. H., Stehli, A., Owens, E. B., Mitchell, J. T., . . . MTA Cooperative Group. (2016). Functional adult outcomes 16 years after childhood diagnosis of attention-deficit/hyperactivity disorder: MTA results. *Journal of the American Academy of Child & Adolescent Psychiatry, 55*(11), 945–952. doi:10.1016/j.jaac.2016.07.774

Hennissen, L., Bakker, M. J., Banaschewski, T., Carucci, S., Coghill, D., Danckaerts, M., . . . ADDUCE Consortium. (2017). Cardiovascular effects of stimulant and non-stimulant medication for children and adolescents with ADHD: A systematic review and meta-analysis of trials of methylphenidate, amphetamines and atomoxetine. *CNS Drugs, 31*(3), 199–215. doi:10.1007/s40263-017-0410-7

Hervas, A., Huss, M., Johnson, M., McNicholas, F., van Stralen, J., Sreckovic, S., . . . Robertson, B. (2014). Efficacy and safety of extended-release guanfacine hydrochloride in children and adolescents with attention-deficit/hyperactivity disorder: A randomized, controlled, phase III trial. *European Neuropsychopharmacology, 24*(12), 1861–1872. doi:10.1016/j.euroneuro.2014.09.014

Hetrick, S. E., McKenzie, J. E., Cox, G. R., Simmons, M. B., & Merry, S. N. (2012). Newer generation antidepressants for depressive disorders in children and adolescents. *Cochrane Database System Review,* 11, CD004851. doi:10.1002/14651858.CD004851.pub3

Hitchcock, C., & Westwell, M. S. (2017). A cluster-randomized, controlled trial of the impact of Cogmed Working Memory Training on both academic performance and regulation of social, emotional, and behavioral challenges. *Journal of Child Psychology & Psychiatry, 58,* 140–150. doi:10.1111/jcpp.12638

Hoekzema, E., Carmona, S., Tremols, V., Gispert, J. D., Guitart, M., Fauquet, J., . . . Villarroya, O. (2010). Enhanced neural activity in frontal and cerebellar circuits after cognitive training in children with attention-deficit/hyperactivity disorder. *Human Brain Mapping, 31*(12), 1942–1950. doi:10.1002/hbm.20988

Holmskov, M., Storebø, O. J., Moreira-Maia, C. R., Ramstad, E., Magnusson, F. L., Krogh, H. B., . . . Simonsen, E. (2017). Gastrointestinal adverse events during methylphenidate treatment of children and adolescents with attention deficit hyperactivity disorder: A systematic review with meta-analysis and Trial Sequential Analysis of randomized clinical trials. *PLoS One, 12*(6), e0178187. doi:10.1371/journal.pone.0178187

Holtmann, M., Sonuga-Barke, E., Cortese, S., & Brandeis, D. (2014). Neurofeedback for ADHD: A review of current evidence. *Child & Adolescent Psychiatric Clinics of North America, 23,* 789–806. doi:10.1016/j.chc.2014.05.006

Hoogman, M., Bralten, J., Hibar, D. P., Mennes, M., Zwiers, M. P., Schweren, L. S. J., . . . Franke, B. (2017). Subcortical brain volume differences in participants with attention deficit hyperactivity disorder in children and adults: A cross-sectional mega-analysis. *Lancet Psychiatry, 4*(4), 310–319. doi:10.1016/S2215-0366(17)30049-4

Houghton, S., Alsalmi, N., Tan, C., Taylor, M., & Durkin, K. (2017). Treating comorbid anxiety in adolescents with ADHD using a cognitive behavior therapy program approach. *Journal of Attention Disorders, 21*(13), 1094–1104. doi:10.1177/1087054712473182

Howard, A. L., Robinson, M., Smith, G. J., Ambrosini, G. L., Piek, J. P., & Oddy, W. H. (2011). ADHD is associated with a "Western" dietary pattern in adolescents. *Journal of Attention Disorders, 15,* 403–411. doi:10.1177/1087054710365990

Hoza, B. (2007). Peer functioning in children with ADHD. *Journal of Pediatric Psychology, 32,* 655–663. doi:10.1093/jpepsy/jsm024

Hoza, B., Martin, C. P., Pirog, A., & Shoulberg, E. K. (2016). Using physical activity to manage ADHD symptoms: The state of the evidence. *Current Psychiatry Reports, 18,* 113. doi:10.1007/s11920-016-0749-3

Hutchinson, S. L., Ghuman, J. K., Ghuman, H. S., Karpov, I., & Schuster, J. M. (2016). Efficacy of atomoxetine in the treatment of attention-deficit hyperactivity disorder in patients with common comorbidities in children, adolescents and adults: a review. *Therapeutic Advances in Psychopharmacology, 6*(5), :317–334. doi:10.1177/2045125316647686

Individuals with Disabilities Education Improvement Act of 2004, PL 108-446, 20 U.S.C. §§ 1400 *et seq.*

Jacka, F. N., Ystrom, E., Brantsaeter, A. L., Karevold, E., Roth, C., Haugen, M., . . . Berk, M. (2013). Maternal and early postnatal nutrition and mental health of offspring by age 5 years: A prospective cohort study. *Journal of the American Academy of Child & Adolescent Psychiatry, 52*(10), 1038–1047. doi:10.1016/j.jaac.2013.07.002

Jacobson, L. J., Ryan, M., Martin, R. B., Ewen, J., Mostofsky, S. H., & Denckla, M. B. (2011). Working memory influences processing speed and reading fluency in ADHD. *Child Neuropsychology, 17,* 209–224. doi:10.1080/09297049.2010.532204

Jahromi, L. B., Kasari, C. L., McCracken, J. T., Lee, L. S., Aman, M. G., McDougle, C. J., . . . Posey, D. J. (2009). Positive effects of methylphenidate on social communication and self-regulation in children with pervasive developmental disorders and hyperactivity. *Journal of Autism & Developmental Disorders, 39,* 395–404. doi:10.1007/s10803-008-0636-9

Jafarinia, M., Mohammadi, M. R., Modabbernia, A., Ashrafi, M., Khajavi, D., Tabrizi, M., . . . Akhondzadeh, S. (2012). Bupropion versus methylphenidate in the treatment of children with attention-deficit/hyperactivity disorder: Randomized double-blind study. *Human Psychopharmacology, 27*(4), 411–418. doi:10.1002/hup.2242

Jain, R., Segal, S., Kollins, S. H., & Khayrallah, M. (2011). Clonidine extended-release tablets for pediatric patients with attention-deficit/hyperactivity disorder. *Journal of the American Academy of Child & Adolescent Psychiatry, 50*(2), 171–179. doi:10.1016/j.jaac.2010.11.005

Janssen, T. W., Bink, M., Geladé, K., van Mourik, R., Maras, A., & Oosterlaan, J. (2016). A randomized controlled trial into the effects of neurofeedback, methylphenidate, and physical activity on EEG power spectra in children with ADHD. *Journal of Child Psychology & Psychiatry & Allied Disciplines, 57,* 633–644. doi:10.1007/s00787-016-0902

Jaselskis, C. A., Cook, Jr., E. H., Fletcher, K. E., & Leventhal, B. L. (1992). Clonidine treatment of hyperactive and impulse children with autistic disorder. *Journal of Clinical Psychopharmacology, 12*(5), 322–327.

Jensen, C. M., & Steinhausen, H. -C. (2015). Comorbid mental disorders in children and adolescents with attention-deficit/hyperactivity disorder in a large nationwide study. *Attention Deficit Hyperactivity Disorders, 7,* 27–38. doi 10.1007/s12402-014-0142-1

Jitendra, A. K., DuPaul, G. J., Someki, F., & Tresco, K. E. (2008). Enhancing academic achievement for children with attention-deficit hyperactivity disorder: Evidence from school-based intervention research. *Developmental Disabilities Research Reviews, 14,* 325–330. doi:10.1002/ddrr.39

Kamp, C. F., Sperlich, B., & Holmberg, H. C. (2014). Exercise reduces the symptoms of attention-deficit/hyperactivity disorder and improves social behavior, motor skills, strength, and neuropsychological parameters. *Acta Paediatrica, 103,* 709–714. doi:10.111/apa.12628

Kaplan, B. J., McNicol, J., Conte, R. A., & Moghadam, H. K. (1989). Dietary replacement in preschool-aged hyperactive boys. *Pediatrics, 83,* 7–17.

Karalunas, S. L., Gustafsson, H. C., Dieckmann, N. E., Tipsord, J., Mitchell, S. H., & Nigg, J. T. (2017). Heterogeneity in developmental aspects of working memory predicts longitudinal attention deficit hyperactivity disorder symptom change. *Journal of Abnormal Psychology, 126,* 774–792. doi:10.1037/abn0000292

Kasper, L. J., Alderson, R. M., & Hudec, K. L. (2012). Moderators of working memory deficits in children with attention-deficit/hyperactivity disorder (ADHD): A meta-analytic review. *Clinical Psychology Review, 32*, 605–617. doi:10.1016/j.cpr.2012.07.001

Kaufman, J., Birmaher, B., Brent, D., Rao, U., Flynn, C., Moreci, P., . . . Ryan, N. (1997). Schedule for Affective Disorders and Schizophrenia for School-Age Children—Present and Lifetime Version (K-SADS-PL): Initial reliability and validity data. *Journal of the American Academy of Child & Adolescent Psychiatry, 36*(7), 980–988. doi:10.1097/00004583-199707000-00021

Kent, J. M., Hough, D., Singh, J., Karcher, K., & Pandina, G. (2013). An open-label extension study of the safety and efficacy of risperidone in children and adolescents with autistic disorder. *Journal of Child and Adolescent Psychopharmacology, 23*(10), 676–686. http://doi.org/10.1089/cap.2012.0058

Kidwell, K. M., Van Dyk, T. R., Lundahl, A., & Nelson, T. D. (2015). Stimulant medications and sleep for youth with ADHD: A meta-analysis. *Pediatrics, 136*(6), 1144–1153. doi:10.1542/peds.2015-1708

Kieling, C., Goncalves, R. R. F., Tannock, R., & Castellanos, F. X. (2008). Neurobiology of attention-deficit/hyperactivity disorder. *Child & Adolescent Psychiatric Clinics of North America, 17*, 285–307. doi:10.1016/j.chc.2007.11.012

Kirk, H., Gray, K., Ellis, K., Taffe, J., & Cornish, K. (2017). Impact of attention training on academic achievement, executive functioning, and behavior: A randomized controlled trial. *American Journal on Intellectual & Developmental Disabilities, 122*, 97–117. doi:10.1352/1944-7558-122.2.97

Kisicki, J. C., Fiske, K., & Lyne, A. (2007). Phase 1, double-blind, randomized, placebo-controlled dose-escalation study of the effects on blood pressure of abrupt cessation versus taper down of guanfacine extended release tablets in adults aged 19 to 24 years. *Clinical Therapeutics, 29*, 1967–1979.

Klein, R. G., Mannuzza, S., Olazagasti, M. A., Roizen, E., Hutchison, J. A., Lashua, E. C., & Castellanos, F. X. (2012). Clinical and functional outcome of childhood attention-deficit/hyperactivity disorder 33 years later. *Archives of General Psychiatry, 69*(12), 1295–1303. doi:10.1001/archgenpsychiatry.2012.271

Kok, F. M., Groen, Y., Fuermaier, A. B. M., & Tucha, O. (2016). Problematic peer functioning in girls with ADHD: A systematic literature review. *PLOS One, 11*, e0165119. doi:10.1371/journal.pone.0165119

Kollins, S. H., Jain, R., Brams, M., Segal, S., Findling, R. L., Wigal, S. B., & Khayrallah, M. (2011). Clonidine extended-release tablets as add-on therapy to psychostimulants in children and adolescents with ADHD. *Pediatrics, 127*(6), e1406–e1413. doi:10.1542/peds.2010-1260

Kraft, J. T., Dalsgaard, S., Obel, C., Thomsen, P. H., Henriksen, T. B., & Scahill, L. (2012). Prevalence and clinical correlates of tic disorders in a community sample of school-age children. *European Journal of Child & Adolescent Psychiatry, 21*, 5–13. doi:10.1007/s00787-011-0223-z

Kratochvil, C. J., Greenhill, L. L., March, J. S., Burke, W. J., & Vaughn, B. S. (2004). The role of stimulants in the treatment of preschool children with attention-deficit hyperactivity disorder. *CNS Drugs, 18*, 957–966. doi:10.2165/00023210-200418140-00001

Kratochvil, C. J., Newcorn, J. H., Arnold, L. E., Duesenberg, D., Emslie, G. J., Quintana, H., . . . Biederman, J. (2005). Atomoxetine alone or combined with fluoxetine for treating ADHD with comorbid depressive or anxiety symptoms. *Journal of the American Academy of Child & Adolescent Psychiatry, 44*, 915–924. doi:10.1097/01.chi.0000169012.81536.38

Kratochvil, C. J., Wilens, T. E., Greenhill, L. L., Gao, H., Baker, K. D., Feldman, P. D., & Gelowitz, D. L. (2006). The effects of long-term atomoxetine treatment for young children with attention-deficit hyperactivity disorder. *Journal of the American Academy of Child & Adolescent Psychiatry, 45*, 919–927. doi:10.1097/01.chi.0000222788.34229.68

Kratochvil, C. J., Vaughan, B. S., Stoner, J. A., Daughton, J. M., Lubberstedt, B. D., Murray, D. W., . . . March, J. S. (2011). A Double-Blind, Placebo-Controlled Study of Atomoxetine in Young Children with ADHD. *Pediatrics*, 127(4), e862–e868. doi:10.1542/peds.2010-0825

Kubas, H. A., Backenson, E. M., Wilcox, G., Piercy, J. C., & Hale, J. B. (2012). The effects of methylphenidate on cognitive function in children with attention-deficit/hyperactivity disorder. *Postgraduate Medicine, 124*(5), 33–48. doi:10.3810/pgm.2012.09.2592

Lahey, B. B., Pelham, W. E., Loney, J., Kipp, H., Ehrhardt, A., Lee, S. S., . . . Massetti, G. (2004). Three-year predictive validity of *DSM-IV* attention deficit hyperactivity disorder in children diagnosed at 4-6 years of age. *American Journal of Psychiatry, 161*(11), 2014–2020. doi:10.1176/appi.ajp.161.11.2014

Lahey, B. B., Pelham, W. E., Loney, J., Lee, S. S., & Willcutt, E. (2005). Instability of the DSM-IV subtypes of ADHD from preschool through elementary school. *Archives of General Psychiatry, 62*, 896–902.

Lamberti, M., Italiano, D., Guerriero, L., D'Amico, G., Siracusano, R., Ingrassia, M., . . . Gagliano A. (2015). Evaluation of acute cardiovascular effects of immediate-release methylphenidate in children and adolescents with attention-deficit hyperactivity disorder. *Neuropsychiatric Disease and Treatment, 11*, 1169–1174. doi:10.2147/NDT.S79866

Langberg, J. M., Arnold, L. E., Flowers, A. M., Epstein, J. N., Altaye, M., Hinshaw, S. P., . . . Hechtman, L. (2010). Parent-reported homework problems in the MTA study: Evidence for sustained improvement with behavioral treatment. *The Journal of Clinical Child and Adolescent Psychology, 39*, 220–233. doi:10.1080/15374410903532700

Lange, K. W., Hauser, J., Lange, K. M., Makulska-Gertruda, E., Nakamura, Y., Reissmann, A., . . . Takeuchi, Y. (2017). The role of nutritional supplements in the treatment of ADHD: What the evidence says. *Current Psychiatry Reports, 19*(2), 8. doi:10.1007/s11920-017-0762-1

Lee, S. S., Humphreys, K. L., Flory, K., Liu, R., & Glass, K. (2011). Prospective association of childhood attention-deficit/hyperactivity disorder (ADHD) and substance use and abuse/dependence: a meta-analytic review. *Clinical Psychology Review, 31*(3):328–341. doi:10.1016/j.cpr.2011.01.006

Lee, S. S., Sibley, M. H., & Epstein, J. N. (2016). Attention-deficit/hyperactivity disorder across development: Predictors, resilience, and future directions. *Journal of Abnormal Psychology, 125*, 151–153. doi:10.1037/abn.0000114

Leffler, J. M., Riebel, J., & Hughes, H. M. (2015). A review of child and adolescent diagnostic interviews for clinical practitioners. *Assessment, 22*(6), 690–703. doi:10.1177/1073191114561253

Lemmon, M. E., Gregas, M., & Jeste, S. S. (2011). Risperidone use in autism spectrum disorders: A retrospective review of a clinic-referred patient population. *Journal of Child Neurology, 26*(4), 428–432. doi:10.1177/0883073810382143

Leonard, M. A., Milich, R., & Lorch, E. P. (2011). The role of pragmatic language use in mediating the relation between hyperactivity and inattention and social skills problems. *Journal of Speech Language & Hearing Research, 54*, 567–579. doi:10.1044/1092-4388(2010/10-0058)

Levy, F., Wimalaweera, S., Moul, C., Brennan, J., & Dadds, M. R. (2013). Dopamine receptors and the pharmacogenetics of side-effects of stimulant treatment for attention-deficit/hyperactivity disorder. *Journal of Child and Adolescent Psychopharmacology, 23*(6), 423–425. doi:10.1089/cap.2013.0006

Lima Lde, A., Feio-dos-Santos, A. C., Belangero, S. I., Gadelha, A., Bressan, R. A., Salum, G. A., . . . Brentani, H. (2016). An integrative approach to investigate the respective roles of single-nucleotide variants and copy-number variants in attention-deficit/hyperactivity disorder. *Scientific Reports, 6*, 22851. doi:10.1038/srep22851

Lipkin, P. H., Goldstein, I. J., & Adesman, A. R. (1994). Tics and dyskinesias associated with stimulant treatment in attention-deficit/hyperactivity disorder. *Archives of Pediatrics & Adolescent Medicine, 148*, 859–861.

Lo-Castro, A., D'Agati, E., & Curatolo, P. (2010). ADHD and genetic syndromes. *Brain and Development, 33*(6), 456–461. doi:10.1016/j.braindev.2010.05.011

Loe, I. M., & Feldman, H. M. (2007). Academic and educational outcomes of children with ADHD. *Ambulatory Pediatrics, 7*(Suppl. 1), 82–90. doi:10.1016/j.ambp.2006.05.005

Loy, J. H., Merry, S. N., Hetrick, S. E., & Stasiak, K. (2017). Atypical antipsychotics for disruptive behavior disorders in children and youths. *Cochrane Database System Review, 8*, CD008559. doi:10.1002/14651858.CD008559.pub3

Lu, Y., Sjölander, A., Cederlöf, M., D'Onofrio, B. M., Almqvist, C., Larsson, H., & Lichtenstein, P. (2017). Association between medication use and performance on higher education entrance tests in individuals with attention-deficit/hyperactivity disorder. *JAMA Psychiatry, 74*(8), 815–822. doi:10.1001/jamapsychiatry.2017.1472

Maayan, L., Paykina, N., Fried, J., Strauss, T., Gugga, S. S., & Greenhill, L. (2009). The open-label treatment of attention-deficit/hyperactivity disorder in 4- and 5-year-old children with beaded methylphenidate. *Journal of Child & Adolescent Psychopharmacology, 19*, 147–153. doi:10.1089/cap.2008.053

Mahone, E. M., Ranta, M. E., Crocetti, D., O'Brien, J., Kaufmann, W. E., Denckla, M. B., & Mostofsky, S. H. (2011). Comprehensive examination of frontal regions in boys and girls with attention-deficit/hyperactivity disorder. *Journal of the International Neuropsychological Society, 17*(6), 1047–1057. doi:10.1017/S1355617711001056

Man, K. K. C., Ip, P., Chan, E. W., Law, S. L., Leung, M. T. Y., Ma, E. X. Y., . . . Wong, I. C. K. (2017). Effectiveness of pharmacological treatment for attention-deficit/hyperactivity disorder on physical injuries: A systematic review and meta-analysis of observational studies. *CNS Drugs, 31*(12), 1043-1055. doi:10.1007/s40263-017-0485-1

Maneeton, N., Maneeton, B., Srisurapanont, M., & Martin, S. D. (2011). Bupropion for adults with attention-deficit/hyperactivity disorder: Meta-analysis of randomized, placebo-controlled trials. *Psychiatry and Clinical Neurosciences, 65*(7), 611–617. doi:10.1111/j.1440-1819.2011.02264.x

Maneeton, N., Maneeton, B., Intaprasert, S., & Woottliluk, P. (2014). A systematic review of randomized controlled trials of bupropion versus methylphenidate in the treatment of attention-deficit/hyperactivity disorder. *Neuropsychiatric Disease and Treatment, 10*, 1439–49. doi:10.1002/hup.2242

Manor, I., Magen, A., Keidar, D., Rosen, S., Tasker, H., Cohen, T., . . . Weizman, A. (2012). The effect of phosphatidylserine containing omega3 fatty-acids on attention-deficit hyperactivity disorder symptoms in children: A double-blind placebo-controlled trial, followed by an open-label extension. *Eurpean Psychiatry, 27*(5), 335–342. doi:10.1016/j.eurpsy.2011.05.004

Marangoni, C., De Chiara, L., & Faedda, G. L. (2015). Bipolar disorder and ADHD: Comorbidity and diagnostic distinctions. *Current Psychiatry Reports, 17*, 67. doi:10.1007/s11920-015-0604-y

Marcus, R. N., Owen, R., Manos, G., Mankoski, R., Kamen, L., McQuade, R. D., . . . Findling, R. L. (2011). Safety and tolerability of aripiprazole for irritability in pediatric patients with autistic disorder: A 52-week, open-label, multicenter study. *Journal of Clinical Psychopharmacology, 72*(9), 1270–1276. doi:10.4088/JCP.09m05933

Martin, N. C., Piek, J. P., & Hay, D. (2006). DCD and ADHD: A genetic study of their shared etiology. *Human Movement Science, 25*, 110–124.

Martinussen, R., Hayden, J., Hogg-Johnson, S., & Tannock, R. (2005). A meta-analysis of working memory in children with attention-deficit/hyperactivity disorder. *Journal of the American Academy of Child and Adolescent Psychiatry, 44*, 377–384. doi:10.1097/01.chi.0000153228.72591.73

May, D. E., & Kratochvil, C. J. (2010). Attention-deficit/hyperactivity disorder: Recent advances in pediatric pharmacotherapy. *Drugs, 70*, 15–40.

Maziade, M., Rouleau, N., Lee, B., Rogers, A., David, L., & Dickson, R. (2009). Atomoxetine and neuropsychological function in children with attention-deficit/hyperactivity disorder: Results of a pilot study. *Journal of Child & Adolescent Psychopharmacology, 19*, 709–718. doi:10.1089/cap.2008.0166

Mazzone, L., Reale, L., Mannino, V., Cocuzza, M., & Vitiello, B. (2011). Lower IQ is associated with decreased clinical response to atomoxetine in children and adolescents with attention-deficit hyperactivity disorder. *CNS Drugs, 25*(6), 503–509. doi:10.2165/11590450-000000000-00000

McBurnett, K., & Pfiffner, L. J. (2009). Treatment of aggressive ADHD in children and adolescents: Conceptualization and treatment of comorbid behavior disorders. *Postgraduate Medicine, 121*, 158–165. doi:10.3810/pgm.2009.11.2084

McCann, D., Barrett, A., Cooper, A., Crumpler, D., Dalen, L., Grimshaw, K., & Stevenson, J. (2007). Food additives and hyperactive behavior in 3-year-old and 8/9-year-old children in the community: A randomised, double-blinded, placebo-controlled trial. *Lancet, 370*, 1560–1567. doi:10.1016/S0140-6736(07)61306-3

McCracken, J. T., McGough, J. J., Loo, S. K., Levitt, J., Del'Homme, M., Cowen, J., . . . Bilder, R. M. (2016). Combined stimulant and guanfacine administration in attention deficit/hyperactivity disorder: A controlled, comparative study. *Journal of the American Academy of Child & Adolescent Psychiatry, 55*(8), 657–666.e1. doi:10.1016/j.jaac.2016.05.015

McDougle, C. J., Scahill, L., Aman, M. G., McCracken, J. T., Tierney, E., Davies, M., & Vitiello, B. (2005). Risperidone for the core symptom domains of autism: Results from the study by the autism network of the research units on pediatric psychopharmacology. *American Journal of Psychiatry, 162*, 1142–1148. doi:10.1176/appi.ajp.162.6.1142

McInnes, A., Humphries, T., Hogg-Johnson, S., & Tannock, R. (2003). Listening comprehension and working memory are impaired in attention-deficit/hyperactivity disorder irrespective of language impairment. *Journal of Abnormal Child Psychology, 31*, 427–443.

McKeown, R. E., Holbrook, J. R., Danielson, M. L., Cuffe, S. P., Wolraich, M. L., & Visser, S. N. (2015). The impact of case definition on attention-deficit/hyperactivity disorder prevalence estimates in community-based samples of school-aged children. *Journal of the American Academy of Child & Adolescent Psychiatry, 54,* 53–61.

McLennan, J. D. (2016). Understanding attention deficit hyperactivity disorder as a continuum. *Canadian Family Physician, 62,* 979–982.

Meinzer, M. C., Pettit, J. W., & Viswesvan, C. (2014). The co-occurrence of attention-deficit/hyperactivity disorder and unipolar depression in children and adolescents: A meta-analytic review. *Clinical Psychology Review, 34,* 595–607. doi:10.1016/j.cpr.2014.10.002

Metin, B., Krebs, R. M., Wiersema, J. R., Verguts, T., Gasthuys, R., van der Meere, J. J., . . . Sonuga-Barke, E. (2015). Dysfunctional modulation of default mode network activity in attention-deficit/hyperactivity disorder. *Journal of Abnormal Psychology, 124*(1), 208–214. doi:10.1037/abn0000013

Middeldorp, C. M., Hammerschlag, A. R., Ouwens, K. G., Groen-Blokhuis, M. M., Pourcain, B. S., Greven, C. U., . . . Boomsma, D. I. (2016). A genome-wide association meta-analysis of attention-deficit/hyperactivity disorder symptoms in population-based pediatric cohorts. *Journal of the American Academy of Child & Adolescent Psychiatry, 55*(10), 896–905 e896. doi:10.1016/j.jaac.2016.05.025

Mikami, A. Y., Jia, M., & Jiwon, J. (2014). Social skills training. *Child & Adolescent Psychiatric Clinics of North America, 23,* 775–788. doi:10.1016/j.chc.2014.05.007

Ming, X., Mulvey, M., Mohanty, S., & Patel, V. (2011). Safety and efficacy of clonidine and clonidine extended-release in the treatment of children and adolescents with attention deficit hyperactivity disorders. *Adolescent Health, Medicine and Therapeutics, 2,* 105–112. doi:10.2147/AHMT.S15672

Miodovnik, A., Harstad, E., Sideridis, G., & Huntington, N. (2015). Timing of the diagnosis of attention-deficit/hyperactivity disorder and autism spectrum disorder. *Pediatrics, 136,* e830–e837. doi:10.1542/peds.2015-1502

Modesto-Lowe, V., Charbonneau, V., & Farahmand, P. (2017). Psychotherapy for adolescents with attention-deficit/hyperactivity disorder: A pediatrician's guide. *Clinical Pediatrics, 56,* 667–674. doi:10.1177/0009922816673308

Moffitt, T. E., Houts, R., Asherson, P., Belsky, D. W., Corcoran, D. L., Hammerle, M., . . . Caspi, A. (2015). Is adult ADHD a childhood-onset neurodevelopmental disorder? Evidence from a four-decade longitudinal cohort study. *American Journal of Psychiatry, 172*(10), 967–977. doi:10.1176/appi.ajp.2015.14101266

Mohammadi, M. R., Hafezi, P., Galeiha, A., Hajiaghaee, R, & Akhondzadeh, S. (2012). Buspirone versus methylphenidate in the treatment of children with attention-deficit/hyperactivity disorder: Randomized double-blind study. *Acta Medica Iranica, 50*(11), 723–738.

Mohan, A., Roberto, A. J., Mohan, A., Lorenzo, A., Jones, K., Carney, M. J., . . . Lapidus, K. A. (2016). The significance of the default mode network (DMN) in neurological and neuropsychiatric disorders: A review. *Yale Journal of Biology and Medicine, 89*(1), 49–57.

Molina, B. S., Hinshaw, S. P., Eugene, A. L., Swanson, J. M., Pelham, W. E., Hechtman, L., . . . MTA Cooperative Group (2013). Adolescent substance use in the multimodal treatment study of attention-deficit/hyperactivity disorder (ADHD) (MTA) as a function of childhood ADHD, random assignment to childhood treatments, and subsequent medication. *Journal of the American Academy of Child & Adolescent Psychiatry, 52*(3), 250–263. doi:10.1016/j.jaac.2012.12.014

Molitor, S. J., Langberg, J. M., & Evans, S. W. (2016). The written expression abilities of adolescents with attention-deficit/hyperactivity disorder. *Research in Developmental Disabilities, 51-51,* 49–59. doi:10.1016/j.ridd.2016.01.005

Monastra, V. J. (2008). Quantitative electroencephalography and attention-deficit/hyperactivity disorder: Implications for clinical practice. *Current Psychiatry Reports, 10,* 432–438. doi:10.1007/s11920-008-0069-3

Montgomery, P., Burton, J. R., Sewell, R. P., Spreckelsen, T. F., & Richardson, A. J. (2013). Low blood long chain omega-3 fatty acids in UK children are associated with poor cognitive performance and behavior: A cross-sectional analysis from the DOLAB study. *PLoS One, 8,* e66697. doi:10.1371/journal.pone.0066697

Mooney, M. A., McWeeney, S. K., Faraone, S. V., Hinney, A., Hebebrand, J., Consortium, I., . . . Wilmot, B. (2016). Pathway analysis in attention deficit hyperactivity disorder: An ensemble approach. *American Journal of Medical Genetics B: Neuropsychiatric Genetics, 171*(6), 815–826. doi:10.1002/ajmg.b.32446

Mostafalou, S., & Abdollahi, M. (2017). Pesticides: An update of human exposure and toxicity. *Archives of Toxicology, 91,* 549–599. doi:10.1007/s00204-016-1849-x

Mrug, S., Molina, B. S., Hoza, B., Gerdes, A. C., Hinshaw, S. P., Hechtman, L., & Arnold, L. E. (2012). Peer rejection and friendships in children with attention-deficit/hyperactivity disorder: Contributions to long-term outcomes. *Journal of Abnormal Child Psychology, 40*(6), 1013–1026. doi:10.1007/s10802-012-9610-2

MTA Cooperative Group. (1999a). A 14-month randomized clinical trial of treatment strategies for attention-deficit/hyperactivity disorder. *Archive of General Psychiatry, 56,* 1073–1086.

MTA Cooperative Group. (1999b). Moderators and mediators of treatment response for children with attention-deficit/hyperactivity disorder. *Archives of General Psychiatry, 56,* 1088–1096.

MTA Cooperative Group. (2004a). National Institute of Mental Health multimodal treatment study of ADHD follow-up: 24-month outcomes of treatment strategies for attention-deficit/hyperactivity disorder. *Pediatrics, 113,* 754–761.

MTA Cooperative Group. (2004b). National Institute of Mental Health multimodal treatment study of ADHD follow-up: Changes in effectiveness and growth after the end of treatment. *Pediatrics, 113,* 762–769.

Murphy, K., Ratey, N., Maynard, S., Sussman, S., & Wright, S. D. (2010). Coaching for ADHD. *Journal of Attention Disorders, 13,* 546–552. doi:10.1177/1087054709344186

Murray, D. W. (2010). Treatment of preschoolers with attention-deficit/hyperactivity disorder. *Current Psychiatry Reports, 12,* 374–381. doi:10.1007/s11920-010-0142-6

Nazar, B. P., Bernardes, C., Peachey, G., Sargeant, J., Mattos, P., & Treasure, J. (2016). The risk of eating disorders comorbid with attention-deficit/hyperactivity disorder: A systematic review and meta-analysis. *International Journal of Eating Disorders, 49,* 1045–1057. doi:10.1002/eat.22643

Nevels, R. M., Dehon, E. E., Alexander, K., & Gontkovsky, S. T. (2010). Psychopharmacology of aggression in children and adolescents with primary neuropsychiatric disorders: A review of current and potentially promising treatment options. *Experimental & Clinical Psychopharmacology, 18,* 184–201. doi:10.1037/a0018059

Newcorn, J. H., Stein, M. A., Childress, A. C., Youcha, S., White, C., Enright, G., & Rubin, J. (2013). Randomized, double-blind trial of guanfacine extended release in children with attention-deficit/hyperactivity disorder: Morning or evening administration. *Journal of the American Academy of Child & Adolescent Psychiatry, 52*(9), 921–930. doi:10.1016/j.jaac.2013.06.006

Nicolescu, R., Petcu, C., Cordeanu, A., Fabritius, K., Schlumpf, M., Krebs, R., . . . Winneke, G. (2010). Environmental exposure to lead, but not other neurotoxic metals, relates to core elements of ADHD in Romanian children: Performance and questionnaire data. *Environmental Research, 110,* 476–483. doi:10.1016/j.envres.2010.04.002

Nigg, J. T., & Holton, K. (2014). Restriction and elimination diets in ADHD treatment. *Child and Adolescent Psychiatric Clinics of North America, 23,* 937–953. doi:10.106/j.chc.2014.05.010

Nigg, J. T., Lewis, K., Edinger, T., & Falk, M. (2012). Meta-analysis of attention-deficit/hyperactivity disorder or attention-deficit/hyperactivity disorder symptoms, restriction diet, and synthetic food color additives. *Journal of the American Academy of Child & Adolescent Psychiatry, 51,* 86–97. doi:10.1016/j.jaac.2011.10.015

Nijmeijer, J. S., Minderaa, R. B., Buitelaar, J. K., Mulligan, A., Hartman, C., & Hoekstra, P. J. (2007). Attention-deficit/hyperactivity disorder and social dysfunctioning. *Clinical Psychology Review, 28,* 692–708. doi:10.1016/j.cpr.2007.10.003

Nikolas, M. A., & Burt, S. A. (2010). Genetic and environmental influences on ADHD symptom dimensions of inattention and hyperactivity: A meta-analysis. *Journal of Abnormal Psychology, 119,* 1–17. doi:10.1037/a0018010

Olfson, M., Crystal, S., Huang, C., & Gerhard, T. (2010). Trends in antipsychotic drug use by very young, privately insured children. *Journal of the American Academy of Child & Adolescent Psychiatry, 49,* 13–23. doi:10.1097/00004583-201001000-00005

Olfson, M., Huang, C., Gerhard, T., Winterstein, A. G., Crystal, S., Allison, P. D., & Marcus, S. C. (2012). Stimulants and cardiovascular events in youth with attention-deficit/hyperactivity disorder. *Journal of the American Academy of Child & Adolescent Psychiatry, 51*(2), 147–156. doi:10.1016/j.jaac.2011.11.008

Osunsanmi, S., & Turk, J. (2016). Influence of age, gender, and living circumstances on patterns of attention-deficit/hyperactivity disorder medication use in children and adolescents with or without intellectual disabilities. *Journal of Child & Adolescent Psychopharmacology, 26*(9), 828–834.

Otasowie, J., Castells, X., Ehimare, U. P., & Smith, C. H. (2014). Trycyclic antidepressants for attention deficit hyperactivity disorder (ADHD) in children and adolescents. *Cochrane Database System Review, 19,* 9. doi:10.1002/14651858.CD006997.pub2

Owens, J. S., Goldfine, M. E., Evangelista, N. M., Hoza, B., & Kaiser, N. M. (2007). A critical review of self-perceptions and the positive illusory bias in children with ADHD. *Clinical Child & Family Psychology Review, 10,* 335–351. doi:10.1007/s10567-007-0027-3

Ozbaran, B., Kose, S., Yuzuguldu, O., Atar, B., & Aydin, C. (2015). Combined methylphenidate and atomoxetine pharmacotherapy in attention deficit hyperactivity disorder. *The World Journal of Biological Psychiatry, 16*(8), 619–624. doi:10.3109/15622975.2015.1051109.

Ozdag, M. F., Yorbik, O., Ulas, U. H., Hamamcioglu, K., & Vural, O. (2004). Effect of methylphenidate on auditory event related potentials in boys with attention deficit hyperactivity disorder. *International Journal of Pediatric Otorhinolaryngology, 68,* 1267–1272. doi:10.1016/j.ijporl.2004.04.023

Palumbo, D., Spencer, T., Lynch, J., CoChien, H., & Faraone, S. V. (2004). Emergence of tics in children with ADHD: Impact of once-daily OROS methylphenidate therapy. *Journal of Child & Adolescent Psychopharmacology, 14,* 185–194. doi:10.1089/1044546041649138

Pastor, P. N., Reuben, C. A., Duran, C. R., & Hawkins, L. D. (2015). Associations between diagnosed ADHD and selected characteristics among children 4-17 years: United States, 2011-2013. *NCHS Data Brief, 201,* 1–8..

Pauls, A. M., O'Daly O. G., Rubia, K., Riedel, W. J., Williams, S. C. R., & Mehta, M. A. (2012). Methylphenidate effects on prefrontal functioning during attentional-capture and response inhibition. *Biological Psychiatry, 72*(2), 142–149. doi:10.1016/j.biopsych.2012.03.028

Pearson, D. A., Santos, C. W., Aman, M. G., Arnold, L. E., Casat, C. D., Mansour, R., . . . Cleveland, L. A. (2013). Effects of extended release methylphenidate treatment on ratings of attention-deficit/hyperactivity disorder (ADHD) and associated behavior in children with autism spectrum disorders and ADHD symptoms. *Journal of Child and Adolescent Psychopharmacology, 23*(5), 337–351. doi:10.1089/cap.2012.0096

Pelham, W. E., & Fabiano, G. A. (2008). Evidence-based psychosocial treatments for attention-deficit/hyperactivity disorder. *Journal of Clinical Child & Adolescent Psychology, 37,* 184–214. doi:10.1080/15374410701818681

Pelham, W. E., Fabiano, G. A., & Massetti, G. M. (2005). Evidence-based assessment of attention-deficit/hyperactivity disorder in children and adolescents. *Journal of Clinical Child and Adolescent Psychology, 34,* 449–476. doi:10.1207/s15374424jccp3403_5

Pelham, W. E., Jr., Fabiano, G. A., Waxmonsky, J. G., Greiner, A. R., Gnagy, E. M., Pelham, W. E., III, . . . Murphy, S. A. (2016). Treatment sequencing for childhood ADHD: A multiple-randomization study of adaptive medication and behavioral interventions. *Journal of Clinical Child & Adolescent Psychology, 45*(4), 396 *NCHS Data Brief,* (415. doi:10.1080/15374416.2015.1105138

Pelsser, L. M. J., Frankena, K., Toorman, J., & Pereira, R. R. (2017). Diet and ADHD, reviewing the evidence: A systematic review of meta-analyses of double-blind placebo-controlled trials evaluating the efficacy of diet interventions on the behavior of children with ADHD. *PLoS ONE, 12,* e0169277. doi:10.1371/journal.pone.0169277

Pelsser, L. M. J., Frankena, K., Toorman, J., Savelkoul, H. F. J., Pereira, R. R., & Buitelar, J. K. (2009). A randomized controlled trial into the effects of food on ADHD. *European Journal of Child & Adolescent Psychiatry, 18,* 12–19.

Perera, H., Jeewandara, K. C., Seneviratne, S., & Guruge, C. (2012). Combined omega3 and omega6 supplementation in children with attention-deficit hyperactivity disorder (ADHD) refractory to methylphenidate treatment: A double-blind, placebo-controlled study. *Journal of Child Neurology, 27,* 747–753. doi:10.1177/0883073811435243

Pham, A. V., & Riviere, A. (2015). Specific learning disorders and ADHD: Current issues in diagnosis across clinical and educational settings. *Current Psychiatry Reports, 17,* 38. doi:10.1007/s11920-015-0584-y

Piek, J. P., & Dyck, M. J. (2004). Sensory-motor deficits in children with developmental coordination disorder, attention-deficit/hyperactivity disorder and autistic disorder. *Human Movement Science, 23,* 475–488. doi:10.1016/j.humov.2004.08.019

Pievsky, M. A., & McGrath, R. E. (2018). The neurocognitive profile of attention-deficit/hyperactivity disorder: A review of meta-analyses. *Archives of Clinical Neuropsychology, 33*(2), 143 *NCHS Data Brief,* (157. doi:10.1093/arclin/acx055

Pingault, J. B., Viding, E., Galera, C., Greven, C. U., Zheng, Y., Plomin, R., & Rijsdijk, F. (2015). Genetic and environmental influences on the developmental course of attention-deficit/hyperactivity disorder symptoms from childhood to adolescence. *JAMA Psychiatry, 72*(7), 651–658. doi:10.1001/jamapsychiatry.2015.0469

Pliszka, S. R. (2000). Patterns of psychiatric comorbidity with attention deficit hyperactivity disorder. *Child & Adolescent Psychiatric Clinics of North America, 9,* 525–540.

Pliszka, S. R., Crismon, M. L., Hughes, C. W., Corners, C. K., Emslie, G. J., Jensen, P. S., . . . Lopez, M. (2006). The Texas children's medication algorithm project: Revision of the algorithm for pharmacotherapy of attention-deficit/hyperactivity disorder. *Journal of the American Academy of Child & Adolescent Psychiatry, 45,* 642–657. doi:10.1097/01.chi.0000215326.51175.eb

Polanczyk, G. V., Salum, G. A., Sugaya, L. S., Caye, A., & Rohde, L. A. (2015). Annual Research Review: A meta-analysis of the worldwide prevalence of mental disorders in children and adolescents. *Journal of Child Psychology & Psychiatry, 56,* 345–365. doi:10.1111/jcpp.12381

Polanczyk, G. V., Willcutt, E. G., Salum, G. A., Kieling, C., & Rohde, L. A. (2014). ADHD prevalence estimates across three decades: An updated systematic review and meta-regression analysis. *International Journal of Epidemiology, 43,* 434–442. doi:10.1093/ije/dyt261

Pollak, Y., Benarroch, F., Kanengisser, L., Shilon, Y., Benpazi, H., Shalev, R. S., & Gross-Tsur, V. (2009). Tourette syndrome–associated psychopathology: Roles of comorbid attention-deficit/hyperactivity disorder and obsessive compulsive disorder. *Journal of Developmental & Behavioral Pediatrics, 30,* 413–419. doi:10.1097/DBP.0b013e3181ba0f89

Popper, C. W. (2000). Pharmacologic alternatives to psychostimulants for the treatment of attention-deficit/hyperactivity disorder. *Child & Adolescent Psychiatric Clinics of North America, 9,* 605–646.

Posey, D. J., Stigler, K. A., Erickson, C. A., & McDougle, C. J. (2008). Antipsychotics in the treatment of autism. *Journal of Clinical Investigation, 118,* 6–14. doi:10.1172/JCI32483

Prevatt, F. (2016). Coaching for college students with ADHD. *Current Psychiatry Reports, 18,* 110. doi:10.1007/s11920-016-0751-9

Pringsheim T., Hirsch, L., Gardner, D. M., et al. (2015). The pharmacological management of oppositional behaviour, conduct problems, and aggression in children and adolescents with attention-deficit hyperactivity disorder, oppositional defiant disorder, and conduct disorder: a systematic review and meta-analysis. Part 1: psychostimulants, alpha-2 agonists, and atomoxetine. Can J Psychiatry, 60(2):42–51. doi:10.1177/070674371506000202

Pringsheim, T., & Steeves, T. (2011). Pharmacological treatment for attention deficit hyperactivity disorder (ADHD) in children with comorbid tic disorders. *Cochrane Database System Review,* 4, CD007990. doi:10.1002/14651858.CD007990.pub2

Punja, S., Shamseer, L., Hartling, L., Urichuk, L., Vandermeer, B., Nikles, J., & Vohra, S. (2016). Amphetamines for attention deficit hyperactivity disorder (ADHD) in children and adolescents. *Cochrane Database System Review, 2,* CD009996. doi:10.1002/14651858.CD009996.pub2

Qiu, A., Crocetti, D., Adler, M., Mahone, E. M., Denckla, M. B., Miller, M. I., & Mostofsky, S. H. (2009). Basal ganglia volume and shape in children with attention deficit hyperactivity disorder. *American Journal of Psychiatry, 166*(1), 74–82. doi:10.1176/appi.ajp.2008.08030426

Quinn, P. D., Chang, Z., Hur, K., Gibbons, R. D., Lahey, B. B., Rickert, M. E., . . . D'Onofrio, B. M. (2017). ADHD medication and substance-related problems. *American Journal of Psychiatry, 174*(9), 877–885. doi:10.1176/appi.ajp.2017.16060686

Quinn, P. O. (2008). Attention-deficit/hyperactivity disorder and its comorbidities in women and girls: An evolving picture. *Current Psychiatry Reports, 10,* 419–423. doi:10.1007/s11920-008-0067-5

Raggi, V. L., & Chronis, A. M. (2006). Interventions to address the academic impairment of children and adolescents with ADHD. *Clinical Child and Family Psychology Review, 9,* 85–111. doi:10.1007/s10567-006-0006-0

Rapaport, J., Buchsbaum, M., Zahn, T. P., Weingartner, H., Ludlow, C., & Mikkelsen, E. J. (1978). Dextroamphetamine: Cognitive and behavioral effects in normal prepubertal boys. *Science, 199,* 560–563. doi:10.1126/science.341313

Rapport, M. D., Orban, S. A., Kofler, M. J., & Friedman, L. M. (2013). Do programs designed to train working memory, other executive functions, and attention benefit children with ADHD? A meta-analytic review of cognitive, academic, and behavioral outcomes. *Clinical Psychology Review, 33,* 1237–1252. doi:10.1016/j.cpr.2013.08.005

Reale, L., Bartoli, B., Cartabia, M., Zanetti, M., Costantino, M. A., Canevini, M. P., Termine, C., & Bonati, M. (2017). Comorbidity prevalence and treatment outcome in children and adolescents with ADHD. *European Child & Adolescent Psychiatry, 26*(12), 1443–1457. doi:10.1007/s00787-017-1005-z

Redmond, S. M. (2016). Language impairment in attention-deficit/hyperactivity disorder context. *Journal of Speech, Language, and Hearing Research, 59,* 133–142. doi:10.1044/2015_JSLHR-L-15-0038

Reed, V. A., Buitelaar, J. K., Anand, E., Day, K. A., Treuer, T., Upadhyaya, H. P., . . . Savill, N. C. (2016). The safety of atomoxetine for the treatment of children and adolescents with attention-deficit/hyperactivity disorder: A comprehensive review of over a decade of research. *CNS Drugs, 30*(7), 603–628. doi:10.1007/s40263-016-0349-0

Rehabilitation Act of 1973, PL 93-112 29 U.S.C. §§ 791 *et seq.*

Reyes, M., Croonenberghs, J., Augustyns, I., & Eerdekens, M. (2006). Long-term use of risperidone in children with disruptive behavior disorders and sub-average intelligence: Efficacy, safety, and tolerability. *Journal of Child & Adolescent Psychopharmacology, 16,* 260–272. doi:10.1089/cap.2006.16.260

Reynolds, C. R., & Kamphaus, R. W. (2015). *Behavior Assessment System for Children, Third Edition (BASC-3).* New York, NY: Pearson.

Riddle, M. A., Yershova, K., Lazzaretto, D., Paykina, N., Yenokyan, G., Greenhill, L., . . . Posner, K. (2013). The Preschool Attention-Deficit/Hyperactivity Disorder Treatment Study (PATS) 6-year follow-up. *Journal of the American Academy of Child & Adolescent Psychiatry, 52*(3), 264–278 e262. doi:10.1016/j.jaac.2012.12.007

Riglin, L., Collishaw, S., Thapar, A. K., Dalsgaard, S., Langley, K., Smith, G. D., . . . Thapar, A. (2016). Association of genetic risk variants with attention-deficit/hyperactivity disorder trajectories in the general population. *JAMA Psychiatry, 73*(12), 1285–1292. doi:10.1001/jamapsychiatry.2016.2817

Ríos-Hernández, A., Alda, J. A., Farran-Codina, A., Ferreira-García, E., & Izquierdo-Pulido, M. (2017). The Mediterranean diet and ADHD in children and adolescents. *Pediatrics, 139*, e20162027. doi:10.1542/peds.2016-2027

Ritz, B. W., & Lord, R. S. (2005). Case study: The effectiveness of a dietary supplement regimen in reducing IgG-mediated food sensitivity in ADHD. *Alternative Therapies, 11*, 72–75.

Rizzo, R., Gulisano, M., Calì, P. V., & Curatolo, P. (2013). Tourette syndrome and comorbid ADHD: Current pharmacological treatment options. *European Journal of Paediatric Neurology, 17*(5), 421–428. doi:10.1016/j.ejpn.2013.01.005

Robin, A. L. (2008). Family intervention for home-based problems of adolescents with attention-deficit/hyperactivity disorder. *Adolescent Medicine, 19*, 268–277.

Robin, A. L. (2014). Family therapy for adolescents with ADHD. *Child & Adolescent Clinics of North America, 23*, 747–756. doi:10.1016/j.chc.2014.06.001

Robinson, K. E., Kaizar, E., Catroppa, C., Godfrey, C., & Yeates, K. O. (2014). Systematic review and meta-analysis of cognitive interventions for children with central nervous system disorders and neurodevelopmental disorders. *Journal of Pediatric Psychology, 39*, 846–865. doi:10.1093/jpepsy/jsu031

Rowland, A. S., Skipper, B. J., Umbach, D. M., Rabiner, D. L., Campbell, R. A., Naftel, A. J., & Sandler, D. P. (2015). The prevalence of ADHD in a population-based sample. *Journal of Attention Disorders, 19*(9), 741–754. doi:10.1177/1087054713513799

Roy, A., Hechtman, L., Arnold, L. E., Swanson, J. M., Molina, B. S. G., Sibley, M. H., . . . MTA Cooperative Group. (2017). Childhood predictors of adult functional outcomes in the Multimodal Treatment Study of Attention-Deficit/Hyperactivity Disorder (MTA). *Journal of the American Academy of Child & Adolescent Psychiatry, 56*(8), 687–695 e687. doi:10.1016/j.jaac.2017.05.020

Rubia, K., Halari, R., Cubillo, A., Smith, A. B., Mohammad, A. M., Brammer, M., & Taylor, E. (2011). Methylphenidate normalizes fronto-striatal underactivation during interference inhibition in medication-naïve boys with attention-deficit hyperactivity disorder. *Neuropsychopharmacology, 36*(8), 1575–1586. doi:10.1038/npp.2011.30

Rubia, K., Alegria, A., & Brinson, H. (2014). Imaging the ADHD brain: disorder-specificity, medication effects and clinical translation. *Expert Review of Neurotherapeutics, 14*(5), 519–538. doi:10.1586/14737175.2014.907526

Rucklidge, J. J. (2010). Gender differences in ADHD. *Psychiatric Clinics of North America, 33*, 357–373.

Rucklidge, J. J., Eggleston, M. J. F., Johnstone, J. M., Darling, K., & Framptom, C. M. (2017). Vitamin-mineral treatment improves aggression and emotional regulation in children with ADHD: A fully blinded, randomized, placebo-controlled trial. *Journal of Child Psychology & Psychiatry, 59*(3), 232–246. doi:10.1111/jcpp.12817

Rucklidge, J. J., Frampton, C. M., Gorman, B., & Boggis, A. (2014). Vitamin-mineral treatment of attention-deficit hyperactivity disorder in adults: Double-blind randomized placebo-controlled trial. *British Journal of Psychiatry, 204*, 306–315. doi:10.1192/bjp.bp.113.132126

Rushton, J. L., Fant, K. E., & Clark, S. J. (2004). Use of practice guidelines in the primary care of children with attention-deficit/hyperactivity disorder. *Pediatrics, 114*, e23–e28. doi:10.1542/peds.114.1.e23

Safren, S. A., Sprich, S., Mimiaga, M. J., Surman, C., Knouse, L., Groves, M., & Otto, M. W. (2010). Cognitive behavioral therapy vs. relaxation with educational support for medication-treated adults with ADHD and persistent symptoms: A randomized controlled trial. *Journal of the American Medical Association, 304*, 875–880. doi:10.1001/jama.2010.1192

Sallee, F. R. (2010). The role of alpha2-adrenergic agonists in attention-deficit/hyperactivity disorder. *Postgraduate Medicine, 122*, 78–87. doi:10.3810/pgm.2010.09.2204

Sallee, F. R., Lyne, A., Wigal, T., & McGough, J. J. (2009). Long-term safety and efficacy of guanfacine extended release in children and adolescents with attention-deficit/hyperactivity disorder. *Journal of Child & Adolescent Psychopharmacology, 19*, 215–226. doi:10.1089/cap.2008.0080

Sasser, T. R., Kalvin, C. B., & Bierman, K. L. (2016). Developmental trajectories of clinically significant attention-deficit/hyperactivity disorder (ADHD) symptoms from Grade 3 through 12 in a high-risk sample: Predictors and outcomes. *Journal of Abnormal Psychology, 125*, 207–219. doi:10.1037/abn0000112

Satterthwaite, T. D., Wolf, D. H., Erus, G., Ruparel, K., Elliott, M. A., Gennatas, E. D., . . . Gur, R. E. (2013). Functional maturation of the executive system during adolescence. *Journal of Neuroscience, 33*(41), 16249–16261. doi:10.1523/JNEUROSCI.2345-13.2013

Sauer, J. M., Ring, B. J., & Witcher, J. W. (2005). Clinical pharmacokinetics of atomoxetine. *Clinical Pharmacokinetics, 44*(6), 571–590.

Savill, N. C., Buitelaar, J. K., Anand, E., Day, K. A., Treuer, T., Upadhyaya, H. P., & Coghill, D. (2015). The efficacy of atomoxetine for the treatment of children and adolescents with attention-deficit/hyperactivity disorder: A comprehensive review of over a decade of clinical research. *CNS Drugs, 29*(2), 131–151. doi:10.1007/s40263-014-0224-9

Sayal, K., Chudal, R., Hinkka-Yli-Salomäki, S., Joelsson, P., & Sourander, A. (2017). Relative age within the school year and diagnosis of attention-deficit hyperactivity disorder: A nationwide population-based study. *Lancet Psychiatry, 4*, 868–875. doi:10.1016/S2215-0366(17)30394-2

Scahill, L., Specht, M., & Page, C. (2014). The prevalence of tic disorders and clinical characteristics in children. *Journal of Obsessive-Compulsive and Related Disorders, 3*, 394–400. doi:10.1016/j.jocrd.2014.06.002

Scahill, L., McCracken, J. T., King, B. H., Rockhill, C., Shah, B., Politte, L., . . . McDougle, C. J. (2015). Extended-release guanfacine for hyperactivity in children with autism spectrum disorder. *American Journal of Psychiatry, 172*(12), 1197–1206. doi:10.1176/appi.ajp.2015.15010055

Schab, D. W., & Trinh, N. T. (2004). Do artificial food colors promote hyperactivity in children with hyperactive syndromes? A meta-analysis of double-blind placebo-controlled trials. *Journal of Developmental & Behavioral Pediatrics, 25*, 423–4334. doi:10.1097/00004703-200412000-00007

Schans, J. V., Cicek, R., de Vries, T. W., Hak, E., & Hoekstra, P. J. (2017). Association of atopic diseases and attention-deficit/hyperactivity disorder: A systematic review and meta-analysis. *Neuroscience & Biobehavioral Reviews, 74*(Pt A), 139–148. doi:10.1016/j.neubiorev.2017.01.011

Schatz, D. B., & Rostain, A. L. (2006). ADHD with comorbid anxiety: A review of the literature. *Journal of Attention Disorders, 10*, 141–149. doi:10.1177/1087054706286698

Scheffler, R. M., Brown, T. T., Fulton, B. D., Hinshaw, S. P., Levine, P., & Stone, S. (2009). Positive association between attention-deficit/hyperactivity disorder medication use and academic achievement during elementary school. *Pediatrics, 123*, 1273–1279. doi:10.1542/peds.28-1597

Schlander, M., Schwarz, O., Rothenberger, A., & Roessner, V. (2011). Tic disorders: Administrative prevalence and co-occurrence with attention-deficit/hyperactivity disorder in a German community sample. *European Journal of Psychiatry, 26,* 370–374. doi:10.1016.j.eurpsy.2009.10.003

Schmidt, M. H., Möcks, P., Lay, B., Eisert, H. -G., Fojkar, R., Fritz-Sigmund, D., . . . Musaeus, B. (1997). Does oligoantigenic diet influence hyperactive/conduct-disordered children—A controlled trial. *European Child & Adolescent Psychiatry, 6,* 88–95. doi:10.1007/BF00566671

Schwartz, S., & Correll, C. U. (2014). The efficacy of atomoxetine for the treatment of children and adolescents with attention-deficit/hyperactivity disorder: Results from a comprehensive meta-analysis and metaregression. *Journal of the American Academy of Child & Adolescent Psychiatry, 53*(2), 174–187. doi:10.1016/j.jaac.2013.11.005

Sciberras, E., Mueller, K. L., Efron, D., Bisset, M., Anderson, V., Schilpzand, E. J., . . . Nicholson, J. M. (2014). Language problems in children with ADHD: A community-based study. *Pediatrics, 133*(5), 793–800. doi:10.1542/peds.2013-3355

Sciberras, E., Mulraney, M., Silva, D., & Coghill, D. (2017). Prenatal risk factors and the etiology of ADHD- Review of existing evidence. *Current Psychiatry Reports, 19,* 1. doi:10.1007/s11920-017-0753-2

Scott, N. G., Ripperger-Suhler, J., Rajab, M. H., & Kjar, D. (2010). Factors associated with atomoxetine efficacy for treatment of attention-deficit/hyperactivity disorder in children and adolescents. *Journal of Child & Adolescent Psychopharmacology, 20,* 197–203. doi:10.1089/cap.2009.0104

Semrud-Clikeman, M. (2012). The role of inattention on academics, fluid reasoning, and visual-spatial functioning in two subtypes of ADHD. *Applied Neuropsychology Child, 1,* 18–29. doi:10.1080/21622965.2012.665766

Seo, J., Lee, B. K., Jin, S. U., Jang, K. E., Park, J. W., Kim, Y. T., . . . Chang, Y. (2015). Altered executive function in the lead-exposed brain: A functional magnetic resonance imaging study. *Neurotoxicology, 50,* 1–9. doi:10.1016/j.neuro.2015.07.002

Shadrin, A. A., Smeland, O. B., Zayats, T., Schork, A. J., Frei, O., Bettella, F., . . . Andreassen, O. A. (2018). Novel loci associated with attention-deficit/hyperactivity disorder are revealed by leveraging polygenic overlap with educational attainment. *Journal of the American Academy of Child & Adolescent Psychiatry, 57*(2), 86–95. doi:10.1016/j.jaac.2017.11.013

Shaffer, D., Fisher, P., Lucas, C. P., Dulcan, M. K., & Schwab-Stone, M. E. (2000). NIMH Diagnostic Interview Schedule for Children Version I (NIMH-DISC-IV): Description, differences from previous versions, and reliability of some common diagnoses. *Journal of the American Academy of Child & Adolescent Psychiatry, 39,* 28–38. doi:10.1097/00004583-200001000-00014

Shang, C. Y., Pan, Y. L., Lin, H. Y., Huang, L. W., & Gau, S. S., (2015). An open-label, randomized trial of methylphenidate and atomoxetine treatment in children with attention-deficit/hyperactivity disorder. *Journal of Child and Adolescent Psychopharmacology, 25*(7), 566–573. doi:10.1089/cap.2015.0035.

Sharif, M. R., Madani, M., Tabatabaei, F., & Tabatabaee, Z. (2015). The relationship between serum vitamin D level and attention deficit hyperactivity disorder. *Iran Journal of Child Neurology, 9,* 48–53. PMID:26664441, PMCID:PMC4670977

Sharp, S.I., McQuillin, A., & Gurling, H.M. (2009). Genetics of attention-deficit hyperactivity disorder (ADHD). *Neuropharmacology, 57(7-8),* 590-600. Doi:10.1016/j.neuropharm, 2009.08.011.

Shaw, P., De Rossi, P., Watson, B., Wharton, A., Greenstein, D., Raznahan, A., . . . Chakravarty, M. M. (2014). Mapping the development of the basal ganglia in children with attention-deficit/hyperactivity disorder. *Journal of the American Academy of Child & Adolescent Psychiatry, 53*(7), 780–789 e711. doi:10.1016/j.jaac.2014.05.003

Shaw, P., Malek, M., Watson, B., Greenstein, D., de Rossi, P., & Sharp, W. (2013). Trajectories of cerebral cortical development in childhood and adolescence and adult attention-deficit/hyperactivity disorder. *Biological Psychiatry, 74,* 599–606. doi:10.1016/j.biopsych.2013.04.007

Shaw, P., & Rabin, C. (2009). New insights into attention-deficit/hyperactivity disorder using structural neuroimaging. *Current Psychiatry Reports, 11,* 393–398. doi:10.1007/s11920-009-0059-0

Shin, J. Y., Roughead, E. E, Park, B. J., & Pratt, N. L. (2016). Cardiovascular safety of methylphenidate among children and young people with attention-deficit/hyperactivity disorder (ADHD): Nationwide self-controlled case series study. *The BMJ, 353,* i2550. doi:10.1136/bmj.i2550

Shillingford, A. J., Glanzman, M., Ittenbach, R., Clancy, R. R., Gaynor, J. W., & Wernovsky, G. (2009). Inattention, hyperactivity and school performance in a population of school-age children with complex congenital heart disease. *Pediatrics, 121,* e759–e767. doi:10.1542/peds.2007-1066

Sibley, M. H., Evans, S. W., & Serpell, Z. N. (2010). Social cognition and interpersonal impairment in young adolescents with ADHD. *Journal of Psychopathology and Behavior Assessment, 32,* 193–202. doi:10.1007/s10862-009-9152-2

Sibley, M. H., Rohde, L. A., Swanson, J. M., Hechtman, L. T., Molina, B. S. G., Mitchell, J. T., . . . Multimodal Treatment Study of Children with ADHD Cooperative Group. (2018). Late-onset ADHD reconsidered with comprehensive repeated assessments between ages 10 and 25. *American Journal of Psychiatry, 175*(2), 140–149. doi:10.1176/appi.ajp.2017.17030298

Simone, A. N., Marks, D. J., Bedard, A. C., & Halperin, J. M. (2018). Low working memory rather than ADHD symptoms predicts poor academic achievement in school-aged children. *Journal of Abnormal Child Psychology, 46*(2), 277–290. doi:10.1007/s10802-017-0288-3

Simonoff, E., Taylor, E., Baird, G., Bernard, S., Chadwick, O., Liang, H., . . . Jichi, F. (2013). Randomized controlled double-blind trial of optimal dose methylphenidate in children and adolescents with severe attention deficit hyperactivity disorder and intellectual disability. *Journal of Child Psychology and Psychiatry, 54*(5), 527–535. doi:10.1111/j.1469-7610.2012.02569.x

Singer, H. S. (2005). Tourette syndrome: From behavior to biology. *Lancet (Neurology), 4,* 149–159. doi:10.1016/S1474-4422(05)70018-1

Sitaram, R., Ros, T., Stoeckel, L., Haller, S., Scharnowski, F., Lewis-Peacock, J., . . . Sulzer, J. (2017). Closed-loop brain training: The science of neurofeedback. *Nature Reviews Neuroscience, 18*(2), 86–100. doi:10.1038/nrn.2016.164

Sjowall, D., Bohlin, G., Rydell, A. -M., & Thorell, L. B. (2017). Neuropsychological deficits in preschool as predictors of ADHD symptoms and academic achievement in late adolescence. *Child Neuropsychology, 23,* 111–128. doi:10.1080/09297049.2015.1063595

Smith, E., Meyer, B. J., Koerting, J., Laver-Bradbury, C., Lee, L., Jefferson, H., . . . Sonuga-Barke, E. J. (2017). Preschool hyperactivity specifically elevates long-term mental health risks more strongly in males than females: A prospective longitudinal study through to young adulthood. *European*

Child & Adolescent Psychiatry, 26(1), 123–136. doi:10.1007/s00787-016-0876-8

Smith, T. F., Schmidt-Kastner, R., McGeary, J. E., Kaczorowski, J. A., & Knopik, V. S. (2016). Pre- and perinatal ischemia-hypoxia, the ischemia-hypoxia response pathway, and ADHD risk. *Behavior Genetics, 46,* 467–477. doi:10.1007/s10519-016-9784-4

Sobel, L. J., Bansal, R., Maia, T. V., Sanchez, J., Mazzone, L., Durkin, K., & Peterson, B. S. (2010). Basal ganglia surface morphology and the effects of stimulant medications in youth with attention deficit hyperactivity disorder. *American Journal of Psychiatry, 167,* 977–986. doi:10.1176/appi.ajp.2010.09091259

Sokolova, E., Oerlemans, A. M., Rommelse, N. N., Groot, P., Hartman, C. A., Glennon, J. C., . . . Buitelaar, J. K. (2017). A Causal and mediation analysis of the comorbidity between attention deficit hyperactivity disorder (ADHD) and autism spectrum disorder (ASD). *Journal of Autism and Developmental Disorders, 47*(6), 1595–1604. doi:10.1007/s10803-017-3083-7

Solanto, M. V., Marks, D. J., Wasserstein, J., Mitchell, K., Abikoff, H., Alvir, J., & Kofman, M. D. (2010). Efficacy of meta-cognitive therapy for adult ADHD. *American Journal of Psychiatry, 167,* 958–968. doi:10.1176/appi.ajp.2009.09081123

Sonuga-Barke, E. J., Brandeis, D., Cortese, S., Daley, D., Ferrin, M., Holtmann, M., . . . European ADHD Guidelines Group. (2013). Nonpharmacological interventions for ADHD: Systematic review and meta-analyses of randomized controlled trials of dietary and psychological treatments. *American Journal of Psychiatry, 170*(3), 275–289. doi:10.1176/appi.ajp.2012.12070991

Sonuga-Barke, E., Brandeis, D., Holtmann, M., & Cortese, S. (2014). Computer-based cognitive training for ADHD: A review of current evidence. *Child & Adolescent Psychiatric Clinics of North America, 23,* 807–824. doi:10.106/j.chc.2014.05.009

Spencer, T. J. (2009). Issues in the management of patients with complex attention-deficit/hyperactivity disorder symptoms. *CNS Drugs, 23*(Suppl. 1), 9–20. doi:10.2165/00023210-200923000-00003

Spencer, T. J., Biederman, J., & Mick, E. (2007). Attention-deficit/hyperactivity disorder: Diagnosis, lifespan, comorbidities and neurobiology. *Journal of Pediatric Psychology, 32,* 631–642. doi:10.1093/jpepsy/jsm005

Spencer, T. J., Kratochvil, C. J., Sangal, R. B., Saylor, K. E., Bailey, C. E., Dunn, D. W., . . . Allen, A. J. (2007). Effects of atomoxetine on growth in children with attention-deficit/hyperactivity disorder following up to five years of treatment. *Journal of Child & Adolescent Psychopharmacology, 17,* 689–700. doi:10.1089/cap.2006.0100

Sprich-Buckminster S., Biederman J., Milberger S., Faraone S. V., & Lehman B. K. (1993). Are prenatal complications relevant to the manifestations of ADD? Issues of comorbidity and familiality. *Journal of the American Academy of Child and Adolescent Psychiatry, 32,* 1032–1037.

Stefanatos, G. A., & Baron, I. S. (2007). Attention-deficit/hyperactivity disorder: A neuropsychological perspective towards *DSM-V. Neuropsychology Review, 17,* 5–38. doi:10.1007/s11065-007-9020-3

Stein, M., Waldman, I., Newcorn, J., Bishop, J., Kittles, R., & Cook, E. (2014). Dopamine transporter genotype and stimulant dose-response in youth with attention-deficit/hyperactivity disorder. *Journal of Child and Adolescent Psychopharmacology, 24*(5), 238–244.

Stergiakouli, E., Martin, J., Hamshere, M. L., Langley, K., Evans, D. M., St Pourcain, B., . . . Davey Smith, G. (2015). Shared genetic influences between attention-deficit/hyperactivity disorder (ADHD) traits in children and clinical ADHD. *Journal of the American Academy of Child & Adolescent Psychiatry, 54*(4), 322–327. doi:10.1016/j.jaac.2015.01.010

Stevens, M. C., Gaynor, A., Bessette, K. L., & Pearlson, G. D. (2016). A preliminary study of the effects of working memory training on brain function. *Brain Imaging & Behavior, 10,* 387–407. doi:10.1007/s11682-015-9416-2

Stevenson, J., Sonuga-Barke, E., McCann, D., Grimshaw, K., Parker, K. M., Rose-Zerilli, M. J., . . . Warner, J. O. (2010). The role of histamine degradation gene polymorphisms in moderating the effects of food additives on children's ADHD symptoms. *American Journal of Psychiatry, 167,* 1108–1115. doi:10.1176/appi.ajp.2010.09101529

Storebø, O. J., Skoog, M., Damm, D., Thomsen, P. H., Simonsen, E., & Gluud, C. (2011). Social skill training for attention deficit hyperactivity disorder (ADHD) in children 5 to 18 years. *Cochrane Database of Systematic Reviews, 12,* CD008223. doi:10.1002/14651858.CD008223.pub2

Storebø, O. J., Ramstad, E., Krogh, H. B., Nilausen, T. D., Skoog, M., Holmskov, M., . . . Gluud, C. (2015). Methylphenidate for children and adolescents with attention deficit hyperactivity disorder (ADHD). *Cochrane Database System Review, 11,* CD009885. doi:10.1002/14651858.CD009885.pub2

Stuhec, M., Munda, B., Svab, B., & Locatelli, I. (2015). Comparative efficacy and acceptability of atomoxetine, lisdexamfetamine, bupropion and methylphenidate in treatment of attention hyperactivity disorder in children and adolescents: A meta-analysis with focus on bupropion. *Journal of Affective Disorders, 178,* 149–159. doi:10.1016/j.jad.2015.03.006

Sudre, G., Choudhuri, S., Szekely, E., Bonner, T., Goduni, E., Sharp, W., & Shaw, P. (2017). Estimating the heritability of structural and functional brain connectivity in families affected by attention-deficit/hyperactivity disorder. *JAMA Psychiatry, 74*(1), 76–84. doi:10.1001/jamapsychiatry.2016.3072

Sullivan, E. L., Nousen, E. K., & Chamiou, K. A. (2014). Maternal high fat diet consumption during the perinatal period programs offspring behavior. *Physiology & Behavior, 123,* 236–242. doi:10.1016/j.physbeh.2012.07.014

Svatkova, A., Nestrasil, I., Rudser, K., Goldenring Fine, J., Bledsoe, J., & Semrud-Clikeman, M. (2016). Unique white matter microstructural patterns in ADHD presentations—a diffusion tensor imaging study. *Human Brain Mapping, 37,* 3323–3336. doi:10.1002/hbm.23243

Swanson, J. M., Arnold, L. E., Molina, B. S. G., Sibley, M. H., Hechtman, L. T., Hinshaw, S. P., . . . Kraemer, H. C. (2017). Young adult outcomes in the follow-up of the multimodal treatment study of attention-deficit/hyperactivity disorder: Symptom persistence, source discrepancy, and height suppression. *Journal of Child Psychology and Psychiatry, 58*(6), 663–678.

Swanson, J., Arnold, L. E., Kraemer, H., Hechtman, L., Molina, B., Hinshaw, S., . . . MTA Cooperative Group. (2008). Evidence, interpretation, and qualification from multiple reports of long-term outcomes in the Multimodal Treatment Study of Children with ADHD (MTA): Part I: Executive summary. *Journal of Attention Disorders, 12*(1), 4–14. doi:10.1177/1087054708319345

Swanson, J., Greenhill, L., Wigal, T., Kollins, S., Steheli, A., Davies, M., . . .Wigel, S. (2006). Stimulant-related reductions of growth rates in the PATS. *Journal of the American Academy of Child & Adolescent Psychiatry, 45,* 1304–1313. doi:10.1097/01.chi.0000235075.25038.5a

Swanson, J. M., Elliott, G. R., Greenhill, L. L., Wigal, T., Arnold, L. E., Vitiello, B., . . . Volkow, N. D. (2007). Effects of stimulants on growth rates across 3 years in the MTA follow-up. *Journal of the American Academy of Child & Adolescent Psychiatry, 46,* 1015–1027. doi:10.1097/chi.0b013e3180686d7e

Swanson, J. M., Schuck, S., Porter, M. M., Carlson, C., Hartman, C. A., Sergeant, J. A., . . . Wigal, T. (2012). categorical and dimensional definitions and evaluations of symptoms of ADHD: History of the SNAP and the SWAN Rating Scales. *International Journal of Educational and Psychological Assessment, 10*(1), 51–70.

Tamm, L., Barnea-Goraly, N., & Reiss, A. L. (2012). Diffusion tensor imaging reveals white matter abnormalities in attention-deficit/hyperactivity disorder. *Psychiatry Research: Neuroimaging, 202,* 150–154. doi:10.1016/j.psychresns.2012.04.001

Tan, B. W. Z., Pooley, J. A., & Speelman, C. P. (2016). A meta-analytic review of the efficacy of physical exercise interventions on cognition in individuals with autism spectrum disorder and ADHD. *Journal of Autism & Developmental Disorders, 46,* 3126–3143. doi:10.1007/s10803-016-2854-x

Tandon, M., & Pergjika, A. (2017). Attention deficit hyperactivity disorder in children. *Child & Adolescent Psychiatric Clinics of North America, 26,* 523–538. http://dx.doi.org/10.1016/j.chc.2017.02.007

Taylor, E. (2017). Attention deficit hyperactivity disorder: Overdiagnosis or diagnosis missed? *Archives of Diseases in Childhood, 102,* 376–379.

ter Laak, M. A., Temmink, A. H., Koeken, A., van't Veer, N. E., Van Hattum, P. R., & Cobbaert, C. M. (2010). Recognition of impaired atomoxetine metabolism because of low CYP2D6 activity. *Pediatric Neurology, 43,* 159–162. doi:10.1016/j.pediatrneurol.2010.04.004

Ter-Stepanian, M., Grizenko, N., Zappitelli, M., & Joober, R. (2010). Clinical response to methylphenidate in children diagnosed with attention-deficit/hyperactivity disorder and comorbid psychiatric disorders. *Canadian Journal of Psychiatry, 55,* 305–312.

Thapar, A. & Cooper, M. (2016). Attention deficit hyperactivity disorder. *Lancet, 387,* 1240–1250.

Thomas, R., Sanders, S., Doust, J., Beller, E., & Glasziou, P. (2015). Prevalence of attention-deficit/hyperactivity disorder: A systemic review and meta-analysis. *Pediatrics, 135,* e994–e1001.

Thompson, A., Maltezos, S., Paliokosta, E., & Xenitidis, K. (2009). Risperidone for attention-deficit hyperactivity disorder in people with intellectual disabilities. *Cochrane Database of Systematic Reviews, 2,* CD007011.

Tsai, M. -H., Hsu, J. -F., & Huang, Y. -S. (2016). Sleep problems in children with attention-deficit/hyperactivity disorder: Current state of knowledge and appropriate management. *Current Psychiatry Reports, 18,* 76. doi:10.1007/s11920-016-0711-4

Turgay, A. (2009). Psychopharmacological treatment of oppositional defiant disorder. *CNS Drugs, 23,* 1–17. doi:10.2165/0023210-200923010-00001

Vaisman, N., Kaysar, N., Zaruk-Adasha, Y., Pelled, D., Brichon, G., Zwingelstein, G., & Bodennec, J. (2008). Correlation between changes in blood fatty acid composition and visual sustained attention performance in children with inattention: Effect of dietary n-3 fatty acids containing phospholipids. *American Journal of Clinical Nutrition, 87*(5), 1170–1180. doi:10.1093/ajcn/87.5.1170

van Lieshout, M., Luman, M., Twisk, J. W., Faraone, S. V., Heslenfeld, D. J., Hartman, C. A., . . . Oosterlaan, J. (2017). Neurocognitive predictors of ADHD outcome: A 6-year follow-up study. *Journal of Abnormal Child Psychology, 45*(2), 261–272. doi:10.1007/s10802-016-0175-3

Vande Voort, J. L., He, J. -P., Jameson, N. D., & Merikangas, K. R. (2014). Impact of the *DSM-5* attention-deficit/hyperactivity disorder (ADHD) age of onset criterion in the U.S. adolescent population. *Journal of the American Academy of Child & Adolescent Psychiatry, 53,* 736–744. https://doi.org/10.1016/j.jaac.2014.03.005

van den Hoofdakker, B. J., Nauta, M. H., van der Veen-Mulders, L., Syteme, S., Emmelkamp, P. M. G., Minderaa, R. B., & Hoekstra, P. J. (2010). Behavioral parent training as an adjunct to routine care in children with attention-deficit/hyperactivity disorder: Moderators of treatment response. *Journal of Pediatric Psychology, 35,* 317–326. doi:10.1093/jpepsy/jsp060

van der Meer, J. M., Oerlemans, A. M., van Steijn, D. J., Lappenschaar, M. G., de Sonneville, L. M., Buitelaar, J. K., & Rommelse, N. N. (2012). Are autism spectrum disorder and attention-deficit/hyperactivity disorder different manifestations of one overarching disorder? Cognitive and symptom evidence from a clinical and population-based sample. *Journal of the American Academy of Child & Adolescent Psychiatry, 51*(11), 1160–1172 e1163. doi:10.1016/j.jaac.2012.08.024

Vélez-Galarraga, R., Guillén-Grima, F., Crespo-Eguílaz, N., & Sánchez-Carpintero, R. (2016). Prevalence of sleep disorders and their relationship with core symptoms of inattention and hyperactivity in children with attention-deficit/hyperactivity disorder. *European Journal of Pediatric Neurology, 20,* 925–937. doi:10.116/j.ejpn.2016.07.004

Vetter, V. L., Elia, J., Erickson, C., Berger, S., Blum, N., Uzark, K., & Webb, C. (2008). Cardiovascular monitoring of children and adolescents with heart disease receiving stimulant drugs. A scientific statement from the American Heart Association Council on Cardiovascular Disease in the Young Congenital Cardiac Defects Committee, American Heart Association Council on Cardiovascular Nursing. *Circulation, 117,* 2407–2423.

Viktorin, A., Rydén, E., Thase, M. E., Chang, Z., Lundholm, C., D'Onofrio, B. M., . . . Landén, M. (2017). The risk of treatment-emergent mania with methylphenidate in bipolar disorder. *American Journal of Psychiatry, 174*(4), 341–348. doi:10.1176/appi.ajp.2016.16040467

Vilgis, V., Silk, T. J., & Vance, A. (2015). Executive function and attention in children and adolescents with depressive disorders: A systematic review. *European Journal of Child & Adolescent Psychiatry, 24,* 365–384.

Villagomez, A. & Ramtekkar, U. (2014). Iron, magnesium, vitamin D, and zinc deficiencies in children presenting with symptoms of attention-deficit/hyperactivity disorder. *Children (Basel), 1,* 261–279. doi:10.3390/children1030261

Visser, S. N., Bitsko, R. H., Danielson, M. L., Gandhour, R., Blumberg, S. J., Schieve, L., & Cuffe, S. (2015). Treatment of attention-deficit/hyperactivity disorder among children with special health care needs. *The Journal of Pediatrics, 166*(6), 1423–1430. doi:10.1016/j.jpeds.2015.02.018

Visser, J. C., Rommelse, N. N. J., Greven, C. U., & Buitelaar, J. K. (2016). Autism spectrum disorder and attention-deficit/hyperactivity disorder in early childhood: A review of unique and shared characteristics and developmental antecedents. *Neuroscience& Biobehavioral Reviews, 65,* 229–263. doi:10.1016/j.neubiorev.2016.03.019

Vitiello, B., Abikoff, H. B., Chuang, S. Z., Kollins, S. H., McCracken, J. T., Riddle, M. A., . . . Greenhill, L. L. (2007).

Effectiveness of methylphenidate in the 10-month continuation phase of the preschoolers with ADHD treatment study (PATS). *Journal of Child & Adolescent Psychopharmacology, 17,* 593–603. doi:10.1089/cap.2007.0058

Vitiello, B., Elliott, G. R., Swanson, J. M., Arnold, L. E., Hechtman, L., Abikoff, H., . . . Gibbons, R. (2012). Blood pressure and heart rate in the multimodal treatment of attention deficit/hyperactivity disorder study over 10 years. *The American Journal of Psychiatry, 169*(2), 167–177. doi.org/10.1176/appi.ajp.2011.10111705

Volkow, N. D., & Swanson, J. M. (2003). Variables that affect the clinical use and abuse of methylphenidate in the treatment of ADHD. *American Journal of Psychiatry, 160,* 1909–1918. doi:10.1176/appi.ajp.160.11.1909

Wang, X., Cao, Q., Wang, J., Wu, Z., Wang, P., Sun, L., . . . Wang, Y. (2016). The effects of cognitive-behavioral therapy on intrinsic functional brain networks in adults with attention-deficit/hyperactivity disorder. *Behaviour Research and Therapy, 76,* 32–39. doi:10.1016/j.brat.2015.11.003

Wang, Y., Huang, L., Zhang, L., Qu, Y., & Mu, D. (2017). Iron status in attention-deficit/hyperactivity disorder: A systematic review and meta-analysis. *PLoS One, 12*(1), e0169145. doi:10.1371/journal.pone.0169145

Warren, A. E., Hamilton, R. M., Belanger, S. A., Gray, C., Gow, R. M., Sanatani, S., . . . Schachar, R. (2009). Cardiac risk assessment before the use of stimulant medications in children and youth: A joint position statement by the Canadian Pediatric Society, the Canadian Cardiovascular Society, and the Canadian Academy of Child and Adolescent Psychiatry. *Canadian Journal of Cardiology, 25,* 625–630. doi:10.1016/S0828-282X(09)70157-6

Waxmonsky, J. G., Waschbusch, D. A., Akinnusi, O., & Pelham, W. E. (2011). A comparison of atomoxetine administered as once versus daily dosing on the school and home functioning of children with attention-deficit/hyperactivity disorder. *Journal of Child & Adolescent Psychopharmacology, 21*(1), 21–32. doi:10.1089/cap.2010.0042

Wehmeier, P. M., Schacht, A., & Barkley, R. A. (2010). Social and emotional impairment in children and adolescents with ADHD and the impact on quality of life. *Journal of Adolescent Health, 46,* 209–217. doi:10.1016/j.jadohealth.2009.09.009

Wehmeier, P. M., Schacht, A., Ulberstad, F., Lehmann, M., Schneider-Fresenius, C., Lehmkuhl, G., Dittmann, R. W., & Banaschewski, T. (2012). Does atomoxetine improve executive function inhibitory control, and hyperactivity? Results from a placebo-controlled trial using quantative measurement technology. *Journal of Clinical Psychopharmacology, 32*(5), 653–60. doi:10.1542/peds.2010-0825

Weiss, M., Murray, C., Wasdell, M., Greenfield, B., Giles, L., & Hechtman, L. (2012). A randomized controlled trial of CBT therapy for adults with ADHD with and without medication. *BMC Psychiatry, 12,* 30. doi:10.1186/1471-244X-12-30

Weiss, M., Panagiotopoulis, C., Giles, L., Gibbins, C., Kuzeljevic, B., Davidson, J., & Harrison, R. (2009). A naturalistic study of predictors and risks of atypical antipsychotic use in an attention-deficit/hyperactivity disorder clinic. *Journal of Child & Adolescent Psychopharmacology, 19,* 575–582. doi:10.1089/cap.2009.0050

Wernicke, J. F., Adler, L., Spencer, T., West, S. A., Allen, A. J., Heiligenstein, J., . . . Michelson, D. (2004). Changes in symptoms and adverse events after discontinuation of atomoxetine in children and adults with attention-deficit/hyperactivity disorder: A prospective, placebo-controlled assessment. *Journal of Clinical Psychopharmacology, 24,* 30–35.

Weyandt, L. L. (2005). Executive function in children, adolescents and adults with attention-deficit/hyperactivity disorder: An introduction to the special issue. *Developmental Neuropsychology, 27,* 1–10. doi:10.1207/s15326942dn2701_1

Wichstrøm, L., Berg-Nielsen, T. S., Angold, A., Egger, H. L., Solheim, E., & Sveen, T. H. (2012). Prevalence of psychiatric disorders in preschoolers. *Journal of Child Psychology & Psychiatry, 53,* 695–705. doi:10.1111/j.1469-7610.2011.02514.x

Wigal, S. B. (2009). Efficacy and safety limitations of attention-deficit/hyperactivity disorder pharmacotherapy in children and adults. *CNS Drugs, 23*(Supplement 1), 21–31. doi:10.2165/00023210-200923000-00004

Wigal, T., Greenhill, L., Chuang, S., McGough, J., Vitiello, B., Skrobala, A., & Stehli, A. -M. (2006). Safety and tolerability of methylphenidate in preschool children with ADHD. *Journal of the American Academy of Child & Adolescent Psychiatry, 45,* 1294–1303. doi:10.1097/01.chi.0000235082.63156.27

Wiggs, K., Elmore, A. L., Nigg, J. T., & Nikolas, M. A. (2016). Pre-and perinatal risk for attention-deficit hyperactivity disorder: Does neuropsychological weakness explain the link? *Journal of Abnormal Child Psychology, 44,* 1473–1485. doi:10.1007/s10802-016-0142-z

Wilens, T. E., Bukstein, O., Brams, M., Cutler, A. J., Childress, A., Rugino, T., Lyne, A., Grannis, K., & Youcha, S. (2012). A controlled trial of extended-release guanfacine and psychostimulants for attention-deficit/hyperactivity disorder. *Journal of the American Academy of Child & Adolescent Psychiatry, 51*(1), 74–85. e2. doi:10.1016/j.jaac.2011.10.012

Wilens, T. E., Haight, B. R., Horrigan, J. P., Hudziak, J. J., Rosenthal, N. E., Connor, D. F., . . . Modell, J. G. (2005). Bupropion XL in adults with attention-deficit/hyperactivity disorder: A randomized, placebo-controlled study. *Biological Psychiatry, 57,* 793–801. doi:10.1016/j.biopsych.2005.01.027

Wilens, T. E., Hammerness, P., Utzinger, L., Schillinger, M., Georgiopoulos, A., Doyle, R. L., . . . Brodziak, K. (2008). An open study of adjunct OROS-methylphenidate in children and adolescents who are atomoxetine partial responders: I. Effectiveness. *Journal of Child & Adolescent Psychopharmacology, 19,* 485–492. doi:10.1089/cap.2008.0125

Wilens, T. E., Robertson, B., Sikirica, V., Harper, L., Young. J. L., Bloomfield, R., . . . Cutler, A. J. (2015). A randomized placebo-controlled trial of guanfacine extended release in adolescents with attention-deficit/hyperactivity disorder. *Journal of the American Academy of Child & Adolescent Psychiatry, 54*(11), 916–925. doi:10.1016/j.jaac.2015.08.016

Willcutt, E. (2012). The prevalence of DSM-IV attention-deficit/hyperactivity disorder: A meta-analytic review. *Neurotherapeutics, 9,* 490–499.

Willcutt, E. G., Doyle, A. E., Nigg, J. T., Faraone, S. V, & Pennington, B. F. (2005).Validity of the executive function theory of attention-deficit/hyperactivity disorder: A meta-analytic review. *Biological Psychiatry, 57,* 1336–1346. doi:10.1016/j.biopsych.2005.02.006

Willcutt, E. G., Pennington, B. F., Olson, R. K., Chabildas, N., & Huslander, J. (2005). Neuropsychological analysis of comorbidity between reading disability and attention-deficit/hyperactivity disorder: In search of the common deficit. *Developmental Neuropsychology, 27,* 35–78. doi:10.1207/s15326942dn2701_3

Williford, A. P., & Shelton, T. L. (2014). Behavior management for preschool children. *Child & Adolescent Psychiatric Clinics of North America, 23,* 717–730. doi:10.1016/j.chc.2014.05.008

Wolraich, M. L., Lambert, W., Doffing, M. A., Bickman, L., Simmons, T., & Worley, K. (2003). Psychometric properties of the Vanderbilt ADHD diagnostic parent rating scale in a referred population. *Journal of Pediatric Psychology, 28,* 559–567. doi:10.1093/jpepsy/jsg046

Wolraich, M. L., McGuinn, L., & Doffing, M. (2007). Treatment of attention deficit hyperactivity disorder in children and adolescents: Safety considerations. *Drug Safety, 30*(1), 17–26. doi:10.2165/00002018-200730010-00003

Wolraich, M. L., McKeown, R. E., Visser, S. N., Bard, D., Cuffe, S., Neas, B., . . . Danielson, M. (2014). The prevalence of ADHD: Its diagnosis and treatment in four school districts across two states. *Journal of Attention Disorders, 18*(7), 563–575. doi:10.1177/1087054712453169

Wolraich, M. L., Wilson, D. B., & White, J. W. (1995). The effect of sugar on behavior or cognition in children. *Journal of the American Medical Association, 274,* 1617–1621. doi:10.1001/jama.274.20.1617

Wood, A. C., Rijsdijk, F., Asherson, P., & Kuntsi, J. (2009). Hyperactive-impulsive symptoms scores and oppositional behaviors reflect alternate manifestations of a single liability. *Behavior Genetics, 39,* 447–460. doi:10.1007/s10519-009-9290-z

Wyciszkiewicz, A., Pawlak, M. A., & Krawiec, K. (2017). Cerebellar volume in attention-deficit/hyperactivity disorder (ADHD): Replication study. *Journal of Child Neurology, 32,* 215–221. doi:10.1177/0883073816678550

Yang, C., Hao, Z., Zhu, C., Guo, Q., Mu, D., & Zhang, L. (2016). Interventions for tic disorders: An overview of systematic reviews and meta analyses. *Neuroscience & Biobehavioral Reviews, 63,* 239–255. doi:10.1016/j.neubiorev.2015.12.013

Yeates, K. O., Armstrong, K., Janusz, J., Taylor, H. G., Wade, S., Stancin, T., & Drotar, D. (2005). Long-term attention problems in children with traumatic brain injury. *Journal of the American Academy of Child & Adolescent Psychiatry, 44,* 574–584. doi:10.1097/01.chi.0000159947.50523.64

Yilmaz, Z., Javaras, K. N., Baker, J. H., Thornton, L. M., Lichtenstein, P., Bulik, C. M., & Larsson, H. (2017). Association between childhood to adolescent attention deficit/hyperactivity disorder symptom trajectories and late adolescent disordered eating. *Journal of Adolescent Health, 61*(2), 140–146. doi:10.1016/j.jadohealth.2017.04.001

Yoncheva, Y. N., Somandepalli, K., Reiss, P. T., Kelly, C., Di Martino, A., Lazar, M., . . . Castellanos, F. X. (2016). Mode of anisotropy reveals global diffusion alterations in attention-deficit/hyperactivity disorder. *Journal of the American Academy of Child & Adolescent Psychiatry, 55*(2), 137–145. doi:10.1016/j.jaac.2015.11.011

Yoshimasu, K., Barbaresi, W. J., Colligan, R. C., Killian, J. M., Voigt, R. G., Weaver, A. L. & Katusic, S.K. (2011). Written-language disorder among children with and without ADHD in a population-based birth cohort. *Pediatrics, 128,* e605. doi:10.1542/peds.2010-2581

Yoshimasu, K., Barbaresi, W. J., Colligan, R. C., Voigt, R. G., Killian, J. M., Weaver, A. L., & Katusic, S. K. (2012). Childhood ADHD is strongly associated with a broad range of psychiatric disorders during adolescence: A population-based birth cohort study. *Journal of Child Psychology and Psychiatry, 53*(10), 1036–1043. doi:10.1111/j.1469-7610.2012.02567.x

Young, S., & Amarasinghe, M. (2010). Practitioner review: Non-pharmacological treatments for ADHD: A lifespan approach. *The Journal of Child Psychology and Psychiatry, 51,* 116–133. doi:10.1111/j.1469-7610.2009.02191.x

Ystrom, E., Gustavson, K., Brandlistuen, R. E., Knudsen, G. P., Magnus, P., Susser, E., . . . Reichborn-Kjennerud, T. (2017). Prenatal exposure to acetaminophen and risk of ADHD. *Pediatrics, 140*(5). doi:10.1542/peds.2016-3840

Zametkin, A. J., Nordahl, T. E., Gross, M., King, A. C., Semple, W. E., Rumsey, J., . . . Cohen, R. M. (1990). Cerebral glucose metabolism in adults with hyperactivity of childhood onset. *New England Journal of Medicine, 323*(20), 1361–1366. doi:10.1056/NEJM199011153232001

CHAPTER 20

Specific Learning Disabilities

Robin P. Church and M.E.B. Lewis

Upon completion of this chapter, the reader will

- Know the historical context for the term *learning disabilities* as well as its definition and implications
- Be aware of key research findings and the biological basis of specific learning disabilities as well as other impairments associated with learning disabilities
- Distinguish among intervention strategies, particularly evidence-based practices used in the assessment and identification of learning disabilities
- Identify the range of outcomes for children and adolescents with learning disabilities
- Recognize the importance of executive function in the diagnosis and treatment of learning disabilities

A great deal of learning involves 1) processing a visual representation of concepts, 2) attaching that perception to language in order to communicate understanding, and 3) demonstrating that understanding with oral or written products. When a child struggles with these subtle and complex perceptual skills, their disabilities in understanding what they are encountering in the classroom impacts their ability to build a "toolbox" for more and more complex learning. This chapter focuses on those children, who represent more than one third of the students identified with disabilities in the United States (National Center for Educational Statistics, 2017; U.S. Department of Education, Office of Special Education Programs, 2016).

Some historical context is important in understanding learning disabilities. In a 1963 conference organized by parents, Samuel Kirk proposed in his keynote address that the term *learning disabilities* be used for otherwise normally developing students who struggle with reading, writing, or math acquisition. Following the conference, the parents of students with such learning disabilities partnered with parents of students with developmental disabilities to mount a national political effort to get educational services for

The authors would like to acknowledge the contribution of Dr. Virginia W. Berninger in the preparation of this chapter. Her insights and research perspectives enriched our presentation of the growing body of research and practice in this most challenging area of need.

their children. Their efforts resulted in the passage of the Education for All Handicapped Children Act in 1975, also known as Public Law 94-142, which guaranteed the civil right of **free appropriate public education (FAPE)** for students with learning disabilities and developmental disabilities (Johnson & Myklebust, 1967; Kirk & Kirk, 1971; Torgesen, 2004).

The *Diagnostic Statistical Manual of Mental Disorders, Fifth Edition* (*DSM-5;* American Psychiatric Association, 2013), is used by medical staff and professionals working in other clinical settings. The *DSM-5* definition of a **learning disorder** (referred to in IDEA 2004 as a specific learning disability, or SLD) is a condition that interferes with the acquisition and use of one or more of the following academic skills: oral language, reading, written language, or mathematics (Clay, 2011; McDonogh, Fanagan, Sy, & Alfonso, 2017). This impairment causes serious difficulties in making daily progress through the general education curriculum at all grade levels. These disorders affect individuals who otherwise demonstrate at least average abilities that are essential for thinking or reasoning. Thus, although intellectual disability, cerebral palsy, seizure disorders, receptive and expressive language disorders, traumatic brain injury, and hearing and vision impairments all can interfere with learning, they are not classified as primary learning disorders.

Recognizing the need for more foundational knowledge to implement FAPE for specific learning disabilities, the 1989 federal Interagency Committee on Learning Disabilities commissioned by the U.S. Congress recommended funding more research on SLDs. This chapter will highlight these findings, which include but are not restricted to the NICHD-funded multi-disciplinary learning disabilities research centers as well as guidelines for applying research findings to practice (Berninger, 2015). In addition, recent research showing that there are multiple types of SLDs is discussed. One important outcome of this research has been a redirection away from a "wait-to-fail" model based on cognitive-achievement discrepancy toward a multi-tiered model of intervention, commonly referred to as response to intervention (RTI) or multitiered systems of support (Vaughn & Fuchs, 2003; Fuchs & Vaughn, 2012; Hughs & Dexter, 2011). This chapter describes learning disabilities not as a single disorder, but as a group of profiles that present differently in different children and need to be fully understood in order for intervention to be effective.

CASE STUDY

Noah is a first grader who has been having trouble learning to read. All of the first-grade teachers in his elementary school provide daily phonological awareness instruction (to help students improve their awareness of phonemes, the sounds that make up syllables and words) for 15 minutes each day during the first 4 months of first grade and daily phonics instruction (teaching students to understand the correspondence between phonemes and written letters and words) for 30 minutes each day during the next 4 months of first grade. This is tier 1 instruction, as part of a 3-tier response to intervention program used by Noah's school to help children with learning problems. During the last 6 weeks of first grade, Noah and his fellow students were individually assessed by the school psychologist on standardized measures of phonological awareness and phonological decoding. This was done by having the students read pseudo words (invented words with plausible English phonology) and then read real words aloud (oral reading). Noah and a number of his peers scored below the 25th percentile on these measures. As such, he was identified as being eligible to receive tier 2 supplementary instruction in second grade in addition to the regular reading program.

Upon entering second grade, Noah received tier 2 supplementary instruction in a small group setting that was provided by trained paraprofessionals. This instruction occurred during regular class time when his classmates were engaged in other kinds of teacher-provided instruction in small groups. Noah's progress was monitored throughout the school year, and at the end of second grade, Noah was again assessed by the school psychologist. His classroom teacher reported that he and several other students who had received tier 2 support were struggling with their written assignments, not just with oral reading. As a result, the psychologist included measures of orthographic awareness (the ability to process and use visual representations of letters and words; e.g., printed words), comprehension, handwriting, spelling, and composition in her assessment along with measures of phonology and decoding. She also reached out to the parents of all the students receiving supplementary reading instruction to obtain developmental, medical, family, and educational histories.

The results of the second-grade RTI assessment were surprising to the teachers and school psychologist. Although most of the 10 children who had received the year of tier 2 supplemental instruction, including Noah, met the RTI criterion for phonological awareness, most did not meet criterion in orthographic awareness (a skill shown in research to be related to handwriting, real word decoding in reading, word encoding in spelling, and composition; Berninger & Richards, 2010). In addition, many of the students still did not meet the RTI criterion for phonological decoding, which requires knowledge and application of correspondences between phonemes (the sounds which compose words) and graphemes (the written representation of phonemes). The students also exhibited individual differences in whether they did or did not meet the RTI criteria in reading comprehension, handwriting, spelling, and timed composition fluency.

Careful examination of the profiles for these students identified three patterns of difficulty. For the first group of students, the most prominent problem was with **dysgraphia,** characterized by 1) impaired legibility and automaticity of letter production, 2) problems with storing and finding ordered letters in long-term memory, and 3) impairments in executive function for planning serial finger movements. Two students with pure dysgraphia profiles were impaired in handwriting rather than reading, but their illegible, slow, nonautomatic letter retrieval and formation interfered with their ability to complete written activities. Thus, a handwriting disability rather than reading disability accounted for their failure to respond to the tier 1 or tier 2 intervention. None of their parents reported oral language problems during the preschool years.

Noah was in the second group of students, whose main problem was with **dyslexia,** characterized by 1) impaired word decoding (reading) and encoding (writing and spelling), 2) difficulties with phonological coding of heard and spoken words, and 3) problems with **orthographic** coding (processing read and written words and retaining them in working memory). These children also had impairments in the integration of phonological and orthographic processing, resulting in both reading and writing deficits. The five students with dyslexia profiles had difficulty translating written pseudo words into oral pseudo words, written real words into oral real words, and spoken words into written words. Two of them (including Noah) also had co-occurring dysgraphia rather than pure dysgraphia. All of these students had difficulty storing and processing written words in their working memory. Several parents of children with dyslexia, including Noah's parents, reported that their children had difficulties with speech articulation during the preschool years, although their language comprehension always seemed fine.

The third group of students had evidence of an oral and written language learning disability (OWL LD). Their difficulties were characterized by 1) impaired listening and reading comprehension and 2) problems with oral and written expression. The three students with OWL LD had difficulty in syntactic coding (the ability to learn grammar and grammatical relationships), which can interfere with sentence processing during listening and reading comprehension as well as sentence production during oral and written expression. Despite their ability to decode and encode (i.e., sounding out words and spelling), they scored poorly on measures of reading comprehension and written composition.

The school psychologist met with Noah's parents to review the results of these assessments. She explained that Noah's reading difficulties were not due to impaired intelligence, but to specific problems with decoding that made it difficult for him to decipher and remember new words, and that he also had additional difficulties with writing. Because of his lack of adequate response to tier 1 and tier 2 interventions, he qualified for tier 3 (special education support) under an individualized education plan (IEP; see Chapter 33). He would receive specialized instruction from a special education teacher, and he would also work with an occupational therapist who, together with his teachers, would help him develop improved writing skills.

Thought Questions:

Why do some students respond to targeted intervention whereas others do not? How can schools meet the challenge of providing adequate shared planning time in the school day for true interdisciplinary collaboration?

DEFINING LEARNING DISORDERS

The Inividuals with Disabilities Education Improvement Act (IDEA) of 2004 defines a specific learning disability as "a disorder in one or more of the basic psychological processes involved in understanding or in using language, spoken or written, which disorder may manifest in imperfect ability to listen, think, speak, read, write, spell, or do mathematical calculations" (§602[26][a]). The term excludes learning problems that are the result of intellectual disability, emotional disturbance, environmental, cultural, or economic disadvantage, or which are a consequence of visual, hearing, or motor disabilities.

This definition is problematic because it fails to define the core features or origins of SLD as illustrated by the case study about Noah and his classmates. The definition does not identify the "basic psychological processes" of learning or how marked an "imperfect ability" to learn must be in order to constitute a disability. It is a definition of exclusion; all other causes for the learning problems must be eliminated. However, it is clear that SLDs can coexist with other conditions, most notably attention-deficit/hyperactivity disorder (ADHD; McNamara, Vervaeke, & Willoughby, 2008; see Chapter 19). Other disabilities identified in IDEA, however, are excluded from the definition of SLD in order to prevent "double dipping" from existing federal programs that deal with and fund those issues. It is clear, however, that a child with a SLD may also have other conditions that affect learning.

Originally, the common approach for diagnosing SLD was to document a severe discrepancy between ability and achievement by demonstrating a significant difference between the child's potential to learn, often expressed as an IQ score, and his or her actual educational achievement (Gregg & Scott, 2000). For at least a decade, other diagnostic approaches, such as the Component Model of Reading and RTI, have supported evidence that this discrepancy approach has poor sensitivity, stability, and specificity in discriminating students with specific reading disability (SRD) from those with low IQ scores and poor reading (Aaron, Joshi, Gooden & Bentum, 2008; Francis et al., 2005; Taylor, Miciak, Fletcher, & Francis, 2017). Calculating the discrepancy between cognitive ability and reading or writing achievement may miss diagnosing a SLD such as oral and written language learning disability (OWL LD) because the nature of the disability lowers the ability to answer questions orally posed by the examiner on verbal cognitive ability tests as well as reading comprehension and written expression. Alternatively, the skill that is impaired, such as handwriting in the case of dysgraphia, may be related to processes other than cognitive abilities (Berninger, 2015; Berninger & Richards, 2010; Berninger & Wolf, 2016).

IDEA 2004 expands the means by which SLD can be determined because it states that "a local education agency shall not be required to take into consideration whether a child has a severe discrepancy between achievement and intellectual ability." It further states that "in determining whether a child has an SLD, a local educational agency may use a process that determines if the child responds to scientific, research-based intervention" (614b, 6, B). This approach, often called RTI, has emerged as common practice.

Planning effective, evidence-based interventions requires an understanding that dyslexia, dysgraphia, dyscalculia (math disability), and OWL LD may be separate or co-occurring deficits within an individual student's performance profile (Geary, 2004; Kamhi & Catts, 2012; Mazzocco, Feigenson, & Halberda, 2011; Silliman & Berninger, 2014). As illustrated for Noah and his fellow students with learning challenges, an examination of the origin of the learning disability profile can provide an evidence-based direction for effective intervention, whereas the discrepancy model does not.

Response to Intervention

Vaughn and Fuchs (2003) advocated redefining learning disability as an inadequate response to instruction. This response to intervention (RTI) approach has proven to be a promising alternative to traditional testing methods for identifying students with specific learning disabilities (Fuchs & Vaughn, 2012). Important benefits of such an approach include 1) identification of students using an at-risk rather than a deficit model, 2) earlier identification and intervention, 3) reduction of identification bias, and 4) a strong focus on student outcome. As shown in the case study at the beginning of this chapter, RTI involves the provision of intensive, systematic instruction for a defined period of time to very small groups of students who are at risk for academic failure (see Box 20.1 for more information on RTI).

Three-Tier Models of Intervention The initial step of RTI involves students receiving instruction in their general education classroom, with their progress being carefully and regularly monitored. Those students who do not progress then receive additional services from a learning or reading specialist. Again, their progress is carefully and regularly monitored. Those who still fail to progress are referred for a special education evaluation (Fuchs, Mock, Morgan, & Young, 2003; Olitsky & Nelson, 2003).

In the most commonly used approach to RTI, and the one used by Noah's school, tier 1 of the model focuses on early intervention based on the National Reading Panel's recommendation for explicit training in phonological awareness and phonological decoding to prevent reading disabilities (National Institute of Child Health and Human Development, 2000). Tier 2 provides additional supplementary instruction in phonological awareness and phonological decoding for those who do not respond to tier 1 instruction; that is, to improve phonological awareness and phonological decoding. Tier 3 provides comprehensive assessment for those who do not respond to tier 2 instruction to determine if they are eligible for special education services (specialized instruction). Typically tier 1 and tier 2 are delivered by trained paraprofessionals (see Box 20.2 for a description of the paraprofessional's role), and tier 3 is delivered by both the school psychologist, who carries out the assessment process, and the special educator, who provides specialized instruction.

In the other main model of RTI, tier 1 children are screened for the skills on which they are weak, and early intervention is then provided for those weaknesses. The screens are based on research showing which skills explain significant and unique variance in not only reading achievement, but also writing achievement and listening and oral language skills related to literacy achievement. For example, Puranik, Wagner, Kim, and Lopez were instrumental in promoting the use of phonological awareness and decoding instruction at tier 1 and tier 2, but they also showed the importance of orthographic awareness and writing instruction (Puranik, Wagner, Kim, & Lopez, 2012). The intervention is then tailored to an

BOX 20.1 EVIDENCE-BASED PRACTICE

Response to Intervention

Response to intervention (RTI) is a multitiered approach to the early identification and support of students with learning and behavioral needs and to closing the achievement gap in at-risk students. The RTI process begins with high-quality instruction and universal screening of all children in the general education classroom.

RTI has also been promoted as an alternative to discrepancy models for identification of students with learning disabilities (Hughes & Dexter, 2011). RTI emphasizes high-quality, scientifically based classroom instruction; ongoing assessment to determine a student's rate of learning; and analysis of these data to determine the level of monitoring and intervention the student needs. The multitiered approach provides increasing levels and intensity of supports. These services may be provided by a variety of personnel, including general education teachers, special educators, and specialists. Progress is closely monitored to assess both the learning rate and level of performance of individual students. Educational decisions about the intensity and duration of interventions are based on individual student response to instruction. RTI is designed for use when making decisions in both general education and special education, creating a well-integrated system of instruction and intervention guided by child outcome data.

For RTI implementation to work well, the following essential components must be implemented with fidelity and in a rigorous manner (Jimmerson, Burns, & VanDerhayden, 2015; McInerney & Elledge, 2013):

- High-quality, scientifically based classroom instruction;
- Ongoing student assessment; and
- Tiered instruction.

BOX 20.2 INTERDISCIPLINARY CARE

The Paraprofessional in the Inclusion Classroom

Since the late 1990s, the structure of the classroom has changed considerably. With the growing use of the inclusion model in general education classrooms, students with special needs with mild to moderate impairments are included in the classrooms of most general education teachers. Some inclusive settings also provide for students with severe disabilities. The range of abilities, disabilities, and disorders within the classroom community can be extensive, with requirements for both physical and instructional accommodations and modifications. The "teacher's aide" is not a new role, but the need for extensive training and continued professional development has become a priority. These individuals are often among the least trained members of the staff in a school, but when well trained and when offered opportunities for collaboration with teachers and related service providers, they can be important partners in the planning, implementation, and monitoring of instruction in the classroom, including the implementation of RTI. Research indicates that these classroom assistants often work in the area of autism, but there is a need for these partners in other settings as well (Moshe, 2017). They can provide instruction to small groups, provide training and oversight in the use of supportive technologies for students, connect with families, assist in creating materials, and participate in some assessments. Teachers have identified the lack of such support as one of the burdens they feel when implementing an inclusion model, and when paraprofessionals have been trained (along with their supervising teacher partners) and participate in team planning, they feel that their skills improve and they seek continued training opportunities (Walker, Douglas, & Chung, 2017). When the partnership of the professional and paraprofessional is established as a co-teaching model, students benefit.

individual student's relative weakness to personalize their early intervention delivered via "differentiated instruction." RTI is evaluated on the basis of whether individual students improve on the skills for which they have received specialized instruction tailored to their weaknesses. Orthographic skills (e.g., naming and coding letters in memory that correspond to phonemes) are also taught at the tier 1 level because considerable research has documented the contribution of orthographic as well as phonological skills to early literacy (for reviews of evidence, see Berninger & Richards, 2010; Henry, Messer, Luger-Klein, & Crane, 2012; Wandell, & Le, 2017). In addition to oral reading (decoding) skills, handwriting and spelling (encoding) skills are also screened and taught if they are found to be weak. At tier 2, the interdisciplinary team engages in a problem-solving consultation for those students who do not respond at tier 1. The goal is to modify the early intervention by introducing new approaches and developing a plan for evaluating their responses to the modified intervention (Berninger, 2007a, 2007b, 2015). For those students who show persisting struggles in response to the tier 2 intervention, a tier 3 comprehensive assessment is conducted with the goal of making an instructionally relevant differential diagnosis that can then be used to design and implement specialized instruction and evaluate a student's response to it. The goal of all tiers in this version of RTI is personalized education based on carefully tailored, intensive instruction and progress monitoring that informs changes in instruction.

Intensive instruction provided daily in a very small group setting, a key component of RTI, is fiscally demanding in that it may impose a staffing burden on a classroom, especially when carried out in a manner supported by research and policy (Fuchs & Fuchs, 2002; Burns, Jimerson, VanDerHeyden, & Deno 2016). Children who make progress at the end of the prescribed time (usually 12–16 weeks) then return to the general education program, reducing needless referrals for evaluation and potential placement in separate, special learning environments. Children who do not make adequate gains receive a second round of intensive intervention (Gortmaker, Daly, McCurdy, Persampieri, & Hergenrader, 2007; Hay, Elias, Fielding-Barnsley, Homel, & Freibery, 2007). Students who do not benefit from an RTI's first two tiers of instruction signal a need for even more intensive forms of educational intervention (Fuchs, Fuchs, & Vaughn, 2014) and should be referred for comprehensive evaluation to determine the specific services and interventions required. There is also direct evidence that significant and widening differences in reading abilities persist between students with reading disabilities who receive intensive summer reading instruction and those who do not (Christodoulou et al., 2017).

Despite widespread support for RTI, challenges to implementation remain. These include reliance on an instructional environment that reflects commitment to fidelity, validity, and collaboration; staff preparation; and the availability of teachers who are well trained in all aspects of instruction. By using scientifically derived interventions for early instructional support, the potential for maintaining those students in the general education environment increases. This is in contrast to the discrepancy model, which is a "wait-to-fail" model in which the student may struggle with learning activities until a discrepancy emerges.

This tiered approach has reduced the numbers of students referred to pullout (outside of the general classroom) or special education services (Berkeley, Bender, Peaster, & Saunders, 2009). In research centers around the nation, studies continue to determine how to more effectively implement this model (Deshler, Mellard, Tollefson, & Byrd, 2005; Kennedy & Deshler, 2010; Moss, Lapp, & O'Shea, 2011; Pullen, Tuckwiller, Konod, Maynard, & Coyne, 2010; Ramaswami, 2010). Although most often described as a three-tier model, some schools identify a fourth, or "specialized" tier, which may provide intervention closer to that provided in special education classes without the express referral for a determination of eligibility for special education. Kavale and Spaulding (2008) reviewed the policy implications for these new regulations and concluded that both RTI and psychometric evaluation are appropriate for the identification of children as having learning disorders, allowing them to receive special education services under an individualized education program (IEP).

The diagnosis of SLD is difficult in students identified as English language learners (ELL) or having limited English proficiency. Some of these students may be experiencing difficulty because of their lack of familiarity with English in its academic and/or social use. Alternatively, some may, in fact, have disabilities in learning in both their native language and English (Barrera, 2006; Blanchett, Klingner, & Harry, 2009; Liu, Ortiz, Wilkinson, Robertson, & Kushner, 2008). For these students, technology, including tablets and laptops with appropriate applications based in their native languages, may afford necessary supports (Jozwik & Douglas, 2017). Although teacher preparation for serving students with SLD has expanded, the preparation of teachers to address the needs of students who may have both a learning disorder and English language proficiency issues needs to be improved (Paneque & Barbetta, 2006).

PREVALENCE

The U.S. Department of Education's National Center for Education Statistics (2018) reported that of the more than 6.4 million students receiving special education services during the 2014–2015 school year, approximately 35%, or 2.2 million, were classified as having SLD. The size of this category has nearly tripled since reporting began in 1977. These statistics represent only those students who are served in the public schools and not those who may be served in private, nonpublic, or homeschool environments. A review of a series of NIH-funded epidemiological studies at the Mayo Clinic showed that one in five otherwise typically developing school-age children and youth has an SLD in reading, writing, or math with or without ADHD (Colligan & Katusic, 2015). In addition, some forms of SLD are underidentified. Writing disabilities in particular have been left behind (Katusic, Colligan, Weaver, & Barbaresi, 2009). Specific language impairment (SLI), which is frequently associated with OWL LD, falls under the eligibility category of communication disorders rather than learning disabilities; as a consequence, students with SLI/OWL LD are often underidentified and not treated for their language learning disabilities (Silliman & Berninger, 2014).

Reporting differences among school districts and states also affect the assessment of the prevalence of SLD. Individual school districts exercise considerable autonomy in defining, describing, and coding disabilities at the time services are determined. When families are persistent in seeking special education services and actively involved in the process of attaining those services, the correct and discrete identification of a child's disability is more certain. In districts in which some disabilities are not specified completely, or include other aspects that contribute to learning difficulties, such as attention or behavior problems, an overembracing term such as *multiple disabilities* may be used. This inexact term camouflages the exact nature of a child's problems with learning and may distort the design of an effective and useful education program. However, without more precise definitions and descriptors in the education law, this type of inexact classification by school teams will continue.

The growing number of individuals identified as being on the autism spectrum has also influenced the overall numbers of individuals identified as being in need of special education (see Chapter 18). Many higher functioning students with autism spectrum disorders (ASD) were formerly classified as having learning disabilities. The overlap of severe learning disorders and higher functioning autism has long been recommended for further study to examine potential links between the two conditions (Williams, Goldstein, Kojkowski, & Minshew, 2008). Although relatively little further research on this has been done, one study (McIntyre et al., 2017) indicates that heterogeneity in reading profiles depends on the level of the ASD. The higher functioning the individual with ASD, the more aligned the profile is to that of an individual with LD. Although this is true of reading profiles, other factors, such as reduced self-regulation of students with ASD, also may have an effect on the independent practice of these skills (Chou, Wehmeyer, Palmer, & Lee, 2017).

The language deficits that may appear in students with SLD or ASD require careful diagnosis and characterization to ensure that interventions can be beneficial and long-term prognosis can be assessed. In a study by Hagberg, Billstedt, Nyden, and Gillberg (2015), adults who had persistent language deficits throughout their school career and into adulthood demonstrated great impairments in daily skills (often with reduced employment) compared with those whose language deficits were only seen in childhood.

ETIOLOGY: BIOLOGICAL AND ENVIRONMENTAL FACTORS

National initiatives such as the Human Genome Project and Decade of the Brain have resulted in an explosion of research on the biological bases of SLDs. Although SLDs and other neurogenetic disorders may share some of the same learning problems at the behavioral level, the underlying genetic and brain bases are not the same as for SLDs such as dysgraphia, dyslexia, OWL LD, and dyscalculia (Berninger, 2015).

Genetics

One reason that not all students respond equally to the same instructional intervention is that the genetic underpinnings are different for language by ear (listening), by mouth (oral expression), by eye (reading), and by hand (written expression). Since the late 1990s, substantial progress has been made in understanding the genetic bases of specific reading disabilities including dyslexia and other language-related SLDs (e.g., Fisher & DeFries, 2002; Olson, Wise, Connors, Rack, & Fulker, 1989; Olson et al., 2013). For example, twin studies have documented both genetic and environmental influences on specific reading disabilities in otherwise typically developing individuals, and unique genetic contributions remain even after students respond to early intervention (Samuelsson et al., 2008). Linkage studies and gene candidate studies have identified relationships between locations in the human genome and specific phenotypes (i.e., behavioral markers of genetic variables). Specific genes may influence response to instruction, and while results for linkage analysis and gene candidate studies have been replicated across multiple research groups, the findings indicate that the genetic bases for specific reading disability are heterogeneous, meaning that multiple gene candidates may underlie the same phenotypic expression. Thus, individuals may differ in the genetic basis for the same observable behavioral difficulties in language learning. This serves to emphasize the complex nature of reading and reading disability.

Research using genetic linkage and association techniques has shown a relationship among specific reading disabilities such as dyslexia and loci on chromosomes 1, 2, 3, 6, 15, and 18 (Raskind, Peter, Richards, Eckert, & Berninger, 2012; Scerri & Schulte-Körne, 2010). The genetic basis of math disabilities has also been studied (Berninger, 2015). In a twin study in which one twin had math disability and the other did not, higher rates of dyscalculia were found in identical than in fraternal twins (Cohen, Kadosh, & Walsh, 2007). There is also evidence that molecular markers differ across dysgraphia, dyslexia, OWL LD, and typical language learners (Abbott, Raskind, Matsushita, Richards, Price, & Berninger, 2017).

Epigenetics research (Cassiday, 2009) is underway that shows that genetic expression at the observable, behavioral level can respond to environmental interaction and input (see Chapter 1). Thus, although genetic anomalies may contribute to the etiology of a SLD at the biological level, the most effective treatment may be environmental (i.e., educational programming). For example, in one study, students with dysgraphia, dyslexia, and OWL LD who completed a special curriculum of computerized instruction showed significant improvement on the biologic impairments associated with their diagnosed SLD (Tanimoto, Thompson, Berninger, Nagy, & Abbott, 2017).

Brain Imaging

Since the Decade of the Brain that began in 1990, there has been an explosion of knowledge about the brain correlates of language and math. A variety of noninvasive imaging methodologies that are safe to use with developing children and youth have been used in research (see Chapter 8). Initially, these studies focused on documenting differences in brain structure and function between typically developing language or math learners and those with an SLD such as dyslexia (e.g., Sandak, Mencl, Frost, & Pugh, 2004; Simos et al., 2002; Turkeltaub, Gareau, Flowers, Zeffiro, & Eden, 2003) or dyscalculia (e.g., Cohen et al., 2007; Dehaene & Cohen, 1995). Subsequent imaging studies have shown how the brain changes in RTI (Berninger & Dunn, 2012; Berninger & Richards, 2010; Gabrieli, 2009) and addressed the issue of whether the brain of students with a SLD, such as SRD, normalized after intervention. Considerable evidence across many research groups now supports the contention that the brain can normalize in response to instruction. One imaging study in particular demonstrated that the brains of students of lower socioeconomic backgrounds are especially responsive to reading interventions (Romeo et al., 2017). This finding is important because SLDs occur in all socioeconomic groups and have a particular impact in children and youth from low-income families who are especially vulnerable to the long-term consequences of SLDs. Understanding brain differences in students with reading disability may also help parents and educators select the best remediation strategy (Wandell & Le, 2017).

CLASSIFYING LEARNING DISORDERS

The section that follows explains and analyzes learning disorders across three classifications: specific reading disability, specific math disability, and specific writing disability.

Specific Reading Disability

SRD, also called developmental dyslexia, is by far the most commonly recognized form of learning disability, accounting for over one third of the special education population (National Center for Educational Statistics, 2017). Theoretically, any defect in the processing or interpretation of written words can lead to a diagnosis of SRD. Efficient reading depends on rapidly, accurately, and fluently decoding and recognizing the phonemes of single words (Talcott et al., 2000; Wolf, Bowers, & Biddle, 2000). Phonological awareness includes 1) phoneme awareness (the understanding that speech is made up of discrete sounds), 2) a metacognitive understanding of word boundaries within spoken sentences, 3) a recognition of syllable boundaries within spoken words, and 4) an ability to isolate these phonemes and establish their location within syllables and words. Phonological awareness manifests in the ability to analyze and manipulate sounds within syllables (e.g., to count, delete, and reorder them). As a child learns to read, specialized areas of the brain and its structures are trained to associate text with the sounds of language (Wandell & Le, 2017). If a child does not realize that syllables and words are composed of phonemes and that these segments can be divided according to their acoustic boundaries, reading will be slow, labored, and inaccurate; in addition, comprehension will be poor. A second possible mechanism may be a defect in phonetic representation in working memory, wherein the child can understand the syntactic structure of a sentence but is unable to maintain it in working memory long enough to comprehend the meaning (Kamil, Pearson, Moje, & Afflerbach, 2010; Mann, 1994).

Poor reading has been linked to phonological processing impairments, but these impairments alone are not sufficient to explain SRD. Wolf and Bowers (1999) proposed three underlying types of specific reading disability: 1) phonological impairment, in which the reader attempts to manage the connection of sound to symbol accurately; 2) disrupted orthographic processing, which results from slow naming speed and influences the acquisition of fluency in both familiar and unfamiliar content; and 3) a combination of both impairments. Individuals who manifest the double impairment, phonological impairments and naming speed impairments, are the poorest readers. This hypothesis has not been universally accepted. Some researchers failed to find a phonological impairment in the absence of a naming-speed impairment and noted that the double-impairment groupings identified individuals with different neuropsychological profiles (Cirino, Israelian, Morris, & Morris, 2005; Waber, Forbes, Wolff, & Weiler, 2004). Others have found little support for the theory that underlies the double-impairment hypothesis, namely that rapid serial processing and temporal integration of letter identities are the primary means by which orthographic codes are formed (Ritchey & Goeke, 2006; Vellutino, Fletcher, Snowling, & Scanlon, 2004; Vukovic & Siegel, 2006). They also question the independence of phonological and rapid naming skills and the specificity of impairments in rapid naming for reading.

The Neural Substrates of Reading Reading is a dynamic process that develops with age and experience. It encompasses a wide variety of skills that develops at varying times. Early instruction focuses on learning to read and targets decoding. Later instruction uses reading to learn, and the focus shifts to comprehension. Beginning, inexperienced readers are focused on decoding and employ a "bottom-up" approach that uses analytic and synthetic processes. They are more focused on sounding out each word they encounter, which can often hinder comprehension. Experienced readers use a "top-down" approach that results in faster, more efficient reading. These readers use context and word recognition to gain meaning. Top-down, or conceptual, approaches assume that the path from text to meaning extends from prior knowledge that is applied to the process of acquiring the sound–symbol connection of reading.

Compensated poor readers recruit additional brain areas to read. Neuroimaging studies in individuals with dyslexia show reduced engagement of the left temporo-parietal cortex for phonological processing of print, altered white matter connectivity, and functional plasticity associated with effective intervention (Fisher & DeFries, 2002; Gabrieli, 2009). Posterior brain systems predominate during early reading acquisition (Simos et al., 2002; Turkeltaub et al., 2003). As individuals become older and are more skilled at reading, they begin to engage parietal and superior temporal areas, with frontal regions coming online last. Individuals who are identified as having dyslexia do not increase activation of the word form area (located in the left occipitotemporal gyrus) even after repeated trials of word exposure. As they grow older, children show the opposite—activation of the anterior system. Anterior activation is not the sole processing difference, however, as individuals with dyslexia also activate their right anterior inferior frontal gyrus as well as the right posterior occipital-temporal region (Sandak et al., 2004). In other words, individuals with dyslexia show abnormalities in brain processing during reading.

Shaywitz and colleagues (2004) have underscored the importance of dysfunction of the left hemisphere brain systems in SRD. They provided a year of intensive reading remediation to a group of individuals with SRD. After the intervention, the individuals made gains in reading fluency, and neuroimaging studies showed increased activation of the anterior and dorsal systems. Another study in adults with a lifetime history of SRD demonstrated that reading remediation in older individuals might be different. This study showed increases in both left and right hemisphere activation following successful reading intervention (Eden et al., 2004).

Specific Math Disability

Specific math disability, also known as dyscalculia, is a complex phenomenon that must be considered in the context of other learning processes and impairments. Three to six percent of individuals have a performance on tests of mathematical ability that is discrepant from their IQ scores (Mazzocco, 2007; Shalev & Gross-Tsur, 2001). This percentage may be higher than the true frequency of a learning disorder in mathematics. Poor performance may be due to a lack of adequate instruction in areas that are covered by the assessment measures.

Another reason for discrepant performance on math tests may relate to impairments in reading or executive function rather than mathematics (Dirks, Spyer, van Lieshout, & de Sonnerville, 2008; Donlan, 2007; Jordan, 2007).

Math disability is commonly seen in the presence of other learning and cognitive disorders. Of individuals with a math disability, approximately 17% have been found to have coexisting SRD and 26% have ADHD (Gersten, Jordan, & Flojo, 2005; Shalev & Gross-Tsur, 2001). In another study that focused on kindergarteners with developmental language disorders, 26% had significantly impaired arithmetic skills (Manor, Shalev, Joseph, & Gross-Tsur, 2001). In addition, Marshall, Schafer, O'Donnell, Elliott, and Handwerk (1999) found that inattention exerts a specific and deleterious effect on the acquisition of arithmetic computation skills. This has led some to defer the diagnosis of math disability in the presence of ADHD until the ADHD is properly managed (Shalev & Gross-Tsur, 2001). Finally, assessment of mathematics encompasses a variety of skills and neuropsychological processes, some of which may be impaired whereas others are relatively spared.

Difficulty with mathematics may manifest in different ways. Counting, basic calculation, problem solving, place values (base-10 concepts), equivalence, measurement, time, relations (as in algebra), and geometry are but some of the ways that mathematics is expressed. Despite the wide range of expression, math disability is specifically defined by deficiencies in fact mastery and calculation fluency (Jordan, Hanich, & Kaplan, 2003). Some of the difficulties that children encounter in mathematics evolve from their earliest encounters with numbers; that is, their number sense and early numeracy. The intuitive understanding of numbers and related concepts such as how numbers grow and diminish with calculation may be viewed as having a parallel to the initial reading skill of phonemic awareness, which includes the earliest awareness of how words are made up of discrete sounds. Research has shown that this initial "gut sense" about numbers may be significant in identifying the origins of math disability (Mazzocco et al., 2011).

Math disability evolves over time. Early presentations exhibit difficulty with retrieval of basic math facts and in computing arithmetic exercises. These have been related to immature counting skills. Older individuals have difficulty in learning arithmetic tables and comprehending the algorithms of adding, subtracting, multiplying, and dividing. These manifest as misuse of signs, forgetting to carry, misplacing digits, or approaching problems from left to right (Shalev, 2004). In another study, 10 to 11 year olds with math disability showed persistently poor math performance on reexamination 6 years later (Shalev et al., 2005).

Visuospatial working memory deficits are often present in those identified with math disability. A broad view of the connection of cognitive, neurobiological, and developmental components is needed, since these elements change throughout development and can create a vulnerability if not recognized (Menon, 2016).

The Neurobiology of Math Neurobiological evidence of math disability is still evolving, and the exact mechanism remains to be delineated. Evidence derived from clinical syndromes, neuroimaging, and genetics suggests a number of brain-based impairments. Although the clinical syndromes point to a major role of the parietal lobe in dyscalculia, the relationship is not simple. Different types of mathematic skills require coordination of different brain functions and, by extension, activation of different brain areas. Complicating this is the finding that people who have difficulty with math will recruit other brain areas and use other psychological mechanisms to compensate for the impairment in brain function.

There is a paucity of studies that focus on the genetics of math disability. Yet, familial occurrences of the disorder have been described. Shalev and Gross-Tsur (2001) found that approximately half of siblings of individuals with math disability also had evidence of math disability. In a study of twins, one of whom had math disability, significantly higher rates of dyscalculia were found in identical twins than in fraternal twins (Cohen et al., 2007).

Several psychological mechanisms have been proposed for math disability. In early research, Rourke and Finlayson (1978) found that individuals with math disability alone showed poor nonverbal skills (visual-spatial and tactile-perceptual), whereas individuals with combined math disability and SRD showed poorer verbal skills (verbal and auditory-perceptual). Geary (2004) has posited three subtypes of math disability based on memory and cognitive impairments: 1) the procedural subtype, 2) the semantic memory subtype, and 3) the visuospatial subtype. Others have associated math disability with executive function and working memory impairments (McLean & Hitch, 1999). Dehaene and Cohen (1995) advocated a "triple-code model" wherein simple arithmetic operations are processed by the verbal system within the left hemisphere and more complex arithmetic procedures that require **subitization** (the ability to perceive at a glance the number of items presented), **cardinality** (the ability to perceive the number of elements in a set or other grouping), and visual representations are bilaterally localized in the brain.

Specific Writing Disability

Specific writing disability, also known as dysgraphia, is a multifaceted and complex deficiency involving the effective and coherent processing of information and transcribing it into written form. Writing is a psychomotor process involving the motor and spatial processes of handwriting, the orthographic coding of letters and symbols, storing and retrieving words, and correct spelling and syntax. In most cases, this deficit occurs together with other developmental disabilities (most commonly dyslexia, attention deficits, and ASD).

Writing difficulties are usually discovered when children are asked to produce written work that demonstrates their progress with reading and requires participation in discussions of subjects learned. Students who become frustrated with the writing process sometimes show fatigue, disengagement, or simply stop writing.

There are stages of writing acquisition that must be understood in order to diagnose the actual origin of the problem—linguistic or motoric. Linguistically, an individual takes in the phonemic and visual components of words and then applies remembered spelling, grammar, and meaning to get the word on paper in a comprehensible format. Motorically, the individual must manage the instrument for writing while remembering and planning the sequence needed to represent letters and other symbols in a defined space (Prunty & Barnett, 2017). Although there is usually a primary cause for the dysgraphia, a student may exhibit both motoric and linguistic symptoms.

The subtypes of specific writing disability are dyslexic dysgraphia, motor dysgraphia, and spatial dysgraphia. Dyslexic dysgraphia is most often seen as illegibility of spontaneously created work; however, given time and a model, copied work improves. Motor dysgraphia stems from poor fine motor control or lack of dexterity. Although copied or spontaneously written material may start out neat and conforming to space, it degrades in longer writing samples (Graham, Collins, & Rigby-Wills, 2017). Sustaining the coordination for the task seems to be a problem. Spatial dysgraphia impacts drawing as well as writing due to the fact that the individual does not perceive space accurately. Written products, both copied and original, are illegible and spread beyond the defined space provided for the task.

Essentially, specific writing disabilities stem from deficits in automatically remembering and mastering the sequences for managing the orthographic "loop"—coding the units of language formation (morphemes, phonemes, and syntax), motor control, sustaining and focusing attention, and self-monitoring production (Berninger & Wolf, 2016).

The Neurobiology of Writing The angular gyrus plays a role in mediating complex language functions, and it connects sensory experiences like touch to spatio-visual experiences that allow recognition of subtle visual distinctions (such as the differences among letters like *g, b, d, p,* and *q*) or punctuation. This ability to note salient features connects to the ability to sustain attention (Nicolson & Fawcett, 2011).

Attention and memory, as executive functions, call on the prefrontal cortex to coordinate the process to allow the student to remember the task assigned, the relevant ideas related to the task, and the organization required to assemble the response to the task orthographically. An area in the middle frontal gyrus (BA6), termed the "graphemic/motor frontal area," supports bridging between orthography and motor programs specific to handwriting (Roux et al., 2009).

IMPAIRMENTS ASSOCIATED WITH SPECIFIC LEARNING DISABILITIES

One quarter to one half of individuals with learning disorders have additional impairments that interfere with school functioning. These may include executive function impairments, ADHD, social cognition impairments, and emotional and behavior disorders. These behavior and emotional problems may be externalizing (e.g., aggression, oppositional-defiant disorder, or conduct disorder) or internalizing (e.g., shyness, depression, or anxiety). Failure to detect and treat these additional impairments is a common reason for failed intervention programs. As comorbid conditions may adversely affect outcome, it may be most appropriate to categorize individuals not only on the basis of their learning impairments, but also according to comorbid conditions.

Memory Impairments

Impairments in the ability to listen, remember, and repeat auditory stimuli have been associated with reading disability. The holding of information in immediate and working memory is essential in learning to read (Berninger & Swanson, 2017). Research shows that children with learning disabilities have deficits in working memory (Peng & Fuchs, 2016) that can affect reading and math performance. Attention components in working memory include 1) focused attention (inhibiting irrelevant information), 2) switching attention (moving from one relevant stimuli to another), 3) sustaining attention over time (maintaining on task behavior), and 4) self-monitoring (having awareness of whether or not you are on task). These contribute uniquely to reading and writing achievement (Berninger & Richards, 2010). A number of studies comparing individuals with equivalent IQ scores but low or high reading abilities have reported impairments in the poor readers on the Digit Span subtest of the Wechsler Intelligence Scale for Children–Fourth Edition (D'Angiulli & Siegel, 2003; Wechsler, 2003). Executive dysfunction coupled with memory impairments may adversely affect a student's ability to choose the appropriate strategy for solving a problem. Working memory, which is based in the area of the prefrontal cortex concerned with short term management of memory and attention, has also been studied and found to be of particular interest (Schuchardt, Maehler, & Hasselhorn, 2008). As a result, the student's ability to use cognitive behavioral techniques may be limited because he or she cannot remember a sequence of problem-solving steps.

Impairments in Executive Functions

According to Pennington (1991), executive functions (see Chapter 13) involve the ability to maintain an appropriate problem-solving set of procedures for attaining a future goal. This includes the ability to 1) inhibit or defer a response; 2) formulate a sequential, strategic plan of action; and 3) encode relevant information in memory for future use. These metacognitive abilities are necessary for organizational skills, planning, future-oriented behavior, maintaining an appropriate problem-solving set of procedures, impulse control, selective attention, vigilance, inhibition, and creativity in thinking. These abilities involve an awareness of what skills, strategies, and resources are needed to perform a task effectively. They also require the ability to use self-regulatory mechanisms to ensure the successful completion of a task, yet students with learning disorders are often impulsive rather than reflective when presented with a problem-solving task. This failure to consider alternative solutions often results in errors or a poor quality solution. Executive functions become essential beginning in Grade 4 in order to complete homework and long-term projects, to sustain attention during lectures, and to set future goals (Berninger, Abbott, & Cook, 2017). Disruption in this organization and control of behavior often manifests as disruption in the classroom. Executive function impairments are also a key feature in ADHD.

Attention-Deficit/Hyperactivity Disorder

Approximately one half of individuals with learning disorders meet criteria for the diagnosis of ADHD, making this the most common comorbid diagnosis. Studies have found that the prevalence of ADHD in individuals with learning disorders is higher than the prevalence of learning disorders in individuals with ADHD (Friedman, Rapport, Orban, Eckrich, & Calub, 2017; Friedman, Rapport, Raiker, Orban, & Eckrich, 2017). The symptoms typically include inattention, impulsivity, and hyperactivity (see Chapter 19). Recent research reviews indicate that the increase in this identified comorbidity may be due to inclusion of students with writing disorders who were previously under-identified relative to students with reading and math disorders (DuPaul, Gormley, & Laracy, 2013).

Impairments in Social Cognition

Impairments in social cognition are noted often in individuals with learning disorders (Bauminger, Edelsztein, & Morash, 2005; Bauminger & Kimhi-Kind, 2008). Such individuals have difficulty understanding complex emotions, tend to be socially isolated, may have few close friends, and infrequently participate in social activities. In turn, they are often overlooked or rejected by their peers because of their odd behavior and poor school or athletic performance. Teachers tend to rate these individuals as having social adjustment difficulties and as being easily led. There may be many reasons for these problems, including poor social comprehension, inability to take the perspective of others, poor pragmatic language skills, an inability to recognize facial expressions, and misinterpretation of body language. This awareness of the intent or perspective of others is called *theory of mind* (see Chapter 18 for a discussion of theory of mind as it relates to ASD) and sheds light on how individuals develop the means to understand the social cues sent by others so that they may develop their own awareness of social situations and form appropriate responses (Bloom & Heath, 2010; Schneider, 2008). The reported prevalence of ASD has increased significantly since 2000, when the CDC reported occurance of one in 150 children, to 2014, when the occurance was reported to be one in 59 children. The child who has a combination of a learning disorder, poor pragmatic language skills, executive function impairments, and impairments in social cognition may be difficult to distinguish from a child who falls on the autism spectrum. It is likely that these conditions will be more closely linked in the future (McIntyre et al., 2017) and may have common genetic and neurobiologic signatures.

Emotional and Behavioral Disorders

Although associated emotional and behavioral impairments may represent endogenous biological conditions, they also may result from the child's experiences of school failure. Although individuals with learning disorders may exhibit conduct disorders, withdrawal, poor self-esteem, and depression, related therapeutic services to address these concomitant disorders are not mandated in federal law. A secondary diagnosis of an emotional disability would have to be in evidence in the student's profile in order for services to be provided to address both the learning disability and related social/emotional responses to the challenges in learning. These individuals are less likely to take pride in their successes and more likely to be overcome by their failures. More than one third of students with learning disorders receive a failing grade in one or more courses each school year. These individuals often exhibit chronic frustration and anxiety (Nielsen et al., in press) as they attempt to meet the demands of skill-based tasks, such as phonological decoding, comprehension, spelling, and math. This school failure, combined with social skills impairments, may lead to peer rejection, poor self-image, and withdrawal from participation in school activities (Abbott et al., 2017; Maag & Reid, 2006). Eventually, these individuals may avoid going to school all together or act out in class in order to obtain the attention they do not receive through good grades. There is a lack of agreement regarding how to best serve students with coexisting emotional/behavioral disorders and SLD, with some experts pointing out that the design of inclusion may exacerbate inner conflicts and frustrations, requiring consideration of more specialized learning settings (Eller, Fisher, Gilchrist, Rozman, & Shockney, 2015). In the United States, the overall dropout rate for individuals with SLD is three times that of all students. In the 2013–2014 school year, 18% of students with SLD dropped out as compared with 6.5% of students overall. Although the dropout rate has decreased since the late 2000s, it remains unacceptably high. During this time period almost half a million students with SLD left high school without a diploma, putting them at high risk for a poor outcome in transitioning to meaningful employment (National Center for Learning Disabilities, 2017).

HEALTH PROBLEMS SIMULATING SPECIFIC LEARNING DISABILITIES

Some individuals who do not have learning disorders may demonstrate learning differences in school as a consequence of another developmental disability, a chronic illness, or psychosocial problems. If these individuals are misdiagnosed as having an SLD, efforts directed solely at treating the learning problem will have limited success. Instead, the underlying problem must be identified and addressed. Once this problem has been treated, the learning problem may well improve or disappear.

For example, if a child has an unidentified sensory impairment, learning is likely to be affected. The provision of hearing aids to a child with hearing loss or of glasses to the child with a refractive error may lead to a significant improvement in school performance (see Chapters 25 and 26). Individuals with epilepsy (see Chapter 22) also may have problems in school resulting either from poorly controlled seizures or from side effects of antiepileptic medication. Modifying the drug regimen may significantly improve both attention and learning. Individuals with psychiatric disorders (see Chapter 27) also may fail in school. The use of psychotropic drugs and psychotherapy, including cognitive behavior therapy (see Chapter 34), often leads to significantly improved school performance, although some of these drugs can have an adverse effect on attention. (For specific information on medication side effects, see Appendix C.)

An increased incidence of learning problems also has been described in individuals with chronic illnesses, such as diabetes, HIV infection, sickle cell disease, cancer, and chronic kidney and liver disease (see Chapter 24). In these situations, a learning disability may exist, but learning difficulties also may result from other causes such as illness, excessive school absences, attention impairments, or depression. A secondary learning problem rather than a learning disability is suggested if learning improves once the medical condition is brought under control (Sexson & Madan-Swain, 1993).

Individuals who were born prematurely have an increased incidence of learning disorders. Acute disorders such as meningitis, encephalitis, and traumatic brain injury (TBI) also can result in the subsequent development of learning problems. Mild TBI is the most common of these and is an increasingly recognized cause of behavior and learning problems in individuals (see Chapter 23). The injury may result in either temporary or permanent neurological impairments. Affected individuals present special challenges in the classroom as a result of the evolving nature of their recovery (Carney & Porter, 2009). During the acute phase, disorders of attention and other executive functions, higher language skills, and behavior are common. Because of this, TBI has been identified as a separate category of disability under IDEA 2004 (see Chapter 33) to distinguish it from specific learning disabilities and other related disorders. However, when recovery is completed, some individuals with TBI may have a residual learning disorder.

Finally, psychosocial influences may affect the child's ability to learn. A child who is hungry cannot pay attention or learn well. A child who comes from a home that does not value learning is at high risk for underachievement in school. A home beset with family problems or abuse is a poor setting in which to encourage the child's school performance. Improvement in these psychosocial areas would likely result in improved school performance but has proven difficult to achieve. Until a complete picture of why students in a particular school are identified as having profiles of underachievement—and until the role of factors such as poverty, prematurity, nutrition, and environmental threats (e.g., lead poisoning and other environmental toxins) are fully understood and addressed—educators will continue to struggle to reconcile disorders of learning and effective instructional practices (see Chapter 42).

What is vital to the improvement of this state of affairs is greater attention to how school teams obtain and use information that identifies learning disabilities and how resources are mobilized to treat the learning disabilities in the school, school district, and community. All existing information should be used in the educational process. Medical and educational assessments by qualified examiners, combined with the assessment data developed by the school, serve as the foundation for developing an effective educational program, which optimizes the use of related services such as speech-language therapy or support from learning specialists in a collaborative effort to serve the student within the most inclusive setting possible (see Chapter 33).

ADDITIONAL CHALLENGES IN THE SCHOOL SETTING

There is a disproportionality of representation of students from various racial and ethnic subgroups in special education (see Chapter 42). This has been linked to gaps in achievement, resulting in the overidentification of these students (Williams, Bryant-Mallory, Coleman, Gottel, & Hall, 2017). Schools serving students with an array of special needs must also consider two additional factors that complicate effective instruction and intervention—the growing number of English language learners and the impact of poverty in some school settings. Roughly 9.4% of students in public school are identified as ELLs (National Center for Educational Statistics, 2017), and of that group, nearly 10% are also identified as having disabilities (Liu, Ward, Thurlow, & Christensen, 2017). This requires attention to accurate assessment of abilities and disabilities so that appropriate intervention to support these students can be provided (Kim & Helphinstine, 2017). This appropriate determination of need will lead to a greater number of students with cultural and linguistic diversity being accurately placed within the inclusive instructional setting (Barrio, 2015; Driver & Powell, 2017).

Poverty and the related factor of homelessness also complicate identifying and serving students, especially when they have learning disabilities. The Condition of Education 2017, a congressionally mandated annual report summarizing the latest data on education in the United States, reports that nearly 20% of children under the age of 18 live in poverty and that 2.5% of the public school population is homeless. This includes students in both urban and rural settings (Barrio, 2017). Because homelessness is closely related to mobility, many children in poverty are moving around so much that accurate assessment of their needs is not possible. Others already identified as needing services often do not receive them due to limited access to records and/or the availability of qualified educators and other specialized providers.

ASSESSMENT PROCEDURES

The assessments used to identify students with an SLD consist of individually administered tests designed to reveal both strengths and challenges so that comprehensive recommendations can be made. A school team, including the parent and student (when appropriate), reviews all assessments and determines the appropriate level of services required to accommodate the student's learning needs. These recommendations are written into the individual education program (IEP) with explicit, measurable goals and objectives, as well as the clear description of how progress will be evaluated (see Chapter 33). Recommendations may include specific programmatic interventions in reading, writing, or mathematics; grouping strategies; or even additional therapeutic interventions from specialists (Fletcher, Lyon, Fuchs, & Barnes, 2007).

The No Child Left Behind (NCLB) Act of 2001 (PL 107-110) has been replaced by the Every Student Succeeds Act of 2015 (PL 114-95; the reauthorization of the Elementary and Secondary Education Act of 1965; see Chapter 33), but the continued emphasis on access to the general education curriculum and high stakes testing as a measure of mastery creates challenges for students with SLD. There have been some victories for families around issues of accommodations and modifications used in instruction and for high stakes testing, but these battles continue to occur.

Psychological, language, and educational tests are the mainstay of assessment in school-age individuals (see Chapter 13). However, a complete medical, behavioral, educational, and social history also should be taken in order to consider confounding variables that may simulate, mask, or worsen a learning disorder (Francis et al., 2005; Lyon, Shaywitz, & Shaywitz, 2003). Simply looking at the discrepancy between potential and actual achievement can lead to misclassification of the students' needs. Evaluators need to use procedures for assessment that provide more information than a simple statistic as an indicator of a student's abilities (Grigorenko, 2009). Global standardized assessment tools, such as IQ tests, are not sensitive enough to allow an instructional program to be tailored to ensure a student's academic growth. Standardized proficiency testing must be combined with authentic assessment, norm-referenced as well as criterion-referenced tests, informal assessment, and portfolio assessment (based on a collection of artifacts that represent the student's work product) to obtain the full picture of how the student is progressing. This permits connecting and applying this information to the content the student is learning. If this does not occur, inappropriate treatment recommendations can result. Labeling a test taker as a "low achiever" does no service to the student. Well-documented strengths and challenges lead to a more serviceable IEP (Liu et al., 2016; Phipps & Beaujean, 2016).

Continued periodic assessment of progress in the class is also required. This periodic "snapshot" of achievement allows the effectiveness of the program to be evaluated and the instructional program to be adjusted. Periodic reassessment of cognitive and executive functions is warranted if the student is failing to progress. In addition, annual assessment of academic subjects is important to determine the progress the child has made and the effectiveness of the program. This aligns with the purpose of RTI as well as the mandates for progress monitoring.

INTERVENTION STRATEGIES

The practice of inclusion has placed most students with learning disabilities into general education classrooms where they have access to the general education curriculum with modifications, accommodations, and supports (see Chapter 33). As a result, interventions and strategies specifically designed for learning disabilities are now embedded into some general education classroom through the Universal Design for Learning (UDL; King-Sears, 2014). UDL provides multiple modes of presentation with a variety of potential responses so that teachers can modify the material for all students. Additionally, computer-assisted instruction (CAI), small group specialized methods, and individual tutoring are now provided within the general education classroom. When available, a special education teacher will collaborate with the general educator to recommend specific strategies or to co-teach certain lessons. The use of evidence-based practices (EBPs) in the general education classroom promise to close the achievement gap for low-performing students, but while gains have been reported, they may be difficult to sustain over time (Fuchs et al., 2015).

The primary goal of intervention is to facilitate the acquisition and expression of the knowledge needed for effective performance in school and subsequently in the workplace. The objectives are to achieve academic competence, treat associated impairments, and prevent adverse mental health outcomes. This requires the cooperation of educators, health care professionals, and families. If individuals with SRD are not provided with an early intervention program composed of instruction in phonological awareness, sound–symbol relations, and contextual reading skills before the third grade, at least three fourths of these students will show little improvement in reading throughout their later school years (Shaywitz & Shaywitz, 2005).

In addition to treating the core learning disorder, intervention strategies need to focus on associated cognitive, attention, language, perceptual, and sensory impairments. Immaturity, lack of motivation, and poor impulse control also must be considered in determining the child's needs for remediation (Bakker, Van Strien, Licht, & Smit-Glaude, 2007). An intervention must recognize the developmental changes that occur as a student gets older. It must be sensitive to the changing demands of the curriculum, the typical developmental challenges faced by the child, and the effects of maturation and intervention on the academic abilities of the student. In addition, successful interventions must not be withdrawn prematurely because of the positive impact they have on developing the self-awareness and self-advocacy skills necessary to combat stigma, to build self-confidence, and to access services and supports in postsecondary school settings or the workplace (Reschly, 2008).

Professionals continue to debate the most effective intervention strategies. A major consideration is whether to teach to the child's abilities (i.e., compensation/circumvention strategies) or the disabilities (i.e., remedial strategies; Liu et al., 2016; Phipps & Beaujean, 2016). Little evidence supports the superiority of one approach over the other. It is generally agreed, however, that there must be a combination of instructional and cognitive interventions (Alexander & Slinger-Constant, 2004).

Instructional Interventions

The following is a review of some interventions in reading, writing, mathematics, and other areas.

Reading In 2000, the National Reading Panel released its report on research-based reading instruction (National Institute of Child Health and Human Development, 2000). The panel identified the following six essential components to a sound reading program: 1) phonemic awareness; 2) phonics skills; 3) fluency, accuracy, speed, and expression; 4) reading comprehension strategies to enhance understanding; 5) teacher education; and 6) computer technology. Once decoding is unlocked, students are able to use these skills to build fluency. The focus can then shift to interventions that support and develop the expansion of vocabulary (for general communication, usage, and technical use) and enhance comprehension. Most states maintain a list of approved evidence-based practices that teachers may draw from in choosing specific interventions. These EBPs are not uniform and vary not only from state to state, but even within different school systems within each state.

Reading proficiency depends on phonological processing and alphabetical mapping. Phonics instruction, however, is different from phonological awareness training (Shaywitz, 2005). Clark and Uhry (1995) defined phonics as a low level of rote knowledge of the association between letters and sounds. Phonological awareness, on the other hand, includes higher level metacognitive understandings of word boundaries within spoken sentences, of syllable boundaries in spoken words, and of how to isolate the phonemes and establish their location within syllables and words. Regardless of the method chosen, the major goal of reading instruction is to improve phonological awareness (the sublexical aspect of reading) so that there is effective word recognition and comprehension of meaning (the lexical aspect of reading). Reading activities focus on helping a child gain print awareness and become attuned to the sound characteristics of language (phoneme awareness) and letter–sound relationships (the alphabetic principle).

Reading instruction in elementary school varies significantly and is influenced by regulation, policy, and budget. The common thread to this instruction includes methods designed to increase skills in acquiring vocabulary, using syntax, and understanding meaning (Alexander & Slinger-Constant, 2004; Schatschneider & Torgesen, 2004). While there is no single model of reading instruction that suffices for all individuals, there are certain components that all agree are essential for good instruction (National Institute of Child Health and Human Development, 2000). In the final analysis, semantic (the meaning of words), syntactic (the rules that govern the ways words combine to form phrases), and graphophonemic (using combined letters and sounds to decode words) systems must be united for successful reading.

Along with knowledge of phonics, efficient reading requires a rapid sight vocabulary (words recognized on sight without sounding them out phonetically). Different word recognition strategies include analysis of sound (phonics or phonetics), analysis for structure (visual configuration), and use of memory skills to recognize words as total entities (whole-word approach). Comprehension strategies center on developing the ability to draw meaning from text and to read fluently. Stevens, Walker, and Vaughn (2016) have provided a synthesis of research showing that repeated reading increases oral reading fluency in students who are competent decoders but need practice in faster, more accurate reading. Multicomponent interventions and assisted reading with audiobooks produced gains in fluency and comprehension and found that repeated reading is still the most effective intervention for improving fluency in students with learning disabilities.

Many students with a reading disability need an adjustment in the curriculum. Some methods of teaching reading, such as Orton-Gillingham, Wilson, and Lindamood Bell, employ multisensory approaches (Birsh, 2011; Ritchey & Goeke, 2006) for the remediation of difficulties in efficient sound–symbol processing. Other approaches include 1) whole language (reinforcing a spectrum of language arts), 2) thematics (utilizing content areas conceptually), 3) literature-based methods (using trade books to build on basal program skills), 4) individualized reading programs (using trade books and alternative literature forms to build personal reading), 5) language experience (having students generate their own reading material), and 6) functional skills (involving the use of materials involved in daily living, e.g., forms, notices, and directions). The increased influence of STEM (science, technology, engineering, and math) has broadened the application of reading and writing skills across the content domains. Unfortunately, teacher preparation programs may not be providing content area teachers with a broad enough understanding of specific learning disabilities and the tools to modify instruction to meet these students' needs.

Despite this, teachers at all levels and in all types of classrooms can give students with SRD tools such as 1) graphic organizers (a visual representation of the material a student is learning that assists the student in brainstorming and/or organizing information to make it easier to understand how ideas connect), 2) anticipation guides (study guides that prepare students to identify the major themes and concepts of a written work,

3) question/answer strategies, 4) think-alouds (explicit modeling in which teachers give an oral description of the cognitive processes they go through as they read with their students), 5) charting and outlining, and 6) induced imagery (teacher guided mental imagery while reading to enhance comprehension). These schemata all help students retain the messages they get through their reading. The intent of these strategies is to provide the reader with ways to chunk or otherwise partition their reading material into segments that they can better understand. The goal of such instructional interventions is movement toward higher levels of critical thinking. By attaining these skills, the student can compete with peers in academic tasks that connect reading to other skills, such as writing and oral discussion.

Reading in Middle School and High School

The mandates of No Child Left Behind, as well as the requirements of school districts for the acquisition of credits toward graduation, have raised the bar for the attainment of a diploma. In addition, a diploma is not acquired by passing courses alone. High school students must demonstrate the ability to pass statewide-standardized measures of mastery of core subjects as well. The path toward independent adulthood, higher education, and continued training in skills needed for employment has a distinct "turn" as students move into middle school and then into high school. As previously stated, in December, 2015, NCLB was replaced by the Every Student Succeeds Act. Although the original provisions of NCLB remain for many aspects of assessment, much of the change relates to the shift of responsibility and accountability for student performance to the individual states. States must show that they have adopted challenging standards in reading, math, and science and that the levels of achievement comport with the standards for admission to higher education institutions as well as with the standards in career and technical education. States may develop alternative assessment standards for students with the most significant cognitive disabilities, but the number of students determined to qualify for this accommodation is limited. In addition, states may choose to administer assessments in annual or multiple interim formats.

The demands of middle school and the pressures of high school programs can be very trying for students with learning disorders. As individuals move from the structure of elementary school to middle and high school, the demands of content reading become an additional burden. The discrete skills of content reading and the related study skills needed for success in secondary education are divided into two approaches. One is a direct instructional approach that separates skills from content, and the other is a functional approach that embeds reading and study skills into the content.

In middle and high school, the reading process must connect with other skills needed for mastering content-related matter in subjects such as social studies, geography, higher level mathematics, and sciences. Study, organizational, and problem-solving skills must blend with the processing skills involved in obtaining meaning from words, sentences, charts, maps, books, poetry, and dramatic or narrative literature. Meaning is easier to teach in the elementary and middle grades than in high school, when it may become buried in nuances of language, such as humor, sarcasm, and metaphor.

The expertise of general educators in middle and high schools is in the content they teach and not in the instructional mechanisms that help students organize, retrieve, and explain text related to that content. In addition, secondary school requires learning multiple content areas in discrete settings with several different teachers. Consequently, the student with SRD may become a "cumulative deficit" reader who makes progress but at a rate that is too slow to maintain adequate academic achievement. The content teacher, therefore, needs to understand not only the demands and organization of his or her content, but also how students must organize that content from lessons so that they can use it in the many forms that secondary school demands (e.g., exams, research papers, and debates).

Writing As much as reading dominates the instructional day of students with SRD, students with disorders of written expression (e.g., dysgraphia) have specific disabilities in processing and reporting information in written form. Writing is firmly connected to reading and spelling because comprehension and exposition of these skills are demonstrated through production of written symbols as indicators of understanding (Berninger & Wolf, 2009; Mason & Graham, 2008). Although writing is a representation of oral language, it also must convey meaning without the benefit of vocal intonation or stress. This makes additional demands on the writer.

Problems in writing may result from either an inability to manipulate a pen and paper to produce a legible representation of ideas or an inability to express oneself on paper. Word processors can assist individuals who have disabilities related to the manipulation of the writing implements (Bain, Baillett, & Moats, 2001; MacArthur, 2009). Remedial and instructional techniques that are helpful with problems of written expression include the use of 1) open-ended sentences; 2) probable passages (a strategy used to draw on a student's prior knowledge of a topic while incorporating writing into a basic reading lesson); 3) journal keeping; 4) modified writing systems, using rebuses in which words are represented by combinations of pictures and individual letters or other symbols; and 5) newspapers and other print media to demonstrate various writing styles and organizational models. Additionally, the ability of the student to maintain and self-regulate attention to spoken and print language sources has an impact on the development of writing and its connection to executive functions (Berninger, Abbot, & Cook, 2017).

Not to be forgotten is the connection of spelling to writing. The developmental stages of spelling need to be explored as teachers approach instruction that connects what is read to the written response of students. These stages include prephonemic, phonemic, transitional, and conventional spelling (Bear & Templeton, 1998). In 1998, the International Reading Association and the National Association for the Education of Young Children (1998) issued a joint position statement that advocated a developmental approach to teaching writing as an outgrowth of the reading process, recommending that students should be moved from the initial, prephonemic, and phonemic attempts at spelling toward correct, conventional spelling of English words. The process must reflect an understanding of the developmental level and needs of the individual student as well.

Content area literacy calls for connections between reading and writing and the development of study skills and organization of written materials so that they are retrievable for later use. Interventions in this area may call for students to share their writing with peers and to examine the writing styles of others. Among the research-based strategies that assist the student with writing disabilities is self-regulated strategy development, a six-step cognitive strategy model designed to make the writing process complete, automatic, and flexible for all subjects (Graham & Harris, 1989; Harris & Pressley, 1991; Reid, 2005; Berninger, Abbott & Cook, 2017).

Writing is also a sociocultural endeavor, representing a cognitive process learned through dialogic interactions, expressing the social and cultural perspectives of the student (Englert, 1992). The difficulties that a student with a learning disorder may have with social perception and awareness of cultural aspects of personal development may influence the written product as well as the writing process.

Mathematics Students with a math disability (i.e., dyscalculia) have an impaired ability to perform basic math operations (i.e., addition, subtraction, multiplication, and division) or may have trouble applying those operations to daily situations (Mazzocco, 2007; Raghubar et al., 2009). Often, however, the problem is in understanding the abstract concepts of mathematical usage (Mabbott & Bisanz, 2008). When students with dyscalculia have only written math problems to solve, the concepts remain vague. When functional applications (e.g., involving money or time) and manipulatives are used, however, the student can connect the concepts to their practical applications and demonstrate greater understanding. For some individuals with this disorder, a calculator may prove helpful. Thus, teaching may focus on the use of money in fast food restaurants (e.g., making change), grocery shopping (e.g., comparing prices per unit of weight), banking (e.g., balancing a checkbook or calculating interest), cooking (e.g., measurement), and transportation (e.g., reading directions and maps and keeping to schedules).

The language aspects of instructing students with a math disability, especially those who also have SRD, have been studied to determine how the reading process influences performance in numeric problem solving (Andersson & Lyxell, 2007; Fuchs & Fuchs, 2002; Powell, Fuchs, Fuchs, Cirino, & Fletcher, 2009; Peng & Fuchs, 2016). In these studies, for students with both reading and math disabilities, problems requiring addition were easier to solve than problems requiring subtraction or problems requiring making change. Powell and colleagues (2009) investigated how much the format of word problems connects to numeric ability and discovered that students with math disability demonstrated an improved ability to solve word problems in math by using diagramming as an intervention (Van Garderen, 2007) to incorporate visuo-spatial reasoning.

The importance of adequate assessment tools in the determination of math disability has been discussed by Lembke and Foegen (2009), whose research in early numeracy (the ability to understand and work with numbers) has posited the relationship of number sense to phonemic awareness in reading. As indicators of math performance among primary grade students, they have identified the skills of quantity discrimination, number identification, and missing number identification as three strong predictors of early mathematical success. Assessment and determination of the possibility of other disabling conditions that might affect learning has also been a concern for researchers, especially the combined impact of reading and math disabilities (Dirks et al., 2008). Limited study has been done on this combined disability effect, although Dirks and colleagues have estimated that more than 7% of students have both SRD and math disabilities.

Powell and colleagues (2009) have demonstrated the effectiveness of an approach that emphasizes problem type for solving mathematical word problems and complex operations (e.g., multiplication). Another approach, emphasizing executive function, involves rehearsal, practice, and mastery of math skills in combination with corrective and positive feedback throughout the process of instruction. A metacognitive approach can give students with dyscalculia hope for greater success and facility in progressing to higher and more complex mathematical operations (Desoete, Roeyers, & Buysse, 2001; Keeler & Swanson, 2001).

The concepts, principles, and procedures that are part of mathematics instruction increase in difficulty through the grades, and so the identification of a math disability may follow the student throughout his or her school career. Geary and Hoard (2005) described the executive functions that are disrupted, namely regulation of attention and the ability to distinguish between relevant and irrelevant numeric associations in solving problems.

For many students with mathematical disabilities, the more abstract levels of mathematics, such as algebra, geometry, and calculus, may remain mysteries forever; however, these students can still gain facility with basic mathematical facts used in daily life (Mercer & Pullen, 2004). Many schools teach students how and when to use calculators so that more complex problems can be simplified or homework checked for accuracy. In addition, computer-assisted instruction in mathematics may provide opportunities for practice and reinforcement.

Other Interventions

Training in Social Cognition The maintenance of self-esteem and the development of social cognition are very important in preventing adverse mental health outcomes in any child. Bandura's (2001) research on social-cognitive theory and self-efficacy has had its impact on general education, but relatively little research has been done on at-risk groups of students, which would include those with learning disabilities. Social and emotional competence is impacted by personal and interpersonal agency, and it influences the outcomes of well-being in these children (Martin, Cumming, O'Neil, & Strnadova, 2017).

Counseling Counseling may be required to treat underlying mental health issues in children with a learning disorder. This can be provided individually or in groups. Family-centered counseling also may be appropriate. Issues to be discussed may include homework, behavior management techniques, parental expectations, and the child's self-esteem. Families also should be provided a source of information about learning disorders, support groups, and their legal rights and responsibilities in the education of their child. In addition to support for families as they get help for their child with learning disorders, these families, especially parents, may need help in addressing their own feelings of grief or powerlessness in assisting their child toward independence in adulthood, higher education, and employment. Innovative therapeutic interventions include movement and dance therapy, art therapy, and music therapy (Unkovich, Butte, & Butler, 2017).

Medication Although learning disorders cannot be "cured" through the use of medication, certain associated impairments that affect learning, such as ADHD (see Chapter 19) and behavior and emotional disorders (see Chapter 27), can be improved with the use of psychoactive drugs. If such drugs are used, their effectiveness must be monitored carefully. Medication should never be a substitute for sound educational programming (see Chapter 38 for a detailed discussion of the role of medications in the treatment of developmental disabilities).

Homework The home and school should be able to function in partnership so that homework does not lead to tension among family members or misunderstanding of the teacher's intent in providing the home assignment. This may require assisting the parent in setting up a workable system and schedule at home. Students with learning disorders often feel that homework is an imposition, providing no personal fulfillment or advancement, so individualization and creative use of assignments is essential for homework to fulfill its reinforcing purpose. Homework should supplement material that was taught during the day (Alvermann & Phelps, 2005).

The improvements and availability of technology to support students in completing assignments have been shown to assist homework completion, especially at the middle and high school levels (King-Sears, Evmenova, & Johnson, 2017). Techniques to facilitate homework performance include the use of coaching models as well as traditional models of home completion. There does not seem to be one particular system of doing homework that emerges as most effective, but research does indicate that the student's perception of the usefulness of the assignment is important (Merriman, Codding, Tryon, & Minami, 2016). There are nonacademic effects of homework on student perceptions of well-being and behavior, particularly for students in high-achieving school settings (Galloway, Conner, & Pope, 2013). Homework should be limited to a specific time allotment. Since 2006, the National Education

Association has recommended 10–20 minutes per day for individuals in kindergarten through second grade and 30–60 minutes per day for individuals in Grades 3–6. Ideally, homework should be completed in a specific area of the home that is quiet, organized, and stocked with needed supplies. Children with learning disabilities may also not bring homework assignments home either to avoid doing them or because they lack the organizational skills to remember the assignment. Many tools are available to assist with this process, including day planners, checklists, iPads, or other technologies. Some schools post homework assignments on the Internet or through other electronic methods—these should assist families in knowing the schedule and content of assignments.

Periodic Reevaluations

The treatment programs for students with learning disabilities are complex, and many potential gaps exist. Furthermore, the child is continually developing, with needs and abilities that change from year to year. Therefore, ongoing monitoring of school progress is essential. The goal of periodic reassessments is to evaluate academic progress, psychosocial issues, and parent–child relationships. Reassessment is also an opportunity to convey new information to the family in an effort to obtain appropriate resources. Finally, it is a time for reassessing the child and revising the educational program. These reevaluations should occur ideally on a yearly basis so that planning for the next school year can occur. Parents and school providers need to be familiar with federal and state policy and regulation on the schedule of assessment and reassessment in order to properly serve the student with learning disabilities as they respond to varied interventions (Silberglitt, Parker, & Muyskens, 2016).

OUTCOME

Academic preparation and interventions have allowed more and more students with SLDs to pursue postsecondary education and to find success in the workplace.

Postsecondary Education

The National Center for Learning Disabilities notes that 68% of high school students with SLD exit with a diploma, compared to 12% who graduate with a certificate of attendance. Unfortunately, they also report that 19% of these students drop out of school before graduating (National Center for Learning Disabilities, 2017). Academic preparation of students with learning disorders is permitting more and more students to pursue postsecondary education. However, having an average of a 10th-grade reading level (Hughes & Smith, 1990; Mason & Mason, 2005) confounds the student with learning disabilities as they attempt the spectrum of academic challenges at the college level. These challenges include writing essays and research papers, completing long and complex reading assignments, taking timed tests, and learning foreign languages (Denckla, 1993; Duquette & Fullarton, 2009; Murray & Wren, 2003).

Some colleges offer adjustments to program loads and schedules, tutorial and other support services, and support technologies that have permitted students with learning disorders to complete college at an increasing rate (Jones, Long, & Finlay, 2007). Among the problems encountered by students with SLD as they enter college is the fact that only 25% identify their special needs to the college, therefore diluting the impact of accommodation or support that may be available. If such accommodations are not obtained early in the postsecondary experience, the risk of not graduating is greatly increased. The completion rate for students with SLD is 41%, compared with a completion rate of 52% for the general population (National Center for Learning Disabilities, 2017).

Employment

Career direction and preparation should be an objective of educational programming beginning in the primary grades. Such training for students with learning disabilities begins with realistic goal setting resulting from a comprehensive assessment of abilities and aptitudes. Without appropriately directed training, students may be unable to support themselves in an independent manner as adults. If career preparation and training services are delayed until adulthood, they are less likely to be effective. The design of these programs becomes part of the student's IEP (see Chapter 33).

A generation ago, the U.S. Department of Labor (1992) published competencies determined to be necessary for employment. This report by the Secretary's Commission on Achieving Necessary Skills (known as the SCANS Report) translated into curriculum areas that deemphasized specific job-related tasks in favor of teaching general competencies that cross all job markets.

Even as adults, some individuals with learning disorders have poor retention of verbal instructions and other problems that may interfere with effectiveness in their jobs. They also may be hesitant to ask questions and seek assistance. Social immaturity, clumsiness, and poor judgment may make social interactions more difficult. The skills taught in career education are those required to overcome these impairments and enhance success in the work environment, be it the classroom or the adult job market. Cooperation, respect, responsibility, teamwork, organization, and ways to seek information to solve one's problems are all part of career education (U.S. Department of Labor, 1992).

According to the National Center for Learning Disabilities report mentioned above, over 46% of students with learning disabilities hold jobs in competitive employment situations. This cannot be judged too critically, however, in light of national trends in employment that might be influenced by economic downturns that affect all potential workers leaving high school. The Bureau of Labor Statistics reports that in 2017 the unemployment rate was 4.8% nationally; however, the unemployment rate for those with a college degree was only 2.5%, while those without a college degree was over 7%. This figure is much increased for young adults with learning disabilities.

SUMMARY

- A specific learning disability is a developmental disorder in which a healthy child of average to above-average intelligence fails to learn adequately in one or more school subjects.
- The underlying cause of these disorders is aberrant brain function, such as impaired phonological decoding in specific reading disability. Neuroimaging, genetic, and neuropsychological studies are providing insight into how the brain guides learning.
- Early detection of learning disorders is important because, if untreated, the child may develop secondary emotional and behavior problems that hinder progress.
- If a learning disorder is suspected, a psychoeducational evaluation should be performed to identify areas of strengths and challenge. Then the education team can develop an individualized education program and appropriate changes in curriculum and supports can be made.
- No single treatment method is ideal for all individuals, so an empiric approach may be needed to find the most useful method. Studies also suggest that the amount of time spent in remediation/practice is very important.
- Career and vocational education should be included in the general educational curriculum and as an individualized transition plan within the IEP.
- Although the individual with SLD usually carries his or her learning impairment into adulthood, the outcome is often good.

ADDITIONAL RESOURCES

LD Online: http://www.ldonline.org

Learning Disabilities Association of America (LDA): http://www.ldanatl.org

National Center for Learning Disabilities (NCLD): http://www.ld.org

Additional resources can be found online in Appendix D: Childhood Disabilities Resources, Services, and Organizations (see About the Online Companion Materials).

REFERENCES

Aaron, P. G., Joshi, R. M., Gooden, R., & Bentum, K. E. (2008). Diagnosis and treatment of reading disabilities based on the Component Model of Reading: An alternative to the discrepancy model of LD. *Journal of Learning Disabilities, 41,* 67–84. doi:10.1177/0022219407310838

Abbott, R., Raskind, W., Matsushita, M., Richards, T., Price, N., & Berninger, V. (2017). Dysgraphia, dyslexia, and OWL LD during middle childhood and early adolescence: Evidence for genetic effects on hallmark phenotypes. *Biomarkers and Genes, 1*(1), 1–10. doi:10.15761/BG.1000103

Alexander, A. W., & Slinger-Constant, A. M. (2004). Current status of treatments for dyslexia: Critical review. *Journal of Child Neurology, 19,* 744–758.

Alvermann, D. E., & Phelps, S. F. (2005). *Content reading and literacy: Succeeding in today's diverse classrooms* (4th ed.). Boston, MA: Allyn & Bacon.

American Psychiatric Association. (2013). *Diagnostic and statistical manual of mental disorders* (5th ed.). Washington, DC: Author.

Andersson, U., & Lyxell, R. (2007). Working memory, deficit in children with mathematical difficulties: A general or specific deficit? *Journal of Experimental Child Psychology, 96,* 197–228. doi:10.1016/j.jecp.2006.10.001

Bain, A., Baillet, L. L., & Moats, L. C. (2001). *Written language disorders: Theory in to practice* (2nd ed.). Austin, TX: PRO-ED.

Bakker, D., Van Strien, J. W., Licht, R., & Smit-Glaude, S. W. D. (2007). Cognitive brain potentials in kindergarten children with subtyped risks of reading retardation. *Annals of Dyslexia, 57*(1), 99–111. doi:10.1007/s11881-007-0005-y

Bandura, A. (2001). Social cognitive theory: An agentic perspective. *Annual Review of Psychology, 52*(1), 1–26.

Barrera, M. (2006). Roles of definitional and assessment models in the identification of new or second language learners of English for special education. *Journal of Learning Disabilities, 39,* 142–156. doi:10.1177/00222194060390020301

Barrio, B. (2015). Fueling disproportionality of culturally and linguistically diverse students in special education: Implications for teacher preparation programs. *Journal of Mestizo and Indigenous Voices, 1*, 1–9.

Barrio, B. (2017). Special education policy change: Addressing the disproportionality of English language learners in special education programs in rural communities. *Rural Special Education Quarterly, (36)*2, 64–72. doi.org/10.1177/8756870517707217

Bauminger, N., Edelsztein, H. S., & Morash, J. (2005). Social information processing and emotional understanding in children with LD. *Journal of Learning Disabilities, 38*, 45–61. doi:10.1177/00222194050380010401

Bauminger, N., & Kimhi-Kind, I. (2008). Social information processing, security of attachment, and emotion regulation in children with learning disabilities. *Journal of Learning Disabilities, 41*, 315–332. doi:10.1177/0022219408316095

Bear, D. R., & Templeton, S. (1998). Explorations in developmental spelling: Foundations for learning and teaching phonics, spelling and vocabulary. *The Reading Teacher, 52*, 222–242.

Berkeley, S., Bender, W. N., Peaster, L. G., & Saunders, L. (2009). Implementation of response to intervention—A snapshot of progress. *Journal of Learning Disabilities, 42*, 85–95. doi:10.1177/0022219408326214

Berninger, V. (2007a). *Process Assessment of the Learner, 2nd Edition. Diagnostic for Reading and Writing (PAL-II RW) administration and scoring manual.* San Antonio, TX: The Psychological Corporation. Now Pearson.

Berninger, V. (2007b). *Process Assessment of the Learner Diagnostic for Math (PAL II-M) administrtion and scoring manual.* San Antonio, TX: Psychological Corporation. Now Pearson.

Berninger, V. W. (2015). *Interdisciplinary frameworks for schools: Best professional practices for serving the needs of all students.* Washington, DC: American Psychological Association, http://dx.doi.org/10.1037/14437-002.

Berninger, V. W., Abbott, R., & Cook, C. R. (2017). Relationships of attention and executive functions to oral language, reading, and writing skills and systems in middle childhood and early adolescence. *Journal of Learning Disabilities, 50*(4), 434–449. doi:10.1177/0022219415617167

Berninger, V., & Dunn, M. (2012). Brain and behavioral response to intervention for specific reading, writing, and math disabilities: What works for whom? In B. Wong & D. Butler (Eds.), *Learning about LD* (4th ed., pp. 59–89). Cambridge, MA: Elsevier/Academic Press.

Berninger, V., & Richards, T. (2010). Inter-relationships among behavioral markers, genes, brain, and treatment in dyslexia and dysgraphia. *Future Neurology, 5*, 597–617. doi:10.2217/fnl.10.22

Berninger, V., & Swanson, H. L. (2017). Role of working memory in the language learning mechanism by ear, mouth, eye, and hand in individuals with and without specific learning disabilities in written language. In T. P. Alloway (Ed.), *Working memory and neurodevelopmental disorders.* Abingdon, United Kingdom: Taylor & Francis Routledge.

Berninger, V. W., & Wolf, B. J. (2016). *Teaching students with dyslexia, dysgraphia, OWL LD, and dyscalculia: Lessons from science and teaching* (2nd ed.). Baltimore, MD: Paul H. Brookes Publishing Co.

Berninger, V. W., & Wolf, B. J. (2009). *Teaching students with dyslexia and dysgraphia: Lessons from teaching and science.* Baltimore, MD: Paul H. Brookes Publishing Co.

Birsh, J. R. (Ed.). (2011). *Multisensory teaching of basic language skills* (3rd ed.). Baltimore, MD: Paul H. Brookes Publishing Co.

Blanchett, W. J., Klingner, J. K., & Harry, B. (2009). The intersection of race, culture, language and disability: Implications for urban education. *Urban Education 44*(4), 389–409. doi:10.1177/0042085909338686

Bloom, E., & Heath, N. (2010). Recognition, expression, and understanding facial expressions of emotion in adolescents with nonverbal and general learning disabilities. *Journal of Learning Disabilities, 43*, 180–192. doi:10.1177/0022219409345014

Bureau of Labor Statistics, U.S. Department of Labor. (2017). Unemployment rate 2.5 percent for college grads, 7.7 percent for high school dropouts, January 2017. Retrieved from https://www.bls.gov/opub/ted/2017/unemployment-rate-2-point-5-percent-for-college-grads-7-point-7-percent-for-high-school-dropouts-january-2017.htm

Burns, M., Jimerson, S., VanDerHeyden, A., & Deno, S. (2016). Toward a unified response-to-intervention model: Multi-tiered systems of support. In S. Jimerson, M. Burns, & A. VanDerHeyden (Eds.), *Handbook of response to intervention* (pp. 719–732). Boston, MA: Springer.

Carney, J., & Porter P. (2009). School reentry for children with acquired central nervous systems injuries. *Developmental Disabilities Research Reviews, 15*(2), 152–158. doi:10.1002/ddrr.57

Cassiday, L. (2009). *Mapping the epigenome. New tools chart. Chemical modifications of DNA and its packaging proteins.* Retrieved from http://www.cen-online.org

Chou, Y., Wehmeyer, M. L., Palmer, S. B., & Lee, J. (2017). Comparisons of self-determination among students with autism, intellectual disability and learning disabilities: A multivariate analysis. *Focus on Autism and Other Developmental Disabilities, 32, 124-132.*

Cirino, P. T., Israelian, M. K., Morris, M. K., & Morris, R. D. (2005). Evaluation of the double-deficit hypothesis in college students referred for learning difficulties. *Journal of Learning Disabilities, 38*, 29–44. doi:10.1177/00222194050380010301

Clark, D. B., & Uhry, J. K. (1995). *Dyslexia: Theory and practice of remedial instruction* (2nd ed.). Timonium, MD: York Press.

Clay, R. A. (2011). Revising the DSM. *Monitor on Psychology, 42*(1), 54.

Cohen, L., Kadosh, R., & Walsh, V. (2007). Dyscalculia. *Current Biology, 17*(22), R946–R947. doi:10.1016/j.cub.2007.08.038

Colligan, R., & Katusic, S. (2015). Overview of epidemiological studies of incidence of learning disabilities with annotated research references from the Mayo Clinic. Rochester, MN. In V. W. Berninger, *Interdiscipinary frameworks for schools: Best professional practices for serving the needs of all students.* Washington, DC: American Psychological Association.

Christodoulou, J. A., Cyr, A., Murtagh, J., Chang, P., Lin, J., Guarino, A. J., . . . Gabrieli, J. D. (2017). Impact of intensive summer reading intervention for children with reading disabilities in early elementary school. *Journal of Learning Disabilities, 50*, 115–127. doi.org/10.1177/0022219415617163

D'Anguilli, A., & Siegel, L. S. (2003). Cognitive functioning as measured by the WISC-R: Do children with learning disabilities have distinctive patterns of performance? *Journal of Learning Disabilities, 36*, 48–58. doi:10.1177/002221940303600 10601.

Dehaene, S., & Cohen, L. (1995). Toward an anatomical and functional model of number processing. *Math Cognition, 1*, 83–120.

Denckla, M. B. (1993). The child with developmental disabilities grown up: Adult residua of childhood disorders. *Neurology Clinics, 11,* 105–125.

Deshler, D. D., Mellard, D. F., Tollefson, J. M., & Byrd, S. E. (2005). Research topics in Responsiveness to intervention: Introduction to the special series. *Journal of Learning Disabilities, 38,* 483–484. doi:10.1177/00222194050380060101

Desoete, A., Roeyers, H., & Buysse, A. (2001). Metacognition and mathematical problem solving in grade 3. *Journal of Learning Disabilities, 34,* 435–449. doi:10.1177/002221940103400505

Dirks, E., Spyer, G., van Lieshout, E. C. D. M., & de Sonneville, L. (2008). Prevalence of combined reading and arithmetic disabilities. *Journal of Learning Disabilities, 41,* 460–473.

Driver, M. K., & Powell, S. R. (2017). Culturally and linguistically responsive schema intervention: Improving word problem solving for English language learners with mathematics difficulty. *Learning Disability Quarterly, 40,* 41–53. doi.org/10.1177/0731948716646730

Donlan, C. (2007). Mathematical development in children with specific language impairments. In D. B. Berch & M. M. M. Mazzocco (Eds.), *Why is math so hard for some children? The nature and origins of mathematical learning difficulties and disabilities* (pp. 151–172). Baltimore, MD: Paul H. Brookes Publishing Co.

DuPaul, G. J., Gormley, M. J., & Laracy, S. D. (2013). Comorbidity of LD and ADHD: Implications of DSM-5 for assessment and treatment. *Journal of Learning Disabilities, 46*(1), 43–51. doi:10.1177/0022219412464351

Duquette, C., & Fullarton, S. (2009). "With an LD you're always mediocre and expect to be mediocre": Perceptions of adults recently diagnosed with learning disabilities. *Exceptionality Education International, 19*(1), 55–71.

Eden, G. F., Jones, K. M., Cappell, K., Gareau, L., Wood, F. B., Zeffiro, T. A., & Flowers, D. L. (2004). Neuronal changes following remediation in adult developmental dyslexia. *Neuron, 44,* 411–422.

Elementary and Secondary Education Act of 1965, PL 89-10, 20 U.S.C. §§ 241 *et seq.*

Eller, M., Fisher, E., Gilchrist, A., Rozman, A., & Shockney, S. (2015). Is inclusion the only option for students with learning disabilities and emotional behavioral disorders? *An Undergraduate Journal in Special Education and Law, 5,* 79–86.

Englert, C. S. (1992). Writing instruction from a sociocultural perspective: The holistic, dialogic, and social enterprise of writing. *Journal of Learning Disabilities, 25,* 153–172. doi:10.1177/002221949202500303

Every Student Succeeds Act of 2015, PL 114-95, S.1177, 114th Cong. (2015). Retrieved from http://edworkforce.house.gov/uploadedfiles/every_student_succeeds_act_-_conference_report.pdf

Fisher, S. E., & DeFries, J. C. (2002). Developmental dyslexia: Genetic dissection of a complex cognitive trait. *Nature Reviews Neuroscience, 3,* 767–780. doi:10.1038/nrn936

Fletcher, J. M., Lyon, G. R., Fuchs, L. S., & Barnes, M. A. (2007). *Learning disabilities: From identification to intervention.* New York, NY: Guilford Press.

Francis, D. J., Fletcher, J. M., Stuebing, K. K., Lyon, G. R., Shaywitz, B. A., & Shaywitz, S. E. (2005). Psychometric approaches to the identification of LD: IQ and achievement scores are not sufficient. *Journal of Learning Disabilities, 38,* 98–108. doi:10.1177/00222194050380020101

Friedman, L. M., Rapport, M. D., Orban, S. A., Eckrich, S. J., & Calub, C. A. (2017). Applied problem-solving in children with ADHD: The mediating roles of working memory and mathematical calculation. *Journal of Abnormal Child Psychology, 46,* 491–504. Advance online publication. doi:10.1007/s10802-017-0312-7

Friedman, L. M., Rapport, M. D., Raiker, J. S., Orban, S. A., & Eckrich, S.J. (2017). Reading comprehension in boys with ADHD: The mediating roles of working memory and orthographic conversion. *Journal of Abnormal Child Psychology, 45,* 273–287. doi:10.1007/s10802-016-0171-7

Fuchs, L. S., & Fuchs, D. (2002). Mathematical problem-solving profiles of students with mathematical disabilities with and without comorbid reading difficulties. *Journal of Learning Disabilities, 35,* 563–573.

Fuchs, L. S., Fuchs, D., Compton, D. L., Wehby, J., Schumacher, R. F., Gersten, R., & Jordan, N. C. (2015). Inclusion versus specialized intervention for very low-performing students: What does access mean in an era of academic challenge? *Exceptional Children, 81,* 134–157. doi:10.1177/0014402914551743

Fuchs, D., Fuchs, L. S., & Vaughn, S. (2014). What is intensive instruction and why is it important? *Teaching Exceptional Children, 46,* 13–18. doi:10.1177/0040059914522966

Fuchs, L. S., & Vaughn, S. (2012). Responsiveness-to-intervention: A decade later. *Journal of Learning Disabilities, 45,* 195–203. doi:10:1177/0022219412442150

Fuchs, D., Mock, D., Morgan, P. L., & Young, C. L. (2003). Responsiveness-to-intervention: Definitions, evidence, and implications for the learning disabilities construct. *Learning Disabilities Research and Practice, 18,* 157–171. doi:10.1111/1540-5826.00072

Gabrieli, J. D. (2009). Dyslexia: A new synergy between education and cognitive neuroscience. *Science, 325*(5938), 280–283. doi:10.1126/science.1171999

Galloway, M., Conner, J., & Pope, D. (2013). Non-academic effects of homework in privileged, high-performing high schools. *The Journal of Experimental Education, 81*(4), 490–510. doi:10.1080/00220973.2012.745469

Geary, D. C. (2004). Mathematics and learning disabilities. *Journal of Learning Disabilities, 37,* 4–15.

Geary, D. C., & Hoard, M. K. (2005). Learning disabilities in arithmetic and mathematics: Theoretical and empirical perspectives. In J. I. D. Campbell (Ed.), *Handbook of mathematical cognition* (pp. 253–267). New York, NY: Psychology Press.

Gersten, R., Jordan, N. C., & Flojo, J. R. (2005). Early identification and interventions for students with mathematics difficulties. *Journal of Learning Disabilities, 38,* 293–304. doi:10.1177/00222194050380040301

Gillingham, A., & Stillman, B. W. (1997). *The Gillingham manual: Remedial training for children with specific disabilities in reading, spelling, and penmanship* (8th ed.). Cambridge, MA: Educators Publishing Service.

Gortmaker. V. J., Daly, E. J., McCurdy, M., Persampieri, M. J., & Hergenrader, M. (2007). Improving reading outcomes for children with learning disabilities using brief experimental analysis to develop parent-tutoring interventions. *Journal of Applied Behavior Analysis, 40,* 203–221. doi:10.1901/jaba.2007.105-05

Graham, S., Collins, A. A., & Rigby-Wills, H. (2017). Writing characteristics of students with learning disabilities and typically achieving peers: A meta-analysis. *Exceptional Children, 83,* 199–218. doi:10.1177/0014402916664070

Graham, S., & Harris, K. R. (1989). Components analysis of cognitive strategy instruction: Effects on learning disabled students' compositions and self-efficacy. *Journal of Educational Psychology, 81*(3) 353–361. doi:10.1037//0022-0663.81.3.353

Gregg, N., & Scott, S. S. (2000). Definition and documentation: Theory, measurement, and the courts. *Journal of Learning Disabilities, 33,* 5–13. doi:10.1177/002221940003300104

Grigorenko, E. L. (2009). Dynamic assessment and response to intervention: Two sides of one coin. *Journal of Learning Disabilities, 42,* 111–132. doi:10.1177/0022219408326207

Hagberg, I., Billstedt, E., Nyden, A., & Gillberg, C. (2015). Asperger syndrome and nonverbal learning difficulties in adult males: Self- and parent-reported autism, attention and executive problems. *European Child and Adolescent Psychiatry, 24*(8), 969–977.

Harris, K. R., & Pressley, M. (1991). The nature of cognitive strategy instruction: Interactive strategy construction. *Exceptional Children, 57,* 392–404.

Hay, I., Elias, G., Fielding-Barnseley, R., Homel, R., & Freibery, K. (2007). Language delays, reading delays, and learning difficulties: Interactive elements requiring multidimensional programming. *Journal of Learning Disabilities, 40*(5), 400–409.

Henry, L. A., Messer, D., Luger-Klein, S., & Crane, L. (2012). Phonological, visual, and semantic coding strategies and children's short-term picture memory span. *Quarterly Journal of Experimental Psychology, 65,* 2033–2053. doi:10.1080/17470218.2012.672997.

Hughes, C. A., & Dexter, D. D. (2011). Response to intervention: A research-based summary. *Theory Into Practice, 50*(1), 4–11. doi:10.1080/00405841.2011.534909

Hughes, C. A., & Smith, J. O. (1990). Cognitive and academic performance of college students with learning disabilities: A synthesis of the literature. *Learning Disabilities Quarterly, 13,* 66–79. doi:10.2307/1510393

Individuals with Disabilities Education Act Amendments (IDEA) of 1997, PL 105-17, 20 U.S.C. §§ 1400 *et seq.*

Individuals with Disabilities Education Improvement Act (IDEA) of 2004, PL 108-446, 20 U.S.C. §§ 1400 *et seq.*

International Reading Association & National Association for the Education of Young Children. (1998). Learning to read and write: Developmentally appropriate practices for young children. *Young Children, 53,* 30–46.

Jimmerson, S. R., Burns, M. K., & VanDerHeyden, A. M. (Eds.). (2015). *Handbook of response to intervention: The science and practice of multi-tiered systems of support.* Springer: NY. doi:10.1007/978-1-4899-7568-3

Johnson, D. J., & Myklebust, H. (1967). *Learning disabilities: Education principles and practice.* Austin, TX: PRO ED.

Jones, F. W., Long, K., & Finlay, W. M. L. (2007). Symbols can improve the reading comprehension of adults with learning disabilities. *Journal of Intellectual Disability Research, 51*(7), 545–550. doi:10.1111/j.1365-2788.2006.00926.x

Jordan, N. C. (2007). Do words count? Connections between mathematics and reading difficulties. In D. B. Berch & M. M. Mazzocco (Eds.), *Why is math so hard for some children? The nature and origins of mathematical learning difficulties and disabilities.* (pp. 107–120). Baltimore, MD: Paul H. Brookes Publishing Co.

Jordan, N. C., Hanich, L. B., & Kaplan, D. (2003). A longitudinal study of mathematical competencies in children with specific mathematics difficulties versus children with comorbid mathematics and reading difficulties. *Child Development, 74,* 834–850. doi:10.1111/1467-8624.00571

Jozwik, S. L. & Douglas, K. H. (2017). Effects of a technology-assisted reading comprehension strategy intervention for English learners with learning disabilities. *Reading Comprehension and Technology, 56,* 42–63.

Kamhi, A. G., & Catts, H. W. (2012). *Perspectives on assessing and improving reading comprehension.* Boston, MA: Allyn & Bacon.

Kamil, M. L., Pearson, P. D., Moje, E. B., & Afflerbach, P. (Eds.). (2010). *Handbook of reading research* (Vol. 4). New York, NY: Routledge.

Katusic, S.K., Colligan, R.C., Weaver, A.L., & Barbaresi, W.J. (2009). The forgotten learning disability—Epidemiology of written language disorder in a population-based birth cohort (1978-1982), Rochester, Minnesota. *Pediatrics, 123,* 1306-1313. Doi 10-1542/peds.2008-2098.

Kavale, K. A. & Spaulding, L. S. (2008). Is response to intervention good policy for specific learning disability? *Learning Disabilities Research & Practice, 23,* 169–179. doi:10.1111/j.1540-5826.2008.00274.x

Keeler, M. K., & Swanson, H. L. (2001). Does strategy knowledge influence working memory in children with math disabilities? *Journal of Learning Disabilities, 34,* 418–434.

Kennedy, M. J., & Deshler, D. D. (2010). Literacy instruction, technology, and students with learning disabilities: Research we have, research we need. *Learning Disabilities Quarterly, 33*(4), 289–298.

Kim, K., & Helphienstine, D. T. (2017). The perils of multilingual students: "I'm not LD, I'm L2 or L3." *Journal of International Students, 7,* 421–428.

King-Sears, M. E. (2014). Introduction to *Learning Disability Quarterly* special series on Universal Design for Learning, part one of two. *Learning Disability Quarterly, 37,* 68–70. doi:10.1177/0731948714528337

King-Sears, M. E., Evmenova, A. S., & Johnson, T. M. (2017). Using technology for accessible chemistry homework for high school students with and without learning disabilities. *Learning Disabilities Research & Practice, 32*(2), 121–131. doi:10.1111/ldrp.12129

Kirk, S. A., & Kirj, W. D. (1971). *Psycholinguistic learning disabilities: Diagnosis and remediation.* Urbana: University of Illinois Press.

Landa, K. G., & Barbetta, P. M. (2017). The effects of repeated readings on the reading performances of Hispanic English language learners with specific learning disabilities. *Journal of International Special Needs Education, 20*(1), 1–13.

Lembke, E., & Foegen, A. (2009). Identifying early numeracy indicators for kindergarten and first grade students. *Learning Disabilities Research and Practice, 24,* 12–20. doi:10.1111/j.1540-5826.2008.01273.

Liu, K. K., Ward, J. M., Thurlow, M. L., & Christensen, L. L. (2017). Large-scale assessment and English language learners with disabilities. *Educational Policy (31)5,* 551–583. doi:10.1177/0895904815613443

Liu, Y., Ortiz, A. A., Wilkinson, C. Y., Robertson, P., & Kushner, M. I. (2008). From early childhood special education to special education resource rooms: Identification, assessment, and eligibility determinations for English language learners with reading-related disabilities. *Assessment for Effective Intervention, 33,* 177–187. doi:10.1177/1534508407313247

Liu, X., Marchis, L., De Biase, E., Breaux, K. C., Courville, T., Pan, X., . . . Kaufman, A. S. (2016). Do cognitive patterns of strengths and weaknesses differentially predict errors on reading, writing, and spelling? *Journal of Psychoeducational Assessment, 35,* 186–205. Doi.org/10.1177/0734282916668996

Lyon, G. R., Shaywitz, S. E., & Shaywitz, B. A. (2003). A definition of dyslexia. *Annals of Dyslexia, 53,* 1–14. doi:10.1007/s11881-003-0001-9

Maag, J. W., & Reid, R. (2006). Depression among students with learning disabilities: Assessing the risk. *Journal of Learning Disabilities, 39,* 3–10. doi:10.1177/00222194060390010201

Mabbott, D. J., & Bisanz, J. (2008). Computational skills, working memory, and conceptual knowledge in older children with mathematics learning disabilities. *Journal of Learning Disabilities, 41,* 15–28. doi:10.1177/0022219407311003

MacArthur, C. A. (2009). Reflections on research on writing and technology for struggling writers. *Learning Disabilities Research & Practice. 24*(2), 93–103. doi:10.1111/j.1540-5826.2009.00283.x

Mann, V. (1994). Phonological skills and the prediction of early reading problems. In N.C. Jordan & J. Goldsmith-Phillips (Eds.), *Learning disabilities: New directions for assessment and intervention* (pp. 67–84). Needham Heights, MA: Allyn & Bacon.

Manor, O., Shalev, R., Joseph, A., & Gross-Tsur, V. (2001). Arithmetic skills in kindergarten children with developmental language disorders. *European Pediatric Neurology Society, 5,* 71–77. doi:10.1053/ejpn.2001.0468

Marshall, R. M., Schafer, V. A., O'Donnell, L., Elliott, J., & Handwerk, M. L. (1999). Arithmetic disabilities and ADHD subtypes: Implications for DSM-IV. *Journal of Learning Disabilities, 32,* 239–247.

Martin, A. J., Cumming, T. M., O'Neill, S. C., & Strnadová, I. (2017) Social and emotional competence and at-risk children's well-being: The roles of personal and interpersonal agency for children with ADHD, emotional and behavioral disorder, learning disability, and developmental disability. In E. Frydenberg, A. Martin, & R. Collie (Eds.), *Social and emotional learning in Australia and the Asia-Pacific.* Singapore: Springer.

Mason, L. H., & Graham, S. (2008). Writing instruction for adolescents with learning disabilities: Programs of intervention research. *Learning Disabilities Research and Practice, 23,* 103–112. doi:10.1111/j.1540-5826.2008.00268.x

Mason, A., & Mason, M. (2005). Understanding college students with learning disabilities. *Pediatric Clinics of North America, 52,* 61–70. doi:10.1016/j.pcl.2004.11.001

Mazzocco, M. M. M. (2001). Math learning disability and math LD subtypes: Evidence from studies of Turner syndrome, fragile X syndrome, and Neurofibromatosis type 1. *Journal of Learning Disabilities, 34,* 520–533. doi:10.1177/002221940103400605

Mazzocco, M. M. M. (2007). Defining and differentiating mathematical learning disabilities and difficulties. In D. B. Berch & M. M. M. Mazzocco (Eds.), *Why is math so hard for some children?* (pp. 29–48). Baltimore, MD: Paul H. Brookes Publishing Co.

Mazzocco, M. M. M., Feigenson, L., & Halberda, J. (2011). Impaired acuity of the approximate number system underlies mathematical learning disability (dyscalculia). *Child Development, 82,* 1224–1237. doi:10.1111/j.1467-8624.2011.01608.x

McInerney, M., & Elledge, A. (2013). *Using a response to intervention framework to improve student learning: A pocket guide for state and district leaders.* Washington, DC: American Institutes for Research.

McLean, J. F., & Hitch, G. J. (1999). Working memory impairments in children with specific arithmetic learning difficulties. *Journal of Experimental Child Psychology, 74*(3), 240–260. doi:10.1006/jecp.1999.2516

McDonogh, E. M., Fanagan, D. P., Sy, M., & Alfonso, V. C. (2017). Specific learning disorder. In S. Goldstein & M. DeVries (Eds.), *Handbook of DSM-5 disorders in children and adolescents* (pp. 77–104). Boston, MA: Springer.

McIntyre, N. S., Solari, E. J., Grimm, R. P., Lerro, L. E., Gonzales, J. E., & Mundy, P. C. (2017). A comprehensive examination of reading heterogeneity in students with high functioning autism: Distinct reading profiles and their relation to autism symptom severity. *Journal of Autism and Developmental Disorders, 47,* 1086–1101.

McNamara, J., Vervaeke, S. L., & Willoughby, T. (2008). Learning disabilities and risk-taking behavior in adolescents: A comparison of those with and without comorbid attention-deficit/hyperactivity disorder. *Journal of Learning Disabilities, 41,* 561–574. doi:10.1177/0022219408326096

Menon, V. (2016). Working memory in children's math learning and its disruption in dyscalculia. *Current Opinion in Behavioral Sciences, 10,* 125–132.

Mercer, C. D., & Pullen, P. C. (2004). *Students with learning disabilities* (6th ed.). Upper Saddle River, NJ: Merrill.

Merriman, D., Codding, R. S., Tryon, G. S., & Minami, T. (2016). The effects of group coaching on the homework problems experienced by secondary students with and without disabilities. *Psychology in the Schools, 53,* 457–470. doi:10.1002/pits.21918

Moshe, A. (2017). Inclusion assistants in general education settings: A model for in-service training. *Universal Journal of Educational Research, 5,* 209–216. doi:10.13189/ujer.2017.050206.

More, C. M., Spies, T. G., Morgan, J. J., & Baker, J. N. (2017). Incorporating English language learner instruction within special education teacher preparation. *Intervention in School and Clinic, 51*(4), 229–237.

Moss, B., Lapp, D., & O'Shea, M. (2011). Tiered texts: Supporting knowledge and language learning for English learners and struggling readers. *English Journal, 100,* 54–60.

Murray, C., & Wren, C. T. (2003). Cognitive, academic, and attitudinal predictors of the grade point averages of college students. *Journal of Learning Disabilities, 36,* 407–415. doi:10.1177/00222194030360050201

National Center for Educational Statistics. (2017). *The condition of education.* Retrieved from https://nces.ed.gov/pubsearch/pubsinfo.asp?pubid=2017144

National Center for Learning Disabilities. (2017). *State of LD.* Retrieved from http://www.ncld.org/social-emotional-and-behavioral-challenges

National Institute of Child Health and Human Development. (2000). *Report of the National Reading Panel: Teaching children to read. An evidence-based assessment of the scientific research literature on reading and its implications for reading instruction.* Retrieved from http://nationalreadingpanel.org/publications.htm

Nicolson, R. I., & Fawcett, A. J. (2011). Dyslexia, dysgraphia, procedural learning and the cerebellum. *Cortex, 47*(1), 117–121. doi:10.1016/j.cortex.2009.08.016

Nielsen, K., Haberman, K., Todd, R., Abbott, R., Mickail, T., & Berninger, V. (in press). Emotional and behavioral correlates of persisting specific learning disabilities in written language (SLDs-WL) during middle childhood and early adolescence. *Journal of Psychoeducational Assessment.* NIHMSID 852098

No Child Left Behind Act of 2001, PL 107-110, 115 Stat. 1425, 20 U.S.C. §§ 6301 *et seq.*

Olitsky, S. E., & Nelson, L. B. (2003). Reading disorders in children. *Pediatric Clinics of North America, 50,* 213–224. doi:10.1016/S0031-3955(02)00104-9

Olson, R., Huslander, J., Christopher, M., Keenan, J. M., Wadsworth, S., Willicutt, E., . . . DeFries, J. (2013). Genetic and environmental influences on writing and their relations to language and reading. *Annals of Dyslexia, 63,* 25–43.

Olson, R., Wise, B., Connors, F., Rack, J., & Fulker, D. (1989). Specific deficits in component reading and language skills: Genetic and environmental influences. *Journal of Learning Disabilities, 22,* 339–348.

Paneque, O. M., & Barbetta, P. M. (2006). A study of teacher efficacy of special education teachers of English language learners with disabilities. *Bilingual Research Journal, 30,* 171–193. doi:10.1080/15235882.2006.10162871

Peng, P., & Fuchs, D. (2016). A meta-analysis of working memory deficits in children with learning difficulties: Is there a difference between verbal domain and numerical domain? *Journal of Learning Disabilities, 49*(1), 3–20.

Pennington, B. F. (1991). Genetics of learning disabilities. *Seminars in Neurology, 11,* 28–34. doi:10.1055/s-2008-1041202

Phipps, L., & Beaujean, A. A. (2016). Review of the patterns of strengths and weaknesses approach in specific learning disabilities. *Research and Practice in the Schools, 4,* 18–28.

Powell, S. R., Fuchs, L. S., Fuchs, D., Cirino, P. T., & Fletcher, J. M. (2009). Do word-problem features differentially affect problem difficulty as a function of students' mathematics difficulty with without reading difficulty? *Journal of Learning Disabilities, 42,* 99–110. doi:10.1177/0022219408326211

Prunty, M., & Barnett, A. L. (2017). Understanding handwriting difficulties: A comparison of children with and without motor impairment. *Journal of Cognitive Neuropsychology, 34,* 205–218. doi:10.1080/02643294.2017.1376630

Pullen, P. C., Tuckwiller, E. D., Konod, T. R., Maynard, K., & Coyne, M. D. (2010). A tiered intervention model for early vocabulary instruction: The effects of tiered instruction for young students at risk for learning disabilities. *Learning Disabilities Research & Practice, 25*(3), 110–123.

Puranic, C. S., Wagner, R. K., Kim, Y., & Lopez, D. (2012). Multivarate assessment of processes in elementary students' written translation. In M. Fayol, D. Alamargot, & V. W. Berninger (Eds.), *Translation of thought to written text while composing: Advancing theory, knowledge research methods, tools, and applications.* New York, NY: Psychology Press.

Raghubar, K., Cirino, P., Barnes, M., Ewing-Cobbs, L., Fletcher, J., & Fuchs, L. (2009). Errors in multi-digit arithmetic and behavioral inattention in children with math difficulties. *Journal of Learning Disabilities, 42,* 356–371.

Ramaswami, R. (2010). Reshaping RTI: Building a better triangle. *T.H.E. Journal, 37*(8), 34–35.

Raskind, W. H., Peter, B., Richards, T., Eckert, M. M., & Berninger, V. W. (2012). The genetics of reading disabilities: From phenotypes to candidate genes. *Frontiers in Psychology, 3,* 601. doi:10.3389/fpsyg.2012.00601

Reid, B. (2005). *Cognitive strategy instruction.* University of Nebraska. Retrieved from http//www.unl.edu/csi/TeachingStrategy.shtml

Reschly, D. J. (2008). Learning disabilities identification: Primary intervention, secondary intervention, and then what? *Journal of Learning Disabilities, 38,* 510–515. doi:10.1177/00222194050380060601

Ritchey, K. D., & Goeke, J. L. (2006). Orton-Gillingham and Orton-Gillingham based reading instruction: A review of the literature. *The Journal of Special Education, 40*(3), 171–183. doi:10.1177/00224669060400030501

Romeo, R. R., Christodoulou, J. A., Halverson, K. K., Murtagh, J., Cyr, A. B., Schimmel, C., . . . Gabrieli, J. D. E. (2017). Socioeconomic status and reading disability: Neuroanatomy and plasticity in response to intervention. *Cerebral Cortex,* 1–16. doi:10.1093/cercor/bhx131

Rourke, B. P., & Finlayson, M. A. J. (1978). Neuropsychological significance of variations in patterns of academic performance: Verbal and visual-spatial abilities. *Journal of Abnormal Child Psychology, 6,* 121–133. doi:10.1007/BF00915788

Roux, F., Dufor, O., Giussani, C., Waman, Y., Draper, L., Longcamp, M., & Demonet, J. (2009). The graphemic/motor frontal area Exner's area revisited. *Annals of Neurology, 66*(4), 537–545. doi:10.1002/ana.21804

Samuelsson, S., Byrne, B., Olson, R., Huslander, J., Wadsworth, S., Corley, R., . . . DeFries, J. C. (2008). Response to early literacy instruction in the United States, Australia, and Scandinavia: A behavioral-genetic analysis. *Learning and Individual Differences, 18,* 289–295.

Sandak, R., Mencl, W. E., Frost, S. J., & Pugh, K. R. (2004). The neurobiological basis of skilled and impaired reading: Recent findings and new directions. *Scientific Studies of Reading, 8,* 273–292. doi:10.1207/s1532799xssr0803_6

Scerri, T. S., & Schulte-Körne, G. (2010). Genetics of developmental dyslexia. *European Child & Adolescent Psychiatry, 19*(3), 179–197. doi:10.1007/s00787-009-0081-0

Schatschneider, C., & Torgesen, J. (2004). Using our current understanding of dyslexia to support early identification and intervention. *Journal of Child Neurology, 19,* 759–765.

Schuchardt, K., Maehler, C., & Hasselhorn, M. (2008). Working memory deficits in children with specific learning disorders. *Journal of Learning Disabilities, 41,* 514–523. doi:10.1177/0022219408317856

Schneider, W. (2008). The development of metacognitive knowledge in children and adolescents: Major trends and implications for education. *Mind, Brain, and Education, 2*(3), 114–121. doi:10.1111/j.1751-228X.2008.00041.x

Sexson, S. B., & Madan-Swain, A. (1993). School reentry for the child with chronic illness. *Journal of Learning Disabilities, 26,* 115–137. doi:10.1177/002221949302600204

Shalev, R. S. (2004). Developmental dyscalculia. *Journal of Child Neurology, 19,* 765–771.

Shalev, R. S., & Gross-Tsur, V. (2001). Developmental dyscalculia. *Pediatric Neurology, 24,* 337–342.

Shalev, R. S., Manor, O., & Gross-Tsur, V. (2005). Developmental dyscalculia: A prospective six-year study. *Developmental Medicine and Child Neurology, 47,* 121–125.

Shaywitz, B. A., Shaywitz, S. E., Blachman, B. A., Pugh, K. R., Fulbright, R. K., Skudlarski, P., . . . Gore, J. C. (2004). Development of left occipitotemporal systems for skilled reading in children after a phonologically based intervention. *Biological Psychiatry, 55,* 926–933. doi:10.1016/j.biopsych.2003.12.019

Shaywitz, S. E. (2005). *Overcoming dyslexia: A new and complete science-based program for reading problems at any level.* New York, NY: Vintage. doi:10.1056/NEJM199201163260301

Shaywitz, S. E., & Shaywitz, B. A. (2005). Dyslexia (specific reading disability). *Biological Psychiatry, 57,* 1301–1309. doi:10.1016/j.biopsych.2005.01.043

Silberglitt, B., Parker, D., & Muyskens, P. (2016) Assessment: Periodic assessment to monitor progress. In S. Jimerson, M. Burns, & A. VanDerHeyden (Eds.), *Handbook of response to intervention* (pp. 271–292). Boston, MA: Springer.

Silliman, E. R., & Berninger, V. W. (2014). Crossdisciplinary dialogue about the nature of oral and written language problems in the context of developmental, academic, and phenotypic profiles. *Topics in Language Disorders, 31,* 6–23.

Simos, P. G., Fletcher, J. M., Foorman, B. R., Francis, D. J., Castillo, E. M., Davis, R. N., . . . Papanicolaou, A. C. (2002). Brain activation profiles during the early stages of reading acquisition. *Journal of Child Neurology, 17,* 159–163. doi:10.1177/088307380201700301

Stevens, E. A., Walker, M. A., & Vaughn, S. (2016). The effects of reading fluency interventions on the reading fluency and reading comprehension performance of elementary students with learning disabilities: A synthesis of the research from 2001 to 2014. *Journal of Learning Disabilities, 50,* 576–590. doi:10.1177/0022219416638028

Talcott, J. B., Witton, C., McLean, M. F., Hansen, P. C., Rees, A., Green, G. G. R., & Stein, J. F. (2000). From the cover: Dynamic sensory sensitivity and children's word decoding skills. *Proceedings of the National Academy of Sciences of the United States of America, 97,* 2952–2957. doi:10.1073/pnas.040546597

Tanimoto, S., Thompson, R., Berninger, V., Nagy, W., & Abbott, R. (2015). Computerized writing and reading instruction for students in grades 4 to 9 with specific learning disabilities affecting written language. *Journal of Computer Assisted Learning, 31,* 671–689. PMC:4743045

Taylor, W. P., Miciak, J., Fletcher, J. M., & Francis, D. J. (2017). Cognitive discrepancy models for specific learning disabilities identification: Simulations of psychometric limitations. *Psychological Assessment, 29*(4), 446–457. doi:10.1037/pas0000356

Torgesen, J. K. (2004) Lessons learned from research on intervention for students who have difficulty learning to read. In P. McCardle & V. Chhabra (Eds), *The voice of evidence in reading research* (pp. 355–382). Baltimore, MD: Paul H. Brookes Publishing Co.

Turkeltaub, P. E., Gareau, L., Flowers D. L., Zeffiro, T. A., & Eden, G. F. (2003). Development of neural mechanisms for reading. *Nature Neuroscience, 6,* 767–773. doi:10.1038/nn1065

Unkovich, G., Butte, C., & Butler, J (Eds.). (2017). *Dance movement psychotherapy with people with learning disabilities.* New York, NY: Routlege.

U.S. Department of Education, National Center for Education Statistics. (2008). *Table 390—Current postsecondary education and employment status, wages earned, and living arrangements of special education students out of secondary school up to 4 years, by type of disability*: 2005. Retrieved from http://nces.ed.gov/progams/digest/d08/tables/dt08_390.asp

U.S. Department of Education, National Center for Education Statistics. (2008). *The condition of education.* Retrieved from https://nces.ed.gov/programs/coe/indicator_cgg.asp

U.S. Department of Education, Office of Special Education Programs. (2016). *38th Annual Report to Congress on the Implementation of the Individuals with Disabilities Education Act.* Washington, DC: Author. Retrieved from http://www.ed.gov/about/reports/annual/osep

U.S. Department of Labor. (1992). *Learning a living: A blueprint for high performance. A SCANS report for AMERICA 2000.* Washington, DC: Secretary's Commission on Achieving Necessary Skills; U.S. Government Printing Office.

Van Garderen, D. (2007). Teaching students with LD to use diagrams to solve mathematical word problems. *Journal of Learning Disabilities, 40*(6), 540–556. doi:10.1177/00222194070400060501

Vaughn, S., & Fuchs, L. S. (2003). Redefining learning disabilities as inadequate response to instruction: The promise and potential problems. *Learning Disabilities Research & Practice, 18,* 137–146. doi:10.1111/1540-5826.00070

Vellutino, F. R., Fletcher, J. M., Snowling, M. J., & Scanlon, D. M. (2004). Specific reading disability (dyslexia): What have we learned in the past four decades? *Journal of Child Psychology and Psychiatry, 45,* 2–40. doi:10.1046/j.0021-9630.2003.00305.x

Vukovic, R. K., & Siegel, L. S. (2006). The double-deficit hypothesis: A comprehensive analysis of the evidence. *Journal of Learning Disabilities, 39,* 25–47. doi:10.1177/00222194060390010401

Waber, D. P., Forbes, P. W., Wolff, P. H., & Weiler, M. D. (2004). Neurodevelopmental characteristics of children with learning impairments classified according to the double-deficit hypothesis. *Journal of Learning Disabilities 37*(5), 451–461. doi:10.1177/00222194040370050

Walker, V. L., Douglas, K. H., & Chung, Y. (2017). An evaluation of paraprofessionals' skills and training needs in supporting students with severe disabilities. *International Journal of Special Education, 32,* 460–471.

Wandell, B. A., & Le, B. A. (2017). Diagnosing the neural circuitry in reading. *Neuron, 96,* 298–311. doi:10.1016/j.neuron.2017.08.007

Wechsler, D. (2003). *Wechsler Intelligence Scale for Children–Fourth Edition (WISC-IV).* San Antonio, TX: Pearson.

Williams, D. L., Goldstein, G., Kojkowski, N., & Minshew, N. J. (2008). Do individuals with higher functioning autism have the IQ profile associated with nonverbal learning disabilities? *Research in Autism Spectrum Disorders, 2*(2), 353–361.

Williams, R. B., Bryant-Mallory, D., Coleman, K., Gotel, D., & Hall, C. (2017). An evidence-based approach to reducing disproportionality in special education and discipline referrals. *Children and Schools, 39*(4), 248–251. doi:10.1093/cf/cdx020

Wolf, M., & Bowers, P. G. (1999). The double-deficit hypothesis for the developmental dyslexias. *Journal of Educational Psychology, 91,* 415–438. doi:10.1037//0022-0663.91.3.415

Wolf, M., Bowers, P., & Biddle, K. (2000). Naming-speed processes, timing, and reading: A conceptual review. *Journal of Learning Disabilities, 33,* 387–407. doi:10.1177/002221940003300409

CHAPTER 21 Cerebral Palsy

Tara L. Johnson, Eric M. Chin, and Alexander H. Hoon, Jr.

Upon completion of this chapter, the reader will

- Understand the definition and causes of cerebral palsy
- Understand how cerebral palsy is diagnosed
- Know the clinical characteristics of the various forms of cerebral palsy
- Know the motor, sensory, cognitive, and medical problems commonly associated with cerebral palsy
- Understand the range of management options available to help children with cerebral palsy reach their full potential
- Be knowledgeable about the medical and functional prognoses for people with cerebral palsy

Many children with cerebral palsy (CP) first come to professional attention because of delays in early motor milestones, particularly rolling, crawling, standing and walking, or signs of early handedness. Most parents know that children begin walking at approximately 1 year of age, and there is an implicit understanding that a child's first steps mark the transition from infancy to toddlerhood. When a young child does not reach this transition at the expected time, alarm bells sound.

CASE STUDY

Jamal is a 15-month-old boy who was seen by his pediatrician for a routine well-child checkup. His mother expressed her worry that Jamal was not yet walking. His pediatrician had previously documented mild delays in motor development at the 12-month office visit. This was attributed to the fact that he was born at 28 weeks' gestation, with a birth weight of 900 grams, following spontaneous labor that was associated with maternal **chorioamnionitis** (an infection of the membranes surrounding the fetus). In the neonatal intensive care unit (NICU), he required ventilatory support for 5 days. At 2 weeks of age, a cranial ultrasound study suggested an abnormality of brain white matter (see Chapter 5).

At his 12-month well-child checkup, his mother noted that Jamal had been sitting for about 2 months. His pediatrician explained that based on age adjustment for prematurity (9 months corrected age), he was only mildly delayed compared with chronological age expectations. Jamal's leg muscles were a little stiff, but his pediatrician knew that many premature infants have mild, temporary abnormalities of muscle tone that often resolve by 15–18 months of age.

On examination at 15 months, Jamal could crawl stiffly on all fours but was not yet pulling up to a standing position. He demonstrated a pronounced tendency to keep his legs stiffly extended with his toes pointed and his feet crossed at the ankles (scissoring). At this point, his pediatrician expressed her concern that Jamal was showing signs of CP.

Thought Questions:

If an infant is suspected of having CP, what are the most important initial steps that should be undertaken regarding medical testing and interventions? What types of accommodations should be considered in the school environment for a child with CP? How does this relate to type of CP and degree of motor impairment?

WHAT IS CEREBRAL PALSY?

CP describes a group of chronic childhood motor impairment disorders defined by specific functional characteristics rather than by the underlying cause. It was first described by William Little, an orthopedic surgeon who treated a child with spastic diplegia, a type of CP (Accardo, 1989). In 2006, CP was defined by an international consensus panel as follows:

> Cerebral palsy describes a group of permanent disorders of the development of movement and posture causing activity limitation that are attributed to nonprogressive disturbances that occurred in the developing fetal or infant brain. The motor disorders of cerebral palsy are often accompanied by disturbances of sensation, perception, cognition, communication, and behavior, by epilepsy, and by secondary musculoskeletal problems. (Rosenbaum et al., 2007, p. 9)

The hallmarks of CP are limitations in mobility and hand use with associated neuromotor abnormalities on physical exam. CP is characterized by impaired control of movement and posture that becomes evident early in life (Jacobsson et al., 2008). There is variability in overall motor function, often with associated impairments in sensation, cognition, communication, oromotor/gastrointestinal dysfunction, bowel/bladder function, and behavior. There may be visual impairment and epilepsy (Bax et al., 2005).

The clinical features of CP are the result of developmental disturbances that occur during early brain development, leading to brain malformation or injury. These disorders most often occur during fetal development or in the perinatal period, but they may also arise during the first years of life. Prematurity, low birth weight, multiple-gestation pregnancy, infection/inflammation, hypoxia-ischemia, and a variety of genetic factors can act in concert, with the end result being CP (Pakula, Van Naarden Braun, & Yeargin-Allsopp, 2009).

Although CP is considered a static ("nonprogressive") disorder, its functional manifestations can "progress" in several different ways. For example, children with early hypotonia (low muscle tone) associated with hypoxic-ischemic encephalopathy (HIE; previously referred to as "birth asphyxia") may develop spasticity or dystonia years later (Scott & Jankovic, 1996). This may be the result of maladaptive plasticity (Johnston, 2009), wherein brain rewiring is misdirected or faulty. As another example, adults with dyskinetic forms of CP (see the Subtypes of Cerebral Palsy section) are prone to developing secondary spinal cord compression from long-term abnormal repetitive head and cervical spine movements. This leads to progressive weakness and loss of function (see Figure 21.1). Finally, there may be progressive orthopedic deformities secondary to spasticity, chronic muscle shortening, and joint dislocations, resulting in loss of motor function.

WHAT CAUSES CEREBRAL PALSY?

The underlying causes and risk factors leading to the development of CP disrupt the development of neuronal networks in the many brain pathways (cortical and subcortical) that control movement. Cortical regions of the brain include the frontal, temporal, parietal, and occipital lobes. Subcortical regions of the brain include the basal ganglia, thalamus, internal capsule, brain stem, and cerebellum (see Chapter 8).

A key concept in understanding the causes of CP is **selective vulnerability** (Johnston, 1998). This term refers to a susceptibility of specific regions and cells to injury during critical time periods in brain development. For example, the brain is structurally formed by approximately 12 weeks, and problems that occur during this time often lead to brain malformations such as holoprosencephaly, absence of the corpus callosum, and lissencephaly (see Chapter 6). From 24–34 weeks' gestation, immature **oligodendrocytes** (brain cells that wrap myelin, a protective lipid-rich covering around axons) are susceptible to injury. Children who are born prematurely typically have spastic forms of CP, characterized by white matter injury around the ventricles, commonly termed periventricular leukomalacia (PVL), which is linked to oligodendrocyte injury.

This is in contrast with full-term infants, where the vulnerability lies in neurons in the basal ganglia and thalamus. A common cause of brain injury in the full-term neonate is perinatal HIE, which is defined as a disruption of blood flow (ischemia) and oxygen supply (hypoxia) to the brain at the time of birth (MacLennan, Nelson, Hankins, & Speer, 2010). Another cause

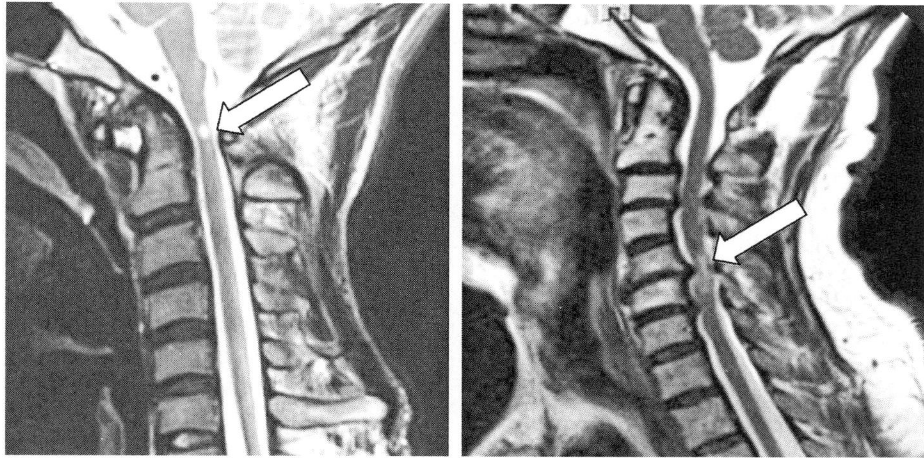

Figure 21.1. The white arrows point to areas of injury in the cervical spinal cord of two adults with dyskinetic (extrapyramidal) cerebral palsy (CP) as a result of cord compression from the chronic stress placed on the cervical spine (C-spine) from repetitive movement. These findings require emergent spinal fusion to stabilize the neck and to prevent the development of acute paralysis. Adults with CP and new neurological findings should have a brain magnetic resonance imaging (MRI) and C-spine MRI.

of brain injury in the neonate is kernicterus, which results from markedly elevated bilirubin levels after birth.

In term infants with HIE or kernicterus, the injury to neurons in these deep gray matter structures is often linked with dyskinetic (dystonic) forms of CP (see Figure 21.2). The recognition of selective vulnerability has led to new treatment approaches in the NICU setting, including the use of hypothermia (lowering body temperature) to ameliorate brain injury in term infants with HIE (Barks, 2008), as well as medications including xenon, erythropoietin, melatonin, and stem cell therapy (Douglas-Escobar & Weiss, 2015).

A common misconception is that most cases of CP result from HIE. It is now clear that birth asphyxia is the cause of CP in only 2%–10% of affected children (Eunson, 2012). This new observation confirms Freud's observation:

> Difficult birth and premature birth are not always accidental happenings, but may frequently be results of a deeper cause, or its expressions, without being the actual etiological factor. Thus it may well be possible that the same pathogenic factors that rendered intrauterine environment abnormal also extended their influence to parturition; abnormal birth is then the final result of abnormal pregnancy. (Freud, 1897)

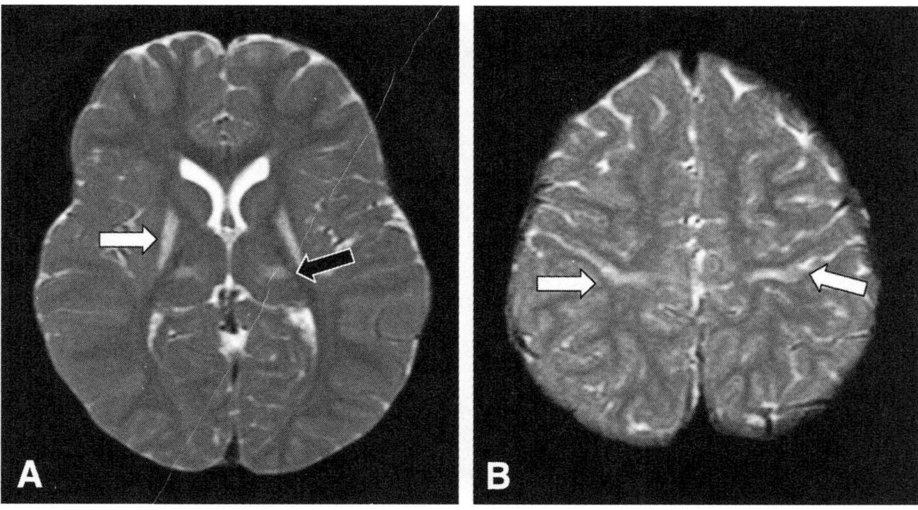

Figure 21.2. The selective vulnerability of specific regions in the brain in infants born at term with asphyxia. A) The white arrow points to injury in the putamen; the black arrow points to injury in the thalamus. B) The white arrows point to injury in the motor cortex. This pattern of injury often leads to dyskinetic (dystonic) cerebral palsy (CP), with limitations in speech and hand use.

A key concept in effectively treating children with CP is the recognition that understanding the underlying cause can serve as a foundation to improve overall management. Understanding the mechanism of injury and the resultant clinical phenotype leads to the recognition of commonly correlated patterns on neurologic examination. For example, prematurity predisposes an infant to PVL, which can result in spastic diplegia, whereas a full-term infant with CP may have basal ganglia involvement, which can result in dyskinetic (athetoid or dystonic) CP.

Approaching diagnosis with an appreciation that neurologic examination findings typically correspond with clinical history enables the identification of other motor disorders that do not fit such patterns. These include rare, but often treatable, genetic disorders such as dopa-responsive dystonia, which can be improved with levodopa (Mink, 2003); mitochondrial disorders (Koene & Smeitink, 2009), some of which can be treated with specially tailored vitamin preparations; and organic acidemias (Seashore, 2009), which may be treatable with special metabolic formulas (see Chapter 16).

Etiology refers to the underlying cause for a disorder, such as CP secondary to brain injury associated with preterm birth. Etiologic diagnosis is also of benefit in establishing both prognosis and recurrence risk of CP or other motor disorders that mimic CP. This knowledge can provide information to families as they contemplate future pregnancies (Hemminki, Li, Sundquist, & Sundquist, 2007). The discovery of genetic etiologies is also emerging, and it may provide insight regarding inherited risk factors for CP (Moreno-De-Luca, Ledbetter, & Martin, 2012).

EPIDEMIOLOGY

In the developed world, CP affects about 2 in 1,000 children (Christenson et al., 2014; Himmelmann, Hagberg, & Uvebrant, 2010). CP is most commonly associated with prematurity and low birth weight. Approximately 50,000 infants who are very low birth weight (less than 1,500 grams) are born in the United States each year, of whom 10%–15% develop spastic CP and 20%–50% develop disorders of higher cortical function, including ADHD, learning disabilities, and intellectual disability (Volpe, 2005). The incidence of CP also increases with decreasing gestation and may occur in up to 28% of infants born before 26 weeks' gestation (Eunson, 2012).

Despite advances in perinatal management over the last 20–30 years, the incidence of CP in term infants has not changed. This is consistent with the understanding that CP in full-term infants most commonly results from prenatal insults or genetic conditions that are independent of, or may operate in conjunction with, factors associated with delivery (Fahey, Maclennan, Kretzschmar, Gecz, & Kruer, 2017).

In developing countries, accurate epidemiological estimates have been difficult to obtain, but overall prevalence appears to be similar to that in developed countries. Small uncontrolled hospital-based studies suggest an increased proportion attributed to perinatal and postneonatal etiologies (e.g., meningitis, kernicterus, trauma, and hypoxic injury) and a decreased proportion associated with prematurity and low birth weight. Accordingly, a greater proportion of quadriplegia has been reported (Colver, Fairhurst, & Pharoah, 2014; Gladstone, 2010).

RISK FACTORS

Infection

Both indirect infections (passed from the mother) and direct infections (of the fetus or newborn infant) have been shown to be associated with CP (Bale, 2009). In term and preterm infants, direct infection of the fetus by viruses such as cytomegalovirus and rubella (Lombardi, Garofoli, & Stronati, 2010) and other infectious agents (e.g., toxoplasmosis, a parasitic infection) has long been a recognized cause of CP. More recently, microcephaly and CP have also been associated with Zika virus (Pessoa et al., 2018). Bacterial meningitis in the newborn also remains a significant cause of CP (Galiza & Heath, 2009).

There is increasing recognition that chorioamnionitis plays a key role in the development of CP in preterm infants (Shatrov et al., 2010). Chorioamnionitis predisposes to premature delivery and may also have direct adverse effects on the fetal brain (Jacobsson, 2004; Yoon, Park, & Chaiworapongsa, 2003). Complex relationships exist among chorioamnionitis, fetal **cytokines** (proteins that regulate the immune response), and other inflammatory factors that, depending on timing, can predispose toward brain injury or can trigger a protective response. The former can lead to cortical or white matter injury in children born preterm (Hagberg et al., 2015).

In the term infant, there is an association among maternal infection, fever, and CP (Nelson & Chang, 2008). Infection during pregnancy may also promote blood hypercoagulation, leading to stroke-like events in the fetus (Leviton & Dammann, 2004; Nelson & Lynch, 2004). Finally, placental abnormalities may contribute to the development of HIE, perinatal stroke, low Apgar scores, and term stillbirth (McIntyre et al., 2015; Wu, 2002).

Prematurity-Related Cerebral Palsy

Premature infants, especially those born prior to 28–32 weeks' gestation or with a birth weight less than 1,500 grams, represent almost half of all individuals with CP (Eunson, 2012). The increased risk of CP in premature infants is related to complex interrelations between destructive and developmental mechanisms (Volpe, 2009).

In premature infants, the two most common types of injury are PVL (see Figure 21.3) and periventricular-intraventricular hemorrhage (PIVH; see Chapter 5). Immaturity of brain development predisposes premature infants to both of these conditions.

In the late 1970s to early 1980s, cranial ultrasound and computed tomography linked CP with brain hemorrhage. In the later 1980s to early 1990s, the advent of magnetic resonance imaging (MRI) vividly confirmed that the major injury was in cerebral white matter. Since the late 2000s, more-detailed MRI studies have shown that the white matter injury is accompanied by diffuse, variable injury in cortical, subcortical, and cerebellar gray matter (Kusters, Chen, Follett, & Dammann, 2009; Reid et al., 2015).

Volpe (2005) demonstrated that the abnormalities in neurons and axons are the result of changes in the normal developmental trajectory of brain development, often initiated by hypoxic-ischemic or infectious/inflammatory cascades of injury. These disturbances may explain the complex patterns of motor, learning, intellectual, and neurobehavioral impairments encountered in affected children.

Finally, in children such as Jamal, there is evidence—using the advanced MRI imaging technique of diffusion tensor imaging (DTI; see Chapter 8), which shows white matter tracts—that functional impairment may result from injury to both sensory and motor cortical pathways (Hoon et al., 2009; Nagae et al., 2007; see Figure 21.4).

Cerebral Palsy in Full-Term Infants

A wide variety of prenatal, perinatal, and genetic factors are linked with CP in full-term infants. These include HIE, congenital brain malformations, coagulation abnormalities, complications related to multiple-gestation pregnancies, and intrauterine infection/inflammation (Jacobsson et al., 2008; Nelson, 2008). Compared with those born prematurely, full-term infants who subsequently develop CP are more likely to be small for gestational age or have malformations inside and outside of the central nervous system (CNS), suggesting problems in early brain development (Krägeloh-Mann et al., 1995).

In full-term infants with severe HIE, who often develop dyskinetic CP, the injury is often in the basal ganglia located deep in the center of the brain (Himmelmann et al., 2009). In the past, high bilirubin levels in the immediate postnatal period resulted in kernicterus, which led to choreoathetoid CP and to hearing impairment. Although kernicterus is rare now in developed countries, more subtle bilirubin-induced neurologic dysfunction continues to be a concern (Shapiro, 2005).

DIAGNOSIS

CP is diagnosed clinically; it is suspected by the presence of delays in motor development and confirmed by distinct abnormalities on neurological examination. Although newborns may have known risk factors for CP (e.g., PVL or HIE), CP cannot be diagnosed at

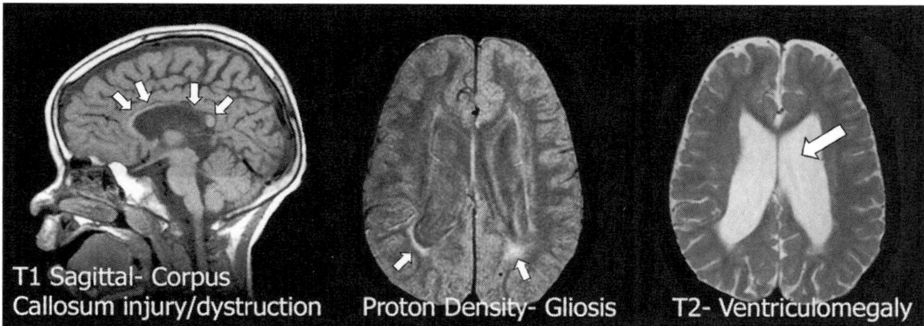

Figure 21.3. This MRI was taken in childhood from a child with periventricular leukomalacia who had spastic quadriplegia. The arrows point to areas of injury or destruction of brain white matter (wiring). The enlarged ventricles (ventriculomegaly) are secondary to loss of surrounding brain tissue. (Adapted with permission from Wolters Kluwer: *Journal of Developmental and Behavioral Pediatrics*. Hoon, A.H., & Melhem, E.R. Neuroimaging: Applications in disorders of early brain development. 21, 291–302. [2000])

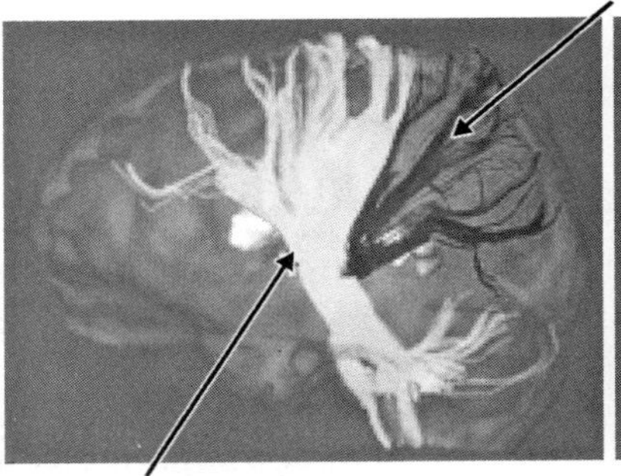

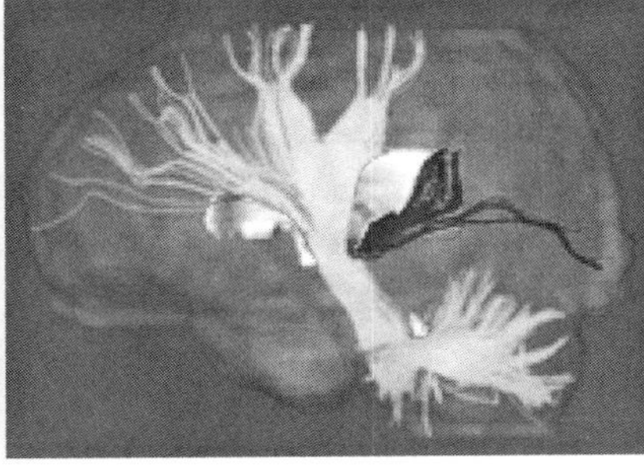
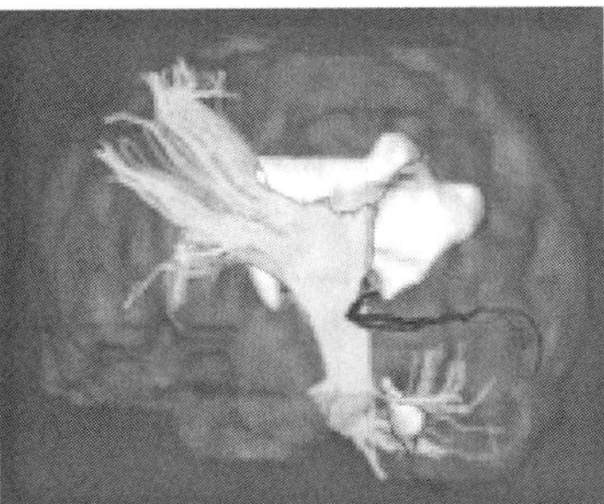

Figure 21.4. Using diffusion tensor imaging (DTI) and tract reconstruction software, three-dimensional images of descending motor pathways (light gray fibers) and thalamocortical sensory tracts (black fibers) are shown in a typically developing child (left panel) and in two children with spastic cerebral palsy in association with periventricular leukomalacia (PVL) (middle and right panels). In the children with PVL, the primary injury is seen as a decrease in black fibers, which transmit sensory information from the thalamus to the cortex. (Adapted with permission from Nagae, L.M., Hoon, Jr., A.H., Stashinko, E., Lin, D., Zhang, W., Levey, E., . . . Mori, S. [2007]. Diffusion tensor imaging in children with periventricular leukomalacia: Variability of injuries to white matter tracts. *AJNR: American Journal of Neuroradiology*, 28[7], pp. 1213–1222.)

birth because the characteristic diagnostic signs are not apparent this early. Using traditional neurological physical exam findings, children with severe forms of CP are usually diagnosed in the first year of life, while those with less severe forms are usually diagnosed during the second year (Aneja, 2004; Palmer, 2004; Russman & Ashwal, 2004).

Early detection of CP is becoming increasingly widespread, with emerging evaluation tools such as Prechtl's General Movement Assessment (General Movements Trust, 2009), which has been shown to be predictive of future motor dysfunction and comorbidities in neonates and infants (Einspieler, Bos, Libertus, & Marschik, 2016; Einspieler & Prechtl, 2005; General Movements Trust, 2009). General movements are a means to evaluate the integrity of the immature nervous system, and they are thought to result from central pattern generators. Such movements include writhing movements, which occur from early fetal life to 6–9 weeks post term, and fidgety movements, which occur from 3–5 months post term. In general, variability of movements is a favorable prognostic sign. Ideally, early detection of CP would promote the institution of intervention at a younger age, and the child would receive increased benefit from the provision of such therapies.

One of the key features of CP is the persistence of primitive reflexes. All infants are born with primitive reflexes. They are called "primitive" because they are present in early life (in some cases, during intrauterine development) and are thought to be controlled by the spinal cord, labyrinths of the inner ear, and the brain stem (the primitive areas of the CNS). Familiar examples of primitive reflexes include the suckling reflex and the hand-grasp reflex in the newborn. As the cortex matures, these reflexes are gradually suppressed and integrated into voluntary movement patterns (see Figure 21.5). The process of integration is usually complete by 12 months of age. In CP, however, these primitive reflex patterns tend to persist beyond early infancy. Among the primitive reflexes, the **asymmetric tonic neck reflex** (Figure 21.6) and the **tonic labyrinthine response** (Figure 21.7) are particularly helpful in the diagnosis of CP.

As primitive reflexes disappear in the typically developing child, **postural reactions** (also known as

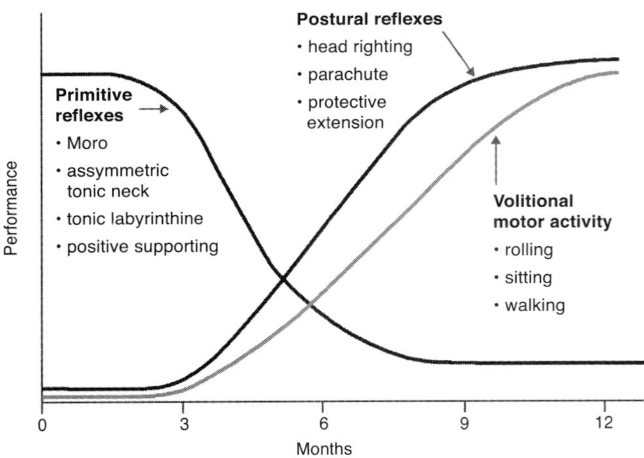

Figure 21.5. The time course of primitive reflexes, postural reflexes, and volitional motor activity in typical motor development. (From Capute, A. J., Accardo, P. J., Vining, E. P. G., Rubenstein, J. E., & Harryman S. [1978]. *Primitive reflex profile*. Baltimore, MD: University Park Press; reprinted by permission.)

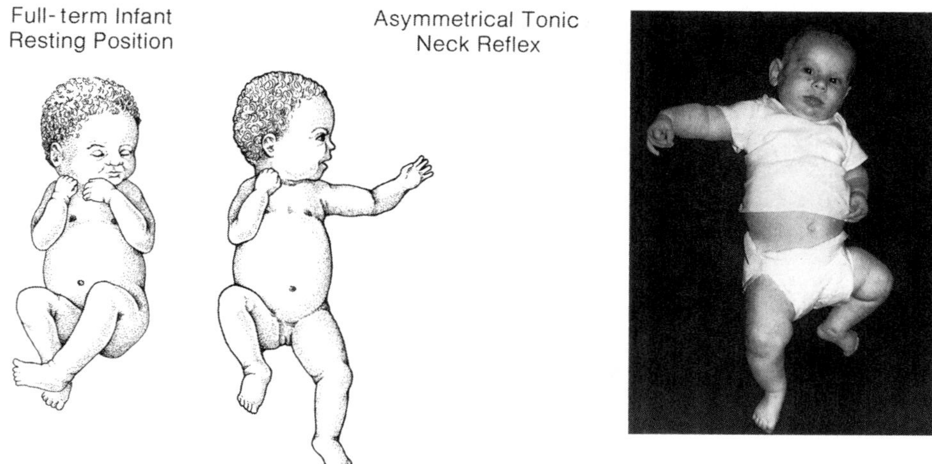

Figure 21.6. The asymmetric tonic neck reflex. In the typical newborn infant, when the head is actively or passively turned to the side, the arm and leg on the same side will extend and the arm and leg on the opposite side will flex, resulting in a "fencing" posture. The opposite pattern occurs when the head is turned to the other side. In typically developing infants, the reflex fades (is integrated) by about 6 months of age and is never obligatory (the infant can break through the pattern with spontaneous movement, even in the newborn period). In children with cerebral palsy, the reflex tends to be more pronounced, persists beyond the expected age, and may be obligatory.

automatic movement reactions) emerge (Figure 21.8). Some of the more important of these reactions are the righting, equilibrium, and protective reactions, which enable the child to develop more complex voluntary movement and better control of posture. The emergence of postural reactions along with the simultaneous disappearance of primitive reflexes are essential precursors for the development of specific motor milestones, such as rolling over and sitting.

In typically developing children, a protective reaction called the parachute response develops by 10–12 months of age. This reaction is manifested by forward extension of the arms when falling forward. Many children with CP have delayed or absent development of postural reactions, including this response, which makes sitting or walking difficult. CP may be viewed as the persistence of primitive reflexes combined with the lack of cortical maturation of postural reactions.

The neurological examination of the motor system is an important tool to characterize an individual's type of CP. Neurological exam findings can be divided into two categories: those that can be seen and those that can be felt (see Figure 21.9). For example, one can observe dystonia, or twisting postures, simply by watching the patient. However, to appreciate spasticity, one must lay hands on the patient and assess the effects of joint motion on resistance to movement (Sanger, Delgado, Gaebler-Spira, Hallett, & Mink, 2003).

Upper Motor Neuron Dysfunction in Cerebral Palsy

The motor impairments in children with CP are secondary to injury in the upper motor neuron (UMN). The UMN system is not a discrete anatomical entity but

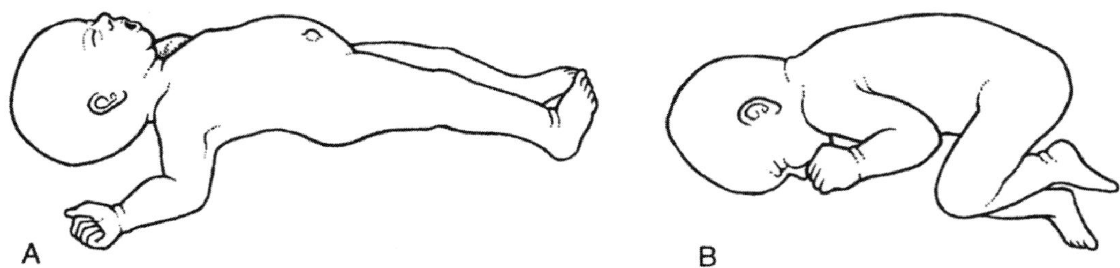

Figure 21.7. The tonic labyrinthine reflex. A) When the child is in the supine position with the head slightly extended, retraction of the shoulders and extension of the legs is observed. B) The opposite occurs when the infant is in the prone position with the head slightly flexed. In typically developing infants, the reflex pattern is barely evident in the newborn period; in children with cerebral palsy, the pattern may dominate posture and movement and may persist throughout life.

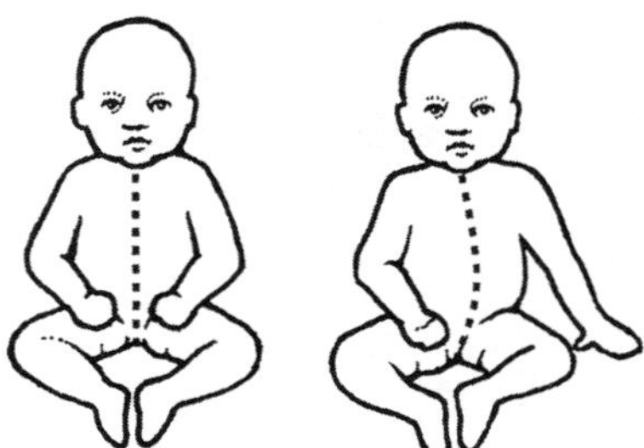

Figure 21.8. Automatic movement responses: the lateral prop reaction. At about 6 months of age, typically developing infants have already developed good postural control of the head and trunk (righting or equilibrium responses) and can stop themselves from falling forward when placed in the sitting position by extending their arms in front of them (forward prop response). By 6 months of age, most infants can also catch themselves when falling to the side by extending the arm on the same side (lateral prop response). This automatic movement reaction is critical for independent sitting and may be delayed or absent in children with cerebral palsy. (From Pellegrino, L., & Dormans, J. P. [1998]. Making the diagnosis of cerebral palsy. In J. P. Dormans & L. Pellegrino [Eds.], *Caring for children with cerebral palsy: A team approach* [p. 39; portion of Figure 2.4]. Baltimore, MD: Paul H. Brookes Publishing Co., Inc.; reprinted by permission.)

refers collectively to the motor control systems based in the brain and spinal cord. The UMN system is distinguished from the lower motor neuron (LMN) system, which refers collectively to the peripheral nerves and the innervated muscles (Figure 21.10; see Chapter 8). The primary components of the UMN system are the **pyramidal tract** (also called the **corticospinal pathways**) and the extrapyramidal system (see Figure 21.11). These systems are differentially affected by disturbances to the developing brain.

UMN dysfunction is characterized by positive and negative signs. Positive signs include spasticity, **hyperreflexia** (increased deep tendon reflexes; e.g., the knee jerk), **clonus** (alternate involuntary muscular contraction and relaxation in rapid succession), **upper limb flexor and lower limb extensor spasms** (spasms of bending of a limb toward or away from the body), and a positive **Babinski sign** (upgoing toe when the sole of the foot is stroked firmly). Negative signs include muscle weakness, loss of manual dexterity, and fatigability. The profile of positive signs tends to vary more from child to child, and this contributes to the classification of the subtypes of CP. It is the negative signs, however, that more directly impede motor function (Sanger et al., 2006).

Seen (Observed)	Felt (Palpated)
Dystonia: twisting postures *Chorea:* dance-like movements *Athetosis:* slow, writhing movements *Ataxia:* gait, titubations (bobbing head movements)	*Spasticity:* velocity-dependent resistance *Rigidity:* co-contraction *Hypotonia:* decreased tone *Muscle consistency:* atrophy in myopathy

Figure 21.9. Elements of the neuromotor examination. The neuromotor examination can be categorized by those findings that can be simply observed and those findings that require palpation. Assessment of movement quality can be characterized by size and speed of movement. Tone is defined as resistance to passive stretch. In spasticity, tone increases as a function of increasing velocity. At high velocities, a clasp-knife phenomenon occurs, with a "catch" that can be felt by the examiner. Rigidity is defined as a lead pipe feel and occurs secondary to co-contraction of opposing muscle groups.

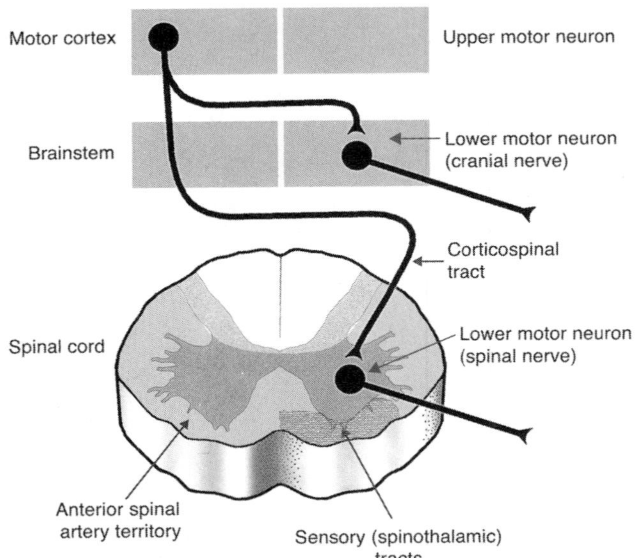

Figure 21.10. The location of upper and lower motor neurons. Low motor neuron dysfunction is associated with peripheral neuropathies. (From Shrestha, S. [2010]. Lesions of upper motor neurons and lower motor neurons. *Medchrome Online Medical Magazine*. Retrieved from http://medchrome.com/basic-science/anatomy/lesions-of-upper-motor-neurons-and-lower-motor-neurons; reprinted by permission.)

Walking

When a child is diagnosed with CP, one of the first questions parents pose is, "Will he or she walk?" In addressing this question, it is important to recognize that "walking" can refer to several levels of ability. A child may be able to walk independently or may need crutches or a walker. A child may be able to walk long distances (community ambulation), short distances only (household ambulation), or solely in the context of therapy (exercise ambulation). In general, children with better motor skills at a younger age (e.g., being able to sit and pull-to-stand before 2 years of age) have a better prognosis for walking than those with less well-developed skills.

Jamal, who we met in the case study at the beginning of this chapter, was sitting independently at 10 months of age, and there was concern that he was not yet walking by 15 months of age. A number of functional assessment systems have been developed to

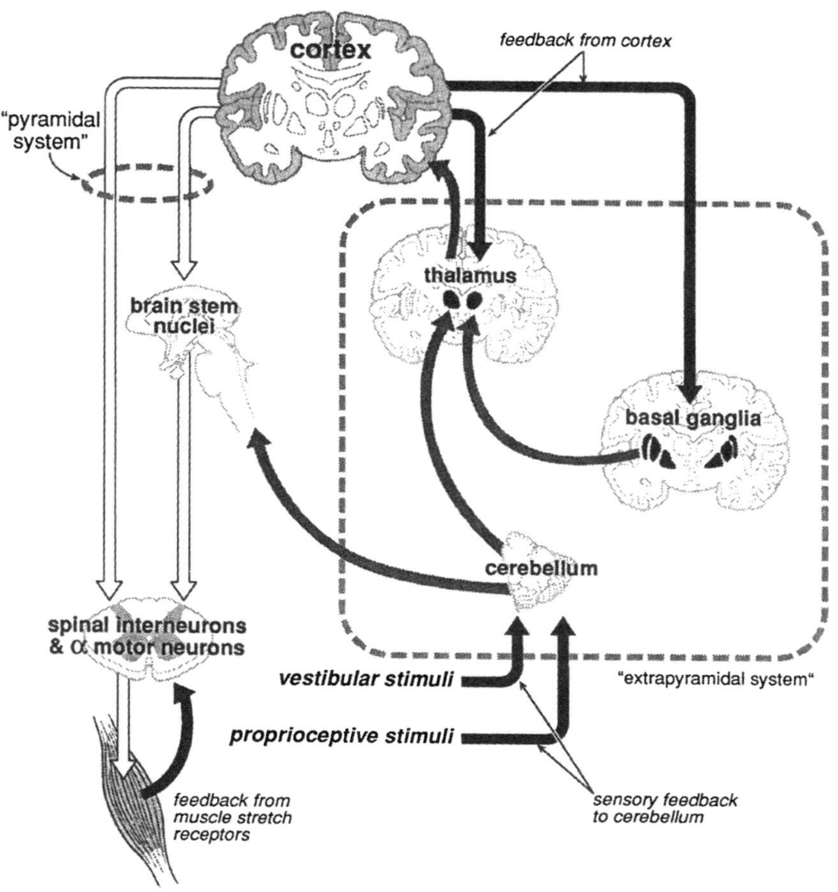

Figure 21.11. The motor control system. The upper motor neuron system consists of the pyramidal and extrapyramidal systems. The pyramidal system connects the motor control center of the cortex to the brainstem and spinal cord and is responsible for the direct control of movement and muscle tone. The extrapyramidal system consists of deep brain structures (especially the basal ganglia and cerebellum) and works primarily by modifying and refining the output of the pyramidal system. The lower motor neuron system consists of neuronal pathways from the spinal cord to the innervated muscles, including nerves that regulate the stretch reflex mechanism. (From Pellegrino, L., & Dormans, J. P. [1998]. Definitions, etiology, and epidemiology of cerebral palsy. In J. P. Dormans & L. Pellegrino [Eds.], *Caring for children with cerebral palsy: A team approach* [p. 10]. Baltimore, MD: Paul H. Brookes Publishing Co., Inc.; reprinted by permission.)

predict walking (Oeffinger et al., 2004; Palisano et al., 1997; see Table 21.1). The Gross Motor Function Classification System—Expanded and Revised (GMFCS–E&R; Palisano, Cameron, Rosenbaum, Walter, & Russell, 2006) is often helpful for planning therapeutic interventions and establishing goals for habilitation. It is more predictive of long-term functional outcome than traditional, impairment-focused classification schemes (Palisano et al., 2007).

The GMFCS can be used to guide prognosis for walking (Rosenbaum et al., 2002; Wood & Rosenbaum, 2000). Children at any level within the classification scheme tend to stay at or move slightly below that level as they reach adolescence and adulthood (Hanna et al., 2009). In general, children at GMFCS levels I or II will have a good prognosis for some degree of independent ambulation and will retain their functionality into adulthood. Children at levels III and IV will have a variable prognosis for walking with some form of assistance and may decline functionally when they reach school age, and children at level V have a poor prognosis for any type of walking.

Precise probability curves for ambulation have been published that allow even more exact predictions of ambulatory potential based on motor functioning at 2½ years of age (Wu, Day, Strauss, & Shavelle, 2004). For example, using these curves, it can be predicted that a child who is able to roll, sit independently, and pull-to-stand at 2½ years of age has a greater than 70% probability of being able to

Table 21.1. Summary of the Gross Motor Function Classification System–Expanded and Revised (GMFCS-E&R)

	Age				
Level	<2 years	2–4 years	4–6 years	6–12 years	12–18 years
I: Walks without limitations	Sits well (hands free to play), crawls and pulls-to-stand; walks between 18 and 24 months without a device	Gets up and down from floor to standing without help; walking is preferred method of mobility	Walks indoors and outdoors; climbs stairs; starting to run/jump	Independent walking, running, jumping, but speed, balance, and coordination are limited; may choose to participate in sports	Independent walking, running, jumping; may choose to participate in sports
II: Walks with limitations	Sits but may need hands for balance; may creep or crawl; may pull-to-stand or cruise	Floor sits, but hard to keep both hands free; mobility by crawling, cruising, or walking with assistive device	Transfers with arm assist; walks without device at home, short distances outside; climbs stairs with railing; no running or jumping	Independent walking but limitations in challenging circumstances; minimal running, jumping	Independent walking but limitations in challenging circumstances; may use hand-held mobility device at school; may use wheeled mobility for long distances
III: Walks using a hand-held mobility device	Sits with low back support; rolls and creeps	Floor sits, often W-sitting, needs help getting to sit; creeping and crawling primary means of mobility; limited assisted standing/walking	Sits in regular chair with pelvic support to allow free hands; walks with device on level surface; transported for long distances	Walks indoors or outdoors with hand-held mobility device; wheeled mobility transport for long distances	Variable use of hand-held mobility device; self-propelled wheel chair or powered mobility at school; powered mobility or wheelchair transport for long distances
IV: Self-mobility with limitations; may use powered mobility	Has head control, but needs trunk support for sitting; rolls to back; may roll to front	Needs hands to maintain sitting; adaptive equipment for sitting/standing; floor mobility only (rolling, creeping, or crawling without reciprocal leg movements)	Adaptive seating needed for maximum hand function; needs assistance for transfers; walks short distances with assistance; power mobility for long distances	Maintains function achieved by ages 4–6 or relies more on power wheelchair for self-mobility; powered mobility or wheelchair transport for long distances	Use wheel mobility in most settings; physical assistance from 1–2 people needed for transfers (may be able to support weight on legs); powered mobility or wheelchair transport for long distances
V: Transported in a manual wheelchair	Limited voluntary control of movement; head and trunk control minimal; needs help to roll	Limited control of movement and posture; all areas of motor function are limited; adaptive equipment does not fully compensate for functional limitations in sitting and standing; no independent mobility (requires transport); some children and youth achieve very limited power mobility with extensive adaptations; older children and youth require 1–2 people or mechanical lift for transfers			

Source: Palisano, Cameron, Rosenbaum, Walter, and Russell (2006).

engage in some form of ambulation by age 7 years. By contrast, a child who can roll but cannot sit or pull-to-stand at 2½ years has only a 25% chance of walking and would most likely do this with the help of an assistive device.

To walk, a child must be able to maintain an upright posture, move forward in a smoothly coordinated manner, and demonstrate protective responses for safety when falling. Even a child with mild CP has difficulty with the neurologic motor control required for ambulation. Common, treatable problems affecting gait include scissoring and an equinus position of the feet. Scissoring occurs because of increased tone in the muscles that control adduction (movement toward the midline) and internal rotation of the hips. Toe walking results from an equinus position of the feet (Figure 21.12) and increased extensor tone in the legs.

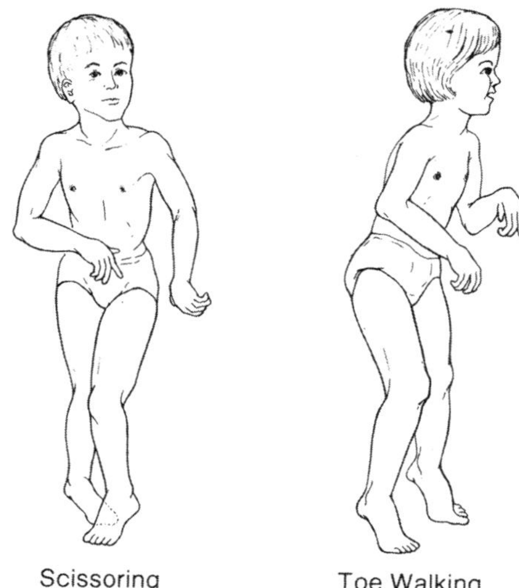

Figure 21.12. Scissoring results from increased tone in the muscles on the inner aspect of the thigh that tend to pull the legs together and turn the legs inward. Toe walking is due to tightness of the calf muscles and Achilles tendon and increased extensor tone in the legs.

Children with CP may also have fine motor impairment, which can be quantified by the Manual Ability Classification System (MACS). A child with MACS level I can handle objects easily and successfully, whereas a child with MACS level V does not handle objects and has severely limited manual dexterity (see Table 21.2; Eliasson et al., 2006).

Children with CP may also have oromotor impairment, which can be quantified by the Eating and Drinking Ability Classification System (EDACS; see Table 21.3). A child with EDACS level I eats and drinks safely and efficiently, while a child with an EDACS level V is unable to eat or drink safely and may require tube feeding for nutritional support (Sellers, Mandy, Pennington, Hankins, & Morris, 2014).

The International Classification of Functioning, Disability, and Health (ICF) is a multidimensional way to classify functioning and disability in the context of medical and environmental domains (WHO, 2001, 2007; see Chapter 32, specifically Figure 32.1). When applying the ICF model to Jamal, the 15-month-old boy with delayed walking, his health condition can be defined as CP and his symptoms are consistent with spastic diplegia secondary to PVL. His body functions and structures can be described as bilateral stiffness and weakness of all extremities, with legs more affected than arms. His *activity* can be described as difficulty with walking, more specifically that he may develop into a child who is a household or community ambulator. One way in which his *participation* may be affected now is the limited options for child care

Table 21.2. Measures of manual dexterity

	Mini-MACS (adapted from Eliasson et al., 2017)	Manual Ability Classification System (MACS) (adapted from Eliasson et al., 2006)
Ages	1–4 years	4–18 years
Level I	***Handles objects easily and successfully.*** At most limitations in the ease of performing manual tasks requiring speed and accuracy.	***Handles objects easily and successfully.*** At most, limitations in the ease of performing manual tasks requiring speed and accuracy. However, any limitations in manual abilities do not restrict independence in daily activities
Level II	***Handles most objects, but with somewhat reduced quality and/or speed of achievement.*** Some actions can only be performed and accomplished with some difficulty and after practice. The child may try an alternative approach, such as using only one hand. The child needs adult assistance to handle objects more frequently compared to children at the same age.	***Handles most objects but with somewhat reduced quality and/or speed of achievement.*** Certain activities may be avoided or be achieved with some difficulty; alternative ways of performance might be used, but manual abilities do not usually restrict independence in daily activities.
Level III	***Handles objects with difficulty. Performance is slow, with limited variation and quality.*** Easily managed objects are handled independently for short periods. The child often needs adult help and support to handle objects.	***Handles objects with difficulty; needs help to prepare and/or modify activities.*** The performance is slow and achieved with limited success regarding quality and quantity. Activities are performed independently if they have been set up or adapted.
Level IV	***Handles a limited selection of easily managed objects in simple actions.*** The actions are performed slowly, with exertion and/or random precision. The child needs constant adult help and support to handle objects.	***Handles a limited selection of easily managed objects in adapted situations.*** Performs parts of activities with effort and with limited success. Requires continuous support and assistance and/or adapted equipment for even partial achievement of the activity.
Level V	***Does not handle objects and has severely limited ability to perform even simple actions.*** At best, the child can push, touch, press, or hold on to a few items in constant interaction with an adult.	***Does not handle objects and has severely limited ability to perform even simple actions.*** Requires total assistance.

Table 21.3. Eating and Drinking Ability Classification System for Individuals with Cerebral Palsy (EDACS; adapted from Sellers et al., 2014)

Level I	Eats and drinks safely and efficiently
Level II	Eats and drinks safely but with some limitations to efficiency
Level III	Eats and drinks with some limitations to safety; maybe limitations to efficiency
Level IV	Eats and drinks with significant limitations to safety
Level V	Unable to eat or drink safely—tube feeding may be considered to provide nutrition

environments that will meet both his cognitive and physical needs. *Environmental factors* may be positive, such as his caring parents; alternatively, they may be barriers, such as stairs in the home. *Personal factors* are that he is a 15-month-old boy, that he has access to early intervention services, and that he is growing up in a stimulating environment.

SUBTYPES OF CEREBRAL PALSY

CP is often divided into specific **phenotypes** (physical appearances) according to the neurological findings and body limbs that are predominantly affected (Koman, Smith, & Shilt, 2004; Figure 21.13). A recognized classification system divides the phenotypes into bilateral (both sides of the body affected) and unilateral (one side affected). This distinction is useful both in evaluating the underlying cause as well as directing management of CP (Rosenbaum, 2007).

Spastic Cerebral Palsy

Spasticity is the abnormal increase in muscle tone resulting from an increased resistance to muscle stretch and lengthening. It restricts voluntary movement and, over time, leads to contractures (Barnes & Johnson, 2008). Spasticity is believed to arise from disruption of the descending pathways involved in motor control, including both pyramidal and parapyramidal pathways. The pyramidal system (i.e., the corticospinal tract) is composed of neurons that extend from the motor cortex to the brainstem and spinal cord. These pathways directly control movement and influence muscle tone and deep tendon reflexes by inhibiting spinal cord mechanisms that direct these processes. In the absence of normal corticospinal inhibition, the spinal cord influences predominate, resulting in spasticity and a positive Babinski sign, two of the hallmarks of spastic CP. The parapyramidal fibers from premotor cortex also contribute to spasticity and UMN signs.

Spastic CP is the most common type of CP (Krägeloh-Mann & Cans, 2009). It is further categorized according to the distribution of limbs involved. In **spastic diplegia,** the legs are more affected than the arms. This is the type of CP most frequently associated with prematurity. In **spastic hemiplegia,** one side of the body is more affected than the other; usually, the arm is more affected than the leg. Because the motor neurons that control one side of the body are located in the opposite cerebral cortex, a right-sided hemiplegia implies injury to the left side of the brain, and vice versa. In **spastic quadriplegia,** all four limbs and usually the trunk and muscles that control the mouth, tongue, and pharynx are affected. The severity of the motor impairment in spastic quadriplegia implies wider cerebral dysfunction and a poorer outcome than for the other forms of spastic CP. Individuals with spastic quadriplegia often have intellectual disability, seizures, sensory impairments, and other medical problems.

Dyskinetic Cerebral Palsy

Children who have CP as a consequence of disturbances in the extrapyramidal system exhibit atypical movements known as **dyskinesias** (CP Family Network, 2012). These include chorea, athetosis, choreoathetosis, and dystonia. Rapid, random, jerky movements are known as **chorea;** slow, writhing movements that appear to flow into one another are called **athetosis.** When seen together, these movements are called **choreoathetosis. Dystonia** refers to repetitive, twisting movements and distorted postures.

Dyskinetic CP (also known as extrapyramidal CP) is characterized by abnormalities in muscle tone that involve the whole body. Changing patterns of tone from hour to hour and day to day are common. These children exhibit increased muscle tone, especially during attempted movement, and normal or decreased tone while asleep. The term athetoid CP characterizes a form of dyskinetic CP that has been associated with kernicterus. Dystonic CP is associated with hypoxic-ischemic encephalopathy as well as with a wide range of genetic disorders. Chorea is the least common form of dyskinetic CP.

Ataxic Cerebral Palsy

Ataxia results from an abnormality in the cerebellum and manifests as the inability to maintain typical

TYPE	Spastic			Dyskinetic	Ataxic
	Unilateral (30%)*	Bilateral (58%)		(7%)	(4%)
SUBTYPE	Hemiplegia	Diplegia	Quadriplegia		
Distribution	Asymmetric; arms/hands often more affected than legs	Symmetric; legs mainly affected, mild difficulties with arms/hands	Both side of the body involved (including head & trunk); may be symmetric or asymmetric	Both sides of the body involved (including head & trunk); symmetric	Both sides of the body involved (including head & trunk); symmetric
Clinical Features	Increased tone Increased reflexes (evidence of *spasticity*) Predominantly one side of the body affected (arm/hand often more than leg) Development of contractures with time	Increased tone Increased reflexes (evidence of *spasticity*) Both sides of the body affected (legs more than arms/hands) Development of contractures with time	Increased tone Increased reflexes (evidence of *spasticity*) Both sides of the body affected with significant variation in the degree of involvement of different limbs Development of contractures with time	Variable tone Reflexes normal or slightly increased Both sides of the body affected Associated with involuntary movements: *athetosis* (slow, writhing movements), *chorea* (rapid, jerking movements) and/or *dystonia* (posturing movements)	Low tone Reflexes normal or slightly increased Both sides of the body affected Associated with *ataxia* (poor balance, tremors, poorly graded voluntary movements)
Periventricular damage	++	+++	++	+	? (insufficient data)
Cortical or deep brain (basal ganglia) damage	++	+	+++	+++	? (insufficient data)
Congenital malformantions	+	+	+	---	++ (especially of the cerebellum)
Infants affected	Mainly Term, some Preterm	Mainly Preterm	Term and Preterm	Mainly Term	Mainly Term

* Percentage of all types of CP; percentages do not include mixed forms of cerebral palsy, or forms for which a subtype is undefined.

Figure 21.13. The subtypes of cerebral palsy (CP). The spastic forms of CP are most common and can involve both sides of the body (diplegia and quadriplegia) or may mainly involve one side of the body (hemiplegia). Diplegia mainly involves the lower extremities and is the most common form of CP associated with periventricular (PV) injury related to prematurity. Quadriplegia involves the whole body and is most often due to hypoxic-ischemic (HI) injury in term infants or PV injury in preterm infants. Hemiplegia may be caused by PV injury but is also commonly caused by prenatal and postnatal stroke (resulting in damage to the cortex on one side). Dyskinetic forms of CP involve the whole body, are associated with involuntary movements, and may be caused by damage to the basal ganglia (deep brain structures) due to HI injury or by newborn jaundice associated with very high levels of bilirubin (kernicterus); it has also been associated with several genetic disorders. Ataxic CP involves the whole body and is associated with problems with balance, tremors, and difficulties with finely graded voluntary movements. The causes of ataxic CP are poorly understood, but it has been associated with congenital abnormalities of the cerebellum. (*Source*: Krägeloh-Mann & Cans, 2009.)

postures and perform typical movements. As a result, movements are jerky and uncoordinated, without the smooth flow of typical motion (CP Family Network, 2012). Ataxic CP is characterized by impairments in voluntary movement, involving balance and position of the trunk and limbs in space. For children who can walk, this is manifested as a wide-based, unsteady gait. Difficulties with controlling the hand and arm during reaching (causing overshooting or past-pointing) and difficulties with the timing of motor movements are also observed. Ataxic CP may be associated with either increased or decreased muscle tone.

Some organizations include hypotonic CP as an additional type (Goldsmith et al., 2016), though a commonly cited consensus definition excludes children with hypotonia as the sole motor finding from the CP diagnosis (Cans et al., 2007).

Mixed Cerebral Palsy

The term *mixed CP* is used when more than one type of motor pattern is present and when one pattern does not clearly predominate over another. The term *total body CP* is sometimes used to emphasize that certain types of CP (dyskinetic, ataxic, mixed, and spastic quadriplegia) involve the entire musculoskeletal system, whereas other forms of spastic CP (e.g., diplegia and hemiplegia) are localized to a particular region of the body.

Although there is some clinical utility in classifying CP on the basis of neuromotor characteristics (e.g., spasticity or dyskinesias), there tends to be a great deal of functional variability within specific subtypes. For example, some children with spastic diplegia may be able to walk independently, whereas others depend on a wheelchair for mobility. As described previously, tools such as the GMFCS have been useful in predicting functional outcomes.

ESTABLISHING THE ETIOLOGY OF CEREBRAL PALSY

In CP, the evaluation for the etiology is often done in parallel with the assessment that establishes the disability or functional diagnosis (Ashwal et al., 2004; National Guideline Alliance, 2017). Establishing the underlying etiology can have important implications for designing treatment and for understanding prognosis and recurrence risk in future children. It also can impact the parental feelings of guilt and responsibility. Information from the medical history and physical examination of a child is critical in establishing an etiology. For example, knowing that a child was born prematurely and has signs of spastic diplegia strongly suggests cerebral white matter injury. Similarly, dystonic CP in the presence of a normal birth history may be associated with a neurogenetic or metabolic disorder (see Chapter 16).

With regard to specialized diagnostic testing, brain imaging is especially helpful (Accardo, Kammann, & Hoon, 2004; Ancel et al., 2006). Seventy to ninety percent of children with CP will have significant diagnostic findings on neuroimaging (Korzeniewski, Birbeck, DeLano, Potchen, & Paneth, 2007). Cranial ultrasound, an inexpensive, noninvasive imaging modality, has utility both in diagnosis and management of the high-risk neonate. Ultrasonography is used for fetal and neonatal screening; it can distinguish large malformations of the brain from abnormalities related to brain hemorrhage or injury (i.e., IVH, PVL).

Brain anatomic MRI is the most helpful imaging technique for establishing the cause of CP (Vermeulen, Wilke, Horber, & Krägeloh-Mann, 2010). Based on an understanding of normal brain development, careful interpretation of MRI studies can show patterns of selective vulnerability in brain structures characteristic of the nature of the insult, gestational timing, and severity (Barkovich, 2005). It should be noted that even a normal MRI can be of benefit, as it may lead to consideration of a potentially treatable metabolic disorder, such as dopa-responsive dystonia (Mink, 2003). Use of advanced MRI techniques such as diffusion weighted imaging, DTI, MR spectroscopy, and functional MRI (see Chapter 8) can provide additional information about brain metabolic function and white matter tract integrity/maturity. Evidence for clinical use of advanced methods (particularly for diffusion MRI) is emerging, but the technical complexity of analysis and interpretation continues to limit widespread routine use (George et al., 2017).

ASSOCIATED IMPAIRMENTS IN CEREBRAL PALSY

Many children with CP have associated impairments. The most common are intellectual disability, visual impairments, hearing impairments, speech-language disorders, seizures, feeding and growth impairments, and behavior-emotional disorders.

Assessment of intellectual functioning in children with CP may be difficult because most tests of cognition require responses that are dependent upon both oromotor and visual-motor skills. Even taking these limitations into account, approximately one half of children with CP have intellectual disability, and many of those with typical intelligence exhibit some degree of learning disability (Nordmark, Hägglund, & Lagergren, 2001). Children with the more severe types of CP are at a greater risk for more significant intellectual disability.

Visual impairments are common and diverse in children with CP. They may be both ocular (e.g., strabismus) and central (i.e., cortical visual impairment; Guzzetta, Mercuri, & Cioni, 2001; see Chapter 25). The premature infant may have severe visual impairment caused by retinopathy of prematurity. Nystagmus, or involuntary oscillating eye movements, may be present in the child with ataxia. Children with hemiplegia may present with homonymous hemianopia, a condition causing loss of one part of the visual field (Jacobson, Rydberg, Eliasson, Kits, & Flodmark, 2010). Strabismus is seen in many children with CP. Finally, children with CP are more prone to hyperopia (farsightedness) than typically developing children (Sobrado, Suarez, & Garcia-Sanchez, 1999).

Hearing, speech, and language impairments are also common, occurring in about 30% of children with CP. Children with CP caused by congenital cytomegalovirus or other intrauterine viral infections often have hearing loss (see Chapter 26). Dyskinetic CP resulting from basal ganglia/thalamus injury is associated with articulation problems because these structures influence tongue and vocal cord movement. In children with CP and typical cognitive development, expressive or receptive language disorders may be present and may evolve into a specific reading disability (see Chapter 20).

Approximately 40% of children with CP develop seizures (Nordmark et al., 2001). Children with more severe intellectual and physical disability are more prone to generalized seizures (Carlsson, Hagberg, & Olsson, 2003). Children whose CP is a consequence of brain malformation, infection, or severe gray matter injury are also at greater risk for generalized seizures (see Chapter 22).

Feeding and growth difficulties also are often present (Samson-Fang et al., 2002). They may be secondary to a variety of problems, including hypotonia, weak suck, poor coordination of the swallowing mechanism, tonic bite reflex, hyperactive gag reflex, and exaggerated tongue thrust. These problems may lead to poor nutrition and, in some cases, require the use of alternative feeding methods, such as tube feeding (see Chapter 29). Medical problems related to poor gastrointestinal motility (including gastroesophageal reflux and constipation) may add to these difficulties.

The combination of poor nutrition and lack of weight-bearing activities also leads to osteopenia (weak bones related to reduced bone mineral density). This places children with CP at increased risk for fractures. Bisphosphonates, which have been used to treat osteoporosis in older adults, have also been shown to be effective in treating osteopenia in CP (Hough, Boyd, & Keating, 2010).

As in other neurodevelopmental disabilities, individuals with CP are affected with psychiatric comorbidities at a rate that is higher than the general population. These include conditions such as anxiety, depression, and adjustment disorders. They also are more likely to have sleep disorders, such as obstructive sleep apnea. In addition, due to their primary condition, they are affected by pain, and thus pain management must be addressed adequately at each health care encounter (Fehlings, 2017).

These associated disorders contribute significantly to the issue of quality of life in individuals with CP (Liptak & Accardo, 2004; Samson-Fang et al., 2002). A comprehensive health plan implemented in the context of a well-defined medical home is a critical component to ensuring that the health needs of children with CP are adequately addressed (Cooley & American Academy of Pediatrics Committee on Children with Disabilities, 2004; see Chapter 41).

COMPREHENSIVE MANAGEMENT FOR INDIVIDUALS WITH CEREBRAL PALSY

Neuroplasticity

A key starting point for discussing management of CP is based on an understanding of neuroplasticity. **Neuroplasticity** refers to the ability of the central nervous system to change in response to environmental stimulation (Wittenberg, 2009). It is characterized by the inherently dynamic biological capacity of the CNS to undergo maturation, change structurally and functionally in response to experience, and adapt following injury (Ismail, Fatemi, & Johnston, 2017). The human brain grows rapidly from conception through early childhood. During this time, typical developmental changes include widespread creation and then destruction of interneuronal connections, or synapses. Experience-dependent and -expectant patterns of synaptic creation and pruning are one major postulated mechanism of early developmental neuroplasticity (Ismail et al., 2017). Neuron- and synapse-level plasticity mechanisms may provide the ability to adapt to environmental changes, to store information in memory (associated with learning), and to recover from brain and spinal cord injury (Johnston, 2009). There is a great deal of information in adults, especially following stroke, supporting the efficacy of neurorehabilitation directed at the plasticity (see Chapter 32).

The child's brain has greater plasticity than the adult brain (Cramer et al., 2011). In CP, as well as in other childhood neurodevelopmental disabilities, the overarching question concerning plasticity involves the nature of the relationship between amount and timing of intervention and resultant outcome (Delgado et al., 2010; Vargus-Adams, 2009).

Overview of Management

Comprehensive management for children with CP includes both accurate diagnosis and effective treatment strategies. Management is based upon the recognition that each child requires a unique combination of medical and rehabilitative interventions that are developed though a team approach and tailored to the family structure and goals. Specialists in orthopedics, neurosurgery, genetics, ophthalmology, gastroenterology, neurology, physical medicine and rehabilitation, psychiatry, and neurodevelopmental pediatrics are all integral to developing a comprehensive medical-surgical treatment plan. Physical and occupational therapists, speech-language pathologists, audiologists, clinical and behavioral psychologists, special education consultants, and social workers are critical team members in developing the rehabilitation and educational plan. An interdisciplinary setting is the ideal approach to management of the child with CP.

It is very important that clinicians and families agree upon specific treatments as well as overall management goals. Typical goals include improvements in function, communication, ease of care, and pain management. Including the child in the decision-making process to the greatest extent possible is critical to successful plan implementation. Treatment should be integrated into the individual families' lifestyles, including other activities and commitments. An important practical consideration is the recognition that a specific medical treatment or therapy may be embraced by one family but rejected by another, even when the overall clinical findings are similar. In the management of CP, effective care coordination and the provision of a medical home are paramount (Figure 21.14).

A family-centered medical home is *not* a building, house, hospital, or home health care service, but rather an approach to providing comprehensive primary care.

In a family-centered medical home the pediatric care team works in partnership with a child and a child's family to assure that all of the medical and nonmedical needs of the child are met.

Through this partnership the pediatric care team can help the family and child access, coordinate, and understand specialty care, educational services, out-of-home care, family support, and other public and private community services that are important for the overall health of the child and family.

The American Academy of Pediatrics (AAP) developed the medical home model for delivering primary care that is accessible, continuous, comprehensive, family-centered, coordinated, compassionate, and culturally effective to *all* children and youth, including those with special health care needs.

Figure 21.14. What is a family-centered medical home? (From National Center for Medical Home Implementation, American Academy of Pediatrics. [n.d.]. *What is a family-centered medical home?* Elk Grove Village, IL: Author. Retrieved from http://medicalhomeinfo.org; reprinted by permission.)

Principles of Management

Management may be divided into rehabilitative, medical, and surgical components (Papavasiliou, 2009). Rehabilitative interventions include conventional therapeutic approaches (physical therapy and occupational therapy), serial casting, orthotic bracing, strength training, aquatherapy, hippotherapy (therapeutic horseback riding), and technology systems such as augmentative communication and power mobility. The focus in physiotherapy has shifted from traditional physical and occupational therapy to approaches combining principles of motor learning and strength and fitness training. In addition to these physical approaches, specialists in social work and psychology who are aware of the effects of motor disability on other aspects of childhood development are of great benefit in fostering social/emotional growth and active participation of the child in the rehabilitation efforts.

In terms of medication, the most commonly used drugs for spasticity and rigidity include baclofen, diazepam, and botulinum toxin (see Appendix C). Carbidopa-levodopa and trihexyphenidyl have been found to be helpful for some children with dystonic CP. Tetrabenazine has been used successfully in selected patients with dyskinetic CP. The purpose of all these medications is to improve motor tone, which enables more physical activity or lessens pain. Orthopedic surgical interventions include tenotomies, tendon transfers, and osteotomies (see Chapter 9). Neurosurgical procedures, including intrathecal baclofen, selective dorsal rhizotomy (SDR), and deep brain stimulation (DBS), may be of benefit in carefully selected patients (Lynn, Turner, & Chambers, 2009).

Early Intervention and Education

A number of studies and reviews support the importance of CP-specific early intervention in optimizing neuroplasticity and reducing deleterious musculoskeletal outcomes. The emergence of earlier, more accurate diagnostic assessment tools (e.g., MRI, Prechtl Qualitative Assessment of General Movements, the Hammersmith Infant Neurological Examination) has allowed identification of high-risk infants in some cases even before 5 months of age (Novak et al., 2017). Task-specific motor training early interventions, which focus on targeting use of the lower-functioning hand in constraint-induced therapy, maximize functional gains and are the new paradigm of care. Beginning therapy as soon as high-risk features are noticed in infants and young children with developmental delay has been a long-standing belief of families and professionals alike, and there is now a growing body of evidence supporting the principles and long-term benefits of early intervention (Novak et al., 2017). One approach would be daily in-home interventions with active parental involvement using activities that are fun and motivational with therapist support (Herskind, Griesen, & Nielsen, 2015). Despite the current focus on early intervention, it should be emphasized to families that no rigid critical period has been identified in broad domains of human development and that experience-dependent (and indeed experience-expectant) plasticity appears to continue through adulthood (Bruer, 2011). Early intervention as currently available should not be seen as a cure, and submaximal early intervention should not be seen as a reason to lose hope.

For most children with CP, the process of rehabilitation begins in the home environment under the Infant and Toddlers program within the Individuals with Disabilities Education Improvement Act of 2004 (IDEA; see Chapter 31), which emphasizes the involvement of parents so that they can learn effective methods of working with their child. Programs are individualized according to the specific needs of the child and the family. While emphasizing home-based services, these programs may also provide consultative and center-based interventions (see Chapter 31).

For many children with CP, entry into preschool represents the first major step into the wider community. Difficulties in accommodating the physical, nutritional, and medical needs of these children must be addressed. For school-age children, although concerns regarding motor function and medical needs continue, an increased attention is focused on learning disabilities, attention and behavior difficulties, intellectual disability, and sensory impairments. For many children, these associated conditions, rather than the motor disability, place them at greatest disadvantage relative to their typically developing peers. Children with CP have traditionally been segregated into classrooms with designations such as "multiply disabled" and "orthopedically impaired," sometimes without proper regard for their intellectual needs. Inclusion is mandated by federal law (IDEA) in general education classrooms and in the least restrictive environment. Inclusive environments, however, require significant collaboration between the general and special education models and work best when a team of educators and paraprofessionals is associated with each classroom (see Chapter 33).

Specific Rehabilitative Techniques

For children with CP, therapy may come in many different forms. Most children receive traditional forms of physical, occupational, and speech therapy. The most common method of motor therapy for the young child is neurodevelopmental therapy (NDT), an approach that is employed by both occupational and physical therapists. It is designed to provide the child with sensorimotor experiences that enhance the development of more typical movement patterns (Campbell, Palisano, & Orlin, 2012; see Chapter 32). NDT is an individualized program of positioning, therapeutic handling, and play, and goals include the normalization of tone and improved control of movement during functional activities.

A promising technique known as constraint-induced therapy, or forced-use therapy, has been introduced to help children with hemiplegic CP (Taub, Ramey, DeLuca, & Echols, 2004; Willis, Morello, Davie, Rice, & Bennett, 2002). The technique involves constraining the more functional arm or hand to force use of the less functional upper extremity. Randomized controlled trials suggest that this technique may be of significant benefit over traditional therapy alone in the short run (Aarts, Jongerius, Geerdink, van Limbeek, & Geurts, 2010). Early initiation of constraint-induced therapy after stroke shows benefit at 12 months, and persistent improvements in motor function are evident as late as 24 months after initial implementation, even if therapy is started over 1 year after the initial insult (Wolf et al., 2010).

Physical exercise is important to strengthen muscles and bones, enhance motor skills, and prevent contractures. In addition, the social and recreational aspects of organized physical activities can be highly beneficial (see Chapter 33). Many popular activities, including swimming, dancing, and horseback riding, can be modified so that children with CP can participate (Meregillano, 2004).

The Special Olympics, founded by Eunice Kennedy Shriver in 1968, has enabled thousands of children and young adults with intellectual disabilities and CP to take part in various sporting events. The rewards of engaging in competitive sports are invaluable for enhancing self-esteem and providing a sense of belonging to a peer group. Parents and professionals should encourage all children to participate in whatever physical activities their interests, motivation, and capabilities allow.

Bracing, Splinting, and Positioning

Therapists make frequent use of braces and splints (collectively referred to as **orthotic** devices) and positioning (seating) devices as aids in the pursuit of functional goals for children with CP. These devices are employed to maintain adequate range of motion, prevent contractures at specific joints, provide stability, and control involuntary movements that interfere with function. For the legs, one of the most commonly prescribed orthotics is a leg brace known as an **ankle-foot orthosis** (AFO). The AFO stabilizes the position of the foot and provides a consistent stretch to the Achilles tendon (see Chapter 32).

A variety of splints can be used to improve hand function. For example, the resting hand splint is commonly used to hold the thumb in an **abducted** (away from the midline) position and the wrist in a neutral or slightly extended position. This helps the child to keep his or her hand open and works to prevent the development of hand deformities. Trunk and body bracing, called a body splint, is made of a flexible, porous material. It controls abnormal tone and involuntary movements by stabilizing the trunk and limbs. Most pediatric braces and splints are custom-made from plastics that are molded directly on the child, and so they must be monitored closely and modified as the child grows or changes abilities.

Positioning devices are used to promote skeletal alignment, to compensate for atypical postures, or to prepare the child for independent mobility. Proper positioning geared toward the age and functional status of the child is often a key intervention in addressing the tone and movement impairments associated with CP. For children who must sit for extended periods of time or who use a wheelchair for mobility, a carefully designed seating system becomes an all-important component of their rehabilitation. Careful attention to functional seating may also have long-term benefits in the prevention of contractures and joint deformities resulting from spasticity (Myhr, von Wendt, Norrlin, & Radell, 1995).

Adaptive Equipment

A wide variety of devices are available to aid mobility. For children who are ambulatory, the use of crutches, walkers, and canes can help in the attainment of walking or in improvement of the quality and range of ambulation. The forearm, or Lofstrand, crutch is used in preference to the familiar under-the-arm crutch. A posterior walker with wheels (i.e., the child is positioned in front of the walker rather than behind) is used in preference to a standard forward-position walker without wheels. Canes are used less commonly.

For children with limited walking skills, wheelchairs are essential for maximizing mobility and function. A wheelchair with a solid seat and back is usually recommended. Some children, however, have difficulty using this type of chair unless modifications are made. The addition of head and trunk supports or a tray may be needed for the child who lacks postural control due to abnormalities in tone. The child with limited head control, feeding difficulties, or low tone may benefit from a high-backed chair that can be tilted back 10–15 degrees (Figure 21.15A). This helps to maintain the child's body and head in proper alignment, and it may help to prevent scoliosis. Special seating cushions or custom-molded inserts that conform to the contours of the body can offer necessary support for the child with orthopedic deformities such as scoliosis.

Motorized (power) wheelchairs can enhance the independence of children who are able to use them. They may be manipulated by hand control, head control, or mouth mechanisms for controlling both speed and direction (Figure 21.15B). These wheelchairs can include leg elevation and tilt-in-space options. They can provide increased independence for individuals who would otherwise be dependent upon others for pressure relief, self-positioning, and lower extremity stretching.

Special supportive strollers are an alternative to wheelchairs for mobility within the community or for the young child whose potential for ambulation has yet to be determined. These are lightweight and collapsible, yet they support the back and keep the hips properly aligned (Figure 21.15C).

Car seats are essential to the safety of all children who ride in automobiles. Several manufacturers offer adapted car seats that meet federal safety guidelines as well as provide proper support for the child with CP.

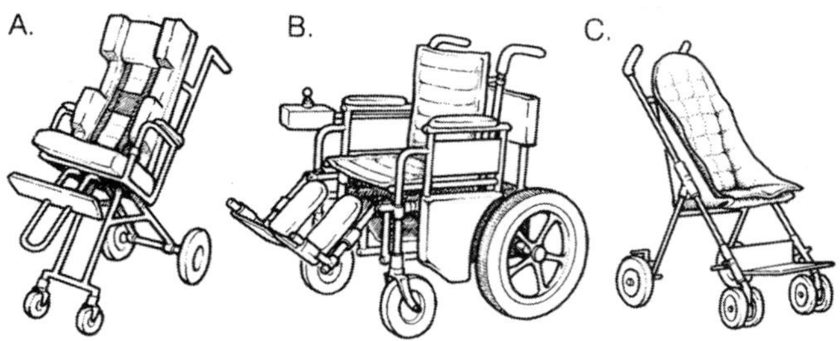

Figure 21.15. Three types of wheelchairs. A) High-backed, tilting chair with lateral inserts and head supports; B) motorized wheelchair with joystick control; and C) supportive collapsible stroller.

Often these models include a base that allows the seat to be used as a stroller or a positioning chair outside of the car. Car beds and special straps are also available for children who have more severe disabilities or who require these special adaptations temporarily (e.g., following surgery).

Assistive Technology/Augmentative and Alternative Communication

Assistive Technology (AT) is an umbrella term describing use of external items to improve functioning for individuals with disabilities. Items or devices used can range from simple, low-technology systems (e.g., communication boards made of cardboard) to customized state-of-the-art computer systems or mechanical aids. **Augmentative and Alternative Communication** (AAC) is a subcategory of AT that provides methods of communication for individuals with impairments in spoken and/or written language. *Augmentative* refers to methods to supplement communication and *alternative* when the child has no speech.

AT devices are often an integral part of the rehabilitation plan for children with CP having complex communication needs (see Chapter 36). Although it is often true that the simplest intervention is the best, the computer is seen as the future of AT. Computers can be used to control the environment, provide a lifeline with the outside world, enable a person to work at home, facilitate artificial speech and sight, and provide entertainment. Recently, there has been a lot of enthusiasm for devices such as the tablets and smartphones for individuals with disabilities, chronic illness, and other impairments due to their relatively low cost and the ease and simplicity of their interfaces, graphics, and applications.

While the tablets and other mobile technologies have opened the doors of communication to individuals who have complex communication needs with measurable short-term benefits, the goals of participation in home, community, and school are more difficult to evaluate and quantify. With open collaboration of all people who are involved in the care of individuals with CP, technology development can proceed in sync with the immediate and broader needs of individuals with CP (McNaughton & Light, 2015).

Neurocognitive Prosthetics

There is an evolving interest in using technology to restore function, which can be attained through neuroprosthetics and neural control interfaces. Neuroprosthetics modulate neural function by directly using implanted electrodes and other hardware in the central nervous system to restore injured special senses or movement (Serruya & Kahana, 2008). Neuroprosthetics currently in use include cochlear and auditory midbrain implants for individuals with profound sensorineural hearing loss (see Chapter 26), and deep brain stimulation used in the management of involuntary movements in dyskinetic forms of CP (see the Neurosurgical Procedures section below).

In contrast, neural-control interfaces can either invasively or noninvasively connect the brain to a computer or machine. Examples of commercially available neural-control interfaces include NeuroSky and Emotiv, by which the users control a computer game with their own "brain waves" as mediated through an electroencephalograph. Other noninvasive techniques include transcranial magnetic stimulation and transcranial direct current stimulation. It is hoped that further advances in neurocognitive prosthetics will improve both communication and mobility for individuals with a wide range of disorders, including CP.

Managing Spasticity and Dystonia

Spasticity and dystonia represent important targets for intervention in CP. The primary goals are to improve function, to prevent or postpone the musculoskeletal complications attendant to these conditions, and to ease the care of the child with significant muscle tightness.

Different treatment modalities work at different levels of brain and spine circuitry (Figure 21.16). Interventions may be employed singly, sequentially, or simultaneously depending on the specific clinical circumstance. As dystonia is caused by disturbances in the extrapyramidal motor control system, pharmacological interventions primarily target the brain and spinal cord. By contrast, the mechanisms that generate spasticity may be affected from the brain to the muscle itself. Therefore, a wider variety of therapeutic modalities are available to modulate the effects of spasticity (see Box 21.1). A potential pitfall in treatment revolves around the relationship between impairment (spasticity or dystonia) and disability. For some children, it is possible to significantly reduce spasticity or dystonia without improving (and in some cases even worsening) functional outcome. Therefore, consultation with experienced professionals who are intimately familiar with a child's particular pattern of skills and impairments is critical to the proper selection of specific interventions (see Box 21.2).

Casting Tone-reducing, or inhibitive, casts are used in some centers as an adjunct to more traditional

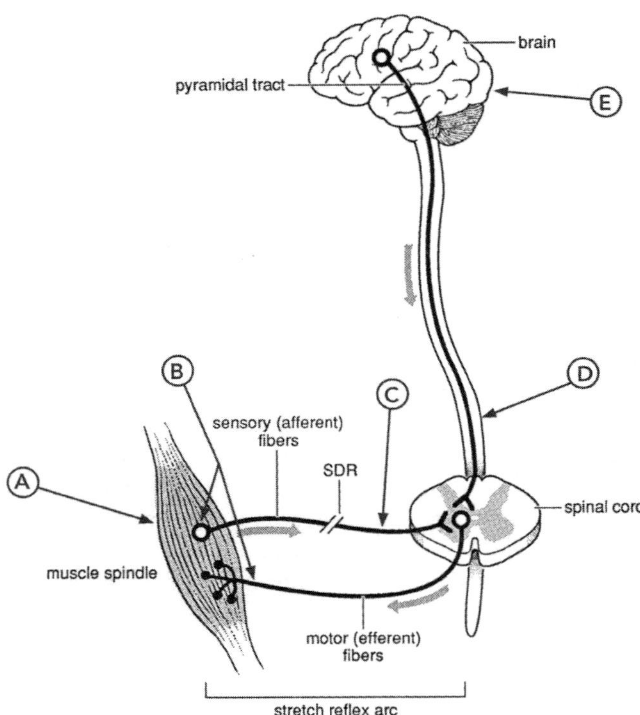

Figure 21.16. Levels of intervention for spasticity and dystonia. A) Inhibitive casting, physical therapy, exercise, and medications such as dantrolene directly affect tone at the muscle level. B) Nerve blocks, motor point blocks, and botulinum toxin work variously at the level of muscle and neuromuscular junction. C) Selective dorsal rhizotomy reduces spasticity by interrupting the sensory component of the stretch reflex arc. D) Medications such as baclofen reduce spasticity at the level of the spinal cord. E) Medications for spasticity, such as diazepam, and medications for dystonia work at the level of the brain. (From Pellegrino, L., & Dormans, J. P. [1998]. Definitions, etiology, and epidemiology of cerebral palsy. In J. P. Dormans & L. Pellegrino [Eds.], *Caring for children with cerebral palsy: A team approach* [p. 46]. Baltimore, MD: Paul H. Brookes Publishing Co., Inc.; adapted by permission.)

methods of managing spasticity (Law et al., 1991). The casts are made for arms or legs and can be either designed for use in immobilization or during weight-bearing activities. Benefits of inhibitive casting include improved gait and weight bearing, increased range of motion, and improved functional hand use. Casts position the limbs so that spastic muscles are in lengthened positions, being gently stretched. Serial application of casts (serial casting) can allow the therapist to increase range of motion gradually in the presence of contractures. After maximal range and position have been achieved, a cast is worn intermittently to maintain the improvement. Casting is now most often used in conjunction with other therapeutic modalities, especially following injection of **botulinum toxin**, sold under the brand name Botox (Glanzman, Kim, Swaminathan, & Beck, 2004; Kay, Rethlefsen, Fern-Buneo, Wren, & Skaggs, 2004; Wasiak, Hoare, & Wallen, 2004).

Nerve Blocks, Motor Point Blocks, and Botulinum Toxin Several injectable agents are available that can be used to target spasticity in particular muscle groups. Certain chemical agents such as diluted alcohol or phenol, which denature muscle and nerve protein at the point of injection, can produce a decrease in muscle tone for months. A **motor point block** with these agents effectively interrupts the nerve supply at the entry site to a spastic muscle without compromising sensation. The main side effect of the procedure is localized pain that may persist for a few days after the injection. Inhibition of spasticity lasts for 4–6 months, and the procedure can be repeated after the initial effect has worn off. This temporary reduction of spasticity allows for more effective application of physical therapy to improve range of motion and function and to potentially postpone orthopedic surgery.

Injectable botulinum toxin was approved as an alternative to motor point blocks in 2000 and has largely supplanted alcohol and phenol (Jefferson, 2004; Mooney, Koman, & Smith, 2003; Morton, Hankinson, & Nicholson, 2004; Pidcock, 2004). Botulinum toxin is produced by the bacterium that causes botulism and is among the most potent neurotoxins known. It works by blocking the nerve-muscle junction. Small quantities can be safely injected directly into spastic muscles without significant spread of the toxin into the bloodstream. The injection results in weakening of the muscle and reduction of spasticity for 3–6 months (the antispasticity effects of the injections dissipate over time). Although botulinum toxin is used mainly to treat spasticity in muscles of the limbs and trunk, other uses have been developed, such as injection of the salivary glands to reduce drooling (Jongerius et al., 2004). Although clarification is still needed regarding the definition of clinical indications and outcomes (Hoare et al., 2010), the use of injectable botulinum toxin has become a mainstay in the management of spasticity in CP and has also found applications for specific types of dystonia (Gordon, 1999; Jefferson, 2004; Mooney et al., 2003). Side effects, including weakness and mild flu-like symptoms, are usually mild and transient. It should be noted, however, that there are very rare reports in which botulism-like clinical pictures, including death, have been reported (Jankovic & Brin, 1991).

Oral Medication A variety of orally administered medications have been used to improve muscle tone in children with spasticity and rigidity (Krach, 2001; Tilton, 2006; see Appendix C).

Several medications used in Parkinson's disease in adults, including carbidopa-levodopa (Sinemet) and

BOX 21.1 EVIDENCE-BASED PRACTICE

Spasticity Treatments

Guidelines: American Academy of Neurology guidelines for spasticity (Delgado et al., 2010) and UK National Guideline Alliance guidelines for spasticity in under-19s (2012; updated without change in 2016)

Treatment	Local or general	Temporary, permanent, or reversible	Recommended settings and level of evidence (see text for detailed indications, contraindications, and considerations)
Oral medications			
Diazepam	General	Temporary	Short-term, as-needed treatment (Delgado et al., 2010) "Consider" for rapid effect, discomfort/pain, spasms, or functional disability (National Guideline Alliance, 2012) Green light ("Effective, do it") rating (Novak et al., 2013)
Oral baclofen			"Consider" for sustained, long-term effect for discomfort/pain, spasms, or functional disability. "Consider" a trial if dystonia is considered to be contributing significantly to problems of posture, function, or pain (National Guideline Alliance, 2012) Overall insufficient data (Delgado et al., 2010) Yellow light ("Uncertain effect; measure outcomes for progress") rating (Novak et al., 2013)
Tizanidine			Overall limited evidence (Delgado et al., 2010) Yellow light ("Uncertain effect; measure outcomes for progress") rating (Novak et al., 2013)
Dantrolene			Overall insufficient data (Delgado et al., 2010) Yellow light ("Uncertain effect; measure outcomes for progress") rating (Novak et al., 2013)
Trihexyphenidyl, Levodopa			"Consider" a trial if dystonia is considered to be contributing significantly to problems of posture, function, or pain (National Guideline Alliance, 2012)
Injectable medication			
Botulinum toxin type A	Local/segmental	Temporary	"Consider" in focal upper or lower extremity spasticity when impeding function, causing pain, disturbing sleep, interfering with other therapies, or for cosmetic purposes (National Guideline Alliance, 2012) Effective and generally safe (Delgado, 2010; Esquenazi et al., 2013) Green light ("Effective, do it") rating (Novak et al., 2013)
Phenol, alcohol, or botulinum toxin type B			Insufficient data (Delgado et al., 2010) Yellow light ("Uncertain effect; measure outcomes for progress") rating (Novak et al., 2013) (alcohol and phenol)
Therapy-based interventions			
Serial casting	Local/segmental	-	Ankles: Green light ("Effective, do it") rating Elsewhere: Yellow light ("Uncertain effect; measure outcomes for progress") rating (Novak et al., 2013)
Orthotics (e.g., AFOs)	Local/segmental	-	Yellow light ("Uncertain effect; measure outcomes for progress") rating (Novak et al., 2013)
Hip bracing	Local/segmental	-	Red light ("Ineffective, don't do it") rating (Novak et al., 2013)

Constraint-induced movement therapy, bimanual training, context-focused therapy, goal-directed/functional training, occupational therapy following botulin toxin injection, home programs for improving motor activity performance and/or self-care	Local/segmental	-	Green light ("Effective, do it") rating (Novak et al., 2013)
Craniosacral therapy, neurodevelopmental therapy, sensory integration			Red light ("Ineffective, don't do it") rating (Novak et al., 2013)
Invasive interventions			
Intrathecal baclofen pump	General	Reversible	"Consider" if persistent difficulties with pain/spasms, posture, function, or ease of care despite noninvasive treatments (National Guideline Alliance, 2012) Yellow light ("Uncertain effect; measure outcomes for progress") rating (Novak et al., 2013)
Orthopedic surgery	Local/segmental	Permanent	"Consider" as an adjunct if concerns regarding hip displacement or spinal deformity to prevent deterioration and improve function (National Guideline Alliance, 2012)
Selective dorsal rhizotomy	Local/segmental	Permanent	"Consider" to improve walking in young people with spasticity and GMFCS II or III (National Guideline Alliance, 2012) Green light ("Effective, do it") rating (Novak et al., 2013)

BOX 21.2 INTERDISCIPLINARY CARE

The Role of the Physical Therapist

In the team approach of caring for children with cerebral palsy (CP), the role of the physical therapist (PT) includes performing a full examination of every body system related to the control of movement, seating/positioning, and mobility. For children with CP, this examination may have a different focus for infants, school-age children, teens, and adults. Routine musculoskeletal examination with specialized examination methods may be applied to determine needs for seating, positioning, gait or standing assistive devices, bracing, and mobility systems such as wheelchairs. The PT's assessment leads to establishing a plan of care with achievable goals.

Common goals of the physical therapist in management of the child with CP		
Examination	Assessment	Treatment
Determining the presence and severity of gross motor delays	Determining a prognosis as it relates to movement, positioning, and mobility	Prescribing bracing, seating or mobility equipment, and adaptive equipment
Determining if movement patterns are typical or impaired	Infants and toddlers: Providing direct services, treatment, and consultation/education	Providing consultative services to child/family, medical team, or program
Contributing to classification (e.g., Gross Motor Function Classification System—Expanded and Revised (GMFCS–E&R; Palisano, Cameron, Rosenbaum, Walter, & Russell, 2006)	School PT: Helping the child gain access to education and social development in school and contributing to the individualized education program (IEP)	Education: Training parents, family, caregivers, and assistants in performing home programs or in implementing aspects of IEP
Screening: Identifying risks, need for preventive intervention, or need for referral to other providers	In some medical settings, the PT consults both the child and the medical team	Prevention: Identifying risk for developing secondary complications of CP and intervening to prevent or manage complications or reduce risk
Monitoring change over time or in response to an intervention		Discharge planning: Determining need for ongoing PT, monitoring needs, and referring to other necessary services or providers

trihexyphenidyl (Artane), have been found to be beneficial for some children with dyskinetic forms of CP (Mink & Zinner, 2009).

Although some specialists prefer trihexyphenidyl, others have reported benefits with levodopa. The medications most commonly used to control spasticity and rigidity are diazepam, baclofen, and dantrolene. Diazepam and its derivative compounds, lorazepam and clonazepam, affect brain control of muscle tone, beginning within 30 minutes after ingestion and lasting about 4 hours. Withdrawal of these drugs should be gradual as physical dependency can develop. Side effects include drowsiness and excessive drooling, which may interfere with feeding and speech. As a result of these side effects, they are less commonly used than oral baclofen.

Baclofen, a GABA B-receptor agonist, was initially used to treat adults with multiple sclerosis and traumatic damage to the spinal cord. It is now commonly used in CP clinics around the world. In children with CP, the most common side effects of the oral form of the medication are drowsiness, nausea, headache, and low blood pressure. About 10% of children treated with baclofen experience side effects that are unpleasant enough to necessitate discontinuation of the medication. Care must be taken when stopping the medication to gradually taper it, as rapid withdrawal can lead to severe side effects, including hallucinations.

Dantrolene works on muscle cells directly, as a calcium channel blocker, to inhibit their contraction. Side effects include drowsiness, muscle weakness, and increased drooling. A rare adverse effect of this drug is severe liver damage, so liver function tests should be performed periodically. Because of this side effect, this medication is used with decreasing frequency.

Although a discussion of the range of side effects associated with oral medications is beyond the scope of this chapter, several generalizations can be made. For example, some medications have easily recognizable side effects, such as sedation from diazepam and seizures from acute baclofen withdrawal. Others may be more subtle, such as cognitive or personality changes with trihexyphenidyl (Carranza-del Rio, Clegg, Moore, & Delgado, 2011).

Periodic drug "holidays" should be considered to determine whether benefits are persistent. As always, clinicians should listen carefully to parental or caregiver concerns about any changes in their children after medication initiation.

Neurosurgical Procedures Intrathecal baclofen is a therapeutic modality that allows for the direct delivery of baclofen into the spinal fluid (i.e., intrathecal) space, where it can inhibit motor nerve conduction at the level of the spinal cord (Disabato & Ritchie, 2003; Fitzgerald, Tsegaye, & Vloeberghs, 2004; Tilton, 2004). A disk-shaped pump is placed under the skin of the abdomen, and a catheter is tunneled below the skin around to the back, where it is inserted through the lumbar spine into the intrathecal space. Baclofen is stored in a reservoir in the disk that can be refilled, and the medication is delivered at a continuous rate that is computer controlled and adjustable. Because the drug is delivered directly to its site of action (the cerebrospinal fluid), a much lower dosage can be used, with a resultant reduced risk of side effects. Improvements in ease of care and comfort are commonly reported. Although functional gains in lower extremity, upper extremity, and even oral/motor function have been observed (Fitzgerald et al., 2004), clear improvements in ambulatory individuals has not been demonstrated (Pin, McCartney, Lewis, & Waugh, 2011). The main disadvantages of intrathecal baclofen are hypotonia (low muscle tone), increased seizures in individuals with known epilepsy, sleepiness, and nausea/vomiting (Gilmartin et al., 2000). Complications related to mechanical failures and infection and the need for intensive and reliable medical follow-up are also significant considerations (Murphy, Irwin, & Hoff, 2002).

Selective dorsal rhizotomy (SDR) is a procedure that reduces spasticity by interrupting the sensory component of the deep tendon reflex, which is exaggerated in children with spastic forms of CP. The surgery reduces spasticity permanently in the legs but not in the arms, so its use is confined mainly to children with spastic diplegia who have good antigravity strength. Although uncertainty exists in regard to long-term functional outcomes in children who undergo this procedure (Koman et al., 2004; Tedroff, Löwing, Jacobson, & Åströmn, 2011), other recent reports have been more encouraging in this regard (Engsberg, Ross, Collins, & Park, 2006; Langerak et al., 2009).

Deep brain stimulation (DBS) is a neurosurgical procedure involving the implantation of a neurostimulator and electrodes that send electrical impulses into brain structures, including the basal ganglia. The impulses are calibrated by an experienced neurologist or technician. While effects are directly mediated by electrical axonal stimulation, there may be additional secondary effects on synaptic plasticity (Herrington, Cheng, & Eskandar, 2016). With careful patient selection, DBS is a promising intervention for children with dyskinetic CP, although improvements are more dramatic in children with genetic forms of dystonia (such as those with DYT1 mutations; Air, Ostrem, Sanger, & Starr, 2011; Elia et al., 2018; Fehlings et al., 2018).

Orthopedic Procedures

Because of the abnormal or asymmetrical distribution of muscle tone, children with CP are susceptible to the development of joint deformities. The most common of these result from permanent shortening or contracture of one or more groups of muscles around a joint, which limits joint mobility. Orthopedic surgery is done to increase the range of motion by lengthening a tendon, cutting through muscle or tendon (release), or moving the point of attachment of a tendon on bone. For example, a partial release or transfer of hyperactive hip adductor muscles (which cause scissoring of the legs) may improve the child's ability to sit and walk and may lessen the chances of a hip dislocation (Hägglund et al., 2005; Stott, Piedrahita, & American Academy for Cerebral Palsy and Developmental Medicine, 2004). A partial hamstring release, involving the lengthening or transfer of muscles around the knee, also may facilitate sitting and walking. A lengthening of the Achilles tendon at the ankle improves toe walking (Figure 21.17).

More complicated orthopedic procedures may be required for correction of a dislocated hip. If this is diagnosed when there is a partial dislocation (called subluxation), release of the hip adductor muscles alone can be effective (Figure 21.18). If the head of the femur (the thigh bone) is dislocated more than one third to one half of the way out of a hip joint socket, a more complex procedure called a varus derotational osteotomy may be necessary. In this operation, the angle of the femur is changed surgically to place the head of the femur back into the hip socket (Figure 21.19). In some cases, the hip socket also must be reshaped to ensure that the hip joint remains functional. Sometimes muscle releases or lengthening are performed at the same time as these procedures.

For ambulatory children with CP, deciding which type of surgery is most likely to improve function is a complex issue. Computerized gait analysis conducted prior to surgical intervention has become increasingly common as an aid in the decision-making process. Precise measurements obtained through motion analysis, force plates, and electromyography offer detailed information relating to specific abnormalities at each lower extremity joint as well as the muscle activity that controls motion through all phases of the gait (Cook, Schneider, Hazlewood, Hillman, & Robb, 2003). Preoperative gait analysis helps to determine exactly which procedures are likely to be successful. Postoperative analysis can provide an objective measure of outcome.

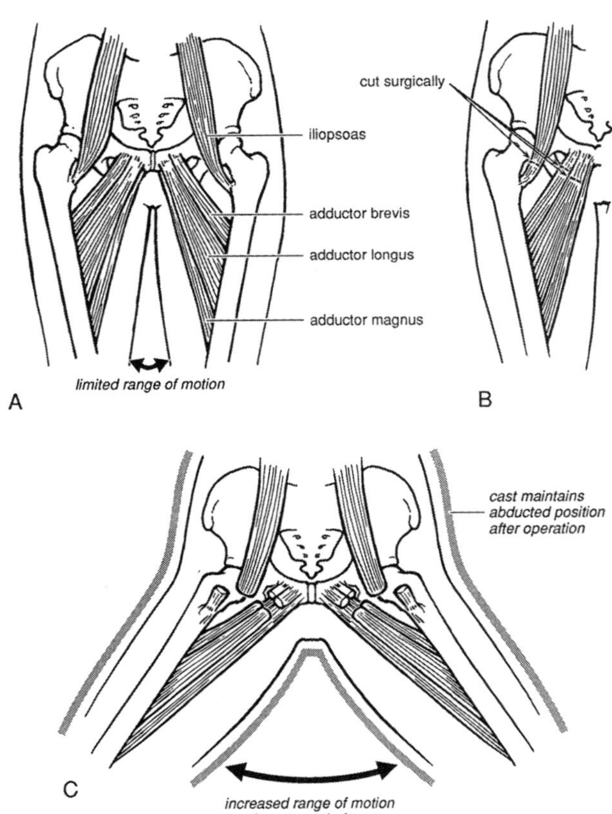

Figure 21.18. Adductor tenotomy. This operation is done to improve scissoring (Figure 24.11) and to prevent hip dislocation caused by contractures of the adductor muscles in the thigh. A) In this procedure, the iliopsoas, adductor brevis, and adductor longus muscles are cut, leaving the adductor magnus intact. B) The child is then placed in a cast for 6–8 weeks to maintain a more open (abducted) position. C) The muscles eventually grow together in a lengthened position, allowing improved sitting and/or walking.

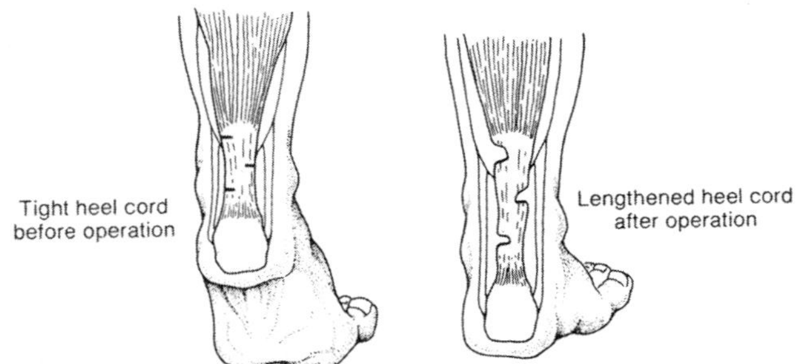

Figure 21.17. Achilles tendon lengthening operation. When the heel cord is tight, the child walks on his or her toes. Surgery lengthens the heel cord and permits a more flat-footed gait.

Scoliosis: Conventional Rods vs. Magnetic Controlled Growing Rods In addition to treating contractures and dislocations, orthopedic surgeons are involved in the treatment of scoliosis (progressive curvature of the spine). Treatment of significant scoliosis

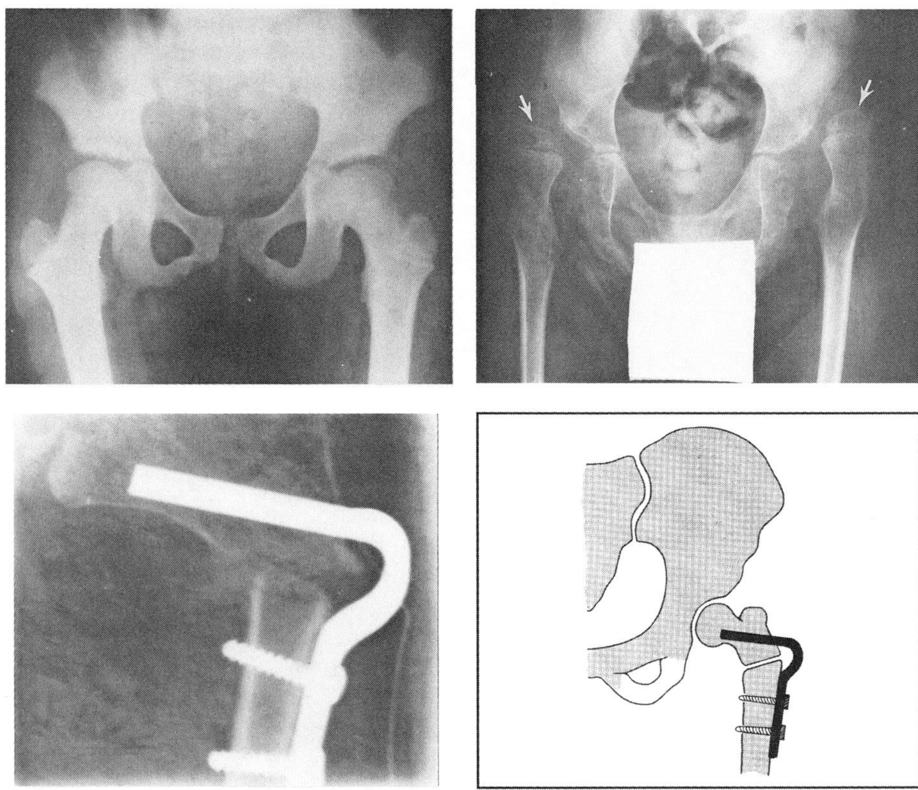

Figure 21.19. Dislocation of the hip. The upper x-rays (frontal view) show a normal hip (left x-ray) and a hip dislocated on both sides (right x-ray). The arrows indicate the points of dislocation. The lower pictures show the results of a varus derotational osteotomy to correct the left-hip dislocation. The femur has been cut and realigned so that it now fits into the hip socket. Pins, which are later removed, hold the bone in place until it heals.

ranges from a molded plastic jacket or a chair insert to surgery that straightens the spine as much as possible.

Children with CP are at increased risk of developing scoliosis, which can lead to medical complications including pulmonary and cardiac sequelae and difficulty with positioning, which can cause pain and secondary skin breakdown. The deformity can also affect the young person's self-esteem. For a number of years orthopedic surgical intervention has involved the placement of spinal rods with fusion of the vertebrae to straighten the spine (Figure 21.20). In the young child who is still growing, this approach requires repeated operations given linear growth over time.

Self-lengthening rods (magnetic controlled growing rods) have been developed for children under 10 years of age with severe spinal curves. These rods allow for vertical growth and correct the spinal deformity. Once placed, these rods can be lengthened noninvasively with an external magnetic device. However, even these rods are not permanent and require replacement as the child grows. As such, they are only beneficial for children too young for spinal fusion. It should also be recognized that this is a new surgical technique—so a precise long term risk-benefit ratio has not yet been determined.

Complementary Health Approaches

When conventional approaches do not lead to the anticipated improvements, families may explore other treatment options, including complementary health approaches (often called complementary and alternative medicine; Oppenheim, 2009; see Chapter 39).

Complementary health approaches includes acupuncture, craniosacral therapy, myofascial release, therapeutic taping, diet and herbal remedies, electrical stimulation, chiropractic treatments, massage, and hyperbaric oxygen therapy. Although there are individual reports and testimonials of dramatic improvements with various alternative therapies, some carry significant risks. Furthermore, rigorous studies have not been conducted to assess efficacy. As with any

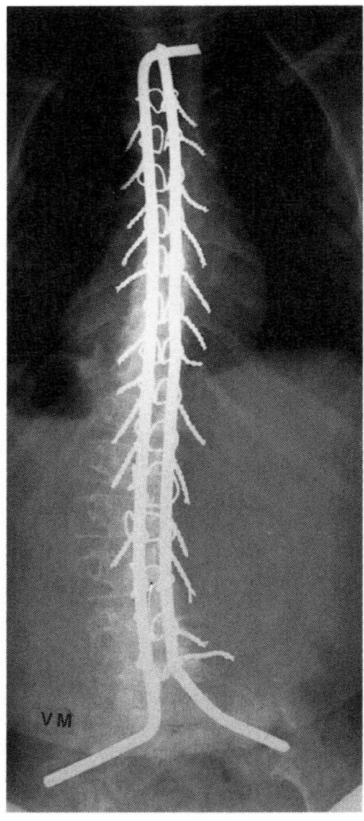

Figure 21.20. Treatment of scoliosis may require spinal fusion. This x-ray shows improved scoliosis following a Luque procedure. During this surgery, the position of the spine is improved using metal hooks, rods, and wires, while bone graft material fuses the spine in position.

treatment, families and clinicians should consider cost, efficacy, and potential side effects before embarking on one of these approaches.

Transition into Adulthood

Adolescence is a critical time in life for all individuals, but for teenagers with CP there are additional challenges (Wood, Kantor, Edwards, & James, 2008). There is the need to transition from pediatric health care providers to those who manage CP in adults, and there are job training, employment, social, recreation, housing, and insurance considerations that require careful planning (see Chapter 40).

Adult Outcomes

Adults with CP are living longer and leading more independent lives than in the past as a result of new treatment options. However, they face challenges, including medical care, accessibility, and vocational opportunities (Tosi, Maher, Moore, Goldstein, & Aisen, 2009; Watson, Parr, Joyce, May, & Le Couteur, 2011).

Although medical care is well established for children with CP, it is more fragmented for adults (Turk, 2009). Adults with CP should look for practitioners who are experienced in the care of chronic disorders and who can provide the additional time that may be required for evaluation. They also need to recognize the importance of preventive care and report any changes in neurological function, as this may represent new impairments secondary to the underlying motor disorder. Adults with CP identify pain as a significant problem and should be encouraged to seek medical care in this circumstance (Vogtle, 2009).

Mobility and the ability to perform activities of daily living should be carefully monitored because some adults experience slow declines over time. Individuals should be provided with instruction in practical matters, such as hiring quality personal aides and caregivers, as well as in self-advocacy and seeking employment opportunities when able.

Although most children with CP will live to adulthood, their projected life expectancy may be less than that of the general population (Hemming, Hutton, Colver, & Platt, 2005; Katz, 2003). For example, an individual with hemiplegic CP probably will have a typical life span, whereas a person with spastic quadriplegia may not live beyond age 40 because of respiratory and nutritional issues (Strauss & Shavelle, 2001). Children with very severe impairments, measured in terms of functional characteristics, have the poorest outcome. Children who cannot lift their heads and are fed via gastrostomy tube may not survive to adulthood (Strauss, Shavelle, & Anderson, 1998).

Excess mortality for people with CP may also be related to comorbid risks such as seizures and aspiration, as well as an increased risk for breast cancer, brain tumors, and circulatory and digestive diseases, most likely related to inadequate medical screening (Murphy, 2010). Unintentional injury rates (e.g., falls) for people with CP are also higher than in the general population (Cooley & American Academy of Pediatrics, 2004; Strauss, Cable, & Shavelle, 1999).

Motor skills and mobility may not be the primary determinant of societal independence; personal characteristics, health status, and environmental factors will also factor into an outcome (Liptak & Accardo, 2004). In fact, the ability to successfully participate in society may be more strongly related to intellectual and interpersonal strengths than to physical abilities. Although approximately one half of individuals with CP have typical intelligence, most still have difficulty leading completely typical lives. This may result from factors ranging from family support and quality of educational programs to availability of community-based training and technical support (Murphy, Molnar, & Lankasky, 1995; Russman & Gage, 1989). In one study of young adults with CP (van der Dussen, Nieuwstraten, Roebroeck, & Stam, 2001), 53% of individuals had some form of secondary education but only 36% subsequently engaged in paid employment. It is hoped that these figures will improve as a result of federal mandates (e.g., the Americans with Disabilities Act of 1990) that define the rights of people with disabilities and are gradually making inroads into societal perceptions of disability. Ultimately, strengthening support to families (Raina et al., 2005), providing ready access to quality medical care, improving special education services, increasing opportunities for employment, and changing attitudes about disabilities in society at large may do as much for children with CP as traditional therapeutic and medical interventions.

ADVOCACY AND AWARENESS

"Nothing about us without us" is a term that is widely utilized to express the belief that the stakeholders should be involved in the decisions that are made about them. In the disability world, this was elegantly expressed by James Charlton in his classic book, *Nothing About Us Without Us: Disability Oppression and Empowerment,* in which he discusses both the problems that people with disabilities face and the solutions in regard to self-determination (Charlton, 2000).

One of the most powerful means to promote self-determination is through social media, which is a collection of computer-mediated tools that promote communication through networks and virtual communities whereby people with similar interests can communicate with each other. It is a powerful way for individuals to share information about common interests. By facilitating communication, these networks can reduce feelings of isolation and provide a means for people to discuss sensitive problems with which only others with similar concerns can relate.

Benefits include a wide audience reach and real-time interactivity and immediacy. With the advent of easily accessible, web-based information on CP diagnosis, management, and care, individuals with CP and their families now have the ability to communicate more freely and participate more actively in medical and rehabilitative decision making and care. There are a number of sites that provide factual information of benefit in this regard. One good example of this is the web site Cerebral Palsy Foundation (http://yourcpf.org/), which provides fact sheets, expert commentaries, resources, videos, news, and blogs.

FUTURE DIRECTIONS

Although advances for individuals with CP never come as quickly as needed or wanted, the future offers hope in a number of areas. These include opportunities for collaborative research, translating basic science into cutting-edge treatments, improved early diagnosis, and improved care in the transition from childhood to adulthood.

Cerebral Palsy Collaborative Research

One of the most encouraging developments is the ongoing work of the international collaboration of centers ("surveillance programs") dedicated to the care of children with CP through the use of registers and surveillance. Currently there are nearly 40 surveillance programs worldwide (Goldsmith et al., 2016). The first large network established in 1998 was the Surveillance for Cerebral Palsy in Europe, now consisting of 24 centers in 20 countries, whose goals are to use epidemiologic data to monitor trends in care, to improve understanding of cause, to promote dissemination of knowledge, and to facilitate research (http://www.scpenetwork.eu/en/cerebral-palsy/). Other groups, including the Australian Cerebral Palsy Register (ACPR), utilize country-wide data to study epidemiology and causes as well as plan for current and future prevention and service provision needs (Australian Cerebral Palsy Register, 2016). In the United States, the Metropolitan Atlanta Developmental Disabilities Surveillance Program has been of great benefit in providing data on CP, as well as intellectual disability, hearing impairment, visual impairment, and autism spectrum disorder (Avchen, Bhasin, & Yeargin-Allsopp, 2006).

Similarly, national collaborative efforts to merge large multicenter data sets for future research will contribute to the advancement of knowledge, including better understanding of variations in clinical care and treatment effect for individuals with CP. The emerging CP Research Network (CPRN) is a new collaborative network of participating CP centers. A core project of CPRN is to develop a U.S.-based CP clinical registry to support future research questions and quality initiatives (CPRN, 2018). Overall, by looking at populations more than individuals, trends can be characterized and large data sets analyzed to create generalizable knowledge.

CP research has been limited in the past by small studies with lack of reproducible results. The recent publication of CP common data elements (CDEs) and outcome measures for children and young people with CP will standardize data collection and assessment. Routine use of these CP CDEs across clinical studies and clinical practice will increase data quality and data sharing, accelerate meta-analysis of studies and clinical trials across centers, and increase the generalizability of results and translation of evidence within clinical practice (NINDS Common Data Elements, 2018; Schiariti et al., 2018).

There is exciting ongoing research targeting brain injury in the high-risk infant, both those that are born preterm and those born at term with HIE. Emerging information has shown that brain cooling for 3 days decreases the risk of death or severe disability in term infants with HIE by a variety of mechanisms, including reducing the metabolic demand of brain cells, reducing inflammation, and decreasing cell death. Current guidelines stop short of recommending widespread adoption of therapeutic hypothermia but focus on maintaining consistent comprehensive care when it is offered (Committee on Fetus and Newborn, 2014). In practice, the use of therapeutic hypothermia is guided by clinical judgment and the specifics of the clinical setting, especially the degree of encephalopathy and hypoxia. Erythropoietin, a cytokine with evidence of neuroprotection in animal models, is also being tested in both preterm and term high-risk infants (Rangarajan & Juul, 2014).

In addition, a promising new therapy for CP secondary to perinatal brain injury is nanomedicine-based treatment. Nanomaterials such as dendrimers, which are very small globular molecules, can provide a vehicle to deliver drugs directly to brain cells that are subject to neuroinflammation and injury. In this way, drugs such as N-acetyl cysteine can potentially be used to promote brain repair and regeneration, hopefully decreasing brain cell injury and enabling typical growth. Currently this is in the research realm and is not used to treat infants (Balakrishnan, Nance, Johnston, Kannan, & Kannan, 2013).

The introduction and now widespread use of advanced genetic testing, including chromosomal microarray and whole-exome sequencing, has provided families and providers etiologic information leading to better prevention, treatment, and family counseling (see Chapter 1). Some of these disorders act through specific genetic mechanisms, while others may predispose infants to acute perinatal events at the time of labor and delivery. Advanced knowledge in this regard can be of benefit in planning for delivery and future pregnancies.

Inborn errors of metabolism (IEMs) are individually rare but collectively common group of genetic diseases with abnormal metabolic pathways, leading to abnormal accumulation of substances and/or reduced ability to make essential compounds with presentations that often mimic CP (see Chapter 16). Effective treatment of IEMs can either be primary or improve function or stabilizing by preventing or slowing further brain injury (Leach, Shevell, Bowden, Stockler-Ipsiroglu, & van Karnebeek, 2014).

Bioengineering advances, especially in robotics, demonstrate promise toward improving function and mobility in children with CP. The field of pediatric neurorehabilitation has rapidly evolved with technological advancements in rehabilitation robotics and computer-assisted systems. For example, preliminary research shows that lower extremity robotic exoskeletons improve crouch gait and may help maintain mobility in children with CP as they age (Lerner, Damiano, & Bulea, 2016).

Advances in Clinical Care

A number of studies and reviews support the importance of CP-specific early intervention to neuroplasticity and prevention of deleterious musculoskeletal outcomes (Novak et al., 2017). Early interventions that focus on task-specific motor training (e.g., constraint-induced therapy) maximize functional gains and are the new paradigm of care. Beginning therapy for infants and young children with developmental delay has been a longstanding belief of families and professionals alike, and there is now a growing body of evidence supporting the principles and long-term benefits of early intervention (Novak et al., 2017). Emerging innovative approaches include tele-rehabilitative tools, combining home-based, goal-directed, task-specific interventions that are fun and motivational with remote monitoring and structuring by therapists and with active parental involvement (Sgandurra et al., 2017).

Opportunities for work, social, and community participation of individuals with disabilities including CP have increased as individuals and families have become self-empowered and more visibly engaged in society. From the professional's perspective, it is very important to "meet people where they are" and address their concerns with recommendations for care as a way to meet their goals. For the person with CP, a partnership with the professional is of tantamount importance to establish and promote goals and outcomes desired by the individual.

SUMMARY

- Cerebral palsy represents a group of chronic motor disorders that result from malformation or injury of the developing brain.
- The impairments associated with CP are variable and nonprogressive, but permanent. These impairments lead to varying degrees of disability that are related to functional mobility, daily living skills, and communication-socialization skills.

- Effective management requires an interdisciplinary strategy that seeks to maximize function and opportunity. Efforts founded on the principles that are articulated in federal legislation will create new opportunities for greater participation and enhanced quality of life for individuals with CP.
- New treatment modalities offer improved quality of life and educational opportunities. The challenge is to provide these opportunities in a changing medical environment, where a premium is not always placed on coordination of care.

ADDITIONAL RESOURCES

CP Resource Center: http://www.cpparent.org

United Cerebral Palsy: http://www.ucp.org

American Academy for Cerebral Palsy and Developmental Medicine (AACPDM): http://www.aacpdm.org/

Additional resources can be found online in Appendix D: Childhood Disabilities Resources, Services, and Organizations (see About the Online Companion Materials).

REFERENCES

Aarts, P. B., Jongerius, P. H., Geerdink, Y. A., van Limbeek, J., & Geurts, A. C. (2010). Effectiveness of modified constraint-induced movement therapy in children with unilateral spastic cerebral palsy: A randomized controlled trial. *Neurorehabilitation and Neural Repair, 24*(6), 509–518.

Accardo, P. J. (1989). William John Little and cerebral palsy in the nineteenth century. *Journal of the History of Medicine and Allied Science, 44*(1), 56–71.

Accardo, J., Kammann, H., & Hoon, A. H., Jr. (2004). Neuroimaging in cerebral palsy. *The Journal of Pediatrics, 145*(Suppl. 2), S19–S27.

Air, E. L., Ostrem, J. L., Sanger, T. D., & Starr, P. A. (2011). Deep brain stimulation in children: Experience and technical pearls. *Journal of Neurosurgery: Pediatrics, 8*(6), 566–574.

Americans with Disabilities Act of 1990, 42 U.S.C. §§ 12101 *et seq*.

Ancel, P. Y., Livinec, F., Larroque, B., Marret, S., Arnaud, C., Pierrat, V., . . . the EPIPAGE Study Group. (2006). Cerebral palsy among very preterm children in relation to gestational age and neonatal ultrasound abnormalities: The EPIPAGE cohort study. *Pediatrics, 117*(3), 828–835.

Aneja, S. (2004). Evaluation of a child with cerebral palsy. *Indian Journal of Pediatrics, 71*(7), 627–634.

Ashwal, S., Russman, B. S., Blasco, P. A., Miller, G., Sandler, A., Shevell, M., & Stevenson, R. (2004). Practice parameter: Diagnostic assessment of the child with cerebral palsy: Report of the Quality Standards Subcommittee of the American Academy of Neurology and the Practice Committee of the Child Neurology Society. *Neurology, 62*(6), 851–863.

Australian Cerebral Palsy Register. (2016). Report of the Australian Cerebral Palsy Register report. Retrieved from https://www.cpregister.com/pubs/pdf/ACPR-Report_Web_2016.pdf

Avchen, R. N., Bhasin, T. K., & Yeargin-Allsopp, M. (2006). Public health impact: Metropolitan Atlanta developmental disabilities surveillance program. *International Review of Research in Mental Retardation, 33*, 149–190.

Balakrishnan, B., Nance, E., Johnston, M. V., Kannan, R., & Kannan, S. (2013). Nanomedicine in cerebral palsy. *International Journal of Nanomedicine, 8*, 4183–4195. doi:10.2147/IJN.S35979

Bale, J. F. (2009). Fetal infections and brain development. *Clinical Perinatology, 36*(3), 639–653.

Barkovich, J. A. (2005). *Pediatric neuroimaging* (4th ed.). Philadelphia, PA: Lippincott Williams & Wilkins.

Barks, J. D. (2008). Current controversies in hypothermic protection. *Seminars in Fetal and Neonatal Medicine, 13*(1), 30–34.

Barnes, M. P., & Johnson, G. R. (2008). *Upper motor neuron syndrome and spasticity*. Cambridge, England: Cambridge University Press.

Bax, M., Goldstein, M., Rosenbaum, P., Leviton, A., Paneth, N., Dan, B., . . . Executive Committee for the Definition of Cerebral Palsy. (2005). Proposed definition and classification of cerebral palsy, April 2005. *Developmental Medicine and Child Neurology, 47*(8), 571–576.

Bruer, J. (2011). *Revisiting 'the myth of the first three years.'* Canterbury, England: Centre for Parenting Culture Studies, Kent University.

Campbell, S. K., Palisano, R. J., & Orlin, M. N. (2012). *Physical therapy for children* (4th ed.). St. Louis, MO: Elsevier/Saunders.

Cans, C., Dolk, H., Platt, M. J., Colver, A., Prasausklene, A., & Rägeloh-Mann, I. K. (2007). Recommendations from the SCPE collaborative group for defining and classifying cerebral palsy. *Developmental Medicine & Child Neurology, 49*(s109), 35–38.

Carlsson, M., Hagberg, G., & Olsson, I. (2003). Clinical and aetiological aspects of epilepsy in children with cerebral palsy. *Developmental Medicine and Child Neurology, 45*(6), 371–376.

Carranza-del Rio, J., Clegg, N. J., Moore, A., & Delgado, M. R. (2011). Use of trihexyphenidyl in children with cerebral palsy. *Pediatric Neurology, 44*(3), 202–206.

Cerebral Palsy Research Network. (2018). *Cerebral palsy research*. Retrieved from http://cprn.org/cerebral-palsy-research/

Charlton, J. I. 2000. *Nothing About Us Without Us: Disability Oppression and Empowerment*. Oakland, CA: University of California Press.

Christensen, D., Van Naarden Braun, K., Doernberg, N. S., Maenner, M. J., Arneson, C. L., Durkin, M. S., . . . Yeargin-Allsopp, M. (2014). Prevalence of cerebral palsy, co-occurring autism spectrum disorders, and motor functioning–Autism and Developmental Disabilities Monitoring Network, USA, 2008. *Developmental Medicine & Child Neurology, 56*(1), 59–65.

Colver, A., Fairhurst, C., & Pharoah, O. D. (2014). Cerebral palsy. *The Lancet, 383*(9924), 1240–1249.

Committee on Fetus and Newborn. (2014). Hypothermia and neonatal encephalopathy. *Pediatrics, 133*(6), 1146–1150.

Cook, R. E., Schneider, I., Hazlewood, M. E., Hillman, S. J., & Robb, J. E. (2003). Gait analysis alters decision-making in cerebral palsy. *Journal of Pediatric Orthopedics, 23*(3), 292–295.

Cooley, W. C., & American Academy of Pediatrics Committee on Children with Disabilities. (2004). Providing a primary care medical home for children and youth with cerebral palsy. *Pediatrics, 114*(4), 1106–1113.

CP Family Network. (2012). *WE MOVE: Worldwide education and awareness for movement disorders.* Retrieved from http://cpfamilynetwork.org/resources/we-move-worldwide-education-awareness-for-movement-disorders/

Cramer, S. C., Sur, M., Dobkin, B. H., O'Brien, C., Sanger, T. D., Trojanowski, J. Q., . . . Vinogradov, S. (2011). Harnessing neuroplasticity for clinical applications. *Brain, 134*(Pt. 6), 1591–1609.

Delgado, M. R., Hirtz, D., Aisen, M., Ashwal, S., Fehlings, D. L., McLaughlin, J., . . . Vargus-Adams, J. (2010). Practice parameter: Pharmacologic treatment of spasticity in children and adolescents with cerebral palsy (an evidence-based review): Report of the Quality Standards Subcommittee of the American Academy of Neurology and the Practice Committee of the Child Neurology Society. *Neurology, 7*(4), 336–343.

Disabato, J., & Ritchie, A. (2003). Intrathecal baclofen for the treatment of spasticity of cerebral origin. *Journal for Specialists in Pediatric Nursing, 8*(1), 31–34.

Douglas-Escobar, M., & Weiss, M. D. (2015). Hypoxic-ischemic encephalopathy: A review for the clinician. *JAMA Pediatrics, 169*(4), 397–403.

Einspieler, C., & Prechtl, H. F. (2005). Prechtl's assessment of General Movements: A diagnostic tool for the functional assessment of the young nervous system. *Mental Retardation and Developmental Disabilities Research Reviews,* 11(1), 61–67.

Einspieler, C., Bos, A. F., Libertus, M. E., & Marschik, P. B. (2016). The General Movement Assessment helps us to identify preterm infants at risk for cognitive dysfunction. *Frontiers in Psychology, 7,* 406.

Elia, A. E., Bagella, C. F., Ferré, F., Zorzi, G., Calandrella, D., & Romito, L. M. (2018). Deep brain stimulation for dystonia due to cerebral palsy: A review. *European Journal of Paediatric Neurology, 22*(2), 308–315. doi:10.1016/j.ejpn.2017.12.002

Eliasson, A., Krumlinde-Sundholm, L., Rösblad, B., Beckung, E., Arner, M., Ohrvall, A., & Rosenbaum, P. (2006). The Manual Ability Classification System (MACS) for children with cerebral palsy: Scale development and evidence of validity and reliability. *Developmental Medicine and Child Neurology, 48*(7), 549–554.

Eliasson, A., Ullenhag, A., Wahlström, U., & Krumlinde-Sundholm, L. (2017). Mini-MACS: Development of the Manual Ability Classification System for children younger than 4 years of age with signs of cerebral palsy. *Developmental Medicine and Child Neurology,* 59(1), 72–78.

Engsberg, J. R., Ross, S. A., Collins, D. R., & Park, T. S. (2006). Effect of selective dorsal rhizotomy in the treatment of children with cerebral palsy. *Journal of Neurosurgery, 105*(Suppl. 1), 8–15.

Esquenazi, A., Albanese, A., Chancellor, M. B., Elovic, E., Segal, K. R., Simpson, D. M., . . . Ward, A. B. (2013). Evidence-based review and assessment of botulinum neurotoxin for the treatment of adult spasticity in the upper motor neuron syndrome. *Toxicon, 67,* 115–128.

Eunson, P. (2012). Aetiology and epidemiology of cerebral palsy. *Paediatrics and Child Health, 22*(9), 361–366.

Fahey, M. C., Maclennan, A. H., Kretzschmar, D., Gecz, J., & Kruer, M. C. (2017). The genetic basis of cerebral palsy. *Developmental Medicine and Child Neurology, 59*(5), 462–469.

Fehlings, D. (2017). Pain in cerebral palsy: a neglected comorbidity. *Developmental Medicine & Child Neurology, 59*(8), 782–783.

Fehlings, D., Brown, L., Harvey, A., Himmelmann, K., Lin, J. P., Macintosh, A., . . . Walters, I. (2018). Pharmacological and neurosurgical interventions for managing dystonia in cerebral palsy: A systematic review. *Developmental Medicine & Child Neurology, 60*(4), 356–366. doi:10.1111/dmcn.13652

Fitzgerald, J. J., Tsegaye, M., & Vloeberghs, M. H. (2004). Treatment of childhood spasticity of cerebral origin with intrathecal baclofen: A series of 52 cases. *British Journal of Neurosurgery, 18*(3), 240–245.

Freud, S. (1968). *Infantile cerebral paralysis.* Coral Gables, FL: University of Miami Press (original work published in 1897).

Galiza, E. P., & Heath, P. T. (2009). Improving the outcome of neonatal meningitis. *Current Opinion in Infectious Disease, 22*(3), 229–234.

General Movements Trust. (2009). *Prechtl's Method on the Qualitative Assessment of General Movements.* Retrieved from www.general-movements-trust.info

George, J. M., Pannek, K., Rose, S. E., Ware, R. S., Colditz, P. B., & Boyd, R. N. (2017). Diagnostic accuracy of early magnetic resonance imaging to determine motor outcomes in infants born preterm: a systematic review and meta-analysis. *Developmental Medicine & Child Neurology, 60*(2), 134–146.

Gilmartin, R., Bruce, D., Storrs, B. B., Abbott, R., Krach, L., Ward, J., . . . Nadell, J. (2000). Intrathecal baclofen for management of spastic cerebral palsy: Multicenter trial. *Journal of Child Neurology, 15*(2), 71–77.

Gladstone, M. (2010). A review of the incidence and prevalence, types and aetiology of childhood cerebral palsy in resource-poor settings. *Annals of Tropical Paediatrics, 30*(3), 181–196.

Glanzman, A. M., Kim, H., Swaminathan, K., & Beck, T. (2004). Efficacy of botulinum toxin A, serial casting, and combined treatment for spastic equinus: A retrospective analysis. *Developmental Medicine and Child Neurology, 46*(12), 807–811.

Goldsmith, S., McIntyre, S., Smithers-Sheedy, H., Blair, E., Cans, C., Watson, L., & Yeargin-Allsopp, M. (2016). An international survey of cerebral palsy registers and surveillance systems. *Developmental Medicine & Child Neurology, 58*(S2), 11–17.

Gordon, N. (1999). The role of botulinum toxin type A in treatment—with special reference to children. *Brain & Development, 21*(3), 147–151.

Guzzetta, A., Mercuri, E., & Cioni, G. (2001). Visual disorders in children with brain lesions: 2. Visual impairment associated with cerebral palsy. *European Journal of Paediatric Neurology, 5*(3), 115–119.

Hagberg, B., Hagberg, G., Beckung, E., & Ubrevant, P. (2001). Changing panorama of cerebral palsy in Sweden. VIII. Prevalence and origin in the birth-year period 1991–94. *Acta Paediatrica, 90*(3), 271–277.

Hagberg, H., Mallard, C., Ferriero, D. M., Vannucci, S. J., Levison, S. W., Vexler, Z. S., & Gressens, P. (2015). The role of inflammation in perinatal brain injury. *Nature Reviews Neurology, 11*(4), 192.

Hägglund, G., Andersson, S., Düppe, H., Lauge-Pedersen, H., Nordmark, E., & Westbom, L. (2005). Prevention of dislocation of the hip in children with cerebral palsy: The first ten years of a population-based prevention programme. *The Journal of Bone and Joint Surgery: British Volume, 87*(1), 95–101.

Hanna, S. E., Rosenbaum P. L., Bartlett, D. J., Palisano, R. J., Walter, S. D., Avery, L., & Russell, D. J. (2009). Stability and decline in gross motor function among children and youth with cerebral palsy aged 2 to 21 years. *Developmental Medicine & Child Neurology, 51*(4), 295–302.

Hemming, K., Hutton, J. L., Colver, A., & Platt, M. J. (2005). Regional variation in survival of people with cerebral palsy in the United Kingdom. *Pediatrics, 116*(6), 1383–1390.

Hemminki, K., Li, X., Sundquist, K., & Sundquist, J. (2007). High familial risks for cerebral palsy implicate partial heritable aetiology. *Pediatric Perinatal Epidemiology, 21*(3), 235–241.

Herrington, T. M., Cheng, J. J., & Eskandar, E. N. (2016). Mechanisms of deep brain stimulation. *Journal of Neurophysiology, 115*, 19–38.

Herskind, A., Greisen, G., & Nielsen, J. B. (2015). Early identification and intervention in cerebral palsy. *Developmental Medicine & Child Neurology, 57*(1), 29–36.

Himmelmann, K., Hagberg, G., & Uvebrant, P. (2010). The changing panorama of cerebral palsy in Sweden. X. Prevalence and origin in the birth-year period 1999–2002. *Acta Paediatrica, 99*(9), 1337–1343.

Himmelmann, K., McManus, V., Hagberg, G., Uvebrant, P., Krägeloh-Mann, I., Cans, C., & SCPE Collaboration. (2009). Dyskinetic cerebral palsy in Europe: Trends in prevalence and refereseverity. *Archives of Disease in Childhood, 94*(12), 921–926.

Hoare, B. J., Wallen, M. A., Imms, C., Villanueva, E., Rawicki, H. B., & Carey, L. (2010). Botulinum toxin A as an adjunct to treatment in the management of the upper limb in children with spastic cerebral palsy (UPDATE). *Cochrane Database of Systematic Reviews, 1*, CD003469.

Hoon, Jr., A. H., Stashinko, E. E., Nagae, L. M., Lin, D. D., Keller, J., Bastian, A., . . . Johnston, M. V. (2009). Sensory and motor deficits in children with cerebral palsy born preterm correlate with diffusion tensor imaging abnormalities in thalamocortical pathways. *Developmental Medicine and Child Neurology, 51*(9), 697–704.

Hough, J. P., Boyd, R. N., & Keating, J. L. (2010). Systematic review of interventions for low bone mineral density in children with cerebral palsy. *Pediatrics, 125*(3), e670–678.

Individuals with Disabilities Education Improvement Act of 2004, 20 U.S.C. §§ 1400 *et seq.*

Ismail, F. Y., Fatemi, A., & Johnston, M. V. (2017). Cerebral plasticity: Windows of opportunity in the developing brain. *European Journal of Paediatric Neurology, 21*(1), 23–48.

Jacobson, L., Rydberg, A., Eliasson, A. C., Kits, A., & Flodmark, O. (2010). Visual field function in school-aged children with spastic unilateral cerebral palsy related to different patterns of brain damage. *Developmental Medicine and Child Neurology, 52*(8), e184–e187.

Jacobsson, B. (2004). Infectious and inflammatory mechanisms in preterm birth and cerebral palsy. *European Journal of Obstetrics, Gynecology, and Reproductive Biology, 115*(2), 159–160.

Jacobsson, B., Ahlin, K., Francis, A., Hagberg, G., Hagberg, H., & Gardosi, J. (2008). Cerebral palsy and restricted growth status at birth: Population-based case-control study. *BJOG: An International Journal of Obstetrics and Gynaecology, 115*(10), 1250–1255.

Jankovic, J., & Brin, M. F. (1991). Therapeutic uses of botulinum toxin. *New England Journal of Medicine, 324*, 1186–1194.

Jefferson, R. J. (2004). Botulinum toxin in the management of cerebral palsy. *Developmental Medicine and Child Neurology, 46*(7), 491–499.

Johnston, M. V. (1998). Selective vulnerability in the neonatal brain. *Annals of Neurology, 44*(2), 155–156.

Johnston, M. V. (2009). Plasticity in the developing brain: Implications for rehabilitation. *Developmental Disabilities Research Reviews, 15*(2), 94–101.

Jongerius, P. H., van den Hoogen, F. J. A., van Limbeek, J., Gabreëls, F. J., van Hulst, K., & Rotteveel, J. J. (2004). Effect of botulinum toxin in the treatment of drooling: A controlled clinical trial. *Pediatrics, 114*(3), 620–627.

Katz, R. T. (2003). Life expectancy for children with cerebral palsy and mental retardation: Implications for life care planning. *Neurorehabilitation, 18*(3), 261–270.

Kay, R. M., Rethlefsen, S. A., Fern-Buneo, A., Wren, T. A. L., & Skaggs, D. L. (2004). Botulinum toxin as an adjunct to serial casting treatment in children with cerebral palsy. *The Journal of Bone and Joint Surgery: American Volume, 86-A*(11), 2377–2384.

Koene, S., & Smeitink, J. (2009). Mitochondrial medicine: Entering the era of treatment. *The Journal of Internal Medicine, 265*(2), 193–209.

Koman, L. A., Smith, B. P., & Shilt, J. S. (2004). Cerebral palsy. *The Lancet, 363*(9421), 1619–1631.

Korzeniewski, S. J., Birbeck, G., DeLano, M. C., Potchen, M. J., & Paneth, N. (2007). A Systematic Review of Neuroimaging for Cerebral Palsy. *Journal of Child Neurology, 23*(2), 216–227.

Krach, L. E. (2001). Pharmacotherapy of spasticity: Oral medications and intrathecal baclofen. *Journal of Child Neurology, 16*(1), 31–36.

Krägeloh-Mann, I., & Cans, C. (2009). Cerebral palsy update. *Brain & Development, 31*(7), 537–544.

Krägeloh-Mann, I., Petersen, D., Hagberg, G., Vollmer, B., Hagberg, B., & Michaelis, R. (1995). Bilateral spastic cerebral palsy—MRI pathology and origin. Analysis from a representative series of 56 cases. *Developmental Medicine and Child Neurology, 37*(5), 379–397.

Kusters, C. D., Chen, M. L., Follett, P. L., & Dammann, O. (2009). "Intraventricular" hemorrhage and cystic periventricular leukomalacia in preterm infants: How are they related? *Journal of Child Neurology, 24*(9), 1158–1170.

Langerak, N. G., Lamberts, R. P., Fieggen, A. G., Peter, J. C., Peacock, W. J., & Vaughan, C. L. (2009). Functional status of patients with cerebral palsy according to the International Classification of Functioning, Disability and Health model: A 20-year follow-up study after selective dorsal rhizotomy. *Archives of Physical Medicine and Rehabilitation, 90*(6), 994–1003.

Law, M., Cadman, D., Rosenbaum, P., Walter, S., Russell, D., & DeMatteo, C. (1991). Neurodevelopmental therapy and upper-extremity inhibitive casting for children with cerebral palsy. *Developmental Medicine and Child Neurology, 33*(5), 379–387.

Leach, E. L., Shevell, M., Bowden, K., Stockler-Ipsiroglu, S., & van Karnebeek, C. D. (2014). Treatable inborn errors of metabolism presenting as cerebral palsy mimics: Systematic literature review. *Orphanet Journal of Rare Diseases, 9*, 197. doi:10.1186/s13023-014-0197-2

Lerner, Z. F., Damiano, D. L., & Bulea, T. C. (2016). A robotic exoskeleton to treat crouch gait from cerebral palsy: Initial kinematic and neuromuscular evaluation. *Conference Proceedings of the IEEE Engineering in Medicine and Biology Society, 2016*, 2214–2217. doi:10.1109/EMBC.2016.7591169

Leviton, A., & Dammann, O. (2004). Coagulation, inflammation, and the risk of neonatal white matter damage. *Pediatric Research, 55*(4), 541–545.

Liptak, G. S., & Accardo, P. J. (2004). Health and social outcomes of children with cerebral palsy. *The Journal of Pediatrics, 145*(Suppl. 2), S36–S41.

Lombardi, G., Garofoli, F., & Stronati, M. (2010). Congenital cytomegalovirus infection: Treatment, sequelae and follow-up. *The Journal of Maternal-Fetal and Neonatal Medicine, 23*(Suppl. 3), 45–48.

Lynn, A. K., Turner, M., & Chambers, H. G. (2009). Surgical management of spasticity in persons with cerebral palsy. *Physical Medicine and Rehabilitation, 1*(9), 834–838.

MacLennan, A., Nelson, K. B., Hankins, G., & Speer, M. (2010). Who will deliver our grandchildren? Implications of cerebral palsy litigation. *JAMA: The Journal of the American Medical Association, 294*(13), 1688–1690.

McIntyre, S., Badawi, N., Blair, E., & Nelson, K. B. (2015). Does aetiology of neonatal encephalopathy and hypoxic-ischaemic encephalopathy influence the outcome of treatment? *Developmental Medicine and Child Neurology, 57*(Suppl. 3), 2–7.

McNaughton, D., & Light, J. (2015). Editorial: What we write about when we write about. *AAC: The Past 30 Years of Research and Future Directions Augmentative and Alternative Communication, 31*(4), 261–270.

Meregillano, G. (2004). Hippotherapy. *Physical Medicine and Rehabilitation Clinics of North America, 15*(4), 843–854.

Mink, J. W. (2003). Dopa-responsive dystonia in children. *Current Treatment Options in Neurology, 5*(4), 279–282.

Mink, J. W., & Zinner, S. H. (2009). Movement disorders II: Chorea, dystonia, myoclonus, and tremor. *Pediatrics in Review, 31*(7), 287–294.

Mooney, J. F., Koman, L. A., & Smith, B. P. (2003). Pharmacologic management of spasticity in cerebral palsy. *Journal of Pediatric Orthopedics, 23*(5), 679–686.

Moreno-De-Luca, A., Ledbetter, D. H., & Martin, C. L. (2012). Genomic insights into the etiology and classification of the cerebral palsies. *Lancet Neurology, 11*(3), 283–292.

Morton, R. E., Hankinson, J., & Nicholson, J. (2004). Botulinum toxin for cerebral palsy: Where are we now? *Archives of Disease in Childhood, 89*(12), 1133–1137.

Murphy, K. (2010). The adult with cerebral palsy. *Orthopedic Clinics of North America, 41*(4), 595–605.

Murphy, N. A., Irwin, M. C., & Hoff, C. (2002). Intrathecal baclofen therapy in children with cerebral palsy: Efficacy and complications. *Archives of Physical Medicine and Rehabilitation, 83*(12), 1721–1725.

Murphy, K., Molnar, G., & Lankasky, K. (1995). Medical and functional status of adults with cerebral palsy. *Developmental Medicine and Child Neurology, 37*(12), 1075–1084.

Myhr, U., von Wendt, L., Norrlin, S., & Radell, U. (1995). Five-year follow-up of functional sitting position in children with cerebral palsy. *Developmental Medicine and Child Neurology, 37*(7), 587–596.

Nagae, L. M., Hoon, Jr., A. H., Stashinko, E., Lin, D., Zhang, W., Levey, E., . . . Mori, S. (2007). Diffusion tensor imaging in children with periventricular leukomalacia: Variability of injuries to white matter tracts. *AJNR: American Journal of Neuroradiology, 28*(7), 1213–1222.

National Guideline Alliance. (2017). *Cerebral palsy in under 25s: Assessment and management*. London, England: National Institute for Health and Care Excellence.

National Guideline Alliance. (2012). Spasticity in under 19s: Management. London, England: National Institute for Health and Care Excellence.

Nelson, K. B. (2008). Causative factors in cerebral palsy. *Clinical Obstetrics and Gynecology, 51*(4), 749–762.

Nelson, K. B., & Chang, T. (2008). Is cerebral palsy preventable? *Current Opinions in Neurology, 21*(2), 129–135.

Nelson, K. B., & Lynch, J. K. (2004). Stroke in newborn infants. *The Lancet Neurology, 3*(3), 150–158.

NINDS. (2018). *Common data elements.* National Institute of Neurological Disorders and Stroke. Retrieved from https://www.commondataelements.ninds.nih.gov/CP.aspx#tab=Data_Standards

Nordmark, E., Hägglund, G., & Lagergren, J. (2001). Cerebral palsy in southern Sweden. II. Gross motor function and disabilities. *Acta Paediatrica, 90*(11), 1277–1282.

Novak, I., Mcintyre, S., Morgan, C., Campbell, L., Dark, L., Morton, N., . . . Goldsmith, S. (2013). A systematic review of interventions for children with cerebral palsy: State of the evidence. *Developmental Medicine & Child Neurology, 55*(10), 885–910.

Novak, I., Morgan, C., Adde, L., Blackman, J., Boyd, R. N., Brunstrom-Hernandez, J., . . . de Vries, L. S. (2017). Early, accurate diagnosis and early intervention in cerebral palsy: Advances in diagnosis and treatment. *JAMA Pediatrics, 171*(9), 897–907.

Oeffinger, D. J., Tylkowski, C. M., Rayens, M. K., Davis, R. F., Gorton, III, G. E., D'Astous, J., . . . Luan, J. (2004). Gross Motor Function Classification System and outcome tools for assessing ambulatory cerebral palsy: A multicenter study. *Developmental Medicine and Child Neurology, 46*(5), 311–319.

Oppenheim, W. L. (2009). Complementary and alternative methods in cerebral palsy. *Developmental Medicine and Child Neurology, 51*(Suppl. 4), 122–129.

Pakula, A. T., Van Naarden Braun, K., & Yeargin-Allsopp, M. (2009). Cerebral palsy: Classification and epidemiology. *Physical Medicine and Rehabilitation Clinics of North America, 20*(3), 425–452.

Palisano, R. J., Cameron, D., Rosenbaum, P. L., Walter, S. D., & Russell, D. (2006). Stability of the Gross Motor Function Classification System. *Developmental Medicine and Child Neurology, 48*(6), 424–428.

Palisano, R., Rosenbaum, P., Bartlett, D., & Livingston, M. (2007). *Gross Motor Function Classification System—Expanded and Revised (GBFCS–E&R).* Retrieved from https://canchild.ca/en/resources/42-gross-motor-function-classification-system-expanded-revised-gmfcs-e-r

Palisano, R., Rosenbaum, P., Walter, S., Russell, D., Wood, E., & Galuppi, B. (1997). Development and reliability of a system to classify gross motor function in children with cerebral palsy. *Developmental Medicine and Child Neurology, 39*(4), 214–223.

Palmer, F. B. (2004). Strategies for the early diagnosis of cerebral palsy. *The Journal of Pediatrics, 145*(Suppl. 2), S8–S11.

Papavasiliou, A. S. (2009). Management of motor problems in cerebral palsy: A critical update for the clinician. *European Journal of Paediatric Neurology, 13*(5), 387–396.

Pessoa, A., van der Linden, V., Yeargin-Allsopp, M., Carvalho, M. D. C. G., Ribeiro, E. M., Braun, K. V. N., . . . Moore, C. A. (2018). Motor abnormalities and epilepsy in infants and children with evidence of congenital Zika virus infection. *Pediatrics, 141*(Suppl. 2), S167–S179.

Pidcock, F. S. (2004). The emerging role of therapeutic botulinum toxin in the treatment of cerebral palsy. *The Journal of Pediatrics, 145*(Suppl. 2), S33–35.

Pin, T. W., McCartney, L., Lewis, J., & Waugh, M. C. (2011). Use of intrathecal baclofen therapy in ambulant children and adolescents with spasticity and dystonia of cerebral origin: A systematic review. *Developmental Medicine and Child Neurology, 53*(10), 885–895.

Raina, P., O'Donnell, M., Rosenbaum, P., Brehaut, J., Walter, S. D., Russell, D., . . . Wood, E. (2005). The health and well-being of caregivers of children with cerebral palsy. *Pediatrics, 115*(6), e626–e636.

Rangarajan, V., & Juul, S. E. (2014). Erythropoietin: emerging role of erythropoietin in neonatal neuroprotection. *Pediatric Neurology, 51*(4), 481–488.

Reid, S. M., Dagia, C. D., Ditchfield, M. R., & Reddihough, D. S. (2015). Grey matter injury patterns in cerebral palsy: Associations between structural involvement on MRI and clinical outcomes. *Developmental Medicine & Child Neurology, 57*(12), 1159–1167.

Rosenbaum, P. L., Walter, S. D., Hanna, S. E., Palisano, R. J., Russell, D. J., Raina, P., . . . Galuppi, B. E. (2002). Prognosis for gross motor function in cerebral palsy: Creation of motor development curves. *JAMA: The Journal of the American Medical Association, 288*(11), 1357–1363.

Rosenbaum, P., Paneth, N., Leviton, A., Goldstein, M., Bax, M., Damiano, D., Dan, B., & Jacobsson, B. (2007). A report: The definition and classification of cerebral palsy April 2006. *Developmental Medicine and Child Neurology, 109*(Suppl.), 8–14.

Russman, B. S., & Ashwal, S. (2004). Evaluation of the child with cerebral palsy. *Seminars in Pediatric Neurology, 11*(1), 47–57.

Russman, B., & Gage, J. (1989). Cerebral palsy. *Current Problems in Pediatrics, 19*(2), 65–111.

Samson-Fang, L., Fung, E., Stallings, V. A., Conaway, M., Worley, G., Rosenbaum, P., . . . Stevenson, R. D. (2002). Relationship of nutritional status to health and societal participation in children with cerebral palsy. *The Journal of Pediatrics, 141*(5), 637–643.

Sanger, T. D., Delgado, M. R., Gaebler-Spira, D., Hallett, M., & Mink, J. M. (2003). Classification and definition of disorders causing hypertonia in childhood. *Pediatrics.*

Sanger, T. D. (2005). Hypertonia in children: How and when to treat. *Child Neurology, 7,* 427.

Sanger, T. D., Chen, D., Delgado, M. R., Gaebler-Spira, D., Hallett, M., & Mink, J. W. (2006). Definition and classification of negative motor signs in childhood. *Pediatrics, 118*(5), 2159–2167.

Schiariti, V., Fowler, E., Brandenburg, J. E., Levey, E., McIntyre, S., Sukal-Moulton, T., . . . Koenig, J. I. (2018). A common data language for clinical research studies: The National Institute of Neurological Disorders and Stroke and American Academy for Cerebral Palsy and Developmental Medicine Cerebral Palsy Common Data Elements Version 1.0 recommendations. *Developmental Medicine and Child Neurology, 60,* 976–986. doi:10.1111/dmcn.13723

Scott, B. L., & Jankovic, J. (1996). Delayed-onset progressive movement disorders after static brain lesions. *Neurology, 46*(1), 68–74.

Seashore, M. R. (2009). The organic acidemias: An overview. *GeneReviews, 1993–2001.* Retrieved from http://www.ncbi.nlm.nih.gov/sites/GeneTests/query

Sellers, D., Mandy, A., Pennington, L., Hankins, M., & Morris, C. (2014). Development and reliability of a system to classify the eating and drinking ability of people with cerebral palsy. *Developmental Medicine and Child Neurology, 56*(3), 245–251.

Serruya, M. D., & Kahana, M. J. (2008). Techniques and devices to restore cognition. *Behavioral Brain Research, 192*(2), 149–165.

Sgandurra, G., Lorentzen, J., Inguaggiato, E., Bartalena, L., Beani, E., Cecchi, F., . . . CareToy Consortium. (2017). A randomized clinical trial in preterm infants on the effects of a home-based early intervention with the "CareToy System." *PLoS One, 2017, 12*(3), e0173521.

Shapiro, S. M. (2005). Definition of the clinical spectrum of kernicterus and bilirubin-induced neurologic dysfunction (BIND). *Journal of Perinatology, 25*(1), 54–59.

Shatrov, J. G., Birch, S. C., Lam, L. T., Quinlivan, J. A., McIntyre, S., & Mendz, G. L. (2010). Chorioamnionitis and cerebral palsy: A meta-analysis. *Obstetrics & Gynecology, 116*(2), 387–392.

Shrestha, S. (2010). Lesions of upper motor neurons and lower motor neurons. *Medchrome Online Medical Magazine.* Retrieved from http://medchrome.com/basic-science/anatomy/lesions-of-upper-motor-neurons-and-lower-motor-neurons/

Sobrado, P., Suarez, J., & Garcia-Sanchez, F. A. (1999). Refractive errors in children with cerebral palsy, psychomotor retardation, and other non-cerebral palsy neuromotor disabilities. *Developmental Medicine and Child Neurology, 41*(6), 396–403.

Stott, N. S., Piedrahita, L., & American Academy for Cerebral Palsy and Developmental Medicine. (2004). Effects of surgical adductor releases for hip subluxation in cerebral palsy: An AACPDM evidence report. *Developmental Medicine and Child Neurology, 46*(9), 628–645.

Strauss, D., & Shavelle, R. (2001). Life expectancy in cerebral palsy. *Archives of Disease in Childhood, 85*(5), 442.

Strauss, D., Cable, W., & Shavelle, R. (1999). Causes of excess mortality in cerebral palsy. *Developmental Medicine and Child Neurology, 41*(9), 580–585.

Strauss, D. J., Shavelle, R. M., & Anderson, T. W. (1998). Life expectancy of children with cerebral palsy. *Pediatric Neurology, 18*(2), 143–149.

Taub, E., Ramey, S. L., DeLuca, S., & Echols, K. (2004). Efficacy of constraint-induced movement therapy for children with cerebral palsy with asymmetric motor impairment. *Pediatrics, 113*(2), 305–312.

Tedroff, K., Löwing, K., Jacobson, D. N., & Åström, E. (2011). Does loss of spasticity matter? A 10-year follow-up after selective dorsal rhizotomy in cerebral palsy. *Developmental Medicine and Child Neurology, 53*(8), 724–729.

Tilton, A. H. (2004). Management of spasticity in children with cerebral palsy. *Seminars in Pediatric Neurology, 11*(1), 58–65.

Tilton, A. H. (2006). Therapeutic interventions for tone abnormalities in cerebral palsy. *NeuroRx, 3*(2), 217–224.

Tosi, L. L., Maher, N., Moore, D. W., Goldstein, M., & Aisen, M. L. (2009). Adults with cerebral palsy: A workshop to define the challenges of treating and preventing secondary musculoskeletal and neuromuscular complications in this rapidly growing population. *Developmental Medicine and Child Neurology, 51*(Suppl. 4), 2–11.

Turk, M. A. (2009). Health, mortality, and wellness issues in adults with cerebral palsy. *Developmental Medicine and Child Neurology, 51*(Suppl. 4), 24–29.

van der Dussen, L., Nieuwstraten, W., Roebroeck, M., & Stam, H. J. (2001). Functional level of young adults with cerebral palsy. *Clinical Rehabilitation, 15*(1), 84–91.

Vargus-Adams, J. (2009). Understanding function and other outcomes in cerebral palsy. *Physical Medicine and Rehabilitation Clinics of North America, 20*(3), 567–575.

Vermeulen, R. J., Wilke, M., Horber, V., & Krägeloh-Mann, I. (2010). Microcephaly with simplified gyral pattern: MRI classification. *Neurology, 74*(5), 386–391.

Vogtle, L. K. (2009). Pain in adults with cerebral palsy: Impact and solutions. *Developmental Medicine and Child Neurology, 51*(Suppl. 4), 113–121.

Volpe, J. J. (2005). Encephalopathy of prematurity includes neuronal abnormalities. *Pediatrics, 116*(1), 221–225.

Volpe, J. J. (2009). The encephalopathy of prematurity—brain injury and impaired brain development inextricably intertwined. *Seminars in Pediatric Neurology, 14*(4), 167–178.

Wasiak, J., Hoare, B., & Wallen, M. (2004). Botulinum toxin A as an adjunct to treatment in the management of the upper limb in children with spastic cerebral palsy. *Cochrane Database of Systematic Reviews, 4*, CD003469.

Watson, R., Parr, J. R., Joyce, C., May, C., & Le Couteur, A. S. (2011). Models of transitional care for young people with complex health needs: A scoping review. *Child Care, Health & Development, 37*(6), 780–791.

Willis, J. K., Morello, A., Davie, A., Rice, J. C., & Bennett, J. T. (2002). Forced-use treatment of childhood hemiparesis. *Pediatrics, 110*(1, Pt. 1), 94–96.

Wittenberg, G. F. (2009). Neural plasticity and treatment across the lifespan for motor deficits in cerebral palsy. *Developmental Medicine and Child Neurology, 51*(Suppl. 4), 130–133.

Wolf, S. L., Thompson, P. A., Winstein, C. J., Phillip Miller, J., Blanton, S. R., Nichols-Larsen, D. S., . . . Sawaki L. (2010). The EXCITE Stroke Trial: Comparing early and delayed constraint-induced movement therapy. *Stroke, 41*(10), 2309–2315.

Wood, D. L., Kantor, D., Edwards, L., & James, H. (2008). Health care transition for youth with cerebral palsy. *Northeast Florida Medicine, 59*(4), 4447.

Wood, E., & Rosenbaum, P. (2000). The gross motor function classification system for cerebral palsy: A study of reliability and stability over time. *Developmental Medicine and Child Neurology, 42*(5), 292–296.

World Health Organization. (2001). *The International Classification of Functioning, Disability and Health (ICF).* Geneva, Switzerland: Author. Retrieved from http://www.who.int/classifications/icf/en/

World Health Organization. (2007). *The International Classification of Functioning, Disability and Health, Children and Youth Version.* Geneva, Switzerland: Author. Retrieved from http://www.who.int/classifications/icf/en/

Wu, Y. W. (2002). Systematic review of chorioamnionitis and palsy. *Mental Retardation and Developmental Disabilities Research Reviews, 8*(1), 25–29.

Wu, Y. W., Day, S. M., Strauss, D. J., & Shavelle, R. M. (2004). Prognosis for ambulation in cerebral palsy: A population-based study. *Pediatrics, 114*(5), 1264–1271.

Yoon, B. H., Park, C. W., & Chaiworapongsa, T. (2003). Intrauterine infection and the development of cerebral palsy. *BJOG: An International Journal of Obstetrics and Gynaecology, 110*(Suppl. 20), 124–127.

CHAPTER 22

Epilepsy

Tesfaye Getaneh Zelleke, Dewi Frances T. Depositario-Cabacar, and William Davis Gaillard

Upon completion of this chapter, the reader will

- Know the signs and symptoms of epilepsy
- Understand the epidemiology and causes of epilepsy
- Understand the basic classification of epilepsy
- Be familiar with common epilepsy syndromes
- Be knowledgeable about the evaluation and treatment of epilepsy
- Be aware of anti-seizure medications and their side effects

Seizures, also referred to as "fits" or "convulsions," are transient disturbances of brain function resulting from an abnormally excessive excitation of cortical neurons. They are seen frequently in childhood. As many as 1 in 10 children will experience at least one seizure before adulthood (Hauser, 1994). The clinical signs and symptoms will vary depending on the location of the epileptic discharge in the cerebral cortex and the extent of spread of the discharge in the brain. Seizures can cause changes in motor movement (e.g., **tonic** [rigid] or **clonic** [uncontrolled jerking] movements), sensation (e.g., a tingling sensation), bodily function (e.g., incontinence), attention (e.g., loss of attention), awareness, and behavior (e.g., loss of consciousness or presence of unusual behaviors such as stereotypic actions).

Seizures can be provoked by an infection (e.g., meningitis or encephalitis), metabolic disturbance (e.g., hypoglycemia), a toxic agent (e.g., pesticides), trauma, or other acute illness. A fever (in children ages 6 months–6 years), an overdose of certain medications (e.g., insulin), meningitis, or a fall in which the child hits his or her head can lead to a seizure (Huang, Chang, & Wang, 1998). Most seizures are either solitary and often provoked events (e.g., a single seizure following a minor head trauma) or limited to a specific and narrow age window (e.g., febrile convulsions).

By contrast, the diagnosis of epilepsy requires two unprovoked seizures that occur at least 24 hours apart. The prevalence of epilepsy in the general pediatric population is 4 to 10 per 1,000 (Berg, 1995). It has variable severity; an individual may experience anywhere from two or three seizures to hundreds over a lifetime. Epilepsy may have a clear origin (e.g., resulting from a malformation of cortical development or perinatal stroke), or it may not have an identifiable cause.

Children with developmental disabilities are at increased risk for epilepsy (Sunder, 1997). For example, it is five times more common in children with cerebral palsy than in typically developing children (Hundozi-Hysenaj & Boshnjaku-Dallku, 2008). With intellectual disability, the risk of developing epilepsy throughout one's lifespan is 15%–20% (Besag, 2002; Forsgren,

Edvinsson, Blomquist, Hiejbel, & Sidenvall, 1990). In addition, if a child has comorbid conditions the risk for epilepsy is increased. For example, autism spectrum disorder (ASD) is associated with a 2% risk of manifesting epilepsy by 5 years of age and an 8% risk by 10 years (Tuchman & Rapin, 2002); however, this risk increases to 35% at 5 years and 67% by 10 years if the child has intellectual disability associated with ASD. In general, the more severe the pathology, the higher the risk of epilepsy (Holmes, 2002; Box 22.1).

The control of epilepsy in children with developmental disabilities tends to be harder to achieve, and medically refractory epilepsy (more than three seizures per year despite treatment with three standard anti-seizure medications [ASMs]) is more common (Airaksinen et al., 2000; Alvarez, Besag, & Iivanainen, 1998). Furthermore, both epilepsy and ASMs may contribute to learning difficulties and to disruptive behavior. Children with epilepsy exhibit a higher incidence of cognitive impairments, attention-deficit/hyperactivity disorder (ADHD), anxiety disorders, and depression.

CASE STUDY

Patricia is a 7-year-old girl who has been referred to the neurology clinic due to "spells." She has been reported by her teachers at school to have staring spells and was thought to have difficulties with attention. Her teacher has noticed that she sometimes submits a written test with unfinished answers. There are also occasions when Patricia feels that she has missed a conversation and is often teased by her classmates. At the neurology clinic, the pediatric neurologist had her hyperventilate by blowing a pinwheel; this elicited a typical spell. To confirm the clinical impression and establish a diagnosis, a sleep-deprived electroencephalogram (EEG) was done, which showed a generalized 3-Hz spike and wave pattern characteristic of absence seizures. Patricia was started on ethosuximide, but she continued to have seizures. Her medication dose was further increased, and she became asymptomatic. A follow-up EEG was normal. Her grades have also improved. She has been doing well for 2 years without any seizures, and the plan is now to discontinue her medication.

Thought Questions:

If a child is having "staring episodes" at school, what observations would help distinguish wandering attention from seizures? How might having epilepsy affect a child's school attendance and performance?

EPILEPSY: DEFINITIONS AND CLASSIFICATION

Epilepsy, derived from the Greek word meaning to *take hold of* or *seize* (Reynolds, 2000), is a neurologic condition in which a person experiences recurrent unprovoked seizures (Hauser, Rich, Lee, Annegers, & Anderson, 1998). Epilepsy has always been defined as two unprovoked seizures occurring more than 24 hours apart. In 2014, a task force expanded this definition by proposing that epilepsy may be defined by any of the following

BOX 22.1 EVIDENCE-BASED PRACTICE

Epilepsy, Autism Spectrum Disorder, and Behavior

Children with autism spectrum disorder (ASD) have an increased incidence of epilepsy (10%–30%; Tuchman, 2013), which is especially prevalent among children who also have concomitant intellectual disability (ID). In addition, children with ASD have an increased incidence of abnormalities on EEG, even in the absence of clinical seizures (20%–30%; Spence & Schneider, 2009). Compared with typically developing children, children with ASD also have increased difficulties with impulsivity, hyperactivity, agitation, mood instability, self-injury, and aggression. A possible link between epilepsy in autism and increased difficulties with behavior has long been a subject of speculation based on the idea that changes in brain function related to seizures might lead to worsening behavior in children with ASD. However, a cross-sectional study involving 2,645 children with ASD found that when controlled for ID, there was no difference in maladaptive behaviors between children with and without epilepsy. In other words, the presence of maladaptive behaviors was most strongly correlated with lower cognitive ability, rather than with epilepsy. The one exception was hyperactivity, which did appear to be increased in the epilepsy group, independent of cognitive level (Viscidi et al., 2014).

The relationship between developmental disabilities such as autism and ID and epilepsy is complex. Future research will help to clarify the nuances of this relationship.

criteria: 1) at least two unprovoked (or reflex) seizures occurring more than 24 hours apart; 2) one unprovoked (or reflex) seizure and a probability of further seizures similar to the general recurrence risk (at least 60%) after two unprovoked seizures, occurring over the next 10 years; or 3) diagnosis of an epilepsy syndrome (see discussion below; Fisher et al., 2014). Unprovoked seizures are seizures that occur spontaneously, without an obvious inciting event (such as a high fever or drug/alcohol withdrawal). Reflex seizures are provoked by specific sensory stimuli (such as flashing lights) or specific movements or activities in specific individuals, and they occur in certain types of epilepsy. The incidence of epilepsy ranges from 41 to 187 out of 100,000 and is highest in the first year of life (Camfield & Camfield, 2015). After a single unprovoked seizure the risk for another seizure is 40%–52% (Berg, 1991). The recurrence risk after two unprovoked seizures is about 80% (Camfield et al., 1985; Hauser et al., 1998; Shinnar et al., 2000). Thirty percent of children with epilepsy will have an incomplete response to medications, and approximately 5%—10% will have intractable epilepsy (i.e., seizures that are frequent despite multiple medications; Ding & Hauser, 2015).

A seizure results from an excessive discharge of a large population of cortical neurons (see Chapter 8). This usually occurs when the excitatory inputs of neurons outweighs the inhibitory inputs. Excessive neuronal firing continues until excitatory neurotransmission is exhausted or the inhibitory networks extinguish it. The seizure usually stops in seconds to minutes, but it may occasionally persist, sometimes requiring urgent medical intervention. When a seizure lasts more than 30 minutes, it is termed *status epilepticus.* The clinical signs and symptoms of the seizure will vary depending on the location of the epileptic discharge in the cerebral cortex and the extent of spread of the discharge in the brain.

Not everyone will have a seizure if presented with the same brain insult because the structural and chemical brain interactions are affected by genetic and acquired factors (Briellmann, Jackson, Tor-boers, & Berkovic, 2001; Frucht, Quigg, Schwaner, & Fountain, 2000). Several factors modulate the predisposition for seizures and the threshold at which they occur. For example, the age of the child and stage of brain development appear to affect the seizure threshold (Moshe, 2000). Some epilepsies are predominantly seen during particular age windows, such as infantile spasms (4–16 months), childhood absence (4–12 years), benign rolandic epilepsy (6–14 years), and juvenile myoclonic epilepsy (8–26 years). The brain undergoes global and regional structural changes over time that involve cortical thickness and myelination (Gage, 2002) as well as changes in brain chemistry and metabolic rates. Changes in normal brain development, structure, or chemistry can affect the subsequent cascade of brain maturation and predispose the child to epilepsy (Lowenstein & Alldredge, 1998). Repair mechanisms following some brain insults can also lead to the formation of abnormal neuronal networks that may generate seizure activity (Cole, 2000). Brain maturation may explain why some children appear to grow into or out of epilepsy (Sillanpää, 2000).

Seizures are disorders of neuronal transmission and brain network interactions. Factors that may predispose a child to have seizures may include 1) injury to brain cells that make them dysfunctional (e.g., traumatic brain injury, stroke, or brain tumors), 2) disruption of brain cell circuits (e.g., tuberous sclerosis and malformations of cortical development), and 3) alterations in intrinsic brain cell excitability (e.g., inherited epilepsies such as severe myoclonic epilepsy and autosomal dominant nocturnal frontal lobe epilepsy).

The clinical signs and symptoms of seizures usually reflect the function of the brain areas from which they arise or to which they propagate. In the 1989 classification scheme (Commission on Classification and Terminology of the International League Against Epilepsy, 1989), seizures were divided into partial (i.e., focal or localized) and generalized depending on the origin and degree of spread of the seizure activity. Partial seizures were further subdivided into simple and complex depending on whether consciousness was altered. In simple partial seizures, there may be 1) a strange sensation called an aura (e.g., an **epigastric** sensation caused by abnormal neuronal discharge in the mesial temporal lobe of the brain), 2) unusual motor activity (e.g., a jerking of the hands, originating from the primary motor cortex of the frontal lobe), or 3) atypical dystonia-like posturing (resulting from spread of the seizure through the basal ganglia). In complex partial seizures, there is propagation to brain structures that alter the state of consciousness (e.g., through the limbic system). As a result, there may be staring, oral automatisms (lip smacking), or fumbling with hands and clothing. When multiple parts of the brain are involved or there is spread of the electrical discharge to both cerebral hemispheres, generalized tonic-clonic activity may result. In the new classification scheme (Berg et al., 2010; Fisher et al., 2017) seizures are described as generalized or focal, with or without impairment of awareness (replacing simple, complex, secondarily generalized, and primary generalized).

The International League Against Epilepsy (ILAE) has divided epilepsies into three categories: focal epilepsy, generalized epilepsy, and epilepsy syndromes. Epilepsy may also be divided into idiopathic, symptomatic, and cryptogenic (Commission on Classification and Terminology of the International League Against Epilepsy, 1989). The term *symptomatic* is used when there is a clear structural brain abnormality (e.g., tuberous sclerosis), an acquired cause of epilepsy (e.g., stroke, tumors, or meningitis), or an associated neurological impairment (e.g., intellectual disability or cerebral palsy). *Idiopathic epilepsies* are assumed to be genetic in origin and comprise about 30% of childhood epilepsies (Hauser & Kurland, 1993). In this form of epilepsy, there are no abnormal neurological and neuroimaging findings, and there may be a family history of seizures. The term *cryptogenic* has been used to refer to epilepsies for which a cause cannot be identified. More recently this classification system has been proposed to be amended to 1) *genetic* (replaces idiopathic), when the epilepsy is secondary to a presumed genetic defect (e.g., SCN1A mutation in Dravet syndrome); 2) *structural or metabolic*, when the epilepsy is due to an acquired brain injury (e.g., brain tumor or stroke), a congenital central nervous system malformation, or an inborn error of metabolism (see Chapters 3 and 16), and 3) *unknown cause* (replaces cryptogenic) when the underlying cause is not identified (Berg et al., 2010).

Children with a first seizure of remote symptomatic etiology (i.e., a seizure that is removed in time following a brain insult) tend to have a higher rate of seizure recurrence (approximately 65%; Berg & Shinnar, 1991; Shinnar et al., 1996). Among those with a remote symptomatic etiology, children with static brain dysfunction since birth, such as intellectual disability or cerebral palsy, tend to have the highest rates of seizure recurrence. In contrast to children with remote symptomatic etiology, children with a first seizure of idiopathic or cryptogenic etiology tend to have lower rates of additional seizures, with an approximate 35% risk (Berg & Shinnar, 1991; Shinnar et al., 1996).

The causes of epilepsy vary with age. Malformations of cortical development, perinatal brain injury, and metabolic disorders are common causes of epilepsy in infancy; genetic and congenital disorders are found in early and later childhood; and hippocampal sclerosis (injury/scarring of the hippocampus; Bazendale & Heaney, 2010), alcohol or drug abuse, and trauma may occur in older children and adolescents (Shorvon, 2000).

Classification of Epilepsy and Epilepsy Syndromes

The diagnosis, treatment, and prognosis of seizure disorders depend on the correct identification of the types of seizures and its epilepsy classification. Childhood epilepsies are classified using variations of the ILAE schema (Commission on Classification and Terminology of the International League Against Epilepsy, 1989).

As mentioned above, the ILAE classifies epilepsy into two major classes: generalized and focal (see Figure 22.1). Other categories include focal-to-bilateral tonic-clonic (a seizure that starts in one side or part of the brain and spreads to both sides), unknown onset, and unclassified (Fisher et al., 2017). Epilepsy syndromes are classified based on the clinical appearance of the seizures, the EEG, and the age of onset. A modified classification system has been developed for some seizures (e.g., neonatal seizures, infantile seizures, and status epilepticus). Another proposed classification system is the 5-axis diagnostic schema, which divides seizures into 1) descriptive ictal terminology, 2) seizure type, 3) syndrome, 4) etiology, and 5) impairment (Engel, 2001). Classifying seizures into different types helps guide further testing, treatment, and estimates of prognosis or outlook.

Occasionally, there is difficulty in classifying epilepsy because 1) the seizure onset is not observed, 2) the focal signs may not be apparent because of the rapid spread of the seizure, or 3) the subtleties of the seizure may be missed because the observers may be so overwhelmed during the event. Fortunately, the interictal (between-seizure) EEG pattern can provide some information on the seizure type (Panayiotopoulos, 1999).

Generalized Seizures

Generalized seizures (those without a clear focal cortical onset) account for more than one third of pediatric epilepsy. They include absence, myoclonic, tonic, clonic, tonic-clonic, and atonic seizures. These seizures have simultaneous bilateral onset, meaning they occur on both sides of the body from the beginning of seizure activity. During generalized seizures, the child may have decreased nonconvulsive motor activity (e.g., the arrest of activity and automatisms seen in absence seizures) or a bilateral synchronous abnormal motor activity (e.g., myoclonic, atonic, or tonic-clonic seizures).

Absence seizures, as described in the case of Patricia, have historically been referred to as "petit mal," and are characterized by brief episodes of impaired consciousness, usually lasting less than 30 seconds, and without **postictal** confusion (confusion immediately following the seizure episode). These seizures may occur numerous times during the day and can affect the child's learning ability by interrupting attention and vigilance. Absence seizures are mediated through the thalamus (see Chapter 8), and onset is usually between 3–12 years of age. The classic EEG pattern shows a 3-Hz generalized spike and wave, which can

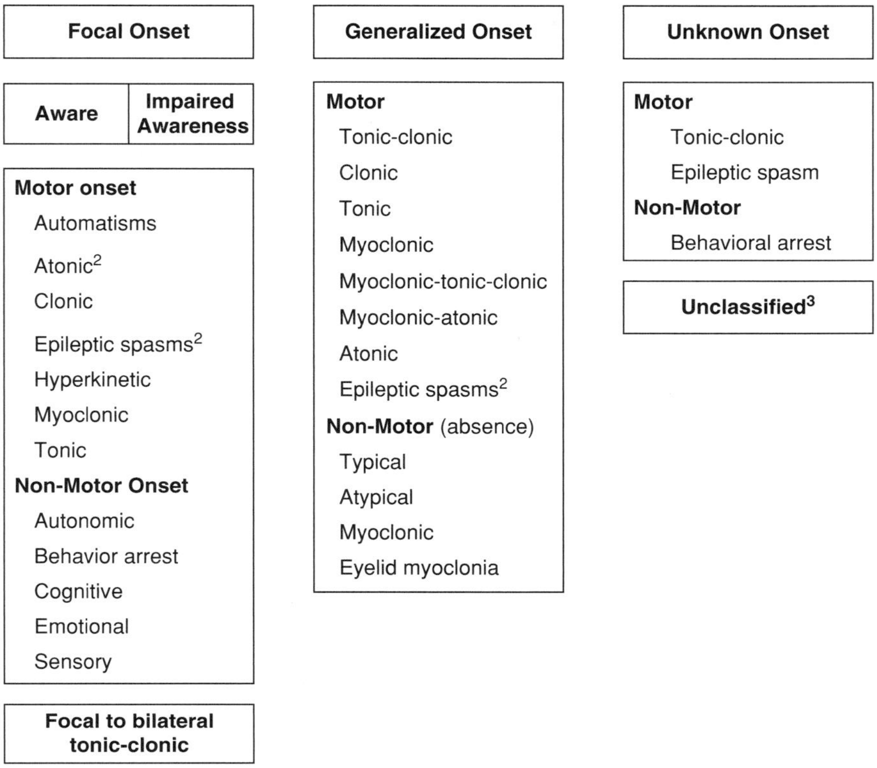

Focal Onset	Generalized Onset	Unknown Onset
Aware / Impaired Awareness	**Motor**	**Motor**
Motor onset	Tonic-clonic	Tonic-clonic
Automatisms	Clonic	Epileptic spasm
Atonic[2]	Tonic	**Non-Motor**
Clonic	Myoclonic	Behavioral arrest
Epileptic spasms[2]	Myoclonic-tonic-clonic	**Unclassified[3]**
Hyperkinetic	Myoclonic-atonic	
Myoclonic	Atonic	
Tonic	Epileptic spasms[2]	
Non-Motor Onset	**Non-Motor** (absence)	
Autonomic	Typical	
Behavior arrest	Atypical	
Cognitive	Myoclonic	
Emotional	Eyelid myoclonia	
Sensory		
Focal to bilateral tonic-clonic		

Figure 22.1. Classification of seizures types.[1] (Fisher R. S., Cross J. H., D'Souza C. et al. [2017] Instruction manual for the ILAE 2017 operational classification of seizure types. Epilepsia doi:10.1111/epi.13671. [Used with permission]). (*Key:* [1]Definitions, other seizure types, and descriptors are listed in the accompanying reference, along with a detailed glossary of term. [2]These could be focal or generalized, with or without alteration of awareness. [3]Due to inadequate information or inability to place in other categories.)

be precipitated by hyperventilation or **photic** (flickering light) stimulation (see Figure 22.2). Sometimes the child may continue to perform a simple automatic activity, such as walking, during the seizure, but is unable to continue a novel task, such as reading aloud. Eye blinking or changes in head and extremity tone may accompany the behavioral arrest (e.g., abruptly stopping reading aloud). Absence seizures cannot be interrupted by verbal or **tactile** (touch) stimulation (Medina et al., 2012). Absence seizures and focal seizures have different features (Table 22.1).

Myoclonic seizures are due to brief contraction of muscles often associated with cortical discharges. They frequently manifest as either a sudden flexion or bending backward of the upper torso and head that lasts less than a second. By contrast, atonic seizures consist of a brief loss of postural tone, which may simulate a fainting spell. While the motor component of both myoclonic and atonic seizures is brief, these seizures often cluster over the course of a few minutes. Atonic seizures that cause an abrupt loss of postural tone are often referred to as "drop" seizures. Consciousness is usually impaired during these events, and affected children make no attempt to protect themselves when they fall as a consequence of the seizure. As a result, there is an increased risk of head injury. Children with these kinds of seizures may need to wear a protective helmet throughout the day. Following these brief seizures, the child immediately regains consciousness, often crying, seemingly not in pain but upset by the sudden disruption.

Tonic-clonic seizures have been referred to historically as "grand mal" seizures. They may originate from a specific area of the cerebral cortex (focal seizures) that secondarily generalizes, or they may arise bilaterally (primary generalized seizure). Clonic motor activity involves repetitive jerking of arms or legs occurring at a regular rate. Tonic activity consists of sustained

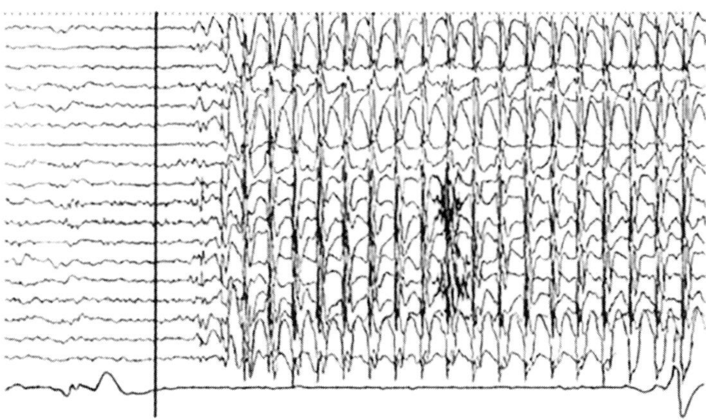

Figure 22.2. Absence seizure.

stiffening/posturing of the extremities. The seizure usually starts with a loss of consciousness, followed by tonic-clonic movements. Respiration may stop briefly, and **cyanosis** (turning blue) and incontinence are common. The EEG shows bilateral spike or polyspike and wave complexes (see below).

Focal Seizures

Focal (formerly termed partial) seizures start in a localized area of the cerebral cortex; they may spread in space and time and may progress to a generalized seizure. They may arise in areas involving motor, sensory, behavioral, autonomic, or cognitive functions (see Figure 22.3). These seizures often begin with an aura and/or an abrupt and unprovoked alteration in behavior. Focal seizures are classified as focal with or without impairment of consciousness or focal-to-bilateral tonic-clonic (Fisher et al., 2017).

A focal seizure without impairment of awareness (previously referred to a simple partial seizure) occurs when the epileptic discharge occurs in a limited region of one cerebral hemisphere and consciousness is maintained. If the event is merely sensory in nature, it is called an aura. If the seizure spreads and results in an alteration of consciousness, it is referred to as a focal seizure with impairment of consciousness (previously referred to as a complex partial seizure). This may or may not progress to secondary generalization, resulting in a tonic-clonic motor seizure.

Focal seizures with impairment of consciousness are usually accompanied by motor movements such as focal motor jerking, motor arrest, or **automatisms.** Automatisms are involuntary movements that may include eye blinking, lip smacking, facial grimacing, groaning, chewing, fidgeting, or buttoning/unbuttoning movements. Occasionally, as a result of impaired awareness, agitation and anxiety may occur in the confused postictal state.

A focal seizure may spread from one portion of the brain to a contiguous area, resulting in the spread of the shaking to other, adjacent, body parts (called a Jacksonian seizure). If there is a focal onset, occasionally tonic or clonic seizures can be followed by a transient weakness on one side of the body called a Todd's paralysis.

Table 22.1. Comparison of focal seizures and absence seizures

	Focal seizures	Absence seizures
Incidence	Common	Uncommon
Duration	30 seconds–5 minutes	Less than 30 seconds
Frequency of occurrence	Occasional	Multiple times daily
Aura	Yes	No
Consciousness	Partial amnesia and confusion	Immediate return to consciousness
EEG pattern	Focal	Generalized

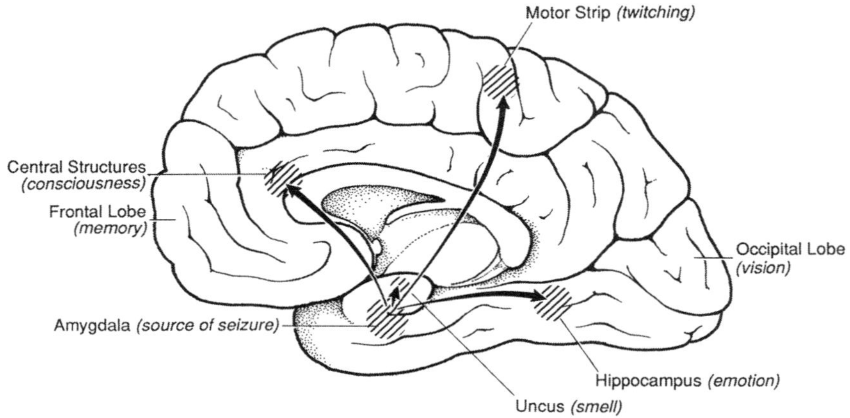

Figure 22.3. Spread of a focal seizure without impairment of consciousness. A seizure may begin anywhere—in this case, the amygdala of the temporal lobe. The initial feature may be the child smelling an unusual odor. The seizure may stop there or project out to the hippocampus, which might trigger feelings of fearfulness or abdominal queasiness. Memory and visual perception may be affected if the frontal or occipital lobe is involved. The seizure might ultimately extend to the motor strip, resulting in twitching of the limb, which may spread to other limbs or to central structures (causing loss of consciousness), thus becoming a complex partial seizure. Finally, the seizure may cross the corpus callosum to the other cerebral hemisphere and thus be converted from a partial to a generalized seizure.

Epilepsy Syndromes

Epilepsy syndromes are seizure disorders that share signs and symptoms, characteristics, specific EEG features, clinical course, prognosis, response to treatment, and sometimes a common pathogenesis or genetic basis (Wolf, 1994). The epilepsy syndromes fall into two broad categories: localization-related epilepsies and generalized-onset syndromes (Table 22.2). Most children with epilepsy have a predominant seizure type at onset that can be defined. However, only about one third can be assigned to a specific epilepsy syndrome using the most recent proposals for epilepsy syndromes (Wirrell, Grossardt, Wong-Kisiel, & Nickels, 2011). A few of the common epilepsy syndromes are discussed below and are organized primarily by age of expression (Table 22.3).

Infantile Spasms Infantile spasms, also known as West syndrome, is characterized by clusters of brief flexor (head, arms, and hip) or extensor (arm and trunk) contractions or spasms, typically associated with distinctive EEG finding, called hypsarrhythmia, and resulting in developmental regression or arrest (Commission on Pediatric Epilepsy of the International League Against Epilepsy, 1992). Infantile spasms are one of the most common forms of epileptic encephalopathy (epilepsy associated with neurocognitive impairment). The peak onset is at 4–7 months of age; 90% of children with this condition have onset before 12 months of age.

An underlying cause or disorder is found in over three quarters of children with infantile spasms (Knupp et al., 2016; Trasmonte & Barron, 1998). Etiologies include neurocutaneous syndromes (especially tuberous sclerosis), metabolic syndromes (e.g., pyridoxine deficiency), genetic syndrome (e.g., Down syndrome), brain malformations of cortical development (e.g., lissencephaly, polymicrogyria, or focal cortical dysplasia), and intrauterine insults (Pellock et al., 2010). Infantile spasms may evolve into Lennox-Gastaut syndrome (LGS) after infancy (see the next section).

A small percentage of children with infantile spasms have a cryptogenic cause (i.e., no identifiable cause). These children tend to respond to therapy (Kivity et al., 2004), have normal development before the spasm onset, and have better epilepsy prognosis and developmental outcomes than children with an identifiable cause.

Early recognition and prompt treatment may improve outcome in infantile spasms. The goal of prompt medical therapy is to normalize the EEG pattern and suppress the seizures. Adrenocorticotropic hormone and vigabatrin are considered to be the first line of treatment (Mackay et al., 2004). However, high-dose prednisolone has also been used successfully as a treatment option (Lux et al., 2004; Pellock et al., 2010). Vigabatrin is specifically used as a first-choice treatment for children with infantile spasms secondary to tuberous sclerosis (Wheless et al., 2007). ASMs have also been used, including valproate, phenobarbital,

Table 22.2. Epilepsy syndromes and other epilepsies, arranged by age of onset

Neonatal period
Benign familial neonatal epilepsy
Early myoclonic encephalopathy
Ohtahara syndrome

Infancy
Epilepsy of infancy with migrating focal seizures
West syndrome
Myoclonic epilepsy in infancy
Benign infantile epilepsy
Benign familial infantile epilepsy
Dravet syndrome
Myoclonic encephalopathy in nonprogressive disorders

Childhood
Febrile seizures plus (can start in infancy)
Panayiotopoulos syndrome
Epilepsy with myoclonic atonic (previously astatic) seizures
Benign epilepsy with centrotemporal spikes
Autosomal dominant nocturnal frontal lobe epilepsy
Late-onset childhood occipital epilepsy (Gastaut type)
Epilepsy with myoclonic absences
Lennox-Gastaut syndrome
Epileptic encephalopathy with continuous spike-and-wave during sleep
Landau-Kleffner syndrome
Childhood absence epilepsy

Adolescence–adult
Juvenile absence epilepsy
Juvenile myoclonic epilepsy
Epilepsy with generalized tonic-clonic seizures alone
Progressive myoclonic epilepsies
Autosomal dominant epilepsy with auditory features
Other familial temporal lobe epilepsies

Less-specific age relationship
Familial focal epilepsy with variable foci (childhood to adult)
Reflex epilepsies
Distinctive constellations

Berg, A. T., Berkovic, S. F., Brodie, M. J., Buchhalter, J., Crosss, J. H., van Emde Boas, W., . . . Scheffer, I. E. (2010). Revised terminology and concepts for organization of seizures and epilepsies: Report of the ILAE Commission on Classification and Terminology, 2005-2009. *Epilepsia*, *51*(4), 676–685.

Table 22.3. Seizure types by age of occurrence

Seizure/epilepsy type	Age of occurrence
Febrile seizures	6 months–6 years
Infantile spasms	4–16 months
Benign rolandic epilepsy	6–14 years (peak at 5–8 years)
Juvenile myoclonic epilepsy	8–26 years (peak at 14 years)
Childhood absence	4–12 years
Lennox-Gastaut syndrome	1–5 years
Juvenile absence epilepsy	7–17 years (peak at 14 years)

lamotrigine, topiramate, and clonazepam, but they are far less effective than steroids and vigabatrin (except for pyridoxine [vitamin B_6] for pyridoxine-dependent seizures; Ito, 1998). In some instances of refractory infantile spasms with focal seizures (called facilitated spasms) or with a single seizure focus identified, epilepsy surgery maybe an option (Shields et al., 1999).

Lennox-Gastaut Syndrome Infantile spasms may evolve into Lennox-Gastaut syndrome (LGS). This disorder is defined by a mixture of seizure types consisting of atypical absence, tonic, drop or atonic, myoclonic, tonic-clonic, and focal seizures with an impairment of awareness. Children with LGS are at an increased risk for frequent falls and injury. The characteristic EEG features include slow background activity, anterior slow spike waves, and multifocal spikes. Both seizure control and resolution of EEG abnormalities appear to be necessary for improved cognitive and behavioral outcome. Unfortunately, the seizures are difficult to control, and most affected children manifest intellectual disability.

Landau-Kleffner Syndrome Landau-Kleffner syndrome, also called acquired epileptic aphasia, is a disorder of childhood characterized by a loss of language skills in association with EEG abnormalities. It is characterized by an **auditory agnosia** (inability to distinguish different sounds in the presence of normal hearing), language regression, and behavioral disturbances that include inattention. These symptoms may develop gradually over months. The EEG pattern shows continuous abnormal epileptiform activity activated by sleep and obscures the normal sleep pattern (Inutsuka et al., 2006; Tassinari et al., 2012). The goal for treatment is normalization of the EEG and control of overt clinical seizures. Several ASMs can be tried, and steroids may be useful. However, while medication may resolve the EEG abnormalities, the aphasia may persist. Prognosis is variable; some children may recover some function after several years, while others are left with permanent speech impairments.

Juvenile Myoclonic Epilepsy Juvenile myoclonic epilepsy (JME) commonly begins during adolescence and is manifested by myoclonic jerks that occur upon awakening. More commonly, these myoclonic jerks are overlooked and, until a generalized tonic clonic occurs, medical attention is not sought. The seizures are exacerbated by alcohol ingestion, sleep deprivation, and photic stimulation. JME is likely genetically mediated, and individuals with JME have typical intelligence. In terms of treatment, ASMs that are effective for generalized rather than focal seizures are indicated, such as valproate and lamotrigine (Montalenti et al., 2001; Wallace, 1998). Previously, individuals with JME were thought to require lifelong treatment with an ASM. However, in a long-term follow-up study, one third of participants experienced seizure remission over time and lifelong ASM treatment was not needed (Camfield & Camfield, 2009).

Benign Epilepsy Syndromes The most common idiopathic benign epilepsy syndrome of childhood is **benign childhood epilepsy with centrotemporal spikes (BECTS),** also referred to as benign Rolandic epilepsy (BRE). This syndrome usually begins at 3–12 years and causes focal seizures without impairment of awareness. The seizures typically start in the region of the cortex that controls mouth and face movements, occur at sleep onset or at arousal, and can generalize. When the seizure starts in sleep, the focal onset is unobserved, so children may appear to be having generalized tonic-clonic seizures (Lerman, 1992). The characteristic EEG abnormality is epileptic spikes that are seen at the centrotemporal areas of the brain (Figure 22.4). Treatment is often not needed, and these syndromes are not associated with long-term sequelae. Some studies, however, have found an increased incidence of language and reading disabilities in affected children (Fejerman et al., 2000).

A second seizure type in this grouping is **benign occipital epilepsy.** It is characterized by visual disturbances and may be accompanied by vomiting, headache, eye blinking, and alteration of consciousness. At times it may be difficult to differentiate from migraine headaches. Unlike BRE, one half of children with benign occipital epilepsy will not outgrow their seizures. **Panayiotopoulus syndrome,** which also exhibits occipital epileptiform discharges, is characterized by brief, paroxysmal, and varying autonomic signs and symptoms.

Febrile Seizures Febrile seizures are the most common seizures occurring at the pediatric age group. They are not considered an epilepsy syndrome because the seizures are provoked. Febrile seizures occur in approximately 5% of children between the ages of 6 months and 5 years (Nelson & Ellenberg, 1978). They generally occur with body temperature elevations above 39° Celsius (102° Fahrenheit). Those that occur with lower temperatures are associated with an increased risk for having recurrent febrile seizures (Berg, Darefsky, Holford, & Shinnar, 1998). Acute illnesses such as upper respiratory illnesses, middle ear infections, and viruses associated with skin rashes (e.g., roseola) are frequent precipitants of febrile seizures.

Febrile seizures occur in two forms: simple febrile seizures, which manifest as a single generalized tonic seizure lasting less than 15 minutes (usually much less than this) and occurring during an acute illness, and complex febrile seizures, which are prolonged, focal, and/or recurrent during a single illness (Shinnar & Glauser, 2002; Seinfeld & Pellock, 2013). Febrile seizures tend to be familial and thus are postulated to have a genetic basis (Audenaert, Van Broeckhoven, & De Jonghe, 2006). In an affected child, the risk for a febrile seizure occurring in a sibling is 10%; if a parent also

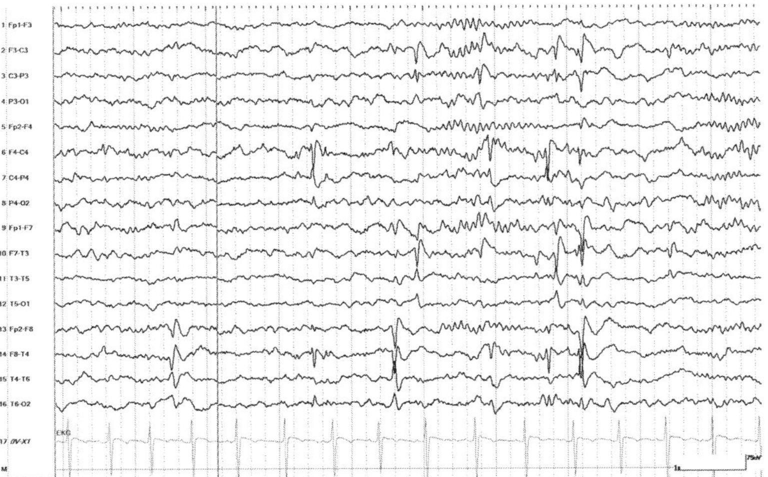

Figure 22.4. Centrotemporal spikes typical of benign childhood epilepsy with centrotemporal spikes (also referred to as benign rolandic epilepsy).

has a history of febrile seizure, the risk for that sibling increases to 50%.

In a child who presents with a febrile seizure, the risk of a subsequent febrile seizure is 30%–50% depending on the child's age at the time of the first seizure, the presence of a family history of febrile seizures, and the degree of fever (Berg et al., 1992). After a simple febrile seizure, the risk of developing epilepsy by school age is 1%; the risk of epilepsy is 2%–3% following a complex febrile seizure (Nelson & Ellenberg, 1976). The risk of developing epilepsy later increases if there is a family history of epilepsy or if the child has a developmental disability such as cerebral palsy, autism, or intellectual disability (Nelson & Ellenberg, 1976). In some studies, a febrile seizure with focal features or febrile status epilepticus has been associated with the development of temporal lobe epilepsy. As many as 30%–50% of adults with refractory temporal lobe epilepsy associated with **mesial temporal sclerosis** (scarring of the hippocampus) have a history of febrile seizures (Bower et al., 2000). By contrast, children with frequent but brief generalized seizures are more likely to have a genetic cause. For example, mutations of the *SCN1A* gene, which mediates neuronal firing, is the underlying cause of the syndrome known as generalized epilepsy with febrile seizures plus, as well as Dravet's syndrome (which is associated with truncation mutations of the SCNIA gene).

For prevention of febrile seizures in susceptible children, parents are taught to treat fever aggressively and promptly with antipyretics (medications for fever, such as acetaminophen). Prophylactic ASMs are usually not recommended since the benefits of intervention do not outweigh the risks of adverse effects from long-term use of medication. Although treatment may prevent subsequent febrile seizures, ASMs do not prevent the development of future epilepsy, and they may interfere with learning and attention (Knudsen, 2000). An alternative to chronic ASMs treatment is acute management with rectal or nasal benzodiazepines at the time of the seizure, which may abort a prolonged febrile seizure or prevent clusters of febrile seizures.

Conditions That Mimic Epilepsy

There are a number of conditions that mimic seizures but are nonepileptic events because they do not involve abnormal discharges of the cortical neurons (see Conditions That May Mimic Epilepsy textbox). They are caused by either physiological or psychological conditions. One study showed that approximately 20% of referrals for video EEG monitoring are not found to have epileptic seizures (Udall et al., 2006). In general, if a behavior can be triggered, interrupted, or modified by external stimuli, then it is probably not a seizure. A few examples are discussed in detail below.

Most random movements seen during sleep are a part of normal sleep activity. These include the random jerks of the extremities or eyes (rapid eye movements) that occur during active sleep, when the child is dreaming. Occasionally, sleep movements can be confused with seizures. **Benign sleep myoclonus of infancy** occurs in newborns and infants during sleep, and these movements disappear on arousal (Pachatz, Fusco, & Vigevano, 1999). It is characterized by a brief arrhythmic twitching of a limb during sleep that may be mistaken for a seizure; the EEG is normal, however, during this behavior.

Other more complex motor behaviors may occur 1–2 hours after sleep onset or occasionally upon arousal. These parasomnias include night terrors, sleep talking, sleep walking, and teeth grinding (Laberge, Tremblay, Vitaro, & Montplaisir, 2000). Rarely, nocturnal frontal lobe seizures are misinterpreted as a parasomnia (see Chapter 28); a video EEG recording is required to distinguish between the two (Lombroso, 2000). During a parasomnia, the eyes are open and the child appears to be awake, but the EEG shows a normal sleep rhythm. These parasomnia episodes may last as long as 15–30 minutes, much longer than a typical seizure, and parents may be unable to end the spell or rouse the child during this time. Rarely, treatment with medication such as diazepam (Valium) is necessary if the behavior is significantly disruptive to family life.

Psychogenic nonepileptic seizures (PNESs) usually present with generalized or subtle motor movements, an abrupt return to consciousness, no post-episode tiredness, and a normal EEG pattern. These spells may occur in an individual with affective and anxiety disorders (Kutluay et al., 2010; Patel, Scott, Dunn, & Garg, 2007). Features that suggest PNES include asynchronous movements that wax and wane, rolling from side to side, pelvic thrusting, eye closure during the spell, and absence of postictal confusion (Avbersek & Sisodiya, 2010). Video EEG monitoring with the goal of capturing the spells is often necessary.

Behaviors such as staring spells and rage attacks can be mistaken for seizures. Brief staring spells (daydreaming or "spacing out") are most commonly a sign of inattention but may resemble absence seizures. Staring spells, however, lack the subtle motor changes seen with absence or focal seizures (Bye, Kok, Ferenschild, & Vles, 2000). In temper tantrums and rage attacks, the child yells, throws himself on the floor, and lashes out at nearby people (Gordon, 1999). This may be associated with sweating, paleness, and dilated pupils. Although a similar dyscontrol syndrome (intermittent explosive disorder) has been seen following frontal or temporal lobe brain injury, ictal (seizure-associated) rage is usually unprovoked, very rare, and not directed toward a person (Pellock, 2015). After a rage attack the child resumes a normal state and may express remorse, while after an ictal event the child does not remember the episode (Pellock, 2015).

Breath-holding spells typically occur in infants between 6–18 months of age and are accompanied by loss of consciousness and generalized convulsions. The child becomes upset and cries vigorously, followed by an arrest in breathing. If the breath holding lasts long enough, it may result in a brief loss of consciousness followed by rapid neurological recovery. In **pallid infantile syncope,** the child faints or convulses after a startling, often minor injury. This presumably results from an exaggerated vasovagal reflex. Occasionally, a prolonged breath-holding or **syncopal** (fainting) episode can be associated with brief generalized convulsions followed by lethargy (Kuhle, Tiefenthaler, Seidl, & Hauser, 2000). There is, however, no epileptic activity on the EEG during these episodes.

Sandifer syndrome, which is associated with sudden arching of the back and rigid posturing of the trunk and upper extremities in infants, is caused by symptomatic gastroesophageal reflux and esophagitis (Frankel, Shalaby, & Orenstein, 2006). It may appear similar to infantile spasms and tonic seizures. The condition is addressed by treating the underlying gastroesophageal reflux with thickened feedings or medications.

Abnormal movements, termed **brainstem release phenomena,** can also be seen in neonates and children who are neurologically disabled. These non-epileptic motor phenomena arise from brainstem centers as a consequence of the reduction of neocortical inhibitory inputs secondary to diffuse encephalopathy (e.g., brain injury in premature infants with intraparenchymal hemorrhage or hypoxic ischemic encephalopathy; see Chapter 5). These movements may include subtle posturing, stiffening, brief deviation of the eyes, cessation of normal motor activity, apnea, or autonomic symptoms (Tharp, 2002). These movements may be difficult to differentiate from seizures; a video EEG may be helpful in distinguishing between the two. Brainstem release phenomena also have features of reflexive behavior, such as being provoked by stimulation and suppressed by gentle restraint (Mizrahi, 2016).

Conditions That May Mimic Epilepsy

- Migraine headaches
- Movement disorders: tic disorders, paroxysmal kinesogenic choreoathetosis
- Breath-holding spells
- Shuddering
- Sandifer's syndrome
- Parasomnias and normal physiological movements in sleep
- Sleep disorders: narcolepsy-cataplexy, night terrors
- Behavioral disorders
- Rage attacks, inattentiveness of ADD
- Panic attacks and hyperventilation
- Psychogenic non-epileptic seizures
- Syncope and other cardiac dysrhythmias/valvular disease/autonomic dysfunction
- Hyperexplexia (exaggerated startle response)
- Brainstem release phenomena
- Gastroesophageal reflux

DIAGNOSIS AND EVALUATION

The diagnosis of epilepsy begins with the clinical history and examination. A detailed description of the suspected seizure is crucial. The history should also include the presence or absence of aura; level of responsiveness during the event; and post-ictal changes, including altered mental status and transient focal neurologic deficits (i.e., Todd's paralysis). Tongue biting and urinary or bowel incontinence during the episode suggests seizure as its cause. Acute seizure precipitants, including infection, trauma, and drugs (illicit or accidental ingestion), need to be explored. The history helps to distinguish seizures from seizure mimics and to classify the seizure type. An infant or young child who turns blue or pale and loses consciousness after being upset or hurt likely has had a breath-holding spell. The presence of an aura or Todd's paralysis suggests a focal seizure. In children who present with a generalized tonic-clonic convulsion, an initial rapid head turn or eye deviation to one side suggests a focal seizure with the epileptogenic focus located in the contralateral brain hemisphere. A staring spell that lasts for a minute or more followed by post-ictal altered mental status (e.g., confusion, lethargy) points to a focal seizure. On the other hand, brief staring spells lasting a few seconds with return to full consciousness immediately afterward suggest absence seizures. Staring could also be a manifestation of non-epileptic events like daydreaming and inattention. About half of non-epileptic events captured on EEG monitoring are staring episodes (Uldall et al., 2006). The physical and neurologic examination may identify an acute illness or an associated neurologic disorder. Attention should be paid to head circumference, the skin exam (looking for evidence of **phakomatoses;** i.e., genetic conditions with characteristic skin findings), and focal neurological deficits.

Routinely performing laboratory tests is not helpful in a well child who has recovered from a brief seizure. Electrolytes should be collected, however, in children younger than 2 years of age to check for abnormal sodium, calcium, and glucose levels. Glucose should be checked in all individuals in status epilepticus and in people who have a history of seizures with fasting. Similarly, performing a **lumbar puncture** (spinal tap) should be reserved for febrile children with prolonged altered consciousness or who have suspected meningitis or encephalitis (De Hertz et al., 2000). In children with continuing neurologic impairment after a seizure, further workup, including lumbar puncture, chemical panel, metabolic tests for inborn errors of metabolism (e.g., plasma amino acids, urine organic acids, lactate, pyruvate), brain imaging (computed tomography [CT]/ magnetic resonance imaging [MRI]), and EEG to rule out nonconvulsive status epilepticus, needs to be considered.

A sleep-deprived EEG is indicated in the workup of all children suspected of having seizures. To perform the EEG several recording electrodes are placed on the scalp at set points over the frontal, central, parietal, temporal, and occipital regions bilaterally. These electrodes record voltage changes from the cortex below. The EEG displays electrical potential differences between neighboring electrodes or between an electrode and a reference. The EEG provides information regarding background brain electrical activity (e.g., generalized or focal slowing, which suggests diffuse or focal cerebral dysfunction, respectively), the presence or absence of epileptic discharges (sharp waves or spike and wave discharges indicating cortical hyperexcitability and, hence, predisposition to seizure), and response to activating procedures (hyperventilation, photic stimulation, and sleep deprivation). Occasionally seizures can be captured or provoked by activating procedures during a routine/standard EEG. The EEG should be recorded during wakefulness and light sleep. Light sleep tends to activate epileptiform discharges and increases the yield of the EEG.

EEG findings, along with the clinical data, help to establish the diagnosis of a specific seizure type. For instance, the finding of 3-Hz generalized spike and wave discharges activated by hyperventilation is diagnostic of absence epilepsy (Figure 22.2). Centrotemporal spike and wave discharges activated in sleep suggest benign childhood epilepsy with centrotemporal spikes (Figure 22.4). The EEG may also provide prognostic information. In children with their first unprovoked seizure who have a normal neurologic examination, the seizure recurrence risk is higher if the EEG is abnormal (Shinnar et al., 1996). In situations where the nature of the events is unclear, continuous video EEG monitoring for 23 hours or longer may be needed to capture and characterize the events. Continuous video EEG is required as part of presurgical evaluation in children for whom epilepsy surgery is being considered (see Box 22.2 for a discussion of the role of the epilepsy specialist, or epileptologist, in the diagnosis and management of complex epilepsy).

Brain imaging with MRI is essential to identify structural lesions that cause seizures. In some epilepsy syndromes such as benign childhood epilepsy with centrotemporal spikes (benign rolandic epilepsy), childhood or juvenile absence epilepsy, and juvenile myoclonic epilepsy, the likelihood of a structural lesion is low and routine neuroimaging is not indicated unless atypical features are present or the clinical course is atypical. Children with simple febrile seizures do

BOX 22.2 INTERDISCIPLINARY CARE

The Epileptologist

An epilepsy specialist (epileptologist) is a neurologist with expertise in epilepsy. For children with epilepsy who do not respond to one or two first-line anti-seizure medications, evaluation by an epilepsy specialist is advisable. The epilepsy specialist will review the seizure history, EEG, and brain MRI. In a child who continued to have seizures after two or more appropriately selected anti-epileptic drugs, the chance of success with another anti-epileptic drug is low. The epilepsy specialist will explore other treatment options, including dietary treatment, surgery, and neuro-modulatory therapies. As the first step the child is admitted to an inpatient video EEG monitoring unit to capture and characterize the child's typical seizures. If surgery is an option to a specific child, the next step is to present and discuss this in a multidisciplinary epilepsy surgical conference. Clinical, EEG, MRI, and neuropsychology findings will be reviewed, and the multidisciplinary team will then determine whether the child is a surgical candidate.

not require routine brain imaging (Subcommittee on Febrile Seizures—American Academy of Pediatrics, 2011). In all other children with recently diagnosed focal or generalized epilepsy and in children younger than 2 years of age, neuroimaging is recommended (Gaillard et al., 2009; Hsieh et al., 2010). The preferred imaging modality is brain MRI because of higher yield and better anatomic detail. High-resolution brain MRI should be performed with epilepsy and age-appropriate protocol (Gaillard et al., 2009). Head CT is usually performed in the emergency room setting; it may identify tumors, bleeding, and calcifications, but it may also provide falsely reassuring negative results.

Functional neuroimaging (see Chapter 8) studies are also used to identify the seizure focus when epilepsy surgery is being considered and a routine MRI is normal. FDG-positron emission tomography (FDG-PET) assesses the interictal brain metabolism. A seizure focus tends to have low metabolism in the interictal period. Interictal and ictal single photon emission computed tomography (SPECT) assesses blood flow to the brain and may therefore be able to identify the seizure focus. Magnetoencephalography (MEG) helps in localizing epileptiform discharges. Functional MRI is a noninvasive technique used to identify functionally critical ("eloquent") brain regions to be spared during epilepsy surgery, such as those that subserve language, motor, sensory, and memory functions (O'Shaughessy, Berl, Moore, & Gaillard, 2008). Magnetic resonance spectroscopy (MRS) performed along with MRI is used to assess the concentration of some chemicals (e.g., N-acetyl aspartic acid, choline, creatine, and lactate) in specific brain regions and is helpful in the workup of certain metabolic disorders (e.g., an abnormal lactate peak may be seen in mitochondrial disorders).

TREATMENT

Once the diagnosis of epilepsy is made and an evaluation is initiated for etiology, then treatment is pursued. ASMs are the first line of treatment in almost all instances of epilepsy. The ideal ASM will control, and hopefully prevent, seizures and correct the underlying epileptogenic tendency without producing adverse effects. However, none of the currently available ASMs meets this standard. The decision to start ASMs treatment in a person with epilepsy is based on balancing the risk of recurrence of seizures, the potential harm involved with occurrence of a seizure, and the adverse effects of ASMs.

The risk of recurrence of seizure after a single unprovoked seizure is 40%–50% (Berg, 2008). It tends to be higher in children with symptomatic causes, an abnormal EEG, a history of febrile seizure, Todd's paralysis, and seizures in sleep (Berg, 2008; Shinnar et al., 1996). About half (53%) of seizure recurrences occur in the first 6 months after the initial seizure, and 88% within 2 years (Shinnar et al., 1996).

The seizure recurrence risk increases to 65%–79% after two unprovoked seizures (Camfield et al., 1985; Hauser et al., 1998). Although initiating ASMs may delay the recurrence of seizures, postponing initiating ASMs until the second seizure does not appear to alter the ultimate prognosis, the risk of brain injury, or the efficacy of ASMs (Arts & Geerts, 2009; Hirtz et al., 2003). A child who has two or more unprovoked seizures should be considered for initiation of ASM. However, treatment should be individualized, and some children with self-limiting epilepsy syndromes like BECTS may not need to be on ASMs even if they have two or more seizures as long as the seizures are infrequent, nocturnal, and manifest as simple partial seizures.

Prehospital Management of Acute Seizures

Children with epilepsy and their families need to be educated about common sense seizure precautions (see the Seizure Precautions: Common Sense Measures textbox). Activities that could potentially result in significant injury or endanger the life of a child who is having a seizure should be avoided.

First aid measures and emergency plans should be discussed with parents and with the school nurse. Children in the midst of a generalized tonic-clonic convulsion ("grand mal seizure") should be placed on a flat surface and turned to one side to prevent aspiration. Tight clothes should be loosened around the neck. No object should be placed between the teeth. The airway should be maintained (for example, by pulling the jaw forward using a jaw-thrust maneuver). Cardiopulmonary resuscitation is usually not needed.

Seizures usually last less than 5 minutes; however, if they persist over 5 minutes they tend to continue for longer periods of time unless there is intervention (Shinnar et al., 2001). If seizure lasts 5 minutes or longer, rectal diazepam gel (Diastat) should be given at home. Intranasal or **buccal** (into-the-cheek) midazolam (Holsti, Dudley, & Shunk, 2010; Scott, Besag, & Neville, 1999) and dissolving clonazepam wafers placed between the cheek and gum (Troeser, Hastriter, & Ng, 2010) are alternatives to rectal diazepam with comparable efficacy and improved ease of use. The family should be educated about the use of the selected emergency medication. Urgent medical attention (i.e., calling 911) is recommended if the child has no known prior seizures, if seizure clusters are unresponsive to medications, if consciousness is not regained following the seizure, or if there is another significant intercurrent illness.

Seizure Precautions: Common Sense Measures

- Take showers instead of baths
- Leave bathroom doors unlocked
- Avoid climbing heights (e.g., trees, ladders)
- Wear a helmet while riding a bicycle or scooter
- Swim in a clear water ONLY with adult supervision
- Ensure parental supervision around hot objects (e.g., stoves) to avoid burn injury

Chronic Management of Epilepsy: Anti-seizure Medications

Mechanisms, Selection, and Use of ASMs

ASMs act on excitatory (glutamate-mediated) and inhibitory (gamma aminobutyric acid [GABA]–mediated) neurotransmission in cortical neurons through one of four mechanisms: 1) modulation of voltage-gated sodium channels (phenytoin, carbamazepine, felbamate, lamotrigine, topiramate, oxcarbazepine, and zonisamide), 2) modulation of calcium channels (ethosuximide, zonisamide, and valproic acid), 3) enhancing GABA action (benzodiazepines, barbiturates, tiagabine, and vigabatrin), and 4) inhibiting glutamate (topiramate and felbamate). Many ASMs exert their effect through multiple mechanisms of action (Sankar & Holmes, 2004). Selection of an ASM is based primarily on seizure type (focal versus generalized), epilepsy syndrome, side effect profile, and comorbidities (Wolfgang, 2007).

ASMs are broadly categorized as narrow spectrum (carbamazepine, gabapentin, lacosamide, oxcarbazepine, phenobarbital, phenytoin, and tiagabine) and broad spectrum (lamotrigine, levetiracetam, rufinamide, topiramate, valproate, and zonisamide). The narrow-spectrum drugs are effective in focal or secondarily generalized epilepsies, while broad-spectrum ASMs are effective in both focal and generalized epilepsies (Asconape, 2010). Table 22.4 shows the selection of ASMs based on seizure type, and the characteristics of individual ASMs can be found in Appendix C. Carbamazepine, oxcarbazepine, leviteracitam, and lamotrigine are first-line drugs in focal seizures with or without secondary generalization, while valproate, lamotrigine, topiramate, and perhaps leviteracitam are first-line drugs in generalized epilepsies (Wheless, Clarke, & Carpenter, 2005; Wilmshurst, Burman, Gaillard, & Cross, 2015; Shih et al., 2017). For Lennox-Gastaut syndrome, additional medication options include rufinamide, clobazam, and felbamate.

Valproate, pregabalin, and carbamazepine are associated with weight gain, while topiramate and zonisamide result in weight loss. When treating individuals who are obese and need to avoid weight gain, topiramate or zonisamide may be preferred choices of ASMs.

Because epilepsy is also comorbid with a range of other neurological conditions and because seizure medications are also effective in a range of other conditions, it is frequently possible to use a single medication to treat epilepsy and its comorbidity. An individual with migraine and epilepsy could be treated for both conditions with topiramate or valproate. Carbamazepine, lamotrigine, and valproate are appropriate choices for individuals with an associated mood disorder. Phenobarbital and topiramate, on the other hand, are associated with depression and are best avoided in people with mood disorders.

The goal of ASM treatment is prevention of seizures while having no or minimal side effects and resulting in an acceptable quality of life (QOL). In children with refractory epilepsy, acceptable seizure control should be defined and agreed upon between the older child, his or her parents, and the health care provider. Many parents will tolerate a few seizures if it means a more alert child with a lower ASM dose and fewer drugs.

Table 22.4. Selection of anti-seizure medications (ASMs) based on seizure types

Seizure type	First-line ASMs
Partial or secondarily generalized epilepsy	Carbamazpine, oxcarbazepin, leviteracitam, lamotrigine
Generalized epilepsy	
Absence	Ethosuximide, lamotrigine, valproate
Juvenile myoclonic epilepsy	Valproate[a], lamotrigine, topiramate
Tonic clonic	Valproate[a], lamotrigine, topiramate
Lennox-Gestaut syndrome	Valproate[a], lamotrigine, topiramate
Infantile spasms	Adrenocorticotropic hormone, vigabatrin[b]

Adapted from Wheless, J. W., Clarke, D., Arzimanoglou, F., & Carpenter, D. (2007). Treatment of pediatric epilepsy: European expert opinion, 2007. *Epileptic Disorders*, 9(4), 353–412.

[a]The risk of valproate-induced hepatic toxicity is high in children less than 2 years of age.

[b]Vigabatrin is the treatment of choice in children with tuberous sclerosis.

ASMs should be started at a low dose and titrated up slowly to the lowest effective dose. Whenever possible, monotherapy is the preferred treatment. **Polypharmacy** (the use of multiple medications) increases the risk of adverse effects and drug interactions. If two or more appropriate ASMs used at reasonable doses have failed an individual with a focal epilepsy, then other treatment modalities (e.g., surgery or the ketogenic diet; see discussion below) should be considered. Once a child is started on ASMs, the child should be monitored for adverse effects. Monitoring drug levels can be useful 1) to assess adherence to treatment, 2) to know the individual's effective therapeutic drug level for future comparisons, 3) to diagnose clinical toxicity, and 4) to adjust dose (Patsalos et al., 2008).

ASM Adverse Effects Prior to 1993, carbamazepine, ethosuximide, phenobarbital, phenytoin, and valproate were the principal ASMs available for use. Since 1993, many new ASMs have been introduced, including felbamate, gabapentin, lacosamide, lamotrigine, levetiracetam, oxcarbazepine, pregabalin, rufinamide, tiagabine, topiramate, zonisamide, and vigabatrin. The newer ASMs as a group have an efficacy comparable to the older drugs in controlling seizures and many have a better side-effect profile.

ASM adverse effects fall in to one of three categories: 1) dose-related adverse effects, 2) idiosyncratic reactions, and 3) chronic adverse effects (Perucca & Meador, 2005). Dose-related adverse effects often impact the central nervous system and manifest as somnolence, dizziness, ataxia, and cognitive impairment. These adverse effects can be minimized by starting with a low dose of ASM and titrating up slowly to the lowest effective dose. Idiosyncratic reactions (rare reactions in specific individuals) include **urticaria** (hives), Stevens-Johnson syndrome (a severe immune reaction associated with blister and peeling of the skin and mucous membranes), hepatitis, and aplastic anemia. Chronic adverse effects like weight change, gingival hyperplasia, hair loss, and abnormal bone metabolism may be seen with prolonged use of ASMs (Perucca & Meador, 2005). When adverse effects occur, the dose of the ASM should be decreased or stopped if the reaction is severe.

ASM-related cognitive adverse effects are especially important in young children who are acquiring new skills, and they may result in long-lasting developmental impairment (Loring & Meador, 2004). ASMs predominantly affect attention and psychomotor speed (Hessen et al., 2006; Lagac, 2006; Loring & Meador, 2004). Although all ASMs may potentially cause cognitive adverse effects, particularly at high doses and in the presence of polypharmacy (Perucca & Meador, 2005), phenobarbital and topiramate seem to be incriminated more often than others (Park & Kwon, 2008). There is concern that the cognitive impairment associated with phenobarbital may be long lasting (Sulzbacher et al., 1999). Cognitive adverse effects of topiramate tend to occur with higher doses, rapid titration, and polypharmacy (Glauser et al., 2007; Park & Kwon, 2008). Leviteracitam is associated with reversible deterioration in behavior and occasionally psychosis. Behavioral adverse effects of leviteracitam are the most common reason for discontinuation of therapy (Egunslola, Choonara, & Sammons, 2016). Perampanil is associated with a higher risk of psychiatric adverse effects including aggression, suicidal ideation, and depression. The risk of these serious psychiatric adverse effects is higher for higher doses and in adolescents as compared with adults (Rugg-Gunn, 2014).

Drug Interactions ASMs that induce hepatic enzymes (e.g., carbamazepine, phenytoin, and phenobarbital) or inhibit hepatic enzymes (e.g., valproate) that are important in drug metabolism (e.g., cytochrome P450 [CYP450] enzymes, glucuronyl transferase, and epoxide hydrolase) may affect the levels of other concomitantly used ASMs or their metabolites as well as other classes of drugs (Perucca & Meador, 2005). Enzyme-inducing ASMs reduce the concentration of other ASMs metabolized by the hepatic enzyme system, in some instances to a significant degree. For example, valproic acid inhibits the metabolism of lamotrigine and may result in higher plasma levels, thus increasing the risk of adverse effects of lamotrigine, especially Stevens-Johnson syndrome. To prevent such adverse effects, lamotrigine should be started at a very low dose, titrated up slowly, and maintained at a relatively lower dose in children taking valproic acid.

Other drugs can also affect the hepatic enzyme systems. Erythromycin and clarithromycin, for instance, inhibit CYP450 enzymes, and as a result, children taking carbamazepine may develop toxicity if either of these antibiotics is concomitantly administered.

Anticipating potential drug interactions, avoiding drug combinations with significant interactions, adjusting doses, monitoring for adverse effects of drugs, and monitoring blood levels of ASMs will help prevent drug toxicity or loss of efficacy due to drug interactions. It is also important to anticipate a significant change in the blood level of ASMs as a concomitantly administered enzyme inducer or inhibitor is discontinued. In children with cancer who require chemotherapy, avoiding enzyme-inducing ASMs and selecting ASMs with little or no hepatic enzyme-inducing effects is desirable, as ASMs may enhance the metabolism of chemotherapeutic agents.

ASMs and Bone Metabolism Chronic use of ASMs may be associated with abnormal bone metabolism. ASMs that induce hepatic cytochrome P450 enzymes accelerate vitamin D metabolism and may cause a vitamin D deficiency (Shellhaas & Joshi, 2010). Laboratory tests (25-OH vitamin D) and imaging studies (DEXA scan) to assess bone metabolism should be monitored in children with prolonged ASM therapy. Multivitamins with calcium and vitamin D are recommended in this group of children.

ASMs in Adolescent Women There are two major concerns in the treatment of adolescent women with epilepsy. One is loss of efficacy of contraception in individuals who are taking certain ASMs (including carbamazepine, phenytoin, phenobarbital, and topiramate, at high dose). These drugs increase the metabolism of estrogen and protein binding of progesterone. In these instances, increasing the estrogen dose and using barrier methods need to be considered to prevent unwanted pregnancy (Zupanc, 2006).

A second concern is **teratogenesis** (adverse effects on the developing fetus; see Chapter 2). Most ASMs are pregnancy category C (teratogenicity in experimental animals, no human studies). With all ASMs, the risk of congenital malformations is higher than the general population (Asconape, 2010), and polytherapy may further increase this risk (Vajda et al., 2016), yet risk-benefit analysis favors continuation of most ASMs during pregnancy. Valproate and phenobarbital, however, tend to be associated with a higher incidence of congenital malformations and are better avoided in pregnancy. Valproate demonstrates a dose-dependent increased risk of major congenital malformations (Tomson et al., 2015), particularly neural tube defects (e.g., spina bifida). Supplementation with folic acid may reduce this risk and is recommended for all women with pregnancy potential (see Chapter 6). Topiramate in polytherapy may also be associated with an increased risk of major congenital malformations (Vajda et al., 2016).

A study that compared the effect of in utero exposure of carbamazepine, lamotrigine, phenytoin, and valproate on IQ at 3 years of age showed that valproate was associated with a significantly increased risk of cognitive impairment and autism (Meador et al., 2010).

Discontinuing ASMs There are a number of concerns about the long-term use of ASMs. These include teratogenicity, poor self-image of being chronically ill, adverse effects of drugs, and cost. As a result, practitioners attempt to stop ASMs after a sufficiently long period of seizure freedom. An EEG is performed when a decision about stopping an ASM is considered; a normal EEG is reassuring, while an abnormal EEG introduces a level of uncertainty about seizure recurrence risk. The risk of seizure recurrence after discontinuation of ASMs in a child who has been seizure free for 2 years or longer is 25%–36% (Caviedes & Herranz, 1998; Shinnar et al., 1994). Children with symptomatic causes and certain developmental disabilities have a lower rate of seizure freedom after discontinuation of ASMs (20%–50%). Medications should be tapered over several months and not abruptly discontinued, as this may precipitate seizures.

Chronic Management of Epilepsy: Other Treatment Options

In the chronic management of epilepsy, pursing other treatment options may be necessary for children who do not respond to appropriate ASMs.

Ketogenic Diet The ketogenic diet mimics the fasting state and is a high-fat, low-carbohydrate, and low-protein diet. It is restrictive. The ketogenic diet is the treatment of choice for glucose transporter deficiency, a condition associated with epileptic encephalopathy resulting from impaired glucose transport to the brain (Klepper, 2008). The ketogenic diet is also used in the treatment of pyruvate dehydrogenase deficiency (a mitochondrial disorder; see Chapter 16). Children with a wide variety of seizure types and syndromes refractory to ASMs benefit from the ketogenic diet. (Freeman, Kossoff, & Hartman, 2007). Urine and blood ketone levels should be monitored to ensure adequate ketosis. Side effects include metabolic acidosis, hypoglycemia, gastrointestinal disturbance, and lethargy in the early stages of initiating the diet. Renal stones, dyslipidemia (abnormalities of lipid metabolism), and failure to thrive are late side effects (Freeman et al., 2007). The diet can be stopped after a child is seizure free for a sufficiently long time in much the same way as discontinuation of ASMs.

Surgical Resection of Epileptic Focus In children with focal epilepsy who have failed two or more appropriate ASMs at an adequate dosage, epilepsy surgery should be considered. After the third medication, the likelihood of additional medications working is only 4%–8%. When a clear focal lesion is present (e.g., mesial temporal sclerosis, focal cortical dysplasia, developmental tumors, or vascular malformations) the likelihood of an excellent outcome from surgery is 80%–85% (50%–60% seizure free, 25%–30% rare seizures; Chern, Patel, Jea, Curry, & Comair, 2010; Englot, Breshears, Sun, Chang, & Auguste, 2013; Englot et al., 2013; Jobst & Cascino, 2015; Rowland et al., 2012). If the

MRI is normal but PET or SPECT scans are abnormal, then there is a 50%–60% likelihood of excellent surgical outcome. If all imaging studies are normal, surgical benefit drops to 25%–30%. **Hemispherectomy** (removing the damage or diseased hemisphere of the brain) is performed for hemimegalencephaly and Rasmussen encephalitis, and occasionally for porencephaly with widespread focal cortical dysplasia.

Palliative Surgery When a seizure focus cannot be identified, or cannot be safely removed surgically due to involvement of eloquent cortex, or when there are multiple seizure foci, then palliative epilepsy surgery may reduce seizure frequency or severity. These procedures rarely result in seizure freedom but may improve quality of life. Disconnecting the corpus callosum (the thick band of nerves connecting the right and left hemispheres of the brain; see Chapter 8) by means of a corpus callosotomy is a treatment option for refractory epilepsy, including atonic (or drop) seizures and secondarily generalized epilepsy (Rosenfeld & Roberts, 2009).

Neuromodulatory Therapies The vagal nerve stimulator provides an intermittent electrical impulse to the left vagus nerve. Approximately 40% of selected individuals may have a 50% reduction in targeted seizures (Mapstone, 2008).

As of 2018, deep brain stimulation and responsive cortical stimulation to abort seizures in response to cortical detection of seizures are being studied in adults but are not yet available for testing in children (Jobst, Darcey, Thadani, & Roberty, 2010).

Nonspecific Interventions Common factors that provoke or exacerbate seizures include sleep deprivation and infections with or without fever. Parents and children should be counseled about good sleep hygiene and the importance of prevention and treatment of infections and fever. Flashing lights provoke seizures in children with photosensitive epilepsy and so should be avoided. Seizures may also be exacerbated around the time of ovulation or menses. Poor adherence to taking ASMs is an important cause of breakthrough seizures, and compliance issues should be discussed with the family.

Vitamins, Minerals, and Complementary and Alternative Medicine Folate supplementation is recommended for females who are taking valproate during their child-bearing years. Pyridoxine (vitamin B_6) is indicated in the treatment of a rare form of epilepsy resulting from pyridoxine dependency or deficiency. Calcium and vitamin D supplementation may be helpful in preventing osteoporosis. Seizures associated with certain inborn errors of metabolism may be treated with vitamins and nutritional supplements.

There is considerable interest from families of children with medically intractable epilepsy about the value of medical marijuana in the treatment of refractory epilepsy. There are limited data indicating improvement in seizure control with cannabidiol (a drug similar, but not identical, to tetrahydrocannabinol, the active substance in medical marijuana) in some epilepsy syndromes. In a recent randomized controlled trial in individuals with Dravet syndrome (a complex epilepsy syndrome and epileptic encephalopathy that presents during the first year of life, cannabidiol resulted in a higher rate of significant seizure reduction as compared to placebo. Adverse effects were mild to moderate and included vomiting, diarrhea, fever, fatigue, somnolence, and abnormal liver function tests (Devinsky et al., 2017). Abnormal liver function tests also tend to be seen in individuals concomitantly taking valproate.

Cannabidiol inhibits or induces the hepatic cytochrome enzyme system, resulting in alteration in blood levels of various medications metabolized by the liver, including ASMs (Brodie & Ben-Menachem, 2017). The interaction between clobazam and cannabidiol is well documented. The blood level of clobazam and its metabolite (N-desmethylclobazam) increase significantly in individuals taking cannabidiol, resulting in excessive sedation. Hence, close monitoring for side effects, drug level monitoring, and adjusting the doses of drugs may be required while on cannabidiol. Although some families consider alternative medicine for the treatment of epilepsy, there is no evidence that the various homeopathic and herbal remedies are effective (Danesi & Adetunji, 1994). It is important to understand that "natural" is not necessarily harmless (see Chapter 39).

MULTIDISCIPLINARY CARE

Addressing the various needs of a child with epilepsy requires a multidisciplinary approach, preferably in a comprehensive epilepsy center. The team includes neurologists, psychiatrists, neuropsychologists, nurses, social workers, and other health professionals.

School Performance and Educational Programs

Children with epilepsy may have cognitive and learning difficulties. A child with absence seizures may start to do poorly as seizure frequency increases. Dosage change or introduction of a new ASM may cause decreased attention and somnolence, which may interfere with the child's school performance. Irritability and aggression may occur as a result of medication adverse effects. Comorbidities such as ADHD may coexist with epilepsy and contribute to poor school performance. Teachers need to be aware of the need for closer monitoring of school performance in children with epilepsy. A child with declining school performance needs a thorough evaluation for possible causes including seizure exacerbation, ASM adverse effects, comorbidities (e.g., ADHD and depression), learning and memory problems, and psychosocial stress. Also, the educational program should be reviewed. Corrective actions may include medication adjustment, treating comorbidities, and designing an individualized education program. Children with epilepsy are eligible to receive special education and related services through the Individuals with Disabilities Education Improvement Act of 2004 (PL 108-446) under the educational classification of "other health impairment" (see Chapter 33).

Having a seizure in the classroom may be a source of anxiety and embarrassment, especially for a child who has tonic-clonic convulsions associated with bladder or bowel incontinence. Educating classmates about epilepsy and what to expect may be helpful. Parents may request a classroom discussion about seizures. The discussion does not have to identify the specific child (Coleman & Fielder, 1999). By contrast, if a child's epilepsy is well controlled and daytime seizures do not occur, a discussion about seizures with classmates may be counterproductive, as the child will be identified as different and subjected to potential stigmatization. For children with poorly controlled seizures associated with incontinence, a towel and fresh change of clothing can be kept in the nurse's office.

Psychosocial Issues

Epilepsy affects health-related quality of life (HRQL) measures through several mechanisms: 1) frequency of seizures, 2) ASM adverse effects, 3) comorbidities (e.g., anxiety, depression, and learning disorders), 4) the presence of an underlying neurologic disorder, 5) social stigma, and 6) the unpredictability of seizures. Even children who have had only a single seizure or children newly diagnosed with epilepsy are more likely to report impaired HRQL, perhaps as a consequence of child and parental anxiety (Modi et al., 2009). Social stigma may affect the child's self-perception, leading to low self-esteem and depression. Parents may react to seizures by overprotecting their child, which may have the unintended consequence of fostering lifelong dependence. Seizures affect the entire family. Mothers of children with epilepsy tend to be at increased risk for depression (Ferro & Speechley, 2009). There also is a significant financial and time burden to the family. The child as well as the whole family needs to be educated about epilepsy and support should be provided.

Children with epilepsy should generally be encouraged to participate in sports. Routine safety precautions should be applied as with any child. However, some sport activities pose a specific danger to the life of a person with epilepsy (e.g., scuba diving, rock climbing, parachuting, and unsupervised swimming) and should be avoided (Fountain & May, 2003).

Family vacations and camping trips should be encouraged, but excess fatigue should be avoided. The family needs to have an adequate supply of ASMs, and the doctor's and pharmacy's contact information should be on hand. Wearing a medical identification bracelet or necklace may be useful if it is acceptable to parents and the child.

Independence should be encouraged as the child enters adulthood. Driving license laws vary from state to state, but generally the individual needs to be seizure free for between 3–12 months before their license can be obtained or reinstated. An altered fertility rate and potential teratogenic effects of ASMs are issues that need to be addressed.

Several organizations advocate and provide resources for individuals with epilepsy, including the American Epilepsy Society, the Epilepsy Foundation, and the International League Against Epilepsy.

OUTCOME

A majority of children (70%–80%) with epilepsy achieve seizure control with the first or second ASM, and about two thirds can be successfully weaned off their ASMs after 2 years of being seizure free (MacDonald et al., 2000). Children with "idiopathic" epilepsy have better long-term outcomes than those with "cryptogenic" epilepsy, who in turn have better long-term outcomes than those with remote symptomatic epilepsy (Sillanpää et al., 2015).

Children who have had a single seizure have comparable intelligence scores to siblings (Sogawa, Masur, O'Dell, Moshe, & Shinnar, 2010). In one prospective study, approximately 74% of children with epilepsy had typical global cognitive function, while the remaining 26% had lower cognitive functioning. Young age at seizure onset, symptomatic cause, epileptic encephalopathy, and continued need for ASM treatment were significant independent risk factors for cognitive impairment (Berg et al., 2008).

The most common causes of mortality in epilepsy are 1) an accident (most often swimming related), 2) the underlying cause of the epilepsy (e.g., brain tumor), and 3) sudden unexpected death in epilepsy (SUDEP). SUDEP is an underappreciated cause of seizure-related deaths (Sillanpää & Shinnar, 2010), and it may be related to post-ictal alterations in respiratory and cardiac function (Harden et al., 2017; Ryvlin et al., 2013). Accurate data on the incidence of SUDEP are lacking. A meta-analysis of studies suggests an incidence of 0.22 out of 1,000 patient-years in childhood, which makes it a very rare occurrence (Harden et al., 2017). Generalized tonic-clonic seizures and nocturnal seizures appear to be risk factors for SUDEP. Other factors that increase the risk of SUDEP include early childhood onset of epilepsy, developmental delay, and refractoriness to multiple ASMs (Morse & Kothare, 2016). Children with Dravet syndrome are also at increased risk of SUDEP (Shmuely, Sisodiya, Gunning, Sander, & Thijs, 2016).

Continued seizures, medication side effects, and depression are associated with poor outcomes, including reduced quality of life, undereducation, unemployment, failure to achieve independence, and difficulties establishing lifelong social bonds (Sillanpää, 2000).

SUMMARY

- Epilepsy is characterized by recurrent seizures that result from abnormal electrical discharges in the brain.
- A seizure is classified as generalized or focal, depending on whether it involves both hemispheres at onset or starts in one hemisphere with or without subsequent spread to the other hemisphere.
- Most epilepsy can be controlled with a single ASM, but there are other treatment options.
- For children with epilepsy associated with multiple disabilities or symptomatic causes, the prognosis is more related to the disabilities and underlying causes than to the epilepsy itself.
- Side effects of medications and comorbidities should be assessed in conjunction with seizure control to optimize quality of life.

ADDITIONAL RESOURCES

American Epilepsy Society: http://www.aesnet.org

Epilepsy Foundation: http://www.efa.org

International League Against Epilepsy: http://www.ilae-epilepsy.org

Additional resources can be found online in Appendix D: Childhood Disabilities Resources, Services, and Organizations (see About the Online Companion Materials).

REFERENCES

Airaksinen, E. M., Matilainene, R., Mononen, T., Mustomen, K., Partanen, J., Jokela, V., & Halonen, P. (2000). A population-based study on epilepsy in mentally retarded children. *Epilepsia, 41,* 1214–1220.

Alvarez, N., Besag, F., & Iivanainen, M. (1998). Use of antiepileptic drugs in the treatment of epilepsy in people with intellectual disability. *Journal of Intellectual Disability Research, 42*(Suppl. 1), 1–15.

Arts, W. F., & Geerts, A. T. (2009). When to start drug treatment for childhood epilepsy: The clinical-epidemiological evidence. *European Journal of Paediatric Neurology, 13,* 93–101.

Asconape, J. J. (2010). The selection of antiepileptic drugs for the treatment of epilepsy in children. *Neurologic Clinics, 28,* 843–852.

Audenaert, D., Van Broeckhoven, C., & De Jonghe, P. (2006). Genes and loci involved in febrile seizures and related epilepsy syndromes. *Human Mutation, 27*(5), 391–401.

Avbersek, A., & Sisodiya, S. (2010). Does the primary literature provide support for clinical signs used to distinguish psychogenic nonepileptic seizures from epileptic seizures? *Journal of Neurology, Neurosurgery, and Psychiatry, 81,* 719.

Bazendale, S., & Heaney, D. (2010). Socioeconomic status, cognition, and hippocampal sclerosis. *Epilepsy & Behavior, 20*(1), 64–67.

Berg A. T., & Shinnar, S. (1991). The risk of seizure recurrence following a first unprovoked seizure: A quantitative review. *Neurology, 41,* 965–972.

Berg, A. T., Shinnar, S., Hauser, W. A., Alemany, M., Shapiro, E. D., Salomon, M. E., & Crain, E. F. (1992). A prospective study of recurrent febrile seizure. *The New England Journal of Medicine, 327*(16), 1122–1127.

Berg, A. T. (1995). The epidemiology of seizures and epilepsy in children. In S. Shinnar, N. Amir, & D. Branski (Eds.), *Childhood seizures* (pp. 1–10). Basel, Switzerland: Karger.

Berg, A. T., Darefsky, A. S., Holford, T. R., & Shinnar, S. (1998). Seizures with fever after unprovoked seizures: An analysis in children followed from the time of a first febrile seizure. *Epilepsia, 39*(1), 77–80.

Berg, A. T., Langfitt, J. T., Testa, F. M., Levy, S. R., DiMario, F., Westerveld, M., & Kulas, J. (2008). Global cognitive function in children with epilepsy: A community-based study. *Epilepsia, 49*(4), 608–614.

Berg, A. T. (2008). Risk of recurrence after a first unprovoked seizure. *Epilepsia, 49*(Suppl. 1), 13–18.

Berg, A. T., Berkovic, S. F., Brodie M. J., Buchhalter, J., Crosss, J. H., van Emde Boas, W., . . . Scheffer, I. E. (2010). Revised terminology and concepts for organization of seizures and epilepsies: Report of the ILAE Commission on Classification and Terminology, 2005-2009. *Epilepsia, 51*(4), 676–685.

Besag, F. M. C. (2002). Childhood epilepsy in relation to mental handicap and behavioral disorders. *Journal of Child Psychology and Psychiatry, 43,* 103–131.

Bower, S. P., Kilpatrick, C. J., Vogrin, S. J., Morris, K., & Cook, M. (2000). Degree of hippocampal atrophy is not related to a history of febrile seizures in patients with proved hippocampal sclerosis. *Journal of Neurology, Neurosurgery and Psychiatry, 69*(6), 733–738.

Briellmann, R. S., Jackson, G. D., Torn-Broers, Y., & Berkovic, S. F. (2001). Causes of epilepsies: Insights from discordant monozygous twins. *Annals of Neurology, 49*(1), 45–52.

Brodie, M. J., & Ben-Menachem, E. (2017). Cannabinoids for epilepsy: What do we know and where do we go? *Epilepsia,* Advance online publication. doi:10.1111/epi.13973

Bye, A. M., Kok, D. J., Frenschild, F. T., & Vies, J. S. (2000). Paroxysmal non-epileptic events in children: A retrospective study over a period of 10 years. *Journal of Paediatrics and Child Health, 36*(3), 244–248.

Camfield, P. R., Camfield, C. S., Dooley, J. M., Tibbles, J. A., Fung, T., & Garner, B. (1985). Epilepsy after a first unprovoked seizure in childhood. *Neurology, 35,* 1657–1660.

Camfield, C. S., & Camfield, P. R. (2009). Juvenile myoclonic epilepsy 25 years after seizure onset, a population based study. *Neurology, 73*(13), e64–e67.

Camfield, P., & Camfield, C. (2015). Incidence, prevalence and aetiology of seizures and epilepsy in children. *Epileptic Disorders, 17*(2), 117–123.

Caviedes, B. E., & Herranz, J. L. (1998). Seizure recurrence and risk factors after withdrawal of chronic antiepileptic therapy in children. *Seizure, 7*(2), 107–714.

Chern, J. J., Patel, A. J., Jea, A., Curry, D. J., & Comair, Y. G. (2010). Surgical outcome for focal cortical dysplasia, an analysis of recent surgical series. *Journal of Neurosurgery: Pediatrics, 6*(5), 452–458.

Cole, A. J. (2000). Is epilepsy a progressive disease? The neurobiological consequences of epilepsy. *Epilepsia, 41*(Suppl. 2), S13–S22.

Coleman, H., & Fielder, A. (1999). Epilepsy education in schools. *Paediatric Nursing, 11*(9), 29–32.

Commission on Classification and Terminology of the International League Against Epilepsy. (1981). Proposed for revised clinical and electroencephalographic classifications of epileptic seizures. *Epilepsia, 22,* 489–501.

Commission on Classification and Terminology of the International League Against Epilepsy. (1989). Proposal for revised classification of epilepsies and epileptic syndromes. *Epilepsia, 30,* 389–399.

Commission on Pediatric Epilepsy of the International League Against Epilepsy. (1992). Workshop on infantile spasms. *Epilepsia, 33,* 195.

Danesi, M. A., & Adetunji, J. B. (1994). Use of alternative medicine by patients with epilepsy: A survey of 265 epileptic patients in a developing country. *Epilepsia, 35*(2), 344–351.

Devinsky, O., Cross, J. H., Laux, L., Marsh, E., Miller, I., Nabbout, R., . . . Cannabidiol in Dravet Study Group. (2017). Cannabidiol in Dravet syndrome study group. Trial of cannabidiol for drug resistant seizures in the Dravet syndrome. *New England Journal of Medicine, 376,* 2011–2020.

Ding, D., & Hauser, W. A. (2015). The natural history of seizures. In E. Wyllie, B. E. Gidal, H. P. Goodkin, T. Loddenkemper, & J. I. Sirven (Eds.), *Wyllie's treatment of epilepsy: Principles and practice* (6th ed., p. 11). Philadelphia, PA: Wolters Kluwer.

Egunsola, O., Choonara, I., & Sammons, H. M. (2016). Safety of lebetiracetam in paediatrics: A systematic review. *PloS One, 11,* e0149686.

Engel, J., Jr. (2001). A proposed diagnostic scheme for people wiht epileptic seizures and with epilepsy: Report of the ILAE Task Force on Classification and Terminology. *Epilepsia, 42*(6), 796–803.

Englot, D. J., Breshears, J. D., Sun, P. P., Chang, E. F., & Auguste, K. I. (2013). Seizure outcomes after resective surgery for extra–temporal lobe epilepsy in pediatric patients. *Journal of Neurosurgery: Pediatrics, 12*(2), 126–133.

Englot, D. J., Rolston, J. D., Wang, D. D., Sun, P. P., Chang, E. F., & Auguste, K. I. (2013). Seizure outcomes after temporal lobectomy in pediatric patients. *Journal of Neurosurgery: Pediatrics, 12*(2), 134–141.

Fejerman, N., Caraballo, R., Tenenbaum, S. N. (2000). Atypical evolutions of benign localization-related epilepsies in children, Are they predictable? *Epilepsia 41*(4), 380–390.

Ferro, M. A., Speechley, K. N. (2009). Depressive symptoms among mothers of children with epilepsy: A review of prevalence, associated factors, and impact on children. *Epilepsia, 50*(1), 2344–2354.

Fisher, R. S., Acevedo, C., Arzimanoglou, A., Bogacz, A., Cross, J. H., Elger, E. E., . . . Wiebe, S. (2014). ILAE official report: A practical clinical definition of epilepsy. *Epilepsia, 55,* 475–482.

Fisher, R. S., Cross, H., D'Souza, C., French, J. A., Haut, S. R., Higurashi, N., . . . Suberi, S. M. (2017). Instruction manual for the ILAE 2017 operational classification of seizure types. *Epilepsia, 58*(4) 531–534 doi:10.1111/epi.13671

Forsgren, L., Edvinsson, S. O., Blomquist, H. K., Heijbel, J., & Sidenvall, R. (1990). Epilepsy in a population of mentally retarded children and adults. *Epilepsy Research, 6,* 234–248.

Fountain, N. B., & May, A. C. (2003). Epilepsy and athletics. *Clinics in Sports Medicine, 22,* 605–616.

Frankel, E. A., Shalaby, T. M., & Orenstein, S. R. (2006). Sandifer syndrome posturing, relation to abdominal wall contractions, gastroesophageal reflux, and fundoplication. *Digestive Diseases and Sciences, 51*(4), 635–640.

Freeman, J. M., Kossoff, E. H., & Hartman, A. L. (2007). The ketogenic diet: One decade later. *Pediatrics, 119,* 535–543.

Frucht, M. M., Quigg, M., Schwaner, C., & Fountain, N. B. (2000). Distribution of seizure precipitants among epilepsy syndromes. *Epilepsia, 41*(12), 1534–1539.

Gage, F. H. (2002). Neurogenesis in the adult brain. *The Journal of Neuroscience, 22*(3), 612–613.

Gaillard, W. D., Chiron, C., Cross, J. H., Harvey, A. S., Kuzniecky, R., Hertz-Pannier, L., . . . ILAE Committee for Neuroimaging, Subcommittee for Pediatric. (2009). Guidelines for imaging infants and children with recent-onset epilepsy. *Epilepsia, 50*(9), 2147–2153.

Glauser, T. A., Dlugos, D. J., Dodson, W. E., Grinspan, A., Wang, S., Wu, S. C., & EPMN-106/INT-28 Investigators. (2007). Topiramate monotherapy in newly diagnosed epilepsy. *Journal of Child Neurology, 22,* 693–699.

Gordon, N. (1999). Episodic dyscontrol syndrome. *Developmental Medicine and Child Neurology, 41*(11), 786–788.

Harden, C., Tomson, T., Gloss, D., Buchhalter, J., Cross, J. H., Donner, E., . . . Ryvlin, P. (2017). Practice guideline summary, sudden unexpected death in epilepsy incidence rates and risk factors: Report of the guideline development, dissemination, and implementation subcommittee of the American Academy of Neurology and the American Epilepsy Society. *Neurology, 88*(17), 1674–1680.

Hauser, W. A., & Kurland, L. T. (1993). Incidence of epilepsy and unprovoked seizures in Rochester, Minnesota, 1935–1984. *Epilepsia 34,* 453–468.

Hauser, W. (1994). The prevalence and incidence of convulsive disorders in children. *Epilepsia, 35*(Suppl 2), S1–S6.

Hauser, W. A., Rich, S. S., Lee, J. R., Annegers, J. F., & Anderson, V. E. (1998). Risk of recurrent seizures after two unprovoked seizures. *New England Journal of Medicine, 338*, 429–434.

Hessen, E., Lossius, M. I., Reinvang, I., & Gjerstad, L. (2006). Influence of major antiepileptic drugs on attention, reaction time, and speed of information processing: Results from a randomized, double blind, placebo-controlled withdrawal study of seizure-free epilepsy patients receiving monotherapy. *Epilepsia, 47*, 2038–2045.

Hirtz, D., Berg, A., Donley, D., Bettis, D., Camfield, C., Camfield, P., . . . Shinnar, S. (2003). Practice parameter: Treatment of the child with a first unprovoked seizure: Report of the Quality Standards Subcommittee of the American Academy of Neurology and the Practice Committee of the Child Neurology Society. *Neurology, 60*(2), 166–175.

Holmes, G. L. (2002). Childhood-specific epilepsies accompanied by developmental disabilities: Causes and effects. In O. Devinsky & L. E. Westbrook (Eds.), *Epilepsy and developmental disabilities* (pp. 23–40). Woburn, MA: Butterworth-Heinemann.

Holsti, M., Dudley, N., & Shunk, J. (2010). Intranasal midazolam vs rectal diazepam for the home treatment of acute seizures in pediatric patients with epilepsy. *Archives of Pediatrics and Adolescent Medicine, 164*(8), 747–753.

Hsieh, D. T., Chang, T., Tsuchida, T. N., Vezina, L. G., Vanderver, A., Siedel, J, . . . Gaillard, W. D. (2010). New onset afebrile seizures in infants: Presenting characteristics. *Neurology, 74*, 150–156.

Huang, C. C., Chang, Y.C., & Wang S. T. (1998). Acute symptomatic seizure disorders in young children—A populations study in Taiwan. *Epilepsia, 39*(9), 960–964.

Hundozi-Hysenaj, H., & Boshnjaku-Dallku, I. (2008). Epilepsy in children with cerebral palsy. *Journal of Pediatric Neurology, 6*, 43–46.

Inutsuka, M., Kobayashi, K., Oka, M., Hattori, J., & Ohtsuka, Y. (2006). Treatment of epilepsy with electrical status epilepticus during slow sleep and its related disorders. *Brain Development, 28*, 281–286.

Ito, M. (1998). Antiepileptic drug treatment of West syndrome. *Epilepsia, 39*(Suppl. 5), 38–41.

Jobst, B. C., & Cascino, G. D. (2015). Resective epilepsy surgery for drug-resistant focal epilepsy: A review. *JAMA, 313*(3), 285–293.

Jobst, B. C., Darcey, T. M., Thadani, V. M., & Roberty, D. W. (2010). Brain stimulation for the treatment of epilepsy. *Epilepsia, 51*(Suppl. 3), 88–92.

Kivity, S., Lerman, P., Ariel, R., Danziger, Y., Mimouni, M., & Shinnar, S. (2004). Long-term cognitive outcomes of a cohort of children with cryptogenic infantile spasms treated with high-dose adrenocorticotropic hormone. *Epilepsia, 45*, 255–262.

Klepper, J. (2008). Glucose transporter deficiency syndrome (GLUTIDS) and the ketogenic diet. *Epilepsia, 49*(Suppl. 8), 46–49.

Knudsen, F. U. (2000). Febrile seizures: Treatment and prognosis. *Epilepsia, 41*(1), 2–9.

Knupp, K. G., Coryell, J., Nickells, K. C., Ryan, N., Leister, E., Loddenkemper, T., . . . Pediatric Epilepsy Research Consortium. (2016). Response to treatment in a prospective national infantile spasms cohort. *Annals of Neurology, 79*(3), 475–484.

Kuhle, S., Tiefenthaler, M., Seidl, R., & Hauser, E. (2000). Prolonged generalized epileptic seizures triggered by breathholding spells. *Pediatric Neurology, 23*(3), 271–273.

Kutluay, E., Selwa, L., Minecan, D., Edwards, J., & Beydoun, A. (2010). Nonepileptic paroxysmal events in a pediatric population. *Epilepsy Behavior, 17*(2), 272–275.

Laberge, L., Tremblay, R. E., Vitaro, F., & Montplaisir, J. (2000). Development of parasomnias from childhood to early adolescence. *Pediatrics, 106*(1, Pt. 1), 67–74.

Lagac, L. (2006). Cognitive side effects of anti-jepileptic drugs, the relevance in childhood epilepsy. *Seizure, 15*, 235–241.

Lerman, P. (1992). Benign partial epilepsy with centrotemporal spikes. In J. Roger, M. Bereau, C. Dravet, P. Genton, C.A. Tassinari, & P. Wolf (Eds.), *Epileptic syndromes in infancy, childhood and adolescence* (pp. 189–200). London, England: John Libbey & Co. Ltd.

Lombroso, C. T. (2000). Pavor nocturnus of proven epileptic origin. *Epilepsia, 41*(9), 1221–1226.

Loring, D. W., & Meadoer, K. J. (2004). Cognitive side effects of antiepileptic drugs in children. *Neurology*, 62, 872–877.

Lowenstein, D. H., & Alldredge, B. K. (1998). Status epilepticus. *The New Journal of Medicine, 338*(14), 970–976.

Lux, A. L., Edwards, S. W., Hancock, E., Johnson, A. L., Kennedy, C. R., Newton, R. W., . . . Osborn, J. P. (2004). The United Kingdom Infantile Spasms Study (UKISS) comparing vigabatrin with prednisolone or tetracosactide at 14 days: A multicentre, randomised controlled trial. *Lancet, 364*, 1773–1778.

Mackay, M. T., Weiss, S. K., Adams-Webber, T., Ashwal, S., Stephens, D., Ballaban-Gill, K., . . . Snead, O. C. III. (2004). Practice parameter, medical treatment of infantile spasms, report of the American Academy of Neurology and the Child Neurology Society. *Neurology, 62*, 1668–1681.

MacDonald, B. K., Johanson, A. L., Goodridge, D. M., Cockerell, O. C., Sander, J. W., & Shorvon, S. D. (2000). Factors predicting prognosis of epilepsy after presentation with seizures. *Archives of Disease in Childhood, 81*(3), 261–262.

Mapstone, T. B. (2008). Vagus nerve stimulation: Current concepts. *Neurosurgery Focus, 25*, B9.

Meador, K. J., Baker, G. A., Browning, N., Clayton-Smith, J., Combs-Cantrell, D. T., Cohen, M., . . . Loring, D. W. (2010). Cognitive function at 3 years of age after fetal exposure to antiepileptic drugs. *New England Journal of Medicine, 360*, 1597–1605.

Medina, M. T., Bereau, M., Hirsch, E., & Panayiotopoulos, C. P. (2012). Childhood absence epilepsy. In M. Bureau, P. Genton, C. Dravet, A. Delgado–Escueta, C. Tassinari, P. Thomas, & P. Wolf (Eds.), *Epileptic syndromes in infancy, childhood and adolescence—With videos* (English and French 5th ed.; p. 255). London, England: John Libbey Eurotext Ltd.

Mizrahi, E. M. (2016). Neonatal seizures. In J. M. Pellock, D. R. Nordli, R. Sankar, & J. W. Wheless (Eds.), *Pellock's pediatric epilepsy: Diagnosis and therapy* (4th ed., p. 489). New York, NY: Demos Medical.

Modi, A. C., King, S. R., Monahan, S. R., Koumoutsos, J. E., Morita, D. A., & Glauser, T. A. (2009). Even a single seizure negatively impacts pediatric health-related quality of life. *Epilepsia, 50*(9), 2110–2116.

Morse, A. M., & Kothare, S. V. (2016). Pediatric sudden unexpected death in epilepsy. *Pediatric Neurology, 57*, 7–16.

Moshe, S. L. (2000). Seizures early in life. *Neurology, 55*(Suppl. 5), S15–S20; discussion, S54–S58.

Montalenti, E., Imperiale, D., Rovera, A., Bergamasco, B., & Benna, P. (2001). Clinical features, EEG findings and diagnostic pitfalls in juvenile myoclonic epilepsy: A series of 63 patients. *Journal of Neuroscience, 184*(1), 65–70.

Nelson, K. B., & Ellenberg, J. H. (1976). Predictors of epilepsy in children who have experienced febrile seizures. *The New England Journal of Medicine, 295*(19), 1029–1033.

Nelson, K. B., & Ellenberg, J. H. (1978). Prognosis in children with febrile seizures. *Pediatrics, 61*(5), 720–727.

O'Shaughnessy, E. S., Berl, M. B., Moore, E. N., & Gaillard, W. D. (2008). Pediatric functional magnetic resonance imaging (fMRI): Issues and applications. *Journal of Child Neurology, 23*, 791–801.

Pachatz, C., Fusco, L., & Vigevano, F. (1999). Benign myoclonus of early infancy. *Epileptic Disorders, 1*(1), 57–61.

Panayiotopoulos, C. P. (1999). *Current problems in epilepsy series: Vol. 15. Benign childhood partial seizures and related epileptic syndromes.* London, England: John Libbey and Co. Ltd.

Park, S. P., & Kwon, S. H. (2008). Cognitive effects of antiepileptic drugs. *Journal of Clinical Neurology 4*, 99–106.

Patel, H., Scott, E., Dunn, D., & Garg, B. (2007). Nonepileptic seizures in children. *Epilepsia, 48*, 2086.

Patsalos, P. N., Berry, D. J., Bourgeois, B. F. D., Cloyd, J. C., Glauser, T. A., Johnnessen, S. I, . . . Perruca, E. (2008). Antiepileptic drugs–Best practice guidelines for the therapeutic drug monitoring: A position paper by the subcommission on therapeutic drug monitoring, ILAE commission on therapeutic strategies. *Epilepsia, 49*(7), 1239–1276.

Pellock, J. M. (2015). Other nonepileptic paroxysmal disorder. In E. Wyllie, B. E. Gidal, H. P. Goodkin, T. Loddenkemper, & J. I. Sirven (Eds.), *Wyllie's treatment of epilepsy: Principles and practice* (6th ed., p. 500). Philadelphia, PA: Wolters Kluwer.

Pellock, J. M., Hrachovy, R., Shinar, S., Baram, T. Z., Bettis, D., Dlugis, D. J., . . . Wheless, J. W. (2010). Infantile spasms: A U.S. consensus report. *Epilepsia, 51*(10), 2175–2189.

Perucca, E., & Meador, K. J. (2005). Adverse effects of antiepileptic drugs. *Acta Neurologica Scandinavia, 112*(Suppl. 181), 30–35.

Reynolds, E. H. (2000). The ILAE/IBE/WHO Global Campaign Against Epilepsy: Bringing epilepsy "out of the shadows." *Epilepsy and Behavior, 1*(4), S3–S8.

Rosenfeld, W. E., & Roberts, D. W. (2009). Tonic and atonic seizures, what's next—VNS or callosotomy? *Epilepsia, 50*(Suppl. 8), 25–30.

Rowland, N. C., Englot, D. J., Cage, T. A., Sughrue, M. E., Barbaro, N. M., & Chang, E. F. (2012). A meta-analysis of predictors of seizure freedom in the surgical management of focal cortical dysplasia. *Journal of Neurosurgery, 116*, 1035–1041.

Rugg-Gunn, F. (2014). Adverse effects and safety profile of perampanel: A review of pooled data. *Epilepsia, 55*(Suppl.1), 13–15.

Ryvlin, P., Nashef, L., Lhatto, S. D., Bateman, L. M., Bird, J., Bleasel, A., . . .Tomson, T. (2013). Incidence and mechanisms of cardiorespiratory arrests in epilepsy monitoring units (MORTEMUS): A retrospective study. *Lancet Neurology, 12*(10), 966–977.

Sankar, R., & Holmes, G. L. (2004). Mechanisms of action for the commonly used antiepileptic drugs, relevance to antiepileptic drug associated neurobehavioral adverse effects. *Journal of Child Neurology, 19*, S6–S14.

Scott, R. C., Besag, F. M., & Neville, B. G. (1999). Buccal midazolam and rectal diazepam for treatment of prolonged seizures in childhood and adolescence, a randomized trial. *Lancet, 353*, 623–626.

Seinfeld, S., & Pellock, J. M. (2013). Recent research on febrile seizures: A review. *Journal of Neurology and Neurophysiology, 4*(165), 19519.

Shellhaas, R. A., & Joshi, S. M. (2010). Vitamin D and bone health among children with epilepsy. *Pediatric Neurology, 42*(6), 385–393.

Shields, W. D., Shewmon, D. A., Peacock, W., LoPresi, C. M., Nakagawa, J., & Yudovin, S. (1999). Surgery for the treatment of medically intractable infantile spasms: A cautionary case. *Epilepsia, 40*(9), 1305–1308.

Shih, J. J., Whitlock, J. B., Chimato, N., Vargas, E., Karceski, S. C., & Frank, R. D. (2017). Epilepsy treatment in adults and adolescents: Expert opinion, 2016. *Epilepsy & Behavior, 69*, 186–222.

Shinnar, S., Berg, A. T., Moshe, S. L., Kang, H., O'Dell, C., Alemany, M., . . . Hauser, W.A. (1994). Discontinuing antiepileptic drugs in children with epilepsy: A prospective study. *Annals of Neurology, 35*(5), 534–545.

Shinnar, S., Berg, A. T., Moshe, S. L., O'Dell, C., Alemany, M., Newstein, D., . . . Hauser, W. A. (1996). The risk of seizure recurrence after a first unprovoked afebrile seizure in childhood: An extended follow-up. *Pediatrics, 98*, 216–225.

Shinnar, S., Berg, A. T., O'Dell, C., Newstein, D., Moshe, S. L., & Hauser, W. A. (2000). Predictors of multiple seizures in a cohort of children prospectively followed from the time of their first unprovoked seizure. *Annals of Neurology, 48*, 140–147.

Shinnar, S., Berg, A. T., Moshe, S. L., & Shinnar, R. (2001). How long do new-onset seizures in children last? *Annals of Neurology, 49*(5), 659–664.

Shinnar, S., & Glauser, T. A. (2002). Febrile seizures. *Journal of Child Neurology, 17*(Suppl. 1), S44–S52.

Shmuely, S., Sisodiya, S. M., Gunning, W. B., Sander, J. W., & Thijs, R. D. (2016). Mortality in Dravet syndrome: A review. *Epilepsy & Behavior, 64*(Pt A), 69–74. doi:10.1016/j.yebeh.2016.09.007

Shorvon, S. (2000). *Handbook of epilepsy treatment.* Malden, MA: Blackwell Science.

Sillanpää, M. (2000). Long term outcome of epilepsy. *Epileptic Disorders, 2*(2), 79–88.

Sillanpää, M., Anttinen, A, Rinne, J. O., Joutsa, J., Sonninen, P., Erkinjuntti, M., . . . Shinnar, S. (2015). Childhood-onset epilepsy five decades later. A prospective population-based cohort study. *Epilepsia, 56*(11), 1174–1183.

Sillanpää, M., & Shinnar, S. (2010). Long-term mortality in childhood-onset epilepsy. *New England Journal of Medicine, 363*(26), 2522–2529.

Sogawa, Y., Masur, D., O'Dell, C., Moshe, S. L., & Shinnar, S. (2010). Cognitive outcomes in children who present with a fist unprovoked seizure. *Epilepsia, 51*(12), 2432–2439.

Spence, S. J., & Schneider, M. T. (2009). The role of epilepsy and epileptiform EEGs in autism spectrum disorders. *Pediatric Research, 65*(6), 599–606. doi:10.1203/PDR.0b013e31819e7168

Subcommittee on Febrile Seizures—American Academy of Pediatrics. (2011). Neurodiagnostic evaluation of the child with simple febrile seizure. *Pediatrics, 127*(2), 389–394.

Sulzbacher, S., Farwell, J. R., Temkin, N., Lu, A. S., & Hirtz, D. J. (1999). Late cognitive effects of early treatment with Phenobarbital. *Clinical Pediatrics 38*, 387–394.

Sunder, T. R. (1997). Meeting the challenge of epilepsy in persons with multiple handicaps. *Journal of Child Neurology, 12*(Suppl. 1), S38–S43.

Tassinari, C. A., Cantalupo, G., Bernardina, B. D., Darra, F., Bureau, M., Cirelli, C., . . . Rubboli, G. (2012). Encephalopathy related to status epilepticus during slow sleep (ESES) including Landau-Kleffner syndrome. In M. Bureau,

P. Genton, C. Dravet, A. Delgado-Escueta, C. Tassinari, P. Thomas, & P. Wolf (Eds.), *Epileptic syndromes in infancy, childhood and adolescence–With videos* (English and French 5th ed., p. 255). London, England: John Libbey Eurotext Ltd.

Tharp, B. (2002). Neonatal seizures and syndrome. *Epilepsia, 43*(Suppl. 3), 2–10.

Tomson, T., Battino, D., Bonizzoni, E., Craig, T., Lindhout, D., Perruca, E., . . . EURAP Study Group. (2015). Dose-dependent teratogenicity of valproate in mono- and polytherapy: An observational study. *Neurology, 85*(10), 866–872.

Trasmonte, J. V., & Barron, T. F. (1998). Infantile spasms: A proposal for a staged evaluation. *Pediatric Neurology, 19*(5), 368–371.

Troeser, M. M., Hastriter, E. V., & Ng, Y. T. (2010). Dissolving oral clonazepam wafers in the acute treatment of prolonged seizures. *Journal of Child Neurology,* Advanced online publication. doi:10.1177/0883073810368312

Tuchman, R. (2013). Autism and social cognition in epilepsy, implications for comprehensive epilepsy care. *Current Opinions in Neurology, 26*(2), 214–218. doi:10.1097/WCO.0b013e32835ee64f

Tuchman, R. F., & Rapin, I. (2002). Epilepsy in autism. *The Lancet Neurology, 1,* 352–358.

Uldall, P., Alving, J., Hansen, L. K., Kiebaek, M., & Buchholt, J. (2006). The misdiagnosis of epilepsy in children admitted to a tertiary epilepsy center with paroxysmal events. *Archives of Disease in Childhood, 91,* 219–221.

Vajda, F. J. E., O'Brien, T. J., Lander, C. M., Garaham, J., & Eadie M. J. (2016). Antiepileptic drug combinations not involving valproate and the risk of fetal malformations. *Epilepsia, 57*(7), 1048–1052.

Viscidi, E. W., Johnson, A. L., Spence, S. J., Buka, S. L., Morrow, E. M., & Triche, E. W. (2014). The association between epilepsy and autism symptoms and maladaptive behaviors in children with autism spectrum disorder. *Autism, 18*(8), 996–1006. doi:10.1177/1362361313508027

Wallace, S. J. (1998). Myoclonus and epilepsy in childhood: A review of treatment with valproate, ethosuximide, lamotrigine and zonisamide. *Epilepsy Research, 29*(2), 147–154.

Wheless, J. W., Clarke, D. F., & Carpenter, D. (2005). Treatment of pediatric epilepsy: Expert opinion, 2005. *Journal of Child Neurology, 20,* S1–S56.

Wheless, J. W., Clarke, D., Arzimanoglou, F., & Carpenter, D. (2007). Treatment of pediatric epilepsy: European expert opinion, 2007. *Epileptic Disorders, 9*(4), 353–412.

Wilmshurst, J. M., Burman, R., Gaillard, W. D., & Cross, J. H. (2015). Treatment of infants with epilepsy, common practices around the world. *Epilepsia, 56*(7), 1033–1046.

Wirrell, E. C., Grossardt, B. R., Wong-Kisiel, L. C. L., & Nickels, K. C. (2011). Incidence and classification of new-onset epilepsy and epilepsy syndromes in children in Olmsted County, Minnesota from 1980 to 2004: A population-based study. *Epilepsy Research, 95,* 110–118.

Wolf, P. (1994). *Epileptic seizures and syndromes.* London, England: John Libbey & Co. Ltd.

Wolfgang, A. A. (2007). Monotherapy in children and infants. *Neurology, 69*(Suppl. 3), S17–S22.

Zupanc, M. L. (2006). Antiepileptic drugs and hormonal contraceptives in adolescent women with epilepsy. *Neurology, 66*(Suppl. 3), S37–S45.

CHAPTER 23 Acquired Brain Injury

Sarah Risen, Scott C. Schultz, and Melissa K. Trovato

Upon completion of this chapter, the reader will

- Describe the different etiologies of acquired brain injury (ABI)
- Explain the incidence, common etiologies, and clinical course of mild, moderate, and severe traumatic brain injury (TBI) in children
- Discuss the management of mild TBI, specifically return-to-learn and return-to-play plans
- Identify clinical features concerning abusive head trauma and describe the subsequent evaluation of this condition
- Understand the nontraumatic causes of ABI
- Understand the key elements of rehabilitation and the outcomes associated with ABI
- Identify the most important strategies for ABI prevention
- Explain why a comprehensive, interdisciplinary team is essential to the acute and long-term care of children with acquired brain injury

Acquired brain injury (ABI) is a nonprogressive insult to the brain after birth resulting in acute, and often chronic, disruption of neurological function. Traumatic brain injury (TBI) is the most common cause of ABI in children, and abusive head trauma (AHT) is the most common cause in infants and toddlers. TBI is classified as mild, moderate, or severe and has a wide spectrum of injury outcomes. Other mechanisms of ABI include anoxic/hypoxic-ischemic brain injury (e.g., cardiac arrest, asphyxiation, and submersion), stroke, infectious (encephalitis/meningitis), autoimmune encephalitis, and other causes.

For all etiologies of ABI, it is important to understand that brain injury in children occurs in the context of a developing brain and therefore can disrupt underlying neurodevelopmental processes by both primary and secondary injury. The clinical symptoms and related management of ABI are generally divided into acute, subacute, and chronic periods. Symptoms at initial presentation may reflect focal regions and/or more diffuse areas of brain dysfunction. Associated symptoms vary by etiology.

Depending on the cause and extent of brain injury, children with ABI may be at risk for long-term impairments or changes in the sensory systems (i.e., vision or hearing), physical function, cognition, language, behavioral and emotional regulation, personality, endocrine function, and sleep regulation. These impairments and changes can adversely affect a child's function at home, in school, and in the community; therefore, a comprehensive multidisciplinary team approach is essential to identify problems and provide strategies to optimize the child's ability to participate in all environments.

CASE STUDY

Johnny was a previously healthy 9-year-old boy who presented to the emergency department (ED) with dizziness and sleepiness after hitting his head on the ground when he fell from play equipment at school. His parents were told by school personnel that he cried immediately (i.e., there was no reported loss of consciousness), but Johnny does not remember climbing on the equipment or the fall. The school nurse noted he seemed confused, and she called his parents, who then brought him to the local hospital.

In the ED, Johnny remained confused and began to have episodes of vomiting. The ED physician ordered a computed tomography (CT) scan of the head given his persistent altered mental status during observation in the ED and onset of emesis. The head CT showed no evidence of skull fracture or internal hemorrhage. His symptoms began to improve after several hours, and he was discharged home with a diagnosis of concussion and recommendations for strict rest (a common recommendation *not* based on up-to-date concussion management evidence, as discussed below) until follow-up evaluation by his primary care physician (PCP).

His parents brought him for follow-up appointments with his PCP several times over the following 3 weeks; she then referred Johnny to the multidisciplinary concussion clinic because of persistent postconcussive symptoms (i.e., daily headache, dizziness, increased sleep, and irritability). Of note, while he had not attempted school work during this time, his parents were concerned that he was not thinking as clearly as before the fall. Four weeks following his concussion, Johnny was seen by the pediatric neurologist, neuropsychologist, and behavior psychologist in a multidisciplinary concussion clinic. At that time, he exhibited the same symptoms; in addition, his parents were concerned that his irritability and behavior were beginning to worsen. He had not been cleared to return to school because his parents were told to wait "until all symptoms resolve" before sending him back or allowing him to return to his normal activities.

On reviewing Johnny's current daily schedule, the team noted that he was sleeping late, eating sporadically, and "resting all day," although his parents noted that lately it has been incredibly challenging to keep him from running around. They felt they were constantly telling him to stop doing things to ensure that he could heal. They shared that Johnny was "bored" at home and wanted to get back to playing baseball. A 45-minute targeted neuropsychological battery revealed overall average to high average cognitive function in most areas but mild weakness in processing speed and working memory.

Johnny and his parents were counseled on concussion and the expected course of recovery. He was provided an individualized return-to-school plan, and lifestyle interventions were emphasized, specifically hydration, regular meals, adequate and consistent sleep (melatonin was recommended for sleep initiation), and avoidance of headache medication overuse. Johnny was taught strategies for activity pacing and developed a daily schedule alternating work, breaks, and preferred activities. Although returning to school full time was emphasized, the benefits of slowly increasing levels of aerobic exercise were also discussed as long as the degree of exertion did not increase concussive symptoms. The team modified a "return-to-play" plan, allowing activity up to (but not beyond) high-aerobic, noncontact activity.

At clinic follow-up 2 weeks later, Johnny and his parents noted a significant reduction in his symptoms, especially his headaches and irritability. He was attending school full days but with accommodations. He was tolerating high-intensity aerobic sports drills without symptoms, and repeat neuropsychological testing revealed improvement in the prior areas of weakness. School accommodations were gradually removed, and he was able to complete all make-up work before his final clinic visit 3 weeks later. At that time (9 weeks following his initial injury), he was asymptomatic, functioning in school without any additional support, and cleared to complete the final stages of the return-to-play plan. Johnny was able to play in the final tournament of his baseball season.

CASE STUDY

Paul is a previously healthy 9-year-old boy who was a belted backseat passenger involved in a motor vehicle collision. The vehicle was hit on the driver's side by a tractor trailer while traveling on the highway. Upon arrival, emergency medical services noted that Paul was unresponsive, and his Glasgow Coma Scale (GCS) score (a quantitative scale to describe a person's level of consciousness) was a 3, the lowest possible score reflecting severe neurological impairment. He was intubated and transported via helicopter to the nearest trauma center.

At the trauma center, a head CT showed a right frontal skull fracture with underlying hemorrhage. He emergently went to the operating room for intracranial pressure (ICP) monitor placement and was admitted to the intensive care unit (ICU). The ICU followed the recommended management guidelines for children with severe TBI. He initially required medications to maintain an adequate blood pressure but then developed intermittent hypertension, tachycardia (elevated heart rate), and hyperthermia (elevated temperature) consistent with paroxysmal sympathetic hyperactivity. While in the ICU, Paul had persistent significantly impaired level of consciousness, requiring a tracheostomy and gastrostomy tube placement 2 weeks after injury. He had increased muscle tone and was seen several days per week by physical and occupational therapy for range of motion exercises and other services.

When Paul became medically stable, he was transferred to the neurology unit for ongoing care. As sedating medications were weaned, he became more responsive. Magnetic resonance imaging (MRI) of his brain completed 4 weeks after injury revealed a large intracranial hematoma in the right frontal lobe and corpus callosum, as well as punctate hemorrhages scattered throughout the left occipital lobe, left frontal lobe, and brainstem, reflecting diffuse axonal injury (DAI).

Paul was then transferred to an inpatient rehabilitation unit. At that time, Paul had spontaneous eye opening and intermittent eye opening to verbal stimuli. After 16 weeks, Paul was inconsistently following simple commands and inconsistently answering yes/no questions with a head nod/shake. Spontaneous movements of his extremities were noted, on the right greater than the left. Paul was discharged from inpatient rehabilitation 24 weeks post injury. He required a ventilator to assist with nighttime breathing due to central sleep apnea and was dependent on a gastrostomy tube for all nutrition.

Paul was then admitted to a day rehabilitation program, where he received intensive physical, occupational, and speech therapy services. At 28 weeks following injury, Paul continued to be in a posttraumatic amnesia (PTA) state (i.e., he was having difficulty learning new information, but he was consistently following commands and able to make choices using eye gaze or reaching with his right hand).

Over the next 6 months, Paul continued to make slow, steady gains, although his cognitive and language functioning remained significantly impaired compared with age-matched peers. He was able to communicate his basic wants and needs with cues, move all his extremities, and walk using a walker and bilateral forearm platforms for 200 feet with minimal assistance. Paul required the use of bilateral ankle-foot orthoses to maintain foot position and provide stability. He was able to feed himself with supervision and required minimal assistance for grooming, bathing, and dressing skills. Paul underwent a modified barium swallow test and was cleared for intake of a regular diet with nectar-thickened liquids. The gastrostomy tube began to be used only for liquid supplementation.

Paul was then transitioned to school with the support of an individualized education program (IEP), developed with the help of an educator from the day program in coordination with the school system. At school, he continued to receive therapy services as well as outpatient physical, occupational, and speech therapy. At 1 year post injury, he continued to make slow progress in all domains.

Thought Questions:

What can parents and teachers do to educate children about the consequences of traumatic brain injury? What can parents and teachers do to assist in the prevention of traumatic head injury in children?

OVERVIEW OF TRAUMATIC BRAIN INJURY

This section provides an overview of TBI, including incidence, causes, pathophysiology (primary and secondary injuries), and initial evaluation.

Incidence

In 2013, approximately 2.8 million Americans sustained a TBI. This represented an increase from 1.6 million in 2007 accounted for by a surge in mild TBI (mTBI)–related ED visits (Taylor, Bell, Breiding, & Xu, 2017). Children younger than 15 years of age sustain an estimated 661,000 TBIs each year, with nearly 1,500 TBI-related deaths occurring in this population. It is important to note that these numbers only account for children with brain injury seen in an ED. As many children may been seen by their pediatrician or a subspecialty provider rather than in the ER, the number of children sustaining at least mild TBIs each year is likely even higher than reported.

Motor vehicle accidents, falls (e.g., from playground equipment), sports injuries (especially football, lacrosse, and hockey), recreational activities (e.g., skiing and surfing), and assault are the common causes of TBI. The precipitants of TBI tend to vary with age. In children younger than 1 year of age, abusive head trauma is the most likely etiology, occurring at a rate of 39.8 per 100,000 children in the United States (Niederkrotenthaler, Xu, Parks, & Sugerman, 2013). The most frequent overall mechanism of injury in children 0–4 and 5–14 years of age is unintentional falls (which includes unknown intent), whereas motor vehicle collisions are most common in adolescents and young adults 15–24 years (Taylor et al., 2017). Figure 23.1 presents the causes of TBI by age group and percentage.

Pathophysiology: Primary and Secondary Injury

TBI results from a direct or indirect biomechanical force exerted on the brain, which is a soft and deformable organ within the rigid skull. Primary brain injury occurs at the moment of impact and can include 1) brain contusions (a localized bruise of brain tissue), 2) vascular injuries causing hemorrhage (bleeding within the brain), 3) skull fractures, and 4) diffuse axonal injury (DAI) (shearing of the nerves that send information between different areas of the brain). A neurometabolic cascade is also triggered at the moment of impact, including widespread release of glutamate (an excitatory neurotransmitter in the brain that can cause injury at high levels), ionic changes, and metabolic alterations. TBI also results in impaired cerebral blood flow and glucose metabolism (Giza & Hovda, 2014). These changes continue to evolve over days and contribute to additional (secondary) brain injury.

Secondary brain injury refers to the cascade of events that occurs in the brain hours to days after the primary injury, resulting in further tissue damage. Secondary injuries include 1) brain swelling/edema, 2) increased intracranial pressure, 3) ischemia or infarctions (diffuse or focal loss of oxygen to the brain or clot related strokes), 4) seizures, 5) alterations in cerebral blood flow, 6) ongoing axonal injury, 7) ongoing metabolic related toxic injury (leading to brain cell death), 8) reduced glucose metabolism, and 9) impaired mitochondrial function (which normally provides energy for brain cells). Additional systemic alterations, such as elevated body temperature, hyperglycemia or hypoglycemia, or hypotension (low blood pressure), have been associated with poorer outcomes, likely compounding the effects of secondary brain injury (Natale, Joseph, Helfaer, & Shaffner, 2000; Vavilala et al., 2003; Young et al., 2017).

Initial Evaluation

Of children presenting to EDs with head trauma, most injuries are mild (upwards of 90%) and do not require acute medical or surgical intervention (Faul, Xu, Wald, & Coronado, 2010). If a child hits his or her head and remains awake, alert, conversant, interactive, and otherwise asymptomatic, close observation and monitoring at home are sufficient. However, a more comprehensive evaluation at an ED is necessary if any of the following signs or symptoms occur:

A

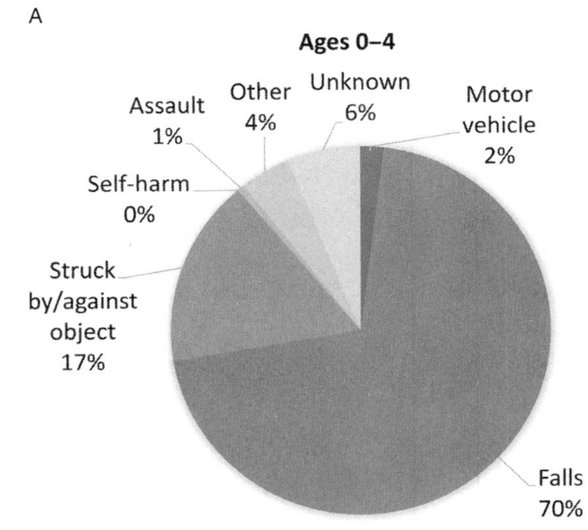

B

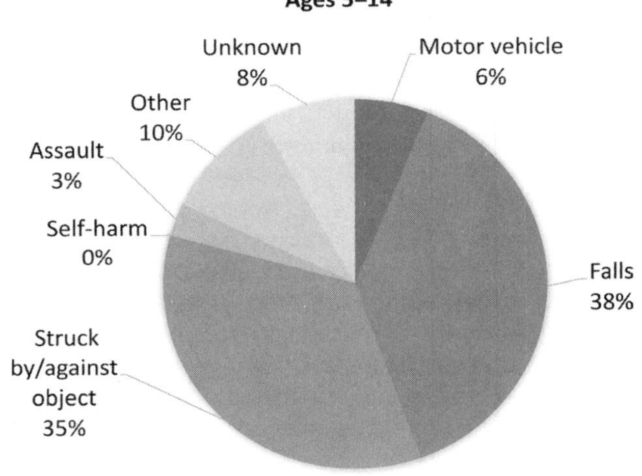

C

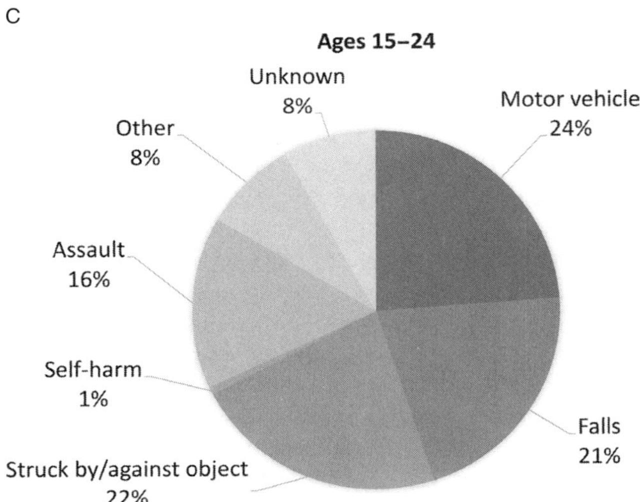

Figure 23.1. Causes of traumatic brain injury by age and percentage. (From Taylor, C. A., Bell, J. M., Breiding, M. J., & Xu, L. [2017]. Traumatic Brain Injury-Related Emergency Department Visits, Hospitalizations, and Deaths—United States, 2007 and 2013. MMWR Surveill Summ, 66[9], 1–16.)

- Any loss of consciousness
- A change in mental status (e.g., difficulty speaking, seizures, confusion, lethargy, excessive sleepiness, or extreme irritability)
- Weakness in the arms or legs
- Complaints of severe headaches that do not abate
- Complaints of changes in hearing or vision
- Nausea and projectile vomiting

In the ED, a neurological examination will be performed. Given the risks of exposure to radiation, it is important to understand that a head CT is not required in the evaluation or diagnosis of concussion in children. Based on the published Pediatric Emergency Care Applied Research Network guidelines for identifying children at risk for concerning injury following head trauma, the ED physician may or may not decide to obtain a head CT (Kupperman et al., 2009). A head CT aids in the evaluation of more severe injury such as bleeding in or around the brain and skull fractures, but it does *not* "diagnose" concussion. In more severe brain injuries, brain MRI provides higher resolution images and is much more effective than CT scans in determining the presence and extent of DAI and other injuries (see Chapter 8). Depending on the clinical progression, results of the physical examination and neuroimaging studies, the child may be discharged home with close observation and follow-up or admitted to the hospital for further care. Children with severe TBIs should be transferred to the nearest Level 1 pediatric trauma center following acute stabilization.

SEVERITY OF TRAUMATIC BRAIN INJURY

There are two common ways to categorize the severity of TBI: the Glasgow Coma Scale (GCS) (Teasdale, 2014; Teasdale & Jennett, 1974) and the duration of post-traumatic amnesia (PTA). The GCS assesses motor response (scored from 1–6), verbal response (1–5), and eye opening (14) within the first 24 hours after brain injury. Following acute resuscitation, if needed, a GCS score of 8 or lower indicates a severe TBI; scores 9–12 indicate a moderate TBI; and scores 13–15 indicate a mild traumatic brain injury. In the acute setting, a person with a score below 8 is said to be comatose (Chung et al., 2006). While a worse outcome across developmental domains is associated with more severe brain injury (and thus a lower GCS score), it is important to note that the prognostic ability of the GCS is limited in children with TBI, and a child with a GCS score of 3–5 can still have meaningful recovery with functional independence (Catroppa, Godfrey, Rosenfeld, Hearps, & Anderson, 2012; Emami et al., 2017; Lieh-Lai et al., 1992).

The duration of posttraumatic amnesia is the length of time for a child to remember events and store new memories. The Children's Orientation and Amnesia Test (Ewing-Cobbs, Levin, Fletcher, Minor, & Eisenberg, 1990) is a widely used tool to assess PTA. In mild TBI the duration of PTA is less than 1 hour, in moderate TBI the duration is between 1 hour and 1 day, and in severe TBI the duration of PTA is longer than 1 day (Wilson, Teasdale, Hadley, Wiedmann, & Lang, 1994). Length of PTA as well as time to follow commands have been shown to be the most consistent and reliable, though weak, predictors of long-term outcome (Davis, Slomine, Salorio, & Suskauer, 2016).

Mild TBI (Concussion)

The term *concussion* (which is an mTBI) continues to receive a significant amount of media attention, especially as it relates to professional football players. In 2013, a little more than 1 million children (from birth to 24 years) were seen in U.S. EDs for brain injury (Taylor et al., 2017). Accounting for children seen by pediatricians, athletic trainers, or other providers, another resource estimates that there are between 1.6 and 3.8 million sports-related concussions (SRCs) in the United States each year (Langlois, Rutland-Brown, & Wald, 2006). Although sports injury is a common and frequently highlighted cause of mTBI, there are many other potential causes, especially falls (e.g., from playground equipment or bicycles), that are actually more common in children less than 12 years of age.

Children seem to be uniquely susceptible to potentially fatal consequences of a second TBI occurring during the acute phase of recovery from an initial concussion, a phenomenon referred to as second impact syndrome (McCrory, Davis, & Makdissi, 2012; McLendon, Kralik, Grayson, & Golomb, 2016). There are now specific laws in all 50 states to protect children by 1) requiring immediate removal of any athlete suspected of having sustained a concussion from participation in sports and 2) prohibiting the child's return to sports until cleared by a qualified professional. The specifics of each law vary by state, but most contain these two components as well as a mandate to educate coaches and/or parents about concussion prior to the start of the season. The application of the laws also vary, with some applicable only to public school athletes and some including community recreational teams.

Diagnosis The most recent Consensus Statement on Concussion in Sport defines SRC as "a traumatic brain injury induced by biomechanical forces."

(McCrory et al., 2017, p. 839). Several common features that may be utilized in clinically defining the nature of a concussive head injury include the following:

- SRC may be caused either by a direct blow to the head, face, neck, or elsewhere on the body with an impulsive force transmitted to the head.
- SRC typically results in the rapid onset of short-lived impairment of neurological function that resolves spontaneously. However, in some cases, signs and symptoms evolve over a number of minutes to hours.
- SRC may result in neuropathological changes, but the acute clinical signs and symptoms largely reflect a functional disturbance rather than a structural injury, and, as such, no abnormality is seen on standard structural neuroimaging studies.
- SRC results in a range of clinical signs and symptoms that may or may not involve loss of consciousness. Resolution of the clinical and cognitive features typically follows a sequential course. However, in some cases symptoms may be prolonged.

The clinical signs and symptoms of SRC cannot be explained by drug, alcohol, or medication use; other injuries (such as cervical injuries, peripheral vestibular dysfunction, etc.); or other comorbidities (e.g., psychological factors or coexisting medical conditions; McCrory et al., 2017).

As illustrated by Johnny in the chapter's initial case study, symptoms of a concussion are typically divided into four overall categories and include (but are not limited to) 1) physical manifestations (confusion, headache, nausea, vomiting, dizziness, hypersensitivity to lights [photophobia] or sounds [phonophobia], loss of balance, and blurry or double vision), 2) changes in sleep (increased or decreased ability to sleep and fatigue), 3) change in emotions/behavior (irritability, increased sadness or nervousness, and increased emotional lability), and 4) changes in cognitive function (difficulty with concentration or memory and responding more slowly than normal). Younger children or those with developmental disabilities may be less likely to express these specific symptoms, and therefore clinical signs (such as increased clinginess, enuresis, appetite changes, nightmares, or other behavior changes) should be considered as proxies for postconcussive symptoms.

There are several validated concussion-related assessments that can be used both on the sideline (for sports-related injuries) and in a clinical setting. The most recent Consensus Statement on Concussion in Sport recommends using the Sports Concussion Assessment Tool, Fifth Edition (SCAT5 and Child SCAT5) as a validated and well-established multimodal concussion assessment tool (Davis et al., 2017).

Management Children with concussion should be evaluated at regular intervals (initially about every 2 weeks) until clinical recovery. This can be done by a provider in one of several disciplines: pediatrics, sports medicine, neurology, or physical medicine and rehabilitation. At each evaluation, ongoing clinical symptoms are assessed. Neither computerized testing nor a neuropsychological evaluation is required in the evaluation of a child with an uncomplicated concussion. A neuropsychologist may complete an assessment focused on functions commonly affected by mTBI. This can provide useful information on the course of cognitive recovery, which may differ from clinical symptom resolution.

Research on mTBI does not support the need for complete rest beyond the acute period following concussion, generally 48 hours (Thomas, Apps, Hoffmann, McCrea, & Hammeke, 2015). There is evidence that supports the avoidance of significant overexertion (i.e., returning immediately to full/nearly full levels of cognitive and physical activity) during the early stages of recovery (i.e., the first few days; Brown et al., 2014). The clinical management of a child with concussion needs to be individualized based on the child's specific symptoms, school and sports circumstances, and response to treatment recommendations. Academic, athletic, and recreational activity management plans need to be modified at each visit based on the child's current status.

After 1–2 days of rest (or at least reduced activity level), a child should transition back to school with appropriate accommodations provided. As concussive symptoms in children can persist for an average of 1–2 months, it is not feasible, and in fact may be harmful, to wait until complete symptom resolution prior to returning to school. Therefore, it is essential for providers to be familiar with common school adjustments and academic accommodations that can optimize a child's return to school and recovery from injury (Box 23.1). The American Academy of Pediatrics (AAP) has published a thorough report on "Returning to Learning" that can help guide a provider who is managing a child after a concussion (Halstead et al., 2013). In addition, the Centers for Disease Control (CDC) Acute Concussion Evaluation (ACE) care plan is accessible online and includes common academic accommodations for providers to modify/recommend in the "Returning to School" section (CDC, 2015).

Just as a stepwise increase in academic activity is recommended, a gradual increase in physical exertion (below a level causing worsening/increase in symptoms) is also advised. For athletes, there are several specific "return-to-play" protocols that providers can access (such as the one outlined in the CDC ACE care plan). For children who are not involved in a formal

BOX 23.1 EVIDENCE-BASED PRACTICE

Returning to School and to Sports Following Concussion/Mild Traumatic Brain Injury (mTBI)

Each year, there are between 1.6 and 3.8 million sports-related concussions in the United States (Langlois, Rutland-Brown, & Wald, 2006). Providers, educators, coaches, and athletic trainers are faced with important decisions regarding when a child should return to school or sports and how to implement an optimal plan to resume these activities.

Return to Learning

In a survey of high school nurses, only half of schools had a plan in place to support the return of a child to school following a concussion, and only two thirds of school nurses had training in concussion (Olympia, Ritter, Brady, & Bramley, 2016). Primary care providers may also be unaware of the needed supports for a child with concussion returning school. In a chart review of primary care providers' initial evaluations of children diagnosed with concussion, only 28% of the pediatricians provided the child/family with return-to-school instructions and only 11% provide recommendations for cognitive rest (Arbogast et al., 2013).

The American Academy of Pediatrics has published "Returning to Learning Guidelines" to assist providers in the development of instructions for schools to optimize the transition back to school for children with concussion (Halstead et al., 2013).

Return to Play

A child who has sustained a concussion should not be "cleared" to return to contact sports before being able to tolerate full days of school without accommodations. (As noted in this chapter, some degree of aerobic activity may enhance concussion recovery, so carefully prescribed noncontact exercise may be permitted prior to full recovery based upon the provider's clinical evaluation and judgment.) Once a provider with expertise in concussion has determined that a child is ready to be cleared to resume sports, the return-to-play protocol guides the child's gradual return to contact sports. However, in a chart review of primary care providers' initial and follow-up evaluations of children diagnosed with concussion, only about 50% of pediatricians provided return-to-activity instructions (Arbogast et al., 2013). Furthermore, one study found that only 15%–40% of high school athletes complied with these return-to-play guidelines, with the athletes that did *not* follow the guidelines returning to contact sports before recommended (Yard & Cornstock, 2009).

Several "return-to-play" guidelines have been published, with all protocols gradually increasing noncontact aerobic exertion prior to returning to contact practice, followed by competitive play (May et al., 2014; McCrory et al., 2012).

Application to Practice

As with other aspects of concussion management, return to play protocols should be individualized, with considerations including the age of the athlete, history of prior concussions, and the specific sport to which they are returning (Canty & Nilan, 2015).

athletics program, it is still recommended to gradually increase physical exertion as tolerated and avoid contact or high-risk activities that could result in another mTBI until the current concussion has fully resolved.

Children with concussion should be symptom-free and able to complete all schoolwork without accommodations (and at preinjury levels of performance) prior to being allowed to return to unrestricted activities, especially contact sports. The decision to allow a return to normal activities may be challenging in the small portion of children with persistent postconcussive symptoms. Children with an atypical or prolonged clinical course, who are unable to tolerate increased cognitive or physical demands despite appropriate accommodations, should be referred to a multidisciplinary clinic with expertise in brain injury for ongoing clinical assessment and management.

Clinical Course Symptom resolution and clinical recovery is expected within 1–2 months in children with concussion (Corwin et al., 2014; Risen, Reesman, Yenokyan, Slomine, & Suskauer, 2017), although a small portion of children report persistent symptoms and require referral to a provider with expertise in brain injury (Barlow et al., 2010; Keenan & Bratton, 2006; Sroufe et al., 2010). Literature supports the strong contribution of premorbid child and family psychological factors to persistent postconcussive symptoms, which may respond well to cognitive behavioral intervention (Bernard, Ponsford, McKinlay, McKenzie, & Krieser, 2016; McNally et al., 2018). This emphasizes the importance of a multidisciplinary treatment team in this population.

Moderate to Severe TBI

In 2013, nearly 50,000 children were admitted to the hospital secondary to TBI and nearly 8,000 children sustained a fatal TBI (Taylor et al., 2017). Though less frequent than mild injuries, moderate and severe TBI are associated with significant and persistent impact on the child and family (Babikian, Merkley, Savage, Giza, & Levin, 2015; Rashid et al., 2014).

Diagnosis Similar to mTBI, moderate to severe TBI results from a biomechanical force transmitted directly or indirectly to the brain; however, children with moderate to severe TBI present with more pronounced neurological deficits (see above for GCS and PTA injury severity classification criteria). As illustrated by Paul, in the second case study at the beginning of this chapter, diagnosis and treatment of moderate to severe TBI begins at the scene of injury or in the ED. After assessment and stabilization of a child's breathing and circulation, a more extensive evaluation of the brain and spine will occur. As noted, the postresuscitation GCS score will help determine the initial severity of brain injury and may guide ongoing acute management. The Brain Trauma Foundation has published guidelines on the acute medical management of severe TBI in children (Kochanek et al., 2012), and adherence to these recommendations has been shown to be associated with improved survival and outcome at discharge from the hospital (O'Lynnger et al., 2016; Vavilala et al., 2014). Throughout a child's hospital course, the goal of treatment is to prevent or limit secondary brain injury.

CT scans of the head and neck, to assess the extent of brain injury and for possible cervical spinal injury, are typically obtained acutely. Children with more severe brain injuries may require a neurosurgical procedure, such as placement of a device to measure ICP. An MRI may be obtained once the child is stabilized to provide further information on the extent of brain damage.

Seizures may occur after a TBI and can increase neurometabolic demand, worsening secondary brain injury. Seizures after TBI are categorized based on the postinjury timing in which they occur. Impact-related seizures are defined as those that occur at the time of injury, usually within minutes of sustaining a TBI (most often an mTBI) but typically do not reflect an increased risk for a long-term seizure disorder (Arndt, Goodkin, & Giza, 2016). Early posttraumatic seizures (EPTS) include immediate posttraumatic seizures (within 24 hours) and delayed EPTS (within the first week following injury; Arndt et al., 2016); they are more common than impact seizures. EPTS have been related to an increased risk for late posttraumatic seizures (Arango et al., 2012) and poorer outcome (Arndt et al., 2013). In children with moderate to severe TBI who undergo continuous electroencephalogram (EEG) monitoring (see Chapter 22), EPTS occurs in roughly 30%, with nearly half having only subclinical seizures (seizure activity detected on EEG but without clinical signs in the child; O'Neil et al., 2015). EPTS are more common in severe TBI, especially with intracranial hemorrhage or depressed skull fractures, abusive head trauma, and in children less than 3 years of age (Arango et al., 2012; Arndt et al., 2016; Bennett, DeWitt, Harlaar, & Bennett, 2017; Liesemer, Bratton, Zebrack, Brockmeyer, & Statler, 2011).

Late posttraumatic seizures (LPTS) occur after the first week of injury and present with greater frequency in older children and young adults (Statler, 2006); however, epileptic spasms have been reported in infants 2 months–2 years following severe TBI (Park & Chugani, 2017). Risk factors for LPTS include abnormal head CT with skull fractures and bleeding in the brain and early posttraumatic seizures (Emanuelson & Uvebrant, 2009; Park & Chugani, 2015). Anti-epileptic prophylaxis (treating with a medication to prevent seizures) has been shown to prevent EPTS but not LPTS (Chang, Lowenstein, & Quality Standards Subcommittee of the American Academy of Neurology, 2003). The risk for ongoing posttraumatic seizures is greatest within the first year following injury but persists even 10 years following TBI, especially in those children with severe TBI (Annegers & Coan, 2000; Christensen et al., 2009). Furthermore, children with severe TBI and posttraumatic epilepsy may be more likely to have intractable epilepsy and be on multiple anti-epileptic medications (Park & Chugani, 2015).

Management Throughout the hospitalization period, efforts should be made to prevent the complications of prolonged bedrest. These problems may include decreased muscle mass and strength, bone loss, skin breakdown, loss of range of motion at joints (contractures), and weight loss. Contractures and skin breakdown may be prevented by appropriate positioning and frequent repositioning. Passive range of motion should be undertaken once the child is medically stable.

Nutrition plays an important role following TBI because of increased daily calorie and protein needs during the healing process (Vavilala, Kernic, et al., 2014; Vavilala, Lujan, et al., 2017). The child may require an alternative means of nutrition, such as a nasogastric tube, to receive calories, liquids, and medication. Gastroesophageal reflux and decreased rate of stomach emptying may also be a problem. Urinary and bowel incontinence is common after severe brain injury, but there may also be urinary retention and constipation, which should be appropriately treated.

Paroxysmal sympathetic hyperactivity (PSH; also known as dysautonomia, diencephalic or thalamic seizures, autonomic or sympathetic storming) occurs in approximately 10% of children with moderate to severe TBI within days to weeks of injury (Kirk et al., 2012; Deepika, Mathew, Kumar, Devi, & Shukla, 2015) and is associated with increased mortality and worse rehabilitation outcomes (Kirk et al., 2012; Pozzi et al., 2014). PSH reflects severe dysregulation of the sympathetic nervous system (SNS) caused by dysfunction of the thalamus or hypothalamus or their connections within the brain (Blackman, Patrick, Buck, & Rust, 2004; see Chapter 8). The diagnosis is based on presence of otherwise unexplained SNS symptoms, including elevated temperature, tachycardia, tachypnea (rapid breathing), hypertension, sweating, and dystonic posturing (abnormal positioning of limbs). PSH typically requires management with medications such as benzodiazepines, beta-blockers like propranolol, or alpha2 agonists like clonidine (Kirk et al., 2012; see Chapter 38).

Clinical Course Following severe TBI, recovery is most rapid during the first year and slows during the following year (Gorman, Barnes, Swank, & Ewing-Cobbs, 2017; Taylor et al., 1999). Recovery is influenced not only by the severity of injury, but also by family factors, including socioeconomic status, resources, and support systems (Anderson, Spencer-Smith, et al., 2009; Catroppa et al., 2012; Keenan & Bratton, 2006). In addition, variability in the rate of recovery and the effects on differing neurodevelopmental domains in children who sustain TBI at different ages suggest an age-dependent neuro-pathophysiological influence on the rate of recovery and neurodevelopmental outcome (Babikian et al., 2015). For many years, it was believed that the younger the age of injury, the better the outcome due to the plasticity of the brain. However, it has been shown that children who sustain a brain injury at an *earlier age* (infants and toddlers) are at increased risk for lasting impairments across all areas compared with older children who sustain a brain injury (Anderson et al., 2009; Andruszkow et al., 2014; Crowe, Catroppa, Babl Rosenfeld, & Anderson, 2012). Yet, stage of development at the time of injury also has an impact on outcome, with differing domains more or less vulnerable at different periods of development. A child may return to the previous developmental level following injury but may have trouble progressing past that stage (Babikian et al., 2015; Giza, Kolb, Harris, Asarnow, & Prins, 2009). This difficulty with progressing into new developmental levels or attaining new developmental milestones has been described as a neurocognitive stall (Babikian et al., 2015; Chapman, 2007). This may be noted in all age groups and is typically manifest as a slowing or lack of further progression in the intellectual, motor, and social development of the child 1 year after injury. Beyond this period of cognitive stall, children will continue to gain skills, though likely at a slower developmental rate.

The outcomes for children who have sustained moderate to severe TBI are variable. Persistent and significant impairments are associated with more severe primary injury, more frequent secondary injuries, a longer ICU stay, and a longer hospital stay (Anderson & Catroppa, 2006; Campbell, Kuehn, Richards, Ventureyra, & Hutchison, 2004). Areas typically affected include language, working memory, executive function, and speed of information processing (Anderson & Catroppa, 2006; Babikian et al., 2015; Campbell et al., 2004). Even with these impairments, a child's preinjury academic skills and global intelligence may remain intact; it is new learning that is most impaired (Babikian et al., 2015). Social, emotional, behavioral, and sleep problems are also common following pediatric TBI and can have a significant impact on a child's daily function.

Abusive Head Trauma

Abusive head trauma (AHT; termed shaken baby syndrome, inflicted head injury, or nonaccidental trauma) is a severe TBI inflicted via abrupt forceful impact and/or violent shaking of infants or young children. Children with AHT most often present emergently with nonspecific signs, such as irritability, vomiting, lethargy, trouble feeding, and apnea (stopping breathing); they may also present with more specific neurological symptoms such as seizures.

AHT is a serious public health concern. In the United States, AHT occurs in 30 to 50 per 100,000 children less than 5 years of age, with the highest rate in children less than 1 year of age (Boop, Axente, Weatherford, & Klimo, 2016; Shanahan, Zolotor, Parrish, Barr, & Runyan, 2013). Importantly, an infant or child who has sustained even a minor abusive injury is at increased risk for future, more severe abuse, including AHT. In a study of infants diagnosed with AHT, nearly one third were previously seen by providers in settings where abuse could have been identified. They often had presented in the past with emesis or bruising or having had prior child protective services (CPS) contact (Letson et al., 2016).

Diagnosis The classic features of AHT are subdural hematoma (SDH; bleeding between the skull and the brain) and retinal hemorrhages (RH; bleeding into the eye seen by an ophthalmologist when examining the back of the eye). As AHT may be inflicted on a child in many different ways (e.g., shaking, blunt force trauma, suffocation, strangulation), these features or other signs of physical injury are not required for the diagnosis of AHT. The diagnosis of AHT is based on the history, physical exam, and medical evaluation. It is essential for providers to recognize all possible red flags of AHT.

In cases of AHT, the cause of injury reported by caregivers is often inconsistent with the clinical findings and the severity of brain injury sustained. For example, although many studies support the benign nature of a fall from a low height (3–4 feet) such as a couch or bed (Lyons & Oates, 1993; Levene & Bonfield, 1991), in a study of infants with traumatic intracranial hemorrhage, children reported by parents to have fallen from a height of less than 3 feet actually had evidence of *more* severe brain injuries (with an increased incidence of SDH, RH, and seizures) and had worse outcomes than those reported by parents to have suffered a variety of other causes. Infants whose parents reported not knowing the mechanism of injury had the *most* severe injuries and outcomes (Amagasa, Matsui, Tsuji, Moriya, & Kinoshita, 2016). The implication is that there would be a higher suspicion of abuse when parents cannot report the mechanism of injury or when the reported mechanism of injury is insufficient to explain the severity of the injury itself. Changes in the history provided by the caregiver upon additional questioning, varying accounts from several caregivers, and other signs of physical abuse (e.g., bruising or patterned marks, such as handprints from slapping, linear marks from an object such as a belt, circular lesions from cigarette burns, etc.) should also raise suspicion for AHT. The hospital's child protective team, which has expertise specifically in the evaluation and diagnosis of abusive injuries in children, should be involved as soon as abuse is suspected.

Management Once the suspicion is raised for AHT by the history, exam, or head CT (i.e., finding SDH), a complete evaluation should be done, including 1) an ophthalmological evaluation looking for RH, 2) a skeletal survey/x-rays for evidence of fractures indicating physical abuse, 3) brain MRI and cervical spine imaging, 4) involvement of the hospital's child protective team, and 5) notification of CPS. If resources allow, continuous EEG monitoring is recommended given the increased frequency of both clinical and subclinical seizures and status epilepticus (persistent seizure activity). Additional laboratory investigation is based on clinical judgment.

While SDH is a cardinal feature of AHT, other intracranial hemorrhages and skull fractures may occur, resulting from direct impact, as well as DAI. Considering the great force needed to inflict AHT and the mechanism of injury, the cervical spinal cord is also vulnerable, especially in ligamentous injury (Choudhary, Ishak, Zacharia, & Dias, 2014), and both AHT and cervical spinal cord injury are associated with bilateral hypoxic-ischemic (reduced oxygen and blood flow delivery) brain injury (Kadom et al., 2014).

Clinical Course AHT has a high mortality rate and is also a major cause of morbidity in young children. In fact, given the unique differences in the infant and young child's nervous system and the major neurodevelopmental changes that occur throughout the first years of life, infants and very young children appear to be particularly vulnerable to effects of brain injury, especially with regard to cognitive development (Anderson, Spencer-Smith et al., 2009). Furthermore, secondary brain injuries, (including seizures, increased ICP, and stroke) are more common in AHT compared with accidental TBI (Ferguson et al., 2017; Hymel, Makoroff, Laskey, Conaway, & Blackman, 2007; Risen, Suskauer, Dematt, Slomine, & Salorio, 2014). The presence of increased morbidity and secondary injuries in AHT emphasizes the importance of strict adherence to the severe TBI guidelines and the use of aggressive neuroprotective strategies (treatment strategies designed to reduce secondary injury) in this population. In addition, children with AHT make similar functional gains during inpatient rehabilitation and following discharge as do children with nonabusive (accidental) head trauma, underscoring the need to ensure ongoing rehabilitation services (Risen et al., 2014).

NONTRAUMATIC ACQUIRED BRAIN INJURY

Common types of nontraumatic ABIs include anoxic/hypoxic-ischemic brain injury, pediatric stroke, infectious encephalitis/meningitis, autoimmune encephalitis, and other causes of ABI (radiation, toxins, etc.). Given the multiple etiologies, it is difficult to determine the overall incidence of ABI in children. While the pathophysiology is unique to each individual cause, the acute disruption in neurological function and potential for chronic neurological impairment are the common bond within ABIs.

Anoxic/Hypoxic-Ischemic Brain Injury

Anoxic (absence of oxygen delivery) and hypoxic-ischemic brain injury are a common cause of ABI encompassing several etiologies, including cardiac arrest (most commonly secondary to respiratory failure in children), submersion (drowning), and asphyxiation (hanging). See Chapter 5 for a discussion of neonatal hypoxic-ischemic encephalopathy.

Hypoxic-ischemic brain injury due to cardiac arrest is most often as a consequence of respiratory failure in children. While certainly less common than in the adult population, it is difficult to determine the overall incidence and epidemiology of nonfatal cardiac arrests in the general pediatric population. Specific populations, such as those with congenital heart disease or certain arrhythmia syndromes, are at high risk for cardiac-mediated arrest. Cardiac arrest may occur in a hospital setting (e.g., in an ED or ICU) or in a community setting; outcomes differ depending on where the event occurs (see below).

Drowning is the most common cause of accidental death in children 1–4 years of age and one of the top five causes of unintentional death in children overall (Borse et al., 2008; Laosse, Gilchrist, & Rudd 2012). Nonfatal drownings occur in approximately 10 of every 100,000 children in the United States, with the highest rate (16 out of every 100,000) in children ages 0–4 years (Felton, Myers, Liu, & Davis, 2015). The highest rates of nonfatal drowning occur in swimming pools (although natural waterways, including freshwater ponds, lakes and streams, and oceans, and bathtubs are other common locations) and among children from minority populations, especially African Americans (Felton et al., 2015).

Asphyxiation/strangulation brain injuries may be intentional (self-inflicted) or unintentional (accidental suffocation). Sadly, hanging/strangulation is the most common mechanism of suicide in school-age children and is especially prevalent among black males with ADHD and young adolescents with depression (Sheftall et al., 2016). Sudden infant death syndrome (also referred to as "sudden unexpected death in infancy") and accidental suffocation during sleep are common causes of hypoxic-ischemic injury and death in infants. Suffocation is 20 to 40 times more likely to occur among infants who sleep in an adult bed than among those who sleep in a crib; by contrast, the risk of suffocation is reduced in infants who sleep in the *same room* (but not the *same bed*) as an adult caregiver (Moon & Task Force on Sudden Infant Death Syndrome, 2016; Scheers, Rutherford, & Kemp, 2003). The importance of prevention efforts for both intentional and unintentional asphyxiation injuries are discussed below.

Independent of etiology, anoxia/hypoxia and ischemia trigger a deleterious neurometabolic cascade, starting with depletion of brain energy reserves and followed by accumulation of harmful metabolites that ultimately trigger neuroinflammation and neuronal cell death. Brain MRI reveals different patterns of hypoxic-ischemic injury depending on the severity of the insult and age (i.e., brain maturity; Huang & Castillo, 2008; White, Zhang, Helvey, & Omojola, 2013). Neuroimaging of milder hypoxic injury in children typically involves the watershed zones and subcortical white matter. Severe hypoxia in postneonatal infants and children up to 2 years of age results in diffuse injury to the gray matter. In contrast to the pattern seen in neonatal injury (see Chapter 5), brain MRI of children 1–2 years of age with hypoxic-ischemic injury may have sparing of the perirolandic cortex and thalami (see Chapter 8). In older children (typically older than 2 years of age), severe hypoxic-ischemic injury imaging patterns appear similar to adults, with vulnerability of the deep gray nuclei, cortex, hippocampi, and cerebellum. Although findings on MRI do not consistently relate to neurological function (Christophe et al., 2002), neuroimaging abnormalities demonstrating diffuse hypoxic-ischemic injury suggest the potential impact on a wide range of neurological functions.

Similar to TBI, it is important to minimize secondary brain injury following anoxia/hypoxia. Continuous EEG monitoring should be considered in children with anoxic/hypoxic-ischemic injury given the increased risk for clinical and subclinical seizures in this population. Furthermore, during the subacute period, children with anoxic/hypoxic-ischemic brain injury are more likely than children with TBI to experience paroxysmal sympathetic hyperactivity. Although there is no specific treatment strategy for anoxic brain injury, a comprehensive, systematic approach similar to TBI is more likely to mitigate further neurological injury.

Although there is a large breadth of literature evaluating neurological outcomes following pediatric TBI, fewer studies have reported outcomes following anoxic/hypoxic-ischemic injury. As of 2018, available studies draw upon samples from inpatient pediatric rehabilitation facilities, which typically reflect the most severely impaired children and do not likely represent the full spectrum of outcomes.

Hypoxic-ischemic brain injury due to cardiac arrest, as mentioned above, is most often a consequence of respiratory failure in children. Although in-hospital cardiac arrest is typically associated with higher survival than out-of-hospital cardiac arrest, the neurological outcomes for both have improved over time. Several factors, including cardiac etiology, bystander performance of cardiopulmonary resuscitation (CPR), duration of CPR, and time to epinephrine administration to restart the heart, have been associated with improved neurological outcome (Anderson et al., 2015; Del Castillo et al., 2014; Forrest, Butt, & Namachivavam, 2017).

Neuropsychological evaluations of children with anoxic brain injury and drowning do suggest a broad spectrum of long-term neurological deficits, including poor coordination and fine motor movements, mild to severe cognitive deficits, and behavioral difficulties (Suominen, Sutinen, Valle, Olkkola, & Lönnqvist, 2014; Thaler et al., 2013). Children with anoxic/hypoxic-ischemic brain injury, however, certainly have the potential to benefit from rehabilitation (discussed later) and to make significant functional gains following hospital discharge.

Pediatric Stroke

Pediatric stroke is another important cause of ABI associated with neurodevelopmental morbidity. Reports on the incidence of stroke from birth to 18 years of age ranges from 1 to 13 per 100,000 children per year (Felling, Sun, Maxwell, Goldenberg, & Bernard, 2017; Roach et al., 2008). Stroke can be categorized as arterial ischemic stroke (loss of blood flow in arteries supplying the brain), venous stroke (secondary to a clot in the brain's venous system), or hemorrhagic stroke (bleeding into the brain substance, ventricles, or subarachnoid space of the brain). In children, stroke can be further categorized by age at the time of stroke, and these categories are associated with different risk factors, presentation, and outcomes.

Perinatal stroke is defined as a stroke that occurs from the prenatal period to 29 days after birth and has unique risk factors related to maternal/pregnancy variables. Any stroke that occurs after 29 days of life is termed childhood stroke. Childhood stroke is also different from strokes in adults, having different risk factors, causes, types, recurrence risk, and outcomes. Unlike adults, a group of risk factors that are not related to lifestyle may predispose children to stroke, including 1) congenital or acquired cardiac disease, 2) prothrombotic states (conditions associated with an increased risk of blood clots), 3) sickle cell disease (see Chapter 24), 4) genetic and metabolic disorders, and 5) cerebral arteriopathies (abnormal development of the arteries of the brain). Almost one half of children with stroke have a known risk factor, and in a systematic review of childhood strokes, nearly one third of ischemic and hemorrhagic strokes had an undetermined cause (Gumer, Del Vecchio, & Aronoff, 2014).

Perinatal stroke may present acutely in the neonatal period with seizures, or present months later (between 4–6 months of age) when asymmetric motor development (weakness on one side of the body) is first recognized. Childhood arterial ischemic stroke may present with the acute onset of focal deficits consistent with the function of the brain region having lost perfusion. Common symptoms include 1) unilateral hemiparesis (weakness) of the face and arm (with or without leg weakness), 2) language or speech difficulties, and 3) ataxia (difficulties with balance); however, they may also include seizures, headache, altered mental status, or a reduced level of awareness. Venous thrombosis is more likely to present with a more gradual onset of diffuse symptoms such as headache, nausea, and vomiting. Acute onset of severe headache typically signals hemorrhagic stroke, which may also be associated with seizures, reduced awareness, and focal signs related to the area of hemorrhage and surrounding edema.

Management of childhood stroke is extrapolated from the literature on the management of adult stroke given the paucity of pediatric stroke treatment trials other than for sickle cell disease (for which intravenous hydration and exchange transfusion are recommended; see Chapter 24). However, while the overarching goal in adult stroke care is rapid diagnosis and management, there is commonly a delay in the diagnosis of stroke in children, and there are questions regarding the optimal treatment of pediatric stroke (see Jordan & Hillis, 2011, and Kirton & deVeber, 2015 for comprehensive reviews on the challenges unique to management of pediatric stroke). Several consensus statements and guidelines review the management of childhood stroke. The American Heart Association guidelines provide recommendations in the management of neonatal and childhood ischemic and hemorrhagic stroke and include recommendations for specific etiologies of stroke (Roach et al., 2008).

The risk of stroke recurrence varies by etiology, most often occurring within the first year following the initial stroke. The overall risk for recurrence of childhood arterial ischemic stroke within 1 year is approximately 7%, but it is significantly increased if cerebral arteriopathy is the underlying etiology. For example, up to 32% of individuals with Moyamoya disease, a progressive cerebral arterial disorder, have recurrent strokes (Fullerton et al., 2016).

Neurodevelopmental sequelae are common, occurring in up to 80% of children with stroke. Motor deficits are the most common and pronounced initial findings, but cognitive, sensory, and emotional/behavioral impairments may emerge over time, reflecting more extensive disruption in neurological function. Gross and fine motor deficits can greatly affect a child's ability to perform daily activities. The trajectory of gross and fine motor recovery following childhood stroke is affected by the age of the child at injury and size of the stroke, with poorer 5-year outcomes in children sustaining arterial ischemic stroke between 1 month and 5 years of age as well as larger and/or bilateral strokes (Cooper et al., 2017; Cooper et al., 2018). Premorbid conditions, often related to the stroke, also affect outcome following stroke. These include children with congenital heart disease and Down syndrome, who may have neurodevelopmental deficits independent of, and then compounded by, a stroke.

Infectious Encephalitis/Meningitis

Infectious encephalitis (inflammation of the brain tissue) and meningitis (inflammation in the membranes surrounding the brain) are broad categories of disease with great variability in age of onset, presenting symptoms, clinical course, laboratory and radiological features, and outcome. More than 100 viruses have been associated with infection of the brain or spinal cord, although herpesviruses, arboviruses (tick or mosquito born), and enteroviruses are the most common. The introduction of vaccinations has changed the nature of bacterial meningitis. While vaccinations have reduced the incidence of *Haemophilus influenzae* type b meningitis by 97% and *Streptococcus pneumoniae* (pneumococcal) meningitis by 34%–62%, there has been a concomitant increase in pneumococcal meningitis caused by serotypes not covered by the vaccine (Kowalsky & Jaffe, 2013). Brain injury due to CNS infection is a consequence of direct invasion of brain tissue by infectious agents, and the subsequent neuroinflammatory response has the potential to induce further brain injury.

Children may present with active infectious symptoms (such as fever, respiratory or gastrointestinal symptoms, and decreased feeding) and neurological symptoms that vary by age of child and etiology (examples include altered mental status, irritability, stiff neck, and seizures). The International Encephalitis Consortium has outlined the definition and diagnostic algorithms for encephalitis, including clinical, laboratory, and imaging features suggestive of specific infections in children (Venkatesan et al., 2013). Evaluation for CNS infection includes a thorough history, physical exam, serum and cerebrospinal fluid (CSF) laboratory studies, and brain MRI. Given the multitude of variables that affect the differential diagnoses in a child presenting with central nervous system infection (such as age, region, and exposure), a pediatric infectious disease provider is often involved in the child's evaluation and treatment decisions. Even with extensive testing, however, the specific infectious cause may not be identified, particularly in presumed viral encephalitis.

The outcome depends on a variety of factors including the child (the "host") and the specific infectious organism (virus or bacterium). Neurodevelopmental sequelae are common following CNS infections and, similar to other mechanisms of ABI, may emerge over time as the child develops. In a meta-analysis of infectious encephalitis in children, Khandaker and colleagues (2016) have reported that long-term neurodevelopmental sequela (i.e., cognitive dysfunction, behavioral abnormalities, and neurological disorders) occur in one half of the affected population, although the outcome varies by etiology with some infections, such as neonatal herpes simplex virus, having the worst outcome. Similarly, at least one half of children with bacterial meningitis have long-term neurodevelopmental disabilities, primarily intellectual and behavioral, and hearing loss is reported in 7%–14% of these children, with 5% having profound hearing loss (Chandran, Herbert, Misurski, & Santosham, 2011; Rodenburg-Volt, Ruytjens, Oostenbrink, Goedegebure, & van der Schroeff, 2016).

Brain injury rehabilitation, early assessment, and long-term neurodevelopmental monitoring is warranted for children following infectious encephalitis and meningitis. In addition, early audiological testing is recommended following bacterial meningitis, with follow-up testing based on clinical symptoms as post-meningitic hearing impairment can improve or worsen over time.

Autoimmune Encephalitis

Autoimmune encephalitis occurs when the body's own immune system mistakenly targets brain tissue, resulting in inflammation and potential brain injury. Acute-disseminating encephalomyelitis (ADEM) is an immune-mediated CNS demyelinating disorder that typically follows a systemic infection by days to weeks. The body's immune system, in an attempt to react to infection, mistakenly targets the tissues of the CNS, especially the white matter (myelin) that insulates nerve cell processes. Encephalopathy (altered mental status) is required for the diagnosis. Other features of ADEM may include focal neurological deficits and seizures as well as a characteristic pattern on brain MRI; however, there are no specific blood or CSF tests for ADEM.

Anti-NMDA receptor encephalitis is the second most common cause of autoimmune encephalitis and is a potentially devastating autoimmune neurological disorder affecting children and young adults. The classical presentation of anti-NMDA receptor encephalitis, described in adults, involves acute behavioral change and psychiatric symptoms followed by seizures, memory deficits, movement disorder, and vital sign lability (Titulauer et al., 2013). However, less is known about the presentation of anti-NMDA receptor encephalitis in children, especially young children. A review of case reports of children less than 3 years of age with anti-NMDA receptor encephalitis suggests that this youngest cohort typically presents with behavioral changes, movement disorders, and speech arrest (Goldberg, Titulaer, de Blank, Sievert, & Ryan, 2014). Therefore, autoimmune encephalitis should be considered in the differential diagnosis of a child presenting with loss of developmental skills (developmental regression).

Across all ages, earlier treatment with immune-modulating therapies is thought to be related to better outcome, and with continued symptom improvement for 12–24 months (Byrne et al., 2015). Bigi, Hladio, Twilt, Dalmau, and Benseler (2015) have provided a comprehensive review of the current known pediatric antibody-associated inflammatory disorders: anti-NMDA receptor encephalitis, Hashimoto encephalitis (also known as steroid-responsive encephalopathy), aquaporin-4, and anti-GAD-65 encephalitis. They note that 27% of affected individuals have ongoing and functionally impairing neurological deficits 2 years following diagnosis. Similar to other etiologies of ABI, these inflammatory brain processes may occur at various stages of neurodevelopment and have the potential to affect ongoing development. As deficits may emerge over time, long-term neurodevelopmental monitoring is recommended in children following autoimmune encephalitis.

Other Causes

Autoimmune disorders (such as systemic lupus erythematosus) may have CNS involvement, sometimes even presenting with neurological or neuropsychiatric symptoms. Toxins (such as chemotherapy and carbon monoxide) and radiation therapy also can induce diffuse brain injury and have long-term neurodevelopmental sequela (see Chapters 2 and 25). Emerging evidence indicates that refractory status epilepticus or persistent seizure activity that does not respond to typical aggressive seizure management (i.e., febrile infection-related epilepsy syndrome and new-onset refractory status epilepticus) triggers a deleterious autoinflammatory response of the immune system in the brain, contributing to both the development of epilepsy and brain injury (Kenney-Jung et al., 2016).

As with any cause of ABI, children with these conditions who experience prolonged hospitalization or severe functional deficits should have intensive inpatient or outpatient brain injury rehabilitation. The potential neurodevelopmental consequences of such diffuse brain injury processes are high and emphasize the importance of vigilant long-term neurodevelopmental monitoring.

REHABILITATION AND OUTCOMES

Once a child with ABI is medically stable and ready for the next level of care, he or she may be transitioned to a rehabilitation hospital for intensive inpatient therapy or may participate in outpatient rehabilitative therapy services depending on the severity of the child's functional impairments. A rehabilitation facility should have the following components of care: 1) expertise in rehabilitation of children, 2) developmentally appropriate treatments, 3) family-centered care, and 4) attention to the child's education and reintegration into the school system. Many rehabilitation hospitals are accredited through the Commission on Accreditation of Rehabilitation Facilities, which sets standards of care for the facilities and offers specialty accreditations for brain injury programs and pediatric specialty programs.

As the child recovers from ABI, functional impairments may become apparent in the following domains: motor (gross and/or fine motor control and balance), sensory (vision or hearing), feeding skills, communication (speech and language), cognition (memory and processing), and behavior (Savage, DePompei, Tyler, & Lash, 2005).

Rehabilitation strives to 1) prevent complications that are caused by immobilization and disuse, 2) increase the use of abilities regained, 3) teach strategies to compensate for impaired or lost function, and 4) alleviate the effect of chronic disability on the process of growth and development (Cope, 1995). The primary goals of rehabilitation for all impairments related to ABI include promotion of recovery, compensation for impairments, and identification and treatment of cognitive and behavioral issues.

Following ABI, the medical team and/or primary care provider help determine the level of care needed. A multidisciplinary intervention including physical therapy, occupational therapy, speech therapy, neuropsychology, special education, and social work may be necessary depending on the severity of the injury and impairments.

Motor Impairments

Motor recovery and functional prognosis following ABI are typically of concern. Studies have shown that motor weakness tends to improve over time and that functional outcomes are good. In TBI, prognosis of motor recovery is related to duration of coma, and significant motor recovery may occur in children who are comatose for less than 3 months (Brink, Imbus, & Woo-Sam, 1980). Evaluating nearly 500 children with ABI admitted to inpatient rehabilitation, 70% regained mobility (7.6 months after injury on average) and functional self-care and mobility skills continued to improve over 5 years following injury (Beretta, Molteni, Galbiati, Stefanoni, & Strazzer, 2017).

Persistent impairments may be noted in strength, balance, speed, and coordination (Beretta et al., 2017), and assessment of hand function reveals decreased fine motor skills, speed, and coordination (Kuhtz-Buschbeck et al., 2003). Constraint-induced movement therapy (i.e., therapy that employs inhibition or constraint of the unaffected limb to encourage use of the impaired limb) is a specific rehabilitation program beneficial for children with unilateral hemiparesis (of any etiology), resulting in positive functional gains in the weaker limb (DeLuca, Trucks, Wallace, & Ramey, 2017).

Motor recovery is also affected by motor impairments related to movement patterns and tone, such as spasticity, dystonia, tremor, and ataxia. Medications or surgery may be used to treat some of these impairments. Medications to treat spasticity and dystonia include baclofen, dantrolene, diazepam, trihexiphenadyl, and tizanidine (see Appendix C). Baclofen may be given orally or directly into the spinal fluid with an intrathecal baclofen pump (Albright & Ferson, 2006). Management of spasticity may also involve localized neuromuscular blockade with botulinum toxins or nerve blocks, such as phenol injections. The effects of botulinum toxins last several months, but repeated injections may be required (Bjornson et al., 2007; Clemenzi et al., 2012; Meholjic-Fetahovic, 2007). Injections should be followed by physical or occupational therapy services to obtain the desired results. Tremor may be treated with propranolol (Inderol) or carbidopa/levodopa (Sinemet). There is, as of 2018, no medicine or surgery that is effective for ataxia.

Orthopedic surgery may be necessary for the treatment of contractures and bony orthopedic deformities. Surgeries may include tendon lengthening, femoral osteotomies (reconfiguring the femur to treat hip spasticity), or spinal fusion for scoliosis.

Sensory Impairments

Both vision and hearing may be affected following ABI. Visual impairments can be due to injury of the optic nerves, impaired visual processing in the brain, or limitation of eye movements resulting from cranial nerve damage. Double vision is common following ABI because of cranial nerve injury. Other impairments may include nystagmus (shaking eye movements caused by cerebellar damage), decreased visual acuity, difficulty with tracking, and visual field cuts. Traumatic injury to the optic nerve is not reversible and can cause blindness (Bodack, 2010; Cockerman et al., 2009). Injury to the occipital lobes, leading to visual cortex damage, can cause cortical blindness (the ability to see but not process visual information; see Chapter 25). Vision assessment by an ophthalmologist or neuro-ophthalmologist is recommended for evaluation of the above impairments.

Sensorineural hearing loss or conductive hearing loss can occur following ABI (especially bacterial meningitis) and is generally unilateral. Hearing loss may be a result of trauma to the middle (conductive) or inner (sensorineural) ear due to traumatic skull base fractures or damage to the central neuronal pathways. Sensorineural loss is more pronounced at the higher hearing frequencies (Lew, Jerger, Guillory, & Henry, 2007; Munjal, Panda, & Pathak, 2010). Given these concerns, audiological evaluation is recommended following ABI. Brainstem auditory-evoked responses can be used for testing children who are unable to participate in traditional behavioral audiometric testing (Lew et al., 2004; see Chapter 26).

Feeding Disorders

ABI can cause **dysphagia** (difficulty in swallowing), which affects oral nutrition and hydration. It can also have a negative impact on a child's ability to protect the airway, leading to an increased risk of aspiration pneumonia (see Chapter 29). The incidence of dysphagia following ABI overall is low; however, it increases markedly with increasing severity of injury. For instance, the incidence of acute dysphagia associated with severe TBI is 68%–76% (Morgan, 2010; Morgan, Mageandran, & Mei, 2010). Associated impairments include atypical tongue movements, poor jaw stability, inefficient chewing, impaired lip closure, and reduced attention and impulsivity during feeding. Signs of aspiration can include coughing after swallowing, wet voice after swallowing, and delayed swallow initiation (Morgan et al., 2010).

A child with dysphagia may require a feeding tube to provide nutrition and hydration. The tube may be a temporary measure, such as a nasogastric tube, or a long-term option, such as a percutaneous (placed through the skin without opening the abdomen) endoscopic gastrostomy (PEG) tube. Children with a PEG tube will receive a standard concentration enteral formula (e.g., Pediasure) to attain maximum nutrition with minimum volume (Cook, Peppard, & Magnuson, 2008).

Given the importance of nutrition on brain injury recovery and ongoing rehabilitation, it is critical to ensure the most optimal method of feeding for a child with ABI.

Communication Skills and Language Impairments

A variety of speech, language, and communication skills can be affected by ABI. Dysarthria (a dysfunction in the motor control of the muscles used for speech that affects articulation and intelligibility) is an especially important sequelae of ABI. The incidence of dysarthria for TBI in children specifically ranges from 2%–60% (Cahill et al., 2005; Morgan et al., 2010). As mentioned above, motor impairment and dysphagia are significantly associated with dysarthria (Morgan et al., 2010).

Language impairments may be expressive (relating to the ability to express thoughts in words and sentences) or receptive (relating to the ability to process and understand language) (see Chapter 17). While basic aspects of speech production (articulation, vocabulary, and grammar) may remain intact following TBI, more complex ("higher-order") language skills and processing are often impaired in children and adolescents with ABI. Daily conversation and real-life, complex communication skills are impaired in children following ABI (Fyrberg, Horneman, Asberg Johnels, Thunberg, & Ahlsen, 2017). The more complex features of language processing are affected by cognitive deficits involving difficulty with judgment related to topic management, turn taking, and pause time (Fyrberg, Marchioni, & Emanuelson, 2007). Individuals with TBI are less appropriate in their use of language and style of speech and have difficulty initiating and sustaining a conversation (Dahlberg et al., 2007). These language and processing deficits often impair a child's social interactions and are related to externalizing (challenging) behaviors (Catroppa & Anderson, 2004). Social isolation may result from these communication impairments.

Language development may be particularly vulnerable to ABI during early childhood. Children who sustained moderate to severe TBI between 4–6 years of age were found to have more significantly impaired verbal abilities and language skills compared with mTBI and children without TBI (Crowe et al., 2014). Speech and language assessment is an important aspect of ongoing neurodevelopmental monitoring following ABI.

Cognitive Impairments

Cognitive impairments are common following ABI. Areas affected may include attention, memory, executive function (planning, initiating, and problem solving), and speed of processing (Babikian et al., 2015; Dikmen et al., 2009). Long-term outcome is correlated with injury severity. The more severe the injury sustained, the worse the outcome across all cognitive domains. Environmental factors unrelated to the injury also have an impact on outcome, including parental occupation, preinjury adaptive abilities, age at time of injury, and preinjury behavior (Anderson et al., 2004).

Preschool children with severe TBI demonstrate slower recovery with poorer cognitive outcome up to 5 years after injury compared with children less severely injured (Anderson et al., 2009; Ylvisaker & Feeney, 2007). Children who are younger at the time of injury may not show the full extent of their cognitive impairments until they reach school age, when the task complexity increases (Anderson & Catroppa, 2005; Babikian et al., 2015; Meekes, Jennekens-Schinkel, & van Schooneveld, 2006).

Cognitive impairments are identified through evaluation by a neuropsychologist that includes tests and questionnaires to assess cognitive, emotional/behavioral, and adaptive functioning (see Chapter 13). The assessment is typically performed in a quiet setting with minimal distractions, and it can be completed while a child is in the hospital or rehabilitation setting or on an outpatient basis. It involves a set of standardized measures to assess language, visuospatial skills, concept formation, reasoning, problem solving, attention, memory, and academic performance. Questionnaires and interviews to assess adaptive and social/emotional functioning are also undertaken.

The results of this testing can be used to assess cognitive strengths and weaknesses (including deficits attributable to ABI effects) and to assist in treatment planning, including educational placement, accommodations, or adjunct therapies (e.g., speech-language therapy, cognitive rehabilitation, executive functioning coaching, and psychotherapy) as necessary (Ylvisaker et al., 2005). Repeat neuropsychological evaluation is recommended as the child reintegrates into the school and community. As the child ages and demands are increased, cognitive impairments may become more apparent and warrant repeat testing and monitoring.

Behavior, Socialization, and Family

Following TBI, changes may be noted in a child's behavioral, emotional, and social interactions. These changes may include adjustment difficulties, psychiatric disorders (including depression and anxiety), disinhibition (lack of restraint manifested as inappropriate social behavior, impulsivity, and poor risk assessment), and social withdrawal (Anderson & Catroppa, 2006; Ylvisaker et al., 2005). Preinjury behavioral and family functioning is also correlated to postinjury function (Anderson et al., 2001).

Management may include medications, counseling, and/or behavioral reinforcement, all of which are tailored to the child's needs (Anderson & Catroppa, 2006; Bates, 2006; Riggio & Wong, 2009; Ylvisaker et al., 2005; see Chapter 27). Behavioral issues and social withdrawal can lead to tension within the family, and social isolation not only affects the child, but can also lead to isolation of the entire family (Kapapa et al., 2010).

Caregivers of children with a severe TBI are also under greater stress and are at higher risk for psychological symptoms (Aitken et al., 2005; Gan & Schuller, 2002). Coping strategies used by families may include denial and disengagement (Stancin, Wade, Walz, Yeates, & Taylor, 2008). Parents and siblings may feel guilt and remorse after the injury. Mothers and fathers often have different coping styles, which may further exacerbate family dysfunction (Wade et al., 2010; see Chapter 37). Prolonged hospitalization may additionally place a financial burden on the family and affect the overall finances and dynamics of the family. Therefore, family support is important in all phases following a TBI, during the acute hospitalization, rehabilitation, and school reintegration. Social workers, psychologists, educators, and other health care professionals may work with the family to assist with resources, family coping and adjustment, discharge planning, and school reentry. Ongoing support groups in the community may be recommended and utilized (Aitken et al., 2005).

School Reentry

One of the main goals following rehabilitation is school and community reintegration. Sustaining an ABI places a child at risk for the presence of long-term academic difficulties, especially following more severe injury. Reading and math abilities may be compromised as well as attention, concentration, and memory (Catroppa et al., 2009; Hawley, Ward, Magnay, & Mychalkiw, 2004). Educational testing as well as neuropsychological testing should be completed to obtain a comprehensive view of the child's impairments (see Chapter 13). Long-term follow-up studies of school-age children with TBI reveal impairments that persist or worsen as the children progress through school (Babikian et al., 2015; Glang et al., 2008).

Special education support is available to those who qualify under one or more of the eligibility categories of the Individuals with Disabilities Education Improvement Act (IDEA) of 2004 (Box 23.2 describes the role of the educational specialist in remediating TBI). TBI is one of the IDEA eligibility categories, and individuals with nontraumatic ABI may qualify under Other Health Impaired. Eligibility in most states requires medical documentation of a TBI or ABI, and physical and intellectual assessments must show a difference between preinjury and postinjury performance. It should be noted that preinjury functioning can be determined by interview and record review.

When a student qualifies, an individualized education program (IEP) is created by a team of individuals, including the parents and representatives from the school or school district (see Chapter 33). The IEP outlines direct services and accommodations needed for the student to be successful in the school environment. Examples include therapy services provided by the school system; a range of classroom settings from self-contained to assistance in the classroom; focused instruction; organizational support; and increased time or strategies to address impairments in attention, organization, or memory. When a child needs accommodations but not direct services, he or she may qualify to receive support and accommodations with a Section 504 plan (Rehabilitation Act of 1973, PL 93-112). These can include reduced work, extended time, check-ins regarding assignments and deadlines, and other organizational supports.

Obtaining an IEP or a Section 504 plan is an important aspect of school reintegration. Without a plan in place, educators may not recognize the impairments and needs of the student. During their training, teachers are rarely exposed to children with ABI; thus, they may not be aware of the potential effects of ABI on learning, memory, and behavior (Glang et al., 2008; Hawley et al., 2004). An IEP or Section 504 plan allows for communication across all school settings regarding the injury and resultant impairments (Hawley et al., 2004). Children with TBI who receive transition support from the hospital are more likely to have an IEP or Section 504 plan in place. Planning for school reentry, transition support, and education of school staff, as well as long-term monitoring, are all important for successful reintegration and school placement.

PREVENTION

Many types of unintentional traumatic injuries are preventable. The leading causes of nonfatal injuries in children are falls; poisoning; burns; and motor vehicle, bicycle, and pedestrian accidents (CDC, 2010). Falls are more common in younger children, bicycle and pedestrian collisions are more common in elementary and middle school–age children, and motor vehicle collisions are more common in adolescents (Mendelson & Fallat, 2007). For each of these brain injury etiologies, there are available prevention strategies. For example, the use of window guards and gates at stairways and

BOX 23.2 INTERDISCIPLINARY CARE

The Education Specialist and Moderate to Severe Traumatic Brain Injury (TBI)

Despite the fact the TBI is known to be associated with neurocognitive sequelae that affect educational outcomes and that the diagnosis of TBI can qualify a child for special education services, schools and teachers are often unprepared to support the needs of children returning to school following moderate to severe TBI (Linden, Braiden, & Miller, 2013).

Not all children with TBI will require special education services, but a significant percentage of children with moderate to severe TBI have some combination of cognitive, learning, language, motor, social, and behavioral difficulties that can impact their ability to learn and perform in school. Children with TBI who are admitted to rehabilitation programs often undergo neuropsychological and educational assessment to evaluate learning strengths and weaknesses and to help guide necessary educational supports as the child returns to school. The educational specialist (ES) serves as a liaison between the medical/rehabilitation and education teams in an effort to optimize the child's transition to school following a TBI. The ES can educate the school staff (and other students if needed) on TBI, assist in development of an individualized education program for the child, monitor the child's progress throughout their schooling, and help adjust educational supports and services as needed.

There are several models for professional training programs for educators of children with TBI that have been implemented and evaluated (Glang et al., 2010). Additionally, thoughtful recommendations have been published to aid the development of a statewide infrastructure for effective educational services for children with TBI (Dettmer, Ettel, Glang, & McAvoy, 2014). In an ideal pediatric TBI program, the services and supports provided by an ES can ease the transition to school and ensure the child's learning environment is appropriate for that specific child. As children are in school 8 hours a day, optimization of a child's educational program and environment can certainly influence the child's ultimate outcome following TBI.

refraining from using infant walkers are strategies for the prevention of falls in infants/toddlers (Schnitzer, 2006). In addition, bicycle helmets are important in the prevention of TBI in children. In fact, biomechanical pediatric skull models have shown that children's bicycle helmets provide a significant reduction in the acceleration and direct compression force, thereby mitigating the risk of more severe TBI (Mattei et al., 2012). Given the high frequency of mTBI in children, methods to prevent concussion in children are essential. Evidence for sport-specific preventive measures to reduce the rate of mTBI in children, such as limited body checking in ice hockey and helmet use when skiing, are emerging, although ongoing research is needed for many potential sport-specific injury prevention strategies (for a comprehensive review, see Emery et al., 2017).

The appropriate use of car seats, boosters, and seat belts has been shown to reduce brain injury in children following a motor vehicle accident (Keenan & Bratton, 2006). The AAP released a policy statement on child passenger safety in 2011 (Durbin & Committee on Injury, Violence, and Poison Prevention, 2011). The statement provides recommendations for best practices, including 1) rear-facing car safety seats for most infants up to 2 years of age, 2) forward-facing car safety seats for most children through 4 years of age, 3) belt-positioning booster seats for most children through 8 years of age, and 4) lap-and-shoulder seat belts for all children who have outgrown booster seats. Children under the age of 13 years should ride in the rear seats of vehicles. Child safety seats decrease the risk of nonfatal injury by approximately 75% (Zaloshnja, Miller, & Hendrie, 2007) and the risk of fatal injury by 28% (Elliott, Kallan, Durbin, & Winston, 2006). Booster seats decrease the risk of nonfatal injury among 4- to 8-year-old children by 45% compared with seat belts (Arbogast, Jermakian, Kallan, & Durbin, 2009). The AAP also recommends that children should not ride in the flatbeds of pickup trucks and that children or teenagers younger than 16 years should not ride an all-terrain vehicle or a lawn mower.

In school-age children, pedestrian injuries typically occur while the child is crossing the road. Strategies that have been utilized to improve street-crossing skills include group education and individualized behavior training. Individualized training appears to be more successful than group training (Schwebel & McClure, 2010). Programs developed to help teach pedestrian safety included the WalkSafe program. This program has been shown to improve pedestrian safety knowledge of school-age children after receiving a 3-day educational experience (Hotz et al., 2009). Children ages 5–14 years have the highest rate of bicycle-related injuries. Head injury accounts for 62% of bicycle-related deaths, 33% of bicycle-related ED visits, and 67% of all bicycle-related hospital admissions (CDC, 1995). Bicycle helmets are effective in decreasing head, brain, and facial injuries when used properly. The risk of TBI is reduced by 60% when wearing a bicycle helmet (Attewell, Glase, & McFadden, 2001; Lee, Schofer, & Koppelman, 2005; Thompson, Rivara, & Thompson, 1999). Helmets and protective gear are also recommended for skating, skateboarding, skiing, snowboarding, scooter riding, horseback riding, and motorcycle riding, as well as participation in contact sports such as football, hockey, and lacrosse (Dellinger & Kresnow, 2010; Jagodzinski & DeMuri, 2005; Schnitzer, 2006).

Motor vehicle collisions are the leading cause of injuries in teenagers. Prevention strategies include limiting nighttime driving, limiting driving with teenage passengers, and developing graduated licensing measures (Williams & Ferguson, 2002). As in younger children, the appropriate use of seat belts is imperative and is the law.

To reduce the risk of drowning in children, providing education on the risk of drowning, offering water safety programs, and mandating the use of pool fencing are effective strategies to reduce the incidence of drowning in children. Isolation fencing (enclosing the pool area only) and the use of a dynamic, secure gate with self-latching lock are especially important (Thompson & Rivara, 2000). The AAP Committee on Injury, Violence, and Poison Prevention published a policy statement on effective strategies to prevent drowning in children (2010).

Increased attention to the epidemiology of intentional asphyxiation related brain injury (hanging injuries) has led to efforts to implement more effective national and local suicide-prevention programs. There are also public health efforts to reduce unintentional asphyxiation injuries, such as educational programs to remove pillows and blankets from infant sleep areas and initiatives to discourage cosleeping. In 2016, the AAP published updated recommendations for a safe sleeping environment (Moon & Task Force on Sudden Infant Death Syndrome, 2016).

The CDC has also published a National Action Plan (2012) outlining a childhood injury prevention framework, a comprehensive program using multiple strategies to prevent unintentional childhood injury. Prevention should be addressed at each well-child visit through parent-focused strategies and through education to teachers and community groups as well as the children themselves. The focus for TBI prevention should be on the appropriate use of seat belts, safe pedestrian behavior, helmet use, prevention of falls, and sports injury prevention. For other etiologies of ABI, the importance of vaccinations, water safety and drowning prevention programs, safe sleeping habits for infants and children, and prompt referral and management for mental health concerns are important preventive measures.

SUMMARY

- ABI encompasses a large group of conditions that result in brain injury with a wide range of severity and outcomes.
- TBI is the most common cause of ABI in children, and AHT is the most common etiology in the youngest children.
- Nontraumatic causes of ABI in children include anoxia/hypoxia-ischemia, stroke, encephalitic/meningitis, and autoimmune disease.
- As ABI occurs during brain development, children are at risk for short- and long-term neurodevelopmental deficits. Persistent functional impairments may involve multiple areas of functioning, including motor, sensory, feeding, communication, cognition, and behavior.
- Restoration and adaptation are the goals of rehabilitation and require a multidisciplinary team including medical professionals, allied health professionals, and education specialists.
- Children should be followed throughout their education to provide academic support and accommodations as needed.
- Most ABIs are preventable. Therefore, brain injury prevention programs are needed, and legislation should be written and enforced to decrease the risk and long-term consequences of ABI.

ADDITIONAL RESOURCES

Brain Injury Association of America: http://www.biausa.org

Traumatic Brain Injury Resource Guide: http://www.neuroskills.com

Additional resources can be found online in Appendix D: Childhood Disabilities Resources, Services, and Organizations (see About the Online Companion Materials).

REFERENCES

Aitken, M. E., Korehbandi, P., Parnell, D., Parker, J. G., Stefans, V., Tompkins, E., & Schultz, E. G. (2005). Experiences from the development of a comprehensive family support program for pediatric trauma and rehabilitation patients. *Archives of Physical Medicine and Rehabilitation, 86,* 175–179.

Albright, A. L., & Ferson, S. S. (2006). Inthrathecal baclofen therapy in children. *Neurosurgery Focus, 2*(2), e3.

Amagasa, S., Matsui, H., Tsuji, S., Moriya, T., & Kinoshita, K. (2016). Accuracy of the history of injury obtained from the caregiver in infantile head trauma. *American Journal of Emergency Medicine, 34*(9), 1863–1867.

AAP Committee on Injury, Violence, and Poison Prevention. (2010). Prevention of drowning. *Pediatrics, 126*(1), 178–185.

Andersen, L. W., Berg, K. M., Saindon, B. Z., Massaro, J. M., Raymond, T. T., Berg, R. A., . . . American Heart Association Get With the Guidelines-Resuscitation, I. (2015). Time to epinephrine and survival after pediatric in-hospital cardiac arrest. *JAMA, 314*(8), 802–810. doi:10.1001/jama.2015.9678

Anderson, V., & Catroppa, C. (2005). Recovery of executive skills following paediatric traumatic brain injury (TBI): A 2 year follow-up. *Brain Injury, 19*(6), 459–470.

Anderson, V., & Catroppa, C. (2006). Advances in postacute rehabilitation after childhood-acquired brain injury: A focus on cognitive, behavioral, and social domains. *American Journal of Physical Medicine & Rehabilitation, 85*(9), 767–778.

Anderson, V. A., Catroppa, C., Haritou, F., Morse, S., Pentland, L., Rosenfeld, J., & Stargatt, R. (2001). Predictors of acute child and family outcome following traumatic brain injury in children. *Pediatric Neurosurgery, 34*(3), 138–148.

Anderson, V., Catroppa, C., Morse, S., Haritou, F., & Rosenfeld, J. V. (2009). Intellectual outcome from preschool traumatic brain injury: A 5-year prospective, longitudinal study. *Pediatrics, 124*(6), e1064–e1071.

Anderson, V. A., Morse, S. A., Catroppa, C., Haritou, F., & Rosenfeld, J. V. (2004). Thirty month outcome from early childhood head injury: A prospective analysis of neurobehavioural recovery. *Brain, 127*(Pt. 12), 2608–2620. doi:10.1093/brain/awh320

Anderson, V., Spencer-Smith, M., Leventer, R., Coleman, L., Anderson, P., Williams, J., . . . Jacobs, R. (2009). Childhood brain insult: Can age at insult help us predict outcome? *Brain, 132*(Pt. 1), 45–56. doi:10.1093/brain/awn293

Andruszkow, H., Deniz, E., Urner, J., Probst, C., Grün, O., Lohse, R., . . . Hildebrand, F. (2014). Physical and psychological long-term outcome after traumatic brain injury in children and adult patients. *Health and Quality of Life Outcomes, 12,* 26.

Annegers, J. F., & Coan, S. P. (2000). The risks of epilepsy after traumatic brain injury. *Seizure, 9,* 453–457.

Arango, J. I., Deibert, C. P., Brown, D., Bell, M., Dvorchik, I., & Adelson, P. D. (2012). Posttraumatic seizures in children with severe traumatic brain injury. *Childs Nervous System, 28*(11), 1925–1929.

Arbogast, K. B., Jermakian, J. S., Kallan, M. J., & Durbin, D. R. (2009). Effectiveness of belt positioning booster seats: An updated assessment. *Pediatrics, 124*(5), 1281–1286.

Arbogast, K. B., McGinley, A. D., Master, C. L., Grady, M. F., Robinson, R. L., & Zonfrillo, M. R. (2013). Cognitive rest and school-based recommendations following pediatric concussion: The need for primary care support tools. *Clinical Pediatrics, 52*(5), 397–402.

Arndt, D. H., Lerner, J. T., Matsumoto, J. H., Madikians, A., Yudovin, S., Valino, H., . . . Giza, C. C. (2013). Subclinical early posttraumatic seizures detected by continuous EEG monitoring in a consecutive pediatrics cohort. *Epilepsia, 54*(10), 1780–1788.

Arndt, D. H., Goodkin, H. P., & Giza, C. G. (2016). Early posttraumatic seizures in the pediatric population. *Journal of Child Neurology, 31*(1), 46–55.

Attewell, R. G., Glase, K., & McFadden, M. (2001). Bicycle helmet efficacy: A meta-analysis. *Accident Analysis and Prevention, 33,* 345–352.

Babikian, T., Merkley, T., Savage, R. C., Giza, C. G., & Levin, H. (2015). Chronic aspects of pediatric traumatic brain injury: Review of the literature. *Journal of Neurotrauma, 32*(23), 1849–1860.

Barlow, K. M., Crawford, S., Stevenson, A., Sandhu, S. S., Belanger, F., & Dewey, D. (2010). Epidemiology of postconcussion syndrome in pediatric mild traumatic brain injury. *Pediatrics, 126*(2), e374–e381.

Bates, G. (2006). Medication in the treatment of the behavioural sequelae of traumatic brain injury. *Developmental Medicine and Child Neurology, 48,* 697–701.

Bennett, K. S., DeWitt, P. E., Harlaar, N., & Bennett, T. D. (2017). Seizures in children with severe traumatic brain injury. *Pediatric Critical Care Medicine, 18*(1), 54–63.

Beretta, E., Molteni, E., Galbiati, S., Stefanoni, G., & Strazzer, S. (2017). Five-year motor functional outcome in children with acquired brain injury. Yet to the end of the story. *Developmental Neurorehabilitation, 21*(7), 449–456. doi:10.1080/17518423.2017.1360408

Bernard, C. O., Ponsford, J. A., McKinlay, A., McKenzie, D., & Krieser, D. (2016). Predictors of post-concussive symptoms in young children: Injury versus non-injury related factors. *Journal of International Neuropsychological Society, 22*(8), 793–803.

Bigi, S., Hladio, M., Twilt, M., Dalmau, J., & Benseler, S. M. (2015). The growing spectrum of antibody-associated inflammatory brain diseases in children. *Neurology, Neuroimmunology, Neuroinflammation, 2*(3), e92.

Bjornson, K., Hays, R., Graubert, C., Price, R., Won, F., McLaughlin, J. F., & Cohen, M. (2007). Botulinum toxin for spasticity in children with cerebral palsy: A comprehensive evaluation. *Pediatrics, 120*(1), 49–58.

Blackman, J. A., Patrick, P. D., Buck, M. L., & Rust, Jr., R. S. (2004). Paroxysmal autonomic instability with dystonia after brain injury. *Archives of Neurology, 61,* 321–328.

Bodack, M. I. (2010). Pediatric acquired brain injury. *Optometry, 81,* 516–527.

Boop, S., Axente, M., Weatherford, B., & Klimo, P. (2016) Abusive head trauma: an epidemiological and cost analysis. *Journal of Neurosurgery Pediatrics, 18*(5), 542–549.

Borse, N. N., Gilchrist, J., Dellinger, A. M., Rudd, R. A., Ballesteros, M. F., & Sleet, D. A. (2008). *CDC childhood injury report: Patterns of unintentional injuries among 0–19 year olds in the United States, 2000-2006.* Atlanta, GA: Centers for Disease Control and Prevention, National Center for Injury Prevention and Control.

Brink, J. D., Imbus, C., & Woo-Sam, J. (1980). Physical recovery after severe closed head trauma in children and adolescents. *Journal of Pediatrics, 97*(5), 721–727.

Brown, N. J., Mannix, R. C., O'Brien, M. J., Gostine, D., Collins, M. W., & Meehan III, W. P. (2014). Effect of cognitive activity level on duration of post-concussion symptoms. *Pediatrics, 133*(2), e299–e304.

Byrne, S., Walsh, C., Hacohen, Y., Muscal, E., Jankovic, J., Stocco, A., . . . King, M. (2015). Earlier treatment of NMDAR antibody encephalitis in children results in a better outcome. *Neurology, Neuroimmunology, and Neuroinflammation, 2*(4), e130.

Cahill, L. M., Murdoch, B. E., & Theodoros, D. G. (2005). Articulatory function following traumatic brain injury in childhood: A perceptual and instrumental analysis. *Brain Injury, 19*(1), 41–58.

Campbell, C. G., Kuehn, S. M., Richards, P. M., Ventureyra, E., & Hutchison, J. S. (2004). Medical and cognitive outcome in children with traumatic brain injury. *The Canadian Journal of Neurological Sciences, 31*(2), 213–219.

Canty, G., & Nilan, L. (2015). Return to play. *Pediatrics in Review, 36*(10), 38–446. doi:10.1542/pir.36-10-438

Catroppa, C., & Anderson, V. (2004). Recovery and predictors of language skills two years following pediatric traumatic brain injury. *Brain & Language, 88*(1), 68–78.

Catroppa, C., Anderson, V. A., Muscara, F., Morse, S. A., Haritou, F., Rosenfeld, J. V., & Heinrich, L. M. (2009). Educational skills: Long-term outcome and predictors following paediatric traumatic brain injury. *Neuropsychological Rehabilitation, 19*(5), 716–732.

Catroppa, C., Godfrey, C., Rosenfeld, J. V., Hearps, S. S., & Anderson, V. A. (2012). Functional recovery ten years after pediatric traumatic brain injury: outcomes and predictors. *Journal of Neurotrauma, 29*(16), 2539–2547.

Centers for Disease Control and Prevention. (1995). Injury control recommendations: Bicycle helmets. *Morbidity and Mortality Weekly Report, 44*(RR-1), 1–18. Retrieved from http://www.cdc.gov/mmwr/pdf/rr/rr4401.pdf

Centers for Disease Control and Prevention. (2006). *Centers for Disease Control Acute Concussion Evaluation (ACE) care plan—school version.* Retrieved from https://www.cdc.gov/headsup/pdfs/providers/ace_care_plan_school_version_a.pdf

Centers for Disease Control and Prevention. (2010). *WISQARS leading causes of nonfatal injury reports.* National Center for Injury Prevention and Control. Retrieved from http://webappa.cdc.gov/sasweb/ncipc/nfilead.html

Centers for Disease Control and Prevention. (2012). *National Action Plan for Child Injury Prevention.* Atlanta, GA: Centers for Disease Control and Prevention, National Center for Injury Prevention and Control.

Centers for Disease Control and Prevention (2015). *Heads up.* Centers for Disease Control and Prevention. Retrieved from https://www.cdc.gov/headsup/providers/discharge-materials.html

Chandran, A., Herbert, H., Misurski, D., & Santosham, M. (2011). Long-term sequelae of childhood bacterial meningitis: an underappreciated problem. *Pediatric Infectious Disease Journal, 30*(1), 3–6.

Chang, B. S., Lowenstein, D. H., & Quality Standards Subcommittee of the American Academy of Neurology. (2003). Practice parameter: Antiepileptic drug prophylaxis in severe traumatic brain injury: Report of the quality standards subcommittee of the American Academy of Neurology. *Neurology, 60*(1), 10–16.

Chapman, S. B. (2007). Neurocognitive stall: A paradox in long term recovery from pediatric brain injury. *Brain Injury Professional, 3*(4), 10–13.

Choudhary, A. K., Ishak, R., Zacharia, T. T., & Dias, M. S. (2014). Imaging of spinal injury in abusive head trauma: a retrospective study. *Pediatric Radiology, 44*(9), 1130–1140.

Christensen, J., Pedersen, M. G., Pedersen, C. B., Sidenius, P., Olsen, J., & Vestergaard, M. (2009). Long-term risk of epilepsy after traumatic brain injury in children and young adults: A population-based cohort study. *Lancet, 373,* 1105–1110.

Christophe, C., Fonteyne, C., Ziereisen, F., Christiaens, F., Deltenre, P., De Maertelaer, V., & Dan, B. (2002). Value of MR imaging of the brain in children with hypoxic coma. *American Journal of Neuroradiology, 23*(4), 716–723.

Chung, C. Y., Chen, C. L., Cheng, P. T., See, L. C., Tang, S. F., & Wong, A. M. (2006). Critical score of Glasgow Coma Scale for pediatric traumatic brain injury. *Pediatric Neurology, 34*(5), 379–387.

Clemenzi, A., Formisano, R., Matteis, M., Gallinacci, L., Cochi, G., Savina, P., & Cicinelli, P. (2012). Care management of spasticity with botulinum toxin-A in patients with severe acquired brain injury: A 1 year follow-up prospective study. *Brain Injury, 26*(7–8), 979–983.

Cockerham, G. C., Goodrich, G. L., Weichel, E. D., Orcutt, J. C., Rizzo, J. F., Bower, K. S., & Schuchard, R. A. (2009). Eye and visual function in traumatic brain injury. *Journal of Rehabilitation Research & Development, 46*(6), 811–818.

Cook, A. M., Peppard, A., & Magnuson, B. (2008). Nutrition considerations in traumatic brain injury. *American Society for Parenteral and Enteral Nutrition, 26*(6), 608–620.

Cooper, A. N., Anderson, V., Greenham, M., Hearps, S., Hunt, R. W., Mackay, M. T., . . . Gordon, A. L. (2018). Motor function daily living skills 5 years after paediatric arterial ischaemic stroke: A prospective longitudinal study. *Developmental Medicine and Child Neurology,* Advance online publication. doi:10.1111/dmcn.13915.

Cooper, A. N., Anderson, V., Hearps, S., Greenham, M., Ditchfield, M., Coleman, L., . . . Gordon, A. L. (2017). Trajectories of motor recovery in the first year after pediatric arterial ischemic stroke. *Pediatrics, 40*(2), pii: e20163870

Cope, N. D. (1995). The effectiveness of traumatic brain injury rehabilitation: A review. *Brain Injury, 9*(7), 649–670.

Corwin, D. J., Zonfrillo, M. R., Master, C. L., Arbogast, K. B., Grady, M. F., Robinson, R. L., . . . Wiebe, D. J. (2014). Characteristics of prolonged concussion recovery in a pediatric subspecialty referral population. *Journal of Pediatrics, 165*(6), 1207–1215.

Crowe, L. M., Anderson, V., Barton, S., Babl, F. E., & Catroppa, C. (2014). Verbal ability and language outcome following traumatic brain injury in early childhood. *Journal of Head Trauma Rehabilitation, 29*(3), 217–223.

Crowe, L. M., Catroppa, C., Babl, F. E., Rosenfeld, J. V., & Anderson, V. (2012). Timing of traumatic brain injury in childhood and intellectual outcome. *Journal of Pediatric Psychology, 37*(7), 745–754.

Davis, G. A., Purcell, L., Schneider, K. J., Yeates, K. O., Gioia, G. A., Anderson, V., . . . Kutcher, J. S. (2017). The Child Sport Concussion Assessment Tool 5th Edition (Child SCAT5): Background and rationale. *British Journal of Sports Medicine, 51*(11), 859–861.

Davis, K. C., Slomine, B. S., Salorio, C. F., & Suskauer, S. J. (2016). Time to follow commands and duration of posttraumatic amnesia predict GOS-E peds scores 1 to 2 years after TBI in children requiring inpatient rehabilitation. *Journal of Head Trauma and Rehabilitation, 31*(2), E39–E47.

Dahlberg, C. A., Cusick, C. P., Hawley, L. A., Newman, J. K., Morey, C. E., Harrison-Felix, C. L., & Whiteneck, G. G. (2007). Treatment efficacy of social communication skills training after traumatic brain injury: A randomized treatment and deferred treatment controlled trial. *Archives of Physical Medicine and Rehabilitation, 88*(12), 1561–1573.

Deepika, A., Mathew, M. J., Kumar, S. A., Devi, B. I., & Shukla, D. (2015). Paroxysmal sympathetic hyperactivity in pediatric traumatic brain injury: A case series of four patients. *Autonomic Neuroscience: Basic and Clinical, 193,* 149–151.

Del Castillo, J., López-Herce, J., Cañadas, S., Matamoros, M., Rodríguez-Núnez, A., Rodríguez-Calvo, A., . . . Iberoamerican Pediatric Cardiac Arrest Study Network (RIBEPCI). (2014). Cardiac arrest and resuscitation in the pediatric intensive care unit: A prospective multicenter multinational study. *Resuscitation, 85*(10), 1380–1386.

Dellinger, A. M., & Kresnow, M. (2010). Bicycle helmet use among children in the United States: The effects of legislation, personal and household factors. *Journal of Safety Research, 41,* 375–380.

DeLuca, S. C., Trucks, M. R., Wallace, D. A., & Ramey, S. L. (2017). Practice-based evidence from a clinical cohort that received pediatric constraint-induced movement therapy. *Journal of Pediatric Rehabilitation Medicine, 10*(1), 37–46.

Dettmer, J., Ettel, D., Glang, A., & McAvoy, K. (2014). Building a statewide infrastructure for effective educational services for students with TBI: Promising practices and recommendations. *Journal of Head Trauma & Rehabilitation, 29*(3), 224–232.

Dikmen, S. S., Corrigan, J. D., Levin, H. S., Machamer, J., Stiers, W., & Weisskopf, M. G. (2009). Cognitive outcome following traumatic brain injury. *Journal of Head Trauma Rehabilitation, 24*(6), 430–438.

Durbin, D. R., & Committee on Injury, Violence, and Poison Prevention. (2011). Child passenger safety. *Pediatrics, 127*(4), 788–793. Reaffirmed November 2014.

Elliott, M. R., Kallan, M. J., Durbin, D. R., & Winston, F. K. (2006). Effectiveness of child safety seats vs. seat belts in reducing risk for death in children in passenger vehicle crashes. *Archives of Pediatrics & Adolescent Medicine, 160*(6), 617–621.

Emami, P., Czorlich, P., Fritzsche, F. S., Westphal, M., Rueger, J. M., Lefering, R., & Hoffmann, M. (2017). Impact of Glasgow Coma Scale score and pupil parameters on mortality rate and outcome in pediatric and adult severe traumatic brain injury: A retrospective, multicenter cohort study. *Journal of Neurosurgery, 126*(3), 760–767.

Emanuelson, I., & Uverbrant, P. (2009). Occurrence of epilepsy during the first 10 years after traumatic brain injury acquired in childhood up to the age of 18 years in the south western Sweden population-based series. *Brain Injury, 23*(7), 612–616.

Emery, C. A., Black, A. M., Kolstad, A., Martinez, G., Nettel-Aguirre, A., Engebretsen, L., . . . Schneider, K. (2017). What strategies can be used to effectively reduce the risk of concussion in sport? A systematic review. *British Journal of Sports Medicine, 51*(12), 978–984.

Ewing-Cobbs, L., Levin, H. S., Fletcher, J. M., Miner, M. D., & Eisenberg, H. M. (1990). The Children's Orientation and Amnesia Test: Relationship to severity of acute head injury and to recovery of memory. *Neurosurgery, 27*(5), 683–691.

Faul, M., Xu, L., Wald, M. M., & Coronado, V. G. (2010). *Traumatic brain injury in the United States: emergency department visits, hospitalizations, and deaths.* Atlanta, GA: Centers for Disease Control and Prevention, National Center for Injury Prevention and Control.

Felling, R. J., Sun, L. R., Maxwell, E. C., Goldenberg, N., & Bernard, T. (2017). Pediatric arterial ischemic stroke: epidemiology, risk factors, and management. *Blood Cells, Molecules, and Diseases, 67,* 23–33.

Felton, H., Myers, J., Liu, G., & Davis, D. W. (2015). Unintentional, non-fatal drowning of children: US trends and racial/ethnic disparities. *BMJ Open, 5*(12), 008444.

Ferguson, M., Sarnaik, A., Miles, D., Shafi, N., Peters, M. J., Truemper, E., . . . Investigators of the Approaches and Decisions in Acute Pediatric Traumatic Brain Injury (ADAPT) Trial. (2017). Abusive head trauma and mortality: An analysis from an international comparative effectiveness study of children with severe traumatic brain injury. *Critical Care Medicine, 45*(8), 1398–1407.

Forrest, A., Butt, W. W., & Namachivayam, S. P. (2017). Outcomes of children admitted to intensive care after out-of-hospital cardiac arrest in Victoria, Australia. *Critical Care & Resuscitation Journal, 19*(2), 150–158.

Fullerton, H. J., deVeber, G. A., Hills, N. K., Dowling, M. M., Fox, C. K., Mackay, M. T., . . . VIPS Investigators. (2016). Inflammatory biomarkers in childhood arterial ischemic stroke: Correlates of stroke cause and recurrence. *Stroke, 47*(9), 2221–2228.

Fyrberg, A., Horneman, G., Asberg Johnels, J., Thunberg, G., & Ahlsen, E. (2017). Communication in children and adolescents after acquired brain injury: An exploratory study. *Journal of Rehabilitation Medicine, 49*(7), 572–578.

Fyrberg, A., Marchioni, M., & Emanuelson, I. (2007). Severe acquired brain injury: Rehabilitation of communicative skills in children and adolescents. *International Journal of Rehabilitation Research, 30,* 153–157.

Gan, C., & Schuller, R. (2002). Family system outcome following acquired brain injury: Clinical and research perspectives. *Brain Injury, 16*(4), 311–322.

Giza, C. C., Kolb, B., Harris, N. G., Asarnow, R. F., & Prins, M. L. (2009). Hitting a moving target: Basic mechanisms of recovery from acquired developmental brain injury. *Developmental Neurorehabilitation, 12*(5), 255–268.

Giza, C. C., & Hovda, D. A. (2014). The new neurometabolic cascade of concussion. *Neurosurgery, 75*(Suppl. 4), S24–S33.

Glang, A., Todis, B., Sublette, P., Brown, B. E., & Vaccaro, M. (2010). Professional development in TBI for educators: The importance of context. *Journal of Head Trauma & Rehabilitation, 25*(6), 426–432.

Glang, A., Todis, B., Thomas, C. W., Hood, D., Bedell, G., & Cockrell, J. (2008). Return to school following childhood TBI: Who gets services? *NeuroRehabilitation, 23*(6), 477–486.

Goldberg, E. M., Titulaer, M., de Blank, P. M., Sievert, A., & Ryan, N. (2014). Anti-N-methyl-D-aspartate receptor mediated encephalitis in infants and toddlers: Case report and review of the literature. *Pediatric Neurology, 50,* 181–184.

Gorman, S., Barnes, M. A., Swank, P. R., & Ewing-Cobbs, L. (2017). Recovery of working memory following pediatric traumatic brain injury: A longitudinal analysis. *Developmental Neuropsychology, 42*(3), 127–145.

Gumer, L. B., Del Vecchio, M., & Aronoff, S. (2014). Strokes in children: A systematic review. *Pediatric Emergency Care, 30*(9), 660–664.

Halstead, M. E., McAvoy, K., Devore, C. D., Carl, R., Lee, M., Logan, K., Council on Sports Medicine and Fitness, & Council on School Health. (2013). Returning to learning following a concussion. *Pediatrics, 132*(5), 948–957.

Hawley, C. A., Ward, A. B., Magnay, A. R., & Mychalkiw, W. (2004). Return to school after brain injury. *Archives of Disease in Childhood, 89,* 136–142.

Hotz, F., de Marcilla, A. G., Lutfi, K., Kennedy, A., Castellon, P., & Duncan, R. (2009). The WalkSafe program: Developing and evaluating the educational component. *The Journal of Trauma Injury, Infection and Critical Care, 66*(Suppl. 3), S3–S9.

Huang, B. Y., & Castillo, M. (2008). Hypoxic-ischemic brain injury: Imaging findings from birth to adulthood. *Radiographics, 28*, 417–439.

Hymel, K. P., Makoroff, K. L., Laskey, A. L., Conaway, M. R., & Blackman, J. A. (2007). Mechanisms, clinical presentations, injuries, and outcomes from inflicted versus noninflicted head trauma during infancy: Results of a prospective, multicentered, comparative study. *Pediatrics, 119*, 922–929.

Individuals with Disabilities Education Improvement Act (IDEA) of 2004, 20 U.S.C. §§ 1400 *et seq.*

Jagodzinski, T., & DeMuri, G. P. (2005). Horse–related injuries in children: A review. *Wisconsin Medical Journal, 104*(2), 50–54.

Jordan, L. C., & Hillis, A. E. (2011). Challenges in the diagnosis and treatment of pediatric stroke. *Nature Reviews: Neurology, 7*(4), 199–208.

Kadom, N., Khademian, Z., Vezina, G., Shalaby-Rana, E., Rice, A., & Hinds, T. (2014). Usefulness of MRI detection of cervical spine and brain injuries in the evaluation of abusive head trauma. *Pediatric Radiology, 44*(7), 839–848.

Kapapa, T., Pfister, U., König, K., Sasse, M., Woischneck, D., Heissler, H. E., & Rickels, E. (2010). Head trauma in children, Part 3: Clinical and psychosocial outcome after head trauma in children. *Journal of Child Neurology, 25*(4), 409–422.

Keenan, H. T., & Bratton, S. L. (2006). Epidemiology and outcomes of pediatric traumatic brain injury. *Developmental Neuroscience, 28*, 256–263.

Kenney-Jung, D. L., Vezzani, A., Kahoud, R. J., LaFrance-Corey, R. G., Ho, M. L., Muskardin, T. W., . . . Payne, E. T. (2016). Febrile infection-related epilepsy syndrome treated with anakinra. *Annals of Neurology, 80*(6), 939–945.

Khandaker, G., Jung, J., Britton, P. N., King, C., Yin, J. K., & Jones, C. A. (2016). Long-term outcomes of infective encephalitis in children: A systematic review and meta-analysis. *Developmental Medicine & Child Neurology, 58*(11), 1108–1115.

Kirk, K. A., Shoykhet, M., Jeong, J. H., Tyler-Kabara, E. C., Henderson, M. J., Bell, M. J., & Fink, E. L. (2012). Dysautonomia after pediatric brain injury. *Developmental Medicine & Child Neurology, 54*(8), 759–764.

Kirton, A., & deVeber, G. (2015). Paediatric stroke: Pressing issues and promising directions. *Lancet Neurology, 14*(1), 92–102.

Kochanek, P. M., Carney, N., Adelson, P. D., Ashwal, S., Bell, M. J., Bratton, S., . . . World Federation of Pediatric Intensive and Critical Care Societies. (2012). Guidelines for the acute medical management of severe traumatic brain injury in infants, children, and adolescents—Second edition. *Pediatric Critical Care Medicine, 13*(Suppl. 1), S1–S82.

Kowalsky, R. H., & Jaffe, D. M. (2013). Bacterial meningitis post-PCV7: Declining incidence and treatment. *Pediatric Emergency Care, 29*(6), 758–766.

Kuhtz-Buschbeck, J. P., Hoppe, B., Gölge, M., Dreesmann, M., Damm-Stünitz, U., & Ritz, A. (2003). Sensorimotor recovery in children after traumatic brain injury: Analyses of gait, gross motor, and fine motor skills. *Developmental Medicine and Child Neurology, 45*(12), 821–828.

Kuppermann, N., Holmes, J. F., Dayan, P. S., Hoyle, J. D., Jr., Atabaki, S. M., Holubkov, R., . . . Pediatric Emergency Care Applied Research Network (2009). Identification of children at very low risk of clinically-important brain injuries after head trauma: A prospective cohort study. *The Lancet, 374*(9696), 1160–1170.

Laosse, O. C., Gilchrist, J., & Rudd, R. A. (2012). Drowning–United States 2005-2009. *Morbidity and Mortality Weekly Report, 61*(19), 344–347.

Langlois, J. A., Rutland-Brown, W., & Wald, M. M. (2006). The epidemiology and impact of traumatic brain injury: A brief overview. *Journal of Head Trauma Rehabilitation, 21*(5), 375–378.

Lee, B. H., Schofer, J. L., & Koppelman, F. S. (2005). Bicycle safety helmet legislation and bicycle-related non-fatal injuries in California. *Accident Analysis and Prevention, 37*(1), 93–102.

Lieh-Lai, M. W., Theodorou, A. A., Sarnaik, A. P., Meert, K. L., Moylan, P. M., & Canady, A. I. (1992). Limitations of the Glasgow Coma Scale in predicting outcome in children with traumatic brain injury. *Journal of Pediatrics, 120*, 195–199.

Letson, M. M., Cooper, J. N., Deans, K. J., Scribano, P. V., Makoroff, K. L., Feldman, K. W., & Berger, R. P. (2016). Prior opportunities to identify abuse in children with abusive head trauma. *Child Abuse and Neglect, 60*, 36–45.

Levene, S., & Bonfield, G. (1991). Accidents on hospital wards. *Archives of Disease in Childhood, 66*, 1047–109.

Lew, H. L., Jerger, J. F., Guillory, S. B., & Henry, J. A. (2007). Auditory dysfunction in traumatic brain injury. *Journal of Rehabilitation Research & Development, 44*(7), 921–928.

Lew, H. L., Lee, E. H., Miyoshi, Y., Chang, D. G., Date, E. S., & Jerger, J. F. (2004). Brainstem auditory-evoked potentials as an objective tool for evaluating hearing dysfunction in traumatic brain injury. *American Journal of Physical Medicine & Rehabilitation, 83*(3), 210–215.

Liesemer, K., Bratton, S. L., Zebrack, M., Brockmeyer, D., & Statler, K. D. (2011). Early post-traumatic seizures in moderate to severe pediatric traumatic brain injury: Rates, risk factors, and clinical features. *Journal of Neurotrauma, 28*, 755–762.

Linden, M. A., Braiden, H. J., & Miller, S. (2013). Educational professionals' understanding of childhood traumatic brain injury. *Brain Injury, 27*(1), 92–102.

Lyons, T. J., & Oates, R. K. (1993). Falling out of bed: A relatively benign occurrence. *Pediatrics, 92*, 125–127.

Mattei, T. A., Bond, B. J., Goulant, C. R., Sloffer, C. A., Morris, M. J., & Lin, J. J. (2012). Performance analysis of the protective effects of bicycle helmets during impact and crush tests in pediatric skull models. *Journal of Neurosurgery Pediatrics, 10*(6), 490–497.

May, K. H., Marshall, D. L., Burns, T. G., Popoli, D. M., & Polikandriotis, J. A. (2014). Pediatric sports specific return to play guidelines following concussion. *International Journal of Sports Physical Therapy, 9*(2), 242–255.

McCrory, P., Davis, G., & Makdissi, M. (2012). Second impact syndrome or cerebral swelling after sporting head injury. *Current Sports Medicine Reports, 11*(1), 21–23.

McCrory, P., Meeuwisse, W., Dvořák, J., Aubry, M., Bailes, J., Broglio, S., . . . Vos, P. E. (2017). Consensus statement on concussion in sport—The 5th international conference on concussion in sport held in Berlin, October 2016. *British Journal of Sports Medicine, 51*(11), 838–847.

McLendon, L. A., Kralik, S. F., Grayson, P. A., & Golomb, M. R. (2016). The controversial second impact syndrome: A review of the literature. *Pediatric Neurology, 62*, 9–17.

McNally, K. A., Patrick, K. E., LaFleur, J. E., Dykstra, J. B., Monahan, K., & Hoskinson, K. R. (2018). Brief cognitive behavioral intervention for children and adolescents with persistent post-concussive symptoms: A pilot study. *Clinical Neuropsychology, 24*(3), 396–412.

Meekes, J., Jennekens-Schinkel, A., & van Schooneveld, M. M. (2006). Recovery after childhood traumatic injury: Vulnerability and plasticity. *Pediatrics, 117*(6), 2330.

Meholjic-Fetahovic, A. (2007). Treatment of the spasticity in children with cerebral palsy. *Bosnia Journal of Basic Science, 7*(4), 363–367.

Mendelson, K. G., & Fallat, M. E. (2007). Pediatric injuries: Prevention to resolution. *Surgical Clinics of North America, 87,* 207–228.

Moon, R. Y., & Task Force on Sudden Infant Death Syndrome. (2016). SIDS and other sleep-related infant deaths: Evidence base of 2016 updated recommendations for a safe infant sleeping environment. *Pediatrics, 138*(5), pii: e20162940

Morgan, A. T. (2010). Dysphagia in childhood traumatic brain injury: A reflection on the evidence and its implications for practice. *Developmental Neurorehabilitation, 13*(3), 192–203.

Morgan, A. T., Mageandran, S. D., & Mei, C. (2010). Incidence and clinical presentation of dysarthria and dysphagia in the acute setting following paediatric traumatic brain injury. *Child: Care, Health, and Development, 36*(1), 44–53.

Munjal, S. K., Panda, N. K., & Pathak, A. (2010). Audiological deficits after closed head injury. *The Journal of Trauma, 68,* 13–18.

Natale, J. E., Joseph, J. G., Helfaer, M. A., & Shaffner, D. H. (2000). Early hyperthermia after traumatic brain injury in children: risk factors, influence on length of stay, and effect on short-term neurological status. *Critical Care Medicine, 28*(7), 2608–2615.

Niederkrotenthaler, T., Xu, L., Parks, S. E., & Sugerman, D. E. (2013). Descriptive factors of abusive head trauma in young children—United States, 2000-2009. *Child Abuse & Neglect, 37*(7), 446–455.

Olympia, R. P., Ritter, J. T., Brady, J., & Bramley, H. (2016). Return to learning after a concussion and compliance with recommendations for cognitive rest. *Clinical Journal of Sports Medicine, 26*(2), 115–119.

O'Lynnger, T. M., Shannon, C. N., Le, T. M., Greeno, A., Chung, D., Lamb, F. S., & Wellons, J. C. (2016). Standardizing ICU management of pediatric traumatic brain injury is associated with improved outcomes at discharge. *Journal of Neurosurgery: Pediatrics, 17*(1), 19–26.

O'Neill, B. R., Handler, M. H., Tong, S., & Chapman, K. E. (2015). Incidence of seizures on continuous EEG monitoring following traumatic brain injury in children. *Journal of Neurosurgery: Pediatrics, 16*(2), 167–176.

Park, J. T., & Chugani, H. T. (2015). Post-traumatic epilepsy in children—experience from a tertial referral center. *Pediatric Neurology, 52*(2), 174–181.

Park, J. T., & Chugani, H. T. (2017). Epileptic spasms in paediatric post-traumatic epilepsy at a tertiary referral centre. *Epileptic Disorders, 19*(1), 24–34.

Pozzi, M., Conti, V., Locatelli, F., Galbiati, S., Radice, S., Citerio, G., Clementi, E., & Strazzer, S. (2014). Paroxysmal sympathetic hyperactivity in pediatric rehabilitation: Clinical factors and acute pharmacological management. *Journal of Head Trauma Rehabilitation, 30*(5), 357–363.

Rashid, M., Goez, H. R., Mabood, N., Damanhoury, S., Yager, J. Y., Joyce, A. S., & Newton, A. S. (2014). The impact of pediatric traumatic brain injury (TBI) on family functioning: A systematic review. *Journal of Pediatric Rehabilitation Medicine, 73*(3), 241–254.

Rehabilitation Act of 1973, 29 U.S.C. §§ 701 *et seq.*

Riggio, S., & Wong, M. (2009). Neurobehavioral sequelae of traumatic brain injury. *Mount Sinai Journal of Medicine, 76,* 163–172.

Risen, S. R., Reesman, J., Yenokyan, G., Slomine, B. S., & Suskauer, S. J. (2017). The course of concussion recovery in children 6-12 years of age: Experience from an interdisciplinary rehabilitation clinic. *Physical Medicine & Rehabilitation, 9*(9), 874–883.

Risen, S. R., Suskauer, S. J., Dematt, E. J., Slomine, B. S., & Salorio, C. F. (2014). Functional outcomes in children with abusive head trauma receiving inpatient rehabilitation compared with children with nonabusive head trauma. *Journal of Pediatrics, 164*(3), 613–619.

Roach, E. S., Golomb, M. R., Adams, R., Biller, J., Daniels, S., Deveber, G., . . . Council on Cardiovascular Disease in the Young. (2008). Management of stroke in infants and children: A scientific statement from a special writing group of the American Heart Association stroke council and the council on cardiovascular disease in the young. *Stroke, 39*(9), 2644–2691.

Rodenburg-Vlot, M. B., Ruytjens, L., Oostenbrink, R., Goedegebure, A., & van der Schroeff, M. P. (2016). Systematic review: Incidence and course of hearing loss caused by bacterial meningitis: in search of an optimal timed audiological follow-up. *Otology & Neurotology, 37*(1), 1–8.

Savage, R. C., DePompei, R., Tyler, J., & Lash, M. (2005). Paediatric traumatic brain injury: A review of pertinent issues. *Pediatric Rehabilitation, 8*(2), 92–103.

Scheers, N. J., Rutherford, G. W., & Kemp, J. S. (2003). Where should infants sleep? A comparison of risk for suffocation of infants sleeping in cribs, adult beds, and other sleeping locations. *Pediatrics, 112*(4):883–889.

Schnitzer, P. G. (2006). Prevention of unintentional childhood injuries. *American Family Physician, 74,* 1864–1869.

Schwebel, D. C., & McClure, L. A. (2010). Using virtual reality to train children in safe street-crossing skills. *Injury Prevention, 16,* e1–e5.

Shanahan, M. E., Zolotor, A. J., Parrish, J. W., Barr, R. G., & Runyan, D. K. (2013). National, regional, and state abusive head trauma: Application of the CDC algorithm. *Pediatrics, 132*(6), e1546–e1553.

Sheftall, A. H., Asti, L., Horowitz, L. M., Felts, A., Fontanella, C. A., Campo, J. V., & Bridge, J. A. (2016). Suicide in elementary school-aged children and early adolescents. *Pediatrics, 138*(4), pii: e20160436

Sroufe, N. S., Fuller, D. S., West, B. T., Singal, B. M., Warschausky, S. A., & Maio, R. F. (2010). Postconcussive symptoms and neurocognitive function after mild traumatic brain injury in children. *Pediatrics, 125*(6), e1331–e1339.

Stancin, T., Wade, S. L., Walz, N. C., Yeates, K. O., & Taylor, H. G. (2008). Traumatic brain injuries in early childhood: Initial impact on the family. *Developmental and Behavioral Pediatrics, 29*(4), 253–261.

Statler, K. D. (2006). Pediatric posttraumatic seizures: Epidemiology, putative mechanisms of epileptogenesis and promising investigational progress. *Developmental Neuroscience, 28*(4–5), 354–363.

Suominen, P. K., Sutinen, N., Valle, S., Olkkola, K. T., & Lönnqvist, T. (2014). Neurocognitive long-term follow-up study on drowned children. *Resuscitation, 85*(8), 1059–1064.

Taylor, C. A., Bell, J. M., Breiding, M. J., & Xu, L. (2017). Traumatic brain injury–related emergency department visits, hospitalizations, and deaths—United States, 2007 and 2013. *MMWR Surveillance Summary, 66*(SS-9), 1–16.

Taylor, H. G., Yeates, K. O., Wade, S. L., Drotar, D., Klein, S. K., & Stancin, T. (1999). Influences on first-year recovery from traumatic brain injury in children. *Neuropsychology, 13*(1), 76–89.

Teasdale, G. (2014). *Glascow Coma Scale*. Retrieved from http://www.glasgowcomascale.org

Teasdale, G., & Jennett, B. (1974). Assessment of coma and impaired consciousness: A practical scale. *The Lancet, 2*, 81–84.

Thaler, N. S., Reger, S. L., Ringdahl, E. N., Mayfield, J. W., Goldstein, G., & Allen, D. N. (2013). Neuropsychological profiles of six children with anoxic brain injury. *Child Neuropsychology, 19*(5), 479–494.

Thomas, D. G., Apps, J. N., Hoffmann, R. G., McCrea, M., & Hammeke, T. (2015). Benefits of strict rest after acute concussion: A randomized controlled trial. *Pediatrics, 135*(2), 213–223.

Thompson, D. C., & Rivara, F. P. (2000). Pool fencing for preventing drowning in children. *Cochrane Database Systematic Review, 2*, CD001047.

Thompson, D. C., Rivara, F. P., & Thompson, R. (1999). Helmets for preventing head and facial injuries in bicyclists. *Cochrane Database of Systematic Reviews, 4*, CD001855.

Titulauer, M. J., McCracken, L., Gabilondo, I., Armangué, T., Glaser, C., Iizuka, T., . . . Dalmau, J. (2013). Treatment and prognostic factors for long-term outcome in patients with anti-NMDA receptor encephalitis: an observational cohort study. *Lancet Neurology, 12*, 157–165.

Vavilala, M. S., Bowen, A., Lam, A. M., Uffman, J. C., Powell, J., Winn, H. R., & Rivara, F. P. (2003). Blood pressure and outcome after severe pediatric traumatic brain injury. *Journal of Trauma*, 55(6), 1039–1044.

Vavilala, M. S., Kernic, M. A., Wang, J., Kannan, N., Mink, R. B., Wainwright, M. S., . . . Pediatric Guideline Adherence and Outcomes Study. (2014). Acute care clinical indicators associated with discharge outcomes in children with severe traumatic brain injury. *Critical Care Medicine, 42*(10), 2258–2266.

Vavilala, M. S., Lujan, S. B., Qiu, Q., Bell, M. J., Ballarini, N. M., Guadagnoli, N., . . . Petroni, G. J. (2017). Intensive care treatments associated with favorable discharge outcomes in Argentine children with severe traumatic brain injury. *PLoS One, 12*(12), e0189296.

Venkatesan, A., Tunkel, A. R., Bloch, K. C., Lauring, A. S., Sejvar, J., Bitnun, A., . . . International Encephalitis Consortium. (2013). Case definitions, diagnostic algorithms, and priorities in encephalitis: consensus statement of the international encephalitis consortium. *Clinical Infectious Disease, 57*(8), 1114–1128.

Wade, S. L., Walz, N. C., Cassedy, A., Taylor, H. G., Stancin, T., & Yeates, K. O. (2010). Caregiver functioning following early childhood TBI: Do moms and dads respond differently? *NeuroRehabilitation, 27*(1), 63–72.

White, M. L., Zhang, Y., Helvey, J. T., & Omojola, M. F. (2013). Anatomical patterns and correlated MRI findings of non-perinatal hypoxic-ischemic encephalopathy. *British Journal of Radiology, 86*(1021), 20120464.

Williams, A. F., & Ferguson, S. A. (2002). Rationale for graduated licensing and the risks it should address. *Injury Prevention, 8*(Suppl. 2), ii9–ii14.

Wilson, J. T., Teasdale, G. M., Hadley, D. M., Wiedmann, K. D., & Lang, D. (1994). Post-traumatic amnesia: Still a valuable yardstick. *Journal of Neurology, Neurosurgery, and Psychiatry, 57*(2), 198–201.

Yard, E. E., & Comstock, R. D. (2009). Compliance with return to play guidelines following concussion in US high school athletes, 2005-2008. *Brain Injury, 23*(11), 888–898.

Ylvisaker, M., Adelson, P. D., Braga, L. W., Burnett, S. M., Glang, A., Feeney, T., . . . Todis, B. (2005). Rehabilitation and ongoing support after pediatric TBI: Twenty years of progress. *Journal of Head Trauma Rehabilitation, 20*(1), 95–109.

Ylvisaker, M., & Feeney, T. (2007). Pediatric brain injury: Social, behavioral, and communication disability. *Physical Medicine and Rehabilitation Clinics of North America, 18*(1), 133–144.

Young, A. M. H., Adams, H., Donnelly, J., Guilfoyle, M. R., Fernandes, H., Garnett, M. R., . . . Hutchinson, P. J. (2017). Glycemia is related to impaired cerebrovascular autoregulation after severe pediatric traumatic brain injury: A retrospective observational study. *Frontiers in Pediatrics, 5*, 205.

Zaloshnja, E., Miller, T. R., & Hendrie, D. (2007). Effectiveness of child safety seats vs. safety belts for children aged 2 to 3 years. *Archives of Pediatrics & Adolescent Medicine, 161*(1), 65–68.

CHAPTER 24

Developmental Disability in Chronic Disease

Nancy J. Roizen and Catherine Scherer

Upon completion of this chapter, the reader will

- Identify developmental disabilities commonly encountered in children with chronic diseases
- Be aware of the biologic factors that contribute to developmental issues in sickle cell disease
- Know the importance of critical congenital heart disease
- Be aware that children with congenital heart disease associated with a genetic syndrome have lower developmental function
- Note the greater degree of developmental problems in the children with end-stage renal disease compared with mild to moderate chronic kidney disease
- Understand the goal of cancer treatment to maximize chances for survival and minimize the impact on long-term cognitive development

In the United States, the epidemiology of many childhood health conditions has shifted from acute to chronic illnesses, with as many as one in three children living with a chronic health condition (Compas, Jaser, Reeslund, Patel, & Yarboi, 2017). Studies show that various chronic health conditions share deficits in cognition for overall intelligence, verbal and nonverbal intelligence, and aspects of executive function (Compas et al., 2017). The pediatric self-report scales of the Patient-Reported Outcomes Measurement Information System (PROMIS), a program of the National Institute of Health developed to improve patient self-report of chronic disease outcomes, have been used to document outcomes in children with chronic disease, including those discussed in this chapter. PROMIS studies reveal that children with higher disease severity, as measured by disease-specific measures and recent hospitalizations, report worse outcomes (DeWalt et al., 2015).

This chapter describes five chronic diseases—sickle cell disease (SCD), congenital heart disease (CHD), chronic kidney disease (CKD), lymphocytic leukemia, and brain cancer—that all have documented increased risk of associated developmental disability. The goal of this chapter is to increase appreciation of these risks and to raise vigilance for and improve the management of developmental problems in children with chronic disease.

SICKLE CELL DISEASE

CASE STUDY

Kisha is a teenager with sickle cell disease (SCD), which was diagnosed by newborn screening. Throughout childhood, she received prophylactic penicillin, special immunizations, and routine well-child care as well as SCD-specific care. In general, her family has been able to manage the painful sickle crises at home, but once or twice a year she has been hospitalized to control more severe episodes. She began taking hydroxyurea (HU), and for the last 3 years she has not been hospitalized. As a child, she was monitored routinely for stroke risk using transcranial Doppler ultrasonography. She has had normal findings, placing her at low risk for stroke. Kisha will be graduating from high school this year and plans to attend college.

Thought Questions:

What are the ways that the medical problems of the chronic diseases described in this chapter impact the development of children? What are the ways that improvements in medical care have improved the functioning of children with these chronic diseases?

Overview

In the United States, sickle cell disease (SCD) occurs in 1 out of 500 African Americans and 1 out of 1,000 to 1,400 Hispanic Americans (National Institutes of Health: National Library of Medicine, 2018). SCD is an autosomal recessive disorder (see Chapter 1) that results in the production of an abnormal hemoglobin, called hemoglobin S (HbS). HbS is caused by a single point mutation in the beta-globin gene. Red blood cells that contain predominantly HbS become sickle shaped in low-oxygen environments, making them susceptible to **hemolysis** (excessive breakdown of red blood cells). Anemia is the result of this shortened red cell life span. In addition, the sickle-shaped red blood cells can cause blockage of the microvasculature, leading to acute and chronic tissue damage including stroke (Meier & Rampersad, 2017).

Diagnosis and Clinical Manifestations

All states now screen newborns for SCD (Meier & Rampersad, 2017). It is a complex, chronic disorder characterized by hemolysis and intermittent **vascular occlusion** (obstruction). This results in acute complications that can rapidly become life-threatening and chronic complications that can lead to damage to multiple body organs. Acute manifestations include bacterial **sepsis** (blood infection), recurrent vaso-occlusive pain crises (VOC), splenic sequestration (accumulation of blood cells in the spleen), aplastic crisis (shutting down of the bone marrow), acute chest syndrome (a pneumonia-like condition), and stroke. Long-term medical consequences of SCD include anemia, restrictive lung disease, pulmonary hypertension, **avascular necrosis** (destruction of bone from microvascular occlusion), and delay in physical growth and sexual maturation (Section on Hematology/Oncology & Committee on Genetics, 2002).

Neurological complications of SCD include headaches and strokes. Among affected children, about 10% will sustain overt strokes (Lopez-Vincent, Ortega-Gutierrez, Amlie-Lefond, & Torbey, 2010; Pegelow et al., 2002), and almost one quarter will have silent strokes before their 18th birthday (Pegelow et al., 2002). An **overt stroke** involves a **focal** (localized) neurologic deficit that lasts for more than 24 hours. It results from an occlusion of one of the cerebral circulation vessels (DeBaun & Vichinsky, 2007). In a **silent stroke,** there is evidence of a cerebral **infarction** (tissue death) on a magnetic resonance imaging (MRI) scan, but a focal neurological deficit will be absent on clinical examination (Ohene-Frempong et al., 1998).

Development and Behavior

Studies demonstrate contributions to deficits in developmental functioning from both biologic and social factors. Neurocognitive functioning through the first year of life, as measured by tests of infant development, generally falls within the typical range (Thompson, Gustafson, Bonner, & Ware, 2002). In infants and toddlers, socioeconomic status (SES) correlates with the cognitive subscales (Schatz, Finke, & Roberts, 2004), but SCD severity (as measured by hemoglobin level) does not correlate with Bayley Scales of Infant Development scores (Drazen, Abel, Gabir, Farmer, & King, 2016). One meta-analysis revealed that even children with no evidence of cerebral infarction had small but detectable decrements on IQ measures over time (4 to 5 points overall; Schatz, Finke, Kellett, & Kramer, 2002). Even among school-age children with SCD who had *not* sustained silent or overt strokes, those with greater cerebral gray matter volume (as measured by MRI) had higher IQs than those with less (Chen et al., 2009).

With regard to special academic services, 58% of children with SCD with silent cerebral infarctions were retained or required special education services, compared with 27% without cerebral infarctions and 6% of siblings without SCD (Schatz, Brown, Pascual, Hsu, & DeBaun, 2001). About one quarter to one third of children with SCD have some type of developmental disability, most frequently affecting the cognitive and academic domains (Schatz & McClellan, 2006).

Children with overt stroke have, on average, a 10- to 15-point drop in IQ scores from prestroke levels (Schatz & McClellan, 2006), while silent strokes impart a milder degree of cognitive impairment (Armstrong et al., 2013). Although cognitive patterns are not consistent across all studies, most show that measures of attention and **executive functioning** (cognitive tasks related to taking in, organizing, processing, and acting on information; see Chapter 13) are adversely affected, leading to an attention-deficit/hyperactivity disorder (ADHD) picture (Schatz & McClellan, 2006).

The impact of SCD on families is similar in many ways to the impact of other severe neurodevelopmental disabilities. Factors related to low SES, concerns about the social stigma, and recurrent, unpredictable medical complications contribute to high levels of family stress (Schatz & McClellan, 2006). Children with SCD who are 12–18 years of age are absent from school an average of 12% of the school year, and more than 35% miss at least a month of school (Schwartz, Radcliffe, & Barakat, 2009).

Behavior challenges in youth with SCD are also increased. Both externalizing behavior problems (e.g., aggression, oppositional defiant disorder, and conduct disorder) and internalizing behaviors (e.g., anxiety and depression) are increased, although children with higher baseline IQs have fewer difficulties (Bakri, Ismail, Elsedfy, Ami, & Ibrahim, 2014; Thompson et al, 2003). By contrast, a longitudinal study of social function revealed no significant differences in measures of friendship or social acceptance when compared with peers (Noll, Kiska, Reiter-Purtill, Gerhardt, & Vannatta, 2010).

Treatment

Early identification through newborn screening, the use of hydroxyurea (HU), and caregiver education on the first line of care have provided a major improvement in the care of children with most SCD genotypes. Penicillin prophylaxis prevents bacterial infections from birth and has dramatically decreased the risk of early death from bacterial sepsis (DeBaun & Vichinsky, 2007; Falletta et al., 1995). With the addition of pneumococcal vaccine, pneumococcal disease has decreased by 70%–90% (Meier & Rampersad, 2017).

HU, a once-daily oral medication, prevents the complications of SCD (see Box 24.1). The 2014 National Heart, Lung, and Blood Institute Evidence Based Management Guidelines for Sickle Cell Disease recommend that all infants 9 months of age and older with SCD be offered HU as a treatment regardless of the frequency or severity of disease (Yawn et al., 2014). Caregiver education has been associated with fewer hospitalizations (Shahine, Badr, Karam, & Abboud, 2015). Family education includes counseling regarding the urgency for prompt evaluation and treatment of febrile illnesses and the acute complications that can cause morbidity and mortality. Although not all children have access, a sickle cell clinic team can provide needed support (see Box 24.2).

Painful vaso-occlusive crises (VOCs) are the most common complaint of older children and adults. Management of VOCs requires a collaborative management plan between the family and the multidisciplinary medical team. Early in the course of managing this problem, comfort measures are used. This is followed by acetaminophen with codeine and short- or long-acting opioids or morphine derivatives. Severe pain episodes require hospitalization and the use of intravenous morphine. The estimated prevalence of opioid addiction in the overall (child and adult) sickle cell population is about 10%, similar to the addiction rate among most chronic pain sufferers in the United States (National Heart, Lung, and Blood Institute, 2017).

Any acute neurological symptoms, including hemiparesis (weakness on one side of the body), akathisia (restless movements), seizures, severe headache, cranial nerve palsy, stupor, or coma, require urgent evaluation for stroke. Strokes are treated acutely with 1) oxygen and blood transfusion therapy, which

BOX 24.1 EVIDENCE-BASED PRACTICE

Hydroxyurea and Sickle Cell Disease

Hydroxyurea (HU) is proving to be a beneficial disease-modifying therapy for sickle cell disease (SCD). HU medication increases HbG and decreases intraerythocytic (red blood cell) HbS concentration, which decreases sickling and hemolysis. In children, HU therapy has decreased vaso-occlusive crises, acute chest syndrome, and transfusions. Children treated with HU are able to spend less time in pain and in the hospital and are not exposed to the damaging side effects of multiple transfusions. In addition, in a large multicenter study, HU was found to have a strong safety profile, and the participants who were treated with HU had similar growth, development, and organ function as the control group (Meier & Rampersad, 2017).

BOX 24.2 INTERDISCIPLINARY CARE

The Sickle Cell Disease Team

The sickle cell disease team can vary, but it generally includes professionals in the following disciplines: pediatric hematology, genetics, nutrition, social work, school intervention specialist, and obstetrics/gynecology. The team also works closely with cardiology and neurology.

together decrease the percent of HbS in the blood by dilution, and 2) exchange transfusion, replacing abnormal blood cells with normal blood cells.

For children like Kisha, primary stroke prevention is key to improved outcomes. Regular screening using transcranial Doppler ultrasound (TCD) which assesses blood velocity in the **cervical** (neck) arteries, has been shown to decrease the incidence of overt stroke by 90% (Enninful-Eghan, Moore, Ichord, Smith-Whitley, & Kwiakowski, 2010). When low velocity is found on TCD, prevention of stroke is accomplished by blood transfusion therapy aimed at keeping the HbS concentration low, thereby decreasing sickling. Continuous transfusions, however, can cause an increased iron load, which is treated with chelation therapy. Studies show that treatment with HU is an acceptable alternative (Meier & Rampersad, 2017).

The only currently available cure for SCD is hematopoietic stem cell transplantation (HSCT). Transplants from matched sibling donors have an overall survival rate of more than 90%. Less than 20% of individuals with SCD have a matched sibling donor. As of 2017, individuals with SCD were being recruited for gene therapy and gene-editing trials (Meier & Rampersad, 2017).

Outcomes

With early identification and the use of disease-modifying therapies, the childhood mortality rate for SCD is close to that of the general population; however, life expectancy has not increased in the past 30 years, remaining at half that of the average American (Lanzkron, Carroll, & Haywood, 2013; Meier & Rampersad, 2017; Piel, Steinberg, & Rees, 2017).

Transfusions, HU, and HSCT presently are the mainstays of therapy. Most SCD centers are developing models to make the transition from pediatric to adult care more successful (see Box 24.2). Adolescents and young adults have increased emergency department visits for acute complications, increased readmission rates, and increased mortality around the time of care transition (Meier & Rampersad, 2017). Improvements in the transition process may translate into improved quality of life with increased life expectancy.

CONGENITAL HEART DISEASE

CASE STUDY

Jose is a 5-year-old boy who was diagnosed with tetralogy of Fallot at 8 days of age, when he presented to the emergency department in cardiogenic shock. He had not had any newborn screening with pulse oximetry because the facility where he was born did not routinely perform it. A temporary shunt procedure was performed in the first days of life, and a definitive repair of his heart condition was completed at 4 months of age. His postoperative course was complicated by a prolonged hospital stay of 3 weeks for respiratory issues as he was weaned from the ventilator. He has been followed by his cardiologist who has been monitoring his right ventricular function, and he recently had a cardiac catheterization because of poor exercise tolerance. He will be starting kindergarten with adapted physical education. His mother has been concerned about his ability to focus in preschool.

Overview

Congenital heart disease (CHD) is one of the most common birth defects. CHDs affect nearly 1% of all births per year in the United States (Best & Rankin, 2016). Gilboa et al. (2016) estimated that 1 million children and 1.4 million adults with CHD live in the United States. CHD includes a wide range of cardiac abnormalities of varying severity, with one out of four children born with CHD having a more severe defect, classified as critical CHD (CCHD). The term CCHD is used when the lesion either causes death or requires a surgical intervention in the newborn period. CHDs are the leading cause of death from birth defects in the first year of life (Patel & Burns, 2013).

Several CCHD lesions have been targeted in newborn screening, including the following:

- *Tetralogy of Fallot,* which involves a ventricular septal defect, an overriding aorta, and some degree of pulmonary stenosis that leads to right ventricle hypertrophy.
- *D-transposition of the great arteries (D-TGA),* in which the aorta is attached to the right side of the heart,

which delivers deoxygenated blood from the body back out to the body, and the pulmonary artery is attached to the left side of the heart, which delivers oxygenated blood from the lungs back to the lungs. (D-TGA is commonly thought of as two circuits of blood running in parallel, rather than the normal flow of blood with the two circuits running in series.)

- *Tricuspid atresia,* in which the tricuspid valve, which connects the right atrium to the right ventricle, does not form. As such, blood cannot flow between those two right heart chambers.
- *Coarctation of the aorta,* which is a severe narrowing of the aorta that makes it more difficult for oxygenated blood from the left side of the heart to circulate out to the body.
- *Total anomalous pulmonary venous return,* in which the pulmonary veins, which return the oxygenated blood from the lungs to the heart, abnormally deliver this blood to the right atrium instead of the left atrium (via abnormal connections or drainage patterns), which leads to mixing of deoxygenated blood returning to the heart with oxygenated blood returning from the lungs.
- *Truncus arteriosus,* which results from abnormal division of the pulmonary and aortic trunks in early fetal development, resulting in a single common outflow tract and valve (called the truncal valve) shared by both the right and left ventricles.
- *Hypoplastic left heart syndrome* (*HLHS;* Yabrodi & Mastropietro, 2016), in which the mitral valve and left ventricle are underdeveloped, resulting in severely limited or absent blood flow out of the left heart chambers and leading to the heart essentially having a single ventricle to pump blood to both the lungs and body. HLHS accounts for 4%–8% of cases of CHD (Benson, Martin, & Lo, 2016) but 23% of cardiac deaths.

Cardiac fetal development has a critical window from 2–7 weeks' gestation (Patel & Burns, 2013; see Chapter 6). The etiology of CHD is usually multifactorial, including both maternal risk factors and genetic abnormalities. Maternal risk factors include hyperglycemia associated with type 2 diabetes mellitus (DM) or gestational DM, obesity, maternal medications, tobacco use, illicit drug use, maternal infections, and environmental toxins (during the 3 months prior to conception through the first trimester). Of children with CHD, 35% have a genetic syndrome. Some of the common genetic syndromes (see Chapter 1 and Appendix B) associated with CHD include Down syndrome, **22q11 deletion syndrome, Noonan syndrome, Turner syndrome, Williams syndrome,** and **VACTERL.** The acronym VACTERL does not refer to an identified genetic cause, but it involves an association of findings that are similar in individuals with the condition, including **V**ertebral, **A**nal, and **C**ardiac defects (40%–80% of patients have CHDs of varying severity), **T**racheo**E**sophageal fistula, **R**enal (kidney) anomalies, and **L**imb abnormalities. Although about 30% of children with hypoplastic left heart syndrome have identified genetic syndromes, nonsyndromic HLHS is genetically variable in its pattern of inheritance (Benson et al., 2016).

Diagnosis and Clinical Manifestations

The initial diagnosis of CHD is established in the fetus via prenatal fetal echocardiograph and in the newborn period via physical examination, pulse oximetry (a noninvasive measure of oxygen saturation), and postnatal transthoracic echocardiography (see Chapter 6). A study by Oster and colleagues (2014) found that 58% of children with CCHD were identified prenatally versus only 20% of children with noncritical CHD. In 2011, the U.S. Health and Human Services Secretary's Advisory Committee on Heritable Disorders in Newborns and Children endorsed the American Academy of Pediatrics/American Heart Association 2009 recommendation to add pulse oximetry to the uniform newborn screening panel to identify CCHD.

A baby with a positive CCHD screen is then evaluated by a pediatric cardiologist with completion of four-extremity blood pressure measurements and then commonly an echocardiogram to further assess cardiac anatomy (Box 24.3). Despite the CCHD screen, some infants with CHD may still be missed, especially those with coarctation of the aorta (Lannering, Bartos, & Mellander, 2015). Infants may present with tachypnea, a concerning heart murmur, poor perfusion/cardiogenic shock, decreased lower extremity pulses, or a hyperactive precordium (front of chest; Lantin-Hermoso et al., 2017). Some experts recommend genetic testing for children with CHD, especially if there is 1) a positive family history of CHD, 2) comorbid congenital malformations, or 3) other significant comorbidities such as developmental disabilities (Marino et al., 2012; Simmons & Brueckner, 2017; Zaidi & Brueckner, 2017).

Development and Behavior

Neurodevelopmental disability is now determined to be "the most common long-term complication of critical CHD and has the most negative impact on quality of life, academic performance, and opportunity for independence as an adult" (Gaynor, 2014, p. 1790).

BOX 24.3 EVIDENCE-BASED PRACTICE

The Impact of Congenital Heart Disease Screening in Newborns

- As mentioned in the case study, Jose's critical congenital heart disease (CCHD) most likely would have been found prior to discharge if a pulse oximetry screening had been done after 24 hours of life, thereby preventing a life-threatening presentation to the emergency department.
- As of December 2017, 36 states have laws requiring newborn screening for CCHD and 12 states have regulations on CCHD.
- Sensitivity of screening for CHD with pulse oximetry ranges from 36%–92% depending on the cardiac defect. Specificity is high, with the percentage for false positives around 0.05%.
- States with mandatory CHD screening have had a 33.4% decrease in early infant deaths from critical congenital heart disease and a 21.4% decrease from other cardiac causes over a period of 6 years. States without screening have had no change in the number of infant deaths from CCHD (Abouk, Grosse, Ailes, & Oster, 2017).

Children with CHD have a 30%–50% risk for neurocognitive deficits including ADHD; deficits in executive function, social skills, motor planning, and visual memory; and difficulty with higher-order integration (Calderon, 2016). The etiology of these deficits is multifactorial and includes genetic, prenatal, and postnatal factors such as age at time of surgical correction and severity of illness; additional risk factors include male sex and disadvantaged SES. In addition, altered cerebral blood flow, impaired oxygen delivery to the central nervous system (CNS), and delayed **folding** (central nervous system development; see Chapter 6) have been found in fetal and newborn studies and are thought to contribute to the risk for neurocognitive deficits (Khalil et al., 2016; Laraja et al., 2017; Miller et al., 2007; Rollins et al., 2017). Smaller brain volumes have been seen as early as 25 weeks' gestation (Kahlil et al., 2016). Preoperatively, 20%–40% of children with CCHD have white matter injury (see Chapter 8), and, postoperatively, 50% have evidence of new white matter injury (Miller et al., 2007).

The white matter injury in infants with CCHD preoperatively is similar to the pattern seen in premature infants and has been termed "encephalopathy of CHD" (Volpe, 2014, p. 963). In children undergoing cardiopulmonary bypass, risk factors for neurodevelopmental delays include genetic disorders, lower birth weight, prematurity, longer duration of intensive care, postoperative seizures, and lower SES (Simmons & Brueckner, 2017). Cardiopulmonary bypass (CPB) carries its own set of significant risks to the infant's developing organs, including nonphysiologic temperatures and perfusion rates, hemodilution, systemic inflammation, and myocardial damage (Lee, Blaine Easley, & Brady, 2008; Pouard & Bojan, 2013; Sturmer et al., 2018). However, it is important to know that despite advances in operative techniques including CPB, neurodevelopmental outcomes have not improved (Gaynor et al., 2015; Marino, 2013).

When compared with peers and siblings without CHD there is an overall 5%–10% decrease in mean IQ in all children with CHD, and the severity of delay correlates to the severity of the CHD. An IQ of less than 70 occurs in 10%–20% of all children with CHD. However, the mean IQs are 90 for nonsyndromic CHD and 70 for syndromic CHD. An IQ of less than 55 is most likely associated with a genetic syndrome or major complication (Figure 24.1; Brosig et al., 2017; Latal, 2016; Naef et al., 2017).

Despite mean IQ scores within the typical range, a high proportion of preschool children with CHD, with or without surgery, are at early cognitive risk. Depending on the severity of the cardiac lesion, early motor delays commonly improve by 3 years of age, but speech, motor, and social-emotional delays can persist. Compared with peers, more children with CHD receive special education (26.9% versus 11.6 %; Riehle-Colarussoet et al., 2015). At school age, children with CHD have more learning disabilities, executive function problems (particularly with organization, planning, and self-monitoring), and socio-emotional delays (Gerstle et al., 2016).

Treatment

The potential benefits of fetal cardiac intervention have been known for many years (Box 24.4). Fetal cardiac interventions can alleviate heart dysfunction, prevent them evolving into hypoplastic left heart syndrome, achieve biventricular outcome, and improve fetal

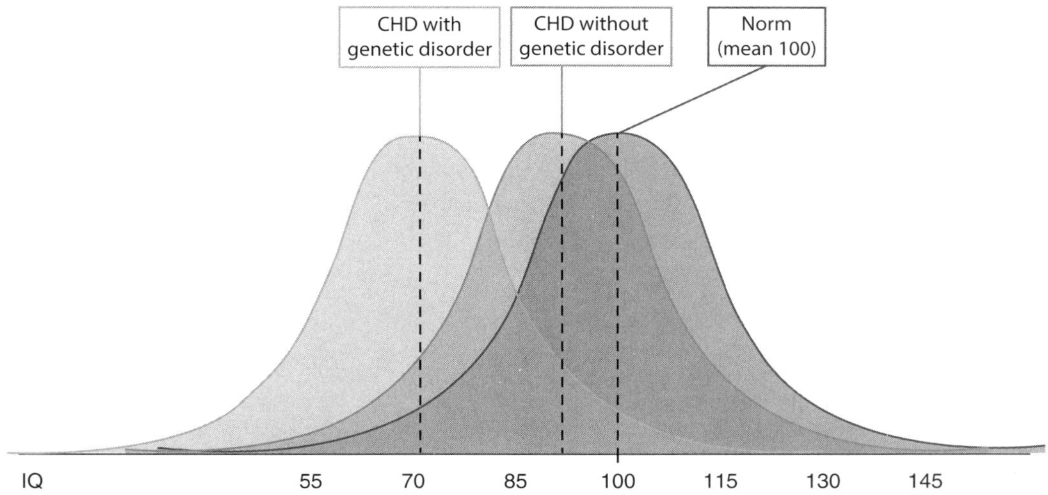

Figure 24.1. IQ range for children with CHD with and without genetic disorders. (Reprinted with permission from Latal, B. [2016]. Neurodevelopmental outcomes of the child with congenital heart disease. *Clinical Perinatology*, *43*, 173–185)

survival. Candidates for clinical fetal cardiac interventions are currently restricted to cases of 1) critical aortic valve stenosis with evolving hypoplastic left heart syndrome, 2) pulmonary atresia with an intact ventricular septum and evolving hypoplastic right heart syndrome, and 3) hypoplastic left heart syndrome with an intact or highly restrictive atrial septum as well as fetal heart block. The therapeutic options include prenatal aortic valvuloplasty (repair of the aortic valve), pulmonary valvuloplasty (repair of the pulmonary valve), creation of interatrial communication, and fetal cardiac pacing.

After identification of CCHD in the newborn, medical stabilization may include the use of prostaglandin E_1 (a potent vasodilator) to keep the **ductus arteriosus** (an artery in the fetus that connects the pulmonary artery to the aorta) open until a surgical procedure or cardiac catheterization can be performed. Children with CCHD are often treated with medication to control congestive heart failure to help optimize growth while awaiting their next procedure(s). Each form of CCHD has a typical type of surgical palliation, but the individual details and timeline for surgery is child specific. For example, infants with D-TGA may require a **balloon atrial septostomy** (a catheter-based procedure) to enlarge the foramen ovale (a fetal connection between the atria; see Figure 6.2 in Chapter 6) until an arterial switch procedure, the currently preferred surgical correction for D-TGA, can be completed (most often within the first 30 days of life). HLHS is commonly treated with a three-stage approach that can include catheter-based and surgical approaches depending on the infant's specific anatomy. These interventions require a team of highly trained professionals (Box 24.5).

Outcomes

With improved surgical techniques, survival rates have increased over the last 20 years, and 80% of children with CHD are living into adulthood. Even children

BOX 24.4 EVIDENCE-BASED PRACTICE

Fetal Cardiac Intervention

Fetal cardiac intervention (FCI) is used in conditions where the fetus is at high risk for prenatal or neonatal death and the intervention may improve survival or alter postnatal disease positively. Pharmacological intervention consists of medication taken orally by the mother or by umbilical vein for fetal arrhythmias. Fetal tachyarrhythmias (a heart rate greater than 160–180 beats per minute) are treated with digoxin and other medications given to the mother. There are also open- and closed-uterus surgical interventions (McElhinney, Tworetzky, & Lock, 2010).

BOX 24.5 INTERDISCIPLINARY CARE

The Congenital Heart Clinic Team

The congenital heart clinic team includes a pediatric cardiologist, pediatric cardiothoracic surgeon, pediatric interventional cardiologist, and pediatric nurse. Because of the common cognitive and motor delays after cardiac surgery, the team also often includes a pediatric neuropsychologist, speech-language pathologist, occupational therapist, and physical therapist.

with HLHS have a 50%–70% survival rate at 5 years and a 10-year survival rate of 40% (Best & Rankin, 2016). In adulthood, children with CHD may have challenges, including educational underachievement, limited employment opportunities, restricted insurability, and diminished quality of life (Latal, 2016). Quality of life may be affected by medical complications and poor exercise tolerance. However, there are many examples of adults with CHD who live independently, succeed in higher education achievement, become gainfully employed, and have families of their own.

CHRONIC KIDNEY DISEASE

CASE STUDY

At 4 months of age, Juanita's pediatrician identified an abdominal mass and evaluation revealed a rare type of renal cancer, which was present in both kidneys. Six years later, after several surgeries, the cancer has not recurred, but renal function of Juanita's remaining kidney is limited, and it is anticipated that as she grows she will eventually need some type of renal replacement therapy (RRT).

Overview

Chronic kidney disease (CKD) involves a progressive and irreversible loss of renal function that occurs over a period of months to years depending on the disease's underlying cause. CKD is defined in stages based on the severity of renal impairment, with Stage I representing a normal glomerular filtration rate (GFR; a measure of kidney function) and Stage 5 reflecting very poor to no kidney function. End stage renal disease (ESRD) is defined as Stage 5 kidney disease requiring treatment with dialysis or kidney transplantation. The incidence and prevalence of CKD in the U.S. pediatric population is unknown as epidemiological information is limited and imprecise. The 2014 data from the annual report published by the United States Renal Data System (2017) noted the pediatric incidence rate of new cases of ESRD per year to be 14 per 1 million children, or affecting about 10,000 children birth to age 19 years in the United States.

In children, CKD can result from **congenital** (present at birth) causes, acquired diseases, or genetic disorders. In young children, the most common causes of CKD are congenital or inherited disorders, including renal **dysplasia** (abnormal growth), obstructive uropathies (flow of urine blocked; e.g., posterior urethral valves), or reflux nephropathy (urine flowing or refluxing backwards to the kidneys). In older children and adolescents, CKD may occur due to acquired glomerular diseases, including focal segmental glomerulosclerosis (scarring of the glomeruli, which filter the blood) and lupus nephritis, a systemic autoimmune disease that can affect the kidneys (Dharnidharka, Fiorina, & Harmon, 2014).

Diagnosis and Clinical Manifestations

Children may be diagnosed with CKD prenatally via ultrasonography or postnatally through abnormalities in the urinalysis or an elevation in serum **creatinine** (the substance produced by muscle tissue that is filtered from the blood by the kidney). Although the early stages of CKD (Stages 1–3) are usually asymptomatic, children may begin to develop mild symptoms of fatigue or decreased appetite in Stage 4 and develop symptoms of **uremia** (accumulated urinary waste products in the blood) in Stage 5. Uremic symptoms include nausea, **anorexia** (loss of appetite), vomiting, weakness, fatigue, pruritis (itchiness), and deficits in neurocognitive function (Vogt & Avner, 2007).

Many complications occur as CKD progresses, and they often begin to manifest in Stage 3 (when kidney function is 30%–60% of normal). Anemia results from decreased production of erythropoietin by the kidney and is associated with decreased exercise tolerance, weakness, pallor, and fatigue. Cardiovascular complications include hypertension, left ventricular hypertrophy (Mitsnefes et al., 2010), and abnormal lipid metabolism. CKD-related bone disease is usually caused by secondary hyperparathyroidism (excessive secretion of parathyroid hormone in response to a low calcium level) and can result in fractures or changes of rickets. Growth impairment is multifactorial and results from metabolic acidosis, anorexia, increased caloric requirements due to chronic illness, metabolic bone disease, and abnormalities in growth hormone metabolism (Vogt & Avner, 2007).

Development and Behavior

Children with CKD are at increased risk for alterations and delays in neurocognitive development. In children and youth like Juanita with mild to moderate CKD, neurocognitive functioning overall is within the average range, but 21%–40% score at least 1 standard deviation (SD) below the mean on measures of IQ, academic achievement, attention regulation, or executive functioning (Hooper et al., 2011). In a more recent study from the same group of 124 preschool children with mild to moderate CKD, median scores were in the average range for developmental level/IQ; attention regulation; and parent ratings of executive function, social-behavior, and adaptive behavior. However, 43% were in the at-risk category for two or more of these measures. None of the disease-related variables of GFR, anemia, hypertension, seizures, and abnormal birth history were associated with outcomes (Hooper et al., 2016).

In a study of 90 children and young adults 8–25 years of age with CKD, compared with unaffected controls, those with CKD had poorer performance in attention, memory, and inhibitory control. Lower performance in multiple domains correlated with decreased estimated GFR, a measure of how well kidneys are functioning (Ruebner et al., 2016). In addition, children with CKD and depression have been found to have lower IQ, lower achievement, and lower scores on quality-of-life measures (Kogon et al., 2016).

Children with ESRD are most significantly impacted by their renal disease. Pollack and colleagues (2016) reported on 18 infants who received hemodialysis (HD); eight (44%) demonstrated significant cognitive disability, and four (22%) had seizures. Madden, Ledermann, Guerrero-Blanco, Bruce, and Trompeter (2003) reported on the cognitive development of 16 surviving children from a cohort of 20 who developed ESRD and required chronic hydroxyrurea prior to 1 year of age. The mean IQ was 86, but scores ranged from 50 to 102. In the children with ESRD, the mean IQ improved following transplantation or dialysis, although it was approximately 8 IQ points below the population norm (Moser, Veale, McAlister, & Archer, 2013).

Children with ESRD and their parents report lower health-related quality of life across all domains, including physical health, psychosocial health, emotional functioning, social functioning, and school functioning when compared with their healthy peers (Goldstein et al., 2006). Another study of 402 children with mild to moderate CKD reported similar findings, with parents and children reporting lower health-related quality of life and poor physical, social, emotional, and school functioning as compared with healthy youth (Gerson et al., 2010).

Treatment

Care of the child with CKD includes efforts to slow progression of the disease, correction of metabolic disturbances intrinsic to CKD, provision of nutritional and hormonal support for growth failure, and preparation for renal replacement therapy (RRT) (Noe & Jones, 2007; see Box 24.6). Strategies to protect kidney function include controlling hypertension with salt and antihypertensive medications, reduction of proteinuria, good hydration, and avoidance of nephrotoxic (toxic to the kidney) drugs. Bone disease may be treated with activated vitamin D, and short stature may benefit from recombinant growth hormone injections. Correction of anemia with iron supplementation and recombinant human erythropoietin may result in decreased fatigue and increased exercise tolerance, cardiovascular improvement, and better neurocognitive outcomes (Vogt & Avner, 2007).

When a child reaches ESRD, RRT (renal transplantation, peritoneal dialysis [PD], or hemodialysis [HD]) be initiated. The ultimate goal for the vast majority of children with ESRD is successful kidney transplantation, although if a transplant is not an option, PD (removing waste products through the child's

BOX 24.6 INTERDISCIPLINARY CARE

The Chronic Renal Disease Team

The chronic renal disease team can vary. The team generally includes three types of registered nurses (RNs)—a general nephrology RN, a transplant coordinator RN, and a dialysis RN—as well as a pediatric nephrologist, a social worker, a dietician, and a psychologist.

surface of their abdominal cavity) or HD (removing waste products from the blood as it passes through a machine) may be offered as a bridge to transplantation. The modality chosen is based on family preference and on technical, social, and compliance issues. Of the 9,767 children and adolescents with ESRD in 2015, the most common RRT was kidney transplant (71.2%), followed by HD (17.8%) and PD (9.7%; U.S. Renal Data System, 2017). From 2010–2015, 36% of children received a kidney transplant within their first year of ESRD.

Outcomes

Neurocognitive functioning in children and youth with mild to moderate CKD is within the average range, but 21% to 40% score at least 1 SD below the mean on measures of IQ, academic achievement, attention regulation, or executive functioning (a score of less than 85; Hooper et al., 2011). Children with ESRD are most affected, with IQ being 8 points below average even after RRT.

Patient survival and graft (transplanted kidney) survival after renal transplantation has markedly improved in recent years. The 5-year survival rate of pediatric renal transplant recipients is now 97%, and 5-year graft (transplanted kidney) survival is 74%–84%. Since patient survival exceeds graft survival, the majority of children who receive kidney transplants will return to dialysis and retransplantation (Holmberg & Jalanko, 2016). The most dramatic improvement in graft survival has been in children 5 years of age or younger. In the pediatric age group, adolescents have the worst long-term graft survival, perhaps as a consequence of poor adherence to medication therapy (Dharnidharka et al., 2014). Of the children who receive their first renal transplant, the 16% who have intellectual disability have equivalent short-term graft and patient survival as children with typical intellectual ability (Wightman et al., 2014).

For children with ESRD, during the years 2010–2014, the 1-year adjusted all-cause mortality rate was 27 per 1,000 patient years, which represented a decrease of 31% from the years 2005–2009. Reduced mortality was reported in almost all age categories, with the greatest point estimate of reduced mortality by 42% in children ages 0–4 years. Across all modalities, the most common causes of death were 1) cardiac arrest (cause unknown), 2) withdrawal from dialysis, and 3) sepsis (overwhelming infection) for children ages 0–21 years. The youngest children had similar reported causes when compared with older children and adolescents (U.S. Renal Data System, 2017).

ACUTE LYMPHOCYTIC LEUKEMIA AND BRAIN CANCER

CASE STUDY

Sarah has trisomy 21 and was born with congenital heart disease, hypothyroidism, and an elevated white blood cell count, which placed her at increased risk for developing a type of leukemia mainly seen in young children with trisomy 21. She has been monitored by pediatric oncology. Around her third birthday, she developed acute megakaryocytic leukemia. Since receiving chemotherapy, she has been in remission and continues on her original developmental trajectory.

Overview

In 2014, 15,780 children in the United States 0–19 years of age were diagnosed with cancer. The most common cancers in children are acute lymphoblastic leukemia (ALL, a blood cell cancer; 20%) and CNS tumors (18%), with medulloblastomas (cerebellar tumors) being the most frequent brain tumors in children. ALL is associated with multiple chromosomal translocations and intrachromosomal rearrangements as well as specific genetic disorders (e.g., Down syndrome; Hunger & Mullighan, 2015). The etiology of brain tumors is not well defined, but 5% of cases are associated with familial and hereditary syndromes (Kuttesch & Ater, 2007).

Diagnosis and Clinical Manifestations

The clinical presentation of ALL includes bruising or bleeding due to thrombocytopenia, pallor and fatigue from anemia, and infection caused by neutropenia (Hunger & Mullighan, 2015). The diagnosis is usually suggested by an abnormal peripheral blood count showing immature malignant blast cells, which is followed by a bone marrow aspiration to establish the diagnosis (Tubergen, Bleyer, Ritchey, & Friehling, 2016). For CNS tumors, the clinical presentation depends on the tumor location, tumor type, and the child's age. The classical symptoms of a brain tumor include persistent and severe headache and vomiting, but brain tumors can also present with disturbances of equilibrium, gait, and coordination (Kuttesch & Ater, 2007). Evaluating a child suspected of having a brain tumor is an emergency; it includes a history, physical examination, ophthalmological examination, and an MRI scan of the brain (Kuttesch & Ater, 2007).

Development and Behavior

Early studies of survivors of childhood ALL determined that cranial radiation therapy was associated with declines in intelligence (Cousens, Waters, Said, & Stevens, 1988) as well as symptoms of ADHD and impaired school performance, especially in arithmetic computation (Butler & Haser, 2006). Studies of chemotherapy-only treatment for childhood ALL also indicate a specific pattern of neuropsychological late effects. Although verbal subtests have not been significantly different between these two groups, perceptual reasoning skills, working memory, and processing speed have been found to be affected in the chemotherapy-only group (please see Chapter 13 for a discussion of the components of neuropsychological testing). The result is that academic progress in both reading and math is impaired. Children who have experienced relapses have poor neurocognitive outcomes, with 20% displaying IQ scores in the range of intellectual disability (Janzen & Spiegler, 2008).

Studies in children treated for CNS tumors with surgery and cranial irradiation therapy have reported declines in intellectual function and in academic achievement (Butler & Haser, 2006). In a study of 120 children treated with surgery and cranial irradiation therapy for medulloblastoma, 42% had a full-scale IQ score of less than 80 at 5 years following treatment and 75% had a full scale IQ of less than 80 at 10 years following treatment (Hoppe-Hirsch et al., 1990). Deficits were observed in memory, attention/concentration, sequencing, processing speed, visual perceptual ability, and language.

Children with brain tumors who require only surgical treatment can have a range of outcomes. Surgery may result in global intellectual ability remaining intact but with deficits in selected or multiple domains. In addition, more than half of children with brain tumors who are treated surgically experienced some form of significant psychological adjustment problem, such as depression, externalizing behaviors, and academic problems (Meyer & Kieran, 2002).

Treatment

Improved survival is due to improvements in efficacy of multi-agent chemotherapy regimens and stratification of treatment intensity according to clinical features. It also correlates with the biologic features of the leukemia cells and the early response to treatment. Treatment of ALL begins with induction therapy using systemic and intrathecal chemotherapy. After achieving remission, the next step in treatment involves the administration of intensive combination chemotherapy to consolidate remission and prevent CNS leukemia. This is followed by an 8-week delayed intensification phase using folinic acid to "rescue" normal tissues from the toxic effects of chemotherapy (Hunger & Mullighan, 2015). After remission, most children enter a maintenance phase of chemotherapy that lasts 2–3 years. About 15%–20% of children have a relapse in the bone marrow and less commonly in the CNS or testes, with cure rates much lower after relapse (Tubergen et al., 2016). Bone marrow transplantation may be part of the treatment regimen if there is relapse.

The foundation for treatment of medulloblastomas is the combination of maximal safe **resection** (surgical removal), chemotherapy, and craniospinal irradiation (Bautista et al., 2017; Kuttesch & Ater, 2007). Several approaches have been taken to decrease irradiation toxicity (Box 24.7). A new approach to decrease irradiation toxicity and increase survival and quality of life, autologous hematopoietic cell transplantation, is being used for initial treatment and recurrent treatment (Box 24.8).

BOX 24.7 EVIDENCE-BASED PRACTICE

Medullobalstoma, Radiation, and Cognition

To decrease neurocognitive deficits in intelligence and academic function related to craniospinal irradiation (CSI) after medulloblastoma surgery, a longitudinal study of risk-adapted (limited) irradiation was conducted. Children with medulloblastoma were divided into average-risk (AR) and high-risk (HR) groups. The children with AR received reduced amounts of CSI. They still had a decline in IQ and less of a decline in academic function, with the most prominent risk factor being younger age. In general, the children in the AR group had less cognitive decline than those in the HR group, suggesting a possible benefit of reduced exposure to CSI, but complex interactions among age, risk, time, and cognitive outcomes were observed, necessitating further study (Mulhern et al., 2005).

BOX 24.8 EVIDENCE-BASED PRACTICE

Autologous Stem Cell Transplantation

Marrow-ablative chemotherapy for malignant brain tumors followed by tandem autologous hematopoietic cell transplantation has shown promising results. This intervention includes multiple (two or three, depending upon protocol) cycles of high-dose chemotherapy that would otherwise be myelo-ablative (completely wipe out someone's ability to make normal blood cells) but that can be effectively rescued by delivering someone's own (autologous) stem cells to help repopulate the bone marrow after the chemotherapy. In children with newly diagnosed malignant brain tumors, overall survival with no irradiation is greatly improved with this technique (Guerra et al., 2017).

Multidisciplinary approaches to treating sequelae include seizure management, physical therapy, endocrine management with tailored hormone and thyroid replacement, customized educational programs, and vocational intervention, all depending on the individual needs of the child (Kuttesch & Ater, 2007; see Box 24.9). Initial studies indicate some success using a cognitive remediation program in which the child is guided through exercises that promote sustained, selective, divided, and executive attention control (Butler et al., 2008; Sohlberg, McLaughlin, Pavese, Heidrich, & Posner, 2000). Treatment with stimulant medication (see Chapters 19 and 38) has also improved performance on tests of attention and on parent and teacher reports (Conklin et al., 2010; Netson et al., 2011).

Outcomes

In children in the United States, cancer is the number one cause of death by disease, accounting for 57% of all deaths by disease. Over the last 40 years, the overall survival rate for cancer improved from 10% to 90%. The overall 5-year childhood cancer survival rate is almost 84%, being 90% for ALL and 74% for CNS cancers. In addition, 60% of children have late effects, including secondary cancers, and 12% do not survive these new cancers (Cure Search for Children's Cancer, 2018).

Children who have undergone cancer treatment are more likely than the general population to repeat a grade in school and to need more learning supports and special education services. Compared with their typically developing peers, children treated for brain tumors are 4 times more likely to repeat a grade, and those receiving cerebral irradiation are 2.5 times as likely to repeat a grade (Barrera, 2005). Compared with siblings, survivors of leukemia and CNS tumors are less likely to finish high school; only those with CNS tumors are also less likely to also complete college (Mitby et al., 2003). Compared with healthy controls, adult survivors of childhood cancers are nearly twice as likely to be unemployed, with those with CNS or brain tumors being nearly five times more likely to be unemployed (De Boer, Verbeek, & Van Dijk, 2006). Minimizing the adverse effects of childhood cancers while maintaining high survival rates with treatment is a goal that has been largely achieved in treatment regimens for ALL but less so in treatment for brain tumors. Improvements in therapy have greatly decreased mortality and morbidity, but advances are needed to achieve optimal neurocognitive outcomes.

SUMMARY

- Children with a spectrum of chronic diseases are more alike than different in the developmental and behavioral challenges that they face.
- Among children with SCD, about 10% will have overt strokes with neurological findings and nearly

BOX 24.9 INTERDISCIPLINARY CARE

The Cancer Team

The clinic cancer team can vary, but typically includes a pediatric oncologist, a pediatric nurse practitioner, a social worker, and a child life specialist (a health care professional who works with children in and outside of the hospital, helping children deal with illness and disability).

one third will have silent strokes with findings on MRIs.

- Children with CHD have a 30%–50% risk for neurocognitive deficits, including ADHD; deficits in executive function, social skills, motor planning, and visual memory; and difficulty with higher-order integration.
- In children and youth with mild to moderate CKD, neurocognitive functioning overall is within the average range, but 21%–40% score at least 1 SD below the mean on measures of IQ, academic achievement, attention regulation, or executive functioning.
- Cancer survivors of ALL and brain tumors frequently have residual cognitive and academic problems as well as ADHD symptoms.

ADDITIONAL RESOURCES

Sickle Cell Disease: National Heart, Lung, & Blood Institute (NHLB) Institute: https://www.nhlbi.nih.gov/health-topics/sickle-cell-disease

National Institute of Diabetes and Digestive and Kidney Diseases: https://www.nhlbi.nih.gov/health-topics/sickle-cell-disease

Children's Oncology Group Link: http://www.survivorshipguidelines.org

Additional resources can be found online in Appendix D: Childhood Disabilities Resources, Services, and Organizations (see About the Online Companion Materials).

REFERENCES

Abouk, R. G., Grosse, S. D., Ailes, E. C., & Oster, M. E. (2017). Association of US state implementation of newborn screening policies for critical congenital heart disease with early infant cardiac deaths. *JAMA, 318*(21), 2111–2118.

Armstrong, F. D., Elkin, T. D., Grown, R. C., Glass, P., Rana, S., Casella, J. F., . . . Baby Hug Investigators. (2013). Developmental function in toddlers with sickle cell anemia. *Pediatrics, 131*, e406–e414.

Bakri, M. H., Ismail, E. A., Elsedfy, G. O., Ami, M. A., & Ibrahim, A. (2014). Behavioral impact of sickle cell disease in young children with repeated hospitalization. *Saudi Journal of Anesthesia, 8*, 504–509.

Barrera, M. (2005). Educational and social late effects of childhood cancer and related clinical, personal and familial characteristics. *American Cancer Society, 104*, 1751–1760.

Bautista, F., Fioravantti, V., de Rojas, T., Carceller, F., Madero, L., Lassaletta, A., . . . Moreno, L. (2017). Medulloblastoma in children and adolescents: A systematic review of contemporary phase I and II clinical trials and biology update. *Cancer Medicine, 6*(11), 2606–2624.

Benson, D. W., Martin, L. J., & Lo, C. W. (2016). Genetics of hypoplastic left heart syndrome. *The Journal of Pediatrics, 173*, 25–31.

Best, K. E., & Rankin, J. (2016). Long-term survival of individuals born with congenital heart disease: A systematic review and meta-analysis. *Journal of the American Heart Association, 5*(9), 1–16.

Brosig, C. L., Bear, L., Allen, S., Hoffmann, R. G., Pan, A., Frommelt, M., . . . Massatto, K. A. (2017). Preschool neurodevelopmental outcomes in children with congenital heart disease. *The Journal of Pediatrics, 183*, 80–86.

Butler, R. W., & Haser, J. K. (2006). Neurocognitive effects of treatment for childhood cancer. *Mental Retardation and Developmental Disabilities Research Reviews, 12*, 184–191.

Butler, R. W., Copeland, D. R., Fairclough, D. L., Mulhern, R. K., Katz, E. R., Kazak, A. E., . . . Sahler, O. J. (2008). A multicenter, randomized clinical trial of a cognitive remediation program for childhood survivors of a pediatric malignancy. *Journal of Consulting and Clinical Psychology, 76*, 367–378.

Calderon, J. (2016). Executive function in patients with congenital heart disease: Only the tip of the iceberg. *The Journal of Pediatrics, 173*, 7–9.

Chen, R., Pawlak, M. A., Flynn, T. B., Krejza, J., Herskovits, E. H., & Melhem, E. R. (2009). Brain morphometry and intelligence quotient measurements in children with sickle cell disease. *Journal of Developmental-Behavioral Pediatrics, 30*, 509–517.

Compas, B. E., Jaser, S. S., Reeslund, K., Patel, N., & Yarboi, J. (2017). Neurocognitive deficits in children with chronic health conditions. *American Psychologist, 72*(4), 326–338.

Conklin, H. M., Reddick, W. E., Ashford, J., Ogg, S. Howard, S. C., Morris, E. B., . . . Khan, R. B. (2010). Long-term efficacy of methylpheniate in enhancing attention regulation, social skills, and academic abilities of childhood cancer survivors. *Journal of Clinical Oncology, 28*, 4465–4472.

Cousens, P., Waters, B., Said, J., & Stevens, M. (1988). Cognitive effects of cranial irradiation of leukaemia: A survey and meta-analysis. *Journal of Child Psychology and Psychiatry, 29*, 839–852.

Cure Search for Children's Cancer. (2018). *Childhood cancer statistics.* Retrieved from https://curesearch.org/Childhood-Cancer-Statistics

DeBaun, M. G., & Vichinsky, E. (2007). Hemoglobinopathies. In R. M. Kliegman, R. E. Behrman, H. B. Jenson, & B. F. Stanton (Eds.), *Nelson textbook of pediatrics* (18th ed., pp. 5–38). Philadelphia, PA: Saunders Elsevier.

De Boer, A. G. E. M., Verbeek, J. H. A. M., & van Dijk, F. J. H. (2006). Adult survivors of childhood cancer and unemployment: A meta-analysis. *Cancer, 107*, 1–11.

DeWalt, D. A., Gross, H. E., Giipson, D. S., Selewske, D. T., DeWitt, E. M., Dampier, C. D., . . . Varni, J. W. (2015). PROMIS pediatric self report scales distinguish subgroups of children within and across six common pediatric chronic health conditions. *Quality of Life Research, 23*(9), 215–2208.

Dharnidharka, V. R., Fiorina, P., & Harmon, W. E. (2014). Kidney transplantation in children. *New England Journal of Medicine, 371*, 549–558.

Drazen, C. H., Abel, R., Gabir, M., Farmer, G., & King, A. A. (2016). Prevalence of developmental delay and contributing factors among children with sickle cell disease. *Pediatric Blood Cancer, 63*, 504–510.

Enninful-Eghan, H., Moore, R. H., Ichord, R., Smith-Whitney, K., & Kwiakowski, J. L. (2010). Transcranial Doppler ultrasonography and prophylactic transfusion program is effective in preventing overt stroke in children with sickle cell disease. *The Journal of Pediatrics, 157,* 479–484.

Falletta, J. M., Woods, G. M., Veter, J. I., Buhanan, G. R., Pegelow, C., Iyer, R. V., . . . Vichinsky, E. (1995). Discontinuing penicillin prophylaxis in children with sickle cell anemia. Prophylactic Penicillin Study II. *Disability Rehabilitation, 127,* 685–690.

Gaynor, J. W. (2014). The encephalopathy of congenital heart disease. *The Journal of Thoracic and Cardiovascular Surgery, 148,* 1790–1791.

Gaynor, J. W., Stopp, C., Wypij, D., Andropoulos, D. B., Atallah, J. Atz, A. M., . . . Newburger, J. W. (2015). Neurodevelopmental outcomes after cardiac surgery in infancy. *Pediatrics, 135,* 816–825.

Gerson, A. C., Wentz, A., Abraham, A. G., Mendley, S. R., Hooper, S. R., Butler, R. W., . . . Furth, S. L. (2010). Health-related quality of life of children with mild to moderate chronic kidney disease. *Pediatrics, 125,* e349–e357.

Gerstle, M., Beebe, D. W., Drotar, D., Cassedy, A., & Marino, B. S. (2016). Executive functioning and school performance among pediatric survivors of complex congenital heart disease. *The Journal of Pediatrics, 173,* 154–159.

Gilboa, S., Devine, O., Kucik, J., Oster, M., Riehle-Colarusso, T., Nembhard, W., . . . Marelli, A. J. (2016). Congenital heart defects in the United States: Estimating the magnitude of the affected population in 2010. *Circulation, 134*(2), 101–109.

Goldstein, S. L., Graham, N., Burwinkle, T., Wardy, B., Farrah, R., & Varni, J. W. (2006). Health-related quality of life in pediatric patients with ESRD. *Pediatric Nephrology, 21,* 846–850.

Guerra, J. A., Dhali, G., Marachelian, A., Castillo, E., Malvar, J., Wong, K., . . . Finlay, J. L. (2017). Marrow-ablative chemotherapy followed by tandem autologous hematopoietic cell transplantation in pediatric patients with malignant brain tumors. *Bone Marrow Transplantation, 52,* 1543–1548.

Holmberg, C., & Jalanko, H. (2016). Long-term effects of paediatric kidney transplantation. *Nature Reviews/Nephrology, 12,* 301–311.

Hooper, S. R., Gerson, A. C., Butler, R. W., Gipson, D. S., Mendley, S. R., Lande, M. B., . . . Warady, B. A. (2011). Neurocognitive functioning of children and adolescents with mild-to-moderate chronic kidney disease. *Clinical Journal of American Society of Nephrology, 6,* 1824–1830.

Hooper, S. R., Gerson, A. C., Johnson, R. J., Mendley, S. R., Shinnar, S., Lande, M. B., et al. (2016). Neurocognitive, social-behavioral, and adaptive functioning in preschool children with mild to moderate kidney disease. *Journal of Developmental & Behavioral Pediatrics, 37,* 231–238.

Hoppe-Hirsch, E., Renier, D., Lellouch-Tubiana, A., Sainte-Rose, C., Pierre-Kahn, A., & Hirsch, J. F. (1990). Medulloblastoma in childhood: Progressive intellectual deterioration. *Childs Nervous System, 6,* 60–65.

Hunger, S. P., & Mullighan, C. G. (2015). Acute lymphoblastic leukemia in children. *New England Journal of Medicine, 373,* 1541–1554.

Janzen, L. A., & Spiegler, B. J. (2008). Neurodevelopmental sequelae of pediatric acute lymphoblastic leukemia and its treatment. *Developmental Disabilities Research Reviews, 14,* 185–195.

Khalil, A., Bennet, S., Thilaganathan, B., Paladini, D., Griffiths, P., & Carvalho, J. S. (2016). Prevalence of prenatal brain abnormalities in fetuses with congenital heart disease: A systematic review. *Ultrasound in Obstetrics & Gynecology, 48*(3), 296–307.

Kogon, A., Matheson, M. B., Flynn, J. T., Gerson, A. C., Warady, B. A., Furth, S. L., . . . CKiD Study Group. (2016). Depressive symptoms in children with chronic kidney disease. *Journal of Pediatrics, 168,* 164–170.

Kuttesch, J. F., & Ater, J. L. (2007). Brain tumors in childhood. In R. M. Kliegman, R. E. Behrman, H. B. Jenson, & B. F. Stanton (Eds.). *Nelson textbook of pediatrics* (18th ed., pp. 2128–2137). Philadelphia, PA: Saunders Elsevier.

Lannering, K., Bartos, M., & Mellander, M. (2015). Late diagnosis of coarctation despite prenatal ultrasound and postnatal pulse oximetry. *Pediatrics, 136*(2), e406–e412.

Lantin-Hermoso, M. R., Berger, S., Blatt, A.B., Richerson, J.E., Morrow, R., . . . Beekman, R. H. (2017). The care of children with congenital heart disease in their primary medical home. *Pediatrics, 140,* 1–10.

Laraja, K., Sadhwani, A., Tworetzky, W., Marshall, A. C., Gauvreau, K., Freud, L., . . . Newburger, J. W. (2017). Neurodevelopmental outcome in children after fetal cardiac intervention for aortic stenosis with evolving hypoplastic left heart syndrome. *The Journal of Pediatrics, 184,* 130–136. e4.

Lanzkron, S., Carroll, C. P., Haywood, C., Jr. (2013). Mortality rates and age at death from sickle cell disease: U.S., 1979–2005. *Public Health Report, 128,* 110–116.

Latal, B. (2016). Neurodevelopmental outcomes of the child with congenital heart disease. *Clinics in Perinatology, 43*(1), 173–185.

Lopez-Vincete, M., Ortega-Gutierrez, S., Amlie-Lefond, C., & Torbey, M. T. (2010). Diagnosis and management of pediatric arterial ischemic stroke. *Journal of Stroke and Cerebrovascular Diseases, 19,* 175–183.

Lee, J. K., Blaine Easley, R., & Brady, K. M. (2008). Neurocognitive monitoring and care during pediatric cardiopulmonary bypass-current and future directions. *Current Cardiology Reviews, 4*(2), 123–139. doi:10.2174/157340308784245766

Madden, S. J., Ledermann, S. E., Guerrero-Blanco, M., Bruce, M., & Trompeter, R. S. (2003). Cognitive and psychosocial outcome of infants dialysed in infancy. *Child: Care, Health & Development, 29,* 55–61.

Marino, B. S. (2013). New concepts in predicting, evaluating, and managing neurodevelopmental outcomes in children with congenital heart disease. *Current Opinion in Pediatrics, 25,* 574–584.

Marino, B. S., Lipkin, P. H., Newburger, J. W., Peacock, G., Gerdes, M., Gaynor, J. W., . . . Mahle, W. T. (2012). Neurodevelopmental outcomes in children with congenital heart disease: Evaluation and management: A scientific statement from the American Heart Association. *Circulation, 126*(9), 1143.

McElhinney, D. B., Tworetzky, W., & Lock, J. E. (2010). Current status of fetal cardiac intervention. *Circulation, 121,* 1256–1263.

Meier, E. R., & Rampersad, A. (2017). Pediatric sickle cell disease: Past successes and future challenges. *Pediatric Research, 81,* 249–258.

Meyer, A. A., & Kieran, M. W. (2002). Psychological adjustment of "surgery-only" pediatric neuro-oncology patients: A retrospective analysis. *Psycho-oncology, 11,* 74–79.

Miller, S. P., McQuillen, P. S., Hamrick, S., Xu, D., Glidden, D. V., Charlton, N., . . . Vigneron, D. B. (2007). Abnormal brain development in newborns with congenital heart disease. *The New England Journal of Medicine, 357*(19), 1928–1938.

Mitby, P. A., Borinson, L. L., Whitton, J. A., Zevon, M. A., Gibbs, I. C., Tersak, J. M., . . . Childhood Cancer Survivor Study Steering Committee. (2003). Utilization of special education services and educational attainment among long-term survivors of childhood cancer: A report from the Childhood Cancer Survivor Study. *Cancer, 97*, 1115–1126.

Mitsnefes, M., Flynn, J., Cohn, S., Samuels, J., Blydt-Hansen, T., Saland, J., . . . CKiD Study Group. (2010). Masked hypertension associated with left ventricular hypertrophy in children with CKD. *Journal of the American Society of Nephrology, 21*, 137–144.

Moser, J. J., Veale, P. M., McAlister, D. L., & Archer, D. P. (2013). A systematic review and quantitative analysis of neurocognitive outcomes in children with four chronic illnesses. *Pediatric Anesthesia, 23*, 1084–1096.

Mulhern, R. K., Palmer, S. L., Merchant, T. E., Wallace, D., Kocak, M., Brouwers, P., . . . Gajjar, A. (2005). Neurocognitive consequences of risk-adapted therapy for childhood medulloblastoma. *Journal of Clinical Oncology, 23*, 5511–5519.

Naef, N., Liamlahi, R., Beck, I., Bernet, V., Dave, H., Knirsch, W., . . . Latal, B. (2017). Neurodevelopmental profiles of children with congenital heart disease at school age. *The Journal of Pediatrics, 188*, 75–86.

National Heart, Lung, and Blood Institute. (2017). *Opioid crisis adds to pain of sickle cell patients.* Retrieved from https://www.nhlbi.nih.gov/news/2017/opioid-crisis-adds-pain-sickle-cell-patients

National Institutes of Health: National Library of Medicine. (2018). *Genetics home reference: Sickle cell disease.* Retrieved from https://ghr.nlm.nih.gov/condition/sickle-cell-disease

Noll, R. B., Kiska, R., Reiter-Purtill, J., Gerhardt, C. A., & Vannatta, K. (2010). A controlled, longitudinal study of the social functioning of youth with sickle cell disease. *Pediatrics, 15*, e1453–1459.

Netson, K. L., Conklin, H. M., Ashford, J. M., Kahalley, L. S., Wu, S., & Xiong, X. (2011). Parent and teacher ratings of attention during a year-long methylphenidate trial in children treatment for cancer. *Journal of Pediatric Psychology, 36*, 438–450.

Noe, H. N., & Jones, D. P. (2007). Care of the child with chronic renal insufficiency and end-stage renal disease. In A. J. Wein (Ed.), *Campbell-Walsh urology* (9th ed., pp. 3230–3232). Philadelphia, PA: Saunders Elsevier.

Ohene-Frempong, K., Weinher, S. J., Sleeper, L. A., Miller, S. T., Embury, S., Moohr, J. W., . . . Gill, F. M. (1998). Cerebrovascular accidents in sickle cell disease: Rates and risk factors. *Blood, 91*, 88–94.

Oster, M. E., Kim, C. H., Kusano, A. S., Cragan, J. D., Dressler, P., Hales, A. R., . . . Correa, A. (2014). A population-based study of the association of prenatal diagnosis with survival rate for infants with congenital heart defects. *The American Journal of Cardiology, 113*(6), 1036–1040.

Patel, S., & Burns, T. (2013). Nongenetic risk factors and congenital heart defects. *Pediatric Cardiology, 34*(7), 1535–1555.

Pegelow, C. H., Macklin, E. A., Moser, F. G., Wang, W. C., Bello, J. A., Miller, S. T., . . . Kinney, T. R. (2002). Longitudinal changes in brain magnetic resonance imaging findings in children with sickle cell disease. *Blood, 99*, 3014–3018.

Piel, F. B., Steinberg, M. H., & Rees, D. C. (2017). Sickle cell disease. *New England Journal of Medicine, 376*, 1561–1573.

Pollack, S., Eisenstein, I., Tarabeih, M., Shasha-Lavski, H., Magen, D., & Zelikovic, I. (2016). Long-term hemodialysis therapy in neonates and infants with end-stage renal disease: A 16-year experience and outcome. *Pediatric Nephrology, 31*, 305–313.

Pouard, P., & Bojan, M. (2013). Neonatal cardiopulmonary bypass. *Seminars in Thoracic and Cardiovascular Surgery: Pediatric Cardiac Surgery Annual, 16*, 59–61.

Riehle-Colarusso, T., Autry, A., Razzaghi, H., Boyle, C. A., Mahle, W. T., Van Naarden Braun, K., . . . Correa, A. (2015). Congenital heart defects and receipt of special education services. *Pediatrics, 136*(3), 496–504.

Rollins, C. K., Asaro, L. A., Akhondi-Asl, A., Kussman, B. D., Rivkin, M. J., Bellinger, D. C., . . . Soul, J. S. (2017). White matter volume predicts language development in congenital heart disease. *The Journal of Pediatrics, 181*, 42–48.

Ruebner, R. L., Laney, N., Kim, J. Y., Hartung, E. A., Hooper, S. R., Radcliffe, J., . . . Furth, S. L. (2016). Neurocognitive dysfunction in children, adolescents, and young adults with CKD. *American Journal of Kidney Disease, 67*, 567–575.

Section on Hematology/Oncology & Committee on Genetics. (2002). Health supervision for children with sickle cell disease. *Pediatrics, 109*, 526–535.

Schatz, J., Brown, R. T., Pascual, J. M., Hsu, L., & DeBaun, M. R. (2001). Poor school and cognitive functioning with silent cerebral infarcts and sickle cell disease. *Neurology, 56*, 1109–1111.

Schatz, J., Finke, R. L., Kellett, J. M., & Kramer, J. H. (2002). Cognitive functioning in children with sickle cell disease: A meta-analysis. *Journal of Pediatric Psychology, 7*, 739–748.

Schatz, J., Finke, R., & Roberts, C. W. (2004). Interactions of biomedical and environmental risk factors for cognitive development: A preliminary study of sickle cell disease. *Journal of Developmental and Behavioral Pediatrics, 5*, 303–310.

Schatz, J., & McCellan, C. B. (2006). Sickle cell disease as a neurodevelopmental disorder. *Mental Retardation and Developmental Disabilities Research Reviews, 12*, 200–207.

Schwartz, L.A., Radcliffe, J., & Barakat, L. P. (2009). Associates of school absenteeism in adolescents with sickle cell disease. *Pediatric Blood Cancer, 52*(1), 92–96.

Shahine R., Badr, L. K., Karam, D., & Abboud, M. (2015). Educational intervention to improve the health outcomes of children with sickle cell disease. *Journal of Pediatric Health Care, 29*, 54–60.

Simmons, M. A., & Brueckner, M. (2017). The genetics of congenital heart disease . . . understanding and improving long-term outcomes in congenital heart disease: A review for the general cardiologist and primary care physician. *Current Opinion, 29*, 520–528.

Sohlberg, M. M., McLaughlin, K. A., Pavese, A., Heidrich, A., & Posner, M. (2000). Evaluation of attention process training and brain injury education in persons with acquired brain injury. *Journal of Clinical Experimental Neuropsychology, 22*(5), 656–676. doi:10.1076/1380-3395(200010)22:5;1-9;FT656

Sturmer, D., Beaty, C., Clingan, S. Jenkins, E., Peters, W., & Ming-Sing, S. (2018). Recent innovations in perfusion and cardiopulmonary bypass for neonatal and infant cardiac surgery. *Translational Pediatrics, 7*, 139–150.

Thompson, Jr., R. J., Armstrong, F. D., Link, C. L., Pegelow, C. H., Moser, F., & Wang, W. C. (2003). A prospective study of the relationship over time of behavior problems, intellectual functioning, and family functioning in children with sickle cell disease: A report from the cooperative study of sickle cell disease. *Journal of Pediatric Psychology, 28*, 59–65.

Thompson, R. J., Gustafson, K. E., Bonner, M. J., & Ware, R. E. (2002). Neurocognitive development of young children with sickle cell disease through three years of age. *Journal of Pediatric Psychology, 27*, 235–244.

Tubergen, D. G., Bleyer, A., Ritchey, A. K., & Friehling, E. (2016). The leukemias. In R. Kliegman, R. R. Behrman, & W. E. Nelson (Eds.), *Nelson textbook of pediatrics* (20th ed., pp. 2437–2455). Philadelphia, PA: Elsevier.

United States Renal Data System. (2017). *2017 annual data report.* Retrieved from https://www.usrds.org/adr.aspx.

Vogt, B. A., & Avner, E. D. (2007). Chronic kidney disease. In R. M. Kliegman, R. E. Behrman, H. B. Jenson, & B. F. Stanton (Eds.), *Nelson textbook of pediatrics* (18th ed., pp. 2210–2213). Philadelphia, PA: Saunders Elsevier.

Volpe, J. J. (2014). Encephalopathy of congenital heart disease–destructive and developmental effects intertwined. *The Journal of Pediatrics, 164,* 962–965.

Wightman, A., Young, B., Bradford, M., Dick, A., Healey, P., McDonald, R., . . . Smith, J. (2014). Prevalence and outcomes of renal transplantation in children with intellectual disability. *Pediatric Transplant, 18,* 714–719.

Yabrodi, M., & Mastropietro, C. W. (2016). Hypoplastic left heart syndrome: From comfort care to long-term survival. *Pediatric Research, 81*(1–2), 142–149.

Yawn, B. P., Buchanan, G. R., Afenyi-Annan, A. N., Ballas, S. K., Hassell, K. L., James, A. H. . . John-Sowah, J. (2014). Management of sickle cell disease: Summary of the 2014 evidence-based report by expert panel members. *Journal of the American Medical Association, 312,* 1033–1048.

Zaidi, S., & Brueckner, M. (2017). Genetics and genomics of congenital heart disease. *Circulation Research, 120,* 923–940.

PART V

Associated Disabilities

CHAPTER 25 Visual Impairment

Heather de Beaufort

Upon completion of this chapter, the reader will

- Know the anatomic sources of childhood visual deficit and conditions related to visual impairment
- Gain an understanding of the prevalence and epidemiology of visual deficits, including in children with disabilities
- Understand the basic evaluation of a child with visual impairment, including the ophthalmologic exam and diagnostic studies
- Recognize some of the ways in which a young person with visual disabilities develops differently from a child whose vision is within the typical range
- Be knowledgeable about treatments used to improve or preserve vision, low-vision aids, and vision therapy
- Be aware of outcomes for children with visual deficits

Impaired vision in childhood can have detrimental effects on physical, neurological, cognitive, and emotional development. A severe visual impairment can cause delays in walking, speech, and language development, as well as in behavior and socialization, if early medical and education interventions are not implemented. Visual impairment can occur as an isolated disability or associated with other developmental disabilities. This chapter explores sources of vision loss, sequelae of vision disorders, and the most common ocular pathology. It reviews the basic pediatric eye exam and common tests used in the workup of vision disorders. Treatments for decreased vision and secondary conditions and low-vision aids for the pediatric population are described. Finally, the effects of blindness on a child's development and outcomes for children with vision impairment are discussed, and relevant educational resources are introduced.

CASE STUDY

Mary is a 12-year-old girl, born prematurely at 24 weeks gestational age, who has cerebral palsy and poor vision with associated **nystagmus**. As a result of her **retinopathy of prematurity** (ROP), she has very high nearsightedness. She requires glasses with extremely thick lenses (–18.50 diopters in her right eye and –24.00 diopters in her left eye), which reduces her visual field. Mary benefits from reading materials with highly contrasted enlarged print on her slant board. Mary wrote the following essay to describe her disabilities and adaptations at school:

> One thing I don't like about homework is that sometimes I can't see the print. I have a slant board, which brings my work closer so I won't have to bend over. Because I feel embarrassed, I don't ask to sit closer to the smart board even if I can't see. Also, I need extended time for assignments and tests. I sometimes use a 'talking' dictionary. My handheld magnifier and distance telescope help me, but I don't always use them because my classmates might make fun of me.

At the ophthalmologist's office, Mary's binocular corrected visual acuity measures 20/60. However, with her compound visual disabilities of **optic atrophy,** myopic degeneration, and nystagmus, Mary requires many learning adaptations.

Thought Questions:

What are multiple ways vision can be compromised, making more comprehensive evaluations important? What are the ways that the various vision specialists can help children with vision impairments?

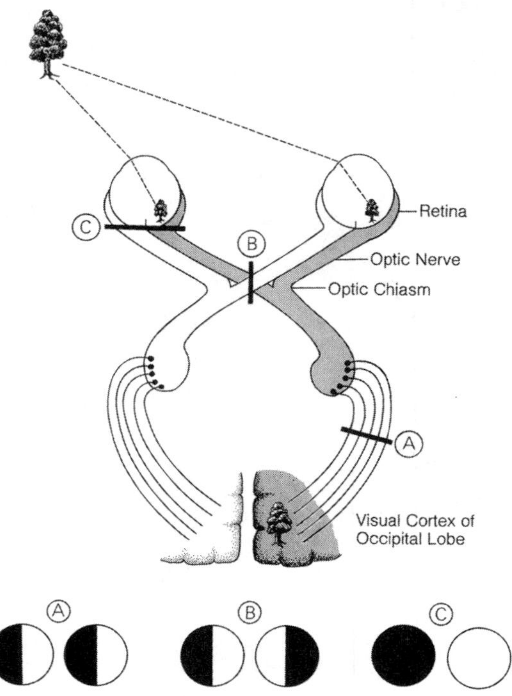

Figure 25.1. The visual pathway. One optic nerve emerges from behind each eye. A portion of the fibers from each crosses at the optic chiasm. An abnormality at various points along the route (upper figure) will lead to different patterns of visual loss (shown as black areas in the lower figures). These are illustrated as A) abnormality at the cortical pathway, B) damage to the optic chiasm, and C) retinal damage.

DEFINITIONS, DESCRIPTIONS, AND CLASSIFICATIONS

Causes of Visual Impairment

In order to see well, one must have a healthy eye, optic nerve, and visual cortex (Figure 25.1). A disturbance in any one of these three areas will result in a loss of vision.

Ocular Vision loss may be due to an abnormality of one of the structures of the eye. Light must pass unhindered through the anterior segment of the eye, like the lens of a camera, and strike a functioning **retina,** like the camera's film, in order for clear images to pass to the optic nerve. For example, if the central **cornea, lens,** or **vitreous** is cloudy or opacified, such as in a **cataract,** light cannot pass through those structures well and vision is degraded. Furthermore, if the retina is abnormal, as seen in retinal detachment or dystrophy, the retinal ganglion cells do not transmit visual information through the optic nerve properly to the visual cortex.

Optic Nerve Next, the optic nerve transmits visual information from the eye to the brain's visual cortex in order for vision to be processed. In the camera analogy, the optic nerve is the USB cord connecting the camera to the computer (or brain) for image processing and storage. Any damage along the length of the optic nerve impairs that transmission of visual information. The optic nerve may never develop properly in utero, as in optic nerve hypoplasia, or it may become damaged due to compression, as in **optic atrophy** or **glaucoma.**

Cerebral/Cortical The final essential component for normal vision is a functioning visual cortex, the section of the brain responsible for visual processing in the occipital lobe. Any pathology in this area, such as stroke or a tumor, will impair vision.

Conditions Related to Impaired Vision and Ocular Pathology

The sections that follow discuss conditions that are related to impaired vision and ocular pathology, including strabismus, nystagmus, abnormal head posture, abnormal color vision, and photophobia.

Strabismus **Strabismus,** or misalignment of the eyes, occurs in about 3%–4% of all children. However, it occurs in 18% of former premature infants and in

55.7% of children with cerebral palsy (Fieβ et al., 2017; Dufresne, Dagenais, & Shevell, 2014). There are three main forms of strabismus: **esotropia** (cross-eyed), in which the eyes turn in; **exotropia** (wall-eyed), in which the eyes turn out (Figure 25.2); or a hyperdeviation, which is a vertical misalignment of the eyes (Granet & Khayali, 2011). Strabismus may be apparent all the time or only intermittently, such as when the child tires. Strabismus is one cause of **amblyopia** or decreased vision in children younger than 9 years of age because the brain ignores the input from the deviated eye to prevent **diplopia,** or double vision. Misalignment of the eyes can result from excessive eye focusing, abnormalities in the nerves supplying the eye muscles or the eye muscles themselves, or damage to the brain regions controlling eye movement (Wright, 2007).

Esotropia can be divided into congenital, accommodative, or other causes (such as secondary to poor vision or acquired from a nerve or brain abnormality). Children with congenital esotropia have crossed eyes from birth or shortly thereafter that require early surgical correction. In accommodative esotropia, a child's eyes cross inward due to moderate or high levels of farsightedness. Excess focusing due to this farsightedness causes convergence. Eyeglasses that correct farsightedness decrease the excessive focusing and thus treat this form of esotropia. Neurological problems such as cerebral palsy may alter the brain's signals to the eye muscles and cause strabismus, which may ultimately require surgical correction. This is also true for the child with hydrocephalus, who may develop strabismus as a result of sixth nerve palsy caused by increased intracranial pressure.

Exotropia may be congenital, sensory, or intermittent in nature. Infants with constant exotropia (persisting after 3 months of age) often have contributing neurologic abnormalities and therefore warrant further evaluation. If there is poor vision in an eye, sensory exotropia may develop; this form may resolve if the vision improves or may require strabismus surgery. Intermittent exotropia is more common in the otherwise-healthy child and is often treated with glasses, patching, convergence exercises, or surgery (Figure 25.2).

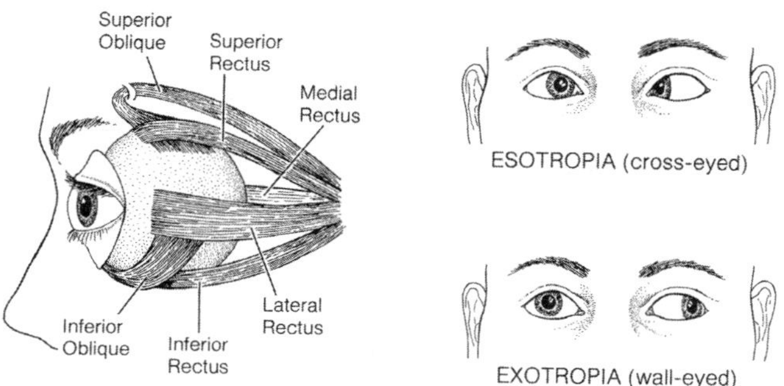

Figure 25.2. The eye muscles (left). Six muscles move the eyeball. A weakness of one of these muscles causes strabismus. In esotropia, the eye turns in, whereas in exotropia, the eye turns out. Esotropia and exotropia of the left eye are illustrated.

Nystagmus By 3–4 months of age a child has developed the ability to fixate on objects. Interruption of this early visual development results in nystagmus, an involuntary back-and-forth (most commonly horizontal) movement of the eyes. Albinism, congenital ocular diseases, and neurologic diseases can all result in nystagmus. Some children have idiopathic infantile nystagmus in which the eyes shake despite normal ocular and neurologic structures. This form is often inherited in an X-linked fashion, and the vision loss secondary to the nystagmus is mild and improves with time. Nystagmus can be latent (only present with occlusion of one eye) or manifest (constant). If the nystagmus is acquired or has atypical features such as rotatory or vertical components, then neurologic evaluation with neuroimaging should be considered, as some brain tumors may present with nystagmus (Papageorgiou, McLean, & Gottlob, 2014).

Abnormal Head Posture Abnormal head postures secondary to an ophthalmologic condition, such as strabismus, **ptosis,** refractive error (especially astigmatism), or nystagmus, is called ocular torticollis. Thus, children with tilted or turned heads should see an ophthalmologist as part of their evaluation. Children with nystagmus turn their head in order to place the eyes where they shake the least and vision is best (the "null point"). In children with strabismus, the eyes may be better aligned in a certain head posture, thus alleviating diplopia. Children with ptosis often lift their chin up to be able to see underneath their lowered upper eyelids.

Abnormal Color Vision Perception of colors can be disturbed for many reasons. Commonly, 1 in 12 males have red-green color deficiency, which is a genetic cause of decreased color perception passed down on the X chromosome. There are also many retinal and optic nerve pathologies that cause decreased color vision, often as an early sign of the disease. Achromotopsia is a serious retinal condition that can cause total loss of color vision.

Photophobia Many congenital and acquired forms of vision loss are associated with sensitivity to light. Severe photophobia can be seen in albinism, aniridia, achromotopsia, and certain corneal dystrophies requiring tinted lenses. It can also be a presenting sign of infantile glaucoma.

Blindness

The definition of blindness from a legal and federal educational perspective is visual acuity of 20/200 or worse in the better eye with correction or a limited visual field that subtends to an angle of not greater than 20 degrees instead of the usual 105 degrees (Individuals with Disabilities Education Improvement Act of 2004, PL 108-446). Individuals with low vision (partially sighted) are defined as having a visual acuity better than 20/200 but worse than 20/70 with correction. Both of these categories are considered visual impairments. People who are legally blind may have considerable useful vision; they may be able to distinguish light and dark, detect objects (20/500 to 20/800), or read enlarged print or regular print using magnification (20/200 to 20/500). Other people who are blind, however, cannot perceive the difference between light and dark. This profound loss of vision even affects circadian rhythms and can disrupt the sleep-wake cycle.

In the educational and rehabilitation fields, blindness is defined functionally as a degree of vision impairment that is so significant that vision cannot be used as the primary channel for learning. A person with low vision can use their vision as a primary channel for learning, but the individual may also need to use other modalities, such as auditory or tactile input, to assist.

PREVALENCE AND EPIDEMIOLOGY

Vision impairment may be due to easily treated causes, such as refractive error and amblyopia, or to more serious structural abnormalities of the eye and brain. Currently, among preschool-age children, 69% of impaired vision is due to uncorrected refractive error and 25% is due to bilateral amblyopia (Varma, Tarczy-Hornoch, & Jiang, 2017).

The leading causes of severe visual impairment in developed countries are cerebral (or cortical) visual impairment (CVI), optic nerve hypoplasia, and inherited retinal disorders. Retinopathy of prematurity (ROP), cataract, glaucoma, and nonaccidental trauma are the most common treatable or avoidable causes of vision loss. Blindness is far more prevalent in developing countries, mostly due to congenital anomalies and corneal opacification secondary to poor nutrition (vitamin A deficiency) and infections such as **trachoma** and onchocerciasis ("river blindness"; Solebo, Teoh, & Rahi, 2017). However, with improvements in nutrition and infectious disease control, there has been a recent shift with causes of visual impairment more mirroring those in developed countries (World Health Organization, 2007).

VISUAL DEFICIT IN CHILDREN WITH DISABILITIES

Many of the causes of developmental disabilities also influence the visual system, especially prematurity, cerebral palsy, brain injury, Down syndrome, and severe hearing loss. In fact, children with disability have a much higher rate of visual impairment (10.5%) than the general population (0.16%), and more than three quarters of visually impaired children have a significant nonophthalmic disorder (Salt & Sargent, 2014). Processes governing eye movement, alignment, visual acuity, and visual perception may mature slowly, partially, or abnormally in these children. Refractive errors, ocular misalignment, and eye movement disorders are especially common. Because of the links between developmental disabilities and vision problems, it is imperative that a pediatric ophthalmologist conduct an examination as part of the overall assessment for a child with a developmental disability. Treatment of these children must address all the disabilities and use all the senses and abilities that remain intact. A multidisciplinary approach involving a range of educational and health care professionals is essential.

ETIOLOGY AND ASSOCIATIONS WITH SPECIFIC DEVELOPMENTAL DISABILITIES

Refractive Error

Light entering the eye is focused by the cornea and lens. Under optimal conditions, light rays are perfectly refracted onto the retina, resulting in a clearly focused image. If the eye is too long or if the refracting mechanisms of the eye are too strong, the focused image falls in front of the retina, blurring the picture. This is called **myopia,** or nearsightedness. If the eye is too short or the refracting mechanisms are too weak, the image is focused behind the retina, also producing a blurred image. In this instance, the person has **hyperopia,** or farsightedness. The other common refractive problem is **astigmatism,** which typically occurs when the surface of the cornea or lens has an elliptical rather than spherical shape. Because of this, light rays entering the eye do not focus on a single point and the image is blurred (see Figure 25.3). A severe refractive error can impair the development of the visual system, affecting the child's interactions with the world. In children with disabilities, even small refractive errors may be corrected to optimize performance.

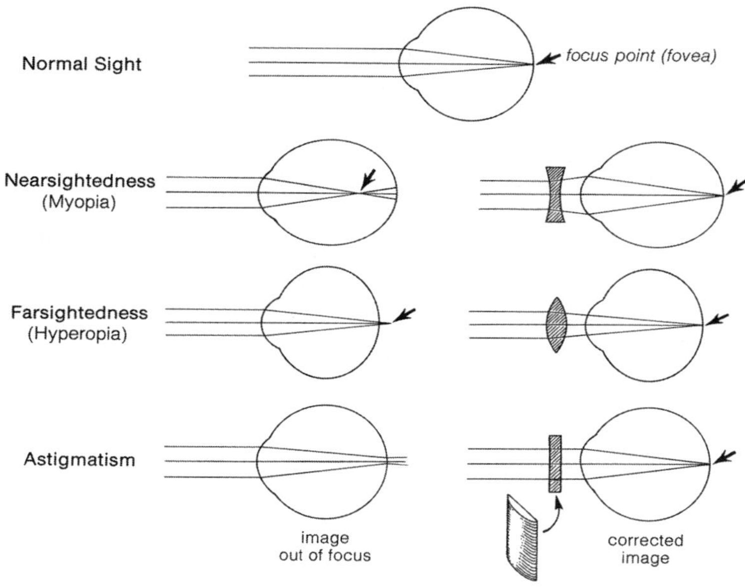

Figure 25.3. Refractive errors. If the eyeball is too long, images are focused in front of the retina (myopia). A concave lens deflects the rays, correcting the problem. If the eyeball is too short, the image focuses behind the retina and is again blurred (hyperopia). A convex lens corrects this. In astigmatism, the eyeball is the correct size, but typically the cornea is misshapen. A cylindrical lens is required to compensate.

Amblyopia

Until around age 9, the visual system remains immature and susceptible to a unique type of visual problem called **amblyopia.** Amblyopia is most often unilateral, in which case a structurally "healthy" eye does not see well because it is "turned off" or ignored by the brain. It is prevalent in 1%–3.5% of children and young adults (Gunton, 2013) and can result from deprivation (something obscuring the vision as seen in ptosis or cataract), strabismus, or refractive etiologies such as anisometropia (difference in refractive error between the two eyes) or high refractive error in both eyes.

Cerebral Visual Impairment

CVI is characterized by visual perceptual deficits due to disorders affecting the visual cortex and associated areas. The ophthalmologic examination may be completely normal, though CVI can occur in conjunction with ocular abnormalities as well. Causes include hypoxic ischemic encephalopathy, central nervous system malformations, neoplasia, infection, metabolic neurodegenerative disease, and underlying genetic causes (Solebo et al., 2017). Children with CVI present a variety of classic behaviors, and visual attention can range from mildly impaired to absent. Early on, parents note that their infant responds to light and dark but may not look directly at the parents' faces, even at 6 months of age. Later, when the child is more alert, the parents observe intermittent or brief visual tracking behavior. The child may "look over" items but not directly at them. Also, these children can see better peripherally if the object or they are moving. Visual function is often noted to improve with time in CVI, and visual stimulation therapies may improve visual function in some patients (Matsuba & Jan, 2006).

Optic Nerve Hypoplasia

In optic nerve hypoplasia (Figure 25.4), a smaller than normal optic nerve with impaired connection to the brain results in decreased vision uncorrectable with glasses. Midline structures in the brain can also be underdeveloped, including the pituitary gland. Children with unilateral or bilateral optic nerve hypoplasia should undergo neuroimaging, especially when there is poor growth, to rule out any abnormality in the pituitary gland that could result in a growth hormone deficiency or other hormonal imbalance. One of the most common causes of visual disability, optic nerve hypoplasia, is often associated with other developmental disabilities.

Optic Nerve Atrophy

Atrophy of the optic nerve (Figure 25.4) is any damage that occurs along the length of the nerve that results in

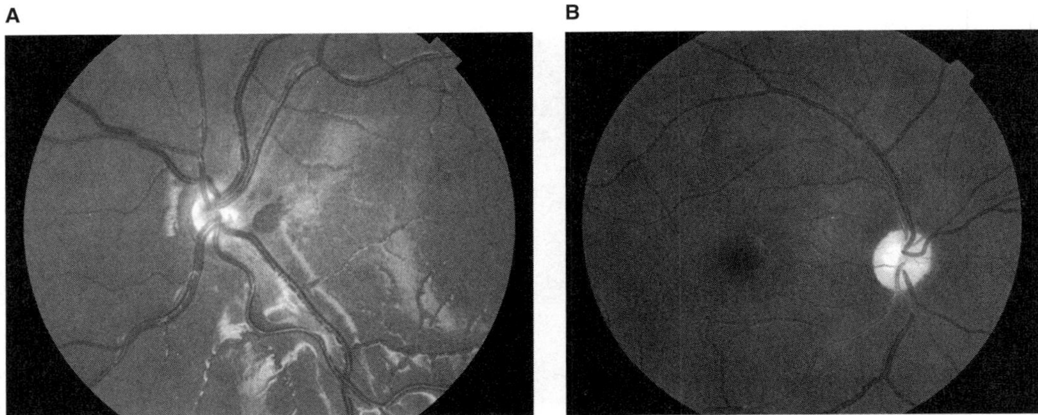

Figure 25.4. Photographs of optic nerve hypoplasia (congenitally small nerve) and optic nerve atrophy (pale, damaged nerve). (Photos courtesy of Carmelina Trimboli.)

decreased central, peripheral, or color vision. There are many causes of optic atrophy, including compression due to a tumor, hydrocephalus or trauma, ischemia, infection, hereditary causes, neurodegenerative etiologies, toxins, and nutritional deficiencies.

Retinopathy of Prematurity

In infants, the most common cause of retinal damage is ROP, as in the case of Mary (see Figure 25.5). The incidence of this condition is increasing as more premature infants worldwide survive due to advances in neonatology care. When an infant is born very early (gestational age 30 weeks or less) or born weighing less than 1,500 grams, it is at increased risk for developing ROP. Excess oxygen exposure to the still developing retinal vasculature, among other factors, can result in abnormal vessel growth and traction retinal detachment. Treatment of severe forms of ROP includes peripheral retinal laser; retinal detachment repair surgery; and, more recently, intraocular injection of antivascular endothelial growth factor, known as Avastin. The neonatology practice of limiting excessive oxygen supplementation can also reduce the risk of ROP (Sternberg & Durrani, 2018).

Despite treatment, children with ROP may have significant visual impairments. Nearly 50% of children

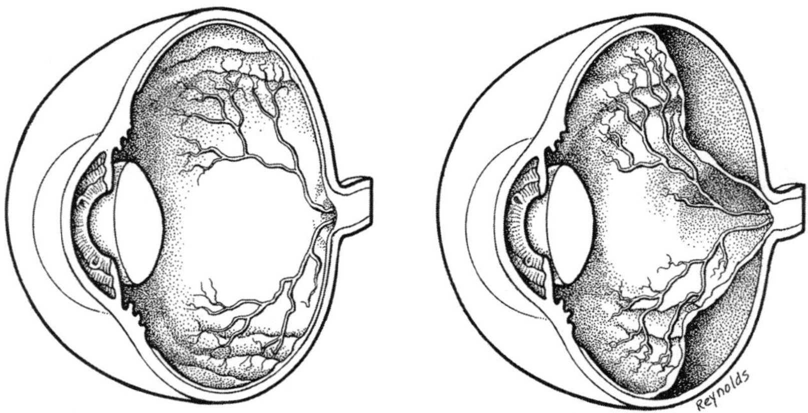

Figure 25.5. Retinopathy of prematurity. Blood vessels in the retina proliferate (left). Eventually they stop growing, leaving a fibrous scar that contracts in the most severe cases and pulls the retina away from the back of the eye, causing blindness (right). (From Batshaw, M. L., & Schaffer, D. B. [1991]. Vision and its disorders. In M.L. Batshaw, *Your child has a disability: A complete source book of daily and medical care* [p. 165]. Baltimore, MD: Paul H. Brookes Publishing Co., Inc. reprinted by permission. Copyright © 1991 by M.L. Batshaw; illustration copyright © 1991 by Lynn Reynolds. All rights reserved.)

born at 27 weeks' gestational age or less have been found to have subnormal visual acuity and/or strabismus (Haugen, Nepstad, Standal, Elgen, & Markestad, 2010). In addition, extremely low birth weight infants (those weighing less than 1,000 grams) are at increased risk of sustaining neurologic insults, such as intracerebral hemorrhage and periventricular leukomalacia, that further impact vision by causing CVI and optic atrophy. Infants born at younger gestational ages also more commonly have neurodevelopmental disabilities (Leversen et al., 2011), which can be compounded by the effects of ROP on vision.

Cataract

Cataract is a defect in lens clarity (see Figure 25.6). Although cataracts primarily develop during adulthood, they also occur in 0.01%–0.15% of children, accounting for about 8% of blindness in children living in developed countries (Liu, 2017). In developed countries, the majority of cataracts do not have a known etiology. However, in developing countries, preventable infections, such as prenatal rubella, account for a large proportion of childhood cataracts (Vinluan, Olveda, Olveda, Chy, & Ross, 2015). A cataract appears as an opacity in the pupil of one or both eyes. If severe and left untreated in childhood, it will cause deprivation amblyopia. All newborns are screened by their pediatrician, and any child with a suspected cataract should see a pediatric ophthalmologist promptly. A cataract may be an isolated abnormality or part of a syndrome or disease, in which case a referral for a genetics evaluation may be warranted. For example, children with certain inborn errors of metabolism (e.g., galactosemia), congenital infections (e.g., rubella), or eye trauma or who are taking certain medications may develop cataracts.

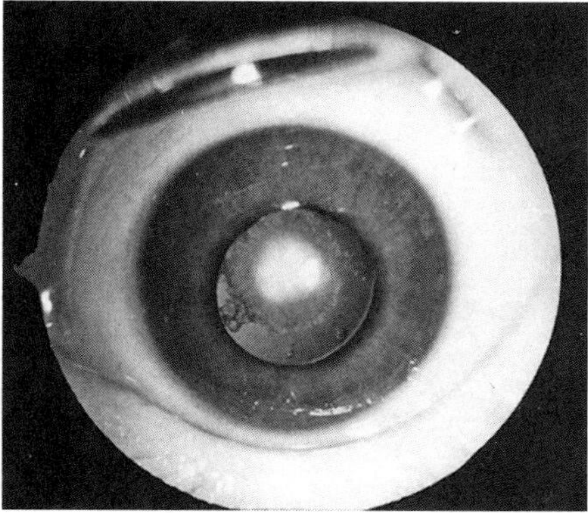

Figure 25.6. Photograph of a cataract; the lens opacity is seen through the pupil.

DIAGNOSIS AND CLINICAL MANIFESTATIONS

Pediatric Ophthalmology Exam

The pediatric eye exam begins in the waiting room. As the child is called to be examined, their visual function and head posture are assessed as they move into the room. Once in the room, a history is obtained from the caregivers and, if possible, the patient. Medical providers must pay close attention to the family ocular history, comorbidities, medications, visual functioning at home and school, and ocular concerns such as photophobia and ocular pain. Generally, depth perception is tested first, either via stereotesting with 3-D glasses or Worth 4 dot testing with red/green glasses. Next, a motility exam is performed at distance and near fixation to determine if strabismus is present. Visual acuity and color vision testing appropriate to the child's age and functioning level are then performed. In infants or nonverbal children, this may involve evaluating a response to light, the ability to fix on and follow an object, an optokinetic reflex with an optokinetic nystagmus spinning drum, and/or preferential looking. An external exam looking at the eyelids and surrounding structures is then performed. Pupils are evaluated with a swinging light test in light and dark conditions. An exam of the anterior segment, or front of the eye, is performed with either a penlight or, in more cooperative patients, a slit lamp to evaluate the cornea, conjunctiva, anterior chamber, iris, and lens. At this point, cycloplegic dilating drops are generally placed in each eye, and the patient must wait 40 minutes while the pupils dilate and accommodation relaxes. The child is then reexamined by the ophthalmologist with a **retinoscope** (a magnifying, streak light source) to determine, using lenses of varying powers, the refractive error. Eyeglasses can then be prescribed as needed. The final portion of the exam is a dilated fundus exam to evaluate the vitreous, retina, and optic nerve in each eye.

Diagnostic Studies

Beyond the pediatric ophthalmology exam, further diagnostic studies include visual field testing, optical coherence tomography (OCT), and visual electrophysiology

Visual Field Testing The visual field test is a method of measuring an individual's scope of vision. Visual field testing maps the peripheral visual fields of each eye individually. Because it is a subjective examination, requiring the patient to understand the testing instructions, it is very difficult to perform for young children or individuals with significant cognitive impairment. This testing is important, however, because visual field deficits can functionally interfere with learning and daily living even when visual acuity is normal.

Optical Coherence Tomography OCT is a more recent form of noninvasive imaging that uses the reflection of light to create high-resolution pictures and measurements of different parts of the eye, including the cornea, iris, retina, and optic nerve, to aid in diagnosis and monitor treatment of certain eye conditions (see Figure 25.7). It has become an invaluable tool for monitoring optic atrophy, as the thickness of the retinal nerve fiber layer, which is decreased in this condition, can be quantitatively measured and monitored over time.

Visual Electrophysiology Electrophysiological testing includes electroretinograms (ERGs) and visual evoked potentials (VEPs) to determine whether the vision problem lies primarily in the eyes or the brain (Almoqbel et al., 2008).

Electroretinogram An ophthalmologist may decide to obtain an ERG when the retina looks normal but vision is absent or very poor, as is sometimes seen in infants with nystagmus. The ERG tests retinal functioning by evaluating the quality of the response of retinal cells (rods and cones) to light stimuli. In ERG testing, modified contact lenses are placed on the corneas of the child after putting in topical anesthetic drops. Depending on the type of equipment used, one to three electrodes are also affixed to the face and/or body. Lights are momentarily flashed in the child's eyes under different conditions while a computer analyzes the information received from the electrodes and from leads attached to the contact lenses. This test may also be performed under anesthesia for children who would not tolerate wearing a contact lens while awake.

Visual Evoked Potential VEP testing is a form of EEG that focuses on the occipital lobe in order to determine if central visual function, from the macula to the occipital lobe, is intact. It is often used in the evaluation of possible CVI. It may also be considered in a patient with poor vision once an ERG indicates that the retina is functioning normally.

Impact on Communication, Psychosocial Skills, and Academics

One might expect severe visual impairment to result in lags in early childhood development. Studies that have examined these issues have indeed found developmental delays, but the delays appear to be dependent on the amount of residual vision and the presence or absence of associated developmental disabilities. The early development of children with vision better than 20/500 and with no other severe associated impairments may approximate that of sighted children. In addition, children with early developmental lags related to more severe visual impairments can catch up with their peers and function in the typical range by school age provided that there are no associated severe disabilities (e.g., cerebral palsy, intellectual disability,

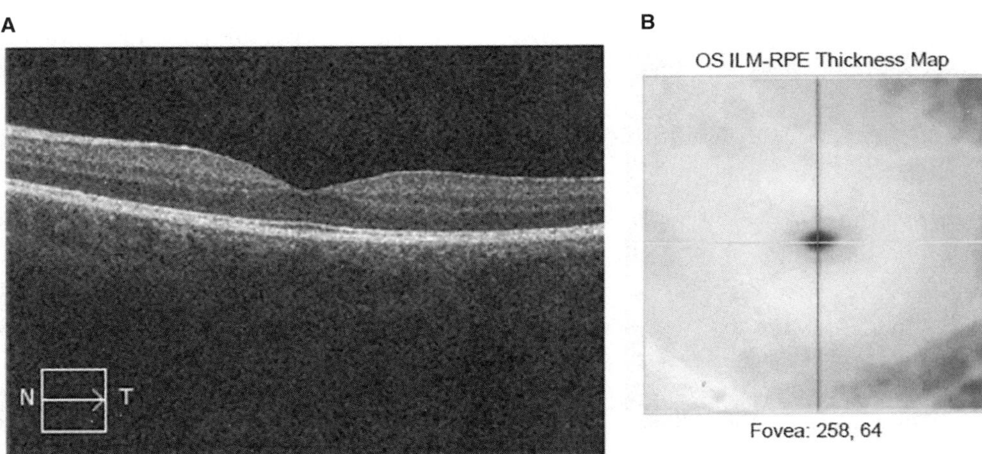

Figure 25.7. OCT image of the central part of the retina called the macula. On the left, the picture shows a slice through the retina with each layer visible. On the right is a color-coded retinal thickness map.

or hearing impairment). Approximately 30% of children with profound visual impairment are at risk of static or regressed cognitive development in the second year of life (Salt & Sargent, 2014). The origin of the visual loss (eye, optic nerve, or brain) does not seem to influence the degree of delay in milestone acquisition. Additionally, most tests of infant development are based primarily on performance of visual skills and may not be optimal in evaluating infants with severe visual impairment as they overestimate delay. Alternative developmental scales that are not visually based should therefore be used to help in evaluation and educational planning (Arzubi & Mambrino, 2010).

Motor Development Initially, an infant who is blind has similar motor activity to sighted infants, but by 2 months of age, they are noted to keep their head bent lower and have abnormal fidgety movements and ataxia. They keep their hands fisted and held at shoulder height until at least 5 months of age, later than sighted peers. Later in infancy, prewalking motor skills such as crawling and standing are also delayed, although the ability to sit occurs at a normal age. Walking, in the absence of other disabilities, is often delayed to 18 to 24 months of age. Visual impairment also affects fine motor skills and balance (Figure 25.8). Given that mobility is the main way that young children explore their environment, an associated motor delay can have an impact on cognitive and social development as well (Cuturi, Aggius-Vella, Campus, Parmiggiani, & Gori, 2016). Decreased motor development in visually impaired children correlates with being less physically fit. There is a higher rate of obesity than in sighted children age 6–12 years, and so promoting a healthy and active lifestyle in children with visual impairment is especially important (Houwen, Hartman, & Visscher, 2010).

Language Development Though infants who are blind may imitate sounds earlier than sighted infants, they may show delays in combining words to express their needs. However, in the child who is blind with average intelligence, speech and language reach typical levels by school age, although speech is accompanied by less body and facial "language" and conversation skills may be less developed. They may ask less questions and use adjectives less. Differences also surface in the use of words and difficulty with pragmatics and pronouns (e.g., saying "you" for "I"; Perez-Pereira & Conti-Ramsden, 1999). See Box 25.1 for more on the tie between language development and vision.

Psychosocial Development Being unable to establish eye contact with parents could have an impact on the infant's attachment and socialization skills. Preverbal communication, which is dependent on visual observation and imitation, could be delayed. It is interesting to note that the child with congenital blindness may be unaware of having an impairment until 4–5 years of age. In the school-age child, however, social skills impairments may be related to social isolation and poor self-image. Therefore, including a child in a program with

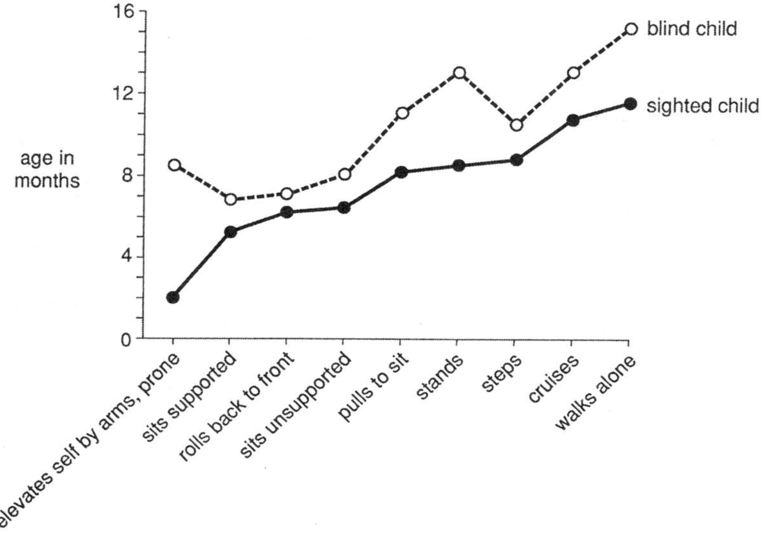

Figure 25.8. Age of attainment of motor skills in sighted and blind children. The motor development of a blind child is delayed. (From *Insights from the Blind: Comparative Studies of Blind and Sighted Infants* by Selma Fraiberg. Copyright © 1997. Reprinted by permission of Basic Books, an imprint of Hachette Book Group, Inc.)

BOX 25.1 EVIDENCE-BASED PRACTICE

Reading Disabilities and Vision

Dyslexia is a language-based reading disability present in approximately 20% of children that is often miscategorized as a vision problem. Though vision impairment may coexist with dyslexia, there is not a higher rate of vision problems among dyslexic children than the general population (Handler & Fierson, 2017). If vision is thought to be a contributing factor to reading difficulty by a child, their parents, or their educators, they should be referred to an ophthalmologist for evaluation and treatment. Dyslexic children should be treated by an educational therapist specializing in the application of phonics. Dyslexia treatments involving behavioral vision therapy, eye muscle exercises, or colored filters or lenses have not been scientifically proven to be efficacious (American Academy of Pediatrics, 2009).

typically developing children should include an agenda to promote socialization (Cochrane, Marella, Keeffe, & Lamoureux, 2011). Vision impairment is also correlated with high rates of mental health issues, especially anxiety, and the diagnosis of psychopathology and subsequent treatment may differ from patients with normal vision (Saisky, Hasid, Ebert, & Kosov, 2014).

MONITORING, SCREENING, AND EVAUATION

As vision impairment (e.g., amblyopia) is the most common potentially treatable disability of childhood, robust screening is necessary to correctly identify affected children and to ensure they are referred for treatment at a young age when vision can still be rehabilitated. With early childhood screening, the risk of persistent amblyopia at 7 years of age is cut in half. Unfortunately, currently less than one in five children receive adequate vision screening. Primary care providers should follow the American Academy of Pediatrics Policy Statement on eye examination guidelines (American Academy of Pediatrics, American Academy of Ophthalmology, American Association for Pediatric Ophthalmology and Strabismus, & American Association of Certified Orthoptists, 2015). Chapter 7 details these age-specific screening guidelines, which include evaluation for the normal and symmetric red reflex from both eyes spontaneously (the red reflex test), the corneal light reflex or cover test of ocular alignment, and developmentally appropriate visual acuity testing. Any child failing a visual screen should be directed to the care of a pediatric ophthalmologist.

Assessing the visual function of children with developmental disabilities is critical in determining the best interventions. It is important to spend time asking the caregivers from their perspective what the child can see or not see, as they observe the child in multiple lighting conditions and in different settings, as well as when the child is rested or tired. Of importance is that their assessment, while not scientific, is more than a one-time snapshot of visual ability. The caregiver's perspective combined with the clinical examination can better capture what the child actually sees, doesn't see, and what accommodations assist him or her to see better. Students who are blind or low vision undergo a formal "functional visual assessment" by a teacher of the visually impaired. This multidisciplinary perspective can be invaluable.

TREATMENT, MANAGEMENT, AND INTERVENTIONS

Refractive Error Correction

Glasses are the most common way refractive error is treated in childhood. If indicated, an ophthalmologist or optometrist (see Boxes 25.2 and 25.3) may prescribe glasses to their pediatric patient to improve vision, treat

BOX 25.2 INTERDISCIPLINARY CARE

Role of the Optometrist

Optometrists are health care professionals who are licensed to evaluate and treat vision changes by prescribing glasses or contact lenses. In some states, they may also treat medical eye conditions by prescribing eye drops. Some subspecialize to become developmental optometrists or low-vision specialists.

BOX 25.3 INTERDISCIPLINARY CARE

Role of Pediatric Ophthalmologist

Pediatric ophthalmologists are physicians who evaluate and treat children with visual or ocular complaints. They may prescribe glasses; treat amblyopia with patching or atropine drops; treat infections or inflammation with eye drops or systemic medications; and perform ocular and orbital surgeries, including strabismus surgery, cataract surgery, and glaucoma surgery. They also treat adults with strabismus despite being pediatric specialists.

amblyopia, or even correct eye crossing, as in accommodative esotropia. Getting a child to wear glasses at all can sometimes be a challenge, but most children adapt well after the first 2 weeks of wear. In certain cases, especially in far-sighted patients, an atropine eye drop may be prescribed in order to facilitate glasses acceptance. A properly fitting frame with a strap or comfort cables around the ears can help. For children with Down syndrome, Specs4us frames have been specifically developed to better fit their facial structure. For patients with severe photophobia, tinting the lenses can significantly improve visual function and comfort.

Contact lenses are less commonly used in childhood due to the difficulty inserting the lens in this population. However, there are certain high refractive error conditions that are best treated with contact lenses because the glasses would be simply too heavy for a child to wear. In aphakic children who have undergone cataract extraction at a young age and lack a lens, they often are prescribed "aphakic" contact lenses of high powers. Contact lenses may also be useful in patients with **aniridia,** or a congenital lack of a normal iris structure resulting in disabling photophobia. These tinted lenses help block excessive amounts of light from entering the eye, making the child with aniridia more comfortable.

There are many children who, due to a medical condition such as autism, do not tolerate wearing glasses at all. There is ongoing research to determine if laser refractive surgery, which is typically reserved for adult patients, is a safe and efficacious way to treat amblyogenic refractive error in this population (Stahl, 2017).

Amblyopia Treatment

Depending on the cause and degree of amblyopia, treatment may involve glasses, patching, or atropine penalization to blur the vision of the better-seeing eye, encouraging the brain to use and develop the vision of the amblyopic eye (Gunton, 2013). Ophthalmic surgery may be needed in cases of deprivational or strabismus amblyopia. If left untreated, amblyopia can lead to lifelong visual impairment. See Box 25.4 to learn more about recent research on amblyopia treatment.

Ophthalmic Surgeries

Surgery is sometimes necessary in order to improve vision or prevent further loss of vision. Cataract surgery may sometimes be performed as young as 1 month of age in order for vision to develop properly. When an eye is deviated and being ignored by the brain, as in strabismic amblyopia, strabismus surgery can help align the eye so that the brain starts using the

BOX 25.4 EVIDENCE-BASED PRACTICE

Amblyopia Treatment

Large-scale, multicentered, randomized trials by the Pediatric Eye Disease and Investigator Group have addressed many questions about amblyopia treatment. Results have shown that amblyopia treatment in general is highly successful, with resolution of amblyopia in approximately 75% of children (younger than 7 years old) when treated with patching or atropine, which were found to be equally equivalent treatment modalities. When either patching or atropine penalization fails to improve vision further, switching to the other treatment modality should be attempted. Surprisingly, almost half of older children (13–17 years of age) with previously untreated amblyopia had improvement (10 or more letters) with treatment despite being several years past the classically defined period of visual development (Gunton, 2013).

eye again. Strabismus surgery may also be performed to straighten a child's head posture in cases of ocular torticollis. Glaucoma surgery is necessary when the eye pressure is elevated to prevent damage to the optic nerve and subsequent blindness if left untreated. When the eyelid is droopy and covering the pupil ("**ptosis**"), vision can only develop properly when the eyelid is surgically elevated. This surgery may be done in infancy, like cataract surgery, so that the vision can develop prior to permanent poor vision and nystagmus setting in after 3 months of age.

Genetic Advances

Clinical trials are currently evaluating targeted gene-replacement therapy for genetic forms of visual impairment in which a normal copy of a patient's defective gene is introduced under the retina by a viral carrier. Clinical studies replacing the *RPE65* gene in patients with retinitis pigmentosa have shown improved visual function, and this is now an available therapy for patients over 12 months of age (Russell et al., 2017). Other forms of inherited blindness, such as Leber's hereditary optic neuropathy, are being studied for possible gene therapy treatments as well.

Low-Vision Aids

If vision remains poor after vision has been optimized through the use of glasses, amblyopia treatment, or indicated surgeries, low-vision aids become essential tools for a child to function well at school and home. Low-vision aids can be divided into three categories; optical, nonoptical, and electronic. For severe vision loss, braille and certain orientation and mobility techniques are essential for education and daily living. (See Box 25.5 to learn about low-vision specialists.)

Optical Optical aids can be divided based on their use for near- or distance-vision activities. For near-vision activities like reading, magnifiers can be single vision spectacle (glasses), handheld, stand, or dome type. Depending on a child's other disabilities, certain magnifiers may work better than others; for instance, if a child has poor motor control, a handheld magnifier may be difficult to use, although a stand or dome magnifier might work well. For distance vision, one may use an extra-short-focus monocular telescope, and these may be either handheld or spectacle mounted. (See Figure 25.9 for examples of low-vision aids.)

Nonoptical Depending on how reduced a patient's vision is, the font size of their work may need to be enlarged. The American Foundation for the Blind recommends using an 18-point or higher font size, nondecorative font styles such as Arial, and bold print, as well as avoiding all caps and italicized letters. Spacing should be at least 1.5 spaces between each line, and reading material on glossy paper should be avoided.

A reading stand or slant board can be very useful for low-vision patients to bring their work closer to their eyes so that they do not have to lean over a flat table. Moreover, a person with low vision may need three times as much light as a person with typical sight. A gooseneck lamp can be useful to bring the light close to the material being viewed. It should be positioned on the same side as the viewing eye if a patient is monocular, and it should not be shining toward the patient's eyes, as that may cause glare.

Glare in some low-vision patients can significantly decrease their visual function. Glasses and contact lenses can be made with varying degrees of tint to improve this. Simple measures like side shields on glasses, wearing a hat, and lighting placement can also reduce glare. Lastly, a typoscope is a piece of durable black plastic with a central cut out section placed over reading material to aid in reading by eliminating glare from the surrounding white page, allowing the user to focus on the desired text. It can be especially useful in patients with hemianopia who have lost half of their visual field.

BOX 25.5 INTERDISCIPLINARY CARE

Role of the Low-Vision Specialist

Low-vision specialists are optometrists or ophthalmologists who work with low-vision patients to evaluate their vision impairment and recommend appropriate optical and nonoptical low-vision aids. They also train their patients how to use each different aid. They may work closely with rehabilitation teachers, orientation/mobility specialists, and occupational therapists to help their patients function visually to the best of their ability.

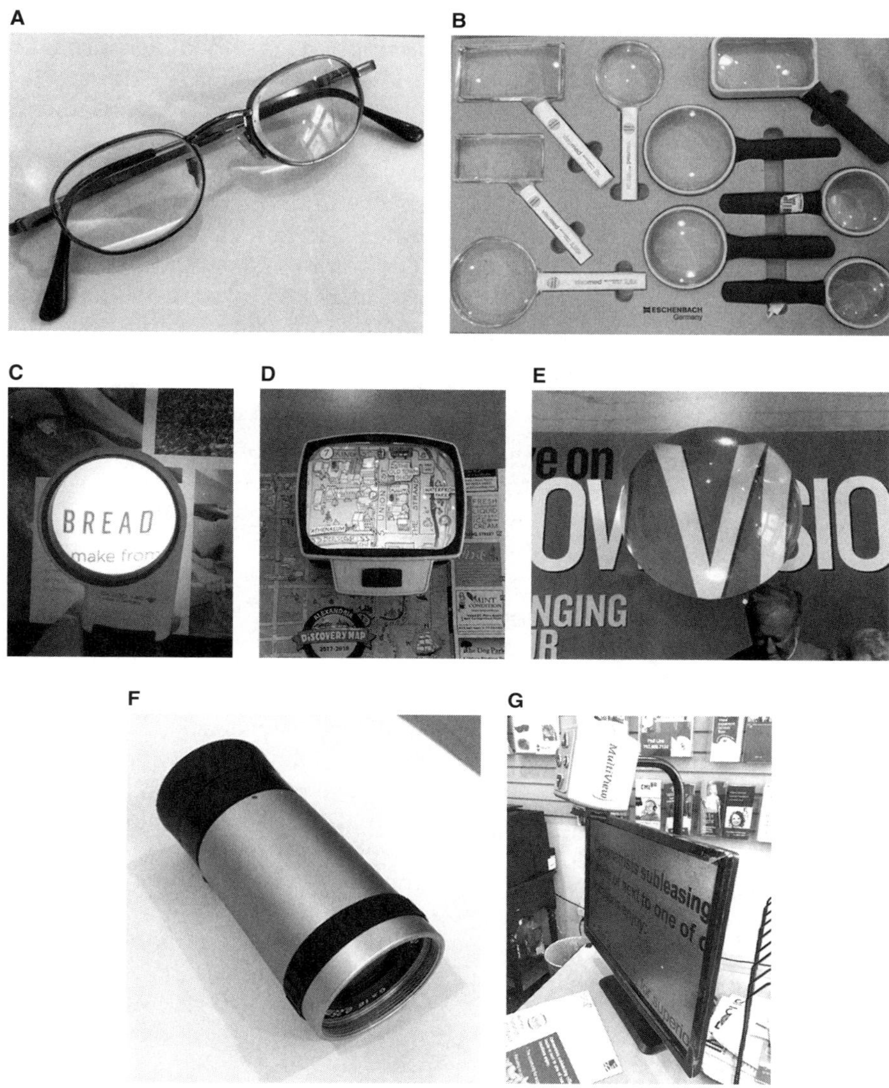

Figure 25.9. Low-vision aids include the following: A) single-vision spectacle magnifier glasses, B) handheld magnifiers, C) handheld magnifier with LED light, D) stand magnifier, E) dome magnifier, F) handheld monocular telescope, G) video magnifier.

Electronic Individuals with severe visual impairment greatly benefit from the omnipresence of computers in today's society. Voice-recognition software permits individuals to input instructions and dictate to computer applications. In addition, there are various devices that "talk," including calculators, clocks, computers, and other assistive technology devices that provide auditory information. Closed-circuit televisions, electronic readers, and high-contrast monitors can be very useful in the education and daily living of the school-age child with low vision. Large-print computer programs, such as ZoomText, enlarge and enhance images and writing on a computer or tablet screen. Screen readers are software programs that convert digital text into speech or braille output (Benedict & Baumgardner, 2009).

Communities are also becoming more accessible to individuals with visual impairment by implementing elevators that announce floors, crosswalk indicators that beep when it is safe to cross the street, and ramps. The use of personal global positioning system (GPS) software is also beneficial, as it supplements use of a mobility cane. A new technology called Aira uses video-equipped smart glasses, artificial intelligence, and live, remote human assistance to help low-vision patients navigate their environment and is being offered in some grocery stores and on college campuses.

Braille Although some children will succeed best with optical aids and devices and large-print books or electronic readers, others, especially those with severe vision loss (20/400 or worse), may succeed best with braille or a combination of learning media referred to as dual media. Braille is a code formed from a series of raised dots on a page that are read from left to right, as print is read visually (Massof, 2009). Readiness for braille begins in kindergarten (Roth & Fee, 2011). Fine motor skills and tactile sensitivity skills are developed first as these are essential in the learning process. When the child is able to recognize small shapes, differentiate between rough and smooth, and follow a line of small figures across a page, the learning of the braille alphabet can begin.

Children with severe visual impairments should also learn to type on a computer. Braille keyboards exist in two forms: a pure braille keyboard and a conventional QWERTY keyboard with braille keys. Digital text can be converted to braille on a refreshable braille display. In addition, a wide variety of books on tape are available from Recording for the Blind & Dyslexic (see http://www.rfbd.org) and from bookstores and libraries. It is critical that a visually impaired child has all of the equipment necessary for learning and independence and that is appropriate for their particular needs. With these tools, children with severe visual impairments are better equipped to succeed in the general education environment.

Orientation and Mobility Techniques As soon as an infant is diagnosed with a severe visual impairment, he or she should be entered into an early intervention program, including working with an orientation and mobility specialist. The focus should be to increase skills in other senses, to improve body concept and awareness, and to promote locomotion and active exploration of the environment (Roman-Lantzy, 2007).

While awake, infants should be placed on their stomach rather than on their back to strengthen neck and trunk muscles. The young child with a severe visual impairment must explore the world through touch and sound. Brain imaging studies have shown that in people who are blind from an early age, the visual cortex can be used for processing tactile and auditory information (Theoret, Merabet, & Pascual-Leone, 2004). Therefore, parents and therapists should place or store textured and sound-producing toys at a height the child can reach. If there is any usable vision, the child should be encouraged to take advantage of it; bright colors should be used, and the child's vision and attention should be directed verbally toward them (Holbrook, McCarthy, & Kamei-Hannan, 2017). It is very important for the parents, teachers, and therapists to verbally cue the child with information prior to being touched/handled in order to eliminate any resistance to touch (tactile defensiveness; Downing & Chen, 2003). The child's name should be used frequently to encourage inclusion in conversations and to ensure that the child will respond to questions in the absence of verbal cues. There also should be a verbal explanation before, during, and after a task is performed (Ferrell, 1984). While the child is moving from one space to another, the purpose of the move and the orientation of the space should be explained.

Orientation encompasses such skills as laterality and directionality. For visually impaired children, there are three main devices used for orientation and mobility training: precanes, powered mobility devices, and virtual reality technology. Precanes can include simple doll strollers or kiddie canes to help a child who is blind navigate their environment, getting auditory and tactile feedback as they move around. Powered mobility devices, frequently used in cerebral palsy, can have utility for children as early as 3 years of age. Virtual reality technology ("BLINDAID") has been developed to train the vision impaired, using auditory, thermal and sensory feedback to improve mobility in a safe but realistic environment. For older children, Ultrabike, which uses ultrasound technology to help the visually impaired cyclist navigate, has been developed (Cuturi et al., 2016).

Vision Therapy

There are many different types of vision therapy available today. Orthoptic vision therapy involves eye exercises to treat eye movement abnormalities, especially convergence insufficiency. A common exercise is a pencil pushup, where a patient focuses on an object as it is brought repeatedly toward their nose in order to improve their ability to converge, or turn, their eyes inward. Behavioral/perceptual vision therapy is performed by developmental optometrists to improve visual perception and processing; however, thus far, this has not been scientifically proven to be effective treatment. Vision therapy for correction of myopia is another recent field within optometry that uses special contact lenses, bifocal glasses, and dilute atropine drops to slow progression of near-sightedness. Its long-term utility is yet unknown. (See Box 25.6 to learn more about the role of the vision therapist.)

BOX 25.6 INTERDISCIPLINARY CARE

Role of the Vision Therapist

Vision therapy is a subset of optometry that can be described as physical therapy for the visual system. It involves an optometrist-led program of certain visual activities to treat certain visual problems. It may include the use of prisms, lenses ("training glasses"), filters, computer programs, balance boards, and metronomes, among other things. There is controversy regarding this field as behavioral vision therapy has been scientifically unproven.

OUTCOMES

Outcomes for the child with severe visual impairment depends on the amount of residual vision, the presence of associated disabilities, the motivation of the child and family, and the skills of the child's teachers and therapists. With severe visual impairment, there may be effects on overall health, self-perception, educational attainment, occupational choices, and other social factors (Davidson & Quinn, 2011). In general, less severe visual impairment and the absence of associated disabilities predict typical development and good outcomes for independence and occupational success. Early intervention and adequate support can help a visually impaired child lead an independent and successful life.

SUMMARY

- Vision impairment arises from a defect in ocular structures, the optic nerve, the visual cortex, or a combination of these areas.
- Vision disorders may result in strabismus (esotropia, exotropia, or vertical eye misalignment), nystagmus, an abnormal head posture, abnormal color vision, or photophobia.
- The most common causes of severe visual impairment include CVI, optic nerve hypoplasia, and inherited retinal disorders.
- Children with developmental disabilities are more likely to have visual impairment.
- Severe visual impairment can have an effect on motor, language, and psychosocial development.
- Vision may be improved with refractive error correction, amblyopia treatment, ophthalmic surgery, or gene replacement therapy.
- Low-vision aids include optical and nonoptical aids, electronic devices, braille, and orientation and mobility techniques.

ADDITIONAL RESOURCES

American Foundation for the Blind (AFB): http://www.afb.org

National Federation of the Blind: http://www.nfb.org

National Library Service for the Blind and Physically Handicapped: http://www.loc.gov/nls.

Additional resources can be found online in Appendix D: Childhood Disabilities Resources, Services, and Organizations (see About the Online Companion Materials).

REFERENCES

Almoqbel, F., Leat, S. J., & Irving, E. (2008). The technique, validity and clinical use of the sweep VEP. *Ophthalmic and Physiological Optics, 5,* 393–403.

American Academy of Pediatrics, American Academy of Ophthalmology, American Association for Pediatric Ophthalmology and Strabismus, & American Association of Certified Orthoptists. (2009). *Policy statement: Learning disabilities, dyslexia, and vision.* Retrieved from http://pediatrics.aappublications.org/content/124/2/837.full

American Academy of Pediatrics, American Academy of Ophthalmology, American Association for Pediatric Ophthalmology and Strabismus, & American Association of Certified Orthoptists. (2015). *Policy statement: Visual system assessment in infants, children, and young adults by pediatricians.* Retrieved from http://pediatrics.aappublications.org/content/early/2015/12/07/peds.2015-3596

Arzubi, E. F., & Mambrino, E. (2010). *A guide to neuropsychological testing for health care professionals.* New York, NY: Springer.

Batshaw, M. L., & Schaffer, D. B. (1991). Vision and its disorders. In M.L. Batshaw, *Your child has a disability: A complete source book of daily and medical care* (pp. 161–178). Baltimore, MD: Paul H. Brookes Publishing Co.

Benedict, R. E., & Baumgardner, A. M. (2009). A population approach to understanding children's access to assistive technology. *Disability Rehabilitation, 31*(7), 582–592.

Cochrane, G. M., Marella, M., Keeffe, J. E., & Lamoureux, E. L. (2011). The Impact of Vision Impairment for Children (IVI_C): Validation of a vision-specific pediatric quality-of-life questionnaire using Rasch analysis. *Investigative Ophthalmology and Visual Science, 52*(3), 1632–1640.

Cuturi, L. F., Aggius-Vella, E., Campus, C., Parmiggiani, A., & Gori, M. (2016). From science to technology: Orientation and mobility in blind children and adults. *Neuroscience & Biobehavioral Reviews, 71*, 240–251.

Davidson, S., & Quinn, G. E. (2011). The impact of pediatric vision disorders in adulthood. *Pediatrics, 127*(2), 334–339.

Downing, J. E., & Chen, D. (2003). Using tactile strategies with students who are blind and have severe disabilities. *TEACHING Exceptional Children, 36*(2), 56–61.

Dufresne, D., Dagenais, L., & Shevell, M. I. (2014). Spectrum of visual disorders in a population-based cerebral palsy cohort. *Pediatric Neurology, 50*(4), 324–328.

Ferrell, K. A. (1984). *Parenting preschoolers: Suggestions for raising young blind and visually impaired children*. New York, NY: AFB Press.

Fieß, A., Kölb-Keerl, R., Schuster, A. K., Knuf, M., Kirchhof, B., Muether, P. S., & Bauer, J. (2017). Prevalence and associated factors of strabismus in former preterm and full-term infants between 4 and 10 years of age. *BMC Ophthalmology, 17*(1). doi:10.1055/s-0043-118852

Fraiberg, S. (1977). *Insights from the blind: Comparative studies of blind and sighted infants*. New York, NY: Basic Books.

Granet, D. B., & Khayali, S. (2011). Amblyopia and strabismus. *Pediatric Annals, 40*(2), 89–94.

Gunton, K. B. (2013). Advances in amblyopia: What have we learned from PEDIG trials? *Pediatrics, 131*(3), 540–547.

Handler, S. M., & Fierson, W. M. (2017). Reading difficulties and the pediatric ophthalmologist. *Journal of American Association for Pediatric Ophthalmology and Strabismus, 21*(6), 436–442.

Haugen, O. H., Nepstad, L., Standal, O. A., Elgen, I., & Markestad, T. (2010). Visual function in 6 to 7 year-old children born extremely preterm: A population-based study. *Acta Ophthalmology,* Advance online publication. doi:10.1111/j.1755-3768.2010.02020.x

Holbrook, M. C., McCarthy, T., & Kamei-Hannan, C. (2017). *Foundations of education*. New York, NY: AFB Press.

Houwen, S., Hartman. E., & Visscher, C. (2010). The relationship among motor proficiency, physical fitness, and body composition in children with and without visual impairments. *Research Quarterly Exercise in Sport, 81*(3), 290–299.

Individuals with Disabilities Education Improvement Act of 2004, PL 108–446, 20 U.S.C. §§ 1400 *et seq.*

Leversen, K. T., Sommerfelt, K., Rønnestad, A., Kaaresen, P. I., Farstad, T., Skranes, J., . . . Markestad, T. (2011). Prediction of neurodevelopmental and sensory outcome at 5 years in Norwegian children born extremely preterm. *Pediatrics, 127*(3), e630–e638.

Liu, Y. (2017). *Pediatric lens diseases*. Singapore: Springer Verlag.

Massof, R. W. (2009). The role of Braille in the literacy of blind and visually impaired children. *Archives in Ophthalmology, 127*(11), 1530–1531.

Matsuba, C. A., & Jan, J. E. (2006). Long-term outcome of children with cortical visual impairment. *Developmental Medicine & Child Neurology, 48*(6), 508.

Papageorgiou, E., Mclean, R. J., & Gottlob, I. (2014). Nystagmus in childhood. *Pediatrics & Neonatology,* 55(5), 341–351.

Perez-Pereira, M., & Conti-Ramsden, G. (1999). *Language development and social interaction in blind children*. Philadelphia, PA: Psychology Press.

Roman-Lantzy, C. (2007). *Cortical visual impairment: An approach to assessment and intervention*. New York, NY: American Foundation for the Blind Press.

Roth, G. A., & Fee, E. (2011). The invention of Braille. *American Journal of Public Health, 101*(3), 454.

Russell, S., Bennett, J., Wellman, J. A., Chung, D. C., Yu, Z., Tillman, A., . . . Maguire, A. M. (2017). Efficacy and safety of voretigene neparvovec (AAV2-hRPE65v2) in patients with RPE65-mediated inherited retinal dystrophy: A randomised, controlled, open-label, phase 3 trial. *The Lancet, 390*(10097), 849–860.

Saisky, Y., Hasid, S., Ebert, T., & Kosov, I. (2014). Issues in psychiatric evaluation of children and adolescents with visual impairment. *Harefuah, 153(2),* 109–112, 125.

Salt, A., & Sargent, J. (2014). Common visual problems in children with disability. *Archives of Disease in Childhood, 99*(12), 1163–1168.

Solebo, A. L., Teoh, L., & Rahi, J. (2017). Epidemiology of blindness in children. *Archives of Disease in Childhood, 102*(9), 853-857.

Stahl, E. D. (2017). Pediatric refractive surgery. *Current Opinion in Ophthalmology, 28*(4), 305–309.

Sternberg, P., & Durrani, A. K. (2018). AJO Centennial: Evolving concepts in the management of retinopathy of prematurity. *American Journal of Ophthalmology, 186,* xxiii–xxxii.

Theoret, H., Merabet, L., & Pascual-Leone, A. (2004). Behavioral and neuroplastic changes in the blind: Evidence for functionally relevant cross-modal interactions. *Journal of Physiology, 98,* 221–233.

Varma, R., Tarczy-Hornoch, K., & Jiang, X. (2017). Visual impairment in preschool children in the United States. *JAMA Ophthalmology, 135*(6), 610.

Vinluan, M. L., Olveda, R. M., Olveda, D. U., Chy, D., & Ross, A. G. (2015). Access to essential paediatric eye surgery in the developing world: A case of congenital cataracts left untreated. *BMJ Case Reports, 2015*(April 22). doi:10.1136/bcr-2014-208197.

Wright, K. W. (2007). *Pediatric ophthalmology for primary care* (3rd ed.). Elk Grove Village, IL: American Academy of Pediatrics.

World Health Organization. (2007). *Global initiative for the elimination of avoidable blindness: Action plan 2006-2011.* Retrieved from http://apps.who.int/iris/handle/10665/43754

CHAPTER 26 Deaf/Hard of Hearing Plus

Susan E. Wiley

Upon completion of this chapter, the reader will

- Recognize that risk factors that contribute to a higher likelihood of hearing loss are more prevalent in children with disabilities than in the general population
- Understand adaptations for testing that are helpful in children who are Deaf/hard of hearing and who are suspected as having a developmental disability
- Identify resources for children who are Deaf/hard of hearing Plus (those with developmental or medical complexities)

Children who are Deaf/hard of hearing (D/HH) are at higher risk than the general population to have developmental disabilities (Boyle et al., 2011; Gallaudet Research Institute, 2011). It is understandable that clinicians and parents may attribute a child's delays to the presence of hearing loss. However, this view can contribute to delays in the identification of developmental needs and can lengthen the time it takes to access broader supports, strategies, and expertise beyond those focusing on deafness. When children experience delays in accessing effective supports, they lose some of the recognized benefits of early intervention (Kennedy et al., 2006). In this chapter, the reader will learn more about factors that place children who are D/HH at greater risk for developmental disabilities, and approaches to the recognition and identification of developmental needs will be discussed. While resources for children who are D/HH with a developmental disability are limited, the chapter will provide guidance on resources for various developmental needs and family support.

CASE STUDY

Abigail is a 9-year-old girl with partial trisomy 9 and intellectual disability. Her family notices that she sits near the television and often asks "What?" when she is spoken to. Her teachers have indicated that she seems more distractible and is not able to get started on work without direct support. When sent for updated vision and hearing testing, Abigail was found to have a bilateral moderately severe sensorineural hearing loss. Upon review of her early history, it was noted that she had received a broad workup, including an evaluation for congenital infections and genetic syndromes at birth because of microcephaly and small-for-gestational-age growth parameters. Genetic testing had revealed a partial trisomy 9; in addition, her urine culture for cytomegalovirus (CMV) was positive. The critical issue in this case is that while Abigail had received an appropriate evaluation at birth, her partial trisomy had overshadowed the other needs related to her care; therefore, she did not receive the hearing monitoring normally recommended for a congenital CMV infection.

Thought Questions:

How are evaluations of hearing and developmental function made more complex when the child has a disability? What factors contribute to failing to notice hearing loss in children with developmental disabilities?

DEFINITIONS, DESCRIPTIONS, AND CLASSIFICATIONS

In the pursuit of the universal use of respectful and person-first language, it is helpful to begin with an understanding of the Deaf culture. *Merriam-Webster's Dictionary and Thesaurus* (2014) includes a number of definitions of the term *culture,* two of which are the following:

1. The customary beliefs, social forms, and material traits of a racial, religious, or social group; also, the characteristic features of everyday existence (such as diversions or a way of life) shared by people in a place or time.
2. The integrated pattern of human knowledge, belief, and behavior that depends upon the capacity for learning and transmitting knowledge to succeeding generations.

In regard to the Deaf community, shared experiences and a shared language are at the foundation of Deaf culture. Furthermore, most individuals who are D/HH have different experiences than their biologic family (Solomon, 2012). In this way, access to a community with similar experiences strengthens the relevance of cultural affiliation for many individuals.

The affiliation with the Deaf community is conveyed with the capital *D* in Deaf. When the lowercase *d* is used, it is indicative of a degree of hearing loss rather than a cultural affiliation. With this framework, Deafness is not viewed as a disability, but rather a unique way of experiencing the world. It is not a problem to fix or something that is missing. When a person has never experienced the world in any different way, it becomes part of his/her identity. This is different than in people who have had hearing much of their life and lose it. For this group of people, hearing loss is more likely viewed as a problem or disability.

There are a number of resources on Deaf culture that can help in beginning to understand this framework (Holcomb, 2012; Holt & Garey, 2007; Humphries & Padden, 1990). Still, it is important to recognize that not all individuals who are D/HH consider themselves members of the Deaf community. These individuals may use the term *hard of hearing* (HH) to describe themselves. Individuals who are HH also have common experiences (Holt & Garey, 2007; Zazove, 1993).

This chapter focuses on *Deaf/hard of hearing Plus,* a term used to convey a respectful perspective for those who are D/HH and have developmental or medical complexities. Candace Lindow-Davies, a mother and active advocate within the national organization Hands and Voices (http://www.cohandsandvoices.org/plus/index.html) helps frame this definition, noting:

> Deaf/HH Plus is meant to be a positive term, not in any way negative or insensitive to the child who has medical issues along with hearing loss. In fact, I see it as an "A+" or "B+," meaning the child carries additional positive qualities. But it is a gift that needs to be carefully unwrapped. And it may not appear to be a gift when you first receive it. Time helps you appreciate, understand and unfold the possibilities. And the "Plus" most often means the child and family has added responsibilities and requires additional expertise. (Lindow-Davies & Kennedy, 2013)

Salient to the discussion of Deaf/HH Plus is the definition of the term *Deaf-blindness.* Deaf-blindness, without explanation, may seem to indicate that a person would have no hearing and no vision. This is not the case. Deaf-blindness is a term that indicates hearing loss of any type or degree and vision impairment that is not correctible. This combination of sensory loss impacts a person's access to communication and learning.

The term *Deaf-blindness* as a label is used to determine service needs across states and educational systems. There is a large discrepancy between census data on Deaf-blindness obtained from U.S. federally funded state Deaf-blind projects and data within special education settings collected by the Office of Special Education Programs (National Center on DeafBlindness, 2016). Data from the 2015 U.S. Department of Education (Office of Special Education Programs 2015 Part B special education child count) identified 1,442 students (3–21 years of age) with an educational category of Deaf-blind. This number is approximately 16% of the 8,979 children (3–21 years of age) identified by the 2016 National Child Center for Deaf-Blindness census.

PREVALENCE AND EPIDEMIOLOGY

D/HH is identified by newborn hearing screening and screening throughout childhood. D/HH occurs at different levels of hearing loss (see Table 26.1). Up to 40%–50% of children who are D/HH have developmental and behavioral needs (Boyle et al., 2011; Chilosi

Table 26.1. Levels of hearing loss by severity

Degree of hearing loss	Hearing loss range (dB HL)
Normal	10–15
Slight	16–25
Mild	26–40
Moderate	41–55
Moderately severe	56–70
Severe	71–90
Profound	91+

From Clark, J. G. (1981). Uses and abuses of hearing loss classification. *ASHA*, *23*, 493–500.

et al., 2010; Gallaudet Research Institute, 2011) that are not a direct result of hearing loss. This rate is higher than in the general population (Table 26.2). Conditions and risk factors associated with hearing loss can also be associated with a risk for developmental disabilities. Examples of risk factors for coexisting developmental disabilities and hearing loss include syndromes, congenital infections, and the need for neonatal intensive care (Joint Committee on Infant Hearing, 2007; see Table 26.2).

While the focus of this chapter is on children who are D/HH Plus, it is important to recognize that hearing loss has often been underrecognized in individuals with intellectual disability (Hey et al., 2014; Russ, Kenney, & Kogan, 2013) and other developmental disabilities. Among a large group of participants in the Special Olympics with intellectual disability who received hearing screening, 60% required follow-up and treatment (Hey et al., 2014). While this included middle ear disease and transient conductive hearing loss, Hey and collaborators noted the importance for ongoing surveillance for fluctuating and progressive hearing loss in children and adults with intellectual disability.

Table 26.2. Percent of the types of disabilities in the Deaf/hard of hearing (HH) and general populations

Type of disability	Within deaf/HH	Within general population
No disability	60%	86%
Cognitive (intellectual disability)	8.3%	0.71%
Cerebral palsy and motor disabilities	8%	0.3%
Blindness and vision impairment	5.6%	0.13%
Attention-deficit/hyperactivity disorder	5.4%	7%
Specific learning disability	8%	4.5%
Autism spectrum disorder	1.7%–7%	1.1%

Sources: Boyle et al. (2011); Gallaudet Research Institute (2011); Reid et al. (2011); Szymanski, Brice, Lam, and Hotto (2012); Thomas, Sanders, Doust, Beller, and Glasziou (2015); and Van Naarden et al. (2015).

In population data on younger children, Russ and colleagues (2013) performed an analysis of the 2005–2006 National Survey of Children with Special Health Care Needs. Within the cross-sectional data on 40,723 children from birth to 17 years of age, 5% of children with an intellectual disability used hearing aids.

There is limited literature describing hearing loss among children with an autism spectrum disorder (ASD). Population data from the Centers for Disease Control and Prevention identified a rate of hearing loss of 1.3 per 1,000 children with ASD who were 8 years old (Kancherla, Van Naarden Braun, & Yeargin-Allsopp, 2013). A systematic review evaluating the prevalence of hearing loss among children with ASD noted challenges with study methodology, sample sizes, and inclusion criteria (Beers, McBoye, Kakande, Dar Santos, & Kozak, 2014). In the studies included in this systematic review, rates of hearing loss in children with ASD ranged from 0%–10%. It is likely that the rate of hearing loss in the general population would be found among children with ASD. Data from the general population suggest that hearing loss (any degree of permanent hearing loss, unilateral or bilateral) occurs in 1 to 3 out of 1,000 children at birth (Boyle et al., 2011; Centers for Disease Control and Prevention, 2010), with an increase of 6 to 12 per 1,000 school-age children (Goman & Lin, 2016).

In children with ASD, it can be challenging to obtain ear-specific and reliable behavioral audiometric information. Fitzpatrick, Lambert, Whittingham, and Leblanc (2014) described a hospital-based group of children with ASD and hearing loss. For children who had not participated in newborn hearing screening, the age of identification of hearing loss ranged from 16 months to over 7 years. This group had evidence of late-onset and progressive hearing loss. Among children who had newborn hearing screening, the age of identification of hearing loss was between 2 to 12 months. To avoid this delay in identifying a hearing loss, Fitzpatrick and colleagues (2014) suggested pursuing definitive hearing testing with auditory brainstem response if behavioral audiometry is not reliable. Conversely, the presence of hearing loss or D/HH can make it challenging to recognize and definitively identify ASD in a child, prompting relatively late ages of identification of ASD in children who are D/HH (Fitzpatrick et al., 2014; Mandell, Novak, & Zubritsky, 2005; Meinzen-Derr et al., 2014; Mood & Shield, 2014).

BOX 26.1 EVIDENCE-BASED PRACTICE

Early Identification of Hearing Loss

A number of early studies (Kennedy et al., 2006; Moeller, 2000; Yoshinaga-Itano et al., 1998) identified the importance of early identification of hearing loss in infants as important to achieve improved language and developmental outcomes. This work greatly accelerated the adoption of universal newborn hearing screening and prompted the development of the 1-3-6 benchmarks for early hearing detection and intervention programs. Outcome is greatly improved if screening is by 1 month of age, identification of hearing loss by 3 months of age, and intervention by 6 months of age (Joint Committee on Infant Hearing, 2007).

Among children with cerebral palsy, various surveys have estimated hearing loss to occur in 4%–13%, with the most commonly cited rate being 12%. Severe to profound hearing loss has been described to occur in 3%–4% of these children (Dufresne, Dagenais, & Shevell, 2014; Reid, Modak, Berkowitz, & Reddihough, 2011).

In children presenting with developmental disabilities, attention problems, or learning difficulties, it is important to pursue a comprehensive evaluation of hearing (and vision), as unidentified hearing loss can interfere with a child's ability to learn and pay attention. Children with mild hearing loss can have difficulty sustaining attention and experience fatigue from processing spoken instruction in the classroom (Đoković et al., 2014; Porter, Sladen, Ampath, Rothpletz, & Bess, 2013). This challenge can mimic difficulties with inattention, prompting an evaluation for ADHD (O'Connell & Casale, 2005). For example, when a child with a hearing loss does not follow through on instructions, this may be associated with the inability to hear and understand the instructions rather than with an issue with inattention. However, children who are D/HH can also have specific learning disabilities and executive functioning disorders (O'Connell & Casale, 2005). It can be challenging to determine the impact of learning and executive functioning deficits on classroom performance in children who are D/HH (Box 26.1).

Complex medical needs and developmental delays may also contribute to the late identification of hearing loss (Chapman et al., 2011; Fitzpatrick, Cesconetto dos Santos, Grandpierre, & Whittingham, 2017; Box 26.2); children who do not pass newborn hearing screening but have no medical complexities receive a confirmed diagnosis of hearing loss more than 2 months earlier than those with medical complexities.

One important reason for identifying a developmental disability in children who are D/HH is that services would broaden to include approaches and supports for the specific learning or behavioral difficulties. The current system supporting the special education needs of children within Part B programming (Individuals with Disabilities Education Improvement Act of 2004) identifies a primary educational label. This can pose problems for children who are D/HH Plus if teams use the educational label as the primary consideration for goals and services. This may limit access to the full breadth of supports a child may need (Borders, Meinzen-Derr, Embury, Bauer, & Wiley, 2015).

The next section will focus primarily on assessment, but there are inherent risks in misclassification and **diagnostic overshadowing** of developmental disabilities in children who are D/HH. Characteristics of developmental disabilities may be attributed to hearing loss (as seen in children with ADHD), and alternatively,

BOX 26.2 EVIDENCE-BASED PRACTICE

Medical and Developmental Complexities

Children with medical and developmental complexities face challenges in the early identification of hearing loss, posing further delays to effective interventions to support optimal development (Chapman et al., 2011; Fitzpatrick et al., 2017). Further work is needed to understand how to ameliorate these gaps in the identification and intervention for children who are Deaf/hard of hearing Plus.

characteristics common in children who are D/HH may be viewed as concerning for an atypical learning pattern. These issues can impact accuracy of the epidemiologic data, a common challenge for low-incidence disabilities.

CAUSES AND ASSOCIATIONS WITH SPECIFIC DEVELOPMENTAL DISABILITIES

As noted earlier, there are overlapping risk factors for developmental disabilities and hearing loss (Joint Committee on Infant Hearing, 2007). In some situations, the cause of hearing loss can indicate a risk for developmental disabilities (such as in symptomatic congenital CMV or in CHARGE syndrome; Ahn & Lee, 2013; see Table 26.3 and Appendix B). In other situations, etiology does not help in understanding the likelihood of developmental concerns beyond that imparted by hearing loss. For example, *GJB2* (connexin) mutations are a common cause of autosomal recessive hearing loss (Gasparini et al., 2000). In early understandings of *GJB2* mutations, it was often reported that children with this genetic etiology of hearing loss were likely to have good developmental outcomes (Sinnathuray et al., 2004). However, over time, reports began to describe children with *GJB2* mutations having coexisting conditions, including other genetic conditions (Kenna et al., 2007; Wiley, Choo, Meinzen-Derr, Hilbert, & Greinwald, 2006).

Table 26.3. Risk factors for hearing loss and known additional developmental risks

Risk factors for hearing loss (Joint Committee for Infant Hearing, 2007)	Known developmental risks beyond hearing loss
NICU stay > 5 days	
ECMO-assisted ventilation	Related to potential CNS injury
Ototoxic medications	Related to underlying condition
Loop diuretics	Related to underlying condition
Hyperbilirubinemia requiring exchange transfusion	Kernicterus
Hypoxic-ischemic events	
In utero infections	*Related to underlying conditions:*
Cytomegalovirus	(Oliver et al., 2009)
Herpes	(Hermansen & Hermansen, 2006)
Rubella	
Syphilis	
Toxoplasmosis	
Postnatal infections	*Related to underlying conditions:*
Herpes encephalitis	(Hermansen & Hermansen, 2006)
Bacterial meningitis	
Other acquired causes of hearing loss	
Head trauma	Related to potential CNS injury (Wade, Zhang, Yeates, Stancin, & Taylor, 2016)
Chemotherapy	Related to toxic effects on CNS (Janzen & Spiegler, 2008)
Craniofacial anomalies	*Related to potential syndromes associated with conditions*
External ear anomalies	
Temporal bone anomalies	
Cleft lip and palate	
Syndrome involving hearing loss	*Specific to syndrome:*
Down syndrome	(Brown, Greer, Aylward, & Hunt, 1990)
Neurofibromatosis	(Hyman, Shores, & North, 2006; Nunes & MacCollin, 2003)
Usher syndrome	(Dammeyer, 2012)
Waardenburg syndrome	(Kiani, Gangadharan, & Miller, 2007)
Neurodegenerative disorders	*Specific to condition:*
Hunter syndrome	(Stapleton et al., 2017)
Sensory motor neuropathies (Freidrich Ataxia, Charcot-Marie Tooth)	(Janzen, Delaney, & Shapiro, 2017; Reetz et al., 2016) (Cornett et al., 2016; Corrado, Ciardi, & Bargigli, 2017)

Key: ECMO, extracorporeal membrane oxygenation.

The co-occurrence of two or more conditions suggests that identifying a known etiology for hearing loss does not protect a child from the presence of other genetic conditions or environmental risks that contribute to the emergence of developmental disabilities.

The coexistence of developmental disorders (such as intellectual disability, ASD, and multiple congenital anomalies) in children who are D/HH is particularly pertinent to the practice of developmental-behavioral pediatrics (see Table 26.4). Focusing only on the hearing loss in the context of the genetic workup in children with developmental disabilities could miss the contribution of other genetic conditions. Developmental-behavioral pediatricians and geneticists are in a position to recognize when a broader genetic workup is indicated. It is appropriate to apply current genetic guidelines for the developmental condition in the general population (Miller et al., 2010) to children who are D/HH when indicated.

DIAGNOSIS AND CLINICAL MANIFESTATIONS

Diagnostic considerations must take into account a recognition of the impact of a child's degree of hearing loss on access to language. Families are faced with making decisions regarding communication approaches early in the time frame of identification of their child's hearing loss. These decisions can include auditory, visual, and/or tactile means (in the case of children who are Deaf-blind). Families experience varying opinions and information related to these decisions (Crow et al., 2014; DesGeorges, 2016; Kushalnagar et al., 2010). As young children grow and develop, differences in language processing may become evident, prompting changes in approaches to building communication skills (Putz, 2012).

Table 26.4. Percent of population with hearing in populations with specific disabilities

Disability	Estimates of percentage of the population with hearing loss
Intellectual disability	5%
Autism spectrum disorder	0.1%
Cerebral palsy	4%–13%

Sources: Dufresne et al. (2014), Fitzpatrick et al. (2014), Mandell et al. (2005), Reid et al. (2011), and Russ et al. (2013).

Appropriate Language Expectations

In children who have had the benefit of early identification and intervention for hearing loss, slow language development as a result of hearing loss should not be considered the norm (Meinzen-Derr et al., 2018; see Box 26.3). Children who receive intervention prior to 6 months of age can achieve language levels within the average range of the general population (Kennedy et al., 2006). Yoshinago-Itano, Sedey, Coulter, and Mehl (1998) found that children identified prior to 6 months of age had language quotients just under 90 compared to a language quotient of approximately 70 for children identified after 2 years of age. Moeller (2000) found a similar impact on receptive vocabulary development, with average standard scores (population mean scores of 95) for children enrolled early in services. This is in distinct contrast to substantially below-average language standard scores (population mean scores of 70) for children who enrolled in services after 35 months of age.

While the attainment of average language abilities among early-identified children who are D/HH seems quite positive, it is imperative to also consider the nonverbal cognitive capabilities when focusing on language development. Children with low-average language skills actually could be exhibiting language underperformance when taking into account their nonverbal cognitive potential (Meinzen-Derr et al., 2014; Meinzen-Derr et al., 2018).

If a child who is D/HH is not making appropriate language progress, there may be a number of contributing factors. No matter what the communication modality chosen (auditory/oral or sign language systems), it is important to have strong access to language information and a language-rich environment.

BOX 26.3 EVIDENCE-BASED PRACTICE

Co-occurrence of Developmental Disabilities

The co-occurrence of a developmental disability in children who are Deaf/hard of hearing (D/HH) is commonly discussed in the literature and supported by existing surveillance systems (Boyle et al., 2011; Chilosi et al., 2010; Gallaudet Research Institute, 2011). This literature suggests a need for a high level of suspicion if a child who is D/HH is not making anticipated developmental progress.

For an auditory/oral approach, it is foundational to have consistent acoustic access through technology (i.e., hearing aids and cochlear implants). Communication environments may need adaptations to ensure that the child is able to have acoustic access to support language development. These adaptations can include addressing the impact of the distance of the speaker to the child and the amount of background noise. Regular technology checks are important, and early recognition of progressive hearing loss can ensure amplification is adjusted accordingly (Barreira-Nielsen et al., 2016).

In families selecting a signing approach, the language competence of those around the child is critical to ensure strong language modeling for supporting language development. When access to language and the rigor of therapeutic interventions are not of concern, but the child is not making expected language progress, there may be the presence of a broader developmental disability or language disorder.

General Assessment Considerations

Assessment of the development of children who are D/HH requires some adaptations and special considerations for testing batteries (Marschark, 2003). Additional factors are also important to consider, including the communication skills of the child, the ability of the clinician to communicate directly with the child, the need and role for an interpreter, and the goals of the evaluation (Reesman et al., 2014).

When possible, evaluators should have a general knowledge of typical development among children who are D/HH (Box 26.4). This allows a context for recognition of atypical learning or behavioral concerns. When this is not possible, partnerships and communication with professionals knowledgeable in deafness can allow for discussions about a specific child's profile; what factors, behaviors, or characteristics could be related to hearing loss; and what may indicate a broader developmental concern.

When assessing/evaluating children who are D/HH and are developing differently, it is helpful to consider how a child accesses and processes information best. There are also situations when a child's "input" for communication and information differs from their preferred "output." For example, children who have good access to sound through amplification may understand spoken language well, yet due to motor difficulties with speech or the presence of a tracheostomy tube, expressive language may be best produced through sign language or the use of technology. In these circumstances, exposing children to the "output" modality is critical to allow continued expressive language growth.

Within the field of complex developmental disabilities, assessment batteries may require adaptations (Goodman, Evans, & Loftin, 2009; National Institutes of Health, 2012; NINDS, 2018). Meaningful information can be elicited from a variety of settings with multiple perspectives (parents, teachers, or therapists). Qualitative information may be more salient than standardized test scores when developing an intervention approach (Box 26.5). For children who are Deaf-blind, specialized expertise is essential in guiding meaningful assessment (National Consortium on Deaf-Blindness, 2009).

Cognitive Abilities It can be helpful to frame an understanding of cognitive development in children who are D/HH by separating the assessment of language from language-based reasoning and focusing on nonverbal reasoning skills. The lack of inclusion of children who are D/HH in normative samples during the development of an assessment tool can limit their utility in children who are D/HH (Reesman et al., 2014). Reesman and colleagues (2014) described various cognitive assessments with guidance on the need for accommodations, interpretation, normative sampling, and potential biases. Tools described include the Bayley Scales of Infant and Toddler Development, Third Edition (Bayley, 2006); the Stanford-Binet Intelligence Scales, Fifth Edition (Roid, 2003); the Leiter International Performance Scale–Revised (Roid & Miller, 1997), the Wechsler Preschool and Primary Scale of Intelligence, Fourth Edition (Wechsler, 2003b);

BOX 26.4 INTERDISCIPLINARY CARE

Importance of Interdisciplinary Team Work for Children Who Are Deaf/Hard of Hearing Plus

A strong and diverse interdisciplinary team is particularly important for assessing children who are Deaf/hard of hearing (D/HH) with a potential developmental disability. A strong understanding of the usual developmental patterns in typically developing D/HH helps team members recognize when a child may be learning and progressing differently.

BOX 26.5 INTERDISCIPLINARY CARE

Importance of Multiple Sources of Information and Perspectives When Considering the Needs of Children Who Are Deaf/Hard of Hearing Plus

Blending expertise from various areas including parents, teachers, interpreters, audiologists, clinicians with expertise in the evaluation and management of children who are Deaf/hard of hearing (D/HH), and clinicians with expertise in the evaluation and management of developmental disabilities will enhance the understanding of a child who is D/HH with a complex learning pattern. With this approach, broader intervention approaches can be implemented, allowing a child who is D/HH Plus the opportunity to make developmental progress.

the Differential Abilities Scales, Second Edition (Elliot, 2007); the Kaufman Assessment Battery for Children, Second Edition (Kaufman & Kaufman, 2004); the Reynolds Intellectual Assessment Scales (Reynolds & Kamphaus, 1998); the Wechsler Nonverbal Scale of Ability (Wechsler & Naglieri, 2006); the Wechsler Intelligence Scale for Children, Fourth Edition (Wechsler, 2003a), the Comprehensive Test of Nonverbal Intelligence (Hammill, Pearson, & Wiederholt, 2009); and the Universal Nonverbal Intelligence Test (Bracken & McCallum, 2016; see Chapter 13).

Autism Spectrum Disorder When evaluating children who are D/HH for ASD, it is important to have a standardized approach that takes into consideration the core features of this social-communication disorder. However, autism-specific assessment tools are very limited regarding validation in children who are D/HH (Mood & Shield, 2014).

ASD symptoms in children who are D/HH may be difficult to categorize on some tools. For example, a child who is D/HH with ASD may not respond to his/her name when called. If the child has amplification and can respond to quiet environmental sounds and the evaluator does not take into consideration the child's ability to perform this skill, this lack of response may be incorrectly ascribed to hearing loss when, in fact, it is due to an ASD. Adaptations may also be required to assess this core social communication. In children who sign, there are ways to gain attention that are different than calling out a name. Responsiveness to these typical strategies, however, can be limited in deaf children with ASD. Atypical language features are evident in children who are D/HH with ASD, such as echolalia in sign language (Shield, Cooley, & Meier, 2017).

Unfortunately, the gold-standard autism assessments, such as the Autism Diagnostic Observation Schedule (Lord et al., 2012); the Autism Diagnostic Interview–Revised (Lord, Rutter, & Le Couteur, 1994), the Childhood Autism Rating Scale (Schopler, Van Bourgondien, Wellman, & Love 2010), the Gilliam Autism Rating Scale (Gilliam, 1995), and the Autistic Behavior Checklist (Krug, Arick, & Almond, 1993), have not been normed or validated in children who are D/HH. Despite these limitations, these tools have been used in describing children who are D/HH and have been diagnosed with ASD (Johansson, Gilberg, & Rastam, 2010; Jure, Rapin, &Tuchman, 1991; Meinzen-Derr et al., 2014; Mood & Shield, 2014; Roper, Arnold, & Monteiro, 2003).

The optimal approach for assessing children who are D/HH and have ASD is to employ a professional trained both in hearing loss and ASD and who can communicate directly with the child irrespective of communication modality. However, meeting this best practice would markedly limit access to assessment. Including professionals knowledgeable in children who are D/HH in the assessment of ASD is encouraged (Szarkowski, Mood, Shield, Wiley, & Yoshinaga-Itano, 2014). When needing to rely on sign language interpreters to facilitate communication, using an interpreter who is familiar with the child's language (such as a school interpreter) and preparing the interpreter with what is needed in the assessment has been a strategy some have used (Szarkowski et al., 2014). The role of interprofessional collaboration cannot be understated in these situations.

Deaf-Blind Children with Deaf-blindness are best assessed through a highly collaborative interdisciplinary team, highlighting a child's functional skills across many domains. Understanding a child's functional vision allows for appropriate visual and tactile adaptations in assessment materials and the testing environment. It is also critical to understand how a child with Deaf-blindness communicates and to have the ability to interpret and respond to the child's communication

(Goodman et al., 2009; National Consortium on Deaf-Blindness, 2009; Riggio & McLetchie, 2008). Each state has a federally funded Deaf-blind project that is a good starting resource for expertise in understanding the complexities of children with Deaf-blindness.

MONITORING, SCREENING, AND EVALUATION

There is a paucity of evidence to guide the use of screening tools to identify developmental difficulties in children who are D/HH. However, it is important to implement ongoing monitoring of progress and recognize when a child is not meeting developmental milestones or when trajectories are diverting from the expected (Wiley & Meinzen-Derr, 2013; Yoshinaga-Itano, Baca, & Seday, 2010; Yoshinaga-Itano, 2014).

Furthermore, as the initial case illustrates, it is important to monitor hearing and vision in children with known developmental disabilities. Continued research in these areas is critical to improve our current approaches to effectively identify developmental disabilities in children who are D/HH and identify hearing loss in children with an existing developmental disability (Chen et al., 2014).

TREATMENT, MANAGEMENT, AND INTERVENTIONS

When considering treatment, management, and interventions for children who are D/HH Plus, the approach to supporting needs related to hearing is not necessarily different than in children who are D/HH (Fitzpatrick et al., 2014; Tharpe, Fin-Szumski, & Bess, 2001). There may be aspects of a specific child's needs that require adaptations to amplification, cochlear implantation, and therapeutic and educational interventions. For example, in a child with cerebral palsy who uses a wheelchair for mobility, positioning may impact the ease of keeping a cochlear implant in place. Families of children who are D/HH with complex needs have indicated an appreciation of access to intervention for hearing (Wiley, Jahnke, Meinzen-Derr, & Choo, 2005). Treatment decisions for a child's specific hearing pattern can be discussed with the family to guide how to apply best available evidence and practice guidelines.

There may be some unique considerations in children who are medically complex. For example, surgical risks, need for ongoing central nervous system imaging, and complex inner ear malformations may contribute to decisions specific to cochlear implantation and other surgically implanted devices (i.e., bone-anchored hearing aids and auditory brainstem implants; Doshi, Schneiders, Foster, Reid, & McDermott 2014; O'Brien et al., 2010; Sennaroğlu et al., 2016). Families and professionals alike are faced with limited outcome data to guide decision making.

Evidence-based treatment options for children who are D/HH Plus are very limited. Traditional interventions used within the field of developmental disabilities that are applied to children who are D/HH Plus are found in only very small case reports. Reports of using the Picture Exchange Communication System (Malandraki & Okalidou, 2007), video modeling (Thrasher, 2014), and augmentative and alternative communication (Lee, Jeong, & Kim, 2013; Meinzen-Derr, Wiley, McAuley, Smith, & Grether, 2017) approaches have been described. Despite the limited evidence in the field, these approaches to build communication in children who are D/HH Plus show promise.

Family-to-family support is important for all families of children who are D/HH and for families of children with developmental disabilities. Due to the unique combination of complexities, it can be challenging to identify mechanisms to meaningfully provide this support for children with D/HH Plus (Myck-Wayne, Robinson & Henson, 2011; Wiley, Gustafson, & Rozniak, 2014).

OUTCOMES

Within the existing literature, there have been two main approaches to understanding outcomes in children who are D/HH Plus. Some authors have described groups of children who are D/HH with a variety of developmental disabilities (cross-categorical), while others have focused on subpopulations of children (i.e., ASD, CHARGE syndrome, or Deaf-blind). The topic of children who are D/HH with ASD is relatively common within the literature. Despite interest in the topic, however, the level of evidence tends to be at a case-description or case-series level, frequently using retrospective chart reviews. Authors rarely describe severity levels or consider the presence of coexisting disabilities, such as an intellectual disability, that could impact language and speech outcomes.

For some coexisting conditions, it is difficult to find specific papers by using a typical query of the literature. A reader may uncover the existence of children with various disabilities (e.g., apraxia of speech within children who are D/HH) when reading the inclusion section of a study and looking at who has been excluded from the analysis. Furthermore, cognitive abilities are often not included in the description of populations of children who are D/HH, prompting difficulties in understanding the complex interplay of disabilities and the impact on specified outcomes.

A limitation of the existing knowledge is the tendency for the literature to compare children who are D/HH Plus with typically developing peers who are D/HH rather than with disability matched or cognitively matched peers (Meinzen-Derr, Wiley, Grether, & Choo, 2011). This poses challenges in guiding families on what to expect related to language and developmental outcomes. Many papers state in their conclusion section that children who are D/HH Plus with implants make progress but at a slower rate than typically developing D/HH children.

Centers vary in their interpretation of outcomes and level of enthusiasm for pursuing specific interventions (i.e., cochlear implantation). In general, reports have described lower long-term adherence with cochlear implant use in children with ASD (Valero et al., 2016) and developmental disabilities (Özdemir et al., 2103) as compared to typically developing implant users. Speech perception and auditory performance among children with disabilities who use cochlear implants have also been described. Some authors have found improvements in objective measures of speech perception, auditory performance, and language skills but at a slower rate and level than typically developing children with implants (Birman, Elliott, & Gibson, 2012; Cruz, Vicaria, Wang, Niparko, & Quittner, 2012; Eshraghi et al., 2015; Mikic et al., 2016).

Within the broader group of children who are D/HH Plus who do not use cochlear implants, early childhood outcomes have been described. In a relatively large group of 119 children with hearing loss and additional disabilities, outcomes were affected by the type of disability (i.e., autism, cerebral palsy, and developmental delay), and level of maternal education affected speech, language, and functional auditory skills (Cupples et al., 2014). They noted that when conditions were not associated with a developmental delay or ASD, outcomes were better predicted by the coexisting condition than by the degree of hearing loss. In addition, a number of authors describe the importance of considering different outcomes, particularly functional and quality-of-life considerations for children who are D/HH Plus (Berrettini et al., 2008; Cejas, Hoffman, & Quittner, 2015; Edwards, Hill, & Mahon, 2012; Wiley et al., 2005; Zaidman-Zait, Curle, Jamieseon, Chia, & Kozak, 2015).

Work with children who are D/HH Plus can present multiple and competing priorities. Families serve as the compass to guide priorities and service delivery models. Building effective teamwork with professionals from a variety of backgrounds and expertise can allow for effective adaptations of intervention strategies to improve a child's outcomes. Using a strengths-based approach is critically important in children who are D/HH and D/HH Plus.

SUMMARY

- Children who are D/HH are at higher risk for developmental disabilities than the general population.
- Children with language delays and developmental disabilities should have hearing and vision evaluated due to risks for sensory impairments.
- The workup in children who are D/HH Plus should include both a hearing-targeted assessment and broader genetic testing based on current guidelines for developmental disabilities.
- Irrespective of communication modality, when children who are D/HH lag behind in their language development, broader developmental concerns should be considered.
- Assessing the breadth of developmental needs in children who are D/HH is enhanced by cross-disciplinary communication and team work.

ADDITIONAL RESOURCES

National Institute on Deafness and Other Communication Disorders/National Institutes of Health: http://www.nidcd.nih.gov/

American Speech-Language-Hearing Association (ASHA): http://www.asha.org

Centers for Disease Control and Prevention: http://www.cdc.gov/hearingloss

Additional resources can be found online in Appendix D: Childhood Disabilities Resources, Services, and Organizations (see About the Online Companion Materials).

REFERENCES

Ahn, J. H., & Lee, K. S. (2013). Outcomes of cochlear implants in children with CHARGE syndrome. *Acta Otolaryngology, 133*(11), 1148–1153.

Barreira-Nielsen, C., Fitzpatrick, E., Hashem, S., Whittingham, J., Barrowman, N., & Aglipay, M. (2016). Progressive hearing loss in early childhood. *Ear and Hearing, 37*(5), e311–e321.

Bayley, N. (2006). *Bayley Scales of Infant and Toddler Development, Third Edition: Administration manual.* San Antonio, TX: Harcourt Assessment.

Beers, A. N., McBoye, M., Kakande, E., Dar Santos, R. C., & Kozak, F. K. (2014). Autism and peripheral hearing loss: A systematic review. *International Journal of Pediatric Otorhinolaryngology, 78*, 96–101.

Berrettini, S., Forli, F., Genovese, E., Santarelli, R., Arslan, E., Chilosi, A. M., & Cipriani, P. (2008). Cochlear implantation in deaf children with associated disabilities: Challenges and outcomes. *International Journal of Audiology, 47*(4), 199–208.

Birman, C. S., Elliott, E. J., & Gibson, W. P. (2012). Pediatric cochlear implants: Additional disabilities prevalence, risk factors, and effect on language outcomes. *Otology & Neurotology, 33*(8), 1347–1352.

Borders, C., Meinzen-Derr, J., Embury, D. C., Bauer, A., & Wiley, S. (2015). Students who are deaf with additional disabilities: Does educational label impact language services? *Deafness & Education International, 17*(4), 204–218.

Boyle, C. A., Boulet, S., Schieve, L. A., Cohen, R. A., Blumbert, S. J., Yeargin-Allsopp, M., . . . Kogan, M. D. (2011). Trends in the prevalence of developmental disabilities in US children, 1997–2008. *Pediatrics, 127,* 1034–1042.

Bracken, B. A., & McCallum, R. S. (2016). *Universal Nonverbal Intelligence Test* (2nd ed.). Austin, TX: PRO-ED.

Brown, F. R., Greer, M. K., Aylward, E. H., & Hunt, H. H. (1990). Intellectual and adaptive functioning in individuals with Down syndrome in relation to age and environmental placement. *Pediatrics, 85*(3), 450–452.

Chapman, D. A., Stempfel, C. C., Bodurtha, J. N., Dodson, K. M., Pandya, A., Lynch, K. B., Kirby, R. S. (2011). Impact of co-occurring birth defects on the timing of newborn hearing screening and diagnosis. *American Journal of Audiology, 20*(2), 132–139.

Cejas, I., Hoffman, M. F., & Quittner, A. L. (2015). Outcomes and benefits of pediatric cochlear implantation in children with additional disabilities: A review and report of family influences on outcomes. *Pediatric Health, Medicine and Therapeutics, 6,* 45–63.

Centers for Disease Control and Prevention. (2010). Identifying infants with hearing loss—United States, 1999-2007. *Morbidity and Mortality Weekly Report, 59,* 220–223.

Chen, H. C., Wang, N. M., Chiu, W. C., Liu, S. Y., Chang, Y. P., Lin, P. Y., . . . Chung, K. (2014). A test protocol for assessing the hearing status of students with special needs. *International Journal of Pediatric Otorhinolaryngology, 78*(10), 1677–1685.

Chilosi, A. M., Comparini, A., Scusa, M. F., Berrettini, S., Forli, F., Battini, R., & Cioni, G. (2010). Neurodevelopmental disorders in children with severe to profound sensorineural hearing loss: A clinical study. *Developmental Medicine & Child Neurology, 52,* 856–862.

Cornett, K. M., Menezes, M. P., Bray, P., Halaki, M., Shy, R. R., Yum, S. W., . . . Burns, J. (2016). Phenotypic variability of childhood Charcot-Marie-Tooth disease. *JAMA Neurology, 73*(6), 645–651.

Corrado, B., Ciardi, G., & Bargigli, C. (2017). Rehabilitation management of the Charcot-Marie-Tooth syndrome: A systematic review of the literature. *Medicine (Baltimore), 95*(17), e3278.

Crowe, K., Fordham, L., McLeod, S., & Ching, T. Y. C. (2014). "Part of our world": Influences on caregiver decisions about communication choices for children with hearing loss. *Deafness & Education International, 16*(2), 61–85.

Cruz, I., Vicaria, I., Wang, N. Y., Niparko, J., & Quittner, A. L. (2012). CDaCI investigative team. Language and behavioral outcomes in children with developmental disabilities using cochlear implants. *Otology & Neurotology, 33*(5), 751–760.

Culture. (2014). In *Merriam-Webster's dictionary and thesaurus* (11th ed.). Springfield, MA: Merriam-Webster.

Cupples, L., Ching, T. Y., Crowe, K., Seeto, M., Leigh, G., Street, L., . . . Thompson, J. (2014). Outcomes of 3-year-old children with hearing loss and different types of additional disabilities. *Journal of Deaf Studies and Deaf Education, J19*(1), 20–39.

Dammeyer, J. (2012). Children with Usher syndrome: Mental and behavioral disorders. *Behavioral and Brain Functions, 27*(8), 16.

DesGeorges, J. (2016). Avoiding assumptions: Communication decisions made by hearing parents of deaf children. *American Medical Association Journal of Ethics, 18*(4), 442–446.

Đoković, S., Gligorović, M., Ostojić, S., Dimić, N., Radić-Šestić, M., & Slavnić, S. (2014). Can mild bilateral sensorineural hearing loss affect developmental abilities in younger school-age children? *Journal of Deaf Studies and Deaf Education, 19,* 484–495.

Doshi, J., Schneiders, S., Foster, K., Reid, A., & McDermott, A. L. (2014). Magnetic resonance imaging and bone anchored hearing implants: pediatric considerations. *International Journal of Pediatric Otorhinolaryngology, 78*(2), 277–279.

Dufresne, D., Dagenais, L., & Shevell, M. I. (2014). Epidemiology of severe hearing impairment in a population-based cerebral palsy cohort. *Pediatric Neurology, 51*(5), 641–644.

Edwards, L., Hill, T., & Mahon, M. (2012). Quality of life in children and adolescents with cochlear implants and additional needs. *International Journal of Pediatric Otorhinolaryngology, 76*(6), 851–857.

Elliott, C. D. (2007). *Differential Abilities Scales* (2nd ed.). San Antonio, TX: Harcourt Assessment.

Eshraghi, A. A., Nazarian, R., Telischi, F. F., Martinez, D., Hodges, A., Velandia, S., . . . Lang, D. (2015). Cochlear implantation in children with autism spectrum disorder. *Otology & Neurotology, 36*(8), e121–e128.

Fitzpatrick, E. M., Lambert, L., Whittingham, J., & Leblanc, E. (2014). Examination of characteristics and management of children with hearing loss and autism spectrum disorders. *International Journal of Audiology, 53*(9), 577–586.

Fitzpatrick, E. M., Cesconetto dos Santos, J., Grandpierre, V., & Whittingham, J. (2017). Exploring reasons for late identification of children with early-onset hearing loss. *International Journal of Pediatric Otorhinolaryngology, 100,* 160–167.

Gallaudet Research Institute. (2011). *Regional and national summary report of data from the 2009-10 annual survey of deaf and hard of hearing children and youth.* Washington, DC: Gallaudet University. Retrieved from http://research.gallaudet.edu/Demographics/2010_National_Summary.pdf

Gasparini, P., Rabionet, R., Barbujani, G., Melghionda S., Petersen, M., Brondum-Nielsen, K., . . . Estivill, X. (2000). High carrier frequency of the 35delG deafness mutation in European populations. Genetic Analysis Consortium of GJB2 35delG. *European Journal of Human Genetics, 8*(1), 19–23.

Gilliam, J. E. (1995). *Gilliam Autism Rating Scale.* Austin, TX: PRO-ED.

Goman, A. M., & Lin, F. R. (2016). Prevalence of hearing loss by severity in the United States. *American Journal of Public Health, 106*(10), 1820–1822.

Goodman, S., Evans, C., & Loftin, M. (2009). *Full position statement paper: Intelligence testing of individuals who are blind or visually impaired.* Louisville, KY: American Printing House for the Blind.

Hammill, D. D., Pearson, N. A., & Wiederholt, J. L. (2009). *Comprehensive Test of Nonverbal Intelligence* (2nd ed.). San Antonio, TX: Pearson Education Inc.

Hermansen, M. C., & Hermansen, M. G. (2006). Perinatal infections and cerebral palsy. *Clinics in Perinatology, 33*(2), 315–333.

Hey, C., Fessler, S., Hafner, N., Lange, B. P., Euler, H. A., & Neumann, K. (2014). High prevalence of hearing loss at Special Olympics: Is this representative of people with intellectual disability? *Journal of Applied Research in Intellectual Disabilities, 27*(2), 125–133.

Holcomb, T. K. (2012). *Introduction to American deaf culture (Professional perspectives on deafness: Evidence and applications)* (1st ed.). New York, NY: Oxford University Press.

Holt, L. R., & Garey, D. [Producers]. (2007). *Through deaf eyes.* Washington, DC: WETA-TV.

Humphries, T. L., & Padden, C. A. (1990). *Deaf in America: Voices from a culture.* Cambridge, MA: Harvard University Press.

Hyman, S. L., Shores, E. A., & North, K. N. (2006). Learning disabilities in children with neurofibromatosis type 1: Subtypes, cognitive profile, and attention-deficit-hyperactivity disorder. *Developmental Medicine and Child Neurology, 48*(12), 973–977.

Individuals with Disabilities Education Improvement Act (IDEA) of 2004, 20 U.S.C. §§ 1400 *et seq.*

Janzen, D., Delaney, K. A., & Shapiro, E. G. (2017). Cognitive and adaptive measurement endpoints for clinical trials in mucopolysaccharidoses types I, II, and III: A review of the literature. *Molecular Genetics and Metabolism, 121*(2), 57–69.

Janzen, L. A., & Spiegler, B. J. (2008). Neurodevelopmental sequelae of pediatric acute lymphoblastic leukemia and its treatment. *Developmental Disabilities Research Reviews, 14*(3), 185–195.

Joint Committee on Infant Hearing. (2007). Year 2007 Position Statement: Principles and guidelines for early hearing detection and intervention programs. *Pediatrics, 120,* 898–921.

Johansson, M., Gillberg, C., & Råstam, M. (2010). Autism spectrum conditions in individuals with Möbius sequence, CHARGE syndrome and oculo-auriculo-vertebral spectrum: Diagnostic aspects. *Research in Developmental Disabilities, 31*(1), 9–24.

Jure, R., Rapin, I., & Tuchman, R. F. (1991). Hearing-impaired autistic children. *Developmental Medicine & Child Neurology, 33*(12), 1062–1072.

Kancherla, V., Van Naarden Braun, K., & Yeargin-Allsopp, M. (2013). Childhood vision impairment, hearing loss and co-occurring autism spectrum disorder. *Disability and Health Journal, 6*(4), 333–342.

Kaufman, A. S., & Kaufman, N. L. (2004). *Kaufman Brief Intelligence Test* (2nd ed.). Torrance, CA: Pearson Western Psychological Services.

Kenna, M. A, Rehm, H. L., Robson, C. D., Frangulov, A., McCallum, J., Yaeger, D., . . . Krantz, I. D. (2007). Additional clinical manifestations in children with sensorineural hearing loss and biallelic GJB2 mutations: Who should be offered GJB2 testing? *American Journal of Medical Genetics Part A, 143A*(14), 1560–1566.

Kennedy, C. R., McCann, D. C., Campbell, M. J., Law, C. M., Mullee, M., Petrou, S., . . . Stevenson, J. (2006). Language ability after early detection of permanent childhood hearing impairment. *New England Journal of Medicine, 354*(20), 2131–2141.

Kiani, R., Gangadharan, S. K., & Miller, H. (2007). Case report: Association of Waardenburg syndrome with intellectual disability, autistic spectrum disorder and unprovoked aggressive outbursts: A new behavioural phenotype? *The British Journal of Developmental Disabilities, 54*(104), 53–62.

Krug, D. A., Arick, J., & Almond, P. (1993) *Autism Screening Instrument for Educational Planning.* Austin, TX: PRO-ED.

Kushalnagar, P., Mathur, G., Moreland, C. J., Napoli, D. J., Osterling, W., Paddon, C., . . . Rathmann, C. (2010). Infants and children with hearing loss need early language access. *Journal of Clinical Ethics, 21*(2), 143–154.

Lee, Y., Jeong, S. W., & Kim, L. S. (2013). AAC intervention using a VOCA for deaf children with multiple disabilities who received cochlear implantation. *International Journal of Pediatric Otorhinolaryngology, 77*(12), 2008–2013.

Lindow-Davies, C., & Kennedy, S. (2013). *What is 'deaf plus'?* Retrieved from http://www.cohandsandvoices.org/plus/index.html

Lord, C., Rutter, M., & Le Couteur, A. (1994). Autism Diagnostic Interview–Revised: A revised version of a diagnostic interview for caregivers of individuals with possible pervasive developmental disorders. *Journal of Autism and Developmental Disorders, 24,* 659–685.

Lord, C., Rutter, M., DiLavore, P. C., Risi, S., Gotham, K., & Bishop, S. L. (2012). *Autism Diagnostic Observation Schedule, Second Edition (ADOS-2).* Torrance, CA: Western Psychological Services.

Malandraki, G., & Okalidou, A. (2007). The application of PECS in a deaf child with autism: A case study. *Focus on Autism and Other Developmental Disabilities, 22,* 23.

Mandell, D. S., Novak, M. M., & Zubritsky, C. D. (2005). Factors associated with age of diagnosis among children with autism spectrum disorders. *Pediatrics, 116*(6), 1480–1486.

Marschark, M. (2003). Cognitive functioning in deaf adults and children. In M. Marschark & P. E. Spencer (Eds.), *Oxford handbook of deaf studies, language, and education* (pp. 464–477). New York, NY: Oxford University Press.

Meinzen-Derr, J., Sheldon, R., Grether, S., Altaye, M., Smith, L., Choo, D. I., . . . Wiley, S. (2018). Language underperformance in young children who are deaf or hard-of-hearing: Are the expectations too low? *Journal of Developmental and Behavioral Pediatrics, 39*(2), 116–125.

Meinzen-Derr, J., Wiley, S., Bishop, S., Manning-Courtney, P., Choo, D. I., & Murray, D. (2014). Autism spectrum disorders in 24 children who are deaf or hard of hearing. *International Journal of Pediatric Otorhinolaryngology, 78*(1), 112–118.

Meinzen-Derr, J., Wiley, S., Grether, S., & Choo, D. (2011). Children with cochlear implants and developmental disabilities: A language skills study with developmentally matched hearing peers. *Research in Developmental Disabilities, 32,* 757–767.

Meinzen-Derr, J., Wiley, S., Grether, S., Phillips, J., Choo, D., Hibner, J., . . . Barnard, H. (2014). Association with functional communication performance and language in children who are deaf or hard-of-hearing. *Journal of Developmental and Behavioral Pediatrics, 35*(3), 197–206.

Meinzen-Derr, J., Wiley, S., McAuley, R., Smith, L., & Grether, S. (2017). Technology-assisted language intervention for children who are deaf or hard-of-hearing: A pilot study of augmentative and alternative communication for enhancing language development. *Disability and Rehabilitation: Assistive Technology, 2*(8), 808–815.

Mikic, B., Jotic, A., Miric, D., Nikolic, M., Jankovic, N., & Arsovic, N. (2016). Receptive speech in early implanted children later diagnosed with autism. *European Annals of Otorhinolaryngology, Head and Neck Diseases, 133*(S1), S36–S39.

Miller, D. T., Adam, M. P., Aradhya, S., Biesecker, L. G., Brothman, A. R., Carter, N. P., . . . Ledbetter, D. H. (2010). Consensus statement: Chromosomal microarray is a first-tier clinical diagnostic test for individuals with developmental disabilities or congenital anomalies. *American Journal of Human Genetics, 86*(5), 749–764.

Moeller, M. P. (2000). Early intervention and language development in children who are deaf and hard of hearing. *Pediatrics, 106*(3), e43.

Mood, D., & Shield, A. (2014). Clinical use of the Autism Diagnostic Observation Schedule–Second Edition with children who are deaf. *Seminars in Speech and Language, 35*(4), 288–300.

Myck-Wayne, J., Robinson, S., & Henson, E. (2011). Serving and supporting young children with a dual diagnosis of hearing loss and autism: The stories or four families. *American Annals of the Deaf, 156*(4), 379–390.

National Center on Deaf-Blindness. (2016). *The 2016 national child count of children and youth who are deafblind.* Retrieved from https://nationaldb.org/reports/national-child-count-2016

National Consortium on Deaf-Blindness, National Center on Deaf-Blindness. (2009). *Authentic assessment.* Retrieved from http://documents.nationaldb.org/products/AuthAssessment.pdf

National Institutes of Health. (2012). *NIH toolkit: Reasonable accommodations guidelines.* Retrieved from http://www.healthmeasures.net/attachments/article/7/NIH%20Toolbox%20 Reasonable%20Accommodations%20Guidelines.pdf

Nunes, F., & MacCollin, M. (2003). Neurofibromatosis 2 in the pediatric population. *Journal of Child Neurology, 18*(10), 718–724.

O'Brien, L. C., Kenna, M., Neault, M., Clark, T. A., Kammerer, B., Johnston, J., . . . Licamell, G. R. (2010). Not a "sound" decision: Is cochlear implantation always the best choice? *International Journal of Pediatric Otorhinolaryngology, 74*(10), 1144–1148.

O'Connell, J., & Casale, K. (2005). Attention deficits and hearing loss: Meeting the challenge. *The Volta Review, 104,* 257–271.

Oliver, S. E., Cloud, G. A., Sánchez, P. J., Demmler, G. J., Dankner, W., Shelton, M., . . . National Institute of Allergy, Infectious Diseases Collaborative Antiviral Study Group. (2009). Neurodevelopmental outcomes following ganciclovir therapy in symptomatic congenital cytomegalovirus infections involving the central nervous system. *Journal of Clinical Virology, S4,* S22–S26.

Özdemir, S., Tuncer, Ü., Tarkan, Ö., Kıroğlu, M., Çetik, F., & Akar, F. (2013). Factors contributing to limited or non-use in the cochlear implant systems in children: 11 years' experience. *International Journal of Pediatric Otorhinolaryngology, 77*(3), 407–409.

Porter, H., Sladen, D. P., Ampah, S. B., Rothpletz, A., & Bess, F. H. (2013). Developmental outcomes in early school-age children with minimal hearing loss. *American Journal of Audiology, 22,* 263–270.

Putz, K. (2012). *The parenting journey: Raising deaf and hard of hearing children.* Cambridge, MA: Barefoot Books.

NINDS. (2018). Cerebral palsy. NINDS common data elements. *National Institute of Neurological Disorders and Stroke.* Retrieved from https://www.commondataelements.ninds.nih.gov/CP.aspx#tab=Data_Standards

Reesman, J. H., Day, L. A., Szymanski, C. A., Witkin, G. A., Kalback, S. R., & Brice, P. J. (2014). Review of intellectual assessment measures for children who are deaf or hard of hearing. *Rehabilitation Psychology, 59*(1), 99–106.

Reetz, K., Dogan, I., Hilgers, R. D., Giunti, P., Mariotti, C., Durr, A., . . . EFACTS Study Group. (2016). Progression characteristics of the European Friedreich's Ataxia Consortium for Translational Studies (EFACTS): A 2-year cohort study. *Lancet Neurology, 15*(13), 1346–1354.

Reid, S. M., Modak, M. B., Berkowitz, R. G., & Reddihough, D. S. (2011). A population-based study and systematic review of hearing loss in children with cerebral palsy. *Developmental Medicine & Child Neurology, 53*(11), 1038–1045.

Reynolds, C. R., & Kamphaus, R. W. (1998). *Reynolds Intellectual Assessment Scales.* Lutz, FL: Psychological Assessment Resources.

Riggio, M., & McLetchie, B. (2008). Assessment. In M. Riggio & B. McLetchie (Eds.), *Deafblindness educational service guidelines* (pp. 35–46). Watertown, MA: Perkins School for the Blind.

Roid, G. H. (2003). *Standford Binet Intelligence Scales* (5th ed.). Rolling Meadows, IL: Riverside Publishing.

Roid, G., & Miller, L. (1997). *Leiter International Performance Scale–Revised.* WoodDale, IL: Stoelting Co.

Roper, L., Arnold, P., & Monteiro, B. (2003). Co-occurrence of autism and deafness: Diagnostic considerations. *Autism, 7*(3), 245–253.

Russ, S. A., Kenney, M. K., & Kogan, M. D. (2013). Hearing difficulties in children with special health care needs. *Journal of Developmental & Behavioral Pediatrics, 34*(7), 478–485.

Schopler, E., Van Bourgondien, M. E., Wellman, G. J., & Love, S. R. (2010). *Childhood Autism Rating Scale* (2nd ed.). San Antonio, TX: Pearson.

Sennaroğlu, L., Colletti, V., Lenarz, T., Manrique, M., Laszig, R., Rask-Andersen, H., . . . Polak, M. (2016). Consensus statement: Long-term results of ABI in children with complex inner ear malformations and decision making between CI and ABI. *Cochlear Implants International, 17*(4), 163–171.

Shield, A., Cooley, F., & Meier, R. P. (2017). Sign language echolalia in deaf children with autism spectrum disorder. *Journal of Speech, Language, and Hearing Research, 60*(6), 1622–1634.

Sinnathuray, A. R., Toner, J. G., Geddis, A., Clarke-Lyttle, A. J., Patterson, C. C., & Hughes, A. E. (2004) Auditory perception and speech discrimination after cochlear implantation in patients with connexin 26 (GJB2) gene-related deafness. *Otology & Neurotology, 25,* 930–934.

Solomon, A. (2012). *Far from the tree: Parents, children and the search for identity.* New York, NY: Simon & Schuster.

Stapleton, M., Kubaski, F., Mason, R. W., Yabe, H., Suzuki, Y., Orii, K. E., . . . Tomatsu, S. (2017). Presentation and treatments for mucopolysaccharidosis type II (MPS II; Hunter syndrome). *Expert Opinion on Orphan Drugs, 5*(4), 295–307.

Szarkowski, A., Mood, D., Shield, A., Wiley, S., & Yoshinaga-Itano, C. (2014). A summary of current understanding regarding children with autism spectrum disorder who are deaf or hard of hearing. *Seminars in Speech and Language, 35,* 241–259.

Szymanski, C. A., Brice, P. J., Lam, K. H., & Hotto, S. A. (2012). Deaf children with autism spectrum disorders. *Journal of Autism and Developmental Disorders, 42*(10), 2027–2037.

Tharpe, A. M., Fino-Szumski, M. S., & Bess, F. H. (2001). Survey of hearing aid fitting practices for children with multiple impairments. *American Journal of Audiology, 10*(1), 32–40.

Thomas, R., Sanders, S., Doust, J., Beller, E., & Glasziou, P. (2015). Prevalence of attention-deficit/hyperactivity disorder: A systematic review and meta-analysis. *Pediatrics, 135*(4), e994–e1001.

Thrasher, A. (2014). Video modeling for children with dual diagnosis of deafness or hard of hearing and autism spectrum disorder to promote peer interaction. *Seminars in Speech and Language, 35*(4), 331–342.

Valero, M. R., Sadadcharam, M., Henderson, L., Freeman, S. R., Lloyd, S., Green, K. M., . . . Bruce, I. A. (2016). Compliance with cochlear implantation in children subsequently diagnosed with autism spectrum disorder. *Cochlear Implants International, 17*(4), 200–206.

Van Naarden Braun, K., Christensen, D., Doernberg, N., Schieve, L., Rice, C., . . . Yeargin-Allsopp, M. (2015). Trends in the prevalence of autism spectrum disorder, cerebral palsy, hearing loss, intellectual disability, and vision impairment, Metropolitan Atlanta, 1991–2010. *PLoS One, 10*(4), e0124120.

Wade, S. L., Zhang, N., Yeates, K. O., Stancin, T., & Taylor, H. G. (2016). Social environmental moderators of long-term functional outcomes of early childhood brain injury. *JAMA Pediatrics, 170*(4), 343–349.

Wechsler, D. (2003a). *Wechsler Intelligence Scale for Children* (4th ed.). San Antonio, TX: Psychological Corporation.

Wechsler, D. (2003b). *Wechsler Preschool and Primary Scale of Intelligence* (4th ed.). San Antonio, TX: Pearson Education, Inc.

Wechsler, D., & Naglieri, J. A. (2006). *Wechsler Nonverbal Scale of Ability*. San Antonio, TX: Pearson Education Inc.

Wiley, S., Choo, D., Meinzen-Derr, J., Hilbert, L. & Greinwald, J. (2006). GJB2 mutations and additional disabilities in a pediatric cochlear implant population. *International Journal of Pediatric Otorhinoiaryngology, 70*(3), 493–500.

Wiley, S., Gustafson, S., & Rozniak, J. (2014). Needs of parents of children who are deaf/hard of hearing with autism spectrum disorder. *The Journal of Deaf Studies and Deaf Education, 19*(1), 40–49.

Wiley, S., Jahnke, M., Meinzen-Derr, J., & Choo, D. (2005). Perceived qualitative benefits of cochlear implants in children with multi-handicaps. *International Journal of Pediatric Otorhinolaryngology, 69*(6), 791–798.

Wiley, S., & Meinzen-Derr, J. (2013). Use of the Ages and Stages Questionnaire in young children who are deaf/hard of hearing as a screening for additional disabilities. *Early Human Development, 89*(5), 295–300.

Wiley, S., Meinzen-Derr, J., Stremel-Thomas, K., Schalock, M., Bashinski, S. M., & Ruder, C. (2013). Outcomes for children with deaf-blindness with cochlear implants: A multisite observational study. *Otology & Neurotology, 34*(3), 507–515.

Yoshinaga-Itano, C. (2014). Principles and guidelines for early intervention after confirmation that a child is deaf or hard of hearing. *Journal of Deaf Studies and Deaf Education, 19*(2), 143–175.

Yoshinaga-Itano, C., Baca, R. L., & Sedey, A. L. (2010). Describing the trajectory of language development in the presence of severe-to-profound hearing loss: A closer look at children with cochlear implants versus hearing aids. *Otology & Neurotology, 31*(8), 1268–1274.

Yoshinaga-Itano, C., Sedey, A. L., Coulter, D. K., & Mehl, A. L. (1998). Language of early- and later-identified children with hearing loss. *Pediatrics, 102*(5), 1161–1171.

Zaidman-Zait, A., Curle, D., Jamieson, J. R., Chia, R., & Kozak, F. K. (2015). Cochlear implantation among deaf children with additional disabilities: Parental perceptions of benefits, challenges, and service provision. *Journal of Deaf Studies and Deaf Education, 20*(1), 41–50.

Zazove, P. (1993). *When the phone rings, my bed shakes*. Washington, DC: Gallaudet University Press.

CHAPTER 27

Behavioral and Psychiatric Disorders

Adelaide S. Robb and Gabrielle Sky Cardwell

Upon completion of this chapter, the reader will

- Understand that individuals with developmental disabilities have a relatively high prevalence of psychiatric disorders
- Be able to describe the types and symptoms of psychiatric disorders among people with developmental disabilities
- Be able to discuss interventions in children who have a dual diagnosis of a developmental disability and a psychiatric disorder

Children with developmental disabilities manifest the same range of psychiatric illnesses that typically developing children do, but they may also face psychiatric illnesses specific to their disorder. The presence of a developmental disability, especially intellectual disability, often alters the symptomatic presentation of psychiatric disorders and makes accurate diagnosis more difficult. Recognition of these problems in children with **dual diagnoses** (a developmental disability and a psychiatric disorder) is crucial for caregivers. When these psychiatric disorders go unrecognized or untreated, affected children can fail in educational and social settings, engage in challenging behaviors at home, and show aggression and self-injury. These comorbid conditions may ultimately determine the child's outcome and placement. Notably, individuals with developmental disabilities who exhibit challenging behaviors such as aggression and self-injury are more likely to have a comorbid psychiatric disorder (Grey, Pollard, McClean, MacAuley, & Hastings, 2010). If the condition is identified early, however, treatment can be started and long-term adverse effects minimized.

It is a challenge for parents and individuals working with children with developmental disabilities to be alert to the possible presence of a psychiatric disorder and obtain early assessment, diagnosis, and treatment. This chapter addresses the identification and treatment of behavioral and psychiatric disorders in children with disabilities; it also discusses developmental transitions and their effect on behavior.

CASE STUDY

Gregory, age 17, has high-functioning autism spectrum disorder (ASD), attention-deficit/hyperactivity disorder (ADHD), and generalized anxiety disorder (GAD). He is in a special educational setting for high school students with high-functioning ASD and attends a special academy for culinary students as part of his academic day. He is being treated with an **antipsychotic medication** (aripiprazole), an antidepressant (bupropion), and a **stimulant** (methylphenidate). He has been stable for a long period with resolution of his previous psychiatric symptoms. The family has been concerned about his weight, which has increased above a BMI of 30 primarily due to excessive eating despite frequent exercise. In consultation with the family, the child psychiatrist began slowly tapering off the antipsychotic medication, which can cause overeating, over a 3-month time period. Once he was off the antipsychotic medication, his psychiatric condition deteriorated. He became irritable and easily angered. He was aggressive at home, with classmates, and with teachers. The school and parents consulted with the psychiatrist, who restarted Gregory on aripiprazole and titrated the dose back up to his prior dose with rapid resolution of his symptoms. He was back to being himself by the end of the second week on aripiprazole. His parents and therapy team are now evaluating other approaches to weight control.

Thought Questions:

At what ages (e.g., preschool age, school age, and adolescence) do the different types of behavioral and psychiatric disorders typically appear or are diagnosed? For the three disorders of interest, what are the main categories of intervention?

PREVALENCE OF PSYCHIATRIC DISORDERS AMONG CHILDREN WITH DEVELOPMENTAL DISABILITIES

In their landmark study of the epidemiology of childhood psychiatric disorders on the Isle of Wight, Rutter, Graham, and Yule (1970) found emotional disturbances in 7%–10% of typically developing children. In contrast, 30%–42% of children with intellectual disability demonstrated psychiatric disorders (Rutter et al., 1970). In a Swedish study, Gillberg et al. (1986) found that 57% of children and adolescents with mild intellectual disability and 64% with severe intellectual disability met diagnostic criteria for a psychiatric disorder. Additional studies have confirmed these results; children with intellectual disabilities have a four- to five-fold higher rate of psychiatric disorders than typically developing peers, and that higher rate does not diminish as the children grow into adolescence (Howlett, Florio, Xu, & Trollor, 2015).

In examining specific neurodevelopmental disorders, it is apparent that patients can have different rates of psychiatric disorders depending on their diagnosis (see Table 27.1). In children with velocardiofacial syndrome (22q11.2 deletion syndrome), the most common behavioral/psychiatric disorders are ADHD (25%–46%); major depressive disorder (12%–20%); and anxiety disorders, including specific phobias (27%–61%; Arnold, Siegel-Bartelt, Cytrynbaum, Teshima, & Schachar, 2001). In adults with 22q11.2 deletion, 32% experienced psychotic symptoms and 41% had depression (Schneider et al., 2014; Swillen & McDonald-McGinn, 2015; Tang et al., 2014). Both boys and girls with fragile X syndrome have higher rates of social anxiety than typically developing peers. Affected girls have higher rates of depression and affected boys have higher rates of aggression (Gross, Hoffmann, Bassell, & Berry-Kravis, 2015; Powis & Oliver, 2014). In children with fragile X syndrome, the rates of anxiety were reported to be as high as 42% when teachers were asked to rate symptoms; parents noted anxiety in 26% of the same children (Sullivan, Hooper, & Hatton, 2007). In girls with fragile X syndrome, the rates of mood disorders were found to be 47%, with major depression representing half of those disorders (Freund, Reiss, & Abrams, 1993). Boys with fragile X syndrome were found to have high rates of manic/hyperactive behaviors, but low rates of depressed mood based on maternal report (Thurman, McDuffie, Hagerman, & Abbeduto, 2014). Rates of bipolar disorder, however, are lower in children with fragile X than in the general population (Hessl et al., 2001). Up to 70% of boys with fragile X syndrome can exhibit self-injurious behavior (SIB; Hall, Barnett, & Hustyi, 2016; see Chapter 15).

Children with trisomy 21 (Down syndrome) have increased rates of behavioral disorders; 20%–40% exhibit aggression and ADHD versus 5%–8% ADHD in typically developing children. Adolescents with trisomy 21 also have increased rates of unspecified psychosis or depression with psychotic features (43% versus 13%) compared to adolescents with other intellectual disorders (Dykens et al., 2015). Adults are at increased risk for dementia and withdrawal depression compared with typically developing adults (Dekker et al., 2015; Esbensen, Johnson, Amaral, Tan, & Macks, 2016; Lautarescu, Holland, & Zaman, 2017; Määttä, Tervo-Määttä, Taanila, Kaski, & Iivanainen, 2014; McCarron, McCallion, Reilly, & Mulryan, 2014). In trisomy 21, conduct disorder (CD) and oppositional defiant disorder (ODD) occur at comparable rates with the general population (12%), whereas autism occurs in about 10% versus a little more than 1% in the general population (Lott, 2012; see Chapter 15).

In children with Prader-Willi syndrome, the occurrence of obsessive-compulsive disorder (OCD) symptoms varies according to the molecular defect. Individuals with long type I 15q deletions have compulsive cleaning (e.g., grooming and showering), whereas those with short type II 15q deletions have academic OCD symptoms (e.g., rereading, erasing, and counting; Zarcone et al., 2007). Prader-Willi is also associated

Table 27.1. Percentages of mental illness by developmental disability

Population	MI	ADHD	ODD	CD	MDD	BPD	SZ/PSY	AXD	PH	GAD	SIB	ASD
General	7–10	5–8	6–10	2–9	3.3–11.2	2–5	1.1	6–25	0.6–15	0.4–1	<1	<1
DD	30–42		48									
Mild ID	57										5	
Severe ID	64											
VCF–child		25–46			12–20			27–61				
VCF–adult					41		32					
FRX								26–42				
FRX–girl					47 mood half MDD							
FRX–boy											58	
TR21		20–40	12	12								10
PWS						15–17						
TS								High SP				
XXYY					50							
FAE				50		33–35						
FAS					18	33–35						
WS	80	65							54	12		

Key: DD, developmental disability; ID, intellectual disability; VCF, velocardiofacial syndrome; FRX, fragile X syndrome; TR21, trisomy 21; PWS, Prader-Willi syndrome; TS, Turner syndrome; FAE, fetal alcohol exposure; FAS, fetal alcohol syndrome; WS, Williams syndrome; MI, mental illness; ADHD, attention-deficit/hyperactivity disorder; ODD, oppositional defiant disorder; CD, conduct disorder; MDD, major depressive disorder; BPD, bipolar disorder; SZ/PSY, schizophrenia/psychotic disorder; AXD, anxiety disorder; PH, phobia; GAD, generalized anxiety disorder; SIB, self-injurious behavior; ASD, autism spectrum disorder; SP, social phobia.

with higher rates of bipolar disorder (15%–17% versus 2%–5% in the typically developing population) and mood disorders (with psychotic features occurring in 28% versus 0.4% in the general population; Butler, Manzardo, & Forster, 2016; Skokauskas, Sweeny, Meehan, & Gallagher, 2012). Adolescents with Turner syndrome have high rates of social phobia, shyness, anxiety, and depression, with anxiety and mood swings becoming evident in adulthood (Saad et al., 2014; Saad, Al-Atram, Baseer, Ali, & El-Houfey, 2015). Almost half of individuals with XXYY syndrome have major depression and are at an increased risk for ADHD (Tartaglia, Ayari, Hutaff-Lee, & Boada, 2012).

In children who have prenatal exposure to alcohol but without features of fetal alcohol syndrome (FAS; see Chapter 2), rates of CD are as high as 50% (Burd, Klug, Martsolf, & Kerbeshian, 2003). For children with FAS, both suicide and depression rates are elevated. Up to half attempt suicide, and major depression is found in approximately 18% of those exposed to alcohol in utero (Burd et al., 2003; O'Connor et al., 2002). For those with fetal alcohol spectrum disorder (including both FAS and prenatal alcohol exposure), rates of bipolar disorder range from 33%–35% (O'Connor et al., 2002). CD and ADHD are also common among these individuals, with pooled prevalence rates of 90.7% and 51.2%, respectively (Popova et al., 2016).

In a comprehensive study of children with Williams syndrome, 80% were found to have one or more psychiatric disorders, the most common being ADHD (65%), followed by specific phobia (54%) and then GAD (12%) (Leyfer, Woodruff-Borden, Klein-Tasman, Fricke, & Mervis, 2006). Recent reviews have also found a high prevalence of anxiety in these individuals (Dankner & Dykens, 2012; Riby et al., 2014; Stinton, Tomlinson, & Estes, 2012; Young, Apfeldorf, Knepper, & Yager, 2009).

CAUSES OF PSYCHIATRIC DISORDERS IN DEVELOPMENTAL DISABILITIES

Children with developmental disabilities are at risk for the same types of psychiatric disorders as typically developing children. In addition, certain maladaptive behavior disorders are found principally among individuals with severe to profound levels of intellectual disability. These behaviors include stereotypic movement disorder (i.e., repetitive, self-stimulating, nonfunctional motor behavior, which may include SIB) and pica (i.e., the persistent ingesting of nonfood items).

In some cases, the cause of a psychiatric disorder in individuals with developmental disabilities is the direct result of a biochemical or genetic abnormality (see Box 27.1). For example, in the inborn error of

BOX 27.1 EVIDENCE-BASED PRACTICE

Genetic Testing to Detect Developmental Disorders

Genetic testing can be used to detect and diagnose developmental disorders in children. For example, fluorescence in situ hybridization was one of the first methods of genetic testing used to diagnose 22q11.2 deletion syndrome. This targeted testing method also led to the discovery that many syndromes previously thought to be unrelated conditions, such as velocardiofacial syndrome, also resulted from 22q11.2 deletion (Driscoll et al., 1993). In recent years other genetic tests have been found effective in detecting 22q11.2 deletion syndrome, such as chromosomal microarray analysis (Lu et al., 2008) and multiplex ligation-dependent probe amplification (Schouten et al., 2002).

metabolism Lesch-Nyhan syndrome (see Appendix B), an abnormality in the dopamine neurotransmitter system causes affected individuals to exhibit a compulsive form of SIB (Mohapatra & Sahoo, 2016; Tewari, Mathur, Sardana, & Bansal, 2017). In other cases, conditions that affect the developing brain are risk factors for a psychiatric disorder. For instance, in 1956, Pasamanick, Rogers, and Lilienfeld hypothesized that prenatal brain injury and exposure to toxins during pregnancy could cause behavior disorders in children. In the years since, several studies have linked prenatal alcohol, tobacco, illicit drug, and chemical exposure to the development of neuropsychological disorders in children. Such studies have been important in identifying and eliminating a potential cause of developmental and psychiatric disorders in children.

In addition to fetal alcohol and drug exposure, congenital infections such as rubella (which is associated with ASD) and perinatal or neonatal hypoxic ischemic encephalopathy (brain disorders due to lack of oxygen or blood flow) are associated with memory and language disorders (see Chapter 17). The increased risk of psychiatric disturbance due to neurobiological disorders may be attributable to factors such as irritability, affective instability, distractibility, and communication impairments (Feinstein & Reiss, 1996). Risks may also increase in the presence of conditions such as epilepsy, developmental language disorders, and sensory impairments, which are independently associated with an increased incidence of psychiatric disorders (Salmon, O'Kearney, Reese, & Fortune, 2016; Van Ool et al., 2016; Van Tricht et al., 2015).

The cause of most psychiatric disorders among children with developmental disabilities is likely to be a complex interaction among biological (including genetic), environmental, medical, and psychosocial factors. For example, a young man who has sustained a significant traumatic brain injury (see Chapter 23) with resulting cognitive impairment may regularly become depressed because of a combination of neurotransmitter changes due to brain injury, a familial predisposition to depression, his parents' grief, and his own despair over loss of previous abilities. Children with severe intellectual disability may develop SIB in response to an ear infection or constipation as they cannot verbally express feeling discomfort.

PSYCHIATRIC DISORDERS OF CHILDHOOD AND ADOLESCENCE

The following sections discuss a number of psychiatric disorders; however, two important disorders, ASD and ADHD, are not discussed here because separate chapters are devoted to them (see Chapters 18 and 19). It should be noted that in the *Diagnostic and Statistical Manual–Fifth Edition (DSM-5),* the American Psychiatric Association (APA, 2013) has proposed several criteria changes for diagnosing a number of disorders covered in this section. These are described as follows: Posttraumatic stress disorder (PTSD) in children needs only two symptoms of negative alterations in cognition and mood and two symptoms in arousal and reactivity. The trauma can be the loss of a parent and can manifest as nonspecific frightening dreams, themes of trauma in play, or reenactment of the trauma. In pediatric eating disorders, less emphasis is placed on the strict diagnostic requirement of being less than 85% of ideal body weight and having amenorrhea. The criteria now focus on previous weight and growth patterns and the impact of starvation on multiple organ systems, not just the reproductive system. A new disorder in children under consideration in *DSM-5* is disruptive mood dysregulation with dysphoria, which is considered a milder condition than the classic combined ODD and bipolar disorder. This proposed disorder describes children with persistent negative mood who have outbursts of rage. Changes to other disorder criteria in *DSM-5* are described in the following sections.

Oppositional Defiant and Conduct Disorders

In order for a child to be diagnosed with ODD, there must be a pattern of negative, hostile, and defiant behaviors (APA, 2013). Children must have angry/irritable moods, defiant/headstrong behaviors, and vindictiveness. In terms of the persistence and frequency used to differentiate normative and symptomatic behavior, there are different standards for children by age. Children younger than age 5 should show these behavior problems most days for at least 6 months, whereas children who are older than age 5 years should show such problems at least once a week for at least 6 months. Developmental level, gender, and culture must also be considered in making the diagnosis. Further, these behaviors must occur outside of a psychotic or mood disorder. They must cause impairments in social, educational, or vocational activities and may occur in one or multiple settings. This diagnosis is usually given to preadolescent children.

To be diagnosed with a CD, an individual must demonstrate a pattern of callous and unemotional behavior in which other people's rights are violated, norms are ignored, or rules are broken, and it must have continued for at least 12 months. The four main problem areas are 1) aggression toward people and animals, 2) destruction of property, 3) deceitfulness or theft, and 4) serious violation of rules. Some examples of aggression include bullying and threatening, starting physical fights, using a weapon in fights, being physically cruel to people or animals, stealing while confronting a victim, and forcing someone into unwanted sexual activity. Destruction includes deliberate fire-setting or vandalism or destruction of property. Deceitfulness or theft includes breaking into a house or car, lying to obtain goods or services, and stealing or shoplifting. Serious violation of rules includes staying out at night (but not overnight) before age 13, running away from home overnight at least twice, and frequent truancy from school before age 13. CDs are rarely diagnosed in preadolescent children. If a child meets criteria for CD, he or she does not receive a concurrent diagnosis of ODD. Both ODD and CD occur at higher rates in children with developmental disabilities than in typically developing children, 48% overall versus 6%–10% ODD and 2%–9% CD in typically developing populations (Hardan et al., 1997). It should be noted that children with an intellectual disability and ADHD have higher rates of ODD and CD than children with ADHD alone (Ahuja, Martin, Langley, & Thapar, 2013).

ODD and CD are often associated with ADHD, and the treatment for one may improve the condition of the other (Kutcher et al., 2004). Treatment of both CD and ODD includes the same behavior management techniques useful in ADHD. Similarly, both disorders may benefit from stimulant and other ADHD medications (Connor, Barkley, & Davis, 2000). Among the latter medications are 1) atomoxetine (Strattera), a norepinephrine reuptake inhibitor that is effective at higher doses for children and adolescents with ADHD comorbid with ODD or CD (Newcorn, Spencer, Biederman, Milton, & Michelson, 2005), and 2) long-acting guanfacine, an α-2 receptor antagonist, which also helps control ADHD with comorbid ODD/CD (Connor et al., 2010). A long-acting form of clonidine, another α-2 receptor antagonist, is now approved for ADHD monotherapy in 6–17 year olds (Jain, Segal, Kollins, & Khayrallah, 2011).

Although all categories of ADHD medication (stimulants, norepinephrine reuptake inhibitors, and α-2 receptor agonists), can help when ADHD is comorbid with ODD/CD, behavioral therapy is the preferred treatment for ODD and CD. Behavioral therapy involves setting consistent limits, behavioral expectations, and consequences (see Chapter 34). This intervention must be consistent at home and school so that the child knows that the rules and expectations are enforced in all settings. For younger children, a positive reinforcement system employing stickers and/or a behavior chart to target being respectful and following directions can cover most daily rules and activities. For older children and adolescents, tokens are commonly used to reinforce appropriate behavior. These can be traded for desired activities, such as an extra 30 minutes of television or free computer time. In this way, adolescents earn and pay for their privileges in the same way that adults earn money to buy what they need or want. Evidence-based treatments for CD often include multisystemic therapy (Henggeller et al., 1986) and wraparound services (Burchard, Bruns, & Burchard, 2002). Both treatments are family focused and offer children support and services in their home, school, and community in order to improve behavior (Suter & Bruns, 2009; Weiss et al., 2013). In this way, treatment not only targets the child's behavior, but also the behavior of his or her peers, family, and even those in other networks, such as his or her school, to offer a more holistic, multidomain approach to treatment.

Impulse Control Disorders

Impulse control disorders include intermittent explosive disorder and hair-pulling disorder. Intermittent explosive disorder is diagnosed after several discrete episodes of failure to resist aggressive impulses, with resultant assaults or destruction of property. The severity of the assault must be out of proportion to the precipitating psychosocial stressor. An example might be a child who is told that he cannot have cake until he has finished his lunch. The child then throws his plate across the room, breaks his chair, and starts kicking his little sister over the incident. Treatment of intermittent explosive disorder in adults includes the use of beta-blockers such as propranolol, certain antiepileptic/mood stabilizing drugs (e.g., valproic acid), and novel antipsychotics (e.g., risperidone; Hässler & Reis, 2010). Children with mild to moderate intellectual disability are more likely to have this disorder than their typically developing peers.

An individual fits the profile for hair pulling disorder, historically called trichotillomania, when it results in noticeable hair loss; this can be anywhere on the body. It should not be associated with an underlying skin or physical condition causing hair loss. Consultation with a dermatologist to rule out skin problems such as tinea capitis (ringworm), which can cause hair loss, may be appropriate. A child with this disorder feels tension that makes the child pull out the hair, which is followed by a sense of relief after doing it. Children who have hair pulling disorder may eat the hair, which can cause bezoars (hair balls) in the stomach or gastrointestinal track that need to be surgically or endoscopically removed. In children with hair loss, it is important to ask the parent and child if the child is pulling out and eating hair. Treatment of this disorder is similar to that for OCD, with the use of selective serotonin reuptake inhibitors (SSRIs; e.g., fluoxetine) and cognitive-behavioral therapy (Johnson & El-Alfy, 2016; Keuthen et al., 2012). This hair pulling is seen as being on the spectrum of OCD in contrast to other forms of self-mutilation, such as self-cutting seen in teenagers, which fall on the mood and personality disorder spectrums.

Anxiety Disorders

Anxiety disorders include the *DSM-IV–Text Revision* classifications GAD, panic disorder, social anxiety disorder, OCD, and PTSD. In *DSM-5*, skin-picking disorder has been added (APA, 2013). Anxiety disorders not discussed in this section include separation anxiety, where children become anxious when away from family or the home, and simple phobias such as being frightened of needle sticks or the dark.

Generalized Anxiety Disorder The diagnosis of GAD requires at least 3 months of excessive anxiety and worry most days about two or more of the following: family, health, finances, or school (APA, 2013). The child has difficulty controlling the worry and has accompanying symptoms, including restlessness, quick fatigue, problems concentrating, irritability, muscle tension, and disturbed sleep. The child also shows marked avoidance of, or marked time and effort spent preparing for, situations with potentially negative outcomes. In addition, the child procrastinates in behavior or decision making due to worries and needs repeated reassurances. The child has problems at home or school because of the anxiety, and the anxiety is unrelated to another psychiatric or medical illness. A recent study found that children with an intellectual disability had significantly higher rates of anxiety than typically developing children (Green, Berkovits, & Baker, 2015). Treatment includes cognitive-behavioral therapy to reduce worry (as discussed in Box 27.2) and at times medication such as SSRIs or serotonin-norepinephrine reuptake inhibitors (Creswell, Waite, & Cooper, 2014; Moskowitz et al., 2017; Strawn, Welge, Wehry, Keeshin, & Rynn, 2015). Several studies have shown that medications are effective for pediatric anxiety disorders. Sertraline, duloxetine, and fluvoxamine have been found to be effective in treating GAD in children (Rynn, Siqueland, & Rickels, 2001; Strawn et al., 2015; Walkup et al., 2001). Fluvoxamine is also effective in treating other anxiety disorders, such as social phobia and separation anxiety disorder (Walkup et al., 2001). More recently, a large National Institute of Mental Health (NIMH) study demonstrated that a combination of sertraline and cognitive-behavioral therapy resulted in a better

BOX 27.2 EVIDENCE-BASED PRACTICE

Cognitive-Behavioral Therapy to Treat Childhood Anxiety

Cognitive-behavioral therapy (CBT) is the most widely studied and commonly used treatment for childhood anxiety (Olatunji, Cisler, & Deacon, 2010). However, few studies have examined the effectiveness of CBT for treating anxiety in children with developmental disabilities. Randomized control trials have found CBT to be effective for treating anxiety in children with autism spectrum disorder (Wood et al., 2009), but further research is needed to determine the effectiveness of CBT to treat anxiety in children with other developmental disabilities.

outcome in childhood anxiety disorders than either treatment alone (Walkup et al., 2008).

Panic Disorder To meet diagnostic criteria for panic disorder, an individual must have one or more panic attacks that include at least four of the symptoms listed in Table 27.2. People with panic disorder have panic attacks that recur; are unexpected; and combine with worry about having more panic attacks, worry about the consequence of an attack (e.g., that the child might die or go crazy), or worry leading to a significant change in behavior due to the attacks (e.g., stopping exercise because of a fast heartbeat, rapid breathing, and sweating—feeling like a heart attack). Since panic attack symptoms can mimic other disorders such as heart problems, stomach disorders, seizures, and asthma, appropriate treatment is often delayed while other medical causes are ruled out. In patients with panic disorder, other family members also may have or have had a history of anxiety disorder or panic attacks as there appears to be a genetic component.

Panic attacks do not usually begin until puberty. Adolescents with panic disorder may begin to avoid certain places or situations such as crowds, public transportation, and other places where a panic attack could occur. This maladaptive change in behavior can lead to avoiding exercise or unfamiliar situations or, in extreme cases, to comorbid agoraphobia (fear of leaving the house). Patients with panic disorder can be treated with high-potency benzodiazepines such as alprazolam and clonazepam alone or in combination with SSRIs (Batelaan, Van Balkom, & Stein, 2012). Patients with panic disorder can also be helped through cognitive-behavioral therapy (Hofmann, Asnaani, Vonk, Sawyer, & Fang, 2012; Kircher et al., 2013). In cognitive-behavioral therapy, patients develop a list of things that are least to most likely to cause a panic attack and then work their way through the list, facing the different issues that cause the attacks. The therapist helps the individual devise strategies to temper or overcome the attacks in real time and observes how the anxiety decreases over time.

Table 27.2. Symptoms of panic disorder

Rapid or racing heartbeat
Sweating, trembling, or shaking
Feeling short of breath or as if being smothered
Feeling as if choking
Chest pain or discomfort
Nausea or abdominal distress
Feeling dizzy, lightheaded, or faint
Feeling of unreality or detachment (like floating or in a dream)
Fear of losing control or going crazy
Fear of dying
Numbness and tingling
Hot flashes or chills

Note: At least four symptoms need to be present during an attack for a diagnosis of panic disorder.

Social Anxiety Disorder A phobia particularly relevant to children is social anxiety disorder, which includes school phobia. In this disorder, there is an intense fear (phobia) of acting in a way or showing anxiety symptoms that will be negatively evaluated. The fear is out of proportion to the actual danger posed by the social situation. For children, social anxiety disorder may result in not only making excuses to avoid going to school, but also practicing *selective mutism* in which the child does not speak at all in school but speaks normally in other situations.

Social phobia involves a marked and persistent fear of one or more social or performance situations in which a person is exposed to strangers or to scrutiny by others and worries about possibly doing something embarrassing. A diagnosis for this disorder involves a child having appropriate relationships with family members and friends but being afraid of other peers and adults. Exposure to the social situation (e.g., a birthday party) provokes anxiety and the child may cry, have a tantrum, freeze, or shrink from situations with unfamiliar people. The child may not be aware that the fear is unreasonable, and the fear must impair social functioning. Social phobia is classified as generalized if it takes place in multiple settings, and the symptoms must last for more than 6 months. Treatment includes cognitive-behavioral therapy to reduce anxiety in social situations, speech-making and acting classes for people with performance anxieties, and the use of SSRIs. Children with extreme cases of social phobia are too frightened to speak in the classroom, eat in the cafeteria, or use the restroom at school. This can markedly impair school performance and should not be dismissed as simple shyness. Some children with a variant of social phobia may, like children with social anxiety disorder, have selective mutism, in which they refuse to speak to unfamiliar people or children; SSRIs and behavioral therapy may be helpful in this case (Bergman, Gonzalez, Piacentini, & Keller, 2013; Mohatt, Bennett, & Walkup, 2014). Girls with fragile X syndrome have high rates of both social phobia (55%) and selective mutism (21%; Wadell, Hagerman, & Hessl, 2013).

Obsessive-Compulsive Disorder A child with OCD has obsessions, compulsions, or both. **Obsessions** are recurrent thoughts, images, or impulses that are experienced as intrusive and inappropriate and cause anxiety or distress. The obsessions are not excessive worries about real-life problems (as in generalized anxiety), and individuals attempt to ignore, suppress, or neutralize the obsessions. Children may not be aware that the obsessions and compulsions are unreasonable; furthermore, children with a developmental disability may not realize that the obsessions are a product of the mind. **Compulsions** are repetitive behaviors (e.g., hand washing) or mental acts (e.g., praying or counting) that are done to neutralize an obsession or as part of following rigid rules. A child with obsessions about germs would have washing compulsions to neutralize the germs. The compulsions are designed to reduce distress or to prevent some dreaded act. For example, a child might refuse to step on green tiles in the school corridor because the child believes his or her mother might die if the child stepped on green tiles. Children, especially younger ones, are more likely to have compulsions without the accompanying obsessions; thus, a child might have an elaborate 2-hour bedtime ritual without self-awareness regarding why their bedtime ritual is that certain way.

Some children develop the rapid onset of OCD after a streptococcal skin or throat infection. This is referred to as pediatric autoimmune neuropsychiatric disorders associated with *Streptococcus* infections or PANDAS (Chiarello, Spitoni, Hollander, Matucci Cerinic, & Pallanti, 2017). The first report of pediatric autoimmune neuropsychiatric disorders associated with streptococcal infections (PANDAS) was published by Swedo and colleagues in 1998. Like adult OCD, PANDAS is associated with basal ganglia dysfunction (Orefici, Cardona, Cox, & Cunningham, 2016). Treatments for PANDAS include treatment of underlying infections with antibiotics, psychotropic medications such as benzodiazepines, and behavioral interventions such as cognitive-behavioral therapy (Thienemann et al., 2017).

Common compulsions in children include ordering and arranging, counting, tapping, touching, and collecting/hoarding. Nearly all children exhibit some or all of such behaviors during development. Therefore, in order to meet criteria for the diagnosis, the obsessions and compulsions must consume more than 1 hour per day and interfere with functioning. The definition also quantifies the level of insight by the child for the irrationality of the OCD as absent, poor, or good insight (APA, 2013). It has been found that poor or absent insight is common among children with OCD, especially in children with intellectual disabilities (Lewin et al., 2010). Individuals with chronic tic disorder may exhibit OCD symptoms, and children with ASD may exhibit OCD-like rigidity and repetitive, compulsive behaviors (see Chapter 18).

Treatment of OCD in children and adolescents includes cognitive-behavioral therapy, which is aimed at experiencing the obsessive thought without carrying out the compulsion designed to reduce the anxiety. This form of therapy is called exposure-and-response prevention. A child with fear of germs would be asked to touch a doorknob and then be forbidden to wash his or her hands. Children have weekly assignments in this therapy. Several medications are also approved for the treatment of OCD in children, including clomipramine, sertraline, fluoxetine, and fluvoxamine (DeVaugh-Geiss et al., 1992; Geller et al., 2001; March et al., 1998; Riddle et al., 2001). One paper in the literature described the difference in outcome among children with OCD who were treated with one of four treatments: sertraline, placebo, cognitive-behavioral therapy, or a combination of medication and therapy (Pediatric OCD Treatment Study Team, 2004). Of the four options, the combination therapy helped the most children, followed by cognitive-behavioral therapy alone, sertraline alone, and then placebo. OCD can be comorbid with other developmental disabilities, especially ADHD and ASD.

Posttraumatic Stress Disorder PTSD is an anxiety disorder that occurs after exposure to a traumatic event in which the person experiences or witnesses an actual or threatened death, serious injury, or (in the case of a child) the loss of a parent or other attachment figure. In children with developmental disabilities, PTSD may occur after physical abuse or after the injury that caused the disability. Children with intellectual disability are particularly at risk for PTSD, as they have more limited coping skills. The child responds to the inciting event with intense fear, helplessness, or horror and may have disorganized or agitated behavior. A child with a diagnosis of PTSD must have symptoms for at least 1 month and have impaired functioning. The symptoms are broken down into three categories: re-experiencing the trauma, avoidance and numbing, and increased arousal. Re-experiencing behavior includes 1) recurrent recollections of the event (in children, this may manifest as a repetitive theme in play), 2) dreams of the event (children may have distressing dreams that are not trauma specific, and children do not necessarily need to be able to remember the content of the dreams), 3) flashbacks of the event (children may reenact the trauma), 4) intense mental distress at physical or mental cues that remind the child of the event, and 5) physiological reactivity on exposure to cues that remind the child of the event. Avoidance behavior includes 1) efforts to avoid thoughts or feelings associated with the trauma, 2) efforts to avoid people and places associated with the trauma, 3) inability to recall important aspects of the trauma, 4) decreased interest or participation in activities, 5) feelings of detachment or estrangement, 6) a restricted range of feelings, and 7) a sense of a shortened future. Symptoms of increased arousal include 1) difficulty sleeping, 2) irritability or angry outbursts, 3) difficulty concentrating, 4) hypervigilance, and 5) an exaggerated startle response. PTSD is characterized by duration, either acute (3 months or less) or chronic (more than 3 months), and by delayed onset (starts 6 months after the trauma).

Treatment of PTSD has included both psychotherapy and SSRIs, and a recent meta-analysis includes a critical review of the published trials (Morina, Koerssen, & Pollett, 2016). The largest controlled trial of the SSRI sertraline in PTSD failed to show that medication was superior to placebo (Robb, Cuea, Sporn, Yang, & Vanderburg, 2010). Other studies have shown that trauma-focused cognitive-behavioral therapy shows the best efficacy in youth with PTSD (Ehlers et al., 2014). Patients must practice talking through the thoughts and events that remind them of the incident that elicited the PTSD. Play therapy, in which a child has a chance to relive and triumph over the trauma, may also help work through the loss. Therapy must be based on the cognitive level of the child.

Skin Picking (Excoriation) Disorder In this anxiety disorder, skin picking results in actual skin lesions. Skin picking also causes clinically significant distress or impairment in social, occupation, or other important areas of function. Medical afflictions (e.g., scabies) and other psychiatric disorders (e.g., psychosis) must be eliminated from consideration to make this diagnosis.

Mood Disorders

Mood disorders that may impact children include major depression and bipolar disorder.

Major Depression Children carrying a diagnosis of major depression must have a 2-week period with at least five of the following symptoms that represent a change from previous functioning: 1) depressed mood by subjective report or as observed by others (children and adolescents may have an irritable mood), 2) decreased interest or pleasure in most activities, 3) significant change in weight or appetite (children may fail to make expected weight gains), 4) insomnia or hypersomnia (excessive sleep), 5) psychomotor agitation or retardation, 6) fatigue or loss of energy, 7) feelings of worthlessness or guilt, 8) decreased concentration or indecisiveness, and 9) recurrent thoughts of death and dying. Symptoms must not be due to bereavement and must cause impairment in the child's daily function.

A review of depression in trisomy 21 showed that although antidepressants, electroconvulsive therapy, and psychotherapy were all effective, many people with Down syndrome and depression were undertreated (Walker, Dosen, Buitelaar, & Janzing, 2011). In addition, depressive symptoms and social relating problems in children with trisomy 21 have been found to persist into adulthood (Foley et al., 2015).

In a review of 257 clinic patients with fragile X disorder with anxiety, mood disorder, ADHD, and aggression, Berry-Kravis, Sumis, Hervey, and Mathur (2012) noted that the patients had success rates that varied by treatment, including a 53% response to antidepressants and 54% response to antipsychotics. Those children with fragile X who failed one medication trial had a 73%–77% of responding to a sequential trial in the same category of medication.

In general, children with major depression can be treated with medication or psychotherapy or a combination of both. Studies have shown that several SSRIs are superior to a placebo in the treatment of depression (Emslie et al., 2002; Wagner et al., 2003; Wagner et al., 2004). An NIMH study found that for adolescents with major depression, placebo and cognitive-behavioral therapy alone were similar in improvement, whereas fluoxetine was better, and fluoxetine plus cognitive-behavioral therapy had the best outcome (Treatment for Adolescents with Depression Study Team, 2004). It also has been shown that treatment with a combination of cognitive-behavioral therapy and fluoxetine results in a significantly lower risk of relapse compared to treatment with fluoxetine only in children with major depression (Kennard et al., 2014).

Bipolar Disorder Bipolar disorder consists of swings between depression and **mania/hypomania.** A manic episode consists of a distinct period of abnormally and persistently elevated, expansive, or irritable mood lasting at least 1 week. The mood disturbance must have three of the following symptoms (four symptoms are necessary if irritable): 1) inflated self-esteem or grandiosity, 2) decreased need for sleep, 3) more talkative or pressured speech or vocalizations (in nonverbal children), 4) flight of ideas (idea moves from topic to topic) or racing thoughts, 5) distractibility, 6) increased goal-directed activity or psychomotor agitation, and 7) excessive involvement in pleasurable activities that have a high potential for painful consequences (e.g., promiscuity, drug use, or spending sprees). Hypomania is a less severe set of symptoms than mania. A patient with hypomania would not need to be hospitalized. They would have symptoms for less than 7 days, would only have two of the manic symptoms, or continue to do well at school and home despite silly, goofy behavior.

Individuals with bipolar disorder are treated with mood stabilizers such as lithium or valproic acid (which is also used as an antiepileptic drug and is not U.S. Food and Drug Administration (FDA) approved for the treatment of bipolar disorder in children or adolescents). The only positive trial of an antiepileptic drug for pediatric bipolar disorder is the add-on trial of lamotrigine in pediatric bipolar disorder manic or depressed episode that was effective in reducing bipolar symptoms in youth over the age of 12 (Findling et al., 2015a). They may also benefit from antipsychotic medication such as risperidone, aripiprazole, olanzapine, quetiapine, and ziprasidone in conjunction with mood stabilizers or as monotherapy (use of antipsychotics alone). All of these medications (except ziprasidone) are FDA approved for the treatment of bipolar disorder with mixed or manic episodes in older children and teenagers. Combination therapy with olanzapine and fluoxetine has also been found to be effective and has been FDA approved for treating bipolar depression in adolescents (Detke, DelBello, Landry, & Usher, 2015). Children with bipolar disorder must have consistent bedtimes and routines to ensure that lack of sleep does not precipitate either a manic or mixed episode.

Psychotic Disorders

Psychotic disorders (sometimes called "psychosis") consist of alterations in thinking or perceptions that are not connected with reality. The primary psychotic disorder is **schizophrenia.** The diagnosis of schizophrenia requires the presence of one or more of the following three symptoms for at least 6 months, with active symptoms for 1 month or less if treated: 1) **delusions** (fixed idiosyncratic false belief; e.g., that someone is following the person), 2) **hallucinations** (sensory perception without an environmental stimulus; e.g., hearing a voice when no one else is present), and 3) disorganized speech (APA, 2013). In children, there will be an associated failure to achieve expected levels of interpersonal relationships and academic achievement.

Patients with a mood disorder or an ASD may have psychotic symptoms that are confused with the formal diagnosis of schizophrenia, as examined in Box 27.3. An individual with ASD must have prominent delusions or hallucinations to meet the schizophrenia diagnosis in addition to ASD. Other medical conditions that can mimic schizophrenia include epilepsy, effects of an illegal drug, and brain tumors. Once the diagnosis of schizophrenia has been confirmed, treatment with antipsychotic drugs will reduce the delusions and hallucinations, thereby improving psychosocial functioning. Six atypical antipsychotic medications for schizophrenia are approved for adolescents 13 years and older: aripiprazole, olanzapine (a second-line drug due to metabolic adverse effects), quetiapine, paliperidone, risperidone, and lurasidone (Findling et al., 2008; Findling et al., 2012; Goldman, Loebel, Cucchiaro, Deng, & Findling, 2017; Haas et al., 2009; Kryzhanovskaya et al., 2009; Singh, Robb, Vijapurkar, Nuamah, & Hough, 2013). Trials of ziprasidone and asenapine for adolescent schizophrenia have failed to show a benefit compared with placebo (Findling et al., 2013; Findling et al., 2015b).

Eating Disorders

The three important types of eating disorders that occur in children with developmental disabilities are rumination, binge eating, and pica. In **rumination,** infants or young children repeatedly regurgitate without nausea or gastrointestinal illness for at least 1 month. Regurgitated food may be rechewed, reswallowed, or spit out. To meet the definition of rumination in the context of intellectual disability or ASD, regurgitation should be sufficiently frequent and severe to warrant

BOX 27.3 EVIDENCE-BASED PRACTICE

Autism Spectrum Disorder and Psychotic Disorders

Autism spectrum disorder (ASD) and psychotic disorders such as schizophrenia have historically been considered related disorders (Kyriakopoulos et al., 2015). The disorders share phenotypic characteristics and neurobiological structural similarities (Cheung et al., 2010). However, the two disorders remain clinically distinct. Therefore, although ASD and schizophrenia may share common etiologies, it is important to understand how these disorders are distinct for effective treatment.

independent clinical attention because it may instead be a self-stimulatory behavior in these children. Treatment includes behavioral interventions and the use of gastrointestinal motility agents (e.g., laxatives; Luiselli, 2015; Woods, Luiselli, & Tomassone, 2013). One study of 55 adolescents with rumination found that patients with a comorbid mental health disorder were less likely to respond to treatment (Alioto, Yacob, Yardley, & Di Lorenzo, 2015).

The second common eating disorder is **binge eating,** whereby the child has recurrent episodes of eating large amounts of food during short periods of time. Binge-eating episodes demonstrate at least three of the following features: 1) eating much more rapidly than normal; 2) eating until feeling uncomfortably full; 3) eating large amounts of food when not feeling physically hungry; 4) eating alone because of embarrassment over how much one is eating; and 5) feeling disgusted with oneself, depressed, or very guilty afterwards. The binge-eating episodes should not occur exclusively during the course of anorexia, bulimia, or avoidant/restrictive food intake, and they must occur on average at least once a week for 3 months (APA, 2013). It should be emphasized that children who do binge risk choking to death. Binge eating is a frequent complication of and contributes to the morbid obesity seen among individuals with Prader-Willi syndrome. Children with a binge-eating disorder need nutritional guidance and counseling, parental and school oversight of meals, limited access to food outside of meals, and an exercise routine. For some children with a severe binge-eating disorder, admission to a long-stay residential setting with strict oversight of meals and activity levels can dramatically change the child's weight and improve the underlying medical condition. Untreated ADHD, especially in girls, has been found to place them at higher risk for binge eating in adolescence and young adulthood (Biederman, 2010).

Pica, the persistent craving and ingesting of nonfood items, is a typical behavior of toddlers. When a child older than 2 years displays pica, however, professionals should explore the possibility that the child has a psychiatric disorder or a nutritional deficiency. Also, pica in older children can also be a typical behavior of individuals with severe to profound intellectual disability. Pica from any cause described above can seriously affect a child's well-being. It can result in toxicity from ingested materials such as medications or lead-containing plaster or paint chips, and it can physically damage the gastrointestinal tract. Behavior management techniques (see Chapter 34) have been found to be the most effective intervention for pica (Williams & McAdam, 2012).

Adjustment Disorders

These disorders involve the development of emotional or behavioral symptoms in response to an identifiable stressor and occur within 3 months of the onset of that stressor. The symptoms or behaviors are clinically significant and cause marked distress, in excess of what would be expected from exposure to the stressor, and are accompanied by significantly impaired social or occupational (academic) functioning. With the exception of an ASD, individuals with adjustment disorders do not have another major psychiatric disorder. Once the stressor ends, the symptoms do not persist for more than 6 months. Adjustment disorder with anxiety has symptoms such as nervousness, worry, or jitteriness or, in children, separation anxiety focused on parents. Adjustment disorder with depressed mood includes depression, tearfulness, or hopelessness as the predominant symptoms. Adjustment disorder with disturbances of conduct presents with significant problematic behaviors such as truancy, vandalism, reckless driving, or fighting. Finally, adjustment disorder with mixed disturbance of emotions and conduct includes anxiety or depression plus conduct symptoms.

Children with developmental disabilities may be at higher risk for adjustment disorders because they have limited coping skills and frequently have medical illnesses or require procedures that produce stress. When children with developmental disabilities enter the hospital for a medical procedure or illness, parents, caregivers, and health care providers must be prepared for exaggerated emotional and behavioral responses to being in the hospital and kept away from their normal routine. Children may cry, have tantrums, or act out, or they may alternatively become quiet and withdrawn, refusing to eat or cooperate with staff. Patience and reassurance will generally help the child navigate the stressful situation and return to his or her baseline emotional and behavioral functioning. Interventions to help prevent and treat these adjustment disorders include allowing parents to stay overnight in the hospital and allowing the child to bring special bedding, pillows, transitional objects (e.g., security blankets), stuffed animals, or favorite books or games to improve the child's comfort in the hospital. Visits to the hospital or treatment center ahead of an admission may also help provide familiarity with new places and people and thus diminish fear. One study found that picture schedules can help to relieve anxiety in children with ASD (Chebuhar, McCarthy, Bosch, & Baker, 2013). Such techniques have been found useful in treating children with intellectual disabilities by facilitating better communication with patients and their families, which reduces stress associated with hospital stays (Oulton, Sell, Kerry, & Gibson, 2015).

Maladaptive Behavior Disorders

Some individuals with severe to profound levels of intellectual disability develop behavioral symptoms that are qualitatively different from those seen in people without developmental disabilities. For instance, studies have shown a higher incidence of aggression and SIB in children with developmental disabilities (Schroeder et al., 2014) and that these behaviors are often persistent (Sandman, Kemp, Mabini, Pincus, & Magnusson, 2012). These symptoms, which include repetitive self-stimulating behavior and SIB, can vary among different genetic syndromes (Arron, Oliver, Moss, Berg, & Burbidge, 2011). It is important to identify these behaviors early in childhood for effective intervention.

Individuals who engage in SIB typically display a specific pattern for producing injury. They may bang their heads, bite their hands, pick at their skin, hit themselves with their fists, or poke their eyes. They may do this once or twice a day in association with tantrums, or as often as several hundred times an hour. Tissue destruction, infection, internal injury, loss of vision, and even death may result. These behaviors may be accompanied by additional repetitive, stereotyped behaviors, such as hand waving and body rocking. When these repetitive behaviors interfere with activities of daily living or result in significant injury to the individual, a diagnosis of *stereotypic movement disorder* with SIB is made.

Although serious SIB occurs in fewer than 5% of people of all ages with intellectual disability, these behaviors cause enormous distress to the individuals and their caregivers. Serious SIB can result in severe bodily injury and may lead to residential placement, separating the individual from the family and other community contacts. Some children with SIB also demonstrate severe aggressive behavior toward their caregivers or peers.

SIB is a puzzling and disturbing phenomenon that prompts asking why these individuals hurt themselves. Although no simple answer exists, there is evidence for both environmental and biological causes in the context of enormous individual variation (Schroeder et al., 2014). Some children exhibit SIB because it elicits a desired environmental outcome (i.e., **operant control;** Loschen & Osman, 1992). For example, a girl who is nonverbal but demonstrates head banging will have that reinforced once she learns that this action captures the attention she craves. Other environmental factors that can reinforce SIB include access to desired items (e.g., food), avoidance of task demands (e.g., chores), and certain sensory effects (e.g., bright lights from eye pressing; Mace & Mauk, 1995). The inference that the sensations produced through self-induced painful stimulation may somehow be gratifying has led to the notion that SIB plays a role in regulating physiologic states such as arousal. Guess and Carr (1991) proposed a biobehavioral model in which the regulation of normal sleep, wake, and arousal patterns is delayed or disturbed in some individuals. These individuals then develop stereotypic movements and SIB as a way to self-regulate arousal in understimulating or overstimulating environments. There is also a relationship between SIB and pain in nonverbal children with severe cognitive impairment. They have been found to increase SIB during an ear infection, constipation, or other conditions associated with pain (Peebles & Price, 2012). Other biological factors are suggested by the increased prevalence of SIB in certain genetic syndromes, including fragile X, de Lange, Lesch-Nyhan, Prader-Willi, and Rett syndromes (see Appendix B; Bailey et al., 2012). Psychiatric disorders such as ASD, depression, mania, and schizophrenia are also risk factors for SIB. General medical conditions and medication side effects can be acute precipitants of SIB. For example, a painful middle-ear infection may lead to head banging. Repetitive or ritualistic behavior also has been found to be associated with increased risk for SIB (Davies & Oliver, 2016; Oliver, Petty, Ruddick, & Bacarese-Hamilton, 2012; Petty, Bacarese-Hamilton, Davies, & Oliver, 2014). Evaluating any individual for the cause of SIB includes examining the roles of reactivity to pain and sensory inputs (Summers et al., 2017).

Although the brain mechanisms underlying most forms of SIB remain unknown, several neurotransmitters are thought to be involved. These include dopamine, which mediates certain reinforcement systems in the brain; serotonin, the depletion of which is sometimes associated with violent behavior; gamma-aminobutyric acid (GABA), an inhibitory neurotransmitter; and opioids, the brain's natural painkillers (Verhoeven et al., 1999). The atypical antipsychotic risperidone has been found to be useful in treating SIB (Zarcone et al., 2001) together with applied behavior analysis. As of 2006, risperidone was FDA approved for the treatment of violent and aggressive behavior, including SIB in individuals with ASD. Also, by 2009 aripiprazole was approved for treating irritability and aggression in children and adolescents with ASD (Robb et al., 2010). Behavioral interventions may also be helpful in treating SIB in children with intellectual disabilities, with early intervention being most effective (Kurtz, Chin, Robinson, O'Connor, & Hagopian, 2015; Schroeder et al., 2014).

VULNERABILITY

Individuals with developmental disabilities are at higher risk for psychiatric disorders than their typically developing peers for a variety of reasons, including 1) higher rates of certain psychiatric disorders in specific syndromes (e.g., ADHD in Williams syndrome or irritability in ASD), 2) impairment in the acquisition of age-dependent coping skills (e.g., some syndromes particularly affect skill development including trisomy 21 and fragile X syndrome), 3) multiple hospital stays for treatment of associated medical problems (e.g., surgical releases of contractures in cerebral palsy), 4) physical differences readily seen by peers who may bully the child (e.g., facial features in trisomy 21, skin lesions in neurofibromatosis, and morbid obesity in Prader-Willi syndrome), and 5) a family history of psychiatric disorders that adds to the genetic risk for mental illness in the child with developmental disability. Children with intellectual disabilities also are more likely to experience victimization and chronic loneliness, which increases their risk for a range of mental health problems (Berg, Shiu, Msall, & Acharya, 2015; Gilmore & Cuskelly, 2014). When assessing patients with developmental disabilities for psychiatric symptoms, the practitioner must also consider changes in school, classmates, and living situations, including family members and pets. These socio-environmental factors can either increase or decrease the risk for mental health problems.

EVALUATION

Psychiatric needs can be met only if parents, teachers, and other staff who work with children with disabilities are aware that emotional disturbances may be present. Ideally, the referral for evaluation should be made to professionals (e.g., psychiatrists, psychologists, behavioral neurologists, developmental-behavioral pediatricians, neurodevelopmental pediatricians, and social workers) with specific training, experience, and expertise in the psychiatric disorders of children with developmental disabilities. The goal of evaluation is to formulate an intervention plan based not only on the psychiatric diagnosis, but also on the developmental level of the child, accompanying medical conditions, the family's strengths and challenges, and the needs and limitations of the settings where the child spends his or her time. Often this requires referral to a specialized tertiary care center with a multidisciplinary team, such as a university hospital. Less experienced mental health professionals who undertake such evaluations should have access to consultation from a specialized center.

The mental health professional first takes a detailed history of the current symptoms and problematic behaviors from parents or other caregivers. For example, recent changes in sleep pattern, appetite, or mood provide important evidence of depression. In addition, an individual and family medical history should be obtained. The family history may reveal, for example, other members with mood or anxiety disorders. A review of the individual's past medical and psychological assessments may indicate prior behavior or psychiatric problems. After taking the history, an interview is conducted posing both structured and open-ended questions to the child and parents. If impairments in communication and cognitive skills are significant, the professional can still gain important information from directly observing the child both alone and with parents (King, DeAntonio, McCracken, Forness, & Ackerland, 1994). Input from the school and other care providers frequently helps clarify the diagnostic issues.

The evaluation should also focus on the social system and setting in which the psychiatric disorder occurs. Thus, the professional should evaluate the current level of family functioning by assessing 1) family members' ability to cope with the child's psychiatric disorder and therapy; 2) their current morale, problem-solving abilities, external social supports, and practical resources (e.g., finances and insurance); 3) the system of beliefs that sustains their efforts; and 4) the stability of the parents' relationship. It is important to understand how individual family members are reacting and adjusting to the child's underlying developmental disability as well as any current mental health problems (see Chapter 37). For example, studies have found that parenting stress can result from and be a cause of child behavior problems and is a risk factor for psychiatric disorders in children with intellectual disabilities (Gallagher & Whiteley, 2013; Neece, Green, & Baker, 2012; Valicenti-McDermott et al., 2015).

Following the comprehensive interview, the child may be referred for psychological testing or behavioral assessment. Although standardized behavior rating scales are available, they are insufficient by themselves as diagnostic tools. A single, structured psychological testing instrument may not be able to cover the range of developmental levels and behavioral baselines exhibited by individuals with developmental disabilities. These instruments are important, however, for confirming or adding to information obtained from the history and interview. They can also be extremely helpful in measuring changes that occur during the course of intervention (Aman, Burrow, & Wolford, 1995; Demb, Brier, Huron, & Tomor, 1994; Linaker & Helle, 1994; Reiss & Valenti-Hein, 1994).

Standardized rating scales may be combined with a functional behavior analysis. This type of combined assessment is most useful regarding children with severe behavioral abnormalities for which specific family or behavior therapies are being considered. One of the more helpful rating scales, the Aberrant Behavior Checklist, can be completed by parents or caregivers; is normed on the developmentally disabled population; and tracks five subscales, including irritability and hyperactivity (Aman et al., 1995; see Box 27.4). This scale can be given at baseline and then tracked over time to evaluate responses to interventions both pharmacologic and behavioral. However, as discussed in Box 27.4, it is important to combine such scales with other evaluations such as behavior analysis. Behavior analysis provides direct observation of the child in a natural setting, yielding a clear description of the abnormal behavior itself and its antecedents and consequences (see Chapter 34). Often, changes in a child's environment such as a new teacher, classmate, or bus driver or other changes in a child's routine can precipitate behavioral symptoms.

It is important to note that many symptoms of a psychiatric disorder can actually be caused by a variety of medical disorders and treatments. For example, hypothyroidism, which is common in individuals with Down syndrome, can cause emotional disturbances that present as anxiety or depression. In excessive (and sometimes therapeutic) dosages, drugs used to treat associated impairments such as epilepsy can cause symptoms of hyperactivity or depression (Stephen, Wishart, & Brodie, 2017). Careful evaluation for medical conditions or drug reactions should be a part of any assessment of new-onset behavioral or psychiatric symptoms.

After the evaluations have been completed, the professional can start formulating an intervention plan based on the psychiatric diagnosis, the child's developmental level, accompanying medical conditions, the family's strengths and challenges, and the needs and limitations of the settings where the child spends his or her time.

TREATMENT

Treatment of psychiatric illness in children and adolescents with developmental disabilities involves some or all of the modalities described in the following sections. Interventions must be tailored to each child's needs at home, at school, and with peers. The treatment modalities utilized may need to be adjusted as the child matures and individual needs change.

Educational Interventions

Educational interventions can include a variety of supports to help a child succeed in the classroom (see Chapter 33). Children may benefit from schoolwide positive-behavior interventions and supports, with an individualized behavior intervention plan being developed if necessary. The education setting can also be a form of support. Children may be placed in smaller self-contained classes or included in the general education class but with extra aides or a one-to-one helper. When the child becomes upset, the aide can help calm the child, avoiding the need to leave the classroom. The child may also benefit from therapy sessions with the school counselor or behavioral psychologist. There should be close collaboration among school personnel, parents, and the child's medical team, as discussed in Box 27.5.

Rehabilitation Therapy

There is evidence that language impairments significantly contribute to the development of certain behavior problems. Some aggressive behaviors and SIBs have been linked to the inability to communicate needs, and teaching functional communication skills has been shown to decrease SIB. In children with trisomy 21,

BOX 27.4 EVIDENCE-BASED PRACTICE

The Aberrant Behavior Checklist

The Aberrant Behavior Checklist (ABC; Aman et al., 1995) is used to identify maladaptive behaviors in children with developmental disabilities. However, recent research on the use of this scale as an outcome measure for clinical trials on fragile X syndrome has found that the ABC subscales may not be sensitive to symptoms of patients with higher-functioning fragile X syndrome (Sansone et al., 2012). Such research should be taken into consideration when using this scale as an outcome measure for children with intellectual disabilities, as it highlights the importance of using rating scales in combination with comprehensive interviews.

BOX 27.5 EVIDENCE-BASED PRACTICE

Children with Intellectual Disabilities in School

McIntyre, Blacher, and Baker (2006) found that children with an intellectual disability showed poor adaptation to school compared with typically developing children and that this led to more maladaptive behavior and decreased social skills, which are both risk factors for psychiatric disorders. These findings highlight the importance of early intervention in educational settings and collaboration with school staff and caregivers of children with intellectual disability.

increased disruptive behaviors often indicate underlying medical concerns or frustration that results from the patient's inability to communicate (Skotko, Davidson, & Weintraub, 2013). Children with fragile X syndrome, ASD, and trisomy 21 are significantly less likely than their typically developing peers to signal noncomprehension in communication, which could lead to further challenges in language and academic development (Martin et al., 2017). Thus, speech-language therapy and training in augmentative and alternative communication systems (see Chapters 17 and 36) may be an important part of the intervention program. Similarly, if the child has a physical disability, pain from contractures, an inability to ambulate, or difficulty reaching for desired objects may lead to behavior and mood alterations. Physical and occupational therapy may improve motor function, with associated improvement in behavior and mood.

Psychotherapy

There is ample evidence that various forms of psychological or behavioral therapy (individual, group, and family) can benefit a child or adolescent with developmental disabilities and psychiatric disorders, if it is adapted to the child's developmental age and communication abilities (Brosnan, 2011; Kok, van der Waa, Klip, & Staal, 2016; McGinnes, 2010; Plant, 2007). Table 27.3 shows different types of psychotherapy and the disorders that they are most useful in treating. The goals of therapy are to relieve symptoms and help the child understand the nature of the disability and associated feelings and to come to recognize and appreciate his or her strengths. Psychotherapy, particularly group work, can also enhance social skills and help the child deal with stigmatization, rejection, peer pressure, and attempts at exploitation (Kasari, Rotheram-Fuller, Locke, & Gulsrud, 2012; Koning, Magill-Evans, Volden, & Dick, 2013; Reichow, Steiner, & Volkmar, 2013; Walton & Ingersol, 2013; White et al., 2013). Regrettably, individuals with developmental disabilities are seriously underserved regarding psychotherapy despite the fact that psychotherapy can provide a supportive relationship, help restore self-esteem, and enhance the child's capacity to recognize and master emotional conflicts and solve problems (Dykens, 2016). Psychotherapy also can be added to behavior therapy and pharmacotherapy when these approaches have not adequately

Table 27.3. Types of psychotherapy and uses in different disorders

Therapy	Behavior	CBT	Social skills	Group	Individual	Supportive/educational	Parent training
ADHD	X		X	X			X
ODD and conduct disorder	X		X	X			X
Generalized anxiety disorder		X			X	X	
Social phobia		X	X	X	X	X	X
Panic disorder		X			X	X	
PTSD		X			X	X	
OCD		X			X		
Major depression		X			X	X	
Bipolar disorder					X	X	X
ASD	X	X	X	X		X	X
Schizophrenia		X	X		X	X	X

Key: CBT, cognitive-behavioral therapy; ADHD, attention-deficit/hyperactivity disorder; ODD, oppositional defiant disorder; PTSD, posttraumatic stress disorder; OCD, obsessive-compulsive disorder; ASD, autism spectrum disorder.

resolved symptoms or improved quality of life. Ideally, the therapist should have expertise in working with individuals with developmental disabilities.

Behavior therapy is perhaps the most widely researched psychotherapeutic intervention for children and adolescents with intellectual disabilities (see Chapter 34). Cognitive-behavioral therapy and family interventions have been successful in children with ASD. There are extensive findings supporting the effectiveness of behavioral approaches in psychiatric disorders (Benjamin et al., 2011; Weisz, Hawley, & Doss, 2004). When used in conjunction with comprehensive assessment, accurate medical and psychiatric diagnoses, and programmatic intervention, behavior therapy is among the most powerful available interventions. As with other forms of psychotherapy and pharmacotherapy, however, it should be implemented only under the supervision of licensed professionals who have been specifically trained in this methodology.

Pharmacotherapy

Medication can play an important role in treating the psychiatric disorders that occur in children with developmental disabilities (Efron et al., 2003). Box 27.6 discusses ongoing research on evidence-based pharmacotherapy for children with intellectual disabilities, and Table 27.4 lists the various medications in each of the diagnostic groups that are described next. (Additional information on uses and side effects of these medications can be found in Appendix C.) It has long been understood that pharmacotherapy is different in children than in adults. Because human growth and development vary among individuals, there is no single method to determining the appropriate dose of medications. Predictions of drug clearance in children based on weight and metabolic rate have been found ineffective (Mahmood, 2006). Therefore, it is important to take individual differences into account and to begin treatment at a low dose when prescribing psychotropic medication to children. This is especially important in children with developmental disabilities as these children are at a greater risk for side effects than typically developing children (Ji & Findling, 2016; Simonoff et al., 2013). Medical providers should begin treatment at a low dose and then slowly titrate the dose up.

An example of this was seen in the aripiprazole pediatric trials. Here the titration was quickest in typically developing adolescents with schizophrenia who could accept increased doses every 2 days to a maximum of 30 mg in less than 2 weeks (Findling et al., 2008). In contrast, for children with irritability associated with ASD, when the dose was increased weekly to a maximum dose of 15 mg over 4 weeks, these children had higher rates of side effects despite a lower maximum dose and more gradual titration schedule than their typically developing peers (Robb et al., 2011). In another study, stimulants given to children with ASD were associated with a higher rate of emotional lability, crying, and other side effects than were seen in typically developing preschool children with ADHD (Nickels et al., 2008).

Antidepressants Antidepressants are used to treat major depression and anxiety disorders including OCD, GAD, and separation anxiety disorder (DeVaugh-Geiss et al., 1992; Emslie et al., 2002; Geller et al., 2001; March et al., 1998; Riddle et al., 2001; Wagner et al., 2003; Wagner et al., 2004). Box 27.7 reviews the current FDA-approved antidepressants. The class of antidepressants most commonly used in children and adolescents is the SSRIs.

In 2004, the FDA required drug companies to start putting "black box" warnings—the FDA's highest level of warning before removing a drug from the market—on the packaging of all categories of antidepressants, as well as atomoxetine for ADHD, aripiprazole for treatment-resistant depression, and quetiapine for bipolar depression, noting the potential risk of suicidality while taking these medications. This requirement

BOX 27.6 EVIDENCE-BASED PRACTICE

Evidence-Based Pharmacotherapy for Children with Intellectual Disabilities

There is limited research on evidence-based pharmacotherapy for children with intellectual disabilities. According to a review by Ji and Findling (2016), antipsychotics such as risperidone seem to be effective in reducing challenging behaviors such as aggression and SIB. Methylphenidate and α-agonists may be effective in treating ADHD symptoms in children with intellectual disabilities. However, antidepressants appear to be poorly tolerated in this population (Ji & Findling, 2016). This information is important to consider when deciding on the best course of treatment for children with intellectual disabilities.

Table 27.4. Medications used to treat psychiatric disorders

	Generic name	Trade name	Type	Uses	Other formulations
Antidepressants	Fluoxetine	Prozac, Sarefem	SSRI	Depression, anxiety, OCD	Liquid and weekly
	Fluvoxamine	Luvox, LuvoxCR	SSRI	OCD	None
	Sertraline	Zoloft	SSRI	Depression, anxiety, OCD	Liquid
	Paroxetine	Paxil, Paxil CR	SSRI	Depression, anxiety, OCD	Liquid (not in CR)
	Citalopram	Celexa	SSRI	Depression	Liquid
	Escitalopram	Lexapro	SSRI	Depression, anxiety	Liquid
	Venlafaxine	Effexor, Effexor XR	SNRI	Depression, anxiety	None
	Duloxetine	Cymbalta	SNRI	Depression, GAD	None
	Buproprion	Wellbutrin, Wellbutrin SR, Wellbutrin XL	Dopaminergic	Depression, ADHD	None
Antihypertensives	Propranolol	Inderal, Inderal LA	Beta blocker	Aggressive behavior	None
	Clonidine	Catapres, Cat-apres-TTS patch	Alpha-2-adrenergic agonist	ADHD, tics, sleeping agent	Weekly skin patch
		Kapvay		Monotherapy or with stimulant	
	Guanfacine	Tenex	Alpha-2-adrenergic agonist	ADHD, tics	None
		Intuniv		Monotherapy or with stimulant	
Antipsychotics	Clozapine	Clozaril	Atypical	Treatment-resistant schizophrenia, bipolar disorder (not FDA approved for acute bipolar mania)	None
	Risperidone	Risperdal, Risperdal M-Tab, Risperdal Consta	Atypical	Schizophrenia, bipolar disorder, aggressive behavior in children with autism spectrum disorder	Liquid, oral dissolving tablets (M-Tab), 2-week injection (Consta)
	Olanzapine	Zyprexa, Zyprexa Zydis, Zyprexa Relprev	Atypical	Schizophrenia, bipolar disorder, acute agitation	Oral dissolving tablets, 2-week injection (Relprev) requires extensive monitoring
	Ziprasidone	Geodon	Atypical	Schizophrenia, bipolar disorder, acute agitation	Daily injection
	Quetiapine	Seroquel	Atypical	Schizophrenia, bipolar disorder (acute mania and bipolar depression)	None
	Aripiprazole	Abilify, Abilify Discmelt	Atypical (plus serotonin agonist)	Schizophrenia, bipolar disorder	Liquid, oral dissolving tablets, daily injection
	Paliperidone	Invega, Invega Sustenna	Atypical	Schizophrenia	4-week injection (Sustenna)
	Asenapine	Saphris	Atypical	Bipolar mixed/manic	Sublingual only
	Lurasidone	Latuda	Atypical	Schizophrenia (bipolar depression pending)	None
	Haloperidol	Haldol, Haldol Decanoate	Typical	Schizophrenia, Tourette syndrome, agitation, severe behavior disorders	Liquid, daily injection, monthly injection
	Pimozide	Orap	Typical	Tourette syndrome	None

(continued)

Table 27.4. *(continued)*

	Generic name	Trade name	Type	Uses	Other formulations
Benzodiazepines	Lorazepam	Ativan	Typical	Anxiety	Liquid, daily injection
	Alprazolam	Xanax, Xanax XR	High potency	Panic, anxiety	None
	Clonazepam	Klonopin, Klonopin Wafers	High potency	Panic, anxiety	Oral dissolving tablets
Mood stabilizers	Lithium carbonate	Lithobid, Eskalith, Eskalith-CR	Mood stabilizer	Bipolar disorder (acute mania and maintenance)	Liquid
	Valproic acid	Depakote, Depakote ER, Depacon, Depakene	Antiepileptic drug	Bipolar disorder	Liquid, intravenous, sprinkles
	Carbamazepine	Tegretol, Tegretol XR, Carbatrol, Equetro	Antiepileptic drug	Bipolar disorder	Chewable tablet, liquid
	Oxcarbazepine	Trileptal	Antiepileptic drug	Not FDA approved yet for bipolar disorder, but used	Liquid
	Lamotrigine	Lamictal	Antiepileptic drug	Bipolar maintenance	Chewable tablets
Stimulants and atomoxetine	Methylphenidate–racemic mixture	Ritalin, Ritalin LA, Metadate CD, Concerta, Daytrana	Synthetic stimulant	ADHD	Sprinkles for Ritalin LA and Metadate CD, transdermal patch (Daytrana)
	Dexmethylphenidate	Focalin, Focalin XR	Synthetic stimulant	ADHD	Sprinkles for XR
	Dextroamphetamine	Dexedrine, Dexedrine ER spansules	Stimulant	ADHD	Chewable generic tablet, ER spansule
	Mixed amphetamine salts	Adderall, Adderall XR	Stimulant	ADHD	Sprinkles for XR
	Modafanil	Provigil, Sparlon	Unknown	ADHD (not FDA approved for ADHD due to concern about Stevens-Johnson syndrome)	None
	Atomoxetine	Strattera	NRI	ADHD, maintenance 6–14 years	None

Key: SSRI, selective serotonin reuptake inhibitor; OCD, obsessive-compulsive disorder; CR, controlled release; SNRI, serotonin norepinephrine reuptake inhibitor; XR, extended release; SR, slow release; XL, extra long; ADHD, attention-deficit/hyperactivity disorder; LA, long acting; TTS, transdermal system; ER, extended release; FDA, Food and Drug Administration; CD, controlled delivery; NRI, norepinephrine reuptake inhibitor. For further information see Appendix C.

BOX 27.7 EVIDENCE-BASED PRACTICE

FDA-Approved Antidepressants for Children

In the 1990s, it became apparent that there were limited data on the use of antidepressants in children that had only been approved by the FDA for adults. In response, the FDA required pharmaceutical companies to provide data on new and existing antidepressants for children (Cheung, Emslie, & Mayes, 2005). Since then, several antidepressants, including fluoxetine (Emslie et al., 2002), sertraline (March et al., 1998), clomipramine (DeVaugh-Geiss et al., 1992), fluvoxamine (Walkup et al., 2001), escitalopram (Wagner et al., 2006), and duloxetine (Emslie et al., 2014) have been FDA approved and found effective to treat disorders such as major depression and anxiety disorders.

resulted in a decrease in SSRI prescriptions and an increase in suicide rates in children and adolescents (Gibbons et al., 2007). Although oversight by regulatory bodies is important to ensure patient safety, this study shows how warnings made by these regulatory bodies may have unintended and potentially harmful effects. More recently the antidepressant black box warning has been revised and expanded to include all those individuals younger than 25 years. The current warning states that these antidepressants may increase suicidal thoughts and actions when first started.

Depression and other mental illnesses are the most important causes of suicidal thoughts and actions, and some people may be at a particularly high risk. Families should watch closely for changes in mood, behavior, and the appearance of suicidal thoughts and actions when starting a child on antidepressants, and clinicians should monitor their young patients for any change in mental state and for indications of suicidal ideas or plans. With these controls in place, antidepressants can continue to be useful in the treatment of pediatric mood and anxiety disorders and remain an important part of treatment for these illnesses (Gibbons et al., 2015; Linden et al., 2016).

In a large study of youth with fragile X syndrome and targeted medication use, the authors tracked target symptoms, medication choice, and age of the patient. Anxiety was the most common symptom being treated in 42% of males and 26% of females. By age 20, 45% of males and 32% of females were taking medication for anxiety (Bailey, Raspa, Bishop, Mallya, & Berry-Kravis, 2012). In a 6-month study of young children ages 2–6 years with fragile X syndrome who were treated with low-dose sertraline (2.5 to 5.0 mg daily) or placebo, they found no difference in the primary outcome on the Mullen Scales of Early Learning for expressive language or clinical global improvement (Hess et al., 2016). However, another 6-month study found that children ages 2–3 years with fragile X syndrome who were treated with low-dose sertraline (2.5 to 5.0 mg daily) showed more improvement in receptive language compared with children who received a placebo (Yoo, Burris, Gaul, Hagerman, & Rivera, 2017). In another recent study of individuals with 22q11.2 syndrome, both antidepressants and antipsychotics were found to be effective in reducing symptoms of depression anxiety or psychotic symptoms (Dori, Green, Weizman, & Gothelf, 2017).

Antihypertensives Beta-blockers such as propranolol are used to treat explosive and aggressive behavior, whereas alpha-2 adrenergic receptor agonists (e.g., clonidine, guanfacine) are used to treat ADHD, tic disorder, and Tourette syndrome. These medications sedate and can also lower blood pressure; thus, they should be used cautiously, especially in children with developmental disabilities associated with comorbid cardiac disorders (Ahmed & Takeshita, 1996). In the past decade, long-acting formulations of these drugs have been approved by the FDA for the treatment of ADHD in children and adolescents as monotherapy and in combination with stimulant medication (Connor et al., 2010; Jain et al., 2011; Kollins et al., 2011).

Antipsychotic Medications Antipsychotic medications have been used in children and adults since the 1950s to treat disorders, such as schizophrenia and bipolar. More recently, antipsychotic medications have been used to treat aggression and SIB in children with intellectual disability or ASD. There is, in fact, more safety data on risperidone in children with intellectual disability and ASD than in their typically developing peers. In 2006, risperidone became the first antipsychotic medication approved by the FDA for the treatment of aggressive behavior in individuals with ASD. Aripiprazole has also been approved for the treatment of irritability and aggression in children 6–17 years showing such symptoms in ASD (Robb, 2010). Although these medications have been found to be generally safe and well tolerated in children (Robb et al., 2011), use of antipsychotics to treat disorders in children remains controversial as it has been suggested that children may be at greater risk for adverse events (Vitiello et al., 2009).

Many of the other novel neuroleptics have also been studied in individuals with ASD. Although novel neuroleptics are much more likely to cause weight gain, metabolic syndrome, and diabetes, they are less likely to cause a movement disorder (Scahill et al., 2016; Wink et al., 2014). Another recent study found that antipsychotic medication may have a reparative effect on the white matter microstructure in individuals with 22q11.2 deletion syndrome (Kates et al., 2015).

Benzodiazepines Benzodiazepines are helpful in reducing anxiety in the short term. However, children with developmental disabilities may have paradoxical reactions to these medications—they may become agitated rather than calm and sleepy (Mancuso, Tanzi, & Gabay, 2004; Rothschild, Shindul-Rothschild, Murray, & Brewster, 2000). Although relatively uncommon, the exact mechanisms and cause of paradoxical reactions remain unclear and children appear to be at increased risk (Mancuso et al., 2004). Because chronic use of these agents can cause chemical and behavioral dependency and may alter seizure control, benzodiazepines should not be used for long-term control of anxiety symptoms.

Mood Stabilizers Mood stabilizers include lithium and antiepileptic medication (Findling et al., 2005). They are most commonly used to treat bipolar disorder and aggressive behaviors (see Box 27.8). Lithium is effective in treating current episodes and in preventing future bipolar episodes (Findling et al., 2015a). It is a salt that is excreted through the kidneys and causes increased thirst and urination. It must be used with caution in combination with certain other drugs that can lead to toxic lithium levels, including nonsteroidal anti-inflammatory drugs (e.g., ibuprofen) and certain anticonvulsants (e.g., topiramate) that are excreted by the kidneys. Lithium toxicity can occur with rapid onset if normal fluid intake is decreased, for example with vomiting, diarrhea, or acute illness; this in turn can result in coma, kidney failure, or the need for dialysis. A recent examination of lithium in mouse and fruit fly models of fragile X syndrome showed reversal of behavioral, physiological, cellular, and molecular phenotypes. This success in the animal model led the group to do a pilot clinical trial of lithium in adult patients with fragile X syndrome and found measurable improvements in behavior and function after 2 months of open-label lithium treatment (Liu & Smith, 2014). The subjects had improvement in ADHD symptoms, aggression, vocalizations, self-abuse, work refusal, outbursts, mood swings, tantrums, and other fragile X syndrome–related behaviors. Another study showed that 18% of males and 11% of females with fragile X syndrome were receiving medication for mood swings; by age 20, the rates were 20% of males and 15% of females (Bailey et al., 2012).

At the time of this book's publication, no antiepileptic medications are approved for the treatment of bipolar disorder in children and adolescents. However, the antipsychotic aripiprazole is approved for bipolar disorder as monotherapy and in combination with both lithium and valproic acid.

Stimulants and Atomoxetine Stimulants of both the amphetamine and methylphenidate classes are first-line treatments for ADHD (see Chapter 19), and, as discussed in Box 27.9, research on the long-term efficacy and safety of such medications is ongoing. Both

BOX 27.8 EVIDENCE-BASED PRACTICE

Lithium to Treat Bipolar I Disorder in Children

Lithium has been approved by the U.S. Food and Drug Administration to treat bipolar I disorder in children over the age of 12. However, there are limited studies that have evaluated its effectiveness and safety in children. Findling and colleagues (2015) found that lithium was superior to placebo in reducing manic symptoms and generally well tolerated in children ages 7–17. However, further research is needed to determine the long-term safety and efficacy of lithium to treat bipolar I disorder in children.

BOX 27.9 EVIDENCE-BASED PRACTICE

Methylphenidate to Treat ADHD in Young Children

Methylphenidate was first created and marketed as Ritalin in 1955 and is now a first-line treatment for attention-deficit/hyperactivity disorder (ADHD). However, whereas ADHD symptoms are often present during the preschool years, little is known about the long-term efficacy and safety of methylphenidate use for children in this age group (Vitiello et al., 2015). The Preschool ADHD Treatment Study (PATS; Greenhill et al., 2006) found immediate-release methylphenidate to be effective in treating ADHD in preschool-age children. A 6-year follow-up study of this population found that two thirds of this group continued using the stimulant medication, one quarter of the children discontinued pharmacotherapy, and 13.4% of the children were taking an antipsychotic medication. In addition, antipsychotic use was associated with the presence of a pervasive developmental disorder (Vitiello et al., 2015). This research adds to the limited data on long-term pharmacological treatment of children diagnosed with and treated for ADHD as preschoolers.

families of drugs now have long-acting preparations available that can improve control of ADHD symptoms throughout the day. Side effects include loss of appetite, insomnia, tics, headache, and gastrointestinal side effects (Pearson et al., 2003). The use of atomoxetine has been studied in children with ADHD (Harfterkamp et al., 2012) and ASD and has been found to control hyperactive/impulsive symptoms with an effect similar to methylphenidate (Clemow, Bushe, Mancini, Ossipov, & Upadhyaya, 2017; Gayleard & Mychailyszyn, 2017; Harfterkamp et al., 2012; Harfterkamp et al., 2013; Savill et al., 2015; Shang, Pan, Lin, Huang, & Gau, 2015).

Polypharmacy One of the biggest concerns as youth with intellectual disability become adults is the risk of polypharmacy, the concurrent use of multiple drugs to treat a disorder. Although there is limited research on its safety and effectiveness, polypharmacy—particularly in antipsychotic medications—is common in children (Comer, Olfson, & Mojtabai, 2010; Toteja et al., 2014).

Once medications are added, it becomes very difficult to remove them even when efficacy is not noted. One study involving a chart audit of 517 patients presenting to a specialized psychiatric outpatient clinic found that 70% of the patients were receiving at least one psychotropic medication and 22% had psychotropic polypharmacy (Lunsky & Modi, 2017). Polypharmacy use was associated with female gender, placement in a supervised residential setting, and having more than two psychiatric diagnoses. Another study of 231 patients found even a higher rate of polypharmacy (45%), especially when associated with a dual diagnosis (Hobden, Samuel, LeRoy, & Lindsay, 2013). Further research is necessary to determine the long-term safety and tolerability of polypharmacy in children. This is important for children with intellectual disabilities, as these individuals are at greater risk of polypharmacy as they enter adulthood.

SUMMARY

- Children with developmental disabilities are at higher risk than their typically developing peers of developing psychiatric and behavioral disorders at some time during their childhood or adolescence.
- By being aware of the possibility of psychiatric disorders that can affect a child's behavior, parents, educators, and clinicians can identify problems early and intervene.
- Early intervention leads to more rapid resolution of difficulties and allows children to function more effectively and happily at home, at school, and in the community.

ADDITIONAL RESOURCES

Behavioral and Mental Health, American Academy of Child and Adolescent Psychiatry (AACAP): http://www.aacap.org

American Psychological Association (APA): http://www.apa.org

Association for Behavior Analysis International (ABA International): http://www.abainternational.org

Additional resources can be found online in Appendix D: Childhood Disabilities Resources, Services, and Organizations (see About the Online Companion Materials).

REFERENCES

Ahmed, I., & Takeshita, J. (1996). Clonidine: A critical review of its role in the treatment of psychiatric disorders. *CNS Drugs, 6*, 53.

Ahuja, A., Martin, J., Langley, K., & Thapar, A. (2013). Intellectual disability in children with attention deficit hyperactivity disorder. *The Journal of Pediatrics, 163*(3), 890–895.

Alioto, A., Yacob, D., Yardley, H. L., & Di Lorenzo, C. (2015). Inpatient treatment of rumination syndrome: Outcomes and lessons learned. *Clinical Practice in Pediatric Psychology, 3*(4), 304.

Aman, M. G., Burrow, W. H., & Wolford, P. L. (1995). The Aberrant Behavior Checklist Community: Factor validity and effect of subject variables for adults in group homes. *American Journal on Mental Retardation, 100*, 293–294.

American Psychiatric Association. (2013). *Diagnostic and statistical manual of mental disorders* (5th ed.). Washington, DC: Author.

Arnold, P. D., Siegel-Bartelt, J., Cytrynbaum, C., Teshima, I., & Schachar, R. (2001). Velo-cardio-facial syndrome: Implications of microdeletion 22q11 for schizophrenia and mood disorders. *American Journal of Medical Genetics Part A, 105*(4), 354–362.

Arron, K., Oliver, C., Moss, J., Berg, K., & Burbidge, C. (2011). The prevalence and phenomenology of self-injurious and aggressive behavior in genetic syndromes. *Journal of Intellectual Disability Research, 55*, 109–120.

Bailey, D. B., Raspa, M., Bishop, E., Mallya, U. G., & Berry-Kravis, E. (2012). Medication utilization for targeted symptoms in children with fragile X syndrome: US survey. *Journal of Developmental and Behavioral Pediatrics, 33*, 62–69.

Bailey, Jr., D. B., Raspa, M., Bishop, E., Mitra, D., Martin, S., Wheeler, A., & Sacco, P. (2012). Health and economic consequences of fragile X syndrome for caregivers. *Journal of Developmental & Behavioral Pediatrics, 33*(9), 705–712.

Batelaan, N. M., Van Balkom, A. J., & Stein, D. J. (2012). Evidence-based pharmacotherapy of panic disorder: An update. *International Journal of Neuropsychopharmacology, 15*(3), 403–415.

Benjamin, C. L., Puleo, C. M., Settipani, C. A., Brodman, D. M., Edmunds, J. M., Cummings, C. M., & Kendall, P. C. (2011). History of cognitive-behavioral therapy in youth. *Child and Adolescent Psychiatric Clinics of North America, 20*(2), 179–189.

Berg, K. L., Shiu, C. S., Msall, M. E., & Acharya, K. (2015). Victimization and depression among youth with disabilities in the US child welfare system. *Child: Care, Health and Development, 41*(6), 989–999.

Bergman, R. L., Gonzalez, A., Piacentini, J., & Keller, M. L. (2013). Integrated behavior therapy for selective mutism: A randomized controlled pilot study. *Behavior Research and Therapy, 51*(10), 680–689.

Berry-Kravis, E., Sumis, A., Hervey, C., & Mathur, S. (2012). Clinic-based retrospective analysis of psychopharmacology for behavior in fragile X syndrome. *International Journal of Pediatrics, 2012*, 1–11. doi:10.1155/2012/843016

Biederman, J., Petty, C. R., Monuteaux, M. C., Fried, R., Byrne, D., Spencer, T., . . . Faraone, S. V. (2010). Adult psychiatric outcomes of girls with attention deficit hyperactivity disorder: 11-year follow-up in a longitudinal case-control study. *American Journal of Psychiatry, 167*, 409–417.

Brosnan, J. (2011). A review of behavioral interventions for the treatment of aggression in individuals with developmental disabilities. *Research in Developmental Disabilities, 32*(2), 437–446.

Burchard, J. D., Bruns, E. J., & Burchard, S. N. (2002). The Wraparound Approach. In B. J. Burns & K. Hoagwood (Eds.), *Community treatment for youth: Evidence-based interventions for severe emotional and behavioral disorders* (pp. 69–90). Oxford University Press.

Burd, L., Klug, M. G., Martsolf, J. T., & Kerbeshian, J. (2003). Fetal alcohol syndrome: Neuropsychiatric phenomics. *Neurotoxicology and Teratology, 25*, 697–705.

Butler, M., Manzardo, A., & Forster, J. (2016). Prader-Willi syndrome: Clinical genetics and diagnostic aspects with treatment approaches. *Current Pediatric Reviews, 12*(2), 136–166.

Chebuhar, A., McCarthy, A. M., Bosch, J., & Baker, S. (2013). Using picture schedules in medical settings for patients with an autism spectrum disorder. *Journal of Pediatric Nursing: Nursing Care of Children and Families, 28*(2), 125–134.

Cheung, A. H., Emslie, G. J., & Mayes, T. L. (2005). Review of the efficacy and safety of antidepressants in youth depression. *Journal of Child Psychology and Psychiatry, 46*(7), 735–754.

Cheung, C., Yu, K., Fung, G., Leung, M., Wong, C., Li, Q., . . . McAlonan, G. (2010). Autistic disorders and schizophrenia: related or remote? An anatomical likelihood estimation. *PloS One, 5*(8), e12233.

Chiarello, F., Spitoni, S., Hollander, E., Matucci Cerinic, M., & Pallanti, S. (2017). An expert opinion on PANDAS/PANS: Highlights and controversies. *International Journal Psychiatry in Clinical Practice, 21*(2), 91–98.

Clemow, D. B., Bushe, C., Mancini, M., Ossipov, M. H., & Upadhyaya, H. (2017). A review of the efficacy of atomoxetine in the treatment of attention-deficit hyperactivity disorder in children and adult patients with common comorbidities. *Neuropsychiatric Disease and Treatment, 13*, 357.

Comer, J. S., Olfson, M., & Mojtabai, R. (2010). National trends in child and adolescent psychotropic polypharmacy in office-based practice, 1996-2007. *Journal of the American Academy of Child & Adolescent Psychiatry, 49*(10), 1001–1010.

Connor, D. F., Barkley, R. A., & Davis, H. T. (2000). A pilot study of methylphenidate, clonidine, or the combination in ADHD comorbid with aggressive oppositional defiant or conduct disorder. *Clinical Pediatrics, 39*(1), 15–25.

Connor, D. F., Findling, R. F., Kollins, S. H., Sallee, F., Lopez, F. A., Lyne, A., & Tremblay, G. (2010). Effects of guanfacine extended release on oppositional symptoms in children aged 6–12 years with attention-deficit/hyperactivity disorder and oppositional symptoms: A randomized, double-blind, placebo-controlled trial. *CNS Drugs, 24*(9), 755–768.

Creswell, C., Waite, P., & Cooper, P. J. (2014). Assessment and management of anxiety disorders in children and adolescents. *Archives of Disease in Childhood, 99*(7), 674–678. doi:10.1136/archdischild-2013-303768

Dankner, N., & Dykens, E. M. (2012). Anxiety in intellectual disabilities: Challenges and next steps. In R. M. Hodnapp (Ed.), *International review of research in developmental disabilities* (Vol. 42, pp. 57–83). Cambridge, MA: Academic Press.

Davies, L. E., & Oliver, C. (2016). Self-injury, aggression and destruction in children with severe intellectual disability: Incidence, persistence and novel, predictive behavioral risk markers. *Research in Developmental Disabilities, 49*, 291–301.

Dekker, A. D., Strydom, A., Coppus, A. M., Nizetic, D., Vermeiren, Y., Naudé, P. J., . . . De Deyn, P. P. (2015). Behavioural and psychological symptoms of dementia in Down syndrome: Early indicators of clinical Alzheimer's disease? *Cortex, 73*, 36–61.

Demb, H. B., Brier, N., Huron, R., & Tomor, E. (1994). The adolescent behavior checklist: Normative data and sensitivity and specificity of a screening tool for diagnosable psychiatric disorders in adolescents with mental retardation and other development disabilities. *Research in Developmental Disabilities, 15,* 151–165.

Detke, H. C., DelBello, M. P., Landry, J., & Usher, R. W. (2015). Olanzapine/fluoxetine combination in children and adolescents with bipolar I depression: A randomized, double-blind, placebo-controlled trial. *Journal of the American Academy of Child & Adolescent Psychiatry, 54*(3), 217–224.

DeVaugh-Geiss, J., Moroz, G., Biederman, J., Cantwell, D., Fontaine, R., Greist, J. H., . . . Landau, P. (1992). Clomipramine hydrochloride in childhood and adolescent obsessive-compulsive disorder: A multicenter trial. *Journal of the American Academy of Child and Adolescent Psychiatry, 31,* 45–49.

Dori, N., Green, T., Weizman, A., & Gothelf, D. (2017). The effectiveness and safety of antipsychotic and antidepressant medications in individuals with 22Q11.2 deletion syndrome. *Journal of Child and Adolescent Psychopharmacology, 27*(1), 83–90.

Driscoll, D. A., Salvin, J., Sellinger, B., Budarf, M. L., McDonald-McGinn, D. M., Zackai, E. H., & Emanuel, B. S. (1993). Prevalence of 22q11 microdeletions in DiGeorge and velocardiofacial syndromes: Implications for genetic counselling and prenatal diagnosis. *Journal of Medical Genetics, 30*(10), 813–817.

Dykens, E. M. (2016). Psychiatric disorders in people with intellectual disabilities: Steps toward eliminating research and clinical care disparities. *International Review of Research in Developmental Disabilities* (Vol. 50, pp. 277–302). Cambridge, MA: Academic Press.

Dykens, E. M., Shah, B., Davis, B., Baker, C., Fife, T., & Fitzpatrick, J. (2015). Psychiatric disorders in adolescents and young adults with Down syndrome and other intellectual disabilities. *Journal of Neurodevelopmental Disorders, 7*(1), 9.

Efron, D., Hiscock, H., Sewell, J. R., Cranswick, N. E., Vance, A. L., Tyl, Y., & Luk, E. S. (2003). Prescribing of psychotropic medications for children by Australian pediatricians and child psychiatrists. *Pediatrics, 111*(2), 372–375.

Ehlers, A., Hackmann, A., Grey, N., Wild, J., Liness, S., Albert, I., . . . Clark, D. M. (2014). A randomized controlled trial of 7-day intensive and standard weekly cognitive therapy for PTSD and emotion-focused supportive therapy. *American Journal of Psychiatry, 171*(3), 294–304.

Emslie, G. J., Heiligenstein, J. H., Wagner, K. D., Hoog, S. L, Brown, E., . . . Jacobson, J. G. (2002). Fluoxetine for acute treatment of depression in children and adolescents: A placebo-controlled, randomized clinical trial. *Journal of the American Academy of Child and Adolescent Psychiatry, 41*(10), 1205–1215.

Emslie, G. J., Prakash, A., Zhang, Q., Pangallo, B. A., Bangs, M. E., & March, J. S. (2014). A double-blind efficacy and safety study of duloxetine fixed doses in children and adolescents with major depressive disorder. *Journal of Child and Adolescent Psychopharmacology, 24*(4), 170–179.

Esbensen, A. J., Johnson, E. B., Amaral, J. L., Tan, C. M., & Macks, R. (2016). Differentiating aging among adults with Down syndrome and comorbid dementia or psychopathology. *American Journal on Intellectual and Developmental Disabilities, 121*(1), 13–24.

Feinstein, C., & Reiss, A. L. (1996). Psychiatric disorder in mentally retarded children and adolescents: The challenges of meaningful diagnosis. *Child and Adolescents Psychiatric Clinics of North America, 5,* 1031–1037.

Findling, R. L., McNamara, N. K., Youngstrom, E. A., Stansbrey, R., Gracious, B. L., Reed, M. D., & Calabrese, J. R. (2005). Double-blind 18-month trial of lithium versus divalproex maintenance treatment in pediatric bipolar disorder. *Journal of the American Academy of Child and Adolescent Psychiatry, 44*(5), 461–469.

Findling, R. L., Robb, A., Nyilas, M., Forbes, R. A., Jin, N., Ivanova, S., . . . Carson, W. H. (2008). A multiple-center, randomized, double-blind, placebo-controlled study of oral aripiprazole for treatment of adolescents with schizophrenia. *American Journal of Psychiatry, 165*(11), 1432–1441.

Findling, R. L., McKenna, K., Earley, W. R., Stankowski, J., & Pathak, S. (2012). Efficacy and safety of quetiapine in adolescents with schizophrenia investigated in a 6-week, double-blind, placebo controlled trial. *Journal of Child and Adolescent Psychopharmacology, 22*(5), 327–342.

Findling, R. L., Cavus, I., Pappadopulos, E., Vanderburg, D. G., Schwartz, J. H., Gundapaneni, B. K., & DelBello, M. P. (2013). Ziprasidone in adolescents with schizophrenia: Results from a placebo-controlled efficacy and long-term open-extension study. *Journal of Child and Adolescent and Psychopharmacology, 23*(8), 531–544.

Findling, R. L., Robb, A., McNamara, N. K., Pavuluri, M. N., Kafantaris, V., Scheffer, R., . . . Rowles, B. M. (2015). Lithium in the acute treatment of bipolar I disorder: A double-blind, placebo-controlled study. *Pediatrics, 136*(5), 885–894.

Findling, R. L., Chang, K., Robb, A., Foster, V. J., Horrigan, J., Krishen, A., . . . DelBello, M. (2015a). Adjunctive maintenance lamotrigine for pediatric bipolar I disorder: A placebo-controlled randomized withdrawal study. *Journal of the American Academy of Child and Adolescent Psychiatry, 54*(12), 1020–1031.

Findling, R. L., Landbloom, R. P., Mackle, M., Pallozzi, W., Braat, S., Hundt, C., . . . Mathews, M. (2015b). Safety and efficacy from an 8 week double-blind trial of a 26 week open-label extension of asenapine in adolescents with schizophrenia. *Journal of Child and Adolescent Psychopharmacology, 25*(5), 384–396.

Foley, K.-R., Bourke, J., Einfeld, S. L., Tonge, B. J., Jacoby, P., & Leonard, H. (2015). Patterns of depressive symptoms and social relating behaviors differ over time from other behavioral domains for young people with Down syndrome. *Medicine, 94*(19), e710. http://doi.org/10.1097/MD.0000000000000710

Freund, L. S., Reiss, A. L., & Abrams, M. T. (1993). Psychiatric disorders associated with fragile X in the young female. *Pediatrics, 91*(2), 321–329.

Gallagher, S., & Whiteley, J. (2013). The association between stress and physical health in parents caring for children with intellectual disabilities is moderated by children's challenging behaviours. *Journal of Health Psychology, 18*(9), 1220–1231.

Gayleard, J. L., & Mychailyszyn, M. P. (2017). Atomoxetine treatment for children and adolescents with attention-deficit/hyperactivity disorder (ADHD): A comprehensive meta-analysis of outcomes on parent-rated core symptomatology. *ADHD Attention Deficit and Hyperactivity Disorders, 9*(3), 149–160.

Geller, D. A., Hoog, S. L., Heiligenstein, J. H., Ricardi, R. K., Tamura, R., Kluszynski, S., . . . Fluoxetine Pediatric, OCD Study Team. (2001). Fluoxetine treatment for obsessive-compulsive disorder in children and adolescents: A placebo-controlled clinical trial. *Journal of the American Academy of Child and Adolescent Psychiatry, 40*(7), 773–779.

Gibbons, R. D., Brown, C. H., Hur, K., Marcus, S. M., Bhaumik, D. K., Erkens, J. A., . . . Mann, J. J. (2007). Early evidence on the effects of regulators' suicidality warnings on SSRI prescriptions and suicide in children and adolescents. *American Journal of Psychiatry, 164*(9), 1356–1363.

Gibbons, R. D., Coca Perraillon, M., Hur, K., Conti, R. M., Valuck, R. J., & Brent, D. A. (2015). Antidepressant treatment and suicide attempts and self-inflicted injury in children and adolescents. *Pharmacoepidemiology and Drug Safety, 24*(2), 208–214.

Gillberg, C., Persson, E., Grufman, M., & Themner, U. (1986). Psychiatric disorders in mildly and severely mentally retarded urban children and adolescents: Epidemiological aspects. *British Journal of Psychiatry, 149*, 68–74.

Gilmore, L., & Cuskelly, M. (2014). Vulnerability to loneliness in people with intellectual disability: An explanatory model. *Journal of Policy and Practice in Intellectual Disabilities, 11*(3), 192–199.

Goldman, R., Loebel, A., Cucchiaro, J., Deng, L., & Findling, R. L. (2017). Efficacy and safety of lurasidone in adolescents with schizophrenia: A 6-week, randomized placebo-controlled study. *Journal of Child and Adolescent Psychopharmacology, 27*(6), 516–525.

Green, S. A., Berkovits, L. D., & Baker, B. L. (2015). Symptoms and development of anxiety in children with or without intellectual disability. *Journal of Clinical Child & Adolescent Psychology, 44*(1), 137–144.

Greenhill, L., Kollins, S., Abikoff, H., McCracken, J., Riddle, M., Swanson, J., . . . Skrobala, A. (2006). Efficacy and safety of immediate-release methylphenidate treatment for preschoolers with ADHD. *Journal of the American Academy of Child & Adolescent Psychiatry, 45*(11), 1284–1293.

Grey, I., Pollard, J., McClean, B., MacAuley, N., & Hastings, R. (2010). Prevalence of psychiatric diagnoses and challenging behaviors in a community-based population of adults with intellectual disability. *Journal of Mental Health Research in Intellectual Disabilities, 3*(4), 210–222.

Gross, C., Hoffmann, A., Bassell, G. J., & Berry-Kravis, E. M. (2015). Therapeutic strategies in fragile X syndrome: from bench to bedside and back. *Neurotherapeutics, 12*(3), 584–608.

Guess, D., & Carr, E. (1991). Emergence and maintenance of stereotypy and self-injury. *American Journal on Mental Retardation, 96*, 299–320.

Haas, M., Unis, A. S., Armenteros, J., Copenhaver, M. D., Quiroz, J. A., & Kushner, S. F. (2009). A 6-week, randomized, double-blind, placebo-controlled study of the efficacy and safety of risperidone in adolescents with schizophrenia. *Journal of Child and Adolescent Psychopharmacology, 19*(6), 611–621.

Hardan, A., & Sahl, R. (1997). Psychopathology in children and adolescents with developmental disorders. *Research in Developmental Disabilities, 18*(5), 369–382.

Hagerman, R. J., Jackson, C., Amiri, K., Silverman, A. C., O'Connor, R., & Sobesky, W. (1992). Girls with fragile X syndrome: Physical and neurocognitive status and outcome. *Pediatrics, 89*(3), 395–400.

Hall, S. S., Barnett, R. P., & Hustyi, K. M. (2016). Problem behaviour in adolescent boys with fragile syndrome: Relative prevalence, frequency and severity. *Journal of Intellectual Disability Research, 60*(12), 1189–1199.

Harfterkamp, M., van de Loo-Neus, G., Minderaa, R. B., van der Gaag, R. J., Escobar, R., Schacht, A., . . . Hoekstra, P. J. (2012). A randomized double-blind study of atomoxetine versus placebo for attention-deficit/hyperactivity disorder symptoms in children with autism spectrum disorder. *Journal of the American Academy of Child & Adolescent Psychiatry, 51*(7), 733–741.

Harfterkamp, M., Buitelaar, J. K., Minderaa, R. B., van de Loo-Neus, G., van der Gaag, R. J., & Hoekstra, P. J. (2013). Long term treatment with atomoxetine for ADHD symptoms in children with ASD: an open label extension study. *Journal of Child Adolescent Psychopharmacology, 23*(1–6), 2013.

Hässler, F., & Reis, O. (2010). Pharmacotherapy of disruptive behavior in mentally retarded subjects: A review of the current literature. *Developmental Disabilities Review, 16*(3), 265–272.

Henggeler, S. W., Rodick, J. D., Borduin, C. M., Hanson, C. L., Watson, S. M., & Urey, J. R. (1986). Multisystemic treatment of juvenile offenders: Effects on adolescent behavior and family interaction. *Developmental Psychology, 22*(1), 132.

Hess, L. G., Fitzpatrick, S. E., Nguyen, D. V., Chen, Y., Gaul, K. N., Schneider, A., . . . Rivera, S. (2016). A randomized, double-blind, placebo-controlled trial of low-dose sertraline in young children with fragile X syndrome. *Journal of Developmental and Behavioral Pediatrics, 37*(8), 619.

Hessl, D., Dyer-Friedman, J., Glaser, B., Wisbeck, J., Barais, R. G., Taylor, A., & Reiss, A. L. (2001). The influence of environmental and genetic factors on behavior problems and autistic symptoms in boys and girls with fragile X syndrome. *Pediatrics, 108*(5), E88.

Hobden, K., Samuel, P., LeRoy, B., & Lindsay, D. (2013). An empirical examination of the prevalence and predictors of polypharmacy in individuals with dual diagnosis. *International Journal of Disability, Community, & Rehabilitation, 12*(1). Retrieved from http://www.ijdcr.ca/VOL12_01/articles/hobden.shtml

Hofmann, S. G., Asnaani, A., Vonk, I. J., Sawyer, A. T., & Fang, A. (2012). The efficacy of cognitive behavioral therapy: A review of meta-analyses. *Cognitive Therapy and Research, 36*(5), 427–440.

Howlett, S., Florio, T., Xu, H., & Trollor, J. (2015). Ambulatory mental health data demonstrates the high needs of people with an intellectual disability: Results from the New South Wales intellectual disability and mental health data linkage project. *Australian & New Zealand Journal of Psychiatry, 49*(2), 137–144.

Jain, R., Segal, S., Kollins, S. H., & Khayrallah, M. (2011). Clonidine extended-release tablets for pediatric patients with attention-deficit/hyperactivity disorder. *Journal of the American Academy of Child and Adolescent Psychiatry, 50*(2), 171–179.

Ji, N. Y., & Findling, R. L. (2016). Pharmacotherapy for mental health problems in people with intellectual disability. *Current Opinion in Psychiatry, 29*(2), 103–125.

Johnson, J., & El-Alfy, A. T. (2016). Review of available studies of the neurobiology and pharmacotherapeutic management of trichotillomania. *Journal of Advanced Research, 7*(2), 169–184.

Kasari, C., Rotheram-Fuller, E., Locke, J., & Gulsrud, A. (2012). Making the connection: Randomized controlled trial of social skills at school for children with autism spectrum disorders. *Journal of Child Psychology and Psychiatry, 53*(4), 431–439.

Kates, W. R., Olszewski, A. K., Gnirke, M. H., Kikinis, Z., Nelson, J., Antshel, K. M., . . . Coman, I. L. (2015). White matter microstructural abnormalities of the cingulum bundle in youths with 22q11.2 deletion syndrome: Associations with medication, neuropsychological function, and prodromal symptoms of psychosis. *Schizophrenia Research, 161*(1), 76–84.

Kennard, B. D., Emslie, G. J., Mayes, T. L., Nakonezny, P. A., Jones, J. M., Foxwell, A. A., & King, J. (2014). Sequential treatment with fluoxetine and relapse-prevention CBT to improve outcomes in pediatric depression. *American Journal of Psychiatry, 171*(10), 1083–1090.

Keuthen, N. J., Rothbaum, B. O., Fama, J., Altenburger, E., Falkenstein, M. J., Sprich, S. E., . . . Welch, S. S. (2012).

DBT-enhanced cognitive-behavioral treatment for trichotillomania: A randomized controlled trial. *Journal of Behavioral Addictions, 1*(3), 106–114.

King, B. H., DeAntonio, C., McCracken, J. T., Forness, S. R., & Ackerland, V. (1994). Psychiatric consultation in severe and profound mental retardation. *American Journal of Psychiatry, 151,* 1802–1808.

Kircher, T., Arolt, V., Jansen, A., Pyka, M., Reinhardt, I., Kellermann, T., . . . Ströhle, A. (2013). Effect of cognitive-behavioral therapy on neural correlates of fear conditioning in panic disorder. *Biological Psychiatry, 73*(1), 93–101.

Kok, L., van der Waa, A., Klip, H., & Staal, W. (2016). The effectiveness of psychosocial interventions for children with a psychiatric disorder and mild intellectual disability to borderline intellectual functioning: A systematic literature review and meta-analysis. *Clinical Child Psychology and Psychiatry, 21*(1), 156–171.

Kollins, S. H., Jain, R., Brams, M., Segal, S., Findling, R. L., Wigal, S. B., & Khayrallah, M. (2011). Clonidine extended-release tablets as add-on therapy to psychostimulants in children and adolescents with ADHD. *Pediatrics, 127*(6), e1406–e1413.

Koning, C., Magill-Evans, J., Volden, J., & Dick, B. (2013). Efficacy of cognitive behavior therapy-based social skills intervention for school-aged boys with autism spectrum disorders. *Research in Autism Spectrum Disorders, 7*(10), 1282–1290.

Kryzhanovskaya, L., Schultz, S. C., McDougle, C., Frazier, J., Dittman, R., Robertson-Plouch, C., . . . Tohen, M. (2009). Olanzapine versus placebo in adolescents with schizophrenia: A 6-week, randomized, double-blind, placebo-controlled trial. *Journal of the American Academy of Child and Adolescent Psychiatry, 48*(1), 60–70.

Kurtz, P. F., Chin, M. D., Robinson, A. N., O'Connor, J. T., & Hagopian, L. P. (2015). Functional analysis and treatment of problem behavior exhibited by children with fragile X syndrome. *Research in Developmental Disabilities, 43,* 150–166.

Kutcher, S., Aman, M., Brooks, S. J., Buitelaar, J., van Daalen, E., Fegert, J., . . . Tyano, S. (2004). International consensus statement on attention-deficit/hyperactivity disorder (ADHD) and disruptive behaviour disorders (DBDs): Clinical implications and treatment practice suggestions. *European Neuropsychopharmacology, 14*(1), 11–28.

Kyriakopoulos, M., Stringaris, A., Manolesou, S., Radobuljac, M. D., Jacobs, B., Reichenberg, A., . . . Frangou, S. (2015). Determination of psychosis-related clinical profiles in children with autism spectrum disorders using latent class analysis. *European Child & Adolescent Psychiatry, 24*(3), 301–307.

Lautarescu, B. A., Holland, A. J., & Zaman, S. H. (2017). The early presentation of dementia in people with Down syndrome: A systematic review of longitudinal studies. *Neuropsychology Review, 27*(1), 31–45.

Lewin, A. B., Bergman, R. L., Peris, T. S., Chang, S., McCracken, J. T., & Piacentini, J. (2010). Correlates of insight among youth with obsessive-compulsive disorder. *Journal of Child Psychology and Psychiatry, 51*(5), 603–611.

Leyfer, O. T., Woodruff-Borden, J., Klein-Tasman, B. P., Fricke, J. S., & Mervis, C. B. (2006). Prevalence of psychiatric disorders in 4–16 year olds with Williams syndrome. *American Journal of Medical Genetics B Neuropsychiatric Genetics, 141B*(6), 615–622.

Linaker, O. M., & Helle, J. (1994). Validity of the schizophrenia diagnosis of the Psychopathology Instrument for Mentally Retarded Adults (PIRMA): A comparison of schizophrenic patients with and without mental retardation. *Research in Developmental Disabilities, 15,* 473–486.

Linden, S., Bussing, R., Kubilis, P., Gerhard, T., Segal, R., Shuster, J. J., & Winterstein, A. G. (2016). Risk of suicidal events with atomoxetine compared to stimulant treatment: A cohort study. *Pediatrics, 137*(5), e20153199.

Liu, Z., & Smith, C. B. (2014). Lithium: A promising treatment for fragile X syndrome. *ACS Chemical Neuroscience, 5,* 477–483.

Loschen, E. L., & Osman, O. T. (1992). Self-injurious behavior in the developmentally disabled: Assessment techniques. *Psychopharmacology Bulletin, 28,* 433–438.

Lott, I. T. (2012). Neurological phenotypes for Down syndrome across the life span. In M. Dierssen & R. Torre (Eds.), *Progress in brain research* (Vol. 197, pp. 101–121). Retrieved from https://www.sciencedirect.com/science/article/pii/B9780444542991000066

Lu, X. Y., Phung, M. T., Shaw, C. A., Pham, K., Neil, S. E., Patel, A., . . . Lalani, S. (2008). Genomic imbalances in neonates with birth defects: high detection rates by using chromosomal microarray analysis. *Pediatrics, 122*(6), 1310–1318.

Luiselli, J. K. (2015). Behavioral treatment of rumination: Research and clinical applications. *Journal of Applied Behavior Analysis, 48*(3), 707–711.

Lunsky, Y., & Modi, M. (2017). Predictors of psychotropic polypharmacy among outpatients with psychiatric disorders and intellectual disability. *Psychiatric Services*, Advance online publication. doi:10.1176/appi.ps.201700032

Mace, F. C., & Mauk, J. E. (1995). Bio-behavioral diagnosis and treatment of self-injury. *Developmental Disabilities Research Reviews, 1*(2), 104–110.

Mahmood, I. (2006). Prediction of drug clearance in children from adults: A comparison of several allometric methods. *British Journal of Clinical Pharmacology, 61*(5), 545–557.

Mancuso, C. E., Tanzi, M. G., & Gabay, M. (2004). Paradoxical reactions to benzodiazepines: Literature review and treatment options. *Pharmacotherapy, 24*(9), 1177–1185.

March, J. S., Biederman, J., Wolkow, R., Safferman, A., Mardekian, J., Cook, E. H., . . . Steiner, H. (1998). Sertraline in children and adolescents with obsessive-compulsive disorder: A multicenter randomized controlled trial. *Journal of the American Medical Association, 280*(20), 1752–1756.

Martin, G. E., Barstein, J., Hornickel, J., Matherly, S., Durante, G., & Losh, M. (2017). Signaling of noncomprehension in communication breakdowns in fragile X syndrome, Down syndrome, and autism spectrum disorder. *Journal of Communication Disorders, 65,* 22–34.

Määttä, T., Tervo-Määttä, T., Taanila, A., Kaski, M., & Iivanainen, M. (2014). Adaptive behaviour change and health in adults with Down syndrome: A prospective clinical follow-up study. In F. Atroshi (Ed.), *Pharmacology and nutritional intervention in the treatment of disease.* doi:10.5772/57461

McCarron, M., McCallion, P., Reilly, E., & Mulryan, N. (2014). A prospective 14-year longitudinal follow-up of dementia in persons with Down syndrome. *Journal of Intellectual Disability Research, 58*(1), 61–70.

McGinnes, M. A. (2010). Abolishing and establishing operation analyses of social attention as positive reinforcement for problem behavior. *Journal of Applied Behavioral Analysis, 43*(1), 119–123.

McIntyre, L. L., Blacher, J., & Baker, B. L. (2006). The transition to school: Adaptation in young children with and without intellectual disability. *Journal of Intellectual Disability Research, 50*(5), 349–361.

Mohapatra, S., & Sahoo, A. J. (2016). Self-injurious behavior in a young child with Lesch-Nyhan syndrome. *Indian Journal of Psychological Medicine, 38*(5), 477.

Mohatt, J., Bennett, S. M., & Walkup, J. T. (2014). Treatment of separation, generalized, and social anxiety disorders in youths. *American Journal of Psychiatry, 171*(7), 741–748.

Morina, N., Koerssen, R., & Pollet, T. V. (2016). Interventions for children and adolescents with posttraumatic stress disorder: A meta-analysis of comparative outcome studies. *Clinical Psychology Reviews, 47,* 41–54.

Moskowitz, L. J., Walsh, C. E., Mulder, E., McLaughlin, D. M., Hajcak, G., Carr, E. G., & Zarcone, J. R. (2017). Intervention for anxiety and problem behavior in children with autism spectrum disorder and intellectual disability. *Journal of Autism and Developmental Disorders, 47*(12), 3930–3948.

Neece, C. L., Green, S. A., & Baker, B. L. (2012). Parenting stress and child behavior problems: A transactional relationship across time. *American Journal on Intellectual and Developmental Disabilities, 117*(1), 48–66.

Newcorn, J. H., Spencer, T. J., Biederman, J., Milton, D. R., & Michelson, D. (2005). Atomoxetine treatment in children and adolescents with attention-deficit/hyperactivity disorder and comorbid oppositional defiant disorder. *Journal of the American Academy of Child & Adolescent Psychiatry, 44*(3), 240–248.

Nickels, K., Katusic, S. K., Colligan, R. C., Weaver, A. L, Voigt, R. G., & Barbaresi, W. J. (2008). Stimulant medication treatment of target behaviors in children with autism: A population-based study. *Journal of Developmental and Behavioral Pediatrics, 29*(2), 75–81.

O'Connor, M. J., Shah, B., Whaley, S., Cronin, P., Gunderson, B., & Graham, J. (2002). Psychiatric illness in a clinical sample of children with prenatal alcohol exposure. *American Journal of Drug and Alcohol Abuse, 28*(4), 743–754.

Olatunji, B. O., Cisler, J. M., & Deacon, B. J. (2010). Efficacy of cognitive behavioral therapy for anxiety disorders: a review of meta-analytic findings. *Psychiatric Clinics, 33*(3), 557–577.

Oliver, C., Petty, J., Ruddick, L., & Bacarese-Hamilton, M. (2012). The association between repetitive, self-injurious and aggressive behavior in children with severe intellectual disability. *Journal of Autism and Developmental Disorders, 42*(6), 910–919.

Orefici, G., Cardona, F., Cox, C. J., & Cunningham, M. W. (2016). Pediatric autoimmune neuropsychiatric disorders associated with streptococcal infections (PANDAS). In J. J. Ferretti, D. L. Stevens, & V. A. Fischetti (Eds.), *Streptococcus pyogenes: Basic biology to clinical manifestations.* Retrieved from https://www.ncbi.nlm.nih.gov/books/NBK333433/

Oulton, K., Sell, D., Kerry, S., & Gibson, F. (2015). Individualizing hospital care for children and young people with learning disabilities: it's the little things that make the difference. *Journal of Pediatric Nursing: Nursing Care of Children and Families, 30*(1), 78–86.

Pasamanick, B., Rogers, M. E., & Lilienfeld, A. M. (1956). Pregnancy experience and the development of behavior disorder in children. *American Journal of Psychiatry, 112*(8), 613–618.

Pearson, D. A., Santos, C. W., Roache, J. D., Casat, C. D., Loveland, K. A., Lachar, D., . . . Cleveland, L. A. (2003). Treatment effects of methylphenidate on behavioral adjustment in children with intellectual disability and ADHD. *Journal of the American Academy of Child and Adolescent Psychiatry, 42*(2), 209–216.

Pediatric OCD Treatment Study Team. (2004). Cognitive-behavior therapy, sertraline and their combination for children and adolescents with obsessive-compulsive disorder: The pediatric OCD treatment study (POTS) randomized controlled trial. *Journal of the American Medical Association, 292*(16), 1969–1976.

Peebles, K. A., & Price, T. J. (2012). Self-injurious behaviour in intellectual disability syndromes: Evidence for aberrant pain signalling as a contributing factor. *Journal of Intellectual Disability Research, 56*(5), 441–452.

Petty, J. L., Bacarese-Hamilton, M., Davies, L. E., & Oliver, C. (2014). Correlates of self-injurious, aggressive and destructive behaviour in children under five who are at risk of developmental delay. *Research in Developmental Disabilities, 35*(1), 36–45.

Plant, K.M. (2007). Reducing problem behavior during care-giving in families of preschool-aged children with developmental disabilities. *Research in Developmental Disabilities, 28*(4), 362–85.

Popova, S., Lange, S., Shield, K., Mihic, A., Chudley, A. E., Mukherjee, R. A., . . . Rehm, J. (2016). Comorbidity of fetal alcohol spectrum disorder: A systematic review and meta-analysis. *The Lancet, 387*(10022), 978–987.

Powis, L., & Oliver, C. (2014). The prevalence of aggression in genetic syndromes: A review. *Research in Developmental Disabilities, 35*(5), 1051–1071.

Reichow, B., Steiner, A. M., & Volkmar, F. (2013). Cochrane review: Social skills groups for people aged 6 to 21 with autism spectrum disorders (ASD). *Evidence-Based Child Health: A Cochrane Review Journal, 8*(2), 266–315.

Reiss, S., & Valenti-Hein, D. (1994). Development of a psychopathology rating scale for children with mental retardation. *Journal of Consulting and Clinical Psychology, 62,* 28–33.

Riby, D. M., Hanley, M., Kirk, H., Clark, F., Little, K., Fleck, R., . . . Allday, M. H. (2014). The interplay between anxiety and social functioning in Williams syndrome. *Journal of Autism and Developmental Disorders, 44*(5), 1220–1229.

Riddle, M. A., Reeve, E. A., Yaryura-Tobias, J. A., Yang, H. M., Claghorn, J. L., Gaffney, G., . . . Walkup, J. T. (2001). Fluvoxamine for children and adolescents with obsessive-compulsive disorder: A randomized, controlled multicenter trial. *Journal of the American Academy of Child and Adolescent Psychiatry, 40*(2), 222–229.

Robb, A. S. (2010). Managing irritability and aggression in autism spectrum disorders in children and adolescents. *Developmental Disabilities Research Reviews, 16*(3), 258–264.

Robb, A. S., Andersson, C., Bellochio, E. E., Manos, G., Rojas-Fernandez, C., Mathews, S., . . . Mankoski, R. (2011) Safety and tolerability of aripiprazole in the treatment of irritability associated with autistic disorder in pediatric subjects (6-17 years old): Results from a pooled analysis of 2 studies. *The Primary Care Companion for CNS Disorders, 13*(1), e1–e9.

Robb, A. S., Cueva, J. E., Sporn, J., Yang, R., & Vanderburg, D. G. (2010). Sertraline treatment of children and adolescents with posttraumatic stress: A double-blind, placebo-controlled trial. *Journal of Child and Adolescent Psychopharmacology, 20*(6), 1–9.

Rothschild, A. J, Shindul-Rothschild, V. A., Murray, M., & Brewster, S. (2000). Comparison of the frequency of behavioral disinhibition on alprazolam, clonazepam, or no benzodiazepine in hospitalized psychiatric patients. *Journal of Clinical Psychopharmacology, 20*(1),7–11.

Rutter, M., Graham, P., & Yule, W. (1970). *A neuropsychiatric study in childhood*. London, England: Spastics International.

Rynn, M. A., Siqueland, L., & Rickels, K. (2001). Placebo-controlled trial of sertraline in the treatment of children with generalized anxiety disorder. *American Journal of Psychiatry, 158*(12), 2008–2014.

Saad, K., Abdelrahman, A. A., Abdel-Raheem, Y. F., Othman, E. R., Badry, R., Othman, H. A., & Sobhy, K. M. (2014).

Turner syndrome: Review of clinical, neuropsychiatric, and EEG status: an experience of tertiary center. *Acta Neurologica Belgica, 114*(1), 1–9.

Saad, K., Al-Atram, A. A., Baseer, K. A. A., Ali, A. M., & El-Houfey, A. A. (2015). Assessment of quality of life, anxiety and depression in children with Turner syndrome: A case-control study. *American Journal of Neuroscience, 6*(1), 8–12.

Salmon, K., O'Kearney, R., Reese, E., & Fortune, C. A. (2016). The role of language skill in child psychopathology: Implications for intervention in the early years. *Clinical Child and Family Psychology Review, 19*(4), 352–367.

Sandman, C. A., Kemp, A. S., Mabini, C., Pincus, D., & Magnusson, M. (2012). The role of self-injury in the organisation of behaviour. *Journal of Intellectual Disability Research, 56*(5), 516–526.

Sansone, S. M., Widaman, K. F., Hall, S. S., Reiss, A. L., Lightbody, A., Kaufmann, W. E., . . . Hessl, D. (2012). Psychometric study of the aberrant behavior checklist in fragile X syndrome and implications for targeted treatment. *Journal of Autism and Developmental Disorders, 42*(7), 1377–1392.

Savill, N. C., Buitelaar, J. K., Anand, E., Day, K. A., Treuer, T., Upadhyaya, H. P., & Coghill, D. (2015). The efficacy of atomoxetine for the treatment of children and adolescents with attention-deficit/hyperactivity disorder: A comprehensive review of over a decade of clinical research. *CNS Drugs, 29*(2), 131–151.

Scahill, L., Jeon, S., Boorin, S. J., McDougle, C. J., Aman, M. G., Dziura, J., . . . Deng, Y. (2016). Weight gain and metabolic consequences of risperidone in young children with autism spectrum disorder. *Journal of the American Academy of Child & Adolescent Psychiatry, 55*(5), 415–423.

Schneider, M., Debbané, M., Bassett, A. S., Chow, E. W., Fung, W. L. A., Van Den Bree, M. B., . . . Antshel, K. M. (2014). Psychiatric disorders from childhood to adulthood in 22q11. 2 deletion syndrome: Results from the International Consortium on Brain and Behavior in 22q11. 2 Deletion Syndrome. *American Journal of Psychiatry, 171*(6), 627–639.

Schouten, J. P., McElgunn, C. J., Waaijer, R., Zwijnenburg, D., Diepvens, F., & Pals, G. (2002). Relative quantification of 40 nucleic acid sequences by multiplex ligation-dependent probe amplification. *Nucleic Acids Research, 30*(12), e57.

Schroeder, S. R., Marquis, J. G., Reese, R. M., Richman, D. M., Mayo-Ortega, L., Oyama-Ganiko, R., & Lawrence, L. (2014). Risk factors for self-injury, aggression, and stereotyped behavior among young children at risk for intellectual and developmental disabilities. *American Journal on Intellectual and Developmental Disabilities, 119*(4), 351–370.

Shang, C. Y., Pan, Y. L., Lin, H. Y., Huang, L. W., & Gau, S. S. F. (2015). An open-label, randomized trial of methylphenidate and atomoxetine treatment in children with attention-deficit/hyperactivity disorder. *Journal of Child and Adolescent Psychopharmacology, 25*(7), 566–573.

Simonoff, E., Taylor, E., Baird, G., Bernard, S., Chadwick, O., Liang, H., . . . Wood, N. (2013). Randomized controlled double-blind trial of optimal dose methylphenidate in children and adolescents with severe attention deficit hyperactivity disorder and intellectual disability. *Journal of Child Psychology and Psychiatry, 54*(5), 527–535.

Singh, J., Robb, A., Vijapurkar, U., Nuamah, I., & Hough, D. (2011). A randomized, double-blind study of paliperidone extended-release in treatment of acute schizophrenia in adolescents. *Biological Psychiatry, 70*(12), 1179–1187.

Skokauskas, N., Sweeny, E., Meehan, J., & Gallagher, L. (2012). Mental health problems in children with Prader-Willi syndrome. *Journal of the Canadian Academy of Child and Adolescent Psychiatry, 21*(3), 194.

Skotko, B. G., Davidson, E. J., & Weintraub, G. S. (2013). Contributions of a specialty clinic for children and adolescents with Down syndrome. *American Journal of Medical Genetics Part A, 161*(3), 430–437.

Stephen, L. J., Wishart, A., & Brodie, M. J. (2017). Psychiatric side effects and antiepileptic drugs: Observations from prospective audits. *Epilepsy and Behavior, 71*(Pt. A), 73–78.

Stinton, C., Tomlinson, K., & Estes, Z. (2012). Examining reports of mental health in adults with Williams syndrome. *Research in Developmental Disabilities, 33*(1), 144–152.

Strawn, J. R., Welge, J. A., Wehry, A. M., Keeshin, B., & Rynn, M. A. (2015). Efficacy and tolerability of antidepressants in pediatric anxiety disorders: A systematic review and meta-analysis. *Depression and Anxiety, 32*(3), 149–157.

Strawn, J. R., Prakash, A., Zhang, Q., Pangallo, B. A., Stroud, C. E., Cai, N., & Findling, R. L. (2015). A randomized, placebo-controlled study of duloxetine for the treatment of children and adolescents with generalized anxiety disorder. *Journal of the American Academy of Child and Adolescent Psychiatry, 54*(4), 283–293.

Sullivan, K., Hooper, S., & Hatton, D. (2007). Behavioral equivalents of anxiety in children with fragile X syndrome: Parent and teacher report. *Journal of Intellectual Disability Research, 51*(1), 54–65.

Summers, J., Shahrami, A., Cali, S., D'Mello, C., Kako, M., Palikucin-Reljin, A., . . . Lunsky, Y. (2017). Self-injury in autism spectrum disorder and intellectual disability: Exploring the role of reactivity to pain and sensory input. *Brain Science, 7*(11), pii: E140. doi:10.3390/brainsci7110140

Suter, J. C., & Bruns, E. J. (2009). Effectiveness of the wraparound process for children with emotional and behavioral disorders: A meta-analysis. *Clinical Child and Family Psychology Review, 12*(4), 336.

Swedo, S. E., Leonard, H. L., Garvey, M., Mittleman, B., Allen, A. J., Perlmutter, S., . . . Lougee, L. (1998). Pediatric autoimmune neuropsychiatric disorders associated with streptococcal infections: Clinical description of the first 50 cases. *American Journal of Psychiatry, 155*(2), 264–271.

Swillen, A., & McDonald-McGinn, D. M. (2015). Developmental Trajectories in 22q11.2 Deletion. *American Journal of Medical Genetics. Part C, Seminars in Medical Genetics, 169*(2), 172–181. http://doi.org/10.1002/ajmg.c.31435

Tang, S. X., Yi, J. J., Calkins, M. E., Whinna, D. A., Kohler, C. G., Souders, M. C., . . . Gur, R. E. (2014). Psychiatric disorders in 22q11. 2 deletion syndrome are prevalent but undertreated. *Psychological Medicine, 44*(6), 1267–1277.

Tartaglia, N. R., Ayari, N., Hutaff-Lee, C., & Boada, R. (2012). Attention-deficit hyperactivity disorder symptoms in children and adolescents with sex chromosome aneuploidy: XXY, XXX, XYY, and XXYY. *Journal of Developmental and Behavioral Pediatrics, 33*(4), 309.

Tewari, N., Mathur, V. P., Sardana, D., & Bansal, K. (2017). Lesch-Nyhan syndrome: The saga of metabolic abnormalities and self-injurious behavior. *Intractable & Rare Diseases Research, 6*(1), 65–68.

Thienemann, M., Murphy, T., Leckman, J., Shaw, R., Williams, K., Kapphahn, C., . . . Elia, J. (2017). Clinical management of pediatric acute-onset neuropsychiatric syndrome: Part I—psychiatric and behavioral interventions. *Journal of Child and Adolescent Psychopharmacology, 27*(7), 566–573.

Thurman, A. J., McDuffie, A., Hagerman, R., & Abbeduto, L. (2014). Psychiatric symptoms in boys with fragile X syndrome: A comparison with nonsyndromic autism spectrum disorder. *Research in Developmental Disabilities, 35*(5), 1072–1086.

Toteja, N., Gallego, J. A., Saito, E., Gerhard, T., Winterstein, A., Olfson, M., & Correll, C. U. (2014). Prevalence and correlates of antipsychotic polypharmacy in children and adolescents receiving antipsychotic treatment. *International Journal of Neuropsychopharmacology, 17*(7), 1095–1105.

Treatment for Adolescents with Depression Study Team. (2004). Fluoxetine, cognitive-behavioral therapy, and their combination for adolescents with depression: Treatment for Adolescents with Depression Study (TADS) randomized controlled trial. *Journal of the American Medical Association, 292*(7), 807–820.

Valicenti-McDermott, M., Lawson, K., Hottinger, K., Seijo, R., Schechtman, M., Shulman, L., & Shinnar, S. (2015). Parental stress in families of children with autism and other developmental disabilities. *Journal of Child Neurology, 30*(13), 1728–1735.

Van Ool, J. S., Snoeijen-Schouwenaars, F. M., Schelhaas, H. J., Tan, I. Y., Aldenkamp, A. P., & Hendriksen, J. G. (2016). A systematic review of neuropsychiatric comorbidities in patients with both epilepsy and intellectual disability. *Epilepsy & Behavior,* 60, 130–137.

Van Tricht, M. J., Nieman, D. H., Koelman, J. T., Mensink, A. J., Bour, L. J., Van der Meer, J. N., . . . De Haan, L. (2015). Sensory gating in subjects at ultra high risk for developing a psychosis before and after a first psychotic episode. *The World Journal of Biological Psychiatry, 16*(1), 12–21.

Verhoeven, W. M., Tuinier, S., van den Berg, Y. W., Coppus, A. M., Fekkes, D., Pepplinkhuizen, L., & Thijssen, J. H. (1999). Stress and self-injurious behavior: Hormonal and serotonergic parameters in mentally retarded subjects. *Pharmacopsychiatry, 32,* 13–20.

Vitiello, B., Correll, C., van Zwieten-Boot, B., Zuddas, A., Parellada, M., & Arango, C. (2009). Antipsychotics in children and adolescents: Increasing use, evidence for efficacy and safety concerns. *European Neuropsychopharmacology, 19*(9), 629–635.

Vitiello, B., Lazzaretto, D., Yershova, K., Abikoff, H., Paykina, N., McCracken, J. T., . . . Wigal, T. (2015). Pharmacotherapy of the Preschool ADHD Treatment Study (PATS) children growing up. *Journal of the American Academy of Child & Adolescent Psychiatry, 54*(7), 550–556.

Wadell, P. M., Hagerman, R. J., & Hessl, D. R. (2013). Fragile X syndrome: Psychiatric manifestations, assessment and emerging therapies. *Current Psychiatry Reviews, 9*(1), 53–58.

Wagner, K.D., Ambrosini, P., Rynn, M., Wohlberg, C., Yang, R., Greenbaum, M. S., . . . Deas, D. (2003). Efficacy of sertraline in the treatment of children and adolescents with major depressive disorder: Two randomized controlled trials. *Journal of the American Medical Association, 290*(8), 1033–1041.

Wagner, K. D., Jonas, J., Findling, R. L., Ventura, D., & Saikali, K. (2006). A double-blind, randomized, placebo-controlled trial of escitalopram in the treatment of pediatric depression. *Journal of the American Academy of Child and Adolescent Psychiatry, 45*(3), 280–288.

Wagner, K. D., Robb, A. S., Findling, R. L., Jin, J., Gutierrez, M. M., & Heydorn, W. E. (2004). A randomized, placebo-controlled trial of citalopram for the treatment of major depression in children and adolescents. *American Journal of Psychiatry, 161*(6), 1079–1083.

Walker, J. C., Dosen, A., Buitelaar, J. K., Janzing, J. G. (2011). Depression in Down syndrome: A review of the literature. *Research in Developmental Disabilities, 32*(5), 1432–1440.

Walkup, J.T., Albano, A. M., Piacentini, J., Birmaher, B., Compton, S. N., Sherrill, J. T., . . . Kendall, P. C. (2008). Cognitive behavioral therapy, sertraline or a combination in childhood anxiety. *The New England Journal of Medicine, 359*(26), 2753–2766.

Walkup, J. T., Labellarte, M. J., Riddle, M. A., Pine, D. S., Greenhill, L., Klein, R., . . . Roper, M. (2001). Fluvoxamine for the treatment of anxiety disorders in children and adolescents. *Journal of the American Medical Association, 344*(17), 1279–1285.

Walton, K. M., & Ingersoll, B. R. (2013). Improving social skills in adolescents and adults with autism and severe to profound intellectual disability: A review of the literature. *Journal of Autism and Developmental Disorders, 43*(3), 594–615.

Weiss, B., Han, S., Harris, V., Catron, T., Ngo, V. K., Caron, A., . . . Guth, C. (2013). An independent randomized clinical trial of multisystemic therapy with non-court-referred adolescents with serious conduct problems. *Journal of Consulting and Clinical Psychology, 81*(6), 1027.

Weisz, J. R., Hawley, K. M., & Doss, A. J. (2004). Empirically tested psychotherapies for youth internalizing and externalizing problems and disorders. *Child and Adolescent Psychiatric Clinics of North America, 13*(4), 729–815.

White, S. W., Ollendick, T., Albano, A. M., Oswald, D., Johnson, C., Southam-Gerow, M. A., . . . Scahill, L. (2013). Randomized controlled trial: Multimodal anxiety and social skill intervention for adolescents with autism spectrum disorder. *Journal of Autism and Developmental Disorders, 43*(2), 382–394.

Wink, L. K., Early, M., Schaefer, T., Pottenger, A., Horn, P., McDougle, C. J., & Erickson, C. A. (2014). Body mass index change in autism spectrum disorders: comparison of treatment with risperidone and aripiprazole. *Journal of Child and Adolescent Psychopharmacology, 24*(2), 78–82.

Williams, D. E., & McAdam, D. (2012). Assessment, behavioral treatment, and prevention of pica: Clinical guidelines and recommendations for practitioners. *Research in Developmental Disabilities, 33*(6), 2050–2057.

Wood, J. J., Drahota, A., Sze, K., Har, K., Chiu, A., & Langer, D. A. (2009). Cognitive behavioral therapy for anxiety in children with autism spectrum disorders: A randomized, controlled trial. *Journal of Child Psychology and Psychiatry, 50*(3), 224–234.

Woods, K. E., Luiselli, J. K., & Tomassone, S. (2013). Functional analysis and intervention for chronic rumination. *Journal of Applied Behavior Analysis, 46*(1), 328–332.

Yoo, K. H., Burris, J. L., Gaul, K. N., Hagerman, R. J., & Rivera, S. M. (2017). Low-dose sertraline improves receptive language in children with fragile x syndrome when eye tracking methodology is used to measure treatment outcome. *Journal of Psychology and Clinical Psychiatry, 7*(6), 00465.

Young, T., Apfeldorf, W., Knepper, J., & Yager, J. (2009). Severe eating disorder in a 28-year-old man with William's syndrome. *American Journal of Psychiatry, 166*(1), 25–31.

Zarcone, J. R., Lindauer, S. E., Morse, P. S., Crosland, K. A., Valdovinos, M. G., McKercher, T. L., . . . Schroeder, S. R. (2001). Effects of risperidone on destructive behavior of persons with developmental disabilities: III. Functional analysis. *American Journal on Mental Retardation, 109,* 310–321.

Zarcone, J., Napolitano, D., Peterson, C., Breidbord, J., Ferraioli, S., Caruso-Anderson, M., . . . Thompson, T. (2007). The relationship between compulsive behaviour and academic achievement across the three genetic subtypes of Prader-Willi syndrome. *Journal of Intellectual Disabilities Research, 51*(Pt. 6), 478–487.

CHAPTER 28

Sleep Disorders

Judith Owens and Miriam Weiss

Upon completion of this chapter, the reader will

- Describe the clinical presentation and management of pediatric insomnia
- Outline a therapeutic approach to delayed sleep–wake phase disorders
- List the common features of disorders of arousal
- List pediatric populations at increased risk for sleep-disordered breathing
- Describe key causal factors in restless leg syndrome/periodic limb movement disorders

Sleep problems and disorders are some of the most common complaints brought to the pediatrician and sometimes the most difficult to resolve. In children with developmental disabilities, these issues tend to be even more common. This chapter discusses a range of sleep disorders including insomnia, circadian rhythm disorders, disorders of arousal, sleep-disordered breathing/obstructive sleep apnea (OSA), and movement-related disorders in sleep.

SLEEP ARCHITECTURE

The three categories of sleep stages include wake, non–rapid eye movement (REM) sleep, and REM sleep. The second category, non-REM sleep, is a time of low brain activity and can be divided into three stages of sleep. Stage 1 of non-REM sleep occurs at sleep–wake transitions, comprises 1%–3% of the total sleep period, and can include a normal phenomenon called hypnic jerks or sleep starts. Stage 1 sleep is the easiest from which to awaken. Stage 2 sleep comprises the majority of the sleep period (approximately 50%) and is distributed across the whole night. Stage 3, deep sleep or slow-wave sleep, from which it is most difficult to awaken, occurs predominantly in the first half of the night and comprises 25% of the sleep period. The third category, REM sleep, also known as dream sleep, occurs largely during the second half of the night and increases in duration and intensity in the early morning hours; it comprises about 25% of the total sleep period.

During the typical four to eight sleep cycles, stages progress from non-REM sleep to REM sleep over about 90–110 minutes, with multiple brief arousals followed by a rapid return to sleep. Younger children have shorter sleep cycles and thus have more frequent arousals during the night. In addition, it should be noted that the normal percentages of the sleep stages listed above are typical for older children and adolescents;

for example, the percentage of slow-wave sleep is much higher in infants and younger children and declines in the second decade of life. Finally, different sleep disorders may be linked to specific sleep stages; for example, partial arousal parasomnias (sleep walking and night terrors) arise out of slow-wave sleep and thus mostly occur in the first part of the night (Mindell & Owens, 2015), and sleep-disordered breathing is often worse during REM sleep.

SLEEPING PATTERNS

The amount and distribution of sleep requirement over 24 hours also changes from infancy to adolescence and with a good deal of individual variability. With advances in circadian science, there is now emphasis on both optimal sleep duration and the timing of the sleep period. The time to sleep, or sleep onset latency, typically remains similar with an average of 15–30 minutes throughout the lifespan. Wake time after sleep onset can range from 10–30 minutes, and there can be as many as two dozen brief awakenings across the night. Newborns through 2 months of age require an average of 14 hours of sleep per 24 hours and 1–2 hours of wake time between day and nighttime sleep periods. By 6 months of age, infants do not require feeding during the sleep period and have consolidated their sleep into a 9- to 12-hour sleep period, optimally between 6:30 p.m. and 6:30 a.m. Infants aged 2–12 months require an average of 12–16 hours of sleep, including naps. Naps decrease from four to two per 24 hours during this age range. Children who are 1–2 years old require an average of 11–14 hours of sleep, including one to two naps averaging 2–3 hours in length, with a shift from two to one nap between 18–24 months. Children who are 3–5 years old require an average of 10–13 hours of sleep, and their naps will decrease from one nap to no naps during this age range. By 5 years of age, the majority of children have given up napping (Crosby, LeBourgeois, & Harsh, 2005). Children 6–9 years of age require an average of 10–12 hours of sleep, with a sleep period between 7:30 p.m. and 7:30 a.m.; 10–12 year olds require 10–11 hours, with a sleep period ranging from 8:30 p.m. to 7:30 a.m.; adolescents ages 13–15 require 9–10 hours of sleep, with a sleep period between 9:30 p.m. and 7:30 a.m.; and 16–20 year olds require 8–9.5 hours of sleep, with an optimal sleep period between 10:30 p.m. and 8:00 a.m. (Mindell & Owens, 2015).

Especially in children with developmental disabilities, more than one sleep disorder can present simultaneously. The following case study illustrates both the complexity of presenting complaints and the importance of taking a complete sleep history.

CASE STUDY

Will is a 10-year-old boy who was born with trisomy 21 (Down syndrome). He has limited expressive language skills, although his family is able to interpret most of his verbalizations. Will is pleasant and loving with others, and he enjoys listening to music, watching videos, and looking through comic books. Will also can be oppositional, although his parents have learned that talking to him in a quiet voice and using simple commands are often effective.

Will was diagnosed several years ago with severe OSA, which was documented on an overnight sleep study (polysomnogram), and he subsequently had an adenotonsillectomy (AT). Unfortunately, his postoperative polysomnogram continued to demonstrate severe OSA. His clinical symptoms included loud snoring, witnessed apneas, gasping, choking, restless sleep, sitting up to sleep, and daytime sleepiness. Will has a positive family history of OSA, environmental allergies, obesity, and mild hypothyroidism.

Some nights, Will refuses to go to bed and instead requests to watch TV in the living room. If he is not allowed to watch TV, he will get very upset, cry, and have a temper tantrum. As a result, his parents often give in and allow him to fall asleep on the couch with the TV on. Other nights he will fall asleep at bedtime but will awaken in the middle of the night and get up to watch TV, walk around the house, or get a snack from the kitchen. His mother is exhausted and does not always stay awake until he falls asleep. She often is not aware of his night wakings until she sees evidence the following morning (e.g., cupboards open and food remnants in the kitchen). She is concerned about possible safety issues resulting from his walking around the home unsupervised in the middle of the night. A behavioral therapist has recently started working with Will and his parents. The therapist has been working on setting appropriate limits with Will, and the parents have been open to these suggestions.

Thought Questions:

What are risk factors for obstructive sleep apnea? What are treatment options for children with obstructive sleep apnea who are not candidates for surgical intervention? What are possible interventions for managing insomnia in children with developmental delay?

INSOMNIA

Insomnia is broadly defined as having persistent difficulties with initiating and/or maintaining sleep despite an adequate opportunity to do so. In the younger child, insomnia typically presents as bedtime resistance and/or frequent night wakings, both of which usually require parental intervention. Older children may also complain of difficulty falling asleep or prolonged night wakings. In these instances, parents may not necessarily be aware of these issues (Meltzer & Mindell, 2014).

Insomnia results in daytime impairments, including daytime sleepiness, irritability and mood disturbances, impaired attention and cognition, behavioral dysregulation, poor school performance, and negative social interactions (American Academy of Sleep Medicine, 2014). Insomnia and poor/insufficient sleep are also associated with negative health outcomes, such as obesity and metabolic dysfunction. There are also mental health consequences, including an increased risk of depression, suicide, and self-harm behaviors (Meltzer & Mindell, 2014). Finally, insomnia has a substantial negative impact on the parents and caregivers in regard to their own sleep, daytime function, and stress levels (Honaker & Meltzer, 2014).

Children with developmental disorders are particularly likely to experience and are prone to the adverse effects of sleep dysfunction. For example, children with autism may experience declines in verbal and socialization skills and poor adaptive functioning. Children with attention-deficit/hyperactivity disorder (ADHD) and sleep problems have an increased frequency of externalizing behaviors, oppositional behavior, and depressive symptoms (Maski & Owens, 2016).

Prevalence and Epidemiology

Insomnia occurs in 26%–32% of typically developing children. The prevalence of insomnia in adolescence is estimated to be between 3% and 12%, with a higher frequency typically reported in girls (American Academy of Sleep Medicine, 2014). The prevalence of insomnia is also significantly higher in special needs populations. For example, the rates of insomnia in children with autism is estimated to be 53%–78% (Malow et al., 2012). The sleep initiation type of insomnia is particularly common in children with ADHD (Miano et al., 2016). Sleep initiation and sleep maintenance are also common sleep concerns in children with cerebral palsy (Angriman, Caravale, Novelli, Ferri, & Bruni, 2015).

Etiology and Associations with Specific Developmental Disabilities

The classic "3 P" model of insomnia in adults has important potential parallels in children, including those with special needs. The first "P," *predisposing* factors, includes 1) genetic predisposition, 2) underlying medical issues (e.g., chronic pain, breathing difficulties, concurrent medications, or immobility; American Academy of Sleep Medicine, 2014), 3) mental health issues, 4) child temperament, and 5) intellectual disability. For instance, co-occurring sleep disorders described later, such as circadian misalignment, restless leg syndrome, and OSA, may be contributory to insomnia. Environmental factors such as limited living space and unstable home situations may also play a role. The second "P," *precipitating* factors, includes stressful life events such as relocation, parental separation, a new infant in the family, the death of a loved one, or even a move to a new school environment. The third "P," *perpetuating* factors, includes 1) parenting practices, such as a caregiver's prolonged presence at sleep onset; 2) reactive co-sleeping (i.e., as a response to sleep or health problems rather than a "lifestyle choice"); and 3) inappropriate limit setting. Additional perpetuating factors that have been linked to sleep disturbance include a later bedtime (after 9 p.m.), caffeine consumption, and electronic use during the sleep period (Honaker & Meltzer, 2014).

Insomnia is particularly likely to be of multifactorial origin for children with developmental disorders, such as autism and ADHD. These factors include 1) behavioral issues intrinsic to autism such as repetitive, self-injurious, and ritualistic behaviors, limited communication skills, and responsiveness to social cues; 2) medical issues (e.g., gastrointestinal problems or seizures); 3) psychiatric comorbidities such as anxiety; and 4) biological/circadian factors, such as alterations in normal melatonin receptors or release (Malow et al., 2012). While children with intellectual disabilities overall have an increased prevalence of sleep problems, they are particularly vulnerable to insomnia (Hollway, Aman, & Butter, 2013).

Several studies have shown that children with ADHD may have a delayed release of evening melatonin, which contributes to prolonged sleep onset. In addition, medications used to treat ADHD, such as extended-release psychostimulants, may play a role in insomnia, although the evidence is mixed. Access to electronic media devices also has to be taken into account, as they emit bright light that can affect the body's production of melatonin, delaying sleep onset. As children with ADHD and autism tend to spend more time with electronic media devices than typically developing children, they may be more prone to the sleep-disrupting effects of these blue light–emitting devices (Maski & Owens, 2016).

While insomnia is overall more common in children with developmental and intellectual disabilities, various presentations of insomnia are especially common in several genetic syndromes (see Appendix B). These notably include Smith-Magenis syndrome and Rett syndrome, as well as Williams syndrome, Angelman syndrome, Down syndrome, and fragile X syndrome. Acquired neurodevelopmental disorders, such as fetal alcohol spectrum disorder and cerebral palsy, also have an increased prevalence of insomnia. Many of these children have multiple sleep complaints that tend to be more severe, more refractory to treatment, and more likely to relapse compared with typically developing children.

Diagnosis and Clinical Manifestations

Insomnia in children is defined as the presence of significant difficulty in initiating or maintaining sleep. Chronic insomnia disorder is defined as symptoms occurring at least three times a week and being present for at least 3 months. Short-term insomnia disorder is present for less than 3 months (American Academy of Sleep Medicine, 2014). Presenting symptoms must also be associated with at least one of the following daytime impairments: fatigue, inattention, difficulty with concentration, memory impairment, mood disturbance, daytime sleepiness, academic concerns, or impairment of relationships with family or peers (American Academy of Sleep Medicine, 2014).

Behavioral insomnia in younger, typically developing children, as well as children with developmental disabilities (i.e., does not result primarily from physical factors such as discomfort or medication), may be further categorized as primarily due to inappropriate sleep onset associations, inadequate caregiver limit setting, or both. In the former situation, the child has learned to fall asleep at bedtime under specific conditions that typically require caregiver presence (i.e., being rocked or fed); in the absence of those same conditions following normal night wakings, the child is unable to fall back to sleep independently (i.e., without caregiver intervention), resulting in prolonged night wakings. Limit-setting issues, often involving inconsistent or even nonexistent bedtimes, lack of a bedtime routine, and failure to enforce appropriate nighttime behavior, can result in bedtime resistance and sleep-onset delay as well as prolonged night wakings.

Monitoring, Screening, and Evaluation

The first step in assessment for sleep problems involves general screening for a variety of sleep disorders during clinical encounters. The BEARS tool (which has both a parent and child report component) can be used in clinical settings to screen for the most common childhood sleep complaints. BEARS is an acronym for **B**edtime problems, **E**xcessive daytime sleepiness, **A**wakenings during the night, **R**egularity and duration of sleep, and **S**noring. It has been shown to elicit more information than a single general question, such as "Does your child have any sleep problems?" (see Figure 28.1; Owens & Dalzell, 2005). Other validated

The "BEARS" instrument is divided into five major sleep domains, providing a comprehensive screen for the major sleep disorders affecting children in the 2-to-18-year-old age range. Each sleep domain has a set of age-appropriate "trigger questions" for use in the clinical interview.
B = Bedtime problems
E = Excessive daytime sleepiness
A = Awakenings during the night
R = Regularity and duration of sleep
S = Snoring

Examples of developmentally appropriate trigger questions:

	Toddler/preschool (2–5 years)	School-age (6–12 years)	Adolescent (13–18 years)
Bedtime problems	Does your child have any problems going to bed? Falling asleep?	Does your child have any problems at bedtime? (P) Do you have any problems going to bed? (C)	Do you have any problems falling asleep at bedtime? (C)
Excessive daytime sleepiness	Does your child seem overtired or sleepy a lot during the day? Does she still take naps?	Does your child have difficulty waking in the morning, seem sleepy during the day, or take naps? (P) Do you feel tired a lot? (C)	Do you feel sleepy a lot during the day? In school? While driving? (C)
Awakenings during the night	Does your child wake up a lot at night?	Does your child seem to wake up a lot at night? Any sleepwalking or nightmares? (P) Do you wake up a lot at night? Have trouble getting back to sleep? (C)	Do you wake up a lot at night? Have trouble getting back to sleep? (C)
Regularity and duration of sleep	Does your child have a regular bedtime and wake time? What are they?	What time does your child go to bed and get up on school days? Weekends? Do you think he/she is getting enough sleep? (P)	What time do you usually go to bed on school nights? Weekends? How much sleep do you usually get? (C)
Snoring	Does your child snore a lot or have difficult breathing at night?	Does your child have loud or nightly snoring or any breathing difficulties at night? (P)	Does your teenager snore loudly or nightly? (P)

(P) Parent-directed question
(C) Child-directed question

Figure 28.1. BEARS sleep screening algorithm. (From Mindell, J. A., & Owens, J. A. (2015). *A clinical guide to pediatric sleep: Diagnosis and management of sleep problems* [3rd ed.]. Philadelphia, PA: Wolters Kluwer/Lippincott Williams & Wilkins; reprinted by permission.)

subjective (caregiver report) measures that can be utilized include several sleep questionnaires validated in different age groups (e.g., the Brief Infant Sleep Questionnaire, the Children's Sleep Habits Questionnaire, or the Children's Night Waking Behavioral Scale; Honaker & Meltzer, 2014). Importantly, the initial assessment should include queries regarding symptoms of other sleep disorders that may co-occur with primary insomnia and affect sleep onset (i.e., restless leg syndrome or circadian-based delayed sleep–wake phase disorder) or sleep maintenance (i.e., periodic limb movement disorder or OSA; Honaker & Meltzer, 2014).

Once a sleep concern has been identified, either through screening or a presenting complaint, a comprehensive sleep history includes an assessment of 1) the sleep environment; 2) bedtime routine; 3) sleep-onset associations (conditions required in order for the child to fall asleep at bedtime); 4) actual bedtime and fall asleep time; 5) **sleep onset latency** (the time to transition from lights out to sleep onset); 6) number, duration, and frequency of night wakings/call outs (important to differentiate full and parasomnia/partial awakenings from sleep; 7) the child's behaviors and parental response to night wakings; and 8) morning wake time.

Bedtimes and wake times should include both the average, range, and weekday/weekend variability. Daytime sleepiness in prepubescent children can be assessed by failure to awaken spontaneously at the required time (e.g., child needs multiple reminders), sleeping later when given the opportunity (e.g., on weekends), and signs of sleepiness (dozing off and yawning). Children older than 10 years of age can report daytime sleepiness and may have short and prolonged naps during the day. Sleepiness may present as well as hyperactivity, poor impulse control, inattention, and oppositional behavior.

A sleep log or diary is an essential tool for identifying variability in sleep patterns and quantifying sleep duration. It also helps circumvent the tendency of caregivers to report "last night's" sleep or "worst night's" sleep parameters. Generally recorded over a 2-week period, sleep logs provide detailed "real-time" information regarding 1) sleep onset latency, 2) number and duration of night wakings, 3) time in bed, 4) total sleep time, 5) sleep efficiency (time asleep/time in bed), 6) morning wake time, 7) nap timing and duration (Honaker & Meltzer, 2014), 8) mid–sleep time (a marker of chronotype), and 9) sleep–wake variability (both night-to-night and social jet lag–variability on weekdays versus weekends). In conjunction with a sleep diary, an actigraph (a sleep validated ambulatory accelerometer) can be worn to quantify these same parameters using a validated computer algorithm for activity. Because older children and caregivers may overestimate sleep parameters (American Academy of Sleep Medicine, 2014), actigraphy can be a helpful tool for more objectively evaluating and monitoring insomnia (de Souza et al., 2003).

A much more extensive evaluation of sleep disorders involves polysomnography, as was done with the patient described in the case study at the beginning of this chapter. This is a comprehensive recording of the biophysiological changes that occur during sleep. The **polysomnogram** monitors brain activity (EEG), eye movements (EOG), muscle activity (EMG), and heart rhythm (ECG) during sleep. It should be noted that although the overnight in-lab polysomnogram is the gold standard for evaluation of OSA (i.e., loud nightly snoring or chronic mouth breathing) or periodic limb movement disorder (repeated flexion of the legs in sleep), it is seldom indicated in the evaluation of insomnia except in cases in which other symptoms suggestive of these other disorders co-exist.

Treatment, Management, and Interventions

Behavioral treatments are highly effective in improving both sleep-initiation and sleep-maintenance insomnia symptoms in children (Honaker & Meltzer, 2014). In younger children, the goals of these treatment strategies are to establish healthy bedtime routines and optimal sleep schedules and to optimize the drive to sleep and normal circadian rhythms. Some examples of evidence-based behavioral interventions in younger children include 1) unmodified extinction (e.g., "crying it out," in which caregivers are instructed to ignore the child's protest behavior), 2) graduated extinction (which involves the parent gradually delaying their response to the crying child while providing reassurance with periodic "check-ins"), and 3) "bedtime fading" (which temporarily delays the child's bedtime to more closely approximate their actual fall asleep time, thus reducing sleep-onset latency and the opportunity for frequent "curtain calls"; Gradisar et al., 2016).

For older children, establishing a reward system for desirable bedtime/nighttime behavior can be very effective (e.g., the Bedtime Pass). Common pitfalls in establishing this program include failure to anticipate 1) an "extinction burst" (i.e., an increase in protest/tantrum behavior for several nights after the intervention is implemented) and 2) the "intermittent reinforcement" paradigm, in which the caregiver's failure to respond in a consistent manner to night wakings, for example, actually prolongs the child's problematic behavior.

Several prospective studies have failed to find significant long-term negative effects (i.e., up to 5 years post-treatment) of these behavioral interventions on cognitive and emotional development, behavior, stress levels, psychosocial functioning, and parent–child relationships

(Price, Wake, Ukoumunne, & Hiscock, 2012). It is also worth emphasizing that these same strategies, with some modifications, can be very effective in addressing insomnia in special needs children (Grigg-Damberger & Ralls, 2013). Behavioral therapy approaches are more extensively discussed in Chapter 34.

Another approach to treatment involves cognitive behavioral therapy for insomnia (CBT-I). This includes implementing a multidimensional treatment approach, including 1) basic principles of good sleep hygiene; 2) restricted time in bed (including avoidance of napping); 3) stimulus control (reversing the conditioned association of being in bed with being awake); and 4) psychoeducation, relaxation techniques, and cognitive therapy (addressing maladaptive cognitions and "catastrophizing" about the consequences of insomnia). CBT-I can be very helpful in older children (especially those with comorbid anxiety) and adolescents (de Bruin, Bögels, Oort, & Meijer, 2015; Maski & Owens, 2016). A child with insomnia and developmental disabilities may also benefit from outpatient visits with a psychologist familiar with sleep disorders and treatment or a psychologist with a certification in behavioral sleep medicine (see Box 28.1).

While sleep-inducing medications are frequently used in clinical practice, especially for children with neurodevelopmental disorders, it should be emphasized that there are currently no medications approved by the U.S. Food and Drug Administration (FDA) for treatment of insomnia in children. The few published pediatric randomized controlled trials of either OTC or prescription sedative/hypnotics have overall demonstrated limited or no efficacy. Furthermore, safety profiles are largely absent for these medications in children. Therefore, medications should be used with caution and only in conjunction with behavioral strategies.

However, while further research is needed, especially regarding long-term safety, several clinical trials in both typically developing children and those with developmental disabilities (i.e., autism and ADHD) have suggested that the synthetic form of the pineal gland hormone melatonin may be an effective treatment for sleep-onset and possibly sleep-maintenance (extended-release formulation) insomnia with few identified adverse effects (Maski & Owens, 2016). It should be noted that over-the-counter preparations of melatonin have been shown to be frequently unreliable in terms of actual concentration, and therefore use of pharmaceutical-grade melatonin is recommended. Further research is needed in identifying precipitants of and risk factors for childhood insomnia and evidence-based behavioral best-fit management options.

Talking Points

1. Insomnia is highly prevalent in children with developmental disorders and can be screened for using validated sleep questionnaires.
2. Utilizing the "3 P" method can help identify factors contributing to insomnia (predisposing, precipitating, and perpetuating factors).
3. Behavioral treatments are highly effective in managing insomnia in children, including those with neurodevelopmental disorders.

CIRCADIAN RHYTHM DISORDERS

Circadian rhythm sleep–wake disorders are caused by alterations of the circadian system or a misalignment of the internal circadian rhythm and societal demands (e.g., early school start time for adolescents). This misalignment most often occurs between an individual's internal rhythm and the required timing of environmental demands such as work or school (American Academy of Sleep Medicine, 2014). Circadian rhythm disorders include 1) delayed sleep–wake phase disorder, 2) advanced sleep–wake phase disorder, 3) irregular sleep–wake rhythm disorder, and 4) non-24-hour sleep–wake rhythm disorder. Symptoms must be present for at least 3 months to receive any of these diagnoses (American Academy of Sleep Medicine, 2014).

An important risk factor for circadian rhythm disorders is a circadian preference or "chronotype" at either

BOX 28.1 INTERDISCIPLINARY CARE

The Role of the Behavioral Psychologist

A behavioral psychologist with certification in behavioral sleep medicine is an essential part of a sleep team. This behavioral psychologist evaluates and treats behavioral, psychological, and physiological factors that contribute to the etiology and complicate the management of sleep disorders. However, due to the limited number of psychologists within this specialty, it is beneficial to align the sleep team with a psychologist who can address behavioral concerns that contribute to sleep disorders.

extreme (i.e., persistent and intractable "eveningness" or, less frequently, "morningness"). The most common presenting symptoms of circadian rhythm sleep–wake disorders are difficulty initiating sleep (delayed sleep phase) in the early evening and difficulty waking in the morning, bedtime time and early morning waking (advanced sleep phase), and highly irregular or rapidly changing sleep patterns. These symptoms are associated with excessive sleepiness and consequent impairment in social, educational, mental, or physical functioning (American Academy of Sleep Medicine, 2014).

Delayed sleep–wake phase disorder involves a significant delay in sleep time and wake time in comparison to the timing required to fulfill educational and social demands (Auger et al., 2015). It occurs most frequently in adolescents and young adults, as there is a well-established biological propensity for a sleep phase delay starting at puberty and ending in the mid-20s for most individuals. Over time, this may lead to chronic tardiness, school avoidance, and poor academic performance, or even dropping out of school. It also may be associated with mood changes and impaired social interactions. Sleep quantity and quality are typically normal when the child is allowed to sleep on his/her own delayed schedule (American Academy of Sleep Medicine, 2014). Some recent evidence, however, suggests that an extreme evening chronotype may in and of itself be associated with physical and mental health impairments and increased risk-taking behaviors (American Academy of Sleep Medicine, 2014; Short, Gradisar, Lack, & Wright, 2013).

Advanced sleep–wake phase disorder includes the early timing of sleep onset and sleep offset. This tends to be more common in young children and is defined as difficulty staying awake during the evening hours and a wake time that is undesirably early in relation to caregiver and family schedules (American Academy of Sleep Medicine, 2014; Auger et al., 2015).

Irregular sleep–wake rhythm disorder is quite rare and is characterized by a recurrent pattern of irregular sleep and wake episodes within a 24-hour period. This is characterized by symptoms of insomnia at night, excessive sleepiness during the day, or both (American Academy of Sleep Medicine, 2014). Sleep and wake episodes are fragmented, with the longest sleep period typically less than 4 hours (American Academy of Sleep Medicine, 2014; Auger et al., 2015).

Non-24-hour sleep–wake rhythm disorder, which occurs largely in blind patients and is very rare in sighted individuals, is diagnosed when the patient does not have a 24-hour dark-light cycle, resulting in sleep–wake patterns that show a progressive delay or advance over subsequent days and nights. These sleep–wake schedules gradually shift, with the child alternately experiencing daytime sleepiness and nighttime insomnia (Auger et al., 2015).

Prevalence and Epidemiology

The prevalence of delayed sleep–wake phase disorder in adolescents and young adults is estimated to be between 7% and 16% (American Academy of Sleep Medicine, 2014). While most adolescents experience a normal biological shift (delay) of several hours, with a propensity for a later bedtime and wake time around pubertal onset, in some individuals this "eveningness" tendency is exaggerated. The prevalence of advanced sleep–wake phase disorder and irregular sleep–wake rhythm disorder in the pediatric population has not been extensively documented but is encountered relatively rarely, even in sleep specialty clinics. The prevalence of non-24-hour sleep–wake rhythm disorder in blind individuals is thought to be over 50%; however, data on prevalence in other pediatric populations has not been well studied (American Academy of Sleep Medicine, 2014).

Etiology and Associations with Specific Developmental Disabilities

There are multiple reasons why children with developmental disabilities are at greater risk for circadian rhythm disorders. Children with ADHD may be at higher risk due to intrinsic delayed melatonin onset (American Academy of Sleep Medicine, 2014). Some children with autism have been found to have underlying alterations in the release and metabolism of melatonin and in melatonin receptors, with resulting irregular sleep patterns and either delays in sleep onset or advances in sleep offset (American Academy of Sleep Medicine, 2014). It should be noted that in addition to a genetic predisposition, environmental factors may exacerbate sleep disorders as previously discussed (American Academy of Sleep Medicine, 2014).

Diagnosis and Clinical Manifestations

A sleep log or diary and actigraphy for at least 2 weeks are necessary for assessing sleep–wake patterns in a child suspected of having a circadian rhythm sleep–wake disorder. The sleep log and actigraphy will show an average mid–sleep time (middle of the sleep period) and delayed sleep onset and offset of greater than 2 hours compared with socially acceptable times (American Academy of Sleep Medicine, 2014) or times that conflict with school or other activities. There are also several scales that are appropriate for use in the pediatric population to assess chronotype, including the Morningness-Eveningness

Scale for Children and the Munich Chronotype Questionnaire (Carskadon, Vieira, & Acebo, 1993; Roenneberg, Wirz-Justice, & Merrow, 2003).

Monitoring, Screening, and Evaluation

The sleep log and actigraphy are used to assess treatment response to changes in sleep–wake patterns during each phase of the management process. Evaluation of daytime sleepiness with surveys such as the Epworth Sleepiness Scale (Johns, 1991), periodic assessment of changes in mood, and logs of school attendance and performance are all important to monitor treatment outcomes.

Treatment, Management, and Interventions

The principle components of management of patients with delayed sleep–wake phase disorder include 1) gradually advancing sleep–wake schedules with progressively earlier morning wake times, 2) avoiding evening video bright light close to bedtime (to avoid suppression of melatonin release), 3) increasing morning light exposure, 4) administering melatonin in the evening, and 5) providing CBT-I.

For patients with delayed sleep–wake phase disorder, referral to a sleep specialist should be considered, especially in cases where there is significant school avoidance or a mood disorder. Typically, patients are instructed to successively advance their wake time first and then bedtime until the target sleep schedule is reached. Chronotherapy or successive *delays* in bedtime and wake time by 2–3 hours each day (done to move the patient "forward around the clock") may be employed in cases of severe phase delay; however, this technique is challenging to implement (Auger et al., 2015). Timed morning light exposure should occur at rise time and then may be moved successively earlier, although some care needs to be exercised when a patient has a severe phase delay. This can be provided by natural light or a "bright" light (2,500 to 10,000 lux) via a commercial light box device. Melatonin may be given as a small "chronobiotic" dose (e.g., 0.5 mg to avoid inducing sleepiness) 5–7 hours before sleep onset and/or as a "hypnotic" dose of 3 to 5 mg 30 minutes before bedtime.

A more systemic approach to the general, biologically based tendency toward eveningness in adolescents involves delaying middle and high school start times to allow for adequate sleep and avoid circadian misalignment (a phenomenon also known as "social jetlag"; Adolescent Sleep Working Group, Committee on Adolescence, & Council on School Health, 2014). Chronic sleep deficiency related to early start times (i.e., earlier than 8:30 a.m.) has been shown to be associated with a multitude of educational, mental health, and physical concerns, including drowsy driving, increased risk for obesity, increase in risk-taking behaviors, depressed mood, and lower academic performance. Delayed start times have been associated with improvements in these health, safety, and functional outcomes (Owens & Weiss, 2017). A number of school districts have moved high school start times later as a result of these findings.

Suggested treatment for advanced sleep–wake phase disorder includes evening light therapy, planned sleep schedules with moving bedtime later, and timed melatonin administration in the morning (Auger et al., 2015). Less well-substantiated treatment options for irregular sleep–wake rhythm disorder and non-24-hour sleep–wake rhythm disorder include melatonin administration in the evening, timed light exposure, and changes in sleep–wake scheduling (Auger et al., 2015).

Circadian rhythm sleep–wake disorders that are caused by rigid and more extreme chronotypes are often chronic conditions that are more difficult to treat, while a weaker chronotype, poor sleep hygiene, and secondary gain (school avoidance or social anxiety) are more amenable to treatment when the child is motivated and the family is supportive. For treatment-resistant cases, referral to a sleep specialist is strongly recommended.

Talking Points

1. Children with developmental disabilities may be at higher risk for circadian rhythm disorders, misalignment of the circadian system, and societal demands due to alterations in release or metabolism of melatonin.
2. Delayed sleep–wake phase disorder can be managed with behavioral interventions, including gradual advancement of sleep–wake schedules, avoiding bright light in the evening, increasing morning light exposure, administering melatonin in the evening, and providing CBT-I.

DISORDERS OF AROUSAL/ PARTIAL AROUSAL PARASOMNIAS

Parasomnias are defined as undesirable events or experiences that occur during entry into, arousal from, or within sleep. Some occur during non-REM, and others occur during REM sleep (when dreaming occurs). Partial arousal parasomnia occurs primarily during non-REM slow-wave sleep; it is referred to as a disorder of arousal or partial arousal and includes confusional arousals, sleepwalking (somnambulism), and sleep terrors. Parasomnias associated with REM sleep include nightmares and sleep paralysis.

As noted earlier, disorders of arousal occur almost exclusively during slow-wave or "deep" sleep and thus usually occur within a few hours after sleep onset. The episodes may vary from a few minutes to as long as 30–40 minutes and are characterized by amnesia for the event. During an episode, children or adolescents may have the appearance of being awake, and most children actively avoid comfort or soothing and are very difficult to awaken. Finally, because the relative percentage of slow-wave sleep is highest in childhood and drops fairly dramatically in the second decade of life, disorders of arousal are most common in young children, and their prevalence declines with increasing age (Mindell & Owens, 2015).

Prevalence and Epidemiology

Confusional Arousals Because confusional arousals may not be recognized or brought to medical attention, the prevalence is difficult to determine but has been estimated to be around 15%–20% in children ages 3–13 years. Onset is typically before age 5 and can occur as early as the first year of life, although they may not be recognized as such. Confusional arousals may co-occur with sleepwalking and sleep terrors.

Sleepwalking Sleepwalking is a common childhood phenomenon. It is estimated that 15%–40% of children sleepwalk on at least one occasion; however only about 3%–4% of children have frequent episodes. As with other disorders of arousal, sleepwalking usually abates by adolescence. Sleepwalking prevalence may be underestimated because episodes may be unobserved or misinterpreted as night wakings (many children have both). Onset of episodes is usually between ages 4–6 years, and peak occurrence is between ages 8–12 years. About one third of sleepwalkers have episodes for about 5 years, and a minority (10%) will continue to sleepwalk for up to 10 years (Mindell & Owens, 2015).

Sleep Terrors Less common than confusional arousals and sleepwalking, sleep terrors are experienced by about 1%–6% of children, primarily during the preschool and elementary school years. They have a similar age of onset as sleepwalking, and both types of events may co-occur in the same child. In fact, the prevalence of sleep terrors in children who sleepwalk is about 10%. The frequency of sleep terror episodes is often highest at the onset; frequency also tends to be higher with younger age of onset. It almost always disappears by adolescence. There appears to be little gender difference in the prevalence of disorders of arousal.

Etiology and Associations with Specific Developmental Disabilities

There is sometimes a suggestion of a genetic component to disorders of arousal. The prevalence is approximately 10 times greater in children with a family history of sleepwalking; 45% if one parent has the disorder, and 60% if both parents are affected versus 5% in the general population. Disorders of arousal appear to be more common in individuals with migraine headaches and Tourette syndrome, possibly related to alterations in serotonin metabolism.

Disorders of arousal occur almost exclusively during slow-wave sleep. Because there is an increased homeostatic drive for slow-wave sleep and insufficient sleep often results in a rebound compensatory increase in slow-wave sleep, not getting enough sleep increases the likelihood that a partial arousal parasomnia episode will occur in a susceptible individual. The classic example is a sleepwalking episode occurring after a sleepover with friends that resulted in reduced sleep; high sleep drive due to changes in the sleep schedule and other sleep disruptors, including another sleep disorder, a different environment, illness, or sleeping with a full bladder, may trigger an episode. Noise, caffeine consumption, or a shift to a lighter stage of sleep may all be event triggers as well. Stress and, in rare cases, trauma may cause partial arousal parasomnia, but they are not primary due to an underlying psychological problem or central nervous system disorder.

Finally, although general disorders of arousal do not appear to be significantly increased in children with developmental disorders, they may have a higher prevalence of concurrent primary sleep disorders, such as OSA and periodic limb movement disorder, which increase arousals and trigger events. It should also be noted that while exceedingly rare, nocturnal seizure disorders should be considered as a differential diagnosis (Maski & Owens, 2016).

Diagnosis and Clinical Manifestations

Confusional arousals involve disorientation and unresponsiveness to the environment. They may start with the child sitting up in bed, involve thrashing around, and be accompanied by agitation and combative behavior. If the child gets out of bed, then it is considered a sleepwalking event.

Sleepwalking episodes can begin with confusional arousals, although they can also begin with a child rising from bed. During sleepwalking episodes, the child appears confused or dazed, the eyes are usually open, and she may mumble or give inappropriate answers to questions. Occasionally, a sleepwalking child may appear agitated. A sleepwalker may engage in a range of behavior, such as urinating in a closet, walking calmly to the parents' bedroom, going downstairs, cooking or eating, and leaving the house or stepping through a window onto a balcony or rooftop. Sleepwalking can occur infrequently or on a nightly basis. Injuries can occur during sleepwalking, ranging from bruises to more serious injuries related to leaving the home.

Sleep terrors are dramatic events and, as such, can be highly distressing to caregivers. The child, however, is totally unaware of his or her behavior, and these episodes are much worse to watch than to experience. Sleep terrors usually have a sudden onset, and the child's appearance during one of these episodes is that of extreme agitation, fright, and confusion, often involving crying and/or screaming. Extreme physiologic arousal is common (i.e., hyperventilation, rapid heart rate, excessive sweating, and dilated pupils). The episodes can occur during any sleep period, including naps, but they are usually in the first third of the night when slow-wave sleep predominates (Mindell & Owens, 2015).

Monitoring, Screening, and Evaluation

Having caregivers track the frequency and timing of events associated with disorders of arousal is critical in establishing the diagnosis and documenting a baseline of severity. This can be done in conjunction with a sleep diary to assess sleep duration. It is often also very helpful to ask parents to video record an event, as the verbal description may not include or distort important details such as the duration of the event and specific behaviors. Overnight polysomnography is not routinely ordered as part of the evaluation because these are episodic events and may not be captured on a single-night study. However, if there is a concern about sleep-disordered breathing, periodic limb movement disorder, or a question of nocturnal seizures as part of the differential diagnosis, an overnight sleep study may be appropriate (Maski & Owens, 2016).

Treatment, Management, and Interventions

With the exception of enhanced safety monitoring procedures in sleepwalking, the management of the different disorders of arousal is quite similar. Caregivers should be instructed to avoid waking the child during an episode, as this may increase agitation and prolong the event. The child should be gently guided back to bed. Avoidance of triggers such as insufficient sleep is key, as are other sleep hygiene measures such as a regular sleep–wake schedule and avoiding caffeine. Safety measures include assuring that the caregiver will wake and observe the child, double-locking doors and windows, ensuring the safety of the sleeping environment (e.g., removing clutter on floors), attaching furniture to walls, and installing alarm systems or a bell attached to the bedroom door to alert caregivers (www.sleepwalkingsafety.com).

Scheduled awakenings are typically recommended only for frequent (i.e., nightly) events. These involve having the parent wake the child approximately 15–30 minutes prior to the time of night that the episode (or first episode in the event of more than one) typically occurs. This can be confirmed with a sleep diary. The caregiver is instructed to awaken the child on a nightly basis, just to the point of arousal (e.g., child changes position or mumbles). These nightly awakenings should be continued for 2–4 weeks.

Pharmacologic treatment is very rarely indicated except in cases of persistent, frequent episodes, particularly when there is a high risk of injury, aggressive behavior, or serious disruption to the family. The primary pharmacologic agents used are potent slow-wave sleep suppressants such as benzodiazepines and tricyclic antidepressants (see Appendix C). They typically require very gradual weaning to avoid a rebound increase in events (Mindell & Owens, 2015).

Outcomes

Most children naturally stop sleepwalking or experiencing sleep terrors during childhood, and almost all cases resolve spontaneously following puberty as a result of the associated dramatic decrease in slow-wave sleep. In those individuals whose episodes persist into adolescence and adulthood, awareness of potential triggers is important (e.g., inadequate and/or disrupted sleep and excessive caffeine consumption).

Talking Points

1. Parasomnias, including confusional arousals, sleepwalking, and sleep terrors, occur almost exclusively in slow-wave sleep within the first few hours after sleep onset and are characterized by disorientation and unresponsiveness and amnesia of the event in the morning by the child.
2. Insufficient sleep and sleep disruptors such as OSA are common contributors to parasomnias.
3. Management includes ensuring the child's safety, avoidance of triggers, and treating underlying disorders such as insufficient sleep or OSA.

SLEEP-DISORDERED BREATHING AND OBSTRUCTIVE SLEEP APNEA

Sleep-disordered breathing in children is characterized by an abnormal respiratory pattern during sleep. It encompasses a broad spectrum of respiratory disorders that occur across development, from neonates through adolescence. Types of obstructive sleep-disordered breathing include "primary" snoring, upper airway resistance syndrome, obstructive hypoventilation, and OSA (Mindell & Owens, 2015).

Primary snoring is typically defined as snoring without associated ventilatory abnormalities. However, habitual snoring indicates the presence of heightened *upper airway resistance,* and there is evidence that this snoring alone can be associated with an increased risk for adverse outcomes.

Obstructive hypoventilation is characterized by snoring, increased respiratory effort, and accumulation of carbon dioxide. *OSA* involves repeated episodes of prolonged partial or complete cessation of airflow due to complete and/or partial obstruction during sleep with continued or increased respiratory effort. These disruptions of airflow result in gas exchange abnormalities (i.e., mild to severe hypoxemia and hypercapnia) that contribute to the triggering of arousals that serve to increase upper airway patency. Intermittent hypoxemia, arousals, and recurrent sympathetic activation are thought to be the most significant contributors to the short- and long-term negative sequelae of OSA that include decrements in cardiovascular, metabolic, and neurocognitive function.

Prevalence and Epidemiology

Overall, it is estimated that about 10% of prepubertal children in the United States habitually snore, with 20% snoring occasionally. The prevalence of OSA is estimated to be in the range of 1%–5% (Marcus et al., 2012). Specific populations, however, appear to have a significantly higher prevalence, including African American children, younger children (ages 2–8 years) and boys (particularly after puberty), children with Down syndrome, and other patients with craniofacial anomalies.

Etiology and Associations with Specific Developmental Disabilities

In general terms, OSA results from an anatomically or functionally narrowed upper airway. This may be due to enlargement of the adenoids and tonsils, environmental allergies with nasopharyngeal edema, congenital syndromes impacting the craniofacial region, gastroesophageal reflux, and obesity (Tan, Gozal, & Kheirandish-Gozal, 2013). Reduced upper airway tone may be present in children with neuromuscular disorders, cerebral palsy, and hypothyroidism, placing them at increased risk for OSA.

Decreased central ventilatory drive may be seen in a wide variety of CNS disorders, especially those affecting the brainstem. Obesity is an increasingly common risk factor for sleep-disordered breathing in the pediatric population. Children with syndromes characterized by obesity, such as Prader-Willi and Beckwith-Wiedemann, are at especially high risk. Children with Down syndrome are also high risk for multiple reasons, including truncal obesity, macroglossia, hypotonia, and hypothyroidism. Other contributory factors to sleep-disordered breathing in children include a history of prematurity, exposure to secondhand smoke, and a positive family history of OSA/snoring. See Table 28.1 for risk factors for pediatric sleep-disordered breathing (Owens, 2009).

Diagnosis and Clinical Manifestations

The core presenting symptoms of sleep-disordered breathing in children include loud habitual snoring with or without observed breathing pauses, chronic mouth breathing, restless sleep, and excessive sweating during sleep. Paradoxical movement of the chest wall and abdominal muscles during sleep may also be noted. It can be helpful for caregivers to videotape their child's breathing during sleep to confirm these observations. Excessive daytime sleepiness is less common in children with sleep-disordered breathing compared

Table 28.1. Risk factors for pediatric sleep disordered breathing

Upper airway obstruction
Upper airway narrowing
Reduced upper airway tone
Adenotonsillar hypertrophy
Craniofacial anomalies
Trisomy 21
Hypotonia/neuromuscular disorders
Chronic allergies, asthma
Gastroesophageal reflux
Repaired cleft palate
Obesity
Family history
Prematurity at birth
Prior adenotonsillectomy

Revised from Owens, J. A. (2009). Neurocognitive and behavioral impact of sleep disordered breathing in children. *Pediatric Pulmonology, 44,* 417–422.

with adults, and it tends to occur in the setting of severe OSA and/or obesity. More common are behavior and academic problems. These include concerns about inattention, hyperactivity, impulsivity, and irritability, which may be the primary presenting complaints in children with OSA. In particular, many of the neurocognitive, mood-related, and behavioral manifestations of sleep-disordered breathing closely resemble those associated with ADHD. Secondary enuresis (bedwetting) and an increase in partial arousal parasomnias are less common associated symptoms (Tan et al., 2013).

Monitoring, Screening, and Evaluation

All children should be routinely screened for symptoms of sleep-disordered breathing during well-child doctor visits; a more focused exam and queries regarding potential risk factors should follow if symptoms are present. As parents do not necessarily associate behavioral and attention problems with OSA, a high index of suspicion should be maintained by the clinician. Children presenting with behavioral, mood, attentional, or academic concerns should be systematically screened for symptoms of and risk factors for OSA. Physical exam findings may include increased body mass index, systemic hypertension, adenoidal facies, "allergic shiners," a small chin, swollen nostril turbinates (a shelf of bone covered by mucosa that protrudes into the breathing passage of the nose)/deviated septum, a high arched palate, and tonsillar enlargement.

The American Academy of Pediatrics (AAP) clinical practice guidelines for diagnosis and management of childhood obstructive sleep apnea syndrome (Marcus et al., 2012) recommend overnight in-lab polysomnography as the "gold standard" for the diagnosis of OSA, given that no combination of history and physical findings has been shown to be reliably predictive of significant pathology. Alternative diagnostic evaluations that are not validated and have various drawbacks but may be helpful in settings in which in-lab nocturnal polysomnography is not readily accessible include nocturnal pulse oximetry or video recordings and a daytime nap (in infants) or ambulatory polysomnogram (Marcus et al., 2012). However, it should be noted that lack of evidence of sleep-disordered breathing resulting from any of these alternative studies in a symptomatic patient may represent a false negative, and thus a full polysomnogram is recommended.

Treatment, Management, and Interventions

There are presently no universally accepted guidelines regarding the indications for treatment and follow up of pediatric sleep-disordered breathing. The decision of whether and how to treat OSA in children is contingent on a number of parameters, including severity of polysomnographic study results, the likely cause of upper airway obstruction, duration of the disease, individual patient variables such as age (adult severity criteria may be applied to children ages 13 or older), and either the presence or risk for comorbid conditions (e.g., cardiovascular disease or metabolic syndrome). In the case of moderate to severe disease, the decision to treat is usually straightforward, and most pediatric sleep experts recommend that any child with an apnea index of greater than 5 per hour should be treated (Mindell & Owens, 2015).

Adenotonsillectomy (AT) is the most common treatment for pediatric OSA, and it, in turn, is the most common indication in the United States for tonsillectomy with or without adenoidectomy (see Box 28.2). It is the first-line treatment in any child with significant adenotonsillar enlargement, even in the presence of additional risk factors such as obesity. In uncomplicated cases, the success rate is about 80% in terms of resolution of symptoms (see Box 28.3). Risk factors for residual OSA include obesity, asthma, craniofacial anomalies, Down syndrome, and more severe sleep apnea. It is recommended that these children should be considered for a repeat postoperative polysomnogram, especially if symptoms persist. Other surgical procedures include removal of enlarged turbinates and nasal septal reconstruction (Marcus et al., 2013).

BOX 28.2 INTERDISCIPLINARY CARE

The Role of the Pediatric Otolaryngologists

Pediatric otolaryngologists provide expertise in the evaluation and surgical management of children with sleep disordered breathing. As adenotonsillar hypertrophy and other forms of nasopharyngeal obstruction are the most common contributors to obstructive sleep in children, collaboration with a pediatric otolaryngologist is essential.

BOX 28.3 EVIDENCE-BASED PRACTICE

The CHAT Study

The Childhood Adenotonsillectomy Trial (CHAT) was a randomized controlled study of adenotonsillectomy versus watchful waiting in children with OSA. Published in 2013, it demonstrated normalization of polysomnographic findings in 79% of children who had an adenotonsillectomy for treatment of OSA with an obstructive apnea hypopnea index of greater than 2 per hour and less than 30 per hour. Interestingly, 46% of the children with OSA assigned to watchful waiting in place of adenotonsillectomy had resolution of polysomnographic abnormalities. There was no change in attention or executive function scores after adenotonsillectomy, but there was evidence of reported improvements in executive function and behavior after adenotonsillectomy as compared with the watchful waiting group.

Evidence-based nonsurgical treatment for OSA in children is largely targeted at reducing the obstruction and increasing upper airway patency and includes 1) weight management; 2) nasal steroids/leukotriene esterase inhibitors (like Singulair used in asthma); 3) positional therapy (avoidance of the supine/back sleeping position); 4) oral appliances (mandibular advancement/palatal expansion; see Box 28.4); and 5) myofunctional therapy, which focuses on exercises to correct improper function of the tongue and facial muscles used for chewing and swallowing in order to improve upper airway patency (Camacho et al., 2015). Continuous or bilevel airway pressure therapies are effective and well tolerated by some children who are not candidates for surgery. Education and gradual exposure to the therapy are recommended to improve tolerance and adherence (see Box 28.5).

BOX 28.4 INTERDISCIPLINARY CARE

Dental Sleep Medicine

Dental sleep medicine is playing an increasingly important role in the management of children with sleep-disordered breathing. Maxillofacial features contributing to obstructive sleep apnea may be correctible with oral appliances such as palatal expanders and mandibular advancement. Myofunctional therapy, often delivered under the supervision of a dental hygienist, uses exercises to target improper function of the tongue and facial muscles used for chewing and swallowing to improve upper airway patency.

BOX 28.5 INTERDISCIPLNARY CARE

Positive Airway Pressure

Positive airway pressure (PAP) may be indicated in the child with obstructive sleep apnea who previously had adenotonsillectomy or does not have indication for tonsillectomy. This therapy is a noninvasive method of providing distending pressure to maintain a patent airway through a nasal or full-face interface securely attached to the head. A multidisciplinary sleep team, including sleep providers, pediatric sleep technicians, and sleep coordinators, can successfully help children use PAP therapy. The family and child require education and evaluation of preparedness for this therapy before initiation. Close follow-up of the child's compliance and tolerance to the PAP therapy device are important parts of the successful use of PAP therapy.

Outcomes

Studies that have examined changes in behavior and neuropsychological functioning in children following treatment for OSA have largely documented significant improvement in both short- and long-term outcomes. These have included decreases in daytime sleepiness and improvements in mood, behavior, academics, and quality of life. However, many studies have failed to find a dose-dependent relationship between OSA in children and specific neurobehavioral/neurocognitive deficits. This has led to speculation that other factors, including individual genetic susceptibility; environmental influences, such as allergen and pollution exposure; and comorbid conditions, such as obesity, shortened sleep duration, and the presence of other sleep disorders, may also influence outcome (Marcus et al., 2013).

Talking Points

1. OSA is characterized by repeated episodes of cessation of airflow due to obstruction resulting in gas exchange abnormalities.
2. In addition to loud snoring, pauses in breathing, and restless sleep, common symptoms in children can include inattention, hyperactivity, impulsivity, and irritability.
3. AT is the most common treatment for OSA; other management options include weight management, medication (i.e., nasal steroids and leukotriene esterase inhibitors), positional therapy, oral appliances, myofunctional therapy, and positive airway pressure.

MOVEMENT DISORDERS IN SLEEP: RESTLESS LEG SYNDROME, PERIODIC LIMB MOVEMENT DISORDER, AND SLEEP-RELATED RHYTHMIC MOVEMENT DISORDER

Restless leg syndrome is a neurologic, sensorimotor disorder characterized by an almost irresistible urge to move the legs. These subjective symptoms of a "need" to move and uncomfortable and unpleasant sensations (**dysesthesias**) occur primarily in the legs, although other body parts (e.g., arms) can also be involved. Some patients with restless leg syndrome, however, do not describe a significant sensory component; instead, they experience the urge to move the legs during periods of inactivity as the primary or sole presenting symptom. The urge to move and sensory components are usually at least partially relieved by movement, including walking, rocking, shaking, stretching, and rubbing, but typically this works only as long as the movements continue. Symptoms usually begin or are exacerbated by rest or inactivity (e.g., lying in bed to fall asleep or riding in a car for prolonged periods). A unique feature of restless leg syndrome is that the timing of symptoms also appears to have a circadian component, in that they often peak in the evening hours (Simakajornboon, Kheirandish-Gozal, & Gozal, 2009).

Periodic limb movement disorder, in contrast, requires a polysomnographic rather than clinical diagnosis and is characterized by movements that meet specific criteria for a sequence of repetitive, brief (0.5–10 seconds), and highly stereotyped limb jerks. They commonly consist of rhythmic extension of the big toe and dorsiflexion at the ankle. Most individuals are unaware of these movements, but caregivers may describe "kicking" movements during sleep. Associated sleep disruption and/or daytime sequelae (i.e., daytime sleepiness and mood or behavioral changes) must be present to qualify as a "disorder" (Gingras, Gaultney, & Picchietti, 2011).

Sleep-related rhythmic movements include head banging, body rocking, and head rolling. These are all characterized by repetitive, stereotypic, and rhythmic movements/behaviors that involve large muscle groups. These behaviors typically occur during sleep–wake transitions or light sleep stages, and the duration ranges from minutes to several hours (Mindell & Owens, 2015).

Prevalence and Epidemiology

The prevalence rate of restless limb syndrome in children is estimated to be between 1% and 6%. A large telephone survey study (pediatric "REST" study) found a prevalence of "definite" restless leg syndrome in about 2% of children; one quarter to one half had moderate to severe symptoms (Picchietti et al., 2013).

Because the diagnosis of periodic limb movement disorder requires a polysomnogram, the pediatric prevalence rates are more difficult to quantify. In survey studies of periodic limb movement symptoms, rates are between 8% and 12% (Crabtree et al., 2003; Marcus et al., 2014; Mindell & Owens, 2015). In adults, restless limb syndrome and periodic disorder limb movement syndrome co-occur at a rate of 80% (American Academy of Sleep Medicine, 2014).

Studies have suggested that approximately two thirds of infants engage in some type of sleep-related rhythmic movements, body rocking being the most common. Onset is typically prior to 1 year of age; by 18 months, the prevalence drops to about one third, and by 5 years, it drops to 5% (Mayer, Wilde-Frenz, & Kurella, 2007).

Etiology and Associations with Specific Developmental Disabilities

Overall, it is estimated that 50%–60% of adult restless leg syndrome patients have a positive family history. "Early-onset" restless leg syndrome, also termed "primary" or "familial" restless leg syndrome, appears to have a particularly strong genetic component. It is estimated that 40%–92% of these cases are familial, and the prevalence of restless leg syndrome in first-degree relatives appears to be six to seven times that in the general population (Mindell & Owens, 2015).

A number of studies have implicated low iron levels in both adults and children as an important factor for the presence and severity of both restless leg syndrome symptoms and periodic leg movements (Allen et al., 2018; Dye, Gurbani, & Simakajornboon, 2018).

The postulated underlying mechanisms relate to the role of iron as a cofactor of tyrosine hydroxylase in a rate-limiting step of the synthesis of dopamine. In turn, dopaminergic dysfunction has been implicated as playing a key role in the genesis of both restless leg syndrome and periodic leg movement disorder. Several pediatric case series have suggested that lower-than-normal ferritin levels (defined as less than 50 ng/mL) are found in some 70%–75% of children with restless leg syndrome (Dosman, Witmans, & Zwaigenbaum, 2012).

Medications including antihistamines (such as diphenhydramine/Benadryl), antidepressants (selective serotonin reuptake inhibitors [SSRIs] and tricyclic antidepressants [TCAs]), neuroleptics, and caffeine can all exacerbate underlying restless leg syndrome. Insufficient sleep, as in any underlying sleep disturbance, may exacerbate restless leg syndrome.

Comorbidity between ADHD and restless leg syndrome/periodic limb movement disorder has been commonly reported. For example, it is estimated that over 40% of children with ADHD have restless leg syndrome symptoms and more than a quarter of children with restless leg syndrome have ADHD symptoms (Spruyt & Gozal, 2011). Several studies in referral populations have also found that periodic limb motion occurs in as many as one fourth of children diagnosed with ADHD. Periodic limb motion is also more common in children with sickle cell disease and Williams syndrome.

The etiology of sleep-related rhythmic movements seems to be related to self-soothing behaviors prior to sleep onset or after night wakings. While often distressing to caregivers and sometimes disruptive to other family members' sleep, these behaviors are for the most part considered benign and do not result in injury. They usually occur in typically developing children and are thus not indicative of underlying neurological issues. However, in situations that involve children with developmental disorders, such as autism or severe intellectual disability, there may be an increased risk for self-injury due to the frequency and intensity of the behavior, and these children are more likely to also engage in the behavior while awake.

Diagnosis and Clinical Manifestations

Although symptoms of restless leg syndrome may start as early as 6–12 months of age and thus are very difficult to identify, even relatively young children are often able to describe the sensory symptoms. In clinical interviews, children may use colorful descriptors such as "soda bubbling through my veins," "tiny nails poking my legs," and "people wrestling in my legs." They may use terms like squeezing, tingling, wiggling, itching, popping, "funny" feelings, shaking, aching, or pulling and tugging of the legs. The motor symptoms may be observed by caregivers as stretching or rubbing the legs together or increased motor activity in the evening. In querying a child, a useful question is, "If you had to lie perfectly still while you were falling asleep, would you be able to do it?" Although somewhat nonspecific, a history of "growing pains" (i.e., recurrent limb discomfort or pain occurring at bedtime and/or during night wakings) is often reported in children with restless leg syndrome and periodic leg movement disorder (Mindell & Owens, 2015).

Difficulties initiating sleep are common in restless leg syndrome, as are reports of restless sleep and twitching or kicking during the night in periodic limb movement disorder. Daytime symptoms may include sleepiness and behavioral complaints. Children with these disorders appear to be at higher risk for mood disorders and decreased quality of life.

Monitoring, Screening, and Evaluation

Screening for symptoms of and risk factors for restless leg syndrome and periodic limb movement disorder is particularly important in children who present with sleep-onset insomnia or unexplained daytime fatigue, a chief complaint of restless sleep, and/or evaluation of ADHD. The physical examination is generally normal (including the neurologic examination) in these children, and, in fact, the presence of abnormal physical findings (e.g., pain or limitation of extremity movement) suggests an alternative orthopedic, rheumatologic, or neuromuscular diagnosis. As noted above, a nocturnal polysomnogram that includes leg muscle EMG leads is needed to confirm the presence of periodic leg movements but is not required for a diagnosis of restless leg syndrome. As a marker of decreased iron stores, serum ferritin levels in both children and adults with restless leg syndrome are commonly low. Studies have also suggested that low vitamin D and B12 levels may exacerbate symptoms in some cases. No specific diagnostic evaluation is required for sleep-related rhythmic movements, although home videotaping may be quite helpful in confirming the diagnosis.

Treatment, Management, and Interventions

The decision of whether and how to treat restless leg syndrome depends on the level of severity (intensity, frequency, and periodicity) of sensorimotor symptoms, the degree of interference with sleep, and the impact of daytime sequelae. Similarly, the decision to specifically treat periodic limb movements should be based on the presence or absence of nocturnal symptoms (restless or nonrestorative sleep) and daytime sequelae.

The management of restless leg syndrome and periodic leg movement disorder may be summarized by the acronym AIMS: **A**voidance of exacerbating substances, such as caffeine, antihistamines, and specific antidepressants; **I**ron supplementation; **M**uscle therapy (moderate exercise up to a few hours before bedtime, walking, stretching, massaging the affected area, and applying hot or cold packs); and **S**leep hygiene (maintaining consistent bedtimes and wake times, having a bedtime routine, and obtaining adequate nighttime sleep). The recommended dose of supplemental iron is typically in the range of 3 to 6 mg/kg per day for a duration of at least 3 months, followed by increased dietary iron intake once an appropriate ferritin level (at least 50 ng/ml) is reached. Concomitant use of ascorbic acid (vitamin C) appears to improve iron absorption, while iron absorption is reduced when combined with calcium. The absence of iron rich foods in a child's diet may be an important contributor to the finding of low ferritin levels, and a brief discussion of iron rich foods or a referral to a nutritionist may confer some long-term benefits. Pharmacologic agents are rarely necessary to treat these disorders in childhood, but consultation with a pediatric sleep specialist or neurologist is recommended. There are no FDA-approved drugs for treatment of restless leg syndrome in children.

Rhythmic movement disorders can be very disruptive and upsetting to families and typically only cause superficial physical sequelae. Various behavioral techniques can be effective in reducing the frequency of these behaviors or eliminating them all altogether. These can include an initial focus on eliminating the behavior both during the day and at bedtime, as well as replacement behavioral techniques and charting and rewards. When children with rhythmic movement disorders have a history of trauma, in utero drug exposure, and/or sensory integration problems, a physical therapy intervention may be effective (e.g., brushing, massage, or weight blankets or vests). Generally, no treatment other than reassurance is needed for sleep-related rhythmic movements unless there is evidence of injury. Caregivers should be encouraged to move the crib away from the wall if the noise is disruptive (padding the bed surfaces is usually not effective to stop the behavior). Ensuring sufficient sleep with a regular sleep–wake schedule may help. Making sure the child's bedtime matches his/her fall asleep time may reduce the need to and opportunity for these behaviors at sleep onset. Reducing ambient household noise (e.g., with a white noise machine or fan) may reduce arousals/night wakings. Pharmacologic treatments that have been used in severe cases include clonazepam, hydroxyzine, and tricyclic antidepressants.

Outcomes

No long-term studies have been conducted on the course of restless movement disorder or periodic limb movement disorder in children or adolescents. It appears, however, that restless limb syndrome that begins in childhood or adolescence has a chronic and progressive course and is likely to be a lifelong disorder. Patients with milder disease may have long periods of remission (or episodic exacerbation, as with pregnancy). Cases of secondary restless limb syndrome and periodic limb movement disorder related to iron deficiency generally remit without recurrence when the underlying condition is resolved.

Sleep-related rhythmic movements disappear in 90% of typically developing children by age 4 years. Children who have developmental disorders with sleep-related rhythmic movements associated with self-injurious behaviors often need more intensive management and follow-up.

Talking Points

1. Restless leg syndrome is a neurological disorder characterized by an irresistible urge to move the legs. It is often accompanied by leg discomfort and is a comorbidity in children with ADHD.

2. Treatment of restless leg syndrome includes avoiding exacerbating substances (such as caffeine and SSRIs), iron supplementation if appropriate, muscle therapy, and good sleep hygiene.

3. Rhythmic movement disorders, including head banging and body rocking, are self-soothing behaviors that occur prior to sleep onset and after night wakings. Although distressing to parents, these behaviors are considered benign and are typically not indicative of underlying neurological issues.

SUMMARY

- Sleep disorders in children with developmental disabilities are extremely common.
- Common presenting complaints such as difficulty initiating or maintaining sleep may be due to a variety of biologically and behaviorally based causes (e.g., behavioral insomnia, restless leg syndrome, and circadian-based phase delay or OSA).
- Practitioners should have a regular systematic approach to screening for sleep problems in these children. Comorbid sleep disorders may further compromise daytime function in children with NDD, including mood and behavioral regulation, attention, and cognition. Conversely, successful treatment may improve functioning in both patients and families.
- Behavioral interventions used to treat insomnia in typically developing children can also be effective strategies in children with NDD.
- Essential questions for identifying sleep problems include snoring, difficulty initiating or maintaining sleep, difficulty waking in the morning, and unplanned episodes of sleep during the day.

ADDITIONAL RESOURCES

Stanford University: https://stanfordhealthcare.org/medical-conditions/sleep/pediatric-sleep-disorders/types.html

American Sleep Association: https://www.sleepassociation.org/sleep-disorders/more-sleep-disorders/children-and-sleep/basics-of-sleep-problems-in-children/

Emedicine: Sleep Disorders: https://www.emedicinehealth.com/sleep_and_sleep_disorders_in_children/article_em.htm#sleep_problems_and_sleep_disorders_symptoms

Additional resources can be found online in Appendix D: Childhood Disabilities Resources, Services, and Organizations (see About the Online Companion Materials).

REFERENCES

Adolescent Sleep Working Group, Committee on Adolescence, & Council on School Health. (2014). School start times for adolescents. *Pediatrics, 134*(3), 642–649. doi:10.1542/peds.2014-1697

Allen, R. P., Picchietti, D. L., Auerbach, M., Cho, Y. W., Connor, J. R., Earley, C. J., . . . Winkelman, J. W. (2018). Evidence-based and consensus clinical practice guidelines for the iron treatment of restless legs syndrome/Willis-Ekbom disease in adults and children: An IRLSSG task force report. *Sleep Medicine, 41,* 27–44.

American Academy of Sleep Medicine. (2014). *International classification of sleep disorders* (3rd ed.). Darien, IL: Author.

Angriman, M., Caravale, B., Novelli, L., Ferri, R., & Bruni, O. (2015). Sleep in children with neurodevelopmental disabilities. *Neuropediatrics, 46*(3), 199–210. doi:10.1055/s-0035-1550151

Auger, R. R., Burgess, H. J., Emens, J. S., Deriy, L. V., Thomas, S. M., & Sharkey, K. M. (2015). Clinical practice guideline for the treatment of intrinsic circadian rhythm sleep-wake disorders: Advanced sleep-wake phase disorder (ASWPD), delayed sleep-wake phase disorder (DSWPD), non-24-hour sleep-wake rhythm disorder (N24SWD), and irregular sleep-wake rhythm disorder (ISWRD). An Update for 2015: An American Academy of Sleep Medicine Clinical Practice Guideline. *Journal of Clinical Sleep Medicine, 11*(10), 1199–1236. doi:10.5664/jcsm.5100

Camacho, M., Certal, V., Abdullatif, J., Zaghi, S., Ruoff, C. M., Capasso, R., & Kushida, C. A. (2015). Myofunctional therapy to treat obstructive sleep apnea: A systematic review and meta-analysis. *Sleep, 38*(5), 669–675. doi:10.5665/sleep.4652

Carskadon, M. A., Vieira, C., & Acebo, C. (1993). Association between puberty and delayed phase preference. *Sleep, 16*(3), 258–262.

Crabtree, V. M., Ivanenko, A., O'Brien, L. M., & Gozal, D. (2003). Periodic limb movement disorder of sleep in children. *Journal of Sleep Research*, *12,* 73–78.

Crosby, B., LeBourgeois, M. K., & Harsh, J. (2005). Racial differences in reported napping and nocturnal sleep in 2- to 8-year-old children. *Pediatrics, 115*(1), 225–232. https://www.ncbi.nlm.nih.gov/pmc/articles/PMC2987587

de Bruin, E. J., Bögels, S. M., Oort, F. J., & Meijer, A. M. (2015). Efficacy of cognitive behavioral therapy for insomnia in adolescents: A randomized controlled trial with internet therapy, group therapy and a waiting list condition. *Sleep, 38*(12), 1913–1926. doi:10.5665/sleep.5240

de Souza, L., Benedito-Silva, A. A., Pires, M. L., Poyares, D., Tufik, S., & Calil, H. M. (2003). Further validation of actigraphy for sleep studies. *Sleep, 26*(1), 81–85.

Dosman, C., Witmans, M., & Zwaigenbaum, L. (2012). Iron's role in paediatric restless legs syndrome—A review. *Paediatrics and Child Health, 17*(4), 193–197.

Dye, T. J., Gurbani, N., & Simakajornboon, N. (2018). Epidemiology and pathophysiology of childhood narcolepsy. *Paediatric Respiratory Reviews, 25,* 14–18. doi:1.1016/j.prrv.2016.12.005

Gingras, J. L., Gaultney, J. F., & Picchietti, D. L. (2011). Pediatric periodic limb movement disorder: Sleep symptom and polysomnographic correlates compared to obstructive sleep apnea. *Journal of Pediatric Sleep Medicine, 7*(6), 603–609A. doi:10.5664/jcsm.1460

Gradisar, M., Jackson, K., Spurrier, N. J., Gibson, J., Whitham, J., Williams, A. S., . . . Kennaway, D. J. (2016). Behavioral interventions for infant sleep problems: A randomized controlled trial. *Pediatrics, 137*(6). doi:10.1542/peds.2015-1486

Grigg-Damberger, M., & Ralls, F. (2013). Treatment strategies for complex behavioral insomnia in children with neurodevelopmental disorders. *Current Opinion in Pulmonary Medicine, 19*(6), 616–625. doi:10.1097/MCP.0b013e328365ab89

Hollway, J. A., Aman, M. G., & Butter, E. (2013). Correlates and risk markers for sleep disturbance in participants of the Autism Treatment Network. *Journal of Autism and Developmental Disorders, 43*(12), 2830–2843. doi:10.1007/s10803-013-1830-y

Honaker, S. M., & Meltzer, L. J. (2014). Bedtime problems and night wakings in young children: An update of the evidence. *Paediatric Respiratory Reviews, 15*(4), 333–339. doi:10.1016/j.prrv.2014.04.011

Johns, M. W. (1991). A new method for measuring daytime sleepiness: The Epworth Sleepiness Scale. *Sleep, 14*(6), 540–545.

Malow, B. A., Byars, K., Johnson, K., Weiss, S., Bernal, P., Goldman, S. E., . . . Sleep Committee of the Autism Treatment Network. (2012). A practice pathway for the identification, evaluation, and management of insomnia in children and adolescents with autism spectrum disorders. *Pediatrics, 130*(Suppl. 2), S106–S124. doi:10.1542/peds.2012-0900I

Marcus, C. L., Brooks, L. J., Draper, K. A., Gozal, D., Halbower, A. C., Jones, J., . . . Spruyt, K. (2012). Diagnosis and management of childhood obstructive sleep apnea syndrome. *Pediatrics, 130*(3), 576–584. doi:10.1542/peds.2012-1671

Marcus, C. L., Moore, R. H., Rosen, C. L., Giordani, B., Garetz, S. L., Taylor, H. G., . . . Childhood Adenotonsillectomy Trial. (2013). A randomized trial of adenotonsillectomy for childhood sleep apnea. *The New England Journal of Medicine, 368*(25), 2366–2376. doi:10.1056/NEJMoa1215881

Marcus, C. L., Traylor, J., Gallagher, P. R., Brooks, L. J., Huang, J., Koren, D., . . . Tapia, I. E. (2014). Prevalence of periodic limb movements during sleep in normal children. *Sleep, 37*(8), 1349–1352. http://doi.org/10.5665/sleep.3928

Maski, K., & Owens, J. A. (2016). Insomnia, parasomnias, and narcolepsy in children: Clinical features, diagnosis, and management. *Lancet Neurolology, 15*(11), 1170–1181. doi:10.1016/S1474-4422(16)30204-6

Mayer, G., Wilde-Frenz, J., & Kurella, B. (2007). Sleep related rhythmic movement disorder revisited. *Journal of Sleep Research, 16*(1), 110–116. doi:10.1111/j.1365-2869.2007.00577.x

Meltzer, L. J., & Mindell, J. A. (2014). Systematic review and meta-analysis of behavioral interventions for pediatric insomnia. *Journal of Pediatric Psychology, 39*(8), 932–948. doi:10.1093/jpepsy/jsu041

Miano, S., Esposito, M., Foderaro, G., Ramelli, G. P., Pezzoli, V., & Manconi, M. (2016). Sleep-related disorders in children with attention-deficit hyperactivity disorder: Preliminary results of a full sleep assessment study. *CAN Neuroscience Therapy, 22*(11), 906–914. doi:10.1111/cns.12573

Mindell, J. A., & Owens, J. A. (2015). *A clinical guide to pediatric sleep: Diagnosis and management of sleep problems* (3rd ed.). Philadelphia, PA: Wolters Kluwer/Lippincott Williams & Wilkins.

Owens, J. A. (2009). Neurocognitive and behavioral impact of sleep disordered breathing in children. *Pediatric Pulmonology, 44*, 417–422.

Owens, J. A., & Dalzell, V. (2005). Use of the 'BEARS' sleep screening tool in a pediatric residents' continuity clinic: A pilot study. *Sleep Medicine, 6*(1), 63–69. doi:10.1016/j.sleep.2004.07.015

Owens, J. A., & Weiss, M. R. (2017). Insufficient sleep in adolescents: causes and consequences. *Minerva Pediatics, 69*(4), 326–336. doi:10.23736/S0026-4946.17.04914-3

Picchietti, D. L., Bruni, O., de Weerd, A., Durmer, J. S., Kotagal, S., Owens, J. A., . . . International Restless Legs Syndrome Study Group. (2013). Pediatric restless legs syndrome diagnostic criteria: An update by the International Restless Legs Syndrome Study Group. *Sleep Medicine, 14*(12), 1253–1259. doi:10.1016/j.sleep.2013.08.778

Price, A. M., Wake, M., Ukoumunne, O. C., & Hiscock, H. (2012). Five-year follow-up of harms and benefits of behavioral infant sleep intervention: Randomized trial. *Pediatrics, 130*(4), 643–651.

Roenneberg, T., Wirz-Justice, A., & Merrow, M. (2003). Life between clocks: Daily temporal patterns of human chronotypes. *Journal of Biological Rhythms, 18*(1), 80–90.

Short, M. A., Gradisar, M., Lack, L. C., & Wright, H. R. (2013). The impact of sleep on adolescent depressed mood, alertness and academic performance. *Journal of Adolescence, 36*(6), 1025–1033. doi:10.1016/j.adolescence.2013.08.007

Simakajornboon, N., Kheirandish-Gozal, L., & Gozal, D. (2009). Diagnosis and management of restless legs syndrome in children. *Sleep Medicine Reviews, 13*(2), 149–156. doi:10.1016/j.smrv.2008.12.002

Spruyt, K., & Gozal, D. (2011). Sleep disturbances in children with attention-deficit/hyperactivity disorder. *Expert Reviews of Neurotherapy, 11*(4), 565–577. doi:10.1586/ern.11.7

Tan, H. L., Gozal, D., & Kheirandish-Gozal, L. (2013). Obstructive sleep apnea in children: A critical update. *Nature and Science of Sleep, 5*, 109–123. doi:10.2147/NSS.S51907

CHAPTER **29**

Feeding and Its Disorders

Peggy S. Eicher

Upon completion of this chapter, the reader will

- Describe the feeding and swallowing process and how it changes as an infant grows and develops
- Define how medical, motor, and interactional problems influence a child's feeding function
- Recognize some of the common feeding problems that occur in children with neuro-developmental challenges and what factors contribute to them
- Identify the basic components of a treatment approach to feeding problems

Feeding a child is one of the most satisfying experiences a caregiver can have. However, when it isn't successful, it can be one of the most frustrating. Feeding problems are very common for children both with and without neuro-developmental challenges. Estimates vary from 25%–50% of typically developing children and up to 80% of children with neuro-developmental challenges will present with a feeding concern (Lukens & Silverman, 2014). Therefore, it is paramount that pediatric care providers are equipped with a working knowledge of the normal feeding process and how medical, motor, and behavioral factors influence it. This will enable them to identify what is contributing to the development and maintenance of the child's feeding problem and thereby most effectively treat it. This chapter first reviews the normal feeding process and the changes that occur during typical growth and development. It then describes the most common feeding problems and how various medical and developmental conditions influence the feeding process to contribute to the development of those feeding problems. Treatment approaches and anticipatory guidance to prevent development of feeding problems will be discussed as well. The challenge in treating feeding problems in children with neuro-developmental challenges is not only the issue of identifying all of the factors interfering with the child's feeding function, but also of understanding how they interrelate.

CASE STUDY

Harry is an 18-month-old boy who was referred for a feeding evaluation because he "can't advance past purées and doesn't chew." He was delivered by C-section at 36 weeks' gestation, weighing 7 pounds. He had mild hyperbilirubinemia for which he received a few days of phototherapy, but he transitioned well in the full-term nursery and was discharged home with his mother. Harry crawled at 12 months and walked at 18 months. He can repeat a few words but does not use them spontaneously. He receives therapies through the early intervention program for his delay in motor and expressive language.

Harry breast-fed for 5 weeks and spit up a lot. With introduction of bottle feeding at 5 weeks, he refused to breast-feed. He transitioned to a predigested formula, although he continued to spit up frequently. His mother tried to introduce spoon feedings at 6 months of age. He gagged and vomited on these no matter what the baby food. She tried crunchy chewables, which he would self-feed but then vomit. He was able to tolerate puréed soup like table food purées at 9 months. By 14 months, he was able to ingest stage 2 baby food but could not tolerate stage 3. He continues to drink milk, but only from a bottle and always while lying down. He will drink water from a soft straw cup. Meals are difficult; he always needs distraction, and it takes over an hour to feed him 6 ounces. His parents find that they have to increase distractions as the meal progresses. Sometimes, his mother will resort to sitting him on the floor and feeding him a pouch of baby food by squeezing the contents into his mouth while he sucks on the spout of the pouch. Harry gags at the sight of other people's food. The easiest meal to feed him is in the middle of the day. He wakes up several times a night crying. Harry passes stools one to three times a day, usually after a bottle and with straining. The stool is typically a playdough-like consistency, with occasional hard pellets. He underwent a gastroesophageal endoscopy and modified barium swallow 3 months ago because of his mother's concerns that he is not chewing. The results of both tests were totally normal.

On evaluation, Harry's weight and length were at the 95th percentile for his age. Oral structures were intact. Lungs were clear to auscultation, with no areas of rhonchi or wheezing. His abdomen was distended, but soft with palpable stool in the left lower quadrant. His muscle tone was in the low normal range throughout. Harry's sitting posture included a posterior pelvic tilt, decreased thoracic extension, bilateral shoulder protraction, and forward head posture. Standing posture included decreased abdominal activation with a mild increase in lumbar lordosis. Harry ambulates as his primary means of mobility with fair coordination but with a wide base of support and arms elevated. He uses decreased trunk rotation and decreased abdominal activation, resulting in his weight being set anterior. Passive range-of-motion limitations were noted in bilateral trunk rotation and trunk extension. Decreased balance and abdominal activation were noted with all gross motor activities, and he had a posterior loss of balance.

During the feeding observation, Harry sat in a high chair without the straps on. In the beginning of the meal, he leaned over the tray to look at and swipe on the iPad that was being used to distract him. As the meal progressed his hips slid farther forward in the chair. His mother spoon-fed him puréed food. Harry's acceptance was poor despite the distraction with the iPad. He continually batted at the spoon with his left hand. When he accepted the spoon, he opened his mouth partially and his tongue was retracted. Only the tip to quarter of the toddler spoon entered his mouth, and he closed his lips to strip the spoon, compressed, and swallowed, moving his tongue minimally. He did not lick his lips. At rest, Harry occasionally rolled his tongue around in his mouth. His swallow appeared intact.

Harry needs intervention for his feeding problem. He does not move his tongue as a means of oral transport, and so advancing texture is not possible. Furthermore, his resistance to opening his mouth prevents his mother from stimulating his tongue with the spoon. Meals are so difficult that only his mother and babysitter can feed him; he will not be able to attend preschool unless this improves. Effective intervention must identify what factors are preventing him from eating more successfully. However, identifying those factors correctly requires familiarity with the normal feeding process and how it changes over the first few years of life.

Thought Questions:

Choose a condition of interest—such as autism spectrum disorder or cerebral palsy—and make note of the medical, developmental, and psychosocial factors that can contribute to the development of feeding disorders. For that condition, how can the different members of the interdisciplinary care team contribute to treatment?

THE FEEDING PROCESS

Swallowing

Swallowing is one of the most complex motor activities that humans perform. It entails the coordinated function of striated and smooth muscles of the head and neck plus the respiratory and gastrointestinal (GI) tracts. Swallowing also requires input from the central, peripheral, and autonomic nervous systems (Erasmus, van Hulst, Rotteveel, Willemsen, & Jongerius, 2012; Leopold & Daniels, 2010; Miller, 1986). Swallowing can be divided into four phases (Figure 29.1). Typically, after the first 4–6 months of life, the oral preparatory (Phase 1) and oral transport (Phase 2) phases become primarily volitional. During these oral phases, food is broken up and formed into a bolus by the tongue; the tongue then transports the bolus to the back of the throat. The pharyngeal transfer phase (Phase 3) begins when the bolus passes the faucial arches (near

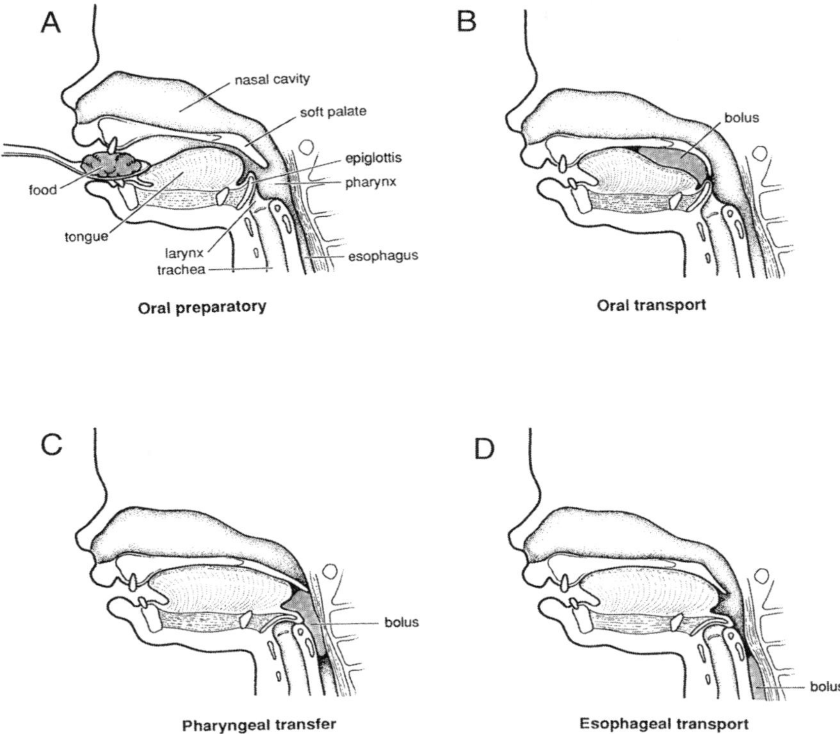

Figure 29.1. A) Phase 1, Oral Preparatory: Food is taken into the mouth, processed to a manageable consistency, and then collected into a small parcel, or bolus. B) Phase 2, Oral Transport: The bolus is then pushed backward by the tongue toward the pharynx. C) Phase 3, Pharyngeal Transfer: As swallowing begins, the epiglottis normally folds over the opening of the trachea to direct food down the esophagus and not into the lungs. D) Phase 4, Esophageal Transport: The peristaltic wave moves the bolus down the esophagus toward the stomach.

the tonsils) and triggers the start of the swallowing cascade. This involves the involuntary sequence of highly coordinated movements of the pharyngeal (throat) and esophageal (tube-to-stomach) muscles. With each swallow, respiration ceases as the soft palate elevates to close off the nasopharynx (entrance to the nasal airway at the back of the mouth). At the same time, forward movement and elevation of the hyoid bone results in 1) tipping of the epiglottis (a projecting piece of cartilage) to cover the trachea (entrance to the lungs) so that food does not slip into the airway and 2) opening the upper esophageal sphincter (UES; the entrance to the esophagus). A wave-like motion (peristalsis) originating in the back wall of the throat propels the bolus past the closed airway, through the open UES, and into the esophagus, marking the start of the esophageal transport phase (Phase 4). During this phase, the bolus is pushed down the esophagus by continuation of the peristaltic wave, which signals the relaxation, or opening, of the lower esophageal sphincter (LES; the entrance to the stomach), allowing the bolus to pass into the stomach. Entrance of the bolus into the stomach and the subsequent closure of the LES mark the end of the esophageal transport phase. These motor movements are synchronized and transmitted through the motor output side of the swallowing center in the brainstem. Sensory information from each level feeds back to the swallowing center to determine whether swallowing should stop, slow down, or continue (Erasmus et al., 2012; Lau, 2016).

The Influence of Growth and Development on the Feeding Process

Developmental Changes in Oral-Motor Skills

The process of swallowing evolves as the nervous system matures and the child experiences successful practice. The oral preparatory phase of swallowing is most influenced by growth and development. Reflexive oral-motor patterns in the infant are integrated into more complex oral-motor patterns that are learned through practice (Sheppard, 2008). Cortical maturation enables more independent and finely graded tongue and jaw movements to develop under increasing volitional control (Leopold & Daniels, 2010). Acquisition of oral-motor skills occurs in a sequential, stepwise progression. Mastery of skills at each level provides the foundation for skills at the next level. Thus, no stage can be skipped without interfering with the foundational skills needed for the next stage (Sheppard, 2008).

Suckling Suckling is the earliest oral pattern. Suckling motions and swallowing activity have been reported in fetuses by 15 weeks' gestation (Nowlan, 2015). Suckling and swallowing are gradually coupled over the course of gestation; the fetus in utero can swallow half an ounce at 20 weeks' gestation and up to 15 ounces each day at 38–40 weeks' gestation. Only following birth and with some practice, however, does the infant develop the rhythmical suck-swallow bursts coordinated with breathing to allow functional feeding. Mature suckling, in which the tongue moves in and out while riding up and down with the jaw, creating a wave-like motion, consists of two components: suction and expression (Lau, 2016). Suction refers to the intraoral negative pressure that pulls liquid into the mouth. Expression corresponds to the compression and/or stripping of the tongue against the hard palate to eject liquid into the mouth. Studies of nutritive sucking in preterm infants have revealed that suckling develops in stages, from the most immature with absent suction and only arrhythmic expression to the most mature with rhythmic bursts of alternating suction/expression (Lau, 2016). They have also identified that the expression component matures before the suction component (Lau, 2016). Infants with an immature suck having only the expression component can be successful with bottle feeding as expression can compress the nipple lying in their mouth. However, breast feeding would be much more difficult because the suction component of suckling enables the infant to latch onto the breast and keep the nipple in the mouth (Lau, 2016).

With further maturation and practice, the tongue exerts increasing force to propel a bolus of food posteriorly to initiate the swallow reflex, and the rate of swallowing increases. Underlying this increased swallowing rate are the maturational changes occurring in three elements of the esophageal phase. First, a well-developed UES and esophageal motility appear around 33–34 weeks' postmenstrual age to enable increased coordination between pharyngeal bolus propulsion and relaxation of the UES and timely transport of the bolus from the pharynx into the esophagus. With maturation of the esophageal body, anterograde peristaltic waves increase and the frequency of nonperistaltic waves decreases (Lau, 2016). The LES functions as a one-way valve to prevent the backward flow or reflux of food up into the esophagus (termed gastroesophageal reflux [GER]; Figure 29.2). The LES controls bolus movement into the stomach and reflux of stomach contents back into the esophagus. Typically, the LES continues to mature over the first 3 months of life with elongation of the esophageal body beneath the diaphragm, allowing development of a mature pressure gradient (Rybak, Pesce, Thapar, & Borrelli, 2017).

For the first 3–4 months of life, suckling is a reflexively driven activity that occurs involuntarily whenever something enters the infant's mouth. With brain maturation, the reflex is integrated and the infant can control initiation of the suckle pattern. Likewise, the ability to stabilize the jaw increases and the tongue dissociates from the jaw, leading to the next stage of sucking.

Sucking During sucking, the lips purse, the jaw opening is smaller and more controlled than in suckling, and the tongue is raised and lowered independently of the jaw. When sucking replaces the anterior/posterior pattern of suckling, usually around 5 months of age, the child can progress to spoon feeding. Because of the predominant up-and-down pattern of sucking, food can be transported to the back of the mouth without first riding out of the mouth on the tongue.

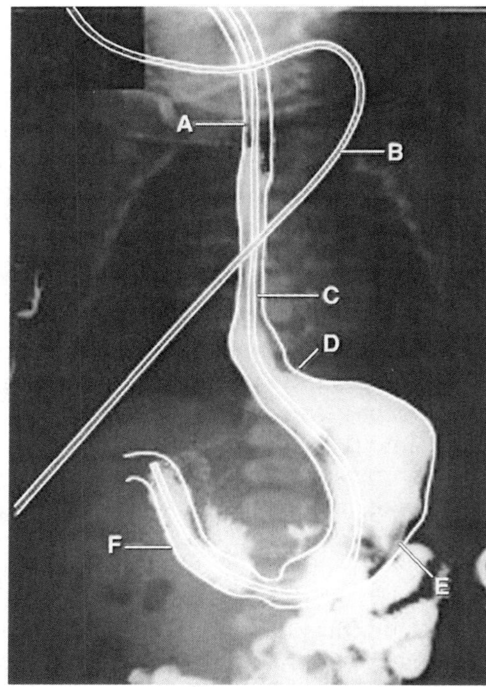

Figure 29.2. Food passes down the esophagus (A), through the lower esophageal sphincter (D), and into the stomach (E) and duodenum (F). If the sphincter does not remain closed after the passage of food, reflux (C) occurs, as shown in this barium study in a child with a nasogastric tube (B) in place.

Munching and Chewing With munching, small pieces of food are broken off, flattened, and then collected for swallowing. Munching consists of a rhythmical bite-and-release pattern with a series of well-graded jaw openings and closings. More important, however, is the emergence of tongue lateralization, which enables the child to move food from side to side and then to regather it in the midline. Actual chewing and grinding food into smaller pieces does not occur until the child acquires a rotary component jaw movement, a capacity that emerges around 9 months of age and is gradually modified via repetition until, by around 2 years of age, it approximates the adult pattern (Gisel, 2008).

Integration with Growth of Oral Structures
Typically, the attainment of new oral-motor skills coincides with the change in oral structures that occurs with growth. The infant, for example, is perfectly equipped for nipple feeding. The cheek fat pads confine the oral cavity while the tongue, soft palate, and epiglottis fill much of the mouth, easing the formation of the vacuum necessary to draw fluids out of the nipple. The larynx (voice box at the entryway to the lungs) is almost tucked under the tongue, necessitating less controlled transport to guide the liquid past the airway and into the esophagus (Bosma, 1986).

With growth, the jaw and palate enlarge in relation to the soft tissue structures, allowing room for the teeth (Figure 29.3). The larger oral cavity is not as efficient for nipple feeding but facilitates spoon entry and lateralization. The larynx descends and moves backward as the neck lengthens. This elongation necessitates increased postural control of the head and neck to enable safe swallowing. Meanwhile, the changes occurring in the child's oral-motor pattern afford the tongue increasing control of collection and propulsion of the food in the mouth and pharynx, enhancing the child's ability to guide the food safely past the airway.

Integration with Psychomotor Development
The ontogeny in oral-motor skills typically corresponds with progression in other areas of development (Table 29.1). The sucking pattern emerges as the child develops gross motor control for righting the head and sitting independently. Munching skills with tongue lateralization typically occurs contemporaneously with a pincer grasp for picking up small pieces, eruption of teeth, and increased trunk control enabling crawling. Desire for inclusion in parents' meals and independence set the stage for introduction of table food pieces and self-feeding (Sheppard, 2008). Interestingly, food neophobia, or the normal "picky" stage that commonly occurs between 1–2 years, is thought to be evolutionarily associated with the gross motor skill of walking as a protective mechanism against the child eating dangerous substances they encounter while mobile (Aldridge, Dovey, Martin, & Meyer, 2010).

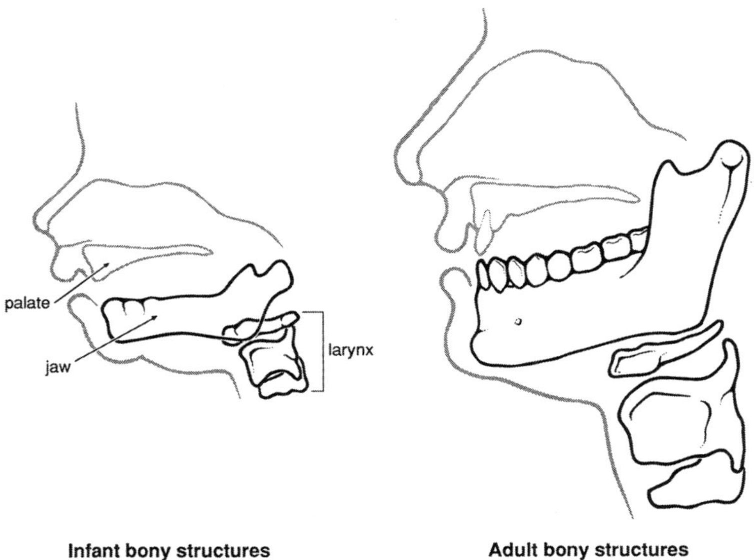

Figure 29.3. The mandible (jaw) enlarges, enabling room for teeth and a larger oral cavity. The larynx descends and moves posteriorly, necessitating increased control of bolus propulsion to guide it past the airway.

Table 29.1. Coordination of developmental milestones with feeding skills

Age	Gross motor	Fine motor	Oral motor	Feeding
Birth–4 months	Increasing head control Push up in prone	Brings hands together at 3 months	Suckle pattern	Nipple feeding
4–7 months	Derotational righting- rolling Sits independently	Reaching Hand to mouth play	Sucking pattern Jaw stability Phasic bite	Initiation of spoon feeds Tongue used to move food back rather than with suction
8–10 months	Lateral props Moves in and out of positions Crawling	Hand raking movements Palmar grasp Pincer grasp	Lateral movement of tongue Crushing jaw movements	Crunchy chewables Moving piece laterally with finger Self-feeding small pieces
10–12 months	Pulls to stand Crawls for mobility	Mature pincer grasp Voluntary release	Controls position of food in mouth with tongue Cup drinking	Soft chewables introduced Holds spoon
12–18 months	Walking	Uses utensils	Rotary chewing	Brings spoon to mouth Increased chewables in meals
18–24 months	Runs	Increasing utensil use Dips food in sauce	Increasing strength and endurance of rotary chew	More self-feeding Avoids new foods

Sources: Arvedson (2006) and Lipkin and Macias (2017).

Interaction with Feeder Because children are dependent on a caregiver for nutrition, the quality of the mealtime interaction with the feeder is tremendously important. Starting with nipple feeding, whether breast or bottle, the American Academy of Pediatrics (n.d.) strongly recommends "responsive feeding" rather than feeding on a schedule. With responsive feeding, infants are fed when they exhibit hunger cues and are allowed to stop feeding when they exhibit signs of being full and satiated. This leads the infant to learn to interpret feelings of hunger and satiety, which enables them to better develop the ability to self-regulate food intake. As the infant grows, the feeder should continue to be sensitive to the infant's cues of hunger and satiety, while establishing a mealtime routine that maximizes the infant's comfort and enables the successful practicing of emerging skills. This approach contributes to making feeding time a pleasant interaction.

Many feeding transitions occur in the first 3 years of life, and a child with a neuro-developmental challenge may have more difficulty during these periods in adjusting to changes in textures, utensils, and settings. This heightens the importance of a stable mealtime environment, interactive communication, and consistent interactions between the caregiver and child. Consistency imparts a sense of familiarity that enables children to be comfortable and more tolerant of mealtimes.

Feeding Problems

Feeding problems are very common in childhood. Children are considered to have feeding difficulties if they are unable or unwilling to eat a similar volume or variety of foods as their peers (Marshall, Hill, Ware, Ziviani, & Dodrill, 2016). The type of feeding problem varies by how much the child eats, what they eat, when they eat, how they eat, and what the caregiver thinks they should be eating. Common feeding issues surround advancing texture, picky eating or food selectivity, food refusal, limited intake, and challenging mealtime behaviors. Because younger children are dependent on a caregiver at mealtimes, the interaction between child and feeder influences whether the child's mealtime function is perceived as a problem or not (Aldridge et al., 2010; Kerzner et al., 2015).

A feeding problem is considered a feeding disorder if the problem exists more than 1 month and/or results in 1) significant weight loss or nutritional deficiency, 2) dependence on tube feeding or nutritional supplements, or 3) impairment in psychosocial functioning and developmental deviation or delay (Phalen, 2013).

Unfortunately, there is not one agreed upon classification system that captures the complexity of the multiple influences on feeding that can contribute to the development of a feeding disorder. Historically, feeding problems were associated with poor growth and classified as organic, with underlying medical issues, or nonorganic, with no physiological cause for the poor growth (Marshall et al., 2016). As there is increased recognition of the many factors influencing pediatric feeding, the field has moved toward a conceptualization of feeding difficulties that recognizes the effects of both biological and behavioral factors and their mutual interaction (Crist & Napier-Phillips, 2001). In 2013, the term **avoidant/restrictive food intake disorder (ARFID)** was introduced in the *Diagnostic and Statistical Manual, Fifth Edition* (American Psychiatric Association, 2013), in an attempt to provide an improved classification for feeding disorders (Phalen, 2013). ARFID entails an intake disturbance in which a child eats too little, eats a limited variety, or has fear of eating, resulting in either faltering growth, nutritional deficiency, dependence on nutritional supplements either orally or by tube, and/or interference with psychosocial functioning. If the feeding disorder is associated with an underlying condition, the presentation of the feeding disorder is more severe than would be expected (Kreipe & Palomake, 2012). Kerzner and colleagues (2015) argue that because of the interaction of the child and feeder and the influence of the feeder's perception of what the child should be eating, a classification scheme must also take into account the feeder's style.

PREVALAENCE AND EPIDEMIOLOGY

Feeding and eating problems affect 25%–40% of healthy, typically developing infants and young children; 40%–70% of children with chronic medical conditions; and up to 80% of children with neuro-developmental disabilities (Lukens & Silverman 2014). The lack of an agreed upon classification scheme has made it difficult to have accurate prevalence estimates. Although "picky" eating can be a normal "phase" before 2 years, it becomes a common problem in children ages 3–11 years, with 13%–22% being reported as food selective (Chatoor, 2002). Up to 40% of these children will continue to be selective into adolescence (Mascola, Bryson, & Agras, 2010). In fact, it is estimated that persistent restriction in food consumption, whether volume or variety, affects up to 5% of children, making it one of the most frequent concerns in pediatrics (Sharp et al., 2016). Epidemiologic studies performed in the United States report that 13%–29% of children and adolescents fit the criteria for avoidant/restrictive food intake disorder (see section on Avoidant/Restrictive Food Intake Disorder) upon initial presentation to eating disorder services. Feeding difficulties, most often food selectivity, are reported to occur in 46%–89% of children on the autism spectrum (Marshall et al., 2016). Children born prematurely, small for gestational age, or with congenital malformations also have an increased risk of feeding disorders, particularly oral-motor problems (Johnson et al., 2016). One study reported that feeding problems occur in 30% of infants born prematurely (Rybak, 2015).

ETIOLOGY AND ASSOCIATIONS WITH SPECIFIC DEVELOPMENTAL DISABILITIES

Feeding problems result from a combination of several factors: anatomical abnormality, motor or sensory dysfunction, medical or psychological conditions, growth abnormality, learning difficulties, and social interaction difficulties (Berlin, Lobato, Pinkos, Cerezo, & LeLeiko, 2011). Because children learn how to eat through practice, anything that impedes successful practice can result in a feeding problem (Sheppard, 2008), and because children with neurodevelopmental challenges have a higher frequency of medical, motor, and learning problems, their risk for feeding problems is greater.

Multiple medical and developmental factors are frequently present in children with feeding problems. Reportedly 48%–85% of children with feeding problems have two or more conditions, and 86%–100% have at least one problem in addition to their feeding difficulties (Berlin et al., 2011). These underlying conditions increase the overall risk of a feeding problem in general rather than for any specific type of feeding problem. Harry, for example, was born preterm, has symptoms consistent with GER, and has developmental delay.

The Influence of Medical Conditions on Feeding

Oral-motor problems in children may have a number of causes, including 1) an anatomical abnormality such as a cleft palate; 2) abnormalities in muscle tone; 3) compensatory postural and breathing patterns resulting from various medical issues, especially respiratory and GI problems; and 4) limited practice of more mature oral-motor patterns. The integration of growth with enlarging structures and increasing neurologic control over posture and oral-motor pattern is so important that delay in gross motor or oral-motor development can decrease feeding efficiency and foster swallowing incompetency (Sheppard, 2008).

Conditions Affecting the Upper Aerodigestive Tract Feeding difficulties may be the first sign of an anatomical defect involving the oral or nasal cavities, pharynx, or esophagus that can adversely affect swallowing. Clefts, such as those in the lip or palate, interfere with sealing off the oral cavity, decreasing the child's efficiency at generating negative pressure and collecting the food in preparation for swallowing. A change in size or shape of an oral structure that affects coordination of the swallowing process can also be a significant problem; for example, enlarged tonsils and adenoids may render the child dependent on his or her mouth as an airway, influencing suck-swallow-breath timing and even coordination if the flow of the food bolus is disrupted by the tonsils. Normal esophageal peristalsis (the involuntary constriction and relaxation of the muscles of the esophagus and intestine, creating wavelike movements that push food forward) is interrupted in children with esophageal atresia or tracheoesophageal fistulae, which are abnormal connections of the esophagus to the respiratory tract. Even after repair of these abnormal connections, the child's swallow will be influenced by the degree of abnormal peristalsis remaining in the esophageal phase of the swallow.

Successful feeding is dependent not only on the anatomy and function of the oral and pharyngeal structures involved in swallowing, but also on the child's medical status, especially with regard to respiration and digestion (Lau, 2016). Sensory information from the lungs, heart, and GI tract goes directly to the swallowing center in the brain. Through this input, a child with breathing difficulty (e.g., wheezing) may start to drool because swallowing frequency slows as a result of the need for increased respiratory rate (Gewolb & Vice, 2006; Khoshoo & Edell, 1999). Current research suggests that the feeding difficulties of preterm infants may relate more to inappropriate swallow–respiration interaction than to the suck–swallow interaction (Fucile, McFarland, Gisel, & Lau, 2012).

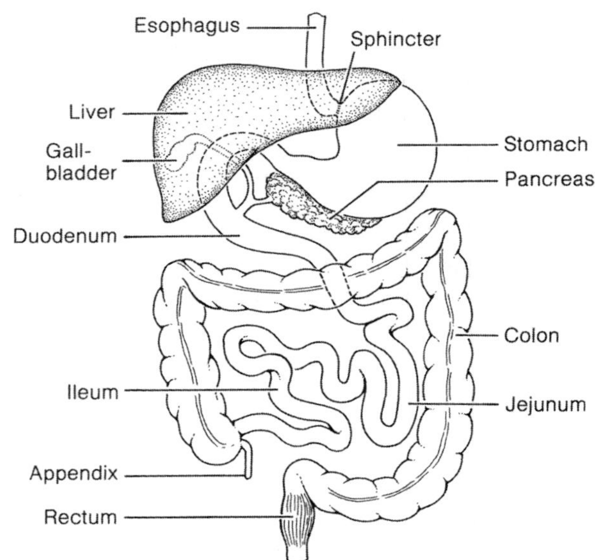

Figure 29.4. After food enters the stomach, it is mixed with acid and is partially digested. Then it passes through the three segments of the small intestine (duodenum, jejunum, and ileum). There, digestive juices are added and nutrients are removed. The remaining water and electrolytes pass through the colon, where water is removed. Voluntary stooling is controlled by the rectal sphincter muscles.

Feedback from the GI Tract

Irritation Input from the GI tract (one long tube that runs from the mouth to the anus) also has a significant impact on the feeding process (Figure 29.4). Chaidez, Hansen, and Hertz-Picciotto (2014) reported that children on the autism spectrum or with other neurodevelopmental challenges are at least three times more likely to experience GI symptoms than typically developing children. Children with feeding problems have high rates of GI problems no matter what other comorbid factors are present (Berlin et al., 2011). Gastroesophageal reflux (GER) is the backward flow of stomach contents up the esophagus. GER can result in vomiting, and if the stomach's contents enter the airway, the reflux can cause coughing, wheezing, and even pneumonia (Rybak et al., 2017). In addition, repeated entry of stomach acid into the esophagus can cause inflammation (esophagitis) that makes eating painful. The child may respond to GER by vomiting, refusing to eat, or taking frequent breaks while eating. GER can result from a number of abnormalities, and some forms can be inherited (Hu et al., 2004). The most common mechanism for GER is transient relaxation of the LES, which occurs with the arrival of the propelled bolus down the esophagus or with increased intragastric pressure, as with burping or stomach distention. Lowered LES resting tone from a head injury or hiatal hernia can also allow reflux of gastric contents (Rybak et al., 2017). LES function can be influenced by meal volume and composition (Kim et al., 2013), and reflux also can result from increased abdominal pressure caused by straining or constipation (Borowitz & Sutphen, 2004).

A child with GER who feels uncomfortable all the time may lose interest in eating or may accept only a few favorite foods (Chaidez et al., 2014). GER can also affect the movement of the tongue, throat, and esophagus, causing the child to choose foods that need less oral preparation and are therefore easier to swallow. The resulting lack of practice with more difficult textures can lead to delayed oral-motor development.

Harry, the child from the opening case study, exemplifies the myriad ways GER can interfere with feeding. Although frequent emesis occurs commonly in the first few months of life, Harry's continued emesis despite transition to a predigested formula that empties faster is consistent with ongoing GER. Other symptoms consistent with GER included gagging at the sight of his parent's food and waking up several times a night. GER explains his difficulty with spoon feedings, in that his ongoing tongue retraction prevents him from using his tongue as a transport surface to propel the food posteriorly. His oral defensiveness prevents his mother from getting the spoon into his mouth to stimulate a more appropriate oral pattern. Thus, the only pattern he practices is nipple compression, which does not enable him to manipulate crunchy chewables, lumps, or even thicker purées. However, he can be successful sucking from the pouches because his mother squeezes the contents into his mouth. He then uses his cheeks and lips to generate enough suction to move the thin purée contents posteriorly.

Vomiting, feeding problems, poor weight gain, and irritability are also characteristics of adverse food reactions, including food allergy and food intolerance. The prevalence of food allergy has been reported as affecting up to 18% of children (Rybak et al., 2017). The most common allergenic foods are cow's milk, hen's eggs, soy, wheat, fish, peanuts, and shellfish (Rybak et al., 2017). Eosinophilic gastroenteropathies are a heterogeneous group of non–IgE-mediated food allergies characterized by feeding intolerance and GER symptoms. Biopsies taken from the lining of the involved area of the GI tract demonstrate increased accumulation of eosinophils, the allergy-reactive white blood cells (Simon, Straumann, Schoepfe, & Simon, 2017). The affected children also frequently have food sensitivity, shown through skin testing, as well as clinical evidence of other allergic disease (Simon et al., 2017). Recent studies support early introduction of some highly allergenic foods to actually help decrease development of food allergies (Ierodiakonou et al., 2016; Perkin et al., 2016; Togias et al., 2017).

Another form of food intolerance is lactose intolerance. Approximately 70% of the world's population has an inherited deficiency of the enzyme lactase, which normally breaks down milk sugar (lactose) to allow its absorption (Vandenplas, 2015). With lactase deficiency, unabsorbed lactose irritates the intestinal wall and causes abdominal discomfort, vomiting, and diarrhea after ingesting milk products. Yet, dairy products are an important, if not the main, source of calcium, vitamin D, and protein for many, rendering their potential elimination challenging. Symptoms of lactose-caused GI irritation can be minimized by staggering milk intake throughout the day, taking lactase pills before ingesting a milk product, or using lactase-containing or lactose-free dairy products.

Dysmotility The phenomenon of "dumping" occurs when the stomach empties too rapidly. Symptoms of dumping include nausea, vomiting, diarrhea, heart palpitations, and weakness (Calabria, Charles, Givler, & De Leon, 2016). Children receiving carbohydrate-based, high-calorie supplements or formulas can have symptoms of dumping, and children who have had a surgical procedure to weaken the pylorus are particularly at risk. Avoidance of dumping requires slowing the rate of stomach emptying or decreasing the concentration of food delivered to the duodenum. This can be accomplished by 1) slowing the feeding rate using continuous feeding, 2) using fat-based instead of carbohydrate-based caloric supplements, or 3) changing to a formula with a lower caloric concentration (Gariepy & Mousa, 2009).

Nausea, vomiting, and bloating may signal delayed stomach emptying (Jericho, Adams, Zhang, Rychlik, & Saps, 2014). Normally, stomach wall contractions mix and push the stomach contents into the duodenum, the upper part of the small intestine. Delayed stomach emptying can be caused by abnormal stomach contractions, a blockage in the pylorus (the sphincter at the junction of the stomach and the duodenum), poor intestinal motility, or a meal heavy in fat or protein.

Digested nutrients get absorbed through the jejunum and ileum (the middle and lower portions of the small intestine), whereas nonabsorbable nutrients, called bulk or fiber, pass to the large intestine, or colon. Although movement from the stomach to the end of the ileum may take only 30–90 minutes, passage through the colon may require 1–7 days. Rapid movement through the colon leads to diarrhea, whereas slower movement causes more water to be absorbed, resulting in hard stools and constipation. Proper bowel evacuation requires adequate fluid, fiber, and coordinated propulsive muscle activity (Dehghani et al., 2015). Overly loose stools may be caused by 1) lactase deficiency, 2) inadequate dietary fiber, 3) dumping, 4) overaggressive use of laxatives or enemas, 5) passage of loose stool around an impaction, 6) disruption in the balance of gut flora, or 7) dietary imbalance via overingestion of fruit juices.

Constipation and/or diarrhea are common problems for children with neurodevelopmental challenges. As an example, almost half of children on the autism spectrum may have either constipation or diarrhea (Holingue, Newill, Lee, Pasricha, & Daniele Fallin, 2017). Chaidez and colleagues (2014) have reported that children with ASD are six times more likely to report diarrhea or constipation than typically developing children. Children with other developmental disabilities are five times more likely than their peers to report constipation (defined as hard stools or a delay or difficulty in defecation that is present for 2 or more weeks; Buie et al., 2010). In addition to aggravating the risk of reflux by increasing intra-abdominal pressure, constipation can be associated with cramping and discomfort that interferes with appetite and contributes to early satiety, sensitivity to foods, and/or swallowing difficulty (Buie et al., 2010; Chaidez et al., 2014). There is some evidence to indicate a direct relationship between reduction of stool in the rectum and decreased abdominal pain with increased appetite, suggesting a communication between rectal fullness and rate of gastric emptying (Boccia et al., 2008). In the case study, Harry has mild constipation in that his stools are hard pellets and come after he drinks a bottle, which in turn may be exacerbating his GER.

Influence of Other Medical Conditions Any medical condition that impairs the function of the respiratory tract or GI tract can influence the feeding and swallowing process. For example, chronic diseases, including asthma, kidney disease, and inborn errors of metabolism (see Chapters 16 and 24), can contribute to the development of a feeding problem. Moreover, these disorders can influence one another. For example, an increase in the effort to breathe can influence GI function by changing the pressure relationship between the chest and abdomen (Ayazi et al., 2011). During an asthma attack, the child generates increased negative lung pressure to breathe; therefore, abdominal pressure is increased relative to chest pressure, increasing the probability of GER. Likewise, GER can contribute to reactive airway narrowing, wheezing, and increased effort to breathe (Jung et al., 2012; Kostovski & Zdraveska, 2015). Thus, a vicious cycle can start fairly easily. Unfortunately, if oral feeding is interrupted for prolonged periods of time for any reason, the child may need to restart feeding at an easier texture, especially if the child has cerebral palsy.

The Interaction of Medical, Sensorimotor, and Psychomotor Conditions

The sensory and motor systems provide both the structural foundation and the sensory information that enable a child to practice and master oral-motor skills. Because the feeding process involves internal activities such as breathing, digestion, and elimination, structural alignment, control, and sensory input affect the feeding process and are in turn affected by it. Abnormal muscle tone, whether high or low, and/or persistent primitive reflex activity (as seen in cerebral palsy; see Chapter 21) interfere with trunk support as well as the appropriate trunk, neck, and head alignment necessary for successful feeding. Likewise, medical conditions can significantly influence posture and alignment. GI discomfort, whether from irritation (as with esophagitis) or distension (as with constipation), compels the child into postures that lessen abdominal pressure. Respiratory conditions that increase the child's effort to breathe lead the child to assume postures that increase the size of the airway. These tend to be extensor positions that interfere with control and alignment through the hips, back, head, and neck. Lack of adequate trunk support and improper alignment greatly hinder rib cage expansion, which ultimately interferes with respiration and increases pressure on the stomach and abdominal cavity. Due to inadequate support and restricted respiration, the shoulders typically elevate, reducing the stability of the base of support for the head and neck. Improper head and neck alignment makes guiding a bolus past the airway more difficult, increasing the risk of aspirating food into the lungs (Alghadir, Zafar, Al-Eisa, & Iqbal, 2017; Larnert & Ekberg, 1995). Improper alignment also limits tongue movement and interferes with oral-motor patterns (Figures 29.5).

For all of these reasons, a child should be seated during feedings with a firm base of support to control positioning of the hips and provided with adequate trunk support to allow neutral positioning of the head and neck. Moreover, the ears and shoulders should be aligned in the same vertical plane as the hips. This may require a slightly reclined position if the child cannot yet sit independently. Some children, in fact, prefer to drink while lying down. Such reclining, if the child has GI problems, may start as a way to stretch out and decrease the pressure on the abdomen or to support the rib cage to facilitate breathing. However, the child then may become dependent on gravity rather than on active tongue transport to move the bolus. As a result, spoon feeding or drinking in an upright position, which requires active oral transport, is not successful.

Harry always lies down to drink his bottle, decreasing his experience using his tongue as the controlling transport surface. Although his mother usually feeds him in a highchair, Harry leans over the tray in the highchair so his head is in a head forward position, which retracts his tongue at rest, making it impossible for his mother to stimulate his tongue with the spoon. Tongue retraction makes it even harder for him to manipulate the food bolus, contributing to his resistance.

Frequently children will avoid certain sensory experiences that cause them discomfort because a sensation is associated with past or current painful, negative stimuli. In regard to feeding, this may involve refusing certain textures, avoiding oral stimulation, or even

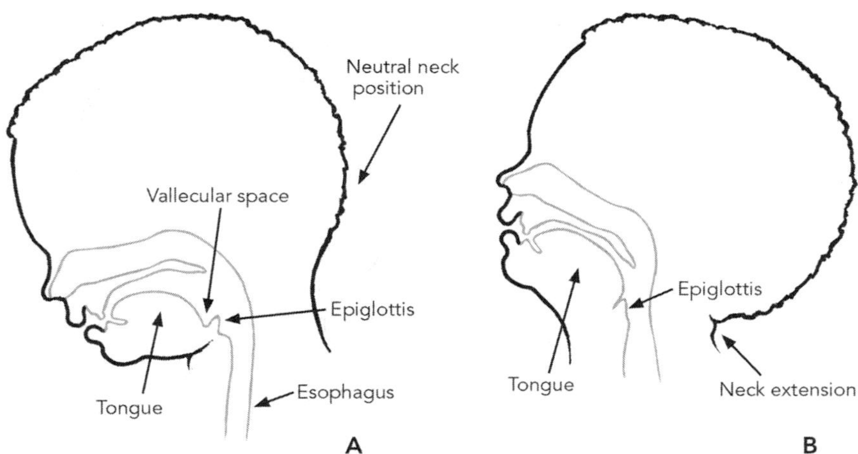

Figure 29.5. A) The child is in a neutral head position with a slight chin tuck. The neutral position allows for open airway while allowing the epiglottis to fall away from the tongue base, opening the vallecular space. This position gives the tongue a strong base of support off of which to move effectively with increased range and control. Widening the vallecular space acts as a "safety net" to catch any early leak of the food bolus from the oral cavity before the swallow. B) The child is in a position of head and neck extension. With neck extension, the tongue base retracts, apposing the epiglottis and eliminating the vallecular space. Tongue retraction decreases control of posterior tongue transport. Moreover, by minimizing the vallecular space, this position decreases the possibility of the vallecular "safety net."

hypersensitivity to the smells or visualization of non-preferred foods. This hypersensitivity may result from an abnormal response of the child's sensory system, but it can be seen also as part of the sensory feedback from a medical condition. For example, a child with GI discomfort may refuse new textures or feel nauseated and anxious at the sight of a spoon or even in response to the smells of other's food, as in Harry's case. In fact, GER can contribute to aspiration by desensitizing the larynx and weakening the laryngeal protective responses (Jadcherla, Hogan, & Shaker, 2010). With treatment of the medical condition, the sensory problems can resolve. A feeding problem may also develop if a medical or developmental condition chronically prevents the child from ingesting an appropriate amount without stress. The child then starts to associate discomfort and pain with feeding and learns to avoid feeding situations. This food avoidance or aversion can continue even after the medical condition has resolved, especially in children who have difficulty interpreting or integrating sensory input from elsewhere in the body.

The child's fine motor and adaptive skills influence the choice of utensils and level of independence at mealtime, and cognitive abilities help to shape how the child interacts with the mealtime environment. Because children are dependent on their caregivers for feeding, and thus for nutrition, effective caregiver–child communication during mealtime is crucial, and an understanding of the child's cognitive level and sensitivity to nonverbal cues prepare the caregiver to effectively communicate with the child. The absence of effective communication increases the likelihood of maladaptive behaviors at mealtime, such as expelling, refusal, or tantrums. If the feeder responds to these maladaptive behaviors by removing the disliked food or ending the meal, the child may repeat the maladaptive behavior the next time a meal is served. If this happens repeatedly the maladaptive behavior becomes a learned response. In Harry's case, he will not even start eating without distraction, and the more difficult he becomes, the more powerful the distraction becomes. He has learned that batting the spoon causes his mother to pull the spoon away and delay the presentation, so batting has become persistent. If he refuses persistently enough, she will even get him out of the chair and feed him without a spoon while he is playing. Refusal gets rewards!

DIAGNOSIS AND CLINICAL MANIFESTATIONS

Diagnosis of what qualifies as a real feeding problem can be difficult in that children go through multiple feeding transitions in the first 2 years of life and may need time to integrate the higher skill, depending on how much practice they get and how motivated they are to eat. However, if the child has had difficulty with previous feeding milestones, the feeding concern is more likely a feeding problem.

Aspiration/Penetration

Aspiration refers to food or a foreign substance entering into the airway (Figures 29.6). It may occur before, during, or after a swallow or as a result of reflux. Everyone aspirates small amounts of food occasionally, but our protective responses—gagging and coughing—help to clear them from the airway. Children with developmental disabilities that affect sensory or motor coordination of the oropharynx, larynx, or trachea, however, are at increased risk for recurrent aspiration (Jadcherla et al., 2010). Furthermore, these children often have impaired protective responses that limit their ability to clear their airway once aspiration occurs. Signs of aspiration are influenced by the age of the child. In infants, it may present as apnea and bradycardia (slowed heart rate) during meals, whereas in older infants and children, it may appear as coughing, congestion, or wheezing. Some children aspirate without a protective response from the body; this is called silent aspiration and is particularly dangerous because it often goes undetected. Recurrent aspiration and resultant accumulation of foodstuffs in the airway cause irritation and inflammation that can lead to pneumonia, bronchitis, or tracheitis (Jadcherla, 2016). If aspiration is suspected, a multidisciplinary feeding team should see the child to evaluate if aspiration is occurring, and, if so, why (Dodrill & Gosa, 2015).

Difficulty Advancing Texture

Coughing and Gagging Coughing and gagging indicate difficulty with swallowing. Both are normal defense mechanisms used to prevent aspiration. Coughing and gagging during the meal may indicate troublesome food textures. For example, if a child gags on lumpy foods but not on purées, it indicates difficulty adequately chewing or transporting the more highly textured food. Harry's ineffective transport pattern contributed to his gagging on lumps and thicker purées. The child who coughs while drinking may have a problem controlling flow through the pharynx and past the airway. If the child coughs or gags at the end of or after a meal but not during the meal, GER should be considered. Persistent coughing or gagging during meals over several weeks is a serious warning sign and requires a swallowing evaluation as soon as possible (Rybak, 2015).

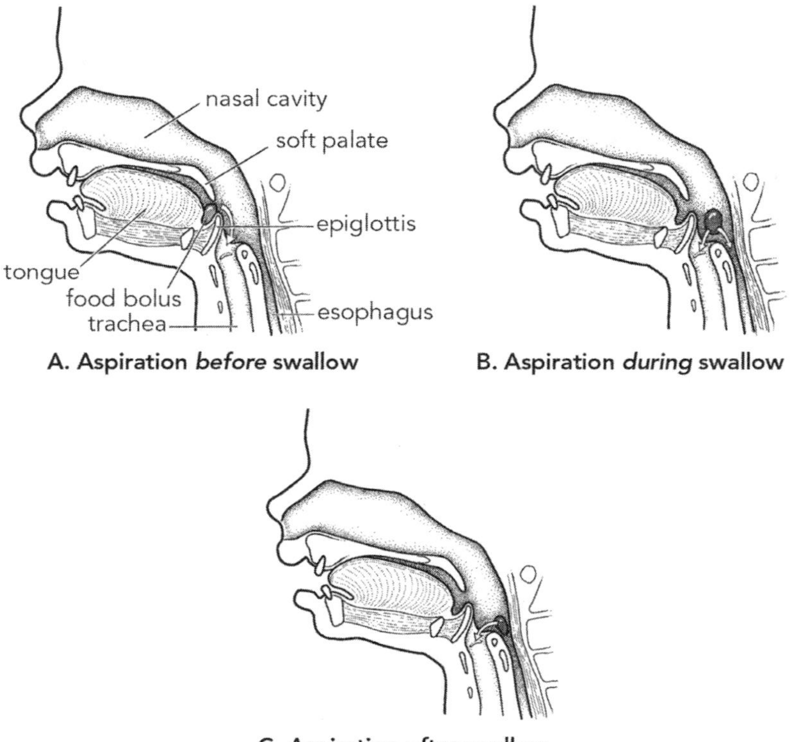

Figure 29.6. A) If a part of the bolus leaks past the soft palate before a swallow is triggered, it can flow past the open epiglottis and into the trachea. B) If the epiglottis is not completely closed as the bolus passes, aspiration can also occur. C) Food residua in the pharynx after a swallow can be carried into the airway with the next breath, resulting in aspiration after the swallow.

Choking Choking occurs when food becomes stuck in the pharynx. This happens most commonly when large pieces of soft solids are given to a child whose munching pattern or suckle transport is inadequate or if the child tends to stuff his or her mouth before swallowing. Cutting foods up into smaller pieces or offering only a couple of pieces at a time may decrease choking. After some practice and with positive reinforcement, the child may be able to gradually increase the size and/or number of chunks accepted. Choking can also occur when there is dysfunction in the UES, as with GER, or when using the mouth as an airway while eating. A full evaluation can help to ascertain the etiology quickly and develop an approach to remediation if needed.

Food Pocketing Food pocketing (holding food in the cheeks or the front of the mouth for prolonged periods) suggests either problematic oral transport or food refusal. Children with difficulty moving their tongue from side to side or those who use an immature central transport pattern often have trouble transporting food back to the midline before a swallow. As a result, mashed food or chunks migrate toward the cheeks. Alternatively, if a child does not want to swallow the food because of its texture or taste, he or she may trap it in the cheeks or under the tongue. Some children with a persistent suckle pattern will move each food bolus to the front of the mouth just behind the front teeth before trying to swallow it. Often this will lead to build up of residue and pooling under the tongue.

Increased Oral Losses Loss of food from the mouth, or "messy eating," may signal an oral-motor problem, whether related primarily to the oral pharyngeal musculature or to the impact of medical or postural conditions on oropharyngeal function. The child may have poor lip closure or jaw instability caused by abnormal tone in the facial muscles. As a consequence, once in the mouth, food may 1) be carried out onto the tongue as a result of a persistent suckle pattern or exaggerated tongue thrust; 2) fall out of the mouth if the child has not practiced an active transport pattern; or 3) be expelled in an attempt to control bolus size, as when there is swallowing difficulty related to GER or throat infection. Sometimes food may be exhaled from the mouth if the oral cavity also serves as the primary airway.

Prolonged Feeding Time

Prolonged feeding time (greater than 30 minutes) usually results from a combination of factors. Oral transport may be slowed by difficulty in collecting food in the mouth or by weakened tongue movements. The suckling pattern of infants with a history of prematurity or cleft palate may utilize more compression than suction. This limits the negative pressure they can generate with which to extract liquid from a nipple and slows the rate of feeding. If pharyngeal transfer is weak or uncoordinated, the child may need more swallows between bites to clear the food bolus from the pharynx. The child may also slow the meal to allow more time for breathing between bites or to complete transport through the esophagus. The child may appear at times to take breaks, or dawdle, during a meal to allow time for gastric emptying. Prolonged feeding time is a difficult problem for both the child and caregiver and signals the need for an evaluation (McCornish et al., 2016). In Harry's case, his mother is unable to get an infant spoonful of food into his mouth because of his oral defensiveness. Furthermore, she is not able to place it on his tongue because his tongue is very retracted.

Avoidant/Restrictive Food Intake Disorder

ARFID, as described earlier in this chapter, is a new diagnostic category that includes food refusal and food selectivity.

Food Refusal Food refusal can be total, in which case the child does not accept and swallow any food, or partial, in which the child eats some food but not enough to sustain adequate growth and nutritional health. Food refusal is most often associated with an ongoing medical problem such as asthma or GER. Because of the resulting lack of practice eating, these children's oral-motor skills are also commonly immature or dysfunctional, which further complicates matters. Food refusal requires a coordinated approach among an interdisciplinary team of physicians and therapists (Dodrill & Gosa, 2015; Lukens & Silverman, 2014; Phalen, 2013; Sharp, Volkert, Scahill, McCracken, & McElhanon, 2017).

Food Selectivity Food selectivity implies that the child will accept only a small number of foods, although he or she may eat large quantities of them. Children with ASD often display selectivity of foods (see Chapter 18). Texture-focused selectivity is most commonly seen in children with cerebral palsy who have oral-motor problems. Selectivity may initially stem from an underlying medical condition but then becomes a learned response perpetuated by environmental or interactional factors even after the instigating factor has been resolved (Clawson & Elliott, 2014; Lukens & Silverman, 2014). Food selectivity is a difficult problem that, like food refusal, requires the coordinated efforts of an interdisciplinary team (Lukens & Silverman, 2014).

MONITORING, SCREENING, AND EVALAUTION

As children learn how to eat through neurologic maturation and successful practice, it is of utmost importance to ask about feeding skills and mealtime interactions at every well-child visit. Following growth parameters can also be helpful, but they are not sensitive to early stages of a feeding problem. Moreover, children may continue to grow normally for some time despite nutritional risk from severe food selectivity or markedly prolonged feeding times that would signal a feeding problem.

Multiple screening tools are available to help differentiate a normal feeding phase from a feeding problem, although there is not one that is universally accepted. Because of the complexity of the feeding process and the multiple influences on it, investigation of a feeding problem should employ a multidisciplinary perspective (Lukens & Silverman, 2014; McCornish et al., 2016; Phalen, 2013). Information is needed regarding how and when the feeding problem started, how it has changed over time, and what interventions have been used. Background information regarding the child's medical, motor, and behavioral history is also important. A thorough evaluation includes the child's medical history, a physical examination, a neurodevelopmental assessment, an oral-pharyngeal evaluation, feeding history, and mealtime observation (McCornish et al., 2016). A nutritional analysis of a 3-day record of the child's intake can provide helpful information regarding the total calories ingested, vitamin and mineral content, and nutritional balance of the diet (McCornish et al., 2016). The information gleaned from the evaluation will identify the feeding problem and the medical, motor, and motivational factors contributing to it (Kerzner et al., 2015).

Diagnostic procedures may be needed to provide further information to support or clarify the clinical impression. Films of the airway can aid in detecting upper airway obstruction. If aspiration of oral feedings is suspected, a modified barium swallow (MBS) with video fluoroscopy is commonly used. In this procedure, the child is placed in the usual feeding position and offered foods to which barium, a milk-like substance visible on x-ray, has been added. The radiologist uses a video fluoroscope to visualize the pharynx and watch how the pharyngeal muscles guide the food bolus past the airway. The texture of the food and liquids can be varied to evaluate how the child's swallowing function changes with different textures. Video fluoroscopy can also give information about airway size and the interface of swallowing and respiration. Flexible endoscopic evaluation of swallowing (FEES) has become more frequently used in evaluating swallowing dysfunction. With FEES, a small endoscope is inserted into the nose and passed to the back of the throat in order to directly visualize the hypopharynx (where the larynx, the entrance to the lungs, sits next to the entrance to the esophagus). The endoscopist can see whether some of the bolus has entered the airway before, during, or after the swallow. The drawback of this procedure is that the area cannot be captured via the camera during a swallow, so the exact mechanism of the aspiration/penetration may not be clear. FEES with sensory testing can yield important information about the sensory thresholds of the area, information that is unavailable from the MBS (Dodrill & Gosa, 2015).

If GI dysmotility is suspected, an upper GI series can be done to rule out anatomical problems. For this procedure, barium is either ingested by the child or infused into the stomach by a nasogastric (NG) tube. As the fluid moves through the esophagus, stomach, and small intestine, the radiologist can identify structural abnormalities (Figure 29.2; Rybak et al., 2017). A second procedure, the milk scan or gastric-emptying study, provides information about height and frequency of GER episodes and assesses the rate of gastric emptying (Figure 29.7; Rybak et al., 2017). During the milk scan, the child swallows a formula to which a small amount of a radioactive tracer has been added, enabling the radiologist to track the milk as it moves through the GI tract. In addition, if the radioactive tracer is found in the lungs after several hours, it suggests that aspiration has occurred during a reflux episode.

The final two tests, the pH probe and gastroesophageal duodenoscopy (endoscopy), are considered the gold standards in the evaluation of GER and esophagitis, respectively (Edeani, Malik, & Kaul, 2017). For the pH probe, an NG-like tube is inserted through the nose and passed down the esophagus to just above the junction of the stomach and esophagus. At the tip of the tube is a small sensor, which detects the pH, or acidity, above the gastroesophageal junction. If acid in the stomach refluxes into the esophagus, the sensor records a sudden drop in the pH level, signaling GER (Figure 29.8). A symptom diary or videotaping of the child's activities and behaviors during the study period enhances the interpretation of the pH changes. A relatively new technology, multiple intraluminal impedance (MII), measures the movement of fluids, solids, and air in the esophagus. MII and pH electrodes should be combined on a single catheter. This combination can detect extremely small amounts of refluxed material, whether or not it is acidic (Edeani et al., 2017). Endoscopy entails passing a fiberoptic tube through the mouth down the

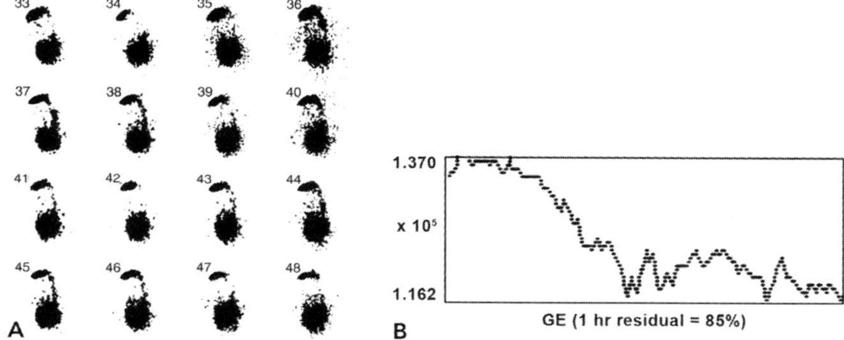

Figure 29.7. In this study, the child is fed a milk formula containing minute amounts of a radioactive label that can be seen on scanning. A) Shown here is a sequence of images taken after the child drinks the milk. The images are generated by a computer from information obtained by the scanner every 120 seconds. The area of radioactivity at the top of each image represents residual formula in the mouth, whereas the lower area of radioactivity is the stomach. Images 34 to 39 show increased activity in the mouth and esophagus, reflecting a reflux episode to the mouth and descending back to the stomach. In images 44 to 48, radioactivity can be seen flowing up from the stomach into the midesophagus, indicating another episode of reflux. A repeat scan after the child was placed on antireflux medication would show an absence of stomach reflux. B) In addition to diagnosing reflux, the milk scan can also evaluate whether the stomach is emptying food into the small intestine at a normal rate. Delayed gastric emptying (GE) increases stomach pressure and the possibility of reflux or vomiting. In the study shown, residual gastric radioactivity decreased by 15% 1 hour after the labeled milk was ingested (decreasing from 1.370×10^5 counters per minute to 1.162×10^5). This 85% 1-hour residual is high, as the normal is 67% or less. Prokinetic agents such as metoclopramide (Reglan) not only decrease gastroesophageal reflux directly, but also indirectly by increasing GE. Following effective medication, the rate of GE would be expected to increase, potentially to normal levels.

esophagus and into the stomach. The child is sedated during this procedure. The gastroenterologist can then look directly at the esophagus and stomach and take small biopsy specimens to look for signs of inflammation, allergy, or infection with organisms such as *Candida* or *Helicobacter pylori* (Edeani et al., 2017).

TREATMENT, MANAGEMENT, AND INTERVENTIONS

Because feeding problems in children with neurodevelopmental challenges usually result from the interaction among multiple factors, managing such problems can be difficult, time consuming, and frustrating (Box 29.1). Effective treatment usually requires intervention from more than one therapeutic discipline, and any plan of intervention must be potentially applicable across all of the child's environments (home, school, and therapist's office) to be truly effective. The treatment team, which should include the child's caregiver, teacher, medical care provider(s), and therapists, needs to prioritize the treatment goals and outline a plan integrating the child's medical, nutritional, and developmental needs (Brackett, Eicher, Kerwin, & Fox, 2012). The primary caregiver, with team input, oversees the plan and monitors progress toward the goals; however, open lines of communication among all team members are crucial. Components of a successful treatment strategy include 1) minimizing negative medical influences, 2) ensuring positioning for feeding, 3) facilitating oral-motor function, 4) improving the mealtime environment, 5) promoting appetite, and 6) using alternative methods of feeding (if needed).

All of these components entail constant monitoring of the child's progress. Recognizing the interactions among the medical, motor, and motivational components enables the team to anticipate changes and treat several components at the same time (Brackett et al., 2012). Obviously, for a feeding program to be successful, the therapists need to be consistent and mindful of how the skills they are forging will affect the child's feeding function.

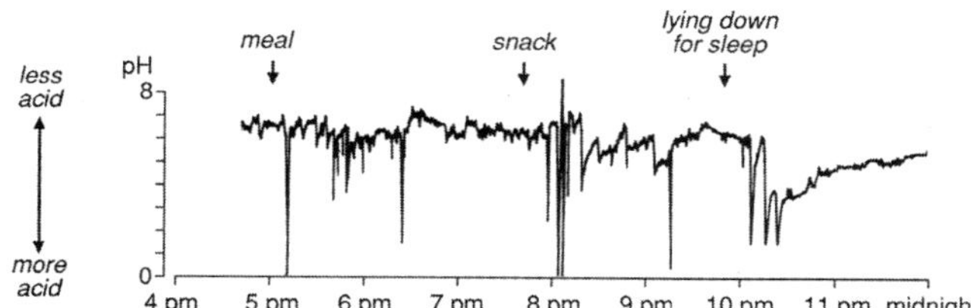

Figure 29.8. A pH probe study is done by passing a tube containing a pH electrode down the esophagus and positioning it just above the stomach. If there is reflux, the pH should drop as the acid contents of the stomach reach the lower esophagus, where the probe is placed. Shown here is an abnormal study with multiple episodes of low pH, occurring about half an hour after feeding and when the child is laid down to sleep. (From Batshaw, M. L. [1991]. *Your child has a disability: A complete sourcebook of daily and medical care* [p. 224]. Baltimore, MD: Paul H. Brookes Publishing Co., Inc.; reprinted by permission. Copyright © 1991 Mark L. Batshaw. Illustration copyright © 1991 by Lynn Reynolds. All rights reserved.)

BOX 29.1 INTERDISCIPLINARY CARE

Family Counselor

The family counselor provides support and recommendations to reduce the stress that affects the whole family because of a child's feeding problem. They also help the family find the strength necessary to carry out the new mealtime protocols and change existing family interaction patterns that are detrimental.

Minimize Negative Medical Influences

Because feeding is a complex skill, a child's feeding function may be very sensitive to even minor medical issues. Thus, parents' and therapists' observations of subtle changes in the child's behaviors, especially during and after feedings, are important and should be shared with medical care providers. Problems with GI irritation and dysmotility can adversely affect respiratory and GI function, as well as the child's level of comfort, and should be treated. For example, Harry is able to drink a bottle sitting up, and his mealtime resistance decreases when he has daily, mushy stools that are not dependent on gastric filling to stimulate evacuation. In fact, his tongue retraction decreases with an improved stooling pattern. Constipation can be remediated by 1) establishing regular toileting times to take advantage of the gastrocolic reflex that occurs after meals; 2) providing adequate fluids to minimize dry, cakey stools; and 3) encouraging active or passive physical exercise. Dietary fiber in the form of fruits, vegetables, and whole-grain foods can also increase movement through the GI tract, although more explicitly fiber-intensive products (e.g., Metamucil or Benefiber) may also be helpful (Tabbers et al., 2014).

When constipation is persistent, additional measures may be needed. To effectively manage persistent constipation, the colon needs to be cleared of stool, and then the child needs to have at least one stool daily with the use of a consistent regimen of appropriate laxatives, if needed, which work to soften the stool and/or stimulate evacuation. Laxatives and suppositories can be used, including milk of magnesia, senna concentrate (Senokot), bisacodyl (Dulcolax), lactulose, polyethylene glycol, or glycerin suppositories (Tabbers et al., 2014). Enemas, such as the Fleet Enema for Children, also may help, but continuous use of enemas can interfere with normal rectal sphincter control and should be avoided. A combination of the discussed approaches may be needed to establish regular bowel movements.

If GI irritation or GER is present, a number of therapeutic modalities are available, including proper positioning, meal modification, medications, and surgery (Rybak et al., 2017). The goal is to minimize gastric irritation and protect the esophagus from reflux of stomach acid, either by reducing the amount of gastric contents or by decreasing stomach acid production. Small, frequent meals help to decrease the volume of food in the stomach at any one time. In addition, studies show that whey-based formulas improve stomach emptying and decrease vomiting in children with certain forms of spastic cerebral palsy (Minor, Ochoa, Storm, & Periman, 2016). Similarly, a change in formula to a different protein source or predigested protein may alleviate irritation in those children with milk or soy protein intolerance (Rybak et al., 2017). Upright positioning and thickened feedings simply rely on gravity to help keep stomach contents from refluxing into the esophagus. Recent research with premature infants shows that side-lying positions can significantly increase the rate of emptying after a feeding, which then can be used to minimize reflux after the meal. As for medications, H2 antagonists (cimetidine [Tagamet], ranitidine [Zantac], and famotidine [Pepcid]), as well as proton pump inhibitors (omeprazole [Prilosec], lansoprazole [Prevacid], and esomeprazole [Nexium]) decrease stomach acidity and thereby lower the risk of reflux-caused inflammation of the esophagus (Rybak et al., 2017). Motility agents such as urecholine (Bethanechol), metoclopramide, and erythromycin increase the tone or movement in the esophageal sphincter and stomach, making it harder for reflux to occur (Rybak et al., 2017).

When GER cannot be controlled by positioning and medication alone, surgery may be needed to prevent problems associated with prolonged reflux. These problems include poor weight gain, recurrent aspiration pneumonia, esophageal stricture, and recurrent apneic episodes (Gariepy & Mousa, 2009). The most common surgical procedure is fundoplication, in which the top of the stomach is wrapped around the opening of the esophagus (Figure 29.9). This decreases reflux while permitting continued oral feeding. An alternative to fundoplication is surgically placing a gastrojejunal (G-J) tube that allows access to the stomach as well

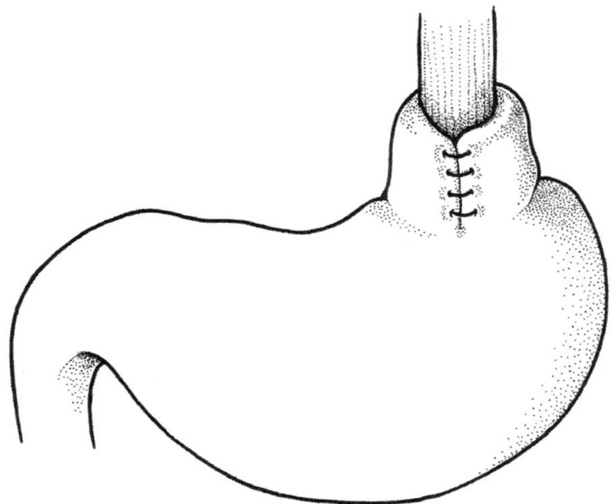

Figure 29.9. In the surgical procedure of fundoplication, the upper stomach is wrapped around the lower esophagus to create a muscular valve that prevents reflux.

as the jejunum, permitting some portion of the feeds to bypass the stomach and thereby decreasing the risk of reflux (Figure 29.10; Gariepy & Mousa, 2009).

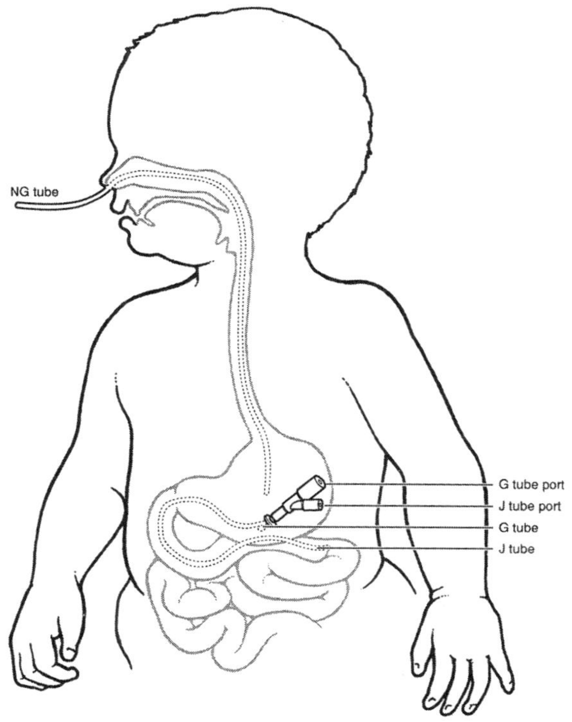

Figure 29.10. The nasogastric (NG) tube is placed through the nostril and into the stomach. An NG tube is helpful when problems with the child's oral function are the primary obstacle to adequate nutrition and are temporary. A gastrojejunal (G-J) tube allows access to the stomach as well as directly into the intestine. The G-J tube has two openings, or ports, and two parts of tubing. The G port connects with the G tube, which empties the stomach. The J port connects with the J tube, which empties into the intestine. A G-J tube can be helpful when the stomach is unable to tolerate the quantity of nutrients needed for adequate growth.

Ensure Proper Positioning for Feeding

Feeding is a flexor activity that requires good breath support. Appropriate positioning maximizes the child's ability to breathe as well as providing the best alignment to optimize function of the muscles involved in the swallowing process (Larnert & Ekberg, 1995). The child should be firmly supported through the hips and trunk to provide a stable base. The head and neck should be aligned in a neutral (upright) position, which decreases extension through the oral musculature while maintaining an open airway (Figure 29.11). Such positioning improves coordination and control of the steps in oral-motor preparation and transport. This, in turn, results in more positive feedback to the child and caregiver as a result of good feeding experiences (Brackett et al., 2012). If the child does not appear comfortable or appropriately supported for feeding in the currently constructed chair, the child's occupational or physical therapist can make changes to improve the support and alignment (Box 29.2). In the case study, Harry is positioned in the highchair with the shoulder straps adjusted snuggly, and the iPad is elevated so that his head is held in a neutral position.

Facilitate Oral-Motor Function

Any technique that eases the child's practice of an oral-motor pattern correctly facilitates oral-motor function. It may consist of oral-motor stimulation or desensitization without food, specific placement of food, or manipulation of the food to make it easier for the child to control. Recent research with premature infants has demonstrated that providing patterned orocutaneous stimulation that mimics the temporal organization of sucking can enhance the premature infant's acquisition of a functional suckle pattern, thereby decreasing the time needed to establish nipple feedings and then attaining full oral feeding (Barlow, Finan, Lee, & Chu, 2008). In older infants, chin support can often facilitate transition of the tongue pattern from a suckle to sucking and later to tongue lateralization (Gisel, 2008). Chewing can be enhanced by placing food between the upper and lower back teeth, which stimulates crushing movements of the jaw as well as lateral movement of the tongue, both of which are needed to master a munching pattern. Another technique is manipulating food textures to facilitate safe, controlled swallowing (Dodrill & Gosa, 2015). Thickening of liquids slows their rate of flow, allowing more time for the child to

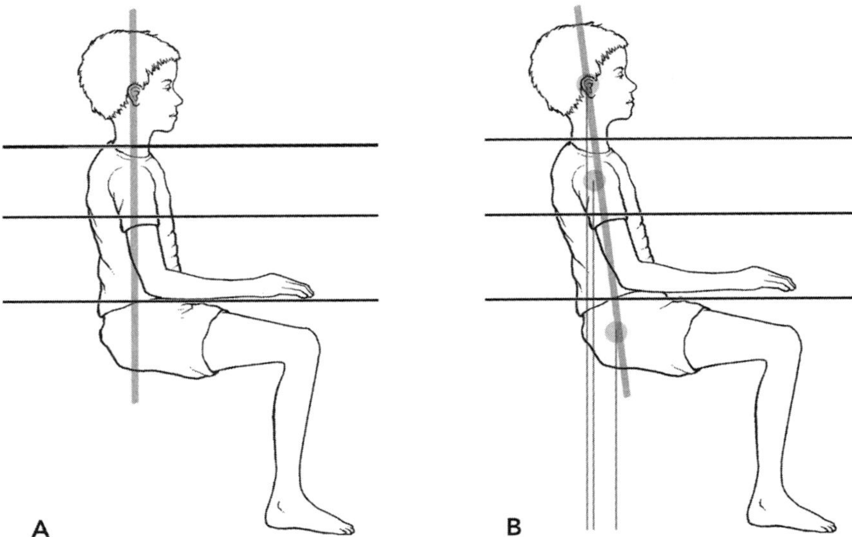

Figure 29.11. A) A child with a neutral pelvis and adequate trunk support to allow neutral positioning of the head and neck. Note how the ears and shoulders align in the same plane as the hips. B) A child supported in a slightly reclined seated position in which the ear, shoulder, and hip remain aligned. This would be a good position for a child who does not have adequate head control to maintain head and neck alignment during a mealtime.

organize and initiate a swallow. Thickening agents (e.g., Thick-It or instant pudding powders) can transform any thin liquid into a nectar-, honey-, or milkshake-like consistency (Box 29.3). In addition, almost any food can be finely chopped or puréed to a texture that the child can more competently manage.

It is important to remember that the primary goal of eating is to achieve adequate nutrition. Thus, when a child is first learning to accept a higher texture of foods, these foods should be presented during snack time, when volumes are smaller. During this transition period, easier textures should be used at mealtimes to ensure consumption of adequate calories for continued growth (Box 29.4). A speech-language pathologist or an occupational therapist can provide information about the child's oral-motor patterns and the appropriate food textures to facilitate improvement in feeding efforts.

Improve the Mealtime Structure

Eating requires more coordination among muscle groups than any other motor activity, including speech. Therefore, it is important to make eating as easy as possible. This can be accomplished by increasing the

BOX 29.2 INTERDISCIPLINARY CARE

Occupational and Physical Therapists

The motor therapists evaluate rib cage mobility and breathing, posture and alignment, and core development and activation in gross motor function, in addition to fine motor skills and sensory functioning. Their input is crucial in optimizing posture and alignment during mealtime as well as appropriate utensil use and necessary adaptations when working on self-feeding. Motor therapy works on ribcage mobilization to enhance respiratory support as well as strengthening activities for the shoulder girdle, trunk rotation, and the core to support optimal posture and alignment for feeding. If the child has sensory issues, such as those manifested by increased sensitivity to different clothing textures, grass, sand, and so on, the occupational therapist can recommend activities to help desensitize the child and therapies to further decrease their hypersensitivity.

BOX 29.3 INTERDISCIPLINARY CARE

Nutritionist/Dietician

The nutritionist helps to evaluate the adequacy of the child's current diet regarding caloric intake and nutritional quality. They can recommend appropriate changes to enhance the child's diet, satisfying the child's caloric and nutrient needs while also providing nutritional balance.

child's focus on the meal and including desirable foods in each meal that are easier to control. The caregiver should let the child know that mealtime is coming so that he or she can prepare for the "work" to be done. This may entail a pre-mealtime routine of going to a special corner of the room and putting on a bib or napkin or performing relaxation therapy, followed by oral stimulation to get the needed muscles ready for eating. Children with feeding difficulties usually eat better in one-to-one situations or in small groups because there are fewer distractions, aiding the ability to focus on the eating process (Clawson & Elliott, 2014). Parental provision of undivided attention also makes mealtimes more reinforcing.

When working on improving or advancing skills, it is important to break the skill down into small tasks that can be practiced with motivation (Sharp et al., 2017; Box 29.5). The child can be successful and ready to couple it with the next step in the process. When a child is eating well and interested in self-feeding, a number of adaptive devices can promote independence in eating. These include bowls with high sides, spoons with built-up or curved handles, and cups with rocker bottoms. The satisfaction that children obtain from eating can be increased by social attention during the meal or earning time for a favorite activity after the meal is completed.

Social interaction is an important part of mealtime as well, although it can be distracting. When peer interaction is the focus, it may be helpful to make the meal small (e.g., a snack) and to provide less challenging foods that do not require as much concentration for the child to successfully eat.

Promote Appetite

Some children have little or no appetite regardless of whether they are receiving enough calories to progress along their growth curve. This may be caused by an underlying medical condition, such as a kidney or metabolic disorder or zinc deficiency, or it may be a sign that a chronic medical condition (e.g., diabetes) is inadequately controlled. Alternatively, some children's appetites may be poor as a consequence of being satiated by their snacking, drinking, or supplemental feedings (Hartdorff et al., 2015). Eating "real" food at mealtimes represents more work to many children with feeding problems than does drinking or grazing on snack foods. Thus, these options can satiate the child and decrease their motivation to eat at mealtimes further. Set meal and snack times in addition to limiting access to fluids for an hour before meals can be helpful to eliminate grazing and promote appetite.

When underlying causes of poor appetite have been addressed, medications to promote appetite may be helpful. Cyproheptadine (Periactin) is a serotonin antagonist that works to increase appetite through two

BOX 29.4 INTERDISCIPLINARY CARE

Speech Therapist

The speech therapist on the team helps to evaluate tongue movement with and without food in the mouth. They facilitate more successful oral motor patterns by manipulating the texture or placement of food in the oral cavity. They may also recommend exercises to work on increasing tolerance to new stimuli in the mouth or stimulating appropriate oral motor patterns. The speech therapist can be very helpful during a modified barium swallow in performing the test with appropriate textures to elucidate the swallowing problem, as well as interpreting the results.

BOX 29.5 INTERDISCIPLINARY CARE

Behavioral Therapist

The behavioral therapist evaluates the antecedents and consequences contributing to the child's interactional behaviors at mealtime. They can recommend structured mealtime protocols to help enlist the child's cooperation to practice more appropriate feeding patterns. In addition, they can provide recommendations for behavioral problems that may be occurring outside of mealtimes.

mechanisms. It has a central effect to increase appetite and also affects the GI tract to enhance volume tolerance (Krasaelap & Madani, 2017; Rodriguez, Diaz, & Nurko, 2013).

There are differing opinions about whether day versus night, or bolus versus continuous, tube feedings are better for promoting appetite (Dsilna, Christensson, Alfredsson, Lagercrantz, & Blennow, 2005; Dsilna, Christensson, Gustafsson, Lagercrantz, & Alfredsson, 2008). Actually, the important thing is to look at how the child is tolerating the tube feedings. If the child retches, gags, vomits, or needs time to recover after tube feedings, he or she is not tolerating them. Sometimes it takes hours for the child to feel comfortable enough to eat orally again. With this in mind, the best tube-feeding schedule to promote a child's appetite is the one that is tolerated without GI discomfort, even if this involves continuous feedings. Once the child's feeding skills have improved, tube feeding volume can be gradually decreased to further promote appetite.

Use Alternative Methods of Feeding

In some cases, oral feeding may not be safe or sufficient to permit adequate nutrition (Mahant, Friedman, Connolly, Goia, & Macarthur, 2009; Quitadamo, Thapar, Staiano, & Borrelli, 2016). For these children, NG tube feedings or the placement of a gastrostomy (G) or G-J feeding tube is required (see Figure 29.10). A commercially prepared enteral formula (e.g., Nutren Jr. or Pediasure) can be used with any of these tubes. Although puréed table food feedings can be given through an NG or a G tube, they are not appropriate for a jejunostomy (J) tube because they will obstruct it. With an NG or a G tube, feedings can be given as single large volumes (boluses) of 3 to 8 ounces every 3–6 hours or as a continuous drip throughout the day or overnight. J-tube feedings must be given continuously, not as a bolus. The advantage of large-volume feedings is that they do not interfere with typical daily activities. The feeding itself takes about 30 minutes. As mentioned previously, however, the large volume may be difficult for the child to tolerate and may lead to vomiting or abdominal discomfort. If this happens, continuous-drip feedings can be instituted. A Kangaroo or similar type of automated pump is then used to deliver the formula at a set rate. Sometimes tube feedings are used to supplement oral feedings. In this case, tube feedings generally are used at night so that the child remains hungry for oral feedings during the day. A nutritionist can recommend the appropriate type of enteral formula as well as the amount of supplementation necessary to provide a nutritionally balanced intake that meets the child's daily caloric needs.

OUTCOMES

Although difficult, feeding problems can be effectively treated if the intervention strategy takes into account the many factors contributing to the feeding problem. In fact, multidisciplinary intervention is now the accepted standard of care for the treatment of pediatric feeding problems (Lukens & Silverman, 2014; Sharp et al., 2017). A recent review of published studies looking at children with complex medical conditions and tube dependence receiving inpatient or day treatment services reported intervention strategies incorporating components from medicine, psychology, speech or occupational therapy, and nutrition. Reportedly, on aggregate at discharge, 71% of these children no longer needed tube feeding, and there was maintenance or continued improvement for 80% of children on follow-up after discharge (Sharp et al., 2017). Thus, there is preliminary evidence to support the positive effects and long-lasting benefits of multidisciplinary treatment. Future research is needed to better define the various types of feeding problems and the disciplinary interventions necessary to most effectively treat them.

SUMMARY

- For children, feeding is complicated by the changes to the swallowing process that typically occur with growth and development.
- Feeding problems are very common for all children, but even more so for children with neurodevelopmental challenges.
- Feeding problems may result from an anatomical, medical, or developmental issue that interferes with successful swallowing. However, the initial problem is often compounded by interaction of ongoing medical, motor, and behavioral issues as time passes.
- More commonly, feeding problems may result from the influence of medical, motor, developmental, and/or interactional factors on the swallowing process, thus interfering with the typical oral-motor progression in the attainment of feeding skills.
- Evaluation of a child with a feeding problem requires an understanding of the normal feeding process and insight from medical, motor (oral, fine, and gross), and behavioral perspectives to accurately identify the factors contributing to the feeding problem.
- Effective intervention requires multidisciplinary input to optimize the child's feeding function while enabling adequate growth, development, and social interaction.

ADDITIONAL RESOURCES

ComeUnity's Resources for Feeding and Growth of Children: http://www.comeunity.com/premature/child/growth/resources.html

New Visions: http://www.new-vis.com

Additional resources can be found online in Appendix D: Childhood Disabilities Resources, Services, and Organizations (see About the Online Companion Materials).

REFERENCES

Aldridge, V. K., Dovey, T. M., Martin, C. I., & Meyer, C. (2010). Identifying clinically relevant feeding problems and disorders. *Journal of Child Health Care, 14*(3), 261–270.

Alghadir, A. H., Zafar, H., Al-Eisa, E. S., & Iqbal, Z. A. (2017). Effect of posture on swallowing. *African Health Sciences, 17*(1), 133–137. doi:10.4314/ahs.v17i1.17

American Academy of Pediatrics. (n.d.). *Is your baby hungry or full? Responsive feeding explained.* Retrieved from http://www.healthychildren.org/English/ages-stages/baby/feeding-nutrition/Pages/Is-Your-Baby-Hungry-or-Full-Responsive-Feeding-Explained.aspx

American Psychiatric Association. (2013). *Diagnostic and statistical manual of mental disorders* (5th ed.). Washington, DC: Author.

Arvedson, J. C. (2006). Swallowing and feeding in infants and young children. *GI Motility Online.* doi:10.1038/gimo17

Ayazi, S., DeMeester, S. R., Hsieh, C. C., Zehetner, J., Sharma, G., Grant, K. S., . . . DeMeester, T. R. (2011). Thoraco-abdominal pressure gradients during the phases of respiration contribute to gastroesophageal reflux disease. *Digestive Diseases and Sciences, 56*(6), 1718–1722. doi:10.1007/s10620-011-1694-y

Barlow, S. M., Finan, D. S., Lee, J., & Chu, S. (2008). Synthetic orocutaneous stimulation entrains preterm infants with feeding difficulties to suck. *Journal of Perinatology, 28,* 541–548.

Berlin, K. S., Lobato, D. J., Pinkos, B., Cerezo, C. S., & LeLeiko, N. S. (2011). Patterns of medical and developmental comorbidities among children presenting with feeding problems: A latent class analysis. *Journal of Developmental and Behavioral Pediatrics, 32,* 41–47.

Boccia, G., Buonavolonta, R., Coccorullo, P., Manguso, F., Fuiano, L., & Staino, A. (2008). Dyspeptic symptoms in children: The result of a constipation-induced cologastric brake? *Clinical Gastroenterology and Hepatology, 6,* 556–560.

Borowitz, S. M., & Sutphen, J. L. (2004). Recurrent vomiting and persistent gastroesophageal reflux caused by unrecognized constipation. *Clinical Pediatrics, 43,* 461–466.

Bosma, J. F. (1986). Development of feeding. *Clinical Nutrition, 5,* 210–218.

Brackett, K., Eicher, P. S., Kerwin, M. L. E., & Fox, C. (2012). An integrated approach to feeding intervention. In K. Van-Dahm (Ed.), *Pediatric feeding disorders: Evaluation and treatment* (pp. 15–33). Framingham, MA: Therapro.

Braun Household Australia. (n.d.). *Feeding milestones.* Retrieved from http://www.braunhousehold.com/en-au/baby-nutrition-centre/feeding-your-baby-toddler/feeding-milestones

Buie, T., Fuchs, G. T., III, Furuta, G. T., Kooros, K., Levy, J., Lewis, J. D., . . . Winter, H. (2010). Recommendations for evaluation and treatment of common gastrointestinal problems in children with ASDs. *Pediatrics, 125,* S19–S29.

Calabria, A. D., Charles, L., Givler, S., & De Leon, D. D. (2016). Postprandial hypoglycemia in children after gastric surgery: Clinical characterization and pathophysiology. *Hormone Research Paediatrica, 85*(2), 140–146. doi:10.1159/000442155, PMCID:PMC4732946, NIHMSID:NIHMS741072

Chaidez, V., Hansen, R. L., & Hertz-Picciotto, I. (2014). Gastrointestinal problems in children with autism, developmental delays or typical development. *Journal of Autism & Developmental Disorders, 44*(5), 1117–1127.

Chatoor, I. (2002). Feeding disorders in infants and toddlers: Diagnosis and treatment. *Child and Adolescent Psychiatry Clinics of North America, 11*(2), 163–183.

Clawson, E. P., & Elliott, C. A. (2014). Integrating evidence-based treatment of pediatric feeding disorders into clinical practice: Challenges to implementation. *Clinical Practice in Pediatric Psychology, 2,* 312–321.

Crist, W., & Napier-Phillips, A. (2001). Mealtime behaviors of young children: A comparison of normative and clinical data. *Journal of Developmental and Behavioral Pediatrics, 22,* 279–286.

Dehghani, S. M., Kulouee, N., Honar, N., Imanieh, M. H., Haghighat, M., & Javaherizadeh, H. (2015). Clinical manifestations among children with chronic functional constipation. *Middle East Journal of Digestive Diseases, 7*(1), 31–35.

Dodrill, P., & Gosa, M. M. (2015). Pediatric dysphagia: Physiology, assessment, and management. *Annals of Nutrition and Metabolism, 66*(Suppl. 5), 24–31.

Dsilna, A., Christensson, K., Alfredsson, L., Lagercrantz, H., & Blennow, M. (2005). Continuous feeding promotes gastrointestinal tolerance and growth in very low birth weight infants. *Journal of Pediatrics, 147,* 43–49.

Dsilna, A., Christensson, K., Gustafsson, A. S., Lagercrantz, H., & Alfredsson, L. (2008). Behavioral stress is affected by the mode of tube feeding in very low birth weight infants. *Clinical Journal of Pain, 24,* 447–455.

Edeani, F., Malik, A., & Kaul, A. (2017). Characterization of esophageal motility disorders in children presenting with dysphagia using high-resolution manometry. *Current Gastroenterology Reports, 19,* 13.

Erasmus, C. E., van Hulst, K., Rotteveel, J. J., Willemsen, M. A. A. P., & Jongerius, P. H. (2012). Swallowing problems in cerebral palsy. *European Journal of Pediatrics, 171*(3), 409–414.

Fucile, S., McFarland, D. H., Gisel, E. G., & Lau, C. (2012). Oral and nonoral sensorimotor interventions facilitate suck-swallow-respiration functions and their coordination in preterm infants. *Early Human Development, 88,* 345–350.

Gariepy, C. E., & Mousa, H. (2009). Clinical management of motility disorders in children. *Seminars in Pediatric Surgery, 18,* 224–238.

Gewolb, I. H., & Vice, F. L. (2006). Maturational changes in the rhythms, patterning, and coordination of respiration and swallow during feeding in preterm and term infants. *Developmental Medicine & Child Neurology, 48,* 589–594.

Gisel, E. G. (2008). Interventions and outcomes for children with dysphagia. *Developmental Disabilities Research Review, 14,* 165–173.

Hartdorff, C. M., Kneepkens, C. M., Stok-Akerboom, A. M., van Kijk-Lokkart, E. M., Engels, M. A., & Kindermann, A. (2015). Clinical tube weaning supported by hunger provocation in fully-tube-fed children. *Journal of Pediatric Gastroenterology and Nutrition, 60,* 538–543.

Holingue, C., Newill, C., Lee, L. C., Pasricha, P. J., & Daniele Fallin, M. (2017). Gastrointestinal symptoms in autism spectrum disorder: A review of the literature on ascertainment and prevalence. *Autism Research,* Advanced online publication. doi:10.1002/aur.1854

Hu, F. Z., Donfack, J., Ahmed, A., Dopico, R., Johnson, S., Post, J. C., & Preston, R. A. (2004). Fine mapping a gene for pediatric gastroesophageal reflux on human chromosome 13q14. *Human Genetics, 114,* 562–572.

Ierodiakonou, D., Garcia-Larsen, V., Logan, A., Groome, A., Cunha, S., Chivinge, J., . . . Boyle, R. J. (2016). Timing of allergenic food introduction to the infant diet and risk of allergic or autoimmune disease. A systematic review and meta-analysis. *JAMA, 316,* 1181–1192.

Jadcherla, S. (2016). Dysphagia in the high-risk infant: Potential factors and mechanisms. *American Journal of Clinical Nutrition, 103*(2), 622S–628S. doi:10.3945/ajcn.115.110106

Jadcherla, S. R., Hogan, W. J., & Shaker, R. (2010). Physiology and pathophysiology of glottic reflexes and pulmonary aspiration: From neonates to adults. *Seminars in Respiratory and Critical Care Medicine, 31*(5), 554–560. doi:10.1055/s-0030-1265896

Jericho, H., Adams, P., Zhang, G., Rychlik, K., & Saps, M. (2014). Nausea predicts delayed gastric emptying in children. *Journal of Pediatrics, 164,* 89–92.

Johnson, S., Matthers, R., Draper, E. S., Field, D. J., Manketelow, B. N., Marlow, N., . . . Boyle, E. M. (2016). Eating difficulties in children born late and moderately preterm at 2 years of age: A prospective population-based cohort study. *American Journal of Clinical Nutrition, 103,* 406–414.

Jung, W. J., Yang, H. J., Min, T. K., Jeon, Y. H., Lee, H. W., Lee, J. S., & Pyun, B. Y. (2012). The efficacy of the upright position on gastro-esophageal reflux and reflux-related respiratory symptoms in infants with chronic respiratory symptoms. *Allergy Asthma Immunology Research, 4*(1), 17–23.

Kerzner, B., Milano, K., MacLean, W. C., Jr., Berall, G., Stuart, S., & Chatoor, I. (2015). A practical approach to classifying and managing feeding difficulties. *Pediatrics, 135,* 344–353.

Khoshoo, V., & Edell, D. (1999). Previously healthy infants may have increased risk of aspiration during respiratory syncytial viral bronchiolitis. *Pediatrics, 104,* 1389–1390.

Kim, H. I., Hong, S. J., Han, J. P., Seo, J. Y., Hwang, K. H., Maeng, H. J., . . . Lee, J. S. (2013). Specific movement of esophagus during transient lower esophageal sphincter relaxation in gastroesophageal reflux disease. *Journal of Neurogastroenterology Motility, 19*(3), 332–337. doi:10.5056/jnm.2013.19.3.332, PMCID:PMC3714411

Kostovski, A., & Zdraveska, N. (2015). PP-16 weak acid reflux a trigger for recurrent respiratory diseases in children. *Journal of Pediatric Gastroenterology and Nutrition, 61*(4), 527. doi:10.1097/01.mpg.0000472244.98097.fd

Krasaelap, A., & Madani, S. (2017). Cyproheptadine: A potentially effective treatment for functional gastrointestinal disorders in children. *Pediatric Annals, 46*(3), e120–e125. doi:10.3928/19382359-20170213-01

Kreipe, R. E., & Palomake, A. (2012). Beyond picky eating: Avoidant/restrictive food intake disorder. *Current Psychiatry Reports, 14,* 421–431.

Larnert, G., & Ekberg, O. (1995). Positioning improves the oral and pharyngeal swallowing function in children with cerebral palsy. *Acta Paediatrica, 84,* 689–692.

Lau, C. (2016). Development of infant oral feeding skills: what do we know? *American Journal of Clinical Nutrition, 103*(Suppl), 616S–621S.

Leopold, N. A., & Daniels, S. K. (2010). Supranuclear control of swallowing. *Dysphagia, 25,* 250–257.

Lipkin, P., & Macias, M. (2017). Developmental milestones for developmental surveillance at preventive care visits. In J. F. Hagan, J. S. Shaw, & P. M. Duncan (Eds.), *Bright futures: Guidelines for health supervision of infants, children, and adolescents* (4th ed., 84–87). Elk Grove Village, IL: American Academy of Pediatrics.

Lukens, C. T., & Silverman, A. H. (2014). Systematic review of psychological intervention for pediatric feeding problems. *Journal of Pediatric Psychology, 38,* 903–917.

Mahant, S., Friedman, J. N., Connolly, B., Goia, C., & Macarthur, C. (2009). Tube feeding and quality of life in children with severe neurological impairment. *Archives of Disease in Children, 94,* 668–673.

Marshall, J., Hill, R. J., Ware, R. S., Ziviani, J., & Dodrill, P. (2016). Clinical characteristics of 2 groups of children with feeding difficulties. *Journal of Parenteral and Gastroenterologic Nutrition, 62,* 161–168.

Mascola, A. J., Bryson, S. W., & Agras, W. S. (2010). Picky eating during childhood: A longitudinal study to age 11 years. *Eating Behavior, 11*(4), 253–257.

McCornish, C., Brackett, K., Kelly, M., Hall, C., Wallace, S., & Powell, V. (2016). Interdisciplinary feeding team: A medical, motor, behavioral approach to complex pediatric feeding problems. *The American Journal of Maternal/Child Nursing, 41*(4), 230–236. doi:10.1097/NMC.0000000000000252, PMID:27710993

Miller, A. J. (1986). Neurophysiological basis of swallowing. *Dysphagia, 1,* 91–100.

Minor, G., Ochoa, J. B., Storm, H., & Periman, S. (2016). Formula switch leads to enteral feeding tolerance improvements in children with developmental delays. *Global Pediatric Health.* Advanced online publication. doi:10.1177/2333794X16681887

Nowlan, N. C. (2015). Biomechanics of foetal movement. *European Cells and Materials, 29,* 1–21. doi:10.22203/eCM.v029a01

Perkin, M. R., Logan, K., Tseng, A., Raji, B., Ayis, S., Peacock, J., . . . EAT Study Team. (2016). Randomized trial of introduction of allergenic foods in breast-fed infants. *New England Journal of Medicine, 374,* 1733–1743.

Phalen, J. A. (2013). Managing feeding problems and feeding disorders. *Pediatrics in Review, 34,* 549–556. doi:10.1542/pir.34-12-549

Quitadamo, P., Thapar, N., Staiano, A., & Borrelli, O. (2016). Gastrointestinal and nutritional problems in neurologically impaired children. *European Journal of Pediatric Neurology, 20*(6), 810–815. doi:10.1016/j.ejpn.2016.05.019

Rodriguez, L., Diaz, J., & Nurko, S. (2013). Edited by WFB: Safety and efficacy of cyproheptadine for treating dyspeptic symptoms in children. *Journal of Pediatrics, 163*(1), 261–267. doi:10.1016/j.jpeds.2012.12.096, PMCID: PMC3661691

Rybak, A. (2015). Organic and nonorganic feeding disorders. *Annals of Nutrition and Metabolism, 66*(S5), 16–22.

Rybak, A., Pesce, M., Thapar, N., & Borrelli, O. (2017). Gastroesophageal reflux in children. *International Journal of Molecular Science, 18*(8), 1671–1687. doi:10.3390/ijms18081671, PMCID:PMC5578061

Sharp, W. G., Stubbs, K. H., Adams, H., Wells, B. M., Lesack, R. S., Criado, K. K., . . . Scahill, L. D. (2016). Intensive manual-based intervention for pediatric feeding disorders: Results from a randomized pilot trial. *Journal of Pediatric Gastroenterology and Nutrition, 62,* 658–663.

Sharp, W. G., Volkert, V. M., Scahill, L., McCracken, C. E., & McElhanon, B. (2017). A systematic review and meta-analysis of intensive multidisciplinary intervention for pediatric feeding disorders: How standard is the standard of care? *Journal of Pediatrics, 181,* 116–124.

Sheppard, J. J. (2008). Using motor learning approaches for treating swallowing and feeding disorders: A review. *Language, Speech, and Hearing Services in Schools, 39,* 227–236.

Simon, D., Straumann, A., Schoepfe, A. M., & Simon, H.-U. (2017). Current concepts in eosinophilic esophagitis. *Allergo Journal International, 26,* 258–266. doi:10.1007/s40629-017-0037-8

Tabbers, M. M., DiLorenzo, C., Berger, M. Y., Faure, C., Langendam, M. W., Nurko, S., . . . Benninga, M. A. (2014). Evaluation and treatment of functional constipation in infants and children: Evidence-based recommendations from ESPGHAN and NASPGHAN. *Journal of Parenteral and Gastroenterologic Nutrition, 58,* 258–274.

Togias, A., Cooper, S. F., Acebal, M. L., Assa'ad, A., Baker, J. R. Jr., Beck, L. A., . . . Boyce, J. A. (2017). Addendum guidelines for the prevention of peanut allergy in the United States: Report of the National Institute of Allergy and Infectious Diseases–Sponsored Expert Panel. *Journal of Allergy & Clinical Immunology, 139,* 29–44.

Vandenplas, Y. (2015). Lactose intolerance. *Asia Pacific Journal of Clinical Nutrition, 24*(Suppl. 1), S9–S13.

PART VI

Interventions

CHAPTER 30

Interdisciplinary Education and Practice

Lewis H. Margolis and Angela McCaffrey Rosenberg

Upon completion of this chapter, the reader will

- Define the attitudes and skills that constitute interdisciplinary education and practice
- Explain the origins and ongoing evolution of interdisciplinary education and practice
- Underscore the value of interdisciplinary practice for the emerging field of children with medical complexity
- Highlight family members as key interdisciplinary partners
- Identify challenges in measuring the effects of interdisciplinary education and practice
- Outline characteristics to advance and sustain interdisciplinary education and practice

In the 21st century, families live in an increasingly complicated and complex world, challenged by globalization (Gerhardt, 2016); demographic shifts, such as changing family composition (Child Trends, 2015); an aging population (Ortman, Velkoff, & Hogan, 2014); increasing cultural diversity (Colby & Ortman, 2015); and a growing prevalence of disabilities (Boyle et al., 2011). At the same time, many basic science and clinical disciplines are becoming more specialized as knowledge and understanding continue to evolve, sometimes at a dramatic pace.

To address the increasing complexity of public health and medical care, national and international entities and scholars have encouraged educators and clinicians to develop programs that enhance the capacity of professionals to collaborate. A variety of groups have suggested that some combination of dedicated interdisciplinary, or interprofessional, education and intentional practice are critical to creating competent professionals. For example, *To Err Is Human*, a report by the Institute of Medicine about patient safety, calls for organizations to "establish interdisciplinary team training programs for providers" (Kohn, Corrigan, & Donaldson, 2000, p. 14). Frenk and colleagues (2010) have promoted a competency-based approach to educating health professionals in which teamwork, or collaboration, is a core competency, and the Interprofessional Education Collaborative (2016) has underscored the need for a seamless transition from education to collaborative practice. In addition, in 2015, the Institute of Medicine convened a committee to move "beyond examining the impact of IPE [interprofessional education] on learners' knowledge, skills, and attitudes to focus on the link between IPE and performance in practice including the impact of IPE on patient and population health and health care delivery system outcomes" (2015, p. 2).

Given the multifaceted aspects of growth and development, as well as the cultural contexts for children, both with and without disabilities, and the families in which they reside and ideally flourish, the professional field of maternal and child health, especially those professional disciplines educated and engaged in the care of children with disabilities, needs to be intentional in advancing collaboration to enhance the well-being of these children and their families.

This chapter traces the institutional development of interdisciplinary approaches and identifies knowledge, attitudes, and skills that define interdisciplinary education and practice. As a way of encouraging the development of this important set of skills, the chapter reviews what still remains a limited body of literature on the effects of interdisciplinary education and practice. It concludes with suggestions for strategies to implement and advance interdisciplinary practice to achieve optimal outcomes for children with disabilities and their families.

CASE STUDY

Imagine that you are a clinician on an interdisciplinary team that provides assessment and rehabilitation services for children with disabilities. You have been on this intact team for 5 years. Your team has had impressive synergy, and, due to similar team processes and approaches, the majority of you get along well. You feel you can often anticipate what your team members will recommend regarding treatment plans, and your own professional input is appreciated.

Overall, this organization has been a positive work environment, but you miss your team leader, who recently retired. She was the central core of the group, hired you, and was an excellent clinician. She set up the team meeting structure and policies by which you operate. Now you have a new team leader, and you are not sure about how she will contribute to the group. She seems to be changing the team structure and processes in ways that you feel are not well thought out. You also have one new team member who is, frankly, difficult, often bringing up seemingly irrelevant issues or ideas that just aren't practical for children. You and other team members have begun to tune out when this person begins to speak.

Today you are having a team meeting about how best to partner with a family in treatment planning. The mother seems challenging to some. The family recently relocated to the area, and the mother brings up how much better the "other state" was in providing services, questioning the quality of some of the services her child is receiving.

Thought Questions:

As a clinical provider or as a student who may be observing, consider a recent team-based clinical encounter that did not seem as effective as you had hoped for or expected. Putting aside whatever complexities and uncertainties of the child's clinical condition that may have complicated the encounter, reflect on the characteristics of the team that may have contributed to your feelings or conclusions. What assumptions may have been made by team members, including the family, that made the encounter less effective? What interdisciplinary skills were in play? Could specific skills have advanced the discussion and plans for the child and family? When your team encounters challenging interdisciplinary situations, do you intentionally seek advice from professionals who think differently than you? If so, what insights have you gained? If not, what prevents you from doing so?

DEFINING INTERDISCIPLINARY EDUCATION AND PRACTICE

Interdisciplinary practice, defined as "collaborative practice that combines the insights of several professional disciplines, consumers, and community members—in designing care or programs" (Margolis, Rosenberg, Umble, & Chewning, 2013, p. 950), is central to the clinical care and policy development for children and youth with special health care needs (CYSHCN). Although the term *interprofessional* has gained ascendancy, this chapter intentionally uses the term *interdisciplinary* because it reflects respect for all of the many different partners who engage in collaboration to advance the well-being of children and their families. The term *interprofessional* places professionals, with all the training and expertise the term implies, at the core of education and practice. This is reflected, for example, in the World Health Organization definition, "when multiple health workers from different backgrounds provide comprehensive services by working with patients, their families, care givers and communities to deliver the highest quality of care across settings" (2010, p. 13). The expertise of parents is at the core of providing high-quality care and services for CYSHCN. According to the National Center for Family/Professional Partnerships of Family Voices (2018),

> Family-centered care is a way of providing services that assures the health and well-being of children and their families through respectful family/professional partnerships. It honors the strengths, cultures, traditions, and expertise that families and professionals bring to this relationship. Family-centered care improves the patient's and family's experience with health care, reduces stress, improves communication, reduces conflict (including lawsuits), and improves the health of children with chronic health conditions.

Roger Schwarz, an internationally recognized expert on team leadership, highlights five assumptions that illuminate and enrich the dynamics of interdisciplinary practice and expand one's lens beyond profession and discipline (Schwarz, 2013). These assumptions underpin what he describes as a mutual learning approach, an approach that strengthens teams of all types and combinations. In considering teams that might work with children with disabilities, these teams could comprise clinicians working to diagnose a challenging condition; partnerships between families and clinicians caring for a child who has a complex social situation; or social workers, educators, and other community service providers working with parents to manage or coordinate the systems of care for a child with special health care needs.

Schwarz's (2013) assumptions about teaming include the following:

1. I have information; so do other people.
2. Each of us sees things that others don't.
3. Differences are opportunities for learning.
4. People may disagree and still have pure motives.
5. I may be contributing to the problem.

These assumptions are highly relevant to engagement with and around the population of children with disabilities. For interdisciplinary practice to be effective, individuals from the many clinical and educational disciplines who interact must recognize that other disciplines, including families and self-advocates, bring their own perspectives and expertise, as well as personal preferences and challenges, which can make the translation of theoretical skills in the clinical practice setting daunting. For example, in the middle of an emotion-laden Individualized Education Program meeting with contrasting views on the continuation of therapies, participants should be aware of personal differences. For example, teams may consider each member's approach to and comfort with change (Discovery Learning, n.d.), conflict style (Killman Diagnostics, n.d.), and use of "thinking" and "feeling" or of "sensing" and "intuition" to understand and approach problems (Myers & Briggs Foundation, n.d.). Evidence suggests that during times of conflict or high emotions, team members should employ knowledge of motivations, personality preferences, and discipline from the perspective of the "other." For example, the reluctance of a team member to make a firm decision related to discontinuation of a therapy may have more to do with their personality preference to remain open to additional information than an unarticulated desire to sabotage the decision.

The second assumption underscores the importance of respect among those who collaborate. The third assumption is perhaps at the very core of the concept of interdisciplinary care: By learning from one another—from parents, from children, from assorted clinical disciplines, or from organizational leaders who oversee services—there is value added to the engagement. The value is truly greater than the sum of the parts in addressing what can often be complicated challenges. The fourth assumption expresses the important role of compassion for one another in collaborative efforts. To be able to step back, be nonjudgmental, and assume the best about one another opens the way for new and creative insights into how to address challenges. The fifth assumption underscores the important skill of self-reflection; that is, the ability to explore within oneself, with humility, the motivations and values behind one's preferences and perspectives.

The Interprofessional Education Collaborative (2016) has outlined four competency domains (see Table 30.1).

The Interdisciplinary Leadership Development Program (ILDP) at the University of North Carolina at Chapel Hill (Dodds et al., 2010) brought together graduate students, parents of children with special health care needs, state MCHB officials, and self-advocates to advance attitudes, beliefs, and skills in interdisciplinary practice. Table 30.2 shows questionnaire items that elicited attitudes and beliefs about interdisciplinary practice and captured the frequency of use of interdisciplinary skills 1–8 years after participation in the ILDP; the items were expressed as 5-point Likert rating scales (Margolis et al., 2013; Rosenberg, Margolis, Umble, & Chewning, 2015). These items reflect both the mutual learning assumptions and interprofessional collaborative competencies described above. The National Center for Interprofessional Practice and Education has become an important repository of tools to describe and assess interprofessional/interdisciplinary efforts (Brandt & Schmitz, 2017).

Engaging with parents on the interdisciplinary team provides an opportunity to reflect upon and employ Schwarz's assumptions as well as the skills and competencies described in Tables 30.1 and 30.2. In the

Table 30.1. Interprofessional education collaborative competency domains with selected competencies

Competency domains	Selected specific competencies
Values/ethics for interprofessional practice	Place the interests of patients and populations at the center of interprofessional health care delivery and population health programs and policies, with the goal of promoting health and health equity across the life span. Respect the unique cultures, values, roles/responsibilities, and expertise of other health professions and the impact these factors can have on health outcomes.
Roles/responsibilities	Communicate one's roles and responsibilities clearly to patients, families, community members, and other professionals. Recognize one's limitations in skills, knowledge, and abilities. Use unique and complementary abilities of all members of the team to optimize health and patient care.
Interprofessional communication	Choose effective communication tools and techniques, including information systems and communication technologies, to facilitate discussions and interactions that enhance team function. Listen actively and encourage ideas and opinions of other team members. Use respectful language appropriate for a given difficult situation, crucial conversation, or interprofessional conflict.
Teams and teamwork	Describe the process of team development and the roles and practices of effective teams. Apply leadership practices that support collaborative practice and team effectiveness. Use available evidence to inform effective teamwork and team-based practices.

From Interprofessional Education Collaborative. (2016). *Core competencies for interprofessional collaborative practice: 2016 update*. Washington, DC: Author.

Table 30.2. Questionnaire items to elicit interdisciplinary practice attitudes and beliefs and determine frequency of interdisciplinary skill use

Attitudes and beliefs about interdisciplinary practice
Providing services in interdisciplinary groups helps professionals become more sensitive to the diverse needs of consumers/patients than providing services as a single discipline.
The benefits of interdisciplinary patient care or program plans are worth the extra time it takes to communicate across disciplines.
The interdisciplinary approach reduces duplication and fragmentation in the delivery of care/services.
Providing services as an interdisciplinary group gets better results for consumers than working as single disciplines.
Interdisciplinary education should be a part of every health professional's preservice training.
I welcome the opportunity to collaborate with members of other disciplines.
I value the contributions of other disciplines to my work.
When I look for my next position, I will purposefully look for an opportunity where collaboration across disciplines is the norm.
Interdisciplinary skills
Assemble interdisciplinary group members appropriate for a given task.
Resolve conflicts in interdisciplinary groups.
Facilitate family–provider partnerships.
Effectively work with consumers with cultural backgrounds different from my own.
Effectively work other professionals with cultural backgrounds different from my own.
Coach coworkers in interdisciplinary practice.
Share ideas from my discipline with members of other disciplines.
Ask for insight or help from members of other disciplines to address a problem.
Use self-reflection to enhance my contributions to interdisciplinary work.
Establish decision-making procedures in an interdisciplinary group.
Develop a shared vision, roles, and responsibilities within an interdisciplinary group.
Critically evaluate information from other disciplines.
Evaluate how well an interdisciplinary group is working together.
Intervene to improve interdisciplinary group function.

(Reprinted with permission from Springer Nature. Maternal and Child Health Journal, 17[5]. Effects of interdisciplinary training on professionals, organizations and systems. 949–958. Margolis, L. H., Rosenberg, A., Umble, K., & Chewning, L. [2012]).

case study, for instance, the mother may have valuable insights into alternative service systems and care practices from her experience living in another state. Team members' expression of interest in her information is not only a chance to learn and build team trust, but may also provide a means to challenge the system status quo. Likewise, instead of dismissing a colleague's seemingly irrelevant discussion points, asking sincere questions will offer insight into his or her rationale and may lead to an improved plan of care for the child and family.

THE GROWTH AND DEVELOPMENT OF INTERDISCIPLINARY PRACTICE

Understanding the importance of bringing together multiple perspectives to advance the well-being of children has been the cornerstone of the evolution of programs and policies in the United States for more than a century. The legislation authorizing establishment of the Children's Bureau in 1912 noted multiple domains, including health, family, courts, and the workplace, pertaining to the welfare of children. Even the restriction on entering households, although intended to address the political concern over the intrusion of the federal government into private family life, expressed respect for families as partners in the care of children.

The Children's Bureau as the Legislative Foundation of Interdisciplinary Practice

The legislation authorizing establishment of the Children's Bureau noted the following:

> The said bureau shall investigate and report to the Secretary of Health and Human Services, upon all matters pertaining to the welfare of children and child life among all classes of our people, and shall especially investigate the questions of infant mortality, the birth rate, orphanage, juvenile courts, desertion, dangerous occupations, accidents and diseases of children, employment, legislation affecting children in the several States and Territories. But no official, or agent, or representative of said bureau shall, over the objection of the head of the family, enter any house used exclusively as a family residence. The chief of said bureau may from time to time publish the results of these investigations in such manner and to such extent as may be prescribed by the Secretary. (Children's Bureau, 1912)

The first training programs supported by the U.S. MCHB in the late 1940s were motivated by the need to develop professionals who could create services that enable children to benefit from the perspectives of multiple disciplines (Athey, Kavanagh, Bagley, & Hutchins, 2000). The move toward interdisciplinary practice gained legislative support with the passage of the Education for All Handicapped Children Act in 1975 (PL 94-142) and with greater emphasis in the Education of the Handicapped Amendments in 1986 (PL 99-457), especially Part C, which established early intervention services. Later amendments (PL 101-476 in 1990) resulted in the widely recognized Individuals with Disabilities Education Act (IDEA), further embedding interdisciplinary practice in legislative policy.

The Importance of an Interdisciplinary Approach to Children with Medical Complexity

According to Cohen and colleagues (2011, p. 529) children with medical complexity (CMC) have "medical fragility" and require "intensive care," two elements that alone demand the collaborative skills and perspectives of many disciplines and family members. The demand for a well-developed competency in interdisciplinary practice is further underscored by the additional phrase, "not easily met by existing health care models."

Advances in diagnosis and treatment have increased survival for children with even the most challenging of conditions. Still, the very low prevalence of CMC, estimated at 0.5% of the population of children (Kuo, Cohen, Agrawal, Berry, & Casey, 2011), should not be misleading, because the rate of increase of this population of children has resulted in tremendous demands. The costs—financial; emotional; and the time and attention of parents, clinicians, and educators—have prompted many models of care. Cohen and colleagues note, however, that "the evidence from examinations of clinical models of effective and efficient provision of health care for CMC remains remarkably limited. Existing care models include medical homes, co-management, and hospital-based and hybrid models that focus on care coordination" (2011, p. 532). Berry, Agrawal, Cohen, and Kuo (2013) and Allshouse, Comeau, Rodgers, and Wells (2018) further highlight the many, as-yet-unanswered, definitional, clinical, financial, health system, and family partnership questions for CMCs. The challenging nature of the conditions, in clinical terms, interpersonal demands, and stresses among institutional stakeholders (e.g., hospitals and insurers), suggests that attention to interdisciplinary competencies should be at the core of these many interactions.

The Role of Families

The intense demands on parents and family members in the care of CMCs and children with developmental disabilities underscore the importance of interdisciplinary skill development for parents as a key discipline. It is crucial to recognize that parents are likely to bring salient insights from the many social determinants (Artiga & Hinton, 2018) that influence their capacities to manage effectively the care of their children. For example, interdisciplinary practitioners must recognize that economic determinants, such as a parent's need to work both a day shift and an evening shift to pay a mortgage, may well impede their ability to follow through with well-meaning therapeutic recommendations for daily exercise regimens or parental social engagement. Similarly, inadequate community infrastructure, such as a lack of available transportation or the availability of affordable respite or child care, may prohibit parent attendance at meetings.

Many federal agencies and professional associations, including the MCHB, Family Voices, the American Academy of Pediatrics (Committee on Hospital Care and Institute for Patient-and Family-Centered Care, 2012), and others (e.g., the Association of University Centers on Disabilities), have articulated the important role of family members as partners with health professionals in providing care for CYSHCN. Indeed, performance measures to document the partnership role of family members have become part of the assessment process for MCHB training and service delivery programs (Maternal and Child Health Bureau, n.d.-a).

Family immersion in interdisciplinary education alongside clinical disciplines can influence their ability to partner both with their peers and health professionals. For example, families that engaged in the ILDP at the University of North Carolina reported enhanced skills in all six dimensions of collaborative family–professional partnerships described by Blue-Banning, Summers, Frankland, Nelson, and Beegle (2004): commitment, equality, trust, respect, communication, and appreciation of diversity of skills. As one parent participant explained:

> I truthfully feel really fortunate that I've been able to help and watch the evolution of family members moving into more of a systems approach, but to also do it with this partnership. It has just been, I can't articulate enough or clearly, the benefit that I think will be derived from this, perhaps not tomorrow, but five years down the road, not only for the graduate students who hopefully one day will go "oh, that's what they were talking about," because we know that experiential learning kicks in, but also for the family members . . . who really are sort of seeing themselves in a different frame and how powerful that is. I can't imagine the benefit any better than that." (Margolis et al., 2017)

As reflected in the case study, the departure of a respected team leader can precipitate a challenging period for team members. However, shifts in leadership are an excellent time to employ interdisciplinary leadership competencies. The new leader's changes in operational procedures, while initially perceived as premature, can pose an opportunity for team re-norming and perhaps expansion of interdisciplinary roles, a reenforcement of the concept of partnership.

MEASURING THE EFFECTS OF INTERDISCIPLINARY EDUCATION AND PRACTICE

On one level, interdisciplinary education involves increasing the understanding of the expertise that assorted disciplines bring to collaborative care. On another level, interdisciplinary education involves developing the capacity to utilize two fundamental insights, independent of discipline, that stem from the following two questions:

- What are my strengths, weaknesses, preferences, and motivations that inform my ability to work collaboratively?
- What are the strengths, weaknesses, preferences, and motivations that inform the ability of my colleagues to work collaboratively?

Evaluation of the ILDP at the University of North Carolina at Chapel Hill involved a collaboration among five training programs—Leadership Education in Neurodevelopmental Disorders (LEND), nutrition, pediatric dentistry, public health, and social work—in which all students participated in conventional courses and projects with interdisciplinary aspects. A subset of these students participated in ILDP workshops on interdisciplinary skills (Dodds et al., 2010). Table 30.3 shows an association between ILDP participation and the frequency of the practice of interdisciplinary skills. In other words, the intentional focus on interdisciplinary practice during the program seemed to enhance the frequency of skill use as far as 8 years afterwards. Qualitative analysis revealed the impact of the ILDP on participants' understanding of their own leadership styles and, equally as important, their abilities to appreciate the preferences and challenges of those with whom they work, which are fundamental to effective

Table 30.3. Effects of individual programs and the Interdisciplinary Leadership Development Program (ILDP) on the frequency of interdisciplinary skill practice

Participants/Skills Frequency[a]	ILDP	Non-ILDP	*P*-value for ILDP attendance	*P*-value for academic program
LEND	3.41	2.87	0.008	0.048
Nutrition	3.08			
Pediatric dentistry	2.79			
M.P.H.	3.27	3.06		
M.S.W./M.S.P.H.	3.08			

Source: Margolis, Rosenberg, Umble, and Chewning (2011).

[a]Very often = 5; Often = 4; Occasionally = 3; Rarely = 2; Never = 1

Key: LEND, Leadership Education in Neurodevelopmental Disabilities; M.P.H., master of public health; MSW/MSPH, master of social work/master of science in public health.

interdisciplinary collaboration (Margolis, Rosenberg, & Umble, 2015).

As noted, most evaluations of interdisciplinary education have been limited to the early levels of the typology described by the Kirkpatrick Model (Kirkpatrick Partners, 2018), specifically reaction, modification of attitudes/perceptions, acquisition of knowledge/skills, and behavioral change (Reeves, Boet, Zierler, & Kitto, 2015). The ILDP evaluation elicited outcomes at the change-in-organizational-practice level. Those who reported having made changes in any of the four domains of organizational practice (i.e., improve a specific program, improve the way an organization works or is structured, develop or improve a partnership, and develop a policy) reported greater mean frequencies in the use of interdisciplinary skills (Margolis et al., 2013).

From the outset, the focus of the ILDP was on understanding others rather than others' disciplines (Margolis et al., 2015). The ILDP seemed to encourage participants to develop a capacity to be curious about what motivates and underlies others' behavior and thinking and about their interests and needs rather than their specific positions when views differ (Schwarz, 2013). The ILDP curriculum, developed around a competency model, seemed to encourage a passion for interdisciplinary/interprofessional practice that may well enhance the effectiveness of the skills that participants acquired. These insights demonstrate that interdisciplinary/interprofessional training involves much more than simply taking courses in other disciplines or with students from other disciplines. The qualitative responses suggest that the ILDP played a meaningful role in the development of interdisciplinary attitudes, beliefs, and use of skills. This should alert training programs to the importance of gathering and analyzing behavioral outcomes (e.g., the frequency with which skills are used) beyond simply inquiring about the perceived value of a particular training or program.

IMPLEMENTING AND SUSTAINING INTERDISCIPLINARY EDUCATION AND PRACTICE

The growing interest in interdisciplinary education has prompted numerous efforts to define structures and processes to advance the practice (Brashers, Owen, & Haizlip, 2015; Hall & Zierler, 2015; Lawlis, Anson, & Greenfield, 2014; Menard & Varpio, 2014; National Center for Interprofessional Practice and Education, 2017; Oandasan & Reeves, 2005a, 2005b). Adapting questions posed by Oandasan and Reeves (2005b), Table 30.4 captures some of the key individual and team characteristics in planning and evaluating interdisciplinary collaborative practice initiatives. Attention to these characteristics can enhance the quality of care and begin to address the need to overcome the tendency to think in silos and to more effectively address differences in clinical opinions.

Adapting lessons from The National Academy of Sciences (NAS) report, *Facilitating Interdisciplinary Research* (National Academy of Sciences, National Academy of Engineering, & Institute of Medicine, 2005, p. 21), Table 30.5 presents a practical tool for programs to reflect on organizational characteristics necessary to advance interdisciplinary practice. Attention to such characteristics can bring a spotlight to practical challenges, such as developing the resources to support interdisciplinary efforts in, for example, care coordination, as well as to facilitate efforts to ensure that all disciplines, including self-advocates, are at the table.

The NAS describes four aspects for successful interdisciplinary research: 1) building bridges, 2) supporting the project, 3) facilities, and 4) organization/administration. Many of these conditions, meant to foster interdisciplinary research among scientists and

Table 30.4. Individual and team considerations in planning and evaluating interdisciplinary education and practice initiatives

Issues	Examples	Considerations
External/internal drivers that influence development	A clinical team makes the case for enhanced interdisciplinary training by noting the contributions of interdisciplinary practice to ongoing quality improvement, responding to the demands of health funders.	Climate of acceptance Current leadership
Potential partners	A recent occupational health graduate joins a clinical practice. After several months of participation in clinical conferences, she shares her observation that voices that could potentially contribute to the quality of care for complex cases are often not at the table. She encourages, for example, that two community organizations, known for their opportunities for families with children with special health care needs may be helpful partners.	Community organizations and individuals Family/friends of patients/clients
Opportunities within the current learning context	A physical therapist on a clinical team reaches out to the local YMCA to explore opportunities to expand its offerings for children with disabilities, such as accessible equipment and activities.	Patient population, practice sites Learner disciplines, training level, timing
Key players in designing intervention	While potential interventions often emerge from the IEP team and family, others such as siblings, extended family-members, and community-based and faith-based organizations may bring useful insights.	Degree of involvement Roles and responsibilities Communication strategies
The need to anticipate and overcome barriers	The interdisciplinary assumption that others may see things differently invites the insights and experiences of others about alternative treatment approaches in addition to potential barriers related to the IEP, based on their unique experiences.	Needs assessment, pre-evaluation
Goal of the activity at interprofessional and profession-specific levels	The members of a clinical team, working with families, share disciplinary insights as to their roles and responsibilities in working toward family-directed goals.	Defining and implementing essential elements of interdisciplinary practice
Specific objectives of activity	Team members establish a practice of regularly giving brief feedback to each other about the use of interdisciplinary skills.	Attitudes, skill development, team building to effect changes in clinical practice Quality of care and population health
Teaching methods and tools to meet objectives	Faculty regularly review literature on methods and activities to advance interdisciplinary continuing education.	Problem-based Practice-based Lab
Evaluation measures	A faculty team plans a series of workshops to introduce the principles of interdisciplinary practice to graduate students in health affairs. While the team will measure satisfaction with the workshops, they also commit to observe and measure interdisciplinary skills among the participants.	Satisfaction, learning of attitudes, knowledge, skills Behaviors that result in short and long term measurable impacts
Sustainability	Graduates of three diverse LEND programs become the directors of clinical training for their respective disciplines at a major medical center. They recognize that in order to realize the benefits of interdisciplinary training and practice, they approach center leadership with proposals and invite a conversation on strategies to raise the necessary resources.	Funding Challenging the culture

Source: Oandasan and Reeves (2005a).

engineers, are applicable to creating positive settings for interdisciplinary education and practice in other fields. For example, *building bridges* includes creating an "environment that encourages faculty/researcher collaboration"; discussing "common problems to solve"; and having "seminars to foster bridges between students, postdoctoral scholars, and investigators at the same institution" (National Academy of Sciences, National Academy of Engineering, & Institute of Medicine, 2005, p. 21).

In *Facilitating Interdisciplinary Research,* the importance of *other institutional policies* is noted. For example, tenure/promotion policies can advance training initiatives if they are recognized as valuable scholarly contributions, or they can impede such training if criteria are limited to narrow, single disciplined–based measures (Hammick, Freeth, Koppel, Reeves, & Barr, 2007).

With regard to governance, the report suggests that a matrix organization may best reflect an interdisciplinary environment. This means that faculty bring to

Table 30.5. Organizational characteristics needed to advance interdisciplinary education and practice: A reflection tool for programs

Characteristic	Definition	Examples
Physical/virtual environment	The virtual and physical environments allow collaborators from different disciplines to meet in a reasonably convenient way, either electronically or in person.	Members of an interdisciplinary group are located in offices with convenient access to one another. Expansion of the web-based clinical platform to assist communicating and sharing of appropriate documents with extended family members and community partners.
Institutional strategic plans	Missions, visions, and goals to support interdisciplinary research and teaching and community engagement	A stated priority in an organization's strategic plan is to further integrate interdisciplinary research, education, and public service. An organization's goal is that all clinicians must participate in at least one interdisciplinary continuing education offering each year.
Financial policies	Institutional financial policies make available monetary and in-kind resources to facilitate interdisciplinary collaboration.	A university policy satisfies the needs of all interdisciplinary partners to share indirect costs on grants. An institutional policy encourages departments such as developmental pediatrics, speech and language pathology, and childhood education to pool financial resources to provide joint training programs.
Other institutional policies	Institutional policies other than financial policies facilitate and support interdisciplinary collaboration.	The dean of a school of nursing promotes a policy to encourage that articles written with colleagues from other disciplines are valued in evaluation for promotion. An occupational therapist paves the way for a physical therapy graduate student to satisfy clinical education requirements related to adaptive equipment use.
Scheduling	A shared calendar that facilitates collaboration across institutional units (e.g., academic programs or departments).	Discipline-specific departments have a common calendar that allows designated blocks of time to be set aside for interdisciplinary education and meetings. A pediatric residency program sets aside a designated block of time for exchange between disciplines (e.g., a journal club).
Governance	Multiple stakeholders, including professionals, clients, families, and/or community members, are active participants in setting the direction of interdisciplinary activities.	The program includes all relevant stakeholder groups on a steering/advisory committee. Family representatives are involved in the revision of clinical and nonclinical curriculum through activities such as completing surveys, participating in planning meetings, and providing ongoing feedback.
Institutional leadership	Relevant institutional leaders, such as deans, chairs, provosts, and clinical program directors acknowledge and support an overall strategic goal of interdisciplinary education, research, and collaboration among schools, departments, and programs.	The chair of a special education department intentionally hires faculty from disciplines such as public health, not normally represented in the department. A dean from a school of medicine supports a partnership with the university's school of public health to offer students dual-degree options between schools.
Champions	Individuals who advocate for, initiate, and maintain clinical or programmatic interdisciplinary collaborations.	A faculty member from a special needs nutrition program initiates a multischool collaborative group to develop an interdisciplinary leadership curriculum. She encourages other faculty to engage in similar initiatives. A psychologist holds a program accountable to ensure that all necessary disciplines are represented on clinical assessment teams.
Culture of collaboration	A culture of interdisciplinary collaboration exists when it is the norm for professionals from different disciplines to value working together. Responsibility is shared in reaching goals, making joint decisions, resolving conflicts, and developing and implementing activities. Trust and respect make it possible to share responsibility in reaching goals.	In response to a community funding opportunity, one of the first question a clinician asks is, "How will I involve my colleagues from other disciplines?" When facing complex family situations, professionals feel comfortable turning to colleagues in other disciplines to provide different perspectives on the situations.
Accountability	Program leaders routinely evaluate whether the programmatic structure, function, and outcomes are consistent with interdisciplinary practice.	In the annual review of a clinical team member, a department head solicits a report about interdisciplinary activities. Clinicians routinely review reports to ensure that the information provided to clients (individuals and caregivers) reflects an interdisciplinary family-centered interpretation of clinical assessments and suggestions for intervention.

(continued)

Table 30.5. *(continued)*

Characteristic	Definition	Examples
Interdisciplinary curricula and instructional methods	Curricular content and instructional objectives are designed to create interdisciplinary thinking and practice among students or trainees. The structure of the training program may include collaborative efforts among disciplines such as joint degrees, courses jointly sponsored and taught, or team teaching by colleagues from varied disciplines.	A program offers an interdisciplinary leadership certificate that includes courses and learning experiences that reflect multiple disciplines. Interdisciplinary clinical teams are used as a teaching forum to advance interdisciplinary knowledge and skills.
Research initiatives and publications	Interdisciplinary research projects and publications integrate the perspectives of investigators from multiple disciplines.	A social work faculty member and a maternal and child health faculty member co-author an article on the role of Title V in domestic violence prevention. A multidisciplinary team authors a paper related to the assessment of children with rare genetic disorders.

the table their different skills or disciplines to focus on collaborating such that their shared expertise can facilitate interdisciplinary training in contrast to enhancing the development of their particular skills in trainees.

In addition, the role of a *culture of collaboration,* a receptive interpersonal and institutional environment where the norms support interdisciplinary efforts, seems more often implicit than explicit in the literature. Commitment to a process of *accountability* is key. *Facilitating Interdisciplinary Research* notes that there should be rewards for academic leaders who encourage interdisciplinary training as well as professional recognition. On the level of programs, there needs to be an explicit effort to articulate goals, review progress, and make changes as indicated, as well as a commitment to accountability across programs and institutions (McHugh, Margolis, Rosenberg, & Humphreys, 2016).

As emphasized by Reeves and colleagues (2015) and the Institute of Medicine (2015), there is an extensive literature on the effects of interdisciplinary training. There are, however, relatively few studies that speak to outcomes; that is, the effects of interdisciplinary care on service delivery and/or patient care. Many studies focus on the development of perceptions and attitudes; knowledge and skills; and, to some degree, behaviors. Table 30.5 suggests that many characteristics of a program or institution must be aligned and addressed. Similarly, at the team level, interactions and meetings about clinical matters should be intentionally attentive to the elements of meaningful interdisciplinary practice.

SUMMARY

- The complex interactions among many systems demand an understanding of interdisciplinary attitudes and a commitment to the skills and competencies that reflect interdisciplinary practice.
- This understanding and commitment build on a valuable and insightful foundation expressed over the years in federal and state policy, programmatic practices, and educational initiatives.
- In spite of the longstanding engagement by families, clinicians, researchers, and policy makers, there must be investment in ongoing efforts to define and evaluate the impact of interdisciplinary education and practice.
- To reach the goals of interdisciplinary practice, the many faculty, programs, and organizations that touch the lives of these children and their families should reflect intentionally on interdisciplinary principles and characteristics as they seek to implement this type of practice.

ADDITIONAL RESOURCES

Physio: Multidisciplinary Care: https://www.physio-pedia.com/Multidisciplinary/Interdisciplinary_Management_in_Cerebral_Palsy

My Child Without Limits: http://www.mychildwithoutlimits.org/plan/early-intervention/multidisciplinary-evaluation-and-assessment/

Association of University Centers on Disabilities (AUCD): https://www.aucd.org/template/page.cfm?id=473

Additional resources can be found online in Appendix D: Childhood Disabilities Resources, Services, and Organizations (see About the Online Companion Materials).

REFERENCES

Allshouse, C., Comeau, M., Rodgers, R., & Wells, N. (2018). Families of children with medical complexity: A view from the front lines. *Pediatrics, 141*(Suppl. 3), S195–S201. doi:10.1542/peds.2017-1284D

Artiga, S., & Hinton, E. (2018). *Beyond health care: The role of social determinants in promoting health and health equity. Issue brief.* San Francisco, CA: Kaiser Family Foundation.

Athey, J., Kavanagh, L., Bagley, K., & Hutchins, V. (2000). *Building the future: The Maternal and Child Health Training Program.* Arlington, VA: National Center for Education in Maternal and Child Health.

Berry, J. G., Agrawal, R. K., Cohen, E., & Kuo, D. Z. (2013). *The landscape of medical care for children with medical complexity.* Overland Park, KS: Children's Hospital Association.

Blue-Banning, M. A., Summers, J. C., Frankland, H. L., Nelson, L., & Beegle, G. (2004). Dimensions of family and professional partnerships: Constructive guidelines for collaboration. *Exceptional Children, 70*(2), 167–185.

Boyle, C., Boulet, S., Schieve, L., Cohen, R., Blumberg, S., & Yeargin-Allsopp, M. (2011). Trends in the prevalence of developmental disabilities in US children, 1997-2008. *Pediatrics, 127,* 1034–1042.

Brandt, B. F., & Schmitz, C. C. (2017). The US National Center for Interprofessional Practice and Education Measurement and Assessment collection. *Journal of Interprofessional Care, 31*(3), 277–281. doi:10.1080/13561820.2017.1286884

Brashers, V., Owen, J., & Haizlip, J. (2015). Interprofessional education and practice guide no. 2: Developing and implementing a center for interprofessional education. *Journal of Interprofessional Care, 29*(2), 95–99. doi:10.3109/13561820.2014.962130

Child Trends. (2015). *Family structure.* Retrieved from https://www.childtrends.org/wp-content/uploads/2015/03/59_Family_Structure.pdf

Children's Bureau. April 9, 1912, ch. 73, § 2, 37 stat. 79.

Cohen, E., Kuo, D. Z., Agrawal, R., Berry, J. G., Bhagat, S. K. M., Simon, T. D., & Srivastava, R. (2011). Children with medical complexity: An emerging population for clinical and research initiatives. *Pediatrics, 127*(3), 529–538. doi:10.1542/peds.2010-0910

Colby, S. L., & Ortman, J. M. (2015). Projections of the size and composition of the U.S. population: 2014 to 2060. *Current Population Reports,* P25-1143.

Committee on Hospital Care and Institute for Patient and Family-Centered Care. (2012). Patient- and family-centered care and the pediatrician's role. *Pediatrics, 129*(2), 394–404. doi:10.1542/peds.2011-3084

Discovery Learning. (n.d.). *Change style indicator.* Retrieved from https://www.discoverylearning.com/store/assessments/change-style-indicator/

Dodds, J., Vann, W., Lee, J., Rosenberg, A., Rounds, K., Roth, M., . . . Margolis, L. H. (2010). The UNC-CH MCH Leadership Training Consortium: Building the capacity to develop interdisciplinary MCH leaders. *Maternal and Child Health Journal, 14*(4), 642–648. doi:10.1007/s10995-009-0483-0

Family Voices. (n.d.). *Our mission.* Retrieved from http://www.familyvoices.org/about?id=0003

Family Voices. (2018). *What is family-centered care?* Retrieved from http://familyvoices.org/familycenteredcare/

Frenk, J., Chen, L., Bhutta, Z. A., Cohen, J., Crisp, N., Evans, T., . . . Zurayk, H. (2010). Health professionals for a new century: Transforming education to strengthen health systems in an interdependent world. *The Lancet, 376*(9756), 1923–1958. doi:10.1016/S0140-6736(10)61854-5

Gerhardt, C. (2016). Globalization and families. In C. L. Shehan (Ed.), *The Wiley-Blackwell encyclopedia of family studies.* Retrieved from https://doi.org/10.1002/9781119085621.wbefs236

Hall, L. W., & Zierler, B. K. (2015). Interprofessional education and practice guide no. 1: Developing faculty to effectively facilitate interprofessional education. *Journal of Interprofessional Care, 29*(1), 3–7. doi:10.3109/13561820.2014.937483

Hammick, M., Freeth, D., Koppel, I., Reeves, S., & Barr, H. (2007). A best evidence systematic review of interprofessional education: BEME Guide No. 9. *Medical Teacher, 29*(8), 735–751. doi:10.1080/01421590701682576

Institute of Medicine. (2015). *Measuring the impact of interprofessional education on collaborative practice and patient outcomes.* Washington, DC: National Academies Press.

Interprofessional Education Collaborative. (2016). *Core competencies for interprofessional collaborative practice: 2016 update.* Washington, DC: Author.

Kilmann Diagnostics. (n.d.). *An overview of the TKI.* Retrieved from http://www.kilmanndiagnostics.com/overview-thomas-kilmann-conflict-mode-instrument-tki

Kirkpatrick Partners. (2018). *Kirkpatrick model.* Retrieved from https://www.kirkpatrickpartners.com/Our-Philosophy/The-Kirkpatrick-Model

Kohn, L. T., Corrigan, J. M., & Donaldson, M. S. (Eds.). (2000). *To err is human: Building a safer health system.* Washington, DC: Institute of Medicine (US) Committee on Quality of Health Care in America. National Academies Press. doi:10.17226/9728

Kuo, D. Z., Cohen, E., Agrawal, R., Berry, J. G., & Casey, P. H. (2011). A national profile of caregiver challenges among more medically complex children with special health care needs. *Archives of Pediatrics & Adolescent Medicine, 165*(11), 1020–1026. doi:10.1001/archpediatrics.2011.172

Lawlis, T. R., Anson, J., & Greenfield, D. (2014). Barriers and enablers that influence sustainable interprofessional education: A literature review. *Journal of Interprofessional Care, 28*(4), 305–310. doi:10.3109/13561820.2014.895977

Margolis, L. H., Fahje Steber, K., Rosenberg, A., Palmer, A., Rounds, K., & Wells, M. (2017). Partnering with parents in interprofessional leadership graduate education to promote family-professional partnerships. *Journal of Interprofessional Care, 31*(4), 497–504. doi:10.1080/13561820.2017.1296418

Margolis, L., Rosenberg, A., & Umble, K. (2015). The relationship between interprofessional leadership education and interprofessional practice: How intensive personal leadership education makes a difference. *Health and Interprofessional Practice, 2*(3), 1–12. doi:10.7710/2159-1253.1071

Margolis, L. H., Rosenberg, A., Umble, K., & Chewning, L. (2011). *Effects of interdisciplinary training on MCH professionals, organizations, and systems.* Retrieved from https://mchb.hrsa.gov/research/project_info.asp?ID=86

Margolis, L. H., Rosenberg, A., Umble, K., & Chewning, L. (2013). Effects of interdisciplinary training on MCH professionals, organizations and systems. *Maternal and Child Health Journal, 17*(5), 949–958. doi:10.1007/s10995-012-1078-8

Maternal and Child Health Bureau. (n.d.-a). *Discretionary grant data collection.* Retrieved from https://mchb.hrsa.gov/data-research-epidemiology/discretionary-grant-data-collection

Maternal and Child Health Bureau. (n.d.-b) *Programs and initiatives, children with special health care needs.* Retrieved from https://mchb.hrsa.gov/maternal-child-health-initiatives/mchb-programs

Maternal and Child Health Bureau. (2018). *Children with special health care needs.* Retrieved from https://mchb.hrsa.gov/maternal-child-health-topics/children-and-youth-special-health-needs

McHugh, M. C., Margolis, L. H., Rosenberg, A., & Humphreys, E. (2016). Advancing MCH interdisciplinary/interprofessional leadership training and practice through a learning collaborative. *Maternal and Child Health Journal, 20*(11), 2247–2253. doi:10.1007/s10995-016-2129-3

Menard, P., & Varpio, L. (2014). Selecting an interprofessional education model for a tertiary health care setting. *Journal of Interprofessional Care, 28*(4), 311–316. doi:10.3109/13561820.2014.893419

Myers & Briggs Foundation. (n.d.). *MBTI basics.* Retrieved from https://www.myersbriggs.org/my-mbti-personality-type/mbti-basics/home.htm?bhcp=1

National Academy of Sciences, National Academy of Engineering, & the Institute of Medicine. (2005). *Facilitating interdisciplinary research.* Washington, DC: National Academies Press.

National Center for Family/Professional Partnerships of Family Voices. (2018). *What is family-centered care?* Retrieved from http://familyvoices.org/familycenteredcare/

National Center for Interprofessional Practice and Education. (2017). *About us.* Retrieved from https://nexusipe.org/

Oandasan, I., & Reeves, S. (2005a). Key elements for interprofessional education. Part 1: The learner, the educator and the learning context. *Journal of Interprofessional Care, 19*(Suppl. 1), 21–38. doi:10.1080/13561820500083550

Oandasan, I., & Reeves, S. (2005b). Key elements of interprofessional education. Part 2: Factors, processes and outcomes. *Journal of Interprofessional Care, 19*(Suppl. 1), 39–48. doi:10.1080/13561820500081703

Ortman, J., Velkoff, V., & Hogan, H. (2014). *An aging nation: The older population in the United States.* Washington, DC: U.S. Census Bureau.

Reeves, S., Boet, S., Zierler, B., & Kitto, S. (2015). Interprofessional education and practice guide no. 3: Evaluating interprofessional education. *Journal of Interprofessional Care, 29*(4), 305–312. doi:10.3109/13561820.2014.1003637

Rosenberg, A., Margolis, L. H., Umble, K., & Chewning, L. (2015). Fostering intentional interdisciplinary leadership in developmental disabilities: The North Carolina LEND experience. *Maternal and Child Health Journal, 19*(2), 290–299. doi:10.1007/s10995-014-1618-5

Schwarz, R. (2013). *Smart leaders, smarter teams: How you and your team get unstuck to get results.* San Francisco, CA: Jossey-Bass.

World Health Organization. (2010). *Framework for action on interprofessional education and collaborative practice.* Geneva, Switzerland: Author.

CHAPTER 31

Early Intervention Services

Toby M. Long

Upon completion of this chapter, the reader will

- Describe the rationale for and history of early intervention services
- Explain the principles of early intervention
- Describe the programs and supports available for young children receiving early intervention services and their families
- Identify the components of federal legislation that support those receiving early intervention services

The availability of **early intervention (EI)** services in virtually every community in the United States shows society's commitment to supporting infants and toddlers with developmental disabilities and their families. EI services are usually provided in the context of federal legislation that defines the structural components and principles governing state-based services for infants and toddlers (from birth to 3 years of age) with disabilities. Services and supports available include **habilitation** therapies, family counseling, early childhood educational services, and others as determined by a **multidisciplinary** team in collaboration with the child's family. This array of services is provided in many settings, in collaboration with a variety of agencies, and utilizes various models of service delivery.

CASE STUDY

Carl is a 6-month-old boy who was born at a gestational age of 26 weeks. After a difficult 4-month hospitalization in the neonatal intensive care unit, he was discharged to his home. **Neurodevelopmental assessment** just prior to discharge showed that his cognitive function was at a newborn level and he had markedly increased tone in his legs. Based on these significant developmental delays/abnormalities, he was referred by his neonatologist to the local EI program. After a comprehensive, multidisciplinary evaluation, he was determined to be eligible for services. An individualized family service plan (IFSP) was then developed. Carl was provided weekly home visits by a physical therapist (for increased tone) and speech-language therapist (for feeding problems). These therapies were also provided at his child care center on a weekly basis. In addition, each provider arranged a home visit with Carl's parents once a month so that they could discuss family concerns and priorities. As a result of the support provided through these interactions, Carl's parents are feeling increasingly confident and competent in caring for him and in supporting his development.

Thought Questions:

How does the primary service provider model of service delivery support the principles of EI? How can EI team members use the description of participation to guide the development of the IFSP?

PRINCIPLES OF EARLY INTERVENTION

The primary goals of EI are to enhance the development of infants and toddlers and minimize the potential for developmental delay by supporting the family to promote their child's optimal development and facilitate the child's participation in family and community activities, (Dunst, Bruder, & Espe-Scherwindt, 2014; Workgroup on Principles and Practices in Natural Environments, 2008). Within those goals, EI focuses on encouraging active participation of families in the intervention by embedding strategies into everyday activities and routines and by delivering services in a manner that is

- Family centered and culturally and linguistically competent;
- Developmentally supportive, strengths based, and helpful for promoting children's participation in their natural environments;
- Comprehensive, coordinated, and team based;
- Individualized, flexible, and responsive to the changing needs of young children and families; and
- Based on the highest quality evidence available.

RESEARCH SUPPORT FOR THE VALUE OF EARLY INTERVENTION

Research over the last 30 years indicates that intervention during early childhood achieves immediate and sustained developmental benefits (Center on the Developing Child at Harvard University, 2010; Spittle, Orton, Anderson, Boyd, & Doyle, 2015). These benefits have also been shown to save money for the community and family over time (Heckman, 2012; also see the textbox on what Heckman has contributed to the evidence in support of EI). Much scientific evidence demonstrates that EI programs generate important benefits for both young children at risk for disability and for those with established disabilities (Dunst et al., 2014; Early Childhood Technical Assistance Center, 2018a). Numerous studies also have identified that a decline in development can be prevented or at least mitigated through providing comprehensive EI programs (Spittle et al., 2015). However, individual responsiveness to EI varies depending on a variety of biological, social, and environmental issues. Consistent evidence for long-term benefits is limited. Current research, in addition to determining the effectiveness of early childhood interventions, focuses on determining which program elements are most effective for which children and under what circumstances. Research also investigates how programs can produce the greatest benefits at the lowest cost.

Return on Investment of EI

James Heckman, a Nobel Prize–winning economist, has demonstrated that high-quality early childhood programs for vulnerable or disadvantaged children can deliver a 13% return on investment (see heckmanequation.org to learn more).

PREVALENCE AND EPIDEMIOLOGY

The Individuals with Disabilities Education Improvement Act (IDEA) of 2004 (PL 108-446) Part C program (Early Intervention Program for Infants and Toddlers with Disabilities) mandates coordinated, multidisciplinary, and interagency systems to deliver specialized EI services, early childhood special education (ECSE), or special education (SE) to all eligible children from birth up to 3 years of age displaying cognitive, behavioral, and/or physical developmental delays or disabilities. In 2015, 357,715 children from birth up to 3 years of age received EI services through Part C of IDEA (3% of the population of children in this age range; U.S. Department of Education, 2017). Children receiving Part C services include those with developmental delays and those with diagnosed conditions.

Overall, approximately 64% of children eligible for Part C services have a developmental delay, 20% have a diagnosed medical condition, and 16% have biomedical and/or environmental risk factors (Hebbeler, Mallik, & Taylor, 2010). In addition, 43% of children receiving services live in households with incomes less than $25,000 a year (Hebbeler et al., 2010). Given the well-established association between disadvantaged status and disability (Ekono, Yang, & Smith, 2016), the system's ability to enroll large numbers of these families is commendable.

COMPONENTS OF PART C OF IDEA: THE INFANTS AND TODDLERS WITH DISABILITIES PROGRAM

Based on research indicating that services provided to young children could prevent or ameliorate biological, social, and environmental risks on development (Spittle et al., 2015), the 1986 amendments to IDEA (then called the Education of the Handicapped Children Act, PL 99-457) established the Infants and Toddlers Program, or EI System. From its inception, this part of the law was meant to be a system of cooperation and collaboration across child-serving systems to provide comprehensive services and supports to families with infants and toddlers with disabilities or delays. The purposes of the Infants and Toddlers Program, or Part C of IDEA, are stated in the supporting legislation as follows:

1. To enhance the development of infants and toddlers with disabilities, to minimize their potential for developmental delay, and to recognize the significant brain development that occurs during a child's first 3 years of life
2. To reduce the educational costs to society, including our nation's schools, by minimizing the need for SE and related services after infants and toddlers with disabilities reach school age
3. To maximize the potential for individuals with disabilities to live independently in society
4. To enhance the capacity of families to meet the special needs of their infants and toddlers with disabilities
5. To enhance the capacity of States and local agencies and service providers to identify, evaluate, and meet the needs of all children, particularly minority, low-income, inner city, and rural children, and infants and toddlers in foster care

Each state must create a system that includes 16 components (see the textbox titled IDEA: Minimum Components of a Statewide, Comprehensive System of Early Intervention Services to Infants and Toddlers with Special Needs). States are required to ensure that those individuals providing the services are appropriately qualified and that a central directory of providers, services, and agencies is available to help identify resources of all kinds relevant to EI. Other structural components are administrative in nature, addressing interagency cooperation, reimbursement, and procedural safeguards. In addition to policies that regulate procedures, financing, and professional standards, five components are specific to providing services: 1) identification and referral, 2) determination of eligibility, 3) development of an IFSP, 4) provision of services, and 5) transition from EI services at age 3. In addition, states are required to report the percentage of infants and toddlers with IFSPs who demonstrate improvement in three outcome areas: social-emotional skills, acquisition and use of knowledge and skills, and the ability to take appropriate action to meet needs.

IDEA: Minimum Components of a Statewide, Comprehensive System of Early Intervention Services to Infants and Toddlers with Special Needs

1. A rigorous definition of the term *developmental delay*
2. Appropriate EI services based on scientifically based research that are, to a practical extent, available to all infants and toddlers with disabilities and their families, including Native American and homeless infants and toddlers
3. Timely and comprehensive multidisciplinary evaluation of the needs of children and family-directed identification of the needs of each family
4. IFSP and service coordination
5. A comprehensive Child Find and referral system
6. A public awareness program, including the preparation and dissemination of information to be given to parents
7. A central directory of services, resources, and research and demonstration projects
8. A comprehensive system of personnel development, including the training of paraprofessionals and primary referral sources
9. Policies and procedures that ensure that personnel are appropriately and adequately prepared and trained
10. A single line of authority in a lead agency designated or established by the governor
11. A policy pertaining to contracting or otherwise arranging for services
12. A procedure for securing timely reimbursement of funds
13. Procedural safeguards
14. A system for compiling data on the EI system
15. A state interagency coordinating council
16. Policies and procedures to ensure that to the maximum extent appropriate, EI services are provided in natural environments except when EI cannot be achieved satisfactorily in a natural environment

Identification and Referral

Under Part C regulations of IDEA (PL 108–446), states are required to establish programs for finding and identifying infants and toddlers who may qualify for EI. These programs and procedures are referred to as Child Find (http://ectacenter.org/topics/earlyid/idoverview.asp). Child Find efforts are most effective when coordinated with other EI programs, such as Medicaid's early and periodic screening, diagnosis, and treatment program. Primary care providers are in a key position to identify young children who are at risk for or who have developmental delays or disabilities (Adams, Tapia, & Council on Children with Disabilities, 2013).

Developmental screening is often the first step in identifying and referring infants and toddlers who could benefit from EI services. When developmental screening occurs in the context of a well-child medical visit, it reinforces the concept that health and development are interrelated. Responding to parental concerns about a child's development has been shown to be as effective in identifying developmental delay as professional opinion and/or standardized screening (Council on Children with Disabilities, Section on Developmental Behavioral Pediatrics, Bright Futures Steering Committee, & Medical Home Initiatives for Children with Special Needs Project Advisory Committee, 2006; Woolfenden et al., 2014). An infant or toddler can be referred to the local EI program directly by anyone (including a relative or friend) who suspects that the child has a developmental delay or disability. Best practice supports referrals to local EI programs that come from parents following discussions with their primary health care providers or from the primary health care provider (Adams et al., 2013). Developmental screening is another option that a state may choose to include as part of its comprehensive Child Find system (IDEA 2004). It should involve the family and other sources of information using a process that is culturally and linguistically sensitive. It should be reliable, valid, cost effective, and time efficient. It should be seen not only as a means of early identification, but also as a service that helps the family understand the child's developmental progress. Several developmental screening tests are commercially available, including 1) the Ages & Stages Questionnaires®, Third Edition (ASQ-3®;Squires & Bricker, 2009); 2) the Denver II (Frankenburg et al., 1992); and 3) the Parents' Evaluations of Developmental Status (Glascoe, 1997).

Determining Eligibility for Early Intervention Services

According to IDEA, each state is required to define criteria by which a child is eligible to receive EI services under Part C. Of note, infants and toddlers who do not meet the eligibility criteria for services under the state-run Part C program can still receive services through other systems, such as directly at a clinic or through a private practitioner.

Current federal regulations describe three categories of eligibility: 1) The child demonstrates a measurable **developmental delay** as defined by each state; 2) the child has a diagnosed physical or mental condition that has a high probability of resulting in developmental delay (e.g., a child with Down syndrome); or 3) professionals who are conducting the evaluation determine that a child demonstrates behaviors indicating atypical development (e.g., a child suspected to have autism) and could benefit from EI services and supports, a process referred to as informed clinical opinion. IDEA indicates that a child meets the definition of developmental delay if he or she has a measurable delay in one or more of five areas: cognitive, physical, communication, social or emotional, and/or adaptive skills. Each state, however, decides how to define the term *measurable delay*. State-specific eligibility criteria can be found online at http://ectacenter.org/~pdfs/topics/earlyid/partc_elig_table.pdf.

A multidisciplinary team, defined by IDEA (34 CFR §303.24) as the involvement of two or more separate disciplines or professions, conducts the eligibility evaluation to determine if a child meets the state-specified eligibility criteria. The process often begins when the family first calls the infant and toddler program for assistance. The program then performs four activities: coordination of a multidisciplinary eligibility evaluation, assessment, development of the IFSP, and commencement of appropriate EI services. These activities must be completed within 45 calendar days from the date that the family provides consent to the initial screening, evaluation, or assessment (§303.310 [b, 2]). After a family is referred, a service coordinator is assigned to partner with the family to plan and coordinate all of the steps leading to the development of a service plan, if appropriate. If the child is found to be eligible, the service coordinator will 1) continue to assist the family in coordinating services across agency lines; 2) serve as the single contact for parents/families to obtain needed help and services; 3) assist families in gaining access to services identified in the IFSP; and 4) help the family through the process of transition to preschool, school, or other appropriate services or exiting the program.

The eligibility evaluation process must be timely, comprehensive, and multidisciplinary. Pertinent records relating to the child's current health status as well as medical history must be reviewed. The evaluation includes assessing the child in five areas of development: physical (including vision, hearing, and gross and fine motor development), cognitive, communication, social-emotional, and adaptive. The multidisciplinary evaluation team must include 1) a family member and

2) two professionals representing different disciplines or one individual who is qualified in more than one discipline or profession (§303.24). For example, the professionals might include an early childhood special educator and a speech-language pathologist or perhaps a motor therapist such as an occupational therapist or a physical therapist. The process must reflect the unique strengths and needs of the child. In addition, family members provide information about concerns, priorities, and resources that may affect their child. (See Box 31.1 on the role that families play on the team.)

In the case study at the beginning of this chapter, Carl was determined to be eligible for EI following his evaluation by a physical therapist and special educator. The assessment indicated that Carl met the specified amount of delay for the state in which he resides in the motor area and in his adaptive skills. In addition, at the time of the evaluation he continued to demonstrate hypertonia in both his legs. The eligibility team also gathered information from the family using a routines-based interview process. All this information was used to develop Carl's IFSP.

Early Intervention Services

Assistive Technology Devices and Services

Audiology

Family training

Health services

Medical services (for diagnostic or evaluation purposes only)

Speech and language pathology

Physical therapy

Occupational therapy

Psychological services

Service coordination

Social work services

Special instruction (also referred to as developmental therapy)

Transportation and related costs

Vision services

Other services as determined by IFSP team

Development of an Individualized Family Service Plan

If the child is found eligible for services through the multidisciplinary child and family evaluation process, a multidisciplinary team, including the parents, develops an IFSP, ensuring that the required services are identified and coordinated and that they relate to the outcomes decided by the team. (See the Early Intervention Services textbox for a list of the services available through Part C). The IFSP can also identify other services if needed to meet the outcomes identified in the IFSP (§303.13 [d]). These services must be provided in natural environments to the maximum extent appropriate to meet the needs of the child. Natural environments are defined in federal regulations as "settings that are natural or normal for an infant or toddler without a disability, and may include the home" (Sec. 303.26). Natural environments are not limited to the home or any other specific place, but they should include activities and routines that offer naturally occurring learning opportunities (Dunst et al., 2014; Law, Darrah, & Pollack, 2011a, 2011b). IDEA describes eight required elements of the IFSP (see the Required Elements of an Individualized Family Service Plan textbox).

Required Elements of an Individualized Family Service Plan

1. A statement of the infant's or toddler's present levels of physical development, cognitive development, communication development, social or emotional development, and adaptive development based on objective criteria

BOX 31.1 INTERDISCIPLINARY CARE

Families Are Critical Team Members

As a member of the multidisciplinary team, the family contributes to the evaluation and assessment process by discussing their concerns for their child, their priorities, and the resources they have available that they find supportive. This information is used to formulate outcomes and identify services and supports that are responsive to the family's needs.

2. A statement of the family's resources, priorities, and concerns relating to enhancing the development of the family's infant or toddler with a disability
3. A statement of the major outcomes expected to be achieved for the infant or toddler and the family, as well as the criteria, procedures, and timelines used to determine the degree to which progress toward achieving the outcomes is being made and whether modifications or revisions of the outcomes or services are necessary
4. A statement of specific EI services necessary to meet the unique needs of the infant or toddler and the family, including the frequency, intensity, and method of delivering services
5. A statement of the natural environments in which EI services should be appropriately provided, including a justification of the extent, if any, to which the services will not be provided in a natural environment
6. The projected dates for initiation of services and the anticipated duration of the services
7. The identification of a service coordinator from the professionals most immediately relevant to the infant's or toddler's or family's needs (or who is otherwise qualified to carry out all applicable responsibilities) who will be responsible for the implementation of the plan and coordination with other agencies and persons
8. The steps to be taken to support the transition of the toddler with a disability to preschool or other appropriate services

Key Principles for Providing Early Intervention Services in Natural Environments

1. Infants and toddlers learn best through everyday experiences and interactions with familiar people in familiar contexts.
2. All families, with the necessary supports and resources, can enhance their children's learning and development.
3. The primary role of a service provider in early intervention is to work with and support family members and caregivers in children's lives.
4. The early intervention process, from initial contacts through transition, must be dynamic and individualized to reflect the child's and family members' preferences, learning styles, and cultural beliefs.
5. IFSP outcomes must be functional and based on children's and families' needs and family-identified priorities.
6. The family's priorities, needs, and interests are addressed most appropriately by a primary provider who represents and receives team and community support.
7. Interventions with young children and family members must be based on explicit principles, validated practices, best available research, and relevant laws and regulations.

Reprinted from Workgroup on Principles and Practices in Natural Environments, OSEP TA Community of Practice: Part C Settings. (2008, March). *Agreed upon mission and key principles for providing early intervention services in natural environments*. Retrieved from http://ectacenter.org/~pdfs/topics/families/Finalmissionandprinciples3_11_08.pdf; reprinted by permission.

Service Provision

According to the mission statement within the statement paper "Agreed Upon Mission and Key Principles for Providing Early Intervention Services in Natural Environments," "Part C early intervention builds upon and provides supports and resources to assist family members and caregivers to enhance children's learning and development through everyday learning opportunities" (Workgroup on Principles and Practices in Natural Environments, 2008, p. 2). This mission is based on seven key principles that underpin family-centered services and supports (see the textbox titled Key Principles for Providing Early Intervention Services in Natural Environments) and that act as guidelines on how EI services should be provided.

The principles of EI promote a flexible system of service provision developed to respond to the team-based outcomes and not just to the diagnosis or the child's level of delay. Contemporary practice models that encompass the principles described above as well as those defined by the Division of Early Childhood Recommended Practices (www.dec-sped.org/dec-recommended-practices) include routines-based intervention (McWilliam, 2016), activity-based intervention (Pretti-Frontczak & Bricker, 2004; Valvano, 2004), context-based learning opportunities (Law et al., 2011b), and participation-based services

(Campbell & Sawyer, 2007). These models all support the following:

1. The critical roles of families as teachers of their children and practitioners as facilitators and teachers of both families and their children (Boyer & Thompson, 2014)
2. The use of common activities and routines as contexts for children's learning (Chai, Zhang, & Bisberg, 2006; Stremel & Campbell, 2007)
3. The need for practice and repetition in order for learning to occur (Ulrich, 2010)

To be successful these models all require that meaningful outcomes be identified and that EI professionals provide a spectrum of consultative and direct services. This approach often departs from the traditional discipline-specific model of a set frequency per week. Meaningful outcomes go beyond specific disciplinary goals to effectively address the child's participation in family and community activities and routines.

Different types of services as well as levels of service may be needed depending on the number of caregivers (e.g., parents, grandparents, and child care providers) and the learning contexts. On the one hand, a biweekly visit with a parent and child who spend the day together at home may suffice to accomplish the desired outcome. On the other hand, a multiple-caregiver situation often requires more frequent contact to demonstrate strategies and allow for more collaboration with key adults. A flexible model might emphasize sequential rather than simultaneous services or varying levels of intensity or frequency. For example, it may be beneficial to "front-load" services, increasing the frequency of services initially and then gradually decreasing them to weekly. Services relate to the accomplishment of the outcome. Each outcome should have distinct services, frequency, intensity, and location identified prior to the implementation of the IFSP. Shifting to a flexible, outcomes-guided model that is family directed increases the likelihood that the recommendations for services will emerge from a thorough analysis of child and family priorities. This individualized, outcomes-driven model contrasts with the traditional model of providing a predetermined group of services by specific disciplines that are driven by a particular disability rather than by the specific needs, priorities, and concerns of the family (Colyvas, Sawyer, & Campbell, 2010; Sheldon & Rush, 2013).

Currently, many state EI programs are implementing a primary service provider (PSP) model. The PSP model promotes assigning one team member to primarily interact with the child, the child's family, and other caregivers (Sheldon & Rush, 2013). The PSP provides EI services for the child and family with consultation, support, and or coaching from other team members. Any member of the IFSP team can be a PSP. Once the outcomes are determined, the team will decide which member of the team would best serve the family as the PSP. Rush and Shelden (2012) recommend that teams consider the characteristics of the parent/family, child, environment, and practitioner when deciding on which team member would be the PSP. As an example, physical therapists are often considered as the PSPs for children with a primary motor disability or delay. However, it is critical that whoever is the PSP should have the knowledge and skills to collaborate with other providers in developing comprehensive, integrated intervention sessions.

Contemporary Practice Models

Contemporary practice models support intervention in a natural environment by stressing the critical roles of the family as the child's teacher and the EI provider as the family's educator. Traditional service delivery is child focused; families often simply observe the service, or the professional teaches the family to execute a specific strategy (Peterson, Luze, Eshbaugh, Jeon, & Kantz, 2007). Intervention strategies that assist families and other caregivers to promote the child's development within the context of naturally occurring learning opportunities are consistent with the concept of natural environments and the intent of family-centered EI (Boyer & Thompson, 2014; Bruder, 2000; Peterson et al., 2007).

By focusing intervention on activities and routines that individual families participate in rather than on locations, the provider takes advantage of natural learning opportunities and family interactions, preferences, and resources. In this participation-based approach, EI professionals intervene with a child by teaching caregivers how to use two primary types of child interventions to promote the child's participation and learning: 1) adapting the environment, materials, or the activity/routine, including the use of assistive technology, and 2) embedding individualized learning strategies within family routines (Colyvas et al., 2010).

Other strategies, such as activity-based interventions (Pretti-Frontczak & Bricker, 2004; Valvano & Rapport, 2006), emphasize that although the intervention is within an activity, routine, or context, the *target* of intervention is the child, promoting his or her skill development. Routines-based intervention stresses the importance of engagement, independence, and social relationships within a naturally occurring child activity (McWilliam, 2010). Because intervention with infants and toddlers is a collaborative process, often including multiple caregivers, caregiver satisfaction or dissatisfaction is also considered. Caregivers must indicate dissatisfaction with the child's performance if they are going to identify functional outcomes from which they can make adaptations or embed a learning strategy. Dunst (2007) promotes the use of contextually mediated practices as an approach to promote the child's acquisition of new skills, competence, and knowledge. Contextually mediated practices use everyday family and community activities (natural environments) as the sources or "context" for learning (see Box 31.2 for more information on contemporary EI).

Transition from Early Intervention Services

Transition is a process that children and families experience as they move from one program or setting to another. Families of young children with developmental delays and disabilities may need to move between home and hospital or from EI to preschool. Under IDEA, young children are no longer eligible to receive EI services at age 3. Thus, the Part C system must begin, if needed, to transition the child from the Part C system at about 2 years, 6 months, to ECSE services, inclusive preschool or childcare programs, or other appropriate services. The 39th Report to Congress on the implementation of IDEA indicates that 60.3% of children exiting Part C were eligible to receive Part B, 619 services during 2014–2015 (U.S. Department of Education, 2017). Careful planning and preparation can ensure that change occurs in a timely and effective manner. Transition planning may also help to alleviate parental stress. To ensure a seamless move from EI to other appropriate services and supports, the IFSP must include a transition plan.

In the case study, Carl received EI services from a physical therapist, receiving intermittent consultation and support from a speech-language pathologist and occupational therapist as needed. As Carl was approaching his third the team began the process of transitioning Carl out of Part C services. By this time, he had received a diagnosis of spastic diplegic cerebral palsy and was using a reverse walker to support his mobility. As his expressive language abilities were not as well developed as his receptive skills, he started using a simple communication device when he was about 2 years of age. Carl was determined to be eligible to receive SE and related services through the Part B 619 program from his local school system. It was planned that starting at age 3 he will attend a school-based Head Start program in his community. His team, consisting of SE, physical therapy, and speech-language pathology professionals, will consult with the classroom teacher on a regular basis, helping the teacher to adapt, accommodate, and or modify her lesson plans as needed to ensure that Carl participates fully in all learning opportunities.

OUTCOMES

It has now been more than 30 years since the establishment of a formal EI system in the United States. Judged by usual standards, this program has been successful. All 50 states and jurisdictions are participating in Part C, meaning that each of the required structural components is in place. Moreover, the number of children served continues to grow annually.

The Department of Education instituted the Early Childhood Outcome system to measure and document outcomes of children and families receiving Part C services. Each state is required to report on the percent of infants and toddlers with IFSPs who demonstrate improved 1) positive social-emotional skills (including social relationships), 2) acquisition and use of knowledge

BOX 31.2 EVIDENCE-BASED PRACTICE

Contemporary Early Intervention

Professionals who provide services to infants and toddlers believe that early childhood intervention positively effects development, health, and family well-being. These positive effects have been documented for decades. Contemporary early childhood intervention builds on this evidence that indicates the following:

- Supportive relationships, adaptive skill building, and positive experiences help young children develop resilience.
- Building the capabilities of adult caregivers helps strengthen the relationships essential to children's lifelong learning, health, and behavior.
- The most important influence on early brain development is the positive interaction between young children and caring adults.

and skills (including early language/communication and early literacy), and 3) use of appropriate behaviors to meet their needs. States are also required to report on the percentage of families participating in Part C who report that EI services have helped their family know their rights, effectively communicate their children's needs, and help their children develop and learn.

Children who exit the system at age 3 are showing clear gains in development. Fifty-nine percent of the children exit with age-appropriate social interaction skills; 50% have age-appropriate skills in knowledge and developmental skills; and 57% use age-appropriate actions to meet their needs (Center for IDEA Early Childhood Data Systems, 2017). The family data also indicate that the Part C system is helpful: Over 89% of families receiving Part C services indicate knowing their rights, 90% report being able to effectively communicate their needs, and over 92% feel confident in helping their child develop and learn (Early Childhood Technical Assistance Center, 2018b).

Although the Part C program is serving many children, states continue to narrow the eligibility criteria (IDEA Infants and Toddlers Coordinators Association, 2017), and children with milder disabilities and less significant delays may actually be the ones who benefit the most from EI services for which they may no longer be eligible to receive (Hebbeler et al., 2010). In addition, evidence exists to suggest that children are receiving fewer services and supports to meet IFSP outcomes (Hebbeler et al., 2010). Although a 2010 study indicated that 63% of the families received an average of 6.5 hours per month of EI services, the 2017 survey of Part C State Coordinators indicates that the average service hours has decreased to about 4 hours per month.

Taken together, it is evident that a comprehensive EI system composed of well-defined structural components can be found in states and communities throughout the United States, providing services and supports to infants and toddlers and their families. However, it is recognized that such a complex and evolving system can be substantially improved to more effectively and efficiently meet the needs of children and families (Boavida, Aguiar, & McWilliam, 2014; Boyer & Thompson, 2014; Dunst, 2007; Tomasellio, Manning, & Dulmus, 2010).

SUMMARY

- EI services for infants and toddlers with disabilities or developmental delay are available in all states and territories.
- Following a multidisciplinary team evaluation to determine eligibility for services, an IFSP is developed.
- Outcomes on the IFSP are created to promote participation in family and community routines
- Services are provided in the natural environment.
- More states are adopting the primary service provider system of service provision.
- Research on the effectiveness of EI has demonstrated the potential for achieving important benefits for infants, toddlers, and their families.

ADDITIONAL RESOURCES

ZERO TO THREE: National Center for Infants, Toddlers, and Families: http://www.zerotothree.org.

Child Development Web: http://www.childdevelopmentweb.com/Information/EIprograms.asp

The Early Childhood Technical Assistance Center: http://www.ectacenter.org

Additional resources can be found online in Appendix D: Childhood Disabilities Resources, Services, and Organizations (see About the Online Companion Materials).

REFERENCES

Adams, R., Tapia, C., & Council on Children with Disabilities. (2013). Early intervention, IDEA Part C services, and the medical home: Collaboration for best practice and best outcomes. *Pediatrics, 132,* e1073–e1088.

Boavida, T., Aguiar, C., & McWilliam, R. A. (2014). A training program to improve IFSP/IEP goals and objectives through the routines-based interview. *Topics in Early Childhood Special Education, 20,* 200–211.

Boyer, V. E., & Thompson, S. D. (2014). Transdisciplinary model and early intervention: Building collaborative relationships. *Young Exceptional Children, 17,* 19–32.

Bruder, M. B. (2000). Family-centered early intervention: Clarifying our values for the new millennium. *Topics in Early Childhood Special Education, 20,* 105–115.

Campbell, P., & Sawyer, L. B. (2007). Supporting learning opportunities in natural settings through participation-based services. *Journal of Early Intervention, 29,* 287–305.

Center for IDEA Early Childhood Data Systems. (2017). *IDEA child outcomes highlights for FFY 2015.* Retrieved from http://ectacenter.org/eco/assets/pdfs/childoutcomeshighlights.pdf

Center on the Developing Child at Harvard University. (2010). *The foundations of lifelong health are built in early childhood.* Retrieved from https://developingchild.harvard.edu/resources/the-foundations-of-lifelong-health-are-built-in-early-childhood/

Chai, A. Y., Zhang, C., & Bisberg, M. (2006). Rethinking natural environment practice: Implications from examining various interpretations and approaches. *Early Childhood Education Journal, 34,* 203–208.

Colyvas, J. L., Sawyer, L. B., & Campbell, P. H. (2010). Identifying strategies early intervention occupational therapists use to teach caregivers. *American Journal of Occupational Therapy, 64*, 776–785.

Council on Children with Disabilities, Section on Developmental Behavioral Pediatrics, Bright Futures Steering Committee, & Medical Home Initiatives for Children With Special Needs Project Advisory Committee. (2006). Identifying infants and young children with developmental disorders in the medical home: An algorithm for developmental surveillance and screening. *Pediatrics, 108*(1), 405–420. (A statement of reaffirmation for this policy was published in *Pediatrics, 134*(5): e1520.)

Dunst, C. J. (2007). Early intervention for infants and toddlers with developmental disabilities. In S. L. Odom, R. H. Homer, M. Snell, & J. Blacher (Eds.), *Handbook of developmental disabilities* (pp. 161–180). New York, NY: Guilford Press.

Dunst, C. J., Bruder, M. B., & Espe-Sherwindt, M. (2014). Family capacity-building in early childhood intervention: Do context and setting matter? *School Community Journal, 24*(1), 37–48.

Early Childhood Technical Assistance Center. (2015). *States' and territories' definitions of/criteria for IDEA Part C eligibility.*

Retrieved from ectacenter.org/~pdfs/topics/earlyid/partc_elig_table.pdf

Early Childhood Technical Assistance Center. (2018a). *IDEA child outcomes highlights for FFY2016*. Retrieved from http://ectacenter.org/eco/pages/childoutcomes-highlights-ffy2016.asp

Early Childhood Technical Assistance Center. (2018b). *IDEA Part C Early Intervention Family Survey Data for FFY2016*. Retrieved from http://ectacenter.org/eco/pages/familyoutcomes-highlights-ffy2016.asp

Ekono, M., Yang, J., & Smith, S. (2016). *Young children in deep poverty*. New York, NY: National Center for Children in Poverty, Mailman School of Public Health, Columbia University.

Frankenburg, W. K., Dodds, J. B., Archer, P., Bresnick, B., Maschka, P., Edelman, N., & Shapiro, H. (1992). *Denver II*. Denver, CO: Denver Developmental Materials.

Glascoe, F. P. (1997). *Parents' Evaluations of Developmental Status (PEDS)*. Nashville, TN: Ellsworth and Vandermeer Press.

Hebbeler, K., Mallik, S., & Taylor, C. (2010). *An analysis of needs and service planning in the Texas early childhood intervention program. Report prepared for Texas Department of Assistive and Rehabilitative Services.* Menlo Park, CA: SRI International.

Heckman, J. (2012). *Invest in early childhood development: Reduce deficits, strengthen the economy: The Heckman Equation.* Retrieved from heckmanequation.org

IDEA Infants and Toddlers Coordinators Association. (2017). *Annual survey: State challenges and responses.* Retrieved from http://ideainfanttoddler.org/pdf/2017-ITCA-State-Challenges-Report.pdf

Individuals with Disabilities Education Improvement Act (IDEA) of 2004, PL 108-446, 20 U.S.C. §§ 1400 *et seq.*

Law, L., Darrah, J., & Pollack, N. (2011a). Focus on function: A cluster, randomized controlled trial comparing child- versus context-focused intervention for young children with cerebral palsy. *Developmental Medicine and Child Neurology, 53*(7), 621–629.

Law, L., Darrah, J., & Pollack, N. (2011b). Context therapy: A new intervention approach for children with cerebral palsy. *Developmental Medicine and Child Neurology, 53*(7), 615–620.

McWilliam, R. A. (2010). *Routines-based early intervention: Supporting young children and their families.* Baltimore, MD: Paul H. Brookes Publishing Co.

McWilliam, R. A. (2016). Early intervention. In B. Reichow, B. A. Boyd, E. E. Barton, & S. L. Odom (Eds.), *Handbook of early childhood special education* (pp. 75–88). Cham, Switzerland: Springer International Publishing.

Peterson, C. A., Luze, G. J., Eshbaugh, E. M., Jeon, H., & Kantz, K. R. (2007). Enhancing parent–child interactions through home visiting: Promising practice or unfulfilled promise. *Journal of Early Intervention, 29*, 119–140.

Pretti-Frontczak, K., & Bricker, D. (2004). *An activity-based approach to early intervention* (3rd ed.). Baltimore, MD: Paul H. Brookes Publishing Co.

Rush, D., & Shelden, M. (2012). *Worksheet for selecting the most likely primary service provider.* Retrieved from http://fipp.org/static/media/uploads/casetools/casetool_vol6_no3.pdf

Sheldon, M., & Rush, D. (2013). Introduction to a primary service provider approach to teaming. In M. Shelden & D. Rush (Eds.), *The early intervention teaming handbook* (pp. 1–26). Baltimore, MD: Paul H. Brookes Publishing Co.

Spittle, A., Orton, J., Anderson, P., Boyd, R., & Doyle, L. (2015). Early developmental intervention programmes provided post hospital discharge to prevent motor and cognitive impairment in preterm infants. *Cochrane Database of Systematic Reviews, 11*, CD005495. doi:10.1002/14651858.CD005495.pub4.

Squires, J., & Bricker, D. (2009). *Ages & Stages Questionnaires®, Third Edition (ASQ-3®): A parent-completed, child-monitoring system.* Baltimore, MD: Paul H. Brookes Publishing Co.

Stremel, K., & Campbell, P. (2007). Implementation of early intervention within natural environments. *Early Childhood Services, 1*, 83–105.Tomasellio, N. M., Manning, A. R., & Dulmus, C. N. (2010). Family-centered early intervention for infants and toddlers with disabilities. *Journal of Family Social Work, 13*, 163–172.

Tomasello, N. M., Manning, A. R., & Dulmus, C. N. (2010). Family-centered early intervention for infants and toddlers with disabilities. *Journal of Family Social Work, 13*(2), 163–172.

Ulrich, B. (2010). Opportunities for early intervention based on theory, basic neuroscience, and clinical science. *Physical Therapy, 91*, 1–13.

U.S. Department of Education. (2017). *Thirty-ninth annual report to Congress on the implementation of the Individuals with Disabilities Education Act, Parts B and C. 2017.* Retrieved from http://www.ed.gov/about/reports/annual/osep

Valvano, J. (2004). Activity-focused motor interventions for children with neurological conditions. *Physical and Occupational Therapy in Pediatrics, 24*, 79–107.

Valvano, J., & Rapport, M. J. (2006). Activity-focused motor interventions for infants and young children with neurological conditions. *Infants and Young Children, 19*, 292–307.

Woolfenden, S., Eapen, V., Williams, K., Hayen, A., Spencer, N., & Kemp, L. (2014). A systemic review of the prevalence of parental concerns measured by the Parents' Evaluation of Developmental Status (PEDS) indicating developmental risk. *BMC Pediatrics*, 231.

Workgroup on Principles and Practices in Natural Environments. (2008). *Agreed upon mission and key principles for providing early intervention services in natural environments.* Retrieved from http://ectacenter.org/~pdfs/topics/families/Finalmissionandprinciples3_11_08.pdf

CHAPTER 32 Rehabilitative Services

Melissa Fleming, Marisa Birkmeier, Mackenzie Brown,
Justin M. Burton, Satvika Garg, and Sarah H. Evans

Upon completion of this chapter, the reader will

- Describe the importance and components of a comprehensive functional assessment in children with developmental disabilities
- Explain the roles of various therapists and pediatric subspecialists involved in the rehabilitative care of children with disabilities
- Identify unique physical and functional treatment approaches to common diagnoses, including cerebral palsy, muscular dystrophy, and spina bifida
- Distinguish diagnosis-specific clinical features that guide physical and functional treatment approaches
- Recognize the variable physical and functional treatment modalities and interventions available to treat children with disabilities
- Identify precautions to consider when providing rehabilitative services to children with these specific diagnoses

The overall goal of treatment for children with physical disabilities is to optimize functional independence with completion of age-appropriate tasks. Individual plans of care should be patient and family centered. In order to achieve this goal, rehabilitation teams use the World Health Organization's International Classification of Functioning, Disability, and Health (ICF) framework for defining health and disability (Figure 32.1). The ICF conceptualizes the unique challenges that children with physical disabilities face, providing practitioners with a framework to develop a comprehensive treatment approach to address the barriers to physical, psychosocial, and emotional health (World Health Organization, 2007).

Interventions used to achieve the goal of functional independence are varied and range from providing durable medical equipment to prescribing medication. Equipment and bracing are used to maximize independence in the least restrictive and most functional manner possible. Pharmaceuticals focus on decreasing symptoms that may be limiting the child's voluntary movements, thereby improving his or her participation in daily care activities.

Most children with physical disabilities will engage in occupational, physical, and/or speech therapy at some point in their development. These specialists provide a supportive and educational environment to optimize developmental goals and improve functional

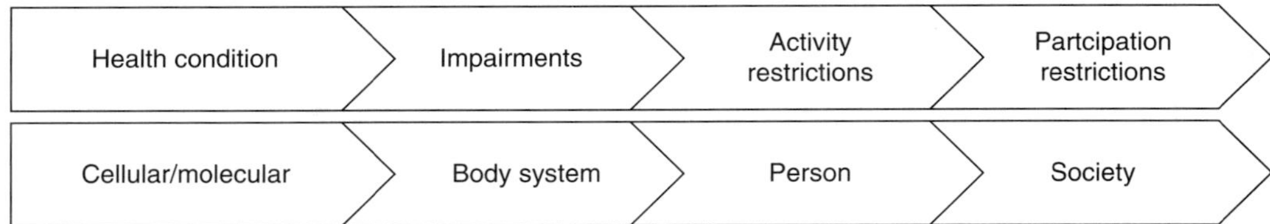

Figure 32.1. The ICF model. A health condition (disease or disorder) exists because of physiologic disturbances at a cellular, molecular, or tissue level. These physiological disturbances cause changes in body function and structure, which can result in an individual experiencing disability (activity restrictions), causing difficulties functioning in societal settings (participation restrictions). Environmental and personal factors further influence and provide a context for changes and differences in function. For example, a 5-year-old boy with joint contractures related to cerebral palsy will have difficulties with mobility and restricted play, which will manifest in specific ways in his particular home, neighborhood, and school. (Adapted from the World Health Organization. [2013]. *International Classification of Functioning, Disability and Health [ICF]: ICF and ICF-Online.* Retrieved from http://apps.who.int/classifications/icfbrowser/)

performance. Within all three therapies, there exists a vast spectrum of techniques and approaches that can vary widely in response to the specific needs of the child and considerations of any related health conditions.

This chapter describes an approach to the assessment of children with physical disabilities, followed by a description of physical and functional treatment approaches for children with commonly encountered diagnoses causing physical disability, focusing on cerebral palsy, muscular dystrophy, and spina bifida. The unique clinical features of each condition that merit a specialized rehabilitative treatment approach are identified, as well as specific precautions and considerations when working with these children.

PRINCIPLES AND PROCESSES OF FUNCTIONAL ASSESSMENT

The clinical assessment, which includes a patient history and physical examination, is the initial component of every patient encounter because it guides diagnosis and treatment. The assessment of children with physical disabilities varies based on both age and developmental skills, which often do not match. Clinicians begin addressing this challenge by gathering a history regarding the child's developmental progress and skills. They also perform a physical examination to evaluate the efficiency with which the child is able to complete these skills and to identify any barriers to progress. Overall, the clinical assessment identifies the child's functional strengths and weaknesses in his or her interactions at home and within the community so that the team of clinicians can optimize the child's participation in society.

A comprehensive assessment considers the child and family as a whole. The ICF, noted above, provides clinicians with a useful framework for conceptualizing the child's level of health and function. It consists of five interacting components: 1) health condition, 2) ability to participate in daily living, 3) required activities, 4) body functions and structures, and 5) environmental and personal factors (World Health Organization, 2013; Table 32.1). The ICF can be very helpful in delineating impairments that limit function, leading the provider to consider appropriate interventions.

In evaluating a child with physical disabilities, the first step is to assess the child's health condition or disease that is the cause of an impairment in function. Examples of impairments include weakness,

Table 32.1. Examples of the World Health Organization's *International Classification of Functioning, Disability, and Health (ICF)* model (2007)

Health condition	Impairments	Activity restrictions	Participation restrictions
Cerebral palsy	Hypertonia	Impaired fine motor skills	Need adaptive driving setup
Duchenne muscular dystrophy	Weakness	Difficulty walking/impaired mobility	Difficulty accessing home and school
Stroke	Hemi-neglect	Impaired navigation around obstacles	Need for supervision and assistance in the community
Burn	Pain and contractures	Limited arm movement	Need for clothing modifications
Pilocytic astrocytoma brain tumor	Hearing impairment	Limited communication	Risk for social isolation and learning issues in school

hypertonia, sensory deficits, contractures, vision and hearing loss, pain, and anxiety. Impairments can lead to "activity restriction," or disability, and to "participation restrictions," or handicaps. Members of the rehabilitation team often use the ICF model to conceptualize how the child's health condition is affecting his or her body and resultant lack of functional independence.

The child with physical disabilities is best treated by an interdisciplinary team of clinicians, a topic that is explored in detail in Chapter 30. The rehabilitation team focuses on specific elements of the child's history and physical development to develop a functional assessment. These are described within the sections that follow.

After assessing the child and determining what impairments are impacting function, the rehabilitation team works with the family (a critical partnership) to develop attainable functional goals and devise a plan to work toward those goals (Table 32.2). Elements of the medical history obtained from the child and family can facilitate diagnosis and lead to the appropriate interventions.

Table 32.2. Medical history

Element of history	Key information	Example questions	Implications
Prenatal and perinatal history	Gestational age at birth, complications during pregnancy or at birth, length of neonatal intensive care unit stay if required, need for perinatal/neonatal surgeries or procedures	Was the child born prematurely? Did the child require a hospital admission after birth?	Prematurity can affect neurodevelopment. Prematurity is a major risk factor for cerebral palsy. Many congenital conditions, such as spina bifida, are detected prenatally.
Developmental history	Timeliness in attaining milestones in domains of gross motor, fine motor, and social/language development	Did the child meet all milestones on time? In which domains does he or she have delays?	Regression of milestones is a concerning finding that requires further investigation. Patterns in attainment of milestones may also indicate pathology.
Family and social history	Review any pertinent familial health conditions and patterns of development in siblings and parents	Did any of the child's siblings exhibit similar delays with milestone achievement?	Assessing the family patterns of development may explain or predict findings, particularly in the child with a genetic disorder.
Cognition and social behavior	Screen for age-appropriate cognition and social engagement, including interaction with family and peers	How does the child interact with his or her siblings and peers? Can he or she sustain attention to activities? Does the school have concerns?	Such screening helps identify if deficits are isolated to motor impairments or if cognition is also affected.
Vision and hearing	History of hearing and vision screens, particularly in children with brain injury or brain tumors	Does the child respond when his or her name is called? Does he or she startle to loud noises? Does he or she track objects appropriately?	Testing to ensure adequate functioning of these systems may be indicated. Interventions such as hearing aids, corrective lenses, or visual therapy/exercises can significantly improve a child's overall level of function when impairments are present. Referral to an audiologist, neuro-optometrist, or vision therapist should be considered if concerns are found.
Speech and language	Screen for impaired production of speech sounds (dysarthria), including intelligibility and quality of speech	Does the child follow basic commands? Can the child make his or her needs and wants known?	Dysarthria can be related to injury of the brain. For example, harsh vocal quality may suggest spastic dysarthria in the setting of an acquired brain injury. Nasal, low-volume speech is typical of flaccid dysarthria associated with conditions such as posterior fossa tumor. Children with dysarthria should be evaluated by a speech therapist. Augmentative and alternative communication may be helpful to improve expressive language in children with significant impairments. Children with dysphonia may benefit from a referral to an otolaryngologist as vocal-fold injections can improve voice quality and volume.

(continued)

Table 32.2. *(continued)*

Element of history	Key information	Example questions	Implications
Feeding/oromotor function	Review diet and feeding habits, screen for any difficulty with swallow and/or managing secretions, assess for any unexpected weight loss/gain	Does the child eat a variable diet? Does the family notice coughing or change in voice when the child eats/drinks? Is there a history of aspiration pneumonia? Does the child tend to drool?	If the child is experiencing difficulty with feeding/swallowing, then evaluation and treatment with a speech therapist is warranted. If the child is unable to eat by mouth safely, alternative routes of nutrition may be recommended, such as through a gastrostomy tube, to prevent aspiration. If the child has difficulty managing secretions, medications, including glycopyrrolate and botulinum toxin injections to the salivary glands, can be considered.
Mobility and other gross motor skills	Level of assistance the child needs to make transitions from lying down to sitting, to standing, and to taking steps; review use of any orthoses, assistive device, or wheeled mobility use	If the child is ambulatory, how does he or she navigate stairs? Does the child trip or fall often? Does he or she wear leg braces? Does he or she use a wheeled mobility device such as a stroller or wheelchair? Does the child require extra head or trunk support?	Such assessment provides important diagnostic information (i.e., frequent tripping and falling can be caused by a gait impairment that requires further diagnostic workup). A thorough assessment of mobility and gross motor skills will help guide treatment to maximize independence with mobility.
Fine motor coordination	Review for age-appropriate fine motor skills, including dexterity with hand use, grip, and skill	Does the child have a hand preference? Does the child hold the hands fisted? Can he or she transfer toys between hands? Can the child use scissors?	Hand preference usually develops between 2–4 years of age; prior to that time, the child should demonstrate functional use of both hands including reaching for objects. Early hand preference (before 18 months) can indicate weakness of the contralateral hand. A "cortical thumb," in which the thumb is tightly adducted into the palm, or hands that are tightly fisted are typical findings in a child with cerebral palsy.
Basic and instrumental activities of daily living (ADLs and IADLs)	Screen for the age-appropriate completion of ADLS and IADLs, including feeding, toileting, and using a computer and phone	Can the child self-feed? Does she use utensils appropriately? How much help does he require for dressing?	Most children can accomplish basic ADLs independently by 6 years of age, or first grade in school. Identifying impairments with completing ADL and IADLs will guide treatment.
Participation in recreation and school	Review child's participation in school and play, including school accessibility, home setup, community spaces, and family/caregiver supports and structures	What extracurricular activities does the child enjoy? Where does the child spend most of his or her time?	This can screen for barriers to participation and offer a variety of adaptive sports programs for children with disabilities that provide great opportunities for exercise and socialization.

Prenatal and Perinatal History

The team should consider if the child was born prematurely. This is known to affect neurodevelopment, and prematurity is a major risk factor for **cerebral palsy.** Was there prenatal testing? Many congenital conditions, including **spina bifida,** are detected prenatally by ultrasound (see Chapter 3).

Developmental History

Asking the family about timeliness in attaining milestones in the domains of gross motor, fine motor, and social/language development is essential. Regression in milestones is a significant finding that requires further investigation. Early attainment of certain milestones may also indicate pathology. For example, early demonstration of a hand preference before the age of 18 months can indicate weakness of the other side. Similarly, early standing due to whole body stiffness can indicate spasticity, as can be seen in cerebral palsy.

Family and Social History

Assessing the health conditions and patterns of development in siblings and parents may help explain or predict findings, particularly in the child with a genetic disorder.

Functional History

The rehab specialist should ask about the child's current level of function in several domains, including the following:

- *Cognition and social behavior:* How does the child interact with his or her family and peers? Can he/she sustain attention to activities? Is the child able to understand age appropriate concepts? Does the school have concerns?
- *Vision and hearing:* Even when the family does not indicate concerns, testing to ensure adequate functioning of these systems may be indicated, particularly in children with brain injury or brain tumors. Interventions such as hearing aids, corrective lenses, or visual therapy/exercises can significantly improve the child's overall level of function when impairments are present. Referral to an audiologist, neuro-optometrist, or vision therapist should be considered if concerns are found (see Chapters 25 and 26).
- *Speech and language:* Does the child understand what is said to him/her? Can the child make needs and wants known? Poor intelligibility due to impaired production of speech sounds, known as dysarthria, can be due to a variety of neurological conditions. For example, an acquired brain injury may result in a spastic or hyperkinetic dysarthria, with a harsh, strangled vocal quality. Breathy, hypernasal, low-volume speech is typical of flaccid dysarthria and is seen in a variety of conditions involving the medulla and associated cranial nerves, including posterior fossa brain tumors. All children with dysarthria should be evaluated by a speech therapist. If intelligibility is so poor that reliable verbal communication is not possible, a speech therapist with experience in augmentative and alternative communication (AAC) may be helpful in developing strategies to improve nonverbal means of expression. Children with dysphonia may benefit from a referral to an otolaryngologist with expertise in dysphonia, as vocal-fold injections can improve voice quality and volume (see Chapter 17).
- *Feeding/oromotor function:* Can the child eat and drink a variety of textures safely? Does the family notice a change in vocal quality, such as a wet voice or coughing when the child drinks? Is there a history of aspiration pneumonia? Does the child tend to drool? If the child has difficulty managing secretions, medications including glycopyrrolate and botulinum toxin injections to the salivary glands can be considered by a physiatrist or other physician. An evaluation and treatment with a speech therapist is also warranted. If the child is unable to eat by mouth safely, the clinician should consider whether a gastrostomy tube placed directly in the stomach is indicated to ensure adequate nutritional intake and whether the child should be prohibited from taking food and fluids by mouth to prevent aspiration (see Chapter 29).
- *Mobility and other gross motor skills:* What level of assistance does the child need to move within the bed, to transition from laying down to sitting to standing, and to take steps? Is the child able to hold his or her head and trunk in an upright, neutral alignment when sitting, or does the child need external support? If the child has a limited ability to ambulate, does he use a wheeled mobility device, such as a stroller or wheelchair? If ambulatory, how does the child navigate stairs? Does he wear any leg braces?
- *Fine motor coordination:* Hand preference usually develops between 2 and 4 years of age; prior to that time, the child should demonstrate functional use of both hands including reaching for objects. A "cortical thumb," in which the thumb is tightly adducted into the palm, or hands that are tightly fisted are typical findings in a child with cerebral palsy (see Chapter 21).
- *Basic and instrumental activities of daily living (ADLs and IADLs):* Basic ADLs are the tasks performed every day to take care of oneself in the home environment, such as feeding, dressing, bathing, personal hygiene and grooming, toileting, and transferring. IADLs are higher level skills needed to live in a community; they include managing money, preparing meals, shopping, taking prescribed medication, using a computer and telephone, and housekeeping skills. Most typically developing children can accomplish basic ADLs independently by 6 years of age or first grade in school.
- *Participation in recreation and school:* It is important to note relevant environmental factors that impact the child's participation in school and play, including school accessibility, home setup, community spaces, and family/caregiver supports and structures. For example, who does the child live with? What community activities do the child and family like to do? What does her day look like? Where does she spend most of her time? What classes or teams does she participate in as an extracurricular activity from school or day care? If none, are there any activities that the child hopes to be involved in the future? There are a variety of adaptive sports

programs for children with disabilities that provide great opportunities for exercise and socialization, such as the Paralympics and Special Olympics.

Physical Exam

The physical exam of the child starts with general observation (see Table 32.3). For example, does the child appear at, above, or below the expected height and weight for age? What is the size and shape of the head, as this often correlates with brain development? Does the abdomen seem distended (constipation is often a challenge in children with limited mobility)?

The focus of the exam is on the neurological and musculoskeletal systems. The neurological exam should include assessment of the child's mental status, cranial nerves, sensation to different modalities, reflexes, coordination (including testing for dysmetria [lack of coordination of movements leading to undershooting or overshooting] and **ataxia**) and the presence of any abnormally patterned or adventitious (unusual) movements.

The musculoskeletal exam should include assessment of the active and passive range of motion around major joints of the limbs and neck, the presence of any abnormal spinal curvature, strength, and muscle tone. Abnormal tone, whether hypertonia or hypotonia, often interferes with development and function. Children with abnormal tone should be referred to a physical medicine and rehabilitation (PM&R) physician for management, including medication and **orthoses** (supports, braces, or splints used to support, align, prevent, or correct the function of limb or joint).

The clinician also needs to test the functional skills that were described during the medical history, considering the following questions:

- How does the child move in the exam room? How does the child transition between surfaces in the room? For example, can he rise from the floor independently?
- Regarding ADLs, can the child take his socks and shoes off and on independently? If given a pen and paper, can he scribble or write in an age-appropriate fashion? Can the child pick up snacks and bring them to his mouth? Does the child demonstrate signs of dysphagia when eating or drinking?
- How does the child interact with his caregiver and others present in the room?

Table 32.3. Physical examination

Elements of physical exam	Key exam features	Implications
General assessment	Weight and height at, above, or below the expected height and weight for age, size and shape of the head, and abdominal distension	Weight and height provide information on development, feeding, and activity level. Head shape correlates with brain development. Abdominal distention may indicate constipation, a common challenge in children with limited mobility.
Neurological assessment	Mental status, cranial nerves, sensation to different modalities, reflexes, coordination (including testing for **dysmetria** [lack of coordination of movements leading to undershooting or overshooting] and **ataxia**), and the presence of any abnormally patterned or **adventitious** (unusual) movements	Quality of movement patterns can provide diagnostic clues. For movement disorders limiting function referral to neurology or a movement disorder specialist may be helpful for pharmaceutical management.
Musculoskeletal assessment	Assessment of the active and passive range of motion around major joints of the limbs and neck, the presence of any abnormal spinal curvature, strength, and muscle tone	Abnormal tone, whether hypertonia or hypotonia, often interferes with development and function. Children with abnormal tone should be referred to a physical medicine and rehabilitation physician for management, including medication therapy and **orthoses** (supports, braces, or splints used to support, align, prevent, or correct the function of limb or joint). For significant contractures, a referral to orthopedic surgery may be warranted.
Functional assessment	Activity in the exam room, including mobility, such as making transitions from the floor to the exam table to sitting; gross motor skills in older, ambulatory children with age-appropriate tasks such as jumping, hopping, and running; activities of daily living, such as age-appropriate scribbling or writing, how the child transfers toys in his or her hands, whether the child can pick up snacks and bring them to his or her mouth, and whether the child helps with removing shoes/socks; and language and communication, including observing interactions between the child and his or her caregiver, such as if the child communicates needs effectively and the vocal quality of speech	Observation of functional tasks performed in the exam room will provide pertinent information for diagnostics purposes, identifying barriers to progress and formulating a treatment plan.

- Does the child have a typical repertoire of play skills for age?
- Does he demonstrate joint attention?
- Can the child communicate needs? What is the vocal quality of speech?

PRINCIPLES OF TREATMENT

Rehabilitative/functional treatment is a unique multimodal treatment approach that uses interdisciplinary teams to address functional impairments from diverse specialty pathways. The focus of functional treatment, as the name implies, is to optimize the child's functional abilities with the overarching goal to increase the child's access to society and their environment. The objective is to identify the child's strengths and maximize those strengths while concurrently recognizing the physical and social barriers limiting progress. Appropriate treatments and services are offered to specifically target the identified impediments. In the case when a barrier cannot be corrected, the goal becomes focused on measures for accommodation. Treatment ranges from therapeutic management on the individual level to recommendations for improving home accessibility and guidance for navigating environmental restrictions. The interdisciplinary approach allows for comprehensive management that extends into the various sectors of the child's life, including home, school, recreation, and family.

The sections that follow outline the physical and functional treatment approaches for children with three commonly encountered diagnoses that cause developmental disability: cerebral palsy, muscular dystrophy, and spina bifida.

CASE STUDY

Thomas is a 5-year-old boy who is followed for spasticity in his lower limbs. He was born prematurely at 28 weeks' gestation. Thomas demonstrated delays in meeting his motor milestones from infancy, although he remained on track with his cognition, language, and communication skills. Given his motor delays, he was referred for early intervention therapy services by his pediatrician at 12 months. When he did begin to walk at 24 months, his parents noted that he consistently walked on his toes, which prompted a referral to the PM&R clinic. On examination, he exhibited bilateral **patellar** (kneecap) hyperreflexia and **clonus** (a series of alternating contractions and partial relaxations of the muscle) in both Achilles tendons, with significant reduction in passive range of motion at the ankles. When walking, he demonstrated toe walking and exaggerated hip **adduction** (movement toward the midline of the body; see Figure 21.12). The rehabilitation team recommended that Thomas undergo botulinum toxin injections to address hypertonia in the legs, to be followed by serial casting at the ankles and a physical therapy course for stretching, strengthening, and improving range of motion and gait biomechanics. After serial casting, he would be fitted for custom ankle-foot-orthotics.

Thomas has cerebral palsy (see Chapter 21), the leading cause of motor impairment and disability in children, especially those born prematurely (see Chapter 5). Specifically, Thomas has spastic diplegic cerebral palsy. For his functional mobility, he is able to walk independently but would likely have some difficulty with uneven surfaces and with keeping up with his peers. His Gross Motor Function Classification System score would be II (see Table 32.4).

Thought Question:

Apply the ICF model to identify Thomas' health condition, impairments, potential activity restrictions, and participation restrictions.

Cerebral Palsy

Therapeutic Approaches The goals of treatment are unique to each patient. Appropriate interventions for cerebral palsy are based on the child's age, functional abilities, pattern of motor deficits, and associated pain/discomfort. Intervention aims to reduce secondary musculoskeletal deformity rather than to treat the primary central neurological deficit, which is currently not possible. Treatment of children with cerebral palsy is best accomplished by a multidisciplinary team (see Box 32.1). Evaluation and ongoing management by physiatrists and therapists are the mainstays in the care of these children.

Rehabilitative Therapy Physical therapy for children with cerebral palsy addresses functional mobility, gross motor skills, postural control, and muscle strengthening/stretching with activities such as partial-body-weight-support gait training. Occupational therapy focuses on ADLs, fine motor skills, stretching, and range of motion. Speech therapy may be beneficial for children when assistance is needed with feeding, communication, and/or cognition. The ideal frequency and duration of therapy are impacted by critical periods of development, times of significant medical changes, and by interventions such as surgical procedures.

Table 32.4. Summary of the Gross Motor Function Classification System

Level	Age: < 2 years	2–4 years	4–6 years	6–12 years
I: Walks without restrictions	Sits well (hands free to play), crawls and pulls-to-stand; walks between 18 and 24 months without a device	Gets up and down from floor to standing without help; walking is preferred method of mobility	Walks indoors and outdoors; climbs stairs; starting to run/jump	Independent walking, running, and jumping, but speed, balance, and coordination are reduced
II: Walks without device; restricted community mobility	Sits but may need hands for balance; may creep or crawl; may pull-to-stand or cruise	Floor sits, but hard to keep both hands free; mobility by crawling, cruising, or walking with assistive device	Transfers with arm assist; walks without device at home and short distances outside; climbs stairs with railing; no running or jumping	Independent walking but limitations in challenging circumstances; minimal running and jumping
III: Walks with assistive device; limited community mobility	Sits with low back support; rolls and creeps	Floor sits, often W-sitting, needs help getting to sit; creeping and crawling primary means of mobility; limited assisted standing/walking	Sits in regular chair with pelvic support to allow free hands; walks with device on level surface; transported for long distances	Walks indoors or outdoors with assistive device; wheelchair mobility or transport for long distances
IV: Limited self-mobility; power mobility	Has head control, but needs trunk support for sitting; rolls to back; may roll to front	Needs hands to maintain sitting; adaptive equipment for sitting/standing; floor mobility only (rolling, creeping, or crawling without reciprocal leg movements)	Adaptive seating needed for maximum hand function; needs assistance for transfers; walks short distances with assistance; power mobility for long distances	Maintains function achieved by ages 4–6 or relies more on power wheelchair for self-mobility
V: Self-mobility severely limited even with assistive devices	Limited voluntary control of movement; head and trunk control minimal; needs help to roll	Limited control of movement and posture; all areas of motor function are limited; adaptive equipment does not fully compensate for functional limitations in sitting and standing; no independent mobility (requires transport); some children achieve very limited power mobility with extensive adaptations		

Adapted from Palisano, R., Rosenbaum, P., Walter, S., Russell, D., Wood, E., & Galuppi, B. (1997). Development and reliability of a system to classify gross motor function in children with cerebral palsy. *Developmental Medicine and Child Neurology, 39*(4), 214–223.

A recent exciting development in the treatment of cerebral palsy has been the use of high-intensity, short-duration constraint-induced movement therapy (CIMT) by physical and occupational therapists in patients with hemiparesis. Here the unaffected limb is restrained with a sling or splint, and intensive therapy is provided to encourage use of the affected arm. CIMT is based on the concept of "neuroplasticity" and the possibility of developing new neuronal synapses and circuits by promoting use of the affected limb (see Box 32.2; DeLuca, Trucks, Wallace, & Ramey, 2017).

BOX 32.1 INTERDISCIPLINARY CARE

Treatment of Cerebral Palsy

When treating children with cerebral palsy, an adaptive approach is necessary. The involvement of physical, occupational, and speech and language therapy, in combination with medical management, is beneficial to facilitate progress in all developmental domains and to reduce the effect of neurological impairments and comorbidities. The team caring for a child with cerebral palsy may include a pediatrician, developmental pediatrician, physiatrist, orthopedic surgeon, neurologist, neurosurgeon, physical therapist, occupational therapist, speech-language pathologist, therapeutic recreation specialist, orthotist, psychologist, social worker, and dietician. Physiatrists will address tone management, pain management, prescription of orthotic devices and durable medical equipment, and evaluation of seating systems.

BOX 32.2 EVIDENCE-BASED PRACTICE

Constraint-Induced Movement Therapy

Constraint-induced movement therapy (CIMT) is a technique to improve upper extremity function utilizing high-intensity therapy while constraining use of the less impaired upper extremity. CIMT is a highly efficacious treatment for children with cerebral palsy based on rigorous clinical trials. CIMT can be successfully implemented in the clinical setting. While CIMT has been designated as the most highly recommended form of intervention for children with hemiparetic cerebral palsy, studies have shown that children across a wide range of etiologies and severity levels have shown positive outcomes (DeLuca et al., 2017).

Promoting General Physical Activity Beyond individualized formal therapy, general physical activity and participation in leisure and recreational activities are important and should be encouraged. Adapted physical education in school, as part of an individualized educational program (see Chapter 33), is helpful in establishing a routine for regular participation. In the United States, adapted physical education is a federally mandated part of special education services under the Individuals with Disabilities Education Improvement Act (IDEA) of 2004 (PL 108-446). In the community, adapted playgrounds can offer additional opportunities for physical activity for children with cerebral palsy. Locating these accessible playgrounds, however, can be challenging (see the Additional Resources section at the end of this chapter). Adapted camps offer additional opportunities for participation in leisure and recreational activities. Competitive sports should also be considered and encouraged when appropriate. For the higher level athletes or those aspiring to reach that level, the Paralympics and related preparatory programs can be explored. The International Paralympic Committee is the governing body for the Paralympic movement and can be a resource, but many countries have their own Paralympic committees. For children with cerebral palsy with cognitive impairment, the Special Olympics can be explored. It is important to note that sociodemographic factors (i.e., household income, parent/caregiver education level, and number of parents) have been found to affect level of participation and are part of the health disparities issues addressed in Chapter 42 (Law et al., 2006).

Orthoses and Rehabilitative Equipment Orthoses or splints are frequently used with a goal of maintaining or increasing range of motion, protecting a joint, stabilizing a joint, or improving functional activity. The most common joints splinted are the ankle and the wrist-hand, but orthoses also are made for the trunk (e.g., dynamic movement orthosis). In addition to orthoses, serial casting, which is the successive application of casts, can be used to increase range of motion. Adaptive equipment can be used to improve functional mobility and/or ADLS. Different examples include wheelchairs, adapted strollers, adapted car seats, positioning chairs, walkers, gait trainers, AAC devices, computer or computer aids, and devices used for environmental control (McMahon et al., 2010). These are further discussed in Chapter 36.

Medication Medication is commonly used in conjunction with therapy, orthoses, and durable medical equipment. Medications for hypertonia are most frequently utilized for spasticity and include baclofen, dantrolene, tizanidine, and benzodiazepines. Of these, baclofen, a gamma-aminobutyric acid B agonist, is used most commonly. Baclofen inhibits overactive neurological signals communicating with the spinal cord. Baclofen and benzodiazepines are used to treat dystonia as well as trihexyphenidyl and carbidopa-levodopa. In addition to oral medication, focal medications in the form of injections are also utilized. Botulinum toxin injections are the most common type of focal treatment. It is injected intramuscularly and acts by inhibiting neurotransmitter release at the neuromuscular junction, which decreases unwanted muscle contraction (see Box 32.3; Copeland et al., 2014; Delgado et al., 2016). Another injectable medication is phenol. Phenol is injected in or near nerves and acts to disrupt signal transmission and conduction to the muscle decreasing unwanted muscle contraction.

Surgery Surgical procedures, primarily neurosurgical or orthopedic, may be recommended. Implantation of an intrathecal baclofen pump is the most common neurosurgical procedure. Rather than administering baclofen by mouth or via an enteral tube, a pump and tubing can be surgically implanted

BOX 32.3 EVIDENCE-BASED PRACTICE

Botulinum Toxin

Botulinum toxin is used frequently to manage hypertonia (spasticity or dystonia) in the pediatric population. The neurotoxin is injected intramuscularly to create a reversible neuromuscular blockade, causing muscle weakness and a reduction in tone. Goals of botulinum toxin injection include improving motor function and decreasing painful muscle spasms. Botulinum injections are effective for improving ease of care and comfort for nonambulatory children with cerebral palsy. Abobotulinumtoxin A (Dysport) is currently the only botulinum toxin A formulation approved by the U.S. Food and Drug Administration for the treatment of lower limb spasticity in pediatric patients ages 2 years and older. Intramuscular abobotulinumtoxin A approval was based on the positive outcomes of a Phase 3 trial that evaluated lower limb spasticity in pediatric patients with cerebral palsy. The results showed that abobotulinumtoxin A was well tolerated and significantly decreased muscle tone (Copeland et al., 2014; Delgado et al., 2016).

to deliver the baclofen directly to the spinal cord (see Box 32.4; Eek et al., 2018; Hasnat & Rice, 2015).

A surgical procedure considered in some children with spastic diplegia is selective dorsal rhizotomy. In this procedure, dorsal spinal nerve rootlets are cut to decrease the overactive spinal reflex and reduce spasticity in the legs. Selection criteria for this procedure are strict because it is irreversible. Deep brain stimulation is an area of interest in children with primarily dystonia or dyskinesia, but evidence for its effectiveness is limited.

Regarding orthopedic intervention, there are various soft-tissue and/or bony procedures commonly performed, including scoliosis surgery, muscle lengthening, contracture release, and tendon transfers. Orthopedic surgery in patients with cerebral palsy is commonly focused on preventing or treating hip subluxation or dislocation (Wynter et al., 2015).

CASE STUDY

Jeffrey is a 4-year-old boy seen because of his mother's concerns related to increased falls and clumsiness in comparison with his peers. Developmentally, he achieved his motor milestones at a slightly slower rate and did not walk independently until 19 months. He has no other significant past medical history. His mother reports that recently he struggles with getting up off the floor and needs extra help climbing the stairs (see Figure 32.2). He has also started to walk on his toes most of the time. Jeffrey has an older cousin on his maternal side with a similar history who now uses a wheelchair, and Jeffrey's mother has a history of early onset cardiomyopathy. His physical examination is significant for calf hypertrophy and proximal muscle weakness. He has a wide-based gait and walks on his toes. He had laboratory testing and was found to have an elevated creatinine kinase level in his blood and a mutation of the dystrophin gene, the genetic defect in Duchenne muscular dystrophy (DMD). He is referred to a neurologist for additional follow-up care.

DMD is the most common progressive childhood neuromuscular disorder (Mah et al., 2014). Chapter 9 provides a full description of typical clinical signs and symptoms, diagnostic testing, and common treatment associated with DMD. This section focuses

BOX 32.4 EVIDENCE-BASED PRACTICE

Intrathecal Baclofen

Intrathecal baclofen can reduce dystonia and spasticity and thus improve skills such as sitting, communication, and fine motor function in patients with cerebral palsy. Studies demonstrate evidence that intrathecal baclofen reduces pain, aids with sleep, and improves ease of care. The original Ashworth scale to evaluate spasticity is the most commonly used outcome measure in studies of intrathecal baclofen (Eek et al., 2018; Hasnat & Rice, 2015).

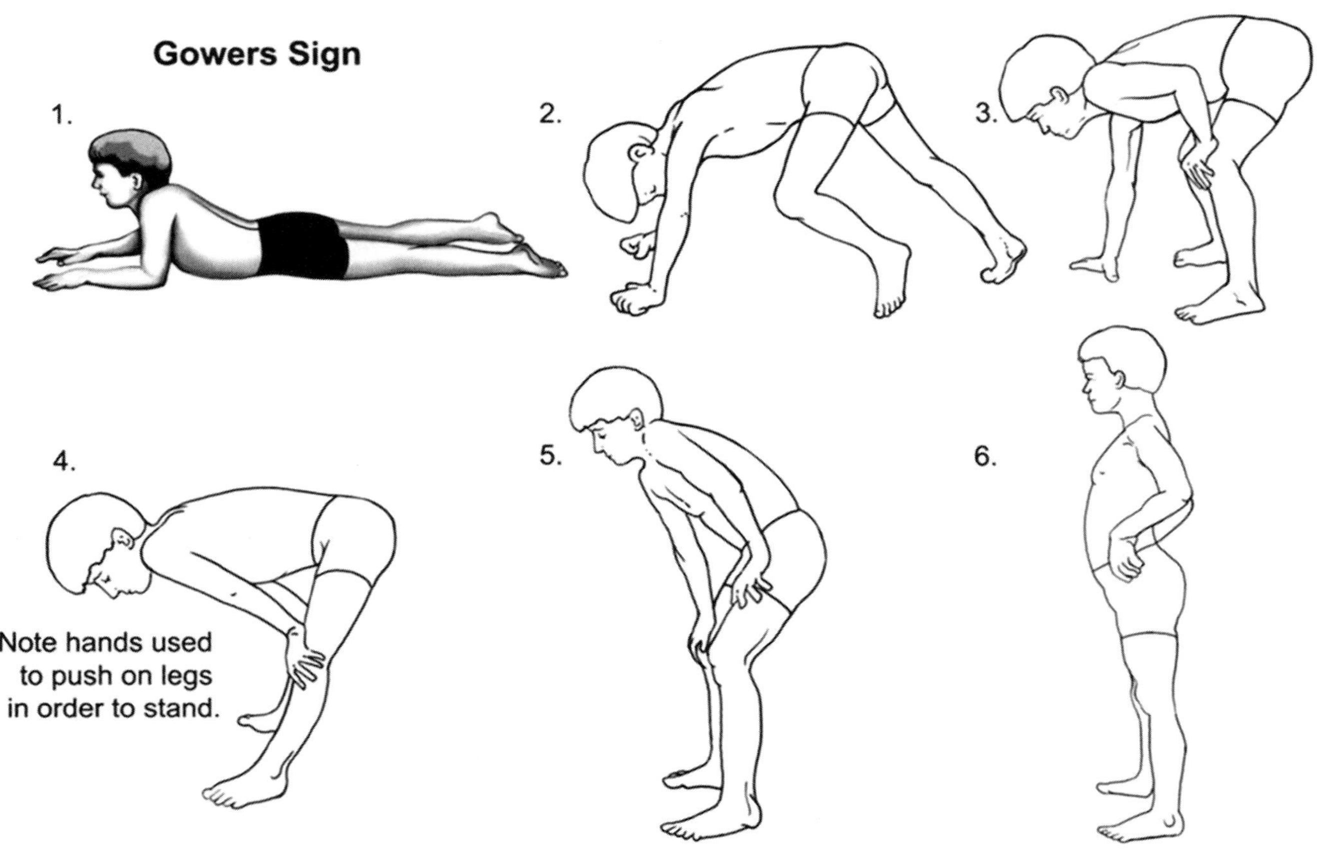

Figure 32.2. Gower's sign.

on the critical need for a rehabilitation team to support children with DMD and their family throughout their lives.

Duchenne Muscular Dystrophy

Therapeutic Approaches In accordance with the World Health Organization's ICF, treatment is focused on preserving and maximizing the child's quality of life and abilities regardless of the stage of the disease. An interprofessional team is critical in the management of a child with DMD. Muscular Dystrophy Association– and Parent Project Muscular Dystrophy–certified care centers are directed by physicians, either physiatrists or neurologists. Treatment focuses primarily on compensatory strategies and the preservation of current function (Birnkrant et al., 2018b; Box 32.5).

BOX 32.5 INTERDISCIPLINARY CARE

Treatment of Muscular Dystrophy

Due to the multisystem involvement of Duchenne muscular dystrophy, optimal management requires an interdisciplinary professional team that works with the patient and the family throughout all phases of the disease process. This team typically includes a neurologist, physiatrist, physical therapist, occupational therapist, speech and language pathologist, orthopedic surgeon, pulmonologist, cardiologist, psychologist, gastroenterologist, and dietician (Birnkrant et al., 2018a).

Rehabilitative Therapy Occupational and physical therapists play key roles as members of the interprofessional team in the management of a child with DMD. Periodic physical assessments aim to monitor the functional progression of the disease and assist with development of an individualized care plan based on the stage of the disease. Therapists focus on maximizing the child's current abilities and maintaining flexibility and strength. Maintenance of strength should never include resistive strengthening exercises or eccentric contractions as these can promote muscle breakdown that cannot be repaired by the body. Treatment strategies emphasize functional training, range of motion, submaximal aerobic exercise programs, splinting for contractures, and recommendations for assistive or adaptive devices for mobility and ADLs (e.g., standard or power wheelchairs; Birnkrant et al., 2018b). Patients are encouraged to avoid unnecessary stair climbing or other activities that stress muscles and require excessive strength. Physiatrists also provide expertise in evaluating equipment and bracing to maximize the child's function. Patients will additionally benefit from periodic evaluation by a speech-language pathologist to monitor and treat challenges with feeding, swallowing, and communication.

Respiratory and pulmonary complications are a major cause of morbidity and mortality in DMD. Cardiologists and pulmonologists are critical team members to follow the child throughout the duration of the disease process. Rehabilitation professionals work closely with the child and family to monitor cardiac and respiratory signs and symptoms to ensure timely follow-up with the appropriate specialist.

Promoting General Physical Activity Patient and family education is critical in guiding a home stretching program, pursuing recreational exercise activities, and modifying school activities. Children with DMD should be instructed to avoid high-resistance strength training and eccentric loading to prevent additional damage to the muscle. Conversely, low-resistance aerobic activity, such as swimming, should be encouraged (Birnkrant et al., 2018b). Recommendations for school may include minimizing stair climbing through the use of elevators and schedule modifications. Preservation of ambulation is critical during the first phase of the disease progression, but it can be saved for mobility in the home or the classroom as well as short-distance ambulation in the community. Treatment strategies include resting/stretching ankle-foot orthoses (AFOs), knee-ankle-foot orthoses for standing and household ambulation (late ambulatory stage), standing frames, and serial casting.

Of note, toe walking is a compensatory strategy for children with DMD due to progressive, proximal muscle weakness. Toe walking should not be discouraged. A balance of recommended interventions should be employed to preserve ambulation without overcorrection of the compensatory mechanisms used by the child to walk (Birnkrant et al., 2018b; Glanzman, Flickinger, Dholakia, Bönnemann, & Finkel, 2011).

Recreational activities are also important for the health and well-being of the child with DMD. Even though individuals with DMD should avoid becoming overly fatigued, this should not limit their participation in recreational activities. They should be encouraged to remain active in the activities they enjoy; they can be transported to the "fun" to preserve energy. Recommendations for sports and recreational activities include cycling, swimming, and other water activities. Participation in recreational teams and events should not stop once the child or adult transitions to a wheelchair for primary mobility. Local and national road races often have a division for duo teams in which one team member will push the other who is in a racing wheelchair. Another activity is Power Soccer, an international team sport for individuals of all genders who use power wheelchairs and cannot play another adaptive sport (Federation Internationale de Powerchair Football Association, 2008).

Orthoses and Rehabilitative Equipment Orthoses or splints are frequently used during rest with a goal of maintaining or increasing range of motion; they are almost never used for boys with DMD during ambulation as they interfere with the ability to obtain a functional posture. Nighttime stretching braces provide a prolonged stretch across the ankle joint and help to maintain length when worn for more than 60 consecutive minutes each day. Recommendations are usually to wear the brace through the night while asleep. Special attention should be paid to adaptive equipment for the bathroom. Grab bars and tub transfer benches make bathing safer when boys are still strong enough to toilet and shower independently. All of the boys will eventually need power wheelchairs, but some will benefit from the use of a manual wheelchair at a younger age to assist with energy conservation during long-distance community ambulation. Lift systems are useful to caregivers when patients require assistance with transfers. As boys become weaker, mobile arm supports and environmental control units can help prolong independence.

Medication Glucocorticosteroids (most commonly prednisone) are currently the most effective pharmacological agents to slow the progressive strength and functional loss and to reduce and stabilize cardiac, respiratory, and musculoskeletal impairments (Birnkrant et al., 2018b; McDonald et al., 2018; Ricotti et al., 2013). Initiation of this therapeutic intervention often occurs after the child demonstrates a plateauing in motor skills, usually around the age of 4 years (Ricotti et al., 2013). Other pharmacological interventions currently under investigation are focused on targeting the primary dystrophin deficit or the secondary pathological mechanisms that result from the lack of dystrophin. Several gene replacement therapies are under evaluation in Phase 1 clinical trials.

Bone health is also of concern related to the side effects from glucocorticosteroid use and overall reduced mobility (Birnkrant et al., 2018a; Guiraud & Davies, 2017). Bone health assessments include urine and serum tests, DEXA scans, and spinal and bone age radiographs, with possible interventions that include supplementation of vitamin D, calcium, and bisphosphonates (Birnkrant et al., 2018a; Guiraud & Davies, 2017; Ricotti et al., 2013).

Lisinopril, an afterload reducer for the circulatory system, is initiated in boys at or about the age of 10 regardless of cardiac function. Early use has been shown to prolong the onset of cardiac failure secondary to cardiomyopathy (Birnkrant et al., 2018a).

Surgery Surgical interventions are indicated to address the development of a progressive scoliosis during the nonambulatory phase. Use of a thoraco-lumbar-sacral orthosis does not slow down the progression of a scoliotic curve. Additional surgical procedures to address contractures and joint deformities for individuals in the nonambulatory phase should be used for specific symptomatic issues, such as positioning in a wheelchair or pain-related issues (Birnkrant et al., 2018b; Hsu & Quinlivan, 2013). Surgical intervention for the preservation of ambulation has mixed outcomes and, if performed, must be closely coordinated by the interprofessional team.

CASE STUDY

Leslie is a 15-year-old girl with a past medical history of having a lumbar myelomeningocele that was closed by a neurosurgeon on her first day of life. She additionally had a ventriculo-peritoneal shunt placed to treat **hydrocephalus** (excessive fluid accumulating in the ventricles of the brain) at 3 months of age. She has been followed in the spina bifida clinic at a children's hospital throughout her life. She catheterizes her bladder every 4 hours to address her **neurogenic** bladder (dysfunction caused by nerve damage) and has a nightly bowel program with an enema for neurogenic bowel. As a young child, Leslie walked with AFOs and a posterior rolling walker. However, she now prefers to use her wheelchair throughout the day. She tells the clinic team that when she uses her chair to get around rather than walking she has more energy for the things she enjoys doing at the end of the school day. She was hospitalized 9 months ago with urosepsis (a potentially life-threatening complication of a urinary infection) related to poor compliance with catheterization. During her hospitalization she developed ischial (pelvic bone) pressure wounds (ulcerations) and is now admitted to the hospital for primary closure of the wounds with plastics surgery. Leslie will be discharged from the acute care hospital to an inpatient rehabilitation facility after surgery. She will work on upper extremity strengthening and safe transfers to prevent surgical wound breakdown and optimization of her bowel and bladder regimen to ensure the wound stays dry and heals appropriately.

Spina Bifida

Spina bifida is the most common birth defect affecting the central nervous system that results in permanent disability. Children with spina bifida present with a spectrum of impairments. Of the neural tube defects, myelomeningocele is the most clinically significant form of spina bifida. Here neural tissue from the developing spinal cord is exposed and degenerates *in utero,* resulting in neurological deficits that vary with the level of the lesion (see Figure 32.3). Disruption of the nerves in the lower spine leads to varying levels of lower extremity paralysis, sensory loss, and bowel and bladder dysfunction. There is a wide range in the level of disability based on multiple factors, including the site of incomplete closure along the spinal cord, the amount of exposed spinal cord, and the timing of surgical intervention (Adzick et al., 2011). In addition, children commonly have further confounding neurologic problems and medical comorbidities that affect their functional independence (Box 32.6).

Therapeutic Approaches Currently, there is no treatment technique to repair or replace damaged nerves in the spinal cord. Thus, treatment for children with spina bifida is aligned with the ICF model to focus on maximizing independence, increasing self-advocacy, and optimizing community participation (see Figure 32.4). In addition, children with spina bifida require frequent surveillance for potential neurological, urologic, skin,

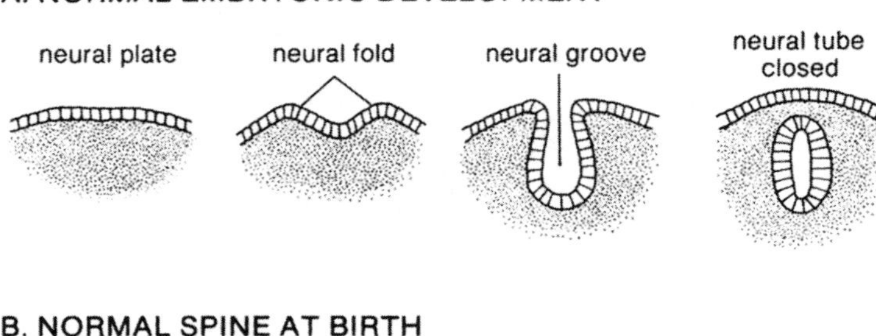

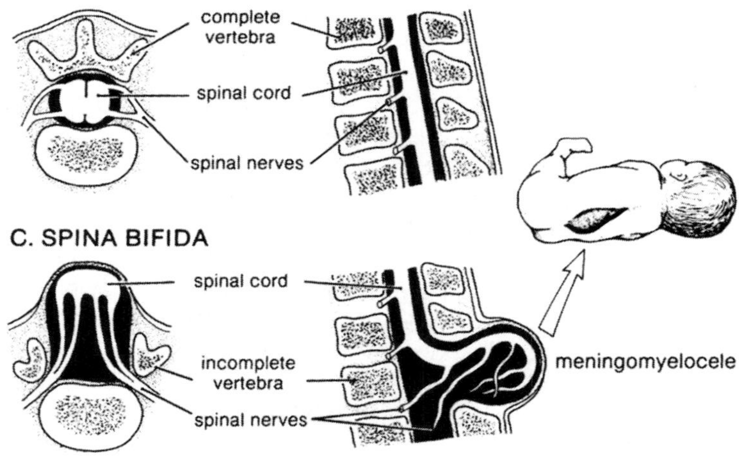

Figure 32.3. Normal neural tube development compared with spina bifida with meningomyelocele. A) The typical formation of the neural tube (i.e., the precursor of the spinal column) during the first month of gestation. B) Complete closure of the neural groove has occurred; the vertebral column and spinal cord appear normal in the cross-section on the left and the longitudinal section on the right. C) Incomplete closure of an area of the spine is called spina bifida and may be accompanied by a meningomyelocele, a sac-like abnormality of the spinal cord. Because nerves do not normally form below this malformation, the child is paralyzed below (or caudal to) that point.

BOX 32.6 INTERDISCIPLINARY CARE

Treatment of Spina Bifida

- Children with spina bifida require close medical management by interdisciplinary teams that include neurosurgeons, physiatrists, orthopedic surgeons, urologists, physical therapists, occupational therapists, dieticians, and social workers.
- Children with spina bifida will benefit from periodic physical and/or occupational therapy throughout their lives. Infants and toddlers have access to home and school-based services through early intervention services, which are part of the Individuals with Disabilities Education Improvement Act (IDEA) of 2004 (PL 108-446).
- A variety of surgical providers are involved in the care of children with spina bifida throughout their lives: Neurosurgeons closely follow patients with spina bifida to screen for and treat possible associated disorders; orthopedic surgeons manage the associated contractures and joint deformities that may occur; and urological surgical interventions are aimed to improve bowel and bladder function and continence.
- The goal when treating children with spina bifida is to maintain stable neurological functioning throughout the patient's lifetime. Rehabilitative specialists and therapists help to monitor neurological functioning.

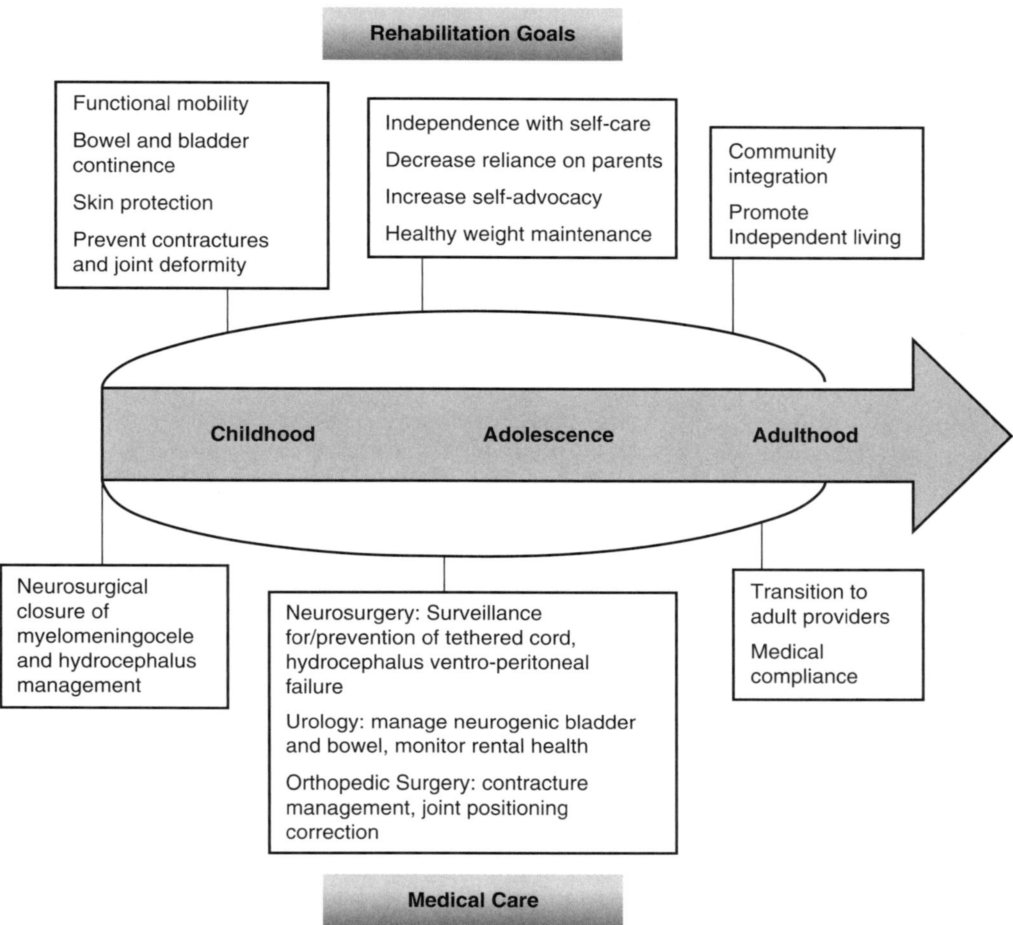

Figure 32.4. Rehabilitation goals.

and musculoskeletal complications that can further limit function and increase morbidity.

When working with children with spina bifida it is important to identify the highest neurologic level of maintained strength and sensation. Once established, this neurological level serves as a functional prognosticator and guides medical decision making, including identification of specific equipment needs and therapy goals. In addition to the preserved level of neurological integrity, independence with mobility and self-care in children with spina bifida is influenced by environmental and physical factors such as contractures, joint deformity, weight, cognitive function, family support, and access to resources.

Rehabilitative Therapy Children with spina bifida benefit from periodic physical and/or occupational therapy throughout their lives. It is not uncommon for patients with spina bifida to reengage with therapy services during critical points in development or after medical or surgical interventions. Habilitative therapy should be initiated early in the patient's life. Home- and school-based services can be accessed through early intervention services.

Occupational and physical therapy support the child in multiple areas, including gross motor development and the advancement of self-care skills. These self-care skills typically include wheelchair transfers, bladder catheterization, skin inspection for pressure ulcers, general hygiene, dressing skills, and donning and doffing orthoses. Exercise regimens focus on active and passive range of motion, stretching, functional strengthening, supported standing programs for weight-bearing benefits, and positioning to maintain good postural alignment. Through development of a home exercise program, therapists will provide the child and family with the skills to be successful in skin care and bowel and bladder management as well as mobility in the home and community.

Promoting General Physical Activity Ambulation potential and functional ability will vary in each child based on the neurological level of the lesion. Additional medical and social variables include cognitive function, weight, access to resources, and comorbidities. Even if community and household ambulation is not possible, therapeutic ambulation has both physiologic and psychologic benefits. Despite the level of the lesion, mobility independence through the use of orthoses and/or mobility equipment such as wheelchairs and scooters is possible and should be encouraged (Apkon et al., 2014; Copp et al., 2015).

Participation in adapted sports is a way for children with spina bifida to optimize their physical and physiological functioning (Shapiro & Malone, 2016). Involvement in sports is also associated with an increase in social support systems and improvements in feelings of self-worth and quality of life (Shapiro & Martin, 2014). In contrast, there is significant risk for weight gain and development of comorbidities due to inactivity in spina bifida patients. Children with varying levels of neurological involvement can participate in a variety of adapted sports activities including parasports such as skiing, tennis, and basketball. Patients with spina bifida, like patients with other spinal cord injuries, who demonstrate impairments in muscle power and range of motion, are still among the most represented athletes in the Paralympics (International Paralympic Committee, 2015).

Orthoses and Rehabilitative Equipment Patients with spina bifida usually need a variety of orthoses and rehabilitative equipment throughout their lives. The type of orthoses and equipment will vary depending on the neurological level of the lesion, clinical presentation, age of the patient, and patient and family needs. Specialized equipment might be needed to achieve these goals, and rehabilitative specialists and therapists can make appropriate equipment and orthotic recommendations. Treatment of individuals with a higher thoracic (chest)–level lesion may emphasize sitting balance and wheelchair mobility, whereas the therapeutic focus for a child with a lower sacral (back)–level lesion may be higher level balance and gait exercises with a goal of participation in sports. Table 32.5 outlines expected functional mobility and equipment needs based on level of impairment. Due to absent sensation below the neurological level of the meningomyelocele, children are at risk for skin breakdown with any ill-fitting orthotics or devices. Therefore, children and families will benefit from education on the need for vigilant skin checks and utilization of pressure relief techniques.

Medication There are no pharmaceutical options to manage the neurological impairments of spina bifida. Pharmaceutical treatments are focused on improving function of and continence of stool and urine. Medications are frequently recommended to decrease bladder storage pressure, improve urinary continence, prevent urinary tract infection, and promote regular bowel movements to prevent constipation. The need for medications to address issues such as increased pain, frequent nausea and vomiting, or increased tone may signal a complication such as shunt failure or tethered cord that needs further workup.

Surgery Surgical interventions for spina bifida usually begin at or even before birth and will continue

Table 32.5. Functional mobility and equipment needs based on level of impairment in children with spina bifida

Motor function	Level of muscle involvement	Expected potential for ambulation	Recommended orthoses for functional or therapeutic ambulation	Durable medical equipment
T12	Abdominal paraspinal	Nonfunctional ambulation; Therapeutic only	RGO	Stander (at young age) Manual wheelchair (may require power assist)
L1	Hip flexors	Household and therapeutic	Long leg: RGO, HKAFO	Manual wheelchair, stander
L2-3	Hip adductors	Household and therapeutic	Long leg: RGO, HKAFO	Manual wheelchair, forearm crutches
L4	Knee extensors	Household +/- community	Short leg: AFO	Manual wheelchair, forearm crutches
L5-S1	Ankle dorsiflexors, ankle invertors, toe extensors	Community ambulation	Short leg: AFO or SMO	+/- Forearm crutches, cane
S2	Ankle plantar flexors	Community ambulation	Foot orthoses	None

Key: RGO, reciprocal gait orthosis; HKAFO, hip-knee-ankle-foot orthosis; AFO, ankle-foot-orthosis; SMO, supra-malleolar orthosis.

BOX 32.7 EVIDENCE-BASED PRACTICE

Randomized Trial of Prenatal Versus Postnatal Repair of Myelomeningocele

A randomized control trial compared outcomes of *in utero* repair of myelomeningocele with standard postnatal repair. Eligible women were assigned to undergo either prenatal surgery before 26 weeks' gestation or standard postnatal repair. The trial was stopped for efficacy of prenatal surgery after the recruitment of 183 of the planned 200 patients. Results revealed that prenatal surgery for myelomeningocele reduced the need for shunting and improved motor outcomes at 30 months but was associated with maternal and fetal risks (Adzick et al., 2011).

throughout the patient's life. A number of surgical specialists are involved in the care of children with spina bifida, including neurosurgeons, orthopedic surgeons, and urologists. An infant with spina bifida will undergo his or her first neurosurgical intervention within 24–48 hours of birth to repair the primary spinal cord defect. Repair of the spinal cord defect during fetal life is now available to appropriate candidates, as studies have shown positive outcomes associated with prenatal myelomeningocele repair by intrauterine surgery for eligible patients (Adzick et al., 2011; see Box 32.7).

Neurosurgery involvement does not stop after closure of the spinal cord defect and is a routine feature in the management of the spina bifida population. Neurosurgeons follow patients with spina bifida closely to screen for and treat possible associated disorders, including Arnold Chiari malformation, hydrocephalus, syringomyelia, and tethered cord (Bowman & McLone, 2010). Orthopedic surgeons manage the associated contractures and joint deformities that may occur from muscular imbalances in the hips, legs, feet, or spine. Goals of urological surgical interventions are to improve bowel and bladder function and continence. Examples include bladder augmentation and Malone antegrade continence enema.

SUMMARY

- The assessment of a child with disabilities relies on both the medical history and physical exam, with an emphasis on gross and fine motor skills as well as cognition, language, and social skills.
- The ICF model of function allows the provider to relate the child's health problem to how it affects their body systems, their personhood, and their interactions with society.
- Loss of skills or milestones is not consistent with cerebral palsy and may indicate a neurodegenerative disorder.
- An early reliable marker for ambulation in the child with cerebral palsy is the ability to sit independently by 2 years of age.
- Avoid progressive resistive strength training and eccentric exercises in patients with DMD to prevent further damage to the muscles.
- Management of respiratory and cardiac complications is paramount for preservation of quality of life and increase in the overall lifespan of an individual with DMD.
- Children with spina bifida require comprehensive surveillance to prevent neurological, urologic, and skin complications that can limit function and increase morbidity.
- Due to absent sensation below the neurological level, children with spina bifida are at risk for skin breakdown and require the incorporation of skin checks and pressure relief techniques into their daily routine.

ADDITIONAL RESOURCES

American Occupational Therapy Association (AOTA): http://www.aota.org

American Physical Therapy Association (APTA): http://www.apta.org

National Rehabilitation Information Center (NARIC): http://www.naric.com

Additional resources can be found online in Appendix D: Childhood Disabilities Resources, Services, and Organizations (see About the Online Companion Materials).

REFERENCES

Adzick, N. S., Thom, E. A., Spong, C. Y., Brock, J. W., Burrows, P. K., Johnson, M. P., . . . Farmer, D. L. (2011). A randomized trial of prenatal versus postnatal repair of myelomeningocele. *New England Journal of Medicine, 364*(11), 993–1004. doi:10.1056/NEJMoa1014379

Apkon, S. D., Grady, R., Hart, S., Lee, A., McNalley, T., Niswander, L., . . . Walker J. O. (2014). Advances in the care of children with spina bifida. *Advances in Pediatrics, 61*(1), 33–74. doi:10.1016/j.yapd.2014.03.007

Birnkrant, D., Bushby, K., Bann, C., Alman, B., Apkon, S., Blackwell, A., . . . Criple, L. (2018a). Diagnosis and management of Duchenne muscular dystrophy, part 2: Respiratory, cardiac, bone health, and orthopaedic management. *The Lancet Neurology, 17* (4), 347–361. doi:10.1016/S1474-4422(18)30025-5

Birnkrant, D., Bushby, K., Bann, Ca., Apkon, S., Blackwell, A., Brumbaugh, D., . . . Clemens, P. (2018b). Diagnosis and management of Duchenne muscular dystrophy, part 1: Diagnosis, and neuromuscular, rehabilitation, endocrine, and gastrointestinal and nutritional management. *The Lancet Neurology, 17* (3), 251–267. doi:10.1016/S1474-4422(18)30024-3

Bowman, R. M., & McLone, D. G. (2010). Neurosurgical management of spina bifida: Research issues. *Developmental Disabilities Research Reviews, 16*(1), 82–87. doi:10.1002/ddrr.100

Copeland, L., Edwards, P., Thorley, M., Donaghey, S., Gascoigne-Pees, L., Kentish, M., . . . Boyd, R. N. (2014). Botulinum toxin A for nonambulatory children with cerebral palsy: A double blind randomized controlled trial. *The Journal of Pediatrics, 165*(1), 140–146.e4. doi:10.1016/j.jpeds.2014.01.050

Copp, A. J., Adzick, N. S., Chitty, L. S., Fletcher, J. M., Holmbeck, G. N., & Shaw, G. M. (2015). Spina bifida. *Nature Reviews. Disease Primers, 1,* 15007. doi:10.1038/nrdp.2015.7

Delgado, M. R., Tilton, A., Russman, B., Benavides, O., Bonikowski, M., Carranza, J., . . . Picaut, P (2016). Abobotulinumtoxin A for equinus foot deformity in cerebral palsy: A randomized controlled trial. *Pediatrics, 137*(2), e20152830–e20152830. doi:10.1542/peds.2015-2830

DeLuca, S. C., Trucks, M. R., Wallace, D. A., & Ramey, S. L. (2017). Practice-based evidence from a clinical cohort that received pediatric constraint-induced movement therapy. *Journal of Pediatric Rehabilitation Medicine, 10*(1), 37–46. doi:10.3233/PRM-170409

Eek, M. N., Olsson, K., Lindh, K., Askljung, B., Påhlman, M., Corneliusson, O., & Himmelmann, K. (2018). Intrathecal baclofen in dyskinetic cerebral palsy: Effects on function and activity. *Developmental Medicine & Child Neurology, 60*(1), 94–99. doi:10.1111/dmcn.13625

Federation Internationale de Powerchair Football Association. (2008). *About FIPFA.* Retrieved from http://fipfa.org/presentation-de-la-fipfa/

Glanzman, A. M., Flickinger, J. M., Dholakia, K. H., Bönnemann, C. G., & Finkel, R. S. (2011). Serial casting for the management of ankle contracture in Duchenne muscular dystrophy. *Pediatric Physical Therapy, 23*(3), 275–279. doi:10.1097/PEP.0b013e318227c4e3

Guiraud, S., & Davies, K. E. (2017). Pharmacological advances for treatment in Duchenne muscular dystrophy. *Current Opinion in Pharmacology, 34,* 36–48. doi:10.1016/j.coph.2017.04.002

Hasnat, M. J., & Rice, J. E. (2015). Intrathecal baclofen for treating spasticity in children with cerebral palsy. *Cochrane Database of Systematic Reviews.* doi:10.1002/14651858.CD004552.pub2

Hsu, J. D., & Quinlivan, R. (2013). Scoliosis in Duchenne muscular dystrophy (DMD). *Neuromuscular Disorders, 23*(8), 611–617. doi:10.1016/j.nmd.2013.05.003

Individuals with Disabilities Education Improvement Act (IDEA) of 2004, PL 108-446, 20 U.S.C. §§ 1400 *et seq.*

International Paralympic Committee. (2015). *IPC athlete classification code.* Retrieved from https://www.paralympic.org/sites/default/files/document/170704160235698_2015_12_17%2BClassification%2BCode_FINAL2_0.pdf

Law, M., King, G., King, S., Kertoy, M., Hurley, P., Rosenbaum, P., . . . Hanna, S (2006). Patterns of participation in recreational and leisure activities among children with complex physical disabilities. *Developmental Medicine and Child Neurology, 48*(5), 337–342. doi:10.1017/S0012162206000740

Mah, J. K., Korngut, L., Dykeman, J., Day, L., Pringsheim, T., & Jette, N. (2014). A systematic review and meta-analysis on the epidemiology of Duchenne and Becker muscular dystrophy. *Neuromuscular Disorders, 24*(6), 482–491. doi:10.1016/j.nmd.2014.03.008

McDonald, C. M., Henricson, E. K., Abresch, R. T., Duong, T., Joyce, N. C., Hu, F., . . . McDonald, C. M. (2018). Long-term effects of glucocorticoids on function, quality of life, and survival in patients with Duchenne muscular dystrophy: A prospective cohort study. *Lancet, 391*(10119), 451–461. pii:S0140-6736(17)32160-8

McMahon, M., Pruitt, D., & Vargus-Adams, J. (2010). Cerebral palsy. In M. A. Alexander & D. J. Matthews (Eds.), *Pediatric rehabilitation, principles and practice* (4th ed., pp. 165–197). New York, NY: Demos Medical Publishing.

Palisano, R., Rosenbaum, P., Walter, S., Russell, D., Wood, E., & Galuppi, B. (1997). Development and reliability of a system to classify gross motor function in children with cerebral palsy. *Developmental Medicine and Child Neurology, 39*(4), 214–223.

Ricotti, V., Ridout, D. A., Scott, E., Quinlivan, R., Robb, S. A., Manzur, A. Y., . . . Scott, E. (2013). Long-term benefits and adverse effects of intermittent versus daily glucocorticoids in boys with Duchenne muscular dystrophy. *Journal of Neurology, Neurosurgery & Psychiatry, 84*(6), 698–705. doi:10.1136/jnnp-2012-303902

Shapiro, D. R., & Malone, L. A. (2016). Quality of life and psychological affect related to sport participation in children and youth athletes with physical disabilities: A parent and athlete perspective. *Disability and Health Journal, 9*(3), 385–391. doi:10.1016/j.dhjo.2015.11.007

Shapiro, D. R., & Martin, J. J. (2014). The relationships among sport self-perceptions and social well-being in athletes with physical disabilities. *Disability and Health Journal, 7*(1), 42–48. doi:10.1016/j.dhjo.2013.06.002

World Health Organization. (2007). *International Classification of Functioning, Disability and Health: Children and Youth Version (ICF-CY).* Geneva: Switzerland: Author.

World Health Organization. (2013). *International Classification of Functioning, Disability and Health (ICF): ICF and ICF-Online, 2013.* Retrieved from http://apps.who.int/classifications/icfbrowser/

Wynter, M., Gibson, N., Willoughby, K. L., Love, S., Kentish, M., Thomason, P., . . . National Hip Surveillance Working Group. (2015). Australian hip surveillance guidelines for children with cerebral palsy: 5-year review. *Developmental Medicine & Child Neurology, 57*(9), 808–820. doi:10.1111/dmcn.12754

CHAPTER 33 Special Education Services

Elissa Batshaw Clair

Upon completion of this chapter, the reader will

- Be aware of the history of special education services
- Be familiar with the Individuals with Disabilities Education Improvement Act of 2004, Every Student Succeeds Act, and other legislation pertaining to education for students with disabilities
- Be knowledgeable about services and supports available for students with disabilities
- Understand the components of an individualized education program
- Understand the roles of a special education teacher

Special education is defined by the Individuals with Disabilities Education Improvement Act (IDEA) of 2004 (PL 108–446) as "specially designed instruction, at no cost to parents, to meet the unique needs of a child with a disability" (§ 602[29]). Special education includes direct educational instruction by a special education teacher; related services such as language therapy, speech therapy, physical therapy, occupational therapy, or social work services; paraprofessional support; or consultation from a special education professional to the general education teacher. All special education services are individualized to provide the instruction necessary to reach each student's goals. IDEA 2004 guarantees a free appropriate public education (FAPE) for all students with disabilities ages 3–21. A zero-reject provision mandates that even students who have severe and multiple impairments have the right to a FAPE in the least restrictive environment (LRE).

Before the enactment of the Education for All Handicapped Children Act of 1975 (PL 94-142), the educational needs of millions of students with disabilities were not being fully met. Students with disabilities did not receive appropriate educational services, were excluded entirely from the public school system and from being educated with their peers, had undiagnosed disabilities that prevented them from having a successful educational experience, or faced a lack of adequate resources within the public school system, requiring them to find services outside of the public school system (PL 108-446 § [601][c][2]).

Since the 1970s, legislation has attempted to address each of these issues. Figure 33.1 summarizes the history of educational law.

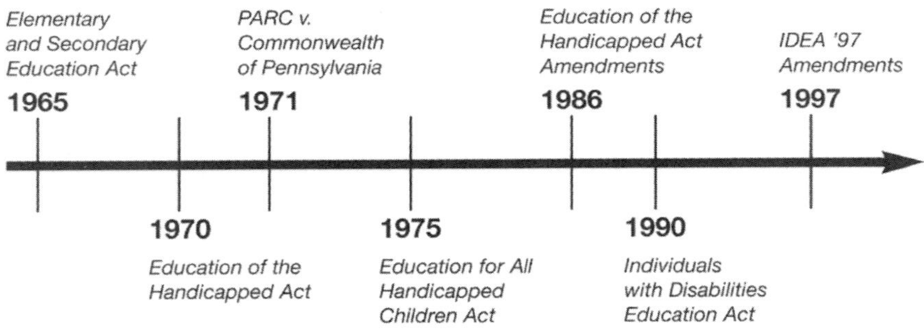

Elementary and Secondary Education Act of 1965 (PL 89-10)	Attempted to correct unequal educational opportunities that resulted from a child's economic condition
Education of the Handicapped Act (EHA) of 1970 (PL 91-230)	Amendment to earlier legislation that established a core grant program for local education agencies (LEAs) to provide services for children with disabilities
Pennsylvania Association of Retarded Citizens (PARC) v. Commonwealth of Pennsylvania (1971)	PARC proved • All children with intellectual disability are capable of benefiting from a program of education and training • Education cannot be defined as only the provision of academic experiences for children • Having undertaken to provide all children with a free appropriate public education (FAPE), the state could not deny students with intellectual disability access to FAPE • The earlier students with intellectual disability are provided education, the better the predictable learning outcomes (Yell, 1998).
Education for All Handicapped Children Act of 1975 (PL 94-142)	• Provided FAPE to all school-age children, regardless of their disability • Was a funded program • Defined the disabilities that would be covered and established guidelines for fair evaluation and assessment
Education of the Handicapped Act Amendments of 1986 (PL 99-457)	• Extended special education services to infants and preschoolers • Developed an individual family service plan (IFSP) for infants and toddlers in early intervention programs (Mercer, 1997)
Individuals with Disabilities Education Act (IDEA) of 1990 (PL 101-476)	• Used person-first language and replaced the word handicap with disability • Arranged for transition planning to occur to help students progress from high school into adulthood (Mercer, 1997) • Emphasized meeting the needs of ethnically and culturally diverse children with disabilities • Indicated early intervention programs to address the needs of children who were exposed prenatally to maternal substance abuse (Mercer, 1997)
Individuals with Disabilities Education Act Amendments of 1997 (IDEA '97; PL 105-17)	• Strengthened the role of parents • Gave increased attention to racial, ethnic, and linguistic diversity to prevent inappropriate identification and mislabeling • Ensured that schools are safe and conducive to learning • Encouraged parents and educators to work out their differences by using nonadversarial means

Figure 33.1. History of educational law prior to the current law, the Individuals with Disabilities Education Improvement Act (IDEA) of 2004 (PL 108-446).

CASE STUDY

Mateo did not walk or speak his first word until 18 months. As a toddler, he received speech therapy in his home once per week in accordance with an **individualized family service plan (IFSP)** provided under Part C (Infants and Toddlers with Disabilities) of IDEA. These services were designed to help Mateo's parents facilitate their son's communication skills. When Mateo entered kindergarten, he was soon identified as having significant delays compared with his classmates and as needing special education services. His parents gave permission for testing, which showed him to be functioning in the range of mild intellectual disability. He was thus eligible for special education services.

An **individualized educational program (IEP)** was developed for Mateo with input from a team consisting of a psychologist, a general education teacher, a special education teacher, a speech-language pathologist, and his parents. The IEP identified the goals for Mateo, the amount of time he would receive special education services, and the **related services** that would be provided to support his educational progress.

The IEP team had a formal discussion that included reviewing information from Mateo's most recent evaluations as well as data collected by teachers and parental input. They determined that the most appropriate placement for Mateo was in an inclusive environment in a class containing students both with and without disabilities. The class was cotaught by a general education and special education teacher. (Ideally this class would be cotaught throughout the entire day, but it is more typical for classes to be cotaught for portions of the day, with only the general education teacher teaching the other portions.) The two teachers worked together to ensure that all students, including Mateo, could have access to the same core curriculum with differentiated instruction and **modifications** to the schoolwork. The team also decided that Mateo would require related services from a speech-language pathologist. Sometimes this therapist would teach a lesson to all or part of the class; at other times, she worked with Mateo individually.

Mateo made good progress in this program and was reassessed regularly so that his IEP could be adjusted. When Mateo was 16 years old, he began the transition planning process mandated by IDEA. With his input during a transition-planning inventory, a **transition IEP** was developed. Mateo was very interested in cooking, often preparing creative meals at home. He chose to attend prevocational food service classes in addition to his academic courses. The high school offered career cluster experiences in culinary arts, and Mateo continued taking vocational classes, honing his skills as a chef. With the help of a job coach provided by the Bureau of Vocational Rehabilitation, Mateo secured a summer job at a local restaurant. He continued in his school program through age 21 because special education legislation offers services through this age for students with disabilities who 1) have not earned all of their credits toward graduation, 2) need additional transition services, or 3) are earning an alternative certificate rather than a general education diploma. Beginning in 11th grade, when Mateo was 17, he worked half days at the restaurant while continuing to attend school part time. At 20 years of age, he enrolled in culinary classes at a community college as part of his ITP. At age 21, he completed his public education, received a diploma, and was subsequently hired full time as an assistant chef at the same restaurant.

Thought Questions:

What are the components and sequence of multitiered systems of support (MTSS)? What are the ways that special education teachers can facilitate learning?

PREVALENCE AND EPIDEMIOLOGY

Eligibility for Special Education

Eligibility for special education services is defined by IDEA 2004. Two other laws, Section 504 of the Rehabilitation Act of 1973 (PL 93-112) and the Americans with Disabilities Act (ADA) of 2008 (PL 110-325), also define avenues for students with disabilities to receive special services. Another law affecting special education but not directly pertaining to eligibility, Every Student Succeeds Act of 2015 (PL 114-95), will be addressed later in this chapter.

Individuals with Disabilities Education Improvement Act of 2004

For a student to receive special education services, he or she must have a physical, cognitive, or behavioral impairment that interferes with the ability to benefit from instruction in the general classroom curriculum. Students who qualify as having a disability under IDEA are provided services through an IEP. The specific disabilities recognized by IDEA Part B Regulations (34 C.F.R § 300.8 [a]) fall under the following categories:

- Intellectual disability
- Hearing impairments (including deafness)
- Speech or language impairments
- Visual impairments (including blindness)
- Emotional disturbances
- Orthopedic impairments
- Autism
- Traumatic brain injury
- Other health impairments (including chronic diseases and attention-deficit/hyperactivity disorder [ADHD] if they impair educational performance)
- Specific learning disabilities
- Deaf-blindness
- Multiple disabilities
- Young child with a developmental delay (ages 3–9)

Autism is the fastest growing of these categories. For the 2009–2010 school year, there were 378,000 students identified with ASD. This accounted for 5.8% of the special education population and 0.8% of the general population. Five years later (2014–2015), there were 576,000 students identified with ASD. This accounted for 8.8% of the special education population and 1.1% of the general population. One area of eligibility that is shrinking is emotional disturbance (ED). Within that same time frame, the number of students qualifying for IEP services as students with ED fell from 420,000 to 349,000, or from 6.5% to 5.3% of the special education population and from 0.9% to 0.7% of total student enrollment (U.S. Department of Education, 2016).

Related Services within Special Education

In addition to the academic services provided by the teacher, students with disabilities are eligible to receive related services. The term **related services** is defined as "transportation and such developmental, corrective, and other supportive services . . . as may be required to assist a student with a disability to benefit from special education" (PL 108-446, § 601[26]). According to IDEA 2004 (PL 108-446, § 602[26]), these services include the following:

- Speech-language pathology and audiology services
- Psychological services
- Physical and occupational therapy
- Recreation, including therapeutic recreation
- Social work services
- Counseling services, including rehabilitation counseling
- Orientation and mobility services, including therapeutic recreation
- Medical services
- Nurse services

Table 33.1 summarizes the types of related services that may be provided for individuals by disability.

Section 504 of the Rehabilitation Act of 1973 and the Americans with Disabilities Act Amendments Act of 2008

The basic concept of IDEA is that of zero reject—in other words, the public school system must accommodate or find alternate accommodations at public expense for every student with a defined disability. If a student does not satisfy the IDEA 2004 criteria for disabilities, he or she may still receive the benefit of access, accommodations, and special services through Section 504 of the Rehabilitation Act of 1973 (PL 93-112) or the ADA of 2008 (PL 110-325), where the objectives and language are similar. These two acts are intended to establish a "level playing field" by eliminating barriers that exclude people with disabilities from participation in the community and workplace. They attempt to eliminate hurdles and discrimination that prevent or hamper participation, whether physical (e.g., steps instead of ramps) or programmatic (e.g., exclusion of a student with HIV from the classroom). The ADA creates access to physical barriers. An example of this is mandating an elevator or lift in a school building if needed for a student with a physical disability. Section 504 of the Rehabilitation Act of 1973 creates access to programmatic needs. An example of this is requiring a place to rest and shortened assignments if needed for a student with cancer who is receiving chemotherapy.

The definition of disability is broader under Section 504 than under IDEA 2004. Although Section 504 covers the majority of students covered by IDEA 2004, the reverse is not the case. Specifically, Section 504 protects people who have a physical or mental impairment that substantially limits one or more major life activities, have a record of such an impairment, or are regarded as having such an impairment. Examples of major life activities include functions such as caring for oneself, performing manual tasks, walking, seeing, hearing, speaking, breathing, learning, and working (34 C.F.R. 104.3[j][2][ii]). Congress further refined this list to include eating, sleeping, standing, lifting, bending, reading, concentrating, thinking, and communicating (U.S. Department of Education, Department of Civil Rights, 2016). In addition, mitigating measures (such as medication, medical supplies, equipment or supplies, low vision devices, mobility devices, prosthetics, hearing aids and cochlear implants, etc., with the exception of ordinary glasses or contact lenses) cannot be considered when determining disability under 504 determinations. For example, the members of the 504 team would not be permitted to determine that, because a student's ADHD medication is effective, that student is not disabled under section 504. As another example, the 504 team cannot determine ineligibility for a student with hearing aids or a cochlear implant because the student is able to process sound well enough to communicate (Office of Civil Rights, 2015).

The following are examples of students who may be covered by Section 504 to receive special services but not by IDEA 2004:

Table 33.1. Examples of disabilities and typical related services provided

	Services									
Disability	Speech-language pathology	Audiology	Behavior support and counseling	Physical therapy	Occupational therapy	Vision (orientation and mobility)	Social work	Assistive technology	Transportation	Medical services
Vision impairment			X		X	X	X	X	X	
Hearing impairment	X	X	X				X	X	X	
Intellectual disability	X		X	X			X	X	X	
Autism	X		X		X		X	X	X	
Other health impairment: Attention-deficit/hyperactivity disorder			X				X	X	X	
Learning disabilities			X				X	X		
Orthopedic impairment: Cerebral palsy	X		X	X	X		X	X	X	X
Traumatic brain injury	X		X	X	X		X	X	X	X

- Students with communicable diseases (e.g., HIV)
- Students with food allergies
- Students with asthma
- Students with attention disorders without significant academic deficiencies
- Students with Tourette syndrome, epilepsy, diabetes, or cancer
- Students with impairments as a result of emotional illness or former misclassification of intellectual disability (Office of Civil Rights, 1995)

Attention-Deficit/Hyperactivity Disorder: IDEA or 504 Students diagnosed with ADHD may require 1) services under IDEA in the category of Other Health Impairment, 2) services under Section 504 of the Rehabilitation Act, or 3) no services that differ from other general education students at their school. Making the decision of whether a student requires an IEP or a 504 plan is individual and based on a team decision after weighing that student's unique strengths and weaknesses. Examples of educational needs that may require accommodations, modifications, or instruction in students with ADHD include the following:

- Difficulty sustaining attention during instruction or when presented with assignments
- Difficulty following multistep directions (working memory)
- Tendency to misplace assignments/supplies
- Difficulty completing long-term assignments (organization)
- Behavior problems (impulsivity, oppositional defiant behavior)

When deciding between an IDEA identification and a 504 plan, the team should consider whether the student needs accommodations, modifications, or specialized instruction to allow him or her access to the general education curriculum. For students whose needs can be served by accommodations, the team may determine that a 504 plan is the most appropriate action. Accommodations for students with ADHD may include shortened assignments without changing the difficulty level; written, multistep directions; or assistance with writing assignments in a daily planner. For students who need specialized instruction, the team may determine that an IEP will most appropriately address deficits in social skills, self-monitoring, accessing memory, regulating alertness, or sustaining effort. For students who require modifications such as lowering the difficulty level of assignments or shortening assignments so that integral portions are omitted, the team may develop an IEP after carefully weighing both options and considering additional factors.

Other Factors That Define Disability

Nondiscriminatory Assessment and Eligibility Public schools are obligated to provide a nondiscriminatory evaluation for any student suspected of having a disability. This includes students enrolled in private schools and students ages 3–5 years who are not yet registered for school. Implementing this requirement varies from state to state. In addition to having access to official preschool Child Find programs (see Chapter 31), generally parents can bring their child to the local school district and request an evaluation. The stated purpose of the initial evaluation is to determine whether a child has a disability and, if present, to establish the student's educational needs (PL 108–446, §§ 612 [a][10][A][ii] and § 614[a] [1][A]).

Parents must consent prior to an evaluation. This consent, however, is not consent for placing the student in a special education program, which must be obtained separately. A student is usually evaluated by a multidisciplinary team consisting of a psychologist and one or more of the following education professionals: speech-language pathologist, occupational therapist, physical therapist, and social worker. The evaluation team should use a comprehensive assessment process to address the student's strengths, interests, goals, and needs in order to determine whether and which special education services are required. The evaluation may include tests of intelligence, academic skills, memory, visual-motor integration, adaptive behavior, reading, math, written expression, social-emotional skills, motor skills, sensory integration, speech, and language. For students whose cognitive functioning is at a preschool level, testing focuses on communication, social, motor, and adaptive skills.

The multidisciplinary team must follow specific guidelines during the student's evaluation. These guidelines were created in response to certain faulty evaluation practices in the past, which led to many students (especially minority students; see Chapter 42) being incorrectly diagnosed and placed in special education. Many minority students who functioned appropriately outside of school were classified as "intellectually disabled" based on a single IQ test. This injustice was first formally recognized with the *Larry P. v. Riles* federal court case in California in 1972. A group of African American students complained that they had been inappropriately placed into special education classes for students with "educatable mental retardation" (EMR) based on intelligence tests that were biased against children of color. The justices ruled that these very common intelligence tests (WISC and Stanford-Binet) were indeed biased and resulted in a disproportionality large percentage of African American students in EMR classes. The court ruled that standardized intelligence tests were no longer to be used in the state of California to determine placement in EMR classes (Bersoff, 1980). With this type of inequity in mind, a number of mandates for nondiscriminatory evaluation procedures were installed as part of IDEA 1990 and continue in IDEA 2004 today. The key mandates are that 1) several tests must be used to determine whether the student has a disability and 2) parental input must be included (PL 108-466, § 614[a][2][A–C] and 614[b][3][A]).

With increasing concerns about the rising number of students classified as having a learning disability, IDEA 2004 prohibits eligibility decisions from being made based on a lack of instruction or as a result of limited English proficiency (PL 108-446, § 614 [b][5][A–C]). Reevaluation of a student with a disability is required to take place no more than once per year or less than once every 3 years unless the parent and local education agency agree that the timelines should be altered.

General Education Legislation Affecting Special Education The Every Student Succeeds Act (ESSA) of 2015, which is a reauthorization of the Elementary and Secondary Education Act of 1965 (PL 94-142), refines IDEA in four areas: 1) alignment of IEP goals to state academic content standards, 2) inclusion in state high-stakes assessment for all students (including the use of alternative assessments based on alternative academic achievement standards, 3) the use of universal design for learning in assessments, and 4) the disaggregation of students with disabilities into a subgroup for accountability purposes. The purpose of these regulations is to ensure that all students with disabilities are educated to the same high standards as their peers without disabilities (Council of Chief State School Officers, 2016).

Endrew F. v. Douglas County In 2017, the Supreme Court changed the provisions of special education with their ruling in the case of *Endrew F. v. Douglas County*. Endrew was a student with autism spectrum disorder whose parents believed that he was not being afforded the opportunity to make progress in his public school. They had unilaterally placed him in a private school (where he was making progress) and were seeking reimbursement for his tuition fees. Prior to this case, school districts were required to provide services that met the "merely more than *de minimis*" standard, meaning that the student must be provided enough services to achieve "some" benefit from their education. This was a result of the 1982 *Board of Education v. Rowley* Supreme Court case. In the case of *Board of Education v. Rowley*, Amy was a student with a hearing impairment. The school system had provided her with a tutor, speech therapist, and an FM unit for the teacher to amplify the teacher's words. Amy's parents wanted the school to provide a sign language interpreter. However, Amy was making adequate progress with the supports provided. The court determined that students with IEPs need only be provided with the services necessary to benefit from their education (*Endrew F. v. Douglas County*, 2017). This 2017 ruling found that the "merely more than *de minimis*" standard did not provide FAPE. Educational institutions are now required to provide "an educational program [that] must be appropriately ambitious in light of [the students] circumstances" (p. 14). For a student to be fully included in the general education classroom, an IEP typically should be "reasonably calculated to enable the student to achieve passing marks and advance from grade to grade" (p. 1). For students who are not included in the general education classroom, the ruling was less clear. However, Justice Roberts wrote that "A student's IEP need not aim for grade-level advancement if that is not a reasonable prospect. But that student's educational program must be appropriately ambitious in light of his circumstances" (*Endrew F. v. Douglas County*, 2017, p. 3).

Racial Disparity One of the goals of IDEA 2004 was to reduce the overrepresentation of minorities in special education. While the reduction of minorities in special education (especially in the area of intellectual disability) remains a goal of the federal government, newer analysis has indicated that discrimination of minorities is through both overrepresentation and underrepresentation in special education (see Chapter 42).

GOALS OF TREATMENT: THE INDIVIDUALIZED EDUCATION PROGAM

An IEP indicates the special educational services a student will receive and the expected achievement with the support of these services over the course of the school year. According to IDEA 2004, these goals must be developed based on 1) the strengths of the student; 2) the concerns of the parents; 3) the results of the most recent evaluation of the student; and 4) the academic, developmental, and functional needs of the student (§ 614[d][3][A]). IEP goals must also align with state grade-level academic content standards. A new

IEP must be written at least once per year and should be modified as often as needed based on an assessment of the student's progress. In addition, an IEP can be amended when changes are necessary (as opposed to rewriting the entire IEP) if the changes are covered within the time frame of the original IEP.

Format and Content

The law is very specific about what must be included in an IEP. According to IDEA 2004, with additions as required by ESSA of 2015 (Council of Chief State School Officers, 2016), an IEP must contain the following items (PL 108-446, § 614 [d][1][A]):

- A statement of the student's present level of academic achievement and functional performance and how the student's disability affects participation in the general curriculum
- A statement of measurable annual goals, including academic and functional goals, which are aligned to state grade-level academic content standards (or alternate academic standards for students with the most significant cognitive disabilities)
- A description of how the student's progress toward the annual goals will be measured
- A statement of the special education, related services, and supplementary aids and services, based on peer-reviewed research to the extent practicable, that will be provided to the student or on behalf of the student
- A statement of modifications or supports for school personnel that will be provided for the student
- An explanation of the extent, if any, to which the student will not participate with students who do not have disabilities in the general education classroom
- A statement of any individual modifications that are needed for the student to participate in statewide or districtwide assessments of student achievement, including information as to if a student will be participating in alternate assessment (based on Alternate Academic Achievement Standards for students with the most significant cognitive disabilities, not to make up more than 1% of the student body)
- A statement of the projected date for the beginning of the services and modifications, along with descriptions and an indication of the anticipated frequency, location, and duration of those services and modifications
- A statement for students 16 years or older of postsecondary goals based on age-appropriate transition assessments related to training; education; employment; and, when appropriate, independent living skills

Personnel

Members of an IEP team include the parent(s); the student (when appropriate); the special education teacher; representatives of related services (such as therapists and social workers); the general education teacher (if the student is likely to participate in the general education environment); the psychologist (see Box 33.1); an interpreter if needed; a representative of the local educational agency, which is normally the school district; and an individual who can interpret evaluation results (PL 108-446, § 614 [d] [1][B] [i–vii]).

Establishment of the Least Restrictive Environment

IDEA 2004 emphasizes that the general education classroom is the appropriate beginning point for planning an IEP. A more restrictive placement should be considered only when participation in the general education classroom is demonstrably not beneficial to the student. Even students with severe cognitive impairments have benefited academically and socially from being educated in an inclusive environment (Williamson, McLeskey, Hoppey, & Rentz, 2006). IDEA clearly states that the need for modifications to the general education curriculum is by itself not a valid reason for placing a student in a more restrictive educational setting. According to the U.S. Department of Education's Office of Special Education and Rehabilitative Services, the appropriate placement of a student should be made based on the

> educational benefits available to the disabled student in a traditional classroom, supplemented with appropriate aids and services, in comparison to the educational benefits to the disabled student from a special education classroom; the non-academic benefits to the disabled student from interacting with nondisabled students; and the degree of disruption of the education of other students, resulting in the inability to meet the unique needs of the disabled student. (1994, p. 7)

Although IDEA 2004 promotes inclusion, FAPE is the primary requirement for the education of students with a disability. For students with severe disabilities, the full continuum of placements, including education

BOX 33.1 INTERDISCIPLINARY CARE

The Role of the School Psychologist

The school psychologist is the gatekeeper to special education, but they have many functions in that role. The school psychologist has the greatest role in the Child Find requirement of the Individuals with Disabilities Education Improvement Act (IDEA) of 2004 (PL 108–446). They are generally the team member that coordinates the evaluation, and they conduct most of the assessments, such as administering tests of intelligence, academics, or emotional functioning. The school psychologist also conducts interviews with parents, teachers, and students, as well as conducts observations of the student in the school environment. In addition, the school psychologist also plays an important preventive role. They work with individual students, families, teachers, and administrators to enable students to be successful in general education and to prevent a placement in special education that could have been avoided. The school psychologist provides counseling to individual students and develops and monitors individual academic and behavioral improvement plans. They connect families to community resources and improve school-family partnerships. The school psychologist works with teachers to facilitate small-group academic and behavioral supports within their classrooms. They work with administrators to facilitate schoolwide multi-tiered systems of support–response to intervention programs for both schoolwide systems of academic growth and positive behavior interventions and support for schoolwide behavioral management.

in separate classrooms or separate schools, may be the most appropriate (Kauffman & Badar, 2016).

There has been a significant decrease in the time students spend in separate settings for special education in the past 2 decades. Between 1989 and 2013, the percentage of students with disabilities receiving services outside of the general education environment for 80% or more of the day was halved, from 69% to 38% (U.S. Department of Education, Office of Special Education and Rehabilitative Services, 2015). Table 33.2 summarizes the different approaches and environments for providing special education services and the distribution of students within these environments.

Development of Annual Goals and Benchmarks or Objectives

IDEA 2004 requires the development of measurable annual goals to enable parents and educators to determine a student's progress. These goals should address both academic and nonacademic concerns and be based on the student's current education and behavior level and aligned to state grade-level academic content standards (or alternate academic standards for students with the most significant cognitive disabilities). The purpose of these goals is to require educational institutions to provide challenging instruction and to hold high expectations for students with disabilities. This is intended to create students who are college or career ready when they transition to adulthood. Parents of students with disabilities are to be informed of their student's progress as often as are parents of students without disabilities. Therefore, if general education report cards are distributed quarterly, reports on goal progress must also be distributed quarterly. Progress toward reaching annual goals does not necessarily require a letter grade but can be performance based or criterion referenced; it can be rated on a spectrum, such as from "no progress" to "goal met." In addition to goals, students who participate in alternative assessments require benchmarks that delineate smaller steps needed to meet the goal (Assistance to States for the Education of Children with Disabilities, 2017).

Example Goals and Benchmarks As an example, a goal for a student named Sally might be, "While participating in a classroom activity, Sally will make one request to an adult or peer using a core vocabulary word (i.e., words that have a functional and academic purpose) through a preferred mode of communication for four out of five classroom activities" (Goalbook, 2017).

Example Short-Term Objectives/Benchmarks

1. By the first quarter, given an object during a classroom activity and a verbal cue, Sally will indicate that the object is liked or disliked (e.g., by smiling or crying) within 5 seconds for four out of five objects.
2. By the second quarter, when presented with a highly preferred object during a classroom activity, Sally

Table 33.2. Different approaches and environments for providing special education services and the distribution of students within these environments

Environment	% of all students with disabilities	Means of service provision
0%–20% of the day spent in a special education setting	All disabilities: 62% Learning disabilities: 69% Speech-language impairment: 87% Emotional disturbance: 45% Intellectual disability: 16% Other health impairments: 64% Autism: 40%	*Co-teaching or general education class with consulting special education teacher or related services provider, services with or without special materials:* A special education teacher or related services provider shares responsibility for teaching with the general education teacher in the general education setting or assists the general education teacher in adapting the general education curriculum to best meet the needs of the child with a disability. A special education professional may also come into the classroom to work directly with the child. *General education with resource services:* The child receives services from a special education teacher and/or related services provider (e.g., physical therapist, occupational therapist, or speech-language pathologist) outside of the general education setting for a small (< 21%) portion of the day.
21%–60% of the day spent in a special education setting	All disabilities: 19% Learning disabilities: 24% Speech-language impairment: 5% Emotional disturbance: 18% Intellectual disability: 27% Other health impairments: 21% Autism: 18%	*General education class with resource services:* The child typically joins a small group of students in a separate classroom (21%–60% of the school day) to work on areas of need, with a special education teacher and/or related services provider.
61%–100% of the day spent in a special education setting	All disabilities: 14% Learning disabilities: 6% Speech-language impairment: 4% Emotional disturbance: 20% Intellectual disability: 49% Other health impairments: 10% Autism: 33%	*Self-contained environment:* The child is educated in a separate special education class for the majority (61%–100%) of the school day but typically has lunch and nonacademic classes with peers without disabilities.
100% of the day spent in a special education setting	All disabilities: 3% Emotional disturbance: 13% Multiple disabilities: 18% Deaf blind: 18%	*Separate day school:* The child attends a school that serves only children with disabilities, and he or she spends no time during the school day with children without disabilities.
	All disabilities: 0.3%	*Separate residential school:* The child attends a live-in special education program.
	All disabilities: 0.4%	*Hospital or home-bound instruction:* The child is unable to attend school and is educated in the hospital during a hospital stay or receives services at home.

Source: U.S. Department of Education, Office of Special Education and Rehabilitative Services (2015).

will independently reach for the object within 3 seconds for four out of five highly preferred objects.

3. By the third quarter, when presented with a preferred object during a classroom activity, Sally will request access to the object by using one core vocabulary word with prompting for four out of five communication opportunities (Goalbook, 2017).

The Transition Individualized Educational Program

An adolescent with a disability needs to start preparing for life in the community (see Chapter 40). According to IDEA 2004, the plans for meeting this goal may include preparing for "postsecondary education, vocational training, integrated employment (including supported employment), competitive employment, continuing and adult education, adult services, independent living, or community participation" (§ 602[30][A]).

Beginning at age 16 (though it is widely recommended to start sooner), a formal transition IEP must be prepared and should be based on the individual student's needs, interests, and choices. It must include the following:

- The development of appropriate measurable postsecondary goals based upon age-appropriate transition assessments related to training; education; employment; and, where appropriate, independent living skills
- The development of a statement of the transition services (including courses of study) needed to assist the student in reaching those goals

Carter, Trainor, Sun, and Owens (2009) recommend that "postsecondary goals be deeply entrenched in values and beliefs about family, community, adulthood and disability" (p. 76). Transition IEPs should be culturally responsive. A transition IEP will map out "instruction, related services, community experiences, the development of employment and other post-school adult living objectives, and, when appropriate, acquisition of daily living skills and functional vocational evaluation" (§ 602[30][C]).

TREATMENT, MANAGEMENT, AND INTERVENTIONS

Multitiered Systems of Support

Multitiered systems of support (MTSS) is a systematic method of delivering increasingly more intensive levels of academic instruction or social/behavioral instruction/support for all students based on need. In this way, struggling students are able to grow academically and behaviorally without the need for a special education designation. The average age that a student is identified as having a specific learning disability in reading is 10 years (or 4th grade). With MTSS, students receive assistance at a much earlier stage in their educational career. The MTSS process is a schoolwide initiative that begins services in kindergarten. Some student's academic and behavioral difficulties are resolved through the MTSS process, and those students are able to avoid placement in special education altogether. Support and instruction is delivered in three tiers: 1) universal, 2) targeted instruction, and 3) intensive interventions. Students who are in Tier 3 and lack progress or students in Tier 3 who require special education levels of service to maintain gains likely need a special education evaluation to determine if they have an identifiable disability. The student's level of progress during tiered instruction is one method that can be used to identify a specific learning disability. MTSS is divided into two systems. The academic segment of MTSS is referred to as response to intervention (RTI). The social/behavioral segment is referred to as positive behavior interventions and supports (PBIS). See Figure 33.2.

Response to Intervention RTI generally includes "universal screening, a high-quality core reading [or other academic] program, progress monitoring, increasingly intensive tiers of intervention, and fidelity of implementation" (Otaiba, Wagner, & Miller, 2014, p. 130).

As with both MTSS systems, RTI is a three-tier model. About 80%–85% of students fall into Tier 1 (universal); these are students who respond to the high-quality, research-based instruction provided in the classroom and perform near grade level or above.

About 10%–15% of students are serviced in Tier 2 (targeted instruction); these are students performing below grade level. Tier 2 students are provided with research-based, small-group instruction in deficit areas in addition to the instruction they receive in the classroom. With this additional instruction, they make progress at a rate that will allow them to catch up with their peers. Some Tier 2 students gain the requisite skills that they were lacking and no longer require additional instruction; these students return to Tier 1. Some Tier 2 students make appropriate progress but require additional instruction to continue their gains; these students remain in Tier 2.

About 5% of students do not progress at a rate that allows them to approximate typical student performance, even with Tier 2 interventions. These students require more intensive services and move to Tier 3 (intensive intervention). In Tier 3, students receive smaller group or individual instruction targeted to meet their unique areas of weakness in addition to the services they receive in Tiers 1 and 2 (Otaiba et al., 2014; Procter, Graves, & Esch, 2012).

RTI also concerns the identification of students with specific learning disabilities (SLD). RTI, in fact, was introduced by IDEA 2004 as an alternate and preferred method for identifying students with SLD.

The Institute of Education Sciences conducted a national study in 2011–2012 of the effectiveness on RTI. The study found that RTI was not an effective intervention; however, this study had serious methodological flaws that call into question its conclusions. For example, the researchers used students who were stronger readers than those who typically receive support, and schools provided small-group instruction to both the experimental and the control group (rather than the typical large-group general education environment). The study also included schools with only one student in the entire school in Tier 2 or 3. Until further research is done, RTI continues to be regarded as an effective intervention for struggling students (Fuchs & Fuchs, 2017; Gersten, Jayanthi, & Dimino, 2017).

Positive Behavioral Interventions and Supports

PBIS includes "key characteristics of (a) school climate, (b) proactive strategies, and (c) systematic, systemwide practices" (Farrell, Collier-Meek, & Pons, 2013, p. 39). It also has three tiers of service. Tier 1 includes explicit teaching of school expectations and routines as well as positive reinforcement (such as tickets that can be turned in for prizes) for following those expectations

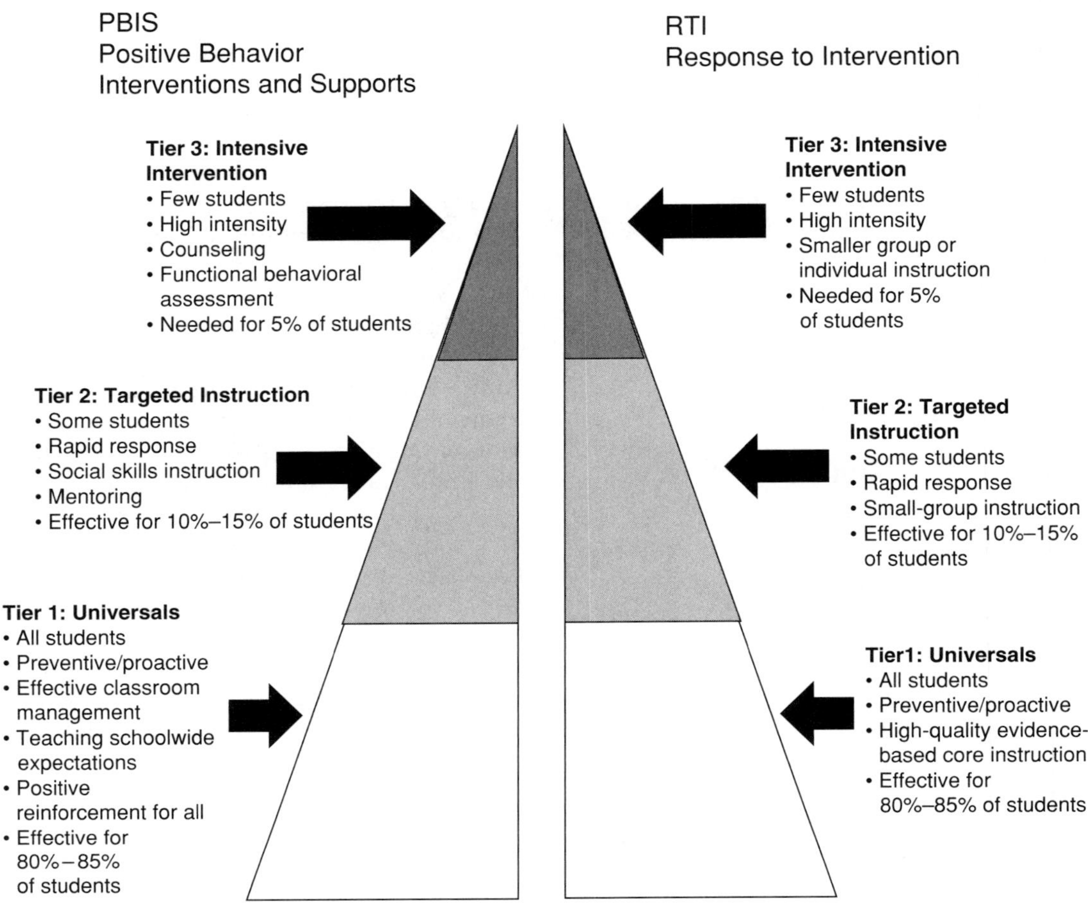

Figure 33.2. Multitiered systems of support.

and routines. Approximately 80%–85% of students behave appropriately under these approaches. Tier 2 interventions are used for the 10%–15% of students who are not progressing with universal supports. These include targeted interventions, such as small-group social skills instruction or check-in/check-out with an adult at the beginning and end of each school day. For the 5% of students not responding to Tier 2 supports, the school will initiate Tier 3. Tier 3 intensive interventions may include counseling and/or wraparound services following a functional behavioral assessment (Farrell et al., 2013; McDaniel, Bruhn, & Mitchell, 2015).

Accommodations and Modifications

Students with disabilities can be supported within the general education curriculum in many ways, among which are accommodations and curriculum modifications. **Accommodations** are changes in the way a student has access to the curriculum or demonstrates learning. Accommodations 1) provide equal access to learning, 2) do not substantially change the instructional level or content, 3) are based on individual strengths and needs, and 4) may vary in intensity or degree. An example of this would be reducing a spelling list that teaches the concept of the *-it* ending from 10 words to 5 words. The student with a disability is responsible for learning the same material as the students without disabilities, although with a reduced output. Other examples include reading directions to the student, providing extended time to complete assignments, providing study aids, giving frequent reminders of rules, using a calculator for solving math word problems, and giving note-taking assistance.

Modifications to curriculum provide material that substantially changes the general education curriculum. An example of this would be requiring less challenging spelling concepts. Here the student is responsible for learning 5 *-it* spelling words, such as *sit,* while his classmates are responsible for learning 10 *-tion* words, such as *conversation.* Modifications should be considered carefully because reducing expectations for students with disabilities can lessen their chance of being college or career ready upon transition to adulthood.

Curriculum modifications in reading may involve approximations of the grade-level curriculum, such as Hi/Lo readers for students with mild reading disabilities. Hi/Lo readers allow access to high-content literature (e.g., *Gulliver's Travels*) at a reduced reading level. Modification for students with more significant disabilities might include accessing a high school reading curriculum through teacher-created digital reading material that boils down classic texts such as *Romeo and Juliet* to key story elements such as "home, family, communicate, love and fight" (Apitz, Ruppar, Roessler, & Pickett, 2017, p. 171). Curriculum modifications may also include supports that allow a child to participate without academic expectations, such as using a calculator for math calculation problems. In contrast, using a calculator to assist in a word problem, with a learning expectation of choosing the correct operation to use to solve the problem, would be considered an accommodation.

Inclusion Practices

A number of practices have been developed to accomplish the goal of inclusion. Inclusion refers to educating people with disabilities alongside people without disabilities. Inclusive classrooms expose all students to the same high standards using universal design for learning, a method of individualizing instruction by matching the means of representation of materials, action and expression of student product, and encouragement of student engagement. In addition to universal design, the inclusive class provides accommodations, modifications, supplementary supports, and collaboration with the special education staff for special needs students (Fuchs et al., 2015).

Co-Teaching

As a co-teacher, the special educator shares the classroom with a general education teacher. The two teachers take joint responsibility for all the students in the class regardless of ability. Co-teaching may take many forms: one teach/one assist, one teach/one observe, station teaching, parallel teaching, alternative teaching, or team teaching (Strieker, Gills, & Zong, 2013). Although not the most effective form, the "one-teach/one-assist" model is the most commonly used approach. Here, while one teacher teaches the entire class, the other helps any students in need. Studies have shown that the most effective method of co-teaching is "team teaching," yet there are barriers to this approach that include poor communication, lack of planning time, and the special education teacher's lack of content mastery (e.g., may not be well trained in math instruction). Solutions to these problems include using technology (such as a shared Google Docs or Dropbox account for lesson planning), active listening, depersonalization, and enhanced communication. The special education teacher might also use self-learning such as the Khan Academy to gain mastery of unfamiliar general education content (Scruggs & Mastropieri, 2017).

High-Leverage Practices in Special Education

The Council for Exceptional Children (2011) has created recommended practices for all special educators in Grades K–12. These 22 high-leverage practices include four aspects of practice: collaboration, assessment, social-emotional-behavioral practices, and instruction. *Collaboration practices* include the following:

- Collaborating with professionals to increase student success
- Collaborating with families to support student learning and secure needed services

Assessment practices include:

- Interpreting and communicating assessment information to stakeholders in order to collaboratively design and implement educational programs
- Using student assessment data to analyze instructional practices and make necessary adjustments

Social/emotional/behavioral practices include:

- Establishing a consistent, organized, and respectful learning environment
- Teaching social behaviors

Instruction practices include:

- Teaching cognitive and metacognitive strategies to support learning and independence
- Providing scaffolded supports
- Teaching students to maintain and generalize new learning across time and settings
- Providing positive and constructive feedback to guide students' learning and behavior
- Using explicit instruction
- Adapting tasks and materials for specific learning goals (McLeskey et al., 2017)

SERVICES PROVIDED BY SPECIAL EDUCATION TEACHERS

Special education teachers provide individualized instruction, supplementary aids, and support designed to meet the needs of students with disabilities. The special education teacher's mission is to instruct and support the student so he or she is able to access the curriculum, benefit from educational instruction, and be college or career ready. Students with disabilities receive the majority of special education services they need from special education teachers, with the remainder of services being provided by related service professionals (as discussed in the section titled Related Services within Special Education). Special education teachers spend the majority of their time directly instructing students with disabilities. The balance of their time is spent creating, adapting, and modifying educational materials; maintaining IDEA documentation; and collaborating with general education teachers (Vannest & Hagan-Burke, 2010). As the IEP manager, the special education teacher is responsible for leading the team in developing the IEP in accordance with the student's needs and the family's input. The special educator also is responsible for assuring that the IEP, once developed, is followed with integrity by the general education staff, paraprofessionals, and related service providers.

Most importantly, special educators are responsible for the direct teaching of academic and functional skills and for providing behavioral supports. In academics, they teach the same material or content (except for students with severe impairments) as is taught in the general education curriculum. However, they provide accommodations and modifications that allow the student to access the material at his or her appropriate instructional level or mode of communication. Even for students with cognitive impairments, academic material can be approximated as an essential skill. As an example, a third-grade core reading skill, "Describe characters in a story (e.g., their traits, motivations, or feelings) and explain how their actions contribute to the sequence of events," can be modified to the essential skill of "Identify the feelings of characters in a story" (Dynamic Learning Maps Alternate Assessment Consortium, 2012, p. 47). Functional skills include daily living skills, social/communicative skills, vocational skills, and/or participation in the community.

THE ROLE OF THE SPECIAL EDUCATION TEACHER IN THE GENERAL EDUCATION CURRICULUM

Although in the past the special educator's role in general education was to support inclusion (for students who qualify for special education services during instruction in the general education classroom), that role is changing. As special education and general education services become more inclusive (see the section titled Response to Intervention), the role of the special educator becomes more complex. Looking to the future, the special educator likely will fill the following roles, as described by Hoover and Patton (2008):

1. Data-driven decision maker
2. Implementer of evidence-based interventions
3. Differentiator of instruction
4. Implementer of socioemotional and behavioral supports
5. Collaborator

The special educator should also be prepared to supervise paraprofessionals and function as a co-teacher in the general education setting.

The Special Education Teacher as Data-Based Decision Maker

Special educators serve as members of problem-solving teams for at-risk students and students with disabilities. The team interprets teacher-generated data to evaluate the amount of progress students are making. The team uses the data to make decisions about the need for instructional changes (Kovaleski & Pedersen, 2009).

The Special Education Teacher as Implementer of Evidence-Based Interventions

Evidence-based interventions are teaching methods that scientific studies have indicated are the most effective. Their use is imperative when working with students with disabilities. Students are identified with educational disabilities because they have not learned effectively when taught with typical instructional methods (Cook, Tankersley, & Landrum, 2009). Commercial evidence-based interventions can be found on the What Works Clearinghouse web site of the U.S. Department of Education (https://ies.ed.gov/ncee/wwc/). The National Center on Intensive Intervention (https://intensiveintervention.org/) provides data-based instructional techniques and interventions to improve outcomes in students with severe and persistent learning and behavior needs. Information about noncommercial evidence-based practices can be found in educational research journals. As an example, publications of the Council for Exceptional Children (a professional organization for special education professionals; https://www.cec.sped.org/) are valuable resources for finding evidence-based interventions.

The Special Education Teacher as Differentiator of Instruction

Differentiated instruction means that the teacher structures instruction to best fit the needs of each student. Instruction can be differentiated in the following areas (Watts-Taffee et al., 2013)

- Content (altering complexity or presentation)
- Process (altering the amount of support as necessary)
- Products (varying methods of demonstrating mastery)
- Learning environment (the physical structure of the room, established learning routines, and culturally inclusive materials)

The Special Education Teacher as Implementer and Facilitator of Social-Emotional and Behavioral Supports

Special educators provide social-emotional and behavioral supports to students through social skills instruction and many other positive behavioral supports and interventions. Social skills instruction can be taught discretely with programs that break down social skills into steps and engage the students in role play. Most programs also have a homework component (the students practice the skill independently) and a self-monitoring component. Examples of such programs include Skill Streaming (McGinnis, 2012) and *The Tough Kids Social Skills Book* (Sheridan, 2010). Social skills can be taught during literacy lessons by incorporating books containing social conflicts or the use of prosocial strategies. In addition to supporting their own students, special educators often serve on schoolwide positive behavior support teams, which provide and monitor schoolwide programs intended to decrease interfering and bullying behaviors.

The Special Education Teacher as Collaborator

As a collaborator, the special education teacher must familiarize the general education teacher with the adaptations and modifications necessary to enable the student to benefit from inclusion. The two teachers then discuss who will be responsible for each aspect of the student's instructional needs. For a student who needs only limited support, the special education teacher might provide content enhancements such as the use of graphic organizers, study guides, or visual displays (Jitendra, Burgess, & Gajria, 2011). The special educator may create adapted tests or check on the student at the end of the day to confirm that all of the homework assignments have been written down. For a student who needs more extensive support, the special education teacher may supply modified assignments that cover the same content as the general education lesson but that are at the student's academic level (see the section titled "Accommodations and Modifications").

The Special Education Teacher as Supervisor of Paraprofessionals

As a supervisor, the special education teacher is responsible for assessing the level of service delivered to students by paraprofessionals. Teachers need to actively manage paraprofessional support by creating a job description so that expectations are clear. Paraprofessionals help provide services but should not engage in instruction, assessment, long-term planning, collaborating and consulting with general educators, or supervising other paraprofessionals. These tasks are the job of the special education teacher. The special education teacher can best maintain quality paraprofessional support by conducting frequent, brief observations with both verbal and written feedback of performance (Douglas, Chapin, & Nolan, 2016; French, 2001). See Box 33.2 for more on special education teachers.

THE SCHOOL–PARENT CONNECTION

One of the keys to positive results for students with disabilities is the teamwork between the school and the family. Educators only see one facet of a student's abilities—his or her performance at school. Parents, conversely, see the whole student. For example, a parent might know of a special interest or enjoyable activity that the educator might provide as a motivator for the student's school performance. Goals and placements also need to be decided jointly by the parents and the special education team. It is encouraging to note that parent attendance at IEP meetings is strong. A federal longitudinal study (the Special Education Elementary Longitudinal Study [SEELS]) found that 90% of parents of students with disabilities attended their students' IEP meeting (SRI International, 2007).

The close partnership between special educators and parents has another direct benefit; the parents understand and appreciate the efforts being

BOX 33.2 EVIDENCE-BASED PRACTICE

Attrition Rates of Special Education Teachers

Rates of attrition among special education teachers remain a perennial concern. Special educators leave the field annually at twice the rate of their general education peers (25% vs. 13%). In addition, teacher burnout has been found to have effects that go beyond the problem of filling classrooms with qualified teachers—it also negatively affects students with disabilities who are working to achieve their goals. Wong, Ruble, Yu, and McGrew (2017) found that high levels of burnout (i.e., a low sense of personal accomplishment directly and emotional exhaustion and depersonalization indirectly) were correlated with lower individualized education program outcomes.

made for their students. SEELS found that 91% of parents believed that IEP goals were challenging and appropriate (SRI International, 2007). In addition, the National Longitudinal Study–2 (NLTS-2) Wave 4 (National Center on Secondary Education and Transition, 2009a) reported that 90% of secondary school parents were satisfied with their student's special education experience.

OUTCOMES

The number of students with disabilities who have graduated from high school increased from 56% in 2006 to 66% in 2016 (National Center for Educational Statistics, 2017). However, many of these students are graduating with alternative diplomas or standards that do not make them college or career ready. Examples of alternative diplomas include certificates for completion, attainment, and attendance or vocational diplomas such as in career or technical education. Some diplomas are granted upon meeting IEP goals (Achieve-National Center on Educational Outcomes, 2016). In addition, although increasing, the 66% rate of graduation among students with disabilities still compares poorly with the 83% graduation rate among their typically developing peers.

Although graduation rates are an important indicator of positive educational outcomes, for many students with disabilities, outcomes are more adequately represented through other means. The NLTS-2 (National Center on Secondary Education and Transition, 2009b) surveyed outcomes of young adults with disabilities in many areas. As an example, 83% liked their job very much or fairly well. Unfortunately, at the time of this writing, the unemployment rate for people with disabilities was 10.5% compared with 4.6% for that of people without disabilities (Department of Labor, 2017). One of the goals of education is to provide students with the tools they need to succeed in life. Individuals who have benefited from their education should feel positively about their future. Table 33.3 represents the percentage of students who feel hopeful about their future, broken down by disability. The results are positive, with over half of students with a wide range of disabilities indicating that they are hopeful about the future a lot or all of the time.

SUMMARY

- Special education and related services are instruction and supplementary supports that are specifically designed to meet the unique educational needs of a student with a disability. These services are mandated by federal law and are provided by special education teachers and related service providers to students with defined disabilities.
- The IEP provides documentation of instruction and support for a student with a disability including goals, accommodations, and modifications. Services are provided within the framework of LRE.
- IDEA 2004 is the federal legislation that describes identification and provision of services for students with disabilities. Section 504 legislation provides coverage for the wider array of students with disabilities who do not qualify under the stricter guidelines of IDEA.
- The MTSS is comprised of three tiered levels of academic and social interventions that support both students with and without an identified disability.
- Special education teachers perform multiple roles, including a data-driven decision maker, an implementer of evidence-based interventions, a differentiator of instruction, an implementer of socioemotional and behavioral supports, and a collaborator.

Table 33.3. How often youth felt hopeful about the future (Item np2V2d): Overall and by primary disability category

	Total	Learning disability	Speech impairment	Mental retardation	Emotional disturbance	Hearing impairment	Visual impairment	Orthopedic impairment	Other health impairment	Autism	Traumatic brain injury	Multiple disabilities	Deaf/ blindness
(1) Never or rarely	14.7%	13.7%	14.5%	22.5%	15.0%	7.2%	4.3%	8.4%	9.6%	17.1%	16.8%	20.5%	7.5%
(2) Sometimes	22.7%	19.5%	30.4%	23.5%	31.1%	23.7%	16.5%	24.3%	25.7%	26.1%	17.7%	16.8%	18.4%
(3) A lot of the time	19.3%	20.8%	19.8%	16.0%	15.4%	28.0%	29.7%	15.0%	14.9%	22.7%	24.6%	14.4%	30.1%
(4) Most or all of the time	43.3%	42.1%	41.1%	31.1%	38.6%	41.2%	49.6%	52.3%	49.8%	33.5%	41.0%	48.0%	44.0%

From National Center on Secondary Education and Transition, Institute on Community Integration. (2009). *NLTS2 Wave 5 Parent/Youth Survey Youth Report of Youth Social Involvement Table 340 Estimates*. Retrieved from http://www.nlts2.org/data_tables/tables/14/np5V2dfrm.html

ADDITIONAL RESOURCES

TASH: http://www.tash.org

Center on Response to Intervention: https://www.rti4success.org/

Positive Behavioral Interventions & Supports (PBIS): https://www.pbis.org/

Intervention Central: http://www.interventioncentral.org/

Additional resources can be found online in Appendix D: Childhood Disabilities Resources, Services, and Organizations (see About the Online Companion Materials).

REFERENCES

Achieve-National Center on Educational Outcomes. (2016). *Diplomas that matter: Ensuring equity of opportunity for students with disabilities.* Retrieved from www.achieve.org/publications/diplomas-that-matter-achieve-nceo

Americans with Disabilities Act of 2008, PL 110-325, 42 U.S.C. §§ 12101 *et seq.*

Apitz, M., Ruppar, A., Roessler, K., & Pickett, K. J. (2017). Planning lessons for students with significant disabilities in high school English classes. *Teaching Exceptional Children, 49,* 168–174.

Assistance to States for the Education of Children with Disabilities, 34 C.F.R. §300.8 (2017). Retrieved from https://ecfr.gov/cgi-bin/text-idx?SID=805f0b2e578921d166c88b99f320353f&mc=true&node=se34.2.300_18&rgn=div8

Assistance to States for the Education of Children with Disabilities and Preschool Grants for Children with Disabilities, 71 Fed. Reg. 46,467 (2006[0]) (to be codified at 34 C.F.R pts 300, 301).

Bersoff, D. N. (1980). Larry P. v. Riles: Legal perspective. *School Psychology Review, 9,* 112–122.

Carter, E. W., Trainor, A. A., Sun, Y., & Owens, L. (2009). Assessing the transition-related strengths and needs of adolescents with high-incidence disabilities. *Exceptional Children, 76,* 74–94.

Cook, B. G., Tankersley, M., & Landrum, T. J. (2009). Determining evidence-based practices in special education. *Exceptional Children, 75,* 365–383.

Council for Exceptional Children. (2011). *Council for Exceptional Children special education professional practice standards.* Retrieved from http://www.cec.sped.org/~/media/Files/Standards/Professional Ethics and Practice Standards/CEC Special Education Professional Practice Standards.pdf

Council of Chief State School Officers. (2016). *ESSA: Key provisions and implications for students with disabilities.* Retrieved from www.ccsso.org/Documents/2016/ESSA_Key_Provisions_Implications_for_SWD.pdf

Department of Labor. (2017). *Persons with disability: Labor force characteristics–2016.* Retrieved from www.bls.gov/news.release/pdf/disabl.pdf

Douglas, S. N., Chapin, S. E., & Nolan, J. F. (2016). Special education teacher's experiences supporting and supervising paraeducators: Implications for Special and General Education Settings. *Teacher Education and Special Education, 39,* 60–74.

Dynamic Learning Maps Alternate Assessment Consortium (2012). *Dynamic learning maps essential elements for language arts.* Retrieved from https://dese.mo.gov/sites/default/files/asmt-dlm-essential-elements-ela.doc

Endrew F. v. Douglas County School District, RE-1 580 U.S. (2017).

Education for All Handicapped Children Act of 1975, PL 94-142, 20 U.S.C. §§ 1400 *et seq.*

Education of the Handicapped Act Amendments of 1986, PL 99-457, 20 U.S.C. §§ 1400 *et seq.*

Education of the Handicapped Act of 1970 (EHA), PL 91-230, 84 Stat. 121-154, 20 U.S.C. §§ 1400 *et seq.*

Elementary and Secondary Education Act of 1965, PL 89-10, 20 U.S.C. §§ 241 *et seq.*

Every Student Succeeds Act of 2015, PL 114-95, 20 U.S.C.

Farrell, A. F., Collier-Meek, M. A., & Pons, S. R. (2013). Embedding positive behavioral interventions and supports in afterschool programs. *Beyond Behavior, 23,* 38–45.

Federal Register. (2006). 34CFR Parts 300 and 301: Assistance to states for the education of children with disabilities and preschool grants for children with disabilities. *Federal Register, Vol. 71,*(No 156), 46647.

Federal Register. (2017). *Title 34 Education: Subtitle B Chapter III Part 300 Subpart A (§ 300.8): Assistance to states for the education of children with disabilities.* Retrieved October 14, 2017, from, https://ecfr.gov/cgi-bin/text-idx?SID=805f0b2e578921d166c88b99f320353f&mc=true&node=se34.2.300_18&rgn=div8

French, N. (2001). Supervising paraprofessionals: A survey of teacher practices. *The Journal of Special Education, 35*(1), 41–53.

Fuchs, D., & Fuchs, L. S. (2017). Critique of the national evaluation of response to intervention: A case for simpler frameworks. *Exceptional Children, 83,* 255–268.

Fuchs, L. S., Fuchs, D., Compton, D. L., Wehby, J., Schumacher, R. F., Gersten, R., & Jordan, N. C. (2015). Inclusion versus specialized intervention for very-low-performing students: What does access mean in an era of academic challenge? *Exceptional Children, 81,* 134–157.

Gersten, R., Jayanthi, M., & Dimino, J. (2017). Too much, too soon? Unanswered questions from national response to intervention evaluation. *Exceptional Children, 83,* 244–254.

Goalbook. (2017). *ELA standard RK.K.3. Goalbook toolkit.* Retrieved from goalbookapp.com/toolkit/v/anchor-page/524e1138-2dfc-4b07-a906-ab684075a1d9

Hoover, J. J., & Patton, J. R. (2008). The role of special educators in a multitiered instructional system. *Intervention in School and Clinic, 43,* 195–202.

Individuals with Disabilities Education Act (IDEA) Amendments of 1997, PL 105-17, 20 U.S.C. §§ 1400 *et seq.*

Individuals with Disabilities Education Act (IDEA) of 1990, PL 101-476, 20 U.S.C. §§ 1400 *et seq.*

Individuals with Disabilities Education Improvement Act (IDEA) of 2004, PL 108-446, 20 U.S.C. §§ 1400 *et seq.*

Jitendra, A. K., Burgess, C., & Gajria, M. (2011). Cognitive strategy instruction of improving expository text comprehension of students with learning disabilities: The quality of evidence. *Exceptional Children, 77,* 135–159.

Kauffman, J. M., & Badar, J. (2016). It's instruction over place—not the other way around! *The Phi Delta Kappan, 44,* 55–59.

Kovaleski, J. F., & Pedersen, J. A. (2009). Best practices in data-analysis teaming. In A. Thomas & J. Grimes (Eds.), *Best practices in school psychology* (pp. 115–130). Bethesda, MD: National Association of School Psychologists.

McDaniel, S. C., Bruhn, A. L., & Mitchell, B. S. (2015). A Tier 2 framework for behavior identification and intervention. *Beyond Behavior, 24,* 10–17.

McGinnis, E. (2012). *Skillstreaming for the elementary school child. A guide for teaching prosocial skills.* Chicago, IL: Research Press.

McLeskey, J., Barringer, M.-D., Billingsley, B., Brownell, M., Jackson, D., Kennedy, M., & Ziegler, D. (2017). High-leverage practices in special education. *Teaching Exceptional Children, 49,* 355–360.

Mercer, C. D. (1997). *Students with learning disabilities.* Upper Saddle River. NJ: Prentice Hall

Morgan, P. L., Farkas, G., Cook, M., Strassfeld, N. M., Hillemeier, M. M., Pun, W. H., & Schussler, D. L. (2017). Are black students disproportionately overrepresented in special education? A best-evidenced synthesis. *Exceptional Children, 83,* 181–198. doi:10.1177/0014402916664042

Morgan, P. L., & Farkas, G. (2016). Evidence of minority underrepresentation in special education and its implications of school psychologists, *Communique, 44,* 6.

Morgan, P. L., Farkas, G., Hillemeier, M. M., Mattison, R., Maczuga, S., Li, H., & Cook, M. (2015). Minorities are disproportionality underrepresented in special education: Longitudinal evidence across five disability conditions. *Educational Researcher, 44,* 278–292. doi:10.3102/0013189X15591157

National Center for Educational Statistics. (2017). *Public high school 4-year adjusted cohort graduation rate (ACGR), by selected student characteristics and state: 2010-11 through 2015-16.* Retrieved from www.nces.ed.gov/programs/digest/d17/tables/dt17_219.46.asp

National Center on Secondary Education and Transition. (2009a). *NLTS2 Wave 4: Parent/Youth Survey: Satisfaction with secondary school experiences.* Retrieved from www.nlts2.org/data_tables/tables/13/np4D6o_cfrm.html

National Center on Secondary Education and Transition. (2009b). *NLTS2 Wave 5 (2009) parent/young adult survey: How young adult usually likes his/her current or most recent job.* Retrieved from https://nlts2.sri.com/data_tables/tables/14/np5T4vfrm.html

National Center on Secondary Education and Transition. (2009). *NLTS2 Wave 5 (2009) parent/young adult survey: Social involvement.* Retrieved from http://www.nlts2.org/data_tables/tables/14/np5V2dfrm.html

Office of Civil Rights. (1995). *The civil rights of students with hidden disabilities under Section 504 of the Rehabilitation Act of 1973.* Retrieved from www2.ed.gov/about/offices/list/ocr/docs/hq5269.html

Office of Civil Rights. (2015). *Frequently asked questions about Section 504 and the education of children with disabilities.* Retrieved from www.2gov/about/offices/list/ocr/504faq.html

Otaiba, S. A., Wagner, R. K., & Miller, B. (2014). "Waiting to fail" redux: Understanding inadequate response to intervention. *Learning Disability Quarterly, 37,* 129–133.

Pennsylvania Association for Retarded Citizens v. Commonwealth of Pennsylvania, 334 F. Supp. 1257 (E.D. Pa. 1971).

Procter, S. L., Graves, S. L., & Esch, R. C. (2012). Assessing African American students for specific learning disabilities: The promises and perils of response to intervention. *The Journal of Negro Education, 81,* 268–282.

Rehabilitation Act of 1973, PL 93-112, 29 U.S.C. §§ 701 *et seq.*

Scruggs, T. E., & Mastropieri, M. A. (2017). Making inclusion work with co-teaching. *Teaching Exceptional Students, 49,* 284–293.

Sheridan, S. M. (2010). *The tough kid social skills book.* Eugene, OR: Pacific Northwest Publishing.

SRI International. (2007). *Special Education Elementary Longitudinal Study (SEELS)* Table *131 & 142.* Retrieved from www.seels.net

Strieker, T., Gills, B., & Zong, G. (2013). Improving pre-service middle school teachers' confidence, competence, and commitment to co-teaching in inclusive classrooms. *Teacher Education Quarterly, 40,* 159–180.

U.S. Department of Education. (2016). *Dear colleague letter: Prevention racial discrimination in special education.* Retrieved from www2.ed.gov/about/offices/list/ocr/letters/colleague-201612-racedisc-special-education.pdf

U.S. Department of Education, Department of Civil Rights. (2016). *Parent and educator resource guide to Section 504 in public elementary and secondary schools.* Retrieved from www2.ed.gov/about/offices/list/ocr/docs/504-resource-guide-201612.pdf

U.S. Department of Education, Office of Special Education and Rehabilitative Services. (1994). *Questions and answers on least restrictive environment (LRE) requirements of the IDEA* Retrieved from www.wrightslaw.com/law/osep/lre.memo.1994.1123.pdf

U.S. Department of Education, Office of Special Education and Rehabilitative Services. (2015). *Table 204.60. Percentage distribution of students 6 to 21 years old served under Individuals with Disabilities Education Act (IDEA), Part B, by educational environment and type of disability.* Retrieved from https://nces.ed.gov/programs/digest/d15/tables/dt15_204.60.asp

U.S. Department of Education, Office of Special Education and Rehabilitative Services. (2016). *Digest of Educational Statistics* Table *204.30: Children 3-21 years old under Individuals with Disabilities Education Act (IDEA), Part B, by type of disability.* Retrieved from https://nces.ed.gov/programs/digest/d16_204.30.asp

Vannest, K. J., & Hagan-Burke, S. C. (2010). Teacher time use in special education. *Remedial and Special Education, 31,* 126–142.

Watts-Taffe, S., Laster, B. P., Broach, L., Marinak, B, Connor, C. M., & Walker-Dalhouse, D. (2013). Differentiated instruction: Making informed teacher decisions. *The Reading Teacher, 66,* 303–314.

Williamson, P., McLeskey, J., Hoppey, D., & Rentz, T. (2006). Educating students with mental retardation in general education classrooms. *Exceptional Children, 72,* 347–362.

Wong, V. W., Ruble, L. A., Yu, Y., & McGrew, J. H. (2017). Too stressed to teach? Teaching quality, student engagement, and IEP outcomes. *Exceptional Children, 83,* 412–427.

Yell, M. L. (1998). *The law and special education.* Upper Saddle River: NJ, Merrill.

CHAPTER 34 Behavioral Therapy

Henry S. Roane, William E. Sullivan, Brian K. Martens, and Michael E. Kelley

Upon completion of this chapter, the reader will

- Describe operant conditioning and its relation to behavioral treatments
- Explain the basic principles underlying behavioral processes
- Understand response measurement and data collection as applied to behaviorally based assessments and treatments
- Identify key components of operational definitions for defining target behaviors and developing a data collection system
- Describe the logical underpinnings of single-case experimental designs and visual inspection of single-case data
- Differentiate among the various types of functional assessments
- Explain the types of behavioral treatments appropriate for challenging behavior exhibited by children with developmental disabilities
- Identify the principal concepts and strategies of behavioral skill instruction for teaching a functional communication response to children with developmental disabilities

This chapter addresses the use of behavioral treatments with children with developmental disabilities. Behavioral treatments for this population are part of a broader group of treatments commonly referred to as "behavioral therapy." All behaviorally based treatments share some core features, such as the use of reinforcement and a focus on environmental determinants of behavior (e.g., antecedents and consequences; Benson, 2016). The focus of this chapter is not on providing an overarching review of behavioral therapy; rather, it describes the appropriate use of behavioral treatments to address behaviors common among children with developmental disabilities.

In particular, this chapter explains the use of behavioral therapy to address two broad areas of functioning that are commonly targeted in this population: challenging behavior and skill development. For example, Dominick, Davis, Lainhart, Tager-Flusberg, and Folstein (2007) surveyed parents concerning the presence of challenging behavior (i.e., atypical eating or sleeping, aggression, self-injury, and tantrums) in a sample of 67 children with autism spectrum disorder

(ASD) and found that 98% of the parents sampled reported at least one type of challenging behavior. By definition, developmental disabilities involve deficits in adaptive and self-help functioning, including academic behavior, thus highlighting the importance of behavioral treatments for skill development. Moreover, the extant literature has consistently shown that behavioral therapies are effective in addressing these concerns (Heyvaert, Saenen, Campbell, Maes, & Onghena, 2014; Roane, Fisher, & Carr, 2016).

This chapter also distinguishes among behavioral treatments to address the phenotypic expression of developmental disabilities and applied behavior analysis (ABA), a specific form of behavioral intervention for ASD. The behavioral treatments discussed herein share a number of common features with ABA therapy, and a discussion of similarities and specific uses for ABA in relation to behavioral therapies can be found elsewhere (Fisher & Zangrillo, 2015; Roane et al., 2016). Thus, while this chapter focuses on the application of behavior analytic principles to the treatment and remediation of behaviors displayed by individuals with developmental disabilities, it does not focus exclusively on ABA as treatment for ASD.

Although the focus of this chapter is on challenging behavior and skill development, behaviorally based treatments can and are often applied to other issues confronted by children with developmental disabilities. In fact, there are a number of studies that describe the use of behavioral therapies, in particular the use of cognitive-behavioral therapy (CBT), for a range of issues encountered by this population. CBT describes psychotherapeutic approaches that posit a malleable relationship among an individual's cognitions, behaviors, and emotions. As such, CBT incorporates a number of strategies aimed to help the individual become aware of their own dysfunctional thoughts, emotional reactions, and maladaptive behavior patterns. Likewise, CBT challenges the individual to analyze and modify problematic thinking and behavior patterns, as well as to adopt alternative ways of perceiving and responding to their environment. Typically, CBT is a short-term intervention that consists of 10–12 sessions of 1 hour per week. Given the brevity of this approach, CBT does not aim to eliminate all challenging or maladaptive behaviors; instead, CBT equips the individual with the tools necessary to continue therapeutic work on their own.

The use of CBT has become increasingly popular, and many CBT programs are considered evidence based in the treatment of a variety of mental health disorders in both adults and children. For example, the National Institute for Clinical Excellence (2011) in the United Kingdom has recommended CBT as the primary treatment for anxiety disorders. However, when discussing the use of CBT with individuals with developmental delays and intellectual disabilities, the collective findings have been mixed. To illustrate this point, Lang, Mahoney, Zein, Delaune, and Amidon (2011) and Lang et al. (2010) conducted two systematic reviews looking at the use of CBT to treat anxiety in individuals diagnosed with ASD. The findings indicated that CBT was effective for individuals with ASD that do not have a comorbid intellectual disability, yet for those with an intellectual disability, CBT had little to no evidence.

Generally speaking, when CBT has been implemented in the pediatric populations, the protocols have been adapted to accommodate the child's unique needs, such as 1) simplifying language, 2) incorporating visual cues, 3) relying on less sophisticated cognitive techniques, 4) increasing the use of positive reinforcement, and 5) incorporating caregivers into treatment. This programmatic adaptation illustrates the concept of *flexibility with fidelity* (Kendall & Beidas, 2007; Kendall, Gosch, Furr, & Sood, 2008). To illustrate this point, Beidas et al. (2010) offered a range of suggestions to modify empirically supported treatments such that the individual's developmental needs are considered. This notion is highly relevant when considering a CBT approach for children with developmental disabilities. Nevertheless, at this time, the evidence for CBT to address maladaptive behavior in children with developmental disabilities still falls short of behavior analytic interventions (Sturmey, 2014). Thus, for the purposes of this chapter, the focus will be on behavior analytic treatments to address challenging behavior in children with developmental disabilities.

As noted above, all forms of behavioral treatments share common core features. The first part of this chapter describes some of these principles, as well as operant conditioning, the theory of learning from which they evolved. The following case study serves to illustrate how behavioral therapy is implemented in practice.

CASE STUDY

Roger is a 7-year-old boy diagnosed with ASD and moderate intellectual disability. Based on the caregiver report, Roger was delayed in meeting the majority of his developmental milestones (i.e., rolling over, sitting up, crawling, walking, and speaking his first words). At the time of the beginning of a formal behavioral therapy program, Roger was able to communicate using two- to three-word phrases and follow single-step commands.

Academically, Roger struggled across most subject areas but had a relative strength in mathematics. He attended public school and was educated in a special education classroom setting with a one-on-one aide to support his behavioral needs. When Roger was 4 years old, it was reported that he began to show aggression toward his parents, teachers, and peers when access to preferred items was restricted or when he was asked to complete academic work other than math. Around this same time, Roger began to display self-injurious behavior (SIB) in the form of head hitting, self-scratching, and eye poking. Typically, his caregivers responded to this behavior by 1) reprimanding him (e.g., "It is not okay to hit Mommy!"), 2) removing him from the situation, or 3) giving him his toys back to calm him down. Over time, his behavior worsened and resulted in Roger being admitted into an outpatient clinic that specialized in the treatment of severe maladaptive behavior.

Thought Questions:

How does the three-term contingency (antecedent, behavior, and consequence) apply to the principals of behavioral therapy? How do the different principals of behavioral therapy apply to a response to serious tantrums?

OPERANT CONDITIONING

The common features of behavioral therapy as applied to the concerns of individuals with developmental disabilities initially arose from the research of American psychologist B. F. Skinner (1957). Skinner was heavily influenced by Darwin's theory of natural selection and applied this theory to understand the manner in which behavior is learned. Specifically, Skinner outlined a process that was referred to as selection by consequences; essentially, behaviors that produce favorable outcomes are likely to persist, whereas behaviors that produce unfavorable outcomes are likely to cease. Thus, the context—or what Skinner referred to as the environment—played a central role in behavior change. For example, in his work with animals (e.g., pigeons and rats), Skinner demonstrated that responses that produced access to food were likely to be repeated and, in many cases, would be completed more rapidly over time.

Skinner's conceptualization of learning was a novel departure from previous theories (e.g., that all learning was essentially reflexive in nature) in that Skinner posited that an organism's behavior "operates" on the environment to produce favorable outcomes and decrease unfavorable outcomes. This theory of learning was thus termed *operant conditioning*.

Basic Principles

Operant conditioning gave rise to a number of principles, concepts, and terms that are prevalent in behavioral therapies for individuals with developmental disabilities. The role of the environment (i.e., the context in which the behavior occurs) was a unique interpretation of how organisms learn. Also, operant conditioning—and by extension, behavioral treatments—conceptualizes behavior by its function (i.e., the purpose it serves) rather than its topography (i.e., what the behavior looks like). This also is a departure from other forms of therapy. In behavioral therapy, treatments are not designed to manage "aggression," per se (i.e., a topographical distinction of the behavior); instead, treatment is designed to address the function of that behavior (e.g., hitting another person to avoid schoolwork).

Three-Term Contingency

Related to a discussion of function is the notion of the three-term contingency, or the A-B-C contingency. That is, operant behavior consists of three components: 1) the **A**ntecedent event that precedes the behavior, 2) the **B**ehavior itself, and 3) the **C**onsequence that follows the behavior. Using a common example, a phone rings (antecedent), which leads the individual to answer the call and say "Hello." Saying "hello" (behavior) is reinforced by a conversation beginning with the caller (consequence). Although this is a simplistic example, it illustrates the extent to which the antecedent, the behavior, and the consequence are linked.

Conceptually, the three-term contingency serves as the basis for most behavioral treatments for individuals with developmental disabilities. Determining what events occasion the occurrence of a particular response (i.e., antecedents) and what events typically follow a response (i.e., consequences) can lead to methods of changing the behavior of interest.

Reinforcement

Reinforcement is a process in which the future likelihood of a behavior increases either by 1) presenting a preferred stimulus (i.e., **positive reinforcement**) or 2) removing a nonpreferred stimulus (i.e., **negative reinforcement**) contingent on a behavior. For example, some children might have a tantrum when preferred items are interrupted or removed, and well-meaning caregivers might respond to this behavior by giving the child attention (e.g., hugs to calm them down) or by giving them back their toys. This represents an example of a positive reinforcement contingency in that having a tantrum produces access to preferred events.

An example of a negative reinforcement contingency might be seen in a child who misbehaves when presented with challenging schoolwork. If the child's behavior is of such severity that it results in removal of the schoolwork or results in the child being sent out of the classroom, the behavior is negatively reinforced by the removal of nonpreferred activities (i.e., schoolwork). An important distinction to understand is that the process of reinforcement always results in an increase in behavior (hence the term *reinforcer,* which means "to strengthen"). This is the case whether the reinforcement process is intentional or unintentional and whether the reinforcing event is providing access to a desirable event or removing (or avoiding) the presentation of an undesirable event.

Extinction

A related principle is **extinction,** which is a process that decreases the occurrence of a behavior through the discontinuation of reinforcement. Using the previous positive reinforcement example, extinction of tantrums would involve the caregiver no longer attending to the child's challenging behavior or not providing the child with preferred toys when the child becomes upset. Extinction is a somewhat gradual behavior change process in which learning occurs over time. In the above scenario, the child will eventually learn that tantrums do not "work" to get a desired response from a caregiver, but the tantrums may actually increase transiently as the child tries to make it "work."

Punishment

Punishment is another process that results in a decrease in behavior. As with reinforcement, punishment is further defined by the presence or absence of a given consequence. Thus, in a positive punishment contingency, behavior results in the presentation of a nonpreferred stimulus. Reprimanding a child is commonly implemented by caregivers as a form of **positive punishment,** meaning the reprimand presented contingent on a behavior is designed to stop that behavior. By contrast, a **negative punishment** contingency is one in which a preferred stimulus is removed contingent upon the occurrence of a behavior. An example of negative punishment could include response cost (e.g., a child throws her toy and her parent then removes the toy for a specific amount of time) or a time-out (e.g., the child is placed in a context in which he cannot access other reinforcers).

Schedule of Reinforcement

Another important principle to consider with the use of reinforcement, extinction, and punishment is the schedule of reinforcement. Simply put, any type of behavior change occurs most rapidly if the programmed contingency is delivered every time the behavior occurs. This is referred to as a continuous schedule of reinforcement. For example, in this chapter's opening case study, if Roger's therapist wanted to teach him to make eye contact, she would immediately and consistently provide praise or access to preferred items every time he made eye contact with her. The use of immediate reinforcement each time the targeted response occurs teaches Roger that there is a positive reinforcement contingency in place for his behavior.

It would be difficult to maintain this level of reinforcement; therefore, to maintain a behavior once it has been acquired, Roger's therapist would move to an intermittent schedule of reinforcement. For example, she might reinforce eye contact after every three occurrences. In addition to using an intermittent schedule, there are a number of other modifications that can be made to promote response maintenance, including varying the amount of reinforcement, altering the requirement of the target response (e.g., only reinforcing longer durations of eye contact), and increasing the number of responses that must occur before reinforcement is delivered. These parameters are discussed later in this chapter.

An important caveat to schedules of reinforcement is the relative consistency or inconsistency with which a contingency is implemented. For example, a therapist used a continuous schedule of reinforcement to teach Roger eye contact and an intermittent schedule to maintain this response. However, mistakes in the delivery of a contingency can also impact learning. Reinforcement, extinction, and punishment have their most robust effects if they are implemented consistently and immediately once they are first introduced into a behavioral treatment. If they are not implemented in this manner, disruptions in the learning process can occur. For example, if extinction is not implemented in a consistent manner (e.g., some responses are reinforced whereas others are not), the child's behavior will not decrease as quickly as intended due to unintentional intermittent reinforcement.

Application to Skill Training

The principles of three-term contingency, reinforcement, and extinction are also critical for understanding skill training and academic instruction from a behavioral perspective. Many behaviors are problematic because they occur too often (i.e., as behavioral excesses). Behavioral excesses are already under control of key antecedent stimuli in the child's environment, have one or more functions or "payoffs" as consequences, and have been learned over time (Martens, Daly, & Ardoin, 2015).

In contrast, skill deficits are behaviors that have not been learned and therefore do not yet have controlling variables in the child's environment. The goals of skill training and academic instruction are to first bring accurate responding and then fast and accurate responding (e.g., saying, "May I have?"") under the control of key stimuli (e.g., a card containing the printed phrase) through the differential reinforcement of correct (but not incorrect) responding in the presence of those stimuli (Martens, Codding, & Sallade, 2017). That is, reinforcement is provided only for correct responses in the presence of the target stimuli; incorrect responses are placed on extinction to make it clear to the learner what response(s) should be exhibited in the presence of the relevant stimuli. When the child consistently says the correct phrase when shown the card, responding has come under stimulus control of the card.

Stimulus control does not happen all at once but strengthens gradually over time as learners are given opportunities to respond with differential reinforcement, modeling, prompting, and error correction (i.e., training). As training progresses, two types of learning take place: how to perform the behavior correctly (e.g., saying the phrase) and when performance of the behavior will be reinforced (e.g., when the card is present). Early in training, a learner's responding becomes more accurate and eventually efficient as a result of prompting, feedback, and reinforcement. Once the learner can perform a skill accurately with a certain amount of assistance (i.e., prompting and error correction), that assistance is withdrawn or gradually faded until the child can perform the skill accurately and independently. Numerous procedures for systematically fading prompts have been reported in the literature to promote learning with no or few errors (e.g., least-to-most prompting and progressive time delay; Alberto & Troutman, 2017).

At the same time that responding is becoming more accurate, key features of stimuli that control responding are becoming more salient, making them easier to detect across learning trials. For example, as one's completion of math facts increases in accuracy, teacher prompts are faded and the learner's behavior comes under the control of the operation presented (e.g., the "A+" sign). Later in training, when nonessential features of the controlling stimuli are varied (e.g., font of the printed text or the presence of a different caregiver) or their context changes (e.g., a different room), strong stimulus control enables the learner to continue responding correctly (i.e., stimulus generalization). Stimulus control and stimulus generalization are therefore the principal concepts of behavioral skill instruction.

MEASUREMENT AND DATA ANALYSIS IN BEHAVIORAL TREATMENTS

The efficacy of behavioral treatments is typically determined at the level of the individual. In contrast, in many health care and social science research studies, the effects of an intervention are assessed at the level of the group. In assessing these effects, descriptive and inferential statistics are employed. However, with most behavioral treatments, the key comparison is not how one group responds relative to another; rather, the variables of interest are changes in the behavior of the individual. To illustrate, in treating Roger's aggression, determining whether a given procedure decreases the amount of aggression he displays relative to no treatment or alternative treatment options would be most instructive. Clinical decision making might be influenced by the literature conducted with groups, but the outcomes are specific to Roger.

Given that behavioral treatments focus on behavior change at the level of the individual, it is important to understand how the effects of an intervention are determined. As noted, behavioral treatments typically differ from group comparisons in this regard. One such difference is the focus of the behavioral treatment. That is, behavioral treatments typically target a particular behavior that can be directly observed. Although these treatments might use indirect measures (e.g., behavior rating scales) as an adjunct measure in determining program effects, the quantification and measurement of client behavior is paramount.

Target Behaviors and Operational Definitions

One of the first steps in behavioral treatment is to determine what behavior will be addressed. The behavior of interest is referred to as the **target behavior,** and the identification of the target behavior is usually determined by the individual, the respective caregivers, and/or other stakeholders in the individual's life. For example, Roger initially was referred to a specialized outpatient clinic for severe aggressive outbursts. Through consultation with his parents and his school, it was determined that his aggression would be the target behavior.

The next step is to define the target behavior. This is an important step because it helps to ensure that all subsequent data collection will address a specific form of the behavior, thereby ensuring consistency across all aspects of behavioral treatment. Thus, an operational definition is developed to quantify the behavior(s) that will be addressed through treatment. Generally, observational definitions should be concise and detailed descriptions that are written in a manner such that anyone who did not know the individual would be able to visualize, imitate, and collect data on the response after reading the definition.

In behavioral treatments, operational definitions focus on observable events. Using Roger as an example, an operational definition for aggression might be "contact between either of Roger's hands, with an open or closed hand, against any part of another person's body from at least 6 inches away." Note that this definition makes no mention of Roger's internal state (e.g., being "angry"); rather, the focus is simply on what behavior can be observed.

Measurement of Target Behavior

Once an operational definition has been developed, it is important to determine the best procedure to measure the occurrence of the behavior. In behavioral treatments, there are generally four ways to measure behavior: 1) how many times it happens (event recording), 2) how long it lasts (duration recording), 3) whether the behavior occurred during a specific observation (interval recording), and 4) what was the outcome of the behavior (permanent product recording).

Each of these measurement systems is associated with various considerations that are linked to the nature of the target behavior. For example, event recording is best used for behaviors that have a discrete beginning and end, such as taking a frequency count on the number of times Roger displays aggression. By contrast, duration and interval recording are better suited for behaviors that are more continuous. For example, when working on Roger's academics, the length of time his buttocks remain in contact with the seat of his chair (i.e., in-seat behavior) is of interest. Finally, permanent product data would provide a record of the outcome of a given behavior. For example, clinicians could measure the number of bruises that Roger's caregivers received from his aggression or the number of math problems that Roger completed in a given teaching session.

Data Collection, Experimental Design, and Data Analysis

Developing an operational definition and determining the appropriate measurement system are the initial steps in developing a behavioral treatment. It is also important to be able to identify the effects of the intervention on an individual level. Here again, behavioral treatments offer a somewhat unique set of procedures to assess intervention effects. Before beginning a treatment, for example, it is recommended to collect sufficient baseline data such that there is a reference point for the occurrence of behavior in the absence of intervention.

There are several considerations for collecting baseline data (e.g., during what context these data will be collected and by whom), but the emphasis is on obtaining information on the "typical" occurrence of behavior. Consequently, it is often necessary to take repeated measures of behavior (i.e., multiple observation) so that a sufficient sample of behavior is obtained. To illustrate, imagine Roger hits his teacher 11 times during reading instruction. Without a frame of reference, it is not possible to determine whether this is a relative improvement or worsening of his behavior. By contrast, if data from reading instruction were gathered over the course of 3 days, revealing 11, 10, and 13 occurrences of aggression, respectively, the clinician has a better understanding of the relative frequency of Roger's aggression in this context.

The collection of baseline data lends itself to a discussion of experimental designs that are used to examine the efficacy of behavioral treatments. A detailed discussion of single-case research designs is beyond the scope of this chapter but is available from a number of other sources (DeRosa, Sullivan, Roane, & Kadey, in press; Kratochwill & Levin, 2015; Perone & Hursh, 2013). Regardless of the design employed, the primary purpose of the single-case design is to demonstrate that implementation of the independent variable (e.g., intervention) is responsible for the change in the dependent variable (e.g., target behavior). This demonstration is also referred to as showing a functional relation.

The demonstration of a functional relation between treatment implementation and behavior change is often determined through the use of visual inspective strategies. Visual inspection is the process of analyzing data in accord with various changes across treatment and nontreatment conditions or when comparing multiple treatments. To do so, data on the target behavior are plotted on an *x-y* ordinate graph so that clinically relevant changes across conditions are readily apparent. These data also serve a predictive function; that is, data plotted for visual inspection should reveal consistent response patterns (assuming effective intervention) so that one can predict a continuation of the behavior pattern with the ongoing implementation of treatment. Alternatively, one could predict behavior change if the intervention were terminated. There are multiple resources available that discuss the critical elements of visual inspection (Bourret & Pietras, 2013; DeRosa et al., in press), the relation between visual inspection and statistical analyses (Baron & Perone, 1998), and methods to enhance reliable visual inspection across multiple clinicians (Fisher, Kelley, & Lomas, 2003; Kahng et al., 2010; Roane, Fisher, Kelley, Mevers, & Bouxsein, 2013).

Thus far, this chapter has covered a number of issues related to basic operant principles, measurement of behavior, and data analysis. Obviously, there are a number of other variables that influence learning and the extent to which behavioral treatments are developed and their effects determined. However, the material noted above serves as the underpinnings to most behavioral treatments for individuals with developmental disabilities. The following sections describe how these basic principles, in concert with other procedures, form the basis of the treatment for challenging behavior and skill acquisition in children with developmental disabilities.

BEHAVIORAL TREATMENT OF CHALLENGING BEHAVIOR

Understanding the role of the environment and the influence of various operant reinforcement contingencies is critical to the development of effective behavioral treatments. Therefore, it is important for a clinician to understand the relative influence of these events on the target behavior. The primary way for determining those relations is through a process called functional assessment.

Assessment of Challenging Behavior

As discussed earlier in this chapter, behavioral treatments address the function of behavior rather than its topography; that is, behavioral treatments are generally developed to address the "purpose" that is served by that target behavior. In 1977, Carr published a seminal paper that described an operant model of SIB that has proven to have application across a wide range of behaviors displayed by individuals with developmental disabilities. Carr's model posited that SIB occurs because it produces outcomes that increase its future likelihood—that is, it occurs because there is a reinforcement contingency in place. Of course, these contingencies typically develop incidentally and over the course of time.

Consider Roger's history of SIB. A well-meaning caregiver might hug or hold Roger during episodes of SIB to either comfort him or prevent the behavior from occurring. Although this might result in a brief termination or decrease in SIB, the ultimate effect of this is that SIB develops a history of producing specific caregiver reactions, which could function to strengthen the behavior through positive reinforcement. A similar scenario could emerge through a child who engages in disruptive behavior (e.g., breaking pencils) when nonpreferred academic material is presented (i.e., negative reinforcement). Carr proposed that some SIB was reinforced by the internal stimulation that it produces or attenuates, which was referred to as a self-stimulatory or automatic reinforcement hypothesis.

Functional assessments are procedures designed to gather information, generate hypotheses about behavioral function, and determine the causal factors contributing to behavior issues. To date, three categories of functional assessments have been presented in the literature:

- Indirect assessment (Kelley, LaRue, Roane, & Gadaire, 2011) describes assessment procedures that are removed in time and place from the occurrence of the challenging behavior. Relevant procedures include interviews; rating scales; and open-ended, question-and-answer forms.
- Descriptive assessment (Martens, DiGennaro, Reed, Szczech, & Rosenthal, 2008) involves direct observation of a target behavior in a relevant setting and data collection on the relevant environmental conditions and target behavior. Although these conditions are fairly unstructured, descriptive assessment involves the direct observation of the target behavior across a variety of contexts (typically in the individual's natural environment), with little to no direct influence over the contingencies that might be impacting the occurrence of the behavior.
- **Functional analysis** (also referred to as an experimental functional assessment) is based on the procedures described by Iwata, Dorsey, Slifer, Bauman, and Richman (1994) and includes the experimental manipulation of environmental variables that putatively influence the occurrence of the target behavior.

The following sections explain each category of functional assessment in more detail.

Indirect Assessment Indirect assessment (Kelley et al., 2011) is a commonly used, eclectic group of procedures employed to quickly and efficiently gather information about a challenging behavior. Indirect assessment may include an initial evaluation in which a therapist gathers demographic information, including the chief areas of complaint. Next, a client may complete a form, on behalf of oneself or another, answering a series of questions, such as ranking the severity of symptoms of ADHD (i.e., by using Conners' rating scales; Conners, 2008). Other scales may provide alternative ratings for statements, such as "My child engages in much more challenging behavior than would be normal in a school." The scale might include a range of potential answers, such as 1) strongly disagree, 2) somewhat disagree, 3) neither agree nor disagree, 4) somewhat agree, and 5) strongly agree. Scoring the ratings can help draw conclusions about why the challenging behavior occurs.

O'Neill and colleagues (1997) developed a comprehensive indirect assessment system, called the Functional Analysis Interview (FAI). It is a structured interview that includes 11 sections that purport to quickly identify putative functions of challenging behavior. The FAI takes approximately 45–90 minutes to finish depending on the amount of information provided by the client. The interview provides a guide for the interviewer across multiple content areas: 1) developing a description of the behavior; 2) identifying settings events, antecedents, and consequences for maladaptive behavior; 3) identifying how efficient the maladaptive behavior is, alternative behavior, and communicative ability; 4) identifying reinforcers; and 5) describing the history of previous interventions. After completing the interview procedures, the interviewer determines the operational definitions of challenging behaviors, environments in which the responses occur, antecedent and consequent conditions influencing the behavior, and other information that will help select an intervention.

Descriptive Assessment Descriptive assessment (Castillo et al., 2018; Lerman & Iwata, 1993; Mace & Lalli, 1991; Martens et al., 2008) procedures control for some significant limitations of indirect assessment techniques. First, indirect assessment relies on accurate recall of past events and faithful ratings of those events. Descriptive assessment, on the other hand, focuses on observation of the behavior in vivo and data collection of the target behavior under naturalistic environmental conditions. Second, indirect procedures are removed in time and place from the occurrence of the target behavior. Descriptive assessment allows for real-time observation of behavior while interacting with the environment.

The primary value of descriptive assessment is in aiding the development of operational definitions of a challenging behavior and generating hypotheses about the behavior's function (Lerman & Iwata, 1993). Descriptive assessments provide information about the conditions under which the target behavior does and does not occur and the order in which a series of challenging behaviors occur (e.g., response class hierarchies); most importantly, it lays the foundation for the development of experimental analysis of the putative variables influencing behavior.

Functional Analysis In 1982, Iwata and colleagues operationalized Carr's (1977) hypotheses in a series of test conditions in a procedure called functional analysis. Specifically, they arranged a number of observations designed to experimentally test a specific reinforcement contingency. In the social disapproval (or attention) condition, the researchers ignored the child unless he or she displayed challenging behavior, in which case they provided attention to the child in the form of statements of concern or disapproval (e.g., saying "Stop that"). This condition assessed the role of positive reinforcement in the occurrence of a challenging behavior.

A second condition, academic demand, was conducted in which the researchers presented academics to the child and provided a break from instructions (in the form of removal of the academic material) contingent on the occurrence of the challenging behavior. This condition assessed the influence of negative reinforcement on the behavior.

An alone condition was also conducted in which the researchers observed a child who was alone in a room through an observation window. In this condition, there were no programmed contingencies in place for the challenging behavior (i.e., the researchers did not respond to the occurrence of the behavior). Sustained occurrences of the behavior in this condition would implicate Carr's self-stimulatory or automatic reinforcement account of challenging behaviors.

Finally, a control condition was contrasted with the above conditions. In the control condition, the child 1) had access to preferred items (to reduce the likelihood of automatically reinforced challenging behavior), 2) had access to adult attention (to reduce the likelihood of positively reinforced challenging behavior), and 3) had no academic demands presented (to reduce the likelihood of negatively reinforced challenging behavior). The relative benefit of this type of functional assessment is that the clinician has direct control over the contingencies that are influencing the behavior, which permits a more detailed level of analysis and hypothesis testing (Vollmer, Roane, & Rone, 2012).

The results of the Iwata and colleagues' (1994) investigation revealed differentiated response patterns across participants (i.e., some individuals displayed the challenging behavior in one condition, whereas others did the same in another condition). These results were important because they validated the hypothesis presented by Carr (1977) regarding the potential role of operant contingencies in the occurrence of a challenging behavior. They also indicated that there were idiosyncratic differences regarding the reason that a challenging behavior occurred across participants. The functional analysis procedure developed by Iwata and colleagues (1994) has been validated in hundreds of studies addressing many different types of challenging behavior (Beavers, Iwata, & Lerman, 2013; Hanley, Iwata, & McCord, 2003). It has also proven to be an adaptable model of assessment, with procedural modifications made to decrease time expenditures (Falcomata, Muething, Roberts, Hamrick, & Shpall, 2016), to develop novel conditions (McCord, Thompson, & Iwata, 2001), and to be implemented in nonclinical settings by individuals other than trained researchers (Martens, Gertz, Werder, & Rymanowski, 2010). Moreover, the advent of functional analysis has resulted in an increased use of reinforcement-based treatments for challenging behaviors and a decreased reliance on punishment-based procedures (Didden, Duker, & Korzilius, 1997). See Box 34.1 for more on the evidence base for functional analysis.

Nevertheless, the functional analysis procedure is not appropriate for all populations or settings. Some limitations of this approach include 1) a temporary worsening of behavior because the individual is contacting reinforcement contingencies that increase the occurrence of that behavior, 2) the use of contrived situations that may not be applicable to the individual's natural environment, and 3) time constraints and necessary expertise in conducting or overseeing the procedure. As a result, a number of alternative procedures have been developed to assess the role of various reinforcement contingencies on the occurrence of challenging behavior (Martens et al., 2008).

Figure 34.1 shows the results of a functional analysis conducted with Roger to identify the reinforcement contingencies that maintained his aggression. A control condition and four test conditions (attention, tangible, demand, and ignore) were implemented in a multi-element, single-case design. The control condition (toy play) consisted of a therapist delivering near continuous attention to Roger, in the absence of any instructions, while he had access to preferred toys. The attention condition involved a therapist diverting their attention away from Roger and delivering attention in the form of reprimands ("No Roger, it's not nice to hit other people!") contingent on aggression.

In the demand condition, the therapist delivered academic instructions to Roger, and, contingent on aggression, a brief break was provided. A tangible condition was also implemented to test for positive reinforcement in the form of tangible items (Vollmer,

BOX 34.1 EVIDENCE-BASED PRACTICE

Functional Analysis

Functional assessment has been identified as a "best practice" to developing treatments for severe maladaptive behavior by the American Academy of Pediatrics (Myers & Johnson, 2007). This assessment approach is based on the analog functional analysis procedure developed by Iwata, Dorsey, Slifer, Bauman, and Richman (1994). In a functional analysis, the individual is exposed to a number of "test" conditions. In each of these conditions, the clinician creates a situation that mimics those from the natural environment that might be associated with an increased probability of severe maladaptive behavior. These test conditions are compared with a control condition that is specifically arranged to promote low levels of maladaptive behavior. The child is exposed to a series of direct observations under the various test (and control) conditions. Those conditions associated with the most elevated and persistent occurrences of maladaptive behavior (compared with the control condition) are indicative of a maintaining reinforcement contingency, or the "function" of the behavior. Treatments are then developed that directly address the function of the behavior.

Beavers, Iwata, and Lerman (2013) reviewed more than 400 published studies that had implemented a functional analysis to identify the reinforcement contingencies that maintained challenging or maladaptive behavior. Although most of those studies (approximately 75%) involved children as participants, the methods were also replicated with adult and geriatric populations. Additional generality for this approach was suggested by the use of functional analysis across individuals with and without intellectual and developmental disabilities, and the studies reviewed addressed a large range of challenging behavior types. Across all reviewed studies, Beavers and colleagues found differentiated results (i.e., one or more test conditions being associated with elevated response levels) in over 90% of cases regardless of age, diagnosis, or type of behavior assessed.

Application to Practice

The functional analysis method is effective for identifying the conditions that are most likely to maintain the occurrence of challenging behavior.

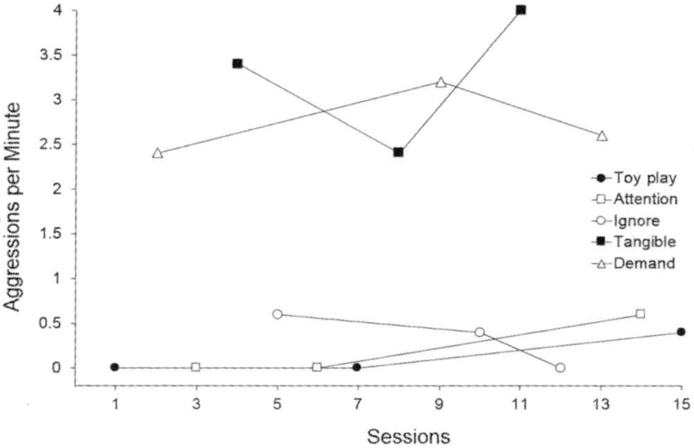

Figure 34.1. Results from Roger's functional analysis displaying aggressions per minute across sessions. Each data path represents the corresponding test (attention, demand, tangible, ignore) and control (toy play) conditions.

Marcus, Ringdahl, & Roane, 1995). Here the therapist restricted access to preferred toys and, following the occurrence of aggression, allowed Roger to continue playing with his toys. Lastly, an ignore condition (similar to Iwata et al.'s alone condition) was conducted in which the therapist was present in the room with Roger but refrained from interacting with him regardless of his behavior.

Outcomes from the functional analysis (Figure 34.1) suggested that Roger's aggression was multiply maintained by both negative reinforcement (i.e., escape from academic instructions) and positive reinforcement (i.e., access to preferred tangible items). For the purpose of this discussion, the focus is on treatments developed to address the positive reinforcement function; procedures for addressing multiple functions and combining interventions are discussed elsewhere (Call, Wacker, Ringdahl, & Boelter, 2005; Neidert, Iwata, & Dozier, 2005; Scheithauer, Mevers, Call, & Shresbury, 2017).

In summary, conducting a functional assessment is a valuable first step in developing an effective behavioral treatment for challenging behaviors displayed by individuals with developmental disabilities. In fact, this approach was deemed a best practice by the American Academy of Pediatrics in its practice guidelines for ASD (Myers & Johnson, 2007). The primary benefit of conducting a functional assessment is that it permits one to test specific hypotheses about the potential contingencies that could be affecting the occurrence of a target behavior, thereby determining the function or purpose that the behavior serves. Once known, behavioral treatments can be developed to specifically intervene on that function.

Treatment of Challenging Behavior

The development of a behavioral treatment typically follows the functional assessment. This link between assessment and treatment is important and somewhat unique, in that the functional assessment informs treatment development by providing information on what environmental variables can be altered in treatment. For example, if the functional analysis indicates a negative reinforcement function, we know that the individual is motivated to use a challenging behavior to avoid nonpreferred activities (e.g., completing adaptive living skills). Given this knowledge, the therapist can develop a treatment that provides access to this reinforcer for some other, appropriate form of behavior. The functional assessment identifies which variable(s) to affect in treatment.

Extinction

Following the logic of intervening on the environmental variables that are identified in the functional assessment, a basic component of many behavioral treatments is **extinction.** Technically speaking, extinction involves interruption of an existing relationship between a response and the maintaining reinforcer. Using Roger's positive-reinforcement function (shown in Figure 34.1) as an example, extinction would be arranged such that Roger's aggression no longer produced access to preferred items. Using this procedure, aggression would no longer "pay off" and, over time, the behavior should decrease. All humans encounter extinction periodically. For example, buying a drink from a vending machine could present an opportunity for extinction. That is, if you put money in the machine and pressed a button for your drink of choice, your behavior would be reinforced by delivery of the drink. If, however, the drink does not appear at the bottom of the machine, your drink selection response would have encountered extinction. Over time, you would quit trying to buy a drink from that particular machine.

Extinction is used as a component of many treatments for challenging behaviors displayed by individuals with developmental disabilities. However, it is rarely used in isolation because extinction alone can result in a number of side effects. Consider the vending machine example. If you place your money in the machine, press the button for drink A, and it does not come out, you tend to engage in a number of other responses. For example, you might press the button for drink A again. You might press that same button repeatedly. After a while, you might vary your responding and press the button for drink B, then drink C, and so on. Some people might become angry and hit the machine or swear aloud. Over time, these behaviors would decrease and you would likely walk away. You might, however, try the machine again the next day or a week later and, if it was still malfunctioning, go through this same series of behaviors. All of these responses are common and are referred to as an **extinction burst.**

When extinction is introduced, there is an increased likelihood of response frequency, response intensity, response variation, and the emergence of emotional behavior or other forms of maladaptive behavior such as aggression. Likewise, the effect of periodically attempting a response that has encountered extinction, such as trying the vending machine after a week, is common and is referred to as **spontaneous recovery.** A review of published data on the use of extinction showed that behaviors resembling an extinction burst only occur in about one third of cases (Lerman & Iwata, 1995).

The potential for extinction bursts is one reason that extinction is rarely implemented as the only component of a behavioral treatment. A second reason is that extinction alone does not permit the development of an alternative response to replace the challenging behavior. Recall the earlier example of using extinction to decrease Roger's aggression. In this case, extinction involved disrupting the relationship between aggression and providing access to preferred activities. That is, Roger's aggression no longer resulted in access to the maintaining reinforcer (access to preferred items). A limitation, however, is that this procedure did not include a mechanism by which Roger could access his preferred activities.

Differential Reinforcement

Differential reinforcement is a broad category of treatments that essentially involve reinforcing behaviors that are alternatives to the challenging behaviors. For example, an individual might be taught to engage in a manual sign to access reinforcement while the challenging behavior is placed on extinction. In Roger's case, this is a treatment procedure by which Roger could access reinforcers.

There are a number of different ways in which a differential reinforcement contingency can be arranged. This section describes three procedures that are used most commonly in the treatment of challenging behaviors for individuals with developmental disabilities: differential reinforcement of other behavior, differential reinforcement of alternative behavior, and differential reinforcement of incompatible behavior.

A **differential reinforcement of other behavior** (DRO) treatment is one in which reinforcement is delivered for the omission of the target behavior for a period of time. For example, in a DRO treatment, a contingency could be arranged such that Roger's aggression was placed on extinction; however, if he did not engage in aggression for a period of time (e.g., 2 minutes), the reinforcer would be delivered. This procedure teaches the individual that challenging behavior "no longer works" and that not engaging in that behavior produces access to reinforcement. Based on this, when using a DRO, there is not a specific contingency to develop other forms of behavior that might serve as alternatives. Given this, a DRA contingency is a viable alternative.

A **differential reinforcement of alternative behavior** (DRA) treatment is one in which an individual is specifically taught an alternative means of access reinforcement. Recall from Figure 34.1 that Roger had a propensity to engage in maladaptive behavior when presented with schoolwork and self-help tasks (i.e., a negative reinforcement function). A DRA procedure for this contingency might involve placing aggression on extinction and reinforcing compliance with academic work (e.g., completion of a task results in a break from work). Therefore, in a DRA treatment, there is a specific response(s) (i.e., alternative behavior) that produces reinforcement and a specific response(s) (i.e., maladaptive behavior) that does not produce access to reinforcement.

Similar to DRA, a differential reinforcement of incompatible behavior (DRI) treatment is one in which a challenging behavior is placed on extinction and the response that is reinforced is one that is incompatible with that behavior. For example, a DRI treatment for aggression might involve extinction for aggression and reinforcement for the individual holding their hands clasped in their lap. DRI procedures have been used less frequently in the behavioral treatment literature relative to DRO and DRA procedures, but they nonetheless present a viable option for the treatment of challenging behavior in individuals with developmental disabilities.

Functional Communication Training

Children with developmental disabilities often do not imitate or ask for information, may exhibit repetitive or stereotypic behavior, may pay little attention to social cues, and may have limited communication skills (Smith, 2001; Wehmeyer, Brown, Percy, Shogren, & Fung, 2017). As a result, these children may fail to acquire or may be delayed in acquiring key or pivotal skills such as functional communication, object discrimination, imitation, simple speech, self-care, and/or playing with peers. Among these skills, functional communication, or expressing one's wants and needs in socially acceptable ways, is critical for children with disabilities and has been identified by teachers as essential for kindergarten readiness (Hustedt, Buell, Hallam, & Pinder, 2018; Lin, Lawrence, & Gorrell, 2003).

Functional communication training (FCT) is an extension of the DRA procedure in which the child is taught a specific communication response (or set of responses) to access the same reinforcer that maintained the challenging behavior. This communication response is also referred to as a "mand" since it is used to "command" or ask for the reinforcer (Skinner, 1957). FCT typically occurs in three stages:

1. A functional analysis is conducted to identify the type of reinforcer maintaining the challenging behavior and the antecedent conditions that increase that reinforcer's value as a motivating operation.
2. A low-effort, socially acceptable communication response (e.g., ask, gesture, card touch, switch, or picture exchange) is taught using differential reinforcement along with modeling, prompting, and error correction.
3. Engagement in the communication response is reinforced while engaging in challenging behavior is placed on extinction in the natural environment.

FCT offers several advantages relative to DRA. Specifically, FCT is appropriate for reducing multiple topographies and functions of challenging behaviors and teaches a communication response that is easily recognized by multiple care providers. It is also common in FCT to promote the generalization of communication using multiple trainers and/or common stimuli (e.g., a printed card) and to promote the maintenance of communication by thinning its reinforcement schedule, introducing a delay between communication and obtaining the reinforcer, or increasing the duration of signaled extinction periods when the reinforcer is unavailable for communication (Fuhrman, Fisher, & Greer, 2016).

CASE STUDY

Because Roger could follow single-step directions, name objects, and communicate vocally in two- to three-word phrases, his behavioral therapy team decided to incorporate FCT into his treatment program and included several of the elements of FCT described previously. Specifically, they taught Roger to say three different communication "frames" ("May I have?," "I would like," and "Can I get?") when presented with a color-coded script (i.e., script training) using the fading procedure of progressive time delay (Betz, Higbee, Kelley, Sellers, & Pollard, 2011; Brodhead, Higbee, Gerencser, & Akers, 2016). The color-coded scripts could then be taken by Roger into different settings as common stimuli, thereby promoting generalization of communication. Also using the presence of the color-coded scripts as stimuli, the team promoted the maintenance of communication by decreasing the amount of time during which the scripts were present as signals for the reinforcement of communication using a multiple-schedule approach (Fuhrman et al., 2016; Greer, Fisher, Saini, Owen, & Jones, 2016). A multiple schedule is a procedure in which two discriminative stimuli are used to signal to the individual the various contingencies that are in place during treatment. That is, during periods when one or more of the color-coded scripts were present, communication was reinforced with access to the item. During other times when the color-coded scripts were not present, communication was not reinforced and Roger had to wait to ask for desired items.

During each script training session, the therapist presented a script (e.g., "May I have?"), immediately modeled it by saying the script for Roger, and gave him 5 seconds to repeat the script. If Roger responded correctly on four of five trials, then the delay between presentation of the script and the model was increased by 3 seconds (i.e., progressive time delay). Training continued until Roger responded correctly before the model on four of five trials over two consecutive sessions for each communication frame.

After Roger was able to say each script accurately, the therapist began script fluency training. Five color-coded copies of each script were created and stacked in random order. Roger was told, "Say the card correctly as fast as you can," and the therapist presented each flash card. Fluency training continued until Roger was no longer able to beat his previous time for saying all 15 flashcard scripts.

Following script acquisition and fluency training, the therapist began teaching Roger to communicate for desired items using the scripts in different situations (i.e., script use). The therapist began each session by placing the corresponding script in front of Roger, displaying a desired item out of reach (e.g., cookie, drink, or toy), and waiting 10 seconds for Roger to use the communication frame to ask for the item. If Roger did not request the item, the therapist prompted a response by saying, "Say the card." Roger was given access to the item after saying the communication response.

To evaluate the effects of FCT on Roger's challenging behavior, the therapist alternated conditions in which the behavior or communication was reinforced using an ABAB single-case reversal design. She then gradually increased the amount of time in which Roger had to wait to ask for his preferred items. The results of this evaluation are presented in Figure 34.2.

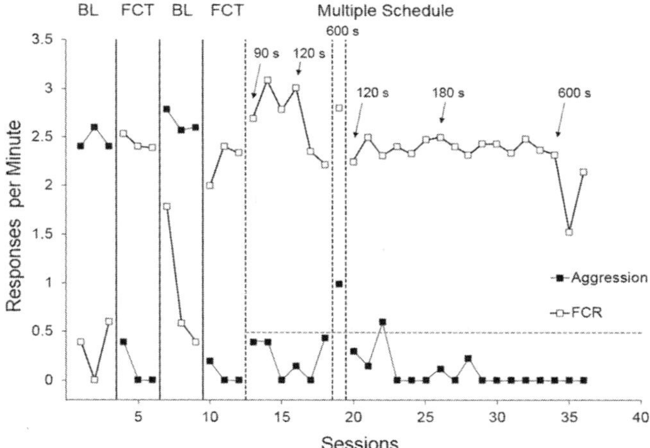

Figure 34.2. Results from Roger's functional communication training (FCT) analysis, displaying aggression (black squares) and functional communication responses (FCR; open squares) per minute across baseline (BL) and FCT sessions. During the multiple-schedule phase, the amount of time before color-coded scripts were presented and FCRs produced reinforcement was gradually increased—that is, i.e., 90 seconds (sec), 120 sec, 180 sec, and 600 sec.

With FCT, it is often necessary to teach an initial form of communication and then expand this repertoire to promote varied responding (see Adami, Falcomata, Muething, & Hoffman, 2017; Brodhead et al., 2016). In this regard, consultation with a speech-language pathologist is helpful (see Box 34.2).

Noncontingent Reinforcement An advantage of FCT is that it teaches a communication response while decreasing the occurrence of challenging behavior. However, there are some cases in which it might be difficult to teach a communication response or other variables impact a caregiver's ability to respond to the individual's communicative behavior (e.g., a caregiver might not always see a manual sign). In this case, noncontingent reinforcement (NCR) is a viable treatment strategy (see Phillips, Iannaccone, Rooker, & Hagopian, 2017). NCR involves the response-independent delivery of reinforcement based on the passage of time.

Although NCR may seem counterintuitive, the approach is effective because it interrupts the relationship between challenging behavior and reinforcement. For example, an NCR procedure for Roger's aggression might be arranged in which aggression was placed on extinction, but every 5 minutes he received access to his preferred activities for a period of time (e.g., 1 minute). This is a response-independent contingency in that Roger would not have to "do" anything to earn the reinforcer, nor would he have to necessarily forgo aggression in this interval as in a DRO; rather, the reinforcer is delivered "for free" based on the passage of time. The rationale for this is one of affecting his motivation to engage in aggression. That is, if he is receiving reinforcer independently, it should decrease his motivation to use aggression to access reinforcement. The adage, "Why buy the cow if the milk is free?" is applicable.

A benefit of NCR to caregivers might be that the caregiver does not have to acknowledge or wait for the child to emit a response; they simply wait for a signal from a timer. This aspect of NCR may make it feasible for some caregivers. NCR does not, however, teach an alternative response (as does DRA and FCT) or have a

BOX 34.2 INTERDISCIPLINARY CARE

Team Members Contributing to the Development of a Functional Assessment and Behavioral Treatment

Role of the medical professional: Identify underlying physical causes of behavior (e.g., self-injury due to eczema, pica due to iron deficiency), medication management, and assessment of the child relative to developmental norms.

Role of the psychologist: Assess and treat comorbid mental health disorders (e.g., anxiety).

Role of the behavior analyst: Identify environmental variables contributing to and maintaining challenging behavior and develop function-matched treatments for challenging behavior and reinforcement-based, skill-acquisition programs.

Role of the speech-language pathologist: Assist in the identification and teaching of communication responses that could serve as functional alternatives to challenging behavior.

Role of the occupational therapist: Assess sensory processing issues and provide strategies to meet the child's unique sensory needs.

Role of the special educator: Identify teaching modifications (instructional and environmental) to facilitate generalization of treatment and identify strategies to incorporate into the classroom.

Role of the social worker: Identify levels of care (e.g., respite services), coordinate care across multidisciplinary providers, and provide family support.

contingency in place to specifically promote decreases in challenging behavior (as does DRO). In addition, there is some risk that the reinforcer delivery in NCR could be incidentally paired with the occurrence of the challenging behavior (Vollmer, Ringdahl, Roane, & Marcus, 1997).

Punishment The role of punishment as a behavior change procedure has been described above. According to practice standards set by individuals who develop behavioral treatments (Van Houten et al., 1988; Vollmer et al., 2011), punishment procedures should only be used 1) when all other evidence-based treatment avenues have been exhausted, 2) when reinforcement-based procedures alone have proven ineffective, or 3) in conjunction with a reinforcement-based procedure.

The use of punishment procedures in the treatment of challenging behaviors displayed by individuals with developmental disabilities has decreased since the development of the functional analysis procedure (Didden et al., 1997). However, some studies suggest that punishment contingencies are necessary in the treatment of some cases of challenging behavior (Hagopian, Fisher, Sullivan, Acquisto, & LeBlanc, 1998; Newcomb & Hagopian, 2018). Also, whereas early studies on the use of punishment involved highly aversive procedures (Lovaas & Simmons, 1969), there has been a general move toward more negative punishment procedures, such as the use of time-out. Although punishment was not used in the case study concerning Roger, recent research shows that a punishment procedure can be necessary to decrease the occurrence of some behaviors exhibited by individuals with ASD and intellectual disabilities (DeRosa, Roane, Bishop, & Silkowski, 2016). As noted by DeRosa and colleagues, punishment was only considered for that individual after a number of reinforcement-based procedures had been ineffective at reducing the participant's rumination to clinically significant levels; this approach is consistent with practice standards regarding the use of punishment.

Generalization of Behavioral Treatments for Challenging Behaviors

Regardless of the treatment approach, an important focus of behavioral treatments should always be programming the environment to ensure that the treatment contingencies are effective across multiple contexts, caregivers, and settings. Stokes and Baer (1977) described nine strategies of generalization that can be used to help ensure that treatments developed in one setting (e.g., a clinic) or implemented by one individual (e.g., a trained clinician) are equally effective across other settings and individuals (e.g., a teacher in a school).

One of the primary procedures used to generalize treatment effects involves the incorporation of natural stimuli into the training (or clinical) environment. For example, it is helpful to incorporate materials that the individual encounters in his or her typical environment. This might include using the actual schoolwork presented in the classroom during treatment in a clinic or arranging the clinic environment to more closely resemble the home environment. For example, a clinical setting might be modified by using more naturalistic furniture (e.g., couches) and using confederate staff members to make the environment more closely resemble the home.

An area of obvious importance in programming for treatment generalization is incorporating the individual's caregivers as treatment agents. There are a number of studies that have examined caregiver-training strategies (Lerman, LeBlanc, & Valentino, 2015). Generally speaking, this involves a gradual program in which caregivers first observe a trained clinician implement the treatment procedures. The clinician and caregiver might then role play the procedures while data are collected on the caregiver's implementation of procedures to ensure they meet criterion levels (e.g., 80% accuracy for implementation). The use of immediate and delayed feedback is also helpful when a caregiver is implementing the treatment. Finally, follow-up in the home either in person or through telehealth (Barretto, Wacker, Harding, Lee, & Berg, 2006; Tomlinson, Gore, & McGill, 2018) is beneficial to ensure program fidelity and long-term maintenance.

SUMMARY

- Operant conditioning views behavior as an interaction between the individual and the environment.
- The core principles of operant conditioning (e.g., reinforcement) form the basis of most behavioral treatments.
- Behavior treatments are individualized and are matched to the function of the individual's challenging behavior.
- Data collection is typically personalized through the use of unique operational definitions, and the effects of interventions are analyzed through single-case experimental designs.
- Functional assessment identifies the environmental variables that are associated with the occurrence and maintenance of challenging behaviors.

- Functional assessment can include an indirect assessment, a descriptive assessment, a functional analysis, or a combination of procedures.
- Following the functional assessment, a treatment is developed that includes operating on the variables identified in the functional assessment. These treatments often involve an extinction component, although extinction is seldom used in isolation.
- Reinforcement-based procedures such as DRO, DRA, DRI, FCT, and NCR are often combined with extinction. Punishment procedures are only necessary in a minority of cases.
- A necessary step throughout the treatment process is to incorporate procedures that will enhance the ability of the treatment to be generalized to other settings and caregivers.
- Other related topics include the use of preference assessments to identify stimuli that can be used as positive reinforcers, stimulus control procedures to teach discrimination across various contingencies, and antecedent-based procedures such as picture schedules or rules.
- Behavioral treatments follow a common process—they are based on a systematic assessment process.

ADDITIONAL RESOURCES

American Academy of Pediatrics/Health Children: https://www.healthychildren.org/English/health-issues/conditions/adhd/Pages/Behavior-Therapy-Parent-Training.aspx

Effective Child Therapy: http://effectivechildtherapy.org/therapies/what-is-behavior-therapy/

Centers for Disease Control and Prevention: https://www.cdc.gov/features/adhd-awareness/index.html

Additional resources can be found online in Appendix D: Childhood Disabilities Resources, Services, and Organizations (see About the Online Companion Materials).

REFERENCES

Alberto, P. A., & Troutman, A. C. (2017). *Applied behavior analysis for teachers* (9th ed.). Upper Saddle River, NJ: Pearson.

Adami, S., Falcomata, T. S., Muething, C. S., & Hoffman, K. (2017). An evaluation of lag schedules of reinforcement during functional communication training: Effects on varied mand responding and challenging behavior. *Behavior Analysis in Practice, 10*(3), 209–213. doi:10.1007/s40617-017-0179-7

Baron, A., & Perone, M. (1998). Experimental design and analysis in the laboratory study of human operant behavior. In K. A. Lattal, M. Perone, K. A. Lattal, & M. Perone (Eds.), *Handbook of research methods in human operant behavior* (pp. 45–91). New York, NY: Plenum Press. doi:10.1007/978-1-4899-1947-2_3

Barretto, A., Wacker, D. P., Harding, J., Lee, J., & Berg, W. K. (2006). Using telemedicine to conduct behavioral assessments. *Journal of Applied Behavior Analysis, 39*(3), 333–340. doi:10.1901/jaba.2006.173-04

Beavers, G. A., Iwata, B. A., & Lerman, D. C. (2013). Thirty years of research on the functional analysis of problem behavior. *Journal of Applied Behavior Analysis, 46*(1), 1–21. doi:10.1002/jaba.30

Beidas, R. S., Benjamin, C. L., Puleo, C. M., Edmunds, J. M., & Kendall, P. C. (2010). Flexible Applications of the Coping Cat Program for Anxious Youth. *Cognitive and Behavioral Practice, 17*(2), 142–153. http://doi.org/10.1016/j.cbpra.2009.11.002

Benson, B. A. (2016). Behavioral approaches. In C. Hemmings & N. Bouras (Eds.), *Psychiatric and behavioral disorders in intellectual and developmental disabilities* (3rd ed., pp. 171–180). New York, NY: Cambridge University Press.

Betz, A. J., Higbee, T. S., Kelley, K. N., Sellers, T. P., & Pollard, J. S. (2011). Increasing response variability of mand frames with script training and extinction. *Journal of Applied Behavior Analysis, 44*, 359–362. doi:10.1901/jaba.2011.44-357

Bourret, J. C., & Pietras, C. J. (2013). Visual analysis in single-case research. In G. J. Madden, W. V. Dube, T. D. Hackenberg, G. P. Hanley, K. A. Lattal, G. J. Madden, . . . K. A. Lattal (Eds.), *APA handbook of behavior analysis* (Vol. 1, pp. 199–217). Washington, DC: American Psychological Association. doi:10.1037/13937-009

Brodhead, M. T., Higbee, T. S., Gerencser, K. R., & Akers, J. S. (2016). The use of discrimination-training procedure to teach mand variability to children with autism. *Journal of Applied Behavior Analysis, 49*, 34–48. doi:10.1002/jaba.280

Call, N. A., Wacker, D. P., Ringdahl, J. E., & Boelter, E. W. (2005). Combined antecedent variables as motivating operations within functional analyses. *Journal of Applied Behavior Analysis, 38*(3), 385–389. http://doi.org/10.1901/jaba.2005.51-04

Carr, E. G. (1977). The motivation of self-injurious behavior: A review of some hypotheses. *Psychological Bulletin, 84*(4), 800. doi:10.1037/0033-2909.84.4.800

Castillo, M. I., Clark, D. R., Schaller, E. A., Donaldson, J. M., DeLeon, I. G., & Kahng, S. (2018). Descriptive assessment of problem behavior during transitions of children with intellectual and developmental disabilities. *Journal of Applied Behavior Analysis, 51*, 99–117. doi:10.1002/jaba.430

Conners, C. K. (2008). *Conners rating scales* (3rd ed.). Toronto, Canada: Multi-Health Systems.

DeRosa, N. M., Roane, H. S., Bishop, J. R., & Silkowski, E. M. (2016). The combined effects of noncontingent reinforcement and punishment on the reduction of rumination. *Journal of Applied Behavior Analysis, 49*, 680–685. doi:10.1002/jaba.304

DeRosa, N. M., Sullivan, W. E., Roane, H. S., & Kadey, H. J. (in press). Single-case experimental designs. In W. W. Fisher, C. C. Piazza, & H. S. Roane (Eds.), *Handbook of applied behavior analysis* (2nd ed.). New York, NY: Guilford.

Didden, R., Duker, P. C., & Korzilius, H. (1997). Meta-analytic study on treatment effectiveness for problem behaviors with individuals who have mental retardation. *American Journal on Mental Retardation, 101*, 387–399.

Dominick, K. C., Davis, N. O., Lainhart, J., Tager-Flusberg, H., & Folstein, S. (2007). Atypical behaviors in children with autism and children with a history of language impairment. *Research in Developmental Disabilities, 28*(2), 145–162. doi:10.1016/j.ridd.2006.02.003

Falcomata, T. S., Muething, C. S., Roberts, G. J., Hamrick, J., & Shpall, C. (2016). Further evaluation of latency-based brief functional analysis methods: An evaluation of treatment utility. *Developmental Neurorehabilitation, 19*(2), 88–94. doi:10.3109/17518423.2014.910281

Fisher, W. W., Kelley, M. E., & Lomas, J. E. (2003). Visual aids and structured criteria for improving inspection and interpretation of single-case designs. *Journal of Applied Behavior Analysis, 36*(3), 387–406. doi:10.1901/jaba.2003.36-387

Fisher, W. W., & Zangrillo, A. N. (2015). Applied behavior analytic assessment and treatment of autism spectrum disorder. In H. S. Roane, J. E., Ringdahl, & T. S. Falcomata (Eds.), *Clinical and organizational applications of applied behavior analysis* (pp. 19–45). San Diego, CA: Elsevier.

Fuhrman, A. M., Fisher, W. W., & Greer, B. D. (2016). A preliminary investigation on improving functional communication training by mitigating resurgence of destructive behavior. *Journal of Applied Behavior Analysis, 49*, 884–899. doi:10.1002/jaba.338

Greer, B. D., Fisher, W. W., Saini, V., Owen, T. M., & Jones, J. K. (2016). Functional communication training during reinforcement schedule thinning: An analysis of 25 applications. *Journal of Applied Behavior Analysis, 49*(1), 105–121. doi:10.1002/jaba.265

Hagopian, L. P., Fisher, W. W., Sullivan, M. T., Acquisto, J., & LeBlanc, L. A. (1998). Effectiveness of functional communication training with and without extinction and punishment: A summary of 21 inpatient cases. *Journal of Applied Behavior Analysis, 31*(2), 211–235. doi:10.1901/jaba.1998.31-211

Hanley, G. P., Iwata, B. A., & McCord, B. E. (2003). Functional analysis of problem behavior: A review. *Journal of Applied Behavior Analysis, 36*, 147–185. doi:10.1901/jaba.2003.36-147

Heyvaert, M., Saenen, L., Campbell, J. M., Maes, B., & Onghena, P. (2014). Efficacy of behavioral interventions for reducing problem behavior in persons with autism: An updated quantitative synthesis of single-subject research. *Research in Developmental Disabilities, 35*, 2463–2476. doi:10.1016/j.ridd.2014.06.017

Hustedt, J. T., Buell, M. J., Hallam, R. A., & Pinder, W. M. (2018). While kindergarten has changed, some beliefs remain the same: Kindergarten's teachers' beliefs about readiness. *Journal of Research in Childhood Education, 32*, 52–66. doi:10.1080/02568543.2017.1393031

Iwata, B. A., Dorsey, M. F., Slifer, K. J., Bauman, K. E., & Richman, G. S. (1994). Toward a functional analysis of self-injury. *Journal of Applied Behavior Analysis, 27*, 197–209. doi:10.1016/0270-4684(82)90003-9

Kahng, S., Chung, K.-M., Gutshall, K., Pitts, S. C., Kao, J., & Girolami, K. (2010). Consistent visual analyses of intrasubject data. *Journal of Applied Behavior Analysis, 43*(1), 35–45. doi:10.1901/jaba.2010.43-35

Kelley, M. E., LaRue, R. H., Roane, H. S., & Gadaire, D. M. (2011). Indirect behavioral assessments: Interviews and rating scales. In W. W. Fisher, C. C. Piazza, & H. S. Roane (Eds.), *Handbook of applied behavior analysis* (pp. 182–190). New York, NY: Guilford.

Kendall, P. C., & Beidas, R. S. (2007). Smoothing the trail for dissemination of evidence-based practices for youth: Flexibility within fidelity. *Professional Psychology: Research and Practice, 38*(1), 13–20. doi:10.1037/0735-7028.38.1.13

Kendall, P. C., Gosch, E., Furr, J. M., & Sood, E. (2008). Flexibility within fidelity. *Journal of the American Academy of Child & Adolescent Psychiatry, 47*(9), 987–993. doi:10.1097/CHI.0b013e31817eed2f

Kratochwill, T. R., & Levin, J. R. (2015). *Single-case research design and analysis (psychology revivals): New directions for psychology and education*. London, United Kingdom: Routledge.

Lang, R., Mahoney, R., Zein, F. E., Delaune, E., & Amidon, M. (2011). Evidence to practice: Treatment of anxiety in individuals with autism spectrum disorders. *Neuropsychiatric Disease and Treatment, 7*(1), 27–30.

Lang, R., Regester, A., Lauderdale, S., Ashbaugh, K., & Haring, A. (2010). Treatment of anxiety in autism spectrum disorders using cognitive behaviour therapy: A systematic review. *Developmental Neurorehabilitation, 13*(1), 53–63. doi:10.3109/17518420903236288

Lerman, D. C., & Iwata, B. A. (1993). Descriptive and experimental analyses of variables maintaining self-injurious behavior. *Journal of Applied Behavior Analysis, 26*(3), 293–319. doi:10.1901/jaba.1993.26-293

Lerman, D. C., & Iwata, B. A. (1995). Prevalence of the extinction burst and its attenuation during treatment. *Journal of Applied Behavior Analysis, 28*(1), 93–94. doi:10.1901/jaba.1995.28-93

Lerman, D. C., LeBlanc, L. A., & Valentino, A. L. (2015). Evidence-based application of staff and caregiver training procedures. In H. S. Roane, J. E., Ringdahl, & T. S. Falcomata (Eds.), *Clinical and organizational applications of applied behavior analysis*. San Diego, CA: Elsevier.

Lin, H. L., Lawrence, F. R., & Gorrell, J. (2003). Kindergarten teachers' views of children's readiness for school. *Early Childhood Research Quarterly, 18*, 225–237. doi:10.1016/S0885-2006(03)00028-0

Lovaas, O. I., & Simmons, J. Q. (1969). Manipulation of self-destruction in three retarded children. *Journal of Applied Behavior Analysis, 2*, 143–157. doi:10.1901/jaba.1969.2-143

Mace, F. C., & Lalli, J. S. (1991). Linking descriptive and experimental analyses in the treatment of bizarre speech. *Journal of Applied Behavior Analysis, 24*(3), 553–562. doi:10.1901/jaba.1991.24-553

Martens, B. K., Codding, R. S., & Sallade, S. J. (2017). School-based instructional support. In J. K. Luiselli (Ed.), *Applied behavior analysis advanced guidebook* (pp. 167–195). London, United Kingdom: Academic Press/Elsevier.

Martens, B. K., Daly, E. J., & Ardoin, S. P. (2015). Applications of applied behavior analysis to school-based instructional intervention. In H. S. Roane, J. L. Ringdahl, & T. S. Falcomata (Eds.), *Clinical and organizational applications of applied behavior analysis* (pp. 125–150). New York, NY: Elsevier.

Martens, B. K., DiGennaro, F. D., Reed, D. D., Szczech, F. M., & Rosenthal, B. D. (2008). Contingency space analysis: An alternative method for identifying contingent relations from observational data. *Journal of Applied Behavior Analysis, 41*(1), 69–81. doi:10.1901/jaba.2008.41-69

Martens, B. K., Gertz, L. E., Werder, L. W., & Rymanowski, J. L. (2010). Agreement between descriptive and experimental analyses of behavior under naturalistic test conditions. *Journal of Behavioral Education, 19*(3), 205–221. doi:10.1007/s10864-010-9110-9

McCord, B. E., Thomson, R. J., & Iwata, B. A. (2001). Functional analysis and treatment of self-injury associated with transitions. *Journal of Applied Behavior Analysis, 34*, 195–210. doi:10.1901/jaba.2001.34-195

Myers, S. M., & Johnson, C. P. (2007). Council on Children with Disabilities. Management of children with autism. *Pediatrics, 120*, 1162–1182. doi:10.1542/peds.2007-2362

National Institute for Clinical Excellence. (2011). *Quick reference guide generalized anxiety disorder and panic disorder (with or without agoraphobia) in adults. Management in Primary, secondary and community care.* London, United Kingdom: Author.

Neidert, P. L., Iwata, B. A., & Dozier, C. L. (2005). Treatment of multiply controlled problem behavior with procedural variations of differential reinforcement. *Exceptionality, 13*(1), 45–53. doi:10.1207/s15327035ex1301_6

Newcomb, E. T., & Hagopian, L. P. (2018). Treatment of severe problem behavior in children with autism spectrum disorder and intellectual disabilities. *International Review of Psychiatry, 30,* 96–109. doi:10.1080/09540261.2018.1435513

O'Neill, R. E., Horner, R. H., Albin, R. W., Sprague, J. R., Storey, K., & Newton, J. S. (1997). *Functional assessment and program development for problem behavior: A practical handbook.* Pacific Grove, CA: Brooks/Cole.

Perone, M., & Hursh, D. E. (2013). Single-case experimental designs. In G. J. Madden, W. V. Dube, T. D. Hackenberg, G. P. Hanley, K. A. Lattal, G. J. Madden, . . . K. A. Lattal (Eds.), *APA handbook of behavior analysis* (Vol. 1, pp. 107–126). Washington, DC: American Psychological Association. doi:10.1037/13937-005

Phillips, C. L., Iannaccone, J. A., Rooker, G. W., & Hagopian, L. P. (2017). Noncontingent reinforcement for the treatment of severe problem behavior: An analysis of 27 consecutive applications. *Journal of Applied Behavior Analysis, 50*(2), 357–376. doi:10.1002/jaba.376

Roane, H. S., Fisher, W. W., & Carr, J. E. (2016). Applied behavior analysis as treatment for autism spectrum disorder. *The Journal of Pediatrics, 175,* 27–32. doi:10.1016/j.jpeds.2016.04.023

Roane, H. S., Fisher, W. W., Kelley, M. E., Mevers, J. L., & Bouxsein, K. J. (2013). Using modified visual inspection criteria to interpret functional-analysis outcomes. *Journal of Applied Behavior Analysis, 46,* 130–146. doi:10.1002/jaba.13

Scheithauer, M. C., Mevers, J. E. L., Call, N. A., & Shrewsbury, A. N. (2017). Using a test for multiply-maintained self-injury to develop function-based treatments. *Journal of Developmental and Physical Disabilities, 29*(3), 443–460. doi:10.1007/s10882-017-9535-3

Skinner, B. F. (1957). *Verbal behavior.* Englewood Cliffs, NJ: Prentice-Hall.

Smith, T. (2001). Discrete trail training in the treatment of autism. *Focus on Autism and Other Developmental Disabilities, 16,* 86–92. doi:10.1177/108835760101600204

Stokes, T. F., & Baer, D. M. (1977). An implicit technology of generalization. *Journal of Applied Behavior Analysis, 10,* 349–367. doi:10.1901/jaba.1977.10-349

Sturmey, P. (2014). *Maladaptive behavior.* In P. Sturmey, R. Didden, P. Sturmey, & R. Didden (Eds.), *Evidence-based practice and intellectual disabilities* (pp. 62–84). Hoboken, NJ: Wiley-Blackwell. doi:10.1002/9781118326077.ch3

Tomlinson, S. R. L., Gore, N., & McGill, P. (2018). Training individuals to implement applied behavior analytic procedures via telehealth: A systematic review of the literature. *Journal of Behavioral Education, 27,* 172-222. doi: 10.1007/s10864-018-9292-0

Van Houten, R., Axelrod, S., Bailey, J. S., Favell, J. E., Foxx, R. M., Iwata, B. A., & Lovaas, O. I. (1988). The right to effective behavioral treatment. *Journal of Applied Behavior Analysis, 21*(4), 381–384. doi:10.1901/jaba.1988.21-381

Vollmer, T. R., Hagopian, L. P., Bailey, J. S., Dorsey, M. F., Hanley, G. P., Lennox, D., . . . Spreat, S. (2011). The association for behavior analysis international position statement on restraint and seclusion. *The Behavior Analyst, 34*(1), 103–110.

Vollmer, T. R., Marcus, B. A., Ringdahl, J. E., & Roane, H. S. (1995). Progressing from brief assessments to extended experimental analyses in the evaluation of aberrant behavior. *Journal of Applied Behavior Analysis, 28*(4), 561–576. doi:10.1901/jaba.1995.28-561

Vollmer, T. R., Ringdahl, J. E., Roane, H. S., & Marcus, B. A. (1997). Negative side effects of noncontingent reinforcement. *Journal of Applied Behavior Analysis, 30,* 161–164. doi:10.1901/jaba.1997.30-161

Vollmer, T. R., Roane, H. S., & Rone, A. B. (2012). Experimental functional analysis. In J. L. Matson (Ed.), *Functional assessment for challenging behaviors* (pp. 125–141). New York, NY: Springer Science + Business Media. doi:10.1007/978-1-4614-3037-7_8

Wehmeyer, M. L., Brown, I., Percy, M., Shogren, K. A., & Fung, W. L. A. (Eds.). (2017). *A comprehensive guide to intellectual and developmental disabilities* (2nd ed.). Baltimore, MD: Paul H. Brookes Publishing Co.

CHAPTER 35 Oral Health

Erik Scheifele, Mitali Y. Patel, Anupama Rao Tate,
and H. Barry Waldman

Upon completion of this chapter, the reader will

- Understand the causes of dental caries (decay) and periodontal disease and become familiar with preventive strategies and treatment
- Become aware of the special oral considerations for children with disabilities
- Appreciate the oral health needs during the transition to adulthood
- Understand the value of a medical-dental home

An individual's oral health is an inseparable part of their overall health and well-being (American Academy of Pediatric Dentistry, 2017–2018a). Individuals with intellectual and developmental disabilities (IDD) are more likely to have unmet dental needs and face substantial challenges in accessing both preventive and routine dental services. Poor oral health can affect an individual's ability to eat, sleep, and function pain free, and it may contribute to systemic illness (Norwood & Slayton, 2013). As the oral health care for those children with developmental disabilities requires specialized knowledge, providers must have an increased awareness, attention, adaptation, and methods of accommodation beyond what are considered routine (American Academy of Pediatric Dentistry, 2017–2018b). Disparities that exist in providing oral health care services for this population have become more evident in recent years (Milano, 2017; Petrovic et al., 2016). Barriers to oral health care may be patient centered, provider centered, financial, or educational (Milano, 2017). Educators and clinicians frequently lack knowledge about the dental needs of children with developmental disabilities, and language, transportation, caregiver beliefs, and cultural beliefs can all affect access to care (American Academy of Pediatric Dentistry, 2017–2018b; see Chapter 41). This chapter focuses on oral health conditions and issues that may be associated with children with IDD.

CASE STUDY

Maggie is a 6-year-old girl with Down syndrome who is nonverbal. Her parents believe she is having oral pain but cannot look in her mouth. She has been eating less and rubbing the right side of her face for the past few days. She is now being examined by her pediatrician. Her parents have tried to prepare their daughter for this experience. However, Maggie gyrates her head and is distracted by bright lights and other stimuli in the pediatrician's office, and the clinician struggles to observe her face, lips, and tonsils. She concludes that everything appears to be "within normal limits." Unfortunately, all too often when it comes to the oral cavity, many pediatricians' examinations tend to be rather cursory, consisting of just a glance at the lips and throat. For most children this sort of examination would be routine and sufficient. Because of the specific risks for dental disease in Down syndrome, however, for Maggie oral-examination procedures warrant special care and the gathering of more information than might be apparent by routine observations. Understanding Maggie's cognitive and functional abilities will help guide communication and instruction at an appropriate level that she can understand. Practices to increase successful interactions include 1) scheduling appointments at the best time of day for the child, 2) minimizing office distractions, 3) providing clear and concise instructions at the appropriate cognitive level, and 4) using tell-show-do instructions to introduce procedures and equipment.

Thought Questions:

What interventions can decrease the development of dental caries? What are ways to enable children with developmental disabilities to receive dental services?

ORAL DEVELOPMENT

Eruption of Teeth

The human face begins growth during the fourth week of embryonic development, with tooth formation originating at approximately 6 weeks of age (Casamassimo, 2013). Although it is commonly said that the first primary tooth should erupt by 6 months of age, the age of eruption actually varies widely, with the first primary tooth coming anywhere between 4 and 17 months of age, while the full complement of primary teeth takes 2–3 years for complete eruption. The first permanent tooth typically emerges around 6 years of age, and most permanent teeth have erupted by 12–13 years of age. Third molars ("wisdom teeth") may erupt between 17–25 years of age.

When a permanent tooth erupts, a primary tooth is usually exfoliated. This does not occur with the first, second, and third permanent molars; however, because they do not have primary teeth counterparts. As noted previously, tooth eruption tables should be evaluated cautiously, especially in children with developmental disabilities, as each child's growth and development is unique. A 6-month discrepancy from the recommended eruption time is not considered unreasonable for any child (Dean, Avery, & McDonald, 2015). Symmetry in eruption and sequence of eruption can be more important than development coinciding with a conventional time schedule. The order in which teeth eruption occurs is more important to monitor rather than the age at which it occurs. What occurs on the right side should occur within a few months on the left, and what occurs in the mandible (lower jaw) should occur in the maxilla (upper jaw) within a reasonable period of time.

Dental Anomalies

Many genetic syndromes associated with developmental disabilities have characteristic developmental dental anomalies. These could include the presence of extra teeth, congenitally absent teeth, unusually shaped teeth, abnormalities in their mineralization, or delays in eruption. These abnormalities may contribute to **malocclusion** (improper interdigitation or alignment of teeth or jaws) and/or to an increased risk for dental caries and periodontal disease. **Anodontia** (the absence of all teeth) is rare, but **oligodontia** (the absence of one or several teeth) can be seen in children with a number of genetic syndromes including Hallermann-Streiff syndrome, chondroectodermal dysplasia, Williams syndrome, Crouzon syndrome, achondroplasia, incontinentia pigmenti, ectodermal dysplasia, and cleft lip and palate (see Appendix A). Disorders affecting development of teeth may also lead to enamel defects and abnormally shaped teeth or contribute to eruption difficulties, as seen in Cornelia de Lange syndrome (Dean et al., 2015). Dentition anomalies also occur in children with chromosomal disorders such as Down syndrome, in children with inborn errors of metabolism such as mucopolysaccharidoses, and in children with inherited disorders of bone formation such as osteogenesis imperfecta (Dean et al., 2015).

Environmental influences can also affect intrauterine tooth development. For example, nutritional deficiencies—especially of calcium; phosphorus; and vitamins A, C, and D—may result in generalized enamel **hypoplasia** (underdevelopment of enamel or enamel irregularities), resulting in defective mineralization of the teeth during their development (Dean et al., 2015).

Developmental tooth anomalies can also occur as a result of childhood illness or its treatment. For example, if a developing fetus or child between 4 months and 8 years of age is exposed to the antibiotic tetracycline, the primary or permanent teeth may have yellow, brown, or gray discoloration when they erupt. Traumatic injury to a tooth can cause a white or brown defect on a single tooth, whereas prematurity and very low birthweight as well as chronic diseases (e.g., liver failure or congenital heart disease) can cause hypoplasia or defects in multiple teeth (Dean et al., 2015). The extent and location of enamel hypoplasia can make teeth more susceptible to caries due to compromised tooth structure.

ORAL DISEASES

There are two basic types of oral disease: dental caries and periodontal disease. Both are usually initiated by specific bacteria and therefore can be considered infectious in nature. In general, they occur more commonly in children with disabilities than in their neurotypical peers.

Dental Caries

Dental caries, often called dental decay or cavities, commonly occurs in children and adolescents and is related to the presence of the bacteria *Streptococcus mutans* and *Lactobacillus acidophilus.* Tooth decay is a multifactorial process that involves the teeth themselves, bacteria, diet, saliva, biofilm, the immune system, biochemistry, and physiology. The "chain of decay" can be seen in Figure 35.1. Bacteria adhering to the teeth break down food, creating acid as a byproduct. The acid damages the integrity of the enamel, and cavitation begins. Tooth breakdown and possible abscess formation can occur when caries is left untreated over a period of time.

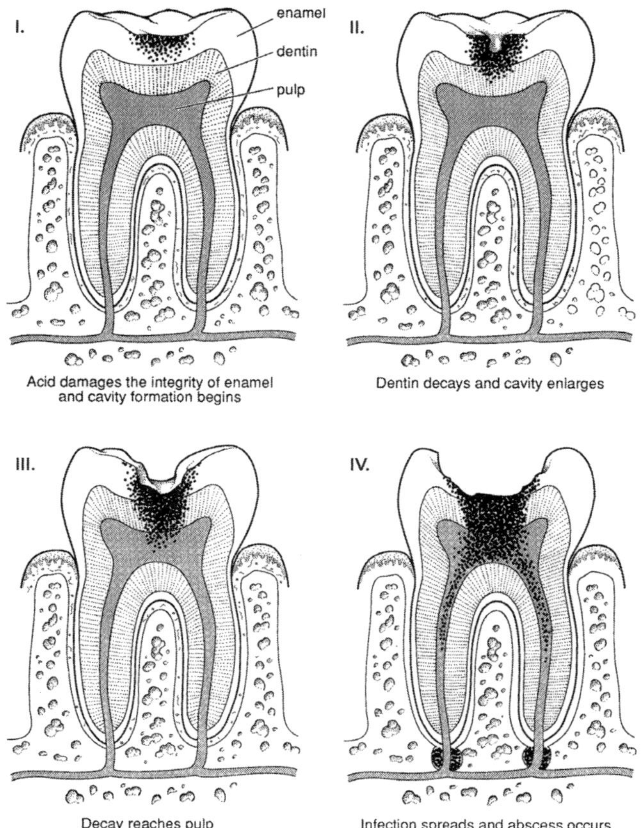

Figure 35.1. In the presence of adverse factors, the chain of decay is as follows: Acid formed from the action of bacteria on carbohydrates damages the enamel, leading to cavity formation. If untreated, the decay eventually affects the dentin and pulp layer of the tooth and may lead to abscess formation.

Bacteria adhere to the teeth in an organized mass called dental **plaque.** Plaque consists of bacteria, bacterial byproducts, **epithelial** cells (from the linings of the lips and mouth), and food particles (Casamassimo, 2013). When plaque becomes calcified, it is called calculus, or **tartar.** Plaque, as well as unremoved tartar, can cause dental decalcification and decay, inflammation, tenderness, and swelling of the gums. This is an early phase of periodontal disease and can lead to loosening of the teeth. The process of decay is characterized by demineralization of enamel and dentin. From 2011 to 2012, the prevalence of dental caries was found to be 37% in 2–8 year old children (Dye, Thornton-Evans, Li, & Iafolla, 2015); the percentage of children ages 5–19 years with untreated dental caries is about 13% (Centers for Disease Control and Prevention, National Center for Health Statistics, 2018).

Caries risk assessment is a tool that can help providers determine and understand the caries disease process in a child, especially risk and susceptibility. Diet, fluoride exposure, oral microflora (bacteria), and a susceptible host are factors, along with behavioral, social, and cultural influences (American Academy of Pediatric Dentistry, 2017–2018a). For young children who are receiving carbohydrate-enriched diets to treat growth and development problems or who require chronic liquid medications that contain sugar, cavities may be rampant. Evidence suggests that the infant formula's impact on the development of early childhood caries depends on the specific properties of the formula. Until more definitive information is available, children should not be allowed to fall asleep with a nursing bottle containing any liquid other than water. The same principle applies to children who are breastfed. Prolonged breast feeding and falling asleep with the nipple in the mouth can promote decay by acid demineralization. In addition, some cultures' practice of dipping pacifiers in sweetened solutions increases the risk of cavities.

In considering the role of bacteria in the tooth decay cycle, it is important to note that children acquire cavity-causing bacteria during the early phases of eruption of their first few teeth. They usually contract the bacteria from their primary caregiver. If that person has a high bacterial count or possesses bacteria that are more efficient in causing cavities, the child is at increased risk for future cavities. Parents can help reduce the risk of bacterial spread by themselves undergoing frequent dental cleanings and restoring carious teeth, thereby reducing their bacterial count.

Periodontal Diseases

Periodontal diseases involve damage to the supporting structures of teeth, such as the **gingiva** (gums) and bony sockets of the teeth. Like caries, gingivitis (the most common and reversible form of periodontal disease) is associated with plaque and specific bacterial organisms. The early signs of periodontal disease involve inflammation and bleeding of the gums; the true impact of these insidious processes can go unrecognized for years. Advanced stages of periodontitis are associated with loss of the bone that supports the tooth. Periodontal disease is caused by both local and systemic factors. Local factors include dental crowding of teeth, poor oral hygiene, dry mouth, and destructive dental habits. Systemic factors include side effects of medications, hormonal alterations, and immune deficiency states. Although the exact cause of this condition is unknown, the overgrowth is generally regarded as an exaggerated response to a local irritant. Overall, gingivitis can be found in up to half of children 4–5 years of age (Casamassimo, 2013). All too often, tooth extraction may be the inevitable solution in cases of advanced periodontal disease and extensive dental decay. Difficulties in patient behavior, the effects of the disability on teeth health, and limited financial resources are some of the variables that lead to the relatively high rate of removal of the teeth in individuals with disabilities.

MALOCCLUSION

Malocclusion can interfere with oral functions such as speech and chewing and can increase the risk of dental caries and periodontal disease. In addition, it can create problems with facial appearance and self-image. Although most malocclusions are minor and require attention only for cosmetic reasons, some may be more severe and debilitating. Individuals with IDD have a higher incidence of malocclusion, with 74% of individuals having a definitive malocclusion (Rada, Bakhsh, & Evans, 2015). In these children, correcting malocclusion by orthodontic therapy to position the teeth properly can also ease routine oral hygiene and thus decrease the risk of dental disease. New technologies such as digital impressions, clear aligners, and specialty equipment have enhanced orthodontic care; however, behavioral challenges and communication issues have kept many providers from attempting to provide orthodontic treatment even if in a limited form to children with IDD (Rada et al., 2015). Difficulties in the maintenance of adequate oral hygiene, the requirement for more dental chair time, and complications of managing associated medical conditions contribute to limited orthodontic care in this population (Blanck-Lubarsch et al., 2014). Other factors affecting access to orthodontic care include financial coverage, provider reimbursement, and finding qualified and willing providers.

ORAL TRAUMA

Uncontrolled head movements, which are characteristic of individuals with cerebral palsy (CP), are a common cause for dental injuries, as the teeth are bumped against hard objects located in the individual's vicinity. As such, movements are equally common in both genders and do not tend to decrease with age. The pattern of injuries to the teeth in individuals with CP differs from the known pattern in a healthy population. In addition, dental and facial trauma can affect both the primary and permanent dentition. Common causes of trauma include motor vehicle accidents, sports injuries, and falls. When the primary dentition is affected by trauma, the underlying permanent dentition can also be affected. A dental injury to the permanent dentition can necessitate numerous procedures and long-term follow-up. Children with special health care needs have a higher prevalence of traumatic dental injury (Al-Batayneh, Owais, Al-Saydali, & Waldman, 2017). Children with CP, for example, are more susceptible to dental trauma in the anterior teeth due to the associated malocclusion, whereas children with conditions associated with developmental disabilities that include difficulty with motor coordination are at risk for dental trauma related to uncontrolled head movements, abrupt movements, and diminished or absent protective reflexes. Patient cooperation and tolerance for dental procedures, the effect of the IDD on the dental and orofacial structures, and long-term care and prognosis can affect treatment of traumatic dental injuries. Lack of dental awareness among parents/caregivers, difficulties in finding a provider, and financial concerns have been cited as reasons for not seeking traumatic dental care (Al-Batayneh et al., 2017). Consideration of these factors may result in the removal of traumatized teeth rather than preservative treatment.

CONTRIBUTING FACTORS TO ORAL CONDITIONS OF INDIVIDUALS WITH DISABILITIES

Oral health is an inseparable part of general health and well-being. Oral diseases can have a direct and devastating impact on the health and quality of life of those with certain special health care needs. Patients with mental, developmental, or physical disabilities who do not have the ability to assume responsibility for or cooperate with preventive oral health practices are at increased risk for oral diseases throughout their lifetime (American Academy of Pediatric Dentistry, 2017–2018a). It is important to understand and explain the role of teeth in eating, speech, growth and development, and aesthetics to patients and their families. An individual child's limitations in being able to articulate the source of oral pain may make it more difficult to prevent, diagnose, and treat dental disease. The actual treatment may also differ because treatment must be adapted to the individual's physical and or cognitive impairment. Therefore, in managing oral health care in the child with a developmental disability, it is important to consider several factors, which are discussed in the following sections.

Regurgitation

Regurgitation (rumination) is often seen in individuals with moderate to profound intellectual disabilities. Swallowing of food, followed by regurgitation, may lead to indigestion, malnutrition, erosion of teeth, and possibly gastroesophageal reflux disease (see Chapter 29). Dental decay may be associated with regurgitation and pouching or pocketing (between cheeks/lips and gums) an accumulation of food.

Physical Limitations

Physical limitations, as seen in CP for example, may affect an individual's ability to carry out personal care, including tooth brushing, rinsing, and flossing. In addition, involuntary movement can make preventive treatment more difficult for caregivers and dental professionals.

Prescription Medication–Induced Decay

Antibiotics, pain, seizure control, and antihistamine oral medications often have a high sugar concentration to mask the taste, which can increase the risk for bacterial growth, acidic biofilm, and dental decay.

Altered Salivary Flow

Psychotropic medications result in decreased salivary flow. This can cause **xerostomia** (dry mouth), salivary gland infections, possible stone formation, and an increased rate of dental decay. In addition, reduced salivary flow is associated with increased burning/soreness of oral mucosal tissues and with difficulty in chewing, speaking, and swallowing. These all can adversely affect food selection and dietary compliance. As an example, children with cystic fibrosis often have thick ropy saliva, which can increase risk of dental decay (Dean et al., 2015).

Food Rewards

Fruit snacks and candy may meet the immediate need to calm and soothe a child or serve as positive reinforcement for behavior, but when combined with other factors, they may dramatically increase decay rates. Frequent intake of sugar-sweetened beverages is also a potential source of tooth decay.

Fractured and Avulsed Teeth

Damaged dentition, particularly of anterior teeth, is often associated with poor ambulatory skills, a history of trauma (accidental or nonaccidental as with seizures or physical abuse), **pica** (eating nonfood items), and self-injurious behavior. Pica may involve chewing on hard, nonedible objects that tend to fracture teeth. Broken and/or discolored teeth can indicate potential infection and should be documented and referred for treatment. Dental and medical professionals should evaluate and report suspected cases of physical abuse when managing oral trauma.

Soft-Tissue Complications

Seizure medication (especially phenytoin) can cause hypertrophy or overgrowth of the gingiva. This can lead to difficulties in delayed **exfoliation** (losing) of primary or eruption of primary and permanent teeth and to periodontal problems. Gingivitis and periodontal disease are more commonly seen in persons with Down syndrome, perhaps because of an immune deficiency (Dean et al., 2015).

Bruxism

Bruxism, or teeth grinding, usually occurs at night. It can be commonly seen in children with athetoid CP. Continued grinding erodes tooth structure and may cause sensitivity requiring dental restoration. Temporomandibular joint disorders can be a long-term pathology noted in the adult patient.

PREVENTION OF DENTAL CARIES AND PERIODONTAL DISEASE

Perhaps the most important component of preventing dental decay begins even before a child's birth. Eliminating or reducing the transmission of cavity-causing bacteria from the mother to the child, particularly during the susceptible period of bacterial colonization as the first teeth are erupting, is key to reducing caries risk. Identifying mothers with high levels of dental decay and educating them on the importance of their own oral health can help change their trajectory of the child's oral health (American Academy of Pediatric Dentistry, 2017–2018c). Once the child's teeth have erupted, the tools for preventive dentistry include establishment of a dental home, brushing, flossing, fluoride application and dental sealants when necessary for permanent teeth.

Brushing and Flossing

Brushing with a fluoridated dentifrice twice daily should be emphasized to help prevent decay and gingivitis. Children younger than 6 years generally have not developed the manual dexterity to effectively remove plaque from their teeth. Young children and those who have IDD that impacts oral hygiene should be encouraged to participate in their own oral hygiene; however, adults must take an active role and assume responsibility for cleaning the teeth and gums.

Power tooth brushes are as effective as manual tooth brushes and may be helpful for those children with physical disabilities. When brushing, a small smear of toothpaste with fluoride is advised for children less than 3 years old. Those who are 3–6 years old should use a small, pea-size amount of toothpaste with fluoride. If bubbles and foam from the toothpaste cause a problem for the child or guardian performing the tooth brushing, an alternative to toothpaste would be to use water. Positioning the child in a supine (reclining) position facilitates good vision, access, and head control and will help the adult performing the brushing. The number of successful positions is as unique as the disability with which the child presents (Casamassimo, 2013; Dean et al., 2015).

Flossing should be performed wherever teeth are in contact with each other, as the toothbrush cannot clean in between the teeth. When dexterity or motor coordination is a problem, floss-holding devices are available and can be used by parents and/or caregivers.

Fluoride

Fluoride makes enamel more resistant to decay and remineralizes incipient carious lesions, making them hard again. Whether present in the municipal water supply, taken as a daily supplement, found in toothpaste, contained in a mouth rinse, or professionally applied, fluoride treatment has been shown to significantly reduce the incidence of dental decay and is an integral part of a preventive program. Studies have demonstrated that fluoride in water can decrease the prevalence of tooth decay by up to 60% (Casamassimo, 2013). Most water filters are charcoal and do not remove fluoride; however, reverse-osmosis home filtration does remove fluoride from water. Bottled water must label its fluoride content if fluoride has been added but not if it is naturally occurring. Based on the child's caries risk, water fluoridation levels, and diet and abilities, specific systemic fluoride supplements may be recommended. It should be noted that excessive systemic fluoride can cause **fluorosis,** a condition in which permanent teeth are discolored or malformed.

Many different fluoride formulations are available, each with specific indicated uses. Some children may benefit from a prescribed fluoride rinse, varnish, paste, or gel that contains higher concentrations of fluoride. Often higher concentrated products, such as fluoride varnish, are applied to reverse the early stages of cavity formation. For children with a high caries risk, varnish applications are recommended every 3 months. Silver diamine fluoride, a professionally applied medicament, can be included as part of a caries management plan for patients for whom traditional restorative treatment is not immediately available.

Diet

In children for whom a diet rich in carbohydrates is medically necessary (e.g., to increase weight gain), the dentist should provide strategies to mitigate the caries risk by altering the frequency of preventive visits (American Academy of Pediatric Dentistry, 2017–2018a). More frequent and intensive oral hygiene regimens may be required. Similarly, children with neuromuscular disorders that result in decreased oral-motor abilities may need an extended period to clear food from their mouths. The increased contact time between teeth and food, especially puréed carbohydrates, places these children at greater risk to develop cavities. Even for neurotypical children, the consistency, frequency, and timing of snacks contribute to the potential for decay. Snacks that are sticky (not just caramels but also fruit snacks) or get stuck in the grooves of teeth (potato chips, or crackers) and those that are eaten frequently between meals have a high potential for causing dental decay.

Dental Sealants

Sealants consist of a plastic coating that is bonded to the biting surface of molars to prevent decay. A long-term reduction of caries in primary and permanent teeth due to the use of sealants has been well documented (Casamassimo, 2013). Many permanent molars have deep grooves that are difficult to keep clean and would benefit from application of sealants. Sealants are technique sensitive and are most effective after full eruption when the tooth can be isolated from saliva and kept dry during placement.

THE DENTAL HOME

Patients with special health care needs who have a dental home (American Academy of Pediatric Dentistry, 2017–2018d) are more likely to receive appropriate preventive and routine care. Ideally, a dental home should be established no later than 12 months of age. The dental home provides an opportunity to provide anticipatory guidance and implement individualized preventive oral health practices to reduce the child's risk of oral disease. As patients reach adulthood, their oral health care needs may extend beyond the scope of the pediatric dentist's training. At this point, patients should be transitioned to a dentist who is knowledgeable about adult oral health needs and able to manage the unique medical needs of the patient.

SPECIAL ISSUES IN DENTAL CARE FOR CHILDREN WITH SPECIFIC DEVELOPMENTAL DISABILITIES

The basic principles of pediatric dental care and oral health apply to all children; however, developmental disabilities may make every day of oral health care a challenge. There are specific dental care issues related to several common developmental disabilities, including Down syndrome, autism, CP, meningomyelocele (spina bifida), and patients who have a seizure disorder. These are discussed in the following sections.

Down Syndrome

In addition to having an intellectual disability, children with Down syndrome have oral findings that may include mouth breathing, open bite and protruding tongue, fissured lips and tongue, **angular cheilitis** (inflammation of the lips), malformed teeth, **microdontia** (very small teeth), midface **hypoplasia** (underdevelopment), small tooth roots, **supernumerary** (extra) teeth, missing teeth, and dental crowding (Dean et al., 2015; Ghaith, Al Halabi, & Alhashmi, 2017; see Chapter 15). Underdevelopment of the midface, hypotonia, dental anomalies, delayed eruption times, and **ectopic** (abnormally placed) eruption may contribute to the development of malocclusion. The incidence of dental caries is similar to or less than that of the general population (Diéguez-Pérez et al., 2016); however, a high incidence of rapid, destructive periodontal disease is commonly experienced (Dean et al., 2015). Children with Down syndrome also have a higher frequency of bruxism (Diéguez-Pérez et al., 2016). **Attrition** (tooth wear) and dental erosion have also been reported to be higher in these children (Dean et al., 2015). Congenital heart disease may also be present, which places these children at increased risk for bacterial endocarditis that may require antibiotic prophylaxis prior to dental procedures.

Autism Spectrum Disorder

The oral and dental conditions of children with autism spectrum disorder (ASD) are similar to other patients (Gandhi & Klein, 2014). In autism, oral health needs are often dictated by the behavior or level of cooperation by a child with sensory integration issues, how the disorder manifests itself in the child's abilities to care for his or her own dental needs, the risk to teeth of self-injurious behavior, and the impact of restricted food preferences on dental health (see Chapter 18). Dental issues related to pica, bruxism, pocketing, and side effects of medication are of particular concern in these children. Children with ASD tend to "pouch" food instead of swallowing it and may prefer soft and sweetened food, which leads to an increased susceptibility to caries (Dean et al., 2015). In addition, the sugar-based food reinforcers that may often be used in applied behavior analysis therapy increase the risk of dental caries. Limiting foods that generate caries should be a goal as well as using reinforcers that have lower carbohydrate content. Children with ASD have a tendency to adhere to strict routines and may require several visits to acclimate the child to the dental environment (Dean et al., 2015). Oral health management and treatment planning are improved with a detailed family-centered approach based on parental preferences and concerns, the patient's challenging behaviors, and related comorbidities (Gandhi & Klein, 2014). A multidisciplinary team approach can be devised involving behavioral, protective stabilization, and pharmacologic management techniques (Gandhi & Klein, 2014).

Cerebral Palsy

For children with CP, the more severe the neurological insult, the higher the risk of dental disease (Jan & Jan, 2016; see Chapter 21). CP can affect oral health significantly, resulting in changes to the oro-facial region's structure; it also can influence the development of parafunctional habits, including feeding problems, difficulty maintaining oral hygiene, and barriers to oral care access (Alhashmi, 2017). A higher prevalence of malocclusion is more likely and commonly includes protrusion of the maxillary anterior teeth and abnormal biting of food. Disharmony between oral muscles is considered a primary cause of the malocclusions (Dean et al., 2015). Low tone of the orofacial musculature and forward thrust of the tongue have been linked to malocclusions (Alhashmi, 2017). **Sialorrhea** (drooling) is commonly secondary to mouth opening and/or swallowing difficulties and can lead to aspiration, skin irritation, and articulation difficulties (Alhashmi, 2017). The increased production of saliva may be related to an irritation such as dental caries or a throat infection (Jan & Jan, 2016). Children with CP are predisposed to finger sucking and mouthing habits, and they frequently experience bruxism, particularly those with severe motor and cognitive deficits (Jan & Jan, 2016). The increased tendency for falling due to difficulty in ambulation, the reduced ability of reflexes to protect against a fall, and the frequent protrusion of the maxillary incisors may also increase these children's risk for dental trauma (Dean et al., 2015). Conflicting data have been reported regarding the incidence of dental caries in patients with CP compared with the general population (Diéguez-Pérez et al., 2016). In addition, for children with CP who are fed through gastrostomy tubes, despite receiving limited or no nutrition by mouth, they are still susceptible to reflux of stomach acid as well as plaque and calculus buildup, placing them at increased risk for aspiration problems and oral disease. Another common problem is gastroesophageal reflux disease (MedicineNet, 2016), which affects dental health and results in dental erosions (Jan & Jan, 2016). Children with CP are also at greater risk of 1) having developmental enamel defects (Jan & Jan, 2016), 2) having a greater frequency of periodontal disease and poor oral hygiene (Alhashmi, 2017; Dean et al., 2015), and 3) developing signs and symptoms of temporomandibular joint disorders (Jan & Jan, 2016). Providers should evaluate each child as an individual and not make assumptions about abilities. Providing dental care in the child's wheelchair or using positioning supports such as pillows or a bean bag in the dental chair will allow the patient to be more comfortable. If brushing teeth after eating is not possible, wiping soft food debris from the mouth using a moistened face cloth or gauze pad provides benefits. In older children, an adapted toothbrush with handle modifications, an electric toothbrush, and floss holders can help maintain good oral hygiene. Involuntary movements and severe bruxism will often make restorative dentistry more difficult; however, empathy and a calm, friendly, professional atmosphere are essential.

Meningomyelocele/Spina Bifida

Individuals with meningomyelocele are at a higher risk for dental caries due to poor oral hygiene, poor nutritional intake, frequent snacking, a carbohydrate-rich diet, and long-term use of sugar-containing medications (Dean et al., 2015; Garg, Utreja, Singh, & Angurana, 2013). The presence of a ventricular shunt in an individual with meningomyelocele and accompanying hydrocephalus may require antibiotic prophylaxis to prevent endocarditis prior to undergoing invasive dental procedures (Garg et al., 2013). As a result of orthopedic deformities, paralysis, genitourinary issues, and associated equipment, a patient might find it difficult to sit in a dental chair throughout an appointment. They may need to be treated in their wheelchair or padded appropriately in the dental chair (Garg & Revankar, 2012). Also, individuals with meningomyelocele have an increased risk of developing an allergic reaction to latex due to repeated exposures and cross-reactive food allergies to foods such as avocados, kiwi fruits, bananas, and chestnuts (Dean et al., 2015). Therefore, proper latex precautions should be taken during all dental appointments and latex-containing dental products should be avoided.

Seizure Disorders

As a result of poor oral hygiene, an increased risk of dental trauma, and side effects of anti-seizure medications, children with seizure disorders may exhibit more dental caries and periodontal issues than their typical piers. Seizure-relate injuries and aspiration risk warrant special dental considerations, such as using fixed prostheses over removable partial appliances (Joshi, Pendyala, Saraf, Choudhari, & Mopagar, 2013). Side effects from anti-seizure medications such as gingival overgrowth, **xerostomia** (dry mouth), and drug interactions may be an issue. Approximately one half of children receiving the anti-seizure medication phenytoin develop gingival overgrowth. Changing or discontinuing the medication may resolve the condition to some degree; however, surgical reduction may be needed (Casamassimo, 2013). Meticulous oral hygiene may prevent or significantly decrease the severity of the condition. Children who suffer from tonic-clonic seizures require special consideration for dental restorations and appliances to prevent the risk of inhalation and damage to appliance and tissues during a seizure (Mehmet, Senem, Sulun, & Humeyra, 2012).

THE CHALLENGE OF PROVIDING DENTAL SERVICES TO INDIVIDUALS WITH DISABILITIES

Children with developmental disabilities are considered to be at a greater risk of developing oral disease and are more likely to have unmet dental needs than typically developing children (Norwood & Slayton, 2013). Not having a medical home is the strongest predictor of having unmet dental needs (McKinney et al., 2014), and individuals with developmental disabilities compared with individuals without developmental disabilities are less likely to have had a preventive dental visit and more likely to receive a lower quality of dental care (Kancherla, Van Naarden, & Yeargin-Allsopp, 2013). In addition, compared with the general population, those with IDD are more likely to have poorer oral hygiene, increased decay, and increased periodontal disease (Binkley et al., 2014). The reasons for this increased risk include 1) cariogenic diets and a preference for carbohydrate-rich foods, 2) medications that are high in sugar (Craig, 2017) or have detrimental side effects such as xerostomia or gingival overgrowth, 3) the inability to clear foods from the oral cavity, 4) physical or cognitive limitations preventing proper oral hygiene, and 5) dependence on a caregiver for oral health care. An inadvertent additional contributing factor to dental disease may be policies promoting community-based living arrangements that increase independence of people with developmental disabilities but decrease direct caregiver support (Norwood & Slayton, 2013). Finally, children with disabilities are now much more likely to survive into adulthood, thus increasing the long-term risk of dental problems (Norwood & Slayton, 2013).

According to a 2012 study, a majority of individuals with developmental disabilities have a usual source of medical care (93%); however, fewer reported having a dentist, and almost two thirds (62%) reported no dental care in the previous year (Morgan et al., 2012). A report from the National Study of Children with Special Health Care Needs (Maternal and Child Health Bureau, 2013) highlighted the finding that dental care was one of the services commonly reported as needed but not received. In addition, despite the trend of the improving condition of children's teeth noted in the 2016 National Survey of Children's Health (Centers for Disease Control and Prevention, 2017), children with developmental disabilities still experience barriers to accessing oral health care. A survey of families of children with special health care needs reported that in the 12 months before the survey, 24% of children needed dental care other than preventive services and 9% were unable to obtain the needed care (Norwood & Slayton, 2013). The families of children with special health care needs also experience higher expenditures for health care when compared with families without special needs children (American Academy of Pediatric Dentistry, 2017–2018b). It should also be noted that the out-of-pocket expenses of dental services are far higher than the costs of other health services for individuals with (and without) special health care needs. For families with limited financial means, this may result in their seeking less dental care. A common cited barrier to oral health care is financing and reimbursement (American Academy of Pediatric Dentistry, 2017–2018a). For many families of children with developmental disabilities, a lack of or inadequate dental insurance is a challenge (Norwood & Slayton, 2013). Many individuals with developmental disabilities utilize federal and state insurance programs to pay for dental and medical services (American Academy of Pediatric Dentistry, 2017–2018d; Centers for Medicare and Medicaid Services, 2014). Even those individuals with private insurance may lack or have restrictions on coverage, especially as they reach adulthood (American Academy of Pediatric Dentistry, 2017–2018b). As reimbursement rates for Medicaid are often below the usual and customary fees, many dentists, including pediatric dentists, do not participate in Medicaid insurance (Norwood & Slayton, 2013), further reducing access to care. It should be noted, however, that medical providers in many states are reimbursed by Medicaid programs for preventive dental care, including fluoride varnish application, so this should be pursued (Norwood & Slayton, 2013). Nonfinancial barriers that inhibit access to oral health care include transportation issues, physical barriers to and within a dentist's office, family time missed from school and work, and difficulty locating providers who participate in the child's insurance plan, mainly Medicaid (American Academy of Pediatric Dentistry, 2017–2018b). Access to care also may be reduced by 1) referring a child too frequently to a dental specialist when an issue could be addressed by the primary provider, 2) not referring when appropriate, and 3) finding a qualified and accepting specialist (Morgan et al., 2012). Overcoming language barriers and developing effective communication are essential for understanding the child and family needs and desires as well as conveying the dentist's attitudes, capabilities, and plans. Additional challenges to access to care are psychosocial factors and cultural beliefs, including oral health beliefs, understanding of caregiver responsibilities, and past dental experiences of the caregiver (American Academy of Pediatric Dentistry, 2017–2018b). Another issue is the competency of the dental office to provide the services required. In the past, dental students received little to no educational experiences in caring for children and adults with disabilities, and despite a 2006 Commission on Dental Accreditation standard that requires dental schools to ensure that their graduates are competent in treating people with special needs, a 2012 study found that students are still inadequately prepared to meet the ongoing treatment needs of individuals with IDD. Complex medical conditions, the need for advanced management techniques such as sedation and general anesthesia, and a lack of facilities equipped to manage these procedures and trained personnel are challenges contributing to the access to care concerns. Pediatric dentists are trained to provide treatment for patients with developmental disabilities; however, there are approximately 5,000 practicing pediatric dentists in the United States as compared with 60,000 general pediatricians. This number of pediatric dentists is too low to meet the treatment needs of this population (Norwood & Slayton, 2013). Oral health education in medical and residency training is very limited. A survey of pediatricians reported that only 36% of practitioners indicated that they had received training in oral health (Norwood & Slayton, 2013). Specialized oral health training is necessary for dental and medical providers in addition to auxiliary personnel in order to be able to address the oral health needs of children with IDD. In addition, the patient-centered care concept of integration of oral health into primary care is thought to increase the effectiveness of care for patients with special health care needs.

Providing patient- and family-centered oral health care for children with disabilities requires an understanding of the disability and associated medical conditions, along with behavioral, social, cultural and financial factors. These concerns may contribute to modifications of a traditional treatment approach (see Box 35.1). There may be commonalities associated with a specific type of disability, but each child's situation is unique, mandating pretreatment planning and proper assessment in order to accommodate the child with special health care needs irrespective of the type of disability (Moore, 2016). A comprehensive assessment of the conditions and circumstances allows for the personalization of the oral health care services for the

BOX 35.1 EVIDENCE-BASED PRACTICE

Silver Diamine Fluoride

Silver diamine fluoride (SDF) application has reemerged as a useful option in caries management for patients with special health care needs. SDF is available in the United States in a 38% formula. It can be utilized to arrest and manage caries in teeth in addition to other measures as part of a caries management plan within a dental home. Due the difficulties and limitations of safely and effectively treating the pediatric population with special health care needs, restorative treatment of dental caries often requires sedation or general anesthesia. SDF can be utilized chairside in uncooperative patients who cannot undergo traditional dental restorations, thereby avoiding sedation or general anesthesia.

SDF involves the application of a liquid to affected teeth, which results in the arrest of caries. Temporary fillings that release fluoride are often used along with SDF. Close monitoring and follow-up with the patient is necessary, as well as possible reapplications. Patient education and reduction of other caries risk factors are also important.

Systemic side effects of SDF application are minimal. The main disadvantage of SDF is the aesthetic result of dark discoloration of teeth after application; however, this is acceptable to many parents as an alternative to sedation or general anesthesia in order to complete restorative treatment (Crystal et al., 2017).

child. This requires intraprofessional and interprofessional collaboration and communication among a team of professionals with the goal of patient- and family-centered care.

As medical management may involve associated medical specialists in addition to a primary care physician, comprehensive dental management may involve a variety of providers as well. Oral health care providers may include a dental hygienist, orthodontist, endodontist, oral surgeon, periodontist, and prosthodontist. Interprofessional relationships are influenced by personal values, expectations, perceptions, and attitudes, as well as intraprofessional and interprofessional conflict, differences in terminology, complexity of care, fear of diluting professional identity, and varying levels of preparation (Quinonez, Kranz, Long, & Rozier, 2014; see Box 35.2). Physicians and dental health care providers may also report different barriers to the coordination of care (Quinonez et al., 2014). An oral health coordinator may assist by reducing the caregiver's barriers to care by providing education and assistance in locating and accessing oral health resources as well as assisting with scheduling and keeping appointments (Binkley, Garrett, & Johnson, 2010). Other professionals such as social workers and child life specialists may assist with reducing barriers and participating in care. Nutritionists are also contributing professionals, as children with special health care needs have risk factors and comorbid conditions requiring nutritional interventions (Academy of Nutrition and Dietetics, 2015).

As children with disabilities present with a variety of dental, medical, and environmental issues, a collaborative team approach helps integrate oral health services into overall patient care. The Interprofessional Education Collaborative Expert Panel reported that professional teams working collaboratively communicate effectively, value each other's perspectives and contributions, understand and appreciate teamwork, and share an ethical code based on fair and high-quality care (Fried, 2013). This improved communication and coordination of care from intraprofessional and interprofessional collaborations suggest that an increase in the quality and safety of oral health care will follow.

Multidisciplinary risk assessment, oral health evaluation, preventive interventions, communication, and education are all considered necessary to provide and maintain access to a broad range of services for this population (Harnagea et al., 2017).

SUMMARY

- Oral health is an inseparable part of general health and well-being.
- Oral health care should include prevention and regular office visits through a dental home.

BOX 35.2 INTERDISCIPLINARY CARE

Oral Health Care Team Providers

Dental hygienist	Provides screening, teeth cleaning, examination, preventive oral health care, and patient education under supervision of a dentist or dental specialist
General dentist	Diagnoses and treats disease and pathology related to the teeth, gums, and oral cavity and provides oral health education and preventive oral health care
Pediatric dentist	Dental specialist that provides primary and comprehensive preventive and therapeutic oral health care for infants and children through adolescence, including those with special health care needs
Orthodontist	Dental specialist that provides diagnosis, prevention, and treatment of malocclusions and neuromuscular and skeletal irregularities of the orofacial region
Endodontist	Dental specialist that provides diagnosis, prevention, and treatment of diseases and pathology of the pulp and associated periradicular conditions
Oral and maxillofacial surgeon	Dental specialist that provides diagnosis and surgical treatment of diseases, injuries, and anomalies of the oral and maxillofacial region
Periodontist	Dental specialist that provides diagnosis, prevention, and treatment of diseases, injuries, and anomalies of the tissues surrounding and supporting the teeth, including the gingiva (gum tissue) and alveolar (tooth supporting) bone
Prosthodontist	Dental specialist that provides diagnosis and treatment of diseases, injuries, and anomalies associated with missing or deficient teeth and/or oral and maxillofacial tissues

Source: American Dental Association (2017).

- Oral health care may prevent and eliminate pain and discomfort.
- Oral health maximizes healthy nutrition, speech, and appearance.

ADDITIONAL RESOURCES

American Academy of Pediatric Dentistry: http://www.aapd.org

American Society of Dentistry for Children: http://www.ucsf.edu/ads/asdc.html

National Institute of Dental and Cranial Facial Research: https://www.nidcr.nih.gov/health-info/developmental-disabilities/more-info

Additional resources can be found online in Appendix D: Childhood Disabilities Resources, Services, and Organizations (see About the Online Companion Materials).

REFERENCES

Academy of Nutrition and Dietetics. (2015). Position of the Academy of Nutrition and Dietetics: Nutrition services for individuals with intellectual and developmental disabilities and special health care needs. *Journal of Academic Nutrition and Dietetics, 115*(4), 593–608.

Al-Batayneh, O. B., Owais, A. I., Al-Saydali, M. O., & Waldman, H. B. (2017). Traumatic dental injuries in children with special healthcare needs. *Dental Traumatology, 33,* 269–275.

Alhashmi, H. (2017). Medical and dental implications of cerebral palsy: Part 2: Oral and dental characteristics: A review. *JSM Dentistry, 5*(2), 108.

American Academy of Pediatric Dentistry. (2017–2018a). Best practices: Caries-risk assessment and management for infants, children, and adolescents. *Pediatric Dentistry, 39*(6), 197–204.

American Academy of Pediatric Dentistry. (2017–2018b). Best practices: Management of dental patients with special health care needs. *Pediatric Dentistry, 39*(6), 229–234.

American Academy of Pediatric Dentistry. (2017–2018c). Best practices: Perinatal and infant oral health care. *Pediatric Dentistry, 39*(6), 208–212.

American Academy of Pediatric Dentistry. (2017–2018d). Policy on dental home. *Pediatric Dentistry, 39*(6), 29–30.

American Dental Association. (2017). *Specialty definitions.* Retrieved from https://www.ada.org/en/ncrdscb/dental-specialties/specialty-definitions

Binkley, C. J., Garrett, B., & Johnson, K. W. (2010). Increasing dental care utilization by Medicaid-eligible children: A dental care coordinator intervention. *Journal of Public Health Dentistry, 70,* 76–84. doi:10.1111/j.1752-7325.2009.00146.x

Binkley, C. J., Johnson, K. W., Abdi, M., Thompson, K., Shamblen, S. R., Young, L., & Zaksek, B. (2014). Improving the oral health of residents with intellectual and developmental disabilities: An oral health strategy and pilot study. *Evaluation and Program Planning, 47,* 54–63. doi:10.1016/j.evalprogplan.2014.07.003

Blanck-Lubarsch, M., Hohoff, A., Wiechmann, D., & Stamm, T. (2014). Orthodontic treatment of children/adolescents with special health care needs: An analysis of treatment length and clinical outcome. *BMC Oral Health, 14,* 67. doi:10.1186/1472-6831-14-67

Casamassimo, P. S. (2013). *Pediatric dentistry: Infancy through adolescence.* St. Louis, MO: Elsevier.

Centers for Disease Control and Prevention. (2017). *Oral and dental health.* Retrieved from https://www.cdc.gov/nchs/fastats/dental.htm

Centers for Disease Control and Prevention, National Center for Health Statistics. (2018). *National Health and Nutrition Examination Survey Data.* Retrieved from https://www.cdc.gov/nchs/data/databriefs/db307.pdf

Centers for Medicare and Medicaid Services. (2014). *EPSDT—A guide for states: Coverage in the Medicaid benefit for children and adolescents.* Retrieved from https://www.medicaid.gov/medicaid/benefits/downloads/epsdt_coverage_guide.pdf

Craig, M. (2017). *Dental care utilization for children with special health care needs in Washington State's access to baby and child dentistry program* (Master's thesis). University of Washington, Seattle. Retrieved from https://digital.lib.washington.edu/researchworks/bitstream/handle/1773/40015/Craig_washington_0250O_17082.pdf?sequence=1

Crystal, Y. O., Marghalani, A. A., Ureles, S. D., Wright, J. T., Sulyanto, R., Divaris, K., . . . Graham, L.(2017). Use of silver diamine fluoride for dental caries management in children and adolescents, including those with special health care needs. *Pediatric Dentistry, 39*(5), E135–E145.

Dean, J. A., Avery, D. R., & McDonald, R. E. (2015). *Dentistry for the child and adolescent.* St. Louis, MO: Elsevier.

Diéguez-Pérez, M., de Nova-Garcia, M-J., Mourelle-Martinez, M. R., & Bartolome`-Villar, B.(2016). Oral health in children with physical (cerebral palsy) and intellectual (Down syndrome) disabilities: Systematic review I. *Journal of Clinical and Experimental Dentistry, 8*(3), e337–e343. doi:10.4317/jced.52922

Dye, B. A., Thornton-Evans, G., Li, X., & Iafolla, T. J. (2015). *Dental caries and sealant prevalence in children and adolescents in the United States, 2011–2012.* National Center for Health Statistics. Retrieved from https://www.cdc.gov/nchs/data/databriefs/db191.pdf

Fried, J. (2013). Interprofessional collaboration: If not now, when? *Journal of Dental Hygiene, 87*(Special Commemorative Issue), 41–43.

Gandhi, R. P., & Klein, U. (2014). Autism spectrum disorders: An update on oral health management. *Journal Evidence Based Dental Practice, 14*(Suppl), 115–126.

Garg, A., & Revankar, A. V. (2012). Spina bifida and dental care: Key clinical issues. *Journal of the California Dental Association, 40*(11), 861–869.

Garg, A., Utreja, A., Singh, S. P., & Angurana, S. K. (2013). Neural tube defects and their significance in clinical dentistry: A mini review. *Journal of Investigative and Clinical Dentistry, 4,* 3–8.

Ghaith, B., Al Halabi, M., & Alhashmi, H. (2017). Dental implications of Down syndrome (DS): Review of the oral and dental characteristics. *JSM Dentistry, 5*(2), 1087. Retrieved from https://www.jscimedcentral.com/Dentistry/dentistry-5-1087.pdf

Harnagea, H., Couturier, Y., Shrivastava, R., Girard, F., Lamothe, L., Bedos, C. P., & Emami, E. (2017). Barriers and facilitators in the integration of oral health into primary care: A scoping review. *BMJ Open, 7,* e016078. doi:10.1136/bmjopen-2017-016078

Jan, B. M., & Jan, M. M. (2016). Dental health of children with cerebral palsy. *Neurosciences, 21*(4), 314–318. doi:10.17712/nsj.2016.4.20150729

Joshi, S. R., Pendyala, G. S., Saraf, V., Choudhari, S., & Mopagar, V. (2013). A comprehensive oral and dental management of an epileptic and intellectually deteriorated adolescent. *Dental Research Journal, 10*(4), 562–567.

Kancherla, V., Van Naarden, B. K., & Yeargin-Allsopp, M. (2013). Dental care among young adults with intellectual disability. *Research in Developmental Disabilities, 34*(5), 1630–1641.

Maternal and Child Health Bureau. (2013). *NS-CSHCN chartbook 2009-2010.* Retrieved from https://mchb.hrsa.gov/cshcn0910/

McKinney, C. M., Nelson, T., Scott, J. M., Heaton, L. J., Vaughn, M. G., & Lewis, C. W. (2014). Predictors of unmet dental need in children with autism spectrum disorder: Results from a national sample. *Academic Pediatrics, 14*(6), 624–631.

MedicineNet. (2016). *GERD (acid reflux, heartburn).* Retrieved from https://www.medicinenet.com/gastroesophageal_reflux_disease_gerd/article.htm

Mehmet, Y., Senem, Ö., Sülün, T., & Hümeyra, K. (2012). Management of epileptic patients in dentistry. *Surgical Science, 3*(1), 47–52.

Milano, M. (2017). Oral healthcare for persons with intellectual or developmental disabilities: Why is there a disparity? *Compendium Continuing Education Dentistry, 38*(10), e5–e8.

Moore, T. A. (2016). Dental care for patients with special needs. *Decisions in Dentistry, 2*(9), 50–53.

Morgan, J. P., Minihan, P. M., Stark, P. C., Finkleman, M. D., Yantsides, C. E., Park, A., . . . Must, A. (2012). The oral health status of 4,732 adults with intellectual and developmental disabilities. *Journal of the American Dental Association, 143*(8), 838–856.

Norwood, K. W. & Slayton, R. L. (2013). Oral health care for children with developmental disabilities. *Pediatrics, 131,* 614–619.

Petrovic, B. B., Peric, T. O., Markovic, D. L. J., Bajkin, B. B., Petrovic, D., Blagojevic, D. B., . . . Vujkov, S. (2016). Unmet oral health needs among persons with intellectual disability. *Research in Developmental Disabilities, 59,* 370–377.

Quinonez, R. B., Kranz, A. M., Long, M., & Rozier, R. G. (2014). Care coordination among pediatricians and dentists: A cross-sectional study of opinions of North Carolina dentists. *BMC Oral Health, 14,* 33. doi:10.1186/1472-6831-14-33

Rada, R., Bakhsh, H. H., & Evans, C. (2015). Orthodontic care for the behavior-challenged special needs patient. *Special Care in Dentistry, 35,* 138–142.

U.S. Department of Health and Human Services. (2017). *Medical expenditure panel survey.* Retrieved from https://MEPS.AHRQ.GOV/MEPSWEB/

CHAPTER 36 Assistive Technology

Larry W. Desch

Upon completion of this chapter, the reader will

- Know the definitions of the terms *assistive technology* and *medical assistive technology*
- Understand the types of conditions that frequently create a need for assistive technology
- Be aware of the major types of both habilitative/rehabilitative and medical assistive technology and know examples of each
- Be able to describe the key legislative and historical issues involving assistive technology
- Know the definition of durable medical equipment (DME) and the limitations that are often put on the purchase of DME by insurance companies and other third parties
- Understand the implications of assistive technology on the socioemotional functioning of children with disabilities and their families
- Understand the basics of proper assessment and training for users of assistive technology
- Know the essentials of funding for assistive technology and the laws dealing with this funding

More than a generation has passed since the technology that we now use on a daily basis, such as personal computers and cell phones, had its origins. Although much has been accomplished, for both able-bodied people and those with disabilities, several problems, such as equitable access and cost, still remain.

The goal of this chapter is to provide necessary information about the major categories of currently available habilitative/rehabilitative and medical assistive technology and the process for evaluating their use and effectiveness. This chapter focuses on "mid-tech" and "high-tech" devices, as many "no-tech" (e.g., hands-on physical therapy) and "low-tech" (e.g., leg braces) devices and methods are discussed in other chapters of this book. Also, the chapter does not address complementary or alternative therapies (see Chapter 39), such as devices using unproven or disproven methodologies like colored lenses for the treatment of dyslexia (American Academy of Pediatrics: Section on Ophthalmology et al., 2009). The devices discussed in this chapter have at least some basic empirical or scientific evidence to document their effectiveness.

Many children with disabilities are able to have more independent function through the use of assistive, adaptive, or augmentative devices. Although definitions for these types of devices vary, there seems to be some consensus emerging. Assistive devices are those that help alleviate the impact of a disability, thus reducing the functional limitations (e.g., tape-recorded lessons for students with a specific reading disability). Adaptive technology substitutes or makes up for the loss of function brought on by a disability (e.g., a sophisticated robotic feeding device provides independence for people with severe spastic quadriplegia). Augmentative devices increase an area of functioning that is deficient, sometimes severely, but for which there are some residual abilities (e.g., a microchip-powered voice output augmentative communication device for a person with severe dysarthria). The term **augmentative devices** currently refers mainly to devices used to improve communication. In this chapter, the term **assistive** is used to encompass all of these terms. This chapter uses this general term for medical devices as well. The term **medical assistive technology** refers to that subset of assistive technology that is used for primarily medical or life-sustaining reasons (e.g., ventilators or feeding pumps). These devices also improve functioning but perhaps in more basic ways (often that are life sustaining).

For many years, assistive technology (sometimes called "AT") has often been thought of as referring only to devices containing microcomputers or other electronics (Desch, 1986). Although such complicated devices may be the only answer for a particular disability-related problem, they represent the higher end of the spectrum of assistive technology that includes low-tech, mid-tech, and high-tech (and everything in between; Desch, 2008). Many people, even professionals working with children with disabilities, do not realize that they may themselves be using assistive technology on a daily basis. For example, a foam or rubber cushion placed over a pencil or pen to help with one's grip and prevent writer's cramp is a low-tech assistive device. However, the use of assistive technology is usually reserved for people with considerably more loss of function due to disability.

Table 36.1 provides examples of assistive devices. Many items on the table that are frequently used are no-tech (e.g., hands-on physical therapy) or low-tech assistive technology—that is, those using low-cost materials and not requiring batteries or other electric sources to

Table 36.1. Types of technology and examples of available devices

Area of disability	Low-tech	Mid-tech	High-tech
Physical	Swivel spoon (and other feeding aids) Wheelchair ramps Adapted playgrounds Most orthotics Grips for pencils	Reciprocating gait orthoses Lightweight wheelchairs Adapted toys	Electronically controlled wheelchairs Environmental control units Robotic therapy devices Functional electric stimulation Voice-input and eye-gaze–input devices
Communication	Simple picture/word boards Eye-gaze picture boards Visual schedule/planner	On/off light for yes/no responses One to multiple digital message recorders Scanning light board	Specialized software on iPad Dedicated speech-generating devices (e.g., Dynavox, Maestro)
Sensory	Magnifying lenses Large-print books Audiobooks	Alerting systems (to movement/ sound) Braille typewriters FM transmitting	Digital hearing aids Cochlear implants Kurzweil 1000 voice-output scanning
Learning	Color-coded notebooks Post-it Notes Flash cards Visual schedule/planner	Talking calculators Electronic spelling/dictionary Tape recorders Audiobooks	Problem-solving software Hypertext learning programs Software for cognitive/attention rehabilitation
Medical assistance	Nasogastric tubes Bladder catheters	Oxygen systems Gastrostomy tubes Indwelling IV tubes	Home continuous positive airway pressure Home ventilators Oxygen monitors Apnea monitors Dialysis machines

operate. Examples include wheelchair ramps, gastrostomy feeding tubes, and printed picture communication boards. Mid-tech devices generally require battery/electrical power or are more complex in their use, such as teletypewriter devices for those who are deaf, home infusion pumps, suction machines, and sophisticated manual wheelchairs. Finally, high-tech devices are those that are complicated and often expensive to own and maintain. Examples include microcomputer-enabled voice output devices, home ventilators, cochlear implants, and electronic wheelchairs.

Assistive devices, across the spectrum, are acquired in one of three ways: 1) direct purchase from a commercial supplier; 2) development of a custom-made device (these can be simple, handmade devices or complex, one-of-a-kind devices made by an engineer or technician for use by one person); or 3) modification of an existing device such as a desktop computer, laptop computer, or telephone (these modifications can also be commercially available items). Some of these modified devices are constructed at rehabilitation centers at a high cost. However, the availability of microprocessing technology has increased such that the purchase of commercial devices or commercial modifications to devices is becoming the most common way to acquire even the most complex, high-tech assistive devices. Where assistive devices can be obtained also varies, from public schools and therapy providers to large university or private rehabilitation centers. Most assistive devices, excluding the medical assistive devices, can be obtained without prescriptions from physicians, although doing so usually precludes their purchase using insurance or other third-party, medical-related funding.

CASE STUDY

Laura is an 8-year-old girl who, according to her mother, "has come a long way" but had a "rough beginning" to her life. Laura and her twin were conceived by in vitro fertilization, were born 6 weeks' premature, and had severe hyperbilirubinemia (jaundice) due to blood group incompatibility. She spent more than a month in the neonatal intensive care unit. Laura had occasional episodes of apnea and bradycardia (periodic breathing arrests accompanied by low heart rate) and was sent home on a cardiorespiratory monitor. At 6 months of age, she had severe **gastroesophageal reflux disease (GERD**; stomach acid moves into the esophagus, causing discomfort) that led to placement of a gastrojejunal tube. This required Laura's parents to learn how to use a feeding pump that would give her formula over several hours. After 2 months, her feedings were able to be changed to oral, and by 1 year, she seemed to be doing fairly well with feeding and in most other areas. At 16 months, however, she often would rock back and forth "for no reason" and was delayed in language. Soon thereafter, Laura was referred to early intervention, had an extensive evaluation by a team of developmental specialists, and was found to have an autism spectrum disorder (ASD). Despite intensive speech/language therapy for 9 months, Laura did not develop much speech and seemed to be getting increasingly frustrated because of her communication difficulties. Laura's speech therapist recommended initially a simple picture-based card system and, later, a computerized speech-generating device. After nearly a year of negotiating with their insurance company and with Laura's school, the parents were finally able to purchase the device. Laura gradually became less irritable and after 6 months of using the speech-generating device, she was beginning to say some words herself. By 6 years of age, she was talking in complete sentences and, as she no longer needed the device, it was donated to the local children's hospital.

Thought Questions:

What are the factors that increase the chances that a particular technology will be used effectively? What are the emotional and financial stresses related to using assistive technology, including those from medical assistive technology?

TECHNOLOGY FOR MEDICAL ASSISTANCE

The Office of Technology Assessment defines a child who receives medical technology assistance as one "who requires a mechanical device and substantial daily skilled nursing care to avert death or further disability" (1987, p. 3). These medical devices replace or augment a vital body function and include respiratory technology assistance (e.g., nasal cannulae for oxygen supplementation, mechanical ventilators, positive airway pressure devices, and artificial airways such as tracheotomy tubes), surveillance devices (e.g., cardiorespiratory monitors and pulse oximeters), nutritive assistive devices (e.g., nasogastric or gastrostomy feeding tubes), equipment for intravenous (IV) therapy (e.g., parenteral nutrition and medication infusion), devices to augment or protect kidney function (e.g., dialysis and urethral catheterization), and ostomies (e.g., gastrostomy and colostomy).

The use of medical technology assistance by children is uncommon—occurring in only about 1 in 1,000 children—and most of these uses are temporary (e.g., following premature birth, injury, or surgery). In a survey of children in Massachusetts who were dependent on technology, more than half (57%) had neurological involvement and 13% had multisystem involvement (Palfrey et al., 1994). The incidence does appear to be increasing, especially in children younger than 3 years of age, primarily as a result of improved survival of very low birth weight infants. Many of these survivors have a high risk for disabilities and chronic illnesses that need complex medical care (Elias & Murphy, 2012; Wise, 2007). More recent statistics on how many children are dependent on technology are difficult to obtain, but estimates in one U.S. state (Utah) has indicated that children on home ventilators represent about 1 in 10,000 children and that this number is likely increasing (Gowans, Keenan, & Bratton, 2007). The types of medical assistive devices that are required in a number of these chronic illnesses are described next, and the principles of device use with children are described in Table 36.2.

Respiratory Support

Infants and children who require respiratory support most often fall into one of two categories: 1) those with problems with their lungs and/or hearts and 2) those with problems with neurological control of breathing and/or weakness of the muscles used to control breathing. As an example of the first category, severe damage to the lungs related to prematurity, called bronchopulmonary dysplasia, can lead to the prolonged need for supplemental oxygen (Jobe & Steinhorn, 2017). Another example is the child with spastic quadriplegic cerebral palsy who may develop a severe scoliosis (curvature of the spine), leading to rib cage distortion and stiffness (see Chapter 21). This chest wall abnormality can cause a decrease in respiratory muscle power and lung function necessitating supplemental oxygen. An example of the second category is neuromuscular disorders, including Duchenne muscular dystrophy (see Chapters 9 and 32) and spinal muscular atrophy (Farrar et al., 2017; Romitti et al., 2015; see Chapter 9).

Children who have chronic respiratory failure require medical technology assistance to maintain normal oxygen levels in the blood, prevent additional lung injury from recurrent infections, and promote optimal growth and development. These goals usually can be accomplished via a combination of oxygen supplementation, noninvasive ventilation using continuous positive airway pressure (CPAP) or bilevel positive airway pressure (BiPAP), chest physiotherapy (CPT), suctioning, and medications (e.g., bronchodilators). When these treatments are ineffective or insufficient, however, mechanical ventilation and tracheostomy tube placement are considered. Equipment that is used to monitor the child's cardiorespiratory status may also be required (e.g., heart rate and blood oxygen monitors). Oxygen is often the single most effective agent in treating the infant or child with chronic lung disease, and supplemental oxygen may be required for months or even years. Oxygen can be administered by nasal cannulae (plastic prongs placed in the nose and connected to a tube that delivers an oxygen/air mixture), face mask, oxygen tent or hood, or an artificial airway (i.e., tracheostomy).

For the child with milder respiratory impairment or obstructive sleep apnea, nasal CPAP may be employed (Amin, Al-Saleh, & Narang, 2016). CPAP can be applied to the child's natural airway via a tight-fitting mask or nasal pillows/cannulae. For more

Table 36.2. Principles for assistive technology device use with children

1. Families are involved in selecting, developing, and implementing assistive technology (AT) devices for children.
2. AT devices should be an integral part of the child's daily routines across the home, child care, school, and other settings.
3. AT devices should be easy to use and adaptable to all of the environments of the child and family.
4. Families are always able to obtain needed AT from providers or a lending library and receive directions for using the device or an activity.
5. AT assessment and interventions should be done using an interdisciplinary team-based manner, with the family and child (if possible) being integral members of the decision-making team.
6. AT should be a consideration for every child during the development of the child's individualized family service plan (in early intervention) or with an individualized education program in school.
7. AT should always be seen as a tool to foster increased learning, functioning, and independence.
8. Providing appropriate AT should be done as early as possible in the child's life. Artificial constraints such as age should rarely be considered.
9. Families and professionals should have access to ongoing opportunities for training to increase knowledge and understanding of AT use and benefits.
10. Families and professionals should have adequate knowledge about funding sources for AT devices and for the training needed for these devices.

Source: Sadao and Robinson (2010).

severe conditions, CPAP is generally given chronically through a tracheostomy tube (Tibballs et al., 2010). If a child is on a mechanical ventilator, positive pressure can be administered between mechanical breaths, in which case the technique is referred to as positive end expiratory pressure (PEEP).

A recent advancement for children with chronic respiratory failure is the use of different types of noninvasive ventilation therapies (Bedi et al., 2018; Castro-Codesai et al., 2018). These often use a more sophisticated method of using CPAP or BiPAP, such as Auto-CPAP, which triggers the delivery of oxygen in response to taking a breath. The main difference between CPAP and BiPAP is that with CPAP a constant positive pressure is present and the patient is breathing spontaneously, whereas with BiPAP a ventilator supplies a pre-set positive pressure during inspiration and there is a lesser pressure delivered during expiration (PEEP). By using BiPAP, the lungs are kept open better, which helps improve gas exchange (e.g., O_2 and CO_2; Morley, 2016). For both CPAP and BiPAP, tight total face masks or tight nasal masks are usually needed because of the pressures that need to be present. The main purpose of using noninvasive ventilation (NIV) is to provide most of the benefits of invasive ventilation (e.g., oxygen through a tracheostomy) without the higher risk of infection and lung injury that can occur with these invasive measures.

Children with respiratory or oral-motor problems also may produce excessive secretions (e.g., saliva) and/or be unable to cough effectively. CPT and suctioning, which can be taught to all caregivers, help clear pulmonary secretions (Krause & Hoehn, 2000). CPT involves the repetitive manual percussion of the chest wall. For infants, this often involves using a handheld vibrator. Secretions are loosened and can then be cleared by coughing or, in children with tracheostomies, by suctioning. Typically, supplemental oxygen is administered before and after suctioning to prevent hypoxia from occurring during the procedure (Flenady & Gray, 2000). Suctioning and CPT are done as often as necessary, usually several times a day. The newest modalities for CPT are the use of automatic devices, such as the high-frequency chest compression vest or devices that cause vibrations of the lungs during breathing (Lee, Button, & Tannenbaum, 2017). A number of recent studies attest to these devices' effectiveness, especially in people who have cystic fibrosis (Dosman & Jones, 2005; Morrison & Milroy, 2017).

A tracheostomy involves the insertion of a plastic tube through a surgically created incision in the cartilage of the trachea, just below the Adam's apple. It is secured around the neck with foam-padded strings. This open airway can then be attached to a mechanical ventilator or to a CPAP device with tubing that provides humidified air or an air/oxygen mixture. If ventilatory support or oxygen is not needed, then a humidifying device (an "artificial nose") is attached to the tracheostomy tube. A speaking valve (e.g., Passy-Muir valve) often is used with the tracheostomy tube to allow more air to go through the vocal cords to allow phonation (Buswell, Powell, & Powell, 2017). The tracheostomy tube also allows the caregiver to have direct access to the airway, permitting suctioning of secretions or removal of other blockages. Children who have tracheostomies may spend part or all of their day connected to a mechanical ventilator that augments or replaces their own respiratory efforts (Edwards et al., 2016; Edwards, O'Toole, & Wallis, 2004).

Monitoring and Surveillance Devices

Children with disorders that affect the heart or lungs are likely to require the use of monitoring or surveillance devices. Although these instruments provide no direct therapeutic benefit, they give early warning of problems and thereby improve care indirectly. The two most common types of electronic surveillance devices are pulse oximeters and cardiorespiratory monitors. They can be used individually or in combination in the hospital and at home.

To avoid giving too much or too little oxygen, **oxygen saturation** (the oxygen-carrying capacity of red blood cells) can be monitored using a device called a pulse oximeter. The pulse oximeter measures oxygen saturation in the arterial blood using a probe that is attached with special tape to one of the child's fingers or toes (Nadkarni, Shah, & Deshmukh, 2000). An alarm can be set to sound below a certain oxygen saturation level. This most commonly occurs when there is low oxygen delivery (e.g., kinked tubing or a low oxygen level in the oxygen tank) or a change in the child's condition (e.g., an increased need for supplemental oxygen because of a respiratory infection). Because this device reflects how well oxygen is being delivered to vital organs, it is an important monitor. Unfortunately, it is quite susceptible to false alarms resulting from probe displacement, movement of the extremity, or electrical interference.

A **cardiorespiratory monitor** has electrodes that are pasted to the child's chest to record heart and respiratory rate (Silvestri et al., 2005). An alarm is part of the system and is set off by rates that are either too high or too low. If the alarm sounds, the caregiver should examine the child's respiratory, cardiovascular, and neurological status. Like the oximeter, the cardiorespiratory monitor can produce false alarms, most commonly resulting from the inadvertent detachment of the chest leads. In the very rare event that the alarm sounds because of a cardiorespiratory arrest (i.e., slowing or stopping of breathing and/or heart rate), cardiopulmonary resuscitation and possibly the use of an automated external defibrillator must be instituted immediately.

Nutritional (Gastrointestinal) Fluid Assistance

Children with cerebral palsy and other chronic neurological conditions are often limited in their ability to take in nutrition by mouth. Despite often needing an increased food intake as a result of their motor-control problems (e.g., dyskinesia), these children may be unable to ingest even a normal intake because of oral-motor impairments, GERD, or food refusal. In these instances, nutritional assistance devices may prove helpful. Tube feedings can be provided in a number of ways. The tube can be temporarily inserted into one nostril and passed into the stomach (**nasogastric tube**) or into the second part of the intestine (**nasojejeunal tube**). When long-term feedings are required, a permanent tube can be placed directly through the skin and into the stomach (**gastrostomy tube,** or **G tube**) or intestine (**jejunostomy tube,** or **J tube**). A G-J tube combines a G tube and a J tube. The J-tube portion travels through the stomach, the duodenum (the first part of the intestine), and into the jejunum to prevent reflux of nutrients. If the child has GERD, the intervention of choice may be the combination of a surgical antireflux procedure (e.g., fundoplication by open or laparoscopic route; see Chapters 21 and 29) and insertion of a G tube or G-J tube. Once the feeding tube is inserted, nutrition can be provided by using a commercially available tube-feeding formula or foods from the family's meals that have been puréed along with fluids.

These types of tubes, especially G tubes, can be inserted using an endoscope and directly through the skin of the abdomen (percutaneous G tube) or by laparoscopic techniques or direct open surgical techniques. Recently, there have been reviews about which technique is the best surgical method of placing these tubes, especially G tubes. The growing consensus has been that, at the present, given no contraindications to a specific technique, the method that the surgeon is most comfortable with is the one that should be used (Baker, Beres, & Baird, 2015).

Intravenous Fluid Assistive Devices

Long-term IV therapy (months to years), generally given through a central venous line, is most often used to provide nutrition and/or to administer medication (Hodgson et al., 2016; McInally, 2005). Total parenteral nutrition involves the provision of a high-calorie, high-protein solution directly into the bloodstream by IV administration. Prolonged IV access may also be needed to provide antibiotics (e.g., when a child has **osteomyelitis,** a deep bone infection) or for cancer chemotherapy. In these situations, a catheter (often called a central line, Hickman line, or Broviac line) may be tunneled into a deep vein under radiological guidance and advanced to a more central position near the heart. This type of catheter averts the need for repeated placement of regular IVs. In addition, a central venous catheter allows the child to receive medication and/or nutrition at home rather than having to remain in the hospital. Central lines are more stable than regular IVs and can be maintained for months or years provided that there is strict adherence to sterile techniques and proper care. For a need of a few week to months (e.g., for short-term parenteral nutrition), a peripherally inserted central catheter (PICC; Kovacich et al., 2016) can be used. For longer term but intermittent use (e.g., chemotherapy), a subcutaneous infusion port can be used (e.g., Mediport). Both of these can be very limiting to a child's movement, and the subcutaneous port needs to be prepared before use with a local anesthetic to lessen the pain of the needle insertion. However, the subcutaneous port greatly decreases the risk of site infections over that of a PICC line (Hodgson et al., 2016; Kovacich et al., 2016).

TECHNOLOGY FOR PHYSICAL DISABILITIES

Children with cerebral palsy or neuromuscular disorders commonly use assistive technology, especially low-tech devices such as ankle-foot orthoses, hand splints, and spinal braces (see Chapters 9, 21, and 32). Mid-tech devices include 1) functional electrical stimulators, which provide neural stimulation to increase mobility; 2) treadmills with support frames to increase strength even in nonambulatory people; and 3) dynamic braces for treatment of a hemiplegic arm. Personal computers, with the appropriate adaptations, can be very useful high-tech tools for people with physical disabilities. Transparent modifications to a computer can be made using add-on equipment and/or specialized software programs (Pousada, Pareira, Groba, Nieto, & Pazos, 2014). These modifications permit most commercially available software programs (including computer games, word-processing programs, and instructional programs) to be used. Transparent modifications do not modify or interfere with either the computer or the standard software program. An example is the keyboard emulator, which is a device such as a joystick that replaces the keyboard (Keates & Robinson, 1999). Keyboard emulators are electronic circuits or switches that function by taking the output from a special keyboard or input device, altering it, and then translating the original signal into a different format that the computer interprets as coming from its own keyboard.

In addition to multiple-use devices, such as computers, many single-application devices have been designed or adapted for people with physical disabilities. Examples range from relatively simple mid-tech feeding devices to elaborate high-tech environmental control units that can turn lights and appliances on and off and can dial a telephone.

TECHNOLOGY FOR SENSORY IMPAIRMENTS

People with sensory impairments have been helped in many ways by assistive devices. For people with visual impairments, there are low-tech magnification devices; mid-tech aids such as alerting systems, laser canes, books on tape, or digital text-to-speech systems; and high-tech systems, such as personal computers with extra-large type on video screens. Various devices using electronic technology have also been developed for people who are blind. These include the Kurzweil 3000™ reading machines that translate printed words to voice-synthesized output and refreshable braille displays (e.g., ALVA BC680™) that provide an alternative access in the form of braille to the text or content displayed on a computer monitor or tablet (Thomas, Barker, Rubin, & Dahlmann-Noor, 2015; see Chapter 25 for more information on assistive technology for people with visual impairments). The near future also holds promise for those with visual impairments as devices using computerized camera systems (such as those in self-driving cars) are being researched with patients. These will serve as methods of augmented reality and will lead to independent accessibility in many places previously deemed too dangerous for someone who is blind or severely visually impaired (Coughlan & Miele, 2017).

Since the mid-1990s, there has been an explosion in the complexity and efficacy of hearing aids for people with hearing impairments. Digital programmable hearing aids have become more available, allowing improved customization for an individual's specific degree and range of hearing loss. Many mid-tech solutions are also available, such as assistive listening devices (infrared or FM transmitters) in movie theaters and classrooms and palm-sized telecommunication devices for use with telephones (Clark & Swanepoel, 2014). Especially for those children whose aided hearing ability is near to normal, there are now software programs available to further improve their speech and language abilities (Meinzen-Derr, Wiley, McAuley, Smith, & Grether, 2017).

For the child with a profound hearing impairment, as well as for their families and others, there have been advances in methods to learn lip reading and sign language by computer modeling programs. In addition, versions of the electronic cochlear implant (CI) have been gradually improving; for most individuals, this device can restore a type of hearing or at least an improved awareness of sounds (Marnane & Ching, 2015; Stern, Yueh, Lewis, Norton, & Sie, 2005). The surgical implantation of CI is not without risks, such as meningitis, and these children need careful follow-up (Rubin & Papsin, 2010; see Chapter 26 for more information on assistive technology for people with hearing impairments).

TECHNOLOGY FOR COMMUNICATION DISABILITIES

Many types of augmentative and alternative communication (AAC) devices exist to assist a person who is unable to use speech for communication (see Table 36.1). Most devices are used for people who have physical disabilities, but AAC has been shown to be quite effective for children who have ASD (Ganz, 2015, Schlosser & Wendt, 2008). Concerns have been raised in the past that using AAC might slow down the acquisition of verbal language, but research has shown that the use of AAC actually increases the development of speech (Binger, Berens, Kent-Walsh, & Taylor, 2008).

Low-tech devices include various lists of words or pictures mounted on durable material. These communication books or boards are used in face-to-face communication; the user points to the selected word or picture to communicate a specific message. A battery-operated scanning communication device using moving lights on pictures is an example of a mid-tech AAC device. Other mid-tech AAC devices include portable voice-output storage units that require direct selection and hold only a few minutes of prerecorded sentences or phrases.

High-tech electronic communication aids, often incorporating single symbols to substitute for groups of words, are becoming more commercially available. Various software companies have started using laptops or tablets as the core part of a communication system, increasing the versatility of these communication aids. Rather than being used only for person-to-person communication, these adapted portables can be used for all types of communication, including letter writing, telecommunications, and e-mail. Adapted computers also can be the foundation for environmental controls, safety systems, and recreation (e.g., Internet access and virtual-reality computer games; Sigafoos et al., 2004; van den Heuvel, Lexis, Gelderblom, Jansens, & de Witte, 2016).

Despite what is portrayed on TV, when compared with high-tech computerized AAC technology, there are significant problems with low-tech and mid-tech devices: 1) they are slow in getting the message across, 2) they provide limited messages (i.e., usually only those about basic needs), and 3) they require face-to-face interaction. Spoken communication among typical individuals is normally performed at such a high speed that patience is needed for conversations between typically communicating people and those using a communication system (especially low-tech systems involving symbols, letters, or word boards). Although these methods are extremely slow, such boards should not be abandoned as they can often be very effective, especially for face-to-face communication. Further, electronic devices are sometimes limited by their need for a power source or the battery life, and most are not suitable for outdoor activities such as going to the beach or walking in the rain. Thus, low-tech solutions such as word and picture boards should always be part of an overall communication system and should be available as a backup to electronic devices, even if one has access to a spare battery or other power source.

TECHNOLOGY FOR COGNITIVE AND LEARNING DISABILITIES

Children who have learning differences have been helped by various assistive technology devices and strategies (Hetzroni & Shrieber, 2004; Perelmutter, McGregor, & Gordon, 2017). Many software programs have been developed since the late 1980s that use computers to assist in reading, math, and other types of special education instruction. These programs range widely in price and utility, and only recently has enough research been performed to begin to determine their effectiveness and generalizability, especially over the long term (Lahm, Bausch, Hasselbring, & Blackhurst, 2001; Liu, Wu, & Chen, 2013). Computer-based instruction, however, has several unique advantages, perhaps the most important of which is the ease of individualization. It is possible to build on children's strengths and talents and develop alternative ways of learning. Very few children in special education have their own personal teacher on a full-time basis; as such, the use of a computer can allow these children to begin to develop independent learning skills. It is crucial to first fully evaluate the educational strengths and needs of a student who has learning difficulties and then apply the assistive technology that can best help the problem. Most of the time, however, low-tech and mid-tech solutions should be considered initially. A high-tech solution is often not the best answer for a specific problem that a child is having in school.

ASSESSMENT FOR ASSISTIVE TECHNOLOGY

The assessment process and the prescribing of any assistive device must be done by a knowledgeable team of professionals. Depending on the type of assistive device to be prescribed, this interdisciplinary team may include a speech-language therapist, a physical therapist, an occupational therapist, a **rehabilitation engineer** (see Box 36.1), a neurodevelopmental pediatrician, a neurologist, a physiatrist or other physician, a special educator, a social worker, and a computer specialist. Also included in the team are the child who will be using the device(s) and his or her family members, who can offer advice that is critical in making final device recommendations. This team approach is essential to properly evaluating the child's motor and intellectual capabilities and narrowing down the devices that may fit within the child's abilities and needs (e.g., educational plans). Much of the research that has been done regarding the effectiveness of a team approach to assistive technology selection is based on adults

BOX 36.1 INTERDISCIPLINARY CARE

Rehabilitation Engineer

A rehabilitation engineer is a person who has college experience and training to be able to apply engineering principles and practices to the design, modification, and manufacturing of assistive technology devices. This individual's main function is to create practical, often individualized, devices in order to help people with various types of disabilities.

with disabilities (e.g., Scherer, Jutai, Fuhrer, Demers, & Deruyter, 2007). A clinical report from the American Academy of Pediatrics, however, is available that provides summarized information about this assessment process in children (Desch, Gaebler-Spira, & Council on Children with Disabilities, 2008).

Figure 36.1 summarizes the assessment process (also see the following section titled Functional Evaluation of the Individual for more information on the assessment tools mentioned in this figure). An important aspect of assessment is consideration of the range of assistive technology that may be useful. The best approach is to begin with the low-tech devices and to move on to mid-tech or high-tech devices only if needed. For example, to get around the home, a child with a severe physical disability may benefit more from ramps and wider doors than from a power wheelchair. The assessment process often involves making educated guesses (based on prior experiences with other people with similar disabilities) and then having the individual try out the chosen devices. A single-subject design methodology is often used to add some objectivity to this device selection process (Zhan & Ottenbacher, 2001). The most complete evaluation possible should be undertaken prior to purchasing the equipment, including testing the device in all settings where it will be used. This avoids buying a device that is unusable or inappropriate.

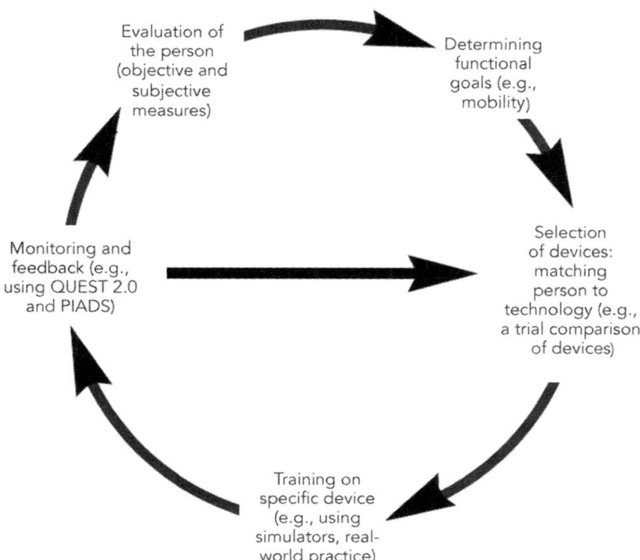

Figure 36.1. The assistive device assessment cycle. (*Key:* QUEST 2.0, Quebec User Evaluation of Satisfaction with Assistive Technology, Version 2.0 [Demers, Weiss-Lambrou, & Ska, 2000]; PIADS, Psychosocial Impact of Assistive Devices Scale [Day, Jutai, & Campbell, 2002; Routhier, Vincent, Morrissette, & Desauliers, 2001].)

Functional Evaluation of the Individual

The ultimate goal for a person using an assistive device is to achieve the highest possible level of functioning. The World Health Organization (2007) has introduced the International Classification of Functioning, Disability and Health-Children and Youth, a system that produces an overall picture of the capabilities of an individual, rather than solely focusing on the disability. A number of other standardized instruments have been developed that can be used to evaluate the current functioning and impact of treatment or intervention, including assistive technology, on children with various types of disabilities. These include the children's version of the Functional Independence Measure (Wong, Au-Yeung, & Law, 2005) and the Pediatric Disability Inventory (Ostensjo, Bjorbaekmo, Carlberg, & Vollestad, 2006).

Without the proper evaluation and ongoing support for the use of assistive devices, a number of studies have shown that there can be a significant amount of assistive devices that are abandoned shortly after they are obtained (Galvin & Scherer, 2004; Martin, Martin, Stumbo, & Morrill, 2011; Phillips & Zhao, 1993; Wessels, Dijcks, Soede, Gelderblom, & De Witte, 2003). To improve utilization, techniques have been developed to predict the successful use of assistive devices. One approach is the Matching Person and Technology (MPT) model (Scherer, 1998a, 2017; Scherer, et al., 2007) that stresses the importance of addressing environmental-, personal-, and technology-related issues. Environmental issues include the family structure and the work or school settings. The personal area includes recognition of functional limitations, motivation, coping skills, and personality traits (e.g., optimism). The technology area includes the characteristics of the assistive device, such as its reliability, ease of use, adaptability, and whether any discomfort or stress is caused by its use. Scherer and colleagues developed an assessment tool, the Assistive Technology Device Predisposition Assessment, which uses the MPT model to facilitate a match between the device and the person to ensure a good long-term result (Scherer, 1998a, 1998b; Scherer & Cushman, 2001). Table 36.3 lists factors that relate to this model. There are also assessment tools that determine the efficacy and satisfaction of the device once in place: the Quebec User Evaluation of Satisfaction with Assistive Technology (QUEST), now called QUEST 2.0 (Brandt, 2005; Demers, Weiss-Lambrou, & Ska, 2000; Demers, Weiss, & Ska, 2002), and the Psychosocial Impact of Assistive Devices Scale (PIADS; Day, Jutai, & Campbell, 2002; Jutai, Fuhrer, Dermers, Scherer, & DeRuyter, 2006). Recently, a number of clinician/researchers have

Table 36.3. Factors associated with abandonment of an assistive device

Possible issues	Possible solutions/preventives
Improper or ineffective training on the use of a device (e.g., single-session training without follow-up and feedback)	Use a multidisciplinary or interdisciplinary team approach to training with the device.
Problems or obstacles in the environment preventing use of a device (e.g., second-floor rooms inaccessible to a power wheelchair user)	Assess *all* potential environments in which the device will be used.
Faults or failures in performance of the device (e.g., assistive device that is too sensitive to movement)	Consider using a rental or loaner device to try out. Become very knowledgeable about the devices being considered.
Device size, weight, or appearance (e.g., assistive device decorated with pink roses given to a boy)	Develop connections with several vendors of devices. Be creative with individualizing the devices (e.g., add colorful stickers).
Motivational factors in the user and/or family members (e.g., depression occurring after traumatic injuries)	Consider cultural factors. Social work or similar evaluations of the client and the family may be needed.
Perceived lack of or minimal need for the device (e.g., decision made not to leave the house rather than to use a wheelchair)	Consider cultural factors and socioeconomic factors (e.g., by social work assessment).
Functional abilities that worsen or improve (e.g., progressive disorder or recovery)	Ensure appropriate medical follow-up of the underlying condition (usually with subspecialists).

Source: Scherer (1998a).

begun to systematically look at methods of assistive technology service delivery, especially to ensure that the person with disability is at the center of the selection process (Federici et al., 2014; Federici & Scherer, 2012; Box 36.2).

Training in the Use of an Assistive Device

Physicians, therapists, and educators who prescribe or recommend electronic assistive devices or assistive devices in general must ensure that the child receives proper training and monitoring for using the device. For some devices and software, demos and simulators are available (e.g., power wheelchair controls and AAC devices), which can help with training before the actual device is ordered (Faria, Reis, & Lau, 2014; Harrison, Derwent, Enticknap, Rose, & Attree, 2002). Simulators are especially helpful in evaluating reaction time, speed, and accuracy, such as in training with people with visual impairments (Todd, Mallya, Majeed, Rojas, & Naylor, 2015).

EFFECTS OF ASSISTIVE TECHNOLOGY ON THE FAMILY AND COMMUNITY

Assistive technology compensates for or builds on the individual skills that each person already possesses. It can lead to increased feelings of success and self-worth and, it is hoped, improved functioning (Guerette, Furumasu, & Tefft, 2013; Wang & Barnard, 2004). For example, several studies have provided evidence for the positive effects of adapted toys on intellectual development (Logan et al., 2017). Although much uncertainty remains about the earliest age at which a child can successfully use an assistive device, some pilot studies suggest children even younger than 5 years of age can benefit. For example, studies demonstrated that children as young as 2 years old can be quite successful in using a power wheelchair and reap considerable social benefits from them (Guerette et al., 2013; Livingstone & Field, 2015). In fact, one study suggests that for children with communicative disabilities, if AAC devices

BOX 36.2 EVIDENCE-BASED PRACTICE

The Importance of Training and Follow-Up Tools

There is increasing evidence that using the assessment and follow-up tools described above in both adults and children with disabilities will lead to much better outcomes. Of course, when dealing with individuals who have varying disabilities, there can be instances of less than ideal results. Training in the use of devices by all involved is critical (see Desideri et al., 2016; Federici et al., 2015; Griffiths & Addison, 2017; Scherer, 2017).

are not being successfully used by first grade, the child will not be an active participant in the classroom setting (Buekelman & Mirenda, 2013).

Although assistive devices can markedly improve function, medical technology can also lead to social isolation. In school, the child is likely to be treated differently because of the accompanying equipment and medical/nursing needs. The presence of a tracheostomy and ventilator can be particularly intimidating. This can be partially offset by educating classmates and teachers and providing psychological counseling for the child. The child and family must also learn to deal with the underlying medical problem that led to the technology dependence. It is generally easier for a child and family to cope with medical technology assistance on a short-term basis, such as when IV antibiotics are necessary to treat a severe infection or when a temporary ostomy is required following abdominal surgery. If the child has a severe chronic disease, however, adaptation to assistive technology is only one issue that the child and family must face (Henderson, Skelton, & Rosenbaum, 2008). Studies have suggested that families fare better if the more significant type of technological assistance, such as mechanical ventilation, lasts less than 2 years. More prolonged periods are associated with an increased risk of parental stress and depression (Amin et al., 2014; Montagnino & Mauricio, 2004). The provision of in-home respite care and family-to-family support systems can be extremely helpful in these situations (Edwards, Morris, Nelson, Panitch, & Miller, 2017).

Despite financial and psychosocial difficulties, children who require chronic and substantial medical technology assistance are being included in their communities today (Feudtner et al., 2005; Seear, Kapur, Wensley, Morrisson, & Behroozi, 2016). A very useful, extensive, and practical book is available from the American Academy of Pediatrics that deals with home care (Libby & Imaizumi, 2009). Home care, especially when ventilator assistance is required, becomes a viable option only after a number of requirements have been met (Carnevale, Alexander, Davis, Rennick, & Troini, 2006; Heaton, Noyes, Sloper, & Shah, 2005):

1. The family must master the child's medical and nursing care.
2. The family needs to select a nursing agency if home nursing services are required and a DME supplier for equipment, disposable supplies, and in-home support (e.g., equipment maintenance and monitoring).
3. The funds to pay for all of these services also must be arranged.
4. Modifications to the family's home may be needed, such as changing existing electrical systems and adding ramps for wheelchair or adapted stroller accessibility.
5. If mechanical ventilation is required, local electric, ambulance, and telephone companies must be notified that a person dependent on life-support technology will be living in the family's home so that the household can be placed on a priority list in the event of a power failure or a medical emergency.

Medical, educational, and therapy (e.g., occupational therapy and physical therapy) services also need to be arranged before discharge from the hospital. A pediatrician or family physician in the community should be identified to provide a medical home. The discharging team should contact this physician prior to the child's hospital discharge to introduce the child and encourage the community physician's active participation in the child's care. If the child requires special rehabilitation therapies after discharge, either center- or home-based providers should be arranged. Educational services also need to be identified, and the child's health care and rehabilitative plans should be written into an individualized family service plan for early intervention services if the child is younger than age 3 or into an individualized education program if the child is preschool or school age (Lipkin, Okamoto, Council on Children with Disabilities, & Council on School Health, 2015). In addition, the school nurse needs to develop an individualized health care plan as well as emergency plans for the child. A center- or school-based educational program offers the child the opportunity to interact with other children in a stimulating environment (Behrmann & Schaff, 2001). These out-of-home experiences should be encouraged if the child's physical condition permits and if appropriate medical or nursing supports are available.

FUNDING ISSUES

Assistive technology can be very expensive depending on the type of equipment required, the extent of the disability, and the professional staffing needs of the child. For medical assistive technology, the two major issues are payment for home nursing care and DME and supplies (including technological assistance). It is sometimes easier to obtain funding for the former than for the latter; however, there is a national shortage of pediatric home care nurses. The primary source of funding for both is insurance, both private and public, and each has restrictions that may affect the provision of medical assistive technology. Every third-party medical payment source has documents that detail which DME will be paid for and under what circumstances. It is crucial that both the providers (e.g., physician) and the family be familiar with this "approved DME listing" as it is difficult to get funding approval for items that are not part of the contract from the insurance carrier.

For assistive technology that can be used in schools, the Individuals with Disabilities Education Improvement Act of 2004 (PL 108-446) as well as other laws (e.g., the Technology-Related Assistance for Individuals with Disabilities Act of 1988 [PL 100-407], the "Tech Act," and the Assistive Technology Act of 2004, PL 108-364 and various legal opinions about these), specifically indicate that funding should be provided for "technological" devices (including software) that are part of a student's IEP. Yet, there are difficulties in actually finding funds to support this, and cooperative efforts among insurance companies, philanthropic agencies, school systems, and parents are often required. Another concern is that often schools will restrict the use of the software or device to the school program (and the student is not able to take it for use at home). However, if even 1 penny of Medicaid money is used by the school to purchase an assistive device for a student, then that student and family have the right to take the device home with them.

For some devices, such as home ventilators, suctioning, or specialized feeding equipment, insurance companies universally recognize that these are medically necessary DME and will pay for them. There continues to be controversy, however, as to whether other assistive devices are medically necessary or whether they are educationally necessary. For example, AAC devices, wheelchairs, or standing frames for children who have cerebral palsy could be used both at home and at school. If a device is shown to be primarily medically necessary, and therefore DME, it may be possible to obtain funding from medical insurance companies. If they are educationally necessary, the school system should purchase the needed devices. As mentioned before, The Tech Act has tried to solve this problem of discriminating between medical and educational use by legally allowing Medicaid funding to be used by the school to purchase the assistive device. The Tech Act further requires that the child be permitted to take home such devices for educationally related purposes. The Tech Act sets a precedent for all types of third-party medical funding to be at least considered for the purchase of essentially all assistive devices.

For years, most forms of private and government medical insurance (e.g., Medicaid) have been willing to pay for the purchase of wheelchairs, and they gradually are beginning to fund other types of assistive devices. Fortunately, AAC devices are increasingly being seen as medically necessary in much the same way as wheelchairs. Physicians are often called upon to send medical necessity letters and prescriptions to funding sources for assistive technology (Cartwright & Council on Children with Disabilities, 2007; Desch et al., 2008; Lipkin et al., 2015; Sneed, May, & Stencel, 2004). This can best be done after the physician consults with the child's therapists and then summarizes current abilities and expected outcomes from using the assistive device. Many assistive devices and their related professional services are relatively new and specialized, and they usually are not included on lists of approved products that are eligible for funding. As a result, many funding agencies need to be properly educated about the potential of these devices to improve functioning and independence for individuals with disabilities. Patience and perseverance are frequently necessary for funding to be secured. Initial denials of payment are almost automatic for some funding sources; however, these denials are usually subject to appeal and reversal. A clinical report from the American Academy of Pediatrics has additional information about the funding process, especially for AAC devices (Desch et al., 2008).

ADVOCACY INFORMATION

Fortunately, increasingly accessible sources of information about assistive technology have been developed. Statewide technological assistance services ("Tech Act sites") are now available in all states, and information from them is becoming more widely accessible. ABLEDATA, which is funded by the National Institute for Disability and Rehabilitation Research, is an example of a large database that holds continuously updated information about assistive technology pertinent to many disabilities. In addition, various organizations dealing with children who have disabilities, such as the Council for Exceptional Children (http://www.cec.sped.org), have developed user-friendly online services that can be used to obtain references and abstracts about many facets of assistive technology, especially in regard to school-related services. On the Internet, there is an increasing number of sites offering resources for people interested in assistive technology, although many of these are thinly veiled advertisements from companies or sites that propose "alternative therapies." Therefore, all web sites must be evaluated critically. Appendix D in the Online Companion Materials provides a list of reputable resources.

SUMMARY

- Most children with disabilities who use assistive technology employ it to make their day-to-day living easier or to improve functioning. However, some children use a medical assistive device that replaces or augments a vital bodily function, such as breathing.
- For the group using rehabilitative assistive technology (e.g., power wheelchairs, AAC, and hearing and vision aids), there is increasing evidence that it is best practice to provide access to appropriate assistive devices at an early age, thereby allowing the children to become proficient in use of the devices by the time they are young adults.
- Improved access to assistive devices also has social implications. As children with disabilities become better able to use their assistive devices or communication devices, they likely will be less isolated and have more contact with their communities as teenagers and adults.
- For children who require medical assistive technology (e.g., respiratory technology devices, surveillance devices, and nutritive assistive devices), the requirement for prolonged medical device assistance (and usually home nursing support) places many financial and emotional stresses on the family. It also leads to considerable challenges for health care professionals and other caregivers, especially in regard to the coordination of care.
- Training of caregivers and others in the use of life-supporting medical technology assistance is best done using a team-approach while the child is hospitalized. Arrangement for financial, nursing, and equipment support is essential before the child goes home.
- The outcome for any child who depends on any type of assistive technology appears to be more a function of the underlying disorder than the type or extent of technology. However, support for the family is essential.

ADDITIONAL RESOURCES

Center for Applied Special Technology (CAST): http://www.cast.org

Independent Living Aids: http://www.independentliving.com

National Center for Technology Innovation (NCTI): http://www.nationaltechcenter.org

Additional resources can be found online in Appendix D: Childhood Disabilities Resources, Services, and Organizations (see About the Online Companion Materials).

REFERENCES

American Academy of Pediatrics: Section on Ophthalmology, Council on Children with Disabilities, American Academy of Ophthalmology, American Association for Pediatric Ophthalmology and Strabismus, & American Association of Certified Orthoptists. (2009). Joint statement—learning disabilities, dyslexia, and vision. *Pediatrics, 124*(2), 837–844.

Amin, R., Al-Saleh, S., & Narang, I. (2016). Domiciliary noninvasive positive airway pressure therapy in children. *Pediatric Pulmonology, 51,* 335–348.

Amin, R., Sayal, P., Syed, F., Chaves, A., Moraes, T. J., & MacLusky, I. (2014), Pediatric long-term home mechanical ventilation: Twenty years of follow-up from one Canadian center. *Pediatric Pulmonology, 49,* 816–824.

Assistive Technology Act Amendments of 2004, PL 108-364, 29 U.S.C. §§ 3001 *et seq.*

Baker, L., Beres, A. L., & Baird, R. (2015). A systematic review and meta-analysis of gastrostomy insertion techniques in children. *Journal of Pediatric Surgery, 50*(5), 718–725.

Bedi, P. K., Castro-Codesai, M. L., Featherstone, R., Al Balawi, M. M., Alkhaledi, B., Kozyrskyj, A. L., . . . MacLean, J.E. (2018). Long-term non-invasive ventilation in infants: A systematic review and meta-analysis. *Frontiers in Pediatrics, 6*(13), 1–25.

Behrmann, M., & Schaff, J. (2001). Assisting educators with assistive technology: Enabling children to achieve independence in living and learning. *Children and Families, 42*(3), 24–28.

Binger, C., Berens, J., Kent-Walsh, J., & Taylor, S. (2008). The effects of aided AAC interventions on AAC use, speech, and symbolic gestures. *Seminars in Speech and Language, 29*(2), 101–111.

Brandt, Å. (2005). Translation, cross-cultural adaptation, and content validation of the QUEST. *Technology and Disability, 17,* 205–216.

Buekelman, D. R., & Mirenda, P. (2013). *Augmentative and alternative communication: Supporting children and adults with complex communication needs* (4th ed.). Baltimore, MD: Paul H. Brookes Publishing Co.

Buswell, C., Powell, J., & Powell, S. (2017), Paediatric tracheostomy speaking valves: Our experience of forty-two children with an adapted Passy-Muir® speaking valve. *Clinical Otolaryngology, 42,* 941–944.

Carnevale, F. A., Alexander, E., Davis, M., Rennick, J., & Troini, R. (2006). Daily living with distress and enrichment: The moral experience of families with ventilator-assisted children at home. *Pediatrics, 117*(1), e48–e60.

Cartwright, J. D., & Council on Children with Disabilities (2007). Provision of educationally related services for children and adolescents with chronic diseases and disabling conditions. *Pediatrics, 119,* 1218–1223.

Castro-Codesai, M. L., Dehaan, R., Featherstone, R., Bedi, P. K., Carrasco, C. M., Katz, S. L., . . . MacLean, J. E. (2018). Long-term non-invasive ventilation therapies in children: A scoping review. *Sleep Medicine Reviews, 37,* 148–158.

Clark, J. L., & Swanepoel, D. W. (2014). Technology for hearing loss—as we know it, and as we dream it. *Disability and Rehabilitation: Assistive Technology, 9*(5), 408–413.

Day, H., Jutai, J., & Campbell, K. A. (2002). Development of a scale to measure the psychosocial impact of assistive devices: Lessons learned and the road ahead. *Disability and Rehabilitation, 24,* 31–37.

Coughlin, J. M., & Miele, J. (2017). AR4VI: AR as an accessibility tool for people with visual impairments. *International Symposium on Mixed and Augmentative Reality (ISMAR-Adjunct),* 288–292.

Demers, L., Weiss-Lambrou, R., & Ska, B. (2000). *Quebec user evaluation of satisfaction with assistive technology: QUEST version 2.0.* Retrieved from http://www.midss.org/sites/default/files/questmanual_final_electronic20version_0.pdf

Demers, L., Weiss, R., & Ska, B. (2002). The Quebec User Evaluation of Satisfaction with Assistive Technology (QUEST 2.0): An overview and recent progress. *Technology and Disability, 14,* 101–105.

Desch, L. W. (1986). High technology for handicapped children: A pediatrician's viewpoint. *Pediatrics, 77,* 71–85.

Desch, L. W. (2008). The spectrum of assistive and augmentative technology for individuals with developmental disabilities. In J. Pasquale & M. Accardo (Eds.), *Capute and Accardo's neurodevelopmental disabilities in infancy and childhood: Vol. 1* (3rd ed., pp. 691–720). Baltimore, MD: Paul H. Brookes Publishing Co.

Desch, L. W., Gaebler-Spira, D., & Council on Children with Disabilities. (2008). Prescribing assistive-technology systems: Focus on children with impaired communication. *Pediatrics, 121*(6), 1271–1280.

Desideri, L., Bizzarri, M., Bitelli, C., Roentgen, U., Gelderblom, G., & de Witte, L. (2016). Implementing a routine outcome assessment procedure to evaluate the quality of assistive technology service delivery for children with physical or multiple disabilities: Perceived effectiveness, social cost, and user satisfaction. *Assistive Technology, 28*(1), 30–40.

Dosman, C. F., & Jones, R. L. (2005). High-frequency chest compression: A summary of the literature. *Canadian Respiratory Journal, 12*(1), 37–41.

Edwards, J. D., Houtrow, A. J., Lucas, A. R., Miller, R. L., Keens, T. G., Panitch, H. B., & Dudley, R. A. (2016). Children and young adults who received tracheostomies or were initiated on long-term ventilation in pediatric ICUs. *Pediatric Critical Care Medicine, 17*(8), e324–e334.

Edwards, J., Morris, M., Nelson, J., Panitch, H. B., & Miller, R. L. (2017). View of directors of home ventilation programs on decisions around long-term ventilation. *American Journal of Respiratory and Critical Care Medicine, 195,* Abstract A2338.

Edwards, E. A., O'Toole, M., & Wallis, C. (2004). Sending children home on tracheostomy dependent ventilation: Pitfalls and outcomes. *Archives of Disease in Childhood, 89*(3), 251–255.

Elias, E. R., & Murphy, N. A. (2012). Home care of children and youth with complex health care needs and technology dependencies. *Pediatrics, 129,* 996–1005.

Faria, B. M., Reis L. P., & Lau, N. (2014). A survey on intelligent wheelchair prototypes and simulators. In A. Rocha, A. Correia, F. Tan, & K. Stroetmann (Eds.), *New perspectives in information systems and technologies, Volume 1. Advances in intelligent systems and computing, 275* (pp. 554-557). Cham, Switzerland: Springer.

Farrar, M. A., Park, S. B., Vucic, S., Carey, K. A., Turner, B. J., Gillingwater, T. H. . . . Keirnan, M. C. (2017). Emerging therapies and challenges in spinal muscular atrophy. *Annals of Neurology, 81,* 355–368.

Federici, S., Corradi, F., Meloni, F., Borsci, S., Mele, M. L., de Sylva, S. D., & Pasqualotto, E. (2014). A person-centered assistive technology service delivery model: A framework for device selection and assignment. *Life Span and Disability, XVIII*(2), 175–198.

Federici, S., Corradi, F., Meloni, F., Borsci, S., Mele, M. L., de Sylva, S. D., & Scherer, M. J. (2015). Successful assistive technology service delivery outcomes from applying a person-centered assessment process: A case study. *Life Span and Disability, XIX*(1), 41–74.

Federici, S., & Scherer, M. J. (2012). *Assistive technology assessment handbook.* Boca Raton, FL: CRC Press.

Feudtner, C., Villareale, N. L., Morray, B., Sharp, V., Hays, R. H., & Neff, J. M. (2005). Technology-dependency among patients discharged from a children's hospital: A retrospective cohort study. *BioMedCentral Pediatrics, 5*(1), 8–15.

Flenady, V. J., & Gray, P. H. (2000). Chest physiotherapy for preventing morbidity in babies being extubated from mechanical ventilation. *Cochrane Database of Systemic Reviews, 2,* CD000283..

Galvin, J. C., & Scherer, M. J. (Eds.) (2004). *Evaluating, selecting and using appropriate assistive technology.* Austin, TX: PRO-ED.

Ganz, J. B. (2015). AAC interventions for individuals with autism spectrum disorders: State of the science and future research directions. *Augmentative and Alternative Communication, 31*(3), 203–214.

Gowans, M., Keenan, H. T., & Bratton, S. L. (2007). The population prevalence of children receiving invasive home ventilation in Utah. *Pediatric Pulmonology, 42,* 231–236.

Griffiths, T., & Addison, A. (2017). Access to communication technology for children with cerebral palsy. *Paediatric and Child Health, 27*(10), 410–475.

Guerette, P., Furumasu, J., & Tefft, D. (2013). The positive effects of early powered mobility on children's psychosocial and play skills. *Assistive Technology, 25*(1), 39–48.

Harrison, A., Derwent G., Enticknap, A., Rose, F. D., & Attree, E. A. (2002). The role of virtual reality technology in the assessment and training of inexperienced powered wheelchair users. *Disability and Rehabilitation, 24,* 599–607.

Heaton, J., Noyes, J., Sloper, P., & Shah, R. (2005). Families' experiences of caring for technology-dependent children: A temporal perspective. *Health and Social Care in the Community, 13*(5), 441–450.

Henderson, S., Skelton, H., & Rosenbaum, P. (2008). Assistive devices for children with functional impairments: Impact on child and caregiver function. *Developmental Medicine and Child Neurology, 50,* 89–98.

Hetzroni, O. E., & Shrieber, B. (2004). Word processing as an assistive technology tool for enhancing academic outcomes of students with writing disabilities in the general classroom. *Journal of Learning Disabilities, 37*(2), 143–154.

Hodgson, K. A., Huynh, J., Ibrahim, L. F., Sacks, B., Golshevsky, D., & Layley, M., . . . Bryant, P. A. (2016). The use, appropriateness and outcomes of outpatient parenteral antimicrobial therapy. *Archives of Diseases of Childhood, 101*(10), 886–893.

Individuals with Disabilities Education Improvement Act (IDEA) of 2004, PL 108-446, 20 U.S.C. §§ 1400 *et seq.*

Jobe, A. H., & Steinhorn, R. (2017). Can we define bronchopulmonary dysplasia? *Journal of Pediatrics, 188,* 19–23.

Jutai, J. W., Fuhrer, M., Dermers, L., Scherer, M., & DeRuyter, F. (2006). Predicting assistive technology device outcomes. *Archives of Physical Medicine and Rehabilitation, 87*(10), e3.

Keates, S., & Robinson, P. (1999). Gestures and multi-modal input. *Behavior and Information Technology, 18*(1), 36–44.

Kovacich, A., Tamma, P., Advani, S., Popoola, V., Colantuoni, E., Gosey, L., & Milstone, A. M. (2016). Peripherally inserted central venous catheter complications in children receiving outpatient parenteral antibiotic therapy (OPAT). *Infection Control & Hospital Epidemiology, 37*(4), 420–424.

Krause, M. F., & Hoehn, T. (2000). Chest physiotherapy in mechanically ventilated children: A review. *Critical Care Medicine, 28,* 1648–1651.

Lahm, E. A., Bausch, M. E., Hasselbring, T. S., & Blackhurst, A. E. (2001). National assistive technology research institute. *Journal of Special Education Technology, 16,* 19–26.

Lee, A. L., Button, B. M., & Tannenbaum, E.-L. (2017). Airway-clearance techniques in children and adolescents with chronic suppurative lung disease and bronchiectasis. *Frontiers in Pediatrics, 5,* 2.

Lipkin, P. H., Okamoto, J., Council on Children with Disabilities, & Council on School Health (2015). The Individuals with Disabilities Education Act (IDEA) for children with special educational needs. *Pediatrics, 136*(6), 31–45.

Libby, R. C., & Imaizumi, O. (Eds.). (2009). *Guidelines for pediatric home health care* (2nd ed.). Itasca, IL: American Academy of Pediatrics.

Liu, G. Z, Wu, N. W., & Chen, Y. W. (2013). Identifying emerging trends for implementing learning technology in special education: A state-of-the-art review of selected articles published in 2008–2012. *Research in Developmental Disabilities, 34*(10), 3618–3628.

Livingstone, R., & Field, D. (2015). The child and family experience of power mobility: A qualitative synthesis. *Developmental Medicine and Child Neurology, 57,* 317–327.

Logan, S. W., Feldner, H. A., Bogart, K. R., Goodwin, B., Ross, S. M., Catena, M. A., & Fine, J. (2017). Toy-based technologies for children with disabilities simultaneously supporting self-directed mobility, participation, and function: A tech report. *Frontiers in Robotics and AI, 4,* 7–15.

Marnane, V., & Ching, T. Y. C. (2015). Hearing aid and cochlear implant use in children with hearing loss at three years of age: Predictors of use and predictors of changes in use. *International Journal of Audiology, 54*(8), 545–551.

Martin, J. K., Martin, L. G., Stumbo, N. J., & Morrill, J. H. (2011). The impact of consumer involvement on satisfaction with and use of assistive technology. *Disability and Rehabilitation, 6,* 225–242.

McInally, W. (2005). Whose line is it anyway? Management of central venous catheters in children. *Paediatric Nursing, 17*(5), 14–18.

Meinzen-Derr, J., Wiley, S., McAuley, R., Smith, L., & Grether, S. (2017). Technology-assisted language intervention for children who are deaf or hard of hearing; a pilot study of augmentative and alternative communication for enhancing language development. *Disability and Rehabilitation: Assistive Technology, 12*(8), 808–815.

Montagnino, B. A., & Mauricio, R. V. (2004). The child with a tracheostomy and gastrostomy: Parental stress and coping in the home—a pilot study. *Pediatric Nursing, 30*(5), 373–380, 401.

Morley, S. L. (2016). Non-invasive ventilation in paediatric critical care. *Paediatric Respiratory Reviews, 20,* 24–31.

Morrison, L., & Milroy, S. (2017). Oscillating devices for airway clearance in people with cystic fibrosis. *Cochrane Database of Systematic Reviews, 5,* CD006842.

Nadkarni, U. B., Shah, A. M., & Deshmukh, C. T. (2000). Non-invasive respiratory monitoring in paediatric intensive care. *Journal of Postgraduate Medicine, 46,* 149–152.

Office of Technology Assessment. (1987). *Technology-dependent children: Hospital versus home care: A technical memorandum* (DHHS Publication No. TM-H-38). Washington, DC: U.S. Government Printing Office.

Ostensjo, S., Bjorbaekmo, W., Carlberg, E. B., & Vollestad, N. K. (2006). Assessment of everyday functioning in young children with disabilities: An ICF-based analysis of concepts and content of the Pediatric Evaluation of Disability Inventory (PEDI). *Disability and Rehabilitation, 28*(8), 489–504.

Palfrey, J. S., Haynie, M., Porter, S., Fenton, T., Cooperman-Vincent, P., Shaw, D., . . . Walker, D. K. (1994). Prevalence of medical technology assistance among children in Massachusetts in 1987 and 1990. *Public Health Reports, 109,* 226–233.

Perelmutter, B., McGregor, K. K., & Gordon, K. R. (2017). Assistive technology interventions for adolescents and adults with learning disabilities: An evidence-based systematic review and meta-analysis. *Computers & Education, 114,* 139–163.

Phillips, B., & Zhao, H. (1993). Predictors of assistive technology abandonment. *Assistive Technology, 5,* 36–45.

Pousada, T., Pareira, J., Groba, B., Nieto, L., & Pazos, A. (2014). Assessing mouse alternatives to access to computer: A case study of a user with cerebral palsy. *Assistive Technology, 26*(1), 33–44.

Romitti, P., Zhu, Y., Puzhankara, S., James, K. A., Nabukera, S. K., Zamba, G. K. D., . . . Bolen, J. (2015). Prevalence of Duchenne and Becker muscular dystrophies in the United States. *Pediatrics, 135*(3), 513–521.

Routhier, F., Vincent, C., Morrissette, M. J, & Desaulniers, L. (2001). Clinical results of an investigation of paediatric upper limb myoelectric prosthesis fitting at the Quebec Rehabilitation Institute. *Prosthetics and Orthotics International, 25(2),* 119–131.

Rubin, L. G., & Papsin, B. (2010). Cochlear implants in children: surgical site infections and prevention and treatment of acute otitis media and meningitis. *Pediatrics, 126*(2), 381–391.

Sadao, K. C., & Robinson, N. B. (2010). *Assistive technology for young children: Creating inclusive learning environments.* Baltimore, MD: Paul H. Brookes Publishing Co.

Scherer, M. J. (1998a). *Matching Person and Technology model and accompanying assessment forms* (3rd ed.). Webster, NY: Institute for Matching Person and Technology.

Scherer, M. J. (1998b). The impact of assistive technology on the lives of people with disabilities. In D. B. Gray, L. A. Quatrano, & M. L. Lieberman (Eds.), *Designing and using assistive technology: The human perspective* (pp. 99-115). Baltimore, MD: Paul H. Brookes Publishing Co.

Scherer, M. (2017). Matching Person and Technology. In M. Maheu, K. Drude, & S. Wright (Eds.), *Career paths in telemental health* (pp. 269–275). Cham, Switzerland: Springer.

Scherer, M. J., & Cushman, L. A. (2001). Measuring subjective quality of life following spinal cord injury: A validation study of the assistive technology device predisposition assessment. *Disabilities and Rehabilitation, 23*(9), 387–393.

Scherer, M. J., Jutai, J., Fuhrer, M., Demers, L., & Deruyter, F. (2007). A framework for modelling the selection of assistive technology devices (ATDs). *Disability & Rehabilitation: Assistive Technology, 2*(1), 1–8.

Schlosser, R. W., & Wendt, O. (2008). Effects of augmentative and alternative communication intervention on speech production in children with autism: A systematic review. *American Journal of Speech Language Pathology, 17*(3), 212–230.

Seear, M., Kapur, A., Wensley, D., Morrisson, K., & Behroozi, A. (2016). The quality of life of home-ventilated children and their primary caregivers plus the associated social and economic burdens: A prospective study. *Archives of Disease in Childhood, 101,* 620–627.

Sigafoos, J., O'Reilly, M. F., Seely-York, S., Weru, J., Son, S. H., Green, V. A., & Lancioni, G. E. (2004). Transferring AAC intervention to the home. *Disability and Rehabilitation, 26*(21-22), 1330–1334.

Silvestri, J. M., Lister, G., Corwin, M. J., Smok-Pearsall, S. M., Baird, T. M., Crowell, D. H., . . . Willinger, M. (2005). Factors that influence use of a home cardiorespiratory monitor for infants: The collaborative home infant monitoring evaluation. *Archives of Pediatrics and Adolescent Medicine, 159*(1), 18–24.

Sneed, R. C., May, W. L., & Stencel, C. (2004). Policy versus practice: Comparison of prescribing therapy and durable medical equipment in medical and educational settings. *Pediatrics, 114*(5), e612–e625.

Stern, R. E., Yueh, B., Lewis, C., Norton, S., & Sie, K. C. (2005). Recent epidemiology of pediatric cochlear implantation in the United States: Disparity among children of different ethnicity and socioeconomic status. *Laryngoscope, 115,* 125–131.

Technology-Related Assistance for Individuals with Disabilities Act Amendments of 1994, PL 103-218, 29 U.S.C. §§ 2201 *et seq.*

Thomas, R., Barker, L., Rubin, G., & Dahlmann-Noor, A. (2015). Assistive technology for children and young people with low vision. *Cochrane Database of Systematic Reviews, 6,* CD011350.

Tibballs, J., Henning R., Robertson, C. F., Massie, J., Hochmann, M., Carter, B., . . . Bryan, D. (2010). A home respiratory support programme for children by parents and layperson carers. *Journal of Paediatrics and Child Health, 46*(1-2), 57–62.

Todd, C., Mallya, S., Majeed, S., Rojas, J., & Naylor, K. (2015) Haptic-audio simulator for visually impaired indoor exploration. *Journal of Assistive Technologies, 9*(2), 71–85.

van den Heuvel, R. J., Lexis, M. A., Gelderblom, G. J., Jansens, R. M., & de Witte, L. P. (2016). Robots and ICT to support play in children with severe physical disabilities: A systematic review. *Disability and Rehabilitation: Assistive Technology, 11*(2), 103–116.

Wang, K. W., & Barnard, A. (2004). Technology-dependent children and their families: A review. *Journal of Advanced Nursing, 45*(1), 36–46.

Wessels, R., Dijcks, B., Soede, M., Gelderblom, G. J., & De Witte, L. (2003). Non-use of provided assistive technology devices, a literature overview. *Technology and Disability, 15,* 231–238.

Wise, P. (2007). The future pediatrician: The challenge of chronic illness. *Journal of Pediatrics, 151,* S6–S10.

Wong, V., Au-Yeung, Y. C., & Law, P. K. (2005). Correlation of Functional Independence Measure for Children (WeeFIM) with developmental language tests in children with developmental delay. *Journal of Child Neurology, 20*(7), 613–616.

World Health Organization. (2007). *International classification of functioning, disability and health–children and youth (ICF-CY).* Geneva, Switzerland: Author.

Zhan, S., & Ottenbacher, K. J. (2001). Single subject research designs for disability research. *Disability and Rehabilitation, 23,* 1–9.

CHAPTER 37 Family Assistance

Michaela L. Zajicek-Farber

Upon completion of this chapter, the reader will

- Understand the impact a developmental disability has on family functioning
- Be knowledgeable about strategies and resources that can help families cope with having a child with a developmental disability
- Learn the principles of family-centered care
- Recognize the influence of societal attitudes, provision of supports, and access to resources on the outcome of children with disabilities

The delivery of family-centered care through interdisciplinary care is essential for the well-being of families of children with disabilities, as a developmental disability has an impact on both the child's development and the functioning of their family throughout the life span (Carr & O'Reilly, 2016; Reichman, Corman, & Noonan, 2008). Families are not all alike, and whether a family has access to needed resources for meeting the needs of their child and how a family handles the day-to-day needs, wants, and stresses of its members influences the well-being, outcomes, and the quality of life of the child with disabilities and their family (Vohra, Madhavan, Sambamoorthi, & St. Peter, 2014). Professionals have come to realize that most families possess strengths and resiliency for guiding their own life course and for grappling with child-rearing issues regardless of the type and degree of their child's disability (Munford, 2016). In addition, more professionals have also come to appreciate the importance of listening to the immediate and long-term needs of the families (Zajicek-Farber, Lotrecchiano, Long, & Farber, 2015). Building a collaborative partnership with families and other medical and nonmedical professionals in the community ensures the optimal care and quality of life for children with disabilities and their families. To be effective in promoting the well-being of families of children with various disabilities, professionals must apply family-centered care in service delivery (Seligman & Darling, 2007), strive to build quality medical homes (Zajicek-Farber, Long, Lotrecchiano, Farber, & Rodkey, 2017), and create effective transdisciplinary partnerships (Cumming & Wong, 2015). This chapter addresses issues that families face throughout their life cycle and the approaches professionals can take to help them.

CASE STUDY

Samantha is an 8-year-old girl with Down syndrome. When Samantha was born, her parents, Monica and Sean, were excited by the prospect of having their first child. Both parents were in their mid-to-late twenties, healthy, and well-connected with their extended families and friends in the community. They were diligent about prenatal care, with Sean often attending prenatal visits with Monica. They were both employed full time, but Monica planned to take a 6-month maternity leave. Following a medically uneventful delivery, they were surprised and distressed to learn that Samantha had Down syndrome.

As a way to cope, Monica spent several hours in her hospital room refusing to see anyone, including Sean or her newborn. Sean left the hospital, trying to figure out what to do. He made calls to his and Monica's parents about the turn of events, and everyone in the family also became upset by the news. To provide quick assistance, the social worker coordinated an interdisciplinary meeting with their obstetrician and the lactation nurse. The obstetrician reviewed the health of their infant and noted that infant Samantha, although currently healthy, had a congenital heart defect that would need to be corrected surgically in the future. The social worker explained her role in supporting new families and provided a folder with a variety of resource information about maternal postpartum care, breastfeeding, infant care, and specific information about raising a child with Down syndrome. The nurse explained how she would provide support to Monica regarding Samantha's feeding. Monica cried as she breastfed Samantha for the first time. In the subsequent days, the social worker met with both parents several times, each time listening and supporting their emotional distress and helping them prioritize their decisions regarding how best to meet with the rest of their family and explain Samantha's condition and needs. Eventually, the social worker and Samantha's pediatrician met together with the parents and one set of grandparents, while the out-of-town grandparents participated by a teleconference, to answer questions about Samantha's condition and care.

The whole family was overwhelmed. Monica and Sean kept asking, "What did we do wrong?" One set of grandparents worried whether they needed to do genetic testing on everyone in their family, and the other set worried whether Samantha would be able to attend regular school and support herself in the future. The social worker and the pediatrician answered many different questions about what the parents and extended family could do to help Samantha to develop in healthy and positive ways and how best to offer their support to Sean and Monica. This intensive meeting served as a precursor to many other meetings coordinated by the social worker.

Over time, the social worker provided direct care and counseling education and guidance with follow-ups, as well as emotional and mental health support and access to instrumental community resources. The social worker was key in providing family-centered case coordination with advocacy and ombudsmanship in collaboration with the pediatrician and other health care disciplines and community services (see Box 37.1). Through partnering with the family and providing ongoing social work and interdisciplinary support and resources, Samantha's

BOX 37.1 INTERDISCIPLINARY CARE

Key Social Work Roles and Services

- Family-centered assistance to help families gain knowledge of their child's condition, figure out the meaning of the symptoms that create a child's disability, and to cope with and adapt to changes of their child's disability and overall psychosocial functioning over time
- Direct and indirect care services to families to help them plan for their own and their children's developmental transitions over their life course
- Assessment of the psychosocial needs of the family and their child for ensuring and promoting healthy development and functioning
- Support with problem-solving by identifying and enhancing family and individual strengths and resiliencies and by removing barriers
- Education, counseling, anticipatory guidance, or therapeutic support services to families or their children to cope with distress and manage various life stressors in healthy ways
- Create access or build supportive resources for all individuals with disabilities in their community
- Collaborate and team with other health care and community providers to build and coordinate quality service delivery and ensure service follow-up
- Research and advocacy to ensure social justice and a healthy quality of life for children with disabilities and their families

parents learned about available supports for families of children with developmental disabilities, including those with Down syndrome.

The parents learned how to establish a medical home for Samantha (see the National Center for Medical Home Implementation: https://medicalhomeinfo.aap.org/Pages/default.aspx) that provided regular primary care and well-child follow-ups, and they also coordinated her ongoing medical needs with the hospital's Down syndrome community clinic and other medical specialists. They gained information on how to access early intervention (EI) services in their community for Samantha's early educational and developmental care (see ZERO TO THREE: https://www.zerotothree.org/resources/83-making-hope-a-reality-early-intervention-for-infants-and-toddlers-with-disabilities; Chapter 31), including nutrition and feeding, speech and language, and optimal ways for promoting parent–child attachment and bonding through play and regular parent–child interaction (see the Centers for Disease Control and Prevention: https://www.cdc.gov/ncbddd/actearly/parents/states.html). They learned about the individual family service plan (IFSP) and later about the individualized education program process used to guide formal education of children with disabilities under the Individuals with Disabilities Act (IDEA) of 2004 (see U.S. Department of Education: https://sites.ed.gov/idea/; Chapter 33). They received information on health insurance options and future life care planning for Samantha (see HealthCare.gov: https://www.healthcare.gov/people-with-disabilities/coverage-options/; U.S. Social Security Administration: https://www.ssa.gov/pubs/EN-05-10026.pdf; Chapter 41). They were provided with connections on how to meet other families of children with Down syndrome (see http://Parent2Parent: www.p2pusa.org/) and with information on services that other families found helpful in caring for their child (see Family Voices: https://www.familyvoices.org/).

The parents learned how to gain emotional and mental health support for coping with the periodic distress often arising around Samantha's developmental transitions, as well as how to support each other as a couple and with their own individual needs. The social worker continued to meet with the family each time they came for Samantha's follow-up at the clinic, coordinated community services, and facilitated access to respite care. The family's social worker noted that over time, the parents' coping and adaptation changed in the context of Samantha's and family members' needs. Samantha's parents' feelings of distress, sorrow, and anger were periodically triggered by life-cycle events, such as when they first enrolled Samantha into a local preschool program that was unfamiliar with the needs of children with Down syndrome or when Sean became temporarily "downsized" in his employment and lost family health insurance. Such feelings were balanced by her parents' ongoing love and commitment to Samantha's well-being and care.

With time, Monica became involved with the local Down syndrome organization and a resource to other parents; Sean became involved in the Special Olympics, assisting Samantha and other children with disabilities to participate in exercise, sports, and other socialization events. Their marriage went through stressful times, and following Samantha's heart repair, they sought marriage counseling that supported their bonds. Subsequently, they had two additional children; the youngest one has recently been identified with autism. Through their religious faith, one side of their extended family has adjusted to the unique needs of their grandchildren and maintains frequent contact; the other side, despite their faith adherence, continues to struggle. Today, Samantha's parents will readily tell you that having a child with disability is "just like having other children, but it's also different and unique." Consider looking at the Abilities web site for more information (www.abilities.com/community/parents-20things.html).

Thought Questions:

How can you can work with families in a family-centered way? How does having a child with a developmental disability affect the various members of the family?

UNDERSTANDING FAMILY SYSTEMS

All families exist within the broader network of their communities and social environmental networks (Walsh, 2015). Bronfenbrenner's (1986) **ecological systems model** illustrates the interactive nature of family existence within a *microsystem, mesosystem, exosystem,* and *macrosystem* (see Figure 37.1). The family, through its matrix of activities, roles, interpersonal relationships, and material and physical characteristics, represents the primary microsystem. Each family interacts with other microsystems, such as child care, schools, employment, health care, and a variety of community programs. In turn, the interactions among microsystems constitute the mesosystem. The functioning of both the microsystems and mesosystem is further influenced by the exosystem and macrosystem. The exosystem represents the policy environment, and the macrosystem comprises the broader societal and cultural beliefs and values that influence all systems.

Within the microsystem, families are viewed as interactive, interdependent, or reactive, and when something happens to one member in the family, the whole family system is affected. Families differ with regard to their membership characteristics and views. Families

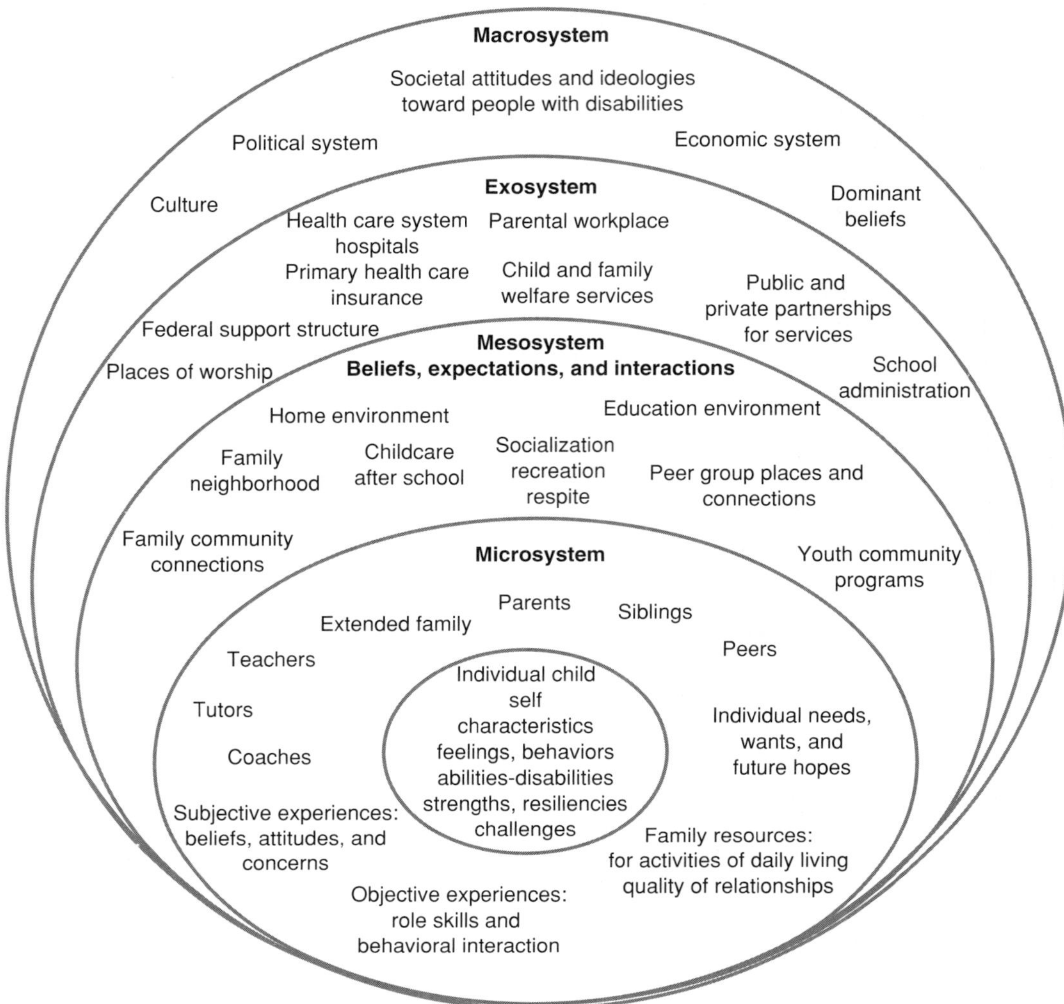

Figure 37.1. The living environment of children with disabilities and their families.

must be considered as configurations that include not only two-parent families, but also step-families, adoptive families, foster families, and intergenerational families. Families may consist of committed individuals who 1) may not be legally married, 2) have gay and lesbian partners, 3) are cohabiting or remarried heterosexual couples, 4) are widowed with children, or 5) are single parents. Families may be adversely affected by an unemployed "breadwinner," a member with a major psychosocial disorder (e.g., substance abuse or mental illness), or a deceased family member whose cultural influence continues to permeate their thinking and behavior (Seligman & Darling, 2007).

A family system transmits traditions, values, ethnic heritage, and spiritual or religious beliefs. In turn, traditions provide members with guidance, strength, comfort, and strategies for coping with the difficulties of daily life (Mackelprang & Salsgiver, 2016). Beliefs, communications, and interactions shape the family's ideological style, relationships, and functional priorities. A family's adherence to their ethnicity, culture, and religious/spiritual rituals; observances in public and private life; and socioeconomic and educational status all influence their cultural style and behavior, including their childrearing beliefs and parenting practices (Hanson & Lynch, 2013). Family beliefs can influence how much they will trust professionals, caregivers, or caregiving institutions and the manner in which the family adapts to their child's disability.

As a family deals with their child's disability, they also confront their beliefs systems about who and what can influence the future course of events (Farber & Maharaj, 2005). Some families believe that this control rests in their own hands (Siman-Tov & Kaniel, 2011), while others believe that control rests in the hands of their religious beliefs, fate, or even pure chance

(Goldstein & Ault, 2015). Family views influence the interpretation of events related to the disability, their help-seeking behavior as a response to the disability, and their approach to caregiving (Xu, 2007). Views and values also influence the family's ability to adapt, negotiate differences, manage stress, and make decisions. In turn, the family's adaptability influences their ability to provide many important supports to their child, including daily care, economic sustenance, housing, education, vocational skill development, socialization, community engagement, recreation, bonds of affection, and spirituality.

Moving through developmental life-cycle transitions can be a major source of stress and challenge for any family, particularly for those raising children with disabilities. Children with disabilities can both positively and negatively affect these and other family functions (Turnbull, Turnbull, Erwin, Soodak, & Shogren, 2015). These life-cycle events begin with the parent's marriage and move through childrearing, management of child schooling and adolescence, launching of young adults, postparenting, and aging. Stress in families is inevitable, but not all family members are impaired by it, and some stress fosters resilience (Valicenti-McDermott et al., 2015). However, accumulated stresses from unmet needs, lack of access to resources, and inadequate management strategies can impair adaptation and result in a crisis in the family's functioning (Neece & Chan, 2017). Fostering family resilience and adaptation is one of the major aims in providing support to families of children with disabilities (Benzies & Mychasiuk, 2009; Pickard & Ingersoll, 2017).

HOW FAMILIES COPE WITH THE DIAGNOSIS

When families are informed of their child's disability, individual members and families as a whole differ widely in their initial responses (Woodman & Hauser-Cram, 2013). Their reaction may depend on 1) the severity of their child's disability, 2) their preparedness for the possibility of this occurring, 3) their prior knowledge about the disability including their own beliefs about why their child might be afflicted with a disability, 4) their experience of interacting with an individual with a similar disability, and 5) the health care professional's manner of delivery of the news (Skotko, Capone, & Kishnanim 2009). The timing, the words used, duration of verbal exchange, and the emotional support that professionals provide greatly influence the family's response to the news (Abbott, Bernard, & Forge, 2013). The impact on the family also depends on their previous life experiences, religious and cultural backgrounds, and age of the child at diagnosis (Vasilopoulou & Nisbet, 2016; White, 2009). Other factors that may influence their reactions include family members' beliefs about individuals with disabilities; knowledge of health treatments; and receptiveness to accepting help from professionals, friends, and other family members (van der Veek, Kraaij, & Garnefski, 2009). In other families, individuals who have had previous experiences with a family member with a disability may be able to adjust more easily to the news, or they may become more distressed depending on that previous experience. Some parents, after years of searching (Watson, Hayes, & Radford-Paz, 2011), may be relieved to finally receive answers and help for their child, but they may also express delayed anger at those who previously reassured them that their child would "grow out of it" (Chiu et al., 2014).

Parental Responses to Diagnosis and Stresses

Responding to the news that a child has a disability is unique, very personal, and often embedded in distress (Alexander & Walendzik, 2016). The most common initial response of parents is some combination of shock, denial, disbelief, guilt, and a sense of loss (Feniger-Schaal & Oppenheim, 2013). Some parents deny their child's diagnosis and visit various professionals, hoping that the conventional wisdom to "get a second opinion" will yield a more optimistic diagnosis or prognosis (Carlsson, Miniscalco, Kadesjo, & Laasko, 2016). Based on the complexity of the child's condition, some parents experience several misdiagnoses before a correct one is given (Mitchell & Holdt, 2014). Families have additional challenges when a child who initially develops typically later acquires a disability. They often have a difficult time accepting that prior aspirations for their child (and potentially for their family) may need to be adjusted. See the textbox titled Common Parental Reactions to Receiving News of their Child's Disability for more on this topic.

When a child's condition is difficult to diagnose, or when professionals are ambiguous or struggle in communicating the diagnosis, parental anxiety rises (Seligman & Darling, 2007). Not having a concrete or well-understood diagnosis is considered very stressful (Madeo, O'Brien, Bernhardt, & Biesecker, 2012). Professionals need to deliver the diagnosis honestly, with compassion, carefully choosing their words, and responding to any questions that parents may have. Professionals also need to understand that the questions parents ask at this juncture are likely to predominantly reflect the answers they are prepared for or emotionally able to hear (Seligman & Darling, 2007). Professionals involved in establishing the diagnosis should provide parents with a written summary that captures the main points to be understood and schedule a follow-up meeting for review of details and answering questions. See the textbox titled Tips for Communicating the Hard News for more on how to best share the diagnosis with families.

After being informed of a diagnosis, parents usually experience a compelling need for information (Gundersen, 2011). While learning to understand the implications of their child's disability, parents experience various intellectual stresses, as they may be required to integrate vast amounts of information about physiology, timing and type of treatments, rationale for treatment approaches, and potential adverse effects and their management (Myers, Mackintosh, & Goin-Kochel, 2009). Families are also often faced with managing instrumental stresses that relate to 1) financing their child's needs; 2) dealing with learning about and administering unfamiliar insurance health policies; and 3) managing the division of labor for providing care for a child with special needs, while still accomplishing household chores and attending to the other family members' needs (Zuckerman et al., 2014). Families strive to normalize their life despite the immediate demands posed by their child's disability, but they come from a wide range of circumstances that may impinge on the child's care. Some families are very knowledgeable about their choices and can financially afford to obtain multiple expert opinions and services. Other families do not have a good understanding of the health care and educational systems or the means to obtain private fee-for-service programs. These problems, often combined with poverty, can directly affect the well-being of both the child and family (Corcoran, Berry, & Hill, 2015).

Specialized medical/therapeutic services and equipment, adapted toys and clothing, and alterations to the household environment can pose substantial financial burdens, which are often overlooked until they urgently surface. Using a **family-centered care** approach in partnering with families involves educating them about their child's condition, making them aware of the resources and entitlements available and helping them examine different treatment choices. Families who are knowledgeable about available resources and assertive in advocating for their child are usually better able to meet their child's needs (Blacher, Knight, Kraemer, & Feinfield, 2016).

Along with intellectual and instrumental stresses, families also struggle with emotional stresses. Uncertainty regarding the diagnosis and prognosis is a major factor contributing to an emotional response to a disability. As the child grows, family responses are subject to periodic exacerbations tied to their child's transitions within their developmental life cycle and to unexpected events (e.g., surgeries or new-onset seizures) that may be tied to the child's condition and health care needs. An uncertainty or ambiguity about a child's diagnosis/prognosis can compromise a parent's sense of control and create distress (Coughlin & Sethares, 2017). Children's ongoing manifestation of severe behavior problems (e.g., hyperactivity, self-injury, or aggression) can challenge parents' coping and leave them exhausted from the need for heightened supervision and sleep deprivation; it can even place them at risk for posttraumatic stress disorder (Stewart, McGillivray, Forbes, & Austin, 2017). Parents of children with rare disorders may feel particularly isolated, as they will not have a community of families dealing with the same condition (Anderson, Elliott, & Zurynski, 2013; Rivard & Mastel-Smith, 2014). For many families and allied health care, educational, and counseling professionals, a useful resource is the magazine *Exceptional Parent* (www.eparent.com), which provides practical advice and up-to-date information on resources and various products useful for families of children and adults with disabilities and special health care needs.

Common Parental Reactions to Receiving News of Their Child's Disability

- Shock, denial, numbness, disbelief, sense of loss for a hoped-for child, and even grief similar to death
- Feelings of crisis, confusion, guilt, shame, and responsibility
- Decreased self-esteem, feelings of devastation, and depression
- Strong anger directed toward the medical staff and professionals involved with the child
- Marital and other family relationships become severely strained
- Family functioning and routines are disrupted and become chaotic

Tips for Communicating the Hard News

- **Prepare and set the stage for a successful conversation:** Arrange to meet in a private setting. Dedicate as much time as you need to have a full conversation with both parents and/or family members. Turn off your cell phone or any pagers. Understand that emotions may be unpredictable. Be ready to listen and to offer emotional and concrete support.

- **Put yourself in the parent's shoes:** Begin by making positive comments about the child's strengths and by reinforcing the parent's skills, love, and dedication to the child. Say things in a kind way. Keep your tone and manner open and available. Be nonjudgmental.
- **Start with the observations, questions, or concerns of the child's parent:** Gently probe and sensitively ask questions that will allow a parent to share their own observations, questions, or concerns first. Then share your own observations in small chunks. Check individual parent's feelings and understanding. Avoid rushing things. Be respectful.
- **Focus on the child's milestones and the need to "rule out" anything serious about the child's condition:** Give the parent something positive to read: Use an example of a developmental checklist of hallmark milestones and any red flags. If you use a web site, make sure that you review the information that the parent will see and read before the meeting.
- **Refer parents and caregivers to other resources:** Give written information summary on the developmental disorder, highlighting the main points. Help parents see the developmental disorder described in writing, whether through literature or on the web. Explain acronyms and avoid medical or other professional technical jargon.
- **Emphasize the importance of early identification and intervention:** Tell the parent that EI is key to help the child and that getting additional assessments of the child's language, behavior, and social interactions with others are just as important as any assessments for medications or procedures. Write down the names and contact information of any services that you recommend, make sure that you know these services well, and help parents prepare for recommended service encounters.
- **Take the time to listen to the parent and observe the child before you do, or say, anything:** Listening is key to being able help parents channel their concerns into words and actions.
- **Set a time for follow-up:** Be confident that sharing your concerns is always the right thing to do, but it takes time to process and absorb any news.

Sources: Centers for Disease Control and Prevention (n.d.) and Informing Families Project (2018).

Parental Depression

It is not unusual that after the initial shock or denial subsides, some family members experience depression (Resch, Elliott, & Benz, 2012). Such an emotional state can result from distress combined with the physical strain (or sheer exhaustion) of following through on the many appointments, procedures, recommendations, and care requirements for children with disabilities (Vonneilich, Lüdecke, & Kofahl, 2016). Other factors contributing to depression may be parental or guardian disagreement over the meaning of the diagnosis/prognosis, assignment of blame, sorting through the choice of treatment options, and/or responsibility in caring for the child (Stewart et al., 2017).

Women may tend to be more at risk for depression (Bailey, Golden, Roberts, & Ford, 2007; Barker et al., 2011). Symptoms of clinical depression include extreme fatigue, restlessness or irritability, insomnia, changes in appetite, and/or loss of sex drive. Professionals should screen for depression in family caregivers and refer them for further evaluation and treatment as needed (Gallagher & Hannigan, 2014). Parents' depression may also be accompanied by anger, which may be directed at a person, an event, their sense of divine intervention, or life in general. If directed at a person, the anger may be focused on the doctor, other professionals, the other partner, other children in the family, or the child with the disability; it may also be self-directed (Heiman & Berger, 2008). Regardless of where the anger is directed, it is important to recognize that such expressions are part of a coping strategy. Anger may well be an appropriate expression of frustration when parents feel their opinions are not being heard or respected. However, it may be inappropriately directed at a "safe" target (e.g., the partner) rather than at the person for whom it is felt (i.e., the professional who communicated the diagnosis). To support the family in managing their coping, the professional can suggest several evidence-based psychotherapeutic approaches to assist the family. Such common evidence-based therapeutic supports include **cognitive-behavioral therapy** (**CBT**; Singer, Ethridge & Aldana, 2007), **mindfulness practice** (Dykens, Fisher, Taylor, Lambert, & Miodrag, 2014), and **interpersonal psychotherapy** (**IPT**; Law, 2011). **Family therapy** can also be effective (Carr, 2014), and **behavior family therapy** is considered particularly useful when children's behaviors overwhelm parenting practices (Harris & Bruey, 2015). **Parent–child interaction therapy (PCTI)** has been used with a variety of families of children with different kinds of disabilities (Crnic, Neece, McIntyre, Blacher, & Baker, 2017), including those with a child with a severe developmental delay (Lesack, Bears, Celano, & Sharp, 2014).

Other therapeutic services are also available when parents struggle with domestic violence, abuse, neglect, or addictions or live in very impoverished environments (Tellegen & Sanders, 2013).

Accessing support from the family and community environment is critical for family well-being (Tint & Weiss, 2016). Families who have strong interpersonal relationships are better able to meet the challenges they encounter. However, sometimes, family or friends may be unable or ill-equipped to provide the needed support. The extended family may not accept the diagnosis or may assign blame to one of the parents, most commonly to the one unrelated to them. Friends may feel uncomfortable in the presence of the child with a disability, and, as a result, they may avoid interactions with the family. Parents may also be embarrassed by their child's disability or unable to manage their child's disruptive or oppositional behaviors and thus rarely venture into the community. They may find it difficult emotionally to see their friends' typically developing children. All of these factors can lead to family social isolation, and, in turn, undermine family management of their parenting (Skotarczak & Lee, 2015).

Family Coping

With time, most parents are able to cope with their child's disability and recognize positive outcomes from the experience. Signs of positive parental adaptions to a child's diagnosis include the following:

- Acknowledgment of emotional struggles in learning the child's diagnosis or condition
- Recognition of and reflection on changes in reactions since learning of the diagnosis
- Halt in the preoccupation with searching for existential reasons for child's condition
- Acknowledgment of the need to move on and go on making the best of life
- Recognition of child's strengths and capabilities in addition to difficulties
- Accurate representation of the range of their child's abilities

In many families, the process of raising a child with a disability increases cohesion, hardiness, and compassion among family members (Beighton & Wills, 2017). For some, it even leads to a more meaningful life (McConnell, Savage, Sobsey, & Uditsky, 2015). With experience and support, parents also become experts in meeting their child's needs. They develop assertiveness in learning to advocate for and obtain what is needed from professionals and agencies to support their child. Their resilience and increasing abilities not only protect but also benefit the child, who may ultimately advance more than what was originally predicted at the time of diagnosis.

For most families, the sadness lessens as they develop routines for care (see the textbox titled Stabilizing Effects of Child and Family Routines), gain access to EI and respite care services, and begin seeing progress in their child's development (Horsley & Oliver, 2015). Naturally occurring family and child routines and meaningful rituals are particularly key in providing stabilizing and predictable structures that guide child behavior and the emotional climate during child development—especially when family life becomes stressful or when children are going through difficult stages or experiences (Boyd, McCarthy, & Sethi, 2014). The need for enhanced support and/or therapy, however, may recur at various developmental stages. The use of **telehealth** (Hinton, Sheffield, Sanders, & Sofronoff, 2017) or electronic and video-based communication is rapidly expanding and can be effectively used to support communication with families (Oberleitner et al., 2011). **Parenting networks** in which parents educate and support one another are often very powerful and may be even more effective in some cases than professional support (Wynter, Hammarberg, Sartore, Cann, & Fisher, 2015).

Stabilizing Effects of Child and Family Routines

"Because our daughter's needs were high, it almost seemed like the family routines we had went out the window. Getting a diagnosis and referrals to services and professionals was a tremendous relief, but then we were so busy that we still lived pretty much in chaos. It's so much better now that we have a routine that we usually stick to. Even if we can't all the time, I feel much better knowing it's there and we can eventually get back to it."

—Parent of child with disability

From Raising Children Network. (2018). *Routines and children with disability.* Retrieved from https://raisingchildren.net.au/disability/family-life/family-management/routines-disability

LONG-TERM EFFECTS ON THE PARENTS

Research on support to families suggests that services benefit families when they are delivered in a family-centered manner and address parent-identified and -prioritized issues (King & Chiarello, 2014). Research on family-centered, help-giving practices (Dunst, Trivette, & Hamby, 2007) shows that to promote positive family functioning, service efforts need to do the following:

- Focus on family-identified needs, goals, aspirations, and plans
- Identify and capitalize on family strengths for harnessing resources
- Strengthen existing social support networks and identify other potential sources
- Use helping behaviors that promote family competencies and strengths
- Use linguistically sensitive communication strategies to convey care and empathy
- Promote collaboration in examining different treatments and service options
- Be proactive in mobilizing resources and exploring options for treatments
- Respect family choices for making decisions
- Engage in follow-up

Conducting an assessment of family strengths and needs is important when trying to determine how much assistance might be provided (Munford, 2016). Different assessment instruments exist for this purpose, including the Family Functioning Style (FFS) scale (Trivette, Dunst, Deal, Hamer, & Propst, 1990), the Parents Need Survey (PNS; Seligman & Darling, 2007), the Family Empowerment Scale (FES; Singh et al., 1995; Vuorenmaa, Halme, Åstedt-Kurki, Kaunonen, & Perälä, 2014), the Family Needs Inventory (FNI; Alsem et al., 2014), the Measure of Processes of Care (MPOC; Cunningham & Rosenbaum, 2014), the Family Support Scale (FSS; Dunst, Jenkins, & Trivette, 1984; Hall & Graff, 2011), the Feetham Family Functioning Survey (FFFS; Roberts & Feetham, 1982), and the Family Quality of Life Scale (FQOL; Hoffman, Marquis, Poston, Summers, & Turnbull, 2006).

Considering the many stresses families experience in childrearing, research has found that having a strong marital relationship, competent parenting and problem-solving skills, financial stability, and supportive social networks leads to more positive outcomes (Marshak & Prezant, 2007; Wang & Singer, 2016). Although some parental relationships are strengthened by challenges in raising a child with a disability, others deteriorate, especially if the relationship was previously troubled (Tomeny, Baker, Barry, Eldred, & Rankin, 2016; Wieland & Baker, 2010). Fostering early assistance through community affiliations and providing effective behavioral interventions in the home can effectively increase family functioning, particularly when families struggle with alcohol abuse or other addictions (Petrenko, 2015).

Parents of children with severe developmental disabilities, chronic behavior problems, and/or medical fragility (e.g., requiring technology assistance to live and function) are at the greatest risk for caregiver burnout and impaired functioning (Ello & Donovan, 2005). Although many families with severely impaired children do well, some have considerable difficulties finding and being included within their community system of care (Overmars-Marx, Thomése, Verdonschot, & Meininger, 2014). As a result, they continue to experience chronic stress (Coughlin & Sethares, 2017), which can lead to depression, physical illness, or posttraumatic stress disorder. When feelings of sadness or grief become chronic and interfere with the parent's ability to function, psychological intervention is indicated (Gordon, 2009). Kazak and colleagues (2005) contend that professionals need to explore how the family has dealt with previous stressors and whether the family members emerged with a sense of competence or insecurity.

Reframing and normalizing are important intervention strategies in helping families cope, particularly those with children whose disability condition requires technological dependence and support (Toly, Musil, & Carl, 2012). **Normalizing** involves communicating that the emotions and struggles experienced are both normal and expected (Rehm & Bradley, 2005). This approach from a professional can help reduce family members' feelings of isolation and stigma (Werner & Shulman, 2015). **Reframing** means reinterpreting a behavior or its context by viewing it through a different lens and focusing on the adaptive and positive aspects rather than negative ones (Neff & Faso, 2015). Family-oriented approaches are particularly effective in altering the counterproductive belief that children with disabilities should be the sole focus of family concerns. When in need, the whole family should take part in the intervention and be supported rather than the child alone (Seligman & Darling, 2007; Wang & Singer, 2016).

There is substantial research regarding how families of children with disabilities encounter barriers to inclusion in their communities and human services, including special education services and health care (Odom, Buysse, & Soukakou, 2011; Wehmeyer, Brown, Percey, Shogren, & Fung, 2017). Such difficulties are often compounded by some families' lower socioeconomic and educational status. Further barriers are also posed by providers' lack of training in providing culturally sensitive services to individuals with developmental disabilities, lack of acceptance of Medicaid payments, and lack of family centeredness in health care service delivery (Magaña, Parish, & Son, 2015; Zajicek-Farber et al., 2017). To ensure that the values, beliefs, and perspectives of families are considered when conducting assessments and in developing and implementing services, Klinger, Blanchett, and Harry (2007) recommend that professionals do the following:

- Become knowledgeable about the impact that race, class, culture, and language have on families' access to services
- Communicate with families and their children (with or without disabilities) in their preferred language using professionally trained interpreter services
- Communicate in a manner that uses common (culturally sensitive) lay words and avoids overreliance on professional jargon
- Recognize that families may have their own individualistic ways of handling things that do not fit one "particular" culture or style
- Use multiple sources for assessment for determining family needs
- Give time and voice to both parents and their children
- Make sure that any printed materials are in the families' preferred language
- Whenever possible, provide services to diverse families within the inclusive context of community services

EFFECTS ON SIBLINGS

The siblings of a child with a disability have unique needs and concerns that may vary with gender, age, birth order, and temperament (Stoneman, 2005), as well as genetic predisposition and family factors (Orsmond & Seltzer, 2009; Tudor, Rankin, & Lerner, 2017). A number of years ago Coleby (1995) found that older male siblings had an increased appreciation for children with disabilities, near-age siblings had less contact with peers, and younger siblings of children with disabilities showed increased anxiety. More recently, Cridland, Jones, Stoyles, Caputi, and Magee (2016) found that older female siblings showed increased behavior challenges, perhaps because of being overburdened with child care responsibilities. Sibling concerns also appeared to reflect such situational variables as whether their own needs were being met, how the parents were handling the diagnosis emotionally, what information the siblings were being told, and how much they understood. More recent studies have also found an increased risk for behavior problems (Platt, Roper, Mandleco, & Freeborn, 2014) and social impairment in siblings (Schwichtenberg, Young, Sigman, Hutman, & Ozonoff, 2010), especially in the presence of demographic risks such as immigrant status and poverty (Macks & Reeve, 2007). Giallo, Gavidia-Payne, Minett, and Kapoor (2012) noted that approximately 30% of siblings of youth with various disabilities may present with emotional or behavioral adjustment problems, although other studies have reported siblings to be well-adjusted (Ward, Tanner, Mandleco, Dyches, & Freeborn, 2016).

It is important to remember that children in general have mixed feelings about their siblings regardless of whether they have a disability (Carrillo, 2012; Schuntermann, 2009). Children may be glad that they do not have a disability but feel simultaneously guilty about this feeling. They may worry that they will "catch" the disability or fantasize that they actually caused it by having bad thoughts about their sibling. Adolescents may question whether they will pass on a similar disability to their future children. Due to the extra care and time required by the child with a disability, the typically developing siblings may think that their parents love their brother or sister more than them. As a consequence, siblings may misbehave to get attention, or alternatively they may isolate themselves, worrying about taxing their overburdened parents (Hartling et al., 2014).

Giallo and Gavidia-Payne (2006) found that parent and family factors were stronger predictors of sibling adjustment difficulties than siblings' own experience with stress and coping. In particular, family socioeconomic status, management of stress, degree of family time and routines, problem-solving and communication, and family hardiness influenced siblings' difficulties. Hence, care must be taken to balance parenting efforts to ensure that both children with and without disabilities are adequately supported (Kramer, Hall, & Heller, 2013).

Despite these concerns, some evidence indicates that siblings of children with disabilities may demonstrate increased maturity, a sense of responsibility, a tolerance for being different, feelings of closeness to the family, and enhanced self-confidence and independence (Taeyoung & Horn, 2010; Walton & Ingersoll, 2015). Some also choose to enter helping professions or become involved in advocacy (Hodapp, Sanderson, Meskis, & Casale, 2017).

Siblings of children with disabilities fare best psychologically when their parents' relationship is stable and supportive, feelings are discussed openly, the disability is explained completely, and the siblings are not overburdened with child care responsibilities (Lobato & Kao, 2005). Parents must remember that children observe them closely and take their lead. Parents' approach to ensuring that all family members' needs are being addressed sets the tone for the entire family.

Children should be informed at an early age about their sibling's disability to ensure that their knowledge is based on facts, not misconceptions. This education must be done in an age-appropriate fashion, with the siblings feeling free to ask questions at any time. By the time the typically developing siblings reach adolescence, parents need to be ready to share with them information about genetic counseling, estate planning, guardianship arrangements, wills, and so forth. It is helpful for siblings to know what resources and options exist. Some siblings may choose to have their sibling with a disability live with them as adults, while others may prefer seeking independent or assisted living arrangements or other choices once their own parents can no longer provide the needed care (McHale, Updegraff, & Feinberg, 2016).

EFFECTS ON THE EXTENDED FAMILY

Having grandchildren creates strong feelings of satisfaction, fulfillment of life's purpose, joy, and comfort, but learning that a grandchild has a disability can lead to mixed feelings (Kolomer, 2008). Just like parents, grandparents can harbor guilt, assign blame, or even reject the child (Lee & Gardner, 2010). In addition, the quality of the relationship grandparents have with their own children affects their acceptance of their grandchild's disability (Findler, 2016). Typically, when a grandchild is born with a disability, grandparents grieve for their own loss of a "normal grandchild" and for their child's loss. Some may experience denial more strongly than do the parents, and their reaction can interfere with the family's adaptation to the disability (Seligman & Darling, 2007). Counseling, support groups for grandparents, and/or information given via the parents can lead them to become more supportive of the family and better able to cope with a child's disability (Kresak, Gallagher, & Kelley, 2014).

Grandparents can also be a strong source of support to the family. They may provide respite care, help out with household chores, and provide financial assistance, yet their support may also come at a cost to their own well-being (Miller, Buys, & Woodbridge, 2012). Other extended family members and friends can also help or hinder the parents' ability to cope. Some may have their own concerns or beliefs that interfere with their ability to be supportive; others may not know what to say or how to be supportive. In these instances, professionals can suggest ways to discuss these issues with family or friends, or create access to other supportive social networks (e.g., advocacy groups for their child's disorder; Vora, 2016).

EFFECTS ON THE CHILD WITH A DISABILITY

Preschool Age

In early childhood, the child with a disability may not recognize that he or she is different from other children. Parents, however, closely scrutinize their child's development (Ray, Pewitt-Kinder, & George, 2009). Educating children in their naturally inclusive environments (Sood, Szymanski, & Schranz, 2015) and encouraging various play interactions serve as early typical learning experiences of young children that are equally important for children with disabilities (Myck-Wayne, 2010). Children's interactions with family members and peers during play serves as a preparation for future school interactions, and how parents manage those interactions is critical (Diamond & Hong, 2010).

Parent education regarding the process and course of their child's early development and a referral to EI and special preschool services are very important at this stage (Noonan & McCormick, 2013). Equally important is obtaining help for parents' management of children's early challenging behaviors (Chai & Lieberman-Betz, 2016). Federal legislation plays a key role in providing services to young children with disabilities. Part C of IDEA addresses the specific needs of infants and toddlers with disabilities (birth–age 3) and their families, and Part B mandates services for children ages 3–5 (Guralnick & Bruder, 2016). Children with disabilities and their parents who participate in EI programs often benefit from accompanying services (Zajicek-Farber et al., 2011). The focus on providing EI leads to interactions between parents and (often) multiple professionals to set up an IFSP, setting the tone for addressing the child's disability in the home and the community (Gatmaitan & Brown, 2016). This process, however, can be overwhelming for parents, and it helps when they work closely with the designated service coordinator or social worker on the interdisciplinary team (Rosenkoetter, Hains, & Dogaru, 2007).

School Age

By school age, most children with disabilities are aware of their abilities and challenges and may need help in dealing with feelings of being different. Weight management (related to being underweight or overweight) in young children with disabilities can present additional challenges for their immediate social participation and long-term health (Emerson & Robertson, 2010, McGillivray, McVilly, Skouteris, & Boganin, 2013), and evaluation of mood and affect in children with developmental disabilities has been a growing area of importance in assessing their well-being (Leffert, Siperstein, & Widaman, 2010). Full acceptance of the child's abilities must first come from the home. If the child is seen as being worthwhile and capable by parents and siblings, his or her self-image is usually positive. This acceptance includes participating in family activities ranging from family events and vacations to religious services; community recreational programs; and, if possible, sports or physical play. This acceptance requires that the child's abilities (or lack thereof) are discussed openly and the child is involved in these discussions in an age-appropriate fashion. Discussing and demonstrating how to handle different situations at home improves the child's ability to cope with social situations in the community. Seeking input and guidance from teachers or school staff who interact regularly with the child can help identify the child's strengths and weaknesses in social interactions (Webb, Greco, Sloper, & Beecham, 2008). In order for school and community inclusion to work well, however, teachers and school personnel and community-relevant individuals must be adequately informed and trained about the specific needs of the child (Ryan & Quinlan, 2018). Research has identified care coordination as a crucial aspect of well-being for children with disabilities and special health care needs and their families (Hillis, Brenner, Larkin, Cawley, & Connolly, 2016).

The child with disabilities gains self-confidence through participation in activities in which he or she can be successful and through interactional experiences with others in their environment (Hong, Kwon, & Jeon, 2014). The philosophy of inclusion is that children who have disabilities can participate in general activities provided that they have or receive appropriate adaptations or assistance. Yet, successful inclusions require not only the philosophical and moral acceptance of the need for societal provision of support to children with disabilities and their families, but also the actual facilitation of access and creation of services for such needed support (Cummings, Sills-Busio, Barker, & Dobbins, 2015). Such an inclusive approach, however, should not preclude participation in specific (targeted) programs, such as the Special Olympics or camp programs for children who have varied abilities or specialized needs (Aggerholm & Moltke Martiny, 2017; D'Eloia & Price, 2016).

Some children with disabilities need encouragement and assistance in building social skills and developing friendships during typical social activities (Rogers, Hemmeter, & Wolery, 2010). Summer camps that welcome children with varied needs provide an avenue to develop important socialization skills and experience independence from parents (Henderson, Whitaker, Bialeschki, Scanlin, & Thurber, 2007). Such participation encourages maturation and skill development for the child with disabilities (Goodwin et al., 2011). Furthermore, by participating in an inclusive environment, children and staff without disabilities learn more about tolerance, acceptance, and what it means to have a disability. In turn, they become more knowledgeable and caring of people with differences and less prone to bias (Siperstein, Glick, & Parker, 2009).

Adolescence

Transitioning to adolescence is an important time for families of youth with disabilities that needs to be anticipated, planned for, and well supported (Burke, Patton, & Taylor, 2016). Adolescence is a challenging period for all children and their families because many biological and social changes are taking place, and it can be a particularly difficult time for adolescents with developmental disabilities and their parents (Mitchell & Hauser-Cram, 2010). For parents, adolescence signals their child's proximity to adulthood and adult responsibilities. It quite naturally elicits anxieties and fears about independence, self-sufficiency, and maturity, especially when the child has a disability (Boehm, Carter, & Taylor, 2015). For adolescents, this is a period of many discoveries about self and others, and many adolescents become preoccupied with comparing themselves to their peers (Kuo, Orsmond, Coster, & Cohn, 2014). This desire for fitting in and peer approval in areas of physical and intellectual development may need to be adjusted because of limitations posed by the disability. Negotiating these differences tends to be less of an issue if the adolescent with a disability has 1) at least one supportive peer friend (with or without a disability), 2) a peer group with diverse members, 3) parents who actively encourage the adolescent's participation and involvement in activities that promote independence, and/or 4) the capacity to adjust to being perceived as being "different" (Zajicek-Farber, 1998).

Research shows that adolescents with developmental disabilities compounded with impaired cognitive functioning, as well as those with an acquired disability (e.g., from a traumatic brain injury), are at an increased risk for experiencing mental health difficulties. These often present as mood upheavals, anxiety, oppositional defiant disorder, inattention, aggression, self-injury, and other behavioral difficulties that compromise the adolescents' functioning and social interactions with others (Green, Berkovits, & Baker, 2015). Effective treatment solutions for addressing the mental and behavioral distress of adolescents with behavioral disabilities is an ongoing area of need. Currently, pharmacology is often considered as the primary means for addressing oppositional behaviors or aggression in adolescents with disabilities (Park et al., 2016). However, pharmacology treatment alone has not always been an effective solution for addressing behavioral distress or aggression of adolescents with disabilities. Willner (2015) has shown that, with the possible exception of risperidone, there is no reliable evidence that antidepressant, neuroleptic, or anticonvulsant drugs are effective treatments for aggression in people with intellectual disabilities.

Others point to the fact that we need more and better understanding of the concept and meaning of mental and behavioral health in adolescents with disabilities. For example, Bermejo, Mateos, and Sánchez-Mateos (2014) have noted that the way in which people with intellectual disability express basic affect to emotional stimuli is very similar to that of the general population in terms of *happy-sad* and *calm-nervous.* However, there are also some real differences in the affective dimensions that have to be considered in our understanding of the emotional life of people with intellectual disability. Bradley, Caldwell, and Korossy reinforced this point by indicating that:

> when people with intellectual and developmental disabilities experience mental distress, or their behaviors appear unusual, attending carefully to their communication in whatever way this occurs is crucial, as their perspectives on what may be causing this distress (or unusual behaviors), may be different from what might be concluded based on traditional psychiatric diagnostic frameworks. (2015, pp. 94–95)

Singh and colleagues (2014) demonstrated that mindfulness-based positive behavior support training can, for example, assist parents to effectively manage the challenging behaviors of their adolescents with autism and increase their positive social interactions without raising parental stress levels. Moskowitz and colleagues (2017) have also shown that when a **cognitive behavioral therapy (CBT)** approach was augmented with **applied behavior analysis (ABA)** and **positive behavior interventions and supports (PBIS)** school-age children with autism and cognitive impairments were able to significantly decrease their level of anxiety and their associated negative behaviors toward self and others. Moskowitz and colleagues (2017) also note that recognizing anxiety in children with disabilities can help parents, teachers, clinicians, and researchers regard challenging behaviors as potential signs of anxiety (i.e., escaping anxiety) rather than noncompliance, disobedience, or defiance (i.e., escaping demand). In this way, identifying anxiety can help prevent challenging behaviors before they occur by reducing anxiety or teaching the child to cope with anxiety.

In sum, active professional vigilance is needed to screen and assess both the mental health of adolescents with developmental disabilities (Emerson, Einfeld, & Stancliffe, 2010) and the ability of the parents or caregivers to cope and manage the given situation (Zajicek-Farber et al., 2015). Research shows that anxiety and other mental health issues have been generally underrecognized in this population (Christensen, Baker, & Blacher, 2013; Rodas, Zeedyk, & Baker, 2016). In addition, adolescents with disabilities are at high risk for being excluded from typical daily activities, which, in turn, influences their emotional well-being. Jin, Yun, and Agiovlasitis (2018) found that children with disabilities enjoyed the same activities as their typically developing peers. Activities allowing children to experience enjoyment (perceived as "fun") have the best chance of ensuring children's engagement and participation. Parents' ability to encourage and promote the child's engagement in the activity by their attitude, emotional responses, and use of resources is crucial for the child's successful participation, particularly in sports or recreational activities (Rimmer,, Rowland, & Yamaki, 2007; Rimmer, 2017).

Adolescents with disabilities who remain more isolated and parent dependent tend to struggle reaching a more independent adulthood and have poorer outcomes (Anaby et al., 2014). In addition, youth with disabilities need to be included in mainstream health promotion activities, including socializations and sex education (Akre, Light, Sherman, Polvinen, & Rich, 2015; Maart & Jelsma, 2010) in a way and at a level at which they feel comfortable and can understand (van der Stege et al., 2014). Management of personal hygiene—and competent health and safety practices in supporting a healthy adolescent intimacy and privacy—requires not only a high quality individualized mentoring of an adolescent with frank and sensitive dialogue, but also an individualized training and education of school staff or any health care providers (Wilson & Frawley, 2016).

Parents (and caregiving staff) also need to be encouraged to give the adolescents with disabilities the necessary freedom to become progressively more independent and take reasonable risks (Munro, Garza, Hayes, & Watt, 2016). Such an approach is best accomplished when parents/caregivers and professionals partner early to promote independence in youth with disabilities (Pleet-Odle et al., 2016). To help parents plan for their adolescents with disabilities' futures, professionals need to support families in the following ways:

- Approach transitions universally by focusing on similarities among transitions at various life stages
- Focus on family services and supports throughout the life span, not just during early childhood or adolescence
- Begin the parental dialogue on envisioning and transition planning early and repeat and review at each transition
- Interact with families respectfully according to their unique cultural-linguistic preferences
- Partner with families to explore role models for their adolescent with disabilities
- Include the adolescent with disabilities in the dialogue with their family as much as possible, but also provide individualized mentoring and training for the youth to promote his or her self-determination in making choices and practicing their social skills
- Explore/create opportunities and provide concrete information for parents to learn about transitioning services from school to adult support services, eligibility, and how to gain access in their community

Allow for time to listen to parental worries or anxieties about their adolescents' future, but continue encouraging and empowering parents to trust their instincts for building support networks and planning for their adolescent's future in all domains: academic, recreational, extracurricular, vocational, spiritual, social and community involvement, and health care.

Young Adulthood

The transition to adulthood is both important and difficult for adolescents with disabilities and their parents (Landmark, Ju, & Zhang, 2010). For these adolescents, leaving school creates many worries and anxiety beyond those of typical adolescents; however, with ongoing discussions regarding their concerns and with early anticipatory planning, they can be supported to transition into young adulthood according to their needs (Young, Dagnan, & Jahoda, 2016). Carter, Austin, and Trainor (2012) found that for adolescents with severe physical or intellectual disabilities, the factors that best predicted the future likelihood of securing a meaningful employment included having hands-on employment experiences (paid or unpaid) during high school years, being involved in more household responsibilities, and having parents with higher expectations for their adolescent's abilities. Ju, Zeng, and Landmark (2017) examined the postsecondary school achievement of students with disabilities and found that self-advocacy, self-awareness, problem-solving, and goal setting/attainment are important individual traits of successful individuals with disabilities. They also noted that related trainings (e.g., self-advocacy training and coaching services) were found to improve social skills and encouraged students to utilize community available disability services and support systems to achieve academic success.

Objective role transitions, such as finishing school, finding full-time paid employment, getting married, and starting a family, have been the most common criteria used to evaluate success in adulthood for typically developing youth. However, these role transitions are also becoming less reliable indicators of adulthood, as changing societal economic (employment-related) and social (educational demands–related) conditions continue to alter the traditional paths to adulthood for all youth and especially those with disabilities (Settersten & Ray, 2010). Therefore, a young adult's ability to cope and become as independent as possible depends not only on the management of the disability, but also on 1) the effectiveness of the family to plan and manage this transition emotionally and financially (see Leonard et al., 2016, and Chapter 40) and 2) the community's willingness and the legal support to determine access to support services for children, adolescents, and adults across their life span (Rattaz, Michelon, Roeyers, & Baghdadli, 2017).

Although some adolescents with disabilities *do* achieve independence, many struggle, and some never attain this goal (Henninger & Taylor, 2013). For young adults who cannot achieve true independence, limited alternatives are available depending on where they live, their family finances, and their individual self-care abilities. Much also depends on the existence of societal supports that may or may not exist for supported employment and inclusion of adults with disabilities into normalized community living and activities (Henninger & Taylor, 2014). Research shows that the quality of life of families of young adults with disabilities improves when they are supported by societal resources that help them plan for long-term guardianship across the life span and adjust to the implications of having an adult child with disability (Lindsay & Hoffman, 2015; Stewart et al., 2014). Such services typically need to include the following:

- Identifying options for an appropriate and possible range of living environments for their young adult or child with disability
- Finding appropriate vocational and/or employment opportunities and services

- Planning for how the adult-age child may navigate transportation and mobility in the community and in personal living environments
- Addressing special or unique issues of socialization, intimacy, sexuality, and procreation
- Recognizing the need for socialization opportunities and community connectedness
- Facilitating transitioning to and coordinating adult health care services
- Managing the continued financial implications of lifelong dependency.

Professional Behavior Using Principles of Family-Centered Care

- Demonstrate respect and sensitivity for the child and family in all types of interactions, including verbal and nonverbal communication.
- Be knowledgeable about and recognize the importance of racial, ethnic, cultural, linguistic, and socioeconomic diversity and these factors' effect on the family's experiences in seeking help and their perception of care and support.
- Actively seek to identify the strengths of each child and family and help the child and family use these strengths to promote their natural resilience and address challenging situations.
- Facilitate a partnering climate and time and encourage the child, the adolescent, and the family to ask questions and express their choices about treatment, care, and support.
- Explore options and potential effects of different choices for treatment and care with both the child and family, encourage their input and feedback, and acknowledge their preferences and choices.
- Assist the family in obtaining interdisciplinary and transdisciplinary input and coordination of care regarding options for treatment and support services.
- Ask about barriers or challenges the child, the adolescent, and the family may be experiencing in their psychosocial adjustment to treatment, care, or receipt of support.
- Engage in anticipatory guidance and provide and share with the child and family the types of available formal and informal support services that might be helpful for ensuring healthy child and family functioning during critical and transitional developmental periods.
- Encourage the separate input and advocacy of the child, the adolescent, and the family in all forms of professional interaction, education, and the development of policies for treatment and program interventions.
- Ensure flexibility in developing organizational policies, procedures, and providers' practices so that all services can be individualized to the diverse needs, beliefs, and cultural values of each child and family.
- Strive to collaborate and partner with families at all levels of health care service delivery.

Sources: National Center for Medical Home Implementation (n.d.); National Early Childhood Technical Assistance Center (n.d.); Zajicek-Farber et al., 2015; and Zajicek-Farber et al., 2017. For more information, see http://www.medicalhomeinfo.org and http://www.nectac.org.

PRINCIPLES OF FAMILY-CENTERED CARE: ROLE OF THE PROFESSIONAL

The textbox titled Professional Behavior Using Principles of Family-Centered Care lists principles of family-centered care that represent the current philosophy guiding the interactions among professionals and the families of children with disabilities (Zajicek-Farber et al., 2015). The goal of family-centered care is to facilitate the best possible outcomes for both the children and their families. To achieve this goal, professionals must initiate a process of service delivery and support that invites and establishes a collaborative relationship based on mutual respect and open communication. When such a family-centered relationship is forged, families come to see the professionals as partners who are flexible in solving problems and in giving constructive feedback. Professionals are also then seen as being respectful of cultural diversity, sensitive to family's linguistic issues, and able to listen to family needs with empathy and compassion. Through this shared focus, both families and professionals can appreciate the unique expertise that each contributes (Zajicek-Farber et al., 2017).

Over time, families of children with disabilities may encounter a bevy of professionals including physicians, nurses, teachers, physical and occupational therapists, psychologists, social workers, and agency or hospital administrators. Individually, and as a group, professionals bear the primary responsibility for explaining the results of developmental evaluations and testing, presenting treatment options, teaching intervention and advocacy strategies, and exploring and accessing available support systems. The initial contact that families have with professionals often takes place during a crisis when they are stressed, confused, and vulnerable, and how professionals respond to them sets the tone for future interactions (Vohra et al., 2014). Wright, Hiebert-Murphy, and Trute (2010) examined professional perceptions and organizational factors that support or hinder the implementation of family-centered practices. These included the organization's culture and climate (e.g., caseload size and activity, supervision, staff training), policy limitations, and availability of collateral services. Other research has found that when the case workers provided emotional support, information, and assistance in identifying and meeting family needs, along with advocacy and service coordination, outcomes for children with disabilities and their families improved (Wright, 2013).

As a result of their training, experience, and expertise, professionals often have strong opinions about what is best for the child and family. Yet, they must remember that individuals with disabilities and their families have the right to choose their own path. Families who make their own choices are better at attaining their goals and addressing their needs (Hiebert-Murphy, Trute, & Wright, 2011). However, when the choices the family makes are perceived as potentially deleterious to the child's well-being, the professional must take responsible and ethical action. For example, it is the professional's responsibility to inform the family of the risks and benefits of validated and nonvalidated therapies, while respecting the family's autonomy. The one exception is when it is believed that the family's actions may be harmful to the child or individual with disabilities. The professional must then contact the local child welfare agency (or protective services) to report the professional's suspicion or knowledge of abuse or neglect. Research unfortunately shows that children, adolescents, and adults with disabilities are more likely to be abused than their peers without disabilities (Byrne, 2017; Euser, Alink, Tharner, IJzendoorn, & Bakermans-Kranenburg, 2016; Rowsell, Clare, & Murphy, 2013; Stalker, Taylor, Fry, & Stewart, 2015).

THE ROLE OF SOCIETY AND COMMUNITY

The family's community and environmental context plays an important role in determining the social inclusion and outcome of its members (Simplican, Leader, Kosciulek, & Leahy, 2015). In today's society, there is a greater acceptance of people with disabilities being members of the community, and there are more educational, vocational, housing, and support services available, including religious participation (Ault, Collins, & Carter, 2013). Federal legislation guarantees equal opportunities for all members of society. Federal funding provides for a protection and advocacy system for people with disabilities in each state. IDEA (2004; PL 108446) mandates free and appropriate educational and rehabilitative services for school-age children. Reaching citizens of all ages with disabilities, the Americans with Disabilities Act (ADA) of 1990 (PL 101-336) focuses on the establishment of rights regarding access to employment, transportation, telecommunications, and public accommodations. Effects of the ADA are visible through the presence of accessible city sidewalks, ramps on buildings, public transportation equipped with wheelchair lifts, accessible computers in libraries, and other technological advances. As a result of these efforts and other laws (e.g., the Assistive Technology Act of 2004), individuals with disabilities and their families are guaranteed the same civil rights as individuals without disabilities (Bausch, Ault, & Hasselbring, 2015). However, advances in technology can have both positive and not-so-positive effects (Ellis & Goggin, 2015). For example, while technological advances have improved the communication options for people with disabilities, such as through social media (Gips, Zhang, & Anderson, 2015), cyberbullying of children, adolescents, and adults with cognitive impairments has become a rising societal concern (Carrington et al., 2017; Hernandez, Brodwin, & Siu, 2017).

Although laws are important, they need to be accompanied by a change in the public's perception and attitudes toward individuals with disabilities (Mackelprang & Salsgiver, 2016). Reducing societal stigma toward disabilities (Lalvani, 2015), increasing social inclusion (Anastasiou & Kauffman, 2013), and ensuring equitable supports for aging parents providing lifelong care for their adult children with developmental disabilities should be ongoing goals for our society (Seltzer, Floyd, Song, Greenberg, & Hong, 2011).

Signs of improvement in societal attitudes, in fact, seem to be emerging. Young adults who have grown up in schools with children with disabilities are more sensitive to and appreciative of their needs and abilities. More individuals with disabilities are now in the workforce. Individuals with disabilities are often portrayed in a positive light in movies, television shows, advertisements, and the news. Adaptive and assistive technologies, including the use of universal design, are slowly removing barriers and increasing overall societal integration of individuals with diverse abilities (Burgstahler, 2015). However, although society has made itself more accessible to and supportive of individuals with disabilities, the future remains challenging and requires ongoing vigilance and advancement (Bumble, Carter, McMillan, & Manikas, 2017).

SUMMARY

- A child's developmental disability impacts the life course of his or her development and also all members in the family.
- Initially, the family goes through periods of grieving and disappointments for the loss of their imagined "typical life" for their child.
- Over time and with support, the family's coping strategies evolve and generally improve.
- Parents learn to master their child's care and become more effective supporters and advocates for their child's health, education, and other needed services.
- Over time, youths with disabilities gain skills to cope and manage their own disability and learn to become self-advocates.
- Each developmental transition brings about challenges and changes that impinge on the adapting and coping of the child with disability and his or her family.
- Working in partnership with the parents and the child with disability, the social worker, along with the medical and nonmedical providers in the community, provides an important role in promoting and supporting the health and psychosocial well-being outcomes of children with disabilities and their families.

ADDITIONAL RESOURCES

Beach Center on Disability: http://www.beachcenter.org

Children's Disabilities Information: http://www.childrensdisabilities.info/prematurity/followup.html

Exceptional Parent: http://www.eparent.com

Family Village: A Global Community of Disability-Related Resources: http://www.familyvillage.wisc.edu

Additional resources can be found online in Appendix D: Childhood Disabilities Resources, Services, and Organizations (see About the Online Companion Materials).

REFERENCES

Abbott, M., Bernard, P., & Forge, J. (2013). Communicating a diagnosis of autism spectrum disorder—a qualitative study of parents' experiences. *Clinical Child Psychology and Psychiatry, 18*(3), 370–382.

Aggerholm, K., & Moltke Martiny, K. M. (2017). Yes we can! A phenomenological study of a sports camp for young people with cerebral palsy. *Adapted Physical Activity Quarterly, 34*(4), 362–381.

Akre, C., Light, A., Sherman, L., Polvinen, J., & Rich, M. (2015). What young people with spina bifida want to know about sex and are not being told. *Child: Care, Health and Development, 41*(6), 963–969.

Alexander, T., & Walendzik, J. (2016). Raising a child with Down syndrome: Do preferred coping strategies explain differences in parental health? *Psychology, 7*(1), 28–39.

Alsem, M. W., Siebes, R. C., Gorter, J. W., Jongmans, M. J., Nijhuis, B. G. J., & Ketelaar, M. (2014). Assessment of family needs in children with physical disabilities: Development of a family needs inventory. *Child: Care, Health and Development, 40*(4), 498–506.

Americans with Disabilities Act (ADA) of 1990, PL 101336, 42 U.S.C. §§ 12101 *et seq.*

Anaby, D., Law, M., Coster, W., Bedell, G., Khetani, M., Avery, L., & Teplicky, R. (2014). The mediating role of the environment in explaining participation of children and youth with and without disabilities across home, school, and community. *Archives of Physical Medicine and Rehabilitation, 95*(5), 908–917.

Anastasiou, D., & Kauffman, J. M. (2013). The social model of disability: Dichotomy between impairment and disability. *The Journal of Medicine and Philosophy: A Forum for Bioethics and Philosophy of Medicine, 38*(4), 441–459.

Anderson, M., Elliott, E. J., & Zurynski, Y. A. (2013). Australian families living with rare disease: Experiences of diagnosis, health services use and needs for psychosocial support. *Orphanet Journal of Rare Diseases, 8*(1), 1–9.

Ault, M. J., Collins, B. C., & Carter, E. W. (2013). Congregational participation and supports for children and adults with disabilities: Parent perceptions. *Intellectual and Developmental Disabilities, 51*(1), 48–61.

Bailey, D. B., Golden, R. N., Roberts, J., & Ford, A. (2007). Maternal depression and developmental disability: Research critique. *Developmental Disabilities Research Reviews, 13*(4), 321–329.

Barker, E. T., Hartley, S. L., Seltzer, M. M., Floyd, F. J., Greenberg, J. S., & Orsmond, G. I. (2011). Trajectories of emotional well-being in mothers of adolescents and adults with autism. *Developmental Psychology, 47*(2), 551–561.

Bausch, M. E., Aut, M. J., & Hasselbring, T. S. (2015). Assistive technology in schools: Lessons learned from the National Assistive Technology Research Institute. In D. L. Edyburn (Ed.), *Efficacy of assistive technology interventions* (pp. 13–50). Boston, MA: Emerald Group Publishing Limited.

Beighton, C., & Wills, J. (2017). Are parents identifying positive aspects to parenting their child with an intellectual disability or are they just coping? A qualitative exploration. *Journal of Intellectual Disabilities, 21*(4), 325–345.

Benzies, K., & Mychasiuk, R. (2009). Fostering family resiliency: A review of the key protective factors. *Child & Family Social Work, 14*(1), 103–114.

Bermejo, B. G., Mateos, P. M., & Sánchez-Mateos, J. D. (2014). The emotional experience of people with intellectual disability: An analysis using the international affective pictures system. *American Journal on Intellectual and Developmental Disabilities, 119*(4), 371–384.

Blacher, J., Knight, E., Kraemer, B., & Feinfield , K. A. (2016). Supporting families who have children with intellectual disability. In A. Carr, C. Linehan, G. O'Reilly, P. Walsh, & J. McEvoy (Eds.), *The handbook of intellectual disability and clinical psychology practice* (2nd ed., pp. 283–310). New York, NY: Routledge.

Boehm, T. L., Carter, E. W., & Taylor, J. L. (2015). Family quality of life during the transition to adulthood for individuals with intellectual disability and/or autism spectrum disorders. *American Journal on Intellectual and Developmental Disabilities, 120*(5), 395–411.

Boyd, B. A., McCarty, C. H., & Sethi, C. (2014). Families of children with autism: A synthesis of family routines literature. *Journal of Occupational Science, 21*(3), 322–333.

Bradley, E., Caldwell, P., & Korossy, M. (2015). "Nothing about us without us": Understanding mental health and mental distress in individuals with intellectual and developmental disabilities and autism through their inclusion, participation, and unique ways of communicating. In J. V. M. Welie (Ed.), *Caring for persons with intellectual and developmental disabilities. Ethical and religious perspectives* (pp. 94–109). Retrieved from https://dspace2.creighton.edu/xmlui/bitstream/handle/10504/65683/2015-32.pdf

Bronfenbrenner, U. (1986). Ecology of the family as a context for human development research perspectives. *Developmental Psychology, 22,* 723–742.

Bumble, J. L., Carter, E. W., McMillan, E. D., & Manikas, A. S. (2017). Using community conversations to expand employment opportunities of people with disabilities in rural and urban communities. *Journal of Vocational Rehabilitation, 47*(1), 65–78.

Burgstahler, S. (2015). Opening doors or slamming them shut? Online learning practices and students with disabilities. *Social Inclusion, 3*(6), 69–79.

Burke, M. M., Patton, K. A., & Taylor, J. L. (2016). Family support: A review of the literature on families of adolescents with disabilities. *Journal of Family Social Work, 19*(4), 252–285.

Byrne, G. (2017). Prevalence and psychological sequelae of sexual abuse among individuals with an intellectual disability: A review of the recent literature. *Journal of Intellectual Disabilities.* Advanced online publication. doi:10.1177/1744629517698844

Carlsson, E., Miniscalco, C., Kadesjö, B., & Laakso, K. (2016). Negotiating knowledge: Parents' experience of the neuropsychiatric diagnostic process for children with autism. *International Journal of Language & Communication Disorders, 51*(3), 328–338.

Carr, A. (2014). The evidence base for couple therapy, family therapy and systemic interventions for adult-focused problems. *Journal of Family Therapy, 36*(2), 158–194.

Carr, A., & O'Reilly, G. (2016). Lifespan development and the family lifecycle. In A. Carr, C. Linehan, G. O'Reilly, P. Walsh, & J. McEvoy (Eds.), *The handbook of intellectual disability and clinical psychology practice* (2nd ed., pp. 45–77). New York, NY: Routledge.

Carrillo, V. (2012). *Growing up with autism: The sibling experience* (Doctoral dissertation). California State University, Long Beach, CA. Retrieved from https://search.proquest.com/openview/47b4ddf38eaa8106cb648c26a6976d60/1?pq-rigsite=gscholar&cbl=18750&diss=y

Carrington, S., Campbell, M., Saggers, B., Ashburner, J., Vicig, F., Dillon-Wallace, J., & Hwang, Y. S. (2017). Recommendations of school students with autism spectrum disorder and their parents in regard to bullying and cyberbullying prevention and intervention. *International Journal of Inclusive Education, 21*(6), 1045–1064.

Carter, E. W., Austin, D., & Trainor, A. A. (2012). Predictors of postschool employment outcomes for young adults with severe disabilities. *Journal of Disability Policy Studies, 23*(1), 50–63.

Centers for Disease Control and Prevention. (n.d.). *Tips for talking with parents about developmental concerns.* Retrieved from cdc.gov/ncbddd/actearly/parents/states.html

Chai, Z., & Lieberman-Betz, R. (2016). Strategies for helping parents of young children address challenging behaviors in the home. *Teaching Exceptional Children, 48*(4), 186–194.

Chiu, Y. N., Chou, M. C., Lee, J. C., Wong, C. C., Chou, W. J., Wu, Y. Y., . . . Gau, S. S. F. (2014). Determinants of maternal satisfaction with diagnosis disclosure of autism. *Journal of the Formosan Medical Association, 113*(8), 540–548.

Christensen, L., Baker, B. L., & Blacher, J. (2013). Oppositional defiant disorder in children with intellectual disabilities. *Journal of Mental Health Research in Intellectual Disabilities, 6*(3), 225–244.

Coleby, M. (1995). The school-aged siblings of children with disabilities. *Developmental Medicine and Child Neurology, 37,* 415–426.

Corcoran, J., Berry, A., & Hill, S. (2015). The lived experience of US parents of children with autism spectrum disorders: A systematic review and meta-synthesis. *Journal of Intellectual Disabilities, 19*(4), 356–366.

Coughlin, M. B., & Sethares, K. A. (2017). Chronic sorrow in parents of children with a chronic illness or disability: An integrative literature review. *Journal of Pediatric Nursing, 37,* 108–116.

Cridland, E. K., Jones, S. C., Stoyles, G., Caputi, P., & Magee, C. A. (2016). Families living with autism spectrum disorder: Roles and responsibilities of adolescent sisters. *Focus on Autism and Other Developmental Disabilities, 31*(3), 196–207.

Crnic, K. A., Neece, C. L., McIntyre, L. L., Blacher, J., & Baker, B. L. (2017). Intellectual disability and developmental risk: Promoting intervention to improve child and family well-being. *Child Development, 88*(2), 436–445.

Cumming, T., & Wong, S. (2015). Changing and sustaining transdisciplinary practice through research partnerships. In P. Gibbs (Ed.), *Transdisciplinary professional learning and practice* (pp. 25–39). New York, NY: Springer International Publishing.

Cummings, K. P., Sills-Busio, D., Barker, A. F., & Dobbins, N. (2015). Parent–professional partnerships in early education: Relationships for effective inclusion of students with disabilities. *Journal of Early Childhood Teacher Education, 36*(4), 309–323.

Cunningham, B. J., & Rosenbaum, P. L. (2014). Measure of processes of care: A review of 20 years of research. *Developmental Medicine & Child Neurology, 56*(5), 445–452.

D'Eloia, M. H., & Price, P. (2016). Sense of belonging: Is inclusion the answer? *Sport in Society, 21*(1), 91–105.

Diamond, K. E., & Hong, S. Y. (2010). Young children's decisions to include peers with physical disabilities in play. *Journal of Early Intervention, 32*(3), 163–177.

Dunst, C. J., Jenkins, V., & Trivette, C. (1984). Family Support Scale: Reliability and validity. *Journal of Individual, Family, and Community Wellness, 1*(4), 45–52.

Dunst, C. J., Trivette, C. M., & Hamby, D. W. (2007). Meta-analysis of family-centered helpgiving practices research. *Developmental Disabilities Research Reviews, 13*(4), 370–378.

Dykens, E. M., Fisher, M. H., Taylor, J. L., Lambert, W., & Miodrag, N. (2014). Reducing distress in mothers of children with autism and other disabilities: A randomized trial. *Pediatrics, 134*(2), e454–e463.

Ellis, K., & Goggin, G. (2015). Disability media participation: Opportunities, obstacles and politics. *Media International Australia, 154*(1), 78–88.

Ello, L. M., & Donovan, S. J. (2005). Assessment of the relationship between parenting stress and a child's ability to functionally communicate. *Research on Social Work Practice, 15*(6), 531–544.

Emerson, E., Einfeld, S., & Stancliffe, R. J. (2010). The mental health of young children with intellectual disabilities or borderline functioning. *Social Psychiatry and Psychiatric Epidemiology, 45*(5), 579–587.

Emerson, E., & Robertson, J. (2010). Obesity in young children with intellectual disabilities or borderline intellectual functioning. *International Journal on Pediatric Obesity, 5*(4), 320–326.

Euser, S., Alink, L. R., Tharner, A., IJzendoorn, M. H., & Bakermans-Kranenburg, M. J. (2016). The prevalence of child sexual abuse in out-of-home care: Increased risk for children with a mild intellectual disability. *Journal of Applied Research in Intellectual Disabilities, 29*(1), 83–92.

Farber, M., & Maharaj, R. (2005). Empowering high-risk families of children with disabilities. *Research on Social Work Practice, 15*(6), 501–515.

Feniger-Schaal, R., & Oppenheim, D. (2013). Resolution of the diagnosis and maternal sensitivity among mothers of children with intellectual disability. *Research in Developmental Disabilities, 34*(1), 306–313.

Findler, L. (2016). Being a grandparent of a child with a disability. In L. Findler & O. Taubman (Eds.), *Grandparents of children with disabilities* (pp. 39–67). New York, NY: Springer International Publishing.

Gallagher, S., & Hannigan, A. (2014). Depression and chronic health conditions in parents of children with and without developmental disabilities: The Growing Up in Ireland cohort study. *Research in Developmental Disabilities, 35*(2), 448–454.

Gatmaitan, M., & Brown, T. (2016). Quality in individualized family service plans: Guidelines for practitioners, programs, and families. *Young Exceptional Children, 19*(2), 14–32.

Giallo, R., & Gavidia-Payne, S. (2006). Child, parent, and family factors as predictors of adjustment for siblings of children with disability. *Journal of Intellectual Disability and Research, 50*, 937–948.

Giallo, R., Gavidia-Payne, S., Minett, B., & Kapoor, A. (2012). Sibling voices: The self-reported mental health of siblings of children with a disability. *Clinical Psychologist, 16*, 36–43.

Gips, J., Zhang, M., & Anderson, D. (2015). Towards a Google Glass based head control communication system for people with disabilities. In C. Stephanidis (Ed.), *The 17th International Conference on Human-Computer Interaction* [Posters' Extended Abstracts] (pp. 399–404). New York, NY: Springer International Publishing. Retrieved from http://www.cs.bc.edu/~gips/GipsZhangAndersonHCI2015withAddendum.pdf

Goldstein, P., & Ault, M. J. (2015). Including individuals with disabilities in a faith community: A framework and example. *Journal of Disability & Religion, 19*(1), 1–14.

Goodwin, D. L., Lieberman, L. J., Johnston, K., & Leo, J. (2011). Connecting through summer camp: Youth with visual impairments find a sense of community. *Adapted Physical Activity Quarterly, 28*(1), 40–55.

Gordon, J. (2009). An evidence-based approach for supporting parents experiencing chronic sorrow. *Pediatric Nursing, 35*(2), 115–119.

Green, S. A., Berkovits, L. D., & Baker, B. L. (2015). Symptoms and development of anxiety in children with or without intellectual disability. *Journal of Clinical Child & Adolescent Psychology, 44*(1), 137–144.

Gundersen, T. (2011). 'One wants to know what a chromosome is': The Internet as a coping resource when adjusting to life parenting a child with a rare genetic disorder. *Sociology of Health & Illness, 33*(1), 81–95.

Guralnick, M. J., & Bruder, M. B. (2016). Early childhood inclusion in the United States: Goals, current status, and future directions. *Infants & Young Children, 29*(3), 166–177.

Hall, H. R., & Graff, J. C. (2011). The relationships among adaptive behaviors of children with autism, family support, parenting stress, and coping. *Issues in Comprehensive Pediatric Nursing, 34*(1), 4–25.

Hanson, M. J., & Lynch, E. W. (2013). *Understanding families: Supportive approaches to diversity, disability, and risk* (2nd ed.). Baltimore, MD: Paul H. Brookes Publishing.

Harris, S. L., & Bruey, C. T. (2015). Families of the developmentally disabled. In I. R. H. Falloon (Ed.), *Handbook of behavioural family therapy* (pp. 181–190). New York, NY: Routledge.

Hartling, L., Milne, A., Tjosvold, L., Wrightson, D., Gallivan, J., & Newton, A. S. (2014). A systematic review of interventions to support siblings of children with chronic illness or disability. *Journal of Paediatrics and Child Health, 50*(10), E26–E38. doi:10.1111/j.1440-1754.2010.01771.x

Heiman, T., & Berger, O. (2008). Parents of children with Asperger syndrome or with learning disabilities: Family environment and social support. *Research in Developmental Disabilities, 29*(4), 289–300.

Henderson, K., Whitaker, L., Bialeschki, M., Scanlin, M., & Thurber, C. (2007). Summer camp experiences. *Journal of Family Issues, 28*(8), 987–1007.

Henninger, N. A., & Taylor, J. L. (2013). Outcomes in adults with autism spectrum disorders: A historical perspective. *Autism, 17*(1), 103–116.

Henninger, N. A., & Taylor, J. L. (2014). Family perspectives on a successful transition to adulthood for individuals with disabilities. *Mental Retardation, 52*(2), 98–111.

Hernandez, E. J., Brodwin, M. G., & Siu, F. W. (2017). Bullying, students with disabilities, and recommendations for prevention of bullying. *Rehabilitation Professional, 25*(1), 51–57.

Hiebert-Murphy, D., Trute, B., & Wright, A. (2011). Parents' definition of effective child disability support services: Implications for implementing family-centered practice. *Journal of Family Social Work, 14*(2), 144–158.

Hillis, R., Brenner, M., Larkin, P., Cawley, D., & Connolly, M. (2016). The role of care coordinator for children with complex care needs: A systematic review. *International Journal of Integrated Care, 16*(2), 12.

Hinton, S., Sheffield, J., Sanders, M. R., & Sofronoff, K. (2017). A randomized controlled trial of a telehealth parenting intervention: A mixed-disability trial. *Research in Developmental Disabilities, 65*, 74–85.

Hodapp, R. M., Sanderson, K. A., Meskis, S. A., & Casale, E. G. (2017). Adult siblings of persons with intellectual disabilities: Past, present, and future. In R. M. Hoddap & D. J. Fiddler (Eds.), *International review of research in developmental disabilities* (Vol. 53, pp. 163–202). Cambridge, MA: Academic Press.

Hoffman, L., Marquis, J., Poston, D., Summers, J. A., & Turnbull, A. (2006). Assessing family outcomes: Psychometric evaluation of the Beach Center Family Quality of Life Scale. *Journal of Marriage and Family, 68*(4), 1069–1083.

Hong, S. Y., Kwon, K. A., & Jeon, H. J. (2014). Children's attitudes towards peers with disabilities: Associations with personal and parental factors. *Infant and Child Development, 23*(2), 170–193.

Horsley, S., & Oliver, C. (2015). Positive impact and its relationship to well-being in parents of children with intellectual disability: A literature review. *International Journal of Developmental Disabilities, 61*(1), 1–19.

Individuals with Disabilities Education Improvement Act of 2004, PL 108-446, 20 U.S.C. §§ 1400 *et seq.*

Informing Families Project. (2018). *Appropriate, accurate information.* Retrieved from http://www.informingfamilies.ie/information-for-professionals.10.html

Jin, J., Yun, J., & Agiovlasitis, S. (2018). Impact of enjoyment on physical activity and health among children with disabilities in schools. *Disability and Health Journal, 11*(1), 14–19.

Ju, S., Zeng, W., & Landmark, L. J. (2017). Self-determination and academic success of students with disabilities in postsecondary education: A review. *Journal of Disability Policy Studies, 28*(3), 180–189.

Kazak, A., Kassam-Adams, N., Schneider, S., Zelikovsky, N., Alderfer, M., & Rourke, M. (2005). An integrative model of pediatric medical traumatic stress. *Journal of Pediatric Psychology, 31*(4), 343–355.

King, G., & Chiarello, L. (2014). Family-centered care for children with cerebral palsy: Conceptual and practical considerations to advance care and practice. *Journal of Child Neurology, 29*(8), 1046–1054.

Klinger, J., Blanchett, W., & Harry, B. (2007). Race, culture, and developmental disabilities. In S. L. Odom, R. H. Horner, M. E. Snell, & J. Blacher (Eds.), *Handbook of developmental disabilities* (pp. 55–75). New York, NY: Guilford.

Kolomer, S. (2008). Grandparents as caregivers. *Journal of Gerontological Social Work, 50*(1), 321–344.

Kramer, J., Hall, A., & Heller, T. (2013). Reciprocity and social capital in sibling relationships of people with disabilities. *Mental Retardation, 51*(6), 482–495.

Kresak, K. E., Gallagher, P. A., & Kelley, S. J. (2014). Grandmothers raising grandchildren with disabilities: Sources of support and family quality of life. *Journal of Early Intervention, 36*(1), 3–17.

Kuo, M. H., Orsmond, G. I., Coster, W. J., & Cohn, E. S. (2014). Media use among adolescents with autism spectrum disorder. *Autism, 18*(8), 914–923.

Lalvani, P. (2015). Disability, stigma and otherness: Perspectives of parents and teachers. *International Journal of Disability, Development and Education, 62*(4), 379–393.

Landmark, L. J., Ju, S., & Zhang, D. (2010). Substantiated best practices in transition: Fifteen plus years later. *Career Development for Exceptional Individuals, 33*(3), 165–176.

Law, R. (2011). Interpersonal psychotherapy for depression. *Advances in Psychiatric Treatment, 17*(1), 23–31.

Lee, M., & Gardner, J. (2010). Grandparents' involvement and support in families with children with disabilities. *Educational Gerontology, 36*(6), 467–499.

Leffert, J. S., Siperstein, G. N., & Widaman, K. F. (2010). Social perception in children with intellectual disabilities: The interpretation of benign and hostile intentions. *Journal of Intellectual Disability Research, 54*(2), 168–180.

Leonard, H., Foley, K. R., Pikora, T., Bourke, J., Wong, K., McPherson, L., . . . & Downs, J. (2016). Transition to adulthood for young people with intellectual disability: The experiences of their families. *European Child & Adolescent Psychiatry, 25*(12), 1369–1381.

Lesack, R., Bears, K., Celano, M., & Sharp, W. G. (2014). Parent–child interaction therapy and autism spectrum disorder: Adaptations with a child with severe developmental delays. *Clinical Practice in Pediatric Psychology, 2*(1), 68–82.

Lindsay, S., & Hoffman, A. (2015). A complex transition: Lessons learned as three young adults with complex care needs transition from an inpatient paediatric hospital to adult community residences. *Child: Care, Health and Development, 41*(3), 397–407.

Lobato, D. J., & Kao, B. T. (2005). Brief report: Family-based group intervention for young siblings of children with chronic illness and developmental disability. *Pediatric Psychology, 30*(8), 678–682.

Maart, S., & Jelsma, J. (2010). The sexual behaviour of physically disabled adolescents. *Disability and Rehabilitation, 32*(6), 438–443.

Mackelprang, R. W., & Salsgiver, R. (2016). *A diversity model approach in human service practice* (3rd ed.). Chicago, IL: Lyceum.

Macks, R. J., & Reeve, R. E. (2007). The adjustment of non-disabled siblings of children with autism. *Journal of Autism and Developmental Disorders, 37,* 1060–1067.

Madeo, A. C., O'Brien, K. E., Bernhardt, B. A., & Biesecker, B. B. (2012). Factors associated with perceived uncertainty among parents of children with undiagnosed medical conditions. *American Journal of Medical Genetics Part A, 158*(8), 1877–1884.

Magaña, S., Parish, S. L., & Son, E. (2015). Have racial and ethnic disparities in the quality of health care relationships changed for children with developmental disabilities and ASD? *American Journal on Intellectual and Developmental Disabilities, 120*(6), 504–513.

Marshak, L. E., & Prezant, F. (2007). *Married with special needs children: A couple's guide to keeping connected.* Bethesda, MD: Woodbine House.

McConnell, D., Savage, A., Sobsey, D., & Uditsky, B. (2015). Benefit-finding or finding benefits? The positive impact of having a disabled child. *Disability & Society, 30*(1), 29–45.

McGillivray, J., McVilly, K., Skouteris, H., & Boganin, C. (2013). Parental factors associated with obesity in children with disability: a systematic review. *Obesity Reviews, 14*(7), 541–554.

McHale, S. M., Updegraff, K. A., & Feinberg, M. E. (2016). Siblings of youth with autism spectrum disorders: Theoretical perspectives on sibling relationships and individual adjustment. *Journal of Autism and Developmental Disorders, 46*(2), 589–602.

Miller, E., Buys, L., & Woodbridge, S. (2012). Impact of disability on families: Grandparents' perspectives. *Journal of Intellectual Disability Research, 56*(1), 102–110.

Mitchell, D. B., & Hauser-Cram, P. (2010). Early childhood predictors of mothers' and fathers' relationships with adolescents with developmental disabilities. *Journal of Intellectual Disabilities Research, 54*(6), 487–500.

Mitchell, C., & Holdt, N. (2014). The search for a timely diagnosis: Parents' experiences of their child being diagnosed with an autistic spectrum disorder. *Journal of Child & Adolescent Mental Health, 26*(1), 49–62.

Moskowitz, L. J., Walsh, C. E., Mulder, E., McLaughlin, D. M., Hajcak, G., Carr, E. G., & Zarcone, J. R. (2017). Intervention for anxiety and problem behavior in children with autism spectrum disorder and intellectual disability. *Journal of Autism and Developmental Disorders, 47*(12), 3930–3948.

Munford, R. (2016). Building strengths and resilience: Supporting families and disabled children. In C. DeMichelis & M. Ferrari (Eds.), *Child and adolescent resilience within medical contexts* (pp. 227–245). New York, NY: Springer International Publishing.

Munro, M. P., Garza, M. M., Hayes, J. R., & Watt, E. A. (2016). Parental perceptions of independence and efficacy of their children with visual impairments. *Journal of Human Services: Training, Research, and Practice, 1*(1), 1–29.

Myck-Wayne, J. (2010). In defense of play: Beginning the dialog about the power of play. *Young Exceptional Children, 13*(4), 14–23.

Myers, B. J., Mackintosh, V. H., & Goin-Kochel, R. P. (2009). "My greatest joy and my greatest heart ache": Parents' own words on how having a child in the autism spectrum has affected their lives and their families' lives. *Research in Autism Spectrum Disorders, 3*(3), 670–684.

National Center for Medical Home Implementation. (n.d.). *Family-centered medical home overview.* Retrieved from http://www.medicalhomeinfo.org/about/medical_home

National Early Childhood Technical Assistance Center. (n.d.). *NECTAC: The National Early Childhood Technical Assistance Center.* Retrieved from http://www.nectac.org

Neece, C. L., & Chan, N. (2017). The stress of parenting children with developmental disabilities. In K. Deater-Deckard & R. Panneton (Eds.), *Parental stress and early child development* (pp. 107–124). New York, NY: Springer International Publishing.

Neff, K. D., & Faso, D. J. (2015). Self-compassion and well-being in parents of children with autism. *Mindfulness, 6*(4), 938–947.

Noonan, M. J., & McCormick, L. (2013). *Teaching young children with disabilities in natural environments.* Baltimore: MD, Paul H. Brookes Publishing Company.

Oberleitner, R., Wurtz, R., Popovich, M. L., Fiedler, R., Moncher, T., Laxminarayan, S., & Reischl, U. (2011). HealthiInformatics: A roadmap for autism knowledge sharing. In L. Bos, D. Carroll, L. Kun, A. Marsh, & L. Roa (Eds.), *Future visions on biomedicine and bioinformatics 2. Medical care and compunetics 2* (pp. 321–326). Berlin/Heidelberg, Germany: Springer.

Odom, S. L., Buysse, V., & Soukakou, E. (2011). Inclusion for young children with disabilities: A quarter century of research perspectives. *Journal of Early Intervention, 33*(4), 344–356.

Orsmond, G., & Seltzer, M. (2009). Adolescent siblings of individuals with an autism spectrum disorder: Testing a diathesis-stress model of sibling well-being. *Journal of Autism and Developmental Disorders, 39*(7), 1053–1065.

Overmars-Marx, T., Thomése, F., Verdonschot, M., & Meininger, H. (2014). Advancing social inclusion in the neighbourhood for people with an intellectual disability: An exploration of the literature. *Disability & Society, 29*(2), 255–274.

Park, S. Y., Cervesi, C., Galling, B., Molteni, S., Walyzada, F., Ameis, S. H., . . . Correll, C. U. (2016). Antipsychotic use trends in youth with autism spectrum disorder and/or intellectual disability: A meta-analysis. *Journal of the American Academy of Child & Adolescent Psychiatry, 55*(6), 456–468.

Petrenko, C. L. (2015). Positive behavioral interventions and family support for fetal alcohol spectrum disorders. *Current Developmental Disorders Reports, 2*(3), 199–209.

Pickard, K. E., & Ingersoll, B. R. (2017). Using the double ABCX model to integrate services for families of children with ASD. *Journal of Child and Family Studies, 26*(3), 810–823.

Platt, C., Roper, S. O., Mandleco, B., & Freeborn, D. (2014). Sibling cooperative and externalizing behaviors in families raising children with disabilities. *Nursing Research, 63*(4), 235–242.

Pleet-Odle, A., Aspel, N., Leuchovius, D., Roy, S., Hawkins, C., Jennings, D., . . . Test, D. W. (2016). Promoting high expectations for postschool success by family members: A "to-do" list for professionals. *Career Development and Transition for Exceptional Individuals, 39*(4), 249–255.

Raising Children Network. (2018). *Routines and children with disability.* Retrieved from https://raisingchildren.net.au/disability/family-life/family-management/routines-disability

Rattaz, C., Michelon, C., Roeyers, H., & Baghdadli, A. (2017). Quality of life in parents of young adults with ASD: EpiTED cohort. *Journal of Autism and Developmental Disorders, 47,* 2826–2837.

Ray, J., Pewitt-Kinder, J., & George, S. (2009). Partnering with families of children with special needs. *Young Children, 64*(5), 16–22.

Rehm, R., & Bradley, J. (2005). Normalization in families raising a child who is medically fragile/technology dependent and developmentally delayed. *Qualitative Health Research, 15*(6), 807–820.

Reichman, N., Corman, H., & Noonan, K. (2008). Impact of child disability on the family. *Maternal and Child Health Journal, 12*(6), 679–683.

Resch, J. A., Elliott, T. R., & Benz, M. R. (2012). Depression among parents of children with disabilities. *Families, Systems, & Health, 30*(4), 291–301.

Rimmer, J. H. (2017). Equity in active living for people with disabilities: Less talk and more action. *Preventive Medicine, 95,* S154–S156.

Rimmer, J. H., Rowland, J. L., & Yamaki, K. (2007). Obesity and secondary conditions in adolescents with disabilities. Addressing the needs of an underserved population. *Journal of Adolescent Health, 41*(3), 224–229.

Rivard, M. T., & Mastel-Smith, B. (2014). The lived experience of fathers whose children are diagnosed with a genetic disorder. *Journal of Obstetric, Gynecologic, & Neonatal Nursing, 43*(1), 38–49.

Roberts, C. S., & Feetham, S. L. (1982). Assessing family functioning across three areas of relationships. *Nursing Research, 31*(4), 231–235.

Rodas, N. V., Zeedyk, S. M., & Baker, B. L. (2016). Unsupportive parenting and internalising behaviour problems in children with or without intellectual disability. *Journal of Intellectual Disability Research, 60*(12), 1200–1211.

Rogers, L., Hemmeter, M., & Wolery, M. (2010). Using a constant time delay procedure to teach foundational swimming skills to children with autism. *Topics in Early Childhood Special Education, 30*(2), 102–111.

Rosenkoetter, S. E., Hains, A. H., & Dogaru, C. (2007). Successful transitions for young children with disabilities and their families: Roles of school social workers. *Children & Schools, 29*(1), 25–34.

Rowsell, A. C., Clare, I. C., & Murphy, G. H. (2013). The psychological impact of abuse on men and women with severe intellectual disabilities. *Journal of Applied Research in Intellectual Disabilities, 26*(4), 257–270.

Ryan, C., & Quinlan, E. (2018). Whoever shouts the loudest: Listening to parents of children with disabilities. *Journal of Applied Research in Intellectual Disabilities, 31*(52), 203–214.

Schuntermann, P. (2009). Growing up with a developmentally challenged brother or sister: A model for engaging siblings based on mentalizing. *Harvard Review of Psychiatry, 17*(5), 297–314.

Schwichtenberg, A. J., Young, G. S., Sigman, M., Hutman, T., & Ozonoff, S. (2010). Can family affectedness inform infant sibling outcomes of autism spectrum disorders? *Journal of Child Psychology and Psychiatry, 51*(9), 1021–1030.

Seligman, M., & Darling, R. B. (2007). *Ordinary families, special children: A systems approach to childhood disability* (3rd ed.). New York, NY: Guilford.

Seltzer, M. M., Floyd, F., Song, J., Greenberg, J., & Hong, J. (2011). Midlife and aging parents of adults with intellectual and developmental disabilities: Impacts of lifelong parenting. *American Journal on Intellectual and Developmental Disabilities, 116*(6), 479–499.

Settersten, Jr., R. A., & Ray, B. (2010). What's going on with young people today? The long and twisting path to adulthood. *The Future of Children, 20*(1), 19–41.

Siman-Tov, A., & Kaniel, S. (2011). Stress and personal resource as predictors of the adjustment of parents to autistic children: A multivariate model. *Journal of Autism and Developmental Disorders, 41*, 879–890.

Simplican, S., Leader, G., Kosciulek, J., & Leahy, M. (2015). Defining social inclusion of people with intellectual and developmental disabilities: An ecological model of social networks and community participation. *Research in Developmental Disabilities, 38*, 18–29.

Singer, G. H., Ethridge, B. L., & Aldana, S. I. (2007). Primary and secondary effects of parenting and stress management interventions for parents of children with developmental disabilities: A meta-analysis. *Developmental Disabilities Research Reviews, 13*(4), 357–369.

Singh, N. N., Curtis, W. J., Ellis, C. R., Nicholson, M. W., Villani, T. M., & Wechsler, H. A. (1995). Psychometric analysis of the Family Empowerment Scale. *Journal of Emotional and Behavioral Disorders, 3*(2), 85–91.

Singh, N. N., Lancioni, G. E., Winton, A. S., Karazsia, B. T., Myers, R. E., Latham, L. L., & Singh, J. (2014). Mindfulness-based positive behavior support (MBPBS) for mothers of adolescents with autism spectrum disorder: Effects on adolescents' behavior and parental stress. *Mindfulness, 5*(6), 646–657.

Siperstein, G., Glick, G., & Parker, R. (2009). Social inclusion of children with intellectual disabilities in a recreational setting. *Intellectual and Developmental Disabilities, 47*(2), 97–107.

Skotarczak, L., & Lee, G. K. (2015). Effects of parent management training programs on disruptive behavior for children with a developmental disability: A meta-analysis. *Research in Developmental Disabilities, 38*, 272–287.

Skotko, B. G., Capone, G. T., & Kishnani, P. S. (2009). Postnatal diagnosis of Down syndrome: Synthesis of the evidence on how best to deliver the news. *Pediatrics, 124*(4), e751–e758.

Sood, D., Szymanski, M., & Schranz, C. (2015). Enriched home environment program for preschool children with autism spectrum disorders. *Journal of Occupational Therapy, Schools, & Early Intervention, 8*(1), 40–55.

Stalker, K., Taylor, J., Fry, D., & Stewart, A. B. (2015). A study of disabled children and child protection in Scotland—a hidden group? *Children and Youth Services Review, 56*, 126–134.

Stewart, D., Law, M., Young, N. L., Forhan, M., Healy, H., Burke-Gaffney, J., & Freeman, M. (2014). Complexities during transitions to adulthood for youth with disabilities: Person–environment interactions. *Disability and Rehabilitation, 36*(23), 1998–2004.

Stewart, M., McGillivray, J. A., Forbes, D., & Austin, D. W. (2017). Parenting a child with an autism spectrum disorder: A review of parent mental health and its relationship to a trauma-based conceptualization. *Advances in Mental Health, 15*(1), 4–14.

Stoneman, Z. (2005). Siblings of children with disabilities: Research themes. *Mental Retardation, 43*(5), 339–350.

Taeyoung, K., & Horn, E. (2010). Sibling-implemented intervention for skill development with children with disabilities. *Topics in Early Childhood Special Education, 30*(2), 80–90.

Tellegen, C. L., & Sanders, M. R. (2013). Stepping Stones Triple P-Positive Parenting Program for children with disability: A systematic review and meta-analysis. *Research in Developmental Disabilities, 34*(5), 1556–1571.

Tint, A., & Weiss, J. A. (2016). Family wellbeing of individuals with autism spectrum disorder: A scoping review. *Autism, 20*(3), 262–275.

Toly, V. B., Musil, C. M., & Carl, J. C. (2012). A longitudinal study of families with technology-dependent children. *Research in Nursing & Health, 35*(1), 40–54.

Tomeny, T. S., Baker, L. K., Barry, T. D., Eldred, S. W., & Rankin, J. A. (2016). Emotional and behavioral functioning of typically-developing sisters of children with autism spectrum disorder: The roles of ASD severity, parental stress, and marital status. *Research in Autism Spectrum Disorders, 32*, 130–142.

Trivette, C., Dunst, C., Deal, A., Hamer, A., & Propst, S. (1990). Assessing family strengths and family functioning style. *Topics in Early Childhood Special Education, 10*(1), 16–35.

Tudor, M. E., Rankin, J., & Lerner, M. D. (2018). A model of family and child functioning in siblings of youth with autism spectrum disorder. *Journal of Autism and Developmental Disorders, 48*(4), 1210–1227.

Turnbull, A. A., Turnbull, H. R., Erwin, E. J., Soodak, L. C., & Shogren, K. A. (2015). *Families, professionals, and exceptionality: Positive outcomes through partnerships and trust* (7th ed.). New York, NY: Pearson.

Valicenti-McDermott, M., Lawson, K., Hottinger, K., Seijo, R., Schechtman, M., Shulman, L., & Shinnar, S. (2015). Parental stress in families of children with autism and other developmental disabilities. *Journal of Child Neurology, 30*(13), 1728–1735.

van der Stege, H. A., Hilberink, S. R., Visser, A. P., & Van Staa, A. (2014). Motivational factors in discussing sexual health with young people with chronic conditions or disabilities. *Sex Education, 14*(6), 635–651.

van der Veek, S., Kraaij, V., & Garnefski, N. (2009). Down or up? Explaining positive and negative emotions in parents of children with Down syndrome: Goals, cognitive coping, and resources. *Journal of Intellectual and Developmental Disabilities, 34*(3), 216–229.

Vasilopoulou, E., & Nisbet, J. (2016). The quality of life of parents of children with autism spectrum disorder: A systematic review. *Research in Autism Spectrum Disorders, 23*, 36–49.

Vohra, R., Madhavan, S., Sambamoorthi, U., & St. Peter, C. (2014). Access to services, quality of care, and family impact for children with autism, other developmental disabilities, and other mental health conditions. *Autism, 18*(7), 815–826.

Vonneilich, N., Lüdecke, D., & Kofahl, C. (2016). The impact of care on family and health-related quality of life of parents with chronically ill and disabled children. *Disability and Rehabilitation, 38*(8), 761–767.

Vora, K. S. (2016). Family members as caregivers of individuals with intellectual disabilities: Caregiving for individuals with intellectual disabilities. In R. T. Gopalan (Ed.), *Handbook of research on diagnosing, treating, and managing intellectual disabilities* (pp. 118–138). Hershey, PA: IGI Global.

Vuorenmaa, M., Halme, N., Åstedt-Kurki, P., Kaunonen, M., & Perälä, M. L. (2014). The validity and reliability of the Finnish Family Empowerment Scale (FES): A survey of parents with small children. *Child: Care, Health and Development, 40*(4), 597–606.

Walsh, F. (2015). *Strengthening family resilience.* New York, NY: Guilford.

Walton, K. M., & Ingersoll, B. R. (2015). Psychosocial adjustment and sibling relationships in siblings of children with autism spectrum disorder: Risk and protective factors. *Journal of Autism and Developmental Disorders, 45*(9), 2764–2778.

Wang, M., & Singer, G. H. (2016). *Supporting families of children with developmental disabilities: Evidence-based and emerging practices.* Oxford, England: Oxford University Press.

Ward, B., Tanner, B. S., Mandleco, B., Dyches, T. T., & Freeborn, D. (2016). Sibling experiences: Living with young persons with autism spectrum disorders. *Pediatric Nursing, 42*(2), 69–76.

Watson, S. L., Hayes, S. A., & Radford-Paz, E. (2011). Diagnose me please! A review of research about the journey and initial impact of parents seeking a diagnosis of developmental disability for their child. *International Review of Research in Developmental Disabilities, 41,* 31–72.

Webb, R., Greco, V., Sloper, P., & Beecham, J. (2008). Key workers and schools: Meeting the needs of children and young people with disabilities. *European Journal of Special Needs Education, 23*(3), 189–205.

Wehmeyer, M. L., Brown, I., Percey, M., Shogren, K. A., & Fung, W. L. A. (2017). *A comprehensive guide to intellectual and developmental disabilities.* Baltimore, MD: Paul H. Brookes.

Werner, S., & Shulman, C. (2015). Does type of disability make a difference in affiliate stigma among family caregivers of individuals with autism, intellectual disability or physical disability? *Journal of Intellectual Disability Research, 59*(3), 272–283.

White, S. E. (2009). The influence of religiosity on well-being and acceptance in parents of children with autism spectrum disorder. *Journal of Religion, Disability & Health, 13*(2), 104–113.

Wieland, N., & Baker, B. (2010). The role of marital quality and spousal support in behaviour problems of children with and without intellectual disability. *Journal of Intellectual Disability Research, 54*(7), 620–633.

Willner, P. (2015). The neurobiology of aggression: Implications for the pharmacotherapy of aggressive challenging behaviour by people with intellectual disabilities. *Journal of Intellectual Disability Research, 59*(1), 82–92.

Wilson, N. J., & Frawley, P. (2016). Transition staff discuss sex education and support for young men and women with intellectual and developmental disability. *Journal of Intellectual & Developmental Disability, 41*(3), 209–221.

Woodman, A. C., & Hauser-Cram, P. (2013). The role of coping strategies in predicting change in parenting efficacy and depressive symptoms among mothers of adolescents with developmental disabilities. *Journal of Intellectual Disability Research, 57*(6), 513–530.

Wright, A. (2013). Managing the successful implementation of family centered care. In B. Trute & D. Hiebert-Murphy (Eds.), *Partnering with parents: Family-centered care practices in children's services* (pp. 287–310). Toronto, Canada: University of Toronto Press.

Wright, A., Hiebert-Murphy, D., & Trute, B. (2010). Professionals' perspectives on organizational factors that support or hinder the successful implementation of family-centered practice. *Journal of Family Social Work, 13,* 114–130.

Wynter, K., Hammarberg, K., Sartore, G. M., Cann, W., & Fisher, J. (2015). Brief online surveys to monitor and evaluate facilitated peer support groups for caregivers of children with special needs. *Evaluation and Program Planning, 49,* 70–75.

Xu, Y. (2007). Empowering culturally diverse families of young children with disabilities: The Double ABCX model. *Early Childhood Education Journal, 34*(6), 431–437.

Young, R., Dagnan, D., & Jahoda, A. (2016). Leaving school: a comparison of the worries held by adolescents with and without intellectual disabilities. *Journal of Intellectual Disability Research, 60*(1), 9–21.

Zajicek-Farber, M. L. (1998). Promoting good health in adolescents with disabilities. *Health and Social Work, 23*(3), 203–213.

Zajicek-Farber, M. L., Long, T. M., Lotrecchiano, G. R., Farber, J. M., & Rodkey, E. (2017). Connections between family centered care and medical homes of children with neurodevelopmental disabilities: Experiences of diverse families. *Journal of Child and Family Studies, 26*(5), 1445–1459.

Zajicek-Farber, M. L., Lotrecchiano, G. R., Long, T. M., & Farber, J. M. (2015). Parental perceptions of family centered care in medical homes of children with neurodevelopmental disabilities. *Maternal and Child Health Journal, 19*(8), 1744–1755.

Zajicek-Farber, M. L., Wall, S., Kisker, E., Luze, G. J., & Summers, J. A. (2011). Comparing service use of Early Head Start families of children with and without disabilities. *Journal of Family Social Work, 14*(2), 159–178.

Zuckerman, K. E., Sinche, B., Mejia, A., Cobian, M., Becker, T., & Nicolaidis, C. (2014). Latino parents' perspectives on barriers to autism diagnosis. *Academic Pediatrics, 14*(3), 301–308.

CHAPTER 38 Pharmacological Therapy

Shogo John Miyagi and Johannes N. van den Anker

Upon completion of this chapter, the reader will

- Understand the role of medication in the treatment of children with disabilities
- Be able to describe the factors for consideration when starting medication in children with disabilities
- Advocate for the safe and effective use of medications in children with disabilities
- Appreciate the issues surrounding the use of complementary and alternative medicine

Pharmacotherapy plays an important and vital role in the treatment of children with developmental disabilities. Medications will not cure a child, but they can help to alleviate symptoms associated with the child's condition. Such medications include anti-epileptic drugs for seizures, stimulant medication for attention-deficit/hyperactivity disorder (ADHD), spasticity medication for cerebral palsy, and enzyme replacement therapy for inborn errors of metabolism. There may be multiple medication options for each condition or symptom, but each drug also has associated adverse effects. Some may be serious, such as hepatic failure, whereas others may be less severe, such as drowsiness. In addition, children metabolize and dispose of drugs differently than adults based on their developmental stage. The pediatric population ranges from premature neonates through adolescents and can vary in weight between 0.5 kg to over 100 kg (de Wildt, Tibboel, & Leeder, 2014). Further complicating the use of medication in children is the relative lack of clinical trial studies of drug efficacy, side effects, and proper dosage in children of different ages and medical complexities (Frattarelli et al., 2014). Yet, it is important to be able to balance the risks and benefits associated with each medication prior to starting pharmacotherapy (Elzagallaai, Greff, & Rieder, 2017). This chapter will highlight important factors to consider when initiating drug therapy in children with disabilities. In addition, the chapter will cover techniques and methods to help parents and families ensure optimal drug therapy for their children.

CASE STUDY

Zachary is a 5-year-old boy who is in kindergarten. His mother expresses concern during their annual well-child visit that he has been disruptive in class and is having difficulty paying attention and following directions. She also notes that he started behaving this way during preschool but that she had attributed this to her son being immature. After further evaluation by the physician, it was concluded that Zachary may have ADHD, the inattention subtype. Upon hearing the diagnosis, the mother asks if methylphenidate would help her son because it has "cured" her friend's 14-year-old daughter who had ADHD. The clinician explains to the mother that behavioral therapy is the first-line treatment and most effective in this age group. The mother pushes the clinician, saying that she is a single mother with two other children and it may be difficult to also include behavioral therapy into her busy family schedule; she asks again for a medication option. The clinician stresses that behavioral therapy is the best treatment option for Zachary and that they can reassess his progress in a few months. The mother agrees to the plan and is connected with a behavioral therapist and a school counselor to develop a behavioral management plan for Zachary as part of a 504 program.

CASE STUDY

Isaac is a 6-month-old boy who was born with cerebral palsy resulting from severe hypoxic-ischemic encephalopathy (HIE; see Chapter 21). On his recent clinic visit, his mother mentioned that Isaac seems to make a fist almost constantly and that it is difficult to unbend his knees and arms when changing his clothes or diaper. Upon further examination, Isaac showed signs of spasticity. To help alleviate this symptom, the physician prescribed baclofen 0.2 mg per kg, three times per day orally (the body weight is 5.5 kg for a total dose of 1.1 mg per dose) and asked the mother to return to the clinic within 2 weeks to see if the baclofen had any beneficial effect. Upon returning, the mother stated that baclofen was showing no effect, positive or negative. The physician gradually increased the dose until Isaac's hypertonicity improved; the final dose was 6 mg (1.1 mg per kg per dose) given three times per day. At the next clinic visit, the mother expressed concern that he was getting too much baclofen because the dose was twice what she had found on the Internet to be typical. The physician reassured her that this dose was acceptable for Isaac as long as he was not experiencing any undesired side effects (e.g., drowsiness). Isaac's mother confirmed he had not had any side effects and therefore she continued Isaac on the prescribed baclofen dose.

Thought Questions:

What are additional factors to consider when initiating a medication trial in a child with developmental disabilities? What resources can provide information on medication?

THE ROLE OF MEDICATIONS

Children with developmental disabilities are frequently treated with drugs, often more than one at the same time. Therefore, it is very important to understand the role of medications in this patient population. Children can be treated prophylactically to prevent exacerbations; for example, glycerol phenylbutyrate is used to prevent hyperammonemic episodes in the management of urea cycle disorders (Berry et al., 2017; see Chapter 16). Medications are also used to treat symptoms associated with certain medical conditions; for Isaac, baclofen was used to treat his spasticity caused by cerebral palsy (Goyal, Laisram, Wadhwa, & Kothari, 2016). Both desired and undesired effects of a medication largely depend upon the concentration of the drug at the site of action (e.g., liver, lung, or brain). This is determined by 1) how the drug is absorbed by the gut (e.g., if taken orally), 2) how it is distributed in the body to different tissues, 3) how it is metabolized (i.e., most often via the liver), and 4) how it is eliminated by the body (i.e., most often via the kidneys). In addition, variations among people can also cause differences in drug concentrations. These differences include age, disease, concomitant medications, and genetics (see Factors Impacting Drug Concentrations; de Wildt et al., 2014; Kearns et al., 2003; van den Anker, 2010). The amount of drug needed for clinical effectiveness varies widely between children and adults and requires individualization of dosing regimens.

WHEN TO START MEDICATIONS

The decision to begin medication(s) takes place when nonpharmacological treatments (if available) have been optimized or exhausted. In the case of Zachary, the decision to start medications for his ADHD has been delayed because he had not yet undergone behavioral therapy. When beginning treatment with medication, it is important to understand 1) the treatment goals, 2) the monitoring parameters, and 3) the risks associated with taking the drug. Treatment goals and end points should be established when starting drug therapy and should be evaluated on a periodic basis during treatment; these can include cessation of symptoms (e.g., baclofen to treat spasticity) or prevention of disease symptoms (e.g., levetiracetam to prevent seizures). Medications also need to be monitored; some can be monitored using a basic clinical examination, whereas others require more intense monitoring such as **therapeutic drug monitoring** (the clinical practice of measuring specific drug concentrations in blood samples at designated intervals to ensure a therapeutic concentration in a patient's bloodstream), liver function tests, complete blood counts, and metabolic panels (Gerlach et al., 2016; Kang & Lee, 2009). **Adverse drug reactions (ADRs),** which are an unintended response to a drug that occurs at standard doses used in the treatment or prevention of a specific disease, can also occur. Some ADRs are dose related (e.g., baclofen and drowsiness), and others are paradoxical (e.g., diphenhydramine causing excitability in some children instead of the intended drowsiness). In addition, children are more prone to ADRs than adults due to differences in drug disposition (Elzagallaai et al., 2017; Garon et al., 2017).

When starting medications in children, the general rule of thumb is "start low and go slow" (Pejovic-Milovancevic et al., 2011, p. 315). This means starting drug therapy at the lowest possible dose and then titrating up slowly until the desired effects are seen. This also minimizes the risk of ADRs. The general rule does not apply during critical illness, such as sepsis or status epilepticus, where aggressive and prompt treatment is necessary. A second important point is that when considering starting additional medications, it is important to first optimize current drug therapy because **polypharmacy** (the use of multiple drugs by a single patient to treat one or more conditions) also increases the risk of ADRs (Dai, Feinstein, Morrison, Zuppa, & Feudtner, 2016). Children with disabilities typically take more medications compared with typically developing children. As a result, attention must be paid to maximize the effects of the medication while minimizing the number of prescribed drugs and attendant risk of side effects (Box 38.1). Therefore, it is important to define treatment goals prior to starting medications to ensure effective drug therapy and understand the risk-benefit ratio of the medication.

FACTORS AFFECTING DRUG CONCENTRATIONS

A number of factors can impact drug concentrations and effectiveness, including developmental pharmacology; drug, disease, and food interactions; and pharmacogenomics. Each of these factors is discussed in the sections that follow.

Developmental Pharmacology

Infants and children are inherently different from adults in terms of behavioral and medical perspectives. The developmental changes in children remarkably affect their **pharmacokinetics** (the absorption, distribution, metabolism, and excretion of drugs; i.e., what the body does to the drug) and **pharmacodynamics** (the biochemical and physiological effects of drugs; i.e., what the drug does to the body; de Wildt et al., 2014; Kearns et al., 2003; Mulla, 2010; van den Anker, 2010). Developmental changes in various organ systems that affect pharmacokinetics (e.g., changes in gastric pH, body fat composition, maturation of the gastrointestinal system, changes in drug metabolizing enzymes in the liver, and renal function changes as the child develops) require medications to be periodically adjusted. Pediatric dosing **nomograms** (charts showing scales for drug dosage) are available for many drugs that are broken down by age groups and body weight (Anderson & Holford, 2013). Developmental changes in pharmacodynamics also play a role in the adjustment of medication as biological systems evolve from birth. This is especially important in the treatment of children with disabilities, because many medications affect the central

BOX 38.1 INTERDISCIPLINARY CARE

Role of the Outpatient Pharmacist in Medication Management

The role of the pharmacist has expanded since the late 1980s, most notably in the area of medication therapy management. Though this has mostly focused on the care of chronic adult conditions (Brahm & Brown, 2004), pharmacists can also play a vital role in the care of children with disabilities (Gray et al., 2017). Outpatient pharmacists in the clinic and retail setting are a valuable resource in helping to optimize medications in these children. Every prescription sent to a pharmacy is verified by a pharmacist: They check to see if 1) the dose is correct and 2) there are no interactions with any other medication the patient is concurrently taking. Pharmacists in this setting also counsel patients and families on the best way to take medications (e.g., take with a fatty meal or avoid taking with calcium-containing products). Finally, they make recommendations to physicians and other health care providers on alternative medication therapies and different formulations, and they can administer vaccinations in the outpatient setting (Abraham, Brothers, Alexander, & Carpenter, 2017; Deshpande, Schauer, Mott, Young, & Cory, 2013). As children who are medically complex live longer, outpatient pharmacists serve as valuable members of the health care team in their optimal management.

nervous system (CNS), which grows rapidly from birth. These changes can cause a paradoxical effect or require higher doses to achieve therapeutic clinical end points (Mulla, 2010). For example, digoxin is used in children with congenital heart disease to prevent arrhythmias, and they require higher doses compared with adults to achieve the same clinical response due to changes in the heart muscle over time (Hastreiter, van der Horst, Voda, & Chow-Tung, 1985; Wells, Young, & Kearns, 1992; Wettrell & Andersson, 1977). Another example is the use of benzodiazepines in preterm infants and neonates. Benzodiazepines are typically used to abort seizures; however, their use in preterm infants and neonates can cause seizures because of developmental changes in the GABA receptor, which is involved in inhibitory signals in the brain (Andersen et al., 2002; Brooks-Kayal & Pritchett, 1993; Chugani, Kumar, & Muzik, 2013). Therefore, the developmental changes in children require periodic monitoring and dose adjustment to maximize efficacy and minimize toxicity.

Drug, Disease, and Food Interactions

Sometimes when there is **polypharmacy,** medications can interact with each other causing **drug–drug interactions,** which are a change in a drug's effect when taken together with another drug due to changes in pharmacokinetics. This can lead to overexposure and toxicity or underexposure and subtherapeutic effects. For example, erythromycin is an antibiotic for treatment of infections and also a commonly used gastrointestinal motility agent for patients with CNS disorders, such as HIE and traumatic brain injury (TBI). Erythromycin can also inhibit an important drug-metabolizing enzyme (CYP3A4) and increase drug levels of medications that use that enzymatic pathway; this may require a decrease in that drug's dose while concomitantly receiving erythromycin (Dai et al., 2016; de Wildt et al., 2014; Zhou, Xue, Yu, Li, & Wang, 2007). Another example is phenobarbital; this medication is frequently used in the treatment of seizures in neonates with HIE and as an adjunctive therapy for pediatric epilepsy (Glauser et al., 2016; National Clinical Guideline Centre [UK], 2012). In addition, phenobarbital can induce multiple drug-metabolizing enzymes, which can lead to decreased concentrations of drugs that utilize those pathways and result in subtherapeutic levels of drugs (de Wildt et al., 2014; Zhou et al., 2007).

There also can be **drug–disease interactions,** which are a change in a drug's effect due to a disease state that affects drug metabolism or absorption. As with drug–drug interactions, these drug–disease interactions can cause either elevated or decreased drug concentrations, which can lead to ADRs or subclinical benefits. Children with disabilities are more frequently hospitalized than their typically developing peers; this is especially relevant because critical illnesses can also affect drug metabolism and thus the efficacy of drugs. For example, older pediatric patients with methylmalonic acidemia (a type of inborn error of metabolism) have impaired renal function; thus, their medications have to be adjusted because of the decreased elimination of drugs through the kidney (Zsengellér et al., 2014). Patients with trisomy 21/Down syndrome often have congenital heart defects that may be associated with a prolonged QT interval on an electrocardiogram (Tisma-Dupanovic et al., 2011). Certain medications can also prolong the QT interval, such as azithromycin for pneumonia. Heart arrhythmias are more likely to occur if patients with an already prolonged QT take medications that can further increase it (Ayad, Assar, Simpson, Garner, & Schussler, 2010; Box 38.2).

BOX 38.2 INTERDISCIPLINARY CARE

Role of the Inpatient Pharmacist

Children with medically complex needs are living longer lives, but they have increased risks of infections and other comorbidities that frequently require hospitalization. For example, children with cerebral palsy are frequently admitted for aspiration pneumonia that can require intravenous antibiotics. In addition to treating their acute problem, medications for their chronic conditions must be continued. One of the responsibilities of a clinical (inpatient) pharmacist is to ensure seamless transitions of care (outpatient to inpatient and vice versa; Zhang, Zhang, Huang, Luo, & Wen, 2012). Also, clinical pharmacists typically will conduct rounds with the interprofessional medical team, intervene on possible adverse drug reactions, recommend dosing for therapeutic drug monitoring, and suggest alternatives when first- or second-line therapies fail. Evidence shows that increased pharmacist presence in the hospital is associated with substantially improved care of critically ill children and that they are a valuable member of the medical team (Dai et al., 2016).

Finally, there can be drug–food interactions, which are a change in a drug's effect due to the interactions with foods, beverages, or supplements. Like the other interactions, certain foods can increase or decrease drug concentrations in the body. Parents may unknowingly be giving medications to their child with food that may negatively impact the effectiveness of the medications (Deng et al., 2017; Schmidt & Dalhoff, 2002). For example, ciprofloxacin is a commonly prescribed antibiotic that is used for respiratory infections, such as aspiration pneumonia. However, calcium in food products (e.g., milk, formula, and even calcium-fortified orange juice) can bind ciprofloxacin and decrease its absorption; this can lead to decreased drug concentrations in the body and treatment failure (Neuhofel, Wilton, Victory, Hejmanowsk, & Amsden, 2002). Children with trisomy 21 are at increased risk for hypothyroidism and need to take levothyroxine to correct their thyroid dysfunction (Lavigne et al., 2017). This drug is best taken on an empty stomach with a small glass of water. If taken with food or another beverage, it can greatly decrease the absorption of levothyroxine and lead to subclinical outcomes (Geer, Potter, & Ulrich, 2015).

In sum, children with disabilities often have chronic conditions that require the long-term use of medications. Medications can have drug–drug, drug–disease, and drug–food interactions, and therefore it is important to routinely assess concomitant medication therapy and drug administration techniques during each clinic visit and patient encounter. Clinical outcomes from medications can be maximized and ADRs can be minimized by taking the time to evaluate how the patients are taking their medications.

Pharmacogenomics

Genes also play an important role in an individual's response to drugs. **Pharmacogenomics,** the study of how genes affect a person's response to drugs, helps us understand genetic variations between people to predict a drug's appropriate dose and clinical effectiveness. Pharmacogenomics helps to explain why a drug may be effective in some people but fail to benefit others. In some cases, patients who fail treatment may also experience serious ADRs. These genetic variations are called **polymorphisms** (the occurrence of multiple phenotypes in a population; Ahmed, Zhou, Zhou, & Chen, 2016; Sissung et al., 2017). For example, children with autism may be prescribed antidepressants to treat repetitive behaviors and social anxiety. However, these drugs can be affected by different polymorphisms of drug-metabolizing enzymes; these polymorphisms can either decrease drug concentrations (and decrease clinical efficacy) or increase drug concentrations (and cause ADRs; Sissung et al., 2017). Another example is with baclofen and the treatment of spasticity. In the case of Isaac, baclofen was effective in treating his symptoms; however, baclofen does not achieve the same clinical response in all patients due to the pharmacogenomic variability in baclofen drug metabolism (McLaughlin et al., 2018).

Pharmacogenomics can also contribute to ADRs. As mentioned earlier, ADRs can either be classified as 1) dose dependent or 2) paradoxical. It is hypothesized that some paradoxical ADRs occur due to drugs binding to off-target receptors; thus, patients with a certain polymorphism may be at more risk for ADRs. For example, carbamazepine is a commonly used drug in the treatment of epilepsy; this medication can cause an ADR called Steven-Johnson syndrome (a severe type of immune-skin reaction where the surface layers of skin and mucous membranes blister and peel). It is strongly associated with the HLA-B*15:02 allele, especially in the ethnic Han Chinese population where this polymorphism is highly present (Garon et al., 2017).

Although there have been many recent advances in pharmacogenomics, there is still a lack of clinical applicability (Chang, McCarthy, & Shin, 2015). Despite this, there is a great potential in improving treatments using pharmacogenomics, especially in the area of behavioral health. Children with disabilities often require these types of medications, and they are administered in a trial-and-error approach to find the medication with the greatest benefit and least side effects. A pharmacogenomics-guided treatment approach can reduce costs and time to achieve effective treatment and outcomes (Valdes & Yin, 2016; Box 38.3).

FACTORS AFFECTING DRUG ADMINISTRATION

The formulations of medications and the routes by which they are administered are important considerations and potential challenges when administering drugs in the pediatric population.

Formulations

In adults, medications are fixed at set doses, typically as single- or multiple-strength pills (e.g., acetaminophen 500-mg tablet; levetiracetam 250-mg, 500-mg, and 750-mg tablets). However, this becomes problematic in pediatrics because 1) not all children can swallow pills and 2) the doses that are available may be too much for the child. Children, with appropriate training, can learn to swallow pills between 6 and 11 years of age (Jones et al., 2017; Meltzer, Welch, & Ostrom, 2006; Patel, Jacobsen,

BOX 38.3 EVIDENCE-BASED PRACTICE

The Case for the Use of Pharmagenomics in the Treatment of Autism

Many medications are used in the treatment of autism. For example, risperidone, an atypical antipsychotic, is commonly used to treat irritability associated with autism, albeit with mixed clinical outcomes (Dean, 2012). This medication also has a significant side effect profile, which includes altered cardiac conduction, decreased blood cell counts, cerebrovascular effects, serum lipid abnormalities, extrapyramidal symptoms (movement disorders), hyperglycemia, hyperprolactinemia, priapism, and weight gain (Taketomo, Hodding, & Kraus, 2017). However, not all children with autism taking risperidone experience these side effects. Recent literature has shown associations between drug concentrations of risperidone and 9-hydroxyrisperidone (a metabolite) and certain polymorphisms of CYP2D6 (a drug-metabolizing enzyme involved in the metabolism of risperidone) and drug transporters (Medhasi, Pasomsub, et al., 2016; Medhasi, Pinthong, et al., 2016; Vanwong et al., 2017). Patients with these polymorphisms have elevated levels of drug and thus may be at an increased risk of adverse events, such as hyperprolactinemia (Hongkaew et al., 2015; Ngamsamut et al., 2016). Another study showed a significant association with nonstable clinical outcomes in children with autism who had the Taq1A T-carriers of the dopamine 2 receptor gene (Nuntamool et al., 2017). Together, these studies support the use of pharmacogenomics when using risperidone.

Jhaveri, & Bradford, 2015). However, there will be some children who will have difficulty with swallowing pills or who cannot physically swallow pills due to their disability (e.g., cerebral palsy). Options for children who cannot swallow pills include liquids (e.g., solutions, suspensions, syrups, emulsions), orally disintegrating tablets, chewable tablets, transdermal patches, intranasal sprays, rectal suppositories or enemas, intravenous injections, nebulized liquids, and inhalers. However, all formulations (dosage forms of the medication) do not exist for each medication (Ivanovska, Rademaker, van Dijk, & Mantel-Teeuwisse, 2014). Another problem is that the child may not like a certain formulation of the drug. For example, the child may not like the taste of chewable or disintegrating tablets, which may be bitter (Batchelor & Marriott, 2015). Or, the child may resist receiving the enema or suppository because he or she feels uncomfortable about getting it rectally. All these issues must be taken into consideration when starting medications for children with disabilities.

Another issue with medications for children with disabilities is the dose. Although it may be possible to use a pill cutter to divide the tablet to achieve the correct dose (e.g., if the levetiracetam dose needed is 125 mg, half of a 250-mg tablet may be used), this technique will not always work when doses are not half or a quarter of a tablet size. Furthermore, medications may not be available as a tablet but only as a formulation that cannot be cut, such as a capsule or an **extended-release** formulation that allows the drug to be slowly released over a period of time (this formulation will lose its effectiveness if it is crushed or cut). As discussed earlier, for non–life-threatening situations, medical professionals should slowly titrate up the dose to maximize the beneficial effect while minimizing ADRs; this may not be possible with tablets. In the case of Isaac, his starting dose of baclofen was 1.1 mg. Baclofen tablets are only available as 5-mg and 10-mg tablets; it would be difficult to cut a 5-mg tablet into a 1.1-mg dose. Instead, his physician would prescribe a liquid formulation that could be easily and accurately measured in a syringe.

Finally, the commercial availability of some formulations presents a challenge. In the case of Isaac, there is a commercially available baclofen oral suspension that he could use (i.e., his family could pick it up at any pharmacy). However, this baclofen suspension became commercially available in 2016. If Isaac had started baclofen before 2016, his parents would have needed to get his baclofen at a **compounding pharmacy** (a special pharmacy that can make drug formulations that are specifically tailored to patients such as liquid suspensions, suppositories, and creams). It is important to note that not all retail pharmacies are compounding pharmacies; this presents a barrier to patient and their families in obtaining these compounded medications, especially in more rural areas. Further complicating the problem is that these compounded medications typically have shorter shelf-lives than commercially available medications (Batchelor & Marriott, 2015; Ivanovska et al., 2014). For example, children with maple syrup urine disease (an inborn error of metabolism, see Chapter 16) are treated with supplements of valine and isoleucine. These amino acids are only commercially available as a powder, and it is often compounded into an oral solution for ease of administration. In addition, the shelf-life of compounded valine and isoleucine oral solutions is only 14 days (United States Pharmacopeia, 2017), which means that the family would need to pick up these medications every 2 weeks from the pharmacy. Formulation issues can present a challenge not only for children with disabilities, but for all children.

Routes of Administrations

Some children with disabilities do not have typical swallowing reflexes (e.g., children with severe cerebral palsy; Martinez-Biarge et al., 2012) or TBI (Popernack, Gray, & Reuter-Rice, 2015). Due to an inability to swallow, they often receive food and medication via **nasogastric tubes** (**NG** tubes; tubes that reach the stomach through the nasal opening) or **gastric tubes** (**G** tubes; tubes that are inserted through the abdomen wall directly into the stomach). This presents a challenge when administering oral medications, especially when it is in a solid form such as a tablet or capsule. Routes of administrations, defined as the path a drug is administered into the body, such as oral, intravenous, transdermal, or inhalation, ultimately determines the formulation of the medication.

To complicate the issue, some formulations are not compatible with certain routes of administration. For example, ciprofloxacin (an antibiotic) is available in a commercially available suspension; however, it can clot NG tubes as it is a thick and grainy solution. Instead of using the commercially available suspension, it is recommended to crush and dissolve a tablet to give through an NG tube (White & Bradnam, 2015). Another issue that can arise is if there is a change in the route of administration (e.g., oral to intravenous). A commonly encountered example is oxcarbazepine, a typically prescribed anti-epileptic drug. This medication is only available as a suspension or tablet; if a child with epilepsy is admitted to the hospital and cannot take anything by mouth, oxcarbazepine needs to be switched to a different drug that can be given intravenously. Another instance where a similar challenge may occur is with hydroxocobalamin (vitamin B12) in children with disorders of intracellular cobalamin metabolism (an inborn error of metabolism). Although this vitamin is available as liquid or tablet, children with these disorders require intramuscular injections due to limited oral absorption (Carrillo, Adams, & Venditti, 2017; Green et al., 2017).

Finally, certain routes of drug administration can cause drug interactions; this is most notable with feeding tubes and children with disabilities who require feeding around the clock. As mentioned earlier, certain medications, such as levothyroxine, can have interactions with other drugs or food. It is recommended to hold feeds for at least 1 to 2 hours before and 30 minutes after drug administration to minimize the interactions with other food or drugs (if applicable). It is also important to flush the tube before and after drug administration to minimize drug binding to the feeding tube (Grissinger, 2013). Like with formulations, being cognizant of the different routes of administration can lead to reducing the risk of treatment failure. In this regard, pharmacists and clinical pharmacologists are important members of the interprofessional team who can provide answers to these types of problems (Boxes 38.1 and 38.2).

OTHER FACTORS TO CONSIDER

Off-Label Use of Drugs

The research and development of the majority of drugs on the markets have focused on adults; consequently, the data proving safety and efficacy for these medications are all based on adult data. These clinical trials often excluded infants, children, adolescents, and pregnant women, as they are considered vulnerable populations. This means that many drugs given to infants, children, and adolescents are used **off label** (an unlabeled use of an approved drug). On label means that the use is listed in the package insert of the drug (i.e., approved by a regulatory agency such as the U.S. Food and Drug Administration). The absence of an indication on the drug label does not necessarily mean it would be wrong to use it in a certain age group or for a particular disorder. However, it means that there may be a lack of sufficient evidence, as determined by a regulatory agency, to be included as an approved use in the label (Frattarelli et al., 2014; Ito, 2017). This concept is especially important because many children with disabilities are often prescribed medications off label, especially in the case of psychotropic medications (Bruni et al., 2018; Kearns & Hawley, 2014; Sharma et al., 2016). When prescribing medications off label, current literature should be used to evaluate the risks and benefits as well as duration of therapy and incidence of adverse effects. It is also important to note that some medications are prescribed off label with minimal evidence because that drug has been entrenched in clinical practice. In the case of Isaac, he was prescribed oral baclofen to treat his hypertonicity. However, there is mixed efficacy regarding the use of oral baclofen in this patient population (Navarrete-Opazo, Gonzalez, & Nahuelhual, 2016). Finally, finding strong evidence can be challenging as it is hard to design clinical trials involving children with disabilities. It may be acceptable to use medications off label, but it is important for the physician to critically evaluate the literature on a periodic basis to see if better treatment options exist.

Use of Complementary Health Approaches

The use of **complementary health approaches (CHA)** is widespread (Tsourounis & Dennehy, 2015), especially among families of children with disabilities and particularly in children less than 1 year of age (Harris, 2005; Provenzi, Barello, Saettini, Scotto di Minico, & Borgatti, 2017; see Chapter 39). CHA are health and wellness therapies that are not typically part of a conventional Western medicine. Complementary medicine are treatments (e.g., megavitamins) combined with conventional medicine, whereas alternative medicine are treatments used in place of conventional medicine. Families may be reluctant to mention the use of CHA to the health care providers because of the negative connotations in the medical community. Further compounding the problem is that many clinicians also do not ask patients and their families regarding CHA use during patient visits (Gaylord & Mann, 2007). As stated earlier, supplements, nutraceuticals, and other CHA-related products can negatively interact with other drugs, either decreasing the efficacy of medications and/or increasing the likelihood of ADRs. For example, Bacopa monnieri, or the waterhyssop, is an Ayurvedic herb that is believed by some to improve cognition and behavior in children and adults (Kean, Downey, & Stough, 2016), and it is sometimes used by families with children with autism. However, this herb can inhibit drug metabolizing enzymes and potentially lead to ADRs when taken with other medications that utilize this pathway (Ramasamy, Kiew, & Chung, 2014). Another issue is evidence of the lack of efficacy of many CHA. CHA are started by families in the belief that they will help their child; some are started as a result of cultural beliefs, whereas others may be started due to word of mouth from other families with the disorder based on anecdotal evidence (Bang et al., 2017; Smolinske, 2017). As an example, a deficiency in omega-3 polyunsaturated fatty acids has been found in some children with autism and ADHD (Agostoni et al., 2017). Parents may give omega-3 fatty acids supplements to their children in the hope of helping neurocognitive development, but current evidence shows a lack of efficacy (Agostoni et al., 2017). Finally, it is important to know that supplements and CHA products are not as tightly regulated by the FDA as medications. This lack of federal oversight can lead to misbranded (not containing ingredients stated), tainted (containing unlisted ingredients), or adulterated products (containing unsafe ingredients; Abdel-Tawab, 2017; Humbert & Kornspan, 2017). Therefore, it is imperative that discussions of CHA use be included in every patient visit to ensure optimal pharmacotherapy outcomes.

Role of Vaccines

Although not typically thought of as a medication, vaccines play an important role in the health and well-being of children with disabilities. Immunization is a cost-effective method that prevents many common childhood diseases and is one of the greatest public health achievements of the 20th century. Although commonly associated with infancy, since 2005 there have also been new adolescent vaccines that have come to the market that are recommended by the Advisory Committee on Immunization Practices of the Centers for Disease Control and Prevention (2017). Children with disabilities experience many adverse health outcomes and are at greater risk for infections (e.g., children with Down syndrome); thus, vaccinations provide an effective and economical health benefit. However, literature suggests that vaccine coverage in adolescents and young male children with disabilities is lagging. Potential strategies for increasing compliance include scheduling vaccinations at existing medical visits, having all members of the health care team be responsible for vaccinations, and approaching the subject of vaccination at every patient encounter (McRee, Maslow, & Reiter, 2017; Reiter & McRee, 2016; Walmsley, 2011). Everything considered, low levels of vaccination coverage in the population are missed opportunities for optimal health outcomes, and all members of the health care team should be actively involved to ensure coordinated care.

Drug Costs and Medical Insurance

In countries where universal health care does not exist, drug expenditures are a significant financial burden for families of children with disabilities. These families have health care costs that are three times higher than families with typically developing children, and they experience much higher out-of-pocket costs (Newacheck & Kim, 2005). These financial barriers can force families to decide between medications and other essential living expenses, such as food and housing (Berkowitz, Seligman, & Choudhry, 2014). However, when families must forgo the purchase of needed medication, it can lead to suboptimal outcomes and costly hospitalizations for their child with disabilities (Coller et al., 2014). Families also can be underinsured and may have high deductibles, which can limit medication purchases (Committee on Child Health Financing, 2014; Szilagyi, 2012). There are mechanisms and assistance available to families to help with out-of-pocket costs such as copay cards, drug assistance programs, and government-subsidized insurance for children (e.g., Children's Health Insurance Program [CHIP]; see

Chapter 41). For that reason, it is important to evaluate the ability of families to obtain medications without significantly affecting their financial situations at every medical visit.

Communication and Medication Adherence

Both written and verbal communication are an important part of health care. Effective communication contributes to **adherence** (also known as compliance; it is the degree to which a patient correctly follows medical advice and/or takes their medication). This can increase patient safety, clinical outcomes, and overall satisfaction (Yin et al., 2010). Once the patient leaves the medical visit, the health care team must rely on the parent and child to ensure appropriate dosing and administration. Therefore, it is imperative that the health care team clearly communicate to the family how to properly take the medication and explain why it is needed (Berrier, 2016). **Health literacy** (the degree to which individuals have the capacity to understand basic health information in order to make appropriate and informed decisions) and parental beliefs also play an important role in adherence. This is especially critical in cases when parents may not fully comprehend the role of their child's medication or when parents hold cultural beliefs that conflict with the prescribed therapy (Cohen, Dillon, Gladwin, & De La Rosa, 2013; Johnston, Seipp, Hommersen, Hoza, & Fine, 2005). For example, parents may withhold drugs because they believe medications cause more harm than good (e.g., parents may refuse anti-epileptic drugs and as a result the child experiences more seizures). Conversely, parents may jump to the conclusion that a medication can cure their children without any further intervention (Schwartz & Axelrad, 2015). In conclusion, open and honest communication between medical providers and families of children with disabilities will promote medication adherence and effective clinical outcomes.

SUMMARY

- Medications should be started when nonpharmacological options have been maximized.
- When starting medications in non–life-threatening situations for children with disabilities, it is best to "start low and go slow." This will help to reduce ADRs.
- There are many factors that can impact drug concentrations. It is important to periodically adjust medications and talk with patients and families about how they are taking their medication.
- Many medications in children with disabilities are often given off label. Critically evaluating the literature prior to and during treatment is important.
- CHA is growing in use. Many of these treatments are benign, but some can cause harm or decrease the efficacy of concomitant medications.
- Medication adherence is the responsibility of the patient, family, and medical team. Assessing adherence on a consistent basis will help to maximize drug outcomes.
- Pharmacists and clinical pharmacologists can be valuable team members in the care of children with disabilities by providing expert drug advice and recommendations.

ADDITIONAL RESOURCES

MyChildWithoutLimits: http://www.mychildwithoutlimits.org/plan/common-treatments-and-therapies/drug-therapy/

Drug InfoNet: http://www.druginfonet.com.

MedlinePlus: https://medlineplus.gov/druginformation.html

Additional resources can be found online in Appendix D: Childhood Disabilities Resources, Services, and Organizations (see About the Online Companion Materials).

REFERENCES

Abdel-Tawab, M. (2017). Do we need plant food supplements? A critical examination of quality, safety, efficacy, and necessity for a new regulatory framework. *Planta Medica, 84*(6-07), 372–393. doi:10.1055/s-0043-123764

Abraham, O., Brothers, A., Alexander, D. S., & Carpenter, D. M. (2017). Pediatric medication use experiences and patient counseling in community pharmacies: Perspectives of children and parents. *Journal of the American Pharmacists Association, 57*(1), 38–46.e2. doi:10.1016/j.japh.2016.08.019

Agostoni, C., Nobile, M., Ciappolino, V., Delvecchio, G., Tesei, A., Turolo, S., . . . Brambilla, P. (2017). The role of omega-3 fatty acids in developmental psychopathology: A systematic review on early psychosis, autism, and ADHD. *International Journal of Molecular Sciences, 18*(12), 2608. doi:10.3390/ijms18122608

Ahmed, S., Zhou, Z., Zhou, J., & Chen, S.-Q. (2016). Pharmacogenomics of drug metabolizing enzymes and transporters: Relevance to precision medicine. *Genomics, Proteomics & Bioinformatics, 14*(5), 298–313. doi:10.1016/j.gpb.2016.03.008

Andersen, D. L., Eckert, A. L., Tsai, V. W.-W., Burke, C. J., Tannenberg, A. E. G., & Dodd, P. R. (2002). GABA(A) receptor sites in the developing human foetus. *Brain Research. Developmental Brain Research, 139*(2), 107–119.

Anderson, B. J., & Holford, N. H. G. (2013). Understanding dosing: Children are small adults, neonates are immature children. *Archives of Disease in Childhood, 98*(9), 737–744. doi:10.1136/archdischild-2013-303720

Ayad, R. F., Assar, M. D., Simpson, L., Garner, J. B., & Schussler, J. M. (2010). Causes and management of drug-induced long QT syndrome. *Proceedings (Baylor University. Medical Center), 23*(3), 250–255.

Bang, M., Lee, S. H., Cho, S.-H., Yu, S.-A., Kim, K., Lu, H. Y., . . . Min, S. Y. (2017). Herbal medicine treatment for children with autism spectrum disorder: a systematic review. *Evidence-Based Complementary and Alternative Medicine, 2017*, 8614680. doi:10.1155/2017/8614680

Batchelor, H. K., & Marriott, J. F. (2015). Formulations for children: Problems and solutions. *British Journal of Clinical Pharmacology, 79*(3), 405–418.

Berkowitz, S. A., Seligman, H. K., & Choudhry, N. K. (2014). Treat or eat: Food insecurity, cost-related medication underuse, and unmet needs. *The American Journal of Medicine, 127*(4), 303–310, e3. doi:10.1016/j.amjmed.2014.01.002

Berrier, K. (2016). Medication errors in outpatient pediatrics. *American Journal of Maternal Child Nursing, 41*(5), 280–286. doi:10.1097/NMC.0000000000000261

Berry, S. A., Longo, N., Diaz, G. A., McCandless, S. E., Smith, W. E., Harding, C. O., . . . Vockley, J. (2017). Safety and efficacy of glycerol phenylbutyrate for management of urea cycle disorders in patients aged 2 months to 2 years. *Molecular Genetics and Metabolism, 122*(3), 46–53. doi:10.1016/j.ymgme.2017.09.002

Brahm, N. C., & Brown, R. C. (2004). Clinical pharmacology services: A pharmacist-based consulting service for the developmentally disabled. *American Journal of Health-System Pharmacy, 61*(5), 487–493.

Brooks-Kayal, A. R., & Pritchett, D. B. (1993). Developmental changes in human gamma-aminobutyric acid: A receptor subunit composition. *Annals of Neurology, 34*(5), 687–693. doi:10.1002/ana.410340511

Bruni, O., Angriman, M., Calisti, F., Comandini, A., Esposito, G., Cortese, S., & Ferri, R. (2018). Practitioner review: Treatment of chronic insomnia in children and adolescents with neurodevelopmental disabilities. *Journal of Child Psychology and Psychiatry, and Allied Disciplines, 59*(5), 489–508. doi:10.1111/jcpp.12812

Carrillo, N., Adams, D., & Venditti, C. P. (2017). Disorders of intracellular cobalamin metabolism. In M. P. Adam, H. H. Ardinger, R. A. Pagon, S. E. Wallace, L. J. Bean, H. C. Mefford, . . . N. Ledbetter (Eds.), *GeneReviews*. Seattle, WA: University of Washington. Retrieved from http://www.ncbi.nlm.nih.gov/books/NBK1328/

Centers for Disease Control and Prevention. (2017). *Immunization schedules.* Retrieved from https://www.cdc.gov/vaccines/schedules/index.html

Chang, M. T., McCarthy, J. J., & Shin, J. (2015). Clinical application of pharmacogenetics: focusing on practical issues. *Pharmacogenomics, 16*(15), 1733–1741. doi:10.2217/pgs.15.112

Chugani, H. T., Kumar, A., & Muzik, O. (2013). GABA(A) receptor imaging with positron emission tomography in the human newborn: A unique binding pattern. *Pediatric Neurology, 48*(6), 459–462. doi:10.1016/j.pediatrneurol.2013.04.008

Cohen, D., Dillon, F. R., Gladwin, H., & De La Rosa, M. (2013). American parents' willingness to prescribe psychoactive drugs to children: A test of cultural mediators. *Social Psychiatry and Psychiatric Epidemiology, 48*(12), 1873–1887. doi:10.1007/s00127-013-0710-2

Coller, R. J., Nelson, B. B., Sklansky, D. J., Saenz, A. A., Klitzner, T. S., Lerner, C. F., & Chung, P. J. (2014). Preventing hospitalizations in children with medical complexity: A systematic review. *Pediatrics, 134*(6), e1628–e1647. doi:10.1542/peds.2014-1956

Committee on Child Health Financing. (2014). High-deductible health plans. *Pediatrics, 133*(5), e1461–e1470. doi:10.1542/peds.2014-0555

Dai, D., Feinstein, J. A., Morrison, W., Zuppa, A. F., & Feudtner, C. (2016). Epidemiology of polypharmacy and potential drug-drug interactions among pediatric patients in ICUs of U.S. children's hospitals. *Pediatric Critical Care Medicine, 17*(5), e218–e228. doi:10.1097/PCC.0000000000000684

de Wildt, S. N., Tibboel, D., & Leeder, J. S. (2014). Drug metabolism for the paediatrician. *Archives of Disease in Childhood, 99*(12), 1137–1142. doi:10.1136/archdischild-2013-305212

Dean, L. (2012). Risperidone therapy and CYP2D6 genotype. In V. Pratt, H. McLeod, L. Dean, A. Malheiro, & W. Rubinstein (Eds.), *Medical genetics summaries*, 357-367. Bethesda, MD: National Center for Biotechnology Information (US). Retrieved from http://www.ncbi.nlm.nih.gov/books/NBK425795/

Deng, J., Zhu, X., Chen, Z., Fan, C. H., Kwan, H. S., Wong, C. H., . . . Lam, T. N. (2017). A review of food-drug interactions on oral drug absorption. *Drugs, 77*(17), 1833–1855. doi:10.1007/s40265-017-0832-z

Deshpande, M., Schauer, J., Mott, D. A., Young, H. N., & Cory, P. (2013). Parents' perceptions of pharmacists as providers of influenza vaccine to children. *Journal of the American Pharmacists Association, 53*(5), 488–495. doi:10.1331/JAPhA.2013.13017

Elzagallaai, A. A., Greff, M., & Rieder, M. J. (2017). Adverse drug reactions in children: The double-edged sword of therapeutics. *Clinical Pharmacology and Therapeutics, 101*(6), 725–735. doi:10.1002/cpt.677

Frattarelli, D. A., Galinkin, J. L., Green, T. P., Johnson, T. D., Neville, K. A., Paul, I. M., . . . American Academy of Pediatrics Committee on Drugs. (2014). Off-label use of drugs in children. *Pediatrics, 133*(3), 563–567. doi:10.1542/peds.2013-4060

Garon, S. L., Pavlos, R. K., White, K. D., Brown, N. J., Stone, C. A., & Phillips, E. J. (2017). Pharmacogenomics of off-target adverse drug reactions. *British Journal of Clinical Pharmacology, 83*(9), 1896–1911. doi:10.1111/bcp.13294

Gaylord, S. A., & Mann, J. D. (2007). Rationales for CAM education in health professions training programs. *Academic Medicine, 82*(10), 927–933. doi:10.1097/ACM.0b013e31814a5b43

Geer, M., Potter, D. M., & Ulrich, H. (2015). Alternative schedules of levothyroxine administration. *American Journal of Health-System Pharmacy, 72*(5), 373–377. doi:10.2146/ajhp140250

Gerlach, M., Egberts, K., Dang, S.-Y., Plener, P., Taurines, R., Mehler-Wex, C., & Romanos, M. (2016). Therapeutic drug monitoring as a measure of proactive pharmacovigilance in child and adolescent psychiatry. *Expert Opinion on Drug Safety, 15*(11), 1477–1482. doi:10.1080/14740338.2016.1225721

Glauser, T., Shinnar, S., Gloss, D., Alldredge, B., Arya, R., Bainbridge, J., . . . Treiman, D. M. (2016). Evidence-based guideline: Treatment of convulsive status epilepticus in children and adults: Report of the Guideline Committee of the American Epilepsy Society. *Epilepsy Currents, 16*(1), 48–61. doi:10.5698/1535-7597-16.1.48

Goyal, V., Laisram, N., Wadhwa, R. K., & Kothari, S. Y. (2016). Prospective randomized study of oral diazepam and baclofen on spasticity in cerebral palsy.

Journal of Clinical and Diagnostic Research, 10(6), RC01–RC05. doi:10.7860/JCDR/2016/17067.7975

Gray, N. J., Shaw, K. L., Smith, F. J., Burton, J., Prescott, J., Roberts, R., . . . McDonagh, J. E. (2017). The role of pharmacists in caring for young people with chronic illness. *The Journal of Adolescent Health, 60*(2), 219–225. doi:10.1016/j.jadohealth.2016.09.023

Green, R., Allen, L. H., Bjørke-Monsen, A.-L., Brito, A., Guéant, J.-L., Miller, J. W., . . . Yajnik, C. (2017). Vitamin B12 deficiency. *Nature Reviews. Disease Primers, 3*, 17040. doi:10.1038/nrdp.2017.40

Grissinger, M. (2013). Preventing errors when drugs are given via enteral feeding tubes. *P&T: A Peer-Reviewed Journal for Formulary Management, 38*(10), 575–576.

Harris, A. B. (2005). Evidence of increasing dietary supplement use in children with special health care needs: Strategies for improving parent and professional communication. *Journal of the American Dietetic Association, 105*(1), 34–37. doi:10.1016/j.jada.2004.10.007

Hastreiter, A. R., van der Horst, R. L., Voda, C., & Chow-Tung, E. (1985). Maintenance digoxin dosage and steady-state plasma concentration in infants and children. *The Journal of Pediatrics, 107*(1), 140–146.

Hongkaew, Y., Ngamsamut, N., Puangpetch, A., Vanwong, N., Srisawasdi, P., Chamnanphon, M., . . . Sukasem, C. (2015). Hyperprolactinemia in Thai children and adolescents with autism spectrum disorder treated with risperidone. *Neuropsychiatric Disease and Treatment, 11*, 191–196. doi:10.2147/NDT.S76276

Humbert, J., & Kornspan, N. (2017, November). *FDA DDI webinar series: Tainted products marketed as dietary supplements* [Video webinar]. Retrieved from https://www.fda.gov/AboutFDA/WorkingatFDA/FellowshipInternshipGraduateFacultyPrograms/PharmacyStudentExperientialProgramCDER/ucm567435.htm

Ito, S. (2017). Drugs for children. *Clinical Pharmacology and Therapeutics, 101*(6), 704–706. doi:10.1002/cpt.675

Ivanovska, V., Rademaker, C. M. A., van Dijk, L., & Mantel-Teeuwisse, A. K. (2014). Pediatric drug formulations: A review of challenges and progress. *Pediatrics, 134*(2), 361–372. doi:10.1542/peds.2013-3225

Johnston, C., Seipp, C., Hommersen, P., Hoza, B., & Fine, S. (2005). Treatment choices and experiences in attention deficit and hyperactivity disorder: Relations to parents' beliefs and attributions. *Child: Care, Health and Development, 31*(6), 669–677. doi:10.1111/j.1365-2214.2005.00555.x

Jones, D. F., McRea, A. R., Jairath, M. K., Jones, M. S., Bradford, K. K., & Jhaveri, R. (2017). Prospective assessment of pill-swallowing ability in pediatric patients. *Clinical Pediatrics*, 9922817724399. doi:10.1177/0009922817724399

Kang, J. S., & Lee, M. H. (2009). Overview of therapeutic drug monitoring. *The Korean Journal of Internal Medicine, 24*(1), 1–10. doi:10.3904/kjim.2009.24.1.1

Kean, J. D., Downey, L. A., & Stough, C. (2016). A systematic review of the Ayurvedic medicinal herb Bacopa monnieri in child and adolescent populations. *Complementary Therapies in Medicine, 29*, 56–62. doi:10.1016/j.ctim.2016.09.002

Kearns, G. L., Abdel-Rahman, S. M., Alander, S. W., Blowey, D. L., Leeder, J. S., & Kauffman, R. E. (2003). Developmental pharmacology–drug disposition, action, and therapy in infants and children. *The New England Journal of Medicine, 349*(12), 1157–1167. doi:10.1056/NEJMra035092

Kearns, M. A., & Hawley, K. M. (2014). Predictors of polypharmacy and off-label prescribing of psychotropic medications: a national survey of child and adolescent psychiatrists. *Journal of Psychiatric Practice, 20*(6), 438–447. doi:10.1097/01.pra.0000456592.20622.45

Lavigne, J., Sharr, C., Elsharkawi, I., Ozonoff, A., Baumer, N., Brasington, C., . . . Skotko, B. G. (2017). Thyroid dysfunction in patients with Down syndrome: Results from a multi-institutional registry study. *American Journal of Medical Genetics, Part A, 173*(6), 1539–1545. doi:10.1002/ajmg.a.38219

Martinez-Biarge, M., Diez-Sebastian, J., Wusthoff, C. J., Lawrence, S., Aloysius, A., Rutherford, M. A., & Cowan, F. M. (2012). Feeding and communication impairments in infants with central grey matter lesions following perinatal hypoxic-ischaemic injury. *European Journal of Paediatric Neurology, 16*(6), 688–696. doi:10.1016/j.ejpn.2012.05.001

McLaughlin, M. J., He, Y., Brunstrom-Hernandez, J., Thio, L. L., Carleton, B. C., Ross, C. J. D., . . . Leeder, J. S. (2018). Pharmacogenomic variability of oral baclofen clearance and clinical response in children with cerebral palsy. *PM&R: The Journal of Injury, Function, and Rehabilitation, 10*(3), 235–243. doi:10.1016/j.pmrj.2017.08.441

McRee, A.-L., Maslow, G. R., & Reiter, P. L. (2017). Receipt of recommended adolescent vaccines among youth with special health care needs. *Clinical Pediatrics, 56*(5), 451–460. doi:10.1177/0009922816661330

Medhasi, S., Pasomsub, E., Vanwong, N., Ngamsamut, N., Puangpetch, A., Chamnanphon, M., . . . Sukasem, C. (2016). Clinically relevant genetic variants of drug-metabolizing enzyme and transporter genes detected in Thai children and adolescents with autism spectrum disorder. *Neuropsychiatric Disease and Treatment, 12*, 843–851. doi:10.2147/NDT.S101580

Medhasi, S., Pinthong, D., Pasomsub, E., Vanwong, N., Ngamsamut, N., Puangpetch, A., . . . Sukasem, C. (2016). Pharmacogenomic study reveals new variants of drug metabolizing enzyme and transporter genes associated with steady-state plasma concentrations of risperidone and 9-hydroxyrisperidone in Thai autism spectrum disorder patients. *Frontiers in Pharmacology, 7*, 475. doi:10.3389/fphar.2016.00475

Meltzer, E. O., Welch, M. J., & Ostrom, N. K. (2006). Pill swallowing ability and training in children 6 to 11 years of age. *Clinical Pediatrics, 45*(8), 725–733. doi:10.1177/0009922806292786

Mulla, H. (2010). Understanding developmental pharmacodynamics: Importance for drug development and clinical practice. *Paediatric Drugs, 12*(4), 223–233. doi:10.2165/11319220-000000000-00000

National Clinical Guideline Centre (UK). (2012). *The epilepsies: The diagnosis and management of the epilepsies in adults and children in primary and secondary care: Pharmacological update of Clinical Guideline 20.* London, England: Royal College of Physicians. Retrieved from http://www.ncbi.nlm.nih.gov/books/NBK247130/

Navarrete-Opazo, A. A., Gonzalez, W., & Nahuelhual, P. (2016). Effectiveness of oral baclofen in the treatment of spasticity in children and adolescents with cerebral palsy. *Archives of Physical Medicine and Rehabilitation, 97*(4), 604–618. doi:10.1016/j.apmr.2015.08.417

Neuhofel, A. L., Wilton, J. H., Victory, J. M., Hejmanowsk, L. G., & Amsden, G. W. (2002). Lack of bioequivalence of ciprofloxacin when administered with calcium-fortified orange juice: A new twist on an old interaction. *Journal of Clinical Pharmacology, 42*(4), 461–466.

Newacheck, P. W., & Kim, S. E. (2005). A national profile of health care utilization and expenditures for children with special health care needs. *Archives of Pediatrics & Adolescent Medicine, 159*(1), 10–17. doi:10.1001/archpedi.159.1.10

Ngamsamut, N., Hongkaew, Y., Vanwong, N., Srisawasdi, P., Puangpetch, A., Chamkrachangpada, B., . . . Sukasem, C. (2016). 9-hydroxyrisperidone-induced hyperprolactinaemia in Thai children and adolescents with autism spectrum disorder. *Basic & Clinical Pharmacology & Toxicology, 119*(3), 267–272. doi:10.1111/bcpt.12570

Nuntamool, N., Ngamsamut, N., Vanwong, N., Puangpetch, A., Chamnanphon, M., Hongkaew, Y., . . . Sukasem, C. (2017). Pharmacogenomics and efficacy of risperidone long-term treatment in Thai autistic children and adolescents. *Basic & Clinical Pharmacology & Toxicology, 121*(4), 316–324. doi:10.1111/bcpt.12803

Patel, A., Jacobsen, L., Jhaveri, R., & Bradford, K. K. (2015). Effectiveness of pediatric pill swallowing interventions: A systematic review. *Pediatrics, 135*(5), 883–889. doi:10.1542/peds.2014-2114

Pejovic-Milovancevic, M., Miletic, V., Popovic-Deusic, S., Draganic-Gajic, S., Lecic-Tosevski, D., & Marotic, V. (2011). Psychotropic medication use in children and adolescents in an inpatient setting. *Psychiatrike = Psychiatriki, 22*(4), 314–319.

Popernack, M. L., Gray, N., & Reuter-Rice, K. (2015). Moderate-to-severe traumatic brain injury in children: Complications and rehabilitation strategies. *Journal of Pediatric Health Care, 29*(3), e1–e7. doi:10.1016/j.pedhc.2014.09.003

Provenzi, L., Barello, S., Saettini, F., Scotto di Minico, G., & Borgatti, R. (2017). Paediatricians should encourage the parents of children with special healthcare needs to disclose their use of complementary and alternative medicine. *Acta Paediatrica, 106*(11), 1883–1884. doi:10.1111/apa.13967

Ramasamy, S., Kiew, L. V., & Chung, L. Y. (2014). Inhibition of human cytochrome P450 enzymes by Bacopa monnieri standardized extract and constituents. *Molecules, 19*(2), 2588–2601. doi:10.3390/molecules19022588

Reiter, P. L., & McRee, A.-L. (2016). Correlates of receiving recommended adolescent vaccines among youth with special health care needs: Findings from a statewide survey. *Vaccine, 34*(27), 3125–3131. doi:10.1016/j.vaccine.2016.04.062

Schmidt, L. E., & Dalhoff, K. (2002). Food-drug interactions. *Drugs, 62*(10), 1481–1502.

Schwartz, D. D., & Axelrad, M. E. (2015). Conceptualizing adherence. In D. D. Schwartz & M. E. Axelrad (Eds.), *Healthcare partnerships for pediatric adherence: Promoting collaborative management for pediatric chronic illness care* (pp. 21–40). New York, NY: Springer International Publishing.

Sharma, A. N., Arango, C., Coghill, D., Gringras, P., Nutt, D. J., Pratt, P., . . . Hollis, C. (2016). BAP position statement: Off-label prescribing of psychotropic medication to children and adolescents. *Journal of Psychopharmacology, 30*(5), 416–421. doi:10.1177/0269881116636107

Sissung, T. M., McKeeby, J. W., Patel, J., Lertora, J. J., Kumar, P., Flegel, W. A., . . . Goldspiel, B. R. (2017). Pharmacogenomics implementation at the National Institutes of Health Clinical Center. *Journal of Clinical Pharmacology, 57*(Suppl. 10), S67–S77. doi:10.1002/jcph.993

Smolinske, S. C. (2017). Dietary supplements in children. *Pediatric Clinics of North America, 64*(6), 1243–1255. doi:10.1016/j.pcl.2017.09.001

Szilagyi, P. G. (2012). Health insurance and children with disabilities. *The Future of Children, 22*(1), 123–148.

Taketomo, C. K., Hodding, J. H., & Kraus, D. M. (2017). *Pediatric & neonatal dosage handbook: An extensive resource for clinicians treating pediatric and neonatal patients.* Hudson, Ohio: Lexi-Comp.

Tisma-Dupanovic, S., Gowdamarajan, R., Goldenberg, I., Huang, D. T., Knilans, T., & Towbin, J. A. (2011). Prolonged QT in a 13-year-old patient with Down syndrome and complete atrioventricular canal defect. *Annals of Noninvasive Electrocardiology, 16*(4), 403–406. doi:10.1111/j.1542-474X.2011.00471.x

Tsourounis, C., & Dennehy, C. (2015). Chapter 50: Introduction to dietary supplements. In D. L. Krinsky, Ferreri, S. P., Hemstreet, B., Hume, A. L., Rollins, C. J., & Tietze, K. J. (Eds.) *Handbook of nonprescription drugs: An interactive approach to self-care* (18th ed.). Washington, DC: American Pharmacists Association.

United States Pharmacopeia. (2017). USP <795> Pharmaceutical compounding—nonsterile preparations. In *Second supplement to USP 40–NF 35* (pp. 675-683). Rockville, MD: The United States Pharmacopeial Convention.

Valdes, R., & Yin, D. T. (2016). Fundamentals of pharmacogenetics in personalized, precision medicine. *Clinics in Laboratory Medicine, 36*(3), 447–459. doi:10.1016/j.cll.2016.05.006

van den Anker, J. N. (2010). Developmental pharmacology. *Developmental Disabilities Research Reviews, 16*(3), 233–238. doi:10.1002/ddrr.122

Vanwong, N., Ngamsamut, N., Medhasi, S., Puangpetch, A., Chamnanphon, M., Tan-Kam, T., . . . Sukasem, C. (2017). Impact of CYP2D6 polymorphism on steady-state plasma levels of risperidone and 9-hydroxyrisperidone in Thai children and adolescents with autism spectrum disorder. *Journal of Child and Adolescent Psychopharmacology, 27*(2), 185–191. doi:10.1089/cap.2014.0171

Walmsley, D. (2011). Routine pediatric immunization, special cases in pediatrics: Prematurity, chronic disease, congenital heart disease: Recent advancements/changes in pediatric vaccines. *Primary Care, 38*(4), 595–609, vii. doi:10.1016/j.pop.2011.07.002

Wells, T. G., Young, R. A., & Kearns, G. L. (1992). Age-related differences in digoxin toxicity and its treatment. *Drug Safety, 7*(2), 135–151.

Wettrell, G., & Andersson, K. E. (1977). Clinical pharmacokinetics of digoxin in infants. *Clinical Pharmacokinetics, 2*(1), 17–31.

White, R., & Bradnam, V. (2015). *Handbook of drug administration via enteral feeding tubes* (3rd ed.). London, England: Pharmaceutical Press.

Yin, H. S., Mendelsohn, A. L., Wolf, M. S., Parker, R. M., Fierman, A., van Schaick, L., . . . Dreyer, B. P. (2010). Parents' medication administration errors: Role of dosing instruments and health literacy. *Archives of Pediatrics & Adolescent Medicine, 164*(2), 181–186. doi:10.1001/archpediatrics.2009.269

Zhang, C., Zhang, L., Huang, L., Luo, R., & Wen, J. (2012). Clinical pharmacists on medical care of pediatric inpatients: A single-center randomized controlled trial. *PloS One, 7*(1), e30856. doi:10.1371/journal.pone.0030856

Zhou, S.-F., Xue, C. C., Yu, X.-Q., Li, C., & Wang, G. (2007). Clinically important drug interactions potentially involving mechanism-based inhibition of cytochrome P450 3A4 and the role of therapeutic drug monitoring. *Therapeutic Drug Monitoring, 29*(6), 687–710. doi:10.1097/FTD.0b013e31815c16f5

Zsengellér, Z. K., Aljinovic, N., Teot, L. A., Korson, M., Rodig, N., Sloan, J. L., . . . Rosen, S. (2014). Methylmalonic acidemia: A megamitochondrial disorder affecting the kidney. *Pediatric Nephrology, 29*(11), 2139–2146. doi:10.1007/s00467-014-2847-y

CHAPTER 39

Complementary Health Approaches

Thomas D. Challman

Upon completion of this chapter, the reader will

- Understand the types of complementary health approaches currently being used in children with disabilities
- Be able to discuss the evidence base for various complementary health approaches
- Understand how to counsel families effectively regarding the use of these therapies

Caregivers of children with disabilities—and the health care practitioners who provide medical care for these children—often hear about therapies, whether via the Internet, social media, or word of mouth, that are promoted as beneficial for some aspect of a child's developmental or behavioral functioning. They may also read about these therapies in peer-reviewed journals (Kemper, Gardiner, & Birdee, 2013; Levy & Hyman, 2017). The evidence base used to justify these therapies is commonly suboptimal; as such, rational strategies are clearly needed to help make sense of this information.

In many medical conditions in which there are no highly effective treatment approaches, therapies that may have limited plausibility and a weak evidence base may gain popularity. This phenomenon has emerged in the field of developmental disabilities because caregivers of children with disabilities have a desire to pursue treatments that they feel might be helpful. Care must be taken, however, to guard against ineffective or pseudoscientific treatments that create the potential for harm—physical, emotional, or financial. Importantly, the ethical principles of beneficence, nonmaleficence, autonomy, justice, and truthfulness need to be included within a framework that caregivers and medical providers use to critically analyze whether a particular nonstandard therapy should be supported or discouraged.

CASE STUDY

Stephen is a 3-year-old boy who presented to his pediatrician at the age of 2 years with language delay, decreased social responsiveness, and various repetitive behaviors. His behavioral and developmental features satisfied criteria for a diagnosis of autism spectrum disorder (ASD). Intervention services were initiated—speech-language therapy and behavioral therapy based on the principles of applied behavior analysis. His pediatrician also ordered fragile X DNA analysis and chromosomal microarray, which were normal. His parents return with additional questions. A friend, who also has a child with ASD, told them about a nutritional supplement and special diet that can improve a child's language skills and social behavior. Stephen's parents did additional reading about these and other therapies on the Internet, and they are looking for guidance about whether to use these therapies in their son.

Thought Question:

How should pediatricians address parents' questions about complementary health approaches?

HISTORY, DEFINITIONS, AND DESCRIPTIONS

Various definitions have been used to try to demarcate nonstandard therapies from conventional or accepted medical practices. The term *complementary and alternative medicine* enjoyed a period of popularity and had various definitions, including the following:

- "Interventions not taught widely in medical schools or generally available at U.S. hospitals" (Eisenberg et al., 1993, p. 246)
- "Diagnosis, treatment and/or prevention which complements mainstream medicine by contributing to a common whole, by satisfying a demand not met by orthodoxy or by diversifying conceptual frameworks of medicine" (Ernst et al., 1995, p. 506)
- "A broad domain of healing resources that encompasses all health systems, modalities, and practices and their accompanying theories and beliefs, other than those intrinsic to the politically dominant health systems of a particular society or culture in a given historical period" (O'Connor et al., 1997, p. 50)
- Practices that are "not presently considered an integral part of conventional medicine" (National Center for Complementary and Alternative Medicine, 2000, p. 8)

More recently, the term **complementary health approaches (CHA)** has been used to describe treatments that fall outside the mainstream of standard medical care and the term **integrative medicine** has been used to describe the concept of using standard and nonstandard therapies in a coordinated manner (National Center for Complementary and Integrative Health, 2016). The National Center for Complementary and Integrative Health (NCCIH), a National Institutes of Health center established for the purpose of studying complementary health approaches, categorizes these practices into two main domains—natural products (including botanical agents, vitamins, minerals, and special diets) and mind–body practices (such as massage therapy, yoga, chiropractic, and acupuncture). It is important to note that any dichotomy between CHA and conventional medicine may be a false one—ultimately, therapies either have some degree of effectiveness or they do not, and what we should be most attentive to is the evidence that supports or refutes the plausibility and efficacy of a particular treatment. A treatment that initially gains popularity as a complementary health approach can, and should with the development of a sufficient body of evidence of effectiveness, migrate into the realm of accepted medical practice—although thus far this has been an infrequent occurrence.

The use of CHA is common among adults and children. The first national survey to determine patterns of use of these therapies showed them to be employed commonly among adults in the United States (Eisenberg et al., 1993), with approximately one third of the respondents reporting the use of at least one nonstandard therapy during the prior year. Subsequent studies have also indicated that the use of nonstandard therapies is common among adults (Barnes, Powell-Griner, McFann, & Nahin, 2004; Posadzki, Watson, Alotaibi, & Ernst, 2013; Stussman, Black, Barnes, Clarke, & Nahin, 2015) and children (Black, Clarke, Barnes, Stussman, & Nahin, 2015; Davis & Darden, 2003; Yussman, Ryan, Auinger, & Weitzman, 2004). In the 2012 National Health Interview Survey, the overall prevalence of CHA use among children ages 4–17 years in the United States was 11.6%. The rate of nonstandard therapy use is increased in children with chronic medical conditions (Adams et al., 2013; Magi et al., 2015), and among children with developmental disabilities or mental health concerns. Estimates of the prevalence of CHA use in children with ASD range from 28%–54% (Akins, Krakowiak, Angkustsiri, Hertz-Picciotto, & Hansen, 2014; Höfer, Hoffmann, & Bachmann, 2017; Perrin et al., 2012; Salomone et al., 2015). Frequent use of CHA has been demonstrated in other developmental or mental health disorders, including 30% in children with non-ASD developmental disabilities (Akins et al., 2014); 28.9% in children with attention-deficit/hyperactivity disorder (ADHD), anxiety, or depression (Kemper et al., 2013); and 26.8% in children with cerebral palsy (Majnemer et al., 2013). In multiple studies, an association between higher levels of parental education and nonstandard therapy use in children has been demonstrated (Akins et al., 2014; Davis, Meaney, & Duncan, 2004; Sawni-Sikand, Schubiner, & Thomas, 2002).

TREATMENT, MANAGEMENT, AND INTERVENTIONS

What Does the Evidence Show?

Scientific evidence has a hierarchy (Oxford Centre for Evidence-Based Medicine, 2009), which is an essential point to remember when weighing evidence for or against the efficacy of specific CHA in the treatment of children with disabilities. As with conventional health practices, CHA should be evaluated with clinical trials that include known doses of intervention, randomization, clinical characterization of patients, and appropriate control groups. These design factors are necessary to interpret studies that are large enough to support statistical interpretation. In this chapter, discussion of specific CHAs relies on reviews and/or meta-analysis rather than case reports.

Natural Products

Natural products include interventions such as herbs and other supplements, vitamins, and special diets.

Supplements and Vitamins Melatonin has been used to target sleep problems in children with developmental disorders, and there is a reasonable amount of published evidence that it is effective for shortening sleep latency and increasing total sleep time in children with disabilities (Schwichtenberg & Malow, 2015; Box 39.1). Omega-3 fatty acids are among the most widely used natural product in the pediatric population. However, evidence is currently inconclusive whether polyunsaturated fatty acids have specific therapeutic benefit in children with ADHD or specific learning disorders (Gillies, Sinn, Lad, Leach, & Ross, 2012; Tan, Ho, & The, 2016). Vitamin B6 and magnesium have also been studied as a treatment for ASD, but the evidence remains inadequate to recommend their use (Nye & Brice, 2009).

Special Diets Various special diets have been promoted in the treatment of ADHD, ASD, and other developmental disorders. The **Feingold diet** (Feingold, 1975) became popular in the 1970s based on the theory that certain food additives contribute to the symptoms of ADHD. Controlled trials of this diet have not shown any clear efficacy. Although some studies have suggested some benefit of an elimination diet (Pelsser et al., 2009; Sonuga-Barke et al., 2013), specific special dietary manipulations are not currently a recommended treatment approach in children with ADHD (American Academy of Pediatrics, Subcommittee on Attention-Deficit/Hyperactivity Disorder, Steering Committee on Quality Improvement and Management, 2011). Likewise, despite the popularity of the gluten- and casein-free diet in children with ASD, the scientific literature currently does not indicate that this diet is efficacious for any of the core symptoms (Hyman et al., 2016; Sathe, Andrews, McPheeters, & Warren, 2017), although it may improve some gastrointestinal symptoms reported in children with ASD (Levy & Hyman, 2017).

Hyperbaric Oxygen Therapy **Hyperbaric oxygen therapy** (HBOT) has also been used as a treatment for children with cerebral palsy, ASD, and other developmental disorders based on the hypothesis that supranormal oxygen concentrations can heal damaged or dormant brain tissue. The biological plausibility of this idea is weak, and experimental evidence that HBOT is beneficial in the treatment of any developmental disability is lacking. Adverse effects of HBOT, such as barotrauma, can occur. The available scientific literature currently does not support the use of HBOT in children with ASD (Xiong, Chen, Luo, & Mu, 2016).

Mind–Body Practices

As defined by the NCCIH, this group of therapeutic approaches include therapies such as biofeedback, acupuncture, massage, meditation, relaxation techniques, spinal manipulation, yoga, and energy-based practices such as Qi Gong and therapeutic touch. Current evidence does not support a clear role for these treatment approaches in the management of children with disabilities.

BOX 39.1 EVIDENCE-BASED PRACTICE

Melatonin for Sleep Problems in Children with Autism Spectrum Disorder (ASD)

Sleep problems, including prolonged sleep latency and nocturnal awakenings, are extremely common in children with developmental disabilities, including ASD. Melatonin, a hormone produced by the pineal gland, has been studied as a possible treatment for these types of sleep disturbances. A number of studies have shown that melatonin can be effective in shortening the sleep latency and increasing the total sleep duration in children with ASD, although the overall degree of these effects is modest. Although behavioral strategies, including good sleep hygiene practices, remain the first-line approach for sleep problems in children with disabilities, clinicians can consider melatonin as an adjunctive treatment.

Source: Cuomo et al. (2017).

Meditation and Massage Short-term improvements in certain behavioral, language, or sensory measures have been observed in some studies of meditation or massage in children with disabilities. A systematic review of studies of massage therapy for children with ASD highlighted the high risk of bias in these studies and suggested that no firm conclusions could be reached regarding the effectiveness of this therapy in this population (Lee, Kim, & Ernst, 2011). Likewise, in a meta-analysis of studies of massage therapy administered to premature infants, benefits on weight gain and length of stay were demonstrated, but there were no clear differences in neurobehavioral functioning (Wang, He, & Zhang, 2013).

Sensory Integration Therapy Sensory integration dysfunction, more recently referred to as sensory processing disorder, was initially proposed as a theory in the 1970s (Ayres, 1972). This theory is based in the notion that inefficient and disorganized responses to sensory input to the brain is linked to many developmental and behavioral symptoms. Although various sensory-based methods are widely used in the treatment of children with developmental disabilities, particularly ASD, the evidence base to support the use of this therapy remains limited. Several small, short-term studies have indicated improvement in certain sensory measures and motor skills among children receiving sensory-related therapies, although statistically significant benefits in other outcomes were not observed and the risk of bias in these studies was generally high (Weitlauf, Sathe, McPheeters, & Warren, 2017; see Chapter 7).

Music Therapy Music therapy, defined as the use of music interventions to accomplish individualized goals within a therapeutic relationship (American Music Therapy Association, n.d.), has also been used in children with ASD and other developmental disabilities. The largest and most rigorous randomized clinical study of improvisational music therapy (compared with enhanced standard care) in children with ASD showed no significant difference in symptom severity, as measured by the Autism Diagnostic Observation Schedule social affect domain scores, over a 5-month follow-up period, and it did not support the use of this therapy for symptom reduction in this population of children (Bieleninik et al., 2017). Further data are needed to support or refute the role of music therapy in children with disabilities.

Electroencephalographic Biofeedback Electroencephalographic (EEG) biofeedback (neurofeedback) has been investigated as a treatment for conditions such as ADHD. In this technique, children try to learn to use brain electrical activity to control a computer interface, with the goal of improving ability to sustain attention. Criticism has been raised about the methodologies of some of the early positive studies of this intervention (Heywood & Beale, 2003; Kline, Brann, & Loney, 2002; Ramirez, Desantis, & Opler, 2001). EEG biofeedback is not presently a well-validated treatment approach in children with ADHD (Cortese et al., 2016), although the technique continues to be studied.

Other mind–body practices, including auditory integration training, vision therapy, craniosacral therapy, chiropractic manipulation, and energy-based practices (including therapeutic touch and acupuncture) also have weak theoretical bases, lack sufficient evidence in the scientific literature, and currently have no role in the management of children with disabilities (see Table 39.1).

Counseling Families Regarding Complementary Health Approaches

Many factors attract families to CHA. There is growing societal acceptance of the promotion of wellness through dietary and mind–body practices, and there is a perception that natural approaches are safer and carry fewer adverse effects compared with conventional medical approaches. Families may also welcome the greater control that pursuing therapies in line with their philosophical beliefs affords. Scientific evidence of efficacy may not be an equally weighted factor for families in their decision to pursue CHA. Caregivers and medical providers should be encouraged to consider the following questions when trying to determine the legitimacy of a nonstandard therapy (Lilienfeld, Lynn, & Lohr, 2014; Nickel, 1996). These relate to the theoretical basis for the therapy, the previous scientific evaluation of the therapy, and the methods by which the therapy is promoted. Although therapies should not automatically be discounted simply because they seem unconventional, affirmative responses to any of the following questions should raise a red flag about the legitimacy of a specific nonstandard therapy:

- Is the treatment based on a theory that is overly simplistic?
- Is the treatment based on proposed forces or principles that are inconsistent with accumulated knowledge from other scientific disciplines?
- Has the treatment changed little over a very long period of time?

Table 39.1. Summary recommendations for the use of complementary health approaches in children with disabilities based on current evidence relying on systematic reviews and meta-analyses

	Mind–body practices	Natural products and other biologically based practices
Sufficient evidence exists to support current use	None	Melatonin to shorten sleep latency
More research is needed	Biofeedback, electroencephalography/electromyography Meditation, relaxation techniques Music therapy Massage Sensory integration therapy Transcranial magnetic stimulation	Omega-3 fatty acids Oxytocin
Current evidence does not support use	Chiropractic Auditory integration therapy Vision therapy, visual perceptual training Reflexology Craniosacral therapy Patterning, Doman-Delacato method Acupuncture Energy therapies: therapeutic touch, Reiki, Qi gong Magnet therapy Homeopathy	Pharmacological doses of vitamins (except for the treatment of known metabolic disorders) Gluten-free, casein-free diet in autism spectrum disorder (ASD) Chelation therapy Secretin for treatment of ASD Hyperbaric oxygen for treatment of ASD or cerebral palsy Antiviral agents Immunoglobulins Stem cell therapy

- Is there an absence of well-designed studies published in the peer-reviewed medical literature, or do proponents imply that it is not feasible to scientifically test the therapy?
- Do proponents of the treatment cherry pick data that support the value of the treatment while ignoring contradictory evidence?
- Do proponents of the treatment assume a treatment is effective until there is evidence to the contrary?
- Do proponents claim that a treatment cannot be studied in isolation but only in combination with a package of other interventions or practices?
- Is the treatment promoted as being free of adverse effects?
- Are anecdotes and testimonials used as a primary marketing strategy?
- Do proponents of the treatment use scientific-sounding, but nonsensical, terminology to describe the treatment?
- Is the treatment promoted for a wide range of physiologically diverse conditions? (Adapted with permission from Challman, T. D., & Myers, S. M. [2018]. Complementary health approaches in developmental and behavioral pediatrics. In *Developmental and behavioral pediatrics* [2nd ed.]. Itasca, IL: American Academy of Pediatrics.)

Ethical principles need to be considered in any analysis of the use of nonstandard therapies. As outlined above, most of these therapies have very limited evidence to show that they are actually helpful in the conditions for which they are promoted. Beneficence requires that providers remain concerned about the welfare of children with disabilities when considering which therapies to provide or endorse. This same principle also applies to conventional medical practices in the care of children with disabilities—many widely prescribed treatments suffer from an inadequate evidence base to support their use. Likewise, all therapies, conventional and nonstandard alike, carry certain risks. Caregivers and health care providers should be especially wary of potentially harmful nonstandard biomedical interventions, such as chelation therapy (Brown, Willis, Omalu, & Leiker, 2006), which is based on an unsupported theory concerning heavy metals in the etiology of ASD and which has no role in ASD treatment (James, Stevenson, Silove, & Williams, 2015). When considering the safety of nonstandard therapies, providers and caregivers must be cognizant of the principle of nonmaleficence, or limiting harm in the quest for achieving an outcome. Whereas direct adverse physical effects from nonstandard biological or manipulative interventions are the most obvious safety concern (Ernst, 2003), attention also needs to be given to other potential negative consequences of nonstandard therapy use, such as increased time and financial demands on a family that lead to inadvertent diversion from interventions that are known to be effective. At times, the principles of beneficence and nonmaleficence can come into conflict with caregivers' autonomy to choose certain treatments. A challenge for health care providers is to balance these principles, with the understanding that children's health and safety should always take highest priority. Whereas not all providers who promote nonstandard therapies support beliefs that discourage medical interventions known to be beneficial (Wardle, Frawley, Steel, & Sullivan, 2016), the ethical principle of justice dictates that access to services that have proven individual or public health value be maintained even if CHA are being utilized.

Expectancy effects such as the **placebo response,** defined as "a genuine psychological or physiological effect, . . . which is attributable to receiving a substance or undergoing a procedure, but which is not due to the inherent powers of that substance or procedure" (Stewart-Williams & Podd, 2004, p. 326), can explain some or all of the apparent positive effects of specific CHA. Although the use of placebos was common in the 19th century and earlier, this practice fell out of favor because of concerns that their use was dishonest and paternalistic (Edwards, 2005). Even now, however, the use of placebos in standard clinical practice is not uncommon (Harris & Raz, 2012), and a possible role in developmental pediatrics has been suggested (Sandler, Glesne, & Bodfish, 2010). However, using CHA solely to harness some degree of placebo effect can be viewed as deceptive and contrary to the ethical principle of truthfulness.

The American Academy of Pediatrics recommends that providers 1) ask families about the use of different therapies; 2) respect the family's perspectives, values, and cultural beliefs regarding treatment approaches; 3) monitor the patient's response to treatment; 4) establish measurable outcomes when nonstandard therapies are being used; and 5) maintain up-to-date knowledge about currently popular nonstandard therapies (American Academy of Pediatrics, 2008). However, there is not a "one-size-fits-all" approach to counseling families about nonstandard therapy use. Therapies for which there is good evidence of inefficacy, or whose potential harm significantly outweighs any theoretical benefit, should be actively discouraged—chelation therapy in ASD is one such example. There may be some therapies that start as nonstandard and unconventional but ultimately demonstrate effectiveness for a condition using rigorous scientific methodology. These therapies should be moved into the domain of accepted medical practice. An additional group of therapies may have some biological plausibility and warrant further scientific investigation. These approaches should not be recommended until an adequate evidence base of effectiveness is developed. Lastly, there may be certain therapies that have meaning for a family in the context of a cultural or religious tradition, and it is reasonable for the provider to support the use of these therapies if there are no unacceptable safety risks. The importance of certain cultural and religious traditions has been offered as an argument for why nonstandard therapies should not be marginalized by the scientific community (Kaptchuk & Eisenberg, 2001). However, the reality is that few currently popular nonstandard therapies in children with disabilities have their origin in cultural or religious beliefs (Akins et al., 2014). Health care providers in the medical home have a duty to discuss the scientific rationale, or lack thereof, for CHA with families and to actively discourage those therapies that lack evidence of effectiveness or possess unacceptable risks.

SUMMARY

- The use of CHA is common in children with disabilities.
- Scientific evidence of the efficacy for most natural products and mind–body practices is weak or absent. Rigorous methodology should be used to test specific interventions to determine whether they have a legitimate role in the management of children with disabilities.
- Strong relationships between families and health care providers in their children's medical homes are necessary to build and maintain trust and communication; this will enable families to feel comfortable discussing CHA and be open to provider advice about the scientific validity of these therapies.

ADDITIONAL RESOURCES

National Center for Complementary and Integrative Health: http://nccih.nih.gov/health/atoz.htm

Therapeutic Research Faculty: http://www.naturaldatabase.therapeuticresearch.com

Additional resources can be found online in Appendix D: Childhood Disabilities Resources, Services, and Organizations (see About the Online Companion Materials).

REFERENCES

Adams, D., Dagenais, S., Clifford, T., Baydala, L., King, W. J., Hervas-Malo, M., . . . Vohra, S. (2013). Complementary and alternative medicine use by pediatric specialty outpatients. *Pediatrics, 131*(2), 225–232.

Akins, R. S., Krakowiak, P., Angkustsiri, K., Hertz-Picciotto, I., & Hansen, R. L. (2014). Utilization patterns of conventional and complementary/alternative treatments in children with autism spectrum disorders and developmental disabilities in a population-based study. *Journal of Developmental & Behavioral Pediatrics, 35*(1), 1–10.

American Academy of Pediatrics (2008). Clinical report: Use of complementary and alternative medicine in pediatrics. *Pediatrics, 122*(6), 1374–1386. Reaffirmed January 2013.

American Academy of Pediatrics, Subcommittee on Attention-Deficit/Hyperactivity Disorder, Steering Committee on Quality Improvement and Management (2011). ADHD: Clinical practice guideline for the diagnosis, evaluation, and treatment of attention-deficit/hyperactivity disorder in children and adolescents. *Pediatrics, 128*(5), 1007–1022.

American Music Therapy Association (n.d.). *What is music therapy?* Retrieved from https://www.musictherapy.org/about/musictherapy/

Ayres, A. J. (1972). *Sensory integration and learning disorders.* Los Angeles, CA: Western Psychological Services.

Barnes, P. M., Powell-Griner, E., McFann, K., & Nahin, R. L. (2004). Complementary and alternative medicine use among adults: United States, 2002. *Advance Data, 343,* 1–19.

Bieleninik, L., Geretsegger, M., Mossler, K., Assmus, J., Thompson, G., Gattino, G., . . . TIME-A Study Team. (2017). Effects of improvisational music therapy vs enhanced standard care on symptom severity among children with autism spectrum disorder: The TIME-A randomized clinical trial. *The Journal of the American Medical Association, 318*(6), 525–535.

Black, L. I., Clarke, T. C., Barnes, P. M., Stussman, B. J., & Nahin, R. L. (2015). Use of complementary health approaches among children aged 4-17 years in the United States: National Health Interview Survey, 2007–2012. *National Health Statistics Report, 78,* 1–19.

Brown, M. J., Willis, T., Omalu, B., & Leiker, R. (2006). Deaths resulting from hypocalcemia after administration of edetate disodium: 2003-2005. *Pediatrics, 118*(2), e534–e536.

Cortese, S., Ferrin, M., Brandeis, D., Holtmann, M., Aggensteiner, P., Daley, D., . . . European ADHD Guidelines Group. (2016). Neurofeedback for attention-deficit/hyperactivity disorder: Meta-analysis of clinical and neuropsychological outcomes from randomized controlled trials [Review]. *Journal of the American Academy of Child & Adolescent Psychiatry, 55*(6), 444–455.

Cuomo, B. M., Vaz, S., Lee, E. A. L., Thompson, C., Rogerson, J. M., & Falkmer, T. (2017). Effectiveness of sleep-based interventions for children with autism spectrum disorder: A meta-synthesis [Review]. *Pharmacotherapy: The Journal of Human Pharmacology & Drug Therapy, 37*(5), 555–578.

Davis, M. P., & Darden, P. M. (2003). Use of complementary and alternative medicine by children in the United States. *Archives of Pediatric and Adolescent Medicine, 157*(4), 393–396.

Davis, M. F., Meaney F. J., & Duncan, B. (2004). Factors influencing the use of complementary and alternative medicine in children. *Journal of Alternative & Complementary Medicine, 10*(5), 740–742.

Edwards, M. (2005). Placebo. *Lancet, 365,* 1023.

Eisenberg, D. M., Kessler, R. C., Foster, C., Norlock, F. E., Calkins, D. R., & Delbanco, T. L. (1993). Unconventional medicine in the United States: Prevalence, costs, and patterns of use. *New England Journal of Medicine, 328,* 246–252.

Ernst, E. (2003). Serious adverse effects of unconventional therapies for children and adolescents: A systematic review of recent evidence [Review]. *European Journal of Pediatrics, 162*(2), 72–80.

Ernst, E., Resch, K. L., Mills, S., Hill, R., Mitchell, A., Willoughby, M., & White, A. (1995). Complementary medicine—a definition. *British Journal of General Practice, 45,* 506.

Feingold, B. F. (1975). *Why your child is hyperactive.* New York, NY: Random House.

Gillies, D., Sinn, J. K. H., Lad, S. S., Leach, M. J., & Ross, M. J. (2012). Polyunsaturated fatty acids (PUFA) for attention deficit hyperactivity disorder (ADHD) in children and adolescents. *Cochrane Database of Systematic Reviews, 7,* CD007986. doi:10.1002/14651858.CD007986.pub2

Harris, C. S., & Raz, A. (2012). Deliberate use of placebos in clinical practice: What we really know. *Journal of Medical Ethics, 38*(7), 406–407.

Heywood, C., & Beale, I. (2003). EEG biofeedback vs. placebo treatment for attention-deficit/hyperactivity disorder: A pilot study. *Journal of Attention Disorders, 7,* 43–55.

Höfer, J., Hoffmann, F., & Bachmann, C. (2017). Use of complementary and alternative medicine in children and adolescents with autism spectrum disorder: A systematic review. *Autism, 21*(4), 387–402.

Hyman, S. L., Stewart, P. A., Foley, J., Cain, U., Peck, R., Morris, D. D., . . . Smith, T. (2016). The gluten-free/casein-free diet: A double-blind challenge trial in children with autism. *Journal of Autism and Developmental Disorders, 46*(1), 205–220.

James, S., Stevenson, S. W., Silove, N., & Williams, K. (2015). Chelation for autism spectrum disorder (ASD). *Cochrane Database of Systematic Reviews, 5,* CD010766. doi:10.1002/14651858.CD010766.pub2

Kaptchuk, T. J., & Eisenberg, D. M. (2001). Varieties of healing. 1: Medical pluralism in the United States. *Annals of Internal Medicine, 135*(3), 189–195.

Kemper, K. J., Gardiner, P., & Birdee, G. S. (2013). Use of complementary and alternative medical therapies among youth with mental health concerns. *Academic Pediatrics, 13*(6), 540–545.

Kline, J. P, Brann, C. N., & Loney, B. R. (2002). A cacophony in the brainwaves: A critical appraisal of neurotherapy for attention-deficit disorders. *The Scientific Review of Mental Health Practice, 1*(1), 44–54.

Lee, M. S., Kim, J. I., & Ernst, E. (2011). Massage therapy for children with autism spectrum disorders: A systematic review. *Journal of Clinical Psychiatry, 72*(3), 406–411.

Levy, S. E., & Hyman, S. L. (2017). Complementary and alternative medicine treatments for children with autism spectrum disorders. *Child and Adolescent Psychiatric Clinics of North America, 24,* 117–143.

Lilienfeld, S. O., Lynn, S. J., & Lohr, J. M. (Eds.). (2014). *Science and pseudoscience in clinical psychology* (2nd ed.). New York, NY: Guilford Press.

Magi, T., Kuehni, C. E., Torchetti, L., Wengenroth, L., Luer, S., & Frei-Erb, M. (2015). Use of complementary and alternative medicine in children with cancer: A study at a Swiss university hospital. *PLoS ONE, 10*(12), e0145787.

Majnemer, A., Shikako-Thomas, K., Shevell, M. I., Poulin, C., Lach, L., Schmitz, N., . . . Group the QUALA. (2013). Pursuit of complementary and alternative medicine treatments in adolescents with cerebral palsy. *Journal of Child Neurology, 28*(11), 1443–1447.

National Center for Complementary and Alternative Medicine. (2000). *Expanding horizons of healthcare: Five year strategic plan 2001-2005.* Washington, DC: U.S. Department of Health and Human Services.

National Center for Complementary and Integrative Health. (2016). *Complementary, alternative, or integrative health: What's in a name?* Retrieved from https://nccih.nih.gov/health/integrative-health#term

Nickel, R. (1996). Controversial therapies for young children with developmental disabilities. *Infants Young Child, 8,* 29–40.

Nye, C., & Brice, A. (2009). Combined vitamin B6-magnesium treatment in autism spectrum disorder. *Cochrane Database of Systematic Reviews, 1,* 00075320-100000000-02514.

O'Connor, B.B., Calabrese, C., Cardeña, E., Eisenberg, D., Fincher, J., Hufford, . . . Zhang, X. (1997). Defining and describing complementary and alternative medicine. Panel on Definition and Description, CAM Research Methodology Conference, April 1995. *Alternative Therapies in Health and Medicine*, 3(2):49-57.

Oxford Centre for Evidence-Based Medicine. (2009). *Oxford Centre for Evidence-Based Medicine–Levels of evidence (March 2009).* Retrieved from http://www.cebm.net/blog/2009/06/11/oxford-centre-evidence-based-medicine-levels-evidence-march-2009

Pelsser, L. M., Frankena, K., Toorman, J, Savelkoul, H. F., Pereira, R. R., & Buitelaar, J. K. (2009). A randomized controlled trial into the effects of food on ADHD. *European Child & Adolescent Psychiatry, 18,* 12–19.

Perrin, J. M., Coury, D. L., Hyman, S. L., Cole, L., Reynolds, A. M., & Clemons, T. (2012). Complementary and alternative medicine use in a large pediatric autism sample. *Pediatrics, 130*(Suppl. 2), S77–S82.

Posadzki, P., Watson, L. K., Alotaibi, A., & Ernst, E. (2013). Prevalence of use of complementary and alternative medicine (CAM) by patients/consumers in the UK: Systematic review of surveys [Review]. *Clinical Medicine, 13*(2), 126–131.

Ramirez, P. M., Desantis, D., & Opler, L. A. (2001). EEG biofeedback treatment of ADD: A viable alternative to traditional medical intervention? [Review]. *Annals of the New York Academy of Sciences, 931,* 342–358.

Salomone E; Charman T; McConachie H; Warreyn P; Working Group 4, COST Action 'Enhancing the Scientific Study of Early Autism'. (2015). Prevalence and correlates of use of complementary and alternative medicine in children with autism spectrum disorder in Europe. *European Journal of Pediatrics, 174*(10), 1277–1285.

Sandler, A. D., Glesne, C. E., & Bodfish, J. W. (2010). Conditioned placebo dose reduction: A new treatment in attention-deficit hyperactivity disorder? *Journal of Developmental & Behavioral Pediatrics, 31*(5), 369–375.

Sathe, N., Andrews, J. C., McPheeters, M. L., & Warren, Z. E. (2017). Nutritional and dietary interventions for autism spectrum disorder: A systematic review. *Pediatrics, 139*(6), e20170346. doi:10.1542/peds.2017-0346

Sawni-Sikand, A., Schubiner, H., & Thomas, R. L. (2002). Use of complementary/alternative therapies among children in primary care pediatrics. *Ambulatory Pediatrics, 2*(2), 99–103.

Schwichtenberg, A. J., & Malow, B. A. (2015). Melatonin treatment in children with developmental disabilities [Review]. *Sleep Medicine Clinics, 10*(2), 181–187.

Sonuga-Barke, E. J., Brandeis, D., Cortese, S. L., Daley, D., Ferrrin, M., Holtmann, M., . . . European ADHD Guidelines Group (2013). Nonpharmacological interventions for ADHD: Systematic review and meta-analyses of randomized controlled trials of dietary and psychological treatments. European ADHD Guidelines Group. *American Journal of Psychiatry, 170,* 275–289.

Stewart-Williams, S., & Podd, J. (2004). The placebo effect: Dissolving the expectancy versus conditioning debate [Review]. *Psychological Bulletin, 130,* 324–340.

Stussman, B. J., Black L. I., Barnes, P. M., Clarke, T. C., & Nahin, R. L. (2015). Wellness-related use of common complementary health approaches among adults: United States, 2012. *National Health Statistics Report, 85,* 1–12.

Tan, M., Ho, J. J., & The, K. (2016). Polyunsaturated fatty acids (PUFAs) for children with specific learning disorders. *Cochrane Database of Systematic Reviews, 9,* CD009398. doi:10.1002/14651858.CD009398.pub3

Xiong, T., Chen, H., Luo, R., & Mu, D. (2016). Hyperbaric oxygen therapy for people with autism spectrum disorder (ASD). *Cochrane Database of Systematic Reviews, 10,* CD010922.

Wang, L., He, J. L., & Zhang, X. H. (2013). The efficacy of massage on preterm infants: A meta-analysis. *American Journal of Perinatology, 30*(9), 731–778.

Wardle, J., Frawley, J., Steel, A., & Sullivan, E. (2016). Complementary medicine and childhood immunization: A critical review [Review]. *Vaccine, 34*(38), 4484–4500.

Weitlauf, A. S., Sathe, N., McPheeters, M. L., & Warren, Z. E. (2017). Interventions targeting sensory challenges in autism spectrum disorder: A systematic review [Review]. *Pediatrics, 139*(6), e20170347.

Yussman, S. M., Ryan, S. A., Auinger, P., & Weitzman, M. (2004). Visits to complementary and alternative medicine providers by children and adolescents in the United States. *Ambulatory Pediatrics, 4*(5), 429–435.

Zollman, C., & Vickers, A. (1999). Complementary medicine in conventional practice. *BMJ, 319,* 901. doi:https://doi.org/10.1136/bmj.319.7214.901

PART VII
Outcomes

CHAPTER 40 Transition from Adolescence to Adulthood

Lisa K. Tuchman and Cara E. Pugliese

Upon completion of this chapter, the reader will

- Be able to describe the importance of planning for the transition to adulthood for youth with intellectual and developmental disabilities (IDD)
- Understand the relationship among neurodiversity, self-advocacy, self-determination, and health outcomes
- Be knowledgeable about the resources and mandated laws available to assist youth with IDD to move from the home to the community and to the adult health care system
- Know the role of employment and postsecondary education in the transition process
- Understand the increased risks of mental health and behavioral issues and how they may affect the transition to adulthood

Individuals with developmental disabilities encounter the same life transitions as their typically developing peers. Perhaps the most challenging of these is the transition to adulthood, which is a period of complex biological, social, and emotional change. This transition involves moving 1) from school to work and/or postsecondary education, 2) into age-appropriate community inclusion, and 3) from child- to adult-oriented health care. This chapter focuses on approaches to ensuring the successful transition of an individual with developmental disabilities from adolescence to adulthood.

CASE STUDY

Elijah is a 22-year-old young man with autism spectrum disorder (ASD) and moderate intellectual disability (ID) who was born prematurely. He completed his public school education 1 year ago. Elijah currently works at a local supermarket. He receives support and guidance from coworkers who were trained by a local job placement program to provide Elijah with natural supports in the workplace. After work, he participates in some recreational and leisure activities with friends. He goes to the gym and swims regularly at the advice of his pediatrician to promote his general health and prevent obesity. However, he has been told that he needs to find a new physician who cares for adults. He has been relying on his parents to help with this endeavor as he has never had to navigate the health system alone and is unsure of next steps. With his increasing job satisfaction and some financial independence, Elijah has expressed a desire to live on his own this past year. He and his parents contacted the local Autism Speaks chapter and, with assistance from advocates, found an apartment and a live-in personal-care attendant. Elijah has recently developed a romantic interest in a young person his same age that he met at his job and hopes he can have a relationship with her. He still goes to his parents' house for family dinners and events at least once a week and spends additional time with his two younger siblings, ages 16 and 18, who come to visit him regularly in his apartment.

Thought Question:

What is the role of his pediatric care providers in preparing Elijah and his family for transition to adulthood, including entry into the adult health care system?

GENERAL PRINCIPLES OF TRANSITION TO ADULTHOOD

There are three basic tenets of successful transition from childhood to adulthood for an individual with intellectual and developmental disabilities (IDD). First, transition is a process, not an event. Planning for transition to adulthood should begin as early as possible in late childhood and early adolescence and take into account the young person's increasing autonomy and capacity for making choices (American Academy of Pediatrics, American Academy of Family Physicians, & American College of Physicians Transitions Clinical Report Authoring Group, 2011). Second, coordination among health care, educational, vocational, and social service systems is essential. Third, self-determination and self-advocacy skills should be fostered throughout the transition process. Standards for transition services call for a youth-centered and strengths-based approach, where the young adult acts autonomously as an informed decision maker during the entire transition process to improve his or her quality of life (Walsh, Jones, & Schonwald, 2017; Wehmeyer & Abery, 2013). Ensuring that a young person understands his or her strengths and challenges and can self-advocate for the accommodations needed to be successful and fulfilled is critical to promoting independence and well-being.

MOVING TOWARD INDEPENDENCE: NEURODIVERSITY, SELF-ADVOCACY, AND SELF-DETERMINATION

Just as people can have significant diversity in their physical abilities—some may use their feet to walk, while others may need a wheelchair or cane—individuals also can have significant differences in their cognitive phenotype or thinking styles. The term *neurodiversity* has been put forward to describe this spectrum. It was first used by ASD rights advocate Judy Singer and journalist Harvey Blume to propose that ASD was more akin to a neurological difference than a disorder (Armstrong, 2015). This term has since spread beyond the ASD rights movement to the broader disability rights community. The concept of neurodiversity originated as a challenge to previously held views of developmental disabilities as inherently pathological, arguing that neurological differences should be viewed as part of one's personal identity, similarly to gender, ethnicity, and sexual orientation (Ripamonti, 2016). The concept of neurodiversity shifts the focus away from a "cure"—of which there are few currently available for many developmental disabilities—and toward accommodations or supports that will help a person achieve his or her goals and lead a fulfilling life. This is analogous to the approach that the deaf community has been pursuing for decades, but it remains controversial as it also converts the concept of a disorder (often with a discrete cause and potential for treatment) to that of normal diversity.

Self-Advocacy and Self-Determination

Both self-advocacy and self-determination are critical skills to foster throughout the life span for successful transition to adulthood. While the concept of **self-advocacy** has many definitions and, in fact, encompasses an entire civil rights movement of and by individuals with IDD, it generally refers to the ability to effectively understand and communicate ones wants and needs (Test, Fowler, Wood, Brewer, & Eddy, 2005). Self-determination is interdependent with self-advocacy and describes the ability to independently set and pursue one's goals (Shogren et al., 2015). It is critical that transitioning adults are able to understand their own strengths and weaknesses to ensure that they can ask for the necessary supports and accommodations needed to achieve their desired goals. Self-determination tends to increase across the life span and is linked to numerous positive outcomes, including more positive employment experiences, independent living, improved community inclusion, and enhanced quality of life for adolescents with IDD (Nota, Soresi, Ferrari, & Wehmeyer, 2011; Wehmeyer, Palmer, Shogren, Williams-Diehm, & Soukup, 2013).

Wehmeyer and Abery (2013) describe self-determined actions as autonomous, self-regulated, psychologically empowered, and self-realized. Students with ID tend to report lower levels of self-determination than students with learning disabilities, ASD, and emotional and behavioral problems (Mumbardó-Adam et al., 2017). This is often due to their having fewer opportunities to make choices in their lives rather than to a lack of capacity to become self-determined (Wehmeyer & Abery, 2013). In fact, research indicates that youth with IDD can become more self-determined when given proper supports and direct instruction (see Wehmereyer & Abery, 2013, for a review). Structured intervention to develop self-determination has been shown to be effective in promoting youths' choice-making, problem-solving, decision-making, goal setting, and self-advocacy skills (Cobb, Lehmann, Newman-Gonchar, & Alwell, 2009). Instruction on self-determination and self-advocacy can be taught and supported through guidance from mentors, professionals, family members, self-advocates, and participation in community mentorship programs.

The skills needed for self-determination can also be explicitly shaped incidentally through real-world learning experiences and by an open and supportive acknowledgement of one's disability (Nota, Ferrari, Soresi, & Wehmeyer, 2007). It is vital that youth with IDD understand that everyone has weaknesses and that they will need to ask for supports and mentorship to be successful in reaching their goals at some point in their lives. This often requires direct instruction by the young adult's support team to have the individual verbally identify situations that require self-advocacy and think out loud in order to explicitly model how he/she can self-advocate or ask for help. Families, teachers, and other well-intentioned people often attempt to protect youth with IDD from failing, but it is essential that they understand that, like everyone else, they have strengths and weaknesses. While those weaknesses are not their fault, it is their responsibility to obtain accommodations to ensure that they can be successful in addressing the challenges they will face. Teaching youth to be strong self-advocates across multiple domains—educational, social, health care, and legal—is critical for them developing successful autonomy. Explicit instruction in self-determination is also vital to teach goal setting, planning, and flexible problem-solving. It is especially important in promoting independence and successful goal attainment when obstacles arise. Families and support individuals also can provide encouragement for the individual with IDD to 1) try new experiences; 2) enhance communication and social interactions; 3) make good choices; and 4) learn about their community so they can become an active, contributing member (supporteddecisionmaking.org).

Ultimately, the focus of transitional care for youth with IDD is to help them realize their full adult potential, which includes belonging to a community where they are respected, valued, and able to contribute. It should also be shaped by their present and future personal goals. Many youth with IDD are disconnected from the community after aging out of the school system. As one example, although nearly 50,000 youth with ASD enter adulthood each year, few have jobs. Youth with ASD from ethnic minorities and low-income groups are further disproportionately affected by poor employment outcomes (Roux, Shattuck, Rast, Rava, & Anderson, 2015). For youth with severe ID, families will usually be able to access services from state departments for developmental disabilities, and the individual is likely to be eligible for long-term services. For youth with mild ID or with typical intelligence but adaptive behavior deficits, adult success or future adult productivity will be dependent on the ability of the individual to learn adaptive and self-advocacy skills.

Teachers and other professionals providing assistance to families can and should begin preparing children with IDD for independence as early as possible. Children as young as 3–5 years of age can begin to incorporate chores into their daily routine. By the developmental age of 6–11 years, children should begin to assume responsibility for their self-care. During adolescence, self-determination skills are focused on identifying and meeting educational/vocational goals and building self-advocacy, including their participation in the **individualized education program** (IEP) process.

MOVING FROM SCHOOL TO WORK

The concept of transition planning originated with schools. As such, education policies are the driving force for almost all aspects of transition. There are five pieces of legislation that outline important educational practices to achieve successful adult outcomes for students with disabilities: 1) the Individuals with Disabilities Education Improvement Act (IDEA) of 2004 (PL 108-446), 2) the School-to-Work Opportunities Act of 1994 (PL 103-239), 3) the Workforce Innovation and Opportunity Act (WIOA) of 2014 (PL 113-128), 4) the Americans with Disabilities Act (ADA) of 1990 (PL 101-336), and 5) the Higher Education Opportunity Act of 2008 (HEOA; PL 110-315). Aspects of these key laws are discussed in the following sections.

Legislation Supporting Transitions for Individuals with Disabilities

The 2004 reauthorization of IDEA in particular has strengthened school-to-work transitions. This legislation established 16 years of age as a clear starting point for transition planning in the IEP. It strengthened the working definition of transition services and redefined transition planning from a statement of needed services to a set of measurable postsecondary goals.

These goals are based upon age-appropriate transition assessments related to training; education; employment; and, where appropriate, independent living skills. This legislation also requires schools to report progress toward meeting transition goals in the IEP. Under IDEA (2004), schools must provide a "summary of performance" to students whose special education eligibility is terminated. This new summary must include information on the student's academic achievement and functional performance and recommendations on how to assist the student in meeting his or her postsecondary goals. While schools are not required to conduct any new assessments or evaluations in order to provide the summary, they must satisfy the disability documentation required under other federal laws, such as the Americans with Disabilities Act and Section 504 of the Rehabilitation Act of 1973 (https://www.ncld.org/archives/action-center/learn-the-law/understanding-section-504). See Chapter 33.

Vocational Rehabilitation

Linking schools with systems of care that serve adults with disabilities, including vocational rehabilitation (VR) agencies, strengthens the transition process. WIOA (2014) specifically aims to increase the access of individuals with disabilities to high-quality workforce services. It prepares them for competitive inclusive employment through mandating training services for individuals with disabilities and structured support for competitive inclusive employment. The WIOA mandates appropriated state funding for transition services to youth with disabilities and supports VR state grant programs engaging employers to improve participant employment outcomes. Each state has a VR agency that provides employment service supports to people with IDD.

Transition planning as mandated by IDEA (2004) stipulates that if necessary, schools are responsible for bringing in representatives from other agencies, such as VR services, to be part of the transition planning process. VR agencies help pay for postsecondary education for qualified young adults. Box 40.1 gives an overview of the support services VR counselors offer. It is important to note that VR counselors are typically assigned to students only during their last 2 years of school but that parents and students can request VR participation as early as age 14 through One-Stop Career Centers (U.S. Department of Labor, 2005) or the school.

Unlike K–12 education, which is universal, adult services and systems are eligibility based and require that individuals meet established requirements, including financial eligibility criteria. Once individuals are determined to be eligible, the VR agency can provide or arrange for a host of training, educational, medical, and other services designed to help these individuals acquire and maintain gainful employment. Similar to the IEP in the school system, all services aim to develop an individualized plan for employment (IPE; previously called an individualized written rehabilitation program), which is directed at meeting the needs of the young person. Although VR counselors can provide direct services, they more often refer the individual to appropriate community-based agencies. Examples of services covered by VR under an IPE include self-advocacy training, the development of employment-readiness skills, adaptive driving evaluation and

BOX 40.1 INTERDISCIPLINARY CARE

What Is a Vocational Counselor?

A vocational counselor is a professional who assists individuals with disabilities with career-related support. These counselors usually have a master's-level degree in mental health or community counseling and have knowledge of available employment opportunities suitable for a wide spectrum of interests and abilities. Rehabilitation counseling is a systematic process supporting individuals with physical, mental, developmental, cognitive, and emotional disabilities to achieve their personal, career, and independent living goals in the most integrated settings possible. The counseling process involves communication, goal setting, and supporting self-advocacy. Vocational counselors can implement individualized psychological, vocational, social, and behavioral interventions. Most often vocational counselors work with nonprofit organizations, schools, or other community-based organizations. Working with clients to identify strengths and areas of challenge can help identify and access employment opportunities that meet the individuals' abilities and strengths. Vocational counselors can also help individuals prepare for interviews, provide resources to hone skills, and support managing expectations. By matching skill sets to jobs, they can help ensure that the individual is successful by finding a job that matches their motivations, goals, and abilities. Many states require that vocational counselors be licensed. For more information, visit http://www.arcaweb.org/.

instruction, identification and procurement of assistive technology, supported employment, and customized employment. One area of concern is that while an increasing number of transition-aged adults with ASD are accessing VR agencies, employment outcomes across the United States have not necessarily improved. These adults frequently remain underemployed, earn wages below the poverty threshold, work fewer hours, and earn lower wages than the total population of transition-aged adults served by the VR (Burgess & Cimera, 2014). There is, however, much variability in the success of different state VR programs. For instance, the Autism Society of North Carolina (a VR vendor specifically for adults with ASD) reports an 87% success rate in obtaining competitive employment in 2011, compared with a mean of 33% across the country for the same year (see Burgess & Cimera, 2014). *Accessing Home and Community Based Services: A Guide for Self-Advocates,* which is authored by the Autistic Self-Advocacy Network and the Autism NOW center, may be a helpful resource (http://autisticadvocacy.org/wp-content/uploads/2014/11/Accessing-HCBS-Guide-v1.pdf).

Moving Toward Postsecondary Education

Individuals with IDD can take a modified path toward postsecondary education. Many families find it helpful to advocate for their child to remain in the school system until age 21 so that he or she can complete standard diploma requirements or take advantage of vocational experiences or community college classes offered by the public school system. Postsecondary education can take many forms. Although traditionally thought of as college, it may be any form of education or training that takes place after a young adult leaves high school, including on-the-job training, specialized coursework, or even courses through postgraduate study.

For youth, it can be helpful to modify the typical college pathway by beginning postsecondary education at a community college and then transferring to a public or private 4-year college. Many students find it beneficial to reduce their work load by taking fewer classes at a time and completing their coursework over an extended period of time. Online courses can also reduce the social burden and allow the student to work at his or her own pace, although these benefits must be balanced with the student's motivation and ability to work independently. All colleges that receive federal funding have a disability support services (DSS) office. Some colleges and universities have developed more robust and comprehensive support programs for students with ASD and other IDD, and it is important to inquire about the level of supports provided at each institution of interest. It also is important to research the quality of each institution's programs and make in-person visits to determine an appropriate fit.

There are many students with ASD and average or above intelligence who identify postsecondary education as a primary goal after completing high school. This is the largest group of individuals with IDD who enter college, and therefore this section discusses their experience in some detail. Many of these incoming students are equipped with the cognitive skills to cope with the academic demand of college but struggle with communication and social interactions, executive function difficulties, maintaining motivation, coping with anxiety and stress, self-advocacy, and sensory overload (Adreon & Durocher, 2007; Alverson, Lindstrom, & Hirano, 2015; Trembath, Germano, Johanson, & Dissanayake, 2012; Van Hees, Moyson, & Roeyers, 2015; White et al., 2016). Sosnowy, Silverman, and Shattuck (2018) conducted interviews with parents and young adults with ASD about their postsecondary college experiences. Parents felt that their adult children often needed more holistic services than are available at most colleges. They indicated their need to take an active role in managing their adult child's daily lives in order for them to succeed in college and that organizing supplemental supports (e.g., help with study skills, organization, and socializing/navigating new relationships with school staff and peers) were necessary for their adult child's success. Students felt that, in addition to academic accommodations (e.g., extended time on tests, tutoring, etc.), they thrived when surrounded by staff who promoted autism acceptance and when they found other students they felt they could relate to. Focus groups with secondary and postsecondary administrators, instructors, and educational/academic support staff revealed challenges that are strikingly similar to those identified by students with ASD and their parents in the areas of executive function (e.g., difficulty understanding the big picture and problems with long-term planning and goal setting), self-advocacy, autonomy and self-sufficiency, and establishment and maintenance of long-lasting interpersonal relationships (Elias, Muskett, & White, 2017; Gobbo & Shmulsky, 2014). When families are visiting colleges, they should consider 1) the level of awareness and acceptance of autism, 2) familiarity with factors that promote success, 3) services and accommodations offered by SSD offices, 4) counseling services offered on campus, and 5) specific autism-related supports or programs that may exist on campus. There are also more formalized fee-based support services, such as the *College Living Experience,* that partner with several academic universities, community colleges, and technical schools to provide wrap-around supports in the areas of academics, social skills, independent living, and career development.

There are other options for postsecondary education such as trade schools, which are typically 2 years or less, that focus on teaching hands-on skills. The Transition and Postsecondary Programs for Students with Intellectual Disability (TPSID) are model demonstration projects funded by the U.S. Department of Education that provide academic enrichment, socialization, independent living skills, and work training after high school exit. These programs are typically noncredit based. Resources such as *Think College*, also funded by the U.S. Department of Education, support evidence-based inclusive higher education options for individuals with IDD by generating and sharing knowledge; guiding institutional change; informing public policy; and engaging with students, professionals, and families (https://thinkcollege.net/tpsid). Data suggest that students with disabilities who spend most of their time in traditional classes and participating in campus culture have better postgraduation employment rates than those who spend most of their time in specialized classes (Grigal, Hart, Smith, & Papay, 2018).

To receive assistance or request accommodations for disability-related needs, a student must take the lead in disclosing his or her disability, providing current documentation of the disability and identifying needed accommodations. Thus, it is up to the student to independently navigate a new system of care and appropriately self-advocate for the accommodations that he or she needs. This requires that the student has a solid foundation in self-advocacy skills. The resource *Navigating College: A Handbook on Self-Advocacy* written for adults with autism provides an introduction to the college experience for students who are interested in postsecondary education (http://autisticadvocacy.org/book/navigating-college/).

Accommodations are established on a case-by-case basis and do not necessarily replicate those provided in the K–12 setting. Examples of accommodations that can be requested of DSS include extra time in test taking, a sign language interpreter, a note taker, and recorded books. Postsecondary education facilities that receive federal funding are required to provide reasonable accommodations to qualified individuals with disabilities under Section 504 of the Rehabilitation Act of 1973 (PL 93-112) and under Titles II and/or III of the ADA. HEOA was enacted in 2008, reauthorizing the Higher Education Act of 1965. This law improves access to postsecondary education for students with IDD by opening up eligibility for Pell grants, supplemental educational opportunity grants, and federal work-study programs and by creating TPSID model demonstration programs and coordinating centers for students with IDD (Smith, 2009).

Entering the Work Force

Work experience is a prerequisite for many jobs. Yet, only 58% of adults with ASD and 74% of adults with other IDD have ever worked between high school and their early 20s. Youth with ASD from ethnic minorities and low-income groups are further disproportionately affected by poor employment outcomes (Roux et al., 2015). Young adults with ASD have far higher rates of disconnection, meaning they never got a job or continued their education after high school, than their peers with other disabilities (Roux et al., 2015), while less than 8% of young adults with a learning disability, emotional disturbance, or speech-language impairment are disconnected, compared with 37% of those with ASD.

VR services should be accessed to facilitate transition-age youth with IDD entering the work force. Adults with ASD who received VR services have been found to have a strong chance of becoming employed once appropriate measures are in place (Jacob, Scott, Falkmer, & Falkmer, 2015). Similar findings have been described for adults with other IDDs, with those receiving VR being 16 times more likely to be employed than those who don't receive these services. Employment rates in 2009 for the 15 million U.S. adults who have a disability were substantially lower than for adults who do not have a disability (16.8% versus 74%). In addition, poverty rates for adults who have a disability are substantially higher than those without disabilities (28.1% versus 10%; von Schrader, Erickson, & Lee, 2010). Even while participating in VR programs, transition-age adults with ASD across the country had yearly earnings below the poverty level for single adults during the 2002–2011 period, with overall mean wages increasing by only $9 from the first to second half of the decade (Burgess & Cimera, 2014).

A plan for paid work experience should be written into a student's IEP starting no later than age 16 years (IDEA, 2004). Job placement choices should be based, when possible, on individual interests, abilities, and postsecondary goals. For example, if a student has set technology-related career goals, an appropriate placement would be one that allows the student to learn to apply these skills in a paid, community-inclusive work setting.

Work Options

Individuals with disabilities who are entering the work force, like those without disabilities, have the option of participating in full-time or part-time competitive employment (Butterworth, Smith, Hall, Migliore, & Winsor, 2009). Community-integrated employment became available for individuals with IDD in the 1980s and rapidly became a preferred option to sheltered vocational workshops (a daytime activity for adults to perform routine tasks like assembly or manufacturing prior to gaining work in a community). However, some families still choose sheltered workshops because they provide consistent hours and long-term stability (Blick, Litz, Thornhill, & Goreczny, 2016). Another option is for the individual to attend an adult day care program that provides care and educational opportunities. While this option is better than spending time at home or in an institution (Campbell, 2012), most individuals with IDD and their families favor community-integrated employment over this and other daytime activities (Dague, 2012; Timmons, Hall, Bose, Wolfe, & Winsor, 2011). A recent study by Blick and colleagues (2016) demonstrated that individuals with IDD who were working in community-based settings reported increased choice and control over their daily activities and greater opportunities for community inclusion, as well as greater involvement in community activities, than adults in sheltered workshops and day care programs.

Competitive Employment An individual engaged in competitive employment is expected to perform essential functions at the same competence level as other employees without disabilities. Individuals with disabilities may request an accommodation under the protections of the ADA that enables them to perform these functions as long as the accommodation does not fundamentally alter the nature of the job. Accommodations covered by ADA include adaptive seating, computer input devices, large-print text, and so forth. To succeed in this **competitive employment** setting, individuals with disabilities must have the same skills requisite for any employee to succeed in the workplace. These skill sets include a knowledge base for the job, appropriate social skills, effective communication skills, and motivation. Individuals with disabilities also must have appropriate independent living skills and the ability to manage their disability-related needs, such as hiring and managing personal-care attendants and arranging transportation services.

Supported Employment **Supported employment** is defined by the Rehabilitation Act Amendments of 1986 (PL 99-506) and 1992 (PL 102-569) as employment in an inclusive setting with ongoing support services for an individual with a disability. Supported employment is a service that can help an individual gain competitive employment in inclusive work settings and provide ongoing support services to help maintain employment. Supported employment programs are generally administered through the state-level Bureaus of Vocational Rehabilitation and state developmental disability agencies. These agencies help people with disabilities through the process of identifying and selecting a service provider who can then help the individual obtain employment by identifying supports through supervisor or coworker assistance (natural supports) or job coaches. A job coach or employment consultant is a person who is hired by the individual or the placement agency. His or her responsibility is to provide specialized on-site training that assists the employee with a disability in learning and performing his or her job and adjusting to the work environment, with the ultimate goal of full inclusion at the worksite (Degeneffe, 2000).

Customized Employment **Customized employment** is a position where a blend of services is provided to increase future employment options for individuals with significant disabilities. These may involve self-employment, entrepreneurship, job carving and restructuring (e.g., an existing job is adjusted so that it contains some, but not all, of the tasks from the original job description), or job sharing (e.g., when two or more people share the tasks of a job). In customized employment, the employer and employee work together to identify a role in the work setting, often creating a new position, to ensure that the employee is a fully integrated team member, that job expectations are in line with the individual's strengths and capabilities, and that the work environment and schedule optimizes success and productivity. The defining aspects of customized employment is the negotiated relationship and the fact that ongoing supports may or may not be necessary for success. Personal agents and customized training are often provided in this work setting (U.S. Department of Labor Office of Disability Employment Policy, 2009). The ideal implementation of customized employment practices replaces the traditional vocational evaluation with a discovery process for individuals with complex disabilities who may not do well in answering questions, completing assessments, and performing tasks that compares individuals to a normative sample. Rather than identifying the employment opportunity that meets the individual's skill sets and strengths with supported employment, customized employment uses a process of discovery, identifying the interests, skills, and abilities of the individual.

Work-Study Employment **Work-study employment** involves part-time work for students that is sanctioned by the school and occurs either on or off campus. Age-appropriate transition assessment information and the student's IEP goals for transition should inform the appropriateness of this type of work. Internship experiences while in school improve employment outcomes (Carter, Austin, & Trainor, 2012; Wehman et al., 2014). Predictors of successful competitive postsecondary employment include paid employment for students while in the high school setting, providing students with direct and explicit instruction on vocational skills, ensuring that students graduate with a high school diploma, and supporting families in having high expectations for their son or daughter to be competitively employed (Southward & Kyzar, 2017).

Volunteering In today's competitive job market, **volunteering** is an opportunity for adolescents to gain valuable insights into the world of work, to develop skills, and to build work-related experience. It can be a positive step toward achievement of full employment or community inclusion goals in the IEP. However, volunteer experiences should not replace paid work experiences when those opportunities are also available, because paid work promotes the individual's self-esteem and pride in their abilities and lessens cultural stereotypes about the employability of individuals with developmental disabilities (Wolf-Branigin, Schuyler, & White, 2007).

Other Prework Options

Some youth with intellectual disabilities may not be ready to make the transition into a work-related setting immediately after exiting the school system (Targett, Wehman, West, Dillard, & Cifu, 2013). For these individuals, other more supportive options are available, such as day treatment/habilitation or work-readiness programs. These programs provide a more intensive level of support and focus on the development of daily living skills rather than job skills. The ultimate goal for any of these programs should remain moving the individual toward some aspect of employment.

MOVING FROM HOME INTO THE COMMUNITY

There are several key financial and legal issues that need to be addressed to ensure that at age 18, or when the individual is ready to move from home to the community, needed resources are available. This involves making sure that 1) there is no loss of income and/or services, 2) family assets are protected, and 3) youth with developmental disabilities are assured of having suitable independent living options. Financial barriers are the most common reason youth with developmental disabilities fail to make the transition to independent living in the community (McPherson et al., 2004).

Financial Options

Supplemental Security Income (SSI) is a monthly payment for individuals with disabilities. To qualify for SSI, individuals must meet both disability and financial eligibility requirements. SSI eligibility is generally determined using adult criteria when adolescents turn 18 years old, with the exception of youth enrolled in a Social Security Administration (SSA) work incentive program. Young people with developmental disabilities may lose their SSI at this time if they fail to meet the adult disability criteria. Conversely, some individuals with disabilities may now qualify for SSI when they had previously been ineligible because individual income, rather than household income, is now used to determine income eligibility. Generally speaking, adults who receive SSI cannot have individual assets greater than $2,000. The SSA, however, does allow several important exceptions to this rule, which are referred to as work incentives (see http://www.SSA.gov/work).

Despite these incentive programs, a significant number of youth with developmental disabilities lose SSI benefits when they become adults. In 2009, adolescents in the 13–17 year age bracket represented 8.8% of SSI recipients. This dropped to 6.9% for young adults in the 18–21 year age bracket (Social Security Office of Retirement and Disability Policy, 2010). Youth who lose SSI benefits when eligibility is redetermined at age 18 should request a second review because more than one third of such requests result in the reinstatement of SSI benefits (American Academy of Pediatrics Council on Children with Disabilities, 2009; Rupp et al., 2005–2006). Some individuals who are found ineligible can continue to receive SSI benefits as long as they participate in approved VR programs. In most states, people who receive SSI automatically also qualify for Medicaid.

Social Security Disability Insurance (SSDI) provides a monthly payment for individuals with disabilities. There are two ways to qualify for SSDI benefits. Workers (including those in sheltered or supported work settings) who have paid into the Social Security system are eligible for SSDI if they are no longer able to work. Monthly SSDI benefits are also usually paid to an adult with developmental disabilities when a parent or guardian meets disability criteria and cannot work. If a parent who is entitled to SSDI benefits cannot work due to disability, retires, or dies and the child has qualifying disability determined prior to age 22, then the child is eligible for the benefits. It is important to know that beneficiaries who receive SSDI for more than 2 years are also eligible for health care coverage under Medicare.

Guardianship and Supported Decision Making

In most states, the natural **guardianship** of parents ends when children reach age 18. At that time, parents no longer have the legal authority to make decisions or sign consent forms for their child unless they submit an application for guardianship at their local probate court. Although every state has its own guardianship law, policy, and practice, the uniting principal across all states is that guardianship is a legal intervention and it is the decision of the court as to whether to appoint a guardian and who that guardian is going to be. The decision regarding the necessity of guardianship should be individualized, and guardianship is not always needed solely because a person has a particular diagnosis, disability, or IQ level. Two prerequisites must exist before a court appoints a guardian: 1) The person must show a lack of capacity (i.e., ability to make and communicate decisions) in important areas of life, such as health care or financial decisions, and 2) there must be a present need for the guardianship above and beyond other less restrictive options. In accord with the principles of self-determination, it is important to evaluate the extent to which an individual can participate in decisions that affect his or her own life (Buchanan & Brock, 1992; Burt, 1996). The National Resource Center for Supported Decision Making emphasizes that capacity can change based on experience, situation, or support needed. When exploring a person's capacity to make decisions, they encourage a careful examination of capacity through the following questions:

- What decisions need to be made?
- What is the person's history of making decisions?
- How has the person utilized help in the decision-making process previously?
- What services has the person enlisted to help with decision making?

Probate courts can appoint someone as a guardian over only that portion of a person's life where he or she shows incompetence and has a need (e.g., a health care guardianship or a conservatorship for finances). Making a decision about guardianship, well in advance of the 18th birthday if possible, is essential to the health transition process. When a youth who has a developmental disability cannot make health care decisions independently, there are several options to consider and procedures to follow in order to obtain legal guardianship. The process of establishing guardianship can be daunting for some families, but it can be necessary for helping caregivers continue to advocate more effectively for their adult children if they need this level of support. Once obtained, guardianship papers should be kept in a wallet so that they can be presented at all health care encounters. Guardianship papers are as important as an insurance card when patients with developmental disabilities enter the adult health care system. The guardian is responsible for notifying relevant schools, agencies, and medical professionals of guardianship and may wish to have documents on file with these groups when appropriate. It is important to note that, ultimately, the decision for guardianship rests with the court. If the court disagrees with decisions made by the appointed guardian, they can take away the rights of that guardian and give it to someone else (National Resource Center for Supported Decision Making, 2016). As such, many families chose to explore other less restrictive options outside of the legal system that grant supported independence to their adult child.

There are several alternatives to guardianship that may be preferable because they increase the individual's autonomy to make decisions, avoid legal "red tape," and acknowledge the individual's needs and rights. In situations where legal guardianship is not indicated, support can be provided informally. Supported decision making is a model that allows individuals with IDD to retain their legal decision-making rights and is recognized as a viable alternative to guardianship. Supported decision making is defined as "practices, arrangements, and agreements that include informal and formal supports from diverse sources (e.g., peers, paid supporters, family, and technological supports, and educational supports" (Uyanik, Shogren, & Blanck, 2017, p. 499). Resources include the National Resource Center for Supported Decision Making (http://supporteddecisionmaking.org), the Center for Public Representation (https://centerforpublicrep.org/initiative/supported-decision-making/), and the Arc Center for Future Planning (https://futureplanning.thearc.org). In supported decision making, a **circle of support** or trusted group of supporters is created from family, friends, and/or community members to help answer questions and discuss options with the individual with IDD. The practices, arrangements, and agreements, however, are ultimately determined by the transitioning young adult (Uyanik et al., 2017; also see centerforpublicrep.org). This circle of support can help discuss the situation or decision to be made with the individual with IDD, provide insights or information about the situation, and help generate or compare options. In this capacity, supported decision making promotes self-determination, autonomy, and control. The individual being supported may wish to give a member of his or her team legal power of attorney to make legal decisions and take care of monetary issues on his or her behalf. There is also the option of using a health care proxy, power of advocate, and Health Insurance Portability and Accountability Act (HIPAA) release as alternatives to legal guardianship. All these documents can be revoked by the individual at any time.

A variant of a circle of support is a **microboard** that is incorporated to include the individual with IDD as the chairperson (Wetherow & Wetherow, 2004). Although these sorts of informal alternatives to guardianship are considered best practice, it should be noted that a legal guardian or a **representative payee** is often required by programs and services, such as SSI and SSDI, in order to disburse funds to an individual with IDD. The paperwork for this should be completed before age 18 to avoid interruption in benefits.

Housing

Finding and securing housing and residential supports for adults with IDD can be challenging for the individual and the family. In one study, 28% of adults with developmental disabilities were found to live in their own home, 58% lived with their families, and 15% resided in publicly funded residential settings (Larson et al.,, 2011). Most new group homes are designed for one to three individuals and are often referred to as **independent residential alternatives** (IRAs), reflecting a trend away from institutional settings of 16 or more people, which was the norm a generation ago. In 2009, the average per-resident expenditures per year were $203,670 in state-operated IRAs (Larson et al., 2011). Home- and community-based services and programs for young adults with developmental disabilities cost substantially less and are in high demand. However, waiting lists are the norm. Over 100,000 individuals with IDD in the United States were waiting for residential services in 2009 (Larson et al., 2011).

Services and programs that assist individuals with community living have increased dramatically since the 1990s as a result of the New Freedom Initiative (Executive Order No. 13217, 2001), the ADA, and the Olmstead decision (*Olmstead v. L.C.*, 527 U.S. 581, 1999). The Olmstead decision interpreted Title II of the ADA to require states to administer their services, programs, and activities "in the most integrated setting appropriate to the needs of qualified individuals with disabilities" (*Olmstead v. L.C.*, 1999). The act holds that states are responsible for integration of individuals with IDD into the community optimizing inclusion in everyday life activities, family relations, and social contacts.

Family Home Many families whose adults have IDD choose for the individual to continue to live at home. Between 1999 and 2009, the number of adults with developmental disabilities living with family members in the United States increased by two thirds, from 355,152 to 599,152 (Larson et al., 2010). The aging of these families, however, is an emerging concern. Approximately one quarter of home-based adults with developmental disabilities live in homes headed by elderly parents, and support systems for aging parents of adults with developmental disabilities are lacking (Heller, Caldwell, & Factor, 2007).

Group Homes The life expectancy for individuals with IDD are comparable to the general population; therefore, demand for residential services is on the rise. The number of people with ID receiving residential services grew from 267,682 in 1988 (Lakin, Prouty, Polister, & Coucouvanis, 2003) to 460,597 in 2011 (Larson, Salmi, Smith, Anderson, & Hewitt, 2013). Stemming from landmark legislation in the 1960s (Community Mental Health Act; PL 88-164) and 1980s (Omibus Budget Reconciliation Act; PL 100-203) and the Olmstead Act, the number of individuals with ID living in state institutions and nursing homes has steadily declined. Concurrently, there has been a rapid growth in the number of small residential settings. The most common form of assisted-living program (outside of the family home) is the group home (Lakin et al., 2010), most of which have on-site counselors who provide supervision and support in daily living skills, employment, and recreation.

Supported Living Services Supported living services (SLSs) provide assistance to adults with developmental disabilities who live in homes in the community that they own or lease. SLSs may include assistance with 1) selecting and moving into a home, 2) choosing personal attendants and housemates, 3) acquiring household furnishings, 4) addressing common daily living activities and emergencies, 5) becoming a participating member in community life, and 6) managing personal financial affairs (Stancliffe & Lakin, 2005).

MOVING FROM PEDIATRIC- TO ADULT-ORIENTED HEALTH CARE

Historically, addressing the health care needs of young adults with IDD mostly fell in the court of pediatrics, as most internists and family practitioners do not receive formal training caring for adults with IDD and are uncomfortable in these settings (Peter, Forke, Ginsburg, & Schwarz, 2009). As the need has grown to provide these services, the health care system has responded by developing resources for adult medical care providers to prepare them to accept adults with IDD into their practices. More education in medical school and graduate medical education programs should focus on meeting the needs of this vulnerable population.

The importance of young adults having a medical home cannot be overemphasized (see Chapter 41; see also Box 40.2). Many practice-based resources are available from the National Health Care Transition Center (http://www.gottransition.org/) and include toolkits for health care providers, parents and families, and the youth with special health care needs. Specific strategies for the successful transition to an adult medical home model are outlined in the joint statement on health care transition put forth in 2011 (American Academy of Pediatrics et al., 2011). In addition, the American College of Physicians developed a toolkit for internal medicine practices that accept youth with special health care needs, including a specific package for youth with IDD available at www.acp.org. Family medicine practices are also well equipped to provide a medical home throughout the life course of individuals with IDD.

Role of Families

Transition planning should consider the needs of the entire family (http://www.p2pusa.org; Taylor, Hodapp, Burke, Waitz-Kudla, & Rabideau, 2017) and include parent training to advocate for youth with IDD (Cheak-Zamora, Teti, Maurer-Batjer, & Koegler, 2017). Improved communication and support for developing self-efficacy are often needed as parents advocate for postsecondary independence while continuing to be primary caregivers. Often this time of transition leads to high levels of stress and anxiety for the caregiver(s) and can adversely impact their own physical and mental health (Betz, Nehring, & Lobo, 2015).

An algorithm for transitioning youths with developmental disabilities to adult health care is outlined in a recent clinical report (American Academy of Pediatrics et al., 2011) that underscores the importance of the patient-centered medical home that provides comprehensive primary care and facilitates partnerships among the individual patient, health care provider, and families (American Academy of Family Physicians et al., 2007). The transition algorithm is driven by a process that includes a longitudinal assessment of readiness, planning, implementation, and documentation of specific transition goals. This algorithm identifies a sequence of four steps of transition-related activities that are ideally, although not necessarily, implemented at specific ages:

Step 1: Discuss the transition policy of the pediatric practice—that is, when the child should transition to adult care (12–13 years of age)

BOX 40.2 EVIDENCE-BASED PRACTICE

Transition from Pediatric to Adult Care

Incomplete transition from pediatric to adult care has been associated with many negative outcomes, including lack of a primary care medical home, foregone care, poor medical outcomes, increased mortality, and difficulty accessing care in a crisis (Acharya, Meza, & Msall, 2017; Lotstein et al., 2013; Tanner et al., 2016). Youth with developmental disabilities are at high risk for not receiving appropriate anticipatory guidance and support around transition planning, and they often require parental/guardian support to navigate the complex adult-oriented health system (McKenzie, Sanders, Bhattacharya, & Bundorf, 2018). Youth of color and non-English speakers are more at risk for being unprepared for health care transition.

There is evidence that adolescent and young adults with increased medical needs who receive specialized hospital-based care coordination during health care transition have improved perception of quality of chronic illness care and reduction in cost and health care utilization (Lemke et al., 2018; Simon et al., 2017). Parental involvement is important to adherence but must be balanced with the need to transfer responsibilities for disease management to the youth. Families remain integral supports for many adults with IDD, but families must learn to balance their advocacy role with their role in supporting the youth's development of self-advocacy skills.

Points to Remember

- Gaps in health care can result in poor health outcomes.
- Evidence supports implementing a structured systematic transition process for improved outcomes.
- Parent involvement is important and necessary but should be balanced with supporting their child's development of self-advocacy skills.

Step 2: Initiate a transition plan jointly with parent and youth (14–15 years of age)

Step 3: Review and update the transition plan (16–17 years of age)

Step 4: Transfer care to adult provider(s) (18–21 years of age)

Written documentation is a key element of the actual transfer of care. It is recommended that adult providers be given a copy of the transition plan as well as documentation of a youth's transition readiness (i.e., self-care and health care navigation skills). They should also be provided with legal documentation (including a signed HIPAA form, a health care proxy, power of attorney, and power of advocate and/or guardianship paperwork) that clearly defines the responsible party for medical decision making. Finally, adult providers should be given a portable medical summary that includes a succinct medical history as well as 1) a list of medical providers; 2) key social service providers; 3) baseline functional and neurologic status; 4) cognitive status, including formal neuropsychological test results and date of administration; 5) condition-specific emergency treatment plans and contacts; and 6) the patient's health education history. The summary should also include an assessment of the individuals' understanding regarding his or her health conditions, treatments, and prognosis. There should be particular attention focused on entry into adult life, including sexuality, family planning, and relevant genetic information. **Medication reconciliation** (where the medication lists are checked for accuracy and to make sure there are no adverse interactions) is recommended at both the giving and receiving end of the transfer from child to adult health care provider. To achieve an effective transfer of care, it is important that there be direct communication between the pediatric and adult providers (The Society for Adolescent Health and Medicine, 2017).

Adherence and Health Literacy

In order to be ready to move into the adult health care system, the adolescent needs 1) to be responsible for taking medications (with supervision when appropriate), 2) to understand and be able to discuss his or her disability, and 3) to use required adaptive equipment or appliances (American Academy of Pediatrics et al., 2011; The Society for Adolescent Health and Medicine, 2017). During the transition process, health care professionals should consider when to start seeing the individual alone (without parents) and when to develop a confidential relationship with the patient.

Health Promotion

Good nutrition, regular exercise, and fostering personal relationships are key parts of maintaining health and quality of life, yet youth with IDD 9–18 years of age spend more time in sedentary activities than their peers and are less fit (Tyler, MacDonald, & Menear, 2014). This problem is amplified when medication that increases appetite and weight gain (e.g., risperdal and olanzapine) is used to manage mood or disruptive behaviors in this population. Early and sustained participation in community-based programs is essential for adolescents and young adults to maintain healthy lifestyles beyond the school years. Lack of physical activity can lead to obesity-related disorders (e.g., type 2 diabetes), which disproportionately affect people with disabilities (Rimmer, 2017).

Leisure activities are very important for young adults with developmental disabilities, as these individuals tend to become socially isolated. People with developmental disabilities requiring extensive to pervasive support (i.e., those with severe to profound intellectual disability) are less likely to participate in leisure activities (Van Naarden Braun, Yeargin-Allsopp, & Lollar, 2009). Therapeutic recreation programs that incorporate social skills training can help individuals with mild-moderate intellectual disability hone their conversation skills, learn to maintain eye contact and use appropriate body language, and become self-advocates (https://www.atra-online.com/page/AboutRecTherapy). Examples of therapeutic recreation programs include the Special Olympics (http://www.specialolympics.org/) and Best Buddies programs (http://www.bestbuddies.org/). For individuals with motor impairments, there is Wheelchair and Ambulatory Sports USA (http://www.wsusa.org/). The National Center on Physical Activity and Disability (http://www.ncpad.org) is a clearinghouse for information promoting physical activity among individuals with disabilities.

Engaging in personal relationships is also a key part of development for all youth. Opportunities for friendships may need to be facilitated, especially once youth are no longer enrolled in school. Companionship, emotional support, and increased self-esteem are all benefits of personal relationships that can increase quality of life.

Sexuality

Sexuality and the formation of romantic relationships are natural aspects of human development and are important for all young adults regardless of gender, orientation, or cognitive level (Ailey, Marks, Crisp, & Hahn, 2003; Pecora, Mesibov, & Stokes, 2016). Many individuals with IDD have the same level of sexual interest as their typically developing peers (Byers, Nichols, & Voyer, 2013; Dewinter, De Graaf, & Begeer, 2017). Youth with IDD can reach biological sexual maturity on a developmental trajectory similar to their typically developing peers, but may lack insight into the socioemotional processes that accompany this development and interest. Core social-communication deficits create a unique burden on these individuals related to sexuality, dating, and friendships and can increase the risk of exploitation due to the difficulty in their recognizing dangerous situations (Brown-Lavoie, Viecili, & Weiss, 2014).

Unfortunately, adolescents with developmental disabilities often do not receive adequate information about sexuality and reproductive health (i.e., sexually transmitted infections, contraception, and reproduction; Brown-Lavoie et al., 2014; Hannah & Stagg, 2016). This places the individual at increased risk to experience sexual victimization and exploitation (Brown-Lavoie et al., 2014). As one example, females with ASD have been found to be at an increased risk for unwanted sexual interactions and adverse sexual experiences compared with their typically developing peers (Pecora et al., 2016). Issues around boundaries, normative sexual feelings, masturbation, relationships, intimacy, and privacy should be addressed early for all youth with IDD. Woodbine Press has a number of excellent books for youth and parents with IDD that discuss puberty, sexuality, and relationships, and *Supporting Teens with Autism on Relationships (STAR)* is a free self-guided skill-building resource that adapts empirically based sexuality education approaches and interventions for parents of children and teens ages 10–18 who have an ASD (http://www.danya.com/autism_pdfs/STAR%20Charting%20the%20 Course%20Parent%20Guide.pdf).

In addition, many youth require significant support around puberty and menses, which can be distressing to many girls with IDD. During pubertal development, typical physical and emotional changes can be difficult for youth with IDD to understand and navigate. For example, approaches to dealing with wearing a bra or sanitary pad, unreciprocated romantic feelings, desire for parenthood, and dating often need parent facilitation. Sexuality is more than sex; it is how a youth feels about his or her developing body.

Another important area of sexuality education is around gender variance. Data suggest that gender variance and varied sexual attraction are more common in adolescents and young adults with developmental disabilities, especially ASD, than in the typically developing population (Van Schalkwyk, Klingensmith, & Volkmar, 2015). One study found that parents of youth with ASD without ID were over seven times more likely to report that their child expressed gender variance than typically developing children and that this occurred equally in females and males (Strang et al., 2016).

Moreover, women with ASD have reported lower rates of heterosexual preference, higher rates of bisexual attraction, and more uncertainty in their attraction toward specific sexes compared with typically developing peers (May et al., 2017). It often can be difficult to define gender dysphoria and transgender identity in individuals with IDD due to social, cognitive, and adaptive limitations. In addition, the gender they identify with may not always match the way they physically present themselves to others. Therefore, parents, health care providers and teachers should pay attention to the development of gender identity at an early age, as gender dysphoria can contribute to fewer meaningful social interactions, significant emotional distress, and poor school performance. The focus should be on acceptance and providing the opportunity for individual exploration of gender-related concerns.

Professionals and parents may either lack the awareness to consider sexuality as part of the adolescent's typical growth and development or are fearful of discussing sensitive issues and acknowledging vulnerability (Murphy, 2005; Tice & Hall, 2008). This results in an information gap that may increase the chances of sexual exploitation and unintended pregnancy. For example, youth with developmental disabilities are four times more likely to be sexually abused or exploited than their typically developing peers (Bowman, Scotti, & Morris, 2010; Dixon, Bergstrom, Smith, & Tarbox, 2010). Lack of knowledge of sexuality, lack of information on exploitation, cognitive deficits, poor social skills, poor self-esteem, and poor body image are some of the factors that place adolescents with developmental disabilities at increased risk (Bowman et al., 2010; Dixon et al., 2010).

Mental Health

Individuals with IDD are also at a higher risk for developing mental health problems than their typically developing peers (see Chapter 27). This so-called "dual diagnosis" affects nearly 40% of children with ID compared with 8% in the general population (Emerson, 2003). While these issues often begin in childhood, they are likely to persist into adulthood and interfere with adaptive functioning (Sukhodolsky, Block, Panza, & Reichow, 2013). Psychosis and behavior disorders, including aggression toward others and self-aggression, are higher than in the general population. The rate for substance abuse, however, is lower than in the general population (Deb, Thomas, & Bright, 2001; Slayter, 2010). The proportion of anxiety and mood disorders are similar to the general population except for in ASD, where 40%–85% of individuals have specific phobias, generalized anxiety, social anxiety, and separation anxiety. This also is true for depression, sleep disorders, seizures, gastrointestinal issues, and multiple other medical and mental health conditions. In addition, individuals from diverse racial and cultural groups may disproportionately miss out on ASD diagnoses and have other labels instead (Bishop-Fitzpatrick & Kind, 2017).

In contrast to ASD, cerebral palsy has not been reported as having increased rates of psychiatric diagnosis, although ascertainment may be problematic. In general, boys and teens with IDD have higher rates of dual diagnosis than girls and younger children. Factors associated with an increased risk of psychopathology include, in addition to age and gender, social deprivation, family composition, number of potentially stressful life events, mental health of the child's caregiver, and family functioning (Emerson, 2003).

However, despite the high reported rates of dual diagnosis, the proper diagnosis of mental illness in a person with IDD remains a challenge. Reiss, Levitan, and Szyszko (1982) termed one major obstacle *diagnostic overshadowing*. This refers to the tendency of clinicians to attribute all the behavioral and emotional problems to the developmental disability itself rather than to a comorbid mental illness. Another problem is that many professionals in the field of mental illness simply do not have training or experience in the field of developmental disabilities (Fletcher, Loschen, Stavrakaki, & First, 2007).

Most service systems for people with developmental disabilities are oriented to chronic care and long-term support, and they provide limited, if any, services for acute mental health crises. Emergency mental health services are typically geared to the needs of the general population. Access to preventive mental health services is problematic as well. Adults with developmental disabilities are seven times more likely to report inadequate emotional support, compared with adults who do not have disabilities (Havercamp, Scandlin, & Roth, 2004).

Behavioral concerns should be investigated rather than ascribed to the individual's developmental disability. It is important to question adolescents and their families about physical symptoms of anxiety and depression, such as altered sleep patterns and appetite. Professionals and educators should also monitor excessive school absences as these may be evidence of a mental health issue.

Studies have also shown a significantly increased prevalence of eating disorders in patients with ASD as compared with healthy control patients (Huke, Turk, Saeidi, Kent, & Morgan, 2013). A restricted food repertoire is common in youth with ASD and can stem from sensory aversions to taste or texture or to cognitive rigidity in trying new or different foods. Screening for disordered eating and referral to a mental health provider and/or nutritionist should be considered for all youth with avoidant or restrictive food intake.

Environmental factors should be considered as precipitants when adolescents with IDD present with new challenging behaviors. For example, it is not unusual for an adolescent with developmental disabilities to experience anxiety when a long-term aide is no longer available at school or when opportunities to socialize diminish with high school graduation. Surgery, a prolonged hospitalization, or medical setbacks can precipitate depressive episodes. It should be emphasized that challenging behaviors occurring across all settings (as opposed to being generated in response to a specific stimulating event or situation) are more likely to be due to organic causes than when they occur in the typical population. Treatments can include psychological, behavioral, pharmacotherapy, and/or environmental interventions. Community-based models of support combined with neuropsychiatric intervention can be a potent therapeutic approach in the management of challenging behaviors in individuals with developmental disabilities (Ferrell, Wolinsky, Kauffman, Flashman, & McAllister, 2004).

SUMMARY

- Health care providers, educators, other professionals, and families should foster the expectation that youth and young adults with IDD will become healthy, happy, active, and productive members of their community.
- Youth with IDD should be provided with opportunities to learn about their strengths, abilities, skills, needs, and interests.
- Youth with IDD should assume responsibility for themselves and understand the difference between the protected worlds of school and home and the worlds of work and adult life. Most of all, they must believe they are capable of success.
- These goals can be accomplished through comprehensive transition planning and advocacy, including self-advocacy, to promote full participation in society.

ADDITIONAL RESOURCES

Going to College: http://www.going-to-college.org/

I'm Determined: http://www.imdetermined.org/

National Gateway to Self Determination: http://www.aucd.org/ngsd/template/index.cfm

National Health Care Transition Center: http://www.gottransition.org

Additional resources can be found online in Appendix D: Childhood Disabilities Resources, Services, and Organizations (see About the Online Companion Materials).

REFERENCES

Acharya, K., Meza, R., & Msall, M. E. (2017). Disparities in life course outcomes for transition-aged youth with disabilities. *Pediatric Annals, 46*(10), e371–e376.

Adreon, D., & Durocher, J. S. (2007). Evaluating the college transition needs of individuals with high-functioning autism spectrum disorders. *Intervention in School and Clinic, 42*(5), 271–279.

Ailey, S. H., Marks, B. A., Crisp, C., & Hahn, J. E. (2003). Promoting sexuality across the life span for individuals with intellectual and developmental disabilities. *Nursing Clinics of North America, 38*(2), 229–352.

Alverson, C. Y., Lindstrom, L. E., & Hirano, K. A. (2015). High school to college: Transition experiences of young adults with autism. *Focus on Autism and Other Developmental Disabilities.* Online publication. doi:10.1177/1088357615611880

American Academy of Pediatrics, American Academy of Family Physicians, & American College of Physicians Transitions Clinical Report Authoring Group. (2011). Supporting the health care transition from adolescence to adulthood in the medical home. *Pediatrics, 128,* 182–200.

American Academy of Pediatrics Council on Children with Disabilities. (2009). Policy statement: Supplemental Security Income (SSI) for children and youth with disabilities. *Pediatrics, 124*(6), 1702–1708.

American Academy of Family Physicians, American Academy of Pediatrics, American College of Physicians, American Osteopathic Association. (2007). *Joint Principles of the Patient-Centered Medical Home.* Accessed https://www.aafp.org/dam/AAFP/documents/practice_management/pcmh/initiatives/PCMHJoint.pdf

American Recovery and Reinvestment Act (ARRA) of 2009, PL 111-5.

Americans with Disabilities Act (ADA) of 1990, PL 101-336, 42 U.S.C. §§ 12101 *et seq.*

Armstrong, T. (2015). The myth of the normal brain: Embracing neurodiversity. *AMA Journal of Ethics, 17*(4), 348–352.

Betz, C. L., Nehring, W. M., & Lobo, M. L. (2015). Transition needs of parents and adolescents and emerging adults with special health care needs and disabilities. *Journal of Family Nursing, 21*(3), 362–412.

Bishop-Fitzpatrick, L., & Kind, A. J. H. (2017). A scoping review of health disparities in autism spectrum disorder. *Journal of Autism and Developmental Disorders, 47*(11), 3380–3391.

Blick, R. N., Litz, K. S., Thornhill, M. G., & Goreczny, A. J. (2016). Do inclusive work environments matter? Effects of community-integrated employment on quality of life for individuals with intellectual disabilities. *Research in Developmental Disabilities, 53,* 358–366.

Bowman, R. A., Scotti, J. R., & Morris, T. L. (2010). Sexual abuse prevention: A training program for developmental disabilities service providers. *Journal of Child Sex Abuse, 19*(2), 119–127.

Brown-Lavoie, S. M., Viecili, M. A., & Weiss, J. A. (2014). Sexual knowledge and victimization in adults with autism spectrum disorders. *Journal of Autism and Developmental Disorders, 44*(9), 2185–2196.

Buchanan, A. E., & Brock, D. W. (1992). *Deciding for others: The ethics of surrogate decision making.* Cambridge, England: Cambridge University Press.

Burt, R. A. (1996). *The suppressed legacy of Nuremberg (Hastings Center Report).* Garrison, NY: The Hastings Center.

Burgess, S., & Cimera, R. E. (2014). Employment outcomes of transition-age adults with autism spectrum disorders: A State of the States Report. *American Journal on Intellectual and Developmental Disabilities, 119*(1), 64–83.

Butterworth, J., Smith, F. A., Hall, A. C., Migliore, A., & Winsor, J. (2009). *State data: The National Report on Employment Services and Outcomes 2009, Institute for Community Inclusion UCEDD.* Boston, MA: University of Massachusetts.

Byers, E. S., Nichols, S., & Voyer, S. D. (2013). Challenging stereotypes: Sexual functioning of single adults with high functioning autism spectrum disorder. *Journal of Autism and Developmental Disorders, 43*(11), 2617–2627.

Campbell, M. (2012). Changing day services: Do you agree? *Journal of Intellectual Disabilities, 16*(3), 205–215.

Carter, E. W., Austin, D., & Trainor, A. A. (2012). Predictors of postschool employment outcomes for young adults with severe disabilities. *Journal of Disability Policy Studies, 23*(1), 50–63.

Cheak-Zamora N. C., Teti, M., Maurer-Batjer, A., & Koegler, E. (2017). Exploration and comparison of adolescents with autism spectrum disorder and their caregiver's perspectives on transitioning to adult health care and adulthood. *Journal of Pediatric Psychology, 42*(9), 1028–1093.

Cobb, B., Lehmann, J., Newman-Gonchar, R., & Alwell, M. (2009). Self-determination for students with disabilities: A narrative metasynthesis. *Career Development for Exceptional Individuals, 32*(2), 108–114.

Dague, B. (2012). Sheltered employment, sheltered lives: Family perspectives of conversion to community-based employment. *Journal of Vocational Rehabilitation, 37*(1), 1–11.

Deb, S., Thomas, M., & Bright, C. (2001). Mental disorder in adults with intellectual disability: Prevalence of functional psychiatric illness among a community-based population aged between 16 and 64 years. *Journal of Intellectual Disability Research, 45,* 495–505.

Degeneffe, C. E. (2000). Supported employment services for persons with developmental disabilities: Unmet promises and future challenges for rehabilitation counselors. *Journal of Applied Rehabilitation Counseling, 31*(2), 41–47.

Dewinter, J., De Graaf, H., & Begeer, S. (2017). Sexual orientation, gender identity, and romantic relationships in adolescents and adults with autism spectrum disorder. *Journal of Autism and Developmental Disorders, 47*(9), 2927–2934. doi:10.1007/s10803-017-3199-9

Dixon, D. R., Bergstrom, R., Smith, M. N., & Tarbox, J. (2010). A review of research on procedures for teaching safety skills to persons with developmental disabilities. *Research into Developmental Disabilities, 31*(5), 985–994.

Elias, R., Muskett, A. E., & White, S. W. (2017). Educator perspectives on the postsecondary transition difficulties of students with autism. *Autism*. Online publication doi:10.1177/1362361317726246

Emerson, E. (2003). Prevalence of psychiatric disorders in children and adolescents with and without intellectual disability. *Journal of Intellectual Disability Research, 47*(1), 51–58.

Exec. Order No. 13217, 66 C.F.R. 33155 (2001).

Ferrell, R. B., Wolinsky, E. J., Kauffman, C. I., Flashman, L. A., & McAllister, T. W. (2004). Neuropsychiatric syndromes in adults with mental retardation: Issues in assessment and treatment. *Current Psychiatry Reports, 6*(5), 380–390.

Fletcher, R., Loschen, E., Stavrakaki, C., & First, M. (Eds.). (2007). *Diagnostic manual—intellectual disability (DM-ID): A textbook of diagnosis of mental disorders in persons with intellectual disability.* Kingston, NY: NADD Press.

Gobbo, K., & Shmulsky, S. (2014). Faculty experience with college students with autism spectrum disorders: A qualitative study of challenges and solutions. *Focus on Autism and Other Developmental Disabilities, 29*(1), 13–22.

Grigal, M., Hart, D., Smith, F. A., & Papay, C. (2018). *Year two student data summary (2016-2017) of the TPSID model demonstration projects.* Boston, MA: University of Massachusetts Boston, Institute for Community Inclusion.

Hannah, L. A., & Stagg, S. D. (2016). Experiences of sex education and sexual awareness in young adults with autism spectrum disorder. *Journal of Autism and Developmental Disorders, 46*(12), 3678–3687.

Havercamp, S. M., Scandlin, D., & Roth, M. (2004). Health disparities among adults with developmental disabilities, adults with other disabilities, and adults not reporting disability in North Carolina. *Public Health Report, 119*(4), 418–426.

Heller, T., Caldwell, J., & Factor, A. (2007). Aging family caregivers: Policies and practices. *Mental Retardation and Developmental Disabilities Research Reviews, 13*(2), 136–142.

Higher Education Opportunity Act of 2008, PL 110-315.

Huke, V., Turk, J., Saeidi, S., Kent, A., & Morgan, J. F. (2013). Autism spectrum disorders in eating disorder populations: A systematic review. *European Eating Disorders Review, 21,* 345–351.

Individuals with Disabilities Education Improvement Act of 2004, PL 108-446, 20 U.S.C. §§ 1400 *et seq.*

Jacob, A., Scott, M., Falkmer, M., & Falkmer, T. (2015). The costs and benefits of employing an adult with autism spectrum disorder: A systematic review. *PLoS ONE, 10*(10), e0139896.

Krahn, G., & Campbell, V. A. (2011). Evolving views of disability and public health: The roles of advocacy and public health. *Disability and Health Journal, 4*(1), 12–18.

Lakin, K. C., Prouty, R., Polister, B., & Coucouvanis, K. (2003). Selected changes in residential service systems over a quarter century, 1977-2002. *Mental Retardation, 41*(4), 303–306.

Larson, S. A., Lakin, C., Salmi, P., Smith, D., Scott, N., & Webster, A. (2011). Children and youth with intellectual or developmental disabilities living in congregate care settings (1977 to 2009): Healthy People 2010 Objective 6.7b Outcomes (Revised). *Intellectual and Developmental Disabilities, 49*(3), 209–213.

Larson, S. A., Salmi, P., Smith, D., Anderson, L. L., & Hewitt, A. (2013). Residential services for persons with intellectual or developmental disabilities: Status and trends through 2011. Minneapolis: University of Minnesota, Research and Training Center on Community Living, Institute on Community Integration.

Lemke, M., Kappel, R., McCarter, R., D'Angelo, L., & Tuchman, L. (2018). Perceptions of health care transition care coordination in patients with chronic illness. *Pediatrics, 141*(5), e20173168.

Lotstein, D. S., Seid, M., Klingensmith, G., Case, D., Lawrence, J. M., Pihoker, C., . . . SEARCH for Diabetes in Youth Study Group. (2013). Transition from pediatric to adult care for youth diagnosed with type 1 diabetes in adolescence. *Pediatrics, 131*(4), e1062–e1070. doi:10.1542/peds.2012-1450.

May, T., Pang, K. C., O'Connell, M. A., & Williams, K. (2017). Typical timing typical pubertal timing in an Australian population of girls and boys with autism spectrum disorder. *Journal of Autism and Developmental Disorders, 47(12),* 3983–3993.

McKenzie, R. B., Sanders, L., Bhattacharya, J., & Bundorf, M. K. (2018). Health care system factors associated with transition preparation in youth with special health care needs. *Population Health Management,* Advanced online publication. doi:10.1089/pop.2018.0027

McPherson, M., Weissman, G., Strickland, B. B., van Dyck, P. C., Blumberg, S. J., & Newacheck, P. W. (2004). Implementing community-based systems of services for children and youths with special health care needs: How well are we doing? *Pediatrics, 113*(Suppl. 5), 1538–1544.

Mumbardó-Adam, C., Guàrdia-Olmos, J., Adam-Alcocer, A. L., Carbó-Carreté, M., Balcells-Balcells, A., Giné, C., & Shogren, K. A. (2017). Self-determination, intellectual disability, and context: A meta-analytic study. *Intellectual and Developmental Disabilities, 55*(5), 303–314.

Murphy, N. (2005) Sexuality in children and adolescents with disabilities. *Developmental Medicine and Child Neurology, 47*(9), 640–644.

National Resource Center for Supported Decision-Making. (2016). *Autonomy, decision-making supports, and guardianship.* Retrieved from http://supporteddecisionmaking.org/news/autonomy-decision-making-supports-and-guardianship

Nota, L., Soresi, S., Ferrari, L., & Wehmeyer, M. (2011). A multivariate analysis of the self determination of adolescents. *Journal of Happiness Studies, 12*(2), 245–266. doi:10.1007/s10902-010-9191-0

Nota, L., Ferrari, L., Soresi, S., & Wehmeyer, M. (2007). Self-determination, social abilities and the quality of life of people with intellectual disability. *Journal of Intellectual Disabilities Research, 51*(11), 850–865.

Olmstead v. L.C., 527 U.S. 581 (1999).

Peter, N. G., Forke, C. M., Ginsburg, K. R., & Schwarz, D. F. (2009) Transition from pediatric to adult care: Internists' perspectives. *Pediatrics, 123*(2), 417–423.

Pecora, L. A., Mesibov, G. B., & Stokes, M. A. (2016). Sexuality in high-functioning autism: A systematic review and meta-analysis. *Journal of Autism and Developmental Disorders, 46*(11), 3519–3556.

Rehabilitation Act Amendments of 1986, PL 99-506, 29 U.S.C. §§ 701 *et seq.*

Rehabilitation Act Amendments of 1992, PL 102-569, 29 U.S.C. §§ 701 *et seq.*

Rehabilitation Act of 1973, PL 93-112, 29 U.S.C. §§ 701 *et seq.*

Reiss, S., Levitan, G. W., & Szyszko, J. (1982). Emotional disturbance and mental retardation: Diagnostic overshadowing. *American Journal of Mental Deficiency, 86*(6), 567–574.

Rimmer, J. H. (2017). Equity in active living for people with disabilities: Less talk and more action. *PrevMED, 95*(Suppl.), S154–S156.

Ripamonti, L. (2016). Disability, diversity, and autism: Philosophical perspectives on health. *The New Bioethics, 22*(1), 56–70.

Roux, A. M., Shattuck, P. T., Rast, J. E., Rava, J. A., & Anderson, K. A. (2015). *National Autism Indicators Report: Transition into young adulthood.* Philadelphia, PA: Life Course Outcomes

Research Program, A. J. Drexel Autism Institute, Drexel University.

Rupp, K., Davies, P. S., Newcomb, C., Iams, H., Becker, C., Mulpuru, S., . . . Miller, B. (2005–2006). A profile of children with disabilities receiving SSI: Highlights from the National Survey of SSI Children and Families. *Social Security Bulletin 2005–2006, 66*(2), 21–48.

School-to-Work Opportunities Act of 1994, PL 103239, 20 U.S.C. 6101 *et seq.*

Section 504 of the Rehabilitation Act, 29 U.S.C. § 794d.

Shogren, K. A., Wehmeyer, M. L., Palmer, S. B., Forber-Pratt, A. J., Little, T. J., & Lopez, S. (2015). Causal agency theory: Reconceptualizing a functional model of self-determination. *Education and Training in Autism and Developmental Disabilities, 50*(3), 251–263.

Simon, T. D., Whitlock, K. B., Haaland, W., Wright, D. R., Zhou, C., Neff, J., . . . Mangione-Smith, R. (2017). Effectiveness of a comprehensive case management service for children with medical complexity. *Pediatrics, 140*(6), e20171641.

Slayter, E. M., (2010). Demographic and clinical characteristics of people with intellectual disabilities with and without substance abuse disorders in a Medicaid population. *Intellectual Developmental Disabilities, 48*(6), 417–431.

Smith, L. S. (2009). Overview of the Federal Higher Education Opportunity Act Reauthorization. In *Think College Insight Brief, Issue No. 1.* Boston, MA: Institute for Community Inclusion, University of Massachusetts, Boston. Retrieved from https://thinkcollege.net/sites/default/files/files/resources/higher%20education%20opportunity%20act%20overview.pdf

Social Security Office of Retirement and Disability Policy. (2010). *Supplement security income.* Table 7.E2—*Percentage distribution of federally administered awards, by sex, age, and eligibility category, 2009.* Retrieved from https://www.ssa.gov/policy/docs/statcomps/supplement/2010/7e.html#table7.e2

Sosnowy, C., Silverman, C., & Shattuck, P. (2018). Parent's and young adults' perspectives on transition outcomes for young adults with autism. *Autism, 22*(1), 29–39.

Southward, J. D., & Kyzar, K. (2017). Predictors of competitive employment for students with intellectual and/or developmental disabilities. *Education and Training in Autism and Developmental Disabilities, 52*(1), 26–37.

Stancliffe, R. J., & Lakin, K. C. (2005). *Costs and outcomes of community services for people with intellectual disabilities.* Baltimore, MD: Paul H. Brookes Publishing Co.

Strang, J. F., Meagher, H., Kenworthy, L., de Vries, A., Menvielle, E., Leibowitz, S. . . . Anthony, L. G. (2016). Initial clinical guidelines for co-occurring autism spectrum disorder and gender dysphoria or incongruence in adolescents. *Journal of Clinical Child & Adolescent Psychology, 47*(1), 105–115.

Sukhodolsky, D. G., Bloch, M. H., Panza K. E., & Reichow, B. (2013). Cognitive-behavioral therapy for anxiety in children with high-functioning autism: A meta-analysis. *Pediatrics, 132*(5), e1341–1350.

Tanner, A. E., Philbin, M. M., DuVal, A., Ellen, J., Kapogiannis, B., & Fortenberry, J. D. (2016). Transitioning adolescents with HIV to adult care: Lessons learned from twelve adolescent medicine clinics. *Journal of Pediatric Nursing, 31*(5), 537–543. doi:10.1016/j.pedn.2016.04.002

Targett, P., Wehman, P., West, M., Dillard, C., & Cifu, G. (2013). Promoting transition to adulthood for youth with physical disabilities and health impairments. *Journal of Vocational Rehabilitation, 39*(2013), 229–239.

Taylor J. L., Hodapp, R. M., Burke, M. M., Waitz-Kudla, S. N., & Rabideau, C. (2017). Training parent of youth with autism spectrum disorder to advocate for adult disability services: Results from a pilot randomized controlled trial. *Journal of Autism and Developmental Disorders, 47*(12), 4025–4031.

Test, D. W., Fowler, C. H., Wood, W. M., Brewer, D. M., & Eddy, S. (2005). A conceptual framework of self-advocacy for students with disabilities. *Remedial Special Education, 26*(1), 43–54.

The Society for Adolescent Health and Medicine. (2017). The use of medication by adolescents and young adults. *Journal of Adolescent Health, 61*(3), 396–399.

Tice, C. J., & Hall, D. M. (2008). Sexuality education and adolescents with developmental disabilities: Assessment, policy, and advocacy. *Journal of Social Work and Disabilities Rehabilitation, 7*(1), 47–62.

Timmons, J. C., Hall, A. C., Bose, J., Wolfe, A., & Winsor, J. (2011). Choosing employment: Factors that impact employment decisions for individuals with intellectual disability. *Intellectual and Developmental Disabilities, 49*(4), 285–299.

Trembath, D., Germano, C., Johanson, G., & Dissanayake, C. (2012). The experience of anxiety in young adults with autism spectrum disorders. *Focus on Autism and Other Developmental Disabilities, 27*(4), 213–224.

Tyler, K., MacDonald, M., & Menear, K. (2014). Physical activity and physical fitness of school-aged children and youth with autism spectrum disorders. *Autism Research and Treatment.* Online publication. doi:10.1155/2014/312163

U.S. Department of Labor. (2005). *Work activity of high school students: Data from the National Longitudinal Survey of Youth 1997.* USDL Reports: 05-732. Retrieved from http://www.bls.gov/nls/nlsy97r6.pdf

U.S. Department of Labor Office of Disability Employment Policy. (2009). *Customized employment: Applying practical solutions for employment success, Vol. II.* Retrieved from https://www.dol.gov/odep/categories/workforce/CustomizedEmployment/practical/index.htm

Uyanik, H., Shogren, K. A., & Blanck, P. (2017). Supported decision-making: Implications from positive psychology for assessment and intervention in rehabilitation and employment. *Journal of Occupational Rehabilitation, 27*(4), 498–506.

Van Hees, V., Moyson, T., & Roeyers, H. (2015). Higher education experiences of students with autism spectrum disorder: Challenges, benefits and support needs. *Journal of Autism and Developmental Disorders, 45*(6), 1673–1688.

Van Naarden Braun, K., Yeargin-Allsopp, M., & Lollar, D. (2009). Activity limitations among young adults with developmental disabilities: A population-based follow-up study. *Research in Developmental Disabilities, 30*(1), 179–191.

Van Schalkwyk, G. I., Klingensmith, K., & Volkmar, F. R. (2015). Gender identity and autism spectrum disorders. *The Yale Journal of Biology and Medicine, 88*(1), 81–83.

von Schrader, S., Erickson, W. A., & Lee, C. G. (2010). *Disability statistics from the Current Population Survey (CPS).* Ithaca, NY: Cornell University Rehabilitation Research and Training Center on Disability Demographics and Statistics (StatsRRTC). Retrieved from www.disabilitystatistics.org

Walsh, C., Jones, B., & Schonwald, A. (2017). Health care transition planning among adolescents with autism spectrum disorder. *Journal of Autism and Developmental Disorders, 47,* 980.

Wehman, P., Schall, C., Carr, S., Targett, P., West, M., & Cifu, G. (2014). Transition from school to adulthood for youth with autism spectrum disorder. *Journal of Disability Policy Studies, 25*(1), 30–40.

Wehman, P., Schall, C., Carr, S., Targett, P., West, M., & Cifu, G. (2014). Transition from school to adulthood for youth with autism spectrum disorder. *Journal of Disability Policy Studies, 25*(1), 30–40.

Wehmeyer, M. L., & Abery, B. H. (2013). Self-determination and choice. *Intellectual and Developmental Disabilities, 51*(5), 399–411.

Wehmeyer, M. L., Palmer, S., Shogren, K., Williams-Diehm, K., & Soukup, J. (2013). Establishing a causal relationship between interventions to promote self-determination and enhanced student self-determination. *Journal of Special Education, 46*(4), 195–210.

Wetherow, D., & Wetherow, F. (2004). *Microboards and microboard association design, development and implementation.* Retrieved from http://www.communityworks.info/articles/microboard.htm

White, S. W., Elias, R., Salinas, C. E., Capriola, N., Conner, C. M., Asselin, S. B., . . . Getzel, E. E. (2016). Students with autism spectrum disorder in college: Results from a preliminary mixed methods needs analysis. *Research in Developmental Disabilities, 56,* 29–40.

Wolf-Branigin, M., Schuyler, V., & White, P. H. (2007). Improving quality of life and career attitudes of youth with disabilities: Experience from the Adolescent Employment Readiness Center. *Research in Social Work Practicum, 17*(3), 324–333.

Workforce Innovation and Opportunity Act (WIOA) of 2014, PL 113-128, 29 U.S.C.

Workforce Investment Act (WIA) of 1998, PL 105-220, 29 U.S.C. §§ 2801 *et seq.*

CHAPTER 41

Medical Home and Health Care Systems

Renee M. Turchi and Angelo P. Giardino

Upon completion of this chapter, the reader will

- Define the terms *children and youth with special health care needs* and *children with medical complexity* and understand the impact of these diagnoses on health care delivery and financing issues
- Describe the complexity involved in developing a medical home that adequately coordinates various services, integration of care, teams, and the risk adjustment for this population
- Discuss trends in alternative payment models and insurance coverage in the provision of health care to these children
- Describe how public health care programs and benefits contribute to these children and their families in achieving patient and family centered care

The federal Maternal and Child Health Bureau (MCHB) defines children and youth with special health care needs (CYSHCN) as "those who have or are at increased risk for a chronic physical, developmental, behavioral or emotional condition and who also require health and related services of a type or amount beyond that required by children generally" (McPherson et al., 1998 p. 138). Based on this definition (Bethell et al., 2015), the National Survey of Children's Health (2016) found an overall national prevalence of 19% of CYSHCN. This is a significant increase from the 2005–2006 estimate of 14% (U.S. Department of Health and Human Services, Health Resources and Services Administration, Maternal and Child Health Bureau, 2007) and 2010 estimate of 15% (U.S. Department of Health and Human Services, Health Resources and Services Administration, Maternal and Child Health Bureau, 2013). One in five U.S. households with children includes at least one CYSHCN (U.S. Department of Health and Human Services, Health Resources and Services Administration, Maternal and Child Health Bureau, 2014). The 2009–10 National Survey of Children with Special Health Care Needs (U.S. Department of Health and Human Services, Health Resources and Services Administration, Maternal and Child Health Bureau, 2013), confirmed that CYSHCN is a diverse group comprised of all races, ethnicities, ages, family incomes, and levels of functional abilities.

Children with medical complexity (CMC) are a subset of CYSHCN; they have multiple chronic conditions often requiring the care of an array of community- and hospital-based providers (Cohen et al., 2011). While CMC have an estimated prevalence of only 0.5%, or 400,000 in the United States (Kuo, Cohen, Agrawal,

Berry, & Casey, 2011), their care accounts for almost one third of annual health care expenditures for children, totaling nearly 100 billion dollars (Cohen et al., 2012; Lassman, Hartman, Washington, Andrews, & Catlin, 2014). CMC have chronic severe health conditions, increased needs for services, major functional limitations, and high health care utilization (Berry et al., 2013).

The term CYSHCN therefore includes an overlapping subgroup of children with developmental disabilities (e.g., cerebral palsy and meningomyelocele), a group of CMC, and a group of typically developing children with complex medical problems (e.g., hemophilia, diabetes, and severe asthma; Davis & Brosco, 2007). Understanding the similarities and differences among the groups can inform clinical decision making, policy development, and resource allocation. (Neff et al., 2014). The need to develop clear definitions of CYSHCN and CMC has fostered research investigating prevalence, quality of care, and health outcomes for this population. However, each group shares similarities around health care structures, processes, policies, and outcomes. Further, there is a cohort of children who fall into multiple groups, as they have both a developmental disability and complex medical problems. Defining this population in pediatric systems is important to deliver effective care across settings in both medical (inpatient/outpatient) and community sectors to best meet the needs of families, to measure outcomes, and to address costs and utilization (Cohen et al., 2018).

It is important to distinguish CMC as a subset of CYSHCN, as cost of care for CMC accounts for nearly one third of all health care spending on children, with high emergency department utilization, hospitalizations, and readmissions (Berry, Toomey, et al., 2013; Neuman et al., 2014). In fact, readmission to the hospital for this population is equivalent to or exceeds that of the elderly (Berry, Hall, et al., 2014; Berry, Toomey, et al., 2013; Cohen et al., 2012).

Thought Questions:

Discuss the role of a medical home for CYSHCN and CMC and how it might impact their overall quality of life. Describe opportunities and challenges in a value-based payment system for CSHCN/CMC. What issues makes financing care for CYSHCN and CMC unique from the perspectives of health care provider, insurer, parent/caregiver, and hospital systems? Examine the various evidence-based models of financing a payment model for CYSHCN.

HEALTH CARE UTILIZATION

Developing an effective health care system that includes a medical home for CYSHCN is the focus of this chapter. The optimal functioning of a high-performing, quality medical home and care coordination system is essential for CYSHCN given the complex array of services required to maintain and improve their functioning. Several of the core features of this system are important for all children (Stille et al., 2010), yet CYSHCN may require an array of services beyond the primary care doctor, including those provided by specialists, therapists, pharmacists, educators, mental health providers, home health care providers, medical equipment providers, and community partners (American Academy of Pediatrics, 2014). Families and clinicians need to invest significant time and effort in coordinating and communicating among providers and across organizations/systems, ensuring that recommendations, financial, insurance, and necessary services are in the care plan (Kuo et al., 2011). Table 41.1a lists a comparison of health care expenditures and utilization between CYSHCN and their peers without disabilities. Table 41.1b lists specific health services utilized by the CYSHCN represented in the 2009–2010 NS-CYSHCN (U.S. Department of Health and Human Services, Health Resources and Services Administration, Maternal and Child Health Bureau, 2013).

To place the utilization of health care services for CYSHCN and CMC in context, Bui and colleagues (2017) examined data from 1996 to 2013. Their study showed that health care spending on all children in the United States increased from $150 billion to $234 billion in that 17-year period (using inflation-adjusted 2015 dollars). The $234 billion accounted for 8.4% of total health care expenditures in 2013 and accounted for 1.42% of the gross domestic product, resulting in a cost of $2,788 per child in the United States that year. The top 10 condition categories and their associated costs were the following:

- Well newborn care in the hospital setting ($27.9 billion)
- Attention-deficit/hyperactivity disorder treatment ($20.6 billion)
- Well dental care, including dental check-ups and orthodontic care ($18.2 billion)
- Asthma care ($9 billion)
- Treatment of oral disorders, including caries, extractions, and oral surgery ($8.7 billion)
- Well child care in the ambulatory setting ($8.5 billion)

Table 41.1a. Comparison of health care expenditures and utilization between children and youth with special health care needs (CYSHCN) and children without disabilities

Category	CYSHCN	Children without disabilities	Comparison
Hospital days	552 days/1,000	90 days/1,000	6 times higher
Physician visits	4.6 visits/year	1.9 visits/year	2 times more visits
Nonphysician professional visits	3 visits/year	0.6 visits/year	5 times more visits
Prescriptions	6.94 medications/year	1.22 medications/year	5 times the number of prescriptions
Home health provider days	1.73 days/year	0.002 days/year	865 times more days
Health care expenditures	$2,335/year	$652/year	3 times the cost
Out-of-pocket expenditures	$352/year	$175/year	2 times the cost

Sources: Agency for Healthcare Research and Quality (2003); Newacheck, Inkelas, and Kim (2004); and Newacheck and Kim (2005).

Table 41.1b. Health care utilization for children and youth with special health care needs (CSHCN) identified in the 2009–2010 National Survey of Children with Special Health Care Needs

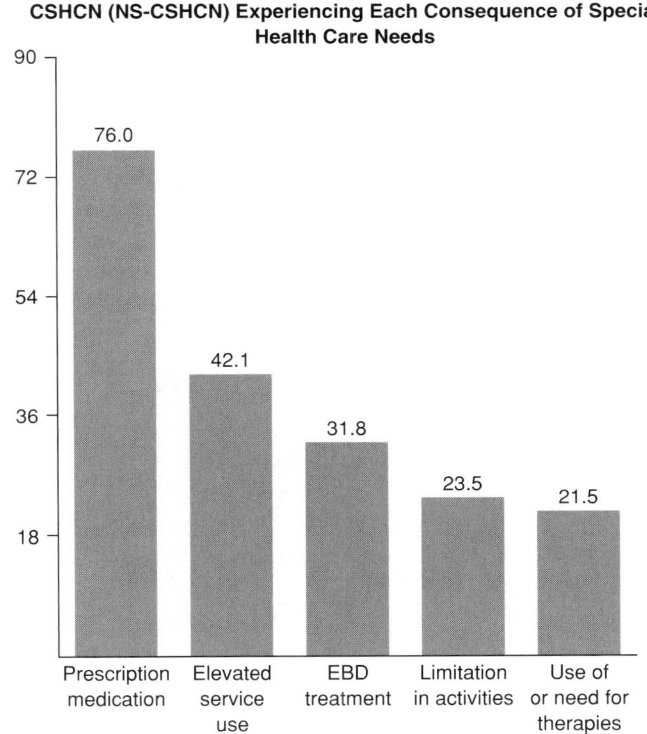

Sample: The presence of a condition expected to last at least 1 year and at least one of the following:

1. The use of or need for prescription medication
2. The use of or need for more medical care, mental health services, or education services than other children of the same age
3. An ongoing emotional, behavioral, or developmental problem that requires treatment or counseling
4. A limitation in the child's ability to do the things that most children of the same age do
5. The use of or need for special therapy, such as physical, occupational, or speech therapy

Description: The need for prescription medication is the most highly utilized service (76% of CYSHCN); followed by the use of or need for extra medical, mental health, or educational services (42.1%); followed by the need for or use of services for ongoing emotional, behavioral, or developmental (EBD) problems (31.8%), limitation in activities (23.5%), and the use of specialized therapies (21.5%). The percentages do not add up to 100 because each child may experience more than one consequence of his or her condition(s).

From U.S. Department of Health and Human Services, Health Resources and Services Administration, Maternal and Child Health Bureau. (2013). Consequences of special needs. In *The National Survey of Children with Special Health Care Needs chartbook 2009–2010.* Rockville, MD: Author. Retrieved from https://mchb.hrsa.gov/cshcn0910/population/pages/hfs/csn.html

- Treatment of upper respiratory infections ($8.4 billion)
- Care for long-term respiratory conditions, such as sleep apnea, allergic rhinitis, and chronic sinusitis ($8.1 billion)
- Treatment of dermatologic conditions, such as cellulitis, cysts, acne, and eczema ($8 billion)
- Emergency treatment of mechanical forces, such as striking an object and cuts ($7.8 billion)

Kogan, Strickland, and Newacheck (2009) estimated that in the first decade of the 21st century, at least 1 in 7 or about 10 million children in the United States had an existing special health care need and had expenditures about three times higher than typically developing children, accounting for 42% of the health care costs spent on child health care (see Tables 41.1a and 41.1b).

Newacheck and Kim (2005) estimated that, on average, out-of-pocket expenses for CYSHCN are about twice what they are for typically developing children. Specifically, of the total cost of services, the following percentages are paid out of pocket by families of CYSHCN:

- 12% of nonphysician services such as physical and occupational therapy
- 14% of physician services
- 30% of prescription costs
- 40% of related services, including vision aids, medical supplies, and other equipment
- 67% of dental services

At least a quarter of families with a CYSHCN and CMC spend at least $1,000 out of pocket per year on expenses related to the CYSHCN/CMC. It should be noted that for lower income families, expenditures of $250 or more are associated with a family perception of a financial burden (Lindley & Mark, 2010). In addition, lower income families experience greater financial burden than those with higher incomes (Newacheck et al., 2004).

An Institute of Medicine report (2001) suggested that the fragmentation of health care in the United States jeopardizes quality of care. To address this concern, all children, whether with a disability or typically developing, should be provided comprehensive health care that is coordinated and occurs within a *medical home* framework and includes care coordination with integration across systems (American Academy of Pediatrics, 2014). However, optimizing care coordination and family engagement through the medical home model requires an integrated assessment, and this should be consistent with the Institute for Healthcare Improvement's Triple Aim framework that focuses on patient outcomes (i.e., population health), patient/family experience, and per-capita costs (Berwick, Nolan, & Whittington, 2008). More recently, Bodenheimer and Sinsky (2014) proposed expansion of the Triple Aim to a Quadruple Aim, adding provider satisfaction and well-being as an essential component of the framework (see Figure 41.1).

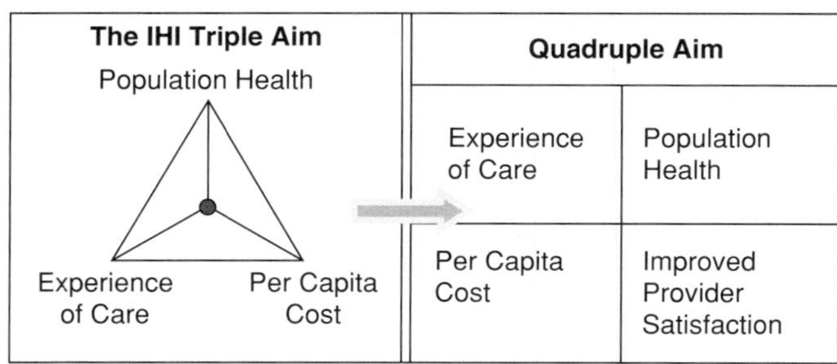

Figure 41.1. The IHI Triple Aim/Quadruple Aim. (Adapted with permission from the Institute for Health Care Improvement [www.ihi.org] and Bodenheimer [2014].)

THE CONCEPT OF THE MEDICAL HOME

The concept of a medical home is not new; it was proposed over 50 years ago by the American Academy of Pediatrics (1967) to help families with care coordination and to improve care. Thirty-five years later, the American Academy of Pediatrics (2002) expanded the statement to include a more comprehensive interpretation of the concept along with operational definitions that would make it easier to recognize care as being consistent with medical home principles. They called for all children to have "a medical home that provides accessible, continuous, comprehensive, family-centered, coordinated, and compassionate health care in an atmosphere of mutual responsibility and trust among clinician, child, and caregiver(s)" (American Academy of Pediatrics, 2002, p. 185). Then, in 2007, the adult and pediatric primary care organizations agreed on core principles, referring to this care model as the patient-centered medical home (American Academy of Family Physicians, 2010). The American Academy of Pediatrics' National Center for Medical Home Implementation (2017) references the medical home policy statement (American Academy of Pediatrics, 2002) in describing the medical home as an approach to providing comprehensive and high-quality primary care. The authors state that the important characteristics of a patient- and family-centered medical home are the following:

- **Accessible:** Care is easy for the child and family to obtain, including geographic access and insurance accommodation.
- **Family centered:** The family is recognized and acknowledged as the primary caregiver and support for the child, ensuring that all medical decisions are made in true partnership with the family.
- **Continuous:** The same primary care clinician cares for the child from infancy through young adulthood (18–21 years), providing assistance and support for transition to adult care.
- **Comprehensive:** Preventive, primary, and specialty care are provided to the child and family.
- **Coordinated:** A care plan is created in partnership with the family and communicated to all health care clinicians and necessary community agencies and organizations.
- **Compassionate:** Genuine concern for the well-being of the child and family are emphasized and addressed.
- **Culturally effective:** The family and child's culture, language, beliefs, and traditions are recognized, valued, and respected.

Notably, a medical home is **not** a building or place—it extends beyond the walls of a clinical practice. Ideally, a medical home builds partnerships with clinical specialists, families, and community resources, and it recognizes the patient's family as the constant in the child's and adolescent's life (National Center for Medical Home Implementation, 2017). This partnership is paramount for children with disabilities, as they require multiple services and systems to maximize their functioning and outcomes.

Health disparities exist regarding access to quality medical homes for CYSHCN among racial and ethnic minorities (Guerrero, Zhou, & Chung, 2018). Addressing issues of cultural and linguistic competency among CYSHCN is essential for practices and programs that provide services and develop policies for CYSHCN (Telfair, Bronheim, & Harrison, 2009). The issue of health care disparities is further discussed in Chapter 42.

Effective primary care has long been recognized as a valuable component for all children in the highly specialized, technology-dependent, tertiary care–based health care delivery system in the United States. Starfield (1992) defined primary care as health care that is 1) first contact, involving an initial physician to whom the family goes to for routine and nonroutine care; 2) community based and accessible; and 3) longitudinal (continuous), coordinated, and comprehensive. In addition, primary care clinicians for children (e.g., community pediatricians, family physicians, and nurse practitioners) provide preventive care, including well-child examinations; immunizations; and vision, hearing, developmental and medical screenings. Primary care also includes personalized care that demonstrates the clinician's knowledge of the patient and family environment, including work, personal, emotional, and—at times—financial concerns. For the child and family, often the primary care team's medical home coordinates care with the pediatric subspecialist(s), the school system, and community providers to ensure comprehensive care. In a few instances, the subspecialist assumes the majority of the responsibilities for the medical home. In some unusual cases, the specialist may also provide well-child care (e.g., for a child with cystic fibrosis who is receiving care at a comprehensive center run by a pulmonologist).

The most recent National Survey of Children's Health (2016) (sponsored and designed by the MCHB at the Health Resources and Services Administration in partnership with the National Center for Health Statistics at the Centers for Disease Control, Child and Adolescent Health Measurement Initiative, and a national technical expert panel) characterizes and describes many aspects of the medical home and systems issues for CYSHCN. The survey demonstrates that the overall prevalence of children with disabilities has increased over time. Figure 41.2 shows how the prevalence of selected developmental disabilities has increased from 2014 to 2016 as well as the overall prevalence of developmental disabilities.

The Patient-Centered Primary Care Collaborative (2017) has examined the effectiveness of both child and adult health care settings based on peer-reviewed literature. They have identified a growing body of literature demonstrating a positive effect of care delivery provided by a patient- and family-centered medical home on cost, quality, and utilization (see Figure 41.3). The results are not unanimous, but the analysis shows that the longer a practice has been operating as a patient- and family-centered medical home and the higher the medical complexity of the patient population being cared for, the more significant positive effects are measured, especially in the cost-savings realm.

Prevalence (percentage) of children ages 3–17 years ever diagnosed with selected developmental disabilities, by year: United States, 2014–2016

Selected developmental disability measure	Estimate (95% confidence interval[1])	Standard error
Autism spectrum disorder		
2014	2.24 (1.90–2.63)	0.18
2015	2.41 (2.01–2.85)	0.21
2016	2.76 (2.29–3.29)	0.25
Intellectual disability		
2014	1.10 (0.89–1.37)	0.12
2015	1.34 (1.03–1.71)	0.17
2016	1.14 (0.87–1.47)	0.15
Other developmental delay		
2014	3.57 (3.11–4.07)	0.24
2015	3.56 (3.07–4.10)	0.26
2016	4.55 (4.00–5.15)	0.29
Developmental disability		
2014	5.76 (5.20–6.37)	0.29
2015	6.04 (5.39–6.75)	0.34
2016	6.99 (6.28–7.76)	0.37

[1]95% confidence interval was calculated using the Korn-Graubard method for complex surveys.

Figure 41.2. Estimated prevalence of children ages 3–7 diagnosed with developmental disabilities in the United States 2014–2016. Note: The linear increase from 2014–2016 is statistically significant ($p < 0.05$). (*Source:* National Center for Health Statistics, 2018.)

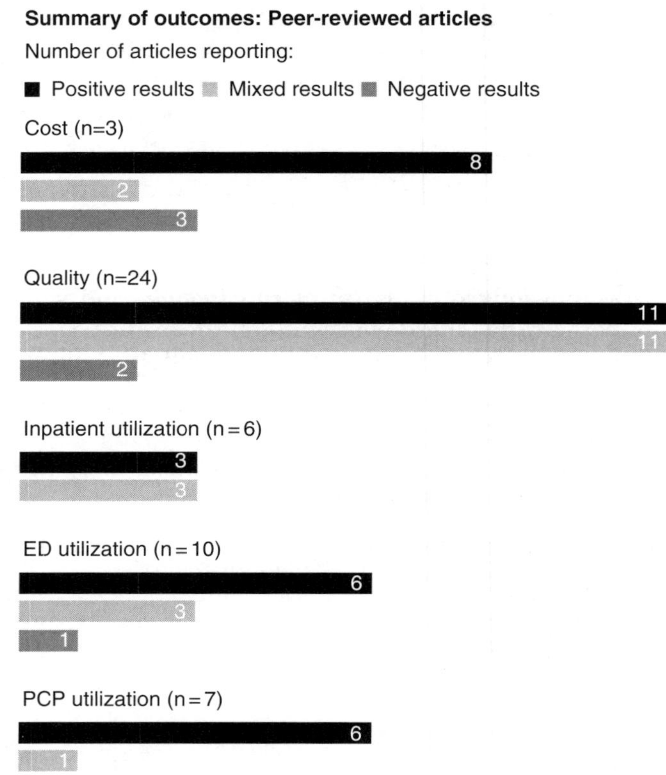

Figure 41.3. The impact patient and family centered medical home has on cost, quality, and utilization. Summary of outcomes: Peer-reviewed articles (From Jabbarpour, Y., De Marchis, E., Bazemore, A., & Grundy, P. [2016.] Impact of Primary Care Practice Transformation on Cost, Quality, and Utilization: A Systematic Review of Research. Executive Summary. Patient-Centered Primary Care Collaborative. Robert Graham Center. P 5. https://www.pcpcc.org/sites/default/files/resources/pcmh_evidence_es_071417%20FINAL.pdf; reprinted by permission.)

THE IMPORTANCE OF COORDINATION OF CARE

Given the many services that may be needed and the number of providers and professionals potentially involved in coordinating the various health care services required by CYSHCN and CMC, coordinating care is important for both the child and family and the health care providers. The child's needs may be complex, and a great deal of time, energy, and skill are required to ensure that the different agencies, institutions, and professionals work effectively together in developing a comprehensive plan of care (American Academy of Pediatrics, 1998, 2014). Effective care coordination and integration are defined as "the set of activities 'in the space between' visits, providers and hospital stays." (American Academy of Pediatrics, 2014, p. e1452.). Integrated care provides effective health care services, from the perspective of the patient and family, across the entire care continuum (American Academy of Pediatrics, 2014). This is particularly relevant for the CYSHCN who often require not only multiple medical specialists, but also medical home team and community partners (e.g., educators, therapists, home health providers, and behavioral and developmental specialists) to communicate and work together to achieve the best outcomes for the child and their family. "Care coordination addresses interrelated medical, social, developmental, behavioral, educational and financial needs to achieve optimal health and wellness outcomes" (Antonelli, McAllister, & Popp, 2009, p. vii). Box 41.1 outlines the framework for highly performing pediatric care coordination. Infrastructure building is needed to create a high-functioning team to effectively integrate care for CYSHCN. There are various models and locations to create these care coordination teams, which necessitate effective resourcing and payment models (Kuo, McAllister, Rossignol, Turchi, & Stille, 2018).

The Agency for Healthcare Research and Quality (2015) notes that while all patients are likely to benefit from the basic elements of care coordination

BOX 41.1 EVIDENCE-BASED PRACTICE

A Framework for Highly Performing Pediatric Care Coordination

Care Coordination Definition

Pediatric care coordination is a patient- and family-centered, assessment-driven, team-based activity designed to meet the needs of children and youth while enhancing the caregiving capabilities of families. Care coordination addresses interrelated medical, social, developmental, behavioral, educational, and financial needs in order to achieve optimal health and wellness outcomes.

Defining Characteristics of Care Coordination

1. Patient and family centered
2. Proactive, planned, and comprehensive
3. Promotes self-care skills and independence
4. Emphasizes cross-organization relationships

Care Coordination Competencies	Care Coordination Functions
1. Develops partnerships	1. Provide separate visits and care coordination interactions
2. Proficient communicator	2. Manage continuous communications
3. Uses assessments for intervention	3. Complete/analyze assessments
4. Facile in care planning skills (PFC)	4. Develop care plans (with family)
5. Integrates all resource knowledge	5. Manage/track tests, referrals, and outcomes
6. Possesses goal/outcome orientation	6. Coach patient/family skills learning
7. Approach is adaptable and flexible	7. Integrate critical care information
8. Desires continuous learning	8. Support/facilitate all care transitions
9. Applies solid team-building skills	9. Facilitate PFC team meetings
10. Adept with information technology	10. Use health information technology for care coordination

From Antonelli, R. C., McAllister, J. W., & Popp, J. (May 2009). *Making Care Coordination a Critical Component of the Pediatric Health System: A Multidisciplinary Framework*. The Commonwealth Fund; reprinted by permission.

(i.e., effective communication and efficient exchange of information among care providers), from a purely efficiency standpoint patient populations with special needs and medical complexity would likely benefit the most from robust care coordination approaches. The following are three key strategies for effective and efficient care coordination:

1. Identify population(s) with needs that are likely to be addressed by care coordination activities
2. Align services directed to the needs of the patient population being served
3. Properly prepare and integrate appropriate personnel to deliver the needed services

It should be noted that the payment aspect for delivering care coordination services remains an unresolved issue and is discussed in more detail below. When care coordination is provided by an insurer or health plan as part of a case management team located in the insurance company, the costs are seen as operational expenses; however, when the health care provider delivers the care coordination services in the high-performing medical home, the additional essential staff and services may not be reimbursable expenses at the practice level.

An American Academy of Pediatrics policy statement on care coordination defines essential characteristics of care coordination as having 1) family-centeredness; 2) a planned, proactive, and comprehensive focus; 3) promotion of self-care skills and independence as a priority; and 4) an emphasis on cross-organizational relationships (American Academy of Pediatrics, 2014). Care coordination addresses primary and specialty medical care, hospital transitions, setting goals with patients and families, and accessing community resources. Taking care coordination one step further fosters care integration that is "the seamless provision of health care services, from the perspective of the patient and family, across the entire care continuum. It results from coordinating the efforts of all providers, irrespective of institutional, departmental, or community-based organizational boundaries" (Antonelli, 2015 p. 6). The Agency for Healthcare Research and Quality provides an instructive graphic to explain the characteristics of care coordination as seen from the perspectives of the patient and family, the health care provider, and the health care system (see Figure 41.4).

According to the 2016 National Survey of Children's Health, slightly less than half (49%) of children were found to be receiving coordinated, ongoing comprehensive care within a medical home. Among the survey respondents indicating a need for care coordination, 72% stated they received needed care coordination. Care coordination can have a favorable impact on the family's experience. An analysis of the NS-CYSHCN in 2005–2006 found that those children who received adequate care coordination had an increased chance of receiving family-centered care, experiencing partnerships with professionals, and indicating satisfaction with services (Turchi et al., 2009).

In an attempt to deal with these issues, insurers, hospitals, and public and private agencies have developed case management programs. The purpose and scope of these programs, however, vary with agency type and often are not focused on the overall coordination of care. As an example, a hospital case management program generally deals with patients at one point in time (i.e., at discharge from a hospital stay) and does not address the patient's needs beyond the hospital episode. Hospitals currently use case managers principally to provide information to payers and assist with discharge planning. In the era of health care reform, however, the case manager's job description may broaden in the context of an accountable care organization (ACO; Watson, 2016). Case managers working for insurers and managed care organizations (MCOs) typically focus more on benefits management and resource utilization and less on care coordination, although some Medicaid MCOs do organize and coordinate a broader package of benefits (Abt Associates, 2000). Many social agencies and public programs provide case management services as these are often mandated by public policy. Title V programs are one of the largest federal block programs, distributing funds to 59 states and jurisdictions. Several of the objectives of Title V funding include, but are not limited to provide "access to preventive and child care services as well as rehabilitative services for children in need of specialized medical services and to provide family-centered, community-based systems of coordinated care for children with special healthcare needs" (U.S. Department of Human Services, 2018). Maternal child health agencies and states submit applications for funds, and, if awarded, they are required to conduct and/or implement needs assessments, reports, and outcomes based on national outcome measures, national performance measures, and evidence-based strategies. While a portion of funds allocated to each entity needs to be spent on CYSHCN, the exact programming and specific efforts are informed by the needs assessments and constituents in each respective agency and state.

Although Medicaid payment for case management may be allocated for a child, families may find that their case manager lacks the necessary medical knowledge or does not communicate adequately with their child's clinicians. Many specialty programs in children's hospitals have nurse specialists who help coordinate the medical care. These specialty-based care coordinators may have comprehensive information about the particular disorder (e.g., diabetes) but may lack knowledge about community- or primary care–level resources and other aspects of comprehensive medical care. This points to the importance of providing care coordination at the community practice (medical home) level. One of the few estimates of the cost of providing care coordination services in a community-based practice suggested that, although substantial, it is not cost prohibitive (Antonelli & Antonelli, 2004).

An important question is whether the increased cost of coordinated care produces better outcomes. There is some evidence to support the value of care coordination in inpatient and family-centered medical homes (Farmer et al., 2011; Long, Bauchner, Sege, Cabral, & Garg, 2012; Mosquera et al., 2014). Effective care coordination may occur in a number of different settings and often is directed toward CYSHCN because they utilize more resources than typically developing children (Kuo et al., 2018). In some studies, findings include fewer emergency department visits, a decreased family financial burden with fewer out-of-pocket expenses, fewer missed days of school and work for the child and caregivers, and improved caregiver-reported satisfaction (Farmer et al., 2011; Long et al., 2012; Mosquera et al., 2014). However, while this may prove cost-effective for the family and insurer, in half the cases, care coordination is often an unreimbursable service for the provider (Antonelli & Antonelli, 2004; Antonelli, Stille, & Antonelli, 2008). It should be noted that even when care coordination is available, many services may not be located in convenient, community-based settings, thus further depleting the family's energy and resources.

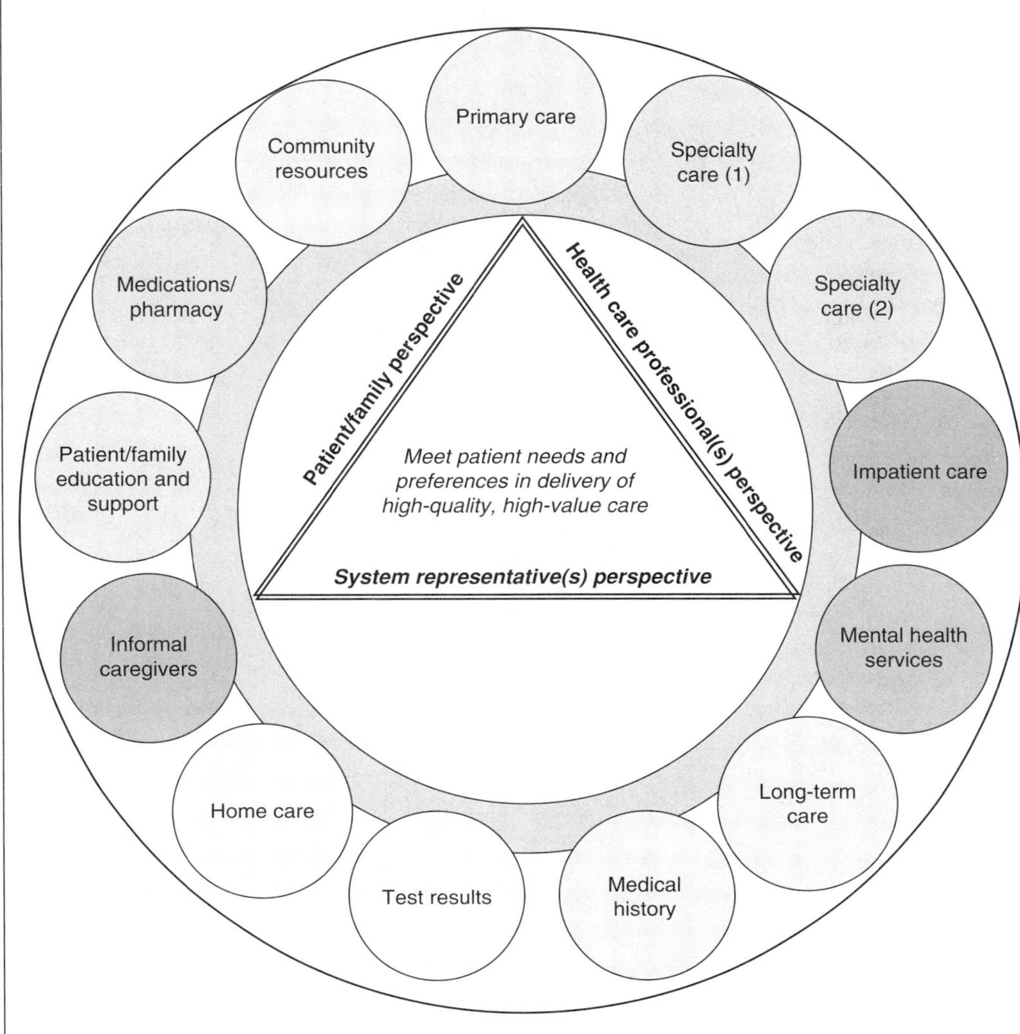

The central *goal* of care coordination is shown in the middle of the diagram.

The 13 small circles represent possible participants, settings, and information important for care delivery and workflow in the clinical setting.

The ring that connects the 13 circles is **CARE COORDINATION**—anything that bridges gaps, i.e., white spaces between the care delivery and workflow circles.

For a given patient at a given point in time, the bridges or *ring* need to form across the applicable *circles,* and through any *gaps* within a given circle, to deliver coordinated care.

Patient/family perspective	**Health care professional(s) perspective**	**System representative(s) perspective**
Care coordination is any activity that helps ensure that the patient's needs and preferences for health services and information sharing across people, functions, and sites are met over time. Patients perceive failures in terms of unreasonable levels of effort required on the part of themselves or their informal caregivers in order to meet care needs during transitions among health care entities.	Clinical coordination involves determining where to send the patient next (e.g., sequencing among specialists), what information about the patient is necessary to transfer among health care entities, and how accountability and responsibility is managed among all health care professionals (doctors, nurses, social workers, care managers, supporting staff, etc.). Care coordination addresses potential gaps in meeting patients' interrelated medical, social, developmental, behavioral, educational, informal support system, and financial needs in order to achieve optimal health, wellness, or end-of-life outcomes, according to patient preferences.	Care coordination is the responsibility of any system of care (e.g., "accountable care organization [ACO]") to deliberately integrate personnel, information, and other resources needed to carry out all required patient care activities between and among care participants (including the patient and informal caregivers). The goal of care coordination is to facilitate the appropriate and efficient delivery of health care services both within and across systems.

Figure 41.4. Care coordination graphic. (From McDonald, K. M., Schultz, E., Albin, L., Pineda, N., Lonhart, J., Sundaram, V., Smith-Spangler, C., Brustrom, J., Malcolm, E., Rohn, L., & Davies, S. Care Coordination Atlas Version 4 [Prepared by Stanford University under subcontract to American Institutes for Research on Contract No. HHSA290-2010-00005I]. AHRQ Publication No. 14-0037- EF. Rockville, MD: Agency for Healthcare Research and Quality. June 2014. [AHRQ Chapter 2, Pg 9].)

Care Planning

The role of the team in care coordination emphasizes the importance of multiple roles, including parents/caregivers, primary care providers, care coordinators, health care specialists, educators, pharmacists, mental health providers, and community partners (Chen et al., 2010; Katkin et al., 2017). The shared responsibility of team members fosters efficiency in planning before, during, and after a patient encounter and includes clinicians, medical assistants, nurses, and office staff (see the textbox titled What Care Planning Involves; Katkin et al., 2017). Staff roles and contributions should be defined and understood by all members (Phillips, Hebish, Mann, Ching, & Blackmore, 2016; see Box 41.2). In addition, practice teams can engage in "huddles" prior to a patient visit where discussions around needed services, planning for the visit, and communication about health events since the patient and family were last in the office are all important (Rodriguez et al., 2015). Often the team can utilize patient registries to identify the CYSHCN who require additional supports, services, or care integration across teams or settings to best serve them and their families (Davis, McFadden, Patterson, & Barkin, 2015). Registries can be created within electronic health records and managed with shared folders among the team. This fosters collaboration with care team members in the community (e.g., therapists, educators in the school system, home health agencies, and behavioral health providers). Training teams and family members about the value and role of care planning is essential. Measuring care coordination activities and experiences across all members of the team can be effective and assist in more efficient time management and patient flow (Ferrari, Ziniel, & Antonelli, 2016).

What Care Planning Involves

- Multiple providers and services across many disciplines
- Summaries and guidelines for current and future health issues to foster communication among all the disciplines caring for the child and his/her family
- Coordination with community partners, home care agencies, and therapists
- Contingency planning for CYSHCN during emergencies and unanticipated health problems
- A summary of medical diagnoses, medications, equipment, specialists, therapists, educational needs, child/youth strengths, transition needs, and contact information

BOX 41.2 INTERDISCIPLINARY CARE

The Role of the Care Coordinator

Role	Location
• Assist patient and families in navigating the health care system and community resources • Develop and maintain care plans and care planning for patients and families • Coordinate patient care services and appointments • Advocate for needed resources and services with agencies and insurance companies • Set goals with patients and families • Ensure patient goals are met and patients/families are satisfied and have consistent comprehensive care • Facilitate effective transitions of care from inpatient to outpatient settings • Foster successful transitions from pediatric- to adult-oriented systems • Collaborate with nonmedical services needed for patients and families (e.g., therapies, education, and behavioral/mental health) • Ensure patient- and family-centered care goals are met and incorporate tenets of medical home and care integration across all aspects of care	• Primary care medical home • Specialty office • Insurance company • Community based • Agencies (e.g., early intervention and behavioral health) **Background/Training** • Nurses • Social workers • Parent partners • Referral coordinator • Curricula available (citations below)

Sources: American Academy of Pediatrics (2014); Boston Children's Hospital (2013); Conway, O'Donnell, and Yates (2017); and Weaver, Che, Petersen, and Hysong, (2018).

- Clearly identified aspects of the child's health that are likely to get better or worse over time for the purpose of future planning
- Clearly noted exacerbations of the chronic condition the child is likely to experience and what acute illnesses he/she may be at enhanced risk for (e.g., flu)
- Clearly identified new co-occuring conditions the child is likely to develop and how they can be avoided or treated early
- Assessment of the family functioning, stress, and social determinants of health
- Discussion of major medical interventions the child and family will likely face over time
- Development of family goals for their child over the next 1, 5, and 10 years

---

Approaching care planning using a patient- and family-centered care lens fosters engagement and ensures efficiency. The publication *Achieving a Shared Plan of Care with Children and Families with Special Health Care Needs* provides a road map for health care teams and families in developing a shared, written plan of care with the support of a high-level, team-based care coordinator (McAllister, 2014). This shared plan of care is informed by family goals and team concerns, merging them into a strategic plan of action to use/follow. Families need to be involved in all aspects of the system "frontlines," from designing systems to implementation, outcome assessment and evaluation, and policy dissemination (Allshouse, Comeau, Rodgers, & Wells, 2018). Outlining and guiding subsequent care coordination activities and contingency planning in an emergency are key aspects to be achieved in partnership with families over time. One study examined the impact of a hospital-based multidisciplinary team's comprehensive needs assessment and the creation of individualized shared care plans on the quality and cost outcomes for CMC and their families. It demonstrated improved family experience of care, but the CMC cohort incurred increased costs with no improvement in functional outcomes compared with the nonintervention cohort (Simon et al., 2017). Given the service needs and multiple providers, patients and families should be engaged as partners at all levels of care coordination and decision making, including goal setting, care planning, care gaps, and assessing their experiences (Cene et al., 2016). Several validated instruments can assist in measuring the patient and caregiver experience (Walker, Stewart, & Grumbach, 2016; Ziniel et al., 2016), and there are existing tools for care coordination activities, including flexible and modifiable care coordination curricula for training health care teams in developing competencies. These skills include care planning, integration with behavioral health, and safe transitions of care, such as transitioning from inpatient to outpatient settings and from the pediatric to the adult sector (Boston Children's Hospital, 2013).

The social determinants of health are defined by the Centers for Disease Control and Prevention (2018, para. 1) as "conditions in the places where people live, learn, work and play that affect a wide range of health risks and outcomes," and they have been shown to be influencers of health outcomes and potential drivers of health care costs (Booske, Athens, Kindig, Park, & Remington, 2010). For example, patients with unmet needs may have increased emergency department utilization and higher rates of no-show appointments (see Chapter 42; Berkowitz et al., 2016; Garg et al., 2013). Screening for social determinants of health within the pediatric medical home model can assist in appropriate resource allocation and ensure that patient and family needs are met (Garg et al., 2007). Screening for social determinants in the population of CYSHCN requires selecting a tool or questions that adequately address the patient population in embedded electronic health records or streamlined systems, communicating appropriately with patients about the social determinants of health, having resources and referral networks to meet the needs of the patients served, and utilizing care integration across systems (both medical and nonmedical) to communicate needs and foster integration (Thomas-Henkel & Schulman, 2017). Community health workers have been identified as a possible resource to assist in interventions with families and have been associated with favorable impacts on health care outcomes (Mathu-Muju, Kong, Brancato, McLeod, & Bush, 2018; Mundorf et al., 2018).

CHANGES IN FINANCING HEALTH CARE FOR CYSHCN

There are several perspectives on what constitutes an optimal health care system for CYSHCN and CMC. For most of its history, the health care system in the United States has utilized a fee-for-service (FFS) model in which the health care provider receives a payment for each unit of service rendered (MacLeod, 2001). In an FFS payment model, the health care provider is compensated for the volume of covered services delivered and not necessarily for the quality or measured outcome of those services. Therefore, a great deal of effort is directed toward counting the specific procedures and services provided during the encounter. In response to skyrocketing costs and general displeasure with the quality of care delivered in the existing FFS system in the United States, reformers have called for a shift from this volume of service, or counting, approach to reimbursement to a model that seeks instead to reimburse for the quality of the care delivered. The ultimate goal is a value-based model that pays for achieving actual positive outcomes for the patient. The equation for value in health care is value = quality / cost. The drive toward paying for quality and outcomes in health care would seem well suited for CYSHCN and CMC, whose health care costs may be as high as three times that of children in the general population (Newacheck & Kim, 2005).

The Centers for Medicare and Medicaid Services (2015) has developed a four-category framework to describe a progressive shift from FFS toward value-based reforms:

1. FFS with no link to quality
2. FFS linked to quality
3. Alternative payment models (APMs) built on an FFS architecture
4. Population-based payment

Figure 41.5 describes the framework and time frame over which the Centers for Medicare and Medicaid Services (CMS) envision the U.S. health care system adopting so-called APMs. CMS is focused initially on the Medicare system, but the expectation is that Medicaid as well as much of the commercial insurance system will likely eventually embrace this effort. In considering the potential benefit of these APMs as they apply to children and adolescents, Dr. Sandra Hassink (2015), then president of the American Academy of Pediatrics, highlighted the longitudinal value of pediatric quality and preventive measures. She noted specifically that the return on investment should not be limited to a benefit plan year since much of the potential benefit may extend beyond that period (e.g., obesity prevention). Clearly, a focus on value of care delivered rather than on the delivery of a volume of services has the potential to be useful in promoting medical homes for CYSHCN and CMC. A value-based approach would likely avoid the challenges of counting and billing for specific services and would instead provide a pathway for the care coordination and related services necessary for ideal care. A value-based approach would likely generate cost savings that can be redirected toward the care coordination so essential to delivering effective medical home care (Agency for Healthcare Research and Quality, 1997). Berry and colleagues (2013) noted a number of examples supporting the value of clinical programs designed to coordinate care and optimize health; Table 41.2 summarizes these promising examples.

One of the principal proposals of health care reform is the development of ACOs. An ACO is defined as follows:

> A group of physicians, other healthcare professionals, hospitals, and other healthcare providers that accept a shared responsibility to deliver a broad set of medical services to a defined set of patients across the age spectrum and who are held accountable for the quality and cost of care provided through alignment of incentives. (American Academy of Pediatrics, 2011, p. 1)

An ACO would be given annual funding on a per-capita basis for providing comprehensive care. In this shared-risk model, if the ACO does not need to expend all the money, it is permitted to keep a portion; however, if it spends more, it is responsible for the financial loss. The foundation of ACOs lies in the primary care medical home and, if adopted, will drive the health care financial discussion in the next decade.

In the current FFS model, care for CYSHCN fosters volume-driven payments that do not adequately support non–face-to-face time, such as care coordination services. Moving toward alternative payment models (e.g., value-based payments, population health, or bundled per-member/per-month models) affords the health care arena an opportunity to explore new payment opportunities for CYSHCN. A shift to a population health framework with high-functioning medical homes and care integration will foster alternative payment models, allowing the care of CYSHCN to best meet their needs. To accomplish this goal, a paradigm shift for this population is needed to include risk stratification (Simon et al., 2014) so that it involves both medical and nonmedical services and communication and coordination with nonmedical partners, addressing the social determinants of health and benchmarking quality for a unique population not fitting into the framework for typically developing children (Langer, Antonelli, Chamberlain, Pan, & Keller, 2018). For example, CYSHCN may have a level of complexity where care coordination reduces the risk of readmissions, but they still may require hospitalizations for some of their intrinsic medical issues. However, addressing effective hand-offs, transitions of care, and post–hospital discharge follow-up may allow for a shared savings for care providers. In addition, utilizing health information exchanges, patient portals, and effective communication may enhance this process. Caring for CYSHCN may also allow for risk-stratified capitation payments to address the added effort and time required to provide high-quality care to this fragile population. These payments could include but not be limited to care coordination, screening, and supporting patient and family engagement, further aligning with the Quadruple Aim (Langer et al., 2018).

Aim: When it comes to improving the way providers are paid, we want to reward value and care coordination rather than volume and care duplication. In partnership with the private sector, the Department of Health and Human Services is testing and expanding new health care payment models that can improve health care quality and reduce its cost.

Payment taxonomy framework

	Category 1 *Fee for services (FFS)–no link to quality*	Category 2 *FFS–link to quality*	Category 3 *Alternative payment models built on FFS architecture*	Category 4 *Population-based payment*
Description	*Payments are based on volume of services and not linked to quality or efficiency.*	*At least a portion of payments vary based on the quality or efficiency of health care delivery.*	*Some payment is linked to the effective management of a population or an episode of care. Payments are still triggered by delivery of services, but there are opportunities for shared savings or 2-sided risk.*	*Payment is not directly triggered by services delivery so volume is not linked to payment. Clinicians and organizations are paid and responsible for the care of a beneficiary for a long period (e.g., greater than 1 year).*
Medicare FFS	Limited in Medicare FFS Majority of Medicare payments are now linked to quality	Hospital value-based purchasing Physicians value-based modifier Readmissions/hospital-acquired condition reduction program	Alternative payment models built on FFS architecture Some payment is linked to the effective management of a population or an episode of care. Payments are still triggered by delivery of services, but there are opportunties for shared savings or 2-sided risk. Accountable care organizations Medical homes Bundled payments Comprehensive primary care initiative Comprehensive Comprehensive end-stage renal disease (ESRD) Medicare–Medicaid financial alignment initiative FFS model	Eligible pioneer accountable care organizations in Years 3–5

Value-based purchasing includes payments made in Categories 2 through 4. Moving from Category 1 to Category 4 involves two shifts: (1) increasing accountability for both quality and total cost of care and (2) a greater focus on population health management as opposed to payment for specific services.

Timeline

Target percentage of Medicare FFS payments linked to quality and alternative payment models in 2016 and 2018

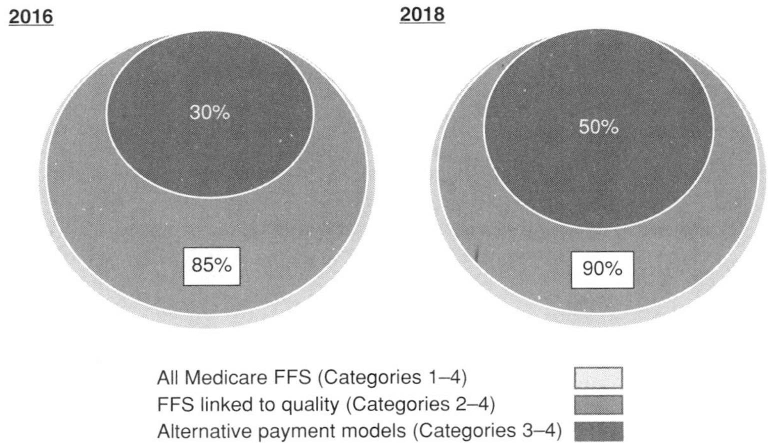

All alternative payment models and payment reforms that seek to deliver better care at lower costs share a common pathway for success: Providers must make fundamental changes in their day-to-day operations that improve quality and reduce costs. Making operational changes will be attractive only if the new alternative payment models and payment reforms are broadly adopted by a critical mass of payers. When providers encounter new payment strategies for one payer but not others, the incentives to fundamentally change are weak. In fact, a provider that alters its system to prevent admissions and succeeds in an alternative payment environment may lose revenue from payers that continue FFS payments.

Figure 41.5. Framework for value-based reimbursement evolution (Agency for Healthcare Research and Quality, 1997; Centers for Medicare and Medicaid Services, 2015).

(continued)

Figure 41.5. *(continued)*

The key elements of value-based purchasing include:

- **Contracts** spelling out the responsibilities of employers as purchasers with selected insurance, managed care, and hospital and physician groups as suppliers.
- **Information** to support the management of purchasing activities.
- **Quality management** to drive continuous improvements in the process of health care purchasing and in the delivery of health care services.
- **Incentives** to encourage and reward desired practices by providers and consumers.
- **Education** to help employees become better health care consumers.

Agency for Healthcare Research and Quality (1997)

Table 41.2. Examples of clinical programs designed to coordinate care and deliver value

Location	Description and citation
Complex Medical Care Program at University of Texas, Houston	Randomized clinical trial of high-risk children with chronic illness (defined as having at least 3 emergency department visits, 2 hospitalizations, or 1 pediatric intensive care unit admission during the previous year, and a 50% or higher estimated risk for hospitalization) treated at a high-risk clinic at the University of Texas, Houston, and randomized to comprehensive care (n = 105) or usual care (n = 96). Enrollment was between March 2011 and February 2013 (when predefined stopping rules for benefit were met), and outcome evaluations continued through August 31, 2013. Mosquera, R. A., Avritscher, E. B., Samuels, C. L., Harris, T. S., Pedroza, C., Evans, P., . . . Moody, S. (2014). Effect of an enhanced medical home on serious illness and cost of care among high-risk children with chronic illness: A randomized clinical trial. *JAMA, 312*(24), 2640–2648.
Two community-based pediatric clinics in Canada staffed with tertiary-care nurse practitioners to coordinate care	Eighty-one patients with medical complexity reported a mean (standard deviation [SD]) decrease in per-member/per-month (PPPM) total health system costs from $244 (SD 981) to $131 (SD 335) without an increase in out-of-pocket costs to families. Fewer inpatient days was the primary reason for the decrease PPPM. Child quality of life improved after enrollment in the clinic intervention. Cohen, E., Lacombe-Duncan, A., Spalding, K., MacInnis J, Nicholas D, Narayanan, U. G., . . . Friedman J. N. (2012). Integrated complex care coordination for children with medical complexity: A mixed-methods evaluation of tertiary care-community collaboration. *BMC Health Services Research, 12*, 366.
Outpatient primary care program for children with medical complexity at Arkansas Children's Hospital	Reported a 1-year decrease in the mean annual cost per-patient-per-month (PPPM) of $1,800 for inpatient care and $6 for emergency department care. Although PPPM cost for outpatient claims and prescriptions increased, the overall cost to Medicaid PPPM decreased by approximately $1,200. Casey, P. H., Lyle, R. E., Bird, T. M., Robbins, J. M., Kuo, D. Z., Brown, A., Tanios, A., & Burns, K. (2011). Effect of hospital-based comprehensive care clinic on health costs for Medicaid-insured medically complex children. *Archives of Pediatric and Adolescent Medicine, 165*(5), 392–398.
A medical home program for children with complex disease at the University of California, Los Angeles	30 CMC were offered a 1-hour intake appointment, 30-minute follow-up visits, access to a family liaison, and a family notebook; they reported a decrease in the average number of emergency department visits from 1.1 (SD 1.7) to 0.5 (SD 0.9) in the 1 year after enrollment. Klitzner, T. S., Rabbitt, L. A., & Chang, R. K. (2010). Benefits of care coordination for children with complex disease: A pilot medical home project in a resident teaching clinic. *Journal of Pediatrics, 156*(6), 1006–1010.
Outpatient consultative program at the Children's Hospital of Wisconsin	Provided intensive care coordination for approximately 230 CMC; reported a $400,000 annual loss to operate the program, while contributing to a 3-year reduction in hospital resource utilization of more than $10 million for its patients. Gordon, J. B., Colby, H. H., Bartelt, T., Jablonski, D., Krauthoefer, M. L., & Havens, P. (2007). A tertiary care-primary care partnership model for medically complex and fragile children and youth with special health care needs. *Archives of Pediatric and Adolescent Medicine, 161*(10), 937–944.
Six primary care pediatric practices in Massachusetts	A care coordination intervention for approximately 150 CMC/CSHCN that included a case manager, parent consultant, and an individualized plan of care was associated with a decrease in hospitalization rate (58%–43%) and a decrease in the rate of parents missing 3 or more weeks of work (26%–14%). The intervention cost $400 per patient. Palfrey, J. S., Sofis, L. A., Davidson, E. J., Liu, J., Freeman, L., & Ganz, M. L. (2004). The Pediatric Alliance for Coordinated Care: Evaluation of a medical home model. *Pediatrics, 113*(Suppl. 5), 1507–1516.

Source: Berry, Agrawal, Cohen, and Kuo (2013).

Insurance Coverage: Public and Private

The federal and state governments provide several other avenues for CYSHCN and CMC and their families to gain access to a range of health care services and funding for these services. These include 1) the Social Security Administration's Supplemental Security Income program that provides income support and/or access to Medicaid; 2) the MCHB's Title V programs, which support systems and provide services in some areas for CYSHCN; and 3) the Individuals with Disabilities Education Improvement Act of 2004 (PL 108-446), which links educational and health care needs with Medicaid funding. However, in practical terms, these programs can have considerable state-to-state variability in eligibility criteria, types of services covered or offered, and amount of care provided.

Where CYSHCN and CMC get their insurance is an important aspect of the financing for their care. According to the Kaiser Family Foundation (Musumeci, 2017), Medicaid and other public health insurance programs cover 44% of CYSHCN and CMC. In addition, publicly funded insurance is the sole source of funding for 36% of CYSHCN and CMC; an additional 8% have public insurance as a supplement to their private coverage. Figure 41.6 arrays the types of health insurance among CYSHCN and CMC.

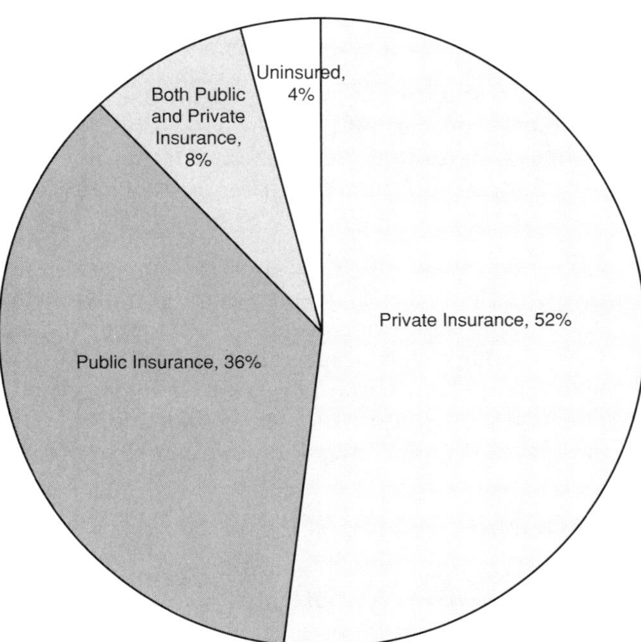

Figure 41.6. Type of health insurance for children with special health care needs. (From Musumeci M. *Medicaid and Children with Special Health Care Needs*. The Henry J. Kaiser Family Foundation Issue Brief. January 2017. http://files.kff.org/attachment/Issue-Brief-Medicaid-and-Children-with-Special-Health-Care-Needs; reprinted by permission.)

The cost trends described above are expected to increase as a function of an increased prevalence of CYSHCN and CMC. For example, between 2001 and 2011, there was a 15.6% increase in children with neurodevelopmental and mental health conditions, accounting for the largest increases in chronic conditions during this time frame (Houtrow, Larson, Olson, Newacheck, & Halfon, 2014).

Wagner (1998) has proposed a chronic care model focusing on patient–provider interactions. The model underscores how favorable outcomes for patients, families, and practice teams ensue when the medical home works in partnership with community resources and policies. Figure 41.7 provides a graphic representation of Wagner's chronic care model, the characteristics of which include the following:

- Providing care in the context of a medical home
- Having processes and incentives to improve the care delivery system
- Having information technology and clinical decision support for clinicians
- Ensuring a focus on effective self-management training and support
- Organizing team activities and practice systems around the unique needs of children, youth, and adults with chronic conditions
- Utilizing appropriate evidence-based guidelines in a measurable manner
- Fostering increased communication between primary care and specialty care providers

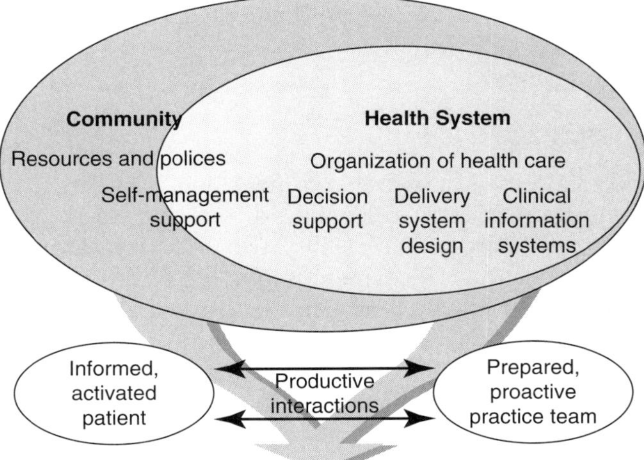

Figure 41.7. Wagner's chronic care model. (From Wagner. [1998]. "Chronic disease management: What will it take to improve care for chronic illness?" *Effective Clinical Practice*, August/September, 1: 2–4; reprinted by permission.)

- Utilizing information systems in a way that produces disease registries, tracking systems, and reminders about important care needs
- Providing care in the environment of a patient- and family-centered medical home

The Centers for Medicare and Medicaid Services, which have federal oversight and responsibility for Medicaid, have established a set of safeguards promoting attention to the unique aspects of caring for CYSHCN and CMC in the current health care environment. To deal with this issue, some states have conceived of "carve-outs" for these children in which the child is handled separately from the general population. CYSHCN also may be eligible for various Medicaid waivers, including 1) the Home and Community-Based Services Waiver, sometimes referred to as a 1915(c) waiver, and 2) the Katie Beckett waiver (Peters, 2005). Both essentially waive, or permit exceptions to, certain federal requirements to provide home- and community-based services as an alternative to institutionalization or continued hospitalization. Such waivers, for example, may permit a family with a CYSHCN or CMC to receive Medicaid in order to access health care services and support for keeping that child at home rather than in a hospital or chronic care facility. One advantage of the waivers is that family income may be exempted from consideration in determining eligibility for Medicaid. The waivers are state-run programs, however, so each state has different approaches to waivers with different eligibility requirements or services. Examples of disorders/diagnoses that may qualify for CYSHCN/CMC waivers include children/youth with intellectual disability, those who are dependent on home nursing services, those with technology dependence or need for mobility aids, and those with autism spectrum disorder (ASD).

Looking to the Future

Classically, the measurable dimensions of health care quality are the structure, the process, and the actual outcomes (Donabedian, 1980). Structure, from a quality and health services perspective, describes aspects of the health care system such as facilities, staffing patterns, and qualifications. Process in this context deals with the policies and procedures that govern aspects of care, such as technical and professional skills, documentation of care, safety practices, and the use of assessment tools. Finally, outcomes deal with the health status of the people served, their health-related knowledge and behavior, and their satisfaction with the care they receive (Monahan & Sykora, 1999). Looking at one special health care need, ASD, the Waisman Center at the University of Wisconsin undertook the National Medical Home Autism Initiative and issued a 47-page document, titled *Medical Home Services for Autism Spectrum Disorders* (2008), which articulates how the medical home concept can be applied to patients and families with ASD. The appendix to this chapter lists five guidelines and addresses recommendations at the family, professional, and governmental levels. See Appendix D in the book's online materials for more valuable resources for both families and professionals to use in assisting CYSHCN and CMC locate and comanage their medical home and the care coordination services they need.

SUMMARY

- Coordinating health care services for CYSHCN and CMC presents a unique challenge to the child's family and health care providers.
- The complexity of the child's needs necessitates time, energy, and skill to coordinate the efforts of different agencies, institutions, and professionals so that they work effectively together in a comprehensive plan of care.
- This coordination is particularly complex because of the labor-intensive nature of the comprehensive case management necessary and because the child's needs may span a range of services, including some that are not traditionally seen as health related.
- Further complicating matters are the many federal and state agencies and programs involved in providing and funding services and the revolutionary changes currently occurring in the health care marketplace.
- All of this points to the importance of each child having a high-quality medical home complete with addressing population health, an interdisciplinary team working with community partners and across systems, patient- and family-centered care, and effective care coordination and integrated care to assist the family in navigating this complex system.

ADDITIONAL RESOURCES

Family Voices Family to Family Health Information Center (HIC): http://www.fv-ncfpp.org/f2fhic/about_f2fhic/

American Academy of Pediatrics Care Coordination Policy Statement: http://pediatrics.aappublications.org/content/early/2014/04/22/peds.2014-0318

National Center for Care Coordination Technical Assistance: https://www.lpfch.org/publication/achieving-shared-plan-care-children-and-youth-special-health-care-needs

Additional resources can be found online in Appendix D: Childhood Disabilities Resources, Services, and Organizations (see About the Online Companion Materials).

REFERENCES

Abt Associates. (2000). *Evaluation of the District of Columbia's demonstration program, "Managed care system for disabled and special needs children": Final report summary.* Retrieved from http://aspe.hhs.gov/daltcp/reports/dc-frs.htm

Agency for Healthcare Research and Quality. (1997). *Theory and reality of value-based purchasing lessons from the pioneer.* Rockville, MD: Author. Retrieved from https://www.ahrq.gov/professionals/quality-patient-safety/quality-resources/tools/meyer/index.html

Agency for Healthcare Research and Quality (2003). *MEPS HC-050: 2000 full year consolidated data file.* Rockville, MD: Author. Retrieved from https://meps.ahrq.gov/data_stats/download_data/pufs/h50/h50doc.pdf

Agency for Healthcare Research and Quality. (2015). *Chartbook on care coordination.* Rockville, MD: Author. Retrieved from http://www.ahrq.gov/research/findings/nhqrdr/2014chartbooks/carecoordination/index.html

Allshouse, C., Comeau, M., Rodgers, R., & Wells, N. (2018). Families of children with medical complexity: A view from the front lines. *Pediatrics, 141*(Suppl. 3), S195–S201.

American Academy of Family Physicians. (2010). *Joint principles statement of accountable care organizations.* Retrieved from https://www.aafp.org/media-center/releases-statements/all/2010/aco-jointprinciples.html

American Academy of Pediatrics. (1967). Pediatric records and a "medical home." In *Standards of child care* (pp. 77–79). Evanston, IL: Author.

American Academy of Pediatrics. (1998). Managed care and children with special health care needs: A subject review (RE9814). *Pediatrics, 102,* 657–660.

American Academy of Pediatrics. (2002). Policy statement: The medical home. *Pediatrics, 110*(1), 184–186.

American Academy of Pediatrics. (2011). *Joint principles of accountable care organizations.* Retrieved from https://www.aap.org/en-us/Documents/practicet_joint_principles_accountable_care_organizations.pdf

American Academy of Pediatrics. (2014). Patient- and family-centered care coordination: A framework for integrating care for children and youth across multiple systems. Council on Children with Disabilities and Medical Home Implementation Advisory Committee. *Pediatrics, 133*(5), e1451–e1460.

Antonelli, R. (2012). *Care integration for children with special health needs: Improving outcomes and managing costs.* Washington, DC: National Governors Association Center for Best Practices.

Antonelli, R. (2015). *Achieving high value outcomes: Using measurement to drive system performance measurement for children and youth with special health care needs.* Retrieved from https://classic.nga.org/files/live/sites/NGA/files/pdf/2015/1511LearningCollaborativeAntonelli.pdf

Antonelli, R. C., & Antonelli, D. M. (2004). Providing a medical home: The cost of care coordination services in a community-based general pediatric practice. *Pediatrics, 113*(5), 1522–1528.

Antonelli, R. C., McAllister, J. W., & Popp, J. (2009). *Making care coordination a critical component of the pediatric health system: A multidisciplinary framework.* New York, NY: The Commonwealth Fund.

Antonelli, R. C., Stille, C. J., & Antonelli, D. M. (2008). Care coordination for children and youth with special health care needs: A descriptive, multisite study of activities, personnel costs, and outcomes. *Pediatrics, 122,* e209–e216.

Berkowitz, S. A., Hulberg, A. C., Hong, C., Stowell, B. J., Tirozzi, K. J., Traore, C. Y., & Atlas S. J. (2016). Addressing basic resource needs to improve primary care quality: A community collaboration programme. *BMJ Quality Safety, 25*(3), 164–172.

Berry, J. G., Agrawal, R. K., Cohen, E., & Kuo, D. Z. (2013). The Landscape of Medical Care for Children with Medical Complexity. Children's Hospital Association, Alexandria, VA, Overland Park, KS, June 2013. Retrieved from http://www.columbia.edu/itc/hs/medical/residency/peds/new_compeds_site/pdfs_new/PL3%20new%20readings/Special_Report_The_Landscape_of_Medical_Care_for_Children_with_Medical_Complexity.pdf

Berry, J. G., Hall, M., Neff, J., Goodman, D. M., Cohen, E., Agrawal, R., Kuo, D., & Feudtner, C. (2014). Children with medical complexity and Medicaid: Spending and cost savings. *Health Affairs (Millwood), 33*(12), 2199–2206.

Berry, J. G., Toomey, S. L., Zaslavsky, A. M., Jha A. K., Nakamura, M. M., Klein, D. J., . . . Schuster, M. A. (2013). Pediatric readmission prevalence and variability across hospitals. *The Journal of the American Medical Association, 309*(4), 372–380.

Berwick, D. M., Nolan, T. W., & Whittington, J. (2008). The Triple Aim: Care, health, and cost. *Health Affairs (Millwood), 27*(3), 759–769.

Bethell, C. D., Blumberg, S. J., Stein, R. E., Strickland, B., Robertson, J., & Newacheck, P. W. (2015). Taking stock of the CYSHCN screener: A review of common questions and current reflections. *Academic Pediatrics, 15*(2), 165–176.

Bodenheimer, T., & Sinsky, C. (2014). From Triple to Quadruple Aim: Care of the patient requires care of the provider. *Annals of Family Medicine, 12*(6), 573–576.

Booske, B. C., Athens, J. K., Kindig, D. A., Park, H., & Remington, P. L. (2010). *Different perspectives for assigning weights to determinants of health.* Madison, WI: University of Wisconsin Population Health Institute.

Boston Children's Hospital. (2013). *Care coordination curriculum.* Retrieved from http://www.childrenshospital.org/integrated-care-program/care-coordination-curriculum

Bui, A. L., Dieleman, J. L., Hamavid, H., Birger, M., Chapin, A., Duber, H. C., . . . Murray, C. J. L. (2017). Spending on children's personal health care in the United States. *JAMA Pediatrics, 171*(2), 183–189.

Cene, C. W., Johnson, B. H., Wells, N., Baker, B., Davis, R., & Turchi, R. (2016). A narrative review of patient and family engagement: The "foundation" of the medical "home." *Medical Care, 54*(7), 697–705.

Centers for Disease Control and Prevention. (2018). *Social determinants of health: Know what affects health.* Retrieved from https://www.cdc.gov/socialdeterminants/index.htm

Centers for Medicare and Medicaid Services. (2015). *Better care, smarter spending, healthier people: Paying providers for value not volume.* Retrieved from https://www.cms.gov/

Newsroom/MediaReleaseDatabase/Fact-sheets/2015-Fact-sheets-items/2015-01-26-3.html

Chen, E. H., Thorn, D. H., Hessler, D. M., Hammer, H., Saba, G., & Bodenheimer, T. (2010). Using the Teamlet Model to improve chronic care in an academic primary care practice. *Journal of General Internal Medicine, 25*(Suppl. 4), S610–S614..

Cohen, E., Berry, J. G., Camacho, X., Anderson, G., Wodchis, W., & Guttmann, A. (2012). Patterns and costs of health care use of children with medical complexity. *Pediatrics, 130*(6), e1463–e1470. PubMed: 23184117

Cohen, E., Berry, J. G., Sanders, L., Schor, E. L., & Wise, P. H. (2018). Status complexicus? The emergence of pediatric complex care. *Pediatrics, 141*(Suppl. 3), S202–S211.

Cohen, E., Kuo, D. Z., Agrawal, R., Berry, J. G., Bhagat, S. K., Simon, T. D., & Srivastava R. (2011). Children with medical complexity: An emerging population for clinical and research initiatives. *Pediatrics, 127*(3), 529–538.

Conway, A., O'Donnell, C., & Yates, P. (2017). The effectiveness of the nurse care coordinator role on patient-reported and health service outcomes: A systematic review. *Evaluation and Health Professions, 1.* doi:163278717734610

Davis, A. M., McFadden, S. E., Patterson, B. L., & Barkin, S. L. (2015). Strategies to identify and stratify children with special health care needs in outpatient general pediatrics settings. *Maternal and Child Health Journal, 19*(6), 1384–1392.

Davis, M. M., & Brosco, J. P. (2007). Being specific about being special: Defining children's conditions and special health care needs. *Archives of Pediatrics and Adolescent Medicine, 161*(10), 1003–1005.

Donabedian, A. (1980). Methods for deriving criteria for assessing the quality of medical care. *Medical Care Research and Review, 37*(7), 653–698.

Farmer, J. E., Clark, M. J., Drewel, E. H., Swenson, T. M., & Ge, B. (2011). Consultative care coordination through the medical home for CYSHCN: A randomized controlled trial. *Maternal and Child Health Journal, 15*(7), 1110–1118.

Ferrari, L. R., Ziniel, S. I., & Antonelli, R. C. (2016). Perioperative care coordination measurement: A tool to support care integration of pediatric surgical patients. *A&A Case Reports, 6*(5), 130–136.

Garg, A., Butz, A. M., Dworkin, P. H., Lewis, R. A., Thompson, R. E., & Serwint, J. R. (2007). Improving the management of family psychosocial problems at low-income children's well child care visits: The WE CARE Project. *Pediatrics, 120*(3), 547–558.

Garg, A., Jack, B., & Zuckerman, B. (2013). Addressing the social determinants of health within the patient-centered medical home: Lessons from pediatrics. *JAMA, 309*(19), 2001–2002. doi:10.1001/jama.2013.1471

Guerrero, A. D., Zhou, X., & Chung, P. J. (2018). How well is the medical home working for Latino and black children? *Maternal and Child Health Journal, 22*(2), 175–183.

Hassink, S. K. (2015). *Letter to Sam Nussbaum, MD. Alternative payment model framework and progress tracking (APM FPT) work group.* Evanston, IL: American Academy of Pediatrics.

Houtrow, A. J., Larson, K., Olson, L. M., Newacheck, P. W., & Halfon, N. (2014). Changing trends of childhood disability, 2001-2011. *Pediatrics, 134*(3), 530–538.

Individuals with Disabilities Education Improvement Act of 2004, PL 108-446, 20 U.S.C. §§ 1400 *et seq.*

Institute for Healhcare Improvement. [2018]. *IHI Triple Aim initiative.* Retrieved from http://www.ihi.org/Engage/Initiatives/TripleAim/Pages/default.aspx

Institute of Medicine. (2001). *Crossing the quality chasm: A new health system for the 21st century.* Washington, DC: National Academies Press.

Jabbarpour, Y., De Marchis, E., Bazemore, A., & Grundy, P. (2016). *Executive summary: Impact of primary care practice transformation on cost, quality, and utilization.* Retrieved from https://www.pcpcc.org/sites/default/files/resources/pcmh_evidence_es_071417%20FINAL.pdf

Katkin, J. P., Kressly, S. J., Edwards, A. R., Perrin, J. M., Kraft, C. A., Richerson, J. E., Tieder, J. S., & Wall, L. (2017). Guiding principles for team based care. Task Force on Pediatric Practice Change. *Pediatrics, 140*(2), pii: e20171489.

Kogan, M. D., Strickland, B. B., & Newacheck, P. W. (2009). Building systems of care: findings from the National Survey of Children With Special Health Care Needs. *Pediatrics, 124*(Suppl. 4), S333–S336.

Kuo, D. Z., Cohen, E., Agrawal, R., Berry, J. G., & Casey, P. H. (2011). A national profile of caregiver challenges among more medically complex children with special health care needs. *Archives of Pediatrics and Adolescent Medicine, 165*(6), 1020–1026.

Kuo, D. Z., McAllister, J. W., Rossignol, L., Turchi, R. M., & Stille, C. J. (2018). Care coordination for children with medical complexity: Whose care is it, anyway? *Pediatrics, 141*(Suppl. 3), S224–S232.

Langer, C. S., Antonelli, R. C., Chamberlain, L., Pan, R. J., & Keller, D. (2018). Evolving federal and state health care policy: Toward a more integrated and comprehensive care-delivery system for children with medical complexity. *Pediatrics, 141*(Suppl. 3), S259–S265.

Lassman, D., Hartman, M., Washington, B., Andrews, K., & Catlin, A. (2014). US health spending trends by age and gender: Selected years 2002–10. *Health Affairs (Millwood), 33*(5), 815–822.

Lindley, L. C., & Mark, B. A. (2010). Children with special health care needs: Impact of health care expenditures on family burden. *Journal of Child and Family Studies, 19*(1), 79–89.

Long, W. E., Bauchner, H., Sege, R. D., Cabral, H. J., & Garg, A. (2012). The value of the medical home for children without special health care needs. *Pediatrics, 129*(1), 87–98.

MacLeod, G. K. (2001). An overview of managed health care. In P. R. Kongstvedt (Ed.), *The managed health care handbook* (4th ed., pp. 3–16). Gaithersburg, MD: Aspen Publishers.

Mathu-Muju, K. R., Kong, X., Brancato, C., McLeod, J., & Bush, H. M. (2018). Utilization of community health workers in Canada's Children's Oral Health Initiative for indigenous communities. *Community Dentistry and Oral Epidemiology,. 46*(2), 185–193.

McAllister, J. (2014). *Achieving a shared plan of care with children and youth with special health care needs.* Palo Alto, CA: Lucile Packard Foundation for Children's Health.

McDonald, K. M., Schultz, E., Albin, L., Pineda, N., Lonhart, J., Sundaram, V., . . . Davies, S. (2014). *Care coordination atlas, Version 4.* AHRQ Publication No. 14-0037-EF. Rockville, MD: Agency for Healthcare Research and Quality.

McPherson, M., Arango, P., Fox, H., Lauver, C., McManus, M., Newacheck, P. W., . . . Strickland, B. (1998). A new definition of children with special health care needs. *Pediatrics, 102*(1, Pt. 1), 137–140.

Medical Expenditure Panel Survey. (2003). *HC-050 documentation, 2000; main data results.* Rockville, MD: Agency for Healtcare Research and Quality. Retrieved from http://www.meps.ahrq.gov/mepsweb/data_stats/download_data/pufs/h50/h50doc.pdf

Monahan, C. A., & Sykora, J. (1999). *Developing and analyzing performance measures: A guide for assessing quality care for children with special health care needs.* Vienna, VA: National Maternal and Child Health Clearinghouse.

Mosquera, R. A., Avritscher, E. B., Samuels, C. L., Harris, T. S., Pedroza, C., Evans, P., . . . Moody, S. (2014). Effect of an enhanced medical home on serious illness and cost of care among high-risk children with chronic illness: A randomized clinical trial. *JAMA, 312*(24), 2640–2648.

Mundorf, C., Shankar, A., Moran, T., Heller, S., Hassan, A., Harville, E., & Lichtveld, M. (2018). Reducing the risk of postpartum depression in a low-income community through a community health worker intervention. *Maternal and Child Health Journal* 22(4), 520–528.

Musumeci, M. (2017). *Medicaid and children with special health care needs.* Retrieved from http://files.kff.org/attachment/Issue-Brief-Medicaid-and-Children-with-Special-Health-Care-Needs

National Center for Health Statistics. (2018). *National Health Interview Survey, 2014–2016.* Retrieved from https://www.cdc.gov/nchs/nhis/about_nhis.htm

National Center for Medical Home Implementation. (2017). *What is medical home?* American Academy of Pediatrics. Retrieved from https://medicalhomeinfo.aap.org/overview/pages/whatisthemedicalhome.aspx

National Survey of Children's Health. (2016). *Child and adolescent health measurement initiative.* Data Resource Center for Child and Adolescent Health. Retrieved from www.childhealthdata.org

Neff, J. M., Clifton, H., Popalisky, J., & Zhou, C. (2014). Stratification of children by medical complexity. *Academic Pediatrics, 15*(2), 191–196. doi:10.1016/j.acap.2014.10.007

Neuman, M. I., Alpern, E. R., Hall, M., Kharbanda, A. B., Shah, S. S., Freedman, S. B., . . . Berry, J. G. (2014). Characteristics of recurrent utilization in pediatric emergency departments. *Pediatrics, 134*(4), e 1025–1031.

Newacheck, P. W., Inkelas, M., & Kim, S. E. (2004). Health services use and health care expenditures for children with disabilities. *Pediatrics, 114*(1), 79–85.

Newacheck, P. W., & Kim, S. E. (2005). A national profile of health care utilization and expenditures for children with special health care needs. *Pediatrics, 159*(1), 10–17.

Patient-Centered Primary Care Collaborative. (2017). The impact of primary care practice transformation on cost, quality, and utilization. Retrieved from https://www.pcpcc.org/sites/default/files/resources/pcmh_evidence_es_071417%20FINAL.pdf

Peters, C. P. (2005). *Children with special care needs: Minding the gaps. Background paper.* National Health Policy Forum. Retrieved from http://www.nhpf.org/library/background-papers/BP_CSHCN_06-27-05.pdf

Phillips, J., Hebish, L. J., Mann, S., Ching, J. M., & Blackmore, C. C. (2016). Engaging frontline leaders and staff in real-time improvement. *Joint Commission Journal on Quality and Patient Safety, 42*(4), 170–183.

Rodriguez, H. P., Meredith, L. S., Hamilton, A. B., Yano, E. M., & Rubenstein, L V. (2015). Huddle up: The adoption and use of structured team communication for VA medical home implementation. *Health Care Management Review, 40*(4), 286–299.

Simon, T. D., Cawthon, M. L., Stanford, S., Popalisky, J., Lyons, D., Woodcox, P., . . . Center of Excellence on Quality of Care Measures for Children with Complex Needs (COE4CCN) Medical Complexity Working Group. (2014). Pediatric medical complexity algorithm: A new method to stratify children by medical complexity. *Pediatrics, 133*(6), e1647–e1654. doi:10.1542/peds.2013-3875

Simon, T. D., Whitlock, K. B., Haaland, W., Wright, D. R., Zhou, C., Neff, J., . . . Mangione-Smith, R. (2017). Effectiveness of a comprehensive case management service for children with medical complexity. *Pediatrics, 140*(6), 1–13.

Social Security Administration (n.d.). *Title V—maternal and child health services block grant.* Retrieved from https://www.ssa.gov/OP_Home/ssact/title05/0500.htm

Starfield, B. (1992). *Primary care: Concept, evaluation and policy.* New York, NY: Oxford University Press.

Stille, C., Turchi, R. M., Antonelli, R., Cabana, M. D., Cheng, T. L., Laraque, D., & Perrin, J. (2010). The family-centered medical home: Specific considerations for child health research and policy. *Academic Pediatrics, 10*(4), 211–217.

Telfair, J., Bronheim, S., & Harrison, S. (2009). Implementation of culturally and linguistically competent policies by state Title V children with special health care needs (CYSHCN) programs. *Maternal and Child Health Journal, 13,* 677.

Thomas-Henkel, C., & Schulman, M. (2017). *Screening for social determinants of health in populations with complex needs: Implementation considerations.* Trenton, NJ: Center for Healthcare Strategies.

Turchi, R. M., Berhane, Z., Bethell, C., Pomponio, A., Antonelli, R., & Minkovitz, C. S. (2009). Care coordination for CYSHCN: Associations with family-provider relations and family/child outcomes. *Pediatrics, 124*(4), S428–S434.

U.S. Department of Human Services. (2018). *Title V maternal and child health services block grant program.* Retrieved from https://mchb.hrsa.gov/maternal-child-health-initiatives/title-v-maternal-and-child-health-services-block-grant-program

U.S. Department of Health and Human Services, Health Resources and Services Administration, Maternal and Child Health Bureau. (2007). *The National Survey of Children with Special Health Care Needs chartbook 2005–2006.* Rockville, MD: Author.

U.S. Department of Health and Human Services, Health Resources and Services Administration, Maternal and Child Health Bureau. (2013). *The National Survey of Children with Special Health Care Needs chartbook 2009–2010.* Rockville, MD: Author.

U.S. Department of Human Services, Health Resources and Services Administration, Maternal and Child Health Bureau. (2014). *Child Health USA 2014.* Rockville, MD: Author.

Wagner, E. H. (1998). Chronic disease management: What will it take to improve care for chronic illness? *Effective Clinical Practice, 1,* 2–4.

Waisman Center. (2008). *Medical home services for autism spectrum disorders.* Retrieved from https://www2.waisman.wisc.edu/cedd/guidelines/pdf/Autism_Flip.pdf

Walker, K. O., Stewart, A. L., & Grumbach, K. (2016). Development of a survey instrument to measure patient experience of integrated care. *BMC Health Services Research, 16,* 193.

Watson, A. (2016). Evaluating and measuring quality and outcomes: A new "essential activity" of case management practice. *Professional Case Management, 21*(1), 51–52.

Weaver, S. J., Che, X. X., Petersen, L. A., & Hysong, S. J. (2018). Unpacking care coordination through a multiteam system lens: A conceptual framework and systematic review. *Medical Care, 56*(3), 247–259.

Ziniel, S. I., Rosenberg, H. N., Bach, A. M., Singer, S. J., & Antonelli, R. C. (2016). Validation of a parent-reported experience measure of integrated care. *Pediatrics, 138*(6), pii: e20160676.

APPENDIX

Waisman Center's Medical Home Services for Patients with Autism Spectrum Disorder (ASD)

Guidelines	Recommendations		
	Individuals with ASD and their family	Professional and training organizations	Government and finance agencies
1. The medical home–primary care practice (MH-PCP) is aware of and implements medical home (MH) principles when caring for children and youth, including those with ASD.	Youth with ASD and their parents serve as teachers and mentors in medical school residency training and continuing education programs and contribute to the development of curriculum and office management tools to help prepare the MH-PCP practice for serving families with ASD.	Accreditation/residency and training programs recognize the importance of the MH principles by including MH practice training as a required component of pre-med, residency, and continuing education curriculum for pediatrics, family medicine, med-peds, and midlevel providers such as nurse practitioners and physician assistants. Board licensing and recertification requirements include MH principles, especially as they relate to the care of patients with ASD and other chronic conditions. Accreditation/residency and training programs include out-of-office/hospital rotations at the community level in service settings and in the homes of children, youth, and families with ASD and other chronic conditions. Professional organizations such as the American Academy of Pediatrics (AAP), the American Academy of Family Physicians (AAFP), and the National Association of Pediatric Nurse Practitioners (NAPNP) provide ongoing continuing medical education training in the principles and implementation of an MD for the care of all children/youth, including those with ASD.	Funders/insurers and other health care payers reimburse MH-PCPs for the extra time required to provide a quality MH to children/youth. This includes the elements of planned care such as care coordination, comanagement with specialists, and collaboration with community agencies required when children have developmental disorders such as ASD.

(continued)

Guidelines	Recommendations		
	Individuals with ASD and their family	Professional and training organizations	Government and finance agencies
2. The MH-PCP is organized in a manner that involves the entire office staff in meeting the complex needs of the patient with ASD and his or her family and offers flexibility in the provision of services.	Youth with ASD and their parents serve as resources and mentors to the MH-PCP administrative and medical staff who schedule appointments and receive ASD families at the office, helping to overcome communication and social barriers (e.g., by providing communication-assisted technology for children or youth who are nonverbal) and address special family needs related to ASD. Families and advocacy groups advocate for improved reimbursement and funding to adequately compensate primary practice providers for the additional time and resources needed to educate and prepare all office staff to serve families with children with ASD, involving the families as mentors and partners with the primary practice.		Accreditation/residency and training programs emphasize the important role of staff at all levels of the practice in serving children with special health care needs such as ASD and prepare staff for their roles in office-based practices.
3. The MH-PCP, in collaboration with subspecialists and community agencies, provides appropriate disorder-specific information (printed, electronic, etc.) on all aspects of ASD, including definition, diagnosis, etiology, genetic, neuropath correlates, and developmental and behavioral characteristics to consumers and other community providers.	Families and advocacy groups serve as resources to MH-PCP professionals and to other families in order to share knowledge and information about their personal experiences with ASD and strategies they have used for treating ASD.	Accreditation/residency and training programs emphasize the importance of education materials to increase knowledge and skills of families and caregivers about all aspects of ASD and teach residents methods for retrieving appropriate evidenced-based and consensus-based materials for distribution to patients' families. Professional organizations such as the AAP, AAFP, and NAPNP engage experts in various fields to develop evidenced-based training materials for distribution to parents by MH-PCPs.	Funders/insurers and other health care payers recognize the need for the additional value of offering materials, information, and training to families.
4. In accordance with the principles of family-centered care, the MH-PCP recognizes parents as valued partners and decision makers in the care of their child and establishes regular, ongoing communication with reciprocal exchange of information. An important component of parent–professional partnerships is listening and acting upon parent concerns about their child's development and/or behavior. The physical health and emotional well-being of the entire family is included and considered in all decision making.	Families in a collaborative partnership with MH-PCP providers are informed about federal, state, and local financing options; insurance benefits; and reimbursement mechanisms for chronic conditions and ASD so that they can fully consider insurance and other financing options in efforts to maximize funding of services for children and youth with ASD.	Accreditation/residency and training programs recognize the importance of training activities in parent–professional partnerships and require all residency programs to implement one of the nationally recognized, parent-led curricula. For pediatricians, this might ideally be done during mandatory developmental pediatric rotations using existing curricula developed by parent advocates (e.g., Delivery of Chronic Care Program now existing in 20 states).	Government recognizes and/or appoints a lead public agency to organize and support a system of electronic communication (such as a web page) as a resource to provide current information on ASD and ASD-related services to parents and professionals statewide. A service agency should support this participation with families who do not have access to the Internet.

Guidelines	Recommendations		
	Individuals with ASD and their family	Professional and training organizations	Government and finance agencies
5. The MH-PCP respects and competently serves the multiple and diverse cultures of children with ASD and their families. The practice is linguistically competent, including having culturally appropriate written materials and translators available.	Families with diverse cultural backgrounds assess materials, educational booklets, and the overall cultural competency of MH-PCP practice. They also participate as trainers in efforts to strengthen cultural competency in serving children and families with ASD from diverse backgrounds.	Professional organizations and other training programs provide professional development for office personnel and support staff that includes training to increase the sensitivity, awareness, and understanding of cultural norms and prepares staff to competently serve a culturally diverse client population.	Funders/insurers and other health care payers compensate primary practices for appropriate on-site translators (including sign language) and other resources to ensure that there is appropriate language proficiency, signage, and written materials in the practice setting.

CHAPTER 42 Racial and Ethnic Disparities

Olanrewaju O. Falusi, Monika Goyal, Elissa Batshaw Clair, Catherine Larsen Coley, Susan Keller, Mary A. Hadley, and Denice Cora-Bramble

Upon completion of this chapter, the reader will

- Describe the complex relationship between childhood disabilities and health and educational disparities
- Recognize successful initiatives to achieve health and educational equity
- Perform a self-assessment of implicit bias
- Incorporate principles of health and educational equity into clinical practice and advocacy efforts

CASE STUDY

Miguel is a 4-year-old Hispanic male recently diagnosed with autism and seeing a speech therapist for the first time. The speech therapist mentions to Miguel's mother, Maria, that she is surprised that he is just starting to receive therapy as most children with autism are diagnosed and start therapy at an earlier age. Maria says she had concerns about his delayed speech and social interactions since he was 2 years old but that their pediatrician was not concerned. Maria confides that she does not feel that the pediatrician spent enough time hearing out her concerns. The pediatrician eventually referred Miguel to a developmental pediatrician when he still had only five words and poor social skills at age 3 years. Miguel has Medicaid insurance coverage and due to a lack of Medicaid-accepting providers in their area, they waited 9 months before seeing a developmental pediatrician who diagnosed him with autism and another 3 months for a speech therapy appointment and special education placement.

Thought Questions

How does a child's race/ethnicity affect his or her access to quality, culturally appropriate health care? How can clinicians examine and address their own implicit or unconscious biases? What factors underlie the racial disproportionality in special education? How can educators examine and address their own implicit or unconscious biases?

DEFINITIONS

As noted in Chapter 12, traditional clinical definitions of disability commonly refer to the individual's functional capacity without explicit regard to the internal (genetic) and external (environmental) factors that may lead to the disability or impact its severity. The National Center for Medical Rehabilitation Research and the World Health Organization (2011) have proposed biopsychosocial models of disability that take into account elements—such as a family's financial limitations or environmental barriers—that may impact a person's ability to achieve optimal function within the disability. A limited, but growing body of literature delves further into the sociocultural factors that may affect the development and treatment of disability and thereby lead to **health disparities** (Bright, Knapp, Hinojosa, Alford, & Bonner, 2016; Schieve, Boulet, Kogan, Van Naarden-Braun, & Boyle, 2011; Spencer & Strazdins, 2015; Thomas, Parish, Rose, & Kilany, 2012).

Although many professionals have an intuitive understanding of the term *health disparity*, there is a lack of consensus on a formal definition of this term (Carter-Pokras & Baquet, 2002; Dehlendorf, Bryant, Huddleston, Jacoby, & Fujimoto, 2010). Most will agree, however, that the term refers to differences in the measures of health and availability of health care across populations. In the United States, the term *health disparities* has generally been assumed to refer to health or health care differences among racial and ethnic groups. For example, the Institute of Medicine (IOM), in their 2002 report on health disparities, "Unequal Treatment," defines disparities in health care as "racial or ethnic differences in the quality of health care that are not due to access-related factors or clinical needs, preferences, and appropriateness of intervention" (2003, p. 4). The IOM has focused its analysis on health care disparities around race and ethnicity at two levels: 1) the operation of health care systems and the legal and regulatory climate in which health care systems function and 2) discrimination at the individual, patient-provider level. The committee further delineated that discrimination refers to differences in care that result from biases, prejudices, stereotyping, and uncertainty in clinical communication and decision making (Institute of Medicine, 2003).

Health equity has been broadly defined as the absence of socially unjust or unfair health disparities (Braveman & Gruskin, 2003). Unlike equality, in which individuals are treated the same, equity ensures groups and individuals have what they need to reach positive outcomes, as depicted in Figure 42.1. Health equity can further be defined as the absence of systematic disparities in health or social determinants of health among social groups who have different levels of underlying social advantage or disadvantage. Inequities in health systematically put groups of people who are already socially disadvantaged at a further disadvantage with respect to their health. This is important because those who are at higher risk of health inequity, racial/ethnic minorities as an example, become part of a vicious cycle, as health is essential to well-being and to overcoming other effects of social disadvantage (Braveman & Gruskin, 2003).

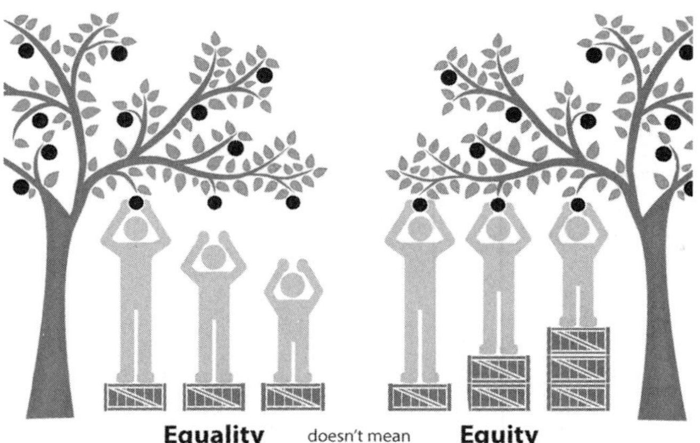

Figure 42.1. Equality versus equity. (From Maine Center for Disease Control and Prevention. [2018]. What is health equity? Retrieved from https://www.maine.gov/dhhs/mecdc/health-equity)

Children with disabilities also comprise a population that often experiences disparities in access to quality care when compared with typically developing children. For example, families of children with disabilities are more likely to encounter delays or frustrations with obtaining needed health, education, and related services, with 35% of families reporting these difficulties (Rosen-Reynoso et al., 2016). From orthopedic disabilities to hearing loss to Down syndrome and intellectual disabilities, families of children with disabilities experience difficulties with respect to transportation, report poorer health status and unmet health and education needs, and are more likely to live in poverty (Boss, Niparko, Gaskin, & Levinson, 2011; Graham, Keys, McMahon, & Brubacher, 2014; Schieve et al., 2011). Although there is a robust body of literature about disparities in health care (Flores & Committee on Pediatric Research, 2010; Institute of Medicine, 2003), published studies focused on health disparities among children with disabilities are much more limited (Houtrow, Okumura, Hilton, & Rehm, 2011; Kuo et al., 2014). When considering health disparities among children with disabilities, racial and ethnic minority children may experience difficulties in two realms: first, they experience a disability, and second, they may experience disparate treatment as a result of membership in an ethnic or racial minority. As a result, minority children with disabilities often experience poorer health status than nonminority children. This chapter will specifically reflect on the complexity of providing health care for racial and ethnic minority children with disabilities who are at the intersection of two disadvantaged populations (Sharby, Martire, & Iversen, 2015). Further, this chapter will review the issue of disparity in regard to the education system for children with disabilities. Health disparities also exist related to gender, rural/urban location, and other factors, but these are beyond the scope of this chapter.

RACIAL AND ETHNIC HEALTH DISPARITIES IN CHILDREN WITH DISABILITIES

Rates of disability, when broadly defined as a limitation in activity, are higher among black children than non-Hispanic white children, but large, nationwide surveys of children with disabilities have found that the racial correlation is diminished or disappears altogether when adjusted for family income and other social factors, suggesting that poverty rather than race is a key factor in having a disability (McManus, Carle, & Rapport, 2014; Newacheck, Stein, Bauman, Hung, & Research Consortium on Children with Chronic Conditions, 2003). However, racial disparities abound in access to care and health outcomes among children with disabilities. For example, minority children with disabilities are less likely to have a medical home (Conrey, Seidu, Ryan, & Chapman, 2013) and to receive resources for transition to adult care (Richmond, Tran, & Berry, 2012). They are also more likely to utilize emergency care than their white counterparts (Raphael, Zhang, Liu, Tapia, & Giardino, 2009). This in turn affects outcomes, as children without a medical home are more likely to have delayed or forgone care and greater unmet health needs. Their parents report worse coping and are more likely to report loss of work time to meet the medical needs of their children (Drummond, Looman, & Phillips, 2012; Okumura, Van Cleave, Gnanasekaran, & Houtrow, 2009; Strickland et al., 2009).

Health disparities persist even when minority children have access to health care. As depicted in Miguel's case, Hispanic children with autism spectrum disorder (ASD) in one study were diagnosed almost 1 year later than white children although parents of both ethnicities voiced their concerns to a health care professional at the same age. The Hispanic children in the study also received fewer specialty services and had higher unmet service needs (McManus et al., 2014). In addition, black children with developmental delay at 24 months who are eligible for services have been found to be five times less likely than their white peers to receive services, largely due to differences in identification and referral. This gap in receipt of services is even more striking if the child only has a developmental delay; that is, if the delay is not associated with a more obvious established condition, such as blindness or extreme prematurity (Feinberg, Silverstein, Donahue, & Bliss, 2011).

The 2009–2010 National Survey of Children with Special Health Care Needs (NS-CSHCN), which analyzed data from telephone interviews of a nationally representative sample of over 40,000 parents of CSHCN, provides a view of how race and ethnicity affect the ability of a child with disabilities to access quality care. Table 42.1 provides an overview of the NS-CSHCN study design and demographics; Figures 42.2 to 42.5 depict key study findings related to race/ethnicity (Data Resource Center for Child and Adolescent Health, 2017; U.S. Department of Health and Human Services, Health Resources and Services Administration, Maternal and Child Health Bureau, 2013). NS-CSHCN analyses demonstrate that black and Hispanic children with ASD, in particular, are more likely to have difficulties or delays in getting services. One analysis found racial disparities in five out of six quality measures of **family-centered care** in children with ASD: 1) The child does not have a personal doctor or nurse, 2) the doctor does not spend enough time with the child, 3) the provider is not sensitive to the family's values or customs, 4) the doctor does not make the child's parents feel like a partner, and 5) the doctor does not provide enough information. (Only "the doctor does not listen carefully" measure

Table 42.1. National Survey of Children with Special Health Care Needs (CSHCN) survey design and demographics at a glance

Survey design and sponsorship	Maternal and Child Health Bureau at the Health Resources and Services Administration in partnership with National Center for Health Statistics at the Centers for Disease Control, Child and Adolescent Health Measurement Initiative, and a National Technical Expert Panel
Data collection	National Center for Health Statistics at the Centers for Disease Control
Geographic areas	Nationwide, all 50 states and the District of Columbia
Periodicity	2001, 2005–2006, 2009–2010, yearly as of 2016–2017
Population sampled	Noninstitutionalized CSHCN in the United States ages 0–17 years
Sample size range	Nationally: between 38,000 and 40,000; State: approximately 750
Representative	Weighted to be representative of the U.S. population of noninstitutionalized CSHCN ages 0–17 years
Topics	Assesses overall health and health status of CSHCN, including medical home, adequate health insurance, access to needed services, and adequate care coordination. Other topics include functional difficulties, transition services, and shared decision making.

Prevalence of CSHCN, by Race/Ethnicity

Non-Hispanic White	Non-Hispanic Black	Hispanic	Asian	American Indian/ Alaska Native	Native Hawaiian Pacific Islander
16.3	17.5	11.2	8.0	13.5	12.3

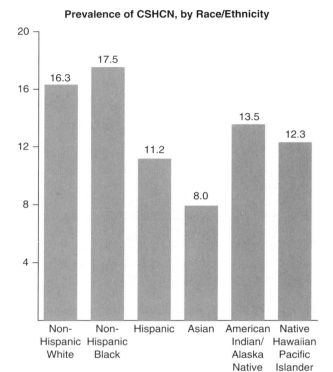

Figure 42.2. National Survey of Children with Special Health Care Needs: Prevalence of CSHCN, by race/ethnicity. (From U.S. Department of Health and Human Services, Health Resources and Services Administration, Maternal and Child Health Bureau. [2013]. *The National Survey of Children with Special Health Care Needs chartbook 2009–2010*. Rockville, Maryland: Author. Retrieved from https://mchb.hrsa.gov/cshcn0910/more/pdf/nscshcn0910.pdf)

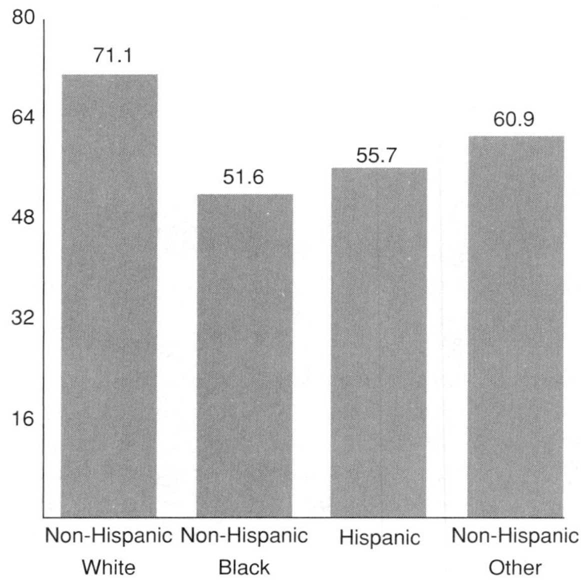

Figure 42.3. National Survey of Children with Special Health Care Needs: Receipt of family-centered care, by race/ethnicity. (From U.S. Department of Health and Human Services, Health Resources and Services Administration, Maternal and Child Health Bureau. [2013]. *The National Survey of Children with Special Health Care Needs chartbook 2009–2010*. Rockville, Maryland: Author. Retrieved from https://mchb.hrsa.gov/cshcn0910/more/pdf/nscshcn0910.pdf)

was similar among all groups.) Hispanic parents in particular reported that their doctors did not spend enough time with their children and that they did not feel that the doctors made them partners in the care of their children. Importantly, these disparities remained when income, insurance, level of education, and the number of parents in the household were included in multivariate analyses (Magaña, Parish, Rose, Timberlake, & Swaine, 2012). Similar analyses have supported these findings that minority children with disabilities are less likely to experience family-centered care (Coker, Rodriguez, & Flores, 2010; Magaña, Parish, & Son, 2015; Montes & Halterman, 2011).

Along with disparities for black and Hispanic families, limited data reveal that American Indian/Alaskan Native CSHCN are more likely to have a greater number of chronic conditions and functional difficulties than white CSHCN and that they are more likely to be affected in their daily activities than white CSHCN (Kenney & Thierry, 2014). Across all races, parents with limited English proficiency—defined by the U.S. Census Bureau as speaking English less than "very well"—are more likely to report that their children with disabilities are uninsured, have no usual source of care, experience long appointment wait times, and lack after-hours care, all of which are known barriers to accessing adequate health care (Eneriz-Wiemer, Sanders, Barr, & Mendoza, 2014; Winitzer, Bisgaier, Grogan, & Rhodes, 2012). Lack of knowledge about the complex U.S. health care system, including the process of specialty referrals and appointments, compounds this problem for immigrant families (Winitzer et al., 2012). In addition, the majority of states place limitations on publicly funded health insurance for noncitizen immigrants, and fear of exposing their undocumented status may also cause immigrant families to avoid accessing needed health care.

RACIAL AND ETHNIC DISPARITIES IN SPECIAL EDUCATION

Health care is not the only area where there are ethnic and racial disparities; it also occurs in education. Thus, it is critical for educators across the spectrum from early education and beyond to recognize and address disparities. All ethnicities are not proportionally represented among students with developmental disabilities. One of the goals of the Individuals with Disabilities Education Improvement Act (IDEA) of 2004 was to reduce the overrepresentation of minorities in special education.

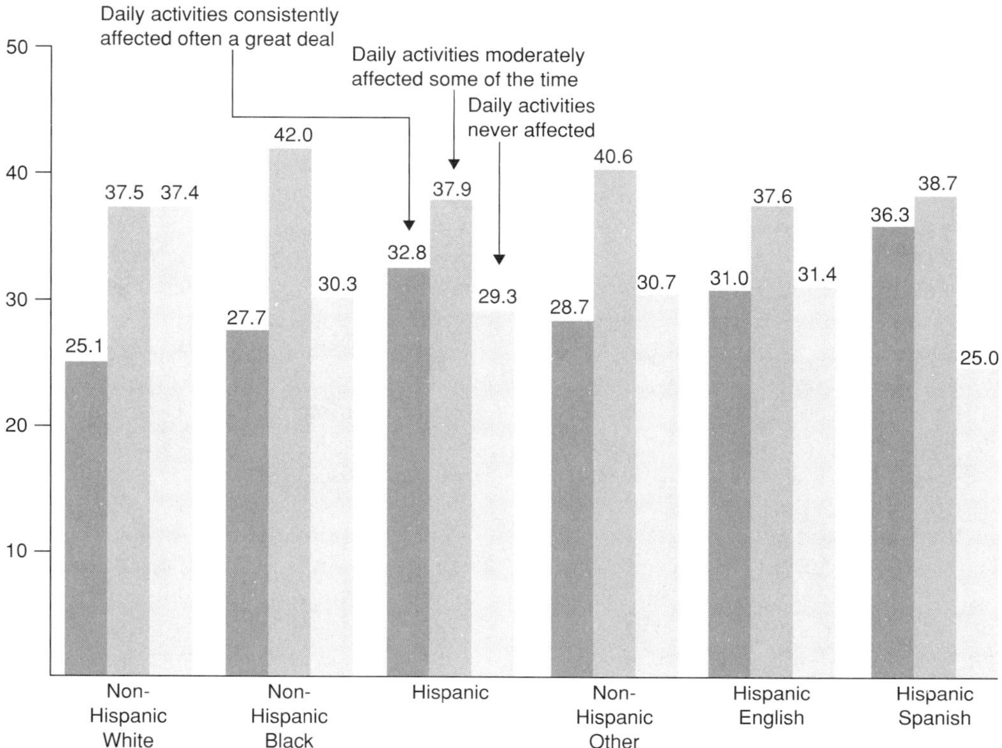

Figure 42.4. National Survey of Children with Special Health Care Needs: Impact of children's conditions on their daily activities, by race/ethnicity and primary language. (From U.S. Department of Health and Human Services, Health Resources and Services Administration, Maternal and Child Health Bureau. [2013]. *The National Survey of Children with Special Health Care Needs chartbook 2009–2010*. Rockville, Maryland: Author. Retrieved from https://mchb.hrsa.gov/cshcn0910/more/pdf/nscshcn0910.pdf)

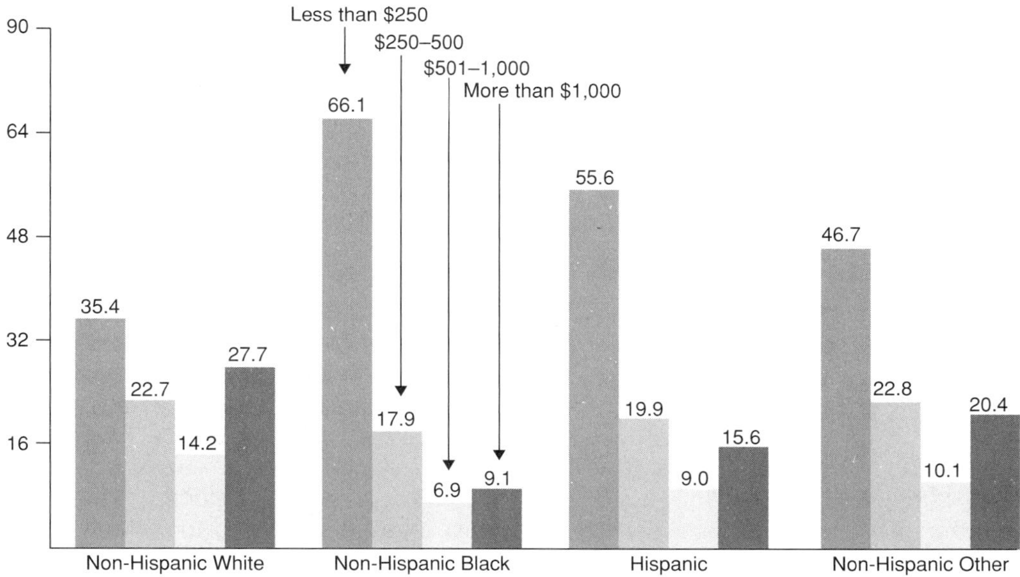

Figure 42.5. National Survey of Children with Special Health Care Needs: Annual out-of-pocket expenses for care of CSHCN, by race/ethnicity. (From U.S. Department of Health and Human Services, Health Resources and Services Administration, Maternal and Child Health Bureau. [2013]. *The National Survey of Children with Special Health Care Needs chartbook 2009–2010*. Rockville, Maryland: Author. Retrieved from https://mchb.hrsa.gov/cshcn0910/more/pdf/nscshcn0910.pdf)

While reduction of the number of minorities in special education remains a goal of the federal government, a more recent analysis has indicated that discrimination of minorities is through both overrepresentation and underrepresentation (U.S. Department of Education, 2016). For example, school staff may overrefer students of color for potential emotional disturbance based on racial stereotypes of violent tendencies or underrefer students for a potential learning disability based on racial stereotypes of lack of motivation among students of color. English language learner students also may be underreferred for evaluation based on a belief that it would not be possible to appropriately evaluate a child who is not proficient in English. Conversely, they may be overidentified due to low performance on assessment measures resulting from the use of inappropriate assessment tools or because of misinterpretation of assessment measures (U.S. Department of Education, National Center for Education and Statistics, 2016). Recent research suggests that underachieving minority students with similar levels of socioeconomic risk factors as their white counterparts (e.g., low birth weight, adolescent mothers, poverty, lead exposure, and inadequate health insurance) are less likely to be identified with a disability and provided with appropriate special education services (Morgan et al., 2015; Morgan & Farkas, 2016; Morgan et al., 2017).

Although black students may be underidentified when compared with similar white students, black students as a group continue to have higher rates of identification than would be expected given their proportion in the general population. However, the gap is narrowing somewhat. In 2008, black students made up 31% of the population with intellectual disability in public schools and 29% of the population with emotional disturbance although they represented only 17% of the overall population. In 2014, they made up 26% of students with intellectual disability and 25% of students with emotional disturbance while representing 18% of total student enrollment (U.S. Department of Education, Office of Special Education and Rehabilitative Services, 2016).

Contrary to common perception, the rate of overrepresentation in special education increases as free lunch status decreases. Black students are more likely to be overidentified in wealthy districts than in districts of poverty. Teachers' classroom management skills, unintentional bias toward the student (including the use of less positive interactions), impressions of families, informal diagnosis of a learning disability or attention-deficit/hyperactivity disorder, external pressure for identification and placement, percentage of minority teachers, student–teacher ratios, and adequate levels of school funding are all contributing factors to overdiagnosis (de Valenzuela, Copeland, Huaqing Qi, & Park, 2006; Skiba, Poloni-Staudinger, Gallini, Simmons, & Feggins-Azziz, 2006; Tenenbaum & Ruck, 2007; van den Bergh, Denessen, Hornstra, Voeten, & Holland, 2010).

Overrepresentation also exists in the area of discipline in school. Both black and Hispanic students are more likely to be suspended than their white classmates. In elementary school, black students are 2.2 times more likely to be suspended than white students; in middle school, that likelihood increases to 3.8 times. Hispanic middle school students are 1.7 times more likely to be suspended (Skiba, Shure, & Williams, 2012). More recent data suggest that black students as a whole are nearly four times more likely to be suspended than white students (U.S. Department of Education, Office for Civil Rights, 2016). Students of color are also disproportionally more likely to be expelled from school regardless of socioeconomic status. In fact, the higher the socioeconomic status of the district, the higher the rates of suspension among students of color (American Psychological Association Zero Tolerance Task Force, 2008; Skiba et al., 2012). This overrepresentation is important because students suspended or expelled are three times more likely than other students to be involved with the juvenile justice system in the next year (The Council of State Governments, 2011).

CASE STUDY

Shontell is a 5-year-old black girl starting kindergarten at a public school. Her teacher, Mrs. Singh, notices that Shontell walks on her toes, has difficulty going up and down stairs, and falls often, especially on the playground. She learned from Shontell's mother, Jasmine, that Shontell was born prematurely. Jasmine worries that Shontell may have cerebral palsy. Due to financial hardships the family has not had stable housing and has had to move often, staying with different friends and family members. Jasmine works whenever she can to support the family, and medical visits take several hours when commuting on public transportation. As a result, Shontell has not had consistent appointments with the same pediatrician, and no official diagnosis has been made. Mrs. Singh shares with Jasmine the availability of school therapy services and the process of beginning an individualized education program (IEP) evaluation. Within the next 60 days, a physical therapist employed by the county school program visits the classroom to evaluate Shontell's balance and strength with functional activities needed to move about the classroom safely and independently. The school team completes the IEP process in partnership with Jasmine, and Shontell begins to receive the recommended in-school services.

ETIOLOGIES AND FEDERAL INITIATIVES

Racial and ethnic health and educational disparities exist among children with disabilities, and the barriers to health and education equity are multifactorial. According to a model developed by Kilbourne and colleagues (Figure 42.6), key potential determinants of health disparities include individual, provider, and health care system factors (Kilbourne, Switzer, Hyman, Crowley-Matoka, & Fine, 2005). In this model, individual (patient)–level factors include race, ethnicity, culture, beliefs, preferences, education and resources, and biologic or genetic factors. Health care provider–level factors include knowledge and attitudes, competing demands, and bias. Providers and educators, in particular, may be vulnerable to unconscious processes such as bias or stereotyping. In the health care field, this, in turn, can adversely impact the clinical encounter, as provider communication and **cultural competence** are additional factors that can contribute to health disparities, as detailed in the Considerations for Clinicians section of this chapter.

Finally, there are structural- and institutional-level factors relating to the health care system that include health services organizations, financing, and delivery as well as health care organization culture and quality improvement (Kilbourne et al., 2005). Institutionalized racism is increasingly recognized as a key factor in the development of health disparities in the United States. Institutionalized racism is defined as "differential access to the goods, services, and opportunities of society by race" and is differentiated from personally mediated prejudice or racism. Institutionalized racism is reflected in norms and laws that have led to discrepancies in access to material conditions and power for certain racial groups over time and is perpetuated in modern-day social structures (Jones, 2000, p. 1212). A history of inequality in access to education, voting rights, housing, and employment contributes to the socioeconomic disparities among races in the United States today. For families struggling with the care of a child with disabilities, multigenerational difficulties due to codified racial discrimination add to the barriers to accessing health care and special education services and feeling empowered through the care process.

Federal policies that support children and families with disabilities—including IDEA 2004, the Americans with Disabilities Act, and Section 504 of the Rehabilitation Act of 1973—aim to reduce these impediments to health care access and to decrease disparities (see Chapter 33). These laws mandate public schools to accommodate or find alternate accommodations for every child with a disability. A child who enters the public school system and has a known or suspected disability would undergo an evaluation to determine placement in special education services, as illustrated

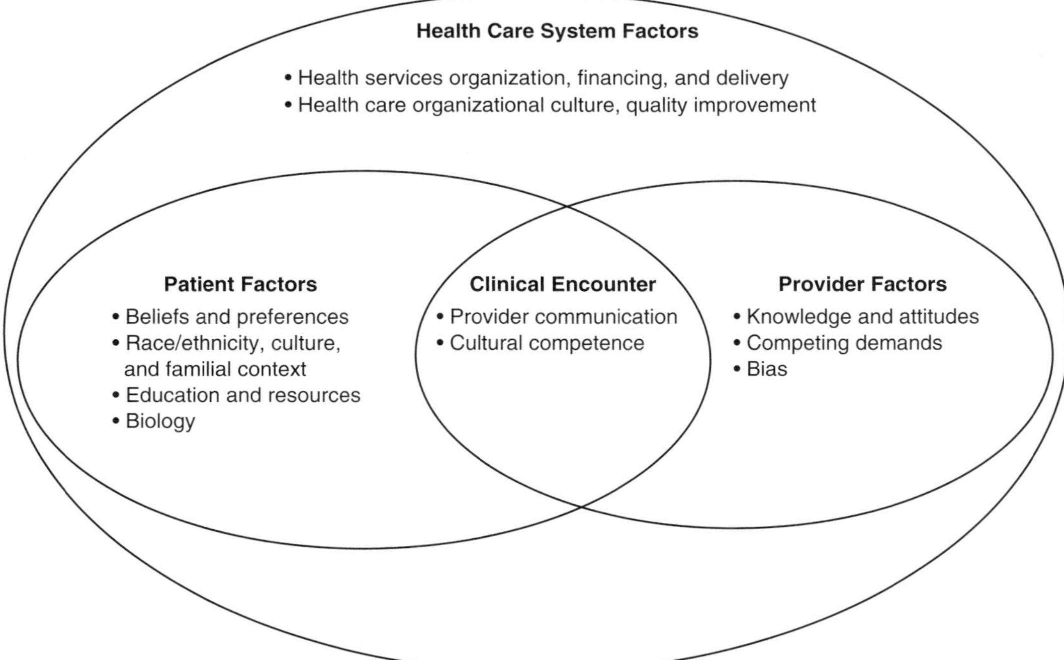

Figure 42.6. Kilbourne model Venn diagram. (From Kilbourne AM, Switzer G, Hyman K, Crowley-Matoka M, and Fine MJ. Advancing Health Disparities Research Within the Health Care System: A Conceptual Framework. Am J Public Health. 2006 December; 96[12]: 2113–2121; reprinted by permission.)

in Shontell's case. In addition, the reauthorization of the IDEA in 2004 specified a goal to reduce the overrepresentation of black youth in special education, particularly in the domains of intellectual disability and emotional disturbance (U.S. Department of Education, National Center for Education Evaluation and Regional Assistance, Institute of Education Sciences, 2011). These federal policies underscore the critical role that individual educators and school systems as a whole can play in reducing disparities. As children typically spend a significant amount of their waking hours in school, learning, emotional, and physical disabilities may be first identified and managed within the school system; this is of particular importance for children who may have limited access to the health care system.

CASE STUDY

Julia is a white occupational therapy student in her first clinical fieldwork placement. She is working in acute care at a large urban children's hospital evaluating and treating children with chronic illness, cancer, and traumatic injury. One day she and her clinical instructor evaluate a child who was severely abused and burned by his father. Afterwards, Julia expresses to her clinical instructor that she is surprised that the child is white. The clinical instructor explains to Julia the concept of **implicit bias** and how assuming the child would be of a minority race implies that people of color are more likely to commit child abuse. He introduces her to an online implicit association test (IAT), which helps her to assess and identify unconscious negative thoughts she holds toward people of color. Through this process, Julia becomes more self-aware and able to recognize ways that she is allowing stereotypes and racial bias to shape her thinking and expectations related to patient care. Because Julia is committed to excellent patient care, she has sought out additional reading and experiences to improve her cultural competence and ability to recognize her own implicit bias.

REDUCING DISPARITIES: CONSIDERATIONS FOR CLINICIANS AND EDUCATORS

The importance of clinician and educator cultural competence cannot be overstated. Skills in cultural competence (knowledge of the norms of other cultures and how to partner with families of various backgrounds), cultural humility (identifying one's own biases and seeking personal growth), and cultural agility (the ability to work effectively across cultures) are all critical for the care and education of diverse populations. These terms are distinguished by nuances, and each has value in various contexts. This chapter uses the term *cultural competence,* which is more commonly used in published studies, and defines it as the skill needed to partner effectively across various cultures while recognizing one's own explicit and implicit biases.

When contemplating how to address health and educational disparities in children with special needs, the Kilbourne model of potential sources of disparities can be helpful. This model addresses patient-level, provider-level, clinical encounter, and health care system factors that contribute to disparities in care (Kilbourne et al., 2005). When extending this model to education and children with disabilities, factors resulting in disparities of care among this vulnerable population include attitudes of health care providers, educators, and the public; physical barriers; miscommunications; income level; ethnic/minority status; insurance coverage; and lack of information tailored to people with disabilities (Sharby et al., 2015). Understanding the factors that contribute to health and educational disparities can inform interventions to achieve health and education equity.

Clinician and educator knowledge and attitudes can contribute to the delivery of unequitable health care and education. Patients cite that providers often lack the necessary time, clinical training, equipment, and resources to provide adequate care for their complex medical needs (Morrison, George, & Mosqueda, 2008). Clinical competency centered on the care of children with disabilities is often inadequate. For instance, when medical students underwent assessments regarding examination skills, they demonstrated significantly more difficulty in both interpersonal skills and physical examination skills when the patient had a disability (Brown, Graham, Richeson, Wu, & McDermott, 2010). However, studies have shown that with increased education, clinician knowledge and attitudes can be modified (Moroz et al., 2010; Symons, Morley, McGuigan, & Akl, 2014). Therefore, the development of curricula for medical schools, programs for other health professionals, and schools of education that focus on increasing the quality of care provided to children with disabilities, particularly regarding communication skills and clinical knowledge, is of paramount importance.

The families of children with disabilities have reported difficulty concentrating on and understanding what their clinician or educator is stating. This barrier may arise especially in cases of intellectual disabilities, hearing impairments, and communication disorders, and it may be further compounded if the clinician or educator is not communicating in a family's native language (O'Day, Killeen, Sutton, & Iezzoni, 2005) or if the recommendations are incompatible with a family's cultural background or socioeconomic status.

If the children and their families believe that clinicians or teachers do not understand them or are uninterested in learning about them and their culture, strengths, and challenges, they will be less likely to seek or continue care, to be open and honest in their communication, and to follow through with recommendations. For instance, the NS-CSHCN demonstrated an association of delayed or foregone care and dissatisfaction with care with parents' perceptions of health care providers' cultural competence (Kerfeld, Hoffman, Ciol, & Kartin, 2011). Health care providers should focus on developing a constructive relationship with the child and his or her family by encouraging them to ask questions and by demonstrating genuine interest in their lives, empathy, and concern for their health. Providing these elements of family-centered care may reduce disparities in health care utilization among minority children with disabilities (Parish, Magaña, Rose, Timberlake, & Swaine, 2012; Box 42.1). Similar approaches can be helpful in the school environment.

Furthermore, clinicians and educators should deliver care recommendations or details of an IEP in a manner that is understandable to children and their families and seek a confirmation of understanding. However, while clinicians or teachers can choose to learn a few key phrases such as "hello" and "thank you" in the languages spoken by one's patients/students to increase rapport, their language skills should be tested and certified before communicating more intensively in those languages (White & Stubblefield-Tave, 2017). Qualified interpreter services should be used with families who have limited English proficiency. It is also important to be sensitive to a family's health and educational literacy, and it may be necessary to provide supplemental materials such as pictures, videos, or low-literacy handouts to the family to promote understanding. Conducting a teach-back, during which the child and his/her family state in their own words the health or educational issues and steps to address the problem at the conclusion of a visit or IEP meeting will help demonstrate whether the clinician/teacher effectively communicated the issues. This represents best practice for communication of health information (White & Stubblefield-Tave, 2017).

Bias in medicine has been previously demonstrated. The Institute of Medicine (now the National Academy of Medicine) has concluded that some evidence suggests that "bias, stereotyping, prejudice, and clinical uncertainty on the part of healthcare providers may be contributory factors to racial and ethnic disparities in healthcare" (Institute of Medicine, 2003, p. 178). Although overt (explicit) discriminatory laws and practices in the United States may have declined in recent decades, covert discrimination and institutional bias are sustained by subtle, implicit (unconscious) attitudes that may influence provider behavior and treatment choices (Hall et al., 2015). As a result, compared with white patients, minority patients may be kept waiting

BOX 42.1 EVIDENCE-BASED PRACTICE

Family-Centered Care

Family-centered care is an evidence-based approach to health care that recognizes that "a partnership among patients, families, and health care professionals is essential to providing quality care" (Coker et al., 2010, p. 1160). As defined by the American Academy of Pediatrics (2003), family-centered care is grounded in a core set of principles, including but not limited to the following:

- Honoring racial, ethnic, cultural, and socioeconomic diversity and its effect on the family's experience and perception of care
- Supporting and facilitating choice for the child and family about approaches to care and support
- Ensuring flexibility in organizational policies, procedures, and provider practices so services can be tailored to the needs, beliefs, and cultural values of each child and family
- Collaborating with families at all levels of health care in the care of the individual child and in professional education, policy making, and program development

Evidence has shown that providing family-centered care in the pediatric setting improves patient outcomes, including reduced patient and parent anxiety, shortens postsurgical recovery times, and increases parents' confidence and problem-solving capacity. In addition, staff in family-centered environments are more likely to provide culturally competent care, report more positive feelings about their patients and their work, and have a lower risk of malpractice lawsuits (American Academy of Pediatrics, 2003; Coker et al., 2010; Magaña et al., 2015).

longer for treatment, may end up having a provider spend less time with them, may be spoken to by providers with a more condescending tone, may receive different treatment plans based on assumptions about adherence capabilities, and so forth (Hall et al., 2015). Some of these same issues exist in the school environment, where the teacher may spend less time with minority parents in conferences or be less positive in their description of the child's performance or behavior.

Tools such as the online IAT (Project Implicit, 2017) provide a validated measure of our implicit biases because they test associative processes that operate automatically and thus are resistant to "faking" or social desirability bias (Dehon et al., 2017). A study of primary care visits examined the relationship between clinician implicit racial bias scores with visit communication through recorded visits and patient ratings of care. In comparison with white patients, when caring for black patients, clinicians with a pro-white bias were more likely to keep patients waiting longer, communicate with verbal dominance, be perceived as less patient centered, and receive poorer ratings of interpersonal care (Cooper et al., 2012). Even well-meaning trainees are not immune to bias. In one study, the vast majority of resident physicians working in an urban pediatric emergency department exhibited pro-white/anti-black racial bias on the child race IAT regardless of their own race, gender, or specialty (Johnson et al., 2017). Unconscious racial bias has also been documented among teachers, with potential effects on student achievement and discipline (Neal, McCray, Webb-Johnson, & Bridgest, 2003; van den Bergh et al., 2010). The IAT has multiple tests regarding race, ethnicity, disability, and many others and is recommended for trainees, practitioners, and educators seeking to examine their own potential biases. The IAT is publicly available at https://implicit.harvard.edu.

Acknowledging biases, both explicit and implicit, is critical to providing equitable care and education. Once providers are able to recognize their own biases, reducing them involves 1) training providers to understand the psychological basis of bias, 2) increasing their internal motivation to address bias in a nonthreatening environment, 3) improving their emotional regulation skills specific to positive interactions, and 4) enhancing providers' self-efficacy in interactions with racially or socially dissimilar patients (Burgess, van Ryn, Dovidio, & Saha, 2007). Along with addressing these unconscious processes, successful training also includes building skills to effectively communicate and negotiate across cultures, languages, and literacy levels (Dykes & White, 2009; Smith et al., 2007). Racial disparities in education can similarly be tempered through interventions such as teacher education in cultural competence; multitiered systems of support, including positive behavioral interventions and supports; and response to intervention (see Chapter 33; Fenning & Sharkey, 2012). These interventions are designed to systematically identify student needs and to provide individualized, high-quality instruction to maximize positive student outcomes.

Finally, clinicians and educators should advocate for institutional and national policies that address disparities and promote equity, including holding their institutions and places of employment accountable for providing culturally and linguistically competent care and education, along with training in cultural competence. This may also involve advocating that a health care institution or school include cultural or racial group analyses and responses to feedback surveys and health/education outcomes data (White & Stubblefield-Tave, 2017). In addition, hiring practices can influence patient-provider and student-teacher rapport, as diversity on clinical and educational teams can reduce unintentional cultural insensitivity (Dykes & White, 2009). Specifically for children with disabilities, employing linguistically competent care coordinators can increase parent satisfaction with care given within the medical home (Hamilton, Lerner, Presson, & Klitzner, 2013). Cultural competence is not only an individual pursuit—it also requires institutional changes in practice. Further research into how federal and state health care financing affects utilization in children with disabilities will be needed to inform legislative advocacy efforts (see Chapter 41).

SUMMARY

- Families with children with disabilities face challenges with accessing quality health care and education, with even greater difficulties reported by racial and ethnic minorities.
- The origins of these disparities are multifactorial, and their effects on health and educational outcomes are an ongoing subject of research, but it is becoming increasingly clear that clinicians and educators can contribute to both raising and reducing barriers to equitable and culturally competent care.
- An initial step toward reducing health and educational disparities is clinician/teacher self-assessment of bias utilizing a tool such as the IAT and bringing these unconscious processes to light.
- Organizational training and ensuring diversity in teams are components of institutional changes that are critical for enhancing cultural competence.

- Ongoing research is needed to track both disability-related and racial/ethnic disparities in order to determine the best practices on the individual, organizational, and national levels that lead to reductions in disparities for the highly vulnerable population of children with disabilities.

ADDITIONAL RESOURCES

Online Implicit Association Test: https://implicit.harvard.edu

Impact of race/racism on health: https://www.youtube.com/watch?v=GNhcY6fTyBM

Child Trends: https://www.childtrends.org/child-trends-5/5-things-know-racial-ethnic-disparities-special-education

Additional resources can be found online in Appendix D: Childhood Disabilities Resources, Services, and Organizations (see About the Online Companion Materials).

REFERENCES

American Academy of Pediatrics. (2003). Family-centered care and the pediatrician's role. *Pediatrics, 112*(3), 691–696.

American Psychological Association Zero Tolerance Task Force. (2008). Are zero tolerance policies effective in the schools? An evidentiary review and recommendations. *The American Psychologist, 63*(9), 852–862. doi:10.1037/0003-066X.63.9.852

Boss, E. F., Niparko, J. K., Gaskin, D. J., & Levinson, K. L. (2011). Socioeconomic disparities for hearing-impaired children in the United States. *The Laryngoscope, 121*(4), 860–866. doi:10.1002/lary.21460

Braveman, P., & Gruskin, S. (2003). Defining equity in health. *Journal of Epidemiology and Community Health, 57*(4), 254–258.

Bright, M. A., Knapp, C., Hinojosa, M. S., Alford, S., & Bonner, B. (2016). The comorbidity of physical, mental, and developmental conditions associated with childhood adversity: A population based study. *Maternal and Child Health Journal, 20*(4), 843–853. doi:10.1007/s10995-015-1915-7

Brown, R., Graham, C., Richeson, N., Wu, J., & McDermott, S. (2010). Evaluation of medical student performance on objective structured clinical exams with standardized patients with and without disabilities. *Academic Medicine, 85*(11), 1766–1771.

Burgess, D., van Ryn, M., Dovidio, J., & Saha, S. (2007). Reducing racial bias among health care providers: Lessons from social-cognitive psychology. *Journal of General Internal Medicine, 22*(6), 882–887. doi:10.1007/s11606-007-0160-1

Carter-Pokras, O., & Baquet, C. (2002). What is a "health disparity"? *Public Health Reports, 117*(5), 426–434. doi:10.1093/phr/117.5.426

Coker, T. R., Rodriguez, M. A., & Flores, G. (2010). Family-centered care for US children with special health care needs: Who gets it and why? *Pediatrics, 125*(6), 1159–1167. doi:10.1542/peds.2009-1994

Conrey, E. J., Seidu, D., Ryan, N. J., & Chapman, D. (2013). Access to patient-centered medical home among Ohio's children with special health care needs. *Journal of Child Health Care: For Professionals Working with Children in the Hospital and Community, 17*(2), 186–196. doi:10.1177/1367493512456111

Cooper, L. A., Roter, D. L., Carson, K. A., Beach, M. C., Sabin, J. A., Greenwald, A. G., & Inui, T. S. (2012). The associations of clinicians' implicit attitudes about race with medical visit communication and patient ratings of interpersonal care. *American Journal of Public Health, 102*(5), 979–987.

Data Resource Center for Child and Adolescent Health. (2017). *National Survey of Children with Special Health Care Needs.* Retrieved from http://www.childhealthdata.org/learn/NS-CSHCN

de Valenzuela, J. S., Copeland, S. R., Huaqing Qi, C., & Park, M. (2006). Examining educational equity: Revisiting the disproportionate representation of minority students in special education. *Exceptional Children, 72*(4), 425–441.

Dehlendorf, C., Bryant, A. S., Huddleston, H. G., Jacoby, V. L., & Fujimoto, V. Y. (2010). Health disparities: Definitions and measurements. *American Journal of Obstetrics and Gynecology, 202*(3), 212–213. doi:10.1016/j.ajog.2009.12.003

Dehon, E., Weiss, N., Jones, J., Faulconer, W., Hinton, E., & Sterling, S. (2017). A systematic review of the impact of physician implicit racial bias on clinical decision making. *Academic Emergency Medicine: Official Journal of the Society for Academic Emergency Medicine, 24*(8), 895–904. doi:10.1111/acem.13214

Drummond, A., Looman, W. S., & Phillips, A. (2012). Coping among parents of children with special health care needs with and without a health care home. *Journal of Pediatric Health Care, 26*(4), 266–275. doi:10.1016/j.pedhc.2010.12.005

Dykes, D. C., & White, A. A., III. (2009). Getting to equal: Strategies to understand and eliminate general and orthopaedic healthcare disparities. *Clinical Orthopaedics and Related Research, 467*(10), 2598–2605. doi:10.1007/s11999-009-0993-5

Eneriz-Wiemer, M., Sanders, L. M., Barr, D. A., & Mendoza, F. S. (2014). Parental limited English proficiency and health outcomes for children with special health care needs: A systematic review. *Academic Pediatrics, 14*(2), 128–136. doi:10.1016/j.acap.2013.10.003

Feinberg, E., Silverstein, M., Donahue, S., & Bliss, R. (2011). The impact of race on participation in Part C early intervention services. *Journal of Developmental and Behavioral Pediatrics, 32*(4), 284–291. doi:10.1097/DBP.0b013e3182142fbd

Fenning, P., & Sharkey, J. D. (2012). Addressing discipline disproportionality with systemic schoolwide approaches. In A. Noltemeyer, & C. McLoughlin (Eds.), *Disproportionality in education and special education* (pp. 199-213). Springfield, IL: Charles C. Thomas Publisher LTD.

Flores, G., & Committee on Pediatric Research. (2010). Technical report—racial and ethnic disparities in the health and health care of children. *Pediatrics, 125*(4), e979–e1020. doi:10.1542/peds.2010-0188

Graham, B. C., Keys, C. B., McMahon, S. D., & Brubacher, M. R. (2014). Transportation challenges for urban students with disabilities: Parent perspectives. *Journal of Prevention & Intervention in the Community, 42*(1), 45–57. doi:10.1080/10852352.2014.855058

Hall, W. J., Chapman, M. V., Lee, K. M., Merino, Y. M., Thomas, T. W., Payne, B. K., . . . Coyne-Beasley, T. (2015). Implicit racial/ethnic bias among health care professionals and its influence on health care outcomes: A systematic review. *American Journal of Public Health, 105*(12), e60–e76.

Hamilton, L. J., Lerner, C. F., Presson, A. P., & Klitzner, T. S. (2013). Effects of a medical home program for children with special health care needs on parental perceptions of care in an ethnically diverse patient population. *Maternal and Child Health Journal, 17*(3), 463–469. doi:10.1007/s10995-012-1018-7

Houtrow, A. J., Okumura, M. J., Hilton, J. F., & Rehm, R. S. (2011). Profiling health and health-related services for children with special health care needs with and without disabilities. *Academic Pediatrics, 11*(6), 508–516.

Institute of Medicine. (2003). Unequal treatment. In B. D. Smedley, A. Y. Stith, and A. R. Nelson (Eds.), *Unequal treatment: Confronting racial and ethnic disparities in health care*. Washington, DC: The National Academies Press. doi:10.17226/10260

Johnson, T. J., Winger, D. G., Hickey, R. W., Switzer, G. E., Miller, E., Nguyen, M. B., . . . Hausmann, L. R. (2017). Comparison of physician implicit racial bias toward adults versus children. *Academic Pediatrics, 17*(2), 120–126. pii:S1876-2859(16)30413-2

Jones, C. P. (2000). Levels of racism: A theoretic framework and a gardener's tale. *American Journal of Public Health, 90*(8), 1212–1215.

Kenney, M. K., & Thierry, J. (2014). Chronic conditions, functional difficulties, and disease burden among American Indian/Alaska Native children with special health care needs, 2009-2010. *Maternal and Child Health Journal, 18*(9), 2071–2079. doi:10.1007/s10995-014-1454-7

Kerfeld, C. I., Hoffman, J. M., Ciol, M. A., & Kartin, D. (2011). Delayed or forgone care and dissatisfaction with care for children with special health care needs: The role of perceived cultural competency of health care providers. *Maternal and Child Health Journal, 15*(4), 487–496. doi:10.1007/s10995-010-0598-3

Kilbourne, A. M., Switzer, G., Hyman, K., Crowley-Matoka, M., & Fine, M. J. (2005). Advancing health disparities research within the health care system: A conceptual framework. *American Journal of Public Health, 96*(12), 2113–2121. doi:10.2105/AJPH.2005.077628

Kuo, D., Goudie, A., Cohen, E., Houtrow, A., Agrawal, R., Carle, A. C., & Wells, N. (2014). Inequities in health care needs for children with medical complexity. *Health Affairs (Millwood), 33*(12), 2190–2198.

Magaña, S., Parish, S. L., Rose, R. A., Timberlake, M., & Swaine, J. G. (2012). Racial and ethnic disparities in quality of health care among children with autism and other developmental disabilities. *Intellectual and Developmental Disabilities, 50*(4), 287–299. doi:10.1352/1934-9556-50.4.287

Magaña, S., Parish, S. L., & Son, E. (2015). Have racial and ethnic disparities in the quality of health care relationships changed for children with developmental disabilities and ASD? *American Journal on Intellectual and Developmental Disabilities, 120*(6), 504–513. doi:10.1352/1944-7558-120.6.504

Maine Center for Disease Control and Prevention. (2018). *What is health equity?* Retrieved from http://www.maine.gov/dhhs/mecdc/health-equity

McManus, B. M., Carle, A. C., & Rapport, M. J. (2014). Classifying infants and toddlers with developmental vulnerability: Who is most likely to receive early intervention? *Child: Care, Health and Development, 40*(2), 205–214. doi:10.1111/cch.12013

Montes, G., & Halterman, J. S. (2011). White-black disparities in family-centered care among children with autism in the United States: Evidence from the NS-CSHCN 2005-2006. *Academic Pediatrics, 11*(4), 297–304. doi:10.1016/j.acap.2011.02.002

Morgan, P. L., Farkas, G., Hillemeier, M. M., Mattison, R., Maczuga, S., Li, H., & Cook, M. (2015). Minorities are disproportionately underrepresented in special education: Longitudinal evidence across five disability conditions. *Educational Researcher, 44*(5), 278–292. doi:10.3102/0013189X15591157

Morgan, P. L., & Farkas, G. (2016). Evidence of minority underrepresentation in special education and its implications for school psychologists. *Communique, 44*(6), 1.

Morgan, P. L., Farkas, G., Cook, M., Strassfeld, N. M., Hillemeier, M. M., Pun, W. H., & Schussler, D. L. (2017). Are black children disproportionately overrepresented in special education? A best-evidence synthesis. *Exceptional Children, 83*(2), 181–198.

Moroz, A., Gonzalez-Ramos, G., Festinger, T., Langer, K., Zefferino, S., & Kalet, A. (2010). Immediate and follow-up effects of a brief disability curriculum on disability knowledge and attitudes of PM&R residents: A comparison group trial. *Medical Teacher, 32*(8), 360–364.

Morrison, E. H., George, V. F., & Mosqueda, L. (2008). Primary care for adults with physical disabilities: Perceptions from consumer and provider focus groups. *Family Medicine, 40*(9), 645–651.

Neal, L. V. I., McCray, A. D., Webb-Johnson, G., & Bridgest, S. T. (2003). The effects of African American movement styles on teachers' perceptions and reactions. *Journal of Special Education, 37*(1), 49–57. doi:10.1177/00224669030370010501

Newacheck, P. W., Stein, R. E., Bauman, L., Hung, Y. Y., & Research Consortium on Children with Chronic Conditions. (2003). Disparities in the prevalence of disability between black and white children. *Archives of Pediatrics & Adolescent Medicine, 157*(3), 244–248. pii:poa20249

O'Day, B., Killeen, M., Sutton, J., & Iezzoni, L. (2005). Primary care experiences of people with psychiatric disabilities: Barriers to care and potential solutions. *Psychiatric Rehabilitation Journal, 28*(4), 339–345.

Okumura, M. J., Van Cleave, J., Gnanasekaran, S., & Houtrow, A. (2009). Understanding factors associated with work loss for families caring for CSHCN. *Pediatrics, 124*(Suppl. 4), S392–S398. doi:10.1542/peds.2009-1255J

Parish, S., Magaña, S., Rose, R., Timberlake, M., & Swaine, J. G. (2012). Health care of Latino children with autism and other developmental disabilities: Quality of provider interaction mediates utilization. *American Journal on Intellectual and Developmental Disabilities, 117*(4), 304–315. doi:10.1352/1944-7558-117.4.304

Project Implicit. (2017). *Implicit association test.* Retrieved from https://implicit.harvard.edu/implicit/

Raphael, J. L., Zhang, Y., Liu, H., Tapia, C. D., & Giardino, A. P. (2009). Association of medical home care and disparities in emergency care utilization among children with special health care needs. *Academic Pediatrics, 9*(4), 242–248. doi:10.1016/j.acap.2009.05.002

Richmond, N. E., Tran, T., & Berry, S. (2012). Can the medical home eliminate racial and ethnic disparities for transition services among youth with special health care needs? *Maternal and Child Health Journal, 16*(4), 824–833. doi:10.1007/s10995-011-0785-x

Rosen-Reynoso, M., Porche, M. V., Kwan, N., Bethell, C., Thomas, V., Robertson, J., . . . Palfrey, J. (2016). Disparities in access to easy-to-use services for children with special health care needs. *Maternal and Child Health Journal, 20*(5), 1041–1053. doi:10.1007/s10995-015-1890-z

Schieve, L. A., Boulet, S. L., Kogan, M. D., Van Naarden-Braun, K., & Boyle, C. A. (2011). A population-based assessment of the health, functional status, and consequent family impact among children with Down syndrome. *Disability and Health Journal, 4*(2), 68–77. doi:10.1016/j.dhjo.2010.06.001

Sharby, N., Martire, K., & Iversen, M. D. (2015). Decreasing health disparities for people with disabilities through improved communication strategies and awareness. *International Journal of Environmental Research and Public Health, 12*(3), 3301–3316. doi:10.3390/ijerph120303301

Skiba, R. J., Shure, L., & Williams, N. (2012). Racial and ethnic disproportionality in suspension and expulsion. In A. Noltemeyer & C. McLoughlin (Eds.), *Disproportionality in education and special education* (pp. 89–118). Springfield, IL: Charles C. Thomas Publisher LTD.

Skiba, R. J., Poloni-Staudinger, L., Gallini, S., Simmons, A. B., & Feggins-Azziz, R. (2006). Disparate access: The disproportionality of African American students with disabilities across educational environments. *Exceptional Children, 72*(4), 411.

Smith, W. R., Betancourt, J. R., Wynia, M. K., Bussey-Jones, J., Stone, V. E., Phillips, C. O., . . . Bowles, J. (2007). Recommendations for teaching about racial and ethnic disparities in health and health care. *Annals of Internal Medicine, 147*(9), 654–665. pii:147/9/654

Spencer, N., & Strazdins, L. (2015). Socioeconomic disadvantage and onset of childhood chronic disabling conditions: A cohort study. *Archives of Disease in Childhood, 100*(4), 317–322. doi:10.1136/archdischild-2013-305634

Strickland, B. B., Singh, G. K., Kogan, M. D., Mann, M. Y., van Dyck, P. C., & Newacheck, P. W. (2009). Access to the medical home: New findings from the 2005-2006 National Survey of Children with Special Health Care Needs. *Pediatrics, 123*(6), e996–1004. doi:10.1542/peds.2008-2504

Symons, A. B., Morley, C. P., McGuigan, D., & Akl, E. A. (2014). A curriculum on care for people with disabilities: Effects on medical student self-reported attitudes and comfort level. *Disability and Health Journal, 7*(1), 88–95.

Tenenbaum, H. R., & Ruck, M. D. (2007). Are teachers' expectations different for racial minority than for European American students? A meta-analysis. *Journal of Educational Psychology, 99*(2), 253–273.

The Council of State Governments. (2011). *Breaking schools' rules: A statewide study of how school discipline relates to students' success and juvenile justice involvement.* Retrieved from csgjusticecenter.org/wp-content/uploads/2012/08/Breaking_Schools_Rules_Report_Final.pdf

Thomas, K. C., Parish, S. L., Rose, R. A., & Kilany, M. (2012). Access to care for children with autism in the context of state Medicaid reimbursement. *Maternal and Child Health Journal, 16*(8), 1636–1644. doi:10.1007/s10995-011-0862-1

U.S. Department of Education. (2016). *Racial and educational disparities in special education.* Table 8 & Table 13. Retrieved from https://www2.ed.gov/programs/osepidea/618-data/LEA-racial-ethnic-disparities-tables/disproportionality-analysis-by-state-analysis-category.pdf

U.S. Department of Education, National Center for Education and Statistics. (2016). *Status and trends in the education of racial and ethnic groups 2016.* Retrieved from https://nces.ed.gov/pubs2016/2016007.pdf

U.S. Department of Education, National Center for Education Evaluation and Regional Assistance, Institute of Education Sciences. (2011). *National assessment of IDEA overview* (NCEE 2011-4026). Retrieved from https://ies.ed.gov/ncee/pubs/20114026/pdf/20114026.pdf

U.S. Department of Education, Office for Civil Rights. (2016). *2013-2014 civil rights data collection: A first look.* Retrieved from https://www2.ed.gov/about/offices/list/ocr/docs/2013-14-first-look.pdf

U.S. Department of Education, Office of Special Education and Rehabilitative Services. (2016). *Digest of educational statistics.* Table 204.30: *Children 3-21 years olds old under individuals with disabilities education act (IDEA), Part B, by race/ethnicity and age group 2000-01- 2013-14.* Retrieved from https://nces.ed.gov/programs/digest/d16/tables/dt16_204.30.asp

U.S. Department of Health and Human Services, Health Resources and Services Administration, Maternal and Child Health Bureau. (2013). *The National Survey of Children with Special Health Care Needs chartbook 2009–2010.* Rockville, Maryland: Author. Retrieved from https://mchb.hrsa.gov/cshcn0910/more/pdf/nscshcn0910.pdf

van den Bergh, L., Denessen, E., Hornstra, L., Voeten, M., & Holland, R. W. (2010). The implicit prejudiced attitudes of teachers: Relations to teacher expectations and the ethnic achievement gap. *American Educational Research Journal, 47*(2), 497–527. doi:10.3102/0002831209353594

White, A. A., III, & Stubblefield-Tave, B. (2017). Some advice for physicians and other clinicians treating minorities, women, and other patients at risk of receiving health care disparities. *Journal of Racial and Ethnic Health Disparities, 4*(3), 472–479. doi:10.1007/s40615-016-0248-6

Winitzer, R. F., Bisgaier, J., Grogan, C., & Rhodes, K. (2012). 'He only takes those type of patients on certain days': Specialty care access for children with special health care needs. *Disability and Health Journal, 5*(1), 26–33. doi:10.1016/j.dhjo.2011.10.002

World Health Organization. (2011). *World report on disability.* Retrieved from http://www.refworld.org/docid/50854a322.html

APPENDIX A Glossary

AAC *See* augmentative and alternate communication.
ABA *See* applied behavior analysis.
abducens nerve The sixth nerve; controls the lateral rectus eye muscle.
abducted Part of the body moved away from the midline.
abduction Moving part of the body away from one's midline.
ABR *See* auditory brainstem response.
abruptio placenta Premature detachment of a normally situated placenta; *also called* placental abruption.
abscesses Localized collections of pus in cavities caused by the disintegration of tissue, usually the result of bacterial infections.
accommodation 1) In special education, a change in how a student gains access to the curriculum or demonstrates his or her learning. This approach does not substantially alter the content or level of instruction (e.g., allowing a student additional time to take a test); 2) the change in the shape of the lens of the eye that allows it to focus on objects at varying distances.
acetabulum The cup-shaped cavity of the hip bone that holds the head of the femur in place, creating a joint.
acetylcholine A neurotransmitter for cholinergic neurons that innervate many tissues, including smooth muscle and skeletal muscle.
acetylcholinesterase (ACHE) An enzyme that stops excitation of a nerve after transmission of an impulse.
acid–base balance In metabolism, the ratio of acidic to basic compounds (or pH).
acidosis Abnormally high levels of acid in the bloodstream. The normal pH is 7.42; acidosis is generally less than pH 7.30.
acquired immunodeficiency syndrome (AIDS) Severe immune deficiency disease caused by human immunodeficiency virus (HIV).
actin Protein involved in muscle contraction.
acute inflammatory peripheral neuropathy The most common form is Guillain-Barre syndrome. It involves an ascending paralysis, with weakness beginning in the feet and hands and migrating toward the trunk. It can cause life-threatening complications, particularly if the breathing muscles are affected or if there is dysfunction of the autonomic nervous system. The disease is usually triggered by an acute infection.
adaptive skills The skills necessary to effectively and independently take care of oneself.
adaptive technology Substitutes or makes up for the loss of function brought on by a disability (e.g., software that permits voice production through a computer for an individual who cannot speak).
adduction Moving a body part, usually a limb, toward the midline.
adenine One of the four nucleotides (chemicals) that comprise DNA.
adenoid Lymphatic tissue located behind the nasal passages.
adenoidectomy The surgical removal of the adenoids.
adenoma sebaceum Benign cutaneous growths, usually seen around the nose, that resemble acne; these occur in individuals with tuberous sclerosis (*see* Appendix B).
adenotonsillectomy Surgical removal of adenoids and tonsils.
adherence Compliance.
adjustment disorders A group of psychiatric disorders, usually of childhood, associated with difficulty adjusting to life changes.
adrenaline A potent stimulant of the autonomic nervous system. It increases blood pressure and heart rate and stimulates other physiological changes needed for a "fight-or-flight" response.
advance directives In children with severe disabilities or diseases, the term is used to define the level of

intervention a parent wants provided in the event of life-threatening emergency or illness in the child.

adverse drug reactions (ADRs) Harmful reaction experienced following the administration of a drug or combination of drugs given at normal doses.

AED *See* automated external defibrillator.

afferent Pertaining to the neural signals sent from the peripheral nervous system to the central nervous system (CNS). Sensory fibers carry signals from muscles, skin, and joints back to the brain.

AFO *See* ankle-foot orthosis.

AFP *See* alpha-fetoprotein.

afterbirth *See* placenta.

agenesis of the corpus callosum Absence of the band of white matter that normally connects the two hemispheres of the brain.

agonist A muscle that works in concert with another muscle to produce movement.

agyria Absence of the normal convolutions on the surface of the brain.

AIDS *See* acquired immunodeficiency syndrome.

alcohol-related neurodevelopmental disorder (ARND) *Previously called* fetal alcohol effects (FAE); refers to the range of neurological and developmental impairments that can affect a child who has been exposed *in utero* to alcohol. The most severe of these effects is fetal alcohol syndrome.

alleles Alternate forms of a gene that may exist at the same site on the chromosome.

alopecia The partial or complete absence of hair from areas of the body where it normally grows.

alpha-fetoprotein (AFP) Fetal protein found in amniotic fluid and serum of pregnant women. Its measurement is used to test for meningomyelocele and Down syndrome in the fetus and is a chemical typically found in the fetal spinal fluid, brain, and spinal cord.

alternative technology *See* adaptive technology.

alveoli Small air sacs in the lungs. Carbon dioxide and oxygen are exchanged through their walls.

amalgam An alloy of mercury and silver used in dental fillings.

amaurosis Blindness with no change in the eye but due to disease of brain, nerve, or spinal cord.

amblyopia Partial loss of sight resulting from disuse atrophy of neural circuitry during a critical period of development, most often associated with untreated strabismus in children.

amino acid Building block of protein needed for normal growth.

amino acid disorders Inborn errors of metabolism resulting from an enzyme deficiency involving amino acids, the building blocks of protein.

amniocentesis A prenatal diagnostic procedure performed in the second trimester in which amniotic fluid is removed by a needle inserted through the abdominal wall and into the uterine cavity.

amniotic fluid Clear fluid that surrounds the fetus during pregnancy, acting as a physical buffer for fetal movements and physical development. It is formed by fetal urine production and lung fluid secretion during fetal respirations.

amygdala A part of the brain involved in sensory procession and emotions.

anaphase The stage in cell division (mitosis and meiosis) when the chromosomes move from the center of the nucleus toward the poles of the cell.

anaphylaxis A life-threatening hypersensitivity response to a medication or food, marked by breathing difficulty, hives, and shock.

anemia Disorder in which the blood has either too few red blood cells or too little hemoglobin.

anencephaly Neural tube defect (NTD) in which either the entire brain or all but the most primitive regions of the brain are missing.

aneuploidy Abnormal number of chromosomes in a cell, for example a human cell having 45 or 47 chromosomes instead of the usual 46.

angiogenesis Development of new blood vessels.

angular cheilitis Inflammation starting at the angles of the mouth and affecting the lips. It is usually caused by nutritional deficiencies, atopic dermatitis, or yeast infection.

ankle-foot orthosis (AFO) An appliance or brace that stabilizes the position of the foot and provides a consistent stretch to the Achilles' tendon.

anodontia The congenital absence of all primary or permanent teeth.

anomalies Birth defects caused by structural abnormalities.

anophthalmia Congenital absence of the eye globes.

anorexia A severe loss of appetite.

anotia Congenital absence of the external ear (auricle).

antagonists Muscles that work at cross-purposes (e.g., the adductor and abductor muscles of the hip oppose each others' actions).

antecedents Events or contextual factors that precede the manifestation of a behavior.

anterior The front part of a structure.

anterior chamber The space between the cornea and lens of the eye.

anterior fontanelle The membrane-covered area on the top of the head; *also called* the "soft spot." It generally closes by 18 months of age.

anterior horn cells Cells in the spinal column that transmit impulses from the pyramidal tract to the peripheral nervous system.

anthropometrics Measurements of the body and its parts.

antibody A protein formed in the bloodstream to fight infection.

anticholinergic medications A group of medications that acts by antagonizing the effects of the neurotransmitter acetylcholine.

anticipation A term used in genetics to denote an expansion in triplet repeats from one generation to the next, leading to a more severe manifestation of the disease (e.g., in fragile X syndrome).

anticonvulsants Medications used for control of seizures.

antidepressants Medications used to control major depression.

antigen A substance that, when introduced into the body, triggers the production of an antibody by the immune system, which will then kill or neutralize the antigen that is recognized as a foreign and potentially harmful invader.

antihistamine A drug that counteracts the effects of histamines, substances involved in allergic reactions.

antipsychotic medications Medications used to treat psychosis; the atypical antipsychotics have also been found to be useful in treating aggression and self-injury in children with severe intellectual disability.

antipyretics Medications used to treat fever.

antiretroviral agents (ARVs) A category of medications used to treat retroviral infections (i.e., HIV/AIDS).

anuria In chronic renal (kidney) failure, the absence of urine production.

anxiety disorders Psychiatric disorders characterized by feelings of anxiety. The disorders include panic attacks, separation anxiety, social anxiety, obsessive-compulsive disorder (OCD), and posttraumatic stress disorder (PTSD).

aorta The major artery, originating in the left ventricle of the heart and supplying oxygenated blood to the body and brain.

Apgar scoring system Scoring system developed by Virginia Apgar to assess neurological status in the newborn infant. Scores range from 0 to 10.

aphasia A class of language disorder that ranges from having difficulty remembering words to being completely unable to speak, read, or write due to damage to the brain.

apical At the tip of a structure.

apnea A lack of spontaneous breathing effort; brief breathing arrests.

apneic Pertaining to an episodic arrest of breathing.

apoptosis Programmed cell death.

applied behavior analysis (ABA) A treatment method, commonly used in autism, that uses behavioral learning theory to change behavior.

appropriate-for-gestational-age The term used when the baby's gestational age findings (e.g., length and weight) after birth match the baby's calendar age.

apraxia The inability to perform coordinated movements or manipulate objects in the absence of a motor or sensory impairment.

aqueous humor The watery fluid in the eyeball that fills the anterior chamber (the space between the lens and the cornea).

arborization A process during neuronal differentiation by which primitive neurons begin to express their distinctive physical and biochemical features.

arachnoid granulations The small whitish villi of the arachnoid membrane, the middle of the three membranes or meninges that surround the brain and spinal cord.

architectonic dysplasias Developmental malformations affecting the neuronal architecture of the brain.

areflexia Lack of deep tendon reflexes.

ARFID *See* avoidant/restrictive food intake disorder.

ARND *See* alcohol-related neurodevelopmental disorder.

arterial blood gas A laboratory profile test of sampled arterial blood, including pH, PaO_2, and $PaCO_2$.

arterial-venous malformation (AVM) Birth defect of blood vessels, most commonly in the brain, that can be associated with a disastrous postthrombotic hemorrhage.

arthritis An inflammatory disease of joints.

arthrogryposis Congenital condition characterized by reduced mobility of multiple joints due to contractures.

articular Referring to the surface of a bone at a joint space.

articulation 1) The formulation of individual speech sounds; 2) the connection at a joint.

articulation disorder A speech disorder involving difficulties in forming specific sounds.

ARVs *See* antiretroviral agents.

ascending infections The transfer of microbes from the maternal genital tract through the cervix and across the amniotic membranes to the fetus.

ASD *See* autism spectrum disorder.

asphyxia Interference with oxygenation of the blood that leads to loss of consciousness and possible brain damage.

aspiration Inhalation of a foreign body, usually a food particle, into the lungs.

aspiration pneumonia Inflammation of the lung(s) caused by inhaling a foreign body, such as food, into the lungs; an infection by the aspiration of food into the lung.

asplenia Nonfunctioning spleen.

assent Agreement to research or treatment, given by a child or minor who is too young to give legally valid informed consent.

assisted reproductive technology (ART) Technology to help human reproduction (e.g., *in vitro* fertilization).

assistive Providing assistance.

assistive devices Any device used to assist in a body function (e.g., a wheelchair).

assistive technology (AT) Technology (often software) to improve communication, movement, independence, and so forth.

astigmatism A condition of unequal curvature of the cornea that leads to blurred vision.

astrocytes Support cells in the central nervous system (CNS) that help form the white matter.

asymmetrical tonic neck reflex (ATNR) A primitive reflex, *also called* the fencer's response, found in infants; usually is no longer evident by 3 months of age. When the neck is turned in one direction, the arm shoots out on the same side and flexes on the opposite side; similar changes occur in the legs.

ataxia An unbalanced gait or movement of any part of the body caused by a disturbance of cerebellar control. Movements are jerky and uncoordinated, without the smooth flow of normal motion.

ataxic Erratic and uncoordinated voluntary movement.

ataxic cerebral palsy A form of dyskinetic cerebral palsy in which the prominent feature is ataxia; characterized by abnormalities of voluntary movement involving balance and position of the trunk and limbs in space (ataxia). Ataxic cerebral palsy may be associated with increased (spastic) or decreased (hypotonic) muscle tone.

athetoid cerebral palsy A form of dyskinetic cerebral palsy associated with athetosis.

athetosis Constant random, slow, writhing involuntary movements of the limbs.

atlantoaxial instability (AAI) Excessive movement at the junction between the atlas (C1) and axis (C2) bones in the upper spine as a result of either a bony or ligamentous abnormality. This is a common finding in Down syndrome.

atlantoaxial subluxation Partial dislocation of the upper spine, a particular risk in Down syndrome.

ATNR *See* asymmetrical tonic neck reflex.

atonic Pertaining to the absence of normal muscle tone.

atopic dermatitis Eczema.

atresia Congenital absence or abnormal narrowing of a body passage or opening.

atria The two upper chambers of the heart.

atrial septal defect A congenital heart defect in which there is lack of closure of the wall separating the two upper chambers of the heart.

attention-deficit/hyperactivity disorder (ADHD) A developmental disorder characterized by impulsivity, hyperactivity, and inattention to a degree that leads to impairment in functioning.

attrition The wearing away by friction or rubbing (e.g., by tooth grinding).

atypical Unusual.

audiometry A hearing test using a device called an audiometer that yields results in the form of a graph showing hearing levels in sound intensity at various wavelengths of sound presented through earphones.

auditory agnosia Inability to distinguish different sounds in the presence of normal hearing.

auditory brainstem response (ABR) A test of central nervous system hearing pathways.

augmentative and alternative communication (AAC) Devices that assist individuals who lack the ability to speak (e.g., a microchip-powered voice output augmentative device for a person with dysarthria).

augmentative devices Devices used to increase an area of functioning that is deficient, sometimes severely, but for which there are some residual abilities.

aura A sensation, usually visual and/or olfactory, marking the onset of a seizure.

auricle The outer ear.

autism spectrum disorder (ASD) A developmental disorder with persistent deficits in social communication and interaction as well as restrictive, repetitive patterns of behavior, interests, and activities.

autoimmune Pertaining to a reaction in which one's immune system attacks other parts of the body.

automated external defibrillator (AED) Portable electronic device that automatically diagnoses the potentially life-threatening cardiac arrhythmias of ventricular fibrillation and ventricular tachycardia in a patient and can provide an electrical impulse to correct the arrhythmia.

automatic movement reactions *See* postural reactions.

automatic reinforcement A behavior that produces internal consequences that can reinforce and thus produce functional relationships that maintain the problem behavior.

automatisms Automatic fine motor movements (e.g., unbuttoning one's clothing–i.e., unconscious) that are part of a seizure.

autonomic Describing the part of the nervous system that regulates certain automatic functions of the body (i.e., heart rate, sweating, and bowel movement).

autonomic nervous system Controls involuntary activities of the cardiovascular, digestive, endocrine, urinary, respiratory, and reproductive systems.

autonomy The ability and/or right to be self-determining; an important concept regarding participating in human trials research.

autosomal dominant Mendelian inheritance pattern in which a single copy of a gene (from either mother or father) leads to expression of the trait.

autosomal recessive Mendelian inheritance pattern in which identical copies of a gene from both mother and father are required to result in the expression of a trait.

autosomes The first 22 pairs of chromosomes. All chromosomes are autosomes except for the two sex chromosomes.

avascular necrosis Destruction of bone from microvascular occlusion.

aversive Pertaining to a stimulus, often unpleasant, that decreases the likelihood a particular response will subsequently occur.

AVM *See* arterial-venous malformation.

avoidant/restrictive food intake disorder (ARFID) Intake disturbance in which a child eats too little, eats a limited variety, or has fear of eating, resulting in either faltering growth, nutritional deficiency, dependence on nutritional supplements, and/ or interference with psychosocial functioning

axon A long, slender projection of a nerve cell, or neuron, that conducts electrical impulses away from the neuron's cell body.

Babinski sign Upgoing toe when the sole of the foot is stroked firmly, often a sign of cerebral palsy outside of the newborn period.

backward chaining Method of teaching a task in which the instructor begins by teaching the last step in a sequence because this step is most likely to be associated with a potent positive reinforcer.

bacteremia Spread of a bacterial organism throughout the bloodstream.

banding In genetics, pertaining to a series of dark and light bars that appear on chromosomes after they are stained. Each chromosome has a distinct banding pattern.

barotrauma Injury related to excess pressure, especially to the lungs or ears.

basal 1) Near the base; 2) relating to a standard or reference point (e.g., basal metabolic rate).

basal ganglia Brain structure at the base of the cerebral hemispheres involved in motor control, cognition, emotions, and learning.

baseline In behavior management, the frequency, duration, and intensity of a behavior prior to intervention.

basilar membrane The thin tissue barrier that extends from the bony shelf of the cochlea to the outer wall and supports the organ of Corti in the inner ear.

behavior Refers to any action that one person can perform and that another person can observe.

behavior family therapy A type of psychotherapy used to modify family function where one or more members is exhibiting behavior problems.

benign childhood epilepsy with centrotemporal spikes (BECTS) *Also called* benign rolandic epilepsy (BRE), it is the most common epilepsy syndrome in childhood. Most children will outgrow the syndrome by 18 years, and treatment with anti-epileptic drugs may not be required.

benign occipital epilepsy A hereditary form of focal epilepsy that involves the occipital lobe of the brain. It occurs during childhood and often does not require antiepileptic drug treatment.

benign rolandic epilepsy (BRE) *See* benign childhood epilepsy with centrotemporal spikes.

benign sleep myoclonus of infancy This form of sleep disorder happens between birth and 6 months and consists of myoclonic jerks that involve limbs, trunk, or the whole body. It occurs in clusters during quiet non-REM sleep and disappears during wakefulness.

beriberi Disease caused by a deficiency of the vitamin B1 (thiamin) and manifested as edema, heart problems, and peripheral neuropathy.

beta-blockers Medications (e.g., propranolol) that were initially used to control high blood pressure and have subsequently been found also to be useful in treating tremor and migraine headache.

binge eating An eating disorder in which there are recurrent episodes of ingesting large amounts of food during short periods of time.

binocular vision The focusing of both eyes on an object to provide a stereoscopic image.

biotin One of the B-complex vitamins needed to activate a number of important enzymatic reactions in the body.

biotinidase deficiency An inborn error of metabolism in which biotin is not released from proteins in the diet during digestion resulting in biotin deficiency. Symptoms include seizures, hypotonia and muscle/limb weakness, ataxia, hearing loss, optic atrophy, skin rashes, and alopecia. If left untreated, the disorder can rapidly lead to coma and death. Treatment involves biotin supplementation. *See* Appendix B.

bipolar disorder A psychiatric disorder manifested by cycles of mania and depression; *previously called* manic-depression.

blastocyst The embryonic group of cells that exists at the time of implantation.

blastomere A cell formed by cleavage of a fertilized egg.

blepharitis Inflammation of the eyelids.

blood PaO_2 A measurement of the partial pressure of arterial oxygen (i.e., the amount of oxygen in the blood).

blood pH Blood acidity; normally around 7.40.

blood poisoning *See* sepsis.

body mass index (BMI) A measurement of the relative percentages of fat and muscle mass in the human body, in which weight in kilograms is divided by height in meters and the result used as an index of obesity.

bolus 1) A small rounded mass of food made ready by tongue and jaw movement for swallowing; 2) a single dose of a large amount of medication given to rapidly attain a therapeutic drug level.

botulinum toxin (Botox) 1) The neurotoxin that produces botulism (food poisoning). 2) Neurotoxin used in the treatment of neuromuscular disorders such as rigidity and spasticity.

botulism Poisoning by botulin toxin and manifested as muscle weakness or paralysis.

BPD *See* bronchopulmonary dysplasia.

brachial plexus Network of nerve fibers, running from the spine through the neck, the axilla (armpit region), and into the arm.

brachialis A muscle in the upper arm.

brachycephaly Tall head shape with flat back part of the skull. Short-headed shape to the skull due to premature closure of the coronal suture.

bradycardia Abnormal slowing of the heart rate, usually to fewer than 60 beats per minute.

braille A system of writing and printing for people who are blind or severely visually impaired.

brainstem The primitive portion of the brain that lies between the cerebrum and the spinal cord.

brainstem release phenomena In infancy abnormal non-epileptic motor phenomena that arise from brainstem centers as a result of the reduction of cortical inhibitory input secondary to an encephalopathy.

branchial arches A series of arch-like thickenings of the body wall in the pharyngeal region of the embryo.

bronchopulmonary dysplasia (BPD) A chronic lung disorder that occurs in a minority of premature infants who previously had respiratory distress syndrome (hyaline membrane disease). It is associated with "stiff" lungs that do not permit adequate exchange of oxygen and carbon dioxide, frequently leads to dependence on ventilator assistance for extended periods, and markedly increases the risk for the child developing asthma in the future.

bronchospasm Acute constriction of the bronchial tube, most commonly associated with asthma.

bruxism Repetitive grinding of the teeth.

buccal Pertaining to the cheek.

bulging fontanel Bulging soft spot on the crown of the head.

bulk Foodstuffs that increase the quantity of intestinal contents and stimulate regular bowel movements. Fruits, vegetables, and other foods containing fiber provide bulk in the diet.

caffeine A central nervous system (CNS) stimulant found in coffee, tea, and cola. It has been used to treat apnea and bradycardia in premature infants.
calcify To become hardened through the laying down of calcium salts.
calculus An abnormal collection of mineral salts on the tooth, predisposing it to decay; *also called* tartar; when plaque becomes calcified.
callus A disorganized network of bone tissue that forms around the edges of a fracture during the healing process.
camptodactyly Deformity of fingers or toes in which they are permanently flexed, frequently the fifth finger.
cancellous Referring to the lattice-like structure in long bones (e.g., the femur).
cardinality The number of basic members in a set.
cardiomegaly Enlarged heart.
cardiopulmonary resuscitation (CPR) An emergency procedure involving manual pumping of the chest combined with rescue breathing that is performed in an effort to preserve intact brain function until further measures are taken to restore spontaneous blood circulation and breathing in a person in cardiac arrest.
cardiorespiratory arrest Slowing or stopping of breathing and/or heart rate.
cardiorespiratory monitor A device used to monitor heart and respiratory rate.
caries Dental decay.
case-control study An observational epidemiologic study of people with a specific disease (or other outcome) of interest and a suitable control (e.g., comparison, reference) group of people without the disease.
catalyze To stimulate a chemical reaction via a compound that is not used up.
cataracts Clouding of the lenses of the eyes.
catheterization Use of a tube to infuse or remove fluids.
caudal Posterior pole of the developing embryo.
caudal agenesis A condition in which there is underdevelopment and fusion of the lower limbs. It is also associated with pelvic and base of the spine anomalies.
caudal regression syndrome Defects that may occur during embryonic life that can result in major malformations of the lower vertebrae, pelvis, and spine.
caudate nucleus Located within the basal ganglia, it is an important part of the brain's learning and memory system.
CBF *See* cerebral blood flow.
cecostomy Surgical formation of a permanent artificial opening into the cecum, the end of the colon.
celiac disease Congenital malabsorption syndrome that leads to the inability to gain weight and the passage of loose, foul-smelling stools. It is caused by intolerance of cereal products that contain gluten (e.g., wheat). Affected individuals should avoid wheat and other grains.
central hypoventilation Shallow breathing leading to low oxygen level resulting from disordered cerebral control of respiration.
central nervous system (CNS) The portion of the nervous system that consists of the brain and spinal cord. It is primarily involved in voluntary movement and thought processes.
central venous line A catheter that is advanced through a peripheral vein to a position directly above the opening to the right atrium of the heart. It is used to infuse long-term medication and/or nutrition.
centrioles Tiny organelles that migrate to the opposite poles of a cell during cell division and align the spindles.
centromere The constricted area of the chromosome that usually marks the point of attachment of the sister chromatids to the spindle during cell division.
cephalocaudal From head to tail; refers to neurological development that proceeds from the head downward.
cephalohematoma A swelling of the head resulting from bleeding of scalp veins. Often found in newborn infants; it is usually not harmful.
cerebellum A cauliflower-shaped brain structure located just above the brainstem beneath the occipital lobes at the base of the skull that is principally involved in muscle tone and coordination of movement. It may also be involved in some cognitive functions such as attention and language as well as in regulating fear and pleasure responses.
cerebral blood flow (CBF) Autoregulated blood flow in the brain.
cerebellar cognitive affective syndrome A syndrome associated with cerebellar injury that includes a combination of impairment of executive functions such as planning, set-shifting, verbal fluency, abstract reasoning, and working memory; difficulties with spatial cognition, including visual-spatial organization and memory; and personality change with blunting of affect or disinhibited and inappropriate behavior.
cerebral contusion A bruise on the cerebral hemispheres.
cerebral hemisphere Either of the two halves of brain substance.
cerebral palsy A disorder of movement and posture due to a nonprogressive defect of the immature brain. *See* Chapter 21.
cerebral vascular accident (CVA) A thrombotic (clot) or hemorrhagic (bleed) stroke that can damage large regions of the brain in the location of a particular blood vessel (artery or vein).
cerebrospinal fluid (CSF) Clear, watery fluid that fills the ventricular cavities within the brain and circulates around the brain and spinal cord.
cerumen Ear wax.
cervical Pertaining 1) to the cervix or 2) to the neck.
cesarean section (C-section) A surgical operation for delivering a baby through incising the uterus.
Charcot–Marie–Tooth disease (CMT) One of the hereditary motor and sensory neuropathies, a group of varied inherited disorders of the peripheral nervous system characterized by progressive loss of muscle tissue and touch sensation across various parts of the body. *See* Chapter 9 and Appendix B.
CHARGE syndrome A syndrome defined by coloboma of the eye, heart defects, atresia of the choanae,

retardation of growth and/or development, genital and/or urinary abnormalities, and ear abnormalities and deafness. These children may have significant vision and hearing impairments. *See* Appendix B.

cheilitis An inflammation of the lips.

chelation therapy The use of an oral, intravenous, or topical medication to remove metal from the body, most commonly used in lead poisoning.

chemotaxis The phenomenon in which cells direct their movements according to certain chemicals in their environment. This is critical to early development (e.g., movement of sperm toward the egg during fertilization) and subsequent phases of development (e.g., migration of neurons or lymphocytes) as well as in normal cellular function.

chemotherapy Drugs used to treat cancer.

chest physiotherapy (CPT) A general term referring to treatments generally performed by respiratory therapists to improve breathing by the indirect removal of mucus from the breathing passages.

Chiari malformation A congenital defect characterized by the downward displacement of the cerebellum through the opening at the base of the skull.

Chiari type II malformation An abnormality, wherein the brainstem and part of the cerebellum are displaced downward toward the neck, rather than remaining within the skull.

childhood apraxia of speech (CAS) A pediatric speech sound disorder in which the precision and consistency of movements underlying speech are impaired in the absence of evident neuromuscular deficits.

choanal atresia Congenital closure of the nasal passage; part of the CHARGE association.

cholelithiasis Gall stones.

cholesteatoma A complication of otitis media in which skin cells from the ear canal migrate through the perforated eardrum into the middle ear, or mastoid region, forming a mass that must be removed surgically.

chorea A disorder marked by involuntary jerky movements of the extremities.

choreoathetosis Movement disorder, characteristic of dyskinetic cerebral palsy, involving frequent involuntary spasms of the limbs; when chorea and athetosis are seen together.

chorioamnionitis An infection of the amniotic sac that surrounds and contains the fetus and amniotic fluid.

chorion The outermost covering of the membrane surrounding the fetus.

chorionic villi Tiny projections that sprout from the chorion to give a maximum area of contact with the maternal blood. Embryonic blood is carried to the villi by the branches of the umbilical arteries and, after circulating through the capillaries of the villi, is returned to the embryo by the umbilical veins. The villi are part of the border between maternal and fetal blood during pregnancy.

chorionic villus sampling (CVS) A prenatal diagnostic procedure done in the first trimester of pregnancy to obtain fetal cells for genetic analysis; minute biopsy of the chorion.

chorioretinitis An inflammation of the retina and choroid that produces severe visual loss.

choroid The middle layer of the eyeball between the sclera and the retina.

choroid plexus Cells that line the walls of the ventricles of the brain and produce cerebrospinal fluid.

chromatids Term given to chromosomes during cell division.

chromosomal microarray analysis (CMA) A genetic test that can detect extra or missing segments of genetic material or DNA.

chromosomes Threadlike strands of DNA and associated proteins in the nucleus of cells that carry the genes transmitting hereditary information.

CI *See* cochlear implant.

ciliary body Located behind the iris, this structure allows drainage out of the eye in the angle where the cornea meets the iris through a spongelike meshwork to Schlemm's canal.

ciliary muscles Small muscles that affect the shape of the lens of the eye, permitting accommodation.

circle of support A group of volunteer advocates, such as family members, friends, and neighbors, who make sure that an individual with a developmental disability has a support system that meets all of his or her needs.

CK *See* creatine kinase.

cleft Term used in reference to a congenital deformity of the lip or palate.

clinical cerebellar cognitive affective syndrome A group of abnormal findings including deficits in spatial processing, working memory, and language associated with cerebellar lesions.

clonus Alternate muscle contraction and relaxation in rapid succession.

clonic Related to clonus.

clubfoot A congenital foot deformity; *also called* talipes equinovarus.

CMV *See* cytomegalovirus.

CNS *See* central nervous system.

coagulation Blood clotting.

coagulopathy Bleeding disorder.

coarctation A congenital narrowing, such as of a blood vessel, most commonly of the aorta.

cochlea The snail-shaped structure in the inner ear containing the hearing organ.

cochlear amplification The positive feedback mechanism within the cochlea involving the outer hair cell that increases the amplitude and frequency selectivity of sound vibrations using electromechanical feedback.

cochlear implant (CI) A device surgically implanted in the cochlea of the ear that permits a form of hearing in individuals with deafness.

codons Triplets of nucleotides that form the DNA code.

cognitive strategy instruction (CSI) CSI teaches metacognitive strategies (thinking about thinking) to improve learning and performance. It is beneficial when teaching more complex material involving problem solving and decision making.

cognitive-behavioral therapy (CBT) A type of psychotherapy that focuses on feelings about behavior.

cohort study An epidemiologic study of subgroups of a population identified with some common characteristic (e.g., an exposure, an ethnic background) that are followed or traced over a period of time for the occurrence of disease.

colic A condition in infancy marked by uncontrollable crying usually caused by abdominal discomfort and often the result of gastroesophageal reflux (GER).

coloboma Congenital cleft in the retina, iris, or other ocular structure.

comorbid A coexisting condition that worsens an underlying disorder.

competent Legally recognized to be able to make decisions for oneself. Minors are presumed to be incompetent, except under certain specified conditions that may vary from state to state.

competing stimuli Stimuli that displace the problem behavior, such as providing food or mouthing toys to children who display pica (eating of nonfood items).

competitive employment To engage in competitive employment, individuals with disabilities must have the same skills requisite for any employee to succeed in the workplace: knowledge base for the job, appropriate social skills, effective communication skills, and motivation. Individuals with disabilities also must have appropriate independent living skills and the skills and abilities to manage their disability-related needs, such as hiring and managing personal care attendants and transportation services.

complementary health approaches (CHA) The use of nonmainstream approaches together with conventional medical approaches; *previously called* complementary and alternative medicine (CAM).

complete learning trials Refers to an opportunity to respond that is controlled by the trainer.

compliance training An important prerequisite to instructional training. The instructor orients the child to attend to the instructor and then issues a developmentally appropriate "do" request.

compounding pharmacy A special pharmacy that can make drug formulations that are specifically tailored to patients such as liquid suspensions, suppositories, and creams.

compulsions Repetitive behaviors (e.g., hand washing) or mental acts (e.g., praying and counting) that are done to neutralize an obsession or as part of following rigid rules

computed tomography (CT) An imaging technique in which x-ray "slices" of a structure are viewed and synthesized by a computer, forming an image. CT scans are less clear than magnetic resonance imaging (MRI) scans but are better at localizing certain tumors and areas of calcification.

concave Having a curved, indented surface.

concussion A clinical syndrome caused by a blow to the head, characterized by transient loss of consciousness.

conductive In reference to hearing the conduction and amplification of sound through the middle ear.

conductive hearing loss Hearing loss resulting from a problem in conducting sound waves anywhere along the route through the outer ear, eardrum, or middle ear.

cones Photoreceptor cells of the eye associated with color vision.

congenital Originating prior to birth.

congenital cytomegalovirus (CMV) One of the most common congenital infections that can result in premature birth, growth restriction, microcephaly, seizures, and hearing loss.

congenital myopathies A group of inherited muscle disorders often associated with mitochondrial dysfunction.

congenital varicella syndrome (VZV) A rare congenital infection resulting from maternal chickenpox during the first two trimesters of pregnancy. The characteristic symptoms in the newborn consist of skin lesions, neurologic defects, and eye and skeletal anomalies.

congenital zika syndrome (CZS) A recently described congenital viral infection resulting in severe microcephaly in affected infants.

conjunctiva The mucous membrane that lines the inner surface of the eyelid and the exposed surface of the eyeball.

consanguinity Familial relationship, such as the marriage of first cousins.

conscience A personal sense, generally intuitive and urgent, of the way one should respond under specific circumstances.

consequences Events or contextual factors that occur subsequent to a behavior and may or may not be causally related to it.

conservatorship A circumstance in which the court declares an individual unable to take care of legal matters and appoints another individual (a conservator) to handle these matters on the individual's behalf.

contiguous gene syndrome A genetic syndrome resulting from defects in a number of adjacent genes.

contingent stimulation Applying punishment following the occurrence of a misbehavior.

contingent withdrawal The removal of access to positive reinforcement following a misbehavior.

continuous positive airway pressure (CPAP) Involves providing a mixture of oxygen and air under continuous pressure; this prevents the alveoli from collapsing between breaths.

continuum A spectrum.

contracture A shortening of muscle fibers and soft tissue around a joint that causes decreased mobility and is almost always irreversible.

contralateral Opposite side.

contusion (of brain) Structural damage limited to the surface layer of the brain caused by trauma.

convex Having a curved, elevated/protruding surface, such as a dome.
cooperative learning An instructional method that includes a range of team-based learning strategies.
cooperative play The developmental stage when young children start to play collaboratively with their peers to achieve a common goal, usually around 4–6 years.
copy number variability (CNV) When the number of copies of a particular gene varies from one individual to the next.
cordocentesis *See* percutaneous umbilical blood sampling (PUBS).
cornea The clear dome that covers and protects the iris of the eye.
corpus callosotomy Surgical procedure in which the corpus callosum is cut to prevent the generalized spread of seizures from one hemisphere to another.
corpus callosum The bridge of white matter connecting the two cerebral hemispheres and permitting the exchange of information between the two hemispheres.
corpus striatum Part of the basal ganglia of the brain, comprising the caudate and lentiform nuclei.
cortex The surface of the cerebral hemisphere, composed principally of neurons and glia.
cortical Pertaining to the cortex or gray matter of the brain.
cortical visual impairment Visual impairment caused by damage to the part of the brain related to vision. Although the eye is normal, the brain cannot properly process the information it receives. The degree of vision loss may be mild or severe and can vary greatly, even from day to day.
corticospinal pathways White matter pathways leading from the brain through the spinal corticospinal tract; *see* pyramidal tract.
cortisol A steroid.
CPR *See* cardiopulmonary resuscitation.
CPT *See* chest physiotherapy.
cranial sutures Fibrous material connecting skull bones.
craniofacial Relating to the skull and bones of the face.
craniosynostosis Premature closure of cranial bones.
creatinine Product produced by muscle tissue and normally filtered from the blood by the kidney.
creatine kinase (CK) An enzyme released by damaged muscle cells. Its level is elevated in muscular dystrophy.
crib death *See* sudden infant death syndrome (SIDS).
Crohn's disease An inflammatory bowel disorder.
crossover The exchange of genetic material between two closely aligned chromosomes during the first meiotic division.
cryotherapy The use of freezing temperatures to destroy tissue.
cryptorchidism Undescended testicles.
crystallized intelligence The part of intellectual functioning that involves the use of knowledge and experience to problem solve.
C-section *See* cesarean section.
CSF *See* cerebrospinal fluid.
CT *See* computed tomography.
cultural competence Knowledge of the norms of other cultures and how to partner with patients of various backgrounds.
customized employment A blend of services designed to increase employment options for individuals with significant disabilities such as self-employment, entrepreneurship, job carving and restructuring, personal agents, and customized training.
CVA *See* cerebral vascular accident.
CVS *See* chorionic villus sampling.
cyanosis A bluish discoloration of the skin resulting from poor circulation or inadequate oxygenation of the blood.
cystic fibrosis An autosomal recessively inherited disorder of the secretory glands leading to malabsorption and lung disease.
cystometrogram (urodynamics) A procedure in which fluid is injected into the bladder and pressure is measured.
cytokines A group of molecules that are either pro- or anti-inflammatory and are part of the human immune system.
cytomegalovirus (CMV) A virus that may be asymptomatic or cause symptoms in adults that may resemble mononucleosis. In the fetus, it can lead to severe abnormalities including microcephaly, seizures, hearing loss, retinitis, and delayed development.
cytoplasm The contents of the cell outside the nucleus.
cytosine One of the four nucleotides (chemicals) that comprise DNA.
cytotoxicity Being toxic to cells.
DAI *See* diffuse axonal injury.
dB *See* decibel.
DDH *See* developmental dislocation of the hip.
debridement The removal of dead tissue (e.g., after a burn or an infection).
decibel (dB) A measure of loudness, used in hearing testing.
decubitus ulcers Bed sores.
delay In developmental disabilities, refers to simply to a slower than expected rate in the acquisition of skills, usually defined with reference to widely accepted developmental milestones.
deletion Loss of genetic material from a chromosome.
delirium An organically based psychosis characterized by impaired attention, disorganized thinking, altered and fluctuating levels of consciousness, and memory impairment. It may be caused by encephalitis, diabetes, or intoxication and is usually reversed by treating the underlying medical problem.
delusions False beliefs, often quite bizarre, that are symptoms of psychosis or drug intoxication.
dementia A progressive neurological disorder marked by the loss of memory, decreased speech, impairment in abstract thinking and judgment, other disturbances of higher cortical function, and personality change (e.g., Alzheimer's disease).

dendrite A short branched extension of a nerve cell, along which impulses received from other cells at synapses are transmitted to the cell body.
dental caries Tooth decay.
dental lamina A thickened band of tissue along the future dental arches in the human embryo.
dental organ The embryonic tissue that is the precursor of the tooth; *also called* tooth bud.
dental plaque Patches of bacteria, bacterial byproducts, and food particles on teeth that predispose them to decay.
dental sealant Plastic substance administered to teeth, most commonly the molars, to increase their resistance to decay.
dentin The principal substance of the tooth surrounding the tooth pulp and covered by the enamel.
deoxyribonucleic acid (DNA) The fundamental component of living tissue. It contains an organism's genetic code.
depolarization The eliminating of the electrical charge of a cell.
depolarizing current An electrical current causing a change in cell membrane voltage.
depressed fracture Fracture of bone, usually the skull, that results in an inward displacement of the bone at the point of impact. It requires surgical intervention to prevent damage to underlying tissue.
deprivation In behavior management, denial of access to a reinforcing item or event.
dermal sinus A cavity lining extending from the skin surface to a deeper structure, most notably the spinal cord.
descriptive analysis Involves the quantitative, direct observation of the individual's behaviors as well as antecedent events and consequences under naturalistic conditions.
descriptive and functional analysis Observation period in behavior management that precedes treatment.
detoxification The conversion of a toxic compound to a nontoxic product.
developmental cerebellar cognitive affective syndrome A syndrome described in children who survive prematurity-related cerebellar injury and have deficits that range from impaired executive function to severe behavioral disturbances that fall on the autism spectrum.
developmental coordination disorder (DCD) A nonprogressive disorder of childhood unassociated with a specific neurologic disorder (e.g., cerebral palsy). It is associated with impairments in skilled motor movements that are appropriate for the child's chronological age and thereby interferes with activities of daily living.
developmental delays Refers to a significant lag in the attainment of milestones in one or more areas of development.
developmental deviance Refers to nonsequential unevenness in the achievement of milestones within one or more streams of development.
developmental disabilities A group of chronic conditions that are attributable to an impairment in physical, cognitive, speech/language, psychological, or self-care areas and that are manifested during the developmental period (younger than 21 years of age).
developmental dislocation of the hip (DDH) A congenital hip dislocation, usually evident at birth, occurring more commonly in girls.
developmental dissociation Refers to a significant difference in developmental rates between two areas.
developmental dysarthria Difficulty with speech due to congenital impairment of oral motor structures or musculature.
developmental milestone A physical, language, or adaptive ability that is achieved by most infants and young children by a certain age.
developmental regression Loss of previously attained milestones.
developmental surveillance The evaluation of a child's developmental performance during the routine provision of health care.
deviate *See* diverge.
dextrose A simple sugar similar to glucose and used to medically correct or prevent low blood sugar.
diagnostic overshadowing A situation where health professionals wrongly presume that present symptoms are a consequence of their patient's underlying condition rather than being a new condition.
diagnostic test A test used to definitively confirm or exclude the presence of a disease or condition in a particular individual.
dialysis A detoxification procedure of the blood (i.e., hemodialysis) or across the peritoneum (i.e., peritoneal dialysis) used to treat kidney failure.
diaphysis The shaft of a long bone lying under the epiphysis.
diastematomyelia A congenital defect in which the spinal cord is divided into halves by a bony or cartilaginous divider, often seen in spina bifida.
diencephalon A part of the forebrain.
differential reinforcement A behavior management technique in which a preferred alternate behavior is positively reinforced while a less preferred behavior is ignored.
differential reinforcement of alternative behaviors (DRA) When the delivery of the reinforcer is contingent on the performance of alternative, more appropriate behaviors.
differential reinforcement of other behaviors (DRO) Consists of the delivery of reinforcers (e.g., attention) contingent on the absence of problem behaviors.
diffuse Spread out.
diffuse axonal injury (DAI) Diffuse injury to nerve cell components, usually resulting from shearing forces. This type of traumatic brain injury is commonly associated with motor vehicle accidents.
diffusion-weighted imaging (DWI) A form of magnetic resonance imaging (MRI) scanning that can identify

with great sensitivity areas of brain, especially white matter, that have suffered an acute injury.

diopters Units of refractive power of a lens (e.g., glasses).

diplegia A form of spastic cerebral palsy, most often found in former premature babies, in which the legs are predominantly affected.

diploid Having paired chromosomes in nondividing cells (i.e., 46 chromosomes in 23 pairs).

diplopia Double vision.

direct instruction (DI) A codified approach to teacher-led instruction that provides explicit instruction with teacher modeling, extensive practice through choral response, brisk pacing, and immediate corrective feedback. The DI technique is very successful for teaching fundamental reading skills and building reading fluency and reading comprehension.

disability Refers to decreased in the ability to perform some action, engage in some activity, or participate in some real-life situation or setting.

discrepancy model In education this is often called the "wait-to-fail" model. As the child ages, they will fall far enough behind to have a significant difference between their ability (IQ) and their achievement.

dislocation The displacement of a bone out of a joint space.

disorders of carbohydrate metabolism Inborn errors of metabolism involving enzyme deficiencies in the breakdown of sugars.

dissociated Not associated with.

dissociation A child may demonstrate an uneven pattern of skills, such that in some areas progress is fairly typical whereas in other areas the child demonstrates a significant departure (delay or deviation) from the expected course.

distal Involving muscles or body segments farther from the center of the body.

distension Abdominal distension is due to an accumulation of air, fluid, or food.

diuretics Medications used to reduce intercellular fluid buildup in the body (edema), especially in the lungs.

diving reflex Named for its presence in diving seals, this also occurs in infants during hypoxic ischemic encephalopathy (HIE) and results in the redistribution of blood away from "nonvital organs" (e.g., kidneys, liver, lungs, intestines, and skeletal muscles) to preserve the perfusion of the "vital organs" (i.e., heart, brain, and adrenal glands). This reflex, if prolonged, may result in insufficient blood supply and damage to the nonvital organs.

DMD *See* Duchenne muscular dystrophy.

DNA *See* deoxyribonucleic acid.

DNR *See* do not resuscitate.

do not resuscitate (DNR) Medical orders that state that, should a patient develop a cardiopulmonary arrest, no attempts at resuscitation would be undertaken; *also called* "No Code" orders.

dominant In genetics, referring to a trait that only requires one copy of a gene to be expressed phenotypically. For example, having brown eyes is a dominant trait, so a child receiving a gene for brown eyes from his or her mother or father (or from both parents) will have brown eyes.

dopamine A neurotransmitter involved in attention deficits (e.g., attention-deficit/hyperactivity disorder [ADHD]) and motor function (e.g., Parkinson's disease).

dorsal Back.

dorsal induction Describes the processes of primary and secondary neurulation during embryogenesis.

dorsiflexion Upward movement of the foot.

dorsolateral Involving both the back and side of a body part.

double effect Principle of a moral argument used to defend certain actions that can be anticipated to have both good and bad outcomes.

double helix The coiled structure of DNA; a structure that resembles a twisted ladder.

drug–disease interaction An event in which a *drug* that is intended for therapeutic use causes harmful effects in a patient because of a *disease* or condition that the patient has.

drug–drug interaction An event in which a *drug* that is intended for therapeutic use causes a side effect in a patient because of an interaction with another *drug* the patient is receiving.

dual diagnosis Refers to a combination of an intellectual disability and psychiatric disorder.

dual discrepancy model The student *both* performs below the level evidenced by classroom peers and shows a learning rate substantially below that of classroom peers.

Duchenne muscular dystrophy (DMD) *See* Appendix B.

ductus arteriosus An arterial connection open during fetal life that diverts the blood flow from the pulmonary artery into the aorta, thereby bypassing the not-yet-functional lungs.

ductus venosus Open during fetal life, it is a shunt that allows oxygenated blood from the placenta to bypass the liver and return to the systemic circulation for distribution to the rest of the body.

duodenal Pertaining to the first section of the small intestine.

duodenal atresia Congenital absence of a portion of the first section of the small intestine; often seen in individuals with Down syndrome.

duodenum The first part of the small intestine; the upper part of the small intestine.

DWI *See* diffusion-weighted imaging.

dynamic In the context of orthotics, capable of active movement.

dysarthria Difficulty with speech due to impairment of oral motor structures or musculature.

dyscalculia Learning disability affecting skills in mathematics.

dyscontrol syndrome Intermittent explosive disorder out of proportion to the event that provokes it.

dysesthesias Abnormal sensation, especially to touch, such as burning or electric shock.

dysgraphia Learning disability in areas of processing and reporting information in written form.
dyskinesia An impairment in the ability to control movements characterized by spasmodic or repetitive motions.
dyskinetic cerebral palsy Type of "extrapyramidal" cerebral palsy often involving abnormality of the basal ganglia and manifesting as rigidity, dystonia, or choreoathetosis.
dyslexia Learning disability affecting reading skills; *also called* specific reading disability.
dysmorphic Unusual physical appearance as a result of a genetic disorder.
dysmorphology The study of birth defects, particularly those affecting the anatomy of the child.
dysmotility Abnormal motility of the gut.
dysostosis An abnormal bony formation.
dysphagia Difficulty in swallowing.
dysphasia Impairment of speech consisting of a lack of coordination and failure to arrange words in proper order due to a central brain lesion.
dysplasia Abnormal tissue development.
dyspraxia Inability to perform coordinated movements despite normal function of the central and peripheral nervous systems and muscles.
dysthymia A mild form of depression characterized by a mood disturbance that is present most of the time and is associated with feelings of low self-esteem, hopelessness, poor concentration, low energy, and changes in sleep and appetite; seen most commonly in adolescents.
dystocia Structural abnormalities of the maternal pelvis that cause a difficult labor or childbirth.
dystonia A disorder of the basal ganglia associated with altered muscle tone leading to contorted body positioning; a movement disorder.
dystonic Contorted body positioning resulting from disorder of the basal ganglia.
dystonic cerebral palsy A form of dyskinetic cerebral palsy, the most prominent feature of which is dystonia.
E. coli *See Escherichia coli.*
Eagle-Barrett syndrome Formerly "prune belly syndrome."
early intervention (EI) *See* Chapter 31.
ECG *See* electrocardiogram.
echocardiography An ultrasonic method of imaging the heart. It can be used to detect congenital heart defects even prior to birth.
echolalic Pertaining to immediate or delayed repetition of a word or phrase said by others; often evident in children with autism spectrum disorder.
echolalia *See* echolalic.
ECMO *See* extracorporeal membrane oxygenation.
ectoderm Outer cell layer in the embryo.
ectodermal dysplasia A diverse group of genetic disorders that involve defects of the hair, nails, teeth, skin, and glands. *See* Appendix B.
ectopia Abnormal congenital or acquired position of a body organ.
ectopic Pertaining to ectopia.
ectopic pregnancy Embryo implanted outside of the uterus.
ectrodactyly Congenital absence of all or parts of digits.
eczema A common skin condition, often occurring in childhood, marked by an itchy inflammatory reaction manifested by tiny blisters with reddening, swelling, bumps, and crusting; *also called* atopic dermatitis.
EDC *See* estimated date of confinement.
EDD Estimated due date; *also called* estimated date of confinement.
edema An abnormal accumulation of fluid in the tissues of the body.
EEG *See* electroencephalogram.
efferent Pertaining to the impulses that go to a nerve or muscle from the central nervous system (CNS); for example, motor fibers transmit impulses from the brain to initiate movement.
effusion A middle-ear infection associated with fluid accumulation.
EI *See* early intervention.
Ehlers-Danlos syndrome *See* Appendix B.
EKG *See* electrocardiogram.
ELBW *See* extremely low birth weight.
electrocardiogram (EKG, ECG) The graphic record of an electronic recording of heart rate and rhythm.
electroencephalogram (EEG) A recording of the electrical activity in the brain that is often used in the evaluation of seizures.
electrolytes Minerals contained in the blood, such as sodium, potassium, and chloride.
electromyography (EMG) A technique for measuring muscle activity and function; recording of electric currents associated with muscle contractions are useful in the diagnosis of a variety of neuromuscular disorders, including anterior horn cell disease, neuropathies, neuromuscular junction disorders, and some myopathies.
electroretinogram (ERG) A graphic record of the electrical activity of the retina.
eloquent cortex The area of the cortex involved in the production of speech.
emancipated minor A teenage minor who is legally free of parental control for giving informed consent to any medical treatment.
embryo The earliest stage of conceptional development after fertilization and during the first 8 weeks of pregnancy. The placenta and most of the primitive organs are formed into the major systems during this time.
embryoblasts The mass of cells inside the early embryo that will eventually give rise to the structures of the fetus.
embryotic period The first 8 weeks of pregnancy.
EMG *See* electromyography.
enamel The calcified outer layer of the tooth.
encephalitis Inflammation of the brain, generally from a viral infection.
encephalocele A neural tube defect characterized by a sac-like protrusion of the brain and the membranes that cover it through an opening in the skull. This defect is

caused by failure of the neural tube to close completely during fetal development.

encephalopathy Disorder or disease of the brain.

enclaves Once considered a viable employment option for individuals with severe disabilities; it brings together groups of individuals with disabilities at one site with a common job coach engaged around a work task.

endocardial cushion defect A congenital heart defect, found often in Down syndrome, where there is a lack of closure of the wall separating the two sides of the heart.

endocarditis Inflammation of the inner lining of the heart.

endochondral ossification Formation of bone from cartilage.

endocrine disruptors Chemicals that may interfere with the body's hormonal system and produce adverse developmental, reproductive, neurological, and immune effects.

endoderm The inner cell layer in the embryo.

enriched environments A type of treatment that focuses on providing stimuli that compete with problem behaviors.

enteral nutrition Feeding directly into the stomach through the nose or mouth to ensure that nutritional requirements are met.

enteric nervous system The subdivision of the autonomic nervous system that controls the gastrointestinal system.

enterobacter A rod-shaped bacteria that can cause gastrointestinal symptoms.

enuresis Involuntary urination especially at night in children.

ependymomas Tumors developing from cells that line both the hollow cavities-ventricles of the brain and the canal containing the spinal cord.

epicanthal folds Crescent-shaped fold of skin on either side of the nose, commonly associated with Down syndrome.

epidemiology The study of the distribution and determinants of disease frequency in specific populations.

epidural anesthesia Pain relief by infusing an anesthetic agent into the epidural space of the spine.

epidural hematoma Localized collection of clotted blood lying between the skull and the outer (dural) membrane of the brain, resulting from the hemorrhage of a blood vessel resting in the dura. This most often results from traumatic head injury.

epigastric Relating to the region around the upper abdomen near the stomach.

epigenetics Changes in gene expression that do not permanently alter the DNA sequence.

epiglottis A lid-like structure that hangs over the entrance to the windpipe and prevents aspiration of food or liquid into the lungs during swallowing.

epilepsy A disorder of the brain characterized by repeated seizures and by the neurobiologic, cognitive, psychological, and social consequences of this condition. *See* Chapter 22.

epiphyses The end plates of long bones where linear growth occurs.

epithelial Pertaining to cells that are found on exposed surfaces of the body (e.g., skin, mucous membranes, and intestinal walls).

equinus Involuntary extension (plantar flexion) of the foot (like a horse); this position is often found in spastic cerebral palsy. It leads to toe walking.

ERG *See* electroretinogram.

erythrocytosis An abnormal increase in the number of circulating red blood cells.

erythropoietin A protein that regulates red blood cell production.

Escherichia coli (E. coli) Bacteria that can cause infections ranging from diarrhea to urinary tract infection to sepsis.

esophageal atresia A congenital defect in which there is a stricture in the esophagus, preventing food from entering the stomach.

esophagus Tube through which food passes from the pharynx to the stomach.

esotropia A form of strabismus in which one or both eyes turn in; "cross-eyed."

estimated date of confinement (EDC) Expected date of delivery; *also called* estimated due date (EDD).

estrogen Female sex hormone.

etiology Refers to the cause of a medical condition.

eustachian tube Connection between oral cavity and middle ear, allowing equilibration of pressure and drainage of fluid.

everted Turned outward.

evidence-based research instruction Defined as "research that involves the application of rigorous, systematic, and objective procedures to obtain reliable and valid knowledge relevant to education activities and programs" (U.S. Department of Education, 2007).

excitotoxic Pertaining to excitotoxins—neurochemicals that can cause neuronal cell death and have been implicated in hypoxic brain damage and acquired immunodeficiency syndrome encephalopathy.

executive function The cognitive tasks related to taking in, organizing, processing, and acting on information. Deficits are present in people with autism spectrum disorder (ASD), learning differences, and attention-deficit/hyperactivity disorder.

exfoliation Refers to the removal of the oldest dead skin cells or the shedding of teeth.

exome The portions of a gene (or the entire genome) that code information for protein synthesis.

exons *See* exome.

exon skipping A novel therapy involving a medication that enables RNA splicing to cause cells to "skip" over faulty sections of genetic code, leading to a truncated but still functional protein despite the genetic mutation.

exotropia A form of strabismus in which one or both eyes turn out; "wall-eyed."

expressive language Communication by spoken language, gesture, signing, or body language.

extended release A form of medication that gradually releases its compound leading to a prolonged period of activity, often 8–12 hours.

extension Movement of a limb at a joint to bring the joint into a more straightened position.

extinction The process through which reinforcement is withheld for a previously reinforced response, resulting in a decrease in the future occurrence of that response; *see* planned ignoring.

extinction burst A transient increase in the frequency and intensity of a challenging behavior before a subsequent reduction occurs.

extracorporeal membrane oxygenation (ECMO) An extreme and invasive life support technique that involves putting a patient onto a heart–lung bypass machine.

extract In the context of medication, a concentrated preparation.

extrapyramidal cerebral palsy *See* dyskinetic cerebral palsy.

extrapyramidal system Areas of the brain involved in subconscious, automatic aspects of motor coordination.

extremely low birth weight (ELBW) Term often used to describe an infant with a birth weight less than 1,000 grams (2 1/4 pounds).

fading Behavioral instruction process by which prompts are withdrawn gradually.

FAE Fetal alcohol effects. *See also* Fetal alcohol spectrum disorder (FASD).

failure to thrive (FTT) Inadequate growth of both weight and height in infancy or early childhood caused by malnutrition, chronic disease, or a congenital anomaly.

false-negative result A test result that indicates that a person does not have a specific disorder when the person actually does have the condition.

false-positive result A test result that indicates that a person has a specific disorder when the person actually does not have the condition.

family-centered care An approach to health care that is based on mutual respect that promotes optimal health outcomes and treatment adherence by encouraging shared decision making in daily patient interactions.

family therapy A type of psychotherapy that involves all members of a nuclear family.

fatty acid oxidation disorders Inborn errors of metabolism involving enzyme deficiencies in the breakdown of fatty acids. *See* Appendix B.

febrile Having an elevated body temperature. A child is considered febrile when registering a fever above 100.4°F (38°C).

FEES Flexible endoscopic evaluation of swallowing.

Feingold diet This diet involves removing synthetic colors, flavors, artificial preservatives, salicylates, and sweeteners from the diet.

femur Long bone in the thigh connecting the hip to the knee.

fencer's response *See* asymmetrical tonic neck reflex (ATNR).

fertilization The entrance of a sperm into the egg, resulting in a conception.

FES *See* functional electrical stimulators.

fetal alcohol effects (FAE) Former term for alcohol-related neurodevelopmental disorder (ARND; *see* Chapter 2).

fetal alcohol spectrum disorders (FASD) Umbrella term for a range of physical and neurodevelopmental disabilities associated with prenatal alcohol exposure.

fetal heart rate (FHR) Normally 120–140 beats per minute and routinely monitored by ultrasound throughout labor to indicate fetal well-being versus fetal distress (i.e., FHR < 100).

fetal heart rate monitoring Monitoring fetal heart rate with ultrasound.

fetal period The time of pregnancy between the 10th week and birth.

FHR *See* fetal heart rate.

fibroma A benign fibrous tumor of connective tissue.

FISH *See* fluorescent *in situ* hybridization.

fissures On the brain, these are deeper than sulci, are first visible during fetal development, and separate each hemisphere into four functional areas or lobes.

flexion Movement of a limb to bend at a joint.

flexor A muscle with the primary function of flexion or bending at a joint.

flexor and extensor spasms Spasms of bending of a limb toward or away from the body.

flora In medicine, bacteria normally residing within a body organ and not causing disease, such as *E. coli* in the intestine.

fluency Aspect of speech, that is, producing speech in a fluid manner.

fluid intelligence The general ability to think abstractly, reason, identify patterns, solve problems, and discern relationships.

fluorescent in situ hybridization (FISH) Technology used to diagnose a number of microdeletion syndromes.

fluorosis A chronic condition caused by excessive intake of fluoride containing compounds, marked by mottling of the teeth.

fMRI *See* functional magnetic resonance imaging.

focal Localized.

focal neurological changes Findings on neurological exams that are abnormal and indicative of a lesion in a particular location in the brain; *also called* focal neurological impairments.

folic acid A vitamin, a deficiency of which during early pregnancy has been linked to neural tube defects.

foramen ovale A tiny window between the right atrium and the left atrium.

forebrain The front portion of the brain during fetal development; *also called* the prosencephalon.

forward chaining A behavior management technique in which the first skill in a sequence is taught first and the last skill is taught last.

fovea *See* fovea centralis.

fovea centralis The small pit in the center of the macula; the area of clearest vision, containing only cones.
frame shift A type of gene mutation in which the insertion or deletion of a single nucleotide leads to the misreading of all subsequent codons as the three base pair reading frame is shifted.
free level In pharmacotherapy, the amount of active drug that is able to produce an effect on the body.
free radicals Chemical compounds, the abnormal accumulation of which has been linked to cancer and neurotoxicity.
frequency Cycles per second, or hertz (Hz), a measure of sound.
frontal lobe Controls both voluntary motor activity and important aspects of cognition.
FTT *See* failure to thrive.
full mutation Having over 200 CGG repeats causing the clinical expression in a triplet repeat disorder such as fragile X syndrome.
functional (experimental) analysis *See* applied behavioral analysis.
functional electrical stimulators (FES) Provide neural stimulation to increase mobility.
functional magnetic resonance imaging (fMRI) A neuroimaging procedure that permits evaluation of the effects of activities, such as reading, on brain function.
fundoplication An operation in which the top of the stomach is wrapped around the opening of the esophagus to correct gastroesophageal reflux disease (GERD).
FXS Fragile X syndrome (*see* Chapter 15).
G tube *See* gastrostomy tube.
GABA *See* gamma-aminobutyric acid.
galactosemia An inborn error of metabolism involving an enzyme deficiency that prevents the breakdown of the sugar galactose, a component of many foods. *See* Appendix B.
gamma-aminobutyric acid (GABA) An amino acid that acts as an inhibitory neurotransmitter.
ganglia Masses of nerve cell bodies.
gastric tube A tube inserted through the abdominal wall that delivers nutrition directly to the stomach.
gastrocolic reflex A trigger that results in an urge to defecate; it generally occurs 30–60 minutes after a meal.
gastroenteritis An acute illness marked by vomiting and diarrhea usually associated with a viral infection (e.g., rotavirus in infants) that generally lasts a few days; *also called* stomach flu.
gastroesophageal duodenoscopy Endoscopy in which a flexible instrument with a light source examines the esophagus, stomach, and small bowel.
gastroesophageal reflux disease (GER/GERD) The backward flow of food into the esophagus after it has entered the stomach; acid reflux.
gastrointestinal (GI) tract The stomach and small intestine.
gastrojejunal (G-J) tube A feeding tube that is inserted through a gastrostomy site and threaded through the stomach and duodenum into the jejunum (the second part of the small intestine).
gastrojejunostomy (G-J) Surgical procedure to prepare for gastrojejunostomy (G-J) tube.
gastroschisis Congenital malformation of the abdominal wall resulting in the protrusion of abdominal organs.
gastrostomy An operation in which an artificial opening is made into the stomach through the wall of the abdomen. This is usually done in order to place a feeding tube into the stomach.
gastrostomy (G) tube A permanent tube placed directly through the skin and into the stomach.
gastrulation stage The phase early in embryonic development during which the single-layered blastula is reorganized into a three-layered structure (the ectoderm, mesoderm, and endoderm).
GBS *See* group B *Streptococcus*.
GDD *See* global developmental delay.
gene A molecular unit of heredity consisting of stretches of DNA and RNA that code for a type of protein or for an RNA chain that has a function in the organism.
gene editing The use of biotechnological approaches to make changes to specific DNA sequences in the genome.
gene therapy The transplantation of normal genes into cells in place of missing or defective ones in order to correct genetic disorders.
genome The complete set of hereditary units (genes) in an organism.
genomic imprinting A condition manifested differently depending on whether the trait is inherited from the mother or father; *also called* uniparental disomy. An example is a deletion in chromosome 15q11–q13, which, when inherited from the mother, results in Angelman syndrome and, when inherited from the father, results in Prader-Willi syndrome. *See* Chapter 1 and Appendix B.
genotype The genetic composition of an individual.
genu varum Bowed legs.
GERD *See* gastroesophageal reflux.
germ cells The cells involved in reproduction (i.e., sperm, eggs).
German measles *See* rubella.
germinal stage Begins with conception and ends when the blastocyst is fully implanted into the uterine wall.
gestational age (GA) The measure of the duration of a pregnancy in weeks, usually taken from the date of the woman's last menstrual period.
GI *See* gastrointestinal tract.
gingiva The gums.
gingivitis Gum inflammation.
G-J tube *See* gastrojejunal tube.
glaucoma Increased pressure within the anterior chamber of the eye that can cause blindness.
glia Cells that compose the white matter and provide a support function for neurons.
glial Pertaining to glia.
global developmental delay (GDD) Significant delays in development of two or more of the following domains:

gross motor/fine motor, speech/language, cognition, social/personal, and activities of daily living (ADL).

globus pallidus A subcortical area of the brain that is a major component of the basal ganglia and is part of the extrapyramidal system.

glossoptosis Downward or backward displacement of the tongue, as in Down syndrome.

glucose A simple sugar that is an important energy source and is a component of many carbohydrates.

glutaminergic neurons Brain cells that release the chemical glutamate, an excitatory neurotransmitter.

gluten-/casein-free diet Involves removing all wheat and milk products from the child's diet.

glycine An amino acid that is a constituent of most proteins and can serve as an excitatory neurotransmitter.

glycogen The chief carbohydrate stored in the body, primarily in the liver and muscles.

GMFCS *See* gross motor function classification system.

goiter Enlargement of the thyroid gland.

Golgi apparatus The intracellular organelle that packages proteins in a form that can be released through the cell membrane and carried throughout the body.

goniometry Use of a hinged measuring tool to determine joint range of motion.

graduated guidance A behavior management technique in which only the level of assistance (guidance) necessary for the child to complete the task is provided.

graft-versus-host disease A mechanism of the body's immune system that destroys foreign proteins. It can be life-threatening when it occurs in a child who has received a bone marrow or organ transplant and has a suppressed immune system. Symptoms include diarrhea, skin breakdown, and shock.

grammar The system of and rules for using units of meaning (morphemes) and syntax in language.

grapheme A unit, such as a letter, of a writing system.

gravida/para The number of times a woman has been pregnant (gravid) and has delivered (parous) a living infant.

grey matter The part of the brain rich in neurons. It comprises the cortex.

gross motor function classification system (GMFCS) An assessment of ambulatory ability for children with cerebral palsy.

group B *Streptococcus* (GBS) Bacteria, causing one of the most common and severe neonatal infections.

guanine One of the four nucleotides (chemicals) that comprises DNA.

guided compliance A behavior management technique involving the use of graduated guidance to teach functional tasks.

Guillain-Barré syndrome An acute inflammatory peripheral neuropathy (*see* Appendix B).

gynecomastia Excessive breast growth in males.

gyri Convolutions of the surface of the brain; *singular*: gyrus.

habilitation The teaching of new skills to children with developmental disabilities. It is called habilitation rather than rehabilitation because these children did not possess these skills previously.

Haemophilus influenzae A bacteria that can cause serious infections in children including meningitis.

hallucinations Sensory perceptions without a source in the external world. These most commonly occur as symptoms of psychosis, drug intoxication, or seizures.

hamartomas A benign (not cancer) growth made up of an abnormal mixture of cells and tissues normally found in the area of the body where the growth occurs.

hand splints A form of low-tech assistive device for children with cerebral palsy or neuromuscular disorder.

haploid Having a single set of human chromosomes (23), as in the sperm or egg.

hCG *See* human chorionic gonadotropin.

health disparities Racial or ethnic differences in the quality of health care that are not due to access-related factors or clinical needs, preferences, and appropriateness of intervention.

health equity The absence of systematic disparities in health or social determinants of health between social groups who have different levels of underlying social advantage or disadvantage.

health literacy The capacity to obtain, process, and understand basic health information and services that are needed to make appropriate decisions about one's own or one's child's health.

hearing loss A condition characterized by a decrease in the ability to hear based on decreased intensity, loudness as measured in decibels (dB), or frequency of sound.

hemangiomas Congenital abnormal masses of blood vessels, such as "birth marks."

hematocrit Percentage of red blood cells in whole blood, normally about 35%–40%.

hematologic Relating to the blood system.

hematopoietic Relating to the formation of red blood cells.

hematuria Blood in the urine.

hemihypertrophy Asymmetric overgrowth of the face or limbs.

hemiplegia Spasticity and weakness on one side of the body.

hemispherectomy Surgical removal of most of one cerebral hemisphere for treatment of intractable generalized seizures.

hemodialysis A detoxification procedure in which an individual's blood is gradually removed through an artery, passed through an artificial kidney machine, and then returned cleansed. It is used most commonly to treat end stage renal disease.

hemoglobin Blood protein capable of carrying oxygen to body tissues.

hemolytic Excessive breakdown of red blood cells.

hemolytic anemia Anemia due to the destruction of red blood cells.

hemostat A small surgical clamp used to constrict a tube or blood vessel.

hepatomegaly Enlarged liver.
hepatosplenomegaly Enlargement of the liver and spleen.
herpes simplex virus (HSV) A virus that can lead to symptoms that range from cold sores to genital lesions to encephalitis; also a cause of fetal malformations and sepsis in early infancy.
hertz (Hz) Cycles per second; a measure of the frequency of sound.
heteroplasmy The presence of multiple kinds of mitochondrial DNA within a single cell or individual.
heterotopia Migration and development of normal neural tissue in an abnormal location in the brain.
heterozygous Carrying two genes that are dissimilar for one trait.
hexosaminidase An enzyme, a deficiency of which leads to Tay-Sachs disease.
HIE *See* hypoxic ischemic encephalopathy.
high-stakes testing One of the most controversial tenets of the No Child Left Behind (NCLB) Act of 2001. Under NCLB, all students, in all schools, in all districts must take standardized assessments to determine whether they are functioning on grade level in the areas of reading/language arts, math, and science, regardless of disability.
high-tech assistive technology A form of assistive technology that is complicated and often expensive to own and maintain.
hippocampus A region of the brain in the floor of each lateral ventricle that has a central role in the formation of memories, emotion, and the rapid learning of new information.
hippotherapy The therapeutic use of horseback riding.
Hirschsprung disease Congenitally enlarged colon.
HMD *See* hyaline member disease.
holoprosencephaly A congenital defect manifest by impaired cleavage of the cerebral hemispheres. *See* Appendix B.
homeobox (HOX) A group of genes involved in early embryonic development.
homeostasis Metabolic equilibrium of the body.
homozygous Carrying identical genes for any given trait.
HOX *See* homeobox.
HSV *See* herpes simplex virus.
human chorionic gonadotropin (hCG) The hormone secreted by the embryo that prevents its expulsion from the uterus. A pregnancy test measures the presence of this hormone in the blood or urine.
hyaline membrane disease (HMD) A disorder characterized by respiratory distress in the newborn period, principally in premature infants; *also called* respiratory distress syndrome (RDS).
hybrid Offspring of parents of different species.
hydrocephalus A condition characterized by the abnormal accumulation of cerebrospinal fluid within the ventricles of the brain. In infants, this leads to enlargement of the head and compression of the brain.
hyperacusis Unusual sensitivity to certain sounds such as a vacuum cleaner, often found in children with autism.
hyperalimentation *See* parenteral feeding.
hyperbaric oxygen therapy (HBOT) Involves breathing 100% oxygen while under increased atmospheric pressure.
hyperbilirubinemia Excess accumulation of bilirubin in the blood, which can result in jaundice, a yellowing of the complexion and/or the whites of the eyes, or kernicterus, the yellow staining of certain central parts of the brain.
hypercholesterolemia Elevated cholesterol levels in blood.
hyperglycemia High blood sugar level as seen in diabetes.
hyperimmune globulin Blood that is especially rich in antibodies against a virus.
hyperkalemia Elevations in levels of potassium in the blood.
hyperopia Farsightedness.
hyperparathyroidism High level of blood parathyroid hormone, which causes abnormalities in calcium and phosphorous metabolism.
hyperphagia Pathological overeating.
hyperreflexia Increased deep tendon reflexes, such as the knee jerk.
hypersynchronous In the context of the central nervous system (CNS), pertaining to the discharge of many neurons at the same time that leads to a seizure.
hypertelorism Widely spaced eyes.
hypertension Elevated blood pressure.
hyperthermia Significantly elevated body temperature.
hyperthyroidism Condition resulting from excessive production of thyroid hormone.
hypertonia Increased muscle tone as seen in spastic cerebral palsy.
hypertrichosis Excessive hair growth.
hypertrophy Overgrowth of a body part or organ.
hypocalcemia Low blood calcium level.
hypogenitalism Having small genitalia.
hypoglycemia Low blood sugar level, usually below a concentration of 40–50 milligrams of glucose per 100 milliliters of blood for a period of time.
hypogonadism Decreased function of sex glands with resultant retarded growth and sexual development.
hypomania Symptoms not severe enough to meet full mania criteria, with being silly not euphoric, talking fast or too much but not pressured, and babbling incoherently.
hypopharynx The area at the back of the throat where the larynx sits next to the entrance to the esophagus.
hypoplasia Defective formation of a tissue or body organ leading it to be small and underdeveloped.
hypoplastic lungs Small lungs that are not fully developed.
hyporeflexia Decreased deep tendon reflexes.
hypospadias A congenital defect in which the opening of the urethra is on the underside, rather than at the end, of the penis.

hypotelorism The presence of an abnormally decreased distance between the two eyes.
hypotension Low blood pressure.
hypothalamus A portion of the brain that directs a number of important bodily functions including many autonomic functions of the peripheral nervous system. Connections with structures of the endocrine and nervous systems enable the hypothalamus to play a vital role in maintaining homeostasis. The hypothalamus also influences various emotional responses.
hypothermia Excessively low body temperature.
hypothyroidism Condition resulting from deficient production of thyroid hormone.
hypotonia Decreased muscle tone.
hypoxemia Seriously low blood oxygen supply to the entire body.
hypoxia A lower-than-normal concentration of oxygen in blood.
hypoxia-ischemia Lack of adequate oxygenation and/or blood circulation.
hypoxic Having reduced oxygen content in body tissues.
hypoxic ischemic encephalopathy (HIE) An acute brain malfunction often resulting in coma caused by acute reduction in the blood flow and the oxygen supply to the brain.
hypsarrhythmia Electroencephalographic (EEG) abnormality seen in infants with infantile spasms. It is marked by chaotic spike–wave activity.
hysterectomy The surgical removal of the uterus.
Hz *See* hertz.
ichthyosis Dry and scaly skin.
ictal Pertaining to a seizure event.
IDDM *See* insulin-dependent diabetes mellitus.
idiopathic Without an identifiable cause.
IEP *See* individualized education program.
IFSP *See* individualized family service plan.
IH *See* learning/instructional hierarchy.
ileostomy A surgically placed opening from the small intestine through the abdominal wall to divert bowel or bladder contents after an operation.
ileum Lower portion of the small intestine.
imaginative play When a child uses their imagination to make believe with role-play scenarios.
imitation training A behavior management technique in which the teacher demonstrates the desired behavior, asks the child to complete the action, and provides positive reinforcement when the task is completed.
immunoglobulin An antibody produced by the body after exposure to a foreign agent, such as a virus.
impact In reference to traumatic head injury, the forcible striking of the head against an object.
imperforate Lacking a normal opening in a body organ. The most common example in childhood is an absent or closed anus.
implantation The attachment and imbedding of the fertilized egg (blastocyst) into the mucous lining of the uterus.
implicit bias Attitudes or stereotypes that affect our understanding, actions, and decisions in an unconscious manner and may be favorable or unfavorable toward a particular social group.
in utero Occurring during fetal development.
***in vitro* fertilization** Fertilization of harvested eggs and allowing them to develop in culture to the blastomere, or eight-cell stage, at which point they are implanted into the uterus of the recipient.
inborn error of metabolism An inherited enzyme deficiency leading to the disruption of normal bodily metabolism (e.g., phenylketonuria [PKU]). *See* Chapter 16.
incidence The rate of occurrence of new cases of a disorder in a population expressed as a function of time.
incidental teaching An ardent attempt to catch the child complying with commands or following instructions in his or her everyday life and to praise (reinforce) the performance.
incisors Front teeth used for cutting.
incus One of the three small bones in the middle ear that help amplify sound.
independent residential alternatives (IRA) Independent living centers; group homes designed for one to three individuals.
indirect assessment Simplest method of gathering information about behavioral function that consist of questionnaires and rating scales that are completed by caregivers.
individualized education program (IEP) A written plan, mandated by federal law, that maps out the objectives and goals that a child receiving special education services is expected to achieve over the course of the school year.
individualized family service plan (IFSP) A written plan detailing early intervention and related services to be provided to an infant or toddler with disabilities in accordance with federal law.
inertial Pertaining to the tendency to keep moving in the same direction as the force that produced the movement.
infantile spasms A seizure type in infancy marked by brief flexor spasms, usually lasting 1–3 seconds.
infarction Obstruction of the blood supply to an organ or region of tissue causing death of the tissue.
inferior In anatomy, below.
inferior vena cava The main vein feeding into the baby's heart.
influenza An acute illness caused by a virus that attacks the respiratory tract.
informed consent The written consent of a person to undergo a procedure or treatment after its risks and benefits have been explained in easily understood language.
inhaled nitric oxide (iNO) A therapeutic gas for treating persistent pulmonary hypertension of the neonate (PPHN). It is mixed with the baby's oxygen supply in miniscule amounts and directly stimulates pulmonary function.

inner ear Comprised of the semicircular canals and cochlea, which form the organs of balance and hearing and are embedded in the temporal bone of the skull.

instructional training A behavior management technique in which the teacher describes the desired behavior, asks the child to perform it, and provides positive reinforcement upon completion of the task.

insulin-dependent diabetes mellitus (IDDM) A disorder in which blood sugar level is high enough to require treatment with insulin.

insult An attack on a body organ that causes damage to it. This may be physical, metabolic, immunological, or infectious.

integrative medicine Refers to a practice that combines conventional and types of complementary and alternative treatments for which there is evidence of safety and effectiveness.

intellectual disability Significantly subaverage general intellectual functioning accompanied by significant limitations in adaptive functioning; *previously called* mental retardation. *See* Chapter 14.

intensity Strength.

interictal In an individual with a seizure disorder, pertaining to the periods when seizures are not occurring.

internal capsule The area of white matter in the brain that separates the caudate nucleus and the thalamus from the lenticular nucleus. The internal capsule contains both ascending and descending axons so it can control distant movement.

interpersonal psychotherapy (IPT) A time-limited psychotherapy that focuses on building interpersonal skills.

interphase The period in the cell life cycle when the cell is not dividing.

interval schedules Provision of reinforcement based on the passage of a certain amount of time relative to the child's performance of a behavior or task.

intervillous space the space between the villi of the placenta containing the vessels of both mother and embryo.

intrathecal The infusion of medication into the spinal space.

intrauterine growth restriction (IUGR) Fetal weight that is below the 10th percentile for gestational age as determined through an ultrasound; *also called* fetal growth restriction or small for gestational age.

intravenous Infusion into a vein.

intraventricular hemorrhage (IVH) A hemorrhage into the cerebral ventricles.

introns The noncoding regions of the genome.

intubation Insertion of a tube through the nose or mouth into the trachea to permit mechanical ventilation.

inversion In genetics, the result of two breaks on a chromosome followed by the reinsertion of the missing fragment at its original site but in the inverted order.

ionic Pertaining to mineral ions, a group of atoms carrying a charge of electricity.

iris The circular, colored membrane behind the cornea that surrounds the pupil.

ischemia A decreased blood flow to an area of the body that leads to tissue death.

isochromosome A chromosome with two copies of one arm and no copy of the other.

isometric contraction Muscular contraction against resistance in which the length of the muscle remains the same.

ITP *See* individualized transition plan.

IUGR *See* intrauterine growth restriction.

IVH *See* intraventricular hemorrhage.

J tube *See* jejunostomy tube.

Jacksonian seizure Spread of focal epileptiform activity to contiguous brain areas resulting in a seizure which starts in one part of the body and involves adjacent body regions as the seizure evolves.

jaundice A yellowing of the complexion and the whites of the eyes resulting from hyperbilirubinemia.

jejunostomy (J) tube A tube placed through the skin of the abdomen and directly into the jejunum to provide nutrition.

jejunum The second portion of the small intestine.

joint attention A precommunication skill in which an adult and a young child share gestures and eye gaze toward the same object or event. This skill is lacking in the young child with autism spectrum disorder.

kangaroo care A method of caring for premature babies in which the infants are held skin-to-skin with the mother throughout the day.

karyotyping Photographing the chromosomal makeup of a cell. In a human, there are 23 pairs of chromosomes in a normal karyotype.

kernicterus A disorder caused by severe jaundice in the newborn, with deposition of the pigment bilirubin in the brain leading to athetoid cerebral palsy, hearing loss, vision problems, and/or intellectual disability.

ketogenic diet Special diet high in fat used to promote the use of ketones as an energy source; used in some children with intractable epilepsy.

ketosis The buildup of acid in the body, most often associated with starvation, inborn errors of metabolism, or diabetes.

Klebsiella pneumoniae A bacteria that can cause pneumonia, especially in immunocompromised individuals.

kyphoscoliosis A combination of humping and curvature of the spine.

kyphosis An excessive anterior (forward) curvature of the spine creating a hump.

labyrinth One of the major components of the inner ear, the other being the cochlea.

lactase Enzyme necessary to digest the milk sugar lactose.

lactic acid Chemical produced in muscles as a result of anaerobic glucose metabolism.

lacrimal gland Gland that produces tears.

lactose Milk sugar composed of glucose and galactose.

laminar Layered.

lanugo Fine body hair found in newborns.

large for gestational age (LGA) Weighing more than 4 kilograms, about 9 or more pounds at birth. This typically occurs in infants of diabetic mothers.
lateral To the side; away from the midline.
lateral ventricles Cavities in the interior of the cerebral hemisphere containing cerebrospinal fluid. They are enlarged with hydrocephalus or with brain atrophy.
laterality Dominance of one side of the brain, eyes, or hands in controlling particular functions.
law of effect Functional relationship between behavior and its consequences.
LBW *See* low birth weight.
learned helplessness Occurs when families, teachers, and other well-intentioned people often protect youth with disabilities from making mistakes and avoid discussing the ramifications of a child's disability as they help them prepare for adulthood.
learning disability A developmental disability characterized by difficulty with certain academic skills such as reading or writing in individuals with typical intelligence. *See* Chapter 20.
learning/instructional hierarchy (IH) Describes behaviors to be learned and mastered, not only by their form but by the level of proficiency with which they are performed.
left ventricular hypertrophy Enlargement of the left side of the heart.
lens The biconvex, translucent body that rests in front of the vitreous humor of the eye and precisely focuses the light rays on the retina.
lentiform nucleus A large, cone-shaped mass of gray matter just lateral to the internal capsule of the brain.
lesions Injuries or loss of function.
leukemias Blood cell cancers.
lexicon The vocabulary of a person.
LGA *See* large for gestational age.
ligament A sheet or band of tough, fibrous tissue connecting bones or cartilage at a joint.
ligamentous laxity Double jointedness; hyperflexibility.
linear fracture Break of a bone in a straight line; refers to a type of skull fracture or fracture of a long bone (arm or leg).
lipid metabolism The creation and/or breakdown of lipids including cholesterol and fat-soluble vitamins.
lipoma A benign, fatty tissue tumor.
lissencephaly A congenital abnormality marked by a "smooth" brain due to incomplete neuronal proliferation and migration and resultant lack of folds (gyri) and grooves (sulci). *See* Appendix B.
listeria monocytogenes The causative agent of listeriosis.
locus Focus or location.
lordosis An excessive posterior (backward) curvature of the spine.
low birth weight (LBW) Term often used to describe an infant with a birth weight less than 2,500 grams (5 1/2 pounds).
lower esophageal sphincter (LES) The muscular valve connecting the esophagus and stomach and normally preventing reflux.
low-tech assistive technology An assistive device that does not require batteries or other electric sources to operate.
lumbar Pertaining to the lower back.
lumbar puncture The tapping of the subarachnoid space to obtain cerebrospinal fluid from the lower back region. This procedure is used to diagnose meningitis and to measure chemicals in the spinal fluid; *also called* a spinal tap.
lumbosacral plexus Nerves arising from the lower back enlargement of the spinal cord and controlling leg movement.
lymphadenopathy Enlargement of lymph nodes.
lymphocyte A type of white blood cell.
lymphoma A cancerous growth of lymphoid tissue.
lyonization The genetic principle discovered by Mary Lyon that there is X chromosome inactivation in females.
lysosome Minute organelle in cells that contains enzymes used to digest potentially toxic material.
macrocephaly Large head size.
macroorchidism Having abnormally large testicles; found in fragile X syndrome.
macrosomia Large body size.
macrostomia Large mouth.
macula The area of the retina that contains the greatest concentration of cones and the fovea centralis, where central vision is processed.
magnetic resonance imaging (MRI) Imaging procedure that uses the magnetic resonance of atoms to provide clear images of interior parts of the body. It is particularly useful in diagnosing structural abnormalities of the brain.
magnetic resonance spectroscopy (MRS) A study that can be done as part of a regular MRI scan. Rather than provide a picture of the brain, it analyzes the presence and amount of certain metabolic components in various brain regions. It is particularly helpful in diagnosing certain inborn errors of metabolism, such as mitochondrial disorders (*see* Appendix B).
major depression A prolonged period of depressed mood.
malformations Abnormally formed body parts.
malignant hyperthermia A life-threatening elevation of body temperature associated with the administration of an anesthetic agent.
malleus One of the three small bones in the middle ear that help amplify sound.
malnutrition Inadequate nutrition for typical growth and development to occur.
malocclusion The improper fitting together of the upper and lower teeth.
mandible Lower jaw bone.
mania A distinct period of abnormally and persistently elevated, expansive, or irritable mood. This mood disturbance is sufficiently severe to cause impairment in function.
manic depression *See* bipolar disorder.
Marfan syndrome Disorder of connective tissue that strengthens the body's structures (*see* Appendix B).

mass spectrometry A technique used for identifying chemical, drug, or metabolic abnormalities in the blood or urine.

mastoiditis Infection of the mastoid air cells that rest in the temporal bone behind the ear. This is an infrequent complication of chronic middle-ear infection.

mature minor A teenage minor who may give consent because the physician judges that he or she understands the nature, purpose, and risks of the proposed treatment; generally limited to minors at least 15 years old where the treatment is for the patient's own benefit and is judged necessary by conservative medical opinion (compare with *emancipated minor*).

maxilla The bony region of the upper jaw.

maxillary hypoplasia Incomplete development of the upper jaw.

MBD *See* metabolic bone disease.

meconium The thick and tarry stool that is formed during fetal life consisting of swallowed amniotic fluid debris, gastrointestinal mucous and green bile secretions from the liver, and sloughed off gastrointestinal epithelial cells; is not normally passed until after birth.

medial Toward the center or midline.

median plane The midline plane of the body. It runs vertically and separates the left and right halves of the body.

medical assistive technology Subset of assistive technology that is used for primarily medical or life-sustaining reasons (e.g., ventilators and feeding pumps).

medical home Involves a trusting partnership between a child, a child's family, and the pediatric primary care team who oversees the child's health and well-being within a community-based system that provides uninterrupted care to support and sustain optimal health outcomes.

medication reconciliation The process of creating an accurate list of all the medications a patient is taking and comparing that list against the physician's admission, transfer, and/or discharge orders to ensure that both match.

medium chain fatty acids Fatty acids that can bypass the normal uptake process and go directly to the liver.

medulloblastomas Cerebellar tumors.

megavitamin therapy The use of more than 10 times the average daily required amount of vitamins; *also called* orthomolecular therapy.

meiosis Reductive cell division occurring only in eggs and sperm in which the daughter cells receive half (23) the number of chromosomes of the parent cells (46).

melanocytes Pigment-forming skin cells.

melatonin A naturally occurring hormone available as an over-the-counter preparation for which there is evidence of efficacy in improving sleep onset in children with disabilities who have sleep problems.

Mendelian traits Dominant and recessive traits inherited according to the genetic principles put forward by Gregor Mendel.

meningeal Related to the meninges, the three membranes enveloping the brain and spinal cord.

meningitis Infection, often bacterial, of the meninges or sac that surround the brain.

meningocele Protrusion of the meninges through a defect in the skull or vertebral column; a neural tube defect.

meningoencephalitis A generalized and often devastating infection of the brain and central nervous system.

meningomyelocoele Protrusion of meninges and malformed spinal cord through a defect in the vertebral column; *also called* myelomeningocele.

menses Menstrual flow.

mental retardation *See* intellectual disability.

mentation Thinking.

mesencephalon Midbrain region.

mesial temporal sclerosis Scarring in the middle temporal lobes of the brain often leading to partial seizures. *See* Chapter 22.

mesoderm Middle cell layer in the embryo.

messenger ribonucleic acid (mRNA) RNA, synthesized from a DNA template during transcription, that mediates the transfer of genetic information from the cell nucleus to ribosomes in the cytoplasm, where it serves as a template for protein synthesis.

metabolic bone disease (MBD) *Previously called* renal osteodystrophy, results from abnormalities in calcium, phosphorous, vitamin D, and parathyroid hormone.

metaphase The stage in cell division in which each chromosome doubles.

metaphyses The ends of the shaft of long bones connected to the epiphyses.

methionine An amino acid.

methylation The attachment of methyl groups to DNA at the cytosine base that turns gene function off.

microboard A non-profit corporation, usually of family members and friends of a person with a disability, created to support that person.

microcephaly Abnormally small head.

microdeletion A microscopic deletion in a chromosome associated with a loss of a small number of contiguous genes; a chromosomal deletion spanning several genes that is too small to be detected under the microscope using conventional cytogenetic methods but can be detected using newer molecular genetic techniques such as microarrays.

microdeletion syndromes Genetic disorders caused by mutations in a small number of contiguous genes, an example being velocardiofacial syndrome; *see also* contiguous gene syndrome.

microdontia Very small teeth.

micrognathia Receding chin.

microphthalmia Small eye.

micropreemie Term often used to describe an infant born weighing less than 800 grams (1.75 pounds) or before 26 weeks.

microswitches Switches used to control computers, environmental control systems, or power wheelchairs that have been adapted so that less pressure than normal is required for activation.

microtia Small ear.

microtrauma Small injuries such as stress cracks or fractures that occur in the growth area or cartilage of growing bones as a result of high impact or overloading.

mid-tech assistive technology An assistive device that generally requires battery/electrical power or is more complex in its use; for example, teletypewriter (TTY) devices for those who are deaf, home-infusion pumps, suction machines, and sophisticated manual wheelchairs.

middle ear The part of the ear that consists of the eardrum and, beyond it, a cavity ending in a chain of three little bones that connect the middle ear to the internal ear.

MII *See* multiple intraluminal impedance.

milligram One thousandth of a gram.

milliliter One thousandth of a liter; equal to about 15 drops.

mindfulness practice The psychological process of bringing one's attention to the internal and external experiences occurring in the present moment, which can be developed through the practice of meditation or other training.

missense mutation Gene error (mutation) resulting from the replacement of a single nucleic acid for another, resulting in a misreading of the DNA code.

mitochondrial myopathy Congenital muscle disorder caused by a mutation in the mitochondrial DNA.

mitosis Cell division in which two daughter cells of identical chromosomal composition to the parent cell are formed. Each contains 46 chromosomes.

mixed cerebral palsy A form of cerebral palsy with spastic and dyskinetic components; this term is used when more than one type of motor pattern is present and when one pattern does not clearly predominate over another.

MOs *See* motivating operations.

modification In special education, a substantial change in the method or scoring scale used to assess a student's academic performance or knowledge (e.g., using a portfolio of work to demonstrate a student's learning).

molded ankle-foot orthoses A plastic insert for the shoe that is used to treat toe walking.

monosomy Chromosome disorder in which one chromosome is absent. The most common example is Turner syndrome, XO (*see* Appendix B).

monosomy X Turner syndrome (*see* Appendix B).

morbidity Medical complication of an illness, procedure, or operation.

moro reflex A primitive reflex elicited when a newborn infant experiences a sudden drop of the head and neck or a loud noise. The infant responds with sudden extension and then flexion of the neck, arms, and legs, and then cries irritably.

morphemes The smallest linguistic units of meaning.

morula The group of cells formed by the first divisions of a fertilized egg.

mosaic trisomy Type of Down syndrome in which the individual has two distinct populations of cells, one containing 46 chromosomes and the other containing 47 chromosomes.

mosaicism The presence of two genetically distinct types of cells in one individual.

MOSF *See* multi-organ system failure.

motivating operations (MOs) Play a central role in the operant learning conceptualization of motivation; produces two effects: 1) a change in the value of a consequence and 2) a corresponding change in the strength of motivation.

motor point block The injection of a denaturing agent into the nerve supply of a spastic muscle. This effectively interrupts the nerve supply at the entry site to a spastic muscle without compromising sensation and results in the return of tone toward normal.

MRI *See* magnetic resonance imaging.

mRNA *See* messenger ribonucleic acid.

MRS *See* magnetic resonance spectroscopy.

MS/MS *See* tandem mass spectrometer.

mucopolysaccharides Product of metabolism that may accumulate in cells and cause a progressive neurological disorder (e.g., Hurler syndrome, *see* Appendix B).

multidisciplinary When referring to developmental disabilities, this term describes an approach involving several professional specialties who assess a patient together and develop/carry out a treatment plan.

multifactorial Describing an inheritance pattern in which environment and heredity interact.

multi-organ system failure (MOSF) This devastating condition can result from the diving reflex during severe hypoxic ischemic encephalopathy (HIE).

multiple intraluminal impedance (MII) A technology that measures the movement of fluids, solids, and air in the esophagus.

multitiered systems of support (MTSS) A systemic, continuous improvement framework in which data-based problem-solving and decision making is practiced across all levels of the educational system for supporting students.

muscle spindles Muscle fibers that are part of the reflex arc that controls muscle contraction.

muscle and tendon structures Muscle and tendons associated with long bones such as the tibia, fibia, and femur that are more susceptible to injury during growth periods.

musculoskeletal Referring to the muscle and bone support system of the body.

mutation A change in the genomic sequence resulting in a variant form that may be transmitted to subsequent generations and may be associated with disease.

myasthenia gravis Neuromuscular disorder involving the muscles and the nerves that control them (*see* Chapter 9).

myelinated Insulating sheath around many nerve fibers in the white matter, increasing the speed at which impulses are conducted.

myelination The production of a coating called myelin around an axon, which quickens neurotransmission; a process that involves elaboration of supportive structures that improve transmission of electrical impulses from one part of the nervous system to another.

myelomeningocele *See* meningomyelocele.

myoclonus Irregular, involuntary contraction of a muscle.

myoglobinuria The spillage of myoglobin, the oxygen-transporting protein of muscle, into the urine. This can occur with trauma, vascular problems, certain drugs and other situations that destroy or damage the muscle, releasing myoglobin into the circulation and thus to the kidneys.

myopathies A muscular disease in which the muscle fibers do not function for any one of many reasons, resulting in muscular weakness. The most common example is muscular dystrophy.

myopia Nearsightedness.

myosin Protein necessary for muscle contraction.

myotonia Abnormal rigidity of muscles when voluntary movement is attempted.

myringotomy The surgical incision of the eardrum, usually accompanied by the placement of pressure-equalization tubes, to drain fluid from the middle ear.

nasal cannula A plastic prong placed in the nose and connected to a tube that delivers an oxygen/air mixture.

nasal pillows A prop attached to an oxygen line to permit the flow of oxygen directly into the nose.

nasogastric (NG) tube A feeding tube placed in the nose and extended into the stomach.

nasojejunal tube A feeding tube placed in the nose and extended through the stomach and into the jejunum.

nasopharynx Posterior portion of the oral cavity above the palate.

NCS *See* nerve conduction studies.

NDT *See* neurodevelopmental therapy.

NEC *See* necrotizing enterocolitis.

necrosis Death of tissue.

necrotizing enterocolitis (NEC) Severe inflammation of the small intestine and colon, most common in premature infants.

negative punishment Involves the contingent removal of a consequence (i.e., positive reinforcer).

negative reinforcement Behavioral phenomenon in which an individual's behavior permits an unpleasant event to be avoided or escaped, with a resultant increase in this behavior in the future.

neonatal intensive care unit (NICU) Hospital unit specializing in providing newborn life support treatments.

neonatal seizure Seizures in newborn infants appear different than in older children. The seizure may manifest as arm and/or leg tonic/clonic movements that seem like bicycling or rowing. Movements may also be more subtle, including spasmodic lip smacking or tongue thrusting, ocular movements such as excessive blinking or prolonged eye opening/staring, or episodes of apnea and bradycardia.

nerve blocks Direct injection of denaturing agents into motor nerves to decrease spasticity.

nerve conduction studies (NCS) Involves placing needle electrodes at various points on the body to test motor and sensory function of the peripheral nerves.

nerve conduction velocity Measure of nerve function.

neuropores The rostral and caudal openings of the neural tube which close around 6 weeks gestational age.

neural crest A band of cells that lie along the length of the neural tube and developing spinal cord.

neural fold During embryonic life, the fold created when the neural plate expands and rises; later it becomes the spinal column.

neural network A network involving many brain regions working in concert to store and use information obtained from the environment.

neural plate Earliest fetal brain mass development derived from the ectodermal germ layer of the embryo in the first 7 weeks of gestation.

neural proliferation A sustained period of vigorous cellular division which peaks between 6 and 22 weeks gestational age, giving rise to precursors of the future neuronal and glial populations of the brain.

neural tube The stage of central nervous system (CNS) development that follows neural plate formation, which subsequently gives rise to the various parts of the brain (i.e., the forebrain folding into the cerebrum and the hindbrain into the cerebellum, brainstem, and spinal cord).

neural tube defects (NTDs) Birth defects of the brain and spina cord (i.e., spina bifida and anencephaly).

neurocutaneous syndromes A group of genetic disorders that lead to growth of tumors in various parts of the body.

neurodevelopmental assessment A comprehensive evaluation of brain systems including neuromotor, learning, attention, speech, language, motor planning, cognition, and behavior.

neurodevelopmental treatment (NDT) An intervention approach used with children with neurologically based motor disabilities such as cerebral palsy.

neurofibromatosis Genetic disorders associated with tumor formation in the brain and other organs. *See* Appendix B.

neurogenesis The birth of neurons.

neurogenic Originating in, starting from, or caused by the nervous system or nerve impulses.

neurulation stage The folding process in human embryos, which includes the transformation of the neural plate into the neural tube.

neuroleptic malignant syndrome A rare toxic reaction to a medication in which there is a potentially life-threatening high fever, most commonly a problem with anesthetic agents.

neuromuscular Affecting both muscles and nerves.

neuron Any of the impulse-conducting cells that constitute the brain, spinal column, and nerves, consisting of a nucleated cell body with one or more dendrites and a single axon; *also called* a nerve cell.

neuronal Pertaining to the neuron.

neuroplasticity The inherently dynamic biological capacity of the central nervous system to undergo maturation, to change structurally and functionally in response to experience, and to adapt following injury.
neuropsychological assessment The administration of a battery of tests to determine a patient's cognitive function.
neuropsychology The study of the structure and function of the brain as it relates to specific psychological processes and behaviors.
neurotoxicant A chemical compound that can damage neurons; *also called* neurotoxin.
neurotransmitter A chemical released at the synapse that permits transmission of an impulse from one nerve to another.
neurulation Sequential central nervous system developmental processes of neuron cell proliferation and the migration of nascent neurons outward from the center of the developing brain to the outer cortex.
neutropenia Low white blood cell count.
next-generation sequencing (NGS) A high-throughput method used to determine a portion of the nucleotide sequence of an individual's genome.
NG tube *See* nasogastric tube.
NICU *See* neonatal intensive care unit.
nomogram A mathematical model that shows relationships between things.
nondisjunction Failure of a pair of chromosomes to separate during mitosis or meiosis, resulting in an unequal number of chromosomes in the daughter cells.
nonsense mutation Gene defect in which a single base pair substitution results in the premature termination of a message and the resultant production of an incomplete and inactive protein; *See* missense mutation.
nonverbal communication The use of gestures, facial expressions, signs, and body positions to communicate.
norepinephrine A neurotransmitter.
normalizing Making conform to a norm or standard.
NTDs *See* neural tube defects.
nuchal translucency measurement The assessment of the size of the translucent space behind the neck of the fetus using ultrasound at between 10 and 14 weeks of pregnancy, reflecting the amount of fluid that has accumulated under the skin of the fetus. It is abnormal in Down syndrome.
nucleotide bases The nucleic acids that form DNA—adenine, guanine, cytosine, and thymine.
nucleus The spheroid body located centrally within a cell and containing the chromosomes.
nutritive assistive devices Devices that assist in providing nutrition to an individual who cannot take oral feeding. These include nasogastric and gastrostomy feeding tubes.
nystagmus Involuntary rapid movements of the eyes (jiggling of the eyes) due to abnormalities in the cerebellum.
object permanence In infant development the ability to understand that objects continue to exist even if they cannot be seen directly.
oblique muscles Eye muscles whose primary function is to rotate the eyes. Their secondary function is to handle moving the eyes horizontally and vertically.
obsessions Recurrent and persistent thoughts and ideas that cannot be suppressed.
obsessive-compulsive disorder (OCD) A psychiatric disorder in which recurrent and persistent thoughts and ideas that cannot be suppressed (obsessions) are associated with repetitive behaviors (compulsions), such as excessive handwashing.
obstructive sleep apnea Recurring brief interruption of breathing during sleep due to obstruction usually of the upper airway.
obstructive uropathy Pathologic condition that blocks urine flow.
occipital lobe The posterior area of the brain where the visual receptive cortex is located.
OCD *See* obsessive-compulsive disorder.
ocular Pertaining to the eye.
oculomotor nerve The third cranial nerve controls the four eye muscles not controlled by the trochlear and abducens nerves.
off label Use of medication for disorders that have not been FDA approved.
oligodendrocytes A type of glial brain cell.
oligodontia The absence of one or several teeth.
oligohydramnios The presence of too little amniotic fluid, which may result in fetal deformities, including clubfoot and hypoplastic lungs.
oliguria Decreased passage of urine.
omphalocele Congenital herniation of abdominal organs through the navel.
onychomycosis A fungal infection of the nails.
oophorectomy Surgical removal of the ovary or ovaries.
operant control Control established and maintained by operant contingencies (i.e., the relationships in effect between the behavior and its consequences).
ophthalmologist Physician specializing in treatment of diseases of the eye.
ophthalmoscope An instrument containing a mirror and a series of magnifying lenses used to examine the interior of the eye.
opiate antagonists A category of medications that block endorphin receptors of the brain.
opisthotonos Abnormal positioning of the body in which the back is arched while the head and feet touch the bed; holding the head arched backward.
optic chiasm Located just before the nerves enter the brain, it is where the crossover of nerve fibers occurs.
optic nerve Transmits visual information from the retina to the brain.
optokinetic Pertaining to movement of the eyes.
oral pharyngeal musculature Muscles in the throat.
oral preparatory phase (phase I) The step preceding swallowing in which food is formed into a bolus in the mouth.
oral transport (phase II) The transport of a bolus of food to the back of the mouth so that it can be swallowed; primarily under volitional control.

organ of Corti A series of hair cells in the cochlea that form the beginning of the auditory nerve.
organelles Small, specialized structures within cells that operate like organs by carrying out specific tasks. Examples include the nucleus, which contains the chromosomes, and mitochondria, which are essential for energy production.
organic acidemias Inborn errors of metabolism involving enzyme deficiencies in the breakdown of organic acids (e.g., methylmalonic aciduria; *see* Appendix B); *also called* organic acid disorders and organic acidurias.
organophosphate pesticides Any of several organic compounds containing phosphorus that are used as pesticides.
ornithine transcarbamylase An enzyme in the urea cycle. An inborn error of metabolism involving a deficiency of this enzyme leads to episodes of encephalopathy.
orocutaneous stimulation This stimulation therapy mimics the temporal organization of sucking and can enhance the premature infant's acquisition of a functional suckle pattern.
oropharynx The part of the pharynx between the soft palate and the upper edge of the epiglottis.
orthographic Relating to the rules that lets us visually represent a language correctly.
orthomolecular therapy *See* megavitamin therapy.
orthopedic Relating to bones or joints.
orthosis Orthopedic device (e.g., a splint or brace) used to support, align, or correct deformities or to improve the function of limbs; *plural*: orthoses; *also called* orthotic.
orthotic Device that supports or corrects the function of a limb or the torso; *also called* orthosis.
orthotist Professional trained in the fitting and construction of splints, braces, and artificial limbs.
osmolarity The concentration of dissolved particles in a liquid.
ossicles The three small bones in the middle ear—the stapes, incus, and malleus.
osteoarthritis Degenerative joint disease.
osteoblasts Cells that produce bony tissue.
osteoclast Cell that absorbs and removes bone.
osteoid The substrate of bone.
osteomyelitis Bone infection.
osteopenia The loss of bony tissue resulting in low bone density.
osteopetrosis A genetic disorder marked by deficient osteoclastic activity. A buildup of bone encroaches on the eye, brain, and other body organs, leading to early death; bone weakness.
osteotomies Surgical cuts through the bone to correct deformities.
ostomy An artificial opening in the abdominal region, for example, for discharge of stool or urine.
otitis media Middle-ear infection.
otoacoustic emissions (OAE) Low-intensity sound energy emitted by the cochlea subsequent to sound stimulation as measured by a microphone coupled to the external ear canal.
otolith organ Part of the ear that contains both the organ of hearing (the cochlea) and the organ of balance (the labyrinth).
ototoxic Toxic to the auditory nerve, leading to hearing impairment.
oval window Connects the middle to the inner ear.
overt strokes Involves a focal (localized) neurological deficit that lasts more than 24 hours and results from an occlusion of one of the large anterior cerebral circulation vessels.
oxidative phosphorylation A chemical reaction occurring in the mitochondrion, resulting in energy production.
oximeter An instrument that measures oxygen saturation in the bloodstream.
oxygen saturation The amount of oxygen bound to hemoglobin in the blood, expressed as a percentage of the maximal binding capacity. The normal range is 95%–100%.
oxygenation The provision of sufficient oxygen for bodily needs.
pachygyria Abnormal convolutions on the surface of brain.
palatal Relating to the palate, the back portion of the roof of the mouth.
palate The roof of the mouth.
pallid infantile syncope Form of breath-holding spell in which the child turns pale and faints follows a frightening or painful experience.
palmar grasp reflex A primitive reflex where when an object is placed in an infant's hand and the palm of the child is stroked, the fingers will close reflexively.
pancreatitis An inflammation of the pancreas.
panic disorder A psychiatric disorder in which the patient has episodes of sudden and irrational fears associated with hyperventilation and palpitations.
Panayiotopoulos syndrome Also known as early-onset occipital epilepsy; is a common childhood epilepsy syndrome with partial seizures.
parallel play Involves children playing adjacent to each other but not trying to influence one another's behavior. Children usually play alone during parallel play but are interested in what other children are doing. This usually occurs after the first birthday.
paraplegia Paralysis of the legs and lower body.
parapodium A reciprocal gait orthosis or a hip-knee-ankle-foot orthosis used in combination with crutches or a walker.
parasomnia Sleep disturbances (i.e., night terrors and sleep walking).
parenchymal Tissue within a body organ.
parent–child interaction therapy (PCIT) A psychological treatment approach for young children with emotional and behavioral disorders that places emphasis on improving the quality of the parent–child relationship and changing parent–child interaction patterns. Children and their caregivers are seen together in PCIT.
parenteral feeding Intravenous provision of high-quality nutrition (i.e., carbohydrates, protein, and fat) used in children with malabsorption, malnutrition, and

short bowel syndrome; *also called* hyperalimentation; parenteral feeding is usually administered in a hospital setting on a short-term basis.

parenting networks Parents who educate and support one another.

paresthesias Numbness with skin sensations, such as burning, prickling, itching, or tingling.

parietal lobe The middle-upper part of the hemisphere of the brain; brain region involved in integrating sensory information and in visual-spatial processing.

Parkinson's disease A progressive neurological disease, usually occurring in older people, associated with tremor, slowed movements, and muscular rigidity.

parotid The salivary gland beside the ear.

paroxysmal Intermittent.

partial graduated guidance Instructor uses minimal physical contact but much praise in helping the child learn a desired task.

parvovirus A group of extremely small DNA viruses. Intrauterine infection with one type of parvovirus increases the risk of miscarriage but has not been shown to result in fetal malformations.

patella Kneecap.

patent ductus arteriosus (PDA) The persistence of a fetal passage permitting blood to bypass the lungs.

patent foramen ovale (PFO) A tiny open window in the atrial wall of the heart passing oxygenated blood from the right atrium into the left atrium, thus bypassing circulation to the fetal lungs *in utero*.

paternalism Imposing a decision on another person for that person's welfare (e.g., the theory that "doctor knows best").

PBIS *See* positive behavior interventions and supports.

PCB *See* polychlorinated biphenyl.

PDA *See* patent ductus arteriosus.

PDD Pervasive developmental disorder (*see* Chapter 18).

penetrance The percentage of people with a particular genetic mutation who express symptoms of the disorder. A disorder shows reduced penetrance when some people with the genetic defect are completely without symptoms.

percutaneous umbilical blood sampling (PUBS) A prenatal diagnostic procedure for obtaining fetal blood for genetic testing; *also called* cordocentesis.

percutaneously Through the skin.

perfusion The passage of blood through the arteries to an organ or tissue.

perinatal transmission Refers to the transmission of a disease-causing agent from mother to baby during the period immediately before and after birth

periodontal disease Disease of the gums and bony structures that surround the teeth.

periosteum Fibrous tissue covering and protecting all bones.

peripheral nervous system The parts of the nervous system other than the brain and spinal cord.

peripheral venous lines Catheters that are placed in a superficial vein of the arm or leg to provide medication.

peristalsis The voluntary constriction and relaxation of the muscles of the esophagus and intestine, creating wavelike movements that push food forward.

peritoneal Referring to the membrane surrounding the abdominal organs.

periventricular leukomalacia (PVL) Injury to part of the brain near the ventricles caused by lack of oxygen; occurs principally in premature infants.

periventricular region The area surrounding the ventricles.

peroxisome A cellular organelle involved in processing fatty acids.

persistent pulmonary hypertension of the newborn/persistent fetal circulation (PPHN/PFC) Persistent high pulmonary blood pressure in the newborn period due to vasoconstriction of the pulmonary arterial blood vessels and resulting in severe hypoxia.

pes cavus High-arched foot.

pes planus Flat feet.

pesticide A chemical used to kill insects.

PET scan *See* positron emission tomography.

petechiae A small purplish spot, usually on the skin, caused by a minute hemorrhage.

PFO *See* patent foramen ovale.

PGD *See* preimplantation genetic diagnosis.

pH probe A small sensor, which detects the pH, or acidity, above the gastroesophageal junction.

phakomatoses Genetic syndromes characterized by benign tumor like nodules of the eye, skin, and brain. The four disorders designated phakomatoses are neurofibromatosis, tuberous sclerosis, Sturge-Weber syndrome, and von Hippel-Lindau disease.

phalanges Bones of the fingers and toes.

pharmacodynamics Explains the drug's effects (i.e., the relationship between the dose of a drug and the individual's response to it).

pharmacogenomics The study of how variations in the human genome affect the individual's response to a particular medication or group of medication.

pharmacokinetics The interactions of a drug and the body in terms of its absorption, distribution, metabolism, and excretion.

pharyngeal Pertaining to the pharynx or back of the throat.

pharyngeal transfer phase (phase III) The transfer of a food bolus from the mouth to the pharynx on its way to being swallowed; begins when the bolus passes the faucial arches (near the tonsils) and triggers the start of the swallowing cascade.

pharynx The back of the throat.

phenothiazines Antipsychotic medications that affect neurochemicals in the brain and are used to control aggressive behavior and psychotic symptoms.

phenotype The physical appearance of a genetic trait.

phenylalanine An amino acid, the elevation of which causes phenylketonuria (PKU).

phenylketonuria (PKU) Birth defect in which a child is born without the ability to break down amino acids called phenylalanine. *See* Chapter 16.

philtrum Vertical groove between nose and mouth.
phobias Irrational fears.
phocomelia Congenitally foreshortened limbs.
phoneme The smallest unit of sound in speech.
phonetic Pertaining to the sounding out of words.
phonological disorder Involves having difficulty learning the sound system of a language and the rules for combining sounds.
phonological processing The use of the sounds of one's language (i.e., phonemes) to process spoken and written language.
phonological processing disorder A developmental disorder in which there is difficulty learning the rules about which sounds go together in specific positions within words when sounds are voiced or voiceless.
phonology The set of sounds in a language and the rules for using them.
photic Relating to light.
photoreceptors Receptors for light stimuli; the rods and cones in the retina.
physes Growth plates of a developing long bone.
physiotherapy Physical therapy.
pica Ingestion of nonfood items.
pincer grasp A pattern emerging at 10–12 months of age whereby an infant can hold a small object between the pads of the opposed thumb and index or middle finger.
pitch The frequency of sounds, measured in cycles per second, or hertz (Hz). Low-pitched sounds have a frequency less than 500 Hz and a bass quality. High-pitched sounds have a frequency greater than 2,000 Hz and a tenor quality.
PKU *See* phenylketonuria (*see* Chapter 16 and Appendix B).
placebo An inactive substance used as a control in a study to determine the effectiveness of a drug.
placebo response A situation where an inactive substance (e.g., sugar, distilled water, or saline solution) improves a patient's condition simply because the person has the expectation that it will be helpful.
placenta The organ of nutritional exchange between the mother and the embryo. It has both maternal and embryonic elements, is disc shaped, and is about 7 inches in diameter. The umbilical cord attaches in the center of the placenta; *also called* the afterbirth; *adjective*: placental.
placenta accreta Abnormal adherence of the chorionic villi to the uterus.
placenta previa Condition in which the placenta is implanted in the lower segment of the uterus, extending over the cervical opening.
placental abruption *See* abruptio placenta; early separation of the placenta from the uterine wall.
planned ignoring A behavior management technique based on withholding positive reinforcement following the occurrence of a nondangerous, nondestructive challenging behavior; *also called* extinction.
plantarflexion A toe-down motion of the foot at the ankle.
plantargrade Flat on the floor.
plaque A semi-hardened accumulation of bacteria adhering to the teeth.
plasma The noncellular content of blood; *also called* serum.
plasmapheresis The removal of blood followed by filtering the plasma and reinfusing the blood products. This procedure is done to remove toxins and antibodies as in Guillain-Barré syndrome.
plasticity The ability of an organ or part of an organ to take over the function of another damaged organ; the ability of the nervous system to change or adapt.
pneumocystis carinii pneumonia Lung infection often seen in immunocompromised individuals, such as those with acquired immunodeficiency syndrome (AIDS).
point mutation A mutation in a single nucleotide (DNA) base leading to a genetic syndrome (e.g., sickle cell disease).
polar body testing Polar bodies are the by-products of the egg's division during meiosis. The two polar bodies are essentially discarded by the egg. By analyzing the polar bodies, it is possible to infer the genetic status of the egg.
polio Viral infection of the spinal cord causing an asymmetrical ascending paralysis, now prevented by vaccination.
polychlorinated biphenyl (PCB) One of a group of organic compounds originally used in industry and now recognized as an environmental pollutant.
polydactyly Extra fingers or toes.
polygenic risk score (PRS) A number based on the variation in multiple genetic loci that serves as a predictor of the risk of developing a specific polygenic disorder such as hypertension.
polyhydramnios The presence of excessive amniotic fluid; often associated with certain fetal anomalies such as esophageal atresia.
polymicrogyria A brain with too many convoluted gyri that are smaller than normal due to abnormal neuronal migration during embryogenesis of the central nervous system.
polymorphism A variation in DNA that is too common (occurs in greater than 1% of the population) to be due to a new mutation.
polypharmacy The concurrent use of multiple medications by a patient.
polysomnogram Procedure performed during sleep that involves monitoring the electroencephalogram (EEG), electrocardiogram (EKG), and respiratory efforts. It is used to investigate individuals with sleep disorders, including sleep apnea; *also called* a sleep study.
polyuria Excessive passage of urine.
POR *See* prevalence odds ratio.
positive behavioral interventions and supports (PBIS) Positive reinforcement used to control undesired behaviors.
positive predictive value The probability that individuals with a positive screening test truly have the disease.

positive pressure ventilation Application of positive pressure to the inspiratory phase when the patient has an artificial airway in place and is connected to a ventilator.

positive punishment Involves the contingent delivery of a consequence (*sometimes termed* an aversive stimulus).

positive reinforcement A method of increasing desired behaviors by rewarding them; exists when the contingent delivery of an outcome produces an increase in the likelihood of the behavior(s) upon which it is contingent.

positive reinforcers Any tangible (e.g., food or toy) or action (e.g., hug) that is reinforcing to an individual and will lead to a subsequent increase in the behavior that preceded it.

positive support reflex (PSR) Primitive reflex present in an infant, in which the child reflexively accepts weight on the feet when bounced, appearing to stand briefly.

positron emission tomography (PET) Imaging study utilizing radioactive-labeled chemical compounds to study the metabolism of an organ, most commonly the brain.

postconceptional age (PCA) Dates the onset of human development from the presumed date of ovulation (i.e., when fertilization occurs).

posterior In back of or the back part of a structure.

postictal Immediately following a seizure episode.

postterm birth Birth after 42 weeks' gestation.

posttraumatic stress disorder (PTSD) Psychiatric disorder in which a previously experienced stressful event is reexperienced psychologically many times and associated with anxiety and fear.

postural reactions Normal reflexlike protective responses of an infant to changes in position; *also called* automatic movement reactions.

PPHN/PFC *See* persistent pulmonary hypertension of the newborn/persistent fetal circulation.

PPV *See* positive pressure ventilation.

pragmatics The study of language as it is used in a social context (e.g., conversation).

precocious puberty A condition in which the changes associated with puberty begin at an unexpectedly early age.

preeclampsia Disorder of late pregnancy characterized by high blood pressure with swelling and/or protein in the mother's urine, seen especially in teenagers and women older than 35 years; *also called* toxemia of pregnancy; blood toxemia of pregnancy.

preference assessments Assessments to identify high-preference stimuli that may be potential reinforcers in a behavior management program.

pregnancy-associated plasma protein A (PAPP-A) A plasma protein that is used as a blood screening test between 8 and 14 weeks' gestation. Diminished levels of the protein suggest an increased risk for Down syndrome, intrauterine growth retardation, preeclampsia, and stillbirth.

preimplantation genetic diagnosis (PGD) Refers to procedures that are performed on embryos prior to implantation. PGD is considered another approach to prenatal diagnosis. When used to screen for a specific genetic disease, it avoids selective pregnancy termination as the method makes it highly likely that the baby will be free of the disease under consideration. PGD is an adjunct to assisted reproductive technology and requires *in vitro* fertilization (IVF) to obtain oocytes or embryos for evaluation.

premolar Teeth in the back of the mouth used for grinding.

premutation A sequence of multiply repeated nucleotides that may produce a disease in one's offspring but may not produce clinically apparent disease in the carrier. The classic example is fragile X syndrome, where CGG repeats of < 200 are considered premutations and repeats of > 200 are full mutations.

prenatal screening Noninvasive (usually maternal blood) tests used to screen for genetic disorders in the fetus.

presbyopia A decrease in the accommodation of the lens of the eye that occurs with aging.

pretend play Make-believe play.

preterm birth Birth prior to 37 weeks' gestation; prematurity.

prevalence The number of cases of a disease that are present in a particular population at a given time.

prevalence odds ratio (POR) The burden or status of a disease in a defined population at a specified time, including all cases of disease in the population whether they are newly diagnosed or previously recognized.

priapism Painful and long-lasting penile erections.

primary neurulation The process by which the neural plate develops a midline groove, the edges of which fold over, converge, and close to form the neural tube.

primitive reflexes Infantile reflexes that tend to fade in the first year of life (i.e., the suck, startle, and root) (*see* Chapter 21).

promotor region A segment of DNA usually occurring upstream from a gene coding region (exon) and acting as a controlling element in the expression of that gene.

prompts Cues (e.g., verbal and visual) that direct the child to participate in a targeted activity.

prone Face down.

prophase The initial stage in cell division when the chromosomes thicken and shorten to look like separate strands.

prophylaxis Use of a preventive agent.

proprioception Ability to sense the position, location, orientation, and movement of body parts.

proptosis Appearance of protruding eyes.

prosencephalon *See* forebrain. The forward-most bulge, gives rise to the left and right cerebral hemispheres.

prosocial Socially acceptable.

prosody The intonation and rhythm of speech.

proteinuria Protein in urine.

proto-declarative pointing Pointing in order to share interest or attention about an object. This developmental milestone typically appears between 9 and 14 months of age.

proto-imperative pointing Pointing in order to use another person to obtain an object. This developmental milestone typically appears between 12 and 14 months of age.

proximal Describing the part nearest the midline or trunk.

proxy consent Consent for treatment or research given by a parent or guardian for a child or an incompetent adult.

pseudohypertrophy Enlarged but weak muscle, as found in muscular dystrophy.

pseudomonas A bacterial infection that most commonly causes pneumonia in immunocompromised patients.

PSR *See* positive support reflex.

psychoeducational Pertaining to the testing of intelligence, academic achievement, and other types of psychological and educational processes.

psychological assessment Incorporates test scores into a broadly based assessment of a child's abilities and functioning; *also called* psychological testing.

psychosis A psychiatric disorder characterized by hallucinations, delusions, loss of contact with reality, and unclear thinking; *adjective*: psychotic.

psychotherapy Nonpharmacological treatment for an individual with an emotional disorder. Various types of psychotherapy range from supportive counseling to psychoanalysis with services usually provided by a psychologist, psychiatrist, or social worker.

ptosis Droopy eyelids.

PTSD *See* posttraumatic stress disorder.

PUBS *See* percutaneous umbilical blood sampling.

pulmonary Pertaining to the lungs.

pulmonary hypertension Increased back pressure in the pulmonary artery leading to decreased oxygenation and right heart failure.

pulmonary vascular obstructive disease This leads to increased back pressure in the arteries that connect the heart to the lungs and results in congestive heart failure.

pulmonary vascular resistance (PVR) Vasoconstriction of the pulmonary blood vessels normally high during fetal life, which should relax immediately upon birth with the first breaths of life.

pulmonary vasodilation Relaxation of the lung's blood vessels soon after birth to establish lung circulation and extinguish fetal circulation.

pulp The soft tissue under the dentin layer in teeth containing blood vessels, lymphatics (lymph vessels), connective tissue, and nerve fibers.

pulse oximeter A device that measures oxygen tension noninvasively.

pulse oximetry screening A newborn screening test that improves detection of critical congenital heart defects.

punishment In behavior management, a procedure or consequence that decreases the frequency of a behavior through the use of a negative stimulus or withdrawal of a preferred activity/object.

pupil The aperture in the center of the iris.

purine A type of organic molecule found in RNA and DNA.

puritis Itchiness.

purpuric Bruising indicating bleeding into the skin.

purpuric skin lesions Bruising.

putamen A part of the lentiform nucleus that is lateral to the globus pallidus in the brain. It is associated with the corpus striatum and receives connections from the suppressor centers of the cortex.

PVL *See* periventricular leukomalacia.

PVR *See* pulmonary vascular resistance.

pyloric stenosis A congenital narrowing of the opening from the stomach to the small bowel.

pylorus The sphincter at the junction of the stomach and the duodenum.

pyramidal tract A nerve tract; *also called* the corticospinal tract, leading from the cortex into the spinal column and involved in the control of voluntary motor movement. Damage to this tract results in spasticity, commonly seen in cerebral palsy.

pyridoxine Vitamin B_6.

quadriplegia Paralysis of all four extremities.

quickening The first signs of life felt by the mother as a result of fetal movements in the fourth or fifth month of pregnancy.

rad A measure of radioactivity.

radial-digital grasp A grasp pattern emerging in the 8th–9th month of age characterized by holding an object between an opposed thumb and fingertips with the object held toward the distal end of these digits so that a space is visible between the thumb and the fingers.

radial-palmar grasp A baby will begin involving the thumb and all fingers, while using more of the thumb side of their hand to grab objects.

radiograph A medical x-ray.

ratio schedules Provision of reinforcement following a set number of correct responses.

real-time ultrasonography The use of sound waves to provide a moving (real-time) image used in fetal monitoring.

rebound A phenomenon in which as a medication dose wears off, a person's behavior or symptoms become worse than when completely off medication.

receptive aphasia Impairment of receptive language due to a disorder of the central nervous system (CNS).

receptive language The cognitive processing involved in comprehending oral, symbolic, or written language.

recessive Pertaining to a trait that is expressed only if the child inherits two copies of the gene; from the Latin word for "hidden."

recti muscles Eye muscles that converge the eyes toward the nose for near activities and diverge the eyes for far ones.

recurrence risk In medical genetics, the chance that an inherited disorder that is present in a family will recur in that family, affecting one or more other members in the future.

red reflex The reddish-orange reflection from the eye's retina that is observed when using an ophthalmoscope or retinoscope.

refracted Bent, toward a focal point.

reframing Reinterpreting a behavior by viewing it from a different lens and focusing on the adaptive and positive aspects rather than negative ones.

regurgitation The involuntary return of partially digested food from the stomach into the mouth.

rehabilitation engineer A specially trained engineer who designs, adapts, and evaluates technological solutions to problems confronting individuals with disabilities.

reinforcer A response to a behavior that increases the likelihood that the behavior will occur in the future.

related services Services (e.g., transportation, occupational and physical therapy) that supplement the special education services provided to a child with a developmental disability.

renal dysplasia Small, abnormal kidneys.

repetitive microtrauma Small injury of lesion that can become problematic if repetitive.

representative payee Often required by programs and services in order to disburse funds to an individual with developmental disabilities.

resonance In linguistics and speech-language pathology, the balance of air flow between the nose and the mouth.

resonance disorders Abnormal amounts of nasality, often caused by structural malformations, such as enlarged adenoids and tonsils, or structural anomalies, such as a deviated septum.

respiratory technology assistance Medical devices used to replace or augment a vital body function.

response to intervention (RTI) Represents a shift in thinking about students who have difficulty learning at the same rate as their peers. Students with learning difficulties are provided supplementary instruction within general education, with special education being the final rung on the ladder of support. RTI also concerns the diagnosis of students with specific learning disabilities (SLD). RTI was introduced by the Individuals with Disabilities Education Improvement Act (IDEA) of 2004 as an alternate and preferred method for diagnosing children with SLD. It is likely that when IDEA is next reauthorized, RTI will be the only acceptable method for diagnosing SLD.

restrictive/repetitive behaviors and interests (RRBIs) Core symptoms of autism spectrum disorder. They include repetitive movements with objects, repeated body movements such as rocking and hand-flapping, ritualistic behavior, sensory sensitivities, and circumscribed interests.

retina The photosensitive nerve layer that lines the back of the eye, senses light, and creates impulses that travel through the optic nerve to the brain.

retinopathy Disorder of the retina.

retinopathy of prematurity (ROP) A disorder involving abnormal blood vessel development in the retina of the eye in a premature infant. It has been linked to excessive provision of oxygen.

retinoscope An instrument used to detect errors of refraction in the eye.

retro-illumination In split-lamp examination of the eye, it is a method of illuminating a structure by using the light that is reflected by the iris or by a lens containing a cataract.

retrospective payment system Pertaining to a fee-for-service health care model in which payment occurs after services are rendered.

retrovirus The class of viruses that includes human immunodeficiency virus (HIV), the causative agent of acquired immunodeficiency syndrome (AIDS).

Rh incompatibility Condition occurring when an Rh+ baby is born to an Rh– mother. This leads to breakdown of red blood cells in the baby and the excessive release of bilirubin, predisposing the Rh+ baby to kernicterus.

rhabdomyolysis Breakdown of muscle tissue.

rhombencephalon The hindbrain region of the embryo.

ribonucleic acid (RNA) A nucleic acid that is an essential component of all cells, composed of a long, usually single-stranded chain of nucleotide units that contain the sugar ribose. It is essential for protein synthesis within the cell.

ribosome Intracellular structure involved in protein synthesis. It reads the genetic code delivered to it by mRNA.

rickets Bone disease resulting from nutritional deficiency of vitamin D.

rights Moral or legal claims by one party against another.

rigid Pertaining to increased tone marked by stiffness.

ring chromosome A ring-shaped chromosome formed when deletions occur at both tips of a normal chromosome with subsequent fusion of the tips, forming a ring.

RNA *See* ribonucleic acid.

rods Photoreceptor cells of the eye associated with low-light vision.

rolandic epilepsy An inherited benign form of epilepsy occurring in children and characterized by sudden episodes of arrested speech and muscular contractions of the side of the face.

rootlets Small branches of nerve roots.

ROP *See* retinopathy of prematurity.

rostral Anterior pole of the developing embryo.

RTI *See* response to intervention.

rubella A viral infection. Generally causes a mild elevation of temperature and skin rash and resolves in a few days. However, when it occurs in a pregnant woman during the first trimester, it can lead to intrauterine infection and severe birth defects; *also called* German measles.

Rubinstein-Taybi syndrome *See* Appendix B.
rumination The regurgitating and chewing again of previously swallowed food.
sacral Relating to the bone at the base of the spine.
SAH *See* subarachnoid hemorrhage.
salicylates Chemicals found in many food substances and in aspirin.
saline A salt solution.
Sally-Ann test A psychological test that measures a person's social cognitive ability to attribute false beliefs to others.
sarcomeres The contractile units of the muscle fiber.
Sarnat neurological score The most popular system for grading the severity of hypoxic ischemic encephalopathy (HIE); it ranges from 1 (mild) to 3 (severe) in neonates.
satiation Having had enough or too much of something.
scala media (SM) Fluid-filled cavity within the cochlea of the ear.
scala tympani (ST) One of the three spirally arranged canals into which the bony canal of the cochlea is partitioned.
scala vestibuli (SV) One of the three spirally arranged canals into which the bony canal of the cochlea is partitioned.
schizencephaly A severely malformed brain with clefts formed because of a neuronal migrational defect during early embryogenesis.
schizophrenia A psychiatric disorder with characteristic psychotic symptoms (i.e., prominent delusions, hallucinations, catatonic behavior, and/or flat affect).
Schlemm's canal The passageway in which the aqueous fluid leaves the eye.
Schwann cell A myelin-secreting glial cell that spirally wraps around an axon of the peripheral nervous system to form the myelin sheath.
sclera The thick, white nontransparent fibrous covering in the eye.
scoliosis Lateral curvature of the spine.
screening test A test designed to screen for, but not definitively diagnose, a particular condition.
SDH *See* subdural hemorrhage.
seborrheic dermatitis Dandruff.
secondary Occurring as a consequence of a primary disorder.
secondary neurulation A series of events at the lower edge of the neural tube in which the caudal eminence develops into the bottom most segments of the spine and elements of the lower intestine.
second-trimester ultrasonography An ultrasound conducted in the 13th–14th week of pregnancy to test for Down syndrome and other congenital anomalies.
secretin Hormone produced in the duodenum that stimulates secretion of pancreatic enzymes.
seizure threshold Tolerance level of the brain for electrical activity. If level of tolerance is exceeded, a seizure occurs.
selective serotonin reuptake inhibitors (SSRIs) Commonly used medications for treatment of depression and anxiety. They act by decreasing reuptake of serotonin from the synaptic cleft, resulting in more serotonin being available for neurotransmission.
selective vulnerability Refers to a susceptibility of specific regions and cells to injury.
self-advocacy People with disabilities taking control of their own lives, including being in charge of their own care in the medical system.
self-injurious behavior (SIB) The intentional, direct injuring of body tissue most often done without suicidal intentions.
semantics The study of and conventions governing meanings of words.
semicircular canals The three bony fluid-filled loops in the bony labyrinth of the internal ear, associated with the sense of balance.
sensorineural Involving the cochlea or auditory nerve.
sensorineural hearing loss Hearing loss caused by damage to the sensory cells and/or nerve fibers of the inner ear.
sensory integration The ability to integrate the senses of touch (tactile), balance (vestibular), and where the body and its parts are in space (proprioceptive).
sensory integration (SI) therapy Therapy that uses controlled sensory stimulation combined with a meaningful adaptive response to achieve changes in learning and behavior. A common method used in occupational therapy.
sensory processing disorder (SPD) A condition in which the brain has trouble receiving and responding to information that comes in through the senses. It is not currently recognized as a distinct medical diagnosis.
separation anxiety Excessive concern about separation, usually of mother from child (e.g., school phobia).
sepsis Infection that has spread throughout the bloodstream and can be life threatening; *also called* blood poisoning.
sequential modification If desired changes in behavior are not observed to occur across settings and behaviors, concrete steps are taken to introduce the effective intervention (e.g., positive reinforcement) to each of the behaviors or settings to which transfer of effects is inadequate.
serotonin reuptake inhibitors A group of psychoactive drugs, an example being fluoxetine (Prozac) used to treat depression.
serum *See* plasma.
sex chromosomes The X and Y chromosomes that determine sex.
sex-linked trait *See* X-linked trait.
SGA *See* small for gestational age.
shadowing Technique in which the instructor keeps his or her hands within an inch of the child's hands as the child proceeds to complete the task.

shared decision making Patient or proxy and physician participate together in committing to a treatment decision.
SI therapy *See* sensory integration therapy.
sialorrhea A condition with marked drooling.
SIB *See* self-injurious behavior or aggressions.
SIDS *See* sudden infant death syndrome.
silent stroke A stroke without any outward symptoms.
single nucleotide polymorphisms (SNPs) DNA sequence variations in the population.
single photon emission computed tomography (SPECT) An imaging technique that permits the study of the metabolism of a body organ, most commonly the brain.
single-gene defect A mutation or error in a single gene leads to disease. Examples include sickle cell disease and phenylketonuria.
SLD *See* spoken language disorder.
sleep apnea Brief periods of arrested breathing during sleep, most commonly found in premature infants and in older children and adults with morbid obesity.
sleep myoclonus Sudden jerking movements of the body associated with various sleep stages that may be confused with a seizure.
sleep onset latency The length of time it takes to transition from full wakefulness to sleep once one goes to bed.
small for gestational age (SGA) Refers to a newborn whose weight is below the 10th percentile for gestational age, often referencing prematurely born infants.
SNPs *See* single nucleotide polymorphisms.
social-emotional reciprocity The back-and-forth flow of social interaction.
social-negative reinforcement The removal of some unwanted or aversive event contingent on a behavior may also result in strengthening of that behavior and may take the form of escape or avoidance from the unwanted event.
social-positive reinforcement Events or stimuli that follow the occurrence of a behavior that may function to strengthen that behavior.
soft neurological signs A group of neurological findings that are normal in young children, but when found in older children suggest immaturities in central nervous system (CNS) development (i.e., difficulty performing sequential finger–thumb opposition, rapid alternating movements).
soft spot *See* anterior fontanelle.
somatic Relating to the body.
somatic nervous system (SNS) Part of the peripheral nervous system associated with the voluntary control of body movements via skeletal muscles and with sensory reception of touch, hearing, and sight.
somatosensory system The part of the sensory system concerned with the conscious perception of touch, pressure, pain, temperature, position, movement, and vibration that arise from the muscles, joints, and skin.
somatotopical Organization of the motor area of the brain so that specific regions of the cortex control movement of different areas of the body.
spastic Pertaining to increased muscle tone in which muscles are stiff and movements are difficult; caused by damage to the pyramidal tract in the brain and spinal cord.
spastic diplegia A form of cerebral palsy primarily seen in former premature infants that is manifested as spasticity of both lower extremities with only mild involvement of upper extremities.
spastic hemiplegia A form of cerebral palsy in which one side of the body demonstrates spasticity and the other side is unaffected.
spastic hypertonicity Increased muscle tone and a positive Babinski response, two of the hallmark features of spastic cerebral palsy.
spastic quadriplegia A form of cerebral palsy in which all four limbs are affected. Increased muscle tone (i.e., spasticity) is caused by damage to the pyramidal tract in the brain.
spasticity Abnormally increased muscle tone.
speaking valve A valve that can be used by children who have tracheostomy tubes to permit vocalizations.
specific language impairment A significant deficit in linguistic functioning that does not appear to be accompanied by deficits in hearing, intelligence, or motor functioning.
specific learning disability Includes disorders that affect the ability to understand or use spoken or written language; it may manifest in difficulties with listening, thinking, speaking, reading, writing, spelling, and/or doing mathematical calculations.
SPECT *See* single photon emission computed tomography.
spectrum of developmental disabilities The various neurological disorders that result from abnormalities in cognitive, motor, and neurobehavioral function.
speech and language disorders Problems in communication and related areas such as oral-motor function.
speech sound disorder (SSD) A communication disorder in which children have difficulty saying words or sounds correctly; an articulation disorder.
spoken language disorder (SLD) Also known as an oral language disorder, represents a significant impairment in the acquisition and use of language across modalities (e.g., speech, sign language, or both) due to deficits in comprehension and/or production across any of the five language domains (i.e., phonology, morphology, syntax, semantics, pragmatics).
splenomegaly Enlarged spleen.
spermatocytes Sperm.
spina bifida A developmental defect of the spine, a neural tube defect; *also called* spinal dysraphism.
spina bifida occulta Generally benign congenital defect of the spinal column not associated with protrusion of the spinal cord or meninges; the most common neural tube defect.
spinal braces A form of low-tech assistive device to children with cerebral palsy or neuromuscular disorder.

spinal cord The thick, whitish cord of nerve tissue that extends from the base of the brain down through the spinal column.
spinal dysraphism *See* spinal bifida.
spinal muscular atrophy Congenital neuromuscular disorder of childhood associated with progressive muscle weakness. *See* Appendix B.
spinal tap *See* lumbar puncture.
spindle In mitosis and meiosis, a weblike figure along which the chromosomes are distributed.
spondyloepiphyseal dysplasia Congenital structural abnormality of vertebral column caused by a lack of mineralization of bone. *See* Appendix B.
spontaneous recovery In behavior management, the recurrence of an undesirable behavior after it has been extinguished.
sporadic In genetics, describing a disease that occurs by chance and carries little risk of recurrence.
SSRIs *See* selective serotonin reuptake inhibitors.
standardized rating scales Questionnaires concerning specific behaviors that have been completed for large samples of children so that norms and normal degrees of variation are known.
stapes One of the three small bones in the middle ear, collectively called the ossicles, that help amplify sound.
Staphylococcus aureus The bacteria resulting in staph infections such as cellulitis.
static encephalopathy Characterized by significantly delayed development, with the acquisition of new skills at a slower rate than is typical.
static Unchanging.
status epilepticus A seizure lasting more than 30 minutes.
stenosis An abnormal narrowing.
stereocilia The sensory (hair) cells of the inner ear.
stereotypic movement disorder Disorder characterized by recurring purposeless but voluntary movements (e.g., hand flapping in children with autism); *also called* stereotypies.
stereotypies *See* stereotypic movement disorder.
steroids 1) Medications used to treat severe inflammatory diseases and infantile spasms; 2) certain natural hormones in the body.
stimulant Medication used to treat attention-deficit/hyperactivity disorder (e.g., methylphenidate).
stomach flu *See* gastroenteritis.
strabismus Deviation of one or both eyes during forward gaze; the loss of this coordinated movement leads to misalignment of the eye; crossed eyes.
stranger anxiety A developmental stage during which a child experiences anxiety when separated from the primary caregiver.
subacute progressive encephalopathy Characterized by a gradual and insidious loss of previously obtained cognitive and motor milestones.
subarachnoid Beneath the arachnoid membrane, or middle layer, of the meninges.
subarachnoid hemorrhage (SAH) Hemorrhage into the fluid-filled space between the arachnoid membrane and the underlying brain that can compress or contuse the underlying brain.
subdural Resting between the outer (dural) and middle (arachnoid) layers of the meninges.
subdural hematoma Localized collection of clotted blood lying in the space between the dural and arachnoid membranes that surround the brain. This results from bleeding of the cerebral blood vessels that rest between these two membranes.
subdural hemorrhage (SDH) Hemorrhage between the tough outer membrane (dura) and the meninges surrounding the brain and spinal cord that can compress or contuse the underlying brain.
subluxation Partial dislocation.
submucosal A supporting layer of loose connective tissue directly under a mucous membrane, (i.e., below the palate).
subplate zone A transient fetal area involved in the development of the cerebral cortex.
substrate A compound acted upon by an enzyme in a chemical reaction.
sucrose A sugar molecule composed of glucose and fructose.
sudden infant death syndrome (SIDS) Diagnosis given to a previously well infant (often a former premature baby) who is found lifeless in bed without apparent cause; *also called* crib death.
sudden unexpected infant death (SUID) Sudden death of an infant, with no obvious cause prior to investigation.
sulci Furrows of the brain; *singular:* sulcus.
superior In anatomy, above.
supernumerary Extra.
supine Lying on the back, face upward.
supported employment Defined by the Rehabilitation Act Amendments of 1986 (PL 99-506) and 1992 (PL 102-569) as employment in an inclusive setting with ongoing support services for an individual with a disability.
suppository Small solid medication shaped for ready introduction into one of the orifices of the body other than the oral cavity, such as the rectum, urethra, or vagina.
surfactant A lipoprotein normally secreted into the alveoli with the first breaths of life that acts like a soap bubble and allows for a significant decrease in the alveolar membrane's surface tension, thus making breathing much easier and the lungs much more flexible immediately after birth.
surveillance The ongoing monitoring of disease in the population.
surveillance devices Devices such as cardiorespiratory monitors and pulse oximeters.
sutures In anatomy, the fibrous joints between certain bones (e.g., skull bones).
synapses The minute spaces separating one neuron from another. Neurochemicals breach this gap.
synaptic pruning The process of elimination of excess axons and dendrites beginning at about 2 years of age and continuing throughout childhood and adolescence.
syncopal episode Fainting spell.

syndactyly Webbed hands or feet.
synophrys Confluent eyebrows.
syntax Word order.
syphilis A sexually transmitted disease that can cause an intrauterine infection in pregnant women and result in severe birth defects.
syringomas Benign sweat gland tumors.
syringomyelia A chronic disease of the spinal cord characterized by the presence of a fluid-filled cavity.
syrinx A pathological tube-shaped cavity in the spinal cord.
systemic Involving the body as a whole.
T-cell lymphocyte population White blood cells responsible for recognizing and chemically encoding into immunologic memory any foreign bacterial substances.
tachycardia Rapid heart rate.
tachypnea Rapid breathing.
tactile Relating to touch.
talipes equinovarus *See* clubfoot.
tandem mass spectrometer (MS/MS) A machine that separates and quantifies ions based on their mass-to-charge ratio. It is used in newborn screening to detect a number of inborn errors of metabolism.
tangential migration Cells migrate parallel to the surface of the brain and perpendicular to the radial glia.
tangibles Rewards given in positive reinforcement procedures (e.g., food or toys).
tardive dyskinesia A potentially severe movement disorder resulting from the long-term use of phenothiazines or other antipsychotic medication.
target behaviors Behaviors selected for assessment and management.
tartar *See* calculus.
TCD *See* transcranial Doppler.
tectorial membrane Attached to the cochlea of the inner ear.
telangiectasia Abnormal cluster of small blood vessels.
telehealth Electronic and video-based communication.
telencephalon The structure in the embryo that turns into the cerebral cortex, subcortical white matter, and basal ganglia.
teletypewriter (TTY) An electronic device for text communication via a telephone line used when one or more of the parties has hearing or speech difficulties.
telophase The final phase in cell division in which the daughter chromosomes are at the opposite poles of the cell and new nuclear membranes form.
temporal lobe Brain region involved in visual and auditory processing. The area of the cortex primarily involved in communication and sensation.
tendons Fibrous cords by which muscles are attached to bone or to one another.
teratogens Agents that can cause malformations in a developing embryo.
testosterone Male sex hormone.
tethered Tied down.
tetraploid Having four copies of each chromosome (i.e., 92 chromosomes). This is incompatible with life.
thalamus Region of the brain situated in the posterior part of the forebrain that relays sensory impulses to the cerebral cortex.
theory of mind The ability to intuit and understand others' thoughts, emotions, and perspectives, particularly when they differ from one's own experience.
therapeutic drug monitoring Management of a patient's medication based on measuring blood concentration of the drug over time.
thickening agents Can transform any thin liquid into a nectar-, honey-, or milkshake-like consistency.
thimerosal A mercury-containing organic compound that was in the past used as a preservative in vaccines.
thoracolumbar kyphosis Curvature of the mid-lower spine in the front to back plane.
thrombocytopenia Low platelet count.
thrombophilia A genetic tendency for one's blood to clot more than normal.
thrush Monilial (fungal) yeast infection of the oral cavity sometimes seen in infants.
thymine One of the four nucleotides (chemicals) that comprise DNA.
thymus A gland in the upper chest which plays a key role in regulating immune responses.
thyrotoxicosis A form of hyperthyroidism leading to severe symptoms.
tics Brief repetitive movements or vocalizations that occur in a stereotyped manner and do not appear to be under voluntary control.
time-in A behavioral procedure which dramatically increases pleasant social and physical contact between the child and caregiver.
time-out A procedure whereby the possibility of positive reinforcement is withdrawn for a brief amount of time following the occurrence of a targeted challenging behavior.
TLR *See* tonic labyrinthine reflex.
tocolysis Use of medications to stop preterm labor.
Todd's paralysis Reversible weakness of one side of the body following a seizure.
tonic Effect of prolonged muscular contraction on tone.
tonic labyrinthine response A primitive reflex found in newborns. Tilting the head back while lying on the back causes the back to stiffen and arch backwards; the legs to straighten, stiffen, and push together; the toes to point; the arms to bend at the elbows and wrists; and the hands to become fisted or the fingers to curl. *Also called* tonic labyrinthine reflex (TLR).
tonic-clonic Spasmodic alteration of muscle contraction and relaxation.
tonotopic organization Pertaining to the spatial arrangement of where sound is perceived, transmitted, or received.
tonotopic tuning Process occurring between 28 and 30 weeks' gestation by which exposure to sounds in the intrauterine environment allows the cochlea to begin fine-tuning its response to different frequencies of sound.

tonotopically Arranged spatially by tone as found in the cochlea of the inner ear.
tooth bud *See* dental organ.
TORCH *See* Appendix B.
torticollis Wry neck in which the neck is painfully tilted to one side; a form of dystonia.
toxemia *See* preeclampsia.
toxoplasmosis An infectious disease caused by a microorganism, which may be asymptomatic in adults but can lead to severe fetal malformations.
Toxoplasmosis gondii A parasite that can cause an intrauterine infection and birth defects.
trachea Windpipe.
tracheal intubation Introducing a tube into the airway to facilitate breathing.
tracheoesophageal fistula A congenital connection between the trachea and esophagus leading to aspiration of food and requiring surgical correction.
tracheomalacia Softening of the cartilage of the trachea.
tracheostomy The surgical creation of an opening into the trachea to permit insertion of a tube to facilitate mechanical ventilation.
tracheostomy tube A catheter that is inserted into the trachea for the purpose of supplying air.
trachoma A bacterial infection causing blindness in developing countries.
transcranial Doppler (TCD) An instrument that emits ultrasonic beams to diagnose vascular disease in the head.
transcription The process in which mRNA is formed from a DNA template.
transition individualized education program (transition IEP) A written plan for an adolescent receiving special education services that maps out his or her postschool education, services, and employment and adult living goals. It is required by federal law (IDEA, 2004) to be part of the student's IEP starting at age 16; *previously called* individualized transition plan (ITP).
transitional (fetal) circulation Circulatory changes occurring at birth in the lungs and around the heart, resulting from pulmonary vasodilation and closure of the ductus arteriosus and the foramen ovale (the two fetal bypasses around the lungs during fetal life).
translation A process where the mRNA moves out of the nucleus into the cytoplasm, where it provides instructions for the production of a protein.
translocation The transfer of a fragment of one chromosome to another chromosome.
transplacental transmission The passage of microbes from the maternal to fetal circulation via the placenta.
tremor A trembling motion.
Treponema pallium Microorganism causing syphilis.
trichotillomania Recurrent pulling out of one's hair.
triplet repeat expansion Abnormal number of copies of identical triplet nucleotides (as occurs in fragile X syndrome; *see* Chapter 15).
triploid Having three copies of each chromosome (i.e., 69 chromosomes), which is generally incompatible with life.
trisomy A condition is which there are three copies of one chromosome rather than two (e.g., trisomy 21, Down syndrome).
trochlear nerve The fourth cranial nerve controls the superior oblique eye muscle.
trophoblast The outermost layer of cells that attaches the fertilized egg to the uterine wall.
TTY *See* teletypewriter.
tubers Benign growths found in the brain of an individual with tuberous sclerosis.
twinning The production of twins.
tympanic membrane (TM) Eardrum.
tympanometry The measurement of flexibility of the tympanic membrane as an indicator of a middle-ear infection or fluid in the middle ear.
tympanostomy A small tube inserted through the tympanic membrane after myringotomy to aerate the middle ear; often used in the treatment of recurrent or persistent otitis media (middle ear infection).
tyrosine An amino acid.
UES *See* upper esophageal sphincter.
umbilical cord prolapse The umbilical cord being born before rather than after the baby, thereby becoming compressed by the fetus during the delivery process and interfering with oxygen flow to the fetus during labor.
undernutrition Inadequate nutrition to sustain normal growth.
uniparental disomy *See* genomic imprinting.
unsaturated fatty acid A type of dietary fat, certain kinds of which have been linked to heart disease.
upper esophageal sphincter (UES) A muscle at the entrance to the esophagus.
urea End product of protein metabolism.
urea cycle disorders A group of inborn errors of metabolism. *See* Appendix B.
uremia The abnormal accumulation of urinary waste products in the blood present in renal (kidney) failure.
ureterostomy Surgical procedure creating an outlet for the ureters through the abdominal wall.
urethra Canal through which urine passes from the bladder.
urodynamics A test that accesses how the bladder and urethra are performing their job of storing and releasing urine.
urticarial Hives.
valgus Condition in which the distal body part is angled away from the midline.
varicella The virus that causes chickenpox and shingles.
varus Condition in which the distal body part is angled toward the midline.
vascular occlusion Blockage of a blood vessel.
vasoconstriction A decrease in the diameter of blood vessels.
vasodilation Relaxation and dilation of blood vessels.
vaso-occlusive episode In sickle cell disease, the sudden restriction of blood flow due to sickle-shaped red blood cells blocking capillaries.

ventilator A machine that provides a mixture of air and oxygen to an individual in respiratory failure.
ventral Front.
ventral induction Describes development of the prosencephalon, its division into two sections, the telencephalon and diencephalon, and cleavage of the telencephalon into two cerebral hemispheres.
ventricles Fluid-filled cavities, especially in the heart or brain.
ventricular septal defect A congenital heart defect in which the wall separating the two lower chambers of the heart does not close during embryonic development.
ventricular system Interconnecting cavities of the brain containing cerebrospinal fluid.
ventriculomegaly Enlargement of the cerebral ventricles, usually seen in hydrocephalus.
ventriculoperitoneal shunt (VP shunt) Surgically placed tube connecting a cerebral ventricle with the abdominal cavity; used to treat hydrocephalus by draining cerebrospinal fluid into the child's abdominal cavity.
ventriculo-subgaleal shunt Implanted as a temporary measure for treatment of hydrocephalus, draining cerebrospinal fluid from the ventricles to the scalp.
vertebral arches The bony arches projecting from the body of the vertebra.
vertex presentation Downward position of infant's head during vaginal delivery.
vertical transmission Mother-to-child transmission of infection, especially in human immunodeficiency virus (HIV).
very low birth weight (VLBW) Term often used to describe an infant with a birth weight less than 1,500 grams (3 1/3 pounds).
vesicles Small bladderlike cavities containing specific chemicals (e.g., neurotransmitters).
vesicostomy The surgical creation of an opening for the bladder to empty its contents through the abdominal wall.
vestibular apparatus (VA) *See* vestibular system.
vestibular system Three ring-shaped bodies located in the labyrinth of the ear that are involved in maintenance of balance and sensation of the body's movement through space.
villi Vascular projections, such as those coming from the embryo that become part of the placenta; *singular:* villus.
visceral Relating to the soft internal organs of the body, especially those contained within the abdominal and thoracic cavities.
vision impairment A condition characterized by a loss of visual acuity, where the eye does not see objects as clearly as usual, or a loss of visual field, where the eye cannot see as wide an area as usual without moving the eyes or turning the head.
visual acuity The clarity of vision.
vitiligo A skin disease marked by patches of lack of pigment.
vitreous humor The gelatinous content of the eye located between the lens and retina.
VLBW *See* very low birth weight.
volunteering An opportunity for adolescents to gain valuable insight into the world of work, to develop skills, and to build work-related experience.
VP shunt *See* ventriculoperitoneal shunt.
watershed area Area of tissue lying between two major arteries and thus poorly supplied by blood.
watershed infarct Injury to brain due to lack of blood flow in the brain tissues between interfacing blood vessels.
whole-exome sequencing (WES) A genomic technique for sequencing all of the protein-coding genes in a genome (known as the exome).
work-study employment Part-time work for students sanctioned by the school either on or off campus.
xerosis Dryness of eyes.
xerostomia Dry mouth.
X-linked trait A trait transmitted by a gene located on the X chromosome; *previously called* sex-linked.
Zika virus A virus that can cause an intrauterine infection and severe microcephaly in an affected baby.
zone of proximal development The distance between the actual developmental level as determined by independent problem solving and the level of potential development under guidance.
zygote Fertilized egg.

APPENDIX **B**

Syndromes and Inborn Errors of Metabolism

Kara L. Simpson

The underlying cause of a developmental disability can be explained in some children by a single genetic or teratogenic mechanism. An understanding of the etiology can shed light on the reason for clinical features such as physical malformations, cognitive impairments, and behavior problems. Making a diagnosis in such cases may be important for physicians to implement appropriate medical management or to provide genetic or prenatal counseling. Other professionals may also find that a diagnosis assists them in the development of more global aspects of the child's care, including educational, physical, occupational, and speech-language therapy. The direct benefit to families includes the ability to gather information specific to their child's condition and to seek out support from other parents and/or affected individuals through support groups, conferences, and the Internet. Finally, attaining a specific diagnosis can lead patients, families, and health care professionals to the appropriate disease-oriented organization, which is often a great source of information and support (not just medical, but also emotional and sometimes financial as well). For all of these reasons, the search for an etiology of a child's developmental disability may focus on syndrome identification.

By definition, a *syndrome* is a recurring, recognizable pattern of structural defects and/or secondary effects that represents a single etiology. Syndromes may have a genetic basis (such as chromosomal or single-gene defects; see Chapter 1), can be environmental (e.g., teratogens; see Chapter 2), or can be complex (caused by more than one genetic and/or environmental factor). Genetic syndromes affect multiple organ systems because the genetic defect is usually contained in every cell of the body. This abnormality may interfere with typical development or cause abnormal differentiation of more than one tissue of the body. Many genetic and teratogenic syndromes are of prenatal onset and are evident at birth, usually because of an unusual appearance (i.e., dysmorphic features) or multiple congenital abnormalities. Syndromes are usually stable conditions, and neurological regression is uncommon. A *sequence* is a situation where a single event leads to a single anomaly that has a cascading effect of local and/or distant deformations and/or disruptions. An *association* is a nonrandom occurrence of anomalies with no consistent etiology.

Unlike most syndromes, *inborn errors of metabolism* are usually not evident at birth. During pregnancy, the mother's normal metabolism usually protects the fetus. After delivery, however, there may be an accumulation of toxic metabolites as a result of an enzyme deficiency. The presentation of inborn errors varies from metabolic crisis and death within days of birth to occasional episodes in response to external factors later in childhood. Some metabolic disorders are treatable, and many in this category of genetic conditions are detectable with newborn screening through biochemical or molecular testing (see Chapters 4 and 17). Others, despite early diagnosis and treatment, still lead to irreversible effects.

Although the clinical features associated with certain syndromes and inborn errors of metabolism have been known for centuries (e.g., Down syndrome and congenital hypothyroidism), the chromosomal and molecular basis of the disorders has only been characterized since the 1960s. An increasing number of genetic and biochemical tests can now be utilized to confirm a clinically suspected diagnosis. This is of particular importance because different therapeutic options (or the opportunity to participate in clinical research trials) may be available to individuals on the basis of a genetic diagnosis, particularly in the cases of molecularly based therapies. In addition, a genetic diagnosis allows for accurate recurrence risk estimates, the possibility of invasive prenatal testing on a subsequent pregnancy, and appropriate genetic counseling for other family members.

Diagnostic testing in patients with developmental delay, intellectual disability, congenital anomalies, and dysmorphic features has evolved significantly in the last several years, with the addition of cytogenetic microarrays based on comparative genomic hybridization (CGH) and single nucleotide polymorphism array analyses, as well as next-generation sequencing (NGS) panels and whole-exome sequencing (WES).

With the array CGH, copy number variants are determined by comparing the hybridization pattern intensities between an individual's DNA and control DNA. Microarrays are considered the first-tier clinical test for those with developmental disabilities, congenital anomalies, and autism spectrum disorder. NGS refers to non-Sanger-based, high-throughput DNA sequencing, which allows for billions of DNA strands to be sequenced in parallel. This allows large panels of genes to be tested simultaneously, which is very useful for syndromes with large numbers of associated genes. WES allows for sequencing of the entire exome, which has been helpful in determining new phenotypes of known syndromes and outlining new syndromes. However, the significance of many of the changes found on WES are not yet known, in addition to the possibility of incidental findings and their impact on a family.

It should be noted that genetic testing is frequently not straightforward and often contains changes of unknown significance. It is recommended that the ordering of any genetic testing be done by genetics teams as they have the appropriate resources to explain the results and consequences to patients (see Wallace, S. E., & Bean, L. J. H. [2017]. Educational materials—genetic testing: Current approaches. In M. P. Adam, H. H. Ardinger, R. A. Pagon, S. E. Wallace, L. J. H. Bean, K. Stephens, & A. Amemiya. [Eds.]. *GeneReviews*. Seattle, WA: University of Washington. Retrieved from https://www.ncbi.nlm.nih.gov/books/NBK279899/).

Research on the cognitive abilities of individuals with genetic syndromes has uncovered specific learning and behavior patterns for many syndromes. These are called behavioral phenotypes, and they can be used to establish rational and attainable educational goals to promote a child reaching his or her full cognitive and functional potential (Battaglia, A. & G. S. Fisch. [2010]. Behavioral phenotypes in neurogenetic syndromes. *American Journal of Medical Genetics Part C: Seminars in Medical Genetics, 154C*[4], 387–485). Insight into an individual's specific condition, the behavioral phenotype, cognitive abilities, and learning strengths and weaknesses can be of particular importance in the classroom. References addressing the cognitive and behavioral abilities of individuals with specific genetic conditions are included in this appendix when possible. Some syndromes, however, are so rare that there are not enough data to outline a behavioral phenotype.

Many excellent resources concerning genetic conditions exist for families and health care professionals caring for children with disabilities. Some useful ones include the following:

- **The Genetic Alliance** is a nonprofit organization with a directory of support groups, foundations, research organizations, patient advocacy groups, and tissue registries. The Genetic Alliance is based in Washington, D.C. (202-966-5557; http://www.geneticalliance.org; e-mail: info@geneticalliance.org).
- **The Genetic and Rare Diseases Information Center** (GARD; 888-205-2311; https://rarediseases.info.nih.gov/diseases) is a program of the National Center for Advancing Translational Sciences (NCATS) and is funded by two parts of the National Institutes of Health (NIH): NCATS and the National Human Genome Research Institute (NHGRI). GARD provides the public with access to current, reliable, and easy-to-understand information about rare or genetic diseases in English or Spanish.
- **GeneReviews** (https://www.ncbi.nlm.nih.gov/books/NBK1116/) is administered by the University of Washington and funded by the National Institutes of Health (NIH), the Health Resources and Services Administration (HRSA), and the U.S. Department of Energy (DOE). GeneReviews provides peer-reviewed articles on genetic conditions that include information on diagnosis, management, and genetic counseling of individuals with specific inherited disorders and their families. It also provides relevant resources specific to each disease.
- **The National Organization for Rare Disorders** (NORD; 203-744-0100, toll-free 800-999-6673; http://www.rarediseases.org) is a nonprofit patient advocacy organization dedicated to orphan diseases (disorders occurring in less than 200,000 individuals in the United States). NORD provides information about diseases, referrals to patient organizations, research grants and fellowships, advocacy for the rare-disease community, and medication assistance programs.

- **The Online Mendelian Inheritance in Man** (OMIM; http://www.ncbi.nlm.nih.gov/omim) catalog describes all known Mendelian disorders and over 12,000 genes, providing clinical, biochemical, genetic, and therapeutic information. OMIM is authored and edited at the McKusick-Nathans Institute of Genetic Medicine, Johns Hopkins University School of Medicine.
- **The Genetics Home Reference**, sponsored by the U.S. National Library of Medicine (http://ghr.nlm.nih.gov/), is an excellent resource for health care professionals, teachers, and families, providing basic information about genetics and searchable disease-specific data.

HOW ENTRIES ARE ORGANIZED

This appendix lists a number of syndromes and inborn errors of metabolism that are often associated with developmental disabilities. Included in each listing are the disease category, principal characteristics, pattern of inheritance, frequency of occurrence (prevalence or incidence), treatment options when available, and recent references that further define the syndrome. Cognitive and behavioral changes are noted for disorders in which common developmental abnormalities are widely accepted as being part of the syndrome or inborn error. When known, the causative gene or chromosome location is listed. In describing the chromosomal location, the first number or letter indicates the chromosome on which there is a genetic change (mutation), and the subsequent letter (*p* or *q*) indicates the short or long arm of the chromosome, respectively. The term *ter* is used when the site is at the terminal end of one arm of the chromosome, and *cen* is used when the site is near the **centromere.** The numbers following the *p* or *q* specify the location on the chromosome. For example, Aarskog-Scott syndrome is located on the short arm of the X chromosome at position 11.21, designated as Xp11.21. The inheritance patterns of genetic traits are listed as autosomal recessive (AR), autosomal dominant (AD), X-linked recessive (XLR), X-linked dominant (XLD), mitochondrial (M), new mutation (NM; i.e., diseases caused by new mutations that arise in the sperm or the egg), or sporadic (SP; i.e., noninherited). Each syndrome has been assigned to a disease category, which is defined next. Although this appendix lists a number of the more commonly recognized syndromes associated with developmental disabilities, it is not intended to be all-inclusive. Specific medical terminology is defined in the Glossary (see Appendix A).

DISEASE CATEGORIES

auditory disorders Diseases that affect hearing.

chromosome abnormality Disorder due to a duplication, loss, or rearrangement of chromosomal material.

chromosome breakage syndromes Syndromes associated with increased rates of chromosomal breakage or instability due to defects in DNA repair mechanisms or genomic instability that leads to chromosomal rearrangements.

connective tissue disorders Disorders that affect the connective tissue, the tissue that helps support, binds together, and protects organs.

contiguous gene defect A disorder due to deletion of multiple genes that are adjacent to one another.

endocrine disorder Disorder affecting the endocrine systems glands and secretions (hormones).

immunodeficiency Disorder affecting the immune system which results in a weakened ability to fight off infections.

inborn errors of metabolism Genetic disorders that disrupt metabolism. Most are due to defects of single genes that code for enzymes that break down substrates. Each inborn error of metabolism has been categorized based on the main type of metabolism affected (e.g., carbohydrate, amino acid, organic acid, lysosomal storage disease, or copper).

imprinting defect Group of disorders where there is a defect in the process of genomic imprinting (where certain alleles are expressed based on the parent of origin).

malformation Birth defect that results from intrinsic defects in genes that control development.

multiple congenital anomalies Structural defects that are present at birth and affect multiple structures and organs.

neurological disorders Disorders mainly affecting the brain, spinal cord, and nerves.

neuromuscular diseases Diseases that affect the muscles and/or the nerves that control them.

ophthalmologic disorders Diseases that affect the eye.

overgrowth syndromes Disorders in which there is an abnormal increase in the size of the body or of a specific body part.

peroxisomal disorders A group of disorders caused by a deficiency in enzymes within the peroxisome (an organelle involved in metabolism of very long-chain fatty acids, biosynthesis of plasmalogens, and energy metabolism), or proteins encoded by genes for normal peroxisome assembly.

skeletal dysplasia A group of disorders characterized by abnormalities of bone and cartilage.

SYNDROMES AND DISORDERS

Aarskog-Scott syndrome (faciodigitogenital syndrome or faciogenital dysplasia) *Disease category:* Multiple congenital anomalies. *Clinical features:* Short stature, brachydactyly (short fingers and toes), widow's peak, broad nasal bridge with small nose, hypertelorism, shawl scrotum, and cryptorchidism (undescended testes); learning disabilities and behavioral problems are present in a subset of patients. *Associated complications:* Ptosis, eye movement problems, strabismus, orthodontic problems, and occasional cleft lip/palate. *Cause:* Mutations in *FGD1* (Xp11.21). *Inheritance:* XLR, with partial expression in some females. *Prevalence:* 1:25,000.

References: Taub, M., & Stanton, A. (2008). Aarskog syndrome: A case report and literature review. *Optometry, 79*(7), 371–377.

Verhoeven, W. M. A. (2012). X-linked Aarskog syndrome: Report on a novel FGD1 gene mutation. Executive dysfunction as part of the behavioural phenotype. *Genetic Counseling, 23*(2), 157.

achondroplasia *Disease category:* Skeletal dysplasia. *Clinical features:* The most common form of short stature, associated with rhizomelic (proximal) shortening of the arms and legs, a large head with typical facial features (including frontal bossing and midface hypoplasia), genu varum (bow legs), and trident appearance of the hands. Hypotonia and motor delay is common. Cognitive development and life span are usually normal, although cervical spinal cord compression and upper airway obstruction increase risk of death in infancy. Newer studies show there may be some impairment of verbal IQ, attention, and executive function. Children with achondroplasia should be monitored for changes in their neurological status, particularly if there are concerns about delayed motor development. *Prevalence:* 1:26,000–1:28,000. *Cause:* 98% of affected individuals have a common point mutation in *FGFR3* (4p16.3). *Inheritance:* AD; 80% of cases are caused by NM.

References: Del Pino, M., Ramos Mejia, R., & Fano, V. (2018). Leg length, sitting height, and body proportions references for achondroplasia: New tools for monitoring growth. *American Journal of Medical Genetics, Part A,,176(4),* 896–906.

Wigg, K., Tofts, L., Benson, S., & Porter, M. (2016). The neuropsychological function of children with achondroplasia. *American Journal of Medical Genetics, Part A, 170,* 2882–2888.

Witt, S., Rohenkohl, A., Bullinger, M., Sommer, R., Kahrs, S., Klingebiel, K. H, . . . Quitmann, J. (2017). Understanding, assessing and improving health-related quality of life of young people with achondroplasia—a collaboration between a patient organization and academic medicine. *Pediatric Endocrinology Review, 15*(Suppl. 1), 109–118.

acrocephalosyndactyly, type I *See* Apert syndrome.

acrocephalosyndactyly, type II *See* Carpenter syndrome.

acrocephalosyndactyly, type V *See* Pfeiffer syndrome.

acrofacial dysostosis (Nager syndrome) *Disease category:* Multiple congenital anomalies. *Clinical features:* Downslanting palpebral fissures, micrognathia (small jaw), midface retrusion (backward movement of the mandible), downward slant of eyelids, high nasal bridge, external ear defects, occasional cleft lip/palate, and asymmetric limb anomalies (hypoplastic thumb or radius [a bone in the lower arm]). *Associated complications:* Scoliosis, severe conductive hearing loss, occasional heart or kidney defects, and typically normal intelligence. *Cause:* Mutations in *SF3B4* (1q21.2). *Inheritance:* AD. *Prevalence:* Rare.

References: Bernier, F. P., Caluseriu, O., Ng, S., Schwartzentruber, J., Buckingham, K. J., Innes, A. M., ... Parboosing, J. S. (2012). Haploinsufficiency of SF3B4, a component of the pre-mRNA spliceosomal complex, causes Nager Syndrome. *American Journal of Human Genetics, 90,* 925–933.

Czeschik, J. C., Voigt, C., Alanay, Y., Albrecht, B., Avci, S., Fitzpatrick, D., . . . Wieczorek, D. (2013). Clinical and mutation data in 12 patients with the clinical diagnosis of Nager syndrome. *Human Genetics, 132,* 885–898.

Petit, F., Escande, F., Jourdain, A. S., Porchet, N., Amiel, J., Doray, B., . . . Holder-Espinasse, M. (2014). Nager syndrome: Confirmation of SF3B4 haploinsufficiency as the major cause. *Clinical Genetics, 86,* 246–251.

adrenoleukodystrophy (X-linked ALD) *Disease category:* Neuromuscular disease (for neonatal form, *see* adrenoleukodystrophy, neonatal form). *Clinical features:* Progressive neurological disorder of white matter resulting from accumulation of very long-chain fatty acids; three main phenotypes are seen in affected males. Those with the childhood cerebral form develop normally until between the ages of 4–8 years. Symptoms initially resemble attention-deficit disorder or hyperactivity. Impairment of cognition, behavior, vision, hearing, and motor function develop following initial symptoms and lead to total disability within 2 years. A second phenotype called adrenomyeloneuropathy (AMN) manifests most commonly in the late twenties, as progressive paraparesis (paralysis), sphincter disturbances, sexual dysfunction, and often impaired adrenocortical function. The third phenotype is known as "Addison disease only" and presents with primary adrenocortical insufficiency between age 2 and adulthood without evidence of neurologic abnormality (but can develop later). *Associated complications:* Progressive intellectual deterioration, seizures, endocrine abnormalities, and conductive hearing loss. *Cause:* Mutations in *ABCD1* (Xq28). The ALD protein product is localized to the peroxisomal membrane. *Inheritance:* XLR, with intrafamilial variability ranging from classical childhood-onset ALD to adult-onset ALD to Addison disease; 93% of affected individuals inherit the *ABCD1* mutation from one parent, and 7% from NM. Approximately 20% of females who are carriers develop neurologic manifestations that resemble AMN but have later onset and milder disease than affected males. *Prevalence:* 1:20,000–1:50,000. *Treatment:* Corticosteroid replacement therapy for adrenal insufficiency (will not alter neurologic symptoms). Bone marrow transplant can provide long-term stability and may reverse some neurologic complications in the early stages. Dietary modifications including "Lorenzo's oil" (oleic acid and erucic acid) have been shown to lower VLCFA levels, but clinical effects are still under investigation.

References: Berger, J., Pujol, A., Aubourg, P., & Forss-Petter, S. (2010). Current and future pharmacological treatment strategies in X-linked adrenoleukodystrophy. *Brain Pathology, 20(4),* 845–856.

Kaga, M., Furushima, W., Inagaki, M., & Nakamura, M. (2009). Early neuropsychological signs of childhood adrenoleukodystrophy (ALD). *Brain & Development, 31,* 558–561.

Pierpont, E., Eisengart, J. B., Shanley, R., Nascene, D., Raymond, G. V., Shapiro, E. G., ... Miller, W. P. (2017). Neurocognitive trajectory of boys who received a hematopoietic stem cell transplant at an early stage of childhood cerebral adrenoleukodystrophy. *JAMA Neurology, 74,* 710–717.

Tran, C., Patel, J., Stacy, H., Mamak, E. G., Faghfoury, H., Raiman, J., . . . Mercimek-Mahmutoglu, S. (2017). Long-term outcome of patients with X-linked adrenoleukodystrophy: A retrospective cohort study. *European Journal of Paediatric Neurology, 21,* 600–609.

Aicardi syndrome *Disease category:* Neurologic. *Clinical features:* Infantile spasms, agenesis (absence) of the corpus callosum, and abnormalities of eyes (specifically chorioretinal lacunae). *Associated complications:* Poorly controlled seizures, visual impairment, cortical malformations, vertebral and rib abnormalities, vascular malformations or malignancy, micropthalmia, hypotonia, microcephaly, and moderate to severe intellectual disability. Survival varies, but mean age of death is about 8.3 years, and median age of death is about 18.5 years. *Cause:* No gene or candidate region on the X chromosome has been definitively identified. *Inheritance:* XLD/NM; previously it has been assumed that mutations are lethal in males as Aicardi syndrome has been seen almost exclusively in females or 47, XXY Klinefelter males. More recently there have been rare reports of 46, XY male patients. *Prevalence:* 1:105,000–1:167,000 in the United States.

References: Kroner, B. L., Preiss, L. R, Ardini, M. A., & Gaillard, W. D. (2008). New incidence, prevalence, and survival of Aicardi syndrome from 408 cases. *Journal of Child Neurology, 23,* 531–535.

Steffensen, T. S., Gilbert-Barness, E., Lacson, A., & Margo, C. E.(2009). Cerebellar migration defects in Aicardi syndrome: An extension of the neuropathological spectrum. *Fetal and Pediatric Pathology, 28,* 24–38.

Aicardi-Goutières syndrome (AGS) *Disease category:* Neurologic. *Clinical features:* Early-onset encephalopathy whose clinical features mimic those of acquired *in utero* viral infection. Normal pregnancy, delivery, and neonatal period in 80% of those affected; 20% present with brain calcifications *in utero* and present at birth with abnormal neurologic findings, hepatosplenomegaly, elevated liver enzymes, and thrombocytopenia. The rest of affected infants present at variable times, usually after a period of normal development. They present with subacute onset of severe encephalopathy characterized by extreme irritability, intermittent sterile pyrexias (fevers), loss of skills, and slowing of head growth. *Associated complications:* Peripheral spasticity, dystonic posturing of upper limbs, truncal hypotonia, poor head control, and seizures. Almost all affected individuals have severe intellectual and physical impairment. *Cause:* Seven causative genes have been found: *TREX1* (3p21.3-p21.2), *RNASEH2B* (13q14.1), *RNASEH2C* (11q13.2), *RNASEH2A* (19p13.13), *ADAR* (1q21.3), and *SAMHD1* (20q11.23). *Inheritance:* The majority of cases are AR, although there are AD/NM mutations in *TREX1*. *Prevalence:* Unknown.

References: Crow, Y., Vanderver, A., Orcesi, S., Kuijpers, T. W., & Rice, G. I. (2014). Therapies in Aicardi-Goutieres syndrome. *Clinical and Experimental Immunology, 175,* 1–8.

Crow, Y., Chase, D. S., Lowenstein Schmidt, J., Szynkiewicz, M., Forte, G. M., Ornall, H. L., . . . Rice, G. I. (2015). Characterization of human disease phenotypes associated with mutations in TREX1, RNASEH2A, RNASEH2B, RANSEH2C, SAMHD, ADAR, and IFIH1. *American Journal of Medical Genetics A, 167,* 296–312.

alcohol-related neurodevelopmental defects (ARND) Previously called fetal alcohol effects (FAE); *see* Chapter 2.

Alexander disease *Disease category:* Neurologic. *Clinical features:* Progressive cortical white matter neurological disorder that mostly affects infants and children and results in early death. General characteristics of the disease include seizures, intellectual disability, white matter abnormalities, and megalencephaly (enlarged head). The neonatal form usually ends in death within 2 years. The infantile form presents by age 2, and affected children survive up to several years. The juvenile form presents between ages 4–10 (and occasionally in the teens), and affected individuals survive until early teens to mid-20s and 30s. An adult form has been described, although with variable presentation. *Associated complications:* Hydrocephalus, demyelination, progressive spasticity, and visual impairment; bulbar signs are present in some patients. *Cause:* Mutations in *GFAP* (17q21). *Inheritance:* Majority of cases are caused by an NM with AD inheritance when passed from an affected individual; rare AD families have been reported. *Prevalence:* Rare.

References: Graff-Radford, J., Schwartz, K., Gavrilova, R. H., Lachance, D. H., & Kumar, N. (2014). Neuroimaging and clinical features in type II (late-onset) Alexander disease. *Neurology, 82,* 49–56.

Green, L., Berry, I. R., Childs, A. M., McCullagh, H., Jose, S., Warren, D., . . . Livingston, J. H. (2017). Whole exon deletion in the GFAP gene is a novel molecular mechanism causing Alexander disease. *Neuropediatrics, 49(2),* 118–122.

Angelman syndrome *Disease category:* Imprinting defect/multiple congenital defect/contiguous gene defect. *Clinical features:* Severe developmental delay or intellectual disability, severe speech impairment, gait ataxia, and unique behavior with an inappropriate happy demeanor that includes frequent laughing, smiling, and excitability. *Associated complications:* Seizures and microcephaly. Behavioral features include hyperactivity, short attention span, hand flapping, feeding problems, chewing/mouthing behaviors, fascination with water, and abnormal food-related behaviors. *Cause:* Deletion of 15q11–q13 on the maternally inherited chromosome, paternal inheritance of both copies of chromosome 15 (uniparental disomy, or UPD), a point mutation in the maternal copy of *UBE3A* or an imprinting defect (due to deletion or epigenetic effect). *Inheritance:* All three causes arise as a result of NM; mutations in the *UBE3A* gene may be passed in an AD fashion. *Prevalence:* 1:10,000–1:20,000.

References: Pelc, K., Cheron, G., & Dan, B. (2008). Behavior and neuropsychiatric manifestations in Angelman syndrome. *Neuropsychiatric Disease and Treatment, 4*(3), 577–584.

Quinn, E. D., & Rowland, C. (2017). Exploring expressive communication skills in a cross-sectional sample of children and young adults with Angelman syndrome. *American Journal of Speech Language Pathology, 26,* 369–382.

Williams, C. A. (2010). The behavioral phenotype of the Angelman syndrome. *American Journal of Medical Genetics Part C: Seminars in Medical Genetics, 154C,* 432–437.

Apert syndrome (acrocephalosyndactyly, type I) *Disease category:* Craniosynostosis. *Clinical features:* Craniosynostosis (premature fusion of the cranial sutures) with misshapen head (turribrachycephalic skull shape), high forehead, and flat occiput (back part of head); hypertelorism with downward slant; moderate-to-severe midface hypoplasia (flat midface) and nasal bridge; severe syndactyly (webbing of fingers or toes); limb anomalies; and cleft palate, hypertelorism, and fused cervical vertebrae. *Associated complications:* Hydrocephalus, varying degrees of intellectual disability, hearing loss, teeth abnormalities, and occasional heart and kidney anomalies. *Cause:* Mutations in *FGFR2* (10q26). *Inheritance:* Majority of cases are caused by an NM, with AD inheritance when passed from an affected individual. *Incidence:* 1:100,000. *Treatment:* Early neurosurgical correction of fused sutures improves appearance and may reduce risk of intellectual disability; plastic/orthopedic surgery for limb anomalies.

References: Breik, O.,Mahindu, A., Moore, M. H., Molloy, C. J., Santoreneos, S., & David, D. J. (2016). Apert syndrome: Surgical outcomes and perspectives. *Journal of Craniomaxillofacial Surgery, 44,* 1238–1245.

Fernandes, M. B., Maximino, L. P., Perosa, G. B., Abramides, D. V., Passos-Bueno, M. R., & Yacubian-Fernandes, A. (2016). Apert and Crouzon syndromes—cognitive development, brain abnormalities, and molecular aspects. *American Journal of Medical Genetics, 170,* 1532–1537.

ARND Alcohol-related neurodevelopmental disorder; *see* Chapter 2.

arthrogryposis multiplex congenita *Disease category:* Neuromuscular disease. *Clinical features:* Nonprogressive joint contractures that begin prenatally; flexion contractures at the fingers, knees, and elbows, with muscle weakness around involved joints. *Associated complications:* Occasional kidney and eye anomalies, cleft palate, defects of abdominal wall, and scoliosis. *Cause:* Multiple; most frequently related to an underlying neuropathy, myopathy (muscle weakness), or *in utero* crowding; may be associated with maternal myasthenia gravis. Nerve conduction studies/electromyography (EMG) and muscle biopsy may be beneficial in determining the basis of the condition (myopathic versus neurogenic). Intelligence is usually normal. *Inheritance:* Usually SP and may be caused by teratogenic exposure; however, both AD and AR inheritance also have been reported. *Incidence:* 1:3,000–1:12,000. *Treatment:* Casting of affected joints or surgery, if indicated.

References: Ma, L., & Yu, X. (2017). Arthrogryposis multiplex congenita: Classification, diagnosis, perioperative care, and anesthesia. *Frontiers of Medicine, 11(1),* 48–53.

Skaria, P., Dhal, A., & Ahmed, A. (2017). Arthrogryposis multiplex congenital in utero: radiologic and pathologic findings. *Journal of Maternal-Fetal & Neonatal Medicine, 27,* 1–10.

ataxia telangiectasia *Disease category:* Chromosome breakage syndrome. *Clinical features:* Slowly progressive ataxia, telangiectasias (dilation of capillaries, especially in the sclera [whites of eye] and behind the earlobe), small cerebellum. immune defects, and elevated alpha-fetoprotein in blood. *Associated complications:* Dystonia or choreoathetosis, dysarthric speech (imperfect articulation due to decreased motor control), increased sensitivity to radiation, increased risk of malignancy (especially leukemia or lymphoma), eye movement abnormalities, finger contractures, and increased risk of sinus and pulmonary infections; intelligence is typically unaffected but may decline with disease progression. Intelligence is typically normal, although learning disabilities are common. Survival is usually past 25 years, and some live into their 50s. *Cause:* Mutations in the *ATM* gene (11q22.3). *Inheritance:* AR. Although those with heterozygous mutations in *ATM* still have an increased risk of cancer. *Prevalence:* 1:40,000–1:100,000 live births in the United States. *Treatment:* Variable responses to amantadine and 4-aminopyridine for myoclonus. IVIG (intravenous immunoglobulin) replacement therapy for those with frequent and severe infections and low IgG levels; aggressive pulmonary hygiene for those with chronic bronchiectasis; steroids temporarily improve neurologic function, but symptoms reappear within days of discontinuation; and avoidance of excessive ionizing radiation.

References: Shaikh, A. G., Marti, S., Tarnutzer, A. A., Palla, A., Crawford, T. O., Zee, D. S., & Straumann, D. (2013). Effects of 4-aminopyridine on nystagmus and vestibule-ocular reflex in ataxia-telangiectasia. *Journal of Neurology, 260 (11),* 2728–2735.

van Os, N. J., Roeleveld, N., Weemaes, C. M., Jongmans, M. C., Janssens, G. O., Taylor, A. M., . . . Willemsen, M. A. (2016). Health risks for ataxia-telangiectasia mutated heterozygotes: A systematic review, meta-analysis and evidence-based guideline. *Clinical Genetics, 90(2),* 105–117.

Bardet-Biedl syndrome (BBS) *Disease category:* Multiple congenital anomalies. *Clinical features:* Retinal dysfunction, polydactyly (extra fingers or toes), obesity, learning disabilities, genital abnormalities, and kidney anomalies. *Associated complications:* Speech delay/disorder, developmental delay, behavioral abnormalities, eye abnormalities, ataxia, diabetes, heart abnormalities, abnormal liver function, specific facial features, and night blindness. *Cause:* Mutations have been found in 23 genes: *CCDC28B* (1p35.2), *SDCCAG8* (1q43-q44), *WDPCP* (2p15), *BBS5* (2q31.1), *LZTFL* (3p21.31), *ARL6* (3q11.2), *BBS7* (4q27), *BBS12* (4q12), *PTHB1* (8q22.1), *TMEM67* (8q22.1), *IFT74* (9p21.2) *TRIM32* (9q33.1), *BBIP1* (10q25.2), *BBS10* (12q21.2), *CEP290* (12q21.32), *TTC8* (14q31.3), *BBS4* (15q24.1), *IBBS2* (16q13), *MKS1* (17q22), *MKK5* (20p12.2), and *IFT27* (22q12.3). *Inheritance:* Generally AR, although in some families, mutations in more than one BBS locus may result in a clinical phenotype of BBS. *Prevalence:* 1:100,000.

References: Castro-Sanchez, S.,Alvarez-Satta, M., Corton, M., Guillen, E., Ayuso, C., & Valverde, D. (2015). Exploring genotype-phenotype relationships in Bardet-Biedl syndrome families. *Journal of Medical Genetics, 52*(8), 503–313.

Esposito, G., Testa, F., Zacchia, M., Crispo, A. A., Di Iorio, V., Capolongo, G., . . . Salvatore, F. (2017). Genetic characterization of Italian patients with Bardet-Biedl syndrome and correlation to ocular, kidney and audio-vestibular phenotype: Identification of eleven novel pathogenic sequence variants. *BMC Medical Genetics, 18*(1), 10.

Batten disease *Disease category:* Neurological disorder. *Clinical features:* Typical development until rapid vision loss begins between 4–10 years; children become completely blind within 2–4 years of the onset of vision loss. Gradual onset of ataxia and myoclonic, generalized tonic-clonic or focal seizures happens between ages 9–18 years. Early death usually occurs by late teens or early 20s, although some patients have lived into their 30s. *Associated complications:* Gradual intellectual decline, spasticity, psychosis, kyphoscoliosis, decline in speech, behavioral problems, and sleep disturbance. *Cause:* Mutations in *CLN3, PPT1, TPP1, CLN9,* and *ATP13A2* are associated with juvenile neuronal ceroid-lipofuscinosis. *Treatment:* Antiepileptic drugs should be selected carefully. Lamotrigine had a favorable effect in studies, and benzodiazopenes may be beneficial for seizures, anxiety, spasticity, and sleep disorders. Trihexyphenyldil has improved dystonia and sialorrhea (drooling). Those with swallowing problems may require gastric tube placement. Some patients with CLN3 disease may need antidepressants and antipsychotic agents. *Inheritance:* AR. *Incidence:*

1.3:100,000 to 7:100,000 live births. Many other forms of neuronal ceroid *lipofuscinosis* exist, including infantile, late infantile, juvenile, and adult forms. Mutations in 13 CLN genes cause various forms of neuronal ceroid lipofuscinosis.

References: Aungaroon, G., Hallinan, B., Jain, P., Horn, P. S., Spaeth, C,. & Arya, R. (2016). Correlation among genotype, phenotype, and histology in neuronal ceroid lipofuscinoses: An individual patient data meta-analysis. *Pediatric Neurology, 60,* 42–48.

Williams, R. E., & Mole, S. E. (2012). New nomenclature and classification scheme for the neuronal ceroid lipofuscinoses. *Neurology, 79*(2), 183–191.

Becker muscular dystrophy (BMD) *See* muscular dystrophy.

Beckwith-Wiedemann syndrome *Disease category:* Overgrowth syndrome/imprinting defect/contiguous gene syndrome. *Clinical features:* Macrosomia (large body size); large organs, especially the tongue; and neonatal hypoglycemia (low blood sugar), embryonal tumors (Wilms tumor, hepatoblastoma, neuroblastoma, rhabdomysoarcoma), omphalocele (congenital defect in abdominal wall containing the intestine), ear creases/pits, and kidney abnormalities. *Associated complications:* Advanced growth for the first 6 years, with advanced bone age, occasional hemihyperplasia (abnormal cell proliferation leading to asymmetrical overgrowth), kidney or adrenal anomalies, and occasional developmental delay or intellectual disability (may be due to untreated hypoglycemia). *Cause:* Abnormal transcription and regulation of genes in the imprinted domain on chromosome 11p15.5, two copies of paternal 11p15.5 (paternal uniparental disomy), methylation abnormalities of gene *KCNQ1OT1 (DMR2)* or *H19 (DMR1),* mutations in *CDKN1C,* or maternal rearrangements involving 11p15.5. *Inheritance:* Majority of cases are caused by an NM with AD inheritance, with variable penetrance when passed from an affected individual. *Incidence:* 1:13,700 live births. *Treatment:* Early treatment of hypoglycemia is critical; surgical repair of omphalocele and regular tumor surveillance.

References: Brioude, F., Kalis, J. M., Mussa, A., Foster, A. C., Bliek, J., Ferrero, G. B., . . . Maher, E. R. (2018). Expert consensus document: Clinical and molecular diagnosis, screening and management of Beckwith-Wiedemann syndrome: An international consensus statement. *Nature Reviews. Endocrinology, 14*(4), 229–249.

Brzezinski, J., Shuman, C., Choufani, S., Ray, P., Stavropoulos, D. J., Basran, R., . . . Weksberg, R.(2017). Wilms tumour in Beckwith-Wiedemann syndrome and loss of methylation at imprinting centre 2: Revisiting tumour surveillance guidelines. *European Journal of Human Genetics,* 25(9), 1031–1039.

biotinidase deficiency (late-onset multiple carboxylase deficiency) *Disease category:* Inborn error of metabolism: cofactor deficiency. *Clinical features:* A disorder characterized by varying degrees of intellectual disability, hypotonia, seizures (often infantile spasms), alopecia, skin rash, delayed myelination, and lactic acidosis; onset of symptoms usually occurs between 2 weeks and 2 years of age. *Associated complications:* Hearing and visual impairment, respiratory difficulties and apnea, and recurrent infections. *Cause:* Defects in various enzymes for biotin transport or metabolism; genetic mutations have been identified in *BTN* (3p25). *Inheritance:* AR. *Incidence:* 1:60,000–1:140,000. *Treatment:* Supplementation with oral biotin; response is better if used early in the course of the disease. When picked up by newborn screen and supplementation given early, children have a completely normal outcome.

References: Porta, F., Pagliardini, V., Celestino, I., Pavanello, E., Pagliardini, S., Guardamagna, O., . . . Spada, M. (2017). Neonatal screening for biotinidase deficiency: A 30-year-single center experience. *Molecular Genetics and Metabolism Reports, 13,* 80–82.

Szymanska, E., Sredzinska, M., Lugowska, A., Pajdowska, M., Rokicki, D., &Tylki-Szymanska, A. (2015). Outcomes of oral biotin treatment in patients with biotinidase deficiency—twenty years follow-up. *Molecular Genetics and Metabolism Reports, 5,* 33–35.

Bloom syndrome *Disease category:* Chromosome breakage syndrome. *Clinical features:* Prenatal and postnatal growth retardation; sparse subcutaneous fat; red, sun-sensitive skin lesion appears on the nose and cheeks after sun exposure; and high incidence of multiple cancers. *Associated complications:* Mild intellectual disability or learning disability, gastroesophageal reflux, common infections, infertility in males, reduced fertility in females, non–insulin-dependent diabetes, immunoglobulin deficiency, and chronic lung disease. *Cause:* Mutations in the *BLM* gene, which encodes the *BLM* RecQ protein on chromosome 15q26.1. *Inheritance:* AR. *Prevalence:* Overall prevalence is rare, although it is seen more commonly in the Ashkenazi Jewish population.

References: Cunniff, C., Bassetti, J. A., & Ellis, N. A. (2017). Bloom's syndrome: Clinical spectrum, molecular pathogenesis, and cancer predisposition. *Molecular Syndromology, 8*(1), 4–23.

Thomas, E. R., Shanley, S., Walker, L., & Eeles, R. (2008). Surveillance and treatment of malignancy in Bloom syndrome. *Clinical Oncology, 20*(5), 375–379.

BMD muscular dystrophy, Becker type *See* muscular dystrophy, Duchenne and Becker types.

Börjeson-Forssman-Lehmann syndrome *Disease category:* Multiple congenital anomalies. *Clinical features:*

Obesity, short stature, postpubertal gynecomastia (breast enlargement in males), large ears, coarse facial appearance, small external genitalia, eye anomalies, tapering fingers, and varying degree of intellectual disability. *Associated complications:* Seizures, abnormal head size ranging from microcephalic to macrocephalic, and hypotonia. *Cause:* Mutations in *PHF6* (Xq26.3). *Inheritance:* XLR, with females less severely affected than males. *Prevalence:* Rare.

References: De Winter, C. F., van Dijk, F., Stolker, J. J., & Hennekam, R. C. (2009). Behavioural phenotype in Borjeson-Forssman-Lehmann syndrome. *Journal of Intellectual Disability Research, 53*(4), 319–328.

Di Donato, N., Isidor, B., Lopez Cazaux, S., Le Caignec, C., Klink, B., Kraus, C., . . . Hackmann, K. (2014). Distinct phenotype of PHF6 deletions in females. *European Journal of Medical Genetics, 57*(2–3), 85–89.

Jahani-Asi, A., Cheng, C., Zhang, C., & Bonni, A. (2016). Pathogenesis of Borjeson-Forssman-Lehmann syndrome: Insights from PHF6 function. *Neurobiological Disorders, 96,* 227–235.

Brachmann de Lange syndrome *See* de Lange syndrome.

Canavan disease (spongy degeneration of central nervous system) *Disease category:* Neurological disorder. *Clinical features:* Progressive neurological disorder consisting of macrocephaly, hypotonia progressing to spasticity with age, visual impairment, and early death. Symptoms begin at 3–6 months of age; children do not develop the ability to sit, walk, or talk. Despite limitations, children are interactive. *Associated complications:* Feeding difficulties with progressive swallowing problems, gastroesophageal reflux, severe intellectual disability, and head lag. *Cause:* Deficiency in the enzyme aspartoacylase caused by a mutation in *ASPA* (17pter–p13). *Inheritance:* AR. *Prevalence:* Rare in most populations; about 1:6,400–1:13,456 in the Ashkenazi Jewish population.

References: Hoshino, H., & Kubota, M. (2014). Canavan disease: Clinical features and recent advances in research. *Pediatric International, 56*(4), 477–483.

Mendes, M. I., Smith, D. E., Pop, A., Lennertz, P., Fernandez Ojeda, M. R., Kanhai, W. A., . . . Salomons, G. S. (2017). Clinically distinct phenotypes of Canavan disease correlate with residual aspartoacylase enzyme activity. *Human Mutation, 38,* 524–531.

Carpenter syndrome (acrocephalosyndactyly, type II) *Disease category:* Craniosynostosis. *Clinical features:* Craniosynostosis, flat nasal bridge, malformed and low-set ears, short digits, syndactyly and/or polydactyly, obesity, and hypogenitalism and/or cryptorchidism. *Associated complications:* Congenital heart defects and hearing loss; 75% have mild intellectual disability. *Cause:* Mutations in *RAB23*. Mutations in *MEGF8* have more recently been linked to a subtype of Carpenter syndrome. *Inheritance:* AR. *Prevalence:* Rare.

References: Jenkins, D., Baynam, G., De Catte, L., Elcioglu, N., Gabbett, M. T., Hudgins, L., . . . Wilkie, A. O. (2011). Carpenter syndrome: Extended RAB23 mutation spectrum and analysis of nonsense-mediated mRNA decay. *Human Mutation, 32*(4), E2069–E2078.

Twigg, S. R. F., Lloyd, D., Jenkins, D., Elcioglu, N. E., Cooper, C. D., Al-Sannaa, N., . . . Wilkie, A. O. (2012). Mutations in multidomain protein MEGF8 identify a Carpenter syndrome subtype associated with defective lateralization. *American Journal of Human Genetics, 91*(5), 897–905.

cerebrohepatorenal syndrome *See* Zellweger syndrome.

CHARGE syndrome *Disease category:* Multiple congenital anomalies. *Clinical features:* CHARGE is an acronym that stands for **C**oloboma (defect in iris or retina), ***H***eart defect, choanal ***A***tresia (congenital blockage of the nasal passages), ***R***etarded growth and development, ***G***enital anomalies, and ***E***ar anomalies with or without hearing loss. *Associated complications:* Hypogenitalism, cryptorchidism, occasional cleft lip/palate, varying degrees of intellectual disability ranging from normal intelligence to profound intellectual disability, behavioral problems, and potentially severe visual and hearing impairments. Survival ranges widely, from 5 days to 46 years. *Cause:* Mutations in *CHD7* and *SEMA3E*. *Inheritance:* Majority of cases are caused by a NM, with evidence of AD inheritance when passed from an affected individual; associated with increased paternal age. Usually SP; approximately 8% of cases are familial. *Prevalence:* 1:8,500–1:12,000; more common in females than males.

References: Hale, C. L., Niederriter, A. N., Green, G .E., & Martin, D. M. (2016). Atypical phenotypes associated with pathogenic CHD7 variants and a proposal for broadening CHARGE syndrome clinical diagnostic criteria. *American Journal of Medical Genetics, Part A, 170A*(2), 344–354.

Legendre, M., Abadie, V., Attie-Bitach, T., Philip, N., Busta, T., Bonneau, D., . . . Gilbert-Dussardier, B. (2017). Phenotype and genotype analysis of a French cohort of 119 patients with CHARGE syndrome. *American Journal of Medical Genetics, Part C: Seminars in Medical Genetics, 175*(4), 417–420.

chondroectodermal dysplasia *See* Ellis-van Creveld syndrome.

chromosome 22q11 deletion syndrome (includes phenotypes previously described as DiGeorge syndrome, velocardiofacial syndrome [VCFS], Shprintzen syndrome, conotruncal anomaly face syndrome, some cases of AD Opitz G/BBB syndrome, and Cayler cardiofacial syndrome) *Disease category:* Multiple congenital anomalies/contiguous gene deletion. *Clinical features:* Congenital heart disease (especially conotruncal malformations, such as tetralogy of Fallot, interrupted aortic arch, ventricular septal defect, and truncus arteriosus), palatal abnormalities, characteristic facial features, learning disabilities, and immune deficiency. *Associated complications:* Feeding problems in infancy, hypocalcemia, kidney anomalies, hearing loss, laryngotracheoesophageal anomalies, growth hormone deficiency, rare seizures, hypernasal speech, psychiatric illness, developmental disabilities (ranging from learning disability to more significant cognitive delays), gross and fine motor delays, and expressive language delayed more significantly than receptive language. *Cause:* 1.5- to 3.0-Mb hemizygous deletion of chromosome 22q11.2. Haploinsufficiency of the *TBX1* gene in particular is responsible for most of the physical malformations. There is evidence that point mutations in the *TBX1* gene can also cause the disorder. *Inheritance:* AD; 93% from NM and 7% from an affected parent; one parent occasionally has a chromosomal rearrangement involving 22q, which increases the risk for recurrence; risk to offspring of affected individuals is 50%. *Prevalence:* 1:6,000 in Caucasians, African Americans, and Asians, and 1:3,800 in the Hispanic population in the United States.

References: Cunningham, A. C., Delport, S., Cumines, W., Busse, M., Linden, D. E. J., Hall, J., . . . van den Bree, M. B. M. (2018). Developmental coordination disorder, psychopathology and IQ in 22q11.2 deletion syndrome. *British Journal of Psychiatry, 212*(1), 27–33.

Swillen, A., & McDonald-McGinn, D. (2015). Developmental trajectories in 22q11.2 deletion. *American Journal of Medical Genetics, Part C: Seminars in Medical Genetics, 169*(2), 172–181.

Cohen syndrome *Disease category:* Multiple congenital anomalies. *Clinical features:* Characteristic facial features including thick hair and eyebrows, long eyelashes, wave-shaped palpebral fissures, bulbous nasal tip, smooth or shortened philtrum, retinal dystrophy, progressive high myopia, acquired microcephaly, global developmental delay and variable intellectual disability, hypotonia, and joint hyperextensibility. *Associated complications:* Short stature, small or narrow hands and feet, truncal obesity appearing in teen years after initial poor weight gain, friendly disposition, neutropenia with recurrent infections, and aphthous ulcers (canker sores). *Cause:* Mutations in *VPS13B* (previously *COH1*) (8q21–q22). *Inheritance:* AR. *Prevalence:* Unknown, although it is overrepresented in certain populations such as the Finnish population and the Amish.

References: Duplomb, L.,Duvet, S., Picot, D., Jego, G., El Chehadeh-Djebbar, S., Marle, N, . . . Thauvin-Robinet, C. (2014). Cohen syndrome is associated with major glycosylation defects. *Human Molecular Genetics, 23*(9), 2391–2399.

El Chehadeh-Djebbar, S., Blair, E., Holder-Espinasse, M., Moncla, A., Frances, A. M., Rio, M., . . . Faivre, L. (2013). Changing facial phenotype in Cohen syndrome: Towards clues for an earlier diagnosis. *European Journal of Human Genetics, 21(7),* 736–742.

congenital facial diplegia *See* Moebius sequence.

Cornelia de Lange syndrome *See* de Lange syndrome.

craniofacial dysostosis *See* Crouzon syndrome.

cri-du-chat syndrome (chromosome 5p– syndrome) *Disease category:* Multiple congenital anomalies/Contiguous gene syndrome. *Clinical features:* Prenatal and postnatal growth retardation, cat-like cry in infancy, hypertelorism with downward slant, microcephaly, low-set ears, micrognathia, single palmar crease, and cognitive deficits ranging from learning difficulties in some patients to moderate or severe intellectual disability in others. Receptive language skills are better than expressive language. *Associated complications:* Severe respiratory and feeding difficulties in infancy, hypotonia, inguinal (groin) hernias, occasional congenital heart defects, sleep disturbance, and hyperactivity. *Cause:* Partial deletion of chromosome 5p15.2; deletions can range from involving only the 5p15.2 band to the entire short arm. There is evidence that deletion of the telomerase reverse transcriptase (*TERT*) gene is specifically involved in the phenotypic changes. *Inheritance:* Usually NM; in 12% of cases a parent carries a balanced translocation. *Prevalence:* 1:20,000–1:50,000.

References: Guala, A., Spunton, M., Tognon, F., Pedrinazzi, M., Medolago, L., Ceruitti Mainardi, P., . . . Danesino, C. (2016). Psychomotor development in cri du chat syndrome: Comparison in two Italian cohorts with different rehabilitation methods. *Scientific World Journal, 2016,* 3125283.

Nguyen, J. M., Qualmann, K. J., Okashah, R., Reilly, A., Alexeyev, M. F., & Campbell, D. J. (2015). 5p deletions: Current knowledge and future directions. *American Journal of Medical Genetics, Part C: Seminars in Medical Genetics, 169*(3), 224–238.

Pituch, K., Green, V. A., Didden, R., Whittle, L., O'Reilly, M. F., Lancioni, G. E., & Sigafoos, J. (2010). Educational priorities for children with cri-du-chat syndrome. *Journal of Developmental and Physical Disabilities, 22*(1), 65–81.

Crouzon syndrome (craniofacial dysostosis) *Disease category:* Craniosynostosis. *Clinical features:* Craniosynostosis, shallow orbits with proptosis (protuberant eyeballs), hypertelorism (widely spaced eyes), strabismus, parrot-beaked nose, short upper lip, maxillary hypoplasia (small upper jaw), and conductive hearing loss. *Associated complications:* Increased intracranial pressure, intellectual disability, seizures, visual impairment, agenesis of the corpus callosum, occasional cleft lip or palate, and obstructive airway problems. Some children with Crouzon have acanthosis nigricans (a skin condition characterized by areas of dark velvety discoloration in body folds and creases). *Cause:* Mutations in *FGFR2* (10q25.3–q26). Those with Crouzon with acanthosis nigricans have mutations in *FGFR3*. *Inheritance:* AD with variable expression; up to 25% may represent new mutations. *Prevalence:* Unknown.

References: Azoury, S. C., Reddy, S., Shukla, V., & Deng, C. X. (2017). Fibroblast growth factor receptor 2 (FGFR2) mutation related syndromic craniosynostosis. *International Journal of Biological Sciences, 13(12),* 1479–1488.

Fischer, S., Tovetjarn, R., Maltese, G., Sahlin, P. E., Tarnow, P., & Kolby, L. (2014). Psychosocial conditions in adults with Crouzon syndrome: A follow-up study of 31 Swedish patients. *Journal of Plastic Surgery and Hand Surgery, 48(4),* 244–247.

de Lange syndrome (Brachmann de Lange syndrome, Cornelia de Lange syndrome) *Disease category:* Multiple congenital anomalies. *Clinical features:* Prenatal growth retardation, postnatal short stature, hypertrichosis (excessive body hair), synophrys (confluent eyebrows), anteverted nostrils, depressed nasal bridge, long philtrum (vertical indentation in the middle area of the upper lip), thin upper lip, microcephaly, low-set ears, limb and digital anomalies, and eye problems (myopia, ptosis, or nystagmus). *Associated complications:* Intellectual disability ranging from mild learning disabilities to severe impairments, behavioral problems, occasional heart defect, gastrointestinal problems, features of autism, self-injurious behavior, and occasional hearing loss. *Cause:* Mutations in *NIPBL* (3q26.3) are found in 60% of cases. Mutations in *SMC1A* (Xp11.22-p11.21), *SMC3* (10q25.2), *RAD21* (8q24.11), and *HDAC8* (Xq13.1) have been identified in a small percentage of individuals. A mild version of Cornelia de Lange has been associated with the *SMC3* gene. *Inheritance:* AD or XL; 99% NM. *Prevalence:* Published estimates range from 1:10,000–1:100,000.

References: Boyle, M. I., Jespersgaard, C., Brondum-Nielsen, K., Bisgaard, A. M., & Tumer, Z. (2015). Cornelia de Lange syndrome. *Clinical Genetics, 88 (1),* 1–12.

Mannini, L., Cucco, F., Quarantotti, V., Krantz, I. D., & Musio, A. (2013). Mutation spectrum and genotype-phenotype correlation in Cornelia de Lange syndrome. *Human Mutation, 34(12),* 1589–1596.

Nelson, L., Crawford, H., Reid, D., Moss, J., & Oliver, C. (2017). An experimental study of executive function and social impairment in Cornelia de Lange syndrome. *Journal of Neurodevelopmental Disorders, 9(1),* 33.

DiGeorge syndrome *See* chromosome 22q11 microdeletion syndromes.

DMD muscular dystrophy, Duchenne type *See* muscular dystrophy, Duchenne and Becker types.

Down syndrome *Disease category:* Chromosome abnormality/multiple congenital anomalies. *Clinical features:* Hypotonia, flat facial profile, upward-slanting palpebral fissures, small ears, small nose with low nasal bridge, single palmar crease, short stature, intellectual disability, and congenital heart disease. *Associated complications:* Atlantoaxial (upper cervical spine) instability; hyperextensible large joints; strabismus; thyroid dysfunction; predisposition toward immune disorders and leukemia; eye abnormalities, including strabismus, nystagmus, cataracts, and glaucoma; narrow ear canals and high incidence of middle-ear infections with potential hearing loss; and neurological abnormalities, including risk of seizures and early-onset Alzheimer's disease. *Cause:* Extra chromosome 21 caused by trisomy, mosaicism, or translocation. *Inheritance:* NM; usually nondisjunction chromosomal abnormality. Recurrence risk in the absence of translocation is 1%–2% in women younger than 35 years and the same as the typical maternal age-related risk in women over 35 years of age at delivery. If translocation is present in parent, recurrence risk is higher and is dependent on sex of carrier parent. *Prevalence:* 1:100,000–1.5:100,000. *Incidence:* 1:800 births. *See* Chapter 15.

References: Godfrey, M., & Lee, N. R. (2018). Memory profiles in Down syndrome across development: A review of memory abilities through the lifespan. *Journal of Neurodevelopmental Disorders, 10(1),* 5.

Mason-Apps, E., Stojanovik, V., Houston-Price, C., & Buckley, S. (2018). Longitudinal predictors of early language in infants with Down syndrome: A preliminary study. *Research in Developmental Disabilities, 81,* 37–51.

Will, E. A., Caravella, K. E., Hahn, L. J., Fidler, D. J., & Roberts, J. E. (2018). Adaptive behavior in infants and toddlers with Down syndrome and fragile X syndrome. *American Journal of Medical Genetics, Part B: Neuropsychiatric Genetics, 177*(3), 358–368.

Dubowitz syndrome *Disease category:* Multiple congenital anomalies. *Clinical features:* Prenatal onset of growth deficiency, postnatal short stature, eczema, sparse hair, mild microcephaly, cleft palate, and dysmorphic facial features, including high forehead, broad nasal bridge, ptosis, and epicanthal folds. *Associated complications:* Intellectual disability, behavioral disturbances, recurrent infections, increased frequency of malignancy, occasional hypospadias (abnormality in the location of the male urethra) or cryptorchidism, and hypoparathyroidism. *Cause:*

Unknown. Likely genetic heterogeneous with phenotypic overlap. *Inheritance:* AR. *Prevalence:* Rare.

References: Huber, R. S., Houlihan, D., & Filter, K. (2011). Dubowitz syndrome: A review and implications for cognitive, behavioral, and psychological features. *Journal of Clinical Medicine Research, 3(4),* 147–155.

Stewart, D. R., Pemov, A., Johnston, J. J., Sapp, J. C., Yeager, M., He, J., . . . Savage, S. A. (2014). Dubowitz syndrome is a complex comprised of multiple, genetically distinct and phenotypically overlapping disorders. *PLOS One, 9*(6), e98787.

Duchenne muscular dystrophy (DMD) *See* muscular dystrophy, Duchenne and Becker types.

Edwards syndrome *See* trisomy 18 syndrome.

EEC syndrome *See* ectrodactyly-ectodermal dysplasia-clefting syndrome.

Ehlers-Danlos syndrome (EDS) *Disease category:* Connective tissue disorder. *Clinical features:* At least 10 distinct forms have been described. All include aspects of skin fragility, easy bruisability, joint hyperextensibility, and hyperelastic skin. The classic (previously type I and II) and hypermobility (previously type III) forms are most commonly described and have similar clinical presentations with the previously mentioned features; the vascular form (previously type IV) is characterized by severe blood vessel involvement with risk of spontaneous arterial rupture; the progeroid (premature aging) form is characterized by wrinkled face, curly/fine hair, scanty eyebrows and eyelashes, and periodontitis in addition to the other usual signs of EDS; type V has been questioned as to whether it is actually a distinct phenotype; the kyphoscoliotic (type VI) form is characterized by eye involvement, including corneal fragility and kyphoscoliosis (curvature of the spine); the arthrochalasia type (type VIIA and VIIB) presents with congenital bilateral hip dislocation; the dermatosparaxis type (previously type VIIC) includes delayed closure of the fontanelles, characteristic facies, edema of the eyelids, blue sclerae, and short stature and fingers; the periodontitis type (previously type VIII) includes periodontal disease; and the cardiac valvular form has the typical signs as well as cardiac valvular defects. *Associated complications:* Hypotonia, delayed gross motor milestones, chronic pain, premature loss of teeth, mitral valve prolapse, intestinal hernias, premature delivery from premature rupture of membranes, scoliosis, and abnormalities of thymus. *Cause:* Each form is associated with an abnormality in the formation of collagen. The classic form is caused by mutations in the *COL5A1* and *COL5A2* genes; the hypermobility form is caused by mutations in the *COL3A1* gene as well as the tenascin XB gene (*TNXB*); the vascular type is caused by mutations in the *COL3A1* gene; the progeroid form is caused by mutations in the *B4GALT7* gene; mutations in the lysyl hydroxylase gene (*PLOD*) cause some cases of kyphoscoliotic form; the arthrochalasia type is caused by mutations in the *COL1A1* and *COL1A2* genes; the dermatosparaxis type is linked to the *ADAMTS2* gene; and the cardiac valvular type is linked to *COL1A2*. A possible new form of EDS was discovered in 2010 that is like the kyphoscoliotic form but without lysyl hydroxylase deficiency; it has been linked to the gene *CHST14*. *Inheritance:* The classic, hypermobility, vascular, arthrochalasia, and periodontitis types are all AD. Progeroid, kyphoscoliotic, dermatospraxis, and cardiac valvular are all AR. *Prevalence:* Classic type is 1:20,000; hypermobility type ranges from 1:5,000–1:20,000; kyphoscoliotic form is estimated at around 1:100,000; vascular type is 1:250,000; and the rest are unknown.

References: Baeza-Velasco, C., Bulbena, A., Polanco-Carrasco, R., & Jaussaud, R. (2018). Cognitive, emotional, and behavioral considerations for chronic pain management in the Ehlers-Danlos syndrome hypermobility-type: A narrative review. *Disability Rehabilitation,* 1–9.

Tinkle, B., Castori, M., Berglund, B., Cohen, H., Grahame, R., Kazkaz, H., & Levy, H. (2017). Hypermobile Ehlers-Danlos syndrome (a.k.a. Ehlers-Danlos syndrome type III and Ehlers-Danlos syndrome hypermobility type): Clinical description and natural history. *American Journal of Medical Genetics, Part C: Seminars in Medical Genetics, 175*(1), 48–69.

Ellis-van Creveld syndrome (chondroectodermal dysplasia) *Disease category:* Ectodermal dysplasia. *Clinical features:* Short-limbed dwarfism (final height 43–60 inches or 109–152 centimeters), polydactyly (extra digits), nail abnormalities, neonatal teeth, underdeveloped and premature loss of teeth, and congenital heart defect in 50%; intelligence is usually not affected. *Associated complications:* Severe cardiorespiratory problems in infancy, specifically atrial septation (producing a common atrium in the heart); hydrocephalus; and severe leg deformities. *Cause:* Mutations in *EVC, EVC 2, WDR35,* and *DYNC2I1. Inheritance:* AR. *Prevalence:* Rare, more common in the Amish population.

References: Caparros-Martin, J. A., De Luca, A., Cartault, F., Aglan, M., Temtamy, S., Otaify, G. A., . . . Ruiz-Perez, V. L. (2015). Specific variants in WDR35 cause a distinctive form of Ellis-van Creveld syndrome by disrupting the recruitment of the EvC complex and SMO into the cilium. *Human Molecular Genetics, 24*(14), 4126–4137.

Niceta, M., Margiotti, K., Digilio, M. C., Guida, V., Bruselles, A., Pizzi, S., . . . Tartaglia, M. (2017). Biallelic mutations in DYNC2LI1 are a rare cause of Ellis-van Creveld syndrome. *Clinical Genetics, 93*(3), 632–639.

facio-auriculo-vertebral spectrum *See* oculo-auriculovertebral spectrum.

faciodigitogenital dysplasia (FGDY) *See* Aarskog-Scott syndrome.

FAE *See* fetal alcohol effects.

familial dysautonomia (Riley-Day syndrome) *Disease category:* Neurological disorder. *Clinical features:* Absent or sparse tears, absence of fungiform papillae (knoblike projections) on the tongue, diminished pain and temperature sensation, postural hypotension, abnormal sweating, episodic vomiting, swallowing disorder, ataxia, and decreased reflexes. *Associated complications:* Feeding difficulties, scoliosis, joint abnormalities, hypertension, hypotonia, delay in motor milestones, and aseptic necrosis of bones (damage to bony tissue unassociated with infection or injury). Neuronal degeneration is progressive. *Cause:* Mutation of the *ELP1* (previously *IKBKAP*) gene (9q31–q33). Two common mutations in the Ashkenazi Jewish population. *Inheritance:* AR. *Prevalence:* Rare; 1:36 carrier frequency in the Ashkenazi Jewish population.

References: Mendoza-Santiesteban, C. E., Palma, J. A., Hedges, T. R., Laver, N. V., Farhat, N., Norcliffe-Kaufmann, L, & Kaufmann, H. (2017). Pathological confirmation of optic neuropathy in familial dysautonomia. *Journal of Neuropathology and Experimental Neurology, 76*(3), 238–244.

Rubin, B. Y., & Anderson, S. L. (2017). IKBKAP/ELP1 gene mutations: Mechanisms of familial dysautonomia and gene-targeting therapies. *Applied Clinical Genetics, 10,* 95–103.

FAS *See* fetal alcohol syndrome.

fetal alcohol effects (FAE) Former term for alcohol-related neurodevelopmental effects (ARND); *see* Chapter 2.

fetal alcohol syndrome (FAS) *See* Chapter 2.

fetal face syndrome *See* Robinow syndrome.

fetal hydantoin syndrome *See* Phenytoin syndrome.

FGDY faciogenital dysplasia *See* Aarskog-Scott syndrome.

***FMR1*-related disorders (fragile X syndrome, fragile X–associated tremor/ataxia syndrome [FXTAS], and *FMR1*-related primary ovarian insufficiency [POI])** *Disease category:* Neurological disorder/triplet repeat expansion. *Clinical features:* Males with full mutations typically have a large head, long face, prominent forehead and chin, protruding ears, behavioral problems such as hyperactivity, hand flapping, hand biting, temper tantrums, and sometimes autism. *Associated complications:* Abnormalities of connective tissue with finger joint hypermobility or joint instability, mitral valve prolapse, and large testes. Females heterozygous for full-mutation alleles can have similar phenotypes as males but with lower frequency and generally milder involvement. Both males and females with premutations are known to develop FXTAS/late-onset progressive cerebellar ataxia and intention tremor; 21% of females who are carriers of premutation alleles develop primary ovarian insufficiency (cessation of menses before age 40). *Cause:* Mutation in *FMR1* gene on Xq27–q28; molecular analysis reveals an increase in cytosine-guanine-guanine (CGG) trinucleotide repeats in the coding sequence of the *FMR1* gene. Normal allele sizes vary from 6 to approximately 55 CGG repeats. Phenotypically unaffected individuals have premutations, with an allele size ranging from 55 to 200, but are at risk for FXTAS and POI. Allele sizes of greater than 200 CGG repeats generally indicate a full mutation with phenotypic expression of the syndrome. *Inheritance:* X-linked with genetic imprinting (full mutations are not inherited from the father) and anticipation (number of repeats may increase in subsequent generations). *Prevalence:* 16:100,000–25:100,000 males; prevalence of females affected with fragile X is presumed to be half the male prevalence. *See also* Chapter 15.

References: Crawford, H., Moss, J., Oliver, C., & Riby, D. (2017). Differential effects of anxiety and autism on social scene scanning in males with Fragile X syndrome. *Journal of Neurodevelopmental Disorders, 9*(1), 9.

Hahn, L. J., Brady, N. C., McCary, L., Rague, L., & Roberts, J. E. (2017). Early social communication in infants with fragile X syndrome and infant siblings of children with autism spectrum disorder. *Research in Developmental Disabilities, 71,* 169–180.

5p– syndrome *See* cri-du-chat syndrome.

45,X *See* Turner syndrome.

47,X *See* XXX, XXXX, and XXXXX syndromes.

fragile X syndrome *See FMR1*-related disorders.

Friedreich ataxia *Disease category:* Neurological disorder/triplet repeat expansion. *Clinical features:* Slowly progressive neurological disorder characterized by limb and gait ataxia, dysarthria, nystagmus, pes cavus (high-arched feet), hearing loss, and kyphoscoliosis (backward curve of the spine). In rare cases, progression is rapid. Onset is usually between ages 10–15. *Associated complications:* Delayed motor milestones, cardiomyopathy (heart muscle weakness), and/or congestive heart failure; increased risk of insulin-dependent diabetes mellitus; and impaired color vision. Cognition is not typically affected; however, difficulties with motor planning, concept formation, visuospatial reasoning, attention/working memory, cognitive flexibility, and reduced speed of information processing are common. *Cause:* Usually homozygous guanine-adenosine-adenosine (GAA) expansions in intron 1 of the frataxin (*FXN*) gene on chromosome 9q13; point mutations in the *FXN* gene have also been identified. Normal alleles are 5–33 GAA repeats; premutation alleles are 34–65 uninterrupted GAA repeats; full disease-causing alleles are 66–1700 GAA repeats. *Inheritance:* AR. *Prevalence:* Approximately 2:100,000–4:100,000. *Treatment:* Supportive care includes physical therapy, orthopedic surgery to correct progressive scoliosis, and close cardiology follow-up. Many different possible treatments are being actively studied.

References: Corben, L. A., Lynch, D., Pandolfo, M., Schulz, J. B., Delatycki, M. B., & Clinical Management Guidelines Writing Group. (2014). Consensus clinical management guidelines for Friedreich ataxia. *Orphanet Journal of Rare Diseases, 9,* 184.

Corben, L. A., Klopper, F., Stagnitti, M., Georgiou-Karistianis, N., Bradshaw, J. L., Rance, G., & Delatycki, M. B. (2017). Measuring inhibition and cognitive flexibility in Friedreich ataxia. *Cerebellum,* 16(4), 757–763.

Sayah, S., Rotge, J. Y., Francisque, H., Gargiulo, M., Czernecki, V., Justo, D., . . . Durr, A. (2017). Personality and neuropsychological profiles in Friederich's ataxia. *Cerebellum, 17*(2), 201–212.

G syndrome *See* Opitz GBB syndrome.

GBS *See* Guillain-Barre syndrome.

galactosemia *Disease category:* Inborn error of metabolism: carbohydrate. *Clinical features:* Jaundice, lethargy, and hypotonia in the newborn period; poor weight gain with vomiting and diarrhea; bleeding diathesis; cataracts; liver dysfunction or failure if disease untreated; varying degrees of intellectual impairment (severe if diseases untreated); visual-perceptual impairments; and verbal dyspraxia. *Associated complications:* Ovarian failure, hemolytic anemia, increased risk of sepsis (particularly *Escherichia coli* in the neonate), cerebellar ataxia, tremors, and choreoathetosis (movement disorders). Implementing a galactose-free diet in the newborn period prevents liver failure, sepsis, severe intellectual disability and death, but even when treated, children still experience some cognitive deficits, speech defects, cataracts, and ovarian failure (females). There is a clinical variant galactosemia (p.Ser135Leu/Ser135Leu genotype) that occurs in African Americans and Africans, which, when treated, does not develop the typical long-term complications including premature ovarian failure. Some newborns have a mild variant of galactosemia (Duarte galactosemia), which is not associated with developmental delays, cataracts, or hepatocellular damage. Nutritional intervention is not usually necessary or is needed only in children under 1 year of age, although there is no uniform standard of care for patients with Duarte galactosemia. *Cause:* Most commonly caused by a deficiency of the enzyme galactose-1-phosphate uridyltransferase or GALT (9p13). It also can be caused by a deficiency of galactokinase (GALK) or galactoepimerase (GALE). (They are all enzymes required for digestion of galactose, a natural sugar found in milk). *Inheritance:* AR. *Prevalence:* 1:10,000–1:30,000 in the United States. *Treatment:* Galactose-free diet.

References: Demirbas, D., Coelho, A. I., Rubio-Gozalbo, M. E., & Berry, G. T. (2018). Hereditary galactosemia. *Metabolism, 83,* 188–196.

Pyhtila, B., Shaw, K. A., Neumann, S. E., & Fridovich-Keil, J. L. (2015). Newborn screening for galactosemia in the United States: Looking back, looking around, and looking ahead. *JIMD Reports, 15,* 79–93.

Gaucher disease *Disease category:* Inborn error of metabolism: lysosomal storage disease. *Clinical features:* Three clinically distinct forms, the most common of which (type 1) has onset in adulthood and includes enlarged spleen and liver, anemia, thrombocytopenia (low platelet count), and bone involvement; it is distinguished by the lack of neurological involvement. Most individuals with type 1 go undiagnosed. Type 2 presents in infancy with an enlarged spleen, hematological abnormalities, bony lesions, abnormalities of skin pigmentation, limited psychomotor development, and a rapidly progressive course. Most children will die within the first 2–4 years of life. Type 3 is more variable, with ataxia, seizures, eye movement disorder, and dementia, with onset before age 2 years but with a more slowly progressive course. There is also a perinatal lethal form associated with ichthyosiform (rough, thick, and scaly skin) or collodion (a tight shiny membrane that resembles plastic wrap) skin abnormalities and nonimmune hydrops fetalis (accumulation of fluid, or edema, in the fetus). *Associated complications:* Rare associated features such as cardiac valvular involvement and Parkinsonian features have been associated with specific genotypes. *Cause:* Accumulation of glucosylceramide due to deficiency of the enzyme beta-glucosidase from mutations in the *GBA* gene on chromosome 1q21. *Inheritance:* AR. *Prevalence:* Rare in the general population; prevalence of type 1 estimated to be approximately 1:855 in the Ashkenazi Jewish population. *Treatment:* Enzyme replacement therapy (ERT) improves rate of bone loss and reduces spleen size but does not seem to affect neurological symptoms; thus, it is generally used only in individuals with type 1. For those where ERT is not an option (due to allergy, hypersensitivity, or poor venous access), substrate reduction therapy is an option. Bone marrow transplantation has been used in those with more severe disease, usually type 3.

References: Ceron-Rodriguez, M., Barajas-Colon, E., Ramirez-Devars, L., Gutierrez-Camacho, C., & Salgado-Loza, J. L. (2018). Improvement of life quality measured by Lansky Score after enzymatic replacement therapy in children with Gaucher disease type 1. *Molecular Genetics & Genomic Medicine, 6*(1), 27–34.

Schwartz, I. V. D., Goker-Alpan, O., Kishnani, P. S., Zimran, A., Renault, L., Panahloo, Z., . . . GOS Study Group. (2017). Characteristics of 26 patients with type 3 Gaucher disease: A descriptive analysis from the Gaucher Outcome Survey. *Molecular Genetics and Metabolism Reports, 14,* 73–79.

globoid cell leukodystrophy *See* Krabbe disease.

glutaric acidemia, type I *Disease category:* Inborn error of metabolism: organic acidemia. *Clinical features:* Macrocephaly, hypotonia, basal ganglia lesions causing a movement disorder (dystonia), and seizures present between 6–18 months of age, interrupting otherwise typical development. This disorder may mimic dyskinetic cerebral palsy. *Associated complications:* Episodic acidosis, vomiting, lethargy, and coma. Intellectual disability is usual if a basal ganglia lesion occurs; otherwise intellectual functioning may remain intact. *Cause:* Mutations in *GCDH* (chromosome 19p13.2) resulting in accumulation of glutaric acid and, to a lesser degree, of 3-hydroxyglutaric and glutaconic acids. *Inheritance:* AR. *Prevalence:* Overall frequency is 1:100,000; 1:30,000 in Sweden; and 1:50,000 in the United States. It is more common in certain ethnic groups such as in the Amish population. *Treatment:* Low-protein diet and supplemental oral carnitine. Early treatment results in significantly improved outcome, and the disorder is on newborn screening panels in many countries.

References: Boy, N., Muhlhausen, C., Maier, E. M., Heringer, J., Assmann, B., Burgard, P., . . . Kolker, S. (2017). Proposed recommendations for diagnosing and managing individuals with glutaric aciduria type I: Second revision. *Journal of Inherited Metabolic Diseases, 40*(1), 75–101.

Brown, A., Crowe, L., Bauchamp, M. H., Anderson, V., & Boneh, A. (2015). Neurodevelopmental profile of children with glutaric aciduria type I diagnosed by newborn screening: A follow-up case series. *JIMD Reports, 18,* 125–134.

glutaric acidemia, type II (multiple acyl-CoA dehydrogenase deficiency) *Disease category:* Inborn error of metabolism: organic acidemia. *Clinical features:* Severe metabolic acidosis, hypoglycemia, and cardiomyopathy; urine with a characteristic odor of sweaty feet, similar to that present in isovaleric acidemia. Dysmorphic facial features (macrocephaly, large anterior fontanelle [soft spot], high forehead, flat nasal bridge, and malformed ears) are seen in one half of cases. This condition also can present later in life with episodic vomiting, acidosis, and hypoglycemia. *Associated complications:* Muscle weakness, liver disease, cataracts, respiratory distress, and kidney cysts. *Cause:* Mutations in at least three different genes—*ETFA, ETFB,* and *ETFDH*—have been identified. No clinical differences with respect to causative gene have been identified. *Inheritance:* AR. *Prevalence:* Rare. *Treatment:* Diet with supplemental riboflavin and carnitine.

References: Olsen, R. K. J., Konarikova, E., Giancaspero, T. A., Mosegaard, S., Boczonadi, V., Matakovic, L., . . . Prokisch, H. (2016). Riboflavin-responsive and nonresponsive mutations in FAD synthase cause multiple acyl-CoA dehydrogenase and combined respiratory-chain deficiency. *American Journal of Human Genetics, 98*(6), 1130–1145.

Van der Westhuzien, F. H., Smuts, I., Honey, E., Louw, R., Schoonen, M., Jonck, L. M., & Dercksen, M. (2018). A novel mutation in ETFDH manifesting as severe neonatal-onset multiple acyl-CoA dehydrogenase deficiency. *Journal of Neurological Science, 384,* 121–125.

glycogen storage diseases (glycogenoses) *Disease category:* Inborn error of metabolism: carbohydrate. *Clinical features:* More than 12 forms of glycogen storage diseases are currently known, all caused by defects in the production or breakdown of glycogen and resulting in a wide spectrum of clinical features. They share varying degrees of liver and muscle abnormalities and can be broken down by whether they primarily affect the muscle (and therefore present with muscle cramps, easy fatigability, and progressive muscle weakness) or the liver (where an enlarged liver and decreased blood sugar are the initial symptoms). In all disease forms, patient organs have excessive glycogen accumulation. Types I (glucose-6-phosphate deficiency), II (Pompe disease, acid alpha-glucosidase deficiency), III (amylo-1, 6-glycosidase deficiency), and VI (hepatic phosphorylase deficiency) are the most common and represent almost 95% of cases. Common clinical features include hypoglycemia, short stature, enlarged spleen, and muscle weakness. *Associated complications:* Hypotonia, kidney abnormalities, gouty arthritis, bleeding abnormalities, hypertension, and respiratory distress; type II disease characteristically has severe cardiac, muscle, and neurological involvement. *Cause:* Deficiencies in the various enzymes involved in the synthesis and degradation of glycogen. There are many genes and chromosome locations associated with glycogenoses. *Inheritance:* All except type IX (previously type VIII) are inherited as AR; type IX is XLR. *Prevalence:* Combined incidence of 1:20,000–1:25,000. *Treatment:* Increased protein intake and overnight tube feeding of cornstarch to maintain normoglycemia have been shown to be useful for supportive care. This treatment also prevents growth and developmental problems and can improve the biochemical abnormalities. Enzyme replacement therapy is available for Pompe disease. Liver transplantation has been attempted in types I, III, and IV, with correction of the biochemical abnormalities but not all sequelae.

References: Desai, A. K., Walters, C. K., Cope, H. L., Kazi, Z. B., DeArmey, S. M., & Kishnani, P. S. (2018). Enzyme replacement therapy with alglucosidease alfa in Pompe disease: Clinical experience with rate escalation. *Molecular Genetics and Metabolism, 123*(2), 92–96.

Roscher, A., Patel, J., Hewson, S., Nagy, L, Feigenbaum, A., Kronick, J., . . . Mercimek-Mahmutoglu, S. (2014). The natural history of glycogen storage disease types VI and IX: Long-term outcome from the largest metabolic center in Canada. *Molecular Genetics and Metabolism, 113,* 171–176.

Rousseau-Nepton, I., Huot, C., Laforte, D., Mok, E., Fenyves, D., Constantin, E., & Mitchell, J. (2017). Sleep and quality of life of patients with glycogen storage disease on standard and modified uncooked cornstarch. *Molecular Genetics and Metabolism, 123*(3), 326–330.

GM2 gangliosidosis, type I *See* Tay-Sachs disease.

Goldenhar syndrome *See* oculo-auriculo-vertebral spectrum.

Guillain-Barré Syndrome (GBS) *Disease category:* Neuromuscular disease. *Clinical features:* GBS is an acute inflammatory demyelinating polyneuropathy. There is pain and the development over one to several days of muscle weakness, with the inability to walk and a loss of deep tendon reflexes. The weakness affects both sides of the body symmetrically, usually starting in the lower extremities. The arms are involved later, with maximum weakness occurring by 3 weeks. Most children with GBS begin to recover 2–3 weeks after the symptoms begin. About 85% of affected children are able to walk within 6 months; however, some have residual weakness. The mortality rate is 3%, and the chance of relapse has been reported as 7% in children. *Cause:* It can follow an upper respiratory or gastrointestinal (GI) viral infection. A specific type of GI infection produced by the bacteria *Campylobacter jejuni* has been particularly associated with GBS. GBS is considered an autoimmune disease. Although rare familial cases have been reported, it is thought to be a multifactorial disease with both genetic and environmental factors contributing to its occurrence. *Incidence:* 0.4–1.7 cases per 100,000 people each year. *Diagnosis*: Spinal fluid analysis and electromyographic evaluation. *Treatment:* Treatment is mostly supportive. About 10%–20% need to be placed on a ventilator. Medical treatment includes the use of intravenous immune globulin (IVIG) and/or plasmapheresis.

References: Ancona, P.,Bailey, M., & Bellomo, R. (2018). Characteristics, incidence and outcome of patients admitted to intensive care unit with Guillain-Barre syndrome in Australia and New Zealand. *Journal of Critical Care, 45,* 58–64.

Van den Bergh, P. Y. K.,Pieret, F., Woodard, J. L., Attarian, S., Grapperon, A. M., Nicholas, G., . . . University of Louvain GBS Electrodiagnosis Study Group. (2018). Guillain-Barre syndrome subtype diagnosis: A prospective multicentric European study. *Muscle Nerve, 58*(2), 23–28.

Hallermann-Streiff syndrome (oculo-mandibulo-dyscephaly with hypotrichosis) *Disease category:* Skeletal dysplasia. *Clinical features:* Proportionate short stature; characteristic facial appearance, including small eyes, small, pinched nose, and small mouth; sparse, thin hair; and frontal bossing (prominent central forehead). *Associated complications:* Various eye abnormalities, including nystagmus, strabismus, cataracts, and/or decreased visual acuity; neonatal teeth and other dental abnormalities; narrow upper airway or tracheomalacia (softening of the tracheal cartilages), with related respiratory difficulty; frequent respiratory infections, snoring, and feeding difficulties; clinical overlap with oculo-dento-digital dysplasia (ODDD) has been suggested; and intellectual disability has been reported in some cases. *Cause:* Unknown, believed to be genetic; one patient has been identified with a homozygous mutation in the *GJA1* gene known to be causative in ODDD. *Inheritance:* Most reported cases are not inherited from an affected parent and are assumed to be caused by an NM. *Prevalence:* Rare.

References: Chen, C. L., Peng, J., Jia, X. G., Liu, Z. W., & Zhao, P. Q. (2017). Hallermann-Streiff syndrome with bilateral microphthalmia, pupillary membranes and cataract absorption. *International Journal of Ophthalmology, 10*(6), 1016–1018.

Epee, E., Beleho, D., Bitang, A. T., Njami, V. A., Bengondo, C., & Ebana Mvogo, C. (2017). A familial study of Hallermann-Streiff-Francois syndrome. *International Medical Case Reports Journal, 10,* 193–201.

hemifacial microsomia *See* oculo-auriculo-vertebral spectrum.

hereditary progressive arthro-ophthalmopathy *See* Stickler syndrome.

holocarboxylase synthetase deficiency *Disease category:* Inborn error of metabolism: cofactor deficiency. *Clinical features:* Disorder of biotin metabolism characterized by seizures, hypotonia, lethargy, coma, skin rash, alopecia (loss of hair from skin areas where it is normally present), and acidosis typically presenting before 3 months. Often, the presenting feature is feeding difficulty or respiratory distress. *Associated complications:* Intellectual disability, hearing impairment, optic atrophy with visual impairment, recurrent infections, and vomiting. *Cause:* Mutations in *HCLS* (21q22.13) causing enzyme deficiencies of holocarboxylase synthetase or 3-methylcrotonyl-CoA carboxylase. *Inheritance:* AR. *Prevalence:* Rare. *Treatment:* Oral biotin supplementation. Prenatal treatment with oral biotin corrects lethargy, hypotonia, and vomiting.

References: Donti, T. R.,Blackburn, P. R., & Atwal, P. S. (2016). Holocarboxylase synthetase deficiency pre and post newborn screening. *Molecular Genetics and Metabolism Reports, 7,* 40–44.

Slavid, T. P., Zaidi, S. J., Neal, C., Nishikawa, B., & Seaver, L. H. (2014). Clinical presentation and positive outcome of two siblings with holocarboxylase synthetase deficiency caused by a homozygous L216R mutation. *JIMD Reports, 12,* 109–114.

holoprosencephaly (HPE) *Disease category:* Malformation. *Clinical features:* This classification encompasses a spectrum of midline defects of the brain and face that occur after failed or abbreviated midline cleavage of the developing brain during the third to fourth week of gestation. The most severe defects are incompatible with life. Individuals who survive have varying degrees of disability, ranging from typical development with hypotelorism (widely spaced eyes) to alobar holoprosencephaly (brain without segmentation into hemispheres) and cyclopia (single central eye). *Associated complications:* Seizures, endocrine abnormalities, micropenis and other genital anomalies, cleft of retinae, and intellectual disability. Facial anomalies are seen in 80% of cases. *Cause:* There are environmental and genetic causes for holoprosencephaly. Infants of diabetic mothers have a 200-fold increase risk for holoprosencephaly. Other, less clearly seen associations in animal models include alcohol and retinoic acid, cholesterol-lowering agents, and maternal hypocholesterolemia; 25%–50% of individuals with HPE have a chromosomal abnormality such as trisomy 13, 18, and triploidy. Copy number variants and large structural chromosomal abnormalities have also been documented. The rest have a pathogenic variant in a single gene; mutations in *SHH* (7q36) is the most common cause, followed by mutations in *ZIC2* (13q32); *SIX3* (2p21); *TGIF1* (18p11.3); and many other rare related genes, including *GLI2* (2q14), *PTCH1* (9q22.3), *DISP1* (1q42), *FGF8* (10q24), *FOXH1* (8q24.3), *NODAL* (10q22.1), *TDGF1* (3p23-p21), *GAS1* (9q21.33), *DLL1* (6q27), and *CDON* (11q24.2). *Inheritance:* May be part of a syndrome or caused by teratogenic exposure; as an isolated birth defect, may be AD or AR. *Prevalence:* 1:250 gestations, but 1:10,000 live births.

References: Dubourg, C., Carre, W., Hamdi-Roze, H., Mouden, C., Roume, J., Abdelmajid, B., . . . David, V. (2016). Mutational spectrum in holoprosencephaly shows that FGF is a new major signaling pathway. *Human Mutation, 37*(12), 1329–1339.

Pucciarelli, V., Bertoli, S., Codari, M., Veggiotti, P., Battezzati, A., & Sforza, C. (2017). Facial evaluation in holoprosencephaly. *Journal of Craniofacial Surgery, 28*(1), e22–e28.

Richieri-Costa, A., Vendramini-Pittoli, S., Kokitsu-Nakata, N. M., Zechi-Ceide, R. M., Alvarez, C. W., & Ribeiro-Bicudo, L. A. (2017). Multisystem involvement in a patient with a PTCH1 mutation: Clinical and imaging findings. *Journal of Pediatric Genetics, 6*(2), 103–106.

Holt-Oram syndrome *Disease category:* Multiple congenital anomalies. *Clinical features:* Upper-limb defect ranging from hypoplastic (incompletely formed), abnormally placed, or absent thumbs to hypoplasia of the radius, ulna, or humerus (arm bones) and complete phocomelia (foreshortened limbs); 75% of affected individuals also have a congenital heart defect (atrial septal defect and ventricular septal defect are most common). *Associated complications:* Occasional abnormalities of chest muscles and vertebral anomalies. *Cause:* Mutations in *TBX5* (12q2). Recent study showed mutations in *SALL4* may also cause Holt-Oram. *Inheritance:* AD with variable expression. *Prevalence:* Approximately 1:100,000.

References: Baban, A., Pitto, L., et al. (2014). Holt-Oram syndrome with intermediate atrioventricular canal defect, and aortic coarctation: functional characterization of a de novo TBX5 mutation. *American Journal of Medical Genetics, Part A, 164A,* 1419–1424.

Li, B., Chen, S., Sun, K., Xu, R., & Wu, Y. (2018). Genetic analyses identified a SALL4 gene mutation associated with Holt-Oram syndrome. *DNA Cell Biology, 37*(4), 398–404. Wall, L. B., Piper, S. L., Nabenicht, R., Oishi, S. N., Ezaki, M., & Goldfarb, C. A. (2015). Defining features of the upper extremity in Holt-Oram syndrome. *Journal of Hand Surgery, 40*(9), 1763–1768.

homocystinuria *Disease category:* Inborn error of metabolism: amino acid. *Clinical features:* Downward dislocation of lens of the eye (ectopia lentis) and/or myopia; tall, slim physique; scoliosis; risk for thromboembolism; and developmental delay/intellectual disability. Two forms have been described, differing in their responsiveness to pyridoxine (vitamin B6).

Associated complications: Behavioral disorders, cataracts or glaucoma, and osteoporosis. *Cause:* Mutations in *CBS* (21q22). *Inheritance:* AR with variable expressivity. *Incidence:* Ranges from 1:65,000 in Ireland to 1:344,000 worldwide. *Treatment:* Folic acid and vitamin B12 supplementation, use of betaine, and dietary restriction of methionine. Pyridoxine is used in the rare individuals who have the pyridoxine-responsive form of the disease. Early treatment with pyridoxine in responsive cases may allow typical intelligence. Treatment with above agents significantly reduces the risk of vascular events.

References: El Bashir, H., Dekair, L., Mahmoud, Y., & Ben-Omran, T. (2015). Neurodevelopmental and cognitive outcomes of classical homocystinura: Experience from Qatar. *JIMD Reports, 21,* 89–95.

Morris, A. A., . Kozich, V., Santra, S., Andria, G., Ben-Omran, T. I., Chakrapani, A. B., . . . Chapman, K. A. (2017). Guidelines for the diagnosis and management of cystathionine beta-synthase deficiency. *Journal of Inherited Metabolic Diseases, 40*(1), 49–74.

Poloni, S., Sperb-Ludwig, F., Borsatto, T., Weber Hoss, G., Doriqui, M. J. R, Embirucu, E. K., . . . Schwartz, I. V. D. (2018). CBS mutations are good predictors for B6-responsiveness: A study based on the analysis of 35 Brazilian classical homocystinuria patients. *Molecular Genetics and Genomic Medicine, 6*(2), 160–170.

Hunter syndrome (MPS II) *See* mucopolysaccharidoses (MPS).

Huntington disease (HD; previously called Huntington chorea), juvenile *Disease category:* Neurologic/triplet repeat expansion. *Clinical features:* Juvenile onset progressive neurological disorder. For cases to be considered juvenile HD, onset must occur by 20 years of age. Children present with dysarthria, clumsiness, hyperreflexia, rigidity, and oculomotor disturbances. *Associated complications:* Joint contractures, swallowing dysfunction, and seizures. *Cause:* Expansion of cytosine-adenine-guanine (CAG) trinucleotide repeat in *HTT* (4p16.3). Normal number of CAG repeats is 11–34; individuals affected with juvenile HD have greater than 60 CAG repeats. *Inheritance:* AD with anticipation (earlier onset with each generation, especially when paternally inherited). Progression in children with paternally inherited disease is more rapid than in children with maternally inherited disease. *Prevalence:* 3:100,000–7:100,000 in populations of western European descent. Less frequent in other populations. Juvenile onset disease accounts for 5%–10% of all cases of HD.

References: Moser, A. D., Epping, E., Espe-Pfeifer, P., Martin, E., Zhorne, L., Mathews, K., . . . Nopoulos, P. (2017). A survey-based study identifies common but unrecognized symptoms in a large series of juvenile Huntington's disease. *Neurodegeneration Disease Management, 7*(5), 307–315.

Quarrell, O., O'Donovan, K. L., Bandmann, O., & Strong, M. (2012). The prevalence of juvenile Huntington's disease: A review of the literature and meta-analysis. *PLoS Currents, 4,* e4f8606b742ef3.

Quarrell, O., Nance, M. A., Nopoulos, P., Paulsen, J. S., Smith, J. A., & Squitieri, F. (2013). Managing juvenile Huntington's disease. *Neurodegeneration Disease Management, 3*(3), 10.2217/nmt.13.18.

Hurler syndrome (MPS IH) *See* mucopolysaccharidoses (MPS).

hypophosphatasia *Disease category:* Skeletal dysplasia. *Clinical features:* A disorder of calcium and phosphate metabolism with symptoms ranging from a severe infantile form (which can be rapidly fatal) to a relatively mild childhood form. A total of six forms of the disease have been described (perinatal lethal, perinatal benign, infantile, childhood, adult, and odonto-hypophosphatasia [dental only]). Features include short stature, bowed long bones, craniosynostosis, and hypocalcemia. *Associated complications:* Seizures, multiple fractures, and premature loss of teeth. The perinatal lethal form presents as short limbs and poor ossification (bone formation) of the skeleton, and affected infants usually die from pulmonary insufficiency. The benign perinatal form is usually identified by prenatal ultrasound, but the skeletal manifestations slowly resolve with an eventual phenotype similar to the childhood or adult types. The childhood form presents with an early loss of secondary teeth, short stature, and delayed walking with a waddling gait. Joint pain and nonprogressive muscle weakness may also be present and the features resemble rickets. *Cause:* Mutations in *ALPL* (1p36). *Inheritance:* AR (severe forms), AR/AD (milder forms). *Incidence:* 1:100,000–1:300,000; incidence of severe infantile form is 1:2500 in Mennonite families from Manitoba, Canada.

References: Kishnani, P. S., Rush, E. T., Arundel, P., Bishop, N., Dahir, K., Fraser, W., . . . Ozono, K. (2017). Monitoring guidance for patients with hypophosphotasia treated with asfotase alfa. *Molecular Genetics and Metabolism, 122*(1-2), 4–17.

Tenorio, J., Alvarez, I., Riancho-Zarrabeitia, L., Martos-Moreno, G. A., Mandrile, G., de la Flor Crespo, M., . . . Lapunzina, P. (2017). Molecular and clinical analysis of ALPL in a cohort of patients with suspicion of hypophosphatasia. *Molecular Genetics and Metabolism, Part A, 173*(3), 601–610.

Whyte, M. P., Wenkert, D., & Zhang, F. (2016). Hypophosphatasia: Natural history study of 101 affected children investigated at one research center. *Bone, 93,* 125–138.

incontinentia pigmenti *Disease category:* Dermatologic disorder. *Clinical features:* Swirling patterns of hyperpigmented skin lesions; tooth abnormalities;

microcephaly; ocular abnormalities; thin, wiry hair; hairless lesions; and intellectual disability in approximately one third of cases. *Associated complications:* Spasticity, seizures, and vertebral or rib abnormalities, as well as strabismus, hydrocephalus, and a history of male miscarriages. *Cause:* Mutations in *IKBKG* (previously *NEMO*) gene (Xq28), skewed X-inactivation. A deletion of exons 4–10 is present in about 80% of affected individuals. *Inheritance:* XLD with lethality in males. Living affected males have been found with the 47, XXY karyotype or somatic mosaicism. *Prevalence:* Rare.

References: Greene-Roethke, C. (2017). Incontinentia pigmenti: A summary review of this rare ectodermal dysplasia with neurologic manifestations, including treatment protocols. *Journal of Pediatric Health Care, 31*(6), e45–e52.

Pizzamiglio, M. R., Piccardi, L., Bianchini, F., Canzano, L., Palermo, L., Fusco, F. . . . Ursini, M. V. (2017). Cognitive-behavioural phenotype in a group of girls from 1.2-12 years old with the Incontinentia Pigmenti syndrome: Recommendations for clinical management. *Applied Neuropsychology, Child, 6*(4), 327–334.

infantile Refsum disease *See* Refsum disease, infantile.

isovaleric acidemia *Disease category:* Inborn error of metabolism: organic acidemia. *Clinical features:* A disorder of organic acid metabolism; an acute, often fatal neonatal form is characterized by acidosis and coma; a chronic form presents with recurrent attacks of ataxia, vomiting, lethargy, and ketoacidosis. Attacks are generally triggered by infection or increased protein load. Urine smell of sweaty feet is characteristic. *Associated complications:* Seizures, intellectual disability if untreated, enlarged liver, vomiting, and hematologic abnormalities. *Cause:* Mutations in *IVD* (15q15.1) lead to deficiency of the enzyme isovaleryl-CoA dehydrogenase. *Inheritance:* AR. *Prevalence:* Rare. *Treatment:* Treatment consisting of a low-protein diet with supplemental oral glycine and carnitine has resulted in a relatively good cognitive outcome.

References: Grunert, S. C.,Wendel, U., Linder, M., Leichsenring, M., Schwab, K. O., Vockley, J., . . . Ensenauer, R. (2012). Clinical and neurocognitive outcome in symptomatic isovaleric academia. *Orphanet Journal of Rare Diseases, 7*, 9.

Zaki, O. K., Priya Doss, C. G., Ali, S. A., Murad, G. G., Elashi, S. A., Ebnou, M. S. A., . . . Zayed, H. (2017). Genotype–phenotype correlation in patients with isovaleric acidaemia: Comparative structural modelling and computational analysis of novel variants. *Human Molecular Genetics, 26*(16), 3105–3115.

Joubert syndrome *Disease category:* Multiple congenital anomalies. *Clinical features:* Structural cerebellar abnormalities ("molar tooth sign" on MRI), hypotonia in infancy that develops into ataxia, abnormal eye movements, retinal dysplasia or coloboma, abnormal breathing pattern, and developmental delay/intellectual disability and behavioral problems; characteristic facial appearance, including large head, prominent forehead, ptosis, epicanthal folds, upturned nose, and tongue protrusion. *Associated complications:* Retinal dystrophy, kidney disease, ocular colobomas, occipital encephalocele, hepatic fibrosis, polydactyly, oral hamartomas (benign tumors), and endocrine abnormalities. Cognitive ability ranges from moderate to severe intellectual disability. *Cause:* Joubert syndrome has been linked to 34 different genes. *Inheritance:* AR or XLR. *Prevalence:* Rare.

References: Bachmann-Gagescu, R.,Dempsey, J. C., Phelps, I. G., O'Roak, B. J., Knutzen, D. M., Rue, T. C., . . . Doherty, D. (2015). Joubert syndrome: A model for untangling recessive disorders with extreme genetic heterogeneity. *Journal of Medical Genetics, 52*, 514–522.

Poretti, A., Snow, J., Summers, A. C., Tekes, A., Huisman, T. A. G. M., Aygun, N., . . . Gunay-Aygun, M. (2017). Joubert syndrome: Neuroimaging findings in 110 patients in correlation with cognitive function and genetic cause. *Journal of Medical Genetics, 54*(8), 521–529.

Summers, A. C., Snow, J., Wiggs, E., Liu, A. G., Toro, C., Poretti, A., . . . Gunay-Aygun, M. (2017). Neuropsychological phenotypes of 76 individuals with Joubert syndrome evaluated at a single center. *American Journal of Medical Genetics, Part A, 173*(7), 1796–1812.

juvenile neuronal ceroid lipofuscinosis *See* Batten disease.

Kabuki syndrome *Disease category:* Multiple congenital anomalies. *Clinical features:* Microcephaly, trapezoid philtrum (area between base of nose and upper lip), prominent posteriorly rotated ears, preauricular pit (small hole/indentation on the ear), long palpebral fissures (the opening between the eye lids), thick eyelashes, ptosis, sparse and broad arched eyebrows, congenital heart defect, hirsutism (excessive hair), café au lait spots, cryptorchidism (undescended testes), small penis, hypotonia, and joint hyperextensibility. *Associated complications:* Cleft palate, recurrent ear infections, hearing loss, aspiration pneumonia, feeding difficulties, malabsorption, anal stenosis (stricture), imperforate anus, scoliosis, congenital hip dislocation, increased susceptibility to infections, seizures, intellectual disability, premature thelarche (breast development), hemolytic anemia, and congenital hypothyroidism. *Cause:* Mutations in *KMT2D* (formerly *MLL2*) (12q13.12) and *KDM6A* (Xp11.3). *Inheritance:* AD/XLR. *Prevalence:* Rare. Prevalence in Japan has been estimated at 1:32,000; birth incidence in Australia and New Zealand has been calculated at 1:86,000.

References: Bogershausen, N., Gatinois, V., Riehmer, V., Kayserili, H., Becker, J., Thoenes, M., . . . Wollnik, B. (2016). Mutation update for Kabuki syndrome genes KMT2D and KDM6A and further delineation of X-linked Kabuki syndrome subtype 2. *Human Mutation, 37*(9), 847–864.

Lehman, N., Mazery, A. C., Visier, A., Baumann, C., Lachesnais, D., Capri, Y., . . . Genevieve, D. (2017). Molecular, clinical and neuropsychological study in 31 patients with Kabuki syndrome and KMT2D mutations. *Clinical Genetics, 92*(3), 298–305.

Lepri, F. R., Cocciadiferro, D., Augello, B., Alfieri, P., Pes, V., Vancini, A., . . . Merla, G. (2017). Clinical and neurobehavioral features of three novel Kabuki syndrome patients with KMT2D mutations and review of literature. *International Journal of Molecular Science, 19*(1), 82.

kinky hair syndrome *See* Menkes syndrome.

Klinefelter syndrome (KS; XXY syndrome) *Disease category:* Chromosomal abnormality. *Clinical features:* Occurs only in males. Males with KS have tall, slim stature; long limbs; relatively small penis and testes; and gynecomastia (breast enlargement) in 40%. *Associated complications:* Intention tremor (involuntary trembling arising when attempting a voluntary, coordinated movement) in 20%–50%, learning disabilities and delayed speech and language development, infertility, behavioral disorders, scoliosis, osteoporosis and reduced muscle strength, and vascular problems; 8% have diabetes mellitus as adults and risk of extragonadal midline germ cell tumors. Patients may appear to have no physical changes prior to puberty with the exception of long legs. *Cause:* Chromosomal nondisjunction resulting in the 47, XXY karyotype. *Inheritance:* NM caused by the presence of an additional X chromosome; about 50% of cases caused by maternal nondisjunction (error in the separation of chromosomes), while 50% are caused by paternal nondisjunction. *Prevalence:* 1:500–1:1,000 newborn males. *Treatment:* Hormone treatment is needed in adolescence for the development of secondary male sex characteristics.

References: Gravholt, C. H.,Chang, S., Wallentin, M., Fedder, J., Moore, P., & Skakkabaek, A. (2018). Klinefelter syndrome-integrating genetics, neuropsychology and endocrinology. *Endocrinology Review, 39*(4), 389–423.

Samango-Sprouse, C., Stapleton, E., Chea, S., Lawson, P., Sadeghin, T., Cappello, C., . . . van Rijn, S. (2018). International investigation of neurocognitive and behavioral phenotype in 47, XXY (Klinefelter syndrome): Predicting individual differences. *American Journal of Medical Genetics, Part A, 176*(4), 877–885.

Van Rijn, S., de Sonneville, L., & Swaab, H. (2018). The nature of social cognitive deficits in children and adults with Klinefelter syndrome (47, XXY). *Genes, Brain, Behavior, 17*(6), e12465.

Klippel-Feil syndrome *Disease category:* Multiple congenital anomalies. *Clinical features:* Cervical vertebral fusion present at birth, hemivertebrae (incomplete development of one side of one or more vertebrae). *Associated complications:* Congenital scoliosis; torticollis (wry neck); low hairline; limited range of motion; sacral agenesis (absence of tailbone); hearing loss; occasional congenital heart defect; extra, fused, or missing ribs; middle-ear abnormalities; genitourinary abnormalities; and pain. *Cause:* Mutations in *GDF6* (8q22.2), *GDF3* (12p13.31), and *MEOX1* (17q21.31). *Inheritance:* AD for those with mutations in *GDF6* and *GDF3*. AR if caused by mutation in *MEOX1*. *Incidence:* Approximately 1:40,000, with a slight female predominance.

References: Kenna, M. A., Irace, A. L, Strychowsky, J. E., Kawai, K., Barrett, D., Manganella, J., & Cunningham, M. J. (2018). Otolaryngologic manifestations of Klippel-Feil syndrome in children. *JAMA Otolaryngology-Head & Neck Surgery,144*(3), 238–243.

Saker, E., Loukas, M., Oskouian, R. J., & Tubbs, R. S. (2016). The intriguing history of vertebral fusion anomalies: The Klippel-Feil syndrome. *Child's Nervous System, 32*(9), 1599–1602.

Klippel-Trenaunay-Weber syndrome (Klippel-Trenaunay syndrome) *Disease category:* Multiple congenital anomalies. *Clinical features:* Asymmetric hypertrophy of limb, face (lips, cheeks, tongue, teeth), or other body parts; hemangiomas (benign congenital tumors made up of newly formed blood vessels); and arteriovenous fistulas. *Associated complications:* Dependent on the area of hypertrophy; complications may affect any organ/body part, including the spinal cord (resulting in weakness or paralysis), kidneys (renal obstruction), and brain (intracranial hypertension). *Cause:* Some have mutations in the *PIK3CA* gene, making it part of the *PIK3CA*-related overgrowth spectrum (PROS). Likely other genes are involved that have yet to be identified. *Inheritance:* Believed to be passed on as an AD trait, where individuals are not affected unless a second, somatic mutation (arising after fertilization) occurs. *Prevalence:* Unknown.

References: Brandigi, E., Torino, G., Messina, M., Molinaro, F., Mazzei, O., Matucci, T., & Lopez Gutierrez, J. C. (2018). Combined capillary-venous-lymphatic malformations without overgrowth in patients with Klippel-Trenaunay syndrome. *Journal of Vascular Surgery: Venous and Lymphatic Disorders, 6*(2), 230–236.

Vahidnezhad, H., Youssefian, L, & Uitto, J. (2016). Klippel-Trenaunay syndrome belongs to the PIK3CA-related overgrowth spectrum (PROS). *Experimental Dermatology, 25*(1), 17–19.

Krabbe disease (globoid cell leukodystrophy) *Disease category:* Progressive neurologic disorder. *Clinical features:* In the classic form, symptoms begin before 6 months of age with irritability, progressive stiffness, optic atrophy, cognitive deterioration, and early death, often before 2 years of age. Approximately 10%–15% of cases have onset of symptoms between 6 months and 17 years of age and have slower disease progression. *Associated complications:* Hypertonicity, opisthotonos (back arching), visual and hearing impairment, episodic unexplained fevers, and seizures; peripheral neuropathy. *Cause:* Deficiency of the galactocerebrosidase enzyme resulting from mutations in *GALC* (14q24.3–q32.1). *Inheritance:* AR. *Incidence:* 1:100,000; may be increased in specific populations such as the Druze kindred in Israel (carrier frequency of 1:6). *Treatment:* Hematopoietic stem cell transplantation seems to improve developmental outcome, although it has a high mortality rate.

References: Kwon, J. M., Matern, D., Kurtzberg, J., Wrabetz, L., Gelb, M. H., Wenger, D. A., . . . Orsini, J. J. (2018). Consensus guidelines for newborn screening, diagnosis and treatment of infantile Krabbe disease. *Orphanet Journal of Rare Diseases, 13*(1), 30.

Wright, M. D., Poe, M. D., DeRenzo, A., Haldal, S., & Escolar, M. L. (2017). Developmental outcomes of cord blood transplantation for Krabbe disease: A 15-year study. *Neurology, 89*(13), 1365–1372.

Landau-Kleffner syndrome (LKS) *Disease category:* Neurologic. *Clinical features:* Normal development until ages 5–8 years, beginning with acquired aphasia (loss of speech) and regression in receptive language ability. Seizures are common in 70% of patients (usually atypical absence seizures). *Associated complications:* EEG abnormalities usually are continuous spike-and-wave in sleep (CSWS). Some patients show autistic features and issues with attention. *Cause:* Mutations in *GRIN2A* (16p13.2) have been found in 4.8%–7.7% of patients. Now considered part of the *GRIN2A*-related speech disorder and epilepsy syndromes. *Inheritance:* AD. *Prevalence:* Unknown. *Treatment:* Treatment of seizures with antiepileptic medications. *See* Chapter 22.

References: Caraballo, R. H., Cejas, N., Chamorro, N., Kaltenmeier, M. C., Fortini, S., & Soprano, A. M. (2014). Landau-Kleffner syndrome: A study of 29 patients. *Seizure, 23*(2), 98–104.

Hughes, J. R. (2011). A review of the relationships between Landau-Kleffner syndrome, electrical status epilepticus during sleep, and continuous spike-waves during sleep. *Epilepsy Behavior, 20,* 247–253.

Riccio, C. A., Vidrine, S. M., Cohen, M. J., Acosta-Cotte, D., & Park, Y. (2017). Neurocognitive and behavioral profiles of children with Landau-Kleffner syndrome. *Applied Neuropsychology. Child, 6*(4), 345–354.

Laurence-Moon-Bardet-Biedl syndrome *See* Bardet-Biedl syndrome.

Leber congenital amaurosis *Disease category:* Ophthalmologic. *Clinical features:* Severe visual impairment or blindness presenting in infancy, usually before the age of 6 months. Electroretinogram (ERG) responses are usually nonrecordable. *Associated complications:* High hypermetropia (farsightedness), photophobia (sensitivity to light), oculodigital sign (poking/rubbing/pressing of the eyes), keratoconus (thinning of the cornea), cataracts, and a variable appearance to the fundus. Rarely has been associated with developmental delay or intellectual disability. *Cause:* Mutations in 24 different genes. *Inheritance:* Mostly AR, rarely AD. *Prevalence:* 2:100,000–3:100,000. *Treatment:* There is an FDA-approved gene therapy medication (Luxturna) for those with mutations in *RPE65*.

References: Kumaran, N., Moore, A. T., Weleber, R. G., & Michaelides, M. (2017). Leber congenital amaurosis/early-onset severe retinal dystrophy: Clinical features, molecular genetics and therapeutic interventions. *British Journal of Ophthalmology, 101(9),* 1147–1154.

Russell, S.,Bennett, J., Wellman, J. A., Chung, D. C., Yu, Z. F., Tillman, A., . . . Maguire, A. M. (2017). Efficacy and safety of voretigene neparvovec (AAV2-hRPE65v2) in patients with RPE65-mediated inherited retinal dystrophy: A randomized, controlled, open-label, phase 3 trial. *Lancet, 390*(10097), 849–860.

Sheck, L., Davies, W. I. L, Moradi, P., Robson, A. G., Jumaran, N., Liasis, A. C., . . . Michaelides, M. (2018). Leber congenital amaurosis associated with mutations in CEP290, clinical phenotype, and natural history in preparation for trials of novel therapies. *Ophthalmology, 125*(6), 894–903.

Lennox-Gastaut syndrome *See* Chapter 22.

Lesch-Nyhan syndrome *Disease category:* Inborn error of metabolism: nucleic acid. *Clinical features:* An inborn error of purine metabolism associated with elevated levels of uric acid in blood and urine. Affected males appear symptom free at birth but then present with hypotonia and developmental delay during the first year of life. Dystonia (abnormal movements) and spasticity develop, accompanied by severe involuntary self-injurious behavior, including biting of fingers, arms, and lips. *Associated complications:* Cognitive impairment, seizures in 50%, hematuria (blood in urine), kidney stones, and ultimate kidney failure without treatment. *Cause:* Defect in enzyme hypoxanthine-guanine phosphoribosyl transferase caused by a mutation in *HPRT* (Xq26–q27.2). *Inheritance:* XLR. Affected females with skewed X-inactivation have been reported. Carrier females are typically unaffected, although some have increased uric acid excretion. *Prevalence:* 1:380,000. *Treatment:* Allopurinol is useful in preventing kidney and joint deposition of uric acid. Spasticity is treated with baclofen or benzodiazepines. Numerous medications have been used in the management of self-injurious behavior without much success.

References: Harris, J. C. (2018). Lesch-Nyhan syndrome and its variants: Examining the behavioral and neurocognitive phenotype. *Current Opinion in Psychiatry, 31*(2), 96–102.

Tewar, N., et al. (2017). Lesch-Nyhan syndrome: The saga of metabolic abnormalities and self-injurious behavior. *Intractable Rare Disease Research, 6*(1), 65–68.

lissencephaly syndrome (e.g., Miller-Dieker syndrome) *Disease category:* Malformation. *Clinical features:* Lissencephaly (LIS) and subcortical band heterotopia (SBH) comprise a spectrum of malformations of cortical development caused by insufficient neuronal migration. Main features of LIS include an abnormally thick cortex and reduced or absent formation of cerebral convolutions ("smooth brain"). SBH consists of abnormal bands of neurons beneath a normal cortex. Some patients with LIS have severe congenital microcephaly, referred to as microlissencephaly. *Associated complications:* Intellectual disability, seizures, dysmorphic features, late tooth eruption, poor weight gain, dysphagia (swallowing difficulty), congenital heart defect, and intestinal atresia (congenital closure). Those with multiple congenital anomalies in addition to LIS fall under the Miller-Dieker and Baraitser-Winter cerebrofrontofacial syndromes and X-linked LIS with abnormal genitalia. *Cause:* 19 genes have been defined to date that cause lissencephaly, the most common being *PAFAH1B1* (previously *LIS1*) and *DCX*. *Inheritance:* NM with AD inheritance when passed from an affected individual or XLR (males are typically more severely affected while females have a milder phenotype); possibly increased recurrence risk if one parent has a balanced chromosomal translocation of chromosome 17p. *Prevalence:* Rare.

References: Di Dinato, N., Chiari, S., Mirzaa, G. M., Aldinger, K., Parrini, E., Olds, C., . . . Dobyns, W. B. (2018). Lissencephaly: Expanded imaging and clinical classification. *American Journal of Medical Genetics, Part A, 173*(6), 1473–1488.

Guerrini, R., & Dobyns, W. B. (2014). Malformations of cortical development: Clinical features and genetic causes. *Lancet Neurology, 13,* 710–726.

Herbst, S. M.,Proepper, C. R., Geis, T., Borggraefe, I., Hahn, A., Debus, O., . . . Hehr, U. (2016). LIS1-associated classic lissencephaly: A retrospective, multicenter survey of the epileptogenic phenotype and response to antiepileptic drugs. *Brain Development, 38*(4), 399–406.

Lowe syndrome (oculocerebrorenal syndrome) *Disease category:* Multiple congenital anomalies. *Clinical features:* Bilateral cataracts at birth, hypotonia, absent deep tendon reflexes, kidney dysfunction (proximal renal tubular dysfunction), and dysmorphic facies. *Associated complications:* Poor weight gain, short stature, vitamin D–resistant rickets, seizures, visual impairment (corrected acuity is usually 20/100), glaucoma, intellectual disability in 75%, behavioral problems, intention tremor, craniosynostosis, and peripheral neuropathy (damage to nerves). Female carriers have characteristic findings in the lens (opacities) of each eye. *Cause:* Abnormal inositol phosphate metabolism caused by mutations in *OCRL1* (Xq26.1). *Inheritance:* XLR, with one third of cases being NM. *Prevalence:* 1:100,000.

References: Bokenkamp, A., & Ludwig, M. (2016). The oculocerebrorenal syndrome of Lowe: An update. *Pediatric Nephrology, 31*(12), 2201–2212.

Recker, F., Zaniew, M., Bockenhauer, D., MIglietti, N., Bokenkamp, A., Moczulska, A., . . . Ludwig, M. (2015). Characterization of 28 novel patients expands the mutational and phenotypic spectrum of Lowe syndrome. *Pediatric Nephrology, 300*(6), 931–943.

mandibulofacial dysostosis *See* Treacher Collins syndrome.

maple syrup urine disease (MSUD) *Disease category:* Inborn error of metabolism: amino acid. *Clinical features:* A disorder of branched chain amino acid metabolism with four identified clinical variants (classic, intermittent, intermediate, and thiamine-responsive); the classic form comprises 75% of cases and is characterized by a maple syrup odor in the cerumen (ear wax) and urine from birth to 7 days of age, severe opisthotonos (spasm with body in a bowed position and head and heels bent backward), hypertonia, hypoglycemia, lethargy, and respiratory difficulties. Symptoms appear within the first 48 hours of life; if untreated, it is most often fatal within 1 month. Untreated survivors have severe intellectual disability and spasticity. The intermittent form presents with periods of ataxia, behavior disturbances, drowsiness, and seizures. Attacks are triggered by infections, excessive protein intake, or other physiological stresses. Individuals with the intermediate form usually demonstrate mild to moderate intellectual disability. *Associated complications:* Acidosis, hypoglycemia, growth retardation, and feeding problems; acute episodes are characterized by muscle fatigue, vomiting, impaired cognitive ability, hyperactivity, sleep disturbance, hallucinations, dystonia, and ataxia. *Cause:* Deficiency in branched-chain alpha keto-acid dehydrogenase caused by mutations in *BCKDHA* (1p31), *BCKDHB* (6p22), and *DBT* (19q13.1). *Prevalence:* 1:185,000; increased prevalence in the Mennonite population, with an incidence of 1:380. *Inheritance:* AR. *Treatment:* High-calorie diet with restriction of leucine and supplementation with isoleucine and valine. If instituted early (within 2 weeks of birth), the prognosis is good for typical intelligence. Thiamine is used in the thiamine-responsive form. Orthotopic liver transplantation is effective for classic MSUD.

References: Abi-Warde, M. T., Roda, C., Arnoux, J. B., Servais, A., Habarou, F., Brassier, A., . . . de Lonlay, P. (2017). Long-term metabolic follow-up and clinical outcome of 25 patients with maple syrup urine disease. *Journal of Inherited Metabolic Disease, 40*(6), 783–792.

Bouchereau, J., Leduc-Leballeur, J., Pichard, S., Imbard, A., Benoist, J.F., Abi Warde, M. T., . . . Schiff, M. (2017). Neurocognitive profiles in MSUD school-age patients. *Journal of Inherited Metabolic Disease, 40*(3), 377–383.

Scott, A. I., Cusmano-Ozog, K., Enns, G. M., & Cowan, T. M. (2017). Correction of hyperleucinemia in MSUD patients on leucine-free dietary therapy. *Molecular Genetics and Metabolism, 122*(4), 156–159.

Marfan syndrome *Disease category:* Connective tissue disorder. *Clinical features:* Tall, thin body; upward dislocation of ocular lens; myopia; spiderlike limbs; and hypermobile joints. Average intelligence is expected, although learning disabilities have been reported in up to 50% of children. *Associated complications:* Aortic dilatation or dissection, congestive heart failure, mitral valve prolapse, emphysema, sleep apnea, pectus excavatum (sunken breastbone), or pectus carinatum (pigeon breastbone), and scoliosis. *Cause:* Mutation in *FBN1* (15q15–q21.3). *Inheritance:* AD with wide clinical variability. *Prevalence:* Estimated to be about 1:5,000. *Treatment:* Use of Losartan, an angiotensin II type 1 receptor blocker has been shown to prevent aortic aneurysm through the inhibition of transforming growth factor beta in mice. Doxycycline has also been shown to normalize aortic vasomotor function and suppress aneurysm growth. Trials continue with both of these medications.

References: Becerra-Munoz, V. M.,Gomez-Doblas, J.J., Porras-Martin, C., Such-Martinez, M., Crespo-Leiro, M.G., Barriales-Villa, R., . . . Cabrera-Bueno, F. (2018). The importance of genotype-phenotype correlation in the clinical management of Marfan syndrome. *Orphanet Journal of Rare Disease, 13*(1), 16.

Saeyeldin, A., Zafar, M. A., Velasquez, C. A., Ip, K., Gryaznov, A., Brownstein, A. J., . . . Elefteriades, J. A. (2017). Natural history of aortic root aneurysms in Marfan syndrome. *Annals of Cardiothoracic Surgery, 6*(6), 625–632.

Maroteaux-Lamy syndrome (MPS VI) *See* mucopolysaccharidoses.

McCune-Albright syndrome (polyostotic fibrous dysplasia) *Disease category:* Endocrine disorder. *Clinical features:* Large café-au-lait spots with irregular borders; fibrous dysplasia of bones (thinning of the bone with replacement of bone marrow with fibrous tissue, producing pain and increasing deformity), bowing of long bones, and premature onset of puberty; advanced bone age. *Associated complications:* Hearing or visual impairment, hyperthyroidism, hyperparathyroidism (increased activity of the parathyroid gland, which controls calcium metabolism), abnormal adrenal function, increased risk of malignancy, and occasional spinal cord anomalies. *Cause:* Postmitotic mutation in the *GNAS1* (20q13) causing a defect in the enzyme adenyl cyclase. *Inheritance:* NM arising after fertilization (somatic mosaic) will be passed in an AD fashion if reproductive organs are involved; theoretically lethal unless present in the mosaic form. *Testing:* Mutations in the *GNAS1* gene were found to only be present in 46% of patients presenting with the classic triad. Other tissue types may need to be tested to confirm the presence of the common mutation. *Prevalence:* Rare. Estimates between 1:100,000–1:1,000,000.

References: Boyce, A. M., Turner, A., Watts, L., Forestier-Zhang, L, Underhill, A., Pinedo-Villanueva, R., . . . Javaid, M. K. (2017). Improving patient outcomes in fibrous dysplasia/McCune-Albright syndrome: An international multidisciplinary workshop to inform an international partnership. *Archives of Osteoporosis, 12*(1), 21.

Majoor, B. C. J., Andela, C. D., Bruggemann, J., van de Sande, M. A. J., Kaptein, A. A., Hamdy, N. A. T, . . . Appelman-Dijkstra, N. M. (2017). Determinants of impaired quality of life in patients with fibrous dysplasia. *Orphanet Journal of Rare Diseases, 12*(1), 80.

MELAS (*m*itochondrial myopathy, *e*ncephalopathy, *l*actic *a*cidosis, and *s*troke-like episodes) *See* mitochondrial disorders.

Menkes syndrome (kinky hair syndrome) *Disease category:* Inborn error of metabolism: copper. *Clinical features:* An inborn error of copper metabolism presenting at age 2–3 months with neurologic changes, "steely" texture of hair, and characteristic face with pudgy cheeks. *Associated complications:* Seizures, feeding difficulties, hypotonia, severe intellectual disability, recurrent infections, visual loss, bony abnormalities with tendency toward easy fracture, thrombosis, and early death. *Cause:* Copper deficiency from decreased absorption and/or missing enzymes caused by mutations in the adenosine triphosphatase *ATP7A* gene at Xq13. *Inheritance:* XLR, although some females may present with variable symptoms. *Prevalence:* 1:100,000. *Treatment:* Treatment with copper-histidine has been found to prevent neurological deterioration when provided before the age of 2 months. Treatment provided after 2 months of age cannot prevent neurologic, connective tissue, or bone complications.

References: Smpokou, P., Samanta, M., Gerry, G. T., Hecht, L., Engle, E. C., & Lichter-Konecki, U. (2015). Menkes disease in affected females: the clinical disease spectrum.

American Journal of Medical Genetics, Part A, 167A(2), 417–420.

Ziatic, S.,Comstra, H. S., Gokhale, A., Petris, M. J., & Faundez, V. (2015). Molecular basis of neurodegeneration and neurodevelopmental defects in Menkes disease. *Neurobiological Disease, 81,* 154–161.

MERRF (*m*yoclonic *e*pilepsy with *r*agged *r*ed *f*ibers) *See* mitochondrial disorders.

metachromatic leukodystrophy (arylsulfatase A deficiency) *Disease category:* Inborn error of metabolism: lysosomal storage disorder. *Clinical features:* Metachromatic leukodystrophy (MLD) is split into three subtypes based on age of onset: late-infantile, juvenile, and adult. The enzyme deficiency results in accumulation of toxins and leads to varying degrees of progressive neurological impairment, ranging from unsteady gait to severe rigidity and choreoathetosis. Muscle weakness, hypotonia, frequent falls, and ataxia are common. Onset of the infantile form is by 2 years of age and usually results in death by age 5 (50%–60% of cases). The juvenile form generally begins between 3–16 years of age, is rarer (20%–30% of cases), and progresses more slowly. The adult form presents after age 16. *Associated complications:* Seizures, abdominal distension, and cognitive deterioration. *Cause:* Mutations in the arylsulfatase A (*ARSA*) gene (22q13.33) cause ASA enzyme deficiency and result in the accumulation of sphingolipid sulfatide. *Inheritance:* AR. *Prevalence:* 1:40,000–1:160,000. *Treatment:* Bone marrow transplantation may have beneficial effects on some tissues types but does not affect lipid storage in the brain. Best results when performed in presymptomatic and very early symptomatic patients with juvenile or adult forms of the disease.

References: Eichler, F. S., Cox, T. M., Crombez, E., Dali, C. I., & Kohlschutter, A. (2016). Metachromatic leukodystrophy: An assessment of disease burden. *Journal of Child Neurology, 31*(13), 1457–1463.

Van Rappard, D. F., Klauser, A., Steenweg, M. E., Boelens, J. J., Bugiani, M., & van der Knaap, M. S. (2017). Quantitative MR spectroscopic imaging in metachromatic leukodystrophy: Value for prognosis and treatment. *Journal of Neurology, Neurosurgery, and Psychiatry, 89*(1), 105–111.

methylmalonic aciduria *Disease category:* Inborn error of metabolism: organic acidemia. *Clinical features:* An organic acidemia with multiple subtypes. In the infantile/non–B12-responsive phenotype (most common form), infants are normal at birth but then develop lethargy, vomiting, dehydration, hepatomegaly, hypotonia, and encephalopathy. There is a rarer intermediate B_{12}-responsive type, which presents in the first few months to years with anorexia, poor weight gain, hypotonia, and developmental delay. The atypical/benign adult subtype is associated with increased urinary excretion of methylmalonic acid but may remain asymptomatic. *Associated complications:* Variable developmental delay, kidney failure, metabolic stroke affecting the basal ganglia, movement disorder with choreoathetosis, dystonia, para/quadriparesis, pancreatitis, growth failure, immune dysfunction, and optic nerve atrophy. *Cause:* Isolated methylmalonic aciduria is found in patients with mutations in the MUT gene (*6p21*), causing partial, mut(-), or complete, mut(0), enzyme deficiency. This form is unresponsive to B_{12} therapy. Various forms of isolated methylmalonic aciduria also occur in a subset of patients with defects in the synthesis of the MUT coenzyme adenosylcobalamin (AdoCbl) and are classified according to complementation group: cblA, caused by mutation in *MMAA* (4q31.1-q31.2), and cblB, caused by mutation in *MMAB* (12q24). Combined methylmalonic aciduria and homocystinuria may be seen in complementation groups cblC, cblD, and cblF. *Inheritance:* AR. *Prevalence:* 1:50,000–1:100,000. *Treatment:* Treatment consists of a low-protein, high-calorie diet and supplemental hydroxocobalamin (B_{12}) injections in those who have a B_{12}-responsive form; carnitine is also given. Liver and liver/kidney transplant have been performed to avoid continued damage to the kidneys, and some success has been reported. Carglumic acid has also been used to lower ammonia with good success.

References: Chu, J.,Pupvac, M., Watkins, D., Tian, X., Feng, Y., Chen, S., . . . Rosenblatt, D. S. (2016). Next generation sequencing of patients with mut methylmalonic aciduria: Validation of somatic cell studies and identification of 16 novel mutations. *Molecular Genetics and Metabolism, 118*(4), 264–271.

Sakamoto, R., Nakamura, K., Kido, J., Masumoto, S., Mitsubuchi, H., Inomata, Y., & Endo, F. (2016). Improvement in the prognosis and development of patients with methylmalonic academia after living donor liver transplant. *Pediatric Transplant, 20*(8), 1081–1086.

Miller-Dieker syndrome *See* lissencephaly syndromes.

mitochondrial disorders (mitochondrial encephalopathies and myopathies) *Disease category:* Inborn error of metabolism/mitochondrial disorders. *Clinical features:* This diverse group of disorders is linked by a common etiology—abnormal function of the mitochondria (energy-producing intracellular structures) or abnormalities in mitochondrial metabolism. Mitochondrial disorders can affect every organ system. Common features include ptosis (droopy eyelids), external ophthalmoplegia (paralysis of the external eye muscles), myopathy, cardiomyopathy, short stature, and hypoparathyroidism. *Associated* *complications:* Seizures, sensorineural hearing loss, optic atrophy, retinitis pigmentosa (pigmentary changes in retina causing loss of peripheral vision and clumping of pigment), cataracts, diabetes, migraine, intestinal pseudo-obstruction, reflux, kidney problems, and exercise intolerance. *Cause:* Genes encoding nuclear DNA and mitochondrial DNA (mtDNA) are known to cause mitochondrial disorders. Mutations in different genes may cause the same symptoms. *Inheritance:* AR, AD, NM, or may be inherited from the mother through mtDNA. *Prevalence:* 1:8,500 for all mitochondrial disorders combined. *Treatment:* Early diagnosis and treatment of diabetes, eye abnormalities, and cardiac disease. Coenzyme Q10 and riboflavin have been used with some reported benefit. Intravenous arginine has shown promise to those with stroke. Six mitochondrial disorders are discussed next.

References: Bindu, P. S., Sonam, K., Govindaraj, P., Govindaraju, C., Chiplunkar, S., Nagappa, M., . . . Taly, A. B. (2018). Outcome of epilepsy in patients with mitochondrial disorders: Phenotype genotype and magnetic resonance imaging correlations. *Clinical Neurology and Neruosurgery, 164,* 182–189.

Ganetzky, R. D., & Falk, M. J. (2018). 8-year retrospective analysis of intravenous arginine therapy for acute metabolic strokes in pediatric mitochondrial disease. *Molecular Genetics and Metabolism, 123*(3), 301–308.

Kearns-Sayre syndrome *Clinical features:* Short stature, progressive external ophthalmoplegia, retinitis pigmentosa, heart block, and cerebellar ataxia. Onset is usually in childhood, before age 20 years, with ptosis, ophthalmoplegia, or both. *Associated complications:* Visual impairment, bilateral hearing loss, myopathy, endocrine abnormalities, diabetes mellitus, hypoparathyroidism, dysphagia, and dementia. *Cause:* Deletions in mtDNA (90% have a 2–10 kb mtDNA deletion). *Inheritance:* Maternal, through mtDNA. *Prevalence*: 1.2:100,000 for large-scale mtDNA deletions. *Treatment:* Generally supportive, symptomatic treatment such as cochlear implant for hearing loss, cardiac pacemaker placement for those with cardiac conduction block, eyelid slings for severe ptosis, and hormone replacement for endocrinopathies. Folinic acid supplementation is suggested for those with low CSF folic acid, although recent papers note a lack of clinical response. Co-enzyme Q10 and L-carnitine are also often used.

References: Grady, J. P.,Campbell, G., Ratnaike, T., Blekely, E. L., Falkous, G., Nesbitt, V., . . . McFarland, R. (2014). Disease progression in patients with single, large-scale mitochondrial DNA deletions. *Brain, 137(Pt. 2),* 323–334.

Khambatta, S., Nguyen, D. L., Beckman, T. J., & Wittich, C. M. (2014). Kearns-Sayre syndrome: A case series of 35 adults and children. *International Journal of Genetics Medicine, 7,* 325–332.

Leber hereditary optic neuropathy (LHON) *Clinical features:* Bilateral central vision loss beginning in young adulthood. Patients usually become legally blind. *Associated complications:* Occasionally seen with multiple sclerosis (usually in women); peripheral neuropathy and movement disorders have all been reported as more common in individuals with LHON. *Cause:* Primarily associated with point mutations in mtDNA. *Inheritance:* Maternal, through mtDNA. Males are four to five times more likely to be affected. *Prevalence:* 1:31,000–1:50,000. *Treatment*: Current treatment is typically supportive with visual aids, occupational rehabilitation, and treatment for raised intraocular pressure for those who have that complication. Gene therapy with AAV2 for those with point mutation G11778A in *MT-ND4* is currently being investigated with good safety data in a Phase 1/2 trial.

References: Caporali, L., Iommarini, L., La Morgia, C., Olivieri, A., Achilli, A., Maresca, A., . . . Carelli, V. (2018). Peculiar combinations of individually non-pathogenic missense mitochondrial DNA variants cause low penetrance Leber hereditary optic neuropathy. *PLoS Genetics, 14(2),* e1007210.

Carelli, V., Carbonelli, M., de Coo, I. F., Kawasaki, A., Klopstock, T., Lagreze, W. A., . . . Barboni, P. (2017). International consensus statement on the clinical and therapeutic management of Leber hereditary optic neuropathy. *Journal of Neuro-Ophthalmology, 37(4),* 371–381.

Leigh syndrome (subacute necrotizing encephalomyopathy) *Clinical features:* Encephalopathy, ophthalmoplegia, optic atrophy, and myopathy. *Associated complications:* Developmental delay and regression, ataxia, spasticity, hypertrophic cardiomyopathy, and early death. Onset usually between 3–12 months of age, often after a viral infection. *Cause:* Mutations in many different nuclear and mitochondrial genes involved in energy metabolism, including respiratory chain complexes I, II, III, IV, and V, as well as tRNA proteins, and pyruvate dehydrogenase complex. *Inheritance:* Maternal, AR, XLR. *Prevalence:* 1:30,000–1:40,000. *Treatment:* Usually includes sodium bicarbonate or sodium citrate for acute exacerbations of lactic acidosis and antiepileptic drugs for seizures. Medications for dystonia include benzhexol, baclofen, tetrabenazine, or gabapentin. Anticongestive therapy may be required for cardiomyopathy. Anecdotal reports suggested that dichloroacetate (DCA) may have had short-term clinical improvement, but a double-blind, placebo-controlled trial in MELAS showed a toxic effect of DCA on peripheral nerves. A vitamin cocktail is often given that includes riboflavin, thiamine, and coenzyme Q10. A ketogenic diet may be used in those with refractory epilepsy.

References: Gerards, M., Sallevelt, S. C., & Smeets, H. J. (2016). Leigh syndrome: Resolving the clinical and genetic heterogeneity paves the way for treatment options. *Molecular Genetics and Metabolism, 117*(3), 300–312.

Sofou, K., de Coo, I. F. M., Ostergaard, E., Isohanni, P., Naess, K., De Meirleir, L., . . . Darin, N. (2018). Phenotype-genotype correlations in Leigh syndrome: New insights from a multicenter study of 96 patients. *Journal of Medical Genetics, 55*(1), 21–27.

MELAS (*m*itochondrial myopathy, *e*ncephalopathy, *l*actic *a*cidosis, and *s*troke-like episodes) *Clinical features:* Migraine headaches, seizures, stroke-like episodes, encephalopathy (degenerative disease of the brain), and myopathy. *Associated complications:* Progressive hearing loss, cortical blindness, ataxia, dementia, lactic acidosis, recurrent vomiting, and hemiparesis. *Cause:* A mutation in mtDNA encoding transfer RNA causes reduced mitochondrial protein synthesis. *Inheritance:* Maternal, through mtDNA. *Treatment:* IV arginine therapy has shown significant therapeutic benefit in pediatric mitochondrial disease stroke subjects in those with MELAS, as well as other diagnoses. Acute hemiplegic stroke was particularly responsive to IV arginine treatment.

References: El-Hattab, A. W., Adesina, A. M., Jones, J., & Scaglie, F. (2015). MELAS syndrome: Clinical manifestations, pathogenesis, and treatment options. *Molecular Genetics and Metabolism, 116*(1-2), 4–12.

Ganetzky, R. D., & Falk, M. J. (2018). 8-year retrospective analysis of intravenous arginine therapy for acute metabolic strokes in pediatric mitochondrial disease. *Molecular Genetics and Metabolism, 123*(3), 301–308.

Kraya, T., Neumann, L., Paelecke-Habermann, Y., Deschauer, M., Stoevesandt, D., Zierz, S., & Watzke, S. (2017). Cognitive impairment, clinical severity and MRI changes in MELAS syndrome. *Mitochondrion, S1567-7249*(17), 30162–30169.

MERRF (*m*yoclonic *e*pilepsy with *r*agged *r*ed *f*ibers) *Clinical features:* Myoclonic epilepsy, ataxia, spasticity, and myopathy. *Associated complications:* Optic atrophy, sensorineural hearing loss, peripheral neuropathy, diabetes, cardiomyopathy, dementia, and lipomas (fatty tumors); characteristic ragged red muscle fibers are seen on muscle biopsy examination. *Cause:* Mutations in mtDNA encoding transfer RNA. *Inheritance:* Maternal, through mtDNA. *Treatment*: Conventional antiepileptic drugs for seizures, physical therapy for impaired motor function, and standard pharmacologic therapy for cardiac symptoms. Typically levetiracetam, clonazepam, zonisamide, and valproic acid have been used for myoclonic epilepsy. Valproate can cause secondary carnitine deficiency, however, and should be avoided or used with L-carnitine supplementation. Coenzyme Q10 and L-carnitine are often given with the idea that they may improve mitochondrial function. Aerobic exercise is thought to be helpful.

References: Altmann, J., Buchner, B., Nadaj-Pakleza, A., Schafer, J., Jackson, S., Lehmann, D., . . . Klopstock, T. (2016). Expanded phenotypic spectrum of the m.8344A>G "MERRF" mutation: Data from the German mitoNET registry. *Journal of Neurology, 263*(5), 961–972.

Finsterer, J., Zarrouk-Mahjoub, S., & Shoffner, J. M. (2017). MERRF classification: Implications for diagnosis and clinical trials. *Pediatric Neurology, 80,* 8–23.

NARP (*n*europathy, *a*taxia, *r*etinitis *p*igmentosa) *Clinical features:* Proximal neurogenic muscle weakness with sensory neuropathy, ataxia, and pigmentary retinopathy. *Associated complications:* Seizures, learning difficulties, dementia, short stature, sensorineural hearing loss, progressive external ophthalmoplegia, and cardiac conduction defects. Often stable, but can have episodic deterioration with viral illness. *Cause:* Mutation in the ATP synthase 6 gene. *Inheritance:* Maternal, through mtDNA. *Treatment*: Similar to Leigh syndrome.

References: Claeys, K. G., Abicht, A., Hausler, M., Kleinle, S., Wiesmann, M., Schulz, J. B., . . . Weis, J. (2016). Novel genetic and neuropathological insights in neurogenic muscle weakness, ataxia, and retinitis pigmentosa (NARP). *Muscle and Nerve, 54*(2), 328–333.

Rawle, M. J., & Larner, A. J. (2013). NARP syndrome: A 20-year follow-up. *Case Reports in Neurology, 5*(3), 204–207.

Moebius sequence/syndrome (congenital facial diplegia) *Disease category:* Multiple congenital anomalies. *Clinical features:* Facial paralysis resulting in an expressionless face and facial weakness (bilateral in 92% of cases and unilateral in 8%) due to palsies of the 6th, 7th, and occasionally 12th cranial nerves; occasional abnormalities of fingers and legs; micrognathia; eye abnormalities, including esotropia ("cross-eyed"), and vision problems, including myopia, astigmatism, and amblyopia (impaired vision); and craniofacial malformations. *Associated complications:* Feeding difficulties, oral motor dysfunction, articulation disorder, occasional tracheal or laryngeal anomalies, gross and fine motor delay and dysfunction, and learning disabilities. *Cause:* Linked to 13q12.2-q13 but no known gene. *Inheritance:* Not well characterized; most reported cases are SP, possibly due to an NM; rare reports of AD cases with variable expressivity. *Prevalence:* 1:50,000.

References: Renault, F., Flores-Guevara, R., Sergent, B., Baudon, J.J., Aouizerate, J., Vazquez, M.P., & Gitiaux, C. (2018). Pathogenesis of cranial neuropathies on Moebius syndrome: Electrodiagnostic orofacial studies. *Muscle and Nerve, 58*(1), 79–83.

Strobel, L., & Renner, G. (2016). Quality of life and adjustment in children and adolescents with Moebius syndrome: Evidence for specific impairments in social functioning. *Research in Developmental Disabilities, 53–54,* 178–188.

monosomy X *See* Turner syndrome.

Morquio syndrome (MPS IV) *See* mucopolysaccharidoses.

MSUD *See* maple syrup urine disease.

mucopolysaccharidoses (MPS) *Disease category:* Inborn error of metabolism: lysosomal storage disorder. *Clinical features:* Glycosaminoglycans accumulate within the lysosomes in these seven distinguishable forms of the disorder, each with two or more subgroups. Features shared by most include coarse facial features, thick skin, hirsutism (excessive hair), corneal clouding, and organomegaly (enlargement of spleen and liver). Growth deficiency, intellectual disability, cardiomyopathy, and skeletal dysplasia are also seen. Intelligence is normal in MPS type IV (Morquio syndrome) and MPS type VI (Marataux-Lamy). The various MPS disorders are differentiated by their clinical features, enzymatic defects, genetic transmission, and urinary mucopolysaccharide pattern. *Inheritance:* All are AR except MPSII (Hunter syndrome), which is XLR. *Prevalence:* Overall estimated to be 1:22,500. MPS I (Hurler, Scheie, and Hurler-Scheie syndromes), MPS II (Hunter syndromes), and MPS III (Sanfilippo syndrome) are discussed next. Others include MPS IV (Morquio syndrome), MPS VI (Maroteaux-Lamy syndrome), and MPS VII (Sly syndrome).

References: Chakroborty, P. P., Patra, S., Biswas, S. N., & Barman, H. (2018). Attenuated form of type II mucopolysaccharidosis (Hunter syndrome): Pitfalls and potential clues in diagnosis. *BMJ Case Reports,* pii: bcr-1018,224392.

Eisengart, J. B., Rudser, K. D., Xue, Y., Orchard, P., Miller, W., Lund, T., . . . Whitley, C. B. (2018). Long-term outcomes of systemic therapies for Hurler syndrome: An international multicenter comparison. *Genetics in Medicine.* doi:10.1038/gim.2018.29

Kuiper, G. A., Meijer, L. L. M., Langereis, E. J., & Wijburg, F. A. (2018). Failure to shorten the diagnostic delay in two ultra-orphan diseases (mucopolysaccharidosis types I and III): Potential causes and implications. *Orphanet Journal of Rare Diseases, 13*(1), 2.

Shapiro, E. G., Escolar, M. L., Delaney, K. A., & Mitchell, J. J. (2017). Assessments of neurocognitive and behavioral function in the mucopolysaccharidoses. *Molecular Genetics and Metabolism, 122S,* 8–16.

MPS I (Hurler syndrome, Scheie syndrome, and Hurler-Scheie syndrome) Previously known as Hurler and Scheie syndrome, these disorders are now denoted as severe MPS I or attenuated MPS I. *Clinical features:* Patients with the severe MPS I are normal at birth, but then gradual coarsening of facial features in early childhood becomes apparent. They also have hypertrichosis (excessive hair), a large skull, organomegaly, prominent lips, corneal clouding, dysostosis (malformed bones), and stiffening of joints. There is progressive intellectual deterioration and spasticity by age 3, and growth typically stops. Death typically occurs by age 10. The attenuated form is characterized by hearing loss, cardiac valvular disease, progressive restriction in range of motion with typical stature, typical intelligence (although some may have learning disabilities), and survival into adulthood. *Associated complications:* Chronic ear infections, hearing loss, occasional hernia, visual impairment, brain cysts, and airway obstruction. *Cause:* Deficiency of enzyme alpha-L-iduronidase caused by mutations in *IDUA* (4p16.3). *Inheritance:* AR. *Incidence:* 1:100,000 for the severe form and 1:500,000 for the attenuated form. *Treatment:* Hematopoietic stem cell transplantation (HSCT) in severe MPS I patients can increase survival, improve facial coarseness and hepatosplenomegaly, improve hearing, and maintain normal heart function (but does not improve skeletal manifestations or corneal clouding). HSCT may slow the course of cognitive decline in those with mild impairment at the time of transplant. Enzyme replacement therapy with Aldurazyme is licensed for treatment of non-CNS manifestations of MPS I and improves liver size, growth, joint mobility, breathing, and sleep apnea in those with attenuated disease.

MPS II (Hunter syndrome) *Clinical features:* Features include short stature; enlarged liver and spleen; coarsening of facial features, with hypertrichosis beginning in early childhood; and hoarse voice. Intellectual disability is mild or absent in the attenuated form of the disease; this subtype is compatible with survival to adulthood. The severe form is highlighted by progressive intellectual deterioration first noted between 2–3 years of age; death occurs before age 15 in most cases and is similar to severe MPS I but with clear corneas. *Associated complications:* Sensorineural hearing loss; retinitis pigmentosa with visual loss; macrocephaly; stiffening of joints, particularly those in the hands; cardiac valve disease; hernia; respiratory insufficiency; chronic diarrhea; and seizures. *Cause:* Deficiency of enzyme iduronate-2-sulfatase caused by mutations in *IDS* (Xq28). *Inheritance:* XLR. *Incidence:* 1:100,000–1:170,000 male births. *Treatment:* Minimal success has been reported with bone marrow transplantation. Enzyme replacement therapy for MPS II is now available (idursulfase/Elaprase). Elaprase does not cross the blood-brain barrier, and thus it is not expected that there would be any effect on CNS disease, although early treatment does improve somatic manifestations.

MPS III (Sanfilippo syndrome) *Clinical features:* Four distinct types representing four different enzyme defects with similar clinical features; clinical features present between 2–6 years in children who otherwise appear typical. There is mild coarsening of facial features, coarse hair and hirsutism, absence of corneal clouding, mild enlargement of the liver, joint stiffness, sleep disorders, and progressive mental deterioration. Deterioration is most rapid in type IIIA; death occurs by 10–20 years in most cases. *Associated complications:* Severe behavioral disturbances by age 4–6 years, dysostosis (defective bone formation), diarrhea in 50%, progressive spasticity and ataxia, precocious puberty, and central breathing are problems with advancing disease. *Cause:* Type IIIA: Deficiency of enzyme heparan sulfatase caused by mutations in *SGSH* (17q25.3). Type IIIB: Deficiency of enzyme alpha-N-acetylglucosaminidase caused by mutations in *NAGLU* (17q21). Type IIIC: Deficiency of enzyme acetyl-CoA: alpha-glucosaminide N-acetyltransferase caused by mutations in *HGSNAT* (8p11.2-p11.1). Type IIID: Deficiency of enzyme N-acetyl-alpha-glucosaminine-6-sulfatase caused by mutations in *GNS* (12q14). *Inheritance:* AR. *Incidence:* 1:73,000–1:280,000. *Treatment:* Treatment is supportive only. Bone marrow transplantation has not been successful.

multiple acyl-CoA dehydrogenase deficiency *See* glutaric acidemia, type II.

muscular dystrophy, Duchenne (DMD) and Becker (BMD) types *Disease category:* Neuromuscular disease. *Clinical features:* Progressive proximal muscular degeneration, muscle wasting, hypertrophy (enlargement) of calves, and cardiomyopathy; onset of symptoms in DMD occurs before 3 years. Loss of ability to walk independently occurs by adolescence in DMD. The onset in BMD is later, and the progression is slower. *Associated complications:* Congestive heart failure, scoliosis, flexion contractures, respiratory compromise, and intestinal motility dysfunction (causing constipation); approximately one third of boys with DMD have learning or intellectual disabilities. *Cause:* Mutations in *DMD* (Xp21.1), which encodes dystrophin. *Inheritance:* XLR, with one third of cases due to an NM. *Incidence:* DMD 1:3,500 male births; BMD 1:20,000 males. There are reports of females with clinical features of DMD as the result of X-chromosome rearrangements involving the *DMD* locus because they have Turner syndrome (i.e., complete or partial absence of an X chromosome) or nonrandom X-chromosome inactivation. *Treatment:* Glucocorticosteroids have been shown to prolong ambulation; prednisone and deflazacort have been shown to improve strength and function. In September 2016, the FDA approved eteplirsen (EXONDYS 51) a phosphorodiamidate morpholino oligomer (PMO) drug that acts to promote dystrophin protein production by restoring the translational reading frame of DMD through specific skipping of exon 51 in defective gene variants. While studies have showed an increase in dystrophin production, more data are needed to show clinical benefit. *See* also Chapter 9.

References: Battini, R., Chieffo, D., Bulgheroni, S., Piccini, G., Pecini, C., Lucibello, S., . . . Mercuri, E. (2018). Cognitive profile in Duchenne muscular dystrophy boys without intellectual disability: The role of executive functions. *Neuromuscular Disorders, 28*(2), 122–128.

Kenji Rowel, Q. L., Maruyama, R., & Yokota, T. (2017). Eteplirsen in the treatment of Duchenne muscular dystrophy. *Drug Design, Development and Therapy, 11,* 533–545.

Landfeldt, E.,Mayhew, A., Straub, V., Lochmuller, H., Bushby, K., & Lindgren, P. (2018). Psychometric analysis of the Pediatric Quality of Life Inventory 3.0 Neuromuscular Module administered to patients with Duchenne muscular dystrophy: A Rasch analysis. *Muscle Nerve, 58*(3), 367–373.

myasthenia gravis *Disease category:* Neuromuscular disease. *Clinical features:* Proximal muscle weakness, facial muscle weakness, difficulty chewing, ptosis, dysarthria, dysphagia, and ventilatory insufficiency. *Cause:* Failure of chemical transmission at the neuromuscular junction. It is an autoimmune disorder in which antibodies interfere with neuromuscular transmission. Although in rare instances genetic in origin, it is most often acquired as an autoimmune disorder. *Incidence:* 1:30,000. *Treatment:* Treatment is directed at removing the offending antibody and increasing the level of acetylcholine in the synaptic cleft. The immunological approach has employed corticosteroid medication, immunoglobulin, plasmapheresis, and the surgical removal of the thymus gland. Transient symptom improvement due to increased neurotransmitter levels in the synaptic cleft is achieved with pyridostigmine (Mestinon). Using these various treatment approaches, individuals with myasthenia can lead quite typical lives.

References: Braz, N. F. T.,Rocha, N. P., Vieira, E. L. M., Barbosa, I. G., Gomez, R. S., Kakehasi, A. M., & Teixeira, A. L. (2018). Muscle strength and psychiatric symptoms influence health-related quality of life in patients with myasthenia gravis. *Journal of Clinical Neuroscience, 50,* 41–44.

Sanders, D. B., Wolfe, G. I., Narayanaswami, P., & MGFA Task Force on MG Treatment Guidance. (2018). Developing treatment guidelines for myasthenia gravis. *Annals of the New York Academy of Sciences, 1412*(1), 95–101.

myotonic dystrophy (Steinert disease) *Disease category:* Neuromuscular disease. *Clinical features:* The most prominent feature is myotonia, a form of dystonia involving increased muscular contractility combined with decreased power to release (e.g., a strong handshake with the inability to release it). Other features include myopathy (muscle weakness), dysarthria, ptosis (drooping eyelids), and frontal balding. The age of onset varies from childhood to adulthood. The congenital form is severe, with neonatal hypotonia, motor delay, intellectual disability, and facial muscle palsy. In the congenital form, feeding difficulties and severe respiratory problems are common. In classic myotonia, symptoms do not begin until around 10 years of age. *Associated complications:* Cataracts, cardiac conduction abnormalities, diabetes, and hypogonadism (reduced hormone secretion in testes/ovaries). *Cause:* Type 1 myotonic dystrophy (DM1) is caused by cytosine-thymine-guanine (CTG) expansion mutations in *DMPK* (19q13). Severity typically increases with the number of CTG repeats. Unaffected people have 5–30 repeat copies. Those with the classical adult form have more than 100 copies, and individuals with the congenital form usually have more than 1,000 copies. The correlation among the number of repeats, severity, and age of onset, however, is not always consistent. Myotonic dystrophy type 2 (DM2) is associated with CCTG repeat expansion in *CNBP* (*ZNF9*) (3q13.3-q24). Normal alleles have up to 30 repeats; those affected have 75–11,000 repeats, with an average of 5,000. *Inheritance:* AD with genetic anticipation (repeat expands in subsequent generations and the onset of symptoms becomes earlier); with rare exception, it is the mother who transmits mutations that expand enough to cause the congenital form. There have been no reported *de novo* mutations in DM2. *Prevalence:* 1:8,000; increased prevalence in certain areas of Quebec.

References: Fontinha, C., Engvall, M., Sjogreen, L., & Kiliaridis, S. (2018). Craniofacial morphology and growth in young patient with congenital or childhood onset myotonic dystrophy. *European Journal of Orthodontics, 40*(5), 544–548.

Okkersen, K.,Buskes, M., Groenewoud, J., Kessels, R. P. C., van Engelen, B., & Raaphorst, J. (2017). The cognitive profile of myotonic dystrophy type 1: A systematic review and meta analysis. *Cortex, 95,* 143–155.

Wahbi, K., Porcher, R., Laforet, P., Fayssoil, A., Becane, H. M., Lazarus, A., . . . Duboc, D. (2018). Development and validation of a new scoring system to predict survival in patients with myotonic dystrophy type 1. *JAMA Neurology, 75*(5), 573–581.

Nager syndrome *See* acrofacial dysostosis.

neonatal adrenoleukodystrophy *See* adrenoleukodystrophy, neonatal form.

neurofibromatosis, type I (NF1) *Disease category:* Neurological disorder. *Clinical features:* Multiple café-au-lait spots, axillary (armpit) and inguinal (groin) freckling, nerve tumors (fibromas) in body and on skin, and Lisch nodules (brown bumps on the iris of the eye). *Associated complications:* Glaucoma, scoliosis, hypertension, attention-deficit/hyperactivity disorder (ADHD), macrocephaly (enlarged head) or hydrocephalus, visual impairments (secondary to optic gliomas), and increased risk of numerous malignant and benign tumors in the nervous system (malignant peripheral nerve sheath tumors in 8%–13% of patients); verbal and nonverbal learning disabilities occur in 30%–65% of patients. *Cause:* Mutation in *NF1* (17q11.2), which codes for neurofibromin protein. *Inheritance:* AD with variable expression. Approximately 50% represent NM. *Prevalence:* 1:3,000.

References: Eijk, S., Mous, S. E., Dieleman, G. C., Dierckx, B., Rietman, A. B., deNijs, P. F. A., . . . Legerstee, J. S. (2018). Autism spectrum disorder in an unselected cohort of children with neurofibromatosis type 1 (NF1). *Journal of Autism and Developmental Disorders, 48*(7), 2278–2285.

Torres Nupan, M. M., Velez, Van Meerbeke, A., Lopez Cabra, C. A., & Herrera Gomez, P. M. (2017). Cognitive and behavioral disorders in children with neurofibromatosis type 1. *Frontiers of Pediatrics, 5,* 227.

neurofibromatosis, type II *Disease category:* Neurological disorder. *Clinical features:* Bilateral vestibular schwannomas (benign tumors of auditory nerve), cranial and spinal tumors, neuropathy, and café-au-lait spots (usually fewer than six); in contrast to type I, no Lisch nodules or axillary freckling are seen. *Associated complications:* Deafness (average age of onset is 20 years), cataracts or other ocular abnormalities, and meningiomas (benign tumor of the meninges); tumor growth rates are variable within the same patients and between patients. *Cause:* Mutation in the tumor-suppressor gene (*NF2*) encoding the merlin protein (22q12.2); genotype/phenotype studies show that nonsense mutations (mutations that create a stop codon) are associated with more severe disease presentation than other types of genetic mutations. *Inheritance:* AD with significant variability between patients; up to 50% may represent NM. *Prevalence:* 1:60,000. *Treatment:* Mortality is lower for patients treated in specialty centers. Microsurgery and radiation therapy are both commonly used. Sirolimus is also in clinical trials for treatment of progressive neurofibromatosis type I–associated plexiform neurofibromas.

References: Cosetti, M. K., Golfinos, J. G., & Roland, J. T., Jr. (2015). Quality of life (AoL) assessment in patients with neurofibromatosis type 2 (NF2). *Otolaryngology-Head and Neck Surgery, 4,* 599–605.

Iwatate, K., Yokoo, T., Iwatate, E., Ichikawa, M., Sato, T., Fujii, M., . . . Saito, K. (2017). Population characteristics and progressive disability in Neurofibromatosis type 2. *World Neurosurgery, 106*, 653–660.

Weiss, B., Widemann, B. C., Wolters, P., Dombi, E., Vinks, A., Cantor, A., . . . Fisher, M. J. (2015). Sirolimus for progressive neurofibromatosis type 1-associated plexiform neurofibromas: A neurofibromatosis Clinical Trials Consortium phase II study. *Neuro-Oncology, 17*(4), 596–603. doi:10.1093/neuonc/nou235

Zhao, F., Wang, B., Yang, Z., Zhou, Q., Li, P., Wang, X., . . . Liu, P. (2018). Surgical treatment of large vestibular schwannomas in patients with neurofibromatosis type 2: Outcomes on facial nerve function and hearing preservation. *Journal of Neuro-Oncology, 138*(2), 417–424.

neuronal ceroid lipofuscinosis, juvenile *See* Batten disease.

Niemann-Pick disease, types A and B (acid sphingomyelinase deficiency) *Disease category:* Inborn error of metabolism: lysosomal storage disorder. *Clinical features:* Acid sphingomyelinase deficiency. Type A is neuronopathic and presents in infancy with poor weight gain, enlarged liver and spleen, and rapidly progressive neurological decline. Death occurs by age 2–3 years. Type B is nonneuronopathic and variable but compatible with survival to adulthood and may cause few or no neurological abnormalities. *Associated complications:* Intellectual disability, ataxia, myoclonus, eye abnormalities, coronary artery disease, and lung disease. Main clinical features of type B are enlargement of the spleen and liver resulting in liver dysfunction, as well as cardiac disease, lipid abnormalities, pulmonary involvement, and growth retardation. *Cause:* Sphingomyelinase enzyme deficiency caused by mutations in *SMPD1* (11p15.4). *Inheritance:* AR. *Prevalence:* 1:250,000; incidence of type A is increased in the Ashkenazi Jewish population, and type B is seen equally in all ethnic groups. *Treatment*: Enzyme replacement therapy (olipudase alfa) is being studied with promising improvement of clinical measures and good tolerability.

References: McGovern, M. M., Avetisyan, R., Sanson, B. J., & Lidove, O. (2017). Disease manifestations and burden of illness in patients with acid sphingomyelinase deficiency (ASMD). *Orphanet Journal of Rare Diseases, 12*(1), 41.

Wasserstein, M. P.,Diaz, G. A., Lachmann, R. H., Jouvin, M. H., Nandy, I., Ji, A. J., & Puga, A. C. (2018). Olipudase alfa for treatment of acid sphingomyelinase deficiency (ASMD): Safety and efficacy in adults treated for 30 months. *Journal of Inherited Metabolic Disease, 41*(5), 829–838.

Noonan syndrome *Disease category:* Multiple congenital anomalies. *Clinical features:* Short stature; characteristic facial features, including a triangular shape, deep philtrum (vertical indentation in the middle area of the upper lip), down-slanting palpebral fissures (opening between the eyelids), ptosis, low-set ears, and a low posterior hairline; a short or webbed neck; congenital heart defects (usually pulmonary valve stenosis or hypertrophic cardiomyopathy); and a shield-shaped chest. One third of cases have mild intellectual disability. *Associated complications:* Sensorineural deafness, malocclusion of teeth, learning disabilities with deficits in verbal learning, attention-deficit/hyperactivity disorder, poor motor coordination, bleeding, and lymphatic abnormalities. *Cause:* Nine genes are linked to Noonan syndrome: *PTPN11* (12q24.13), *SOS1* (2p22.12), *RAF1* (3p25.2), *KRAS* (12p12.1), *NRAS* (1p13.2), *RIT1* (1q22), *BRAF* (7q34), *SOS2* (14q21.3), and *LZTR1* (22Q11.21). *Inheritance:* AD, 25%–50% NM. Recent report of AR mutations in *LZTR1*. *Prevalence:* 1:1,000–1:2,500. *Treatment:* Human growth hormone has been used to treat short stature in some patients with Noonan syndrome.

References: Croonen, E. A.,Essink, M., van der Burgt, I., Draaisma, J.M., Noordam, C., & Nijhuis-van der Sande, M. W. G . (2017). Motor performance in children with Noonan syndrome. *American Journal of Medical Genetics, Part A, 173*(9), 2235–2345.

Johnston, J. J., van der Sagt, J. J., Resenfeld, J. A., Pagnamenta, A. T., Alswaid, A., Baker, E. H., . . . Biescker, L. G. (2018). Autosomal recessive Noonan syndrome associated with biallelic LZTR1 variants. *Genetics in Medicine.* doi:10.1038/gim.2017.249

Perrino, F., Licchelli, S., Serra, G., Piccini, G., Caciolo, C., Pasqualetti, P., . . . Vicari, S. (2018). Psychopathological features in Noonan syndrome. *European Journal of Paediatric Neurology, 22*(1), 170–177.

oculo-auriculo-vertebral spectrum (facioauriculovertebral spectrum, Goldenhar syndrome, hemifacial microsomia) *Disease category:* Multiple congenital anomalies. *Clinical features:* Unilateral external ear deformity ranging from absence of an ear to microtia (tiny ear), preauricular (earlobe) tags or pits, middle-ear abnormality with variable hearing loss, facial asymmetry with a small size unilaterally, macrostomia (wide mouth), occasional cleft palate, and microphthalmia (abnormally small eyes), or eyelid coloboma. *Associated complications:* Vertebral anomalies, occasional heart and kidney defects, and intellectual disability in 10%. *Cause:* Unknown. Recent array-CGH studies on a cohort of patients were unable to identify a recurrent chromosomal abnormality. *Inheritance:* Genetically heterogeneous; may be SP in some cases resulting from gestational maternal diabetes; cases with clear AR and AD inheritance have been reported. *Prevalence:* 1:45,000 in Northern Ireland, presumably less common in other populations. *Incidence:* 1:3,000–1:25,000.

References: Beleza-Meireles, A., Hart, R., Clayton-Smith, J., Oliveira, R., Reis, C. F., Venancio, M., . . . Tassabehji, M. (2015). Oculo-auriculo-vertebral spectrum: clinical and molecular analysis of 51 patients. *European Journal of Medical Genetics, 58*(9), 455–465.

Bogusiak, K., Puch A., & Arkuszewski, P. (2017). Goldenhar syndrome: Current perspectives. *World Journal of Pediatrics, 13*(5), 405–415.

Bragagnolo, S., Colovati, M. E. S., Souza, M. Z., Dantas, A. G., F de Soares, M. F., Melaragno, M. I., & Perez, A. B. (2018). Clinical and cytogenomic findings in OAV spectrum. *American Journal of Medical Genetics, Part A, 176*(3), 638–648.

oculocerebrorenal syndrome *See* Lowe syndrome.

oculo-mandibulo-dyscephaly with hypotrichosis *See* Hallermann-Streiff syndrome.

Opitz GBB syndrome (Opitz-Frias syndrome and Opitz oculo-genito-laryngeal syndrome; previously separate and called G syndrome and BBB syndrome [G refers to the surname of the original patient described]) *Disease category:* Multiple congenital anomalies. *Clinical features:* Hypertelorism (widely spaced eyes), hypospadias (opening of the urethra on the underside of the penis), imperforate (without an opening) anus, dysphagia, bifurcated (divided) nasal tip, broad nasal bridge, widow's peak, occasional cleft lip/palate, and mild to moderate intellectual disability in two thirds of affected individuals. *Associated complications:* Gastroesophageal reflux; esophageal dysmotility (poor movement of food through the esophagus); hoarse cry; occasional congenital heart defect; agenesis (absence) of corpus callosum; platelet abnormalities; and structural cerebellar anomalies, including Dandy-Walker malformation. *Cause:* Mutation in *MID1* (Xp22.3) is known to cause the X-linked form. Mutation in *SPECC1L* (22q11.23) causes the AD form. Deletion of 22q11.2 has also been linked and may result in 22q11 deletion syndrome as well. *Inheritance:* AD and XLR; in both the AD and XLR forms, symptoms are more severe in males than in females. *Prevalence:* 1:50,000–1:100,000 in the X-linked form.

References: Kruszka, P., Li, D., Harr, M. H., Wilson, N. R., Swarr, D., McCormick, E. M., . . . Zackai, E. H. (2015). Mutations in SPECC1L, encoding sperm antigen with calponin homology and coiled-coil domains 1-like, are found in some cases of autosomal dominant Opitz G/BBB syndrome. *Journal of Medical Genetics, 52*(2), 104–110.

Maia, N., Nabais Sa, M. J., Tkachenko, N., Soares, G., Margues, I., Rodrigues, B., . . . Jorge, P. (2017). Two novel pathogenic MID1 variants and genotype-phenotype correlation reanalysis in X-linked Opitz G/BBB syndrome. *Molecular Syndromology, 9*(10), 45–51.

Winter, J., Basilicata, M. F., Stemmler, M. P., & Krauss, S. (2016). The MID1 protein is a central player during development and disease. *Frontiers in Biosciences, 21*, 664–682.

osteogenesis imperfecta (OI) *Disease category:* Connective tissue disorder. *Clinical features:* There are multiple types of OI. Type I is characterized by typical height or mild short stature, bone fragility, and blue sclera. Type II usually presents with severe bone deformity and death in the newborn period. Type III is characterized by progressive bone deformity, short stature, triangular face, severe scoliosis, and dental abnormalities. Type IV is clinically similar to type I but presents with normal sclerae, milder bone deformity, variable short stature, and dental abnormalities. Type V is similar to type IV but with hyperplastic callus formation at fracture sites (excessive collection of partly calcified tissue, formed in the blood clot around the site of a healing fracture), calcification of the interosseous membrane between the radius and ulna (the fibrous joint between the two bones of the forearm), and the presence of a radiopaque metaphyseal band adjacent to the growth plates (zone of increased bone density found at the ends of long bones). Type VI is characterized by severe bone deformity, with a moderate short stature and a fish-scale pattern of bone deposition. Type VII causes moderate bone deformations and a mild short stature, with a shortening of the long bones (humerus and femur). *Associated complications:* Increased prevalence of fractures (may be confused with physical abuse) that decreases after puberty, scoliosis, mitral valve prolapse, and occasionally progressive adolescent-onset hearing loss. *Cause:* There are now 19 different genes associated with OI. Mutations in *COL1A1* (17q21-22) and *COL1A2* (7q21-22) represent 80% of OI cases. The other genes include *IFITM5, SERPINF1, CRTAP, LEPRE1, PP1B, SERPINH1, FKBP10, PLOD2, BMP1, SP7, TMEM38B, WNT1, CREB3L1, SPARC,* and *MBTPS2* . *Inheritance:* AD, AR, XLR. *Prevalence:* 1:30,000. *Treatment:* Cyclic intravenous pamidronate therapy to increase bone mineral density. *See* Chapter 9.

References: Forlino, A., & Marini, J. C. (2016). Osteogenesis imperfecta. *The Lancet, 387*(10028), 1657–1671.

Palomo, T., Vilaca, T., & Lazaretti-Castro, M. (2017). Osteogenesis imperfecta: Diagnosis and treatment. *Current Opinion in Endocrinology, Diabetes, and Obesity, 24*(6), 381–388.

Pavone, V., Mattina, T., Pavone, P., Falsaperla, R., & Testa, G. (2017). Early motor delay: An outstanding, initial sign of osteogenesis imperfecta type 1. *Journal of Orthopaedic Case Reports, 7*(3), 63–66.

Trejo, P., & Rauch, F. (2016). Osteogenesis imperfecta in children and adolescents—new developments in diagnosis. *Osteoporosis International, 27*(12), 3427–3437.

pentasomy X *See* XXXXX syndrome.

Pfeiffer syndrome (acrocephalosyndactyly, type V) *Disease category:* Craniosynostosis. Three subtypes of Pfeiffer syndrome have been described with a range of clinical severity. *Clinical features:* Mild craniosynostosis (premature fusion of fibrous sutures on the skull) with brachycephaly (flat head), flat midface, broad thumbs and toes, hypertelorism (widely spaced eyes), and partial syndactyly (fusion of digits). *Associated complications:* Hydrocephalus, airway obstruction due to midface hypoplasia (underdevelopment), hearing impairment, seizures, and occasional intellectual disability. *Cause:* Mutations in *FGFR1* and *FGFR2* (8p11.2–p11.1 and 10q26). *Inheritance:* AD, with many cases due to NM. *Prevalence:* 1:100,000.

References: Giancotti, A, D'Ambrosio, V., Marchionni, E., Squarcella, A., Aliberti, C., La Torre, R., . . . PECRAM Study Group. (2017). Pfeiffer syndrome: literature review of prenatal sonographic findings and genetic diagnosis. *Journal of Maternal Fetal Neonatal Medicine. 30,* 2225–2231.

Maliepaard, M., Mathijssen, I. M., Oosterlaan, J., & Okkerse, J. M. (2014). Intellectual, behavioral, and emotional functioning in children with syndromic craniosynostosis. *Pediatrics, 133*(6), e1608–1615.

phenylketonuria (PKU) *Disease category:* Inborn error of metabolism: amino acid. *Clinical features:* Inborn error of amino acid metabolism without acute clinical symptoms; intellectual disability, microcephaly, abnormal gait, and seizures may develop in untreated individuals. Treated individuals have still been found to have mild cognitive deficits, especially in executive function. Pale skin and blond hair are common features. *Associated complications:* Behavioral disturbances, cataracts, skin disorders, and movement disorders. *Cause:* Classically caused by a deficiency of the enzyme phenylalanine hydroxylase, which is associated with a mutation in *PAH* (12q24.1). *Inheritance:* AR. *Prevalence:* 1:10,000 among Caucasians in the United States. *Treatment:* Early identification is available through newborn screening. A phenylalanine-restricted, low-protein diet should be continued for life and especially in females during childbearing years. Returning to a regular diet even in adulthood may cause reduction of IQ. Specialized formulas are available for individuals who need to be on the restricted diet. Sapropterin dihydrochloride (Kuvan), a synthetic formulation of the cofactor tetrahydrobiopterin (BH4) is approved to reduce blood phenylalanine levels in patients with hyperphenylalaninemia due to tetrahydrobiopterin-responsive PKU. *See* also Chapter 16.

References: De Felice, S., Raomani, C., Geberhiwot, T., MacDonald, A., & Palermo, L. (2018). Language processing and executive functions in early treated adults with phenylketonuria. *Cognitive Neuropsychology, 28,* 1–23.

Hawks, Z. W., Strube, M. J., Johnson, N. X., Grange, D. K., & White D. A. (2018). Developmental trajectories of executive and verbal processes in children with phenylketonuria. *Developmental Neuropsychology, 12,* 1–12.

phenytoin syndrome (fetal hydantoin syndrome) *Disease category:* Malformation. *Clinical features:* Intrauterine growth restriction with microcephaly and minor dysmorphic craniofacial features and limb defects, including hypoplastic nails and distal phalanges (underdeveloped nails and digits). *Associated complications:* Growth problems and developmental delay or intellectual disability. *Cause:* Maternal ingestion of phenytoin (Dilantin) during pregnancy. *Prevalence:* About one third of children whose mothers are taking this drug during pregnancy have features of phenytoin syndrome. *Treatment:* Surgical correction of cranial facial and limb defects when required and feasible.

Reference: Hegde, A.,Kaur, A., Sood, A., Dhanorkar, M., Varma, H.T., Singh, G., . . . Kumar, P. (2017). Fetal hydantoin syndrome. *Journal of Pediatrics, 188,* 304.

Pierre-Robin sequence *Disease category:* Malformation. *Clinical features:* Micrognathia (undersized jaw), cleft palate, and glossoptosis (downward displacement of tongue). *Associated complications:* Neonatal feeding problems, apnea or respiratory distress, upper airway obstruction, and gastrointestinal reflux. *Cause:* Impaired closure of the posterior palatal shelves early in embryonic development; this defect can be an isolated finding or can be associated with trisomy 18, Stickler syndrome, or certain other syndromes. *Inheritance:* AR. *Prevalence:* Unknown. *Treatment:* Surgical procedure can be used to correct micrognathia, which alleviates many of the feeding and respiratory problems.

References: Butow, K. W., Zwahlen, R. A., Morkel, J. A., & Naidoo, S. (2016). Pierre Robin sequence: Subdivision, data, theories, and treatment—Part 3: Prevailing controversial theories related to Pierre Robin sequence. *Annals of Maxillofacial Surgery, 6*(1), 38–43.

Van Nunen, D. P. F.,van den Boogaard, M. H., & Breugem, C. C. (2018). Robin sequence: Continuing heterogeneity in nomenclature and diagnosis. *Journal of Craniofacial Surgery, 29*(4), 985–987.

PKU *See* phenylketonuria.

polyostotic fibrous dysplasia *See* McCune-Albright syndrome.

Prader-Willi syndrome (PWS) *Disease category:* Multiple congenital anomalies/imprinting defect/contiguous gene. *Clinical features:* Short stature; poor weight gain in infancy; hyperphagia (abnormally increased appetite); almond-shaped eyes; viscous (thick) saliva; hypotonia, particularly in the neck region; hypogonadism with cryptorchidism; small hands and feet; and hypopigmentation. *Associated complications:* Mild to moderate intellectual disability, behavior problems (tantrums, obsessive-compulsive disorder, rigidity, food stealing, and skin picking), obstructive sleep apnea, high pain threshold, osteoporosis, neonatal temperature instability, and type 2 diabetes. *Cause:* PWS is caused by a lack of expression of the paternally derived region of 15q11.2-q13. Approximately 65%–75% have a microdeletion, and 20%–30% have maternal uniparental disomy. Other mechanisms include unbalanced chromosome rearrangements and an imprinting defect with a deletion in the imprinting center. *Inheritance:* NM with AD inheritance when passed from an affected individual, although most individuals with PWS do not reproduce. *Prevalence:* 1:10,000–1:30,000. *Treatment:* Weight management and close supervision to minimize food stealing. No medications are currently able to control hyperphagia, but there are several clinical trials of new medications underway. Growth hormone treatment normalizes height.

References: Bonnot, O., Cohen, D., Thuilleaux, D., Consoli, A., Cabal, S., & Tauber, M. (2016). Psychotropic treatments in Prader-Willi syndrome: A critical review of published literature. *European Journal of Pediatrics, 175*(1), 9–18.

Butler, M. G., Kimonis, V., Dykens, E., Gold, J. A., Miller, J., Tamura, R., & Driscoll, D. J. (2018). Prader-Willi syndrome and early-onset morbid obesity NIH rare disease consortium: A review of natural history study. *American Journal of Medical Genetics, Part A, 176*(2), 368–375.

Ishii, A., Ihara, H., Ogata, H., Sayama, M., Gito, M., Murakami, N., . . . Nagai, T. (2017). Autistic, aberrant, and food-related behaviors in adolescents and young adults with Prader-Willi Syndrome: The effects of age and genotype. *Behavioral Neurology, 2017,* 4615451.

propionic acidemia *Disease category:* Inborn error of metabolism: organic acidemia. *Clinical features:* A disorder of organic acid metabolism characterized by episodes of vomiting, lethargy, and coma; hypotonia, bone marrow suppression, enlarged liver, and characteristic facies with puffy cheeks and exaggerated Cupid's bow upper lip. *Associated complications:* Impaired antibody production, intellectual disability, seizures, abnormalities of muscle tone, lack of appetite, prolonged drowsiness, cardiomyopathy, optic atrophy, hearing loss, premature ovarian failure, autism, anxiety, acute psychosis, and hematologic abnormalities. *Cause:* Deficiency of the enzyme propionyl-CoA carboxylase (PCC) caused by mutations in *PCCA* (13q32) and *PCCB* (3q21–q22). *Inheritance:* AR. *Incidence:* Varies widely worldwide. Highest in Greenlandic Inuits (1:1000) and in certain Saudi tribes (1:2,000–1:5,000). In the United States, the live-birth incidence is 1:105,000–1:130,000. *Treatment:* Treatment consists of a diet low in valine, isoleucine, threonine, and methionine, with a supplement of carnitine. A commercial formula meeting these requirements (Propimex) is available. Hemofiltration and peritoneal dialysis have been used with some success in patients in metabolic crisis. Some success has been documented in treating hyperammonemia (elevated plasma ammonia level) in propionic acidemia patients with N-carbamylglutamate (carglumic acid). Liver transplantation has been used in some cases and is considered an option for patients who continue to experience episodes of hyperammonemia despite maximal medical treatment.

References: Arrizza, C., De Gottardi, A., Foglia, E., Baumgartner, M., Gautschi, M., & Nuoffer, J. M. (2015). Reversal of cardiomyopathy in propionic academia after liver transplant: A 10-year follow-up. *Transplant International, 28*(12), 1447–1450.

De la Batie, C. D., Barbier, V., Roda, C., Brassier, A., Arnoux, J.B., Valayannopoulos, V., . . . Ouss, L. (2017). Autism spectrum disorders in propionic academia patients. *Journal of Inherited Metabolic Diseases, 41*(4), 623–629.

Wongkittichote, P., Ah Mew, N., & Chapman, K. A. (2017). Propionyl-CoA carboxylase: A review. *Molecular Genetics and Metabolism, 122*(4), 145–152.

retinitis pigmentosa *Disease category:* Ophthalmologic. *Clinical features:* A group of diseases associated with retinal degeneration, constricted visual fields, and progressive blindness; initial symptom is night blindness occurring in adolescence or adult life and loss of peripheral vision. *Associated complications:* May occur as an isolated condition or as part of over 30 syndromes (e.g., Usher syndrome, Bardet-Biedl Syndrome, and mitochondrial disorders). *Cause:* More than 80 different genes have been identified to date. *Inheritance:* AD in 30%–40% of cases, AR in 50%–60%, and XLR in 5%–15%. A genetic cause is yet to be identified in the remainder. A rare digenic form where individuals are heterozygous for mutations in two genes also exists. Recurrence risk depends on cause and family history. *Incidence:* 1:3,500–1:4,000 in the United States and Europe.

References: Dias, M. F., Joo, K., Kemp, J. A., Fialho, D. L., da Silva Cunha, A. Jr., Woo, S. J., & Kwon, Y .J. (2017). Molecular genetics and emerging therapies for retinitis pigmentosa: Basic research and clinical perspectives. *Progress in Retinal and Eye Research, 63,* 107–131.

Li, S., Yang, M., Liu, W., Liu, Y., Zhang, L, Yang, Y., . . . Zhu, X. (2018). Targeted next-generation sequencing reveals novel RP1 mutations in autosomal recessive retinitis pigmentosa. *Genetic Testing and Molecular Biomarkers, 22*(2), 109–114.

Rett syndrome (Rett's disorder) *Disease category:* Progressive neurologic disorder. *Clinical features:* Typical development until 6–9 months of age, followed by progressive encephalopathy. Features of autism, loss of purposeful hand use (with characteristic wringing of hands), hyperventilation, ataxia, and spasticity. *Associated complications:* Postnatal onset of microcephaly and seizures. *Cause:* Mutations in *MECP2* (Xq28). Mutations in *CDKL5* (Xp22.13) have been found in individuals with what has been characterized as the early-onset seizure variant of Rett. Mutations in *FOXG1* (14q12) are associated with the congenital form. *Inheritance:* XLD with severe neonatal encephalopathy or lethality in males who have *MECP2*-related Rett . *Prevalence:* 1:10,000 among females.

References: Clarkson, T., LeBlanc, J., DeGregorio, G., Vogel-Farley, V., Barnes, K., Kaufmann, W. E., & Nelson, C. A. (2017). Adapting the Mullen scales of early learning for a standardized measure of development in children with Rett syndrome. *Intellectual Developmental Disabilities, 55*(6), 419–431.

Fabio, R. A., Billeci, L., Crifaci, G., Troise, E., Tortorella, G., & Pioggia, G.(2016). Cognitive training modifies frequency EEG bands and neuropsychological measures in Rett syndrome. *Research in Developmental Disabilities, 53–54,* 73–85.

Tokaji, N.,Ito, H., Kohmoto, T., naruot, T., Takahashi, R., Goji, A., . . . Imoto, I. (2018). A rare male patient with classic Rett syndrome caused by MeCP2_e1 mutation. *American Journal of Medical Genetics, Part A, 176(3),* 699–702.

Riley-Day syndrome *See* familial dysautonomia.

Robinow syndrome (fetal face syndrome) *Disease category:* Skeletal dysplasia. *Clinical features:* Slight to moderate short stature, short forearms, macrocephaly with frontal bossing (prominent central forehead); flat facial profile with apparent hypertelorism; small, upturned nose; hypogenitalism; micrognathia; small face; tented upper lip with occasional clefting of the lower lip; hypertrophy (overgrowth) of the gums; deficiency of the lower eyelid, giving the appearance of protruding eyes (exophthalmos); and congenital heart defects. *Associated complications:* Vertebral or rib anomalies, dental malocclusion, genital hypoplasia, inguinal (groin) hernia, enlarged liver and spleen, and developmental delay in 15% of cases. The AR form appears to be more severe, with the kidney anomalies, congenital heart defects, vertebral defects, rib fusions, scoliosis, and cognitive delays occurring more commonly in that form. The AR form has clefting of the distal phalanges (mainly thumbs), which the AD form does not. *Cause:* Mutations in *ROR2* (9q22), *DVL1* (1p36.33), *WNT5A* (3p14.3), and *DVL3* (3q27.1). *Inheritance:* AD, AR. *Prevalence:* Rare.

References: Altunkas, A., Sarikaya, B., Aktas, F., Ozmen, Z., Sonmezgoz, F., Acu, B., . . . Firat, M. M. (2016). Vertebral anomalies accompanying Robinow syndrome. *Spine Journal, 16*(5), e341–e342.

White, J. J., Mazzeu, J. F., Coban-Akdemir, Z., Bayram, Y., Bahrambeigi, V., Hoischen, A., . . . Carvalho, C. M. B. (2018). WNT signaling perturbations underlie the genetic heterogeneity of Robinow syndrome. *American Journal of Human Genetics, 102*(1), 27–43.

Rubinstein-Taybi syndrome *Disease category:* Multiple congenital anomalies. *Clinical features:* Growth retardation, broad thumbs and toes, maxillary hypoplasia (small upper jaw), high-arched palate, down-slanted palpebral fissures (eyelids), prominent nose, pouting lower lip, short upper lip, and occasional agenesis of corpus callosum (absence of the white matter band connecting the two cerebral hemispheres). *Associated complications:* Apnea, constipation, reflux, feeding difficulties, hypotonia, cardiac defects, kidney anomalies, ophthalmologic problems, keloid (scar) formation, glaucoma, cryptorchidism (undescended testes), moderate to severe intellectual disability (IQ scores range from 25–79 and average 36–51), and behavior problems. *Cause:* 70% have mutation or microdeletion of *CREBBP* (16p13.3), and 10% have mutations in *EP300* (22q13). *Inheritance:* Most cases are due to an NM with AD inheritance when passed from an affected individual. *Prevalence:* 1:100,000 to 1:125,000.

References: Cazalets, J. R.,Bestaven, E., Doat, E., Baudier, M. P., Gallot, C., Amestoy, A., . . . Lacombe, D. (2017). Evaluation of motor skills in children with Rubinstein-Taybi syndrome. *Journal of Autism and Developmental Disorders, 47*(11), 3321–3332.

Lopez, M., Garcia-Oguiza, A., Armstrong, J., Garcia-Cobaleda, I., Garcia-Minaur, S., Santos-Simarro, F., . . . Dominguez-Garrido, E. (2018). Rubinstein-Taybi 2 associated to novel EP300 mutations: Deepening the clinical and genetic spectrum. *BMC Medical Genetics, 19*(1), 36.

Russell-Silver syndrome (Silver-Russell syndrome) *Disease category:* Imprinting defect/multiple congenital anomalies. *Clinical features:* Short stature (beginning with intrauterine growth retardation); skeletal asymmetry with hemihypertrophy (enlargement of one side of the body) in 60%; triangular facies, beaked nose, thin upper lip, narrow, high-arched palate, blue sclerae, occasional café-au-lait spots, and fifth-finger clinodactyly; genital anomalies in males; and motor and cognitive developmental delay and learning disabilities. *Associated complications:* Delayed fontanelle (soft spot) closure, hypocalcemia (low blood calcium level) in neonatal period with sweating and rapid breathing, increased risk of fasting hypoglycemia (low blood sugar level) as a toddler, feeding difficulties, precocious sexual development, and vertebral anomalies. *Cause:* 30%–60% of patients have a hypomethylation of the imprinting control region

1 (ICR1) in 11p15.5, affecting the expression of *H19* and *IGF2*; 5%–10% of patients carry a maternal uniparental disomy of chromosome 7. Chromosomal rearrangements have also been reported. There is still a large proportion of patients with an unknown cause. *Inheritance:* NM with AD inheritance when passed from an affected individual; maternal uniparental disomy; AR in rare cases. Recurrence risk is generally low but can be increased in cases of familial epimutations or chromosomal rearrangements. *Incidence:* 1:30,000–1:100,000.

References: Tumer, Z., et al. (2018). Structural and sequence variants in patients with Silver-Russell syndrome or similar features-curation of a disease database. *Human Mutation, 39*(3), 345–364.

Wakeling, E. L., Brioude, F., Lokulo-Sdipe, O., O'Connell, S. M., Salem, J., Bliek, J., . . . Netchine, I. (2017). Diagnosis and management of Silver-Russell syndrome: First international consensus statement. *Nature Reviews Endocrinology, 13*(2), 105–124.

Wollmann, H. A., & Ranke, M. B. (2017). Patients with Silver-Russell-syndrome from birth to adulthood: Diagnosis, development and medical care. *Pediatric Endocrinology Review, 15(Suppl. 1),* 85–91.

Saethre-Chotzen syndrome *Disease category:* Craniosynostosis. *Clinical features:* Short stature; brachycephaly (foreshortened skull); acrocephaly (peaked cranium); radioulnar synostosis (fusion of lower arm bones); syndactyly (fusion) of the second and third fingers and/or of the third and fourth toes; fifth-finger clinodactyly (incurving); craniosynostosis (early fusion of the skull sutures); small ears; and flat facies, with a long pointed nose, low hairline, and facial asymmetry; and shallow asymmetric eye orbits with hypertelorism (widely spaced eyes). *Associated complications:* Late closing fontanelles (soft spot of forehead), deafness, strabismus, proptosis, and lacrimal (tear) duct abnormalities. *Cause:* Mutations in *TWIST* (7p21). *Inheritance:* AD. *Prevalence:* 1:25,000–1:50,000.

References: Altiner, S.,Karabulut, H. G., Yarabas, K., Tukun, A., Collet, C., Kocaay, P., . . . Ilgin Ruhi, H. (2017). A novel TWIST1 gene mutation in a patient with Saethre-Chotzen syndrome. *Clinical Dysmorphology, 26*(3), 175–178.

Tahiri, Y., Bastidas, N., McDonald-McGinn, D. M., Birgfeld, C., Zackai, E. H., Taylor, J., & Bartlett, S. P. (2015). New pattern of sutural synostosis associated with TWIST gene mutation and Saethre-Chotzen syndrome: Peace sign synostosis. *Journal of Craniofacial Surgery, 26*(5), 1564–1567.

Sandifer syndrome (SS) *Disease Category:* Neurological *Clinical Features:* Sudden-onset dystonic movements with arching of the back, rigid posturing, torticollis (wry neck), laterocollis, (uncontrolled tilting of the neck from side to side), or retrocollis (uncontrolled backward tilting of the head). Children are often misdiagnosed with seizures or a movement disorder. *Cause:* Rare complication of gastroesophageal reflux disease (GERD). *Treatment:* Symptoms generally improve after antireflux medication and/or Nisssen fundoplication, a surgical procedure in which the upper portion of the stomach is wrapped around the lower end of the esophagus to prevent reflux. Amino-acid based formula was successful in two patients refractory to other therapies.

References: Bamji, N., Berezin, S., Bostwick, H., & Medow, M. S. (2015). Treatment of Sandifer syndrome with an amino acid-based formula. *American Journal of Perinatology* Reports, *5*(1), e41–e52

Cafarotti, A., Bascietto, C., Salvatore, R., Breda, L., & Chiarelli, F. (2014). A 6-month-old-boy with uncontrollable dystonic posture of the neck. Sandifer syndrome. *Pediatric Annals, 43*(1), 17–19.

Sanfilippo syndrome (MPS III) *See* mucopolysaccharidoses.

Scheie syndrome (MPS V) *See* mucopolysaccharidoses.

Severe combined immunodeficiency (SCID) *Disease category*: Immunodeficiency. *Clinical Features*: Low to absent T and natural killer (NK) lymphocytes and nonfunctional B lymphocytes, failure to thrive, oral/diaper candidiasis (a fungal infection, also called thrush), absent tonsils and lymph nodes, recurrent infections, and persistence of infections despite conventional treatment. *Associated complications*: Rashes, diarrhea, cough, congestion, fever, pneumonia, sepsis, and other severe bacterial infections. *Cause:* Mutations in *IL2RG* (Xq13.1), adenosine deaminase deficiency due to mutations in *ADA* (20q13.12), mutations in *RAG1* (11p12), *RAG2* (11p12), *JAK3* (19p13.11), *IL7R* (5p13.2), *PTPRC* (1q31.3-q32.1), *DCLRE1C* (10p13), *CD3D* (11q23.3), *CD3E* (11q23.3), *CD247* (1q24.2), *PRKDC* (8q11.21), *AK2* (1P35.1), *CORO1A* (16p11.2). *Inheritance*: AR, XLR. *Prevalence*: 1:50,000–1:100,000. *Treatment*: Bone marrow transplant prior to the development of symptoms. Interim management includes treatment of infections and use of immunoglobulin infusions and antibiotics, particularly prophylaxis against *Pneumocystis jiroveci* and fungal infection. Newborn screening currently tests for SCID, allowing for earlier treatment.

References: Haddad, E., Logan, B. R., Griffith, L. M., Buckley, R. H., Parrott, R.E ., Prockop, S. E., . . . Notarangelo, L. D. (2018). SICD genotype and 6-month posttransplant CD4 count predict survival and immune recovery. *Blood, 132*(17), 1737–1749.

Heimall, J., & Cowan, M. J. (2017). Long term outcomes of severe combined immunodeficiency: therapy implications. *Expert Review of Clinical Immunology, 13*(11), 1029–1040.

Silver-Russell syndrome *See* Russell-Silver syndrome.

Sly syndrome (MPS VII) *See* mucopolysaccharidoses.

Smith-Lemli-Opitz syndrome *Disease category:* Inborn error of metabolism-cholesterol synthesis. *Clinical features:* Microcephaly, short nose with upturned nostrils, low serum cholesterol, syndactyly of second and third toes, genitourinary abnormalities, kidney anomalies, and lung malformations. *Associated complications:* Intrauterine growth restriction, postnatal growth retardation, hypotonia, moderate to severe intellectual disability, motor and language delay, seizures, feeding difficulties and vomiting, photosensitivity, and occasional congenital heart defect. Behavioral problems include irritability, sleep disturbance, and self-injurious behavior. *Cause:* Defect in cholesterol metabolism (conversion of 7-DHC to cholesterol) caused by mutations in *DHCR7* (11q12–q13). Clinical features result from deficiency of cholesterol as well as toxic accumulation of 7-DHC. *Inheritance:* AR. *Prevalence:* 1:20,000–1:40,000. *Treatment:* Dietary modifications, including cholesterol supplementation. Simvastin has been shown to be well tolerated and to improve the dehydrocholesterol–to–total sterol ratio and irritability symptoms.

References: Eroglu, Y., Nguyen-Driver, M., Steiner, R.D., Merkens, L., Merkens, M., Roullet, J. B., . . . Freeman, K. A. (2017). Normal IQ is possible in Smith-Lemli-Opitz syndrome. *American Journal of Medical Genetics, Part A, 173*(8), 2097–2100.

Wassif, C. A., Kratz, L, Sparks, S. E., Wheeler, C., Bianconi, S., Gropman, A., . . . Porter, F. D. (2017). A placebo-controlled trial of simvastatin therapy in Smith-Lemli-Opitz syndrome. *Genetics in Medicine, 19*(3), 297–305.

Smith-Magenis syndrome (SMS) *Disease category:* Multiple congenital anomalies/contiguous gene syndrome. *Clinical features:* Feeding difficulties; poor weight gain; hypotonia; hyporeflexia; lethargy; distinctive facial features; developmental delay; cognitive impairment and significant behavioral abnormalities, including sleep disturbance; stereotypies, such as a "self-hug" and "lick and flip" (licking their fingers and flipping pages of books and magazines); and self-injurious behavior, including self-hitting and self-biting. *Associated complications:* Skeletal anomalies, short stature, brachydactyly (short fingers and toes), ophthalmologic abnormalities, otolaryngologic abnormalities, peripheral neuropathy, and cardiac and kidney anomalies. *Cause:* Microdeletion at chromosome 17p11.2 or mutations, including the gene *RAI1*. *Inheritance:* Most cases represent new mutations with AD inheritance when passed from an affected individual. *Prevalence:* 1:25,000.

References: Falco, M., Amabile, S., & Acquavivia, F. (2017). RAI1 gene mutations: Mechanisms of Smith-Magenis syndrome. *Applied Clinical Genetics, 10,* 85–94.

Nag, H. E., Nordgren, A., Anderlid, B. M., & Naerland, T. (2018). Reversed gender ratio of autism spectrum disorder in Smith-Magenis syndrome. *Molecular Autism, 9,* 1.

Wilde, L., & Oliver, C. (2017). Brief report: Contrasting profiles of everyday executive functioning in Smith-Magenis syndrome and Down syndrome. *Journal of Autism and Developmental Disorders, 47*(8), 2602–2609.

Sotos syndrome *Disease category:* Overgrowth syndrome. *Clinical features:* An overgrowth syndrome characterized by a distinctive head shape, macrocephaly (enlarged head), downslanting eyes, flat nasal bridge, accelerated growth with advanced bone age, high forehead, hypertelorism (widely spaced eyes), and prominent jaw. *Associated complications:* Increased risk of abdominal tumors, hypotonia, marked speech delay, congenital heart defects, and varying degrees of cognitive impairment. *Cause:* Mutations and deletions in *NSD1* (5q35.3), *APC2* (19p13.3), and *NFIX* (19p13.13.). *Inheritance:* AD with the majority of cases due to an NM. *Prevalence:* 1:14,000.

References: Lane, C., Milne, E., & Freeth, M. (2016). Cognition and behaviour in Sotos syndrome: A systematic review. *PLoS One, 11*(2), e0149189.

Lane, C., Milne, E. & Freeth, M. (2018). The cognitive profile of Sotos syndrome. *Journal of Neuropsychology.* doi:10.1111/jnp.12146

spongy degeneration of central nervous system *See* Canavan disease.

Stickler syndrome (hereditary progressive arthro-ophthalmopathy) *Disease category:* Connective tissue disorder. *Clinical features:* Flat facies, myopia, cleft of hard or soft palate, and spondyloepiphyseal dysplasia (disorder of bone growth that results in dwarfism, characteristic skeletal abnormalities, and occasionally problems with vision and hearing). *Associated complications:* Hypotonia, hyperextensible joints, occasional scoliosis, risk of retinal detachment, cataracts, arthropathy (joint disease) in late childhood or adulthood, and occasional hearing loss or cognitive impairment. *Cause:* Mutations in type 2, type 9, and type 11 procollagen genes (*COL2A1, COL9A1, COL11A1,* and *COL11A2*), which have been linked to chromosomes 12q13.11–q13.2, 6q13, 1p21, and 6p21.3, respectively. *Inheritance:* AD with variable expression, AR (*COL9A1* mutations). *Prevalence:* 1:7,500–1:9,000.

References: Higuchi, Y.,Hasegawa, K., Yamashita, M., Tanaka, H., & Tsukahara, H. (2017). A novel mutation in the COL2A1 gene in a patient with Stickler syndrome type 1: A case report and review of the literature. *Journal of Medical Case Reports, 11*(1), 237.

Reddy, D. N., Yonekawa, Y., Thomas, B. J., Nudleman, E. D., & Williams, G.A. (2016). Long-term surgical outcomes of retinal detachment in patients with Stickler syndrome. *Clinical Ophthalmology, 10,* 1541–1544.

Sturge-Weber syndrome *Disease category:* Multiple congenital anomalies. *Clinical features:* Flat facial "port wine stains," seizures, glaucoma, and intracranial vascular abnormality. *Associated complications:* Hemangiomas (benign congenital tumors made up of newly formed blood vessels) of meninges; may be progressive in some cases, with gradual visual or cognitive impairment and recurrent stroke-like episodes, hemiparesis, hemiatrophy (atrophy affecting one side of the body), and hemianopia (decreased vision in one eye). *Cause:* Mutation in *GNAQ* (9p21.2). *Inheritance:* Somatic mosaicism. *Incidence:* 1:50,000. *Treatment:* Pharmacologic therapies can be used to treat seizures, surgical intervention can be used for glaucoma, and laser therapy can be used to remove vascular facial features.

References: Bosnyak, E.,Behen, M. E., Guy, W. C., Asano, E., Chugani, H. T., & Juhasz, C. (2016). Predictors of cognitive functions in children with Sturge-Weber syndrome: A longitudinal study. *Pediatric Neurology, 61,* 38–45.

Luat, A. F., Behen, M. E., Chugani, H. T., & Juhasz, C. (2018). Cognitive and motor outcomes in children with unilateral Surge-Weber syndrome: Effect of age at seizure onset and side of brain involvement. *Epilepsy and Behavior, 80,* 202–207.

Shirley, M. D.,Tang, H., Gallione, C. J., Baugher, J. D., Frelin, L. P., Cohen, B., . . . Pevsner, J. (2013). Sturge-Weber syndrome and port-wine stains caused by somatic mutation in GNAQ. *New England Journal Medicine, 368,* 1971–1979.

subacute necrotizing encephalomyopathy Leigh syndrome; *see* mitochondrial disorders.

sulfatide lipidosis *See* metachromatic leukodystrophy.

TAR syndrome *See* thrombocytopenia-absent radius syndrome.

Tay-Sachs disease (GM2 gangliosidosis, type I) *Disease category:* Inborn error of metabolism: lysosomal storage disease. *Clinical features:* A lysosomal storage disorder leading to a progressive neurological condition characterized by deafness, blindness, and seizures; development is typical for the first several months of life. Subsequently, there is an increased startle response, hypotonia followed by hypertonia, a cherry-red spot in the maculae, and optic nerve atrophy. There is rapid decline and fatality by age 5 years. An adult form of this enzyme deficiency presents with ataxia. *Associated complications:* Feeding abnormalities and aspiration. *Cause:* Deficiency of the enzyme hexosaminidase A caused by mutation in *HEXA* (15q23–q24). *Inheritance:* AR. *Prevalence:* 1:112,000; 1:3,600 in the Ashkenazi Jewish population (although extensive genetic counseling of carriers identified through carrier screening programs has led to a reduction of this disorder by more than 90% in this population); increased frequency in the Cajun and French Canadian populations.

References: Jarnes Utz, J. R., Kim, S., King, K., Ziegler, R. Schema, L., Redtree, E. S., & Whitley, C. B. (2017). Infantile gangliosidoses: Mapping a timeline of clinical changes. *Molecular Genetics and Metabolism, 121*(2), 170–179.

Nestrasil, I., Ahmed, A., Utz, J. M., Rudser, K., Whitley, C. B., & Jarnes-Utz, J.R. (2018). Distinct progression patterns of brain disease in infantile and juvenile gangliosidoses: Volumetric quantitative MRI study. *Molecular Genetics and Metabolism, 123*(2), 97–104.

Stepien, K. M., Lum, S. H., Wraith, J. E., Hendriksz, C. J., Church H. J., Priestman, D., . . . Wynn, R. (2017). Haematopoietic stem cell transplantation arrests the progression of neurodegenerative disease in late-onset Tay-Sachs disease. *JIMD Reports, 41,* 17–23.

tetrasomy X *See* XXXX syndrome.

thrombocytopenia-absent radius syndrome (TAR syndrome) *Disease category:* Multiple congenital anomalies. *Clinical features:* Radial aplasia (absence of one of the lower arm bones) with normal thumbs; thrombocytopenia (platelet deficiency) is present in all cases and symptomatic in 90% of cases; and 50% of patients have dysmorphic features, including micrognathia (small jaw) and low posteriorly rotated ears. *Associated complications:* Knee joint abnormalities, neonatal foot swelling, occasional congenital heart or kidney defect, gastrointestinal bleeding, and occasional intracerebral bleeding. *Cause:* Compound heterozygous for a mutation in *RBM8A* and a minimal 200-kb deletion at 1q21.1. *Inheritance:* AR. In 25%–50% of cases, the deletion is *de novo*. *Prevalence:* 1:100,000–1:200,000. *Treatment:* Platelet infusions.

References: Manukjan, G., Bosing, H., Schmugge, M., Strauss, G., & Schulze, H. (2017). Impact of genetic variants on haematopoiesis in patients with thrombocytopenia absent radii (TAR) syndrome. *British Journal of Haematology, 179*(4), 606–617.

Nicchia, E.,Giordano, P., Greco, C., De Rocco, D., & Savoia, A. (2016). Molecular diagnosis of thrombocytopenia-absent radius syndrome using next-generation sequencing. *International Journal of Laboratory Hematology, 38*(4), 412–418.

Tourette syndrome (Gilles de la Tourette syndrome) *Disease category:* Neurological disorder. *Clinical features:* Chronic vocal or motor tics (irrepressible, repetitive, and nonrhythmic movements and vocalizations) present for at least 1 year, obsessive-compulsive disorder (OCD), and attention-deficit/hyperactivity disorder (ADHD). Age of onset is typically between 3–8 years of age, with onset of motor tics most often preceding vocal tics. The course of the tics is waxing and waning, and peak symptom intensity is usually in late childhood (mean age 10 years). Fluctuation occurs in adolescence, and by early adulthood there is often significant improvement. *Associated complications:* Learning difficulties, language-based learning problems, habit disorders such as trichotillomania (chronic hair pulling), pathologic nail biting and skin picking, mood disorders such as bipolar disorder and major depressive disorder, and anxiety. *Cause:* Unknown; *SLITRK1* has been implicated as a candidate gene but studies have not been conclusive. Environmental factors are thought to be involved as well since the concordance rate is not 100% between monozygotic twins. Likely genetically heterogeneous. *Inheritance:* Unknown, thought to be AD. *Prevalence:* 0.3%–1% of the population. Males are affected more often than females, with an approximate four-to-one ratio. *Treatment:* Typical and atypical neuroleptics such as haloperidol and pimozide, alpha adrenergic agonists such as clonidine, habit reversal therapy, surgical intervention for a small subset with intractable Tourette disorder, and repetitive transcranial magnetic stimulation. New agents such as valbenazine, delta-9-tetrahydrocannabinol, and ecopipam are being investigated. Deep brain stimulation has shown improvement in symptoms but also has a large percentage of adverse events.

References: Cravedi, E., Deniau, E., Giannitelli, M., Xavier, J., Hartmann, A., & Cohen, D. (2017). Tourette syndrome and other neurodevelopmental disorders: A comprehensive review. *Child Adolescent Psychiatry and Mental Health, 11,* 59.

Martinez-Ramirez, D., Jiminez-Shahed, J., Leckman, J. F., Porta, M., Servello, D., Meng, F. G., . . . Okun, M. S. (2018). Efficacy and safety of deep brain stimulation in Tourette syndrome: The International Tourette Syndrome Deep Brain Stimulation Public Database and Registry. *JAMA Neurology, 75*(3), 353–359.

Quezada, J., & Coffman, K. A. (2018). Current approaches and new developments in the pharmacological management of Tourette syndrome. *CNS Drugs, 32*(1), 33–45.

TP63-related disorders *Disease category:* Ectodermal dysplasia. *Clinical features:* TP63-related disorders comprise six phenotypes, including ankyloblepharon-ectodermal defects-cleft lip/palate syndrome, Acro-dermo-ungual-lacrimal-tooth (ADULT) syndrome, ectrodactyly, ectodermal dysplasia, cleft lip/palate syndrome 3 (EEC3), limb-mammary syndrome, split-hand/foot malformation type 4 (SHFM4), and isolated cleft lip/cleft palate (orofacial cleft 8). Individuals have varying combinations of ectrodactyly (split hands or feet), ectodermal dysplasia (abnormal skin development), sparse hair, cleft lip and palate, and lacrimal (tear) duct abnormalities; intelligence is not usually affected. *Associated complications:* Occasional kidney or genital anomalies, hearing impairment, hypodontia (underdeveloped teeth), hypoplastic (underdeveloped) breasts, alopecia (areas of hair loss), hypospadias (opening of the urethra is on the underside of the penis), and lymphoma associated with *EEC3* only. *Cause:* Mutations in *TP63* (3q27). *Inheritance:* AD with variable penetrance and expressivity; 30% have an affected parent, and 70% have a *de novo* mutation. *Prevalence:* Unknown.

References: Kawasaki de Araujo, T., Lutosa-Mendes, E., Dos Santos, A. P., Coelho Molck, M., Mazzariol Volpe-Aquino, R., & Gil-da-Silva-Lopes, V. L. (2017). ADULT phenotype and rs16864880 in the *TP63* gene: Two new cases and review of the literature. *Molecular Syndromology, 8*(4), 201–205.

Wenger, T., Li, D., Harr, M. H., Tan, W. H., Pellegrino, R., Stark, Z., . . . Bhoj, E. J., (2018). Expanding the phenotypic spectrum of TP63-related disorders including the first set of monozygotic twins. *American Journal of Medical Genetics, Part A, 176*(1), 75–81.

Treacher Collins syndrome (mandibulofacial dysostosis) *Disease category:* Multiple congenital anomalies. *Clinical features:* Characteristic facial appearance with malformation of external ears, small chin, flattened midface, and cleft palate. *Associated complications:* Conductive or mixed (conductive and sensorineural) hearing loss, defects of middle and inner ear, respiratory and feeding problems, and apnea; intelligence is average in 95% of cases. *Cause:* 78%–93% of patients have mutations in *TCOFI* (5q32–q33), approximately 8% have mutations in *POL1C* (6p21.1) or *POLR1D* (13q12.2). *Inheritance:* AD; 60% NM. AR occurs in a very small proportion of patients (1%). *Incidence:* 1:10,000–1:50,000. *Treatment:* Surgical repair of most malformations.

References: Kadakia, S., Helman, S. N., Badhey, A. K., Saman, M., & Ducic, Y. (2014). Treacher Collins syndrome: The genetics of a craniofacial disease. *International Journal of Pediatric Otorhinolaryngology, 78*(6), 893–898.

Vincent, M., Genevieve, D., Ostertag, A., Marlin, S., Lacombe, D., Martin-Coignard, D., . . . Collet, C. (2016).

Treacher Collins syndrome: A clinical and molecular study based on a large series of patients. *Genetics in Medicine, 18*(1), 49–56.

trisomy 13 syndrome (Patau syndrome) *Disease category:* Chromosome abnormality/multiple congenital anomalies. *Clinical features:* Microphthalmia (abnormally small eyes), coloboma (notches or gaps in one of several parts of the eye), corneal opacity, cleft lip and palate, polydactyly (extra digits), scalp defects, dysmorphic features, low-set ears, and flexion deformity of fingers. *Associated complications:* Cardiac defects, kidney and gastrointestinal tract anomalies, eye abnormalities, visual impairment, sensorineural hearing loss, profound intellectual disability, and cerebral palsy; 50% die within the first month of life. *Cause:* Nondisjunction (usually in maternal meiosis I) resulting in an extra chromosome 13; rarely parental translocation. *Inheritance:* NM; usually nondisjunction chromosomal abnormality; may recur in families in presence of parental translocation. *Incidence:* 1:15,000–1:20,000 births.

References: Kitase, Y., Hayakawa, M., Kondo, T., Saito, A., Tachibana, T., Oshiro, M., . . . Sato, Y. (2017). Factors related to home health-care transition in trisomy 13. *American Journal of Medical Genetics, Part A, 173*(10), 2635–2640.

Kosiv, K. A.,Gossett, J. M., Bai, S., & Collins R. T. (2017). Congenital heart surgery on in-hospital mortality in trisomy 13 and 18. *Pediatrics, 140*(5), e20170772.

trisomy 18 syndrome (Edwards syndrome) *Disease category:* Chromosome abnormality/Multiple congenital anomalies. *Clinical features:* Prenatal onset of growth retardation, low-set ears, clenched fists, "rocker-bottom" feet, congenital heart defects, microphthalmia, coloboma, and corneal opacity; 30% die within first month of life, 50% die by the second month, and only 10% survive their first year. *Associated complications:* Feeding problems, aspiration pneumonia, conductive hearing loss, and profound intellectual disability. *Cause:* Nondisjunction resulting in extra chromosome 18. *Inheritance:* NM; usually a nondisjunction chromosomal abnormality. May recur in families in the presence of parental translocation. *Incidence:* 1:7,500 births.

References: Meyer, R. E., Liu, G., Gilboa, S. M., Ethen, M. K., Aylsworth, A. S., Powell, C. M., . . . National Birth Defects Prevention Network. (2016). Survival of children with trisomy 13 and trisomy 18: A multi-state population-based study. *American Journal of Medical Genetics, part A, 170A*(4), 825–837.

Spierson, H., et al. (2018). Trisomy 18: Palliative surgical intervention. *Archives of Disease in Childhood,103*(10), 1001.

trisomy 21 *See* Down syndrome; *see* also Chapter 15.

trisomy X *See* XXX syndrome.

tuberous sclerosis complex *Disease category:* Neurologic. *Clinical features:* Hypopigmented areas on skin, adenoma sebaceum (acne-like facial lesions), infantile spasms, iris depigmentation, retinal defects, calcium deposits in brain, benign tumor of the kidneys, and pulmonary lesions. *Associated complications:* Seizures, mild to moderate intellectual disability, tumors of the heart, increased risk of malignancy, hypoplastic tooth enamel and dental pits, kidney cysts, and hypertension. *Cause:* Mutations in *TSC1* (16p13) and *TSC2* (9q34); 10% of patients have no variant identified. *Inheritance:* AD with variable expressivity; two thirds of cases are NM. *Incidence:* 1:5,800. *Treatment*: mTOR inhibitors have shown improvement for multiple symptoms. Vigabatrin and other antiepileptics are used for seizures.

References: Gibson, T. T., & Johnston, M. V. (2017). New insights into the pathogenesis and prevention of tuberous sclerosis-associated neuropsychiatric disorders (TAND). *F1000Research, 6,* pii, F1000 Faculty Rev-859.

Peron, A.,Vignoli, A., Briola, F., Morenghi, E., Tansini, L, Alfano, R. M., . . . TSC Study Group of the San Paolo Hospital of Milan. (2018). Deep phenotyping of patients with tuberous sclerosis complex and no mutation identified in TSC1 and TSC2. *European Journal of Medical Genetics, 61*(7), 403–410.

Turner syndrome (45,X; monosomy X) *Disease category:* Chromosome abnormality. *Clinical features:* Affecting females only, the physical features include short stature, broad chest with widely spaced nipples, short neck with low hairline and extra skin at nape ("webbed" appearance), and "puffy" hands and feet. *Associated complications:* "Streak" ovaries causing infertility and delayed puberty, congenital heart defect (often coarctation of aorta), small ear canals, eye involvement (strabismus, ptosis, nystagmus, and cataracts), chronic otitis media in 90% with frequent hearing loss, hypothyroidism, and kidney disease; intelligence is usually average, but the prevalence of learning disabilities is high. *Cause:* Nondisjunction chromosome abnormality resulting in one copy of the sex chromosome. *Inheritance:* NM; usually nondisjunction chromosomal abnormality. *Prevalence:* 1:4,000. *Incidence:* 1:2,000. *Treatment:* Growth hormone has been used successfully to increase eventual adult height. Hormone replacement therapy is needed to initiate puberty (*see* also Chapter 1).

References: Gravholt, C. H., Andersen, N. H., Conway, G. S., Dekkers, O. M., Geffner, M. E., Klein, K. O., . . . International Turner Syndrome Consensus Group. (2017). Clinical practice guidelines for the care of girls and women with Turner syndrome: Proceedings from the 2016 Cincinnati International Turner Syndrome Meeting. *European Journal Endocrinology, 177*(3), G1–G70.

Noordman, I., Duijnhouwer, A., Kapusta, L, Kempers, M., Roeleveld, N., Schokking, M. . . . van Alfen-van der

Velden, J. (2018). Phenotype in girls and women with Turner syndrome: Association between dysmorphic features, karyotype and cardio-aortic malformations. *European Journal Medical Genetics, 61*(6), 301–306.

Reis, C. T., de Assumpcao, M. S., Guerra-Junior, G., & de Lemos-Marini, S. H. V. (2018). Systematic review of quality of life in Turner syndrome. *Quality of Life Research, 27*(8), 1985–2006.

urea cycle disorders *Disease category:* Inborn error of metabolism: amino acid. *Clinical features:* This group of disorders results from defects in any of the first five enzymes in the urea cycle (CPSI, OTC, ASS, ASL, and ARG) or the cofactor producer (NAGS), which break down the excess nitrogen from protein degradation. Severe deficiencies or complete absence of the first four enzymes results in the accumulation of ammonia and other precursor metabolites during the first few days of life. Infants often appear normal initially but rapidly develop lethargy, vomiting, anorexia, hyperventilation or hypoventilation, hypothermia, seizures, neurologic posturing, cerebral edema/encephalopathy, and coma. Partial urea cycle enzyme deficiencies are milder, and ammonia accumulation may be triggered by illnesses or stress at almost any time of life, thus delaying diagnosis by months to years. Deficiency of the fifth enzyme in the pathway causes arginase deficiency, which does not typically have the same frequency of hyperammonemic episodes but results in seizures, intellectual disability, and severe spasticity. Citrin deficiency and hyperornithinemia, hyperammonemia, and homocitrullinuria (HHH) syndrome also occur due to defects in two transporters. *Associated complications:* Loss of appetite, cyclical vomiting, lethargy, behavioral abnormalities, delusions, hallucinations, and psychosis can occur during hyperammonemic episodes. Developmental delay, attention-deficit/hyperactivity disorder, and intellectual disability are common, especially in those patients who have had significantly elevated ammonia levels. Liver failure occurs in some patients. *Cause:* Mutations or deletions involving the genes encoding the enzymes and the cofactor and transporter proteins of the urea cycle. *Inheritance:* AR, except OTC, which is X-linked. *Prevalence:* 1:30,000, although undiagnosed partial defects may make the number much higher. *Treatment:* Hemodialysis for rapidly lowering ammonia levels, ammonia scavenging medications (intravenous for acute hyperammonemia and oral for daily use), restricted-protein diet to reduce excess nitrogen, amino acid supplementation, and liver transplantation in those with recurrent hyperammonemia or significant liver disease. Gene therapy is currently being studied for OTC deficiency.

References: Kido, J., Matsumoto, S., Momosaki, K., Sakamoto, R., Mitsubuchi, H., Endo, F., & Nakamura, K. (2017). Liver transplantation may prevent neurodevelopmental deterioration in high-risk patients with urea cycle disorders. *Pediatric Transplantation, 21*(6), e12987.

Waisbren, S. E., Cuthbertson, D., Burgard, P., Holbert, A., McCarter, R., Cederbaum, S., & Members of the Urea Cycle Disorders Consortium. (2018). Biochemical markers and neuropsychological functioning in distal urea cycle disorders. *Journal of Inherited Metabolic Disease, 41*(4), 657–667.

Usher syndrome *Disease category:* Auditory/ophthalmologic. *Clinical features:* Approximately 10 subtypes exist; all have progressive sensorineural deafness, nystagmus, retinitis pigmentosa, and central nervous system defects (e.g., loss of sense of smell, vertigo, and epilepsy). Type 1 is characterized by profound hearing loss, absent vestibular function, and retinitis pigmentosa (eye disease characterized by black pigmentation and gradual degeneration of the retina) in childhood. Individuals with type 2 have normal vestibular function and less severe hearing loss, with onset of retinitis pigmentosa in the second decade. Type 3 can be differentiated by the presence of a progressive loss of hearing. *Associated complications:* Ataxia, psychosis, cataracts, and occasional cognitive impairment; more than 50% of adults with a combination of congenital blindness and deafness have Usher syndrome. *Cause:* Six genes have been linked to type I: *MYO7A, USH1C, CDH23, PCDH15,* USH1G, and *CIB2.* Three genes are associated with type II: USH2A, *WHRN,* and *ADGRV1CLRN1. HARS* has been linked to type III. *Inheritance:* AR. *Prevalence:* 3.2:100,000–6.2:100,000. *Treatment:* Cochlear implants may be beneficial for some individuals with type 1, while hearing aids are effective for individuals with type 2.

References: Bonnet, C., Riahi, Z., Chantot-Bastauraud, S., Smagghe, L, Letexier, M., Marcaillou, C., . . . Petit, C. (2016). An innovative strategy for the molecular diagnosis of Usher syndrome identifies causal biallelic mutations in 93% of European patients. *European Journal of Human Genetics, 24*(12), 1730–1736.

Magliulo, G., Iannella, G., Gagliardi, S., Iozzo, N., Plateroti, R., Mariottini, A., & Torricelli, F. (2017). Usher's syndrome type II: A comparative study of genetic mutations and vestibular system evaluation. *Otolaryngology Head Neck Surgery, 157*(5), 853–860.

VATER/VACTERL association *Disease category:* Multiple congenital anomalies. *Clinical features:* VATER is a nonrandom group of malformations that co-occur, including vertebral defects (**V**), anal atresia (imperforate anus) (**A**), tracheoesophageal fistula (a problem with the connection between the trachea and esophagus) (**TE**), and kidney anomalies (**R**).

VACTERL is an expanded definition that includes cardiac malformations (**C**) and limb anomalies (**L**). Diagnosis is made if three of seven defects are present. *Associated complications:* Poor weight gain, ear anomalies, facial clefting, respiratory complications, genitourinary anomalies, and radial (lower arm bone) and other limb defects. Intelligence is usually not affected. *Cause:* Likely genetically heterogeneous, and multiple candidate genes are being investigated. *Inheritance:* Usually SP, no recognized genetic or teratogenic cause; rare families with AR pattern. *Prevalence:* 1.6:10,000.

References: Chen, Y., Liu, Z., Chen, J., Zuo, Y., Liu, S., Chen, W., . . . Wu, Z. (2016). The genetic landscape and clinical implications of vertebral anomalies in VACTERL association. *Journal of Medical Genetics, 53*(7), 431–437.

Hilger, A. C., Halbritter, J., Pennimpede, T., van der Ven, A., Sarma, G., Braun, D.A., . . . Hildebrandt, F. (2015). Targeted re-sequencing of 29 candidate genes and mouse expression studies implicate *ZIC3* and *FOXF1* in human VATER/VACTERL association. *Human Mutation, 36*(12), 1150–1154.

Zhang, R., Marsch, F., Kause, F., Degenhardt, F., Schmiedeke, E., Marzheuser, S., . . . Reutter, H. (2017). Array-based molecular karyotyping in 115 VATER/VACTERL and VATER/VACTERL-like patients identifies disease-causing copy number variations. *Birth Defects Research, 109*(13), 1063–1069.

velocardiofacial syndrome (VCFS) *See* chromosome 22q11 microdeletion syndromes.

von Recklinghausen disease *See* neurofibromatosis, type I.

Waardenburg syndrome *Disease category:* Auditory/pigmentary. Four clinical subtypes exist with types I and II accounting for the majority of cases. *Clinical features:* Widely spaced eyes (type I), heterochromia (irises of different colors), white hair forelock, nonprogressive sensorineural hearing loss, and musculoskeletal abnormalities (type III). Types I and II have virtually identical clinical features, with the only distinguishing characteristic being telecanthus (an abnormally long distance from the inside corner of the eye to the nose), which is found in type I but not in type II. Type III has telecanthus (increased distance between the corners of the eyes) and upper limb abnormalities. Type IV (also known as Waardenburg-Shah syndrome) has the additional feature of Hirschsprung disease (a condition with congenital missing nerve cells in the muscles of the colon, leading to difficulty passing stool). *Associated complications:* Impaired vestibular function leading to ataxia, premature graying, vitiligo (patches of skin depigmentation), and occasional glaucoma. *Cause:* Types I and III: mutations in *PAX3* (2q35); type II: mutations in *MITF* (3p14.1–p12.3), *WS2B* (1p21-p13.3), *WS2C* (8p23), *SNAI2* (8q11.21), and *SOX10* (22q13.1); type IV: mutations in *EDNRB* (13q22), *EDN3* (20q13), and *SOX10* (22q13). *Inheritance:* AD, AR. *Prevalence:* 1:20,000–1:40,000.

References: Van Nierop, J. W., Snabel, R. R., Langereis, M., Pennings, R. J., Admiraal, R. J., Mylanus, E. A., & Kunst, H. P. (2016). Paediatric cochlear implantation in patients with Waardenburg syndrome. *Audiology & Neurotology, 21*(3), 187–194.

Wang, X. P., Liu, Y. L., Mei, L. Y., He, C. F., Niu, Z. J., Sun, J., . . . Zhang, H. (2018). Wnt signaling pathway involvement in genotypic and phenotypic variations in Waardenburg syndrome type 2 with MITF mutations. *Journal of Human Genetics, 63*(5), 639–646.

Weaver syndrome *Disease category:* Multiple congenital anomalies: overgrowth. *Clinical features:* Tall stature, distinctive chin with dimple, hypertelorism (widely spaced eyes), macrocephaly (enlarged head), retrognathia (a type of malocclusion), downslanting palpebral fissures (opening between the eyelids), long philtrum, and a depressed nasal bridge; hoarse, low-pitched cry; and deep-set nails. *Associated complications:* Accelerated growth with advanced bone age, hypertonia, camptodactyly (permanently flexed fingers), variable intellectual disability, poor coordination, and umbilical hernia. *Cause:* Mutations in *EZH2* (7q36.1) and *EED* (11q14,2). *Inheritance:* AD. *Prevalence:* Unknown.

References: Cooney, E., Bi, W., Schlesinger, A. E., Vinson, S., & Potocki, L. (2017). Novel EED mutation in patient with Weaver syndrome. *American Journal of Medical Genetics, Part A, 173*(2), 541–545.

Imagawa, E., Higashimoto, K., Sakai, Y., Numakura, C., Okamoto, N., Matsunaga, S., . . . Matsumoto, N. (2017). Mutations in genes encoding polycomb repressive complex 2 subunits cause Weaver syndrome. *Human Mutation, 38*(6), 637–648.

Williams syndrome *Disease category:* Multiple congenital anomalies/contiguous gene. *Clinical features:* Characteristic "elfin" facies (full lips and cheeks and fullness of area around the eyes), short stature, starlike pattern to iris, hoarse voice, communication delays in early childhood followed by increasing verbal abilities later in life, friendly, talkative, extroverted personality, congenital heart defect, and often supravalvular aortic stenosis. *Associated complications:* Hypercalcemia (increased blood calcium level), stenosis (stricture) of blood vessels, kidney anomalies, hypertension, joint contractures, and mild to moderate intellectual disability (but with characteristic strength in verbal abilities). *Cause:* Microdeletion of a segment of chromosome 7q11.23 consisting of approximately 28 genes. *Inheritance:* AD; all cases are the result of NM (sporadic deletions). *Prevalence:* 1:7,500–1:8,000.

References: Diez-Itza, E., Martinez, V., Perez, V., & Fernandez-Urguiza, M. (2017). Explicit oral narrative intervention for students with Williams syndrome. *Frontiers in Psychology, 8*, 2337.

Rossi, N. F., & Giacheti, C. M. (2017). Association between speech-language, general cognitive functioning and behaviour problems in individuals with Williams syndrome. *Journal of Intellectual Disability Research, 61*(7), 707–718.

Van Den Heuvel, E., Manders, E., Swillen, A., & Zink, I. (2016). Developmental trajectories of structural and pragmatic language skills in school-aged children with Williams syndrome. *Journal of Intellectual Disability Research, 60*(10), 903–919.

Wilson disease *Disease category:* Inborn error of metabolism: copper. *Clinical features:* Liver dysfunction, jaundice, Kayser-Fleischer ring (dark ring that appears to encircle the iris of the eye due to copper deposition) in cornea, and low serum ceruloplasmin (an enzyme that is important in the regulation of copper in the body). *Associated complications:* Movement disorders, dysphagia (difficulty swallowing) or other oral-motor dysfunctions, and behavioral disturbances; if left untreated, death from liver failure within 1–3 years of onset. *Cause:* Mutations in the copper metabolism gene *ATP7B* (13q14.3–q21.1), which lead to intracellular accumulation of copper in the liver. *Inheritance:* AR. *Prevalence:* 1:30,000; as high as 1:10,000 in China, Japan, and Sardinia. *Treatment:* Administration of copper-chelating agents in conjunction with a low-copper diet. Liver transplant is used in those who fail to respond to medical therapy.

References: Aggarwal, A., & Bhatt, M. (2018). Advances in treatment of Wilson disease. *Tremor and Other Hyperkinetic Movements, 8*, 525.

Socha, P., Janczyk, W., Dhawan, A., Baumann, U., D'Antiga, L., Tanner, S., . . . Debray, D. (2018). Wilson's disease in children: A position paper by the Hepatology Committee of the European Society for Paediatric Gastroenterology, Hepatology and Nutrition. *Journal of Pediatric Gastroenterology Nutrition, 66*(2), 334–344.

Wolf-Hirschhorn syndrome *Disease category:* Multiple congenital anomalies/contiguous gene. *Clinical features:* Hypertelorism (widely spaced eyes); characteristic broad, beaked nose ("Greek warrior helmet appearance"), downturned mouth, short philtrum (vertical groove between the base of the nose and the border of the upper lip), microcephaly, marked intrauterine growth retardation and premature birth, ear anomalies, and severe intellectual disability with reductions in receptive and expressive language. *Associated complications:* Hypotonia, psychomotor delays, growth delay, kidney anomalies, hypodontia (decreased number of teeth) resulting in feeding problems, seizures, and occasional heart defect or cleft palate. *Cause:* Heterozygous deletion of the Wolf-Hirschorn syndrome critical region (WHSCR) on 4p16.3. *Inheritance:* Occurs as a result of a NM; recurrence risk is greater if parent has a balanced translocation. *Prevalence:* 1:50,000.

References: Battaglia, A., Carey, J. G., & South S. T. (2015). Wolf-Hirschhorn syndrome: A review and update. *American Journal of Medical Genetics, Part C Seminars in Medical Genetics, 169*(3), 216–223.

Nag, H. E., Bergsaker, D. K., Hunn, B. S., Schmidt, S., & Hoxmark, L. B. (2017). A structured assessment of motor function, behavior, and communication in patients with Wolf-Hirschhorn syndrome. *European Journal Medical Genetics, 60*(11), 610–617.

X-linked ALD *See* adrenoleukodystrophy.

XXX (trisomy X; 47,XXX); XXXX (tetrasomy X); and XXXXX (pentasomy X) syndromes *Disease category:* Chromosome abnormality. *Clinical features:* Females with XXX syndrome generally have above-average stature but otherwise typical physical appearance; 70% have significant learning disabilities. Language delay/problems are also present in some girls. Significant malformations have been described in some patients, including gonadal dysgenesis (nonfunctional ovaries), a dysmorphic facial appearance, atrophic or dysplastic (absent or shrunken) kidneys, and vaginal and uterine malformations. XXXX syndrome is associated with a mildly unusual facial appearance, behavioral problems, and moderate intellectual disability. XXXXX syndrome presents with severe intellectual disability and multiple physical defects. *Associated complications:* Infertility and delayed pubertal development. *Cause:* Nondisjunction during meiosis. *Inheritance:* NM; usually nondisjunction chromosomal abnormality, may recur in families in the presence of parental translocation. *Incidence:* 1:800 live-born females.

References: Demirhan, O.,Tanriverdi, N., Yilmaz, M .B., Kocaturk-Sel, S., Inandiklioglu, N., Luleyap, U., . . . Dur, O. (2015). Report of a new case with pentasomy X and novel clinical findings. *Balkan Journal of Medical Genetics, 18*(1), 85–91.

Samango-Sprouse, C., Keen, C., Mitchell, F., Sadeghin, T., & Gropman, A. (2015). Neurodevelopmental variability in three young girls with a rare chromosomal disorder, 48, XXXX. *American Journal of Medical Genetics, Part A, 167A*(10), 2251–2259.

van Rijn, S., Barneveld, P., Descheemaeker, M. J., Giltay, J., & Swaab, H. (2018). The effect of early life stress on the cognitive phenotype of children with an extra X chromosome (47,XXY/47,XXX). *Child Neuropsychology, 24*(2), 277–286.

Wigby, K.,D'Epagnier, C., Howell, S., Reicks, A., Wilson, R., Cordiro, L., & Tartaglia, N. (2016). Expanding the phenotype of triple X syndrome: A comparison of prenatal versus postnatal diagnosis. *American Journal of Medical Genetics, Part A, 170*(11), 2870–2881.

XXY syndrome *See* Klinefelter syndrome.

XYY syndrome *Disease category:* Chromosome abnormality. *Clinical features:* Subtle findings, including a tall stature, severe acne, and large teeth. *Associated complications:* Poor fine-motor coordination; learning disabilities; language delay; varying degrees of behavioral disturbances, including tantrums and aggression; and increased risk for autism. *Cause:* Extra Y chromosome resulting from nondisjunction. *Inheritance:* NM; usually nondisjunction chromosomal abnormality, may recur in families in presence of parental translocation. *Prevalence:* 1:1,000.

References: Ross, J. L., Roeltgen, D. P., Kushner, H., Zin, A. R., Reiss, A., Bardsley, M. Z., . . . Tartaglia, N.(2012). Behavioral and social phenotypes in boys with 47,XYY syndrome or 47,XXY Klinefelter syndrome. *Pediatrics, 129*(4), 769–778.

Ross, J. L., Tartaglia, N., Merry, D. E., Dalva, M., & Zinn, A. R. (2015). Behavioral phenotypes in males with XYY and possible role of increased *NLGN4Y* expression in autism features. *Genes, Brain, and Behavior, 14*(2), 137–144.

Samango-Sprouse, C., Stapelton, E. J., Lawson, P., Mitchell, F., Adeghin, T., Powell, S., & Gropman, A. L. (2015). Positive effects of early androgen therapy on the behavioral phenotype of boys with 47,XXY. *American Journal of Medical Genetics, Part C Seminars in Medical Genetics, 169*(2), 150–157.

Zellweger spectrum disorder (ZSD) *Disease category:* Peroxisomal disorder (*see* adrenoleukodystrophy [X-linked ALD] for the childhood form). *Clinical features:* A disorder of peroxisome biogenesis and an intermediate presentation of the Zellweger syndrome spectrum. Peroxisomes are minute organelles in certain cells that are involved in the processing of long-chain fatty acids. ZSD can present in the neonatal period but generally comes to attention later in childhood because of developmental delays, hearing loss, or visual impairment. The condition is slowly progressive, and hearing and vision worsen with time. Some individuals may develop progressive degeneration of myelin, a leukodystrophy, which may lead to loss of previously acquired skills and eventually death. *Associated complications:* Intellectual disability, cataracts, visual and auditory impairment, liver dysfunction, hypotonia, and hemorrhage/intracranial bleeding. *Cause:* Mutations in 13 different *PEX* genes, resulting in the absence of peroxisomes, have been identified. *Inheritance:* AR. *Prevalence:* 1:50,000–1:80,000, with variation among populations.

References: Braverman, N. E., Raymond, G. V., Rizzo, W. B., Moser, A. B., Wilkinson, M. E., Stone, E. M., . . . Bose, M. (2016). Peroxisome biogenesis disorders in the Zellweger spectrum: An overview of current diagnosis, clinical manifestations, and treatment guidelines. *Molecular Genetics and Metabolism, 117,* 313–321.

Klower, F. C. C., Berendse, K., Ferdinandusse, S., Wanders, R. J., Engelen, M., Y Poll-The, B. T. (2015). Zellweger spectrum disorders: Clinical overview and management approach. *Orphanet Journal of Rare Diseases, 10,* 151.

APPENDIX **C**

Commonly Used Medications

Dimitrios A. Savva, Shogo John Miyagi, and
Johannes N. van den Anker

This appendix contains information about commonly used medications but is not meant to be used to prescribe medication. The generic name of each drug is in capital letters. The trade name is in parentheses; not all preparations are included. The drug categories, uses, standard applications, and common side effects are listed. Commonly used medications are listed in alphabetical order by generic drug name (see Table C.1), drug class (see Table C.2), and brand name (see Table C.3). Please note that uses and standard applications may change during the life of this edition and that additional side effects may be discovered. Specific drug interactions and contraindications such as hepatic or renal (kidney) insufficiency are not included; use of any medication should be discussed with a health care provider familiar with the individual's medical background.

REFERENCES

IBM Corporation (2018). *Micromedex* [Electronic version]. Greenwood Village, CO: Truven Health Analytics. Retrieved from http://www.micromedexsolutions.com/

Taketomo, C. K., Hodding, J. H., & Kraus, D. M. (Eds.) (2017). *Pediatric and neonatal dosage handbook* (24th ed.). Cleveland, OH: Lexicomp.

Table C.1. Commonly used medications, alphabetized by generic drug name

Medication	Category	Use(s)	Standard applications	Side effects
ACETAMINOPHEN (Tylenol)	Analgesic, Antipyretic	Used to treat fever and pain	**CAP, LIQ, TAB, SUPP, IV:** 10–15 mg/kg/dose three to four times daily; max 75 mg/kg/day or 3,000 mg/day	Rash, hepatotoxicity, renal dysfunction
ACETAZOLAMIDE (Diamox)	Anticonvulsant, diuretic, carbonic anhydrase inhibitor	Used to treat metabolic alkalosis, glaucoma, edema, pseudotumor cerebri	**CAP, LIQ, TAB, IV:** 5 mg/kg/dose three to four times daily	Flushing, skin reaction/rash, electrolyte imbalance
ACYCLOVIR (Zovirax)	Antiviral agent	Used primarily to treat or prevent infections caused by herpes simplex viruses or varicella	**CAP, LIQ, TAB, TOP, IV:** Doses vary with clinical situation	Renal dysfunction, headache, gastrointestinal irritation, hepatotoxicity
ALBUTEROL (Ventolin)	Beta 2 agonist bronchodilator	Asthma	**INH:** Dose varies with clinical situation	Increased heart rate, hypokalemia, shakiness, excitability
ALPRAZOLAM (Xanax, Xanax XR)	Benzodiazepine	Anxiety, panic attacks	**TAB, LIQ:** <18 yo: Initial dose of 0.125 mg/dose three times daily; safety and efficacy in children <18 yo are not known ≥18 yo: Initial dose of 0.25–0.5 mg/dose three times daily; max 4 mg/day	Drowsiness, fatigue, depression, decreased salivation, dysarthria, ataxia, addictive potential Avoid abrupt withdrawal
AMITRIPTYLINE (Elavil)	Tricyclic antidepressant	Depression, migraine prophylaxis, neuropathic pain, anxiety	**TAB, IV:** ≥12 yo: 0.33–0.5 mg/kg/dose three times daily; not recommended for children <12 yo Chronic pain management: Initial dose of 0.1 mg/kg/dose once daily, increase to max 2 mg/kg/dose	Sedation, dry mouth, blurred vision, dizziness, urinary retention, confusion, cardiac arrhythmia (rarely)
AMOXICILLIN (Amoxil)	Antibiotic, penicillin	Treatment of susceptible infections most commonly acute otitis media, upper or lower respiratory tract	**CAP, CHEW, TAB, LIQ:** Doses vary with clinical situation	Diarrhea, rash, nausea, allergic reactions
AMOXICILLIN/CLAVULANIC ACID (Augmentin, Augmentin ES, XR)	Antibiotic, penicillin	Treatment of susceptible infections most commonly acute otitis media, upper or lower respiratory tract	**TAB, LIQ, CHEW:** Doses vary with clinical situation Use 600 mg or 42.9 mg per 5 mL suspension formulation with high doses	Diarrhea, rash, nausea
AMPHETAMINE salts (Adderall, Adderall XR)	Stimulant	Attention-deficit/hyperactivity disorder, narcolepsy	**CAP, TAB, LIQ:** One to three times daily; not recommended for <3 yo 3–5 yo: Initial dose of 2.5 mg/dose once daily; increase of 2.5 mg/week until optimal response ≥6 yo: Initial dose of 5 mg/dose once or twice daily; increase of 5 mg/week until optimal response; extended release is dosed once daily	Insomnia, loss of appetite, emotional instability, addictive potential, arrhythmia, visual disturbances Caution in seizure and cardiac patients
ARIPIPRAZOLE (Abilify)	Antipsychotic, atypical	Bipolar disorder, agitation, psychosis, Tourette syndrome, autism spectrum disorder	**TAB:** Initial dose of 2 mg/dose once daily, increase of 5 mg/week until optimal response; max 30 mg/day	Nausea, weight gain, akathisia, somnolence, extrapyramidal effects, fatigue, blurred vision

Medication	Category	Use(s)	Standard applications	Side effects
ATOMOXETINE (Strattera)	Norepinephrine reuptake inhibitor, selective	Attention-deficit/hyperactivity disorder	**CAP:** Initial dose of 0.5 mg/kg/dose once daily, increase after minimum of 3 days to 1.2 mg/kg/day; can divide dose into twice daily; max 1.4 mg/kg/day or 100 mg/day	Headache, palpitations, decreased appetite, abdominal pain, nausea, vomiting, weight loss, hepatotoxicity
AZITHROMYCIN (Zithromax)	Antibiotic, macrolide	Drug used against staphylococcal infections, strep throat, community acquired pneumonia, acute otitis media	**TAB, LIQ, IV:** 10 mg/kg/dose once daily on Day 1 (max 500 mg), then 5 mg/kg/dose once daily on Days 2–5 (max 250 mg)	Hepatotoxicity, nausea, vomiting, diarrhea, dermatitis, fever, drug–drug interactions
BACLOFEN (Lioresal)	Skeletal muscle relaxant	Spasticity of cerebral or spinal origin	**TAB, LIQ, IT:** Oral: Initial dose of 5 mg two or three times daily; increase of 5 mg every 4–7 days; max 30–80 mg/day Intrathecal: 50–600 mcg/day delivered by implantable pump	Drowsiness, muscle weakness, constipation, dizziness, paresthesia Avoid abrupt withdrawal
BENZTROPINE (Cogentin)	Anticholinergic	Movement disorders associated with antipsychotics such as haloperidol	**TAB, IV:** Initial dose of 0.02–0.05 mg/kg/dose; increase of 0.5 mg/dose twice daily; max 6 mg/day	Gastrointestinal upset, drowsiness, dizziness, blurred vision, dry mouth, difficult urination, constipation, tachycardia
BOTULINUM TOXIN A (Botox)	Antispasticity agent	Spasticity in cerebral palsy and spinal cord injury, strabismus, migraines	**IM:** 4 units/kg divided between affected limbs every 2–3 months; injections are administered by a qualified practitioner	Diffuse skin rash, paralysis with overdose, muscle weakness
BUDESONIDE (Pulmicort, Rhinocort)	Corticosteroid	Maintenance and prophylactic treatment of asthma, rhinitis, nasal polyps, Crohn's disease	**INH:** Doses vary with clinical situation	Nausea, cough, oral candidiasis, hoarseness, dry mouth, epistaxis
BUPROPION (Wellbutrin, SR, XL, Zyban)	Antidepressant (dopamine re-uptake inhibitor)	Depression, attention-deficit/hyperactivity disorder, smoking cessation	**TAB:** Safety and efficacy in <18 yo have not been established; limited evidence >6 yo: 6 mg/kg/day; max 300 mg/day	Decreased seizure threshold, nausea, agitation, anxiety, insomnia, decreased appetite, tachycardia Increased suicidal risks in children and adolescents
BUSPIRONE (Buspar)	Antianxiety agent	Anxiety, aggression, depression, attention-deficit/hyperactivity disorder	**TAB:** Safety and efficacy in children <18 yo have not been established	Chest pain, ringing in the ears, dizziness, drowsiness, restlessness, dyskinesia
CALCIUM CARBONATE	Antacid, electrolyte supplement	Relief of acid indigestion, calcium supplementation	**CAP, TAB, LIQ:** Doses vary based on clinical scenario	Abdominal pain, constipation, nausea, vomiting
CALCIUM GLUCONATE	Electrolyte supplement	Treatment of hypocalcemia and conditions secondary to hypocalcemia or hyperkalemia	**CAP, TAB, LIQ, IV:** Doses vary based on clinical scenario	IV: Arrhythmia, heat waves, bradycardia Oral: Constipation

(continued)

Table C.1. *(continued)*

Medication	Category	Use(s)	Standard applications	Side effects
CARBAMAZEPINE (Tegretol, Tegretol XR)	Anti-seizure medication	Epilepsy-partial, generalized or mixed seizures, bipolar disorder, neuralgia, agitation	**CAP, TAB, LIQ, CHEW:** <6 yo: Initial dose of 10–20 mg/kg/day divided two to three times daily; max 35 mg/kg/day 6–12 yo: Initial dose of 200 mg/dose twice daily, increase of 200 mg/week; max 1,200 mg/day	Unsteady gait, double vision, drowsiness, slurred speech, dizziness, tremor, headache, nausea, drug interactions, aplastic anemia, agranulocytosis, rash
CARNITINE (Carnitor)	Nutritional supplement	Primary and secondary carnitine deficiency, especially in inborn errors of metabolism	**TAB, LIQ, IV:** 12.5–25 mg/kg/dose every 6 hours; max 3,000 mg/day	Nausea, vomiting, abdominal cramps, diarrhea, body odor, chest pain, headaches, hypertension with IV
CEFDINIR (Omnicef)	Antibiotic, cephalosporin	Wide spectrum of coverage; used to treat acute otitis media, sinusitis, skin infections, community-acquired pneumonia	**CAP, LIQ:** 7 mg/kg/dose twice daily or 14 mg/kg/dose once daily; max 600 mg/day	Headache, rash, abdominal pain, nausea, vomiting
CEFPODOXIME	Antibiotic, cephalosporin	Wide spectrum of coverage; used to treat acute otitis media, sinusitis, skin infections, community-acquired pneumonia	**TAB, LIQ:** 5 mg/kg/dose every 12 hours for 5–10 days; max 200 mg/dose	Headache, rash, abdominal pain, nausea, vomiting
CEPHALEXIN (Keflex)	Antibiotic cephalosporin	Used to treat susceptible infections of the respiratory tract, skin, and urinary tract; prophylaxis against infective endocarditis	**CAP, TAB, LIQ:** Doses vary based on clinical scenario	Headache, rash, nausea, vomiting, diarrhea, hypersensitivity
CETIRIZINE (Zyrtec)	Antihistamine, alpha/beta agonist decongestant	Allergies, itching	**TAB, LIQ, CHEW:** 6–12 mo: 2.5 mg daily 12 mo–2 yo: 2.5 mg once daily 2–5 yo: 5 mg once daily >6 yo: 10 mg daily	Dry mouth, headache, nausea, somnolence
CHLORPROMAZINE (Thorazine)	Antipsychotic, typical	Psychosis, anxiety, aggression, intractable hiccups, nausea/vomiting, hyperexcitable behavior	**TAB, LIQ, IV:** Doses vary based on clinical scenario	Drowsiness, tardive dyskinesia, hypotensive, weight gain, lower seizure threshold, depletion of white blood cells, rash
CHLOROTHIAZIDE (Diuril)	Diuretic, thiazides	Diuresis	**TAB, LIQ, IV:** IV: 2.5–5 mg/kg/dose twice daily Oral: 5–20 mg/kg/dose twice daily	Electrolyte imbalances
CIPROFLOXACIN (Cipro)	Antibiotic, fluoroquinolone	Treatment/prophylaxis of susceptible infections, (i.e., urinary tract infections, lower respiratory tract infections)	**TAB, LIQ, IV:** 10–20 mg/kg/dose twice daily; max 500 mg/dose	Hepatotoxicity, diarrhea, abdominal pain Avoid with calcium-containing products
CITALOPRAM (Celexa)	Antidepressant (selective serotonin reuptake inhibitors)	Depression, panic disorder, obsessive-compulsive disorder	**TAB, LIQ:** 7–11 yo: 10 mg/dose once daily; increase of 5 mg every 2 weeks; max 40 mg/day ≥12 yo: 20 mg/dose once daily, increase of 10 mg every 2 weeks; max 40 mg/day	Somnolence, insomnia, nausea, dry mouth, increased sweating, agitation, restlessness Increased suicidal risks in children and adolescents

Medication	Category	Use(s)	Standard applications	Side effects
CLARITHROMYCIN (Biaxin, XL)	Antibiotic, macrolides	Wide-spectrum drug used against staphylococcal infection, strep throat, and mycoplasma infections	**TAB, LIQ:** 7.5 mg/kg/dose twice daily; max 500 mg/dose	Stomach upset, diarrhea, nausea, cardiac arrhythmias, drug interactions
CLOMIPRAMINE (Anafranil)	Tricyclic antidepressant	Obsessive-compulsive disorder, trichotillomania	**CAP:** Initial dose of 10–25 mg/day; max 3 mg/kg/day or 200 mg/day	Drowsiness, dry mouth, blurred vision, flushing, constipation, central nervous system depression
CLONAZEPAM (Klonopin)	Benzodiazepine	Seizures, infantile spasms, anxiety, panic disorders	**TAB, ODT:** Initial dose of 0.005–0.1 mg/kg/dose twice daily; max 20 mg/day	Sedation, hyperactivity, confusion, depression Avoid abrupt withdrawal
CLONIDINE (Catapres, Kapvay)	Alpha-2 adrenergic agonist	Hypertension, attention-deficit/hyperactivity disorder, Tourette syndrome, pain management	**TAB, TDP:** Doses vary based on clinical scenario	Dry mouth, sedation, hypotension, drowsiness, and skin reactions with patch Avoid abrupt withdrawal
CLORAZEPATE (Tranxene)	Benzodiazepine	Adjunctive therapy for partial seizures, anxiety	**TAB:** Initial dose of 3.75–7.5 mg/dose twice daily; increase of 3.75 mg/week; max 60 mg/day	Hypotension, drowsiness, dizziness (*see also side effects of* DIAZEPAM)
CLOTRIMAZOLE (Lotrimin, Mycelex)	Antifungal, topical, oral	Antifungal, *Candida albicans* infections	**TAB, TOP:** Cream: Apply twice daily for 2–4 weeks Oral: 10 mg/dose three to five times daily	Skin irritation, peeling, nausea, and vomiting with oral
CLOZAPINE (Clozaril, Fox Aclo)	Atypical antipsychotic	Refractory schizophrenia	**TAB:** Initial dose of 12.5–25 mg/dose once or twice daily	Hypotension, seizure, weight gain, sedation, extrapyramidal effects, agranulocytosis Patients must be registered prior to starting the medication
COLLOIDAL OATMEAL (Aveeno)	Skin treatment	Dry skin, itching	**TOP:** Add to bath or apply as needed	Allergic reaction
CORTICOTROPIN (Acthar, ACTH)	Corticosteroid, systemic	Infantile spasms and Lennox-Gastaut syndrome; many off-label uses	**IV, IM, SQ:** Doses vary based on clinical scenario	Glucose in urine, hypertension, cataracts, brittle bones, altered behavior, immunosuppression
CYPROHEPTADINE (Periactin)	Histamine (H_1) antagonist	Allergies, migraines, appetite stimulation, spasticity, urticaria	**TAB, LIQ:** 0.25 mg/kg/day divided two to three times daily; max 16 mg/day	Weight gain, nausea, gastrointestinal irritation, dry mouth, somnolence
DANTROLENE SODIUM (Dantrium)	Skeletal muscle relaxant	Spasticity in cerebral palsy or spinal cord injury, malignant hyperthermia prevention	**CAP, LIQ, IV:** Initial dose of 0.5 mg/kg/dose twice daily; increase of 0.5 mg/kg/dose every week; max 2 mg/kg/dose two to four times daily Malignant hyperthermia: 2.5 mg/kg/dose	Weakness, drowsiness, lethargy, dizziness, tingling sensation, nausea, diarrhea, hepatotoxicity

(continued)

Table C.1. *(continued)*

Medication	Category	Use(s)	Standard applications	Side effects
DESIPRAMINE (Norpramin)	Tricyclic antidepressant	Depression, anxiety, attention-deficit/hyperactivity disorder, neuropathic pain	**TAB:** Not recommended in <12 yo; 0.5–2.5 mg/kg/dose twice daily; max 150 mg/day	Hypotension, dizziness, constipation, somnolence, dry mouth, blurred vision Increased suicidal risks in children and adolescents
DEXAMETHASONE (Decadron)	Corticosteroid, glucocorticoid	Anti-inflammatory or immunosuppressive used in multiple diseases like airway edema, chemotherapy nausea/vomiting, asthma exacerbation, cerebral edema, croup, bronchopulmonary dysplasia	**TAB, LIQ, IV:** Doses vary based on clinical scenario	Short-term use: headache, mood changes, hypertension or edema Long-term use: osteoporosis, weight gain, increased risk of infection, Cushing's syndrome, glaucoma and thinning skin
DEXTROAMPHETAMINE (Dexedrine, Dextrostat, ProCentra)	Stimulant	Attention-deficit/hyperactivity disorder, narcolepsy	**CAP, LIQ, TAB:** Initial dose of 2.5–5 mg once daily; max 40 mg/day	Insomnia, restlessness, decreased appetite, irritability, headache, abdominal cramps, decreased appetite, potential for abuse
DIAZEPAM (Valium, Diastat)	Benzodiazepine	Sedation, aggression, anxiety, spasticity, seizures, status epilepticus	**TAB, LIQ, IV, SUPP:** Doses vary based on clinical scenario	Sedation, weakness, depression, ataxia, memory disturbance, difficulty handling secretions and chewing/swallowing foods, paradoxical reactions (e.g., anxiety, agitation), respiratory and cardiac depression, rash, low white blood cell count
DIPHENHYDRAMINE (Benadryl)	Antihistamine	Sedation, allergies, hives, extrapyramidal symptoms, motion sickness	**CAP, TAB, TOP, LIQ, IV:** Not recommended <2 yo; 5 mg/kg/day divided three to four times daily; max 300 mg/day	Sedation, insomnia, dry mouth, dizziness, euphoria, gastrointestinal upset, paradoxical excitation
DULOXETINE (Cymbalta)	Antidepressant (norepinephrine serotonin reuptake inhibitor)	Depression, neuropathy, fibromyalgia, anxiety	**CAP:** ≥7 yo: Initial dose of 30 mg/dose once daily; increase to 60 mg after 2 weeks; max 120 mg/day	Dry mouth, nausea, diaphoresis, headache, insomnia, fatigue Increased suicidal risks in children and adolescents
DUODERM	Skin treatment	Skin ulcers/sores, second-degree burns, minor abrasions	**TOP:** Apply topically to site	Allergic reaction to tape or gel formula
ERYTHROMYCIN (E.E.S.)	Antibiotic, prokinetic agent	Used against staphylococcal infection, strep throat, and mycoplasma infections; used for gastro dysmotility, acne	**CAP, TAB, LIQ, IV, TOP:** Doses vary based on clinical scenario	Nausea, vomiting, diarrhea, cardiac dysrhythmias, drug interactions Topical: Skin dryness, peeling, skin irritation
ESCITALOPRAM (Lexapro)	Antidepressant (selective serotonin reuptake inhibitors)	Depression, anxiety, obsessive-compulsive disorder, panic disorder	**TAB, LIQ:** >12 yo: Initial dose of 10 mg/dose once daily; max 20 mg/day	QTc prolongation Increased suicidal risks in children and adolescents
ESOMEPRAZOLE (Nexium)	Proton pump inhibitor	Treatment or relief of ulcers, gastroesophageal reflux disease (GERD), erosive esophagitis associated with GERD	**TAB, CAP, LIQ:** Doses vary based on clinical scenario	Abdominal pain, diarrhea, nausea, flatulence, increased appetite, taste changes, headache

Medication	Category	Use(s)	Standard applications	Side effects
ETHOSUXIMIDE (Zarontin)	Anti-seizure medication	Absence seizures	**CAP, LIQ:** 10 mg/kg/dose twice daily usual dose; max 1.5 g/day	Sedation, unsteady gait, anorexia, rash, stomach distress, blood dyscrasias
FAMOTIDINE (Pepcid)	H_2 antagonist	Gastroesophageal reflux, ulcers	**CAP, TAB, LIQ, IV:** 0.5 mg/kg/dose twice daily with meals; max 80 mg/day	Headache, dizziness, constipation, diarrhea
FELBAMATE (Felbatol)	Anti-seizure medication	Lennox-Gastaut syndrome; also effective in generalized and secondary generalized seizures, partial seizures	**TAB, LIQ:** 15–45 mg/kg/day divided three to four times daily	Anorexia, vomiting, insomnia, headache, rash, risk of life-threatening hepatitis and aplastic anemia
FERROUS SULFATE (Fer-In-Sol)	Nutritional supplement	Iron supplementation	**TAB, LIQ:** 1–3 mg/kg/dose twice daily	Constipation, dark stools, stomach cramps
FEXOFENADINE (Allegra)	Antihistamine	Treat allergies	**TAB, LIQ, CAP, ODT:** 6 mo–2 yo: 15 mg twice daily 2–11 yo: 30 mg twice daily ≥12 yo: 180 mg daily	Dizziness, headache
FLUCONAZOLE (Diflucan)	Antifungal	Treatment or prophylaxis of susceptible fungal infections, including oral and vaginal *C. albicans* infections	**TAB, LIQ, IV:** Doses vary based on clinical scenario	Dizziness, headache, rash, nausea, hepatotoxicity, drug interactions
FLUOXETINE (Prozac)	Antidepressant (selective serotonin reuptake inhibitor)	Depression, self-injurious behavior, Tourette syndrome, obsessive-compulsive disorder, anxiety, bulimia, panic disorder	**TAB, CAP, LIQ:** Safety and efficacy in children have not been established	Anxiety, agitation, sleep disruption, decreased appetite, seizures Increased suicidal risks in children and adolescents
FLUTICASONE (Flonase)	Corticosteroid	Used for asthma, allergic rhinitis	**INH, INS:** Doses vary based on clinical scenario	Throat irritation, upper respiratory tract infections, oral thrush
FOSPHENYTOIN (Cerebyx)	See PHENYTOIN; intravenous substitute for phenytoin	See PHENYTOIN	See PHENYTOIN	See PHENYTOIN
FUROSEMIDE (Lasix)	Diuretic, loop	Diuresis	**TAB, LIQ, IV:** 1 mg/kg/dose given one to four times daily; max 6 mg/kg/dose	Electrolyte abnormalities
GABAPENTIN (Neurontin)	Anti-seizure medication	Adjunctive therapy in partial and secondarily generalized seizures, neuropathic pain	**CAP, TAB, LIQ:** 3–15 mg/kg/dose divided three times daily; max 2,400 mg/day	Sedation, dizziness, unsteady gait, emotional instability Avoid abrupt withdrawal
GLYCEROL PHENYLBUTYRATE (Ravicti)	Urea cycle disorder agent	Chronic management of urea cycle disorders	**LIQ:** Doses vary depending on scenario	Headache, skin rash, abdominal pain
GLYCOPYRROLATE (Robinul)	Anticholinergic	Decreases drooling in cerebral palsy	**TAB, IV:** Oral: 40–100 mcg/kg/dose every 3–4 hours as needed Injection: 4–10 mcg/kg/dose every 3–4 hours as needed	Rapid heart rate, orthostatic hypotension, drowsiness, blurred vision, dry mouth, constipation

(continued)

Table C.1. *(continued)*

Medication	Category	Use(s)	Standard applications	Side effects
GUANFACINE (Tenex, Intuniv)	Alpha-2 agonist	Hypertension, attention-deficit/hyperactivity disorder, Tourette syndrome	**TAB:** Doses vary depending on scenario	Dry mouth, sedation, hypotension, headache, nausea Avoid abrupt withdrawal
HALOPERIDOL (Haldol)	Antipsychotic, typical	Self-injurious behavior, Tourette syndrome, severe agitation, psychosis	**TAB, LIQ, IV, IM:** Doses vary depending on scenario	Extrapyramidal effects, hypotension, nausea, vomiting, electrocardiogram changes, neuroleptic malignant syndrome, lower seizure threshold in epilepsy, anticholinergic effects, tardive dyskinesia
HYDROCORTISONE (Cortizone)	Corticosteroid, topical	Eczema, dermatitis	**TOP:** Apply thin film two to four times daily	Skin irritation, dryness, rash
HYDROCORTISONE/ POLYMYXIN B/ NEOMYCIN (Cortisporin)	Corticosteroid + antibiotic, topical	Steroid-responsive skin conditions with secondary infection	**TOP:** Apply sparingly and massage into skin two or three times daily	Local irritation
IBUPROFEN (Advil, Motrin)	Nonsteroidal anti-inflammatory (NSAID)	Inflammatory diseases and rheumatoid disorders including juvenile rheumatoid arthritis, mild to moderate pain, fever, dysmenorrhea, migraines; also used for PDA closure in neonates	**CAP, TAB, LIQ, IV:** Doses vary depending on scenario	Gastrointestinal irritation, rash, dizziness, increased bleeding risk Caution in ulcer and renal patients
IMIPRAMINE (Tofranil, Janimine)	Tricyclic antidepressant	Depression, enuresis, neuropathy	**CAP, TAB:** Doses vary depending on scenario	Dry mouth, drowsiness, constipation, electrocardiogram abnormalities, increased blood pressure, urinary retention Increased suicidal risks in children and adolescents
INDOMETHACIN (Indocin)	NSAID	Inflammatory diseases and rheumatoid disorders; also used for PDA closure in neonates	**CAP, LIQ, IV:** 1–4 mg/kg/day; max 200 mg/day	Gastrointestinal irritation, rash, dizziness, increased bleeding risk Caution in ulcer and renal patients
ISOTRETINOIN (Accutane, Claravis)	Skin treatment	Severe acne	**CAP:** 0.2–1 mg/kg/dose twice daily	Dry mucous membranes, photosensitivity, dry skin, retinoid dermatitis, teratogen Patients must be registered prior to starting the medication
LAMOTRIGINE (Lamictal)	Anti-seizure medication	Adjunct or monotherapy for a variety of seizures, bipolar disorder	**TAB, LIQ:** Doses vary depending on scenario	Sedation, dizziness, ataxia, headaches, nausea, vomiting, severe and potentially life-threatening skin reactions
LANOLIN/PETROLATUM/ VITAMINS A & D (A&D Ointment)	Skin treatment	Diaper rash	**TOP:** Apply thin film at each diaper change	Allergic reaction

Medication	Category	Use(s)	Standard applications	Side effects
LANSOPRAZOLE (Prevacid)	Proton pump inhibitor	Treatment or relief of ulcers, GERD; adjuvant therapy in the treatment of *Helicobacter pylori*–associated gastritis	**TAB, CAP, LIQ, ODT:** Doses vary depending on scenario	Abdominal pain, nausea, flatulence, increased appetite, headache, fatigue, rash
LEVOALBUTEROL (Xopenex)	See ALBUTEROL	See ALBUTEROL	**INH:** Doses vary depending on scenario	See ALBUTEROL
LEVOCARNITINE	See CARNITINE	See CARNITINE	See CARNITINE	See CARNITINE
LEVETIRACETAM (Keppra)	Anti-seizure medication	Adjunctive therapy in a variety of seizure types, migraine prophylaxis	**TAB, LIQ , IV:** Initial dose of 10 mg/kg/dose twice daily; max 60 mg/kg/day or 3,000 mg/day	Somnolence, nausea, anorexia, dizziness, behavior changes, irritability
LEVOFLOXACIN (Levaquin)	Antibiotic, fluoroquinolone	See CIPROFLOXACIN	**TAB, LIQ, IV:** 8–10 mg/kg/dose once daily	See CIPROFLOXACIN
LEVOTHYROXINE (Synthroid, Levoxyl, Unithroid)	Thyroid product	Hypothyroidism	**TAB, IV:** <1 yo: 6–15 mcg/kg/dose once daily 1–5 yo: 5–6 mcg/kg/dose once daily 6–12 yo: 4–5 mcg/ kg/dose once daily >12 yo: 2–3 mcg/kg/dose once daily	Heart palpitations, nervousness, tremor, excessive sweating, diarrhea, weight loss
LINDANE (Kwell)	Antiparasitic, topical	Scabies and lice	**TOP:** Doses vary depending on scenario	Seizure risk in small children with overuse
LISDEXAMFETAMINE (Vyvanse)	Stimulant	Attention-deficit/hyperactivity disorder	**CAP, CHEW:** 6–17 yo: 20–70 mg once daily in the morning; start 20–30mg each morning	Appetite suppression, insomnia, tachycardia, anxiety, headache, irritability
LITHIUM CARBONATE (Eskalith, Lithobid)	Antipsychotic	Mood stabilizer, bipolar disorder, depression	**CAP, TAB, LIQ:** 15–60 mg/kg/day divided in three to four doses; max 1,800 mg/day	Sedation, confusion, seizures, rash, hypothyroidism, diarrhea, muscle weakness, gastrointestinal irritation, renal dysfunction, tremor
LOPERAMIDE (Imodium)	Antidiarrheal	Treatment of acute diarrhea, traveler's diarrhea	**CAP, LIQ, TAB:** Doses vary depending on scenario	Abdominal cramps, constipation, nausea
LORATADINE (Claritin)	Antihistamine H_1 antagonist	Allergies, urticaria	**CAP, TAB, LIQ:** 2–5 yo: 5 mg daily ≥6 yo: 10 mg daily	Sedation, dry mouth, headache
LORAZEPAM (Ativan)	Benzodiazepine	Anxiety, status epilepticus, agitation, sedation, antiemetic	**TAB, LIQ, IV, IM:** 0.05 mg/kg/dose every 4–8 hours as needed; max 4 mg/dose	Sedation, weakness, depression, unstable gait, memory disturbance
MAGNESIUM HYDROXIDE/ALUMINUM HYDROXIDE (Mylanta)	Antacid, laxative	Antacid for reflux; also helps treat constipation	**LIQ:** 2–4 teaspoons with meals and at bedtime	Abdominal pain, constipation, nausea, vomiting Caution in renal patients

(continued)

Table C.1. *(continued)*

Medication	Category	Use(s)	Standard applications	Side effects
METHYLPHENIDATE/ DEXMETHYLPHENIDATE (Concerta, Daytrana, Metadate, Metadate CD, Metadate ER, Methylin, Methylin ER, Ritalin, Focalin, Focalin XR)	Stimulant	Attention-deficit/hyperactivity disorder	**CAP, LIQ, TAB, TDP:** Doses vary depending on scenario	Appetite suppression, insomnia, arrhythmia, anxiety, headache, irritability
METHYLPREDNISOLONE (Solu Medrol)	Corticosteroid	Reduction of airway inflammation during acute asthma attacks, inflammatory conditions, many others	**TAB, IV:** 0.5 mg/kg/dose to 1 mg/kg/dose four times daily; max 60 mg/day	Headache, mood changes, hypertension or edema, osteoporosis, weight gain, increased risk of infection, Cushing's syndrome, glaucoma, thinning skin
METOCLOPRAMIDE (Reglan)	Prokinetic agent	Antireflux, increases gastric emptying	**TAB, LIQ, ODT, IV:** 0.025–0.125 mg/kg/dose divided four times daily; max 10 mg/dose	Dystonia, drowsiness, sedation, anxiety, leukopenia, muscle stiffness, tardive dyskinesia
MICONAZOLE (2%; e.g., Monistat)	Antifungal, topical	Antifungal, *C. albicans* infections	**TOP:** Apply twice daily	Skin irritation, peeling, pruritis
MINERAL OIL (e.g., Alpha Keri [dry skin], Fleet mineral oil enema [constipation])	Skin treatment, laxative	Emollient for dry skin; oral liquid or enema for constipation	**LIQ, TOP:** Doses vary depending on scenario	Allergic reaction (topical), nausea, and diarrhea (oral)
MINERAL OIL/PETROLATUM/LANOLIN (Nivea, Lubriderm)	Skin treatment	Emollient for dry skin, constipation	**TOP:** Apply as needed	Allergic reaction
MONTELUKAST (Singulair)	Leukotriene receptor antagonist	Asthma, allergies	**TAB, CHEW, LIQ:** 6 mo–5 yo: 4 mg daily 6–14 yo: 5 mg daily >15 yo: 10 mg daily	Headache, altered behavior, eosinophilia
MUPIROCIN (2%; Bactroban)	Antibiotic, topical	Antibiotic for impetigo, secondary infections of skin ulcers, burns	**TOP:** Apply sparingly three times daily; may cover with gauze	Burning, itching, pain at site of application
NALOXONE (Narcan)	Opioid antagonist	Opiate antagonist for treatment of self-injurious behavior	**IV, INS:** Doses vary depending on clinical scenario	Dependent on formulation given
NALTREXONE (Revia)	Opioid antagonist	Opiate antagonist for treatment of self-injurious behavior	**TAB:** Safety and efficacy in <18 yo have not been established	None in opioid-free individuals
NORTRIPTYLINE (Pamelor, Aventyl)	Tricyclic antidepressant	Depression, neuropathic pain, nocturnal enuresis, attention-deficit/hyperactivity disorder	**CAP, TAB, LIQ:** Doses vary depending on scenario	Dry mouth, drowsiness, constipation, electrocardiogram abnormalities, mania, sedation Increased suicidal risks in children and adolescents

Medication	Category	Use(s)	Standard applications	Side effects
NYSTATIN (Mycostatin)	Antifungal	Treatment of yeast and thrush infections in the mouth and gastrointestinal tract	**TOP, LIQ:** Doses vary depending on scenario	Diarrhea, redness, skin irritation, gastro-intestinal upset
OLANZAPINE (Zyprexa)	Antipsychotic, atypical	Treatment of the manifestations of psychotic disorders, Tourette syndrome, anorexia nervosa, autism spectrum disorder	**TAB, CAP, IV, IM:** Initial dose of 2.5 mg/dose once daily, max 20 mg/day	Edema, weight gain, hyperglycemia, somnolence, orthostatic hypotension, increase in lipids, dizziness, tremor Increased suicidal risks in children and adolescents
OMEPRAZOLE (Prilosec)	Proton pump inhibitor	Treatment or relief of ulcers, GERD; adjuvant therapy in the treatment of *H. pylori*–associated gastritis	**LIQ, CAP, TAB:** Doses vary depending on scenario	Abdominal pain, diarrhea, nausea, flatulence, increased appetite, taste changes, headache
OXCARBAZEPINE (Trileptal)	Anti-seizure medication	Generalized tonic-clonic, complex partial, and simple partial seizures as both adjunctive and monotherapy	**TAB, LIQ:** 4–5 mg/kg/dose twice daily; max 2,400 mg/day	Ataxia, dizziness, gastrointestinal irritation, headache, somnolence, tremor, vision disturbances, hyponatremia
OXYBUTYNIN (Ditropan)	Antispasmodic agent, urinary	Antispasmodic for neurogenic bladder	**TAB, LIQ:** 0.2 mg/kg/dose two to four times daily; max 15 mg/day	Palpitations, drowsiness, dizziness, insomnia, dry mouth, nausea, vomiting, constipation, urinary hesitancy or retention, blurred vision, decreased tears, decreased sweating
PAROXETINE (Paxil)	Antidepressant (selective serotonin reuptake inhibitor)	Depression, obsessive-compulsive disorder, anxiety disorders, self-injurious behavior	**TAB, LIQ:** 10–20 mg/dose once daily; max 60 mg/day	Somnolence, headache, insomnia, nausea, constipation, decreased appetite, sexual dysfunction Increased suicidal risks in children and adolescents
PENICILLIN (Pen-VK)	Antibiotic	Treats strep throat	**TAB, LIQ:** 6.25–12.5 mg/kg/dose, four times daily	Allergic reactions, diarrhea, nausea
PERMETHRIN (Nix, Elimite)	Antiparasitic, topical	Scabies and lice	**TOP:** Doses vary depending on scenario	Pruritis, hypersensitivity, burning, stinging, rash
PETROLATUM/MINERAL OIL/WAX/ALCOHOL (Eucerin)	Skin treatment	Emollient for dry skin, itching	**TOP:** Apply as needed	Allergic reaction
PHENOBARBITAL (Luminal)	Anti-seizure medication	Generalized tonic-clonic, simple partial, and secondarily generalized seizures	**CAP, TAB, LIQ, IV:** 0.5–25 mg/kg/dose twice daily	Paradoxical hyperactivity, sedation, learning difficulties, behavioral difficulties, irritability, unsteady gait, respiratory depression
PHENYTOIN (Dilantin)	Anti-seizure medication	Generalized tonic-clonic and complex partial seizures	**CAP, CHEW, LIQ, IV:** Doses vary depending on scenario	Swelling of gums, excessive hair growth, rash, coarsening of facial features, possible adverse effects on learning and behavior, nystagmus and unsteady gait with toxic levels, blood dyscrasias, decreased bone density

(continued)

Table C.1. *(continued)*

Medication	Category	Use(s)	Standard applications	Side effects
POLYETHYLENE GLYCOL 3350 (MiraLax)	Laxative	Treatment of acute and chronic constipation	**POWDER:** 17 yo and older: Dissolve one capful (17 g) in 4–8 oz. of liquid; take once daily Younger than 17 yo: Dose adjusted under the advice of a qualified medical practitioner	Nausea, cramping, flatulence, diarrhea, rash
PREDNISOLONE (Prelone)	Corticosteroid, systemic	Reduction of airway inflammation during acute asthma attacks, inflammatory conditions, nephrotic syndrome	**TAB, LIQ:** Doses vary depending on scenario	Headache, mood changes, hypertension or edema, osteoporosis, weight gain, increased risk of infection, Cushing's syndrome, glaucoma, thinning skin
PREDNISONE (Deltasone)	Corticosteroid, systemic	Reduction of airway inflammation during acute asthma attacks, inflammatory conditions	**TAB, LIQ:** Doses vary depending on scenario	Headache, mood changes, hypertension or edema, osteoporosis, weight gain, increased risk of infection, Cushing's syndrome, glaucoma, thinning skin
PREGABALIN (Lyrica)	Anticonvulsant	Fibromyalgia, neuropathic pain, partial-onset seizures	**CAP, LIQ:** Safety and efficacy in <18 yo have not been established	Dizziness, drowsiness, blurred vision
PRIMIDONE (Mysoline)	Anti-seizure medication	Generalized tonic-clonic and complex partial seizures	**TAB, LIQ:** Doses vary depending on scenario	Drowsiness, dizziness, nausea, vomiting, leucopenia, systemic lupus like syndrome, nystagmus, personality change (*see also side effects of* PHENOBARBITAL)
QUETIAPINE (Seroquel)	Antipsychotic, atypical	Bipolar disorder, psychosis, depression, autism spectrum disorder	**TAB, LIQ:** >10 yo: 25 mg twice daily; max 600 mg/day	Hypertension or hypotension, hyperlipidemia, weight gain, gastrointestinal irritation, somnolence, tremor, extrapyramidal effects, dizziness, asthenia Increased suicidal risks in children and adolescents
RANITIDINE (Zantac)	Histamine H_2 antagonist	Gastroesophageal reflux, ulcers	**CAP, TAB, LIQ, IV:** Doses vary depending on scenario	Headache, dizziness, constipation, diarrhea
RISPERIDONE (Risperdal)	Antipsychotic, atypical	Self-injurious behavior, psychosis, Tourette syndrome, aggression, pervasive developmental disorders	**TAB, LIQ:** 0.25–0.5 mg/dose twice daily; max 10 mg/day	Hypotension, sedation, dizziness, movement disorder, headache, constipation, weight gain, urinary retention, agranulocytosis, hyperprolactinemia, gynecomastia
SELENIUM SULFIDE (2.5%; Selsun Blue)	Skin treatment	Scalp conditions (dandruff or seborrhea)	**TOP:** Apply to wet scalp twice a week as needed	Skin irritation, dry or oily scalp, hair loss, and discoloration
SERTRALINE (Zoloft)	Antidepressant (selective serotonin reuptake inhibitors)	Depression, anxiety, obsessive-compulsive disorder, posttraumatic stress syndrome	**TAB, LIQ:** Safety and efficacy in <18 yo have not been established Initial dose of 25–50 mg/dose once daily; max 200 mg/day	Somnolence, headache, agitation, sleep disruption, decreased appetite, nausea, diarrhea, tremors, sweating, seizures Increased suicidal risks in children and adolescents

Medication	Category	Use(s)	Standard applications	Side effects
SODIUM PHENYLBUTYRATE (Buphenyl)	Hyperammonemia treatment; ammonium detoxicant	Adjunct for urea cycle disorder	**TAB, TOP:** Doses vary depending on scenario	Metabolic abnormalities, abdominal pain, nausea, vomiting
THEOPHYLLINE (Theo-Dur, Uniphyl)	Respiratory agent	Bronchodilator; may be used in conjunction with other treatments for acute or chronic asthma	**CAP, TAB, LIQ, IM, IV:** Doses vary depending on scenario	Nausea, vomiting, stomach pain, gastroesophageal reflux, anorexia, nervousness, tachypnea
THIORIDAZINE (Mellaril)	Antipsychotic, typical	Self-injurious behavior, psychosis	**TAB, LIQ:** Doses vary depending on scenario	Drowsiness, hypotension, movement disorder, electrocardiogram abnormalities, retinal abnormalities, QTc prolongation
THIOTHIXENE (Navane)	Antipsychotic, typical	Self-injurious behavior, psychosis	**CAP, LIQ:** ≥12 yo: 2 mg/dose three times daily; max 30 mg/day	Tardive dyskinesia, neuroleptic malignant syndrome, rapid heart rate, hypotension, drowsiness, bone marrow suppression
TIAGABINE (Gabitril)	Anti-seizure medication	Adjunct for partial seizures	**TAB:** ≥12 yo: Initial dose of 4 mg once daily; max 32 mg/day	Dizziness, headache, sleepiness, central nervous system depression, memory disturbance, unsteady gait, emotionality, tremors, abdominal pain
TOLNAFTATE (Tinactin)	Antifungal, topical	Antifungal, ringworm	**TOP:** Apply small amount of cream or powder to affected area two to three times a day for 2–4 weeks	Skin irritation
TOPIRAMATE (Topamax)	Anti-seizure medication	Refractory partial seizures, Lennox-Gastaut syndrome, migraine prophylaxis	**TAB, CAP:** Initial dose of 0.5–1.5 mg/kg/dose twice daily; max 15 mg/kg/day	Edema, language problems, abnormal coordination, depression, difficulty concentrating, fatigue, dizziness, unsteady gait, sleepiness, weight loss, somnolence, weakness, nystagmus
TRIHEXYPHENIDYL (Artane)	Anticholinergic, drug-induced dystonic reactions	Dystonia reactions in cerebral palsy	**TAB, LIQ:** ≥2 yo: Initial dose of 0.05–0.1mg/kg/dose twice daily	Tachycardia, skin rash, agitation, confusion, gastrointestinal disturbances, blurred vision
TRIAMCINOLONE (Kenalog)	Corticosteroid	Eczema, dermatitis	**TOP:** Apply thin film two to four times daily	Skin irritation, rash, dryness
TRIMETHOPRIM/SULFAMETHOXAZOLE (TMP/SMX) (Bactrim, Septra)	Antibiotic	Treatment or prophylaxis of susceptible infections, including urinary tract infections, otitis media, and sinusitis	**TAB, LIQ, IV:** 4–10 mg/kg/dose of TMP twice daily	Bone marrow suppression, allergic reactions, photosensitivity, gastrointestinal irritation, rash
VALPROIC ACID (Depakene, Depacon, Depakote)	Anti-seizure medication, mood stabilizer	Myoclonic, simple absence, and generalized tonic-clonic seizures, Lennox-Gastaut syndrome, infantile spasms; also used to treat aggression and mood disorders, bipolar disorder, impulsive aggression, intermittent explosive disorder, migraine prophylaxis	**CAP, LIQ, TAB, IV:** Doses vary depending on scenario	Hair loss, weight loss or gain, abdominal distress, tremor, agranulocytosis, low platelet count, teratogen, hepatotoxicity, pancreatitis

(continued)

Table C.1. *(continued)*

Medication	Category	Use(s)	Standard applications	Side effects
VENLAFAXINE (Effexor, Effexor XR)	Antidepressant (norepinephrine-selective reuptake inhibitors)	Depression, anxiety, attention-deficit/hyperactivity disorder, panic disorder	**TAB, CAP:** Initial dose of 12.5 mg/dose once daily, max 75 mg/day	Hypertension, diaphoresis, weight loss, gastrointestinal irritation, insomnia, tremor, dizziness, somnolence, headache Increased suicidal risks in children and adolescents
ZINC OXIDE (Desitin)	Skin treatment	Diaper rash	**TOP:** Apply three or four times daily after diaper change or bath	Allergic reaction
ZINC OXIDE/COD LIVER OIL/LANOLIN/ PETROLATUM (Caldesene ointment)	Skin treatment	Diaper rash	**TOP:** Apply three or four times daily after diaper change or bath	Allergic reaction
ZIPRASIDONE (Geodon)	Antipsychotic, atypical	Bipolar disorder, psychosis, agitation, Tourette syndrome	**CAP, IV, IM:** Doses vary depending on scenario	Orthostatic hypotension, gastrointestinal irritation, hyperglycemia, weight gain, extrapyramidal effects, insomnia, somnolence, QTc prolongation, blood dyscrasias
ZONISAMIDE (Zonegran)	Anti-seizure medication	Adjunctive therapy in partial seizures, infantile spasms, and Lennox-Gastaut syndrome	**CAP:** ≥16 yo: 50 mg/dose twice daily; max 400 mg/day	Somnolence, dizziness, ataxia, loss of appetite, gastrointestinal discomfort, headache, agitation/irritability, confusion, rash, visual disturbances

Key: CAP, capsule; CHEW, chewable; IM, intramuscular injection; INH, inhalation; INS, intranasal; IT, intrathecal; IV, intravenous; LIQ, liquid suspension or solution; ODT, oral dissolvable tablet; SQ, subcutaneous injection; SUPP, suppository; TAB, tablet; TDP, transdermal patch; TOP, topical creams, ointments, or powders; mo, month(s) old; yo, year(s) old.

Table C.2. Commonly used medications, alphabetized by drug class

Drug class	Generic name	Brand name
Acne	ISOTRETINOIN	Accutane, Claravis
Attention-deficit/hyperactivity disorder	AMPHETAMINE SALTS	Adderall
	ATOMOXETINE	Strattera
	BUPROPION	Wellbutrin
	CLONIDINE ER	Kapvay
	DEXTROAMPHETAMINE	Dexedrine, Dextrostat, ProCentra
	GUANFACINE ER	Intuniv
	LISDEXAMFETAMINE	Vyvanse
	METHYLPHENIDATE/DEXMETHYLPHENIDATE	Concerta, Daytrana, Focalin, Metadate, Methylin, Ritalin
Analgesic	ACETAMINOPHEN	Tylenol
Antacid	CALCIUM CARBONATE	Calcium carbonate
	MAGNESIUM HYDROXIDE/ALUMINUM HYDROXIDE	Mylanta
Anti-anxiety	BUSPIRONE	Buspar
Antibiotic	AMOXICILLIN	Amoxil
	AMOXICILLIN/CLAVULANIC ACID	Augmentin
	AZITHROMYCIN	Zithromax
	CEFDINIR	Omnicef
	CEFPODOXIME	Cefpodoxime
	CEPHALEXIN	Keflex
	CIPROFLOXACIN	Cipro
	CLARITHROMYCIN	Biaxin
	ERYTHROMYCIN	E.E.S
	HYDROCORTISONE/POLYMYXIN B/NEOMYCIN (TOPICAL)	Cortisporin
	LEVOFLOXACIN	Levaquin
	MUPIROCIN (TOPICAL)	Bactroban
	PENICILLIN	Pen-VK
	TRIMETHOPRIM/SULFAMETHOXAZOLE (TMP/SMX)	Bactrim, Septra
Anticholinergic	BENZTROPINE	Cogentin
	GLYCOPYRROLATE	Robinul
	TRIHEXYPHENIDYL	Artane
Anticonvulsant/ anti-seizure medication	ACETAZOLAMIDE	Diamox
	CARBAMAZEPINE	Tegretol
	ETHOSUXIMIDE	Zarontin
	FELBAMATE	Felbatol
	FOSPHENYTOIN	Cerebyx
	GABAPENTIN	Neurontin
	LAMOTRIGINE	Lamictal
	LEVETIRACETAM	Keppra
	OXCARBAZEPINE	Trileptal
	PHENOBARBITAL	Luminal
	PHENYTOIN	Dilantin
	PREGABALIN	Lyrica
	PRIMIDONE	Mysoline

(continued)

Table C.2. *(continued)*

Drug class	Generic name	Brand name
	TIAGABINE	Gabitril
	TOPIRAMATE	Topamax
	VALPROIC ACID	Depakote, Depakene, Depacon
	ZONISAMIDE	Zonegran
Antidepressant	AMITRIPTYLINE	Elavil
	BUPROPION	Wellbutrin
	CITALOPRAM	Celexa
	CLOMIPRAMINE	Anafranil
	DESIPRAMINE	Norpramin
	DULOXETINE	Cymbalta
	ESCITALOPRAM	Lexapro
	FLUOXETINE	Prozac
	IMIPRAMINE	Tofranil, Janimine
	NORTRIPTYLINE	Pamelor, Aventyl
	PAROXETINE	Paxil
	SERTRALINE	Zoloft
	VENLAFAXINE	Effexor
Antidiarrheal	LOPERAMIDE	Imodium
Antifungal	FLUCONAZOLE	Diflucan
	CLOTRIMAZOLE	Lotrimin, Mycelex
	MICONAZOLE	Monistat
	NYSTATIN	Mycostatin
	TOLNAFTATE	Tinactin
Antihistamine/allergy relief	CETIRIZINE	Zyrtec
	CYPROHEPTADINE	Periactin
	DIPHENHYDRAMINE	Benadryl
	FEXOFENADINE	Allegra
	LORATADINE	Claritin
Antihypertensive	CLONIDINE	Catapres
	GUANFACINE	Tenex
Antiparasitic	LINDANE	Kwell
	PERMETHRIN	Nix, Elimite
Antipsychotic	ARIPIPRAZOLE	Abilify
	CHLORPROMAZINE	Thorazine
	CLOZAPINE	Clozaril, Fox Aclo
	HALOPERIDOL	Haldol
	LITHIUM CARBONATE	Lithobid, Eskalith
	OLANZAPINE	Zyprexa
	QUETIAPINE	Seroquel
	RISPERIDONE	Risperdal
	THIORIDAZINE	Mellaril
	THIOTHIXENE	Navane
	ZIPRASIDONE	Geodon

(continued)

Table C.2. *(continued)*

Drug class	Generic name	Brand name
Antipyretic	ACETAMINOPHEN	Tylenol
Antireflux	ESOMEPRAZOLE	Nexium
	FAMOTIDINE	Pepcid
	LANSOPRAZOLE	Prevacid
	METOCLOPRAMIDE	Reglan
	OMEPRAZOLE	Prilosec
	RANITIDINE	Zantac
Antispasticity/muscle relaxant	BACLOFEN	Lioresal
	BOTULINUM TOXIN A	Botox
	DANTROLENE SODIUM	Dantrium
	OXYBUTYNIN	Ditropan
Antiviral	ACYCLOVIR	Zovirax
Appetite stimulator	CYPROHEPTADINE	Periactin
Benzodiazepine	ALPRAZOLAM	Xanax
	CLONAZEPAM	Klonopin
	CLORAZEPATE	Tranxene
	DIAZEPAM	Valium, Diastat
	LORAZEPAM	Ativan
Bronchodilators	ALBUTEROL	Ventolin
	LEVALBUTEROL	Xopenex
	THEOPHYLLINE	Theo-Dur, Uniphyl
Corticosteroids	BUDESONIDE	Pulmicort, Rhinocort
	CORTICOTROPIN	Acthar, ACTH
	DEXAMETHASONE	Decadron
	FLUTICASONE	Flonase
	HYDROCORTISONE	Cortizone
	HYDROCORTISONE/POLYMYXIN B/NEOMYCIN (TOPICAL)	Cortisporin
	METHYLPREDNISOLONE	Solu Medrol
	PREDNISOLONE	Prelone
	PREDNISONE	Deltasone
	TRIAMCINOLONE	Kenalog
Diuretic	ACETAZOLAMIDE	Diamox
	CHLOROTHIAZIDE	Diuril
	FUROSEMIDE	Lasix
Electrolyte supplementation	CALCIUM CARBONATE	Calcium carbonate
	CALCIUM GLUCONATE	Calcium gluconate
Laxative	MAGNESIUM HYDROXIDE/ALUMINUM HYDROXIDE	Mylanta
	MINERAL OIL	Fleet mineral oil enema
	POLYETHYLENE GLYCOL 3350	MiraLax
Leukotriene receptor antagonist	MONTELUKAST	Singulair
Nonsteroidal anti-inflammatory drugs (NSAIDs)	IBUPROFEN	Advil, Motrin
	INDOMETHACIN	Indocin

(continued)

Table C.2. *(continued)*

Drug class	Generic name	Brand name
Nutritional supplementation	CARNITINE	Carnitor
	FERROUS SULFATE	Fer-In-Sol
	LEVOCARNITINE	Carnitor
Opioid antagonist	NALOXONE	Narcan
	NALTREXONE	Revia
Prokinetic agents	ERYTHROMYCIN	E.E.S
	METOCLOPRAMIDE	Reglan
Proton pump inhibitors	ESOMEPRAZOLE	Nexium
	LANSOPRAZOLE	Prevacid
	OMEPRAZOLE	Prilosec
Skin treatment	COLLOIDAL OATMEAL	Aveeno
	DUODERM	DuoDERM
	ISOTRETINOIN	Accutane, Claravis
	LANOLIN/PETROLATUM/VITAMINS A & D	A&D Original Ointment
	MINERAL OIL	Alpha Keri
	MINERAL OIL/PETROLATUM/LANOLIN	Nivea, Lubriderm
	PETROLATUM/ALCOHOL/MINERAL OIL/WAX	Eucerin
	SELENIUM SULFIDE	Selsun Blue
	ZINC OXIDE	Desitin
	ZINC OXIDE/COD LIVER OIL/PETROLATUM/LANOLIN	Caldesene ointment
Stimulants	AMPHETAMINE SALTS	Adderall, Adderall XR
	DEXTROAMPHETAMINE	Dexedrine, Dextrostat, ProCentra
	METHYLPHENIDATE/DEXMETHYLPHENIDATE	Concerta, Daytrana, Focalin, Metadate, Methylin, Ritalin
	LISDEXAMFETAMINE	Vyvanse
Thyroid product	LEVOTHYROXINE	Synthroid, Levoxyl, Unithroid
Urea cycle disorder	GLYCEROL PHENYLBUTYRATE	Ravicti
	SODIUM PHENYLBUTYRATE	Buphenyl
Urology	OXYBUTYNIN	Ditropan

Table C.3. Commonly used medications, alphabetized by brand name

Brand name	Generic name
A&D Original Ointment	LANOLIN/PETROLATUM/VITAMINS A and D
Abilify	ARIPIPRAZOLE
Accutane	ISOTRETINOIN
ACTH	CORTICOTROPIN
Acthar	CORTICOTROPIN
Adderall	AMPHETAMINE SALTS
Advil	IBUPROFEN
Allegra	FEXOFENADINE
Alpha Keri	MINERAL OIL
Amoxil	AMOXICILLIN
Anafranil	CLOMIPRAMINE

(continued)

Table C.3. *(continued)*

Brand name	Generic name
Artane	TRIHEXYPHENIDYL
Ativan	LORAZEPAM
Augmentin	AMOXICILLIN/CLAVULANIC ACID
Aveeno	COLLOIDAL OATMEAL
Aventyl	NORTRIPTYLINE
Bactrim	TRIMETHOPRIM/SULFAMETHOXAZOLE (TMP/SMX)
Bactroban 2%	MUPIROCIN
Benadryl	DIPHENHYDRAMINE
Biaxin	CLARITHROMYCIN
Botox	BOTULINUM TOXIN A
Buphenyl	SODIUM PHENYLBUTYRATE
Buspar	BUSPIRONE
Caldesene ointment	ZINC OXIDE/COD LIVER OIL/LANOLIN/PETROLATUM
Carnitor	LEVOCARNITINE
Catapres	CLONIDINE
Celexa	CITALOPRAM
Cerebyx	FOSPHENYTOIN
Cipro	CIPROFLOXACIN
Claravis	ISOTRETINOIN
Claritin	LORATADINE
Clozaril	CLOZAPINE
Cogentin	BENZTROPINE
Concerta	METHYLPHENIDATE
Cortizone	HYDROCORTISONE
Cortisporin	HYDROCORTISONE/POLYMYXIN B/NEOMYCIN
Cymbalta	DULOXETINE
Dantrium	DANTROLENE SODIUM
Daytrana	METHYLPHENIDATE
Decadron	DEXAMETHASONE
Deltasone	PREDNISONE
Depacon	VALPROIC ACID
Depakene	VALPROIC ACID
Depakote	VALPROIC ACID
Desitin	ZINC OXIDE
Dexedrine	DEXTROAMPHETAMINE
Dextrostat	DEXTROAMPHETAMINE
Diamox	ACETAZOLAMIDE
Diastat	DIAZEPAM (RECTAL)
Diflucan	FLUCONAZOLE
Dilantin	PHENYTOIN
Ditropan	OXYBUTYNIN
Diuril	CHLOROTHIAZIDE
DuoDERM	DUODERM

(continued)

Table C.3. *(continued)*

Brand name	Generic name
Effexor	VENLAFAXINE
Elavil	AMITRIPTYLINE
Elimite	PERMETHRIN
E.E.S.	ERYTHROMYCIN
Eskalith	LITHIUM CARBONATE
Eucerin	PETROLATUM/ALCOHOL/MINERAL OIL/WAX
Felbatol	FELBAMATE
Fer-In-Sol	FERROUS SULFATE
Fleet Mineral Oil Enema	MINERAL OIL
Flonase	FLUTICASONE
Focalin	DEXMETHYLPHENIDATE
Fox Aclo	CLOZAPINE
Gabitril	TIAGABINE
Geodon	ZIPRASIDONE
Haldol	HALOPERIDOL
Imodium	LOPERAMIDE
Indocin	INDOMETHACIN
Intuniv	GUANFACINE ER
Janimine	IMIPRAMINE
Kapvay	CLONIDINE ER
Keflex	CEPHALEXIN
Keppra	LEVETIRACETAM
Klonopin	CLONAZEPAM
Kwell	LINDANE
Lamictal	LAMOTRIGINE
Lasix	FUROSEMIDE
Levaquin	LEVOFLOXACIN
Lexapro	ESCITALOPRAM
Lioresal	BACLOFEN
Lithobid	LITHIUM CARBONATE
Lotrimin	CLOTRIMAZOLE
Lubiderm	MINERAL OIL/PETROLATUM/LANOLIN
Luminal	PHENOBARBITAL
Lyrica	PREGABALIN
Mellaril	THIORIDAZINE
Metadate	METHYLPHENIDATE
Methylin	METHYLPHENIDATE
MiraLax	POLYETHYLENE GLYCOL 3350
Monistat 2%	MICONAZOLE
Motrin	IBUPROFEN
Mycelex	CLOTRIMAZOLE
Mycostatin	NYSTATIN
Mylanta	MAGNESIUM HYDROXIDE/ALUMINUM HYDROXIDE

(continued)

Table C.3. *(continued)*

Brand name	Generic name
Mysoline	PRIMIDONE
Narcan	NALOXONE
Navane	THIOTHIXENE
Neurontin	GABAPENTIN
Nexium	ESOMEPRAZOLE
Nivea	MINERAL OIL/PETROLATUM/LANOLIN
Nix	PERMETHRIN
Norpramin	DESIPRAMINE
Omnicef	CEFDINIR
Pamelor	NORTRIPTYLINE
Paxil	PAROXETINE
Pen-VK	PENICILLIN
Pepcid	FAMOTIDINE
Periactin	CYPROHEPTADINE
Prelone	PREDNISOLONE
Prevacid	LANSOPRAZOLE
Prilosec	OMEPRAZOLE
ProCentra	DEXTROAMPHETAMINE
Prozac	FLUOXETINE
Pulmicort	BUDESONIDE
Ravicti	GLYCEROL PHENYLBUTYRATE
Reglan	METOCLOPRAMIDE
Revia	NALTREXONE
Rhinocort	BUDESONIDE
Risperdal	RISPERIDONE
Ritalin	METHYLPHENIDATE
Robinul	GLYCOPYRROLATE
Selsun Blue 2.5%	SELENIUM SULFIDE
Septra	TRIMETHOPRIM/SULFAMETHOXAZOLE (TMP/SMZ)
Seroquel	QUETIAPINE
Singulair	MONTELUKAST
Solu Medrol	METHYLPREDNISOLONE
Strattera	ATOMOXETINE
Synthroid	LEVOTHYROXINE
Tegretol	CARBAMAZEPINE
Tenex	GUANFACINE
Theo-Dur	THEOPHYLLINE
Thorazine	CHLORPROMAZINE
Tinactin	TOLNAFTATE
Tofranil	IMIPRAMINE
Topamax	TOPIRAMATE
Tranxene	CLORAZEPATE
Triamcinolone	TRIAMCINOLONE

(continued)

Table C.3. *(continued)*

Brand name	Generic name
Trileptal	OXCARBAZEPINE
Tylenol	ACETAMINOPHEN
Uniphyl	THEOPHYLLINE
Valium	DIAZEPAM
Ventolin	ALBUTEROL
Vyvanse	LISDEXAMFETAMINE
Wellbutrin	BUPROPION
Xanax	ALPRAZOLAM
Xopenex	LEVALBUTEROL
Zantac	RANITIDINE
Zarontin	ETHOSUXIMIDE
Zithromax	AZITHROMYCIN
Zoloft	SERTRALINE
Zonegran	ZONISAMIDE
Zovirax	ACYCLOVIR
Zyban	BUPROPION
Zyprexa	OLANZAPINE
Zyrtec	CETIRIZINE

Index

Page numbers followed by *f* and *t* indicate figures and tables, respectively.